| midazolam HCl | morphine sulfate | nalbuphine HCl | pentazocine lactate | pentobarbital Na | perphenazine | phenobarbital Na | prochlorperazine edisylate | promazine HCl | promethazine HCl | ranitidine HCl | scopolamine HBr | secobarbital Na | sodium bicarbonate | thiethylperazine maleate | thiopental Na | |
|---|---|---|---|---|---|---|---|---|---|---|---|---|---|---|---|---|
| Y | P | Y | P | P | Y | | P | P | P | Y | P | | | | | atropine sulfate |
| Y | Y | | Y | N | Y | | Y | | Y | | Y | | | Y | | butorphanol tartrate |
| Y | P | | P | N | Y | | P | P | P | N* | P | | | | N | chlorpromazine HCl |
| Y | Y | Y | Y | N | Y | | Y | Y | Y | | Y | N | | | | cimetidine HCl |
| | | | | | | | | | | | | | | | | codeine phosphate |
| | | | | | | | | | | Y | | | | | | dexamethasone sodium phosphate |
| N | P | | P | N | Y | | N | N | N | Y | P | | | | N | dimenhydrinate |
| Y | P | Y | P | N | Y | | P | P | P | Y | P | | | | N | diphenhydramine HCl |
| Y | P | Y | P | N | Y | | P | P | P | | P | | | | | droperidol |
| Y | P | | P | N | Y | | P | P | P | Y | P | | | | | fentanyl citrate |
| Y | Y | Y | N | N | | | Y | Y | Y | Y | Y | N | N | | N | glycopyrrolate |
| | N* | | N | | | P(5) | | N | | | | | | | | heparin Na |
| Y | | Y | Y | | | | N* | | Y | Y | Y | | | Y | | hydromorphone HCl |
| Y | P | Y | P | N | Y | | P | P | P | N | P | | | | | hydroxyzine HCl |
| Y | N | | P | N | Y | | P | P | P | Y | P | | | | N | meperidine HCl |
| Y | P | | P | | P | | P | P | P | Y | P | | N | | | metoclopramide HCl |
| | Y | Y | | N | N | | N | Y | Y | N | Y | | | Y | | midazolam HCl |
| Y | | | P | N* | Y | | P* | P | P* | Y | P | | | | N | morphine sulfate |
| Y | | | | N | | | Y | | N* | Y | Y | | | Y | | nalbuphine HCl |
| | P | | | N | Y | | P | Y | Y | Y | P | | | | | pentazocine lactate |
| N | N* | N | N | | N | | N | N | N | N | P | | Y | | Y | pentobarbital Na |
| N | Y | | Y | N | | | Y | | Y | Y | Y | | | N | | perphenazine |
| | | | | | | | | | | N | | | | | | phenobarbital Na |
| N | P* | Y | P | N | Y | | | P | P | Y | P | | | | N | prochlorperazine edisylate |
| Y | P | | Y | N | | | P | | P | | P | | | | | promazine HCl |
| Y | P* | N* | Y | N | Y | | P | P | | Y | P | | | | N | promethazine HCl |
| N | Y | Y | Y | N | Y | N | Y | | Y | | Y | | | Y | | ranitidine HCl |
| Y | P | Y | P | P | Y | | P | P | P | Y | | | | | Y | scopolamine HBr |
| | | | | | | | | | | | | | | | | secobarbital Na |
| | | | Y | | | | | | | | | | | | N | sodium bicarbonate |
| Y | | Y | | | N | | | | Y | Y | | | | | | thiethylperazine maleate |
| | N | | | Y | | | N | | N | | Y | | N | | | thiopental Na |

*21st Edition*

# Nursing 2001

# DRUG

# HANDBOOK®

SPRINGHOUSE CORPORATION
SPRINGHOUSE, PENNSYLVANIA

## Staff

**Senior Publisher**
Donna O. Carpenter

**Editorial Director**
William J. Kelly

**Clinical Director**
Ann M. Barrow, RN, MSN

**Design Director**
John Hubbard

**Art Director**
Elaine Kasmer Ezrow

**Senior Associate Editor**
Karen C. Comerford

**Clinical Project Editor**
Eileen Cassin Gallen, RN, BSN

**Editors**
Naina Chohan, Rita M. Doyle,
Patricia Nale

**Clinical Editors**
Christine M. Damico, RN, MSN, CPNP;
Lori Musolf Neri, RN, MSN, CCRN,
CPNP; Kimberly A. Zalewski, RN, MSN,
CEN; Theresa Fulginiti, RN, BSN, CEN

**Copy Editors**
Colleen P. Coady, Leslie Dworkin,
Joy Epstein

**Designers**
Arlene Putterman (associate art director),
Joseph John Clark, Don Knauss

**Electronic Production Services**
Diane Paluba (manager), Joyce Rossi
Biletz (technician)

**Manufacturing**
Deborah Meiris (director), Patricia K.
Dorshaw (manager), Otto Mezei (book
production manager)

**Editorial Assistants**
Arlene P. Claffee, Carol A. Caputo

**Indexer**
Barbara Hodgson

# Contents

## Nutritional Drugs

## Miscellaneous Categories

## Appendices and Index

# Contributors and consultants

*At the time of publication, the contributors and consultants held the following positions.*

**Steven R. Abel,** RPh, PharmD
Professor and Head
Department of Pharmacy Practice
Purdue University School of Pharmacy
and Pharmacal Sciences
West Lafayette, Ind.

**Steven R. Benson,** PharmD, BCPS
Clinical Education Consultant
Pfizer, Inc.
St. Paul, Minn.

**James B. Caldwell,** PharmD
Clinical Pharmacy Coordinator
Anne Arundel Medical Center
Annapolis, Md.

**James M. Camamo,** PharmD
Clinical Pharmacist, Medication
Information and Policy Development
University Medical Center
Tucson, Ariz.

**Lawrence Carey,** PharmD
Clinical Pharmacist Supervisor
Jefferson Home Infusion Service
Philadelphia

**Andy Clark,** RPh
Clinical Pharmacist
Nash General Hospital
Rocky Mount, N.C.

**Michael R. Cohen,** RPh, MS
President, Institute for Safe
Medication Practices
Huntingdon Valley, Pa.

**Linda M. Dean,** CRNP, MSN, ANP, ACRN
Director of Clinical Education
MCP Hahnemann University
Philadelphia

**Jennifer L. Defilippi,** PharmD, BCPP
Clinical Psychiatric Specialist
Central Texas Veterans Health
Care System
Waco, Tex.

**David M. DiPersio,** PharmD, BCPS
Clinical Pharmacist, Critical Care
Vanderbilt University Medical Center
Nashville, Tenn.

**Teresa S. Dunsworth,** PharmD, BCPS
Associate Professor of Clinical
Pharmacy
West Virginia University
School of Pharmacy
Morgantown

**Steven Gelone,** PharmD
Infectious Disease Clinical Specalist
Temple University School of Pharmacy
Philadelphia

**S. Kim Genovese,** MSN, MSA, RN,C, CARN
Associate Professior of Nursing
Purdue University
Westville, Ind.

**Mary Jo Gerlach,** RN, MSNEd
Assistant Professor, Adult Nursing
Medical College of Georgia
School of Nursing
Athens

**Theresa B. Germano,** RPh
Clinical Pharmacist
Chestnut Hill Hospital
Philadelphia

**Mildred D. Gottwald,** PharmD
Assistant Clinical Professor
University of California
Department of Clinical Pharmacy
San Francisco

**Ronald L. Greenberg,** PharmD, BCPS
Clinical Pharmacy Specialist
Fairview Ridges Hospital
Burnsville, Minn.

**Tatyana Gurvich,** PharmD
Clinical Pharmacologist
Glendale Adventist Family Practice
Residency Program
Glendale, La.

**Barbara S. Kannewurf,** PharmD
Clinical Pharmacist, Cardiology
University of Washington
Medical Center
Seattle

**Maureen Ketz,** PharmD
Clinical Pharmacist
Mt. Carmel Medical Center
Columbus, Ohio

**Debra A. Kosko,** RN, MN, FNP-C
Faculty, Advanced Practice Nursing
Johns Hopkins University
School of Nursing
Baltimore

**Randall A. Lynch,** RPh, PharmD
Assistant Director, Pharmacy Services
Presbyterian Medical Center/University
of Pennsylvania Health System
Philadelphia

**Catherine Todd Magel,** EdD, RN,C
Assistant Professor
Villanova (Pa.) University
College of Nursing

**Dawna Martich,** RN, MSN
Clinical Trainer
Diabetes Treatment Centers of America
Pittsburgh

**George Melko,** PharmD
Manager, Regulatory Affairs
Astra-Zeneca Pharmaceuticals
Wayne, Pa.

**Kevin ODell,** PharmD
Senior Pharmacotherapy Specialist
Paynesville, Minn.

**William O'Hara,** PharmD
Clinical Team Leader
Thomas Jefferson University Hospital
Philadelphia

**Staci Pacetti,** PharmD
Infectious Disease Pharmacy Resident
Temple University School of Pharmacy
Philadelphia

**Beth Logsdon Pangle,** PharmD, BCNSP
Pediatric Clinical Pharmacy Specialist
Cook Children's Medical Center
Fort Worth, Tex.

**Larry A. Pfeifer,** RPh, MS
Director, Pharmacy Services
National Hansen's Disease Program
Baton Rouge, La.

**Michele L. Phelps,** RN, BSN
Research Nurse
Johns Hopkins Hospital
Baltimore

**David Pipher,** RPh, PharmD
Director of Pharmacy
Forbes Regional Hospital
Monroeville, Pa.

**Ruthie Robinson,** RN, MSN, CCRN, CEN
Staff Nurse, St. Elizabeth Hospital
Emergency Room
Instructor, Nursing
Lamar University
Beaumont, Tex.

**Judy L. Smetzer,** RN, BSN
Director, Risk Management Services
Institute for Safe Medication Practices
Huntingdon Valley, Pa.

**Gary Smith,** RPh, PharmD
Manager, Clinical Pharmacy Services
Fairview Physician Associates
Edina, Minn.

**Dawn M. Specht,** RN, MSN, CEN, CCRN
Clinical Nurse Specialist
Critical Care/Neuroscience
Cooper Health System
Camden, N.J.

**Mary A. Stahl,** RN, CS, MSN, CCRN
Clinical Nurse Specialist
Saint Luke's Hospital
Kansas City, Mo.

**Joseph F. Steiner,** RPh, PharmD
Professor and Director of
Pharmacy Practice
University of Wyoming
School of Pharmacy
Laramie

**Lori Summerson,** RN, BSN, OCN
Clinical Trials Research Nurse
Johns Hopkins Oncology Center
Baltimore

**Catherine Ultrino,** RN, MS, OCN
Assistant Nurse Manager
Boston Medical Center

**Eva M. Vasquez,** PharmD, FCCP, BCPS
Assistant Professor
College of Pharmacy
University of Illinois at Chicago

*Nursing2001 Drug Handbook* was created by pharmacists and nurses to provide the nursing profession with drug information that zeroes in on precisely what nurses need to know. With that goal clearly in mind, *Nursing2001 Drug Handbook* emphasizes clinical aspects of drugs without attempting to replace detailed pharmacology texts. Also, the book is designed to make the content readily accessible and applicable in any clinical setting.

### Features in this edition
The 2001 edition contains many features to enhance nursing knowledge and skills:
• Charts that show the route, onset, peak, and duration of each drug.
• "Elderly" dosage and "Adjust-a-dose" information that details possible dosage adjustments necessary in specific patient populations.
• Monographs on 62 new FDA approved drugs.
• An "Alert" logo in the Nursing Considerations section that now includes cautionary tips for avoiding common medication errors, such as confusing drug names that sound alike or using incorrect administration routes.
• An interactions section that includes interactions with other drugs, herbs, food, and lifestyle behaviors.
• Instructions for preparing and administering I.V. drugs that are highlighted in each appropriate entry.
• Appendices covering dialyzable drugs and therapeutic drug monitoring guidelines that enhance the usefulness of this book.
• Free NDH2001*Plus!* CD-ROM (inside the back cover) that lets you take 10 continuing education tests (and earn 35.5 contact hours), instantly identify common capsules and tablets by their drug imprint codes, learn about potentially dangerous drug interactions, and print out patient-teaching instructions for 200 commonly used drugs and herbs.

NDH2001*Plus!* CD-ROM also links you directly to **NDHnow.com,** the *Nursing2001 Drug Handbook* web site that provides drug updates; important drug news; patient-teaching for administration techniques, supportive measures, and newly approved drugs; clinical pearls on various topics; access to the bookstore; notification of career opportunities; and links to other helpful information.

### Introductory chapters
Chapter 2 explains, in a general way, how drugs work. It also discusses adverse reactions and gives general guidelines about drug use in pregnancy and the presence of drugs in breast milk. Chapters 3 and 4 address the unique problems of administering drugs to children and elderly patients and offer guidelines to minimize problems in these areas. Chapter 5 considers drug therapy as it relates to the nursing process.

### Therapeutic class chapters
Chapters 6 to 98 classify all drugs according to their approved therapeutic uses. Chapter 99, new for *NDH2001*, discusses 25 of the most commonly used herbal medicines because you need to know how a patient's use of herbs can affect assessment, monitoring, and patient teaching.

Drugs with multiple therapeutic uses are classified according to their most common use; they are also listed (with a cross-reference to the major drug entry) in drug groups that share their secondary applications. For example, nadolol, a beta blocker, is described in the chapter that covers antianginals because its major therapeutic application is the management of angina pectoris. Because the drug is less commonly used to treat hypertension, it is also listed among the generic drugs grouped as antihypertensives, with a cross-reference to Chapter 22, Antianginals.

Such classification by therapeutic use offers several advantages. It helps the reader identify an unknown drug by its clinical application alone. It also automatically identifies all other drugs that share the same use and provides easy comparison of their dosages and effects. In this way, it quickly identifies potential pharmacotherapeutic alternatives for patients who can't tolerate or who fail to respond to a particular drug.

Each chapter, representing a major therapeutic use, begins with an alphabetical list of the generic drugs described in that chapter. This is followed by a list of selected combination products in which these drugs are found. Specific information on each drug includes brand names and is arranged under the following headings: *Controlled Substance Schedule (where applicable), Pregnancy Risk Category, How Supplied, Action, Indications & Dosage, Adverse Reactions, Interactions, Effects on Diagnostic Tests, Contraindications, Nursing Considerations, I.V. Administration (where applicable),* and *Patient teaching.*

In each drug entry, the generic name is followed by an alphabetized list of its brand names. A brand name followed by an open diamond ( ◇ ) indicates a drug preparation that doesn't need a prescription. Brands that are specifically Canadian are designated with a dagger (†); those that are specifically Australian are followed by a double dagger (‡); and those that are specifically British are followed by a section mark (§). A brand name with no symbol is available in the United States, Canada, and possibly Australia and the United Kingdom (U.K.). The mention of a brand name in no way implies endorsement of that product or guarantees its legality.

*Alcohol and tartrazine content*
Many liquid drug preparations for oral use contain alcohol. Although the slight sedative effect that alcohol produces is not harmful in most patients—and can sometimes be beneficial—alcohol ingestion can be undesirable and even dangerous. Oral drugs that contain alcohol should be given cautiously, if at all, to patients who are

• concomitantly taking potent CNS depressants such as barbiturates.
• taking drugs that may produce a disulfiram-type reaction (such as chlorpropamide or metronidazole).
• taking disulfiram as part of a treatment program for their alcoholism. Such patients, upon ingestion of alcohol, will exhibit severe signs or symptoms that may include blurred vision, confusion, dyspnea, flushing, sweating, and tachycardia.

To help prevent inadvertent exposure to alcohol, the text signals alcohol content with a single asterisk (*) after each brand name of a liquid preparation that may contain it. In many of the preparations so marked, the alcohol content is small. Nevertheless, these drugs should be avoided by patients susceptible to adverse effects after exposure to alcohol.

Tartrazine dye, also known as FD&C Yellow No. 5, is a common coloring agent in some foods and drugs. Usually harmless, it can provoke a severe reaction in susceptible persons. For this reason, most drug manufacturers have begun to eliminate tartrazine from their products, but many drugs still contain it.

The incidence of tartrazine sensitivity is about 1 in 10,000 in the general population but somewhat higher in persons with asthma or sensitivity to aspirin. The reason for this is unknown. The most common signs and symptoms of tartrazine sensitivity are urticaria, rhinorrhea, asthma, and angioedema. Acutely sensitive persons may develop allergic vascular purpura, tachycardia, dyspnea, and chest pain. These allergic signs or symptoms typically subside spontaneously upon discontinuation of the drug but may require treatment with antihistamines or epinephrine.

Tartrazine may be present in drugs that are yellow, turquoise, green, and maroon. This text signals tartrazine content with a double asterisk (**) after each brand name that may contain it. If you suspect tartrazine sensitivity in a patient receiving such a drug, inform the doctor and contact the manufacturer to determine which dosage forms contain tartrazine.

*Controlled substance schedules*

If a drug is a controlled substance, that is indicated (example: Controlled Substance Schedule II). Drugs regulated under the jurisdiction of the Controlled Substances Act of 1970 are divided into the following groups, or schedules:

• Schedule I (C-I): High abuse potential and no accepted medical use—for example, heroin, marijuana, and LSD.

• Schedule II (C-II): High abuse potential with severe dependence liability—for example, narcotics, amphetamines, dronabinol, and some barbiturates.

• Schedule III (C-III): Less abuse potential than schedule II drugs and moderate dependence liability—for example, nonbarbiturate sedatives, nonamphetamine stimulants, anabolic steroids, and limited amounts of certain narcotics.

• Schedule IV (C-IV): Less abuse potential than schedule III drugs and limited dependence liability—for example, some sedatives, antianxiety agents, and nonnarcotic analgesics.

• Schedule V (C-V): Limited abuse potential. Primarily small amounts of narcotics, such as codeine, used as antitussives or antidiarrheals. Under federal law, limited quantities of certain C-V drugs may be purchased without a prescription directly from a pharmacist if allowed under specific state statutes. The purchaser must be at least age 18 and must furnish suitable identification. All such transactions must be recorded by the dispensing pharmacist.

*Pregnancy risk category*

Each systemically absorbed drug has been assigned a pregnancy risk category based upon available clinical and preclinical information. The Pregnancy Risk Category parallels the five Pregnancy Categories (A, B, C, D, and X) assigned by the FDA to reflect a drug's potential to cause birth defects. Although drugs are best avoided during pregnancy, this rating system permits rapid assessment of the risk-benefit ratio should drug administration to a pregnant woman become necessary. Drugs in category A are generally considered safe to use in pregnancy; drugs in category X are generally contraindicated.

• A: Adequate studies in pregnant women have failed to show a risk to the fetus.

• B: Animal studies have not shown a risk to the fetus, but controlled studies have not been conducted in pregnant women; or animal studies have shown an adverse effect on the fetus, but adequate studies in pregnant women have not shown a risk to the fetus.

• C: Animal studies have shown an adverse effect on the fetus, but adequate studies have not been conducted in humans. The benefits from use in pregnant women may be acceptable despite potential risks.

• D: The drug may cause risk to the human fetus, but the potential benefits of use in pregnant women may be acceptable despite the risks (such as in a life-threatening situation or a serious disease for which safer drugs can't be used or are ineffective).

• X: Studies in animals or humans show fetal abnormalities, or adverse reaction reports indicate evidence of fetal risk. The risks involved clearly outweigh potential benefits.

• NR: Not rated.

*How supplied*

This section lists the preparations available for each drug (for example, tablets, capsules, solutions for injection), specifying available dosage forms and strengths. Dosage strengths specifically available in Canada are designated with a dagger (†), those available in Australia with a double dagger (‡), and those in the U.K. with a section mark (§). Preparations that do not require a prescription are marked with an open diamond (◊).

*Action*

This section succinctly describes the mechanism of action—that is, how the drug provides its therapeutic effect. For example, although all antihypertensives lower blood pressure, they don't all do so by the same pharmacologic process.

Also included in chart form is the onset, peak (described in terms of effect or peak blood level), and duration of drug action for each route of administration, if data are available or applicable. Values listed are for patients with normal renal function, unless specified otherwise.

## Indications & dosage
This section lists general dosage information for adults, children, and elderly patients, as applicable. Dosage instructions reflect current clinical trends in therapeutics and can't be considered as absolute or universal recommendations. For individual application, dosage instructions must be considered in light of the patient's clinical condition. The logo for "Adjust-a-dose" appears in this section.

## Adverse reactions
This section lists adverse reactions to each drug by body system. The most common adverse reactions (those experienced by at least 10% of people taking the drug in clinical trials) are in *italic* type; less common reactions are in roman type; life-threatening reactions are in ***bold italic*** type; and reactions that are common *and* life-threatening are in BOLD CAPITAL LETTERS.

## Interactions
This section lists each drug's confirmed, *clinically significant* interactions with other drugs (additive effects, potentiated effects, and antagonistic effects); herbs (herbal preparations have the potential to significantly affect the anticipated action of a drug); foods, with specific suggestions for avoiding dangerous drug or food interactions (for example, by reducing doses or monitoring food intake); and lifestyle (such as alcohol use or smoking). Drug interactions are listed under the drug that is adversely affected. For example, magnesium trisilicate, an ingredient in antacids, interacts with tetracycline to cause decreased absorption of tetracycline. Therefore, this interaction is listed under tetracycline. To check on the possible effects of using two or more drugs simultaneously, refer to the interaction entry for each of the drugs in question.

## Effects on diagnostic tests
This section lists significant interference with a diagnostic test or its result, either by a drug's direct effects on the test itself or by systemic effects that cause misleading test results.

## Contraindications
This section lists any conditions, especially diseases, in which the use of the drug is undesirable.

## Nursing considerations
This section lists recommendations for cautious use, followed by other useful information, such as monitoring techniques and suggestions for prevention and treatment of adverse reactions. Also included are suggestions for patient comfort and for preparing, administering, and storing each drug.

An "Alert" logo signals cautionary tips, including how to avoid medication errors, such as confusing drug names that sound alike or using incorrect administration route.

Guidelines for properly reconstituting and mixing I.V. drugs along with tips for added safety appear under the "I.V. administration" subhead.

The "Patient teaching" section focuses on explaining the drug's purpose, promoting compliance, and ensuring proper use and storage of the drug. It also includes instructions for preventing or minimizing adverse reactions.

## Photoguide to tablets and capsules
To make drug identification easier for nurses and to enhance patient safety, *Nursing2001 Drug Handbook* offers a full-color photoguide to the most commonly prescribed tablets and capsules. Shown in actual size, the drugs are arranged alphabetically for quick reference, along with their most common dosage strengths. A page reference to the text monograph appears with each drug shown.

## Common abbreviations

| | | | |
|---|---|---|---|
| ACE | angiotensin-converting enzyme | IPPB | intermittent positive-pressure breathing |
| ADH | antidiuretic hormone | IU | international unit |
| AIDS | acquired immunodeficiency syndrome | I.V. | intravenous |
| | | kg | kilogram |
| ALT | alanine transaminase | L | liter |
| AST | aspartate transaminase | LD | lactate dehydrogenase |
| AV | atrioventricular | M | molar |
| b.i.d. | twice daily | $m^2$ | square meter |
| BPH | benign prostatic hyperplasia | MAO | monoamine oxidase |
| BSA | body surface area | mcg | microgram |
| BUN | blood urea nitrogen | mEq | milliequivalent |
| cAMP | cyclic adenosine mono-phosphate | mg | milligram |
| | | MI | myocardial infarction |
| CBC | complete blood count | ml | milliliter |
| CK | creatine kinase | $mm^3$ | cubic millimeter |
| CMV | cytomegalovirus | Na | sodium |
| CNS | central nervous system | NaCl | sodium chloride |
| COPD | chronic obstructive pul-monary disease | ng | nanogram |
| | | NSAID | nonsteroidal anti-inflammatory drug |
| CSF | cerebrospinal fluid | | |
| CV | cardiovascular | OTC | over-the-counter |
| CVA | cerebrovascular accident | PABA | para-aminobenzoic acid |
| $D_5W$ | dextrose 5% in water | PCA | patient-controlled analgesia |
| DIC | disseminated intravascular coagulation | P.O. | by mouth |
| | | P.R. | by rectum |
| dl | deciliter | p.r.n. | as needed |
| DNA | deoxyribonucleic acid | PT | prothrombin time |
| ECG | electrocardiogram | PTT | partial thromboplastin time |
| EEG | electroencephalogram | PVC | premature ventricular contraction |
| EENT | eyes, ears, nose, throat | | |
| FDA | Food and Drug Administra-tion | q | every |
| | | q.i.d. | four times daily |
| g | gram | RBC | red blood cell |
| G | gauge | RDA | recommended daily allowance |
| GFR | glomerular filtration rate | | |
| GGT | gamma-glutamyltransferase | REM | rapid eye movement |
| GI | gastrointestinal | RNA | ribonucleic acid |
| gtt | drops | RSV | respiratory syncytial virus |
| GU | genitourinary | SA | sinoatrial |
| G6PD | glucose-6-phosphate dehy-drogenase | S.C. | subcutaneous |
| | | SIADH | syndrome of inappropriate antidiuretic hormone |
| $H_1$ | histamine$_1$ | | |
| $H_2$ | histamine$_2$ | S.L. | sublingual |
| HIV | human immunodeficiency virus | sp. | species |
| | | $T_3$ | triiodothyronine |
| h.s. | at bedtime | $T_4$ | thyroxine |
| I.D. | intradermal | t.i.d. | three times daily |
| I.M. | intramuscular | U | units |
| INR | international normalized ratio | USP | United States Pharmacopeia |
| | | WBC | white blood cell |

# 2

# Drug actions, reactions, and interactions

Administration of any drug provokes a series of physicochemical events within the body. The first event, when a drug combines with cellular drug receptors, is known as the drug action. What follows as a result of this action is the drug effect. Depending on the number of different cellular drug receptors affected by a given drug, a drug effect can be local, systemic, or both. Obviously, a local effect follows application to the skin; however, transdermal absorption can produce systemic effects. Moreover, local effects can follow systemic absorption. For example, the antipeptic ulcer drug cimetidine acts solely by blocking histamine receptor cells in the parietal cells of the stomach. This is known as a local drug effect because the drug action is sharply limited to one area and does not spread to other parts of the body. However, diphenhydramine produces a systemic effect in that it blocks histamine receptors in widespread areas of the body. Thus, local drug effects are specific to a limited number of organ systems, whereas systemic drug effects are generalized and affect different and diverse organ systems.

## Drug properties
Drug absorption, distribution, metabolism, and excretion make up a drug pharmacokinetic profile. This branch of pharmacology also describes a drug's onset of action, peak concentration level, duration of action, and bioavailability.

### Absorption
Before a drug can act within the body, it must be absorbed into the bloodstream—usually after oral administration, the most commonly used route. Before a drug contained in a tablet or capsule can be absorbed, the dosage form must disintegrate—that is, break into smaller particles. Then these smaller particles can dissolve in gastric juices. Only after dissolving can a drug be absorbed. Most absorption of orally administered drugs oc-curs in the small intestine, where the mucosal villi provide extensive surface area. Once absorbed and circulated in the bloodstream, the drug is bioavailable, or ready to produce a drug effect. Whether such absorption is complete or partial depends on several factors: the drug's physicochemical effects, its dosage form, its route of administration, its interactions with other substances in the GI tract, and various patient characteristics. These same factors also determine the speed of absorption. Thus, oral solutions and elixirs, which bypass the need for disintegration and dissolution, are usually absorbed more rapidly. Some tablets have enteric coatings that prevent disintegration in the acidic environment of the stomach; others may have coatings of varying thickness that delay release of the drug.

Drugs administered I.M. must first be absorbed through the muscle into the bloodstream. Rectal suppositories must dissolve to be absorbed through the rectal mucosa. Drugs administered I.V., which are injected directly into the bloodstream, are completely and immediately bioavailable.

### Distribution
After absorption, a drug moves from the bloodstream into various fluids and tissues within the body; this is distribution. Individual patient variations can greatly alter the amount of drug that is distributed throughout the body. For example, in an edematous patient, a given dose must be distributed to a larger volume than in a nonedematous patient; the amount of drug must sometimes be increased to account for this. Remember, the dose should be decreased when the edema is corrected. Conversely, in an extremely dehydrated patient, the drug will be distributed to a much smaller volume, so the dose must then be decreased. The total area to which a drug is distributed is known as volume of distribution. Patients who are particu-

larly obese may present another problem when considering drug distribution. Some drugs—such as digoxin, gentamicin, and tobramycin—are not well distributed to fatty tissue. Therefore, dosing based on actual body weight may lead to overdose and serious toxicity. In some cases, dosing must be based on lean body weight, or adjusted body weight, which may be estimated from actuarial tables that give average weight range for height.

## Metabolism

Most drugs are metabolized in the liver. Hepatic diseases may affect one or more of the metabolic functions of the liver. Therefore, in patients with hepatic disease, the metabolism of a drug may be increased, decreased, or unchanged. Clearly, all patients with hepatic disease must be monitored closely for drug effect and toxicity.

The rate at which a drug is metabolized varies with the individual. In some patients, drugs are metabolized so quickly that their blood and tissue levels prove therapeutically inadequate. In others, the rate of metabolism is so slow that ordinary doses can produce toxic results.

## Excretion

The body eliminates drugs by metabolism (usually hepatic) and excretion (usually renal). Drug excretion refers to the movement of a drug or its metabolites from the tissues back into circulation and from the circulation into the organs of excretion, where they are removed from the body. Although most drugs are excreted by the kidneys, some drugs can be eliminated via the lungs, exocrine glands (sweat, salivary, or mammary), liver, skin, and intestinal tract. Drugs may also be removed artificially by direct intervention, such as peritoneal dialysis or hemodialysis.

## Other modifying factors

An important factor that influences a drug's action and effect is its *binding to plasma proteins,* especially albumin, and other tissue components. Because only a free, unbound drug can act in the body, such binding greatly influences effectiveness and duration of effect. Protein-binding can be influenced by malnutrition, renal failure, and other protein-bound drugs. When protein-binding is altered, drug dosing may need to be modified.

The *patient's age* is another important factor. Elderly patients usually have decreased hepatic function, less muscle mass, diminished renal function, and decreased serum albumin. Consequently, they need lower doses and sometimes longer dosage intervals to avoid toxicity. With similar consequences, neonates have underdeveloped metabolic enzyme systems and inadequate renal function. They need highly individualized dosages and careful monitoring.

*Underlying disease* can also markedly affect drug action and effect. For example, acidosis may cause insulin resistance. Genetic diseases, such as G6PD deficiency and hepatic porphyria, may turn drugs into toxins with serious consequences. Patients with G6PD deficiency may develop hemolytic anemia when given sulfonamides or a number of other drugs. A genetically susceptible patient can develop an acute porphyria attack if given a barbiturate. Also, patients who have highly active hepatic enzyme systems (for example, rapid acetylators), when treated with isoniazid, can develop hepatitis from the rapid intrahepatic buildup of a toxic metabolite.

## Drug administration issues

Factors related to the administration of a drug can also influence a drug's action within the body. The dosage form of a drug is important. Some tablets and capsules are too large to be easily swallowed by ill patients. Although an oral solution may be substituted, it produces higher drug blood levels than a tablet because the liquid is more easily and completely absorbed. When a potentially toxic drug (such as digoxin) is given, the increased amount absorbed could cause toxicity. Sometimes a change in dosage form requires a change in dosage itself.

Routes of administration are not therapeutically interchangeable. For example, diazepam is readily absorbed orally but is slowly and erratically absorbed I.M. On the other hand, gentamicin must be given parenterally because oral administration yields blood levels inadequate to treat systemic infections.

Improper storage can alter a drug's potency. Most drugs should be stored in tight containers protected from direct sunlight and extremes in temperature and humidity that can cause them to deteriorate. Some may require special storage conditions, such as refrigeration. Drugs should not be stored in the bathroom because of the constantly changing environment.

The timing of drug administration can be important. Sometimes, giving an oral drug during or shortly after mealtime decreases the amount of drug absorbed. This is not clinically significant with most drugs and may in fact be desirable with irritating drugs such as aspirin. But penicillins and tetracyclines should not be scheduled for administration at mealtimes because certain foods can inactivate them. If in doubt about the effect of food on a certain drug, check with the pharmacist.

Consider the patient's age, height, and weight. The doctor will need this information when calculating the dosage for many drugs. It should be accurately recorded on the patient's chart. This chart should also include current laboratory data, especially renal and liver function studies, so the doctor can adjust the dosage as needed.

Watch for metabolic changes. Monitor for physiologic changes (depressed respiratory function, acidosis, or alkalosis) that might alter drug effect.

Know the patient's history. Whenever possible, obtain a comprehensive family history from the patient or his family. Ask about past reactions to drugs, possible genetic traits that might alter drug response, and the current use of other drugs. Multiple drug therapy can cause drug interactions that can dramatically change the effects of many drugs.

## Adverse reactions

Any drug effect other than what is therapeutically intended can be called an adverse reaction. It may be expected and benign, or unexpected and potentially harmful. Mild, but *predictable,* adverse reactions are sometimes called adverse effects. Drowsiness caused by antihistamines is an example of this. During hay fever season, a patient may have to contend with this drowsiness to get relief from hay fever symptoms. In such a case, the dosage may be adjusted up or down to balance therapeutic effects with adverse effects.

An adverse reaction may be tolerated for a necessary therapeutic effect, or it may be hazardous and unacceptable and require discontinuation of the drug. Some adverse reactions subside with continued use. As an example, the drowsiness associated with paroxetine and the orthostatic hypotension associated with prazosin usually subside after several days, as the patient develops a tolerance to these effects. But many adverse reactions are dosage-related and lessen or disappear only if the dosage is reduced. Although most adverse reactions are not therapeutically desirable, an occasional one can be put to clinical use. An outstanding example of this is the drowsiness associated with diphenhydramine, which makes it clinically useful as a mild hypnotic.

*Hypersensitivity,* a term sometimes used interchangeably with drug allergy, is the result of an antigen-antibody immune reaction that occurs in the body when a drug is given to a susceptible patient. One of the most dangerous of all drug hypersensitivities is penicillin allergy. In its most severe form, penicillin anaphylaxis can rapidly become fatal.

Rarely, idiosyncratic reactions occur. These are highly unpredictable, individual, and unusual. Probably the best known idiosyncratic drug reaction is the aplastic anemia caused by the antibiotic chloramphenicol. This reaction appears in only 1 out of 40,000 patients, but when it does occur, it can be fatal. A more common idiosyncratic reaction is extreme sensitivity to very low doses of a drug, or insensitivity to higher-than-normal doses.

To deal with adverse reactions correctly, you need to be alert to even minor changes in the patient's clinical status. Such minor changes may be an early warning of pending toxicity. Listen to the patient's complaints about his reactions to a drug and consider each objectively. You may be able to reduce adverse reactions in several ways. Obviously, dosage reduction can help. But in many cases so does a simple rescheduling of the same dose. For example, pseudoephedrine may produce stimulation that will be no problem if it's given early in the day. Similarly, the drowsiness that occurs with antihistamines or tranquilizers can be totally harmless if the dose is given at bedtime. Most important, your patient needs to be told what adverse reactions to expect, so that he won't become worried or even stop taking the drug on his own. Of course, the patient should report adverse reactions to the doctor.

Recognizing drug allergies or serious idiosyncratic reactions can sometimes be lifesaving. Ask each patient about drugs he is taking or has taken in the past and what, if any, unusual reactions he experienced from taking them. If a patient claims to be allergic to a drug, ask him to tell you exactly what happens when he takes it. He may be calling a harmless adverse effect such as upset stomach an allergic reaction, or he may have a true tendency toward anaphylaxis. In either case, you and the doctor need to know this. Of course, you must record and report clinical changes throughout the patient's hospital stay. If you suspect a severe adverse reaction, withhold the drug until you can check with the pharmacist and the doctor.

### Toxic reactions

Chronic drug toxicities are generally caused by the cumulative effect and resulting buildup of the drug in the body. These effects may be extensions of the desired therapeutic effect. For example, glyburide will normalize blood sugar when given in usual doses but can produce undesired hypoglycemia if given in larger doses.

Drug toxicities typically occur when drug blood levels rise as a result of impaired metabolism or excretion. For example, blood levels of theophylline rise when hepatic dysfunction impairs metabolism of the drug. Similarly, digoxin toxicity can follow impaired renal function because digoxin is eliminated from the body almost exclusively by the kidneys

(via glomerular filtration). Of course, toxic blood levels also follow excessive dosage. Tinnitus is usually a sign that the safe dose of aspirin has been exceeded.

Most drug toxicities are predictable and dosage-related; fortunately, most are also readily reversible once the dosage is adjusted. So be sure to monitor patients carefully for physiologic changes that might alter drug effect. Watch especially for impaired hepatic and renal function. Warn the patient about signs of pending toxicity, and tell him what to do if a toxic reaction occurs. Also, be sure to emphasize the importance of taking a drug exactly as prescribed. Warn the patient about serious problems that could arise if he changes the dose or the schedule for taking it.

### Drug interactions

A drug interaction occurs when one drug administered with or shortly after another drug alters the effect of one or both drugs. Usually the effect of one drug is increased or decreased. For instance, one drug may inhibit or stimulate the metabolism or excretion of the other, or it may release another from plasma protein-binding sites, freeing it for further action.

Combination therapy is based on drug interaction. One drug, for example, may be given to potentiate another. Probenecid, which blocks the excretion of penicillin, is sometimes given with penicillin to maintain adequate blood levels of penicillin for a longer period. In many cases, two drugs with similar actions are given together precisely because of the additive effect that results. For instance, aspirin and codeine, both analgesics, are commonly given in combination because together they provide greater pain relief than either alone.

Drug interactions are sometimes used to prevent or antagonize certain adverse reactions. Hydrochlorothiazide and spironolactone, both diuretics, are commonly administered in combination because the former is potassium-depleting, whereas the latter is potassium-sparing.

Not all drug interactions are beneficial. Multiple drugs can interact to produce effects that are undesirable and sometimes hazardous. Harmful drug interactions decrease efficacy or increase toxicity. For example, in a patient taking both diuretics and lithium, the diuretics may cause an increase in serum levels of lithium, resulting in lithium toxicity. Such a drug effect is known as antagonism. Drug combinations that produce these effects should be avoided if possible. Another kind of inhibiting effect occurs when a tetracycline is administered with calcium- or magnesium-containing drugs or foods (such as antacids or milk). These bind with tetracycline in the GI tract and cause inadequate absorption of tetracycline.

The CD-ROM at the back of *NDH2001 Drug Handbook* reinforces these drug facts by offering scrollable lists of drug names and interacting agents, with possible effects and clinical tips.

## Drugs and pregnancy

Ever since the thalidomide tragedy of the late 1950s—when thousands of malformed infants were born after their mothers used this mild sedative-hypnotic during pregnancy—use of drugs during pregnancy has been a source of serious medical concern and controversy. To identify drugs that may cause such teratogenic effects, preclinical drug studies always include tests on pregnant laboratory animals. These tests point out gross teratogenicity but do not clearly establish safety. Because different species react to drugs in different ways, animal studies do not rule out possible teratogenic effects in humans. For example, the preliminary studies on thalidomide gave no warning of teratogenic effects, and it was subsequently released for general use in Europe.

What about the placental barrier? Once thought to protect the fetus from drug effects, the placenta isn't much of a barrier at all. Except for drugs with exceptionally large molecular structure, almost every drug administered to a pregnant woman crosses the placenta and enters the fetal circulation. An example of a drug with a large molecular size is heparin, the injectable anticoagulant. Theoretically, then, heparin could be used in a pregnant woman without fear of harming the fetus—but even heparin carries a warning for cautious use in pregnancy. Conversely, just because a drug crosses the placenta doesn't necessarily mean it's harmful to the fetus.

Actually, only one factor—stage of fetal development—seems clearly related to exaggerated risk during pregnancy. During two stages of pregnancy—the first and the third trimesters—the fetus is especially vulnerable to damage from maternal use of drugs. During these times, *all* drugs should be given with extreme caution.

The most sensitive period for drug-induced fetal malformation is the first trimester, when fetal organs are differentiating (organogenesis). During this time, *all* drugs, except those labeled as category A or B, should be withheld unless doing so would jeopardize the mother's health. Theoretically, during this sensitive time, even aspirin could harm the fetus. So, strongly advise your patient to avoid *all* self-prescribed drugs during early pregnancy. Fetal sensitivity to drugs is also of special concern during the last trimester. The reason? At birth, when separated from his mother, the neonate must rely on his own metabolism to eliminate any remaining drug. Because his detoxifying systems are not fully developed, any residual drug may take a long time to be metabolized—and thus may induce prolonged toxic reactions. Consequently, drugs should be used only when absolutely necessary during the last 3 months of pregnancy.

Of course, in many circumstances, pregnant women must continue to take certain drugs. For example, a woman with a seizure disorder that is well controlled with an anticonvulsant should continue to take the drug even during pregnancy. Similarly, a pregnant woman with a bacterial infection must receive antibiotics. In such cases, the potential risk to the fetus is outweighed by the mother's need. The relative risk to the fetus is expressed by the drug's pregnancy risk category (see Chapter 1, HOW TO USE *NURSING2001 DRUG HANDBOOK*).

Following these general guidelines can prevent indiscriminate and potentially harmful use of drugs in pregnancy:

● Before a drug is prescribed for a woman of childbearing age, she should be asked the date of her last menstrual period and whether she may be pregnant. If a drug is a known teratogen (for example, isotretinoin), some manufacturers may recommend special precautions to ensure that the drug not be given to a female of childbearing age until pregnancy is ruled out and that contraceptives are used throughout the course of therapy.

● Especially during the first and the third trimesters, a pregnant patient should avoid all drugs except those essential to maintain the pregnancy or maternal health.

● Topical drugs are not exempt from the warning against indiscriminate use during pregnancy. Many topically applied drugs can be absorbed in large enough amounts to be harmful to the fetus.

● When a pregnant patient needs a drug, the doctor should prescribe the safest possible drug in the lowest possible dose to minimize any harmful effect to the fetus.

● Every pregnant patient should check with her doctor before taking a drug.

## Drugs and lactation

Most drugs a breast-feeding mother takes appear in breast milk. Drug levels in breast milk tend to be high when blood levels are high—generally, shortly after taking each dose. Therefore, the mother should be advised to breast-feed *before* taking medication, not *after*.

Nevertheless, with few exceptions, a mother who wishes to breast-feed may continue to do so with her doctor's permission. However, breast-feeding should be temporarily interrupted and replaced with bottle-feeding when the mother must take tetracyclines, chloramphenicol, sulfonamides (during first 2 weeks postpartum), oral anticoagulants, iodine-containing drugs, or antineoplastics.

To protect her infant, a breast-feeding mother should avoid taking drugs indiscriminately. If she needs to take a drug, she should first check with her doctor to be sure of taking the safest drug at the lowest dose.

## Patient education

The following general guidelines will help to ensure that the patient gets maximal therapeutic benefits and avoids adverse reactions, accidental overdose, or potentially harmful changes in effectiveness.

● Tell the patient to store drugs in their original containers, at room temperature (unless directed otherwise), and in places that are not accessible to children or exposed to sunlight. Avoid storage in the bathroom medicine cabinet, in the kitchen close to heat, or in the glove compartment or trunk of an automobile, where extremes of temperature and humidity will cause drugs to deteriorate.

● Instruct the patient to learn the brand name and generic name of all drugs he is taking and to inform his regular health care professionals about their use. Before a patient takes a drug, tell him to report unusual reactions experienced in the past, allergies to foods and other substances, special medical problems, and drugs taken over the last few weeks, including OTC or herbal drugs.

● Inform the patient to always read the label before taking a drug, to take it exactly as prescribed, and never to share prescription drugs.

● Instruct the patient to check the expiration date before taking the drug.

● Warn the patient not to change brands of a drug without medical approval to avoid potentially harmful changes in effectiveness. Certain generic preparations are not equivalent in effect to brand-name preparations of the same drug.

● Caution the patient never to mix different drugs in a single container, remove a drug from its original container, or remove the label. Relying on memory to identify a drug and specific directions for its use is hazardous.

● Instruct the patient to safely discard drugs that are outdated or no longer needed and to keep discarded drugs out of the reach of children and pets.

● Advise the patient to inform the doctor about use of drugs before undergoing surgery (including dental surgery).

• Stress the importance of informing the doctor about adverse reactions experienced during drug therapy.

• Instruct the patient to call the doctor, poison control center, or pharmacist immediately if he or someone else has taken an overdose. The patient should keep handy their phone numbers and other emergency numbers, and he should have syrup of ipecac available at home to induce vomiting, but only if advised to do so by these professionals.

• Advise the patient to have all prescriptions filled at the same pharmacy so that the pharmacist can identify and warn against potentially harmful drug interactions. Also, tell the patient to inform the pharmacist and doctor of OTC or herbal drugs being taken.

• Tell the patient to have a sufficient supply of drugs when traveling. He should carry them with him and not stow them in his luggage.

# 3

# Drug therapy in children

Providing drug therapy to children and adolescents is challenging. Physiologic differences, including those in vital organ maturity and body composition, between children and adults can significantly influence a drug's effectiveness.

## Physiologic changes affecting drug action

A child's absorption, distribution, metabolism, and excretion processes undergo profound changes that affect drug dosage. To ensure optimal drug effect and minimal toxicity, consider these factors when administering drugs to a child.

### Absorption

Drug absorption in children depends on the form of the drug; its physical properties; other drugs or substances such as food, taken simultaneously; physiologic changes; and concurrent disease.

The pH of neonatal gastric fluid is neutral or slightly acidic and becomes more acidic as the infant matures, affecting drug absorption. For example, nafcillin and penicillin G are better absorbed in an infant than in an adult because of low gastric acidity.

Various infant formulas or milk products may increase gastric pH and impede absorption of acidic drugs. If possible, give a child oral drugs on an empty stomach.

Gastric emptying time and transit time through the small intestine—which is longer in children than in adults—can affect absorption. Also, intestinal hypermotility (as in diarrhea) can diminish the drug's absorption.

A child's comparatively thin epidermis allows increased absorption of topical drugs.

### Distribution

As with absorption, changes in body weight and physiology during childhood can significantly influence a drug's distribution and effects. In a premature infant, body fluid makes up about 85% of total body weight; in a full-term infant, 55% to 70%; and in an adult, 50% to 55%. Extracellular fluid (mostly blood) constitutes 40% of a neonate's body weight, compared with 20% in an adult. Intracellular fluid remains fairly constant throughout life and has little effect on drug dosage.

Extracellular fluid volume influences a water-soluble drug's concentration and effect because most drugs travel through extracellular fluid to reach their receptors. Children have a larger proportion of fluid to solid body weight, so their distribution area is proportionally greater.

Because the proportion of fat to lean body mass increases with age, the distribution of fat-soluble drugs is more limited in children than adults. As a result, a drug's lipid or water solubility affects the dosage for a child.

### Binding to plasma proteins

As the result of a decrease in albumin concentration or intermolecular attraction between drug and plasma protein, many drugs are less bound to plasma proteins in infants than in adults.

Furthermore, preparations that bind plasma proteins may displace endogenous compounds, such as bilirubin or free fatty acids. Conversely, an endogenous compound may displace a weakly bound drug. For example, displacement of bound bilirubin can cause a rise in unbound bilirubin, which can lead to increased risk of kernicterus at normal bilirubin levels.

Because only an unbound, or free, drug has a pharmacologic effect, an alteration in ratio of a protein-bound to an unbound active drug can greatly influence its effect.

Several diseases and disorders, such as nephrotic syndrome and malnutrition, can also decrease plasma protein and increase the concentration of an unbound drug, intensifying the drug's effect or producing toxicity.

*Metabolism*

A neonate's ability to metabolize a drug depends on the integrity of the hepatic enzyme system, the intrauterine exposure to the drug, and the nature of the drug itself.

Certain metabolic mechanisms are underdeveloped in neonates. Glucuronidation is a metabolic process that renders most drugs more water soluble, thereby facilitating renal excretion. This process is insufficiently developed to permit full pediatric doses until the infant is age 1 month; therefore, the use of chloramphenicol in a neonate may cause gray baby syndrome, illustrating the infant's inability to metabolize the drug. Use of chloramphenicol in neonates requires decreased dosage (25 mg/kg/day) and monitoring of blood levels.

Conversely, intrauterine exposure to drugs may induce precocious development of hepatic enzyme mechanisms, increasing the infant's capacity to metabolize potentially harmful substances.

Older children can metabolize some drugs (theophylline, for example) more rapidly than adults. This ability may come from their increased hepatic metabolic activity. Doses larger than those recommended for adults may be required.

Also, preparations given concurrently to a child may alter hepatic metabolism and induce production of hepatic enzymes. Phenobarbital, for example, can induce hepatic enzyme production and accelerate metabolism of drugs given concurrently.

*Excretion*

Renal excretion of a drug is the net effect of glomerular filtration, active tubular secretion, and passive tubular reabsorption. Because so many drugs are excreted in the urine, the degree of renal development or presence of renal disease can profoundly affect a child's dosage requirements. If a child is unable to excrete a drug renally, drug accumulation and possible toxicity may result unless the dosage is reduced.

Physiologically, an infant's kidneys differ from an adult's in that they have a high resistance to blood flow and receive a smaller proportion of cardiac output; exhibit incomplete glomerular and tubular development and short, incomplete loops of Henle (a child's glomerular filtration reaches adult values between ages 2½ and 5 months; his tubular secretion may reach adult values between 7 and 12 months); have a low glomerular filtration rate (penicillins are eliminated by this route); demonstrate a decreased ability to concentrate urine or reabsorb various filtered compounds; and have a reduced ability of the proximal tubules to secrete organic acids.

Both children and adults have diurnal variations in urine pH that correlate with sleep-awake patterns.

## Special administration considerations

Biochemically, a drug displays the same mechanisms of action in all individuals. However, the response of a drug can be affected by a child's age and size as well as the maturity of the target organ. To ensure optimal drug effect and minimal toxicity, consider the following factors when administering drugs to pediatric patients.

*Adjusting dosages for children*

When calculating children's dosages, don't use formulas that modify adult dosages: A child is not a scaled-down version of an adult. Pediatric dosages should be calculated on the basis of either body weight (mg/kg) or body surface area (mg/m²).

Reevaluate dosages at regular intervals to ensure necessary adjustments as the child develops. Although body surface area provides a useful standard for adults and older children, don't use it in premature or full-term infants. Use the body weight method instead. Don't exceed the maximum adult dosage when calculating amounts per kilogram of body weight (except with certain drugs such as theophylline, if indicated).

Obtain an accurate maternal drug history—prescription and nonprescription drugs, vitamins, and herbs or other health foods taken during pregnancy. Drugs passed through breast milk can also have adverse effects on the breast-feeding infant. Before a drug is prescribed for a breast-feeding mother, the potential effects on the infant should be investigated.

For example, sulfonamides given to a breast-feeding mother for a urinary tract infection appear in breast milk and may cause kernicterus at lower-than-normal levels of unconjugated bilirubin. Also, high concentrations of isoniazid appear in breast milk. Because this drug is metabolized by the liver, an infant's immature hepatic enzyme mechanisms cannot metabolize the drug, and the infant may suffer CNS toxicity.

### Administering oral drugs

If the patient is an infant, administer the drug in liquid form if possible. For accuracy, measure and give the preparation by oral syringe; never use a vial or cup. Lift the patient's head to prevent aspiration of the drug, and press down on his chin to prevent choking. You may also place the drug in a nipple and allow the infant to suck the contents.

If the patient is a toddler, explain how you're going to give him the drug. If possible, have the parents enlist the child's cooperation. Don't mix the drug with food or call it "candy," even if it has a pleasant taste. Let the child drink liquid drug from a calibrated medication cup rather than from a spoon: It's easier and more accurate. If the preparation is available only in tablet form, crush it and mix it with a compatible syrup. (Check with the pharmacist to verify that the tablet can be crushed without compromising its effectiveness.)

If the patient is an older child who can swallow a tablet or capsule by himself, have him place the drug on the back of his tongue and swallow it with water or fruit juice. Remember, milk or milk products may interfere with drug absorption.

### Administering I.V. infusions

In infants, use a peripheral vein or a scalp vein in the temporal region for I.V. infusions. The scalp vein is safest in that the needle is not likely to be dislodged; however, the head must be shaved around the site. Temporary disfigurement may also result from the needle and infiltrated fluids. For these reasons, the scalp veins are not used as commonly today as they were in the past.

The extremities are the most accessible insertion sites; however, because patients tend to move about, take these precautions:

• Protect the insertion site to prevent catheter or needle dislodgment.
• Use a padded arm board to minimize dislodgment. Remove the arm board during range-of-motion exercises.
• Place the clamp out of the child's reach; if extension tubing is used to allow the child greater mobility, securely tape the connection.
• Provide a simple explanation to the child who must be restrained while asleep to allay anxiety and maintain trust.

During an I.V. infusion to a child, monitor flow rate and check the child's condition and insertion site at least hourly— more frequently if indicated.

Titrate the flow rate only while the patient is composed; crying and emotional upset can constrict blood vessels. Flow rate may vary if a pump isn't used. Flow should be adequate because some drugs (calcium, for example) can be irritating at low flow rates. Infants, small children, and children with compromised cardiopulmonary status are particularly vulnerable to fluid overload with I.V. drug administration. To prevent this problem and help ensure that a limited amount of fluid is infused in a controlled manner, use a volume-control set (a volume-control device in the I.V. tubing) and an infusion pump or a syringe. Do not place more than 2 hours of I.V. fluid at a time in the volume-control set.

### Administering I.M. injections

I.M. injections are preferred when the drug cannot be given by other parenteral routes and rapid absorption is necessary.

The vastus lateralis muscle is the preferred injection site in children under age 2, whereas the ventrogluteal area or gluteus medius muscle can be used in older children. To select the correct needle size, consider the patient's age, muscle mass, and nutritional status and the drug's viscosity; record and rotate injection sites. Explain to the patient that the injection will hurt, but that the medication will help him. Restrain him during the injection, if needed, and comfort him afterward.

### Administering topical drugs and inhalants

Use eardrops warmed to room temperature; cold drops can cause considerable pain and possibly vertigo. To administer drops, turn the patient on his side, with the affected ear up. If he is younger than age 3, pull the pinna down and back; if he is age 3 or older, pull the pinna up and back.

Avoid using inhalants in young children; obtaining their cooperation is difficult. Before attempting to administer a drug through a metered-dose nebulizer to an older child, explain the inhaler to him. Then have him hold the nebulizer upside down and close his lips around the mouthpiece. Have him exhale, pinch his nostrils shut and, when he starts to inhale, release one dose of the drug into his mouth. Tell the patient to continue inhaling until his lungs feel full. Most inhaled drugs are not useful if taken orally; therefore, if you doubt the patient's ability to use the inhalant correctly, don't use it. Such devices as spacers or assist devices may help; check with the pharmacist or health care provider.

Use topical corticosteroids with caution because chronic steroid use in children has been associated with delayed growth. When topical corticosteroids are used on the diaper area of infants, avoid covering this area with plastic or rubber pants, which will act as an occlusive dressing and enhance systemic absorption.

### Administering parenteral nutrition

Administer I.V. nutrition to patients who can't or won't take adequate food orally and patients with hypermetabolic conditions who need supplementation. The latter group includes premature infants and children who have burns or other major trauma, intractable diarrhea, malabsorption syndromes, GI abnormalities, emotional disorders (such as anorexia nervosa), and congenital abnormalities.

Before fat emulsions are administered to infants and children, however, potential benefits must be weighed against possible risks. Fats—supplied as 10% or 20% emulsions—are administered both peripherally and centrally. Their use is limited by the child's ability to metabolize them. An infant or a child with a diseased liver cannot efficiently metabolize fats, for example.

Some fats, however, must be supplied both to prevent essential fatty acid deficiency and to permit normal growth and development. A minimum of calories (2% to 4%) must be supplied as linoleic acid—an essential fatty acid found in lipids. In infants, fats are essential for normal neurologic development.

Nevertheless, fat solutions may decrease oxygen perfusion and may adversely affect children with pulmonary disease. This risk can be minimized by supplying only the minimum fat needed for essential fatty acid requirements and not the usual intake of 40% to 50% of the child's total calories.

Fatty acids can also displace bilirubin bound to serum albumin, causing a rise in free, unconjugated bilirubin and an increased risk of kernicterus. However, fat solutions may interfere with some bilirubin assays and cause falsely elevated levels. To avoid this complication, a blood sample should be drawn 4 hours after infusion of the lipid emulsion; or if the emulsion is introduced over 24 hours, the blood sample should be centrifuged before the assay is performed.

# 4

# Drug therapy in elderly patients

If you're administering drug therapy in elderly patients, you'll want to understand physiologic and pharmacokinetic changes that may alter appropriate drug dosage or cause common adverse reactions or compliance problems.

## Physiologic changes affecting drug action

As a person ages, gradual physiologic changes occur. Some of these age-related changes may alter the therapeutic and toxic effects of drugs.

### Body composition

Proportions of fat, lean tissue, and water in the body change with age. Total body mass and lean body mass tend to decrease; the proportion of body fat tends to increase.

Varying from person to person, these changes in body composition affect the relationship between a drug's concentration and distribution in the body.

For example, a water-soluble drug such as gentamicin is not distributed to fat. Because there's relatively less lean tissue in an elderly person, more drug remains in the blood.

### Gastrointestinal function

In elderly patients, decreases in gastric acid secretion and GI motility slow the emptying of stomach contents and the movement of intestinal contents through the entire tract. Furthermore, research suggests that elderly patients may have more difficulty absorbing drugs. This is a particularly significant problem with drugs that have a narrow therapeutic range, such as digoxin, in which any change in absorption can be crucial.

### Hepatic function

The liver's ability to metabolize certain drugs decreases with age. This decrease is caused by diminished blood flow to the liver, which results from the age-related decrease in cardiac output and from the diminished activity of certain liver enzymes. When an elderly patient takes such sleep medications as flurazepam, the liver's reduced ability to metabolize the drug may produce a hangover effect the next morning.

Decreased hepatic function may cause more intense drug effects owing to higher blood levels, longer-lasting drug effects owing to prolonged blood levels, and a greater incidence of drug toxicity.

### Renal function

Although an elderly person's renal function is usually sufficient to eliminate excess body fluid and waste, the ability to eliminate some drugs may be reduced by 50% or more.

Many drugs commonly used by elderly patients, such as digoxin, are excreted primarily through the kidneys. If the kidneys' ability to excrete the drug is decreased, high blood levels may result. Digoxin toxicity, therefore, is relatively common in elderly patients who are not receiving a reduced digoxin dosage that accommodates decreased renal function.

Drug dosages can be modified to compensate for age-related decreases in renal function. Aided by laboratory tests such as BUN and serum creatinine, doctors may adjust drug dosages so that the patient receives the expected therapeutic benefits without the risk of toxicity. Observe the patient for signs or symptoms of toxicity. A patient taking digoxin, for example, may experience anorexia, nausea, vomiting, or confusion.

## Special administration considerations

Aging is usually accompanied by a decline in organ function that can profoundly affect drug distribution and clearance. This physiologic decline is likely to be exacerbated by a disease or chronic disorder. Together, these factors can significantly increase the risk of adverse reactions, drug toxicity, and noncompliance.

Be aware of these changes when administering a drug to an elderly patient.

### Adverse reactions

Compared with younger people, elderly patients experience twice as many adverse drug reactions relating to greater drug consumption, poor compliance, and physiologic changes.

Signs and symptoms of adverse drug reactions—confusion, weakness, and lethargy—are often mistakenly attributed to senility or disease. If the adverse reaction isn't identified, the patient may continue to receive the drug. Furthermore, he may receive unnecessary additional drugs to treat complications caused by the original drug. This regimen can sometimes result in a pattern of inappropriate and excessive drug use.

Although any drug can cause adverse reactions, most of the serious reactions in the elderly are caused by relatively few drugs. Be particularly alert for toxicities resulting from diuretics, antihypertensives, digoxin, corticosteroids, sleeping aids, and OTC drugs.

### Diuretic toxicity

Because total body water content decreases with age, normal dosages of potassium-wasting diuretics, such as hydrochlorothiazide and furosemide, may result in fluid loss and even dehydration in an elderly patient.

These diuretics may deplete serum potassium, causing weakness in the patient, and they may raise blood uric acid and glucose levels, complicating preexisting gout and diabetes mellitus.

### Antihypertensive toxicity

Many elderly people experience lightheadedness or fainting when using antihypertensives, partly in response to atherosclerosis and decreased elasticity of the blood vessels. Antihypertensives can lower blood pressure too rapidly, resulting in insufficient blood flow to the brain, which could cause dizziness, fainting, or even stroke.

Consequently, dosages of antihypertensives must be carefully individualized. In elderly patients, too-aggressive treatment of high blood pressure may do more harm than good, so treatment goals should be reasonable. Although bringing blood pressure down to 135/90 mm Hg is appropriate, it needs to be done more slowly in elderly patients than in younger patients.

### Digoxin toxicity

As the body's renal function and rate of excretion decline, digoxin levels in the blood may build to toxic levels, causing nausea, vomiting, diarrhea, and—most serious—cardiac arrhythmias. Try to prevent severe toxicity by monitoring serum levels and by observing the patient for early signs and symptoms, such as appetite loss, confusion, or depression.

### Corticosteroid toxicity

Elderly patients on corticosteroids may experience short-term effects, including fluid retention and psychological manifestations ranging from mild euphoria to acute psychotic reactions. Long-term toxic effects such as osteoporosis can be especially severe in elderly patients who have been taking prednisone or related steroidal compounds for months or even years. To prevent serious toxicity, carefully monitor patients on long-term regimens. Observe them for subtle changes in appearance, mood, and mobility; signs of impaired healing; and fluid and electrolyte disturbances.

### Anticoagulant effects

Elderly patients taking anticoagulants have an increased risk of bleeding, especially when they take NSAIDs at the same time (many do). Observe the INR carefully, and monitor the patient for bruising and other signs of bleeding.

### Sleeping aid toxicity

Sedatives or such sleeping aids as flurazepam may cause excessive sedation or residual drowsiness. Keep in mind that ingestion of alcohol may exaggerate such depressant effects, even if the sleeping aid was taken the previous evening. These drugs should be used sparingly in elderly patients.

## OTC drug toxicity

When aspirin, aspirin-containing analgesics, and other OTC NSAIDs (such as ibuprofen, ketoprofen, and naproxen) are used in moderation, toxicity is minimal, but prolonged ingestion may cause GI irritation—even ulcers—and gradual blood loss resulting in severe anemia. Prescription NSAIDs may cause similar problems, especially in the elderly. Although anemia from chronic aspirin consumption can affect all age-groups, elderly patients may be less able to compensate because of their already reduced iron stores.

Laxatives may cause diarrhea in elderly patients who are extremely sensitive to such drugs as bisacodyl. Chronic oral use of mineral oil as a lubricating laxative may result in lipid pneumonia from aspiration of small residual oil droplets in the patient's mouth.

## Noncompliance

Poor compliance can be a problem with patients of any age. A significant number of hospitalizations result from noncompliance to medical regimen. However, in elderly patients, specific factors linked to aging—such as diminished visual acuity, hearing loss, forgetfulness, the common need for multiple drug therapy, and various socioeconomic factors—can combine to make compliance a special problem. About one-third of elderly patients fail to comply with their prescribed drug therapy. They may fail to take prescribed doses or to follow the correct schedule, or they may take drugs prescribed for previous disorders, discontinue drugs prematurely, or indiscriminately use drugs that are to be taken as needed. Elderly patients may also have multiple prescriptions for the same drug and, therefore, inadvertently take an overdose.

Review the patient's drug regimen with him. Make sure he understands the dose amount, the time and frequency of doses, and why he is taking the drug. Also, explain how he should take each drug—that is, with food or water or by itself.

Give the patient whatever help you can to avoid drug therapy problems. Suggest that he use drug calendars, pill sorters, or other aids to help him comply, and refer him to the doctor or pharmacist if he needs further information.

# 5

## Drug therapy and the nursing process

The nursing process guides nursing decisions about drug administration to ensure the patient's safety and meet medical and legal standards. This five-step process provides thorough assessment, appropriate nursing diagnosis, effective planning, correct interventions, and constant evaluation.

### Assessment

During assessment, the nurse focuses on direct data collection by:
• obtaining a drug history from the patient, parent, spouse, or companion
• reviewing the patient's medical history
• performing a physical examination
• obtaining and interpreting relevant laboratory or diagnostic test results.

Data collection begins at admission to the hospital or in an outpatient setting with specific questions about the patient's background, including allergies, medical history, habits, socioeconomic status, lifestyle and beliefs, and sensory deficits. These aspects of the patient's background can significantly influence drug therapy.

*Allergies*
The patient's allergy profile includes reactions to both drugs and food. Information about allergic reactions must specify the drug; a description of the reaction; its situation, time, and setting; and other contributing factors such as concurrent use of stimulants, tobacco, alcohol, or illegal drugs, or a significant change in nutritional patterns. Asking the patient to describe his allergic reaction is especially important to help determine if the patient reacts adversely or simply dislikes taking the drug.

Allergies to foods can also affect drug therapy. For example, allergies to shellfish can contraindicate use of drugs that contain iodine or are by-products of shellfish. Allergies to eggs are significant in patients who are to receive vaccines, which are commonly derived from chick embryos.

*Prescription drugs*
The patient's prescription drug history should explore the following:
• reason for using the drug
• patient's knowledge of the appropriate dosage
• patient's knowledge about determining effectiveness of the drug (if appropriate), potential adverse effects, what to do about adverse effects, and when to contact the doctor
• route of administration
• pattern of administration at home
• cognitive status.

Note any special monitoring the patient must perform, such as blood glucose monitoring before insulin administration or checking radial pulse rate before taking digoxin. Make sure the patient is performing such procedures correctly and that the results are within acceptable limits.

Discuss the effects of drug therapy with the patient and determine if new symptoms or unpredicted adverse reactions have developed. Noting the patient's pattern of administration may provide insight into why a particular drug regimen succeeds or fails.

*OTC drugs and herbal medicines*
A comprehensive drug history should also list OTC drugs and herbal medicines the patient is taking.

Many OTC drugs can inhibit or potentiate the effects of a prescribed drug. For example, aspirin potentiates the anticoagulant effects of warfarin.

OTC drugs include a wide range of products, from aspirin, nutritional supplements, and homeopathic remedies to various sprays and cleaning agents. The patient may not think of these as drugs, so the nurse may have to name types of products to get an accurate response.

Dosage and frequency of use are just as important as the type of OTC product. One aspirin tablet taken once a day may have no effect on concomitant drug therapy; however, a higher dosage (such as that used for arthritis) could profoundly influence therapy.

Just like OTC drugs, herbal medicines can affect how a prescribed drug acts in the body. Chamomile can potentiate the effects of an anticoagulant, for example, and goldenseal can interfere with the action of an antihypertensive.

Ask open-ended questions to allow the patient to provide information that may otherwise be missed.

*Medical history*
In gathering the medical history, note chronic diseases or disorders the patient may have and record the following information for each:
• date of diagnosis
• initial prescribed treatment
• current treatment
• doctor in charge.

Careful attention to this part of the medical history can uncover one of the most important problems with drug therapy—conflicting and incompatible drug regimens. The patient who does not have a primary health care provider to oversee and coordinate all care may seek the care of several specialists who may prescribe drug treatment without knowing what other drugs the patient is taking. Contacting the patient's pharmacist may be beneficial in obtaining a detailed list of medications. A carefully detailed medical history can uncover such problems. The nurse who identifies such conflicting or overlapping drug regimens must call them to the appropriate doctor's attention and then teach the patient about the importance of informing caregivers about all drugs he is taking.

*Habits*
Carefully consider dietary habits and the nontherapeutic use of drugs.

Certain foods can directly influence the effectiveness of many drugs. For example, a person who is taking the anticoagulant warfarin should not increase his intake of green leafy vegetables because they contain levels of vitamin K that can antagonize the drug's anticoagulant effect.

Nontherapeutic use of drugs (including alcohol, caffeine, tobacco, and illegal drugs) can profoundly affect a patient's health and impair the effectiveness of drug therapy. For the patient who uses alcohol, note the frequency of use, the amount, and the type of alcohol consumed. Carefully document the intake of stimulants such as caffeine because they significantly affect a patient's CV status and nervous system. Record the type of stimulant, the frequency of intake, and the amount consumed.

For the patient who uses tobacco, document the following information:
• number of years the patient has used tobacco (this is often written as pack years; for example, 2 packs per day for 20 years equals a 40 pack year history)
• kind of tobacco the patient smokes (cigarettes, cigars, or pipe) or chews
• how many cigarettes or cigars the patient smokes per day or how much and how long he chews tobacco daily
• brand of tobacco the patient smokes or chews.

Defining the patient's use of illegal drugs may be difficult. However, the nurse who suspects such use should encourage the patient to discuss it honestly, emphasizing that these drugs have profound effects that may cause serious drug interactions. If the patient admits using illegal drugs, document the drug, the amount and frequency of use, and the route of administration.

*Socioeconomic status*
Note the patient's age, educational level, occupation, and insurance coverage. These factors may be significant to compliance and to an effective plan of care. The patient's age, for example, can determine whom to include in the care (parents or other family members) and the level of information that is appropriate for teaching the patient.

Knowing the patient's educational background and occupation helps you select interventions at an appropriate level, plan a drug regimen that fits the patient's daily routine, and encourage compliance. Knowing the patient's insurance status may help you anticipate the need for financial assistance and counseling. Remember that noncompliance commonly results from inability to afford drugs.

*Lifestyle and beliefs*
Support systems, marital status, child-bearing status, attitudes toward health and health care, use of the health care system, and daily patterns of activities all affect the plan of care and patient compliance. For example, an 18-year-old single parent who is a high-school dropout on medical assistance and has no family support will probably require more teaching and support to gain a commitment and compliance than a 40-year-old affluent professional who has family support, can understand why he needs the drug, and can readily pay for it.

*Sensory deficits*
Sensory deficit can significantly shape an appropriate plan of care. For example, impaired vision, paralysis of one or more extremities, loss of a limb, or loss of sensation in an extremity can impair the patient's ability to administer a subcutaneous injection, break a scored tablet, or open a drug container. Color blindness may cause difficulty in distinguishing between two drugs. Hearing impairment can complicate effective patient instruction. A sensory deficit requires careful consideration in any plan of prescribed drug therapy.

*Clinical status*
Two other factors can profoundly influence drug therapy: the patient's cognitive status and the systemic effects of the prescribed drugs. A patient's intact cognitive abilities ensure that he can understand and implement the actions necessary for compliance. During the interview, note if the patient is alert and oriented, if he is able to interact appropriately with people, and if his conversation is appropriate. Consider whether the patient can think clearly and express his thoughts coherently. Finally, check both short- and long-term memory because the patient needs both to follow a specified drug regimen. If such evaluation identifies a cognitive deficit, determine the probable cause, which can range from a transient drug-related effect to permanent neurologic impairment, and then determine if the patient can carry out the prescribed regimen. If not, the nurse must find another way to ensure that the patient receives the prescribed therapy.

After completing the drug history, perform a physical examination to assess those body systems that may be affected by a particular drug the patient is taking or that may be prescribed. Every drug has a desired effect on a body system, but it may have an undesired effect on another. For example, chemotherapeutic drugs destroy cancerous cells, but they also affect normal cells and typically cause the patient to experience hair loss, diarrhea, or nausea. Therefore, examine the patient for expected drug effects; also, closely monitor the patient for potentially harmful adverse effects.

## Nursing diagnosis
Using information gathered during assessment, define potential or actual drug-related problems by formulating each in a relevant nursing diagnosis. The most common problem statements related to drug therapy are *Knowledge deficit, Noncompliance,* and *Altered health maintenance.*

## Planning
Nursing diagnoses provide the framework for planning interventions and outcome criteria (patient goals).

*Outcome criteria*
Outcome criteria state the desired patient behaviors or responses that should result from nursing care. Such criteria should be measurable and objective, concise, realistic for the patient, and attainable by nursing management. They should also express patient behavior in terms of expectations and specify a time frame. If possible, include the patient when making the plan. Patients are more likely to adhere to regimens if they feel they are an active member of the decision-making team. A typical outcome statement is "Before discharge, the patient verbalizes major adverse effects related to his chemotherapy."

## Intervention

After developing the outcome criteria, the nurse determines the interventions needed to help the patient reach the desired behavior or goals. Drug-related interventions may focus on patient teaching for a drug's action, adverse effects, scheduling, steps to avoid or treat a drug reaction, or drug administration techniques.

Appropriate interventions related to drug therapy also include administration procedures and techniques, legal and ethical concerns, patient teaching, and concerns related to special groups of patients (elderly, pediatric, pregnant, or breast-feeding patients). Such interventions may be independent nursing actions, such as turning a bedridden patient every 2 hours, or nursing actions that require a doctor's order.

## Evaluation

The final component of the nursing process, evaluation, is a formal and systematic process for determining the effectiveness of nursing care. This process enables the nurse to determine whether outcome criteria were met and thereby make informed decisions about subsequent interventions. For example, if the patient experienced relief of headache within 1 hour after the nurse administered an analgesic, as needed, the outcome criterion was met. If the headache was the same or worse, the outcome criterion was not met and requires a new assessment. The reassessment may result in a new plan of care, or may yield new data that invalidate the nursing diagnosis or suggest new nursing interventions that are more specific or more acceptable to the patient. This assessment could lead to a higher dosage, a different analgesic, or a reevaluation of the cause.

Evaluation enables the nurse to design and implement a revised plan of care, to continuously reevaluate outcome criteria, and to plan again until each nursing diagnosis is successfully completed.

# 6

## Amebicides and antiprotozoals

**atovaquone**
**chloroquine hydrochloride**
  (See Chapter 9, ANTIMALARIALS.)
**chloroquine phosphate**
  (See Chapter 9, ANTIMALARIALS.)
**metronidazole**
**metronidazole hydrochloride**
**pentamidine isethionate**

### COMBINATION PRODUCTS
HELIDAC: metronidazole 250 mg (with povidone), tetracycline 500 mg, bismuth subsalicylate 262.4 mg (with povidone)

---

atovaquone
Mepron, Wellvone§

*Pregnancy Risk Category C*

### HOW SUPPLIED
*Suspension:* 750 mg/5 ml

### ACTION
Unknown. Appears to interfere with electron transport in protozoal mitochondria, inhibiting enzymes needed for the synthesis of nucleic acids and adenosine triphosphate.

| Route | Onset | Peak | Duration |
|-------|-------|------|----------|
| P.O. | Unknown | 1 hr-days | Unknown |

### INDICATIONS & DOSAGE
*Acute, mild to moderate* Pneumocystis carinii *pneumonia in patients who can't tolerate co-trimoxazole—*
**Adults:** 750 mg P.O. b.i.d. with food for 21 days.
❋ *NEW INDICATION: Prevention of* P. carinii *pneumonia in patients who can't tolerant co-trimoxazole—*
**Adults and adolescents ages 13 to 16:** 1,500 mg (10 ml) P.O. daily with food.

### ADVERSE REACTIONS
**CNS:** *headache, insomnia,* asthenia, anxiety, dizziness.
**CV:** hypotension.

**EENT:** *cough,* sinusitis, rhinitis, taste perversion, *oral candidiasis.*
**GI:** *nausea, diarrhea, vomiting,* constipation, *abdominal pain,* anorexia, dyspepsia.
**Hematologic:** anemia, **neutropenia.**
**Hepatic:** elevated liver function tests.
**Metabolic:** hypoglycemia, hyponatremia.
**Skin:** *rash,* pruritus, *diaphoresis,* sweating.
**Other:** *fever, pain.*

### INTERACTIONS
**Drug-drug.** *Rifabutin, rifampin:* decreases atovaquone's steady-state concentration. Avoid concurrent use.

### EFFECTS ON DIAGNOSTIC TESTS
None reported.

### CONTRAINDICATIONS
Contraindicated in patients with hypersensitivity to drug.

### NURSING CONSIDERATIONS
• Use cautiously in breast-feeding patients. Drug has appeared in breast milk.
• Because drug is highly bound to plasma protein (over 99.9%), also use cautiously with other highly protein-bound drugs.
• *Alert:* Because of risk of other concurrent pulmonary infections, monitor patient closely during therapy.

☑ **Patient teaching**
• Instruct patient to take drug with meals because food enhances absorption significantly.

---

metronidazole
Apo-Metronidazole†, Flagyl, Flagyl ER, Metrogyl‡, Novo-Nidazol†, Protostat, Trikacide†

metronidazole hydrochloride
Flagyl IV RTU, Novo-Nidazol†

*Pregnancy Risk Category B*

---

Reactions may be *common,* uncommon, ***life-threatening***, or COMMON AND LIFE-THREATENING.

## HOW SUPPLIED
*Tablets:* 200 mg‡, 250 mg, 375 mg, 400 mg‡, 500 mg
*Tablets (extended-release):* 750 mg
*Oral suspension (benzoyl metronidazole):* 200 mg/5 ml‡
*Injection:* 500 mg/100 ml ready to use
*Powder for injection:* 500-mg single-dose vials

## ACTION
A direct-acting trichomonacide and amebicide that works at both intestinal and extraintestinal sites. It is thought to enter the cells of microorganisms that contain nitroreductase. Unstable compounds are then formed that bind to DNA and inhibit synthesis, causing cell death.

| Route | Onset | Peak | Duration |
|-------|-------|------|----------|
| P.O. | Unknown | 2 hr | Unknown |
| I.V. | Immediate | 1 hr | Unknown |

## INDICATIONS & DOSAGE
*Amoebic hepatic abscess—*
**Adults:** 500 to 750 mg P.O. t.i.d. for 5 to 10 days.
**Children:** 30 to 50 mg/kg daily (in three divided doses) for 10 days.
*Intestinal amebiasis—*
**Adults:** 750 mg P.O. t.i.d. for 5 to 10 days.
**Children:** 30 to 50 mg/kg daily (in three divided doses) for 10 days.
   Therapy for adults or children is followed by oral iodoquinol.
*Trichomoniasis—*
**Adults:** 250 mg P.O. t.i.d. for 7 days or 2 g P.O. in single dose (may give the 2-g dose in two 1-g doses, each on the same day); 4 to 6 weeks should elapse between courses of therapy.
**Children:** 5 mg/kg P.O. t.i.d. for 7 days.
*Refractory trichomoniasis—*
**Adults:** 250 mg P.O. b.i.d. for 10 days. Or, 500 mg P.O. b.i.d. for 7 days.
*Bacterial infections due to anaerobic microorganisms—*
**Adults:** loading dose is 15 mg/kg I.V. infused over 1 hour (about 1 g for a 70-kg [154-lb] adult). Maintenance dose is 7.5 mg/kg I.V. or P.O. q 6 hours (about 500 mg for a 70-kg adult). First maintenance dose should be given 6 hours after loading dose. Maximum dose not to exceed 4 g daily.

*Prevention of postoperative infection in contaminated or potentially contaminated colorectal surgery—*
**Adults:** 15 mg/kg I.V. infused over 30 to 60 minutes and completed about 1 hour before surgery. Then, 7.5 mg/kg I.V. infused over 30 to 60 minutes at 6 and 12 hours after initial dose.
*Bacterial vaginosis—*
**Adults:** 500 mg P.O. b.i.d. for 7 days.

## ADVERSE REACTIONS
**CNS:** vertigo, *headache,* ataxia, dizziness, syncope, incoordination, confusion, irritability, depression, weakness, insomnia, *seizures,* peripheral neuropathy.
**CV:** flattened T wave, edema.
**EENT:** rhinitis, sinusitis, pharyngitis, metallic taste.
**GI:** abdominal cramping or pain, stomatitis, epigastric distress, *nausea,* vomiting, anorexia, diarrhea, constipation, proctitis, dry mouth.
**GU:** darkened urine, polyuria, dysuria, cystitis, decreased libido, dyspareunia, dryness of vagina and vulva, vaginal candidiasis, *vaginitis,* genital pruritus.
**Hematologic:** transient leukopenia, *neutropenia,* thrombophlebitis after I.V. infusion.
**Musculoskeletal:** fleeting joint pains.
**Respiratory:** upper respiratory infection.
**Skin:** flushing, rash.
**Other:** fever, overgrowth of nonsusceptible organisms, especially *Candida.*

## INTERACTIONS
**Drug-drug.** *Cimetidine:* increased risk of metronidazole toxicity because of inhibited hepatic metabolism. Monitor closely.
*Disulfiram:* acute psychoses and confusional states. Don't use within 2 weeks of last disulfiram dose.
*Lithium:* increased lithium levels resulting in possible toxicity. Monitor serum lithium levels closely.
*Oral anticoagulants:* increased anticoagulant effects. Monitor closely.
*Phenobarbital, phenytoin:* decreased metronidazole effectiveness. Total phenytoin clearance may be reduced. Monitor closely.
**Drug-lifestyle.** *Alcohol use:* disulfiram-like reaction (nausea, vomiting, headache,

---

cramps, flushing). Don't use together or for 3 days after completion of drug therapy.

**EFFECTS ON DIAGNOSTIC TESTS**
Metronidazole may interfere with the chemical analyses of aminotransferases and triglycerides, leading to falsely decreased values.

**CONTRAINDICATIONS**
Contraindicated in patients with hypersensitivity to drug or other nitroimidazole derivatives and during the first trimester of pregnancy.

**NURSING CONSIDERATIONS**
• Use cautiously in patients with history of blood dyscrasia or CNS disorder and in those with retinal or visual field changes. Also use cautiously in patients with hepatic disease or alcoholism and in conjunction with hepatotoxic drugs.
• Monitor liver function tests carefully in elderly patients. If test results are altered, metronidazole levels should be monitored closely to prevent toxicity.
• Drug is contraindicated in the first trimester of pregnancy. However, if indicated during pregnancy for trichomoniasis, be aware that the 7-day regimen is preferred over the 2-g, single-dose regimen.
• Give oral form with meals.
• Observe for edema, especially in patients receiving corticosteroids; Flagyl I.V. RTU (ready to use) may cause sodium retention.
• Record number and character of stools when used to treat amebiasis. Metronidazole should be used only after *Trichomonas vaginalis* infection has been confirmed by wet smear or culture, or *Entamoeba histolytica* has been identified. Asymptomatic sexual partners of patients being treated for *T. vaginalis* infection should be treated simultaneously to avoid reinfection.

**I.V. administration**
• No preparation is needed for Flagyl I.V. RTU. To prepare lyophilized vials of metronidazole, add 4.4 ml of sterile water for injection, bacteriostatic water for injection, sterile normal saline for injection, or bacteriostatic normal saline for injection. Reconstituted drug contains 100 mg/ml. Add contents of vial to 100 ml of $D_5W$, lactated Ringer's injection, or normal saline for a final concentration of 5 mg/ml. The resulting highly acidic solution must be neutralized before administering. Carefully add 5 mEq sodium bicarbonate for each 500 mg metronidazole; carbon dioxide gas will form and may need to be vented.
• *Alert:* Infuse drug over at least 1 hour. Don't give I.V. push.
• Don't refrigerate the neutralized diluted solution because precipitation may occur. If Flagyl I.V. RTU is refrigerated, crystals may form. These disappear after the solution warms to room temperature.

**☑ Patient teaching**
• Instruct patient to take oral form with food to minimize GI upset, although extended-release tablets should be taken at least 1 hour before or 2 hours after meals.
• Inform patient that sexual partners should be treated simultaneously to avoid reinfection.
• Instruct patient in proper hygiene.
• Tell patient to avoid alcohol or alcohol-containing medications during therapy and for at least 3 days after therapy is completed.
• Tell patient metallic taste and dark or red-brown urine may occur.

---

**pentamidine isethionate**
NebuPent, Pentacarinat, Pentam 300

*Pregnancy Risk Category C*

**HOW SUPPLIED**
*Injection, aerosol:* 300-mg vial

**ACTION**
Unknown. Believed to interfere with biosynthesis of DNA, RNA, phospholipids, and proteins in susceptible organisms.

| Route | Onset | Peak | Duration |
|-------|-------|------|----------|
| I.V. | Unknown | 1 hr | Unknown |
| I.M., inhalation | Unknown | 0.5 hr | Unknown |

## INDICATIONS & DOSAGE

Pneumocystis carinii *pneumonia—*
**Adults and children:** 3 to 4 mg/kg I.V. or I.M. once daily for 14 to 21 days.
*Prevention of* P. carinii *pneumonia in high-risk patients—*
**Adults:** 300 mg by inhalation (using a Respirgard II nebulizer) once q 4 weeks.

## ADVERSE REACTIONS

**CNS:** confusion, hallucinations, *fatigue, dizziness,* headache.
**CV: *hypotension, ventricular tachycardia,*** *chest pain.*
**EENT***:* burning in throat (with inhaled form), *pharyngitis.*
**GI:** *nausea, metallic taste, decreased appetite, vomiting,* diarrhea, abdominal pain, anorexia, pancreatitis.
**GU:** *elevated BUN and serum creatinine levels,* **acute renal failure.**
**Hematologic: *leukopenia, thrombocytopenia,*** anemia.
**Hepatic:** elevated AST and ALT levels.
**Metabolic: *hypoglycemia,*** hyperglycemia, hypocalcemia.
**Musculoskeletal:** myalgia.
**Respiratory:** *cough, bronchospasm, shortness of breath,* pneumothorax, *congestion.*
**Skin:** rash, ***Stevens-Johnson syndrome.***
**Other:** *night sweats, chills,* edema, *sterile abscess, pain, induration at injection site.*

## INTERACTIONS

**Drug-drug.** *Aminoglycosides, amphotericin B, capreomycin, cisplatin, colistin, methoxyflurane, polymyxin B, vancomycin:* increased risk of nephrotoxicity. Monitor closely.
*Antineoplastics:* additive bone marrow suppression. Use together cautiously.

## EFFECTS ON DIAGNOSTIC TESTS

None reported.

## CONTRAINDICATIONS

Contraindicated in patients with a history of an anaphylactic reaction to drug.

## NURSING CONSIDERATIONS

• Use cautiously in patients with hypertension, hypotension, hypoglycemia, hypocalcemia, leukopenia, thrombocy-

topenia, anemia, diabetes, pancreatitis, Stevens-Johnson syndrome, or hepatic or renal dysfunction.
• Administer aerosol form only by Respirgard II nebulizer. Dosage recommendations are based on the particle size and delivery rate of this device. To administer aerosol, mix contents of one vial in 6 ml sterile water for injection. Do not use normal saline solution. Do not mix with other drugs.
• Don't use low-pressure (less than 20 pounds per square inch [psi]) compressors. The flow rate should be 5 to 7 L/minute from a 40- to 50-psi air or oxygen source.
• For I.M. injection, reconstitute drug with 3 ml of sterile water for a solution containing 100 mg/ml; administer deeply. Expect patient to report pain and induration at injection site.
• Monitor blood glucose, serum calcium, serum creatinine, and BUN levels daily. After parenteral administration, blood glucose level may decrease initially; hypoglycemia may be severe in 5% to 10% of patients. This may be followed by hyperglycemia and type 1 diabetes mellitus, which may be permanent because of pancreatic cell damage.
• In patients with AIDS, pentamidine may produce less severe adverse reactions than co-trimoxazole.

### ⚡ I.V. administration
• Reconstitute drug with 3 ml of sterile water for injection; then dilute in 50 to 250 ml of D₅W. Infuse over at least 60 minutes.
• *Alert:* To minimize risk of hypotension when drug is given I.V., infuse drug slowly with patient lying down. Closely monitor blood pressure.

### ✓ Patient teaching
• Instruct patient to use the aerosol device until the chamber is empty, which may take up to 45 minutes.
• Warn patient that I.M. injection is painful.
• Instruct patient to complete the full course of pentamidine therapy, even if feeling better.

**mebendazole**
**pyrantel pamoate**
**thiabendazole**

## COMBINATION PRODUCTS
None.

---

## mebendazole
Vermox

*Pregnancy Risk Category C*

### HOW SUPPLIED
*Tablets (chewable):* 100 mg

### ACTION
Selectively and irreversibly inhibits uptake of glucose and other nutrients in susceptible helminths.

| Route | Onset | Peak | Duration |
|-------|-------|------|----------|
| P.O. | Unknown | 2-4 hr | Variable |

### INDICATIONS & DOSAGE
*Pinworm—*
**Adults and children over age 2:** 100 mg P.O. as a single dose; repeated if infection persists 2 to 3 weeks later.
*Roundworm, whipworm, hookworm—*
**Adults and children over age 2:** 100 mg P.O. b.i.d. for 3 days; repeated if infection persists 3 weeks later.

### ADVERSE REACTIONS
**CNS:** *seizures.*
**GI:** occasional, transient abdominal pain and diarrhea in massive infection and expulsion of worms.
**Skin:** urticaria.
**Other:** fever.

### INTERACTIONS
**Drug-drug.** *Carbamazepine, hydantoins:* reduced plasma mebendazole levels, potentially decreasing its effect. Monitor closely.
*Cimetidine:* increased plasma mebendazole levels. Monitor closely.

### EFFECTS ON DIAGNOSTIC TESTS
None reported.

### CONTRAINDICATIONS
Contraindicated in patients with hypersensitivity to drug.

### NURSING CONSIDERATIONS
• Tablets may be chewed, swallowed whole, or crushed and mixed with food.
• Administer drug to all family members, as prescribed, to decrease the risk of spreading the infection.
• Dietary restrictions, laxatives, or enemas aren't necessary.
• Safe use in children under age 2 hasn't been established.

### ☑ Patient teaching
• Teach patient about personal hygiene, especially good hand-washing technique. Advise him to refrain from preparing food for others.
• To avoid reinfection, teach patient to wash perianal area daily, to change undergarments and bedclothes daily, and to wash hands and clean fingernails before meals and after bowel movements.

---

## pyrantel pamoate
Antiminth, Combantrin†, Pin-Rid, Pin-X, Reese's Pinworm Medicine

*Pregnancy Risk Category C*

### HOW SUPPLIED
*Tablets:* 62.5 mg
*Capsules (soft-gel):* 180 mg
*Oral suspension:* 50 mg/ml

### ACTION
Blocks neuromuscular action, paralyzing the worm and causing its expulsion by normal peristalsis.

| Route | Onset | Peak | Duration |
|-------|-------|------|----------|
| P.O. | Variable | 1-3 hr | Variable |

---

Reactions may be *common,* uncommon, *life-threatening,* or COMMON AND LIFE-THREATENING.

## INDICATIONS & DOSAGE
*Roundworm, pinworm—*
**Adults and children ages 2 and older:**
11 mg/kg P.O. as a single dose. Maximum dose is 1 g. For pinworm, dose should be repeated in 2 weeks.

## ADVERSE REACTIONS
**CNS:** headache, dizziness, drowsiness, insomnia.
**GI:** anorexia, nausea, vomiting, gastralgia, abdominal cramps, diarrhea, tenesmus.
**Hepatic:** transient elevation of AST.
**Skin:** rash.
**Other:** fever, weakness.

## INTERACTIONS
**Drug-drug.** *Piperazine salts:* possible antagonism. Don't give together.

## EFFECTS ON DIAGNOSTIC TESTS
None reported.

## CONTRAINDICATIONS
Contraindicated in patients with hypersensitivity to drug.

## NURSING CONSIDERATIONS
• Use cautiously in patients with severe malnutrition or anemia or in patients with hepatic dysfunction.
• Dietary restrictions, laxatives, or enemas aren't needed.
• Drug should be given to all family members.

☑ **Patient teaching**
• Inform patient that pyrantel may be taken with food, milk, or fruit juices. Shake suspension well.
• Teach patient about personal hygiene, especially good hand-washing technique. To avoid reinfection, teach patient to wash perianal area daily, to change undergarments and bedclothes daily, and to wash hands and clean fingernails before meals and after bowel movements.
• Advise patient to refrain from preparing food for others.
• Tell patient to take entire dose as prescribed.

# thiabendazole
Mintezol

*Pregnancy Risk Category C*

## HOW SUPPLIED
*Tablets (chewable):* 500 mg
*Oral suspension:* 500 mg/5 ml

## ACTION
Unknown. Appears to inhibit the helminth-specific enzyme fumarate reductase.

| Route | Onset | Peak | Duration |
|-------|---------|--------|----------|
| P.O. | Unknown | 1-2 hr | Unknown |

## INDICATIONS & DOSAGE
*Cutaneous infestations with larva migrans (creeping eruption)—*
**Adults and children:** 25 mg/kg P.O. b.i.d. for 2 to 5 days. Maximum dose is 3 g daily. If lesions persist 2 days after completion of a 2-day course of therapy, course is repeated.
*Roundworm, threadworm, whipworm—*
**Adults and children:** 25 mg/kg P.O. in two doses daily for 2 successive days.
*Trichinosis—*
**Adults and children:** 25 mg/kg P.O. in two doses daily for 2 to 4 successive days.

## ADVERSE REACTIONS
**CNS:** impaired mental alertness, impaired coordination, numbness, *seizures, drowsiness, fatigue,* giddiness, *headache,* dizziness.
**CV:** *hypotension,* flushing.
**EENT:** tinnitus, blurry vision, dry mouth and eyes, xanthopsia.
**GI:** *anorexia, nausea, vomiting,* diarrhea, epigastric distress, cholestasis.
**GU:** hematuria, enuresis, crystalluria, malodorous urine.
**Hematologic:** *leukopenia.*
**Hepatic:** jaundice, transient elevations of AST levels, *parenchymal liver damage.*
**Skin:** *rash, pruritus, erythema multiforme, Stevens-Johnson syndrome.*
**Other:** lymphadenopathy, fever, chills, *angioedema, anaphylaxis.*

## INTERACTIONS
**Drug-drug.** *Theophylline:* may impair hepatic metabolism of theophylline, increasing risk of toxicity. Monitor patient closely.

## EFFECTS ON DIAGNOSTIC TESTS
None reported.

## CONTRAINDICATIONS
Contraindicated in patients with hypersensitivity to drug.

## NURSING CONSIDERATIONS
• Use cautiously in patients with hepatic or renal dysfunction, severe malnutrition, and anemia, and in patients who are vomiting.
• Drug should be administered to all family members, as prescribed, to prevent risk of spreading infection.
• Dietary restrictions, laxatives, or enemas aren't necessary. However, supportive therapy is indicated for anemic, dehydrated, or malnourished patients.

### ☑ Patient teaching
• Teach patient to take drug after meals. For oral suspension, shake before measuring dose. For tablets, advise patient to chew before swallowing.
• Advise patient to avoid hazardous activities such as driving because drug may cause drowsiness.
• Teach patient about personal hygiene, especially good hand-washing technique. To avoid reinfection, teach patient to wash perianal area daily, change undergarments and bedclothes daily, and wash hands and clean fingernails before meals and after bowel movements. Tell him not to prepare food for others during infestation.

## Antifungals

amphotericin B
amphotericin B cholesteryl
  sulfate complex
amphotericin B lipid complex
amphotericin B liposomal
fluconazole
flucytosine
griseofulvin microsize
griseofulvin ultramicrosize
itraconazole
ketoconazole
nystatin
terbinafine hydrochloride

**COMBINATION PRODUCTS**
None.

### amphotericin B
Amphocin, Amphotericin B for
Injection, Fungilin‡, Fungizone
Intravenous

*Pregnancy Risk Category B*

**HOW SUPPLIED**
*Tablets:* 100 mg‡
*Oral suspension:* 100 mg/ml‡
*Lozenges:* 10 mg‡
*Powder for injection:* 50 mg

**ACTION**
Binds to sterol in the fungal cell membrane, altering cell permeability and allowing leakage of intracellular components. Fungal cell death occurs in part as a result of membrane permeability changes.

| Route | Onset | Peak | Duration |
|-------|-------|------|----------|
| P.O. | Unknown | Unknown | Unknown |
| I.V. | Immediate | Unknown | Unknown |

**INDICATIONS & DOSAGE**
*Systemic fungal infections (histoplasmosis, coccidioidomycosis, blastomycosis, cryptococcosis, disseminated candidiasis, aspergillosis, phycomycosis, zygomycosis), meningitis—*

**Adults:** initially, a test dose of 1 mg in 20 ml of $D_5W$ infused I.V. over 20 to 30 minutes may be recommended. If tolerated, daily dose is then initiated as 0.25 to 0.3 mg/kg daily by slow I.V. infusion (0.1 mg/ml) over 2 to 6 hours. Dose is gradually increased to maximum 1 mg/kg daily. If drug is discontinued for 1 week or more, drug is resumed with initial dose and increased gradually.
*Infections of the GI tract due to* Candida albicans—
**Adults:** 100 mg P.O. q.i.d. for 2 weeks.
*Oral and perioral candidal infections—*
**Adults:** 1 lozenge q.i.d. for 7 to 14 days. Lozenge should dissolve slowly.

**ADVERSE REACTIONS**
**CNS:** *headache,* peripheral neuropathy, *malaise, **seizures.***
**CV:** hypotension, ***arrhythmias, asystole,*** hypertension, tachycardia, flushing, *phlebitis, thrombophlebitis.*
**EENT:** hearing loss, tinnitus, transient vertigo, blurred vision, diplopia.
**GI:** *anorexia, weight loss, nausea, vomiting, dyspepsia, diarrhea, epigastric pain, cramping,* melena, steatorrhea, ***hemorrhagic gastroenteritis.***
**GU:** *abnormal renal function with hypokalemia, azotemia, hyposthenuria, renal tubular acidosis, nephrocalcinosis; **permanent renal impairment;*** anuria; oliguria; increased BUN and serum creatinine.
**Hematologic:** *normochromic anemia, normocytic anemia, **thrombocytopenia, leukopenia, agranulocytosis,*** eosinophilia, leukocytosis.
**Hepatic:** hepatitis, jaundice, ***acute liver failure,*** elevated alkaline phosphatase, ALT, AST, GGT, LD, and bilirubin levels.
**Metabolic:** hypokalemia, hypoglycemia, hyperglycemia, hyperuricemia, hypomagnesemia.
**Musculoskeletal:** arthralgia, myalgia.
**Respiratory:** dyspnea, tachypnea, bronchospasm, wheezing.

**Skin:** maculopapular rash, pruritus (without rash).

**Other:** tissue damage with extravasation, *fever, chills, generalized pain,* **anaphylactoid reaction,** pain at injection site.

## INTERACTIONS

**Drug-drug.** *Antineoplastics (mechlorethamine):* may cause renal toxicity, bronchospasm, and hypotension. Use cautiously.

*Cardiac glycosides:* increased risk of digitalis toxicity in potassium-depleted patients. Monitor closely.

*Corticosteroids:* enhanced potassium depletion. Monitor serum potassium levels.

*Flucytosine:* synergistic effect; may cause increased toxicity of flucytosine. Monitor closely.

*Other nephrotoxic drugs (such as antibiotics, pentamidine):* may cause additive renal toxicity. Administer these drugs cautiously.

*Thiazides:* may intensify electrolyte depletion, especially potassium. Monitor for hypokalemia.

**Drug-herb.** *Gossypol:* enhanced or increased risk of renal toxicity when administered together. Avoid concomitant use.

## EFFECTS ON DIAGNOSTIC TESTS
None reported.

## CONTRAINDICATIONS
Contraindicated in patients with hypersensitivity to drug.

## NURSING CONSIDERATIONS
• Use cautiously in patients with impaired renal function.

• *Alert:* Note that different amphotericin B preparations are not interchangeable and that dosages will vary.

• *Alert:* To reduce severe adverse reactions, patient may receive premedication with antipyretics, antihistamines, antiemetics, or small doses of corticosteroids and be given an alternate-day schedule. For severe reactions, discontinue drug and notify doctor.

• Monitor fluid intake and output; report change in urine appearance or volume. Monitor BUN and serum creatinine (or creatinine clearance) at least weekly. Kidney damage is typically reversible if drug is stopped at first sign of dysfunction.

• Obtain liver and renal function studies weekly, if ordered. Drug may be stopped if alkaline phosphatase or bilirubin levels increase. If BUN exceeds 40 mg/100 ml, or if serum creatinine level exceeds 3 mg/100 ml, doctor may reduce or stop drug until renal function improves. Monitor CBC weekly.

• Monitor potassium levels closely, and report signs of hypokalemia. Check calcium and magnesium levels twice weekly, as ordered.

## ◩ I.V. administration
• Be prepared to give initial test dose as prescribed. Monitor patient's pulse, respiratory rate, temperature, and blood pressure for at least 4 hours.

• Use an infusion pump and in-line filter with mean pore diameter larger than 1 micron. Rapid infusion may cause CV collapse.

• Choose I.V. sites in distal veins. If veins become thrombosed, alternate administration sites.

• Monitor vital signs every 30 minutes; fever, shaking chills, and hypotension may appear 1 to 2 hours after start of I.V. infusion and should subside within 4 hours of stopping drug.

• Give antibiotics separately; don't mix or piggyback them with amphotericin B.

• Amphotericin B appears to be compatible with limited amounts of heparin sodium, hydrocortisone sodium succinate, and methylprednisolone sodium succinate.

• Store the dry form at 35.6° to 46.4° F (2° to 8° C). Protect from light. Reconstitute amphotericin B with 10 ml of sterile water only. To avoid precipitation, don't mix with solutions containing sodium chloride, other electrolytes, or bacteriostatic agents (such as benzyl alcohol). Don't use if solution contains precipitate or foreign matter.

• Reconstituted solution is stable for 1 week under refrigeration or 24 hours at room temperature. It has 8-hour stability in room light.

---

☑ **Patient teaching**
• Warn patient of possible discomfort at I.V. site and of other potential adverse reactions. Instruct the patient to report signs and symptoms of hypersensitivity immediately.
• Inform patient that therapy may take several months. Stress importance of compliance and recommended follow-up.

## amphotericin B cholesteryl sulfate complex
Amphotec

*Pregnancy Risk Category B*

### HOW SUPPLIED
*Injection:* 50 mg/20 ml, 100 mg/50 ml

### ACTION
Binds to sterols in cell membranes of sensitive fungi, resulting in leakage of intracellular contents and causing cell death due to changes in membrane permeability. The spectrum of activity includes *Aspergillus fumigatus, Candida albicans, Coccidioides immitis,* and *Cryptococcus neoformans.*

| Route | Onset | Peak | Duration |
|-------|-------|------|----------|
| I.V. | Unknown | 3 hr | Unknown |

### INDICATIONS & DOSAGE
*Invasive aspergillosis in patients in whom renal impairment or unacceptable toxicity precludes use of amphotericin B deoxycholate in effective doses and in those with invasive aspergillosis in whom prior amphotericin B deoxycholate therapy has failed—*
**Adults and children:** 3 to 4 mg/kg/day I.V. Dilute in $D_5W$ and administer by continuous infusion at 1 mg/kg/hour. Perform a test dose before commencing new courses of treatment; infuse a small amount of drug (10 ml of final preparation containing 1.6 to 8.3 mg of drug) over 15 to 30 minutes and monitor for next 30 minutes. Can shorten infusion time to 2 hours or lengthen infusion time based on patient tolerance.

### ADVERSE REACTIONS
**CNS:** abnormal thinking, anxiety, agitation, confusion, depression, dizziness, hallucinations, headache, hypertonia, neuropathy, nervousness, paresthesia, psychosis, *seizures,* somnolence, speech disorder, stupor, asthenia.
**CV:** *arrhythmias, atrial fibrillation, bradycardia, cardiac arrest, heart failure, hemorrhage,* hypertension, *hypotension,* phlebitis, chest pain, orthostatic hypotension, *shock, supraventricular tachycardia,* syncope, *tachycardia,* vasodilation, *ventricular extrasystoles.*
**EENT:** amblyopia, deafness, epistaxis, eye hemorrhage, pharyngitis, tinnitus, rhinitis, sinusitis.
**GI:** anorexia, diarrhea, dry mouth, GI hemorrhage, gingivitis, glossitis, hematemesis, melena, mouth ulceration, *nausea,* oral candidiasis, stomatitis, *vomiting,* weight gain or loss, abdominal pain.
**GU:** albuminuria, dysuria, glycosuria, *increased creatinine,* increased BUN, hematuria, oliguria, urinary incontinence or urine retention, *renal failure.*
**Hematologic:** anemia, coagulation disorders, ecchymosis, hypochromic anemia, leukocytosis, *leukopenia,* petechiae, decreased prothrombin, *thrombocytopenia.*
**Hepatic:** jaundice, *abnormal liver function test results, hepatic failure.*
**Metabolic:** acidosis, dehydration, *hypokalemia,* hypocalcemia, hypoglycemia, hypoproteinemia, hyperglycemia, hypervolemia, hypophosphatemia, hyponatremia, hyperkalemia, hyperlipemia, hypernatremia, *hyperbilirubinemia,* hypomagnesemia.
**Musculoskeletal:** arthralgia, myalgia, neck or back pain.
**Respiratory:** *apnea,* asthma, dyspnea, hemoptysis, hyperventilation, hypoxia, increased cough, lung or respiratory disorders, pleural effusion, *pulmonary edema.*
**Skin:** acne, pruritus, rash, sweating, skin discoloration, nodule, ulcer, urticaria.
**Other:** *allergic reaction,* alopecia, *anaphylaxis, chills,* edema, *fever,* peripheral or facial edema, infection, mucous membrane disorder, pain or reaction at injection site, *sepsis.*

---

*Liquid contains alcohol.    **May contain tartrazine.    †Canada    ‡Australia    §U.K.    ◊OTC

## INTERACTIONS

**Drug-drug.** *Antineoplastics:* may enhance renal toxicity, bronchospasm, and hypotension. Use cautiously.

*Cardiac glycosides:* can enhance potassium excretion and may potentiate digitalis toxicity. Monitor serum potassium closely.

*Corticosteroids:* enhanced potassium depletion, which could predispose patient to cardiac dysfunction. Monitor electrolytes.

*Cyclosporine, tacrolimus:* may possibly increase serum creatinine levels. Monitor renal function.

*Flucytosine:* toxicity may be increased by amphotericin. Use together cautiously.

*Imidazoles (clotrimazole, fluconazole, ketoconazole, miconazole):* may antagonize effects of amphotericin, although their significance has not been determined. Monitor closely.

*Nephrotoxic drugs (such as aminoglycosides, pentamidine):* may enhance renal toxicity. Monitor renal function closely.

*Skeletal muscle relaxants:* amphotericin B–induced hypokalemia may enhance the effects of skeletal muscle relaxants. Monitor serum potassium closely.

## EFFECTS ON DIAGNOSTIC TESTS
None reported.

## CONTRAINDICATIONS
Contraindicated in patients with hypersensitivity to drug or its components unless the benefits outweigh risks.

## NURSING CONSIDERATIONS
• It's unknown if drug appears in breast milk. Because of the potential for serious adverse reactions in breast-fed infants, a decision should be made to discontinue breast-feeding or to stop treatment, taking into account the importance of drug to the mother.
• Monitor intake and output; report changes in urine appearance or volume.
• Monitor renal and hepatic function tests, serum electrolytes (especially potassium, magnesium, and calcium), CBC, and PT.
• *Alert:* Note that different amphotericin B preparations aren't interchangeable and that dosages will vary.

## ◻ I.V. administration
• Store unopened vials at room temperature. Reconstitute 50-mg vial with rapid addition of 10 ml of sterile water for injection, and 100-mg vial with rapid addition of 20 ml sterile water. Shake vial gently. Don't use diluent other than sterile water for injection. Reconstituted drug is clear or opalescent liquid and is stable for 24 hours refrigerated. Discard partially used vials. Don't administer undiluted drug.
• For infusion, add to bag of $D_5W$ to final concentration of approximately 0.6 mg/ml. Drug is incompatible with saline, electrolyte solutions, and bacteriostatic agents. Don't filter or use an in-line filter and don't freeze.
• Infuse drug over at least 2 hours. Don't mix with other drugs. If administered through an existing I.V. line, flush line with $D_5W$ before infusion or use a separate line.
• *Alert:* Monitor vital signs every 30 minutes during initial therapy. Acute infusion-related reactions (fever, chills, hypotension, nausea, tachycardia) usually occur 1 to 3 hours after starting I.V. infusion. These reactions are usually more severe after initial doses and usually diminish with subsequent doses. If severe respiratory distress occurs, stop infusion immediately and don't treat further with drug.
• Pretreatment with antihistamines and corticosteroids or reducing the rate of infusion (or both) may reduce the acute infusion-related reactions.

## ☑ Patient teaching
• Instruct patient to immediately report symptoms of hypersensitivity.
• Warn patient of possible discomfort at I.V. site.
• Advise patient of potential adverse effects, such as fever, chills, nausea, and vomiting. Tell patient that these can be severe with initial treatment but usually subside with repeated doses.

---

## amphotericin B lipid complex
Abelcet

*Pregnancy Risk Category B*

### HOW SUPPLIED
*Suspension for injection:* 100 mg/20-ml vial

### ACTION
Binds to sterols of fungal cell membranes. Fungal cell damage or death is due to increased membrane permeability and leakage of intracellular contents.

| Route | Onset | Peak | Duration |
|-------|-------|------|----------|
| I.V. | Unknown | Unknown | Unknown |

### INDICATIONS & DOSAGE
*Invasive fungal infections, including As-pergillus sp. and Candida sp., in patients who are refractory to or intolerant of conventional amphotericin B therapy—*
**Adults and children:** 5 mg/kg daily I.V. as a single infusion administered at rate of 2.5 mg/kg/hour.

### ADVERSE REACTIONS
**CNS:** headache, pain.
**CV:** chest pain, *cardiac arrest,* hypertension, hypotension.
**GI:** abdominal pain, diarrhea, *GI hemorrhage,* nausea, vomiting.
**GU:** *increased serum creatinine level, kidney failure.*
**Hematologic:** anemia, *leukopenia, thrombocytopenia.*
**Hepatic:** bilirubinemia.
**Metabolic:** hypokalemia.
**Respiratory:** dyspnea, respiratory disorder, *respiratory failure.*
**Skin:** rash.
**Other:** *chills, fever,* infection, MULTIPLE ORGAN FAILURE, *sepsis.*

### INTERACTIONS
**Drug-drug.** *Antineoplastics:* increased risk of renal toxicity, bronchospasm, and hypotension. Use cautiously.
*Cardiac glycosides:* increased risk of digitalis toxicity due to amphotericin B–induced hypokalemia. Monitor serum potassium levels closely.
*Clotrimazole, fluconazole, itraconazole, ketoconazole, miconazole:* may antagonize amphotericin B. Monitor closely.
*Corticosteroids, corticotropin:* enhanced hypokalemia, which may lead to cardiac toxicity. Monitor serum electrolyte levels and cardiac function.
*Cyclosporine:* increased renal toxicity. Monitor closely.
*Flucytosine:* increased risk of flucytosine toxicity due to increased cellular uptake or impaired renal excretion. Use cautiously.
*Nephrotoxic drugs (such as aminoglyco-sides, pentamidine):* increased risk of renal toxicity. Use cautiously. Monitor renal function closely.
*Skeletal muscle relaxants:* enhanced effects of skeletal muscle relaxants resulting from amphotericin B–induced hypokalemia. Monitor serum potassium levels closely.
*Zidovudine:* increased myelotoxicity and nephrotoxicity. Monitor renal and hematologic function.

### EFFECTS ON DIAGNOSTIC TESTS
None reported.

### CONTRAINDICATIONS
Contraindicated in patients with hypersensitivity to amphotericin B or its components.

### NURSING CONSIDERATIONS
• Use cautiously in patients with renal impairment. The need for dosage adjustment should be based on overall clinical status of patient. Renal toxicity is more common at higher dosages.
• *Alert:* Note that different amphotericin B preparations aren't interchangeable and dosages will vary.
• Premedicate patient with acetaminophen, antihistamines, and corticosteroids, as ordered, to prevent or lessen severity of infusion-related reactions, such as fever, chills, nausea, and vomiting, which occur 1 to 2 hours after start of infusion.
• Don't give leukocyte transfusions with drug because acute pulmonary toxicity has been reported with concurrent administration.

• Monitor serum creatinine and electrolyte levels (especially magnesium and potassium), liver function, and CBC during therapy, as ordered.
• It's unknown if drug appears in breast milk; therefore, a decision to administer drug or discontinue breast-feeding should be made.

### ⬛ I. V. administration
• To prepare, shake vial gently until there is no yellow sediment. Using aseptic technique, withdraw calculated dose into one or more 20-ml syringes, using an 18-gauge needle. More than one vial will be required. Attach a 5-micron filter needle to the syringe and inject the dose into an I.V. bag of D₅W. One filter needle can be used for up to four vials of amphotericin B lipid complex. The volume of D₅W should be sufficient to yield a final concentration of 1 mg/ml.
• For pediatric patients and patients with cardiovascular disease, recommended final concentration is 2 mg/ml.
• Don't mix with saline or infuse in same I.V. line as other drugs. Don't use an in-line filter.
• Discard any unused drug; it doesn't contain a preservative.
• Use an infusion pump and administer by continuous infusion at a rate of 2.5 mg/kg/hour. If infusion time exceeds 2 hours, mix contents by shaking infusion bag every 2 hours.
• If infusing through an existing I.V. line, flush first with D₅W.
• If severe respiratory distress occurs, discontinue infusion, provide supportive therapy for anaphylaxis, and notify doctor. Drug shouldn't be reinstituted in this situation.
• Monitor vital signs closely. Fever, shaking chills, and hypotension may appear within 2 hours of initiating infusion. Slowing infusion rate may decrease incidence of infusion-related reactions.
• Infusions are stable for up to 48 hours if refrigerated (36° to 46° F [2° to 8° C]) and up to 6 hours at room temperature.

### ☑ Patient teaching
• Inform patient that fever, chills, nausea, and vomiting may occur during infusion

and that these reactions usually subside with subsequent doses.
• Instruct patient to report any redness or pain at infusion site.
• Teach patient to recognize and report any symptoms of acute hypersensitivity such as respiratory distress.
• Warn patient that therapy may take several months.
• Tell patient to expect frequent laboratory testing to monitor kidney and liver function.

---

## amphotericin B liposomal
AmBisome

*Pregnancy Risk Category B*

### HOW SUPPLIED
*Injection:* 50-mg vial

### ACTION
Antifungal activity is derived from amphotericin B, which binds to the sterol component of a fungal cell membrane, leading to alterations in cell permeability and cell death.

| Route | Onset | Peak | Duration |
|-------|-------|------|----------|
| I.V. | Unknown | Unknown | Unknown |

### INDICATIONS & DOSAGE
*Empirical therapy for presumed fungal infection in febrile, neutropenic patients—*
**Adults and children:** 3 mg/kg I.V. infusion daily.
*Systemic fungal infections due to Aspergillus sp., Candida sp., or Cryptococcus sp. refractory to amphotericin B deoxycholate or in patients in whom renal impairment or unacceptable toxicity precludes use of amphotericin B deoxycholate—*
**Adults and children:** 3 to 5 mg/kg I.V. infusion daily.
*Visceral leishmaniasis in immunocompetent patients—*
**Adults and children:** 3 mg/kg I.V. infusion daily on days 1 to 5, 14, and 21. A repeat course of therapy may be beneficial if initial treatment fails to achieve parasitic clearance.

---

Reactions may be *common,* uncommon, **life-threatening,** or COMMON AND LIFE-THREATENING.

*Visceral leishmaniasis in immunocompromised patients—*
**Adults and children:** 4 mg/kg I.V. infusion daily on days 1 to 5, 10, 17, 24, 31, and 38. Expert advice regarding further treatment is recommended if initial therapy fails or patient experiences relapse.

## ADVERSE REACTIONS
**CNS:** *anxiety, confusion, headache, insomnia, asthenia.*
**CV:** *chest pain, hypotension, tachycardia, hypertension, edema.*
**EENT:** *epistaxis, rhinitis.*
**GI:** *nausea, vomiting, abdominal pain, diarrhea,* **GI hemorrhage,**
**GU:** *hematuria, elevated creatinine and BUN levels.*
**Hepatic:** *elevated ALT and AST levels, increased alkaline phosphatase level, bilirubinemia.*
**Metabolic:** *hyperglycemia, hypernatremia, hypocalcemia, hypokalemia, hypomagnesemia.*
**Musculoskeletal:** *back pain.*
**Respiratory:** *increased cough, dyspnea, hypoxia, pleural effusion, lung disorder, hyperventilation.*
**Skin:** *pruritus, rash, sweating.*
**Other:** *chills, infection, flushing,* **anaphylaxis,** *pain,* **sepsis,** *fever, blood product infusion reaction.*

## INTERACTIONS
**Drug-drug.** *Antineoplastics:* may enhance potential for renal toxicity, bronchospasm, and hypotension. Use cautiously.
*Cardiac glycosides:* increased risk of digitalis toxicity due to amphotericin B–induced hypokalemia. Monitor serum potassium level closely.
*Clotrimazole, fluconazole, ketoconazole, miconazole:* may induce fungal resistance to amphotericin B. Use together cautiously.
*Corticosteroids, corticotropin:* may potentiate potassium depletion, which could result in cardiac dysfunction. Monitor serum electrolyte levels and cardiac function.
*Flucytosine:* may increase flucytosine toxicity by increasing cellular reuptake or impairing renal excretion of flucytosine. Use cautiously.
*Other nephrotoxic drugs, such as antibiotics, antineoplastics:* may cause additive nephrotoxicity. Administer cautiously. Monitor renal function closely.
*Skeletal muscle relaxants:* enhanced effects of skeletal muscle relaxants resulting from amphotericin B–induced hypokalemia. Monitor serum potassium levels.

## EFFECTS ON DIAGNOSTIC TESTS
None reported.

## CONTRAINDICATIONS
Contraindicated in patients with hypersensitivity to drug or its components.

## NURSING CONSIDERATIONS
● Use cautiously in patients with impaired renal function, in elderly patients, and in pregnant women.
● Patients concomitantly receiving chemotherapy or bone marrow transplantation are at greater risk for additional adverse reactions, including seizures, arrhythmias, and thrombocytopenia.
● Don't give leukocyte transfusions with drug because acute pulmonary toxicity has been reported with concurrent administration.
● *Alert:* Note that different amphotericin B preparations aren't interchangeable and dosages will vary.
● To lessen risk or severity of adverse reactions, premedicate patient with antipyretics, antihistamines, antiemetics, or corticosteroids, as ordered.
● Monitor BUN and serum creatinine and electrolyte levels (particularly magnesium and potassium), liver function, and CBC.
● Therapy may take several weeks to months.
● Monitor for signs of hypokalemia (ECG changes, muscle weakness, cramping, drowsiness).
● Patients treated with amphotericin B liposomal had a lower incidence of chills, elevated BUN, hypokalemia, hypertension, and vomiting than patients treated with conventional amphotericin B.
● It's unknown if drug appears in human milk. Because of potential for serious ad-

verse reactions in breast-fed infants, a decision should be made whether to discontinue breast-feeding or discontinue drug, taking into account importance of drug to mother.

### 🖐 I.V. administration
• Reconstitute each 50-mg vial of amphotericin B liposomal with 12 ml of sterile water for injection to yield a solution of 4 mg amphotericin B/ml.
• *Alert:* Don't reconstitute with bacteriostatic water for injection and don't allow bacteriostatic agent in solution. Don't reconstitute with saline or add saline to reconstituted concentration or mix with other drugs.
• After reconstitution, shake vial vigorously for 30 seconds or until particulate matter is dispersed.
• Withdraw calculated amount of reconstituted solution into a sterile syringe and inject through a 5-micron filter into the appropriate amount of $D_5W$ to further dilute to a final concentration of 1 to 2 mg/ml. Lower concentrations (0.2 to 0.5 mg/ml) may be appropriate for pediatric patients to provide sufficient volume of infusion.
• An existing I.V. line must be flushed with $D_5W$ before infusion of drug. If this isn't feasible, drug should be administered through a separate line.
• Use a controlled infusion device and an in-line filter with a mean pore diameter larger than 1 micron. Initially, infuse drug over at least 2 hours. Infusion time may be reduced to 1 hour if treatment is well tolerated. If patient experiences discomfort during infusion, duration of infusion may be increased.
• Observe patient closely for adverse reactions during infusion. If anaphylaxis occurs, stop infusion immediately, provide supportive therapy, and notify doctor.
• Store unopened vial at 36° to 46° F (2° to 8° C). Once reconstituted, store concentrate for up to 24 hours at 36° to 46° F. Don't freeze.

### ✅ Patient teaching
• Teach patient signs and symptoms of hypersensitivity, and stress importance of reporting them immediately.

• Warn patient that therapy may take several months; teach personal hygiene and other measures to prevent spread and recurrence of lesions.
• Instruct patient to report any adverse reactions that occur while receiving drug.
• Instruct patient to watch for and report signs of hypokalemia (muscle weakness, cramping, drowsiness)
• Advise patient that frequent laboratory testing will be necessary.

## fluconazole
Diflucan

*Pregnancy Risk Category C*

### HOW SUPPLIED
*Tablets:* 50 mg, 100 mg, 150 mg, 200 mg
*Powder for oral suspension:* 10 mg/ml, 40 mg/ml
*Injection:* 200 mg/100 ml, 400 mg/200 ml

### ACTION
Inhibits fungal cytochrome P-450 (responsible for fungal sterol synthesis) and weakens fungal cell walls.

| Route | Onset | Peak | Duration |
|-------|-------|------|----------|
| P.O. | Unknown | 1-2 hr | 30 hr |
| I.V. | Immediate | Immediate | Unknown |

### INDICATIONS & DOSAGE
*Oropharyngeal candidiasis—*
**Adults:** 200 mg P.O. or I.V. on first day, followed by 100 mg once daily. Therapy should last at least 2 weeks.
**Children:** 6 mg/kg P.O. or I.V. on first day, followed by 3 mg/kg daily for 2 weeks.
*Esophageal candidiasis—*
**Adults:** 200 mg P.O. or I.V. on first day, followed by 100 mg once daily. Higher doses (up to 400 mg daily) have been used, depending on patient's condition and tolerance of treatment. Patients should receive drug for at least 3 weeks and for 2 weeks after symptoms resolve.
**Children:** 6 mg/kg P.O. or I.V. on first day followed by 3 mg/kg daily for at least 3 weeks, and for at least 2 weeks after symptoms resolve. Doses up to 12 mg/kg may be used based on clinical judgment.

---

*Vulvovaginal candidiasis—*
**Adults:** 150 mg P.O. for one dose only or 50 mg P.O. daily for 3 days.
*Systemic candidiasis—*
**Adults:** 400 mg P.O. or I.V. on first day, followed by 200 mg once daily. Treatment should continue for at least 4 weeks and for 2 weeks after symptoms resolve.
**Children:** 6 to 12 mg/kg/day P.O. or I.V.
*Cryptococcal meningitis—*
**Adults:** 400 mg P.O. or I.V. on first day, followed by 200 mg once daily. Higher doses (up to 400 mg daily) may be used. Treatment should continue for 10 to 12 weeks after CSF cultures are negative.
**Children:** 12 mg/kg/day P.O. or I.V. on first day, followed by 6 mg/kg daily for 10 to 12 weeks after CSF culture is negative.
*Prevention of candidiasis in bone marrow transplant—*
**Adults:** 400 mg P.O. or I.V. once daily. Start prophylaxis several days before anticipated agranulocytosis. Continue therapy for 7 days after neutrophil count rises above 1,000 cells/mm$^3$.
*Suppression of relapse of cryptococcal meningitis in patients with AIDS—*
**Adults:** 200 mg P.O. or I.V. daily.
**Children:** 3 to 6 mg/kg/day P.O. or I.V.
**Adjust-a-dose:** For renally impaired patients, if creatinine clearance is 11 to 50 ml/minute, dosage is reduced by 50%. Patients receiving regular hemodialysis treatment should receive the usual dose after each dialysis session.

### ADVERSE REACTIONS
**CNS:** headache, dizziness.
**EENT:** taste perversion.
**GI:** *nausea*, vomiting, abdominal pain, diarrhea, dyspepsia.
**Hematologic:** *leukopenia, thrombocytopenia.*
**Hepatic:** *hepatotoxicity* (rare), elevated liver enzymes.
**Skin:** rash, *Stevens-Johnson syndrome* (rare).
**Other:** *anaphylaxis.*

### INTERACTIONS
**Drug-drug.** *Cyclosporine, phenytoin, theophylline:* may increase plasma concentrations of these drugs. Monitor serum cyclosporine or phenytoin levels.
*Isoniazid, oral sulfonylureas, phenytoin, rifampin, valproic acid:* increased incidence of elevated hepatic transaminases. Monitor closely.
*Oral antidiabetics (glipizide, glyburide, tolbutamide):* may increase plasma concentrations of these drugs. Monitor for enhanced hypoglycemic effect.
*Rifampin:* enhanced metabolism of fluconazole. Monitor for lack of response.
*Warfarin:* increased risk of bleeding. Monitor PT and INR.
*Zidovudine:* zidovudine activity may be increased. Monitor closely.
**Drug-food.** *Caffeine:* may increase caffeine plasma levels. Ofloxacin or lomefloxacin are alternative drugs.

### EFFECTS ON DIAGNOSTIC TESTS
None reported.

### CONTRAINDICATIONS
Contraindicated in patients with hypersensitivity to drug.

### NURSING CONSIDERATIONS
• Use cautiously in patients with hypersensitivity to other antifungal azole compounds; no data exist regarding cross-sensitivity.
• Periodically monitor liver function during prolonged therapy, as ordered.
• If patient develops mild rash, monitor closely. Discontinue drug if lesions progress, and notify doctor.
• The incidence of adverse reactions appears to be greater in HIV-infected patients.

🔲 **I.V. administration**
• Don't remove protective overwrap from I.V. bags until just before use to ensure product sterility. The plastic container may show some opacity from moisture absorbed during sterilization. This doesn't affect the drug and diminishes over time. Don't add other drugs to the I.V. bag.
• *Alert:* Administer by continuous infusion at a rate not to exceed 200 mg/hour. Use an infusion pump. To prevent air embolism, don't connect in series with other infusions. Don't add other drugs to the solution.

---

*Liquid contains alcohol.    **May contain tartrazine.    †Canada    ‡Australia    §U.K.    ◊OTC

☑ **Patient teaching**
- Tell patient to take drug as directed, even after he feels better.
- Instruct patient to report adverse reactions promptly.

---

## flucytosine
## (5-fluorocytosine, 5-FC)
Ancobon, Ancotil‡

*Pregnancy Risk Category C*

### HOW SUPPLIED
*Capsules:* 250 mg, 500 mg

### ACTION
Unknown. Appears to penetrate fungal cells and cause defective protein synthesis.

| Route | Onset | Peak | Duration |
|-------|-------|------|----------|
| P.O. | Unknown | 1-2 hr | Unknown |

### INDICATIONS & DOSAGE
*Severe fungal infections due to susceptible strains of* Candida *(including septicemia, endocarditis, urinary tract and pulmonary infections) and* Cryptococcus *(meningitis, pulmonary infection, and possible urinary tract infection)—*
**Adults:** 50 to 150 mg/kg daily P.O. in four equally divided doses q 6 hours.

### ADVERSE REACTIONS
**CNS:** headache, vertigo, sedation, fatigue, weakness, confusion, hallucinations, psychosis, ataxia, hearing loss, paresthesia, parkinsonism, peripheral neuropathy.
**CV:** *cardiac arrest,* chest pain.
**GI:** nausea, vomiting, diarrhea, abdominal pain, dry mouth, duodenal ulcer, *hemorrhage,* ulcerative colitis, anorexia.
**GU:** azotemia, elevated creatinine and BUN levels, crystalluria, *renal failure.*
**Hematologic:** anemia, *leukopenia, bone marrow suppression, thrombocytopenia,* eosinophilia, *agranulocytosis, aplastic anemia.*
**Hepatic:** elevated liver enzymes, elevated serum alkaline phosphatase, jaundice.
**Metabolic:** hypoglycemia, hypokalemia.
**Respiratory:** *respiratory arrest,* dyspnea.
**Skin:** occasional rash, pruritus, urticaria, photosensitivity.

### INTERACTIONS
**Drug-drug.** *Amphotericin B:* synergistic effects and possibly enhanced toxicity when used together. Monitor closely.

### EFFECTS ON DIAGNOSTIC TESTS
Flucytosine causes falsely elevated creatinine values on iminohydrolase enzymatic assay.

### CONTRAINDICATIONS
Contraindicated in patients with hypersensitivity to drug.

### NURSING CONSIDERATIONS
- Use with extreme caution in patients with impaired hepatic or renal function or bone marrow suppression.
- Administer capsules over 15 minutes to reduce adverse GI reactions.
- Monitor blood, liver, and renal function studies frequently during therapy; obtain susceptibility tests weekly, as ordered, to monitor drug resistance.
- If possible, regularly perform blood level assays of drug, as ordered, to maintain flucytosine at therapeutic level (25 to 120 mcg/ml). Higher blood levels may be toxic.
- Monitor fluid intake and output; report marked changes.

☑ **Patient teaching**
- Inform patient that therapeutic response may take weeks or months.
- Instruct patient to report adverse reactions promptly.

---

## griseofulvin microsize
Fulcin‡, Fulvicin-U/F, Grifulvin V, Grisactin 500, Grisovin‡, Grisovin, Grisovin FP†

## griseofulvin ultramicrosize
Fulvicin P/G, Grisactin Ultra, Griseostatin‡, Gris-PEG

*Pregnancy Risk Category C*

### HOW SUPPLIED
**griseofulvin microsize**
*Tablets:* 250 mg, 500 mg
*Capsules:* 125 mg, 250 mg

---

Reactions may be *common*, uncommon, *life-threatening*, or COMMON AND LIFE-THREATENING.

*Oral suspension:* 125 mg/5 ml
**griseofulvin ultramicrosize**
*Tablets:* 125 mg, 165 mg, 250 mg,
330 mg

## ACTION
Arrests fungal cell activity by disrupting
mitotic spindle structure.

| Route | Onset | Peak | Duration |
|-------|---------|--------|----------|
| P.O. | Unknown | 4-8 hr | Unknown |

## INDICATIONS & DOSAGE
*Ringworm infections of skin, hair, nails
(tinea corporis, tinea capitis, tinea cruris)
when due to* Trichophyton, Microsporum,
*or* Epidermophyton—
**Adults:** 500 mg of microsize P.O. daily in
single or divided doses. Severe infections
may require up to 1 g daily. Or, 330 to
375 mg ultramicrosize P.O. daily in single
or divided doses. Duration of therapy is 2
to 8 weeks depending on site of infection.
*Tinea pedis, tinea unguium—*
**Adults:** 0.75 to 1 g of microsize P.O. daily. Or, 660 to 750 mg of ultramicrosize
P.O. daily in divided doses. Duration of
therapy is 4 weeks to 1 year.
**Children:** 11 mg/kg/day of microsize
P.O. Or, 7.3 mg/kg/day of ultramicrosize
P.O.

## ADVERSE REACTIONS
**CNS:** headache (in early stages of treatment), fatigue (with large doses), occasional mental confusion, impaired performance of routine activities, psychotic
symptoms, dizziness, insomnia, paresthesia of hands and feet (after extended therapy).
**EENT:** transient decrease in hearing, oral
thrush.
**GI:** nausea, vomiting, flatulence, diarrhea, epigastric distress, *bleeding.*
**GU:** proteinuria, menstrual irregularities.
**Hematologic:** leukopenia, *agranulocytosis,* porphyria.
**Hepatic:** *hepatic toxicity.*
**Skin:** *rash, urticaria,* photosensitivity, angioedema.
**Other:** hypersensitivity reactions, lupus
erythematosus.

## INTERACTIONS
**Drug-drug.** *Coumarin anticoagulants:*
decreased effectiveness. Monitor PT and
INR when used concurrently.
*Cyclosporine:* decreased serum cyclosporine levels. Monitor closely.
*Oral contraceptives:* decreased effectiveness. Suggest alternative methods of contraception.
*Phenobarbital:* decreased griseofulvin
blood levels due to decreased absorption
or increased metabolism. Avoid using together or administer griseofulvin t.i.d.
**Drug-food.** *High-fat meals:* increased absorption. Administer together.
**Drug-lifestyle.** *Alcohol use:* may cause
tachycardia, diaphoresis, and flushing.
Avoid alcohol consumption.
*Sun exposure:* may increase risk of photosensitivity reaction. Avoid unprotected
sun exposure.

## EFFECTS ON DIAGNOSTIC TESTS
None reported.

## CONTRAINDICATIONS
Contraindicated in patients hypersensitive
to drug and in those with porphyria or hepatocellular failure. Also contraindicated
in pregnant patients or women who intend
to become pregnant during therapy.

## NURSING CONSIDERATIONS
• Use cautiously in penicillin-sensitive patients.
• *Alert:* Because of potential toxicity, drug
is used only when topical treatment fails.
• Obtain laboratory tests, as ordered, to
confirm diagnosis. Continue drug until
clinical and laboratory examinations confirm eradication.
• *Alert:* Because griseofulvin ultramicrosize is dispersed in polyethylene glycol, it
is absorbed more rapidly and completely
than microsize preparations and is effective at one-half to two-thirds the usual
griseofulvin dose. Don't interchange
preparations.
• Administer drug after a high-fat meal to
enhance absorption and minimize GI distress.
• Assess hematologic, renal, and hepatic
function periodically during prolonged
therapy, as ordered.

• Discontinue drug in patients who experience agranulocytosis.
• Effective treatment of tinea pedis may require concomitant use of a topical drug.
• Safety in children under age 2 hasn't been established.

☑ **Patient teaching**
• Tell patient to take drug after a high-fat meal.
• Advise patient that prolonged treatment may be needed to control infection and prevent relapse, even if symptoms abate in first few days of therapy.
• Tell patient to keep skin clean and dry and to maintain good hygiene.
• Instruct patient to avoid intense sunlight. Unprotected sun exposure may cause photosensitivity reactions.

---

## itraconazole
Sporanox

*Pregnancy Risk Category C*

### HOW SUPPLIED
*Capsules:* 100 mg
*Oral solution:* 10 mg/ml

### ACTION
Interferes with fungal cell-wall synthesis by inhibiting the formation of ergosterol and increasing cell-wall permeability that makes the fungus susceptible to osmotic instability.

| Route | Onset | Peak | Duration |
|-------|-------|------|----------|
| P.O. | Unknown | 3-4 hr | Unknown |

### INDICATIONS & DOSAGE
*Pulmonary and extrapulmonary blastomycosis, nonmeningeal histoplasmosis—*
**Adults:** 200 mg P.O. daily. Dosage increased as needed and tolerated in 100-mg increments to a maximum of 400 mg daily. Doses that exceed 200 mg daily should be given in two divided doses. Treatment should continue for a minimum of 3 months. In life-threatening illness, a loading dose of 200 mg t.i.d. is given for 3 days.
*Aspergillosis—*
**Adults:** 200 to 400 mg P.O. daily.

*Onychomycosis (fungal nail disease) from dermatophytes of the toenail—*
**Adults:** 200 mg P.O. once daily for 12 consecutive weeks.
*Onychomycosis of the fingernail—*
**Adults:** initially, 200 mg P.O. b.i.d. for 1 week; after 3 weeks, dosage is repeated.
*Oropharyngeal candidiasis—*
**Adults:** 200 mg swished in mouth vigorously and swallowed daily, for 1 to 2 weeks.
*Oropharyngeal candidiasis in patients unresponsive to fluconazole tablets—*
**Adults:** 100 mg swished in mouth vigorously and swallowed b.i.d., for 2 to 4 weeks.
*Esophageal candidiasis—*
**Adults:** 100 to 200 mg swished in mouth vigorously and swallowed daily, for a minimum treatment of 3 weeks. Treatment should continue for 2 weeks after symptoms resolve.

### ADVERSE REACTIONS
**CNS:** headache, dizziness, somnolence, fatigue, malaise.
**CV:** hypertension.
**GI:** *nausea,* vomiting, diarrhea, abdominal pain, anorexia.
**GU:** albuminuria, impotence.
**Hepatic:** impaired hepatic function.
**Metabolic:** hypokalemia.
**Skin:** rash, pruritus.
**Other:** edema, fever, decreased libido.

### INTERACTIONS
**Drug-drug.** *Antacids, $H_2$-receptor antagonists, phenytoin, rifampin:* possible lowered itraconazole plasma levels. Avoid concomitant use.
*Cisapride:* inhibited metabolism of these drugs, resulting in elevated blood levels and risk of serious cardiac toxicity. Never administer together.
*Cyclosporine, digoxin, tacrolimus:* possible increased plasma levels of these drugs. Monitor plasma levels closely.
*Isoniazid:* may decrease plasma levels of itraconazole. Monitor closely.
*Oral anticoagulants:* possible enhanced anticoagulant effects. Monitor PT and INR closely.

---

Reactions may be *common,* uncommon, *life-threatening,* or COMMON AND LIFE-THREATENING.

*Oral antidiabetics:* similar antifungals have caused hypoglycemia. Monitor blood glucose levels closely.

**EFFECTS ON DIAGNOSTIC TESTS**
None reported.

**CONTRAINDICATIONS**
Contraindicated in patients with hypersensitivity to drug; in those receiving astemizole, cisapride, triazolam, or midazolam (orally); and in breast-feeding patients.

**NURSING CONSIDERATIONS**
• Use cautiously in patients with hypochlorhydria because they may not absorb drug readily. Because hypochlorhydria can accompany HIV infection, use cautiously in HIV-infected patients.
• Use cautiously in patients receiving other highly bound medications because drug and its metabolites are more than 99% bound to plasma proteins.
• Perform baseline liver function tests, as ordered, and monitor periodically.

☑ **Patient teaching**
• Teach patient to recognize and report signs and symptoms of liver disease (anorexia, dark urine, pale stools, unusual fatigue, or jaundice).
• Tell patient to take capsule with food to ensure maximal absorption.
• Instruct patient not to use interchangeably with itraconazole capsules.
• Tell patient that oral solution should be used 10 ml at a time.
• Advise patient to take solution without food.
• Inform patient to report all medications to doctor to avoid potential drug interactions.

---

**ketoconazole**
Nizoral

*Pregnancy Risk Category C*

**HOW SUPPLIED**
*Tablets:* 200 mg
*Oral suspension:* 100 mg/5 ml†

**ACTION**
Inhibits purine transport and DNA, RNA, and protein synthesis; increases cell-wall permeability, making the fungus more susceptible to osmotic pressure.

| Route | Onset | Peak | Duration |
|-------|-------|------|----------|
| P.O. | Unknown | 1-2 hr | Unknown |

**INDICATIONS & DOSAGE**
*Systemic candidiasis, chronic mucocandidiasis, oral thrush, candiduria, coccidioidomycosis, blastomycosis, histoplasmosis, chromomycosis, and paracoccidioidomycosis; severe cutaneous dermatophyte infections resistant to therapy with topical or oral griseofulvin—*
**Adults and children over 40 kg (88 lb):** initially, 200 mg P.O. daily in a single dose. Dose may be increased to 400 mg once daily in patients who don't respond.
**Children ages 2 and older:** 3.3 to 6.6 mg/kg P.O. daily as a single dose.

**ADVERSE REACTIONS**
**CNS:** headache, nervousness, dizziness, somnolence, photophobia, *suicidal tendencies,* severe depression.
**GI:** *nausea, vomiting,* abdominal pain, diarrhea.
**GU:** impotence, gynecomastia with tenderness.
**Hematologic:** *thrombocytopenia,* hemolytic anemia, *leukopenia.*
**Hepatic:** elevated liver enzymes, *fatal hepatotoxicity.*
**Metabolic:** hyperlipidemia.
**Skin:** pruritus.
**Other:** fever, chills.

**INTERACTIONS**
**Drug-drug.** *Antacids, anticholinergics, H₂ blockers:* decreased absorption of ketoconazole. Wait at least 2 hours after ketoconazole dose before administering these drugs.
*Anticoagulants:* effects may be enhanced. Monitor INR, PT, and PTT and adjust as needed.
*Cisapride:* may cause ventricular arrhythmias. Avoid use together.
*Cyclosporine:* may increase cyclosporine plasma levels. Monitor serum levels.

---

*Liquid contains alcohol.   **May contain tartrazine.   †Canada   ‡Australia   §U.K.   ◇OTC

*Isoniazid, rifampin:* increased ketoconazole metabolism. Monitor for decreased antifungal effect.
*Paclitaxel:* metabolism inhibited. Use together cautiously.
*Theophylline:* may decrease theophylline plasma levels. Monitor serum levels.
**Drug-herb.** *Yew:* inhibits ketoconazole metabolism. Avoid use together.

**EFFECTS ON DIAGNOSTIC TESTS**
None reported.

**CONTRAINDICATIONS**
Contraindicated in patients with hypersensitivity to drug.

**NURSING CONSIDERATIONS**
• Use cautiously in patients with hepatic disease and in those who are taking other hepatotoxic drugs.
• Because of the potential for serious hepatotoxicity, don't use ketoconazole for less serious conditions, such as fungus infections of the skin or nails.
• Monitor for elevated liver enzymes and nausea that does not subside as well as for unusual fatigue, jaundice, dark urine, or pale stool—all signs or symptoms of possible hepatotoxicity.
• Note that much larger doses (up to 800 mg/day) can be used to treat fungal meningitis and intracerebral fungal lesions.

☑ **Patient teaching**
• Instruct patient with achlorhydria to dissolve each tablet in 4 ml aqueous solution of 0.2 N hydrochloric acid, sip mixture through a glass or plastic straw (to avoid contact with teeth), and end procedure by drinking a glass of water because ketoconazole requires gastric acidity for dissolution and absorption.
• Make sure patient understands that treatment should be continued until all tests indicate that active fungal infection has subsided. If drug is discontinued too soon, infection will recur. Minimum treatment for candidiasis is 7 to 14 days; for other systemic fungal infections, 6 months; for resistant dermatophyte infections, at least 4 weeks.

• Reassure patient that nausea, common early in therapy, will subside. To minimize, divide daily dose into two doses or take it with meals.

---

## nystatin
Mycostatin*, Nadostine†, Nilstat, Nystat-Rx, Nystex*

*Pregnancy Risk Category NR*

**HOW SUPPLIED**
*Tablets:* 500,000 U
*Oral suspension:* 100,000 U/ml; 50, 150, or 500 million U; 1 or 2 billion U
*Powder:* 50, 150, or 500 million U; 1, 2, or 5 billion U
*Troches:* 200,000 U
*Vaginal suppositories:* 100,000 U

**ACTION**
Unknown. Probably binds to sterols in fungal cell membrane, altering cell permeability and allowing leakage of intracellular components.

| Route | Onset | Peak | Duration |
|---|---|---|---|
| P.O., topical | Unknown | Unknown | Unknown |

**INDICATIONS & DOSAGE**
*GI infections—*
**Adults:** 500,000 to 1 million U as oral tablets t.i.d.
*Oral, vaginal, and intestinal infections due to* Candida albicans (Monilia) *and other* Candida *species—*
**Adults:** 400,000 to 600,000 U oral suspension q.i.d. for oral candidiasis.
**Children and infants ages 3 months and older:** 250,000 to 500,000 U oral suspension q.i.d.
**Neonates and premature infants:** 100,000 U oral suspension q.i.d.
*Vaginal infections—*
**Adults:** 100,000 U, as vaginal tablets, inserted high into vagina, daily or b.i.d. for 14 days.

**ADVERSE REACTIONS**
**GI:** transient nausea, vomiting, diarrhea.

---

Reactions may be *common,* uncommon, *life-threatening,* or COMMON AND LIFE-THREATENING.

**INTERACTIONS**
None significant.

**EFFECTS ON DIAGNOSTIC TESTS**
None reported.

**CONTRAINDICATIONS**
Contraindicated in patients with hypersensitivity to drug.

**NURSING CONSIDERATIONS**
• Nystatin is not effective against systemic infections.
• Vaginal tablets can be used by pregnant patients up to 6 weeks before term to treat maternal infection that may cause thrush in neonates.
• For treatment of oral candidiasis (thrush): After the mouth is clean of food debris, have the patient hold suspension in mouth for several minutes before swallowing. When treating infants, swab medication on oral mucosa. Immunosuppressed patients are sometimes instructed by the doctor to suck on vaginal tablets (100,000 U) because this provides prolonged contact with oral mucosa.

☑ **Patient teaching**
• Advise patient to continue medication for at least 2 days after symptoms disappear. Consult doctor for exact length of therapy.
• Instruct patient to continue therapy during menstruation.
• Explain that predisposing factors of vaginal infection include use of antibiotics, oral contraceptives, and corticosteroids; diabetes; reinfection by sexual partner; and tight-fitting pantyhose. Encourage patient to use cotton (not synthetic) underwear.
• Instruct patient in careful hygiene for affected areas, including cleaning perineal area from front to back after defecation.
• Advise patient to report redness, swelling, or irritation.
• Tell patient that overusing mouthwash or wearing poorly fitting dentures, especially in older patients, may promote infection.

## terbinafine hydrochloride
Lamisil

*Pregnancy Risk Category B*

**HOW SUPPLIED**
*Tablets:* 250 mg

**ACTION**
Inhibits squalene epoxidase, a key enzyme in sterol biosynthesis of fungi. This enzyme inhibition results in a deficiency of ergosterol and a corresponding accumulation of sterol within the fungal cell.

| Route | Onset | Peak | Duration |
|-------|-------|------|----------|
| P.O. | Unknown | 2 hr | Unknown |

**INDICATIONS & DOSAGE**
*Fingernail onychomycosis due to dermatophytes (tinea unguium)—*
**Adults:** 250 mg P.O. once daily for 6 weeks.
*Toenail onychomycosis due to dermatophytes (tinea unguium)—*
**Adults:** 250 mg P.O. once daily for 12 weeks.

**ADVERSE REACTIONS**
**CNS:** *headache.*
**EENT:** taste disturbances, visual disturbances.
**GI:** diarrhea, dyspepsia, abdominal pain, nausea, flatulence.
**Hepatic:** hepatobiliary dysfunction (including cholestatic jaundice).
**Hematologic:** *neutropenia,* decrease in absolute lymphocyte counts.
**Skin:** rash, pruritus, urticaria, *Stevens-Johnson syndrome, toxic epidermal necrolysis.*
**Other:** *hypersensitivity reactions, anaphylaxis.*

**INTERACTIONS**
**Drug-drug.** *Cimetidine:* decreases drug clearance by one-third. Avoid concomitant use.
*Cyclosporine:* drug increases clearance of cyclosporine. Monitor serum levels.
*Rifampin:* increases terbinafine clearance by 100%. Monitor patient.

---

*Liquid contains alcohol.  **May contain tartrazine.  †Canada  ‡Australia  §U.K.  ◊OTC

**Drug-food.** *Caffeine:* I.V. caffeine clearance is decreased. Use cautiously together.

**EFFECTS ON DIAGNOSTIC TESTS**
None reported.

**CONTRAINDICATIONS**
Contraindicated in patients with hypersensitivity to drug.

**NURSING CONSIDERATIONS**
• Drug is not recommended in patients with preexisting liver disease or renal impairment (creatinine clearance below 50 ml/minute), or in pregnant or breast-feeding patients.
• Monitor CBC and hepatic enzymes in patients receiving drug for over 6 weeks. Drug should be discontinued if hepatobiliary dysfunction or cholestatic hepatitis develops.
• Safety in children has not been established.
• *Alert:* Don't confuse terbinafine with terbutaline.

☑ **Patient teaching**
• Inform patient that successful treatment of nail infections may not be observed for 10 weeks for toenail infections and 4 weeks for fingernail infections.

# 9

## Antimalarials

chloroquine hydrochloride
chloroquine phosphate
doxycycline
   (See Chapter 14, TETRACYCLINES.)
**hydroxychloroquine sulfate**
**mefloquine hydrochloride**
**primaquine phosphate**
**pyrimethamine**
**pyrimethamine with sulfadoxine**

**COMBINATION PRODUCTS**
None.

---

### chloroquine hydrochloride
Aralen HCl, Chlorquin‡

### chloroquine phosphate
Aralen Phosphate, Avloclor§,
Chlorquin‡

*Pregnancy Risk Category C*

### HOW SUPPLIED
**chloroquine hydrochloride**
*Injection:* 50 mg/ml (40-mg/ml base)
**chloroquine phosphate**
*Tablets:* 250 mg (150-mg base), 500 mg
(300-mg base)
*Injection:* 5 mg (200-mg base)

### ACTION
Unknown. May bind to and alter the properties of DNA in susceptible parasites.

| Route | Peak | Onset | Duration |
|-------|------|-------|----------|
| P.O. | Unknown | 1-3 hr | Unknown |
| I.M. | Unknown | 0.5 hr | Unknown |

### INDICATIONS & DOSAGE
*Acute malarial attacks due to* Plasmodium vivax, P. malariae, P. ovale, *and susceptible strains of* P. falciparum—
**Adults:** initially, 600 mg (base) P.O.; then
300 mg at 6, 24, and 48 hours. Or 160 to
200 mg (base) I.M. initially, repeated in 6
hours p.r.n. Switch patient to oral therapy
as soon as possible.

**Children:** initially, 10 mg (base)/kg P.O.;
then 5 mg (base)/kg at 6, 24, and 48 hours
(don't exceed adult dose). Or 5 mg
(base)/kg I.M. initially, repeated in 6
hours p.r.n. Don't exceed 10 mg (base)/
kg/24 hours. Switch patient to oral therapy as soon as possible.
*Malaria prophylaxis—*
**Adults and children:** 5 mg (base)/kg P.O.
(not to exceed 300 mg) weekly on the
same day (begun 1 to 2 weeks before
probable exposure and continued for 4 to
6 weeks after leaving endemic area). If
treatment begins after exposure, initial
dose is doubled (10 mg/kg) in two divided
doses P.O. 6 hours apart.
*Extraintestinal amebiasis—*
**Adults:** 1 g (600-mg base) chloroquine
phosphate P.O. daily for 2 days; then
500 mg (300-mg base) daily for 2 to 3
weeks. Treatment is usually combined
with an intestinal amebicide. When oral
therapy is unfeasible, administer 4 to 5 ml
chloroquine hydrochloride (200 to 250
mg; 160- to 200-mg base) I.M. daily for
10 to 12 days. Resume oral therapy as
soon as possible.
**Children:** 16.7 mg/kg chloroquine phosphate (10-mg/kg base) P.O. once daily for
2 to 3 weeks. Maximum dose is 500 mg
chloroquine phosphate (300-mg base)
daily.

### ADVERSE REACTIONS
**CNS:** mild and transient headache, psychic stimulation, *seizures,* dizziness, neuropathy.
**CV:** hypotension, ECG changes.
**EENT:** blurred vision; difficulty in focusing; reversible corneal changes; typically
irreversible, sometimes progressive or delayed retinal changes such as narrowing
of arterioles; macular lesions; pallor of
optic disk; optic atrophy; patchy retinal
pigmentation, typically leading to blindness, ototoxicity (nerve deafness, vertigo,
tinnitus).
**GI:** anorexia, abdominal cramps, diarrhea, nausea, vomiting, stomatitis.

---

*Liquid contains alcohol.     **May contain tartrazine.     †Canada     ‡Australia     §U.K.     ◊OTC

**Hematologic:** *agranulocytosis, aplastic anemia,* hemolytic anemia, *thrombocytopenia.*

**Skin:** pruritus, lichen planus eruptions, skin and mucosal pigmentary changes, pleomorphic skin eruptions.

## INTERACTIONS

**Drug-drug.** *Cimetidine:* decreased hepatic metabolism of chloroquine. Monitor for toxicity.

*Kaolin, magnesium and aluminum salts:* decreased GI absorption. Separate administration times.

**Drug-lifestyle.** *Sun exposure:* may exacerbate drug-induced dermatoses. Tell patient to avoid excessive sun exposure.

## EFFECTS ON DIAGNOSTIC TESTS
None reported.

## CONTRAINDICATIONS
Contraindicated in patients with hypersensitivity to drug, retinal or visual field changes, or porphyria.

## NURSING CONSIDERATIONS
• Use with extreme caution in patients with severe GI, neurologic, or blood disorders.
• Use cautiously in patients with hepatic disease or alcoholism because drug concentrates in the liver, and in those with G6PD deficiency or psoriasis because drug may exacerbate these conditions.
• *Alert:* Drug dosage may be discussed in mg or mg-base; be aware of the difference.
• Ensure that baseline and periodic ophthalmic examinations are performed. Check periodically for ocular muscle weakness after long-term use.
• Assist patient with obtaining audiometric examinations before, during, and after therapy, especially if therapy is long-term.
• Monitor CBC and liver function studies periodically during long-term therapy as ordered; if a severe blood disorder not attributable to the disease develops, drug may need to be discontinued.
• *Alert:* Monitor patient for possible overdose, which can quickly lead to toxic symptoms: headache, drowsiness, visual disturbances, CV collapse, and seizures, followed by cardiopulmonary arrest. Children are extremely susceptible to toxicity; avoid long-term treatment.

☑ **Patient teaching**
• To enhance compliance for prophylaxis, advise patient to take drug immediately before or after meals on same day each week.
• Instruct patient to avoid excessive sun exposure to prevent exacerbation of drug-induced dermatoses.
• Tell patient to report adverse reactions promptly, especially blurred vision, increased sensitivity to light, or muscle weakness.

---

## hydroxychloroquine sulfate
Plaquenil Sulfate

*Pregnancy Risk Category C*

## HOW SUPPLIED
*Tablets:* 200 mg (155-mg base)

## ACTION
Unknown. May bind to and alter the properties of DNA in susceptible organisms.

| Route | Onset | Peak | Duration |
|-------|-------|------|----------|
| P.O. | Unknown | 2-4.5 hr | Unknown |

## INDICATIONS & DOSAGE
*Suppressive prophylaxis of malaria attacks due to* Plasmodium vivax, P. malariae, P. ovale, *and susceptible strains of* P. falciparum—

**Adults:** 400 mg ( 310-mg base) P.O. weekly on same day of week (begin 1 to 2 weeks before entering endemic area and continue for 4 weeks after leaving endemic area). If not started before exposure, initial dose is doubled to 800 mg (620-mg base) in two divided doses.

**Children:** 5 mg/kg (base) P.O. weekly on same day of week (begin 1 to 2 weeks before entering endemic area and continue for 4 weeks after leaving endemic area). Don't exceed adult dose. If not started before exposure, initial dose is doubled to 10 mg/kg (base) in two divided doses.

---

Reactions may be *common,* uncommon, *life-threatening,* or COMMON AND LIFE-THREATENING.

*Acute malarial attacks—*
**Adults:** initially, 800 mg (sulfate) P.O.; then 400 mg after 6 to 8 hours; then 400 mg daily for 2 days (total 2 g sulfate salt).
**Children:** 13 mg/kg (sulfate) P.O.; then 6.5 mg/kg 6 hours later; then 6.5 mg/kg daily for 2 days.
*Lupus erythematosus (chronic discoid and systemic)—*
**Adults:** 400 mg (sulfate) P.O. daily or b.i.d., continued for several weeks or months, depending on response. For prolonged maintenance dose, 200 to 400 mg (sulfate) daily.
*Rheumatoid arthritis—*
**Adults:** initially, 400 to 600 mg (sulfate) P.O. daily. When good response occurs (usually in 4 to 12 weeks), dosage is cut in half.

## ADVERSE REACTIONS
**CNS:** irritability, nightmares, ataxia, *seizures,* psychosis, vertigo, nystagmus, dizziness, hypoactive deep tendon reflexes, lassitude, skeletal muscle weakness, headache.
**CV:** T wave inversion or depression, widening of the QRS complex.
**EENT:** blurred vision; difficulty in focusing; reversible corneal changes; typically irreversible, sometimes progressive or delayed retinal changes such as narrowing of arterioles; macular lesions; pallor of optic disk; optic atrophy; visual field defects; patchy retinal pigmentation, commonly leading to blindness, ototoxicity.
**GI:** anorexia, abdominal cramps, diarrhea, nausea, vomiting.
**Hematologic:** *agranulocytosis, leukopenia, thrombocytopenia, hemolysis in patients with G6PD deficiency, aplastic anemia.*
**Skin:** pruritus, lichen planus eruptions, skin and mucosal pigmentary changes, pleomorphic skin eruptions, worsened psoriasis.
**Other:** weight loss, alopecia, bleaching of hair.

## INTERACTIONS
**Drug-drug.** *Cimetidine:* decreased hepatic metabolism of hydroxychloroquine. Monitor for toxicity.

*Kaolin, magnesium and aluminum salts:* decreased GI absorption. Separate administration times.

## EFFECTS ON DIAGNOSTIC TESTS
None reported.

## CONTRAINDICATIONS
Contraindicated in patients with retinal or visual field changes, porphyria, or hypersensitivity to drug and in long-term therapy for children.

## NURSING CONSIDERATIONS
• Use with extreme caution in patients with severe GI, neurologic, or blood disorders.
• Use cautiously in patients with hepatic disease or alcoholism because drug concentrates in liver, and in those with G6PD deficiency or psoriasis because drug may exacerbate these conditions.
• *Alert:* Drug dosage may be discussed in mg or mg-base; be aware of the difference.
• Ensure that baseline and periodic ophthalmic examinations are performed. Check periodically for ocular muscle weakness after long-term use.
• Assist patient with obtaining audiometric examinations before, during, and after therapy, especially if therapy is long-term.
• Monitor CBC and liver function studies periodically during long-term therapy, as ordered; if severe blood disorder not attributable to disease develops, drug may need to be discontinued.
• *Alert:* Monitor patient for possible overdose, which can quickly lead to toxic signs or symptoms: headache, drowsiness, visual disturbances, CV collapse, and seizures, followed by cardiopulmonary arrest. Children are extremely susceptible to toxicity; long-term treatment should be avoided.

☑ **Patient teaching**
• To enhance compliance for prophylaxis, advise patient to take hydroxychloroquine immediately before or after meals on same day each week.
• Instruct patient to report adverse reactions promptly.

## mefloquine hydrochloride
Lariam

*Pregnancy Risk Category C*

### HOW SUPPLIED
*Tablets:* 250 mg

### ACTION
Unknown. Antimalarial action may be related to drug's ability to form complexes with hemin; may also act by raising intravesicular pH in parasite acid vesicles.

| Route | Onset | Peak | Duration |
|-------|-------|------|----------|
| P.O. | Unknown | 7-24 hr | Unknown |

### INDICATIONS & DOSAGE
*Acute malaria infections due to mefloquine-sensitive strains of* Plasmodium falciparum *or* P. vivax—
**Adults:** 1,250 mg P.O. as a single dose. Patients with *P. vivax* infections should receive subsequent therapy with primaquine or other 8-aminoquinolines to avoid relapse after treatment of the initial infection.
*Malaria prophylaxis—*
**Adults:** 250 mg P.O. once weekly. Prophylaxis should be initiated 1 week before entering endemic area and continued for 4 weeks after returning. If patient returns to an area without malaria after a prolonged stay in an endemic area, prophylaxis should end after three doses.

### ADVERSE REACTIONS
**CNS:** dizziness, syncope, headache, psychotic manifestations, hallucinations, confusion, anxiety, fatigue, vertigo, depression, *seizures.*
**EENT:** tinnitus, visual disturbances.
**GI:** anorexia, vomiting, *nausea,* loose stools, diarrhea, abdominal discomfort or pain.
**Hematologic:** decreased hematocrit, *leukopenia,* and *thrombocytopenia.*
**Hepatic:** transient elevations of transaminases.
**Musculoskeletal:** myalgia.
**Skin:** rash.
**Other:** fever, chills.

### INTERACTIONS
**Drug-drug.** *Beta blockers, quinidine, quinine:* ECG abnormalities and cardiac arrest may occur. Avoid concomitant use.
*Chloroquine, quinine:* increased risk of seizures. Avoid concomitant use.
*Valproic acid:* decreased valproic acid blood levels and loss of seizure control at start of mefloquine therapy. Monitor anticonvulsant blood levels.

### EFFECTS ON DIAGNOSTIC TESTS
None reported.

### CONTRAINDICATIONS
Contraindicated in patients with hypersensitivity to mefloquine or related compounds.

### NURSING CONSIDERATIONS
• Use cautiously in patients with cardiac disease or seizure disorders.
• Because the health risks from concomitant administration of quinine and mefloquine are great, mefloquine therapy shouldn't begin sooner than 12 hours after the last dose of quinine or quinidine.
• Patients with *P. vivax* infections are at high risk for relapse because the drug does not eliminate the hepatic phase (exoerythrocytic parasites). Follow-up therapy with primaquine is advisable.
• Monitor liver function tests periodically as ordered.
• If overdose is suspected, induce vomiting or perform gastric lavage as appropriate because of potential for cardiotoxicity. Mefloquine has produced cardiac actions similar to quinidine and quinine.

### ☑ Patient teaching
• Advise patient to take drug on the same day of the week when using it for prophylaxis.
• Tell patient not to take drug on an empty stomach and always to take it with a full glass (at least 8 oz [240 ml]) of water.
• Advise patient to use caution when performing activities that require alertness and coordination because dizziness, disturbed sense of balance, and neuropsychiatric reactions may occur.
• Instruct patient taking mefloquine prophylactically to discontinue drug and to

---

Reactions may be *common,* uncommon, *life-threatening,* or COMMON AND LIFE-THREATENING.

notify doctor if signs or symptoms of impending toxicity, such as unexplained anxiety, depression, confusion, or restlessness, occur.
• Advise patient undergoing long-term therapy to have periodic ophthalmic examinations because drug may cause ocular lesions.

## primaquine phosphate

*Pregnancy Risk Category C*

### HOW SUPPLIED
*Tablets:* 15 mg (base)

### ACTION
Unknown. May bind to and alter the properties of DNA in susceptible parasites.

| Route | Onset | Peak | Duration |
|-------|-------|------|----------|
| P.O. | Unknown | 1-3 hr | Unknown |

### INDICATIONS & DOSAGE
*Radical cure of relapsing vivax malaria, eliminating symptoms and infection completely; prevention of relapse—*
**Adults:** 15 mg (base) P.O. daily for 14 days. (A 26.3-mg tablet provides 15 mg of base.) Begin therapy during the last 2 weeks of, or following, a course of suppression with chloroquine or comparable agent.
**Children:** 0.5 mg/kg/day (0.3-mg base/kg/day; maximum 15-mg base/dose) P.O. for 14 days.

### ADVERSE REACTIONS
**GI:** nausea, vomiting, epigastric distress, abdominal cramps.
**Hematologic:** decreases or increases in WBC counts, decreases in RBC counts, **hemolytic anemia** (in G6PD deficiency), methemoglobinemia (in NADH methemoglobin reductase deficiency).

### INTERACTIONS
**Drug-drug.** *Magnesium and aluminum salts:* decreased GI absorption. Separate administration times.
*Quinacrine:* enhanced toxicity of primaquine. Don't use together.

### EFFECTS ON DIAGNOSTIC TESTS
None reported.

### CONTRAINDICATIONS
Contraindicated in patients with systemic diseases in which agranulocytosis may develop (such as lupus erythematosus or rheumatoid arthritis) and in those taking bone marrow suppressants and potentially hemolytic drugs. Concomitant administration of quinacrine and primaquine is contraindicated.

### NURSING CONSIDERATIONS
• Use cautiously in patients with previous idiosyncratic reaction (manifested by hemolytic anemia, methemoglobinemia, or leukopenia), in those with a family or personal history of favism, and in those with erythrocytic G6PD deficiency or NADH methemoglobin reductase deficiency.
• *Alert:* Drug dosage may be discussed in mg or mg-base; be aware of the difference.
• Administer drug with meals.
• Keep in mind that when administering drug, a fast-acting antimalarial (such as chloroquine) is used to reduce possibility of drug-resistant strains.
• Obtain frequent blood studies and urine examinations, as ordered, in light-skinned patients taking more than 30 mg (base) daily, dark-skinned patients taking more than 15 mg (base) daily, and patients with severe anemia or suspected sensitivity.
• Monitor patient for sudden fall in hemoglobin level or erythrocyte or leukocyte count, or marked darkening of the urine, which suggest impending hemolytic reactions. Discontinue drug immediately and notify doctor.

### ☑ Patient teaching
• Instruct patient to take drug with meals to minimize stomach upset. If stomach upset (nausea, vomiting, or stomach pain) persists, tell patient to notify doctor.
• Tell patient to stop drug therapy and notify doctor immediately if marked darkening of urine occurs.
• Stress importance of completing full course of therapy.

---

*Liquid contains alcohol. **May contain tartrazine. †Canada ‡Australia §U.K. ◊OTC

## pyrimethamine
Daraprim

## pyrimethamine with sulfadoxine
Fansidar

*Pregnancy Risk Category C*

### HOW SUPPLIED
**pyrimethamine**
*Tablets:* 25 mg
**pyrimethamine with sulfadoxine**
*Tablets:* pyrimethamine 25 mg, sulfadoxine 500 mg

### ACTION
Inhibits the enzyme dihydrofolate reductase, thereby impeding reduction of dihydrofolic acid to tetrahydrofolic acid. Sulfadoxine competitively inhibits use of PABA.

| Route | Onset | Peak | Duration |
|-------|-------|------|----------|
| P.O. | Unknown | 1.5-8 hr | 2 wk |

### INDICATIONS & DOSAGE
*Malaria prophylaxis and transmission control (pyrimethamine)—*
**Adults and children ages 10 and older:** 25 mg P.O. weekly.
**Children ages 4 to 10:** 12.5 mg P.O. weekly.
**Children under age 4:** 6.25 mg P.O. weekly.

Needs to be continued in all age-groups for at least 6 to 10 weeks after leaving endemic areas.
*Acute attacks of malaria (Fansidar)—*
**Adults and children ages 14 and older:** 2 to 3 tablets as a single dose, either alone or in sequence with quinine or primaquine.
**Children ages 9 to 13:** 2 tablets.
**Children ages 4 to 8:** 1 tablet.
**Children under age 4:** ½ tablet.
*Malaria prophylaxis (Fansidar)—*
**Adults and children ages 14 and older:** 1 tablet weekly, or 2 tablets q 2 weeks.
**Children ages 9 to 13:** ¾ tablet weekly, or 1 ½ tablets q 2 weeks.
**Children ages 4 to 8:** ½ tablet weekly, or 1 tablet q 2 weeks.

**Children under age 4:** ¼ tablet weekly, or ½ tablet q 2 weeks.
*Acute attacks of malaria (pyrimethamine)—*
**Adults and children ages 15 and older:** 50 mg P.O. daily for 2 days; then once weekly, with doses as described above.
**Children under age 15:** 25 mg P.O. daily for 2 days; then once weekly, with doses as described above.

Not recommended alone in nonimmune patients; drug should be used with faster-acting antimalarials such as chloroquine for 2 days to initiate transmission control and suppressive cure.
*Toxoplasmosis (pyrimethamine)—*
**Adults:** initially, 50 to 75 mg P.O. with 1 to 4 g sulfadiazine; continue for 1 to 3 weeks. Reduce after 3 weeks by half and continue for 4 to 5 weeks.
**Children:** initially, 1 mg/kg/day P.O. (not to exceed 100 mg) in two equally divided doses for 2 to 4 days; then 0.5 mg/kg daily for 4 weeks, along with 100 mg sulfadiazine/kg P.O. daily, divided q 6 hours.

### ADVERSE REACTIONS
**CNS:** headache, peripheral neuritis, mental depression, *seizures,* ataxia, hallucinations, fatigue.
**CV:** *arrhythmias,* allergic myocarditis.
**EENT:** scleral irritation, periorbital edema.
**GI:** anorexia, vomiting, atrophic glossitis.
**Hematologic:** *agranulocytosis, aplastic anemia,* megaloblastic anemia, *leukopenia, thrombocytopenia, pancytopenia.*
**Skin:** *Stevens-Johnson syndrome,* generalized skin eruptions, urticaria, pruritus, photosensitivity.

*Note:* Adverse drug reactions related to sulfadiazine are similar to sulfonamides.

### INTERACTIONS
**Drug-drug.** *Co-trimoxazole, methotrexate, sulfonamides:* increased risk of bone marrow suppression. Don't use together.
*Lorazepam:* increased risk of hepatotoxicity. Avoid concomitant use.
*PABA:* decreased antitoxoplasmic effects. May require dosage adjustment.

**EFFECTS ON DIAGNOSTIC TESTS**
None reported.

**CONTRAINDICATIONS**
Pyrimethamine is contraindicated in patients with hypersensitivity to drug and in those with megaloblastic anemia due to folic acid deficiency. Fansidar is contraindicated in patients with porphyria.

Repeated use of Fansidar is contraindicated in patients with severe renal insufficiency, marked parenchymal damage to the liver, blood dyscrasias, known hypersensitivity to pyrimethamine or sulfonamides, or documented megaloblastic anemia due to folate deficiency. Also contraindicated in infants under age 2 months and in pregnant (at term) and breast-feeding women.

**NURSING CONSIDERATIONS**
• Use cautiously in patients with impaired hepatic or renal function, severe allergy or bronchial asthma, G6PD deficiency, or seizure disorders (smaller doses may be needed), and after treatment with chloroquine.
• Obtain twice-weekly blood counts, including platelets, as ordered, for the patient with toxoplasmosis because dosages used approach toxic levels. If signs of folic acid or folinic acid deficiency develop, dosage should be reduced or discontinued while the patient receives parenteral folinic acid (leucovorin) until blood counts become normal.
• When used to treat toxoplasmosis in patients with AIDS, therapy may be lifelong.
• Fansidar should be used only in areas where chloroquine-resistant malaria is prevalent and only if the traveler plans to stay longer than 3 weeks.

☑**Patient teaching**
• Instruct patient to take drug with meals.
• Inform patient with toxoplasmosis of importance of frequent laboratory studies and compliance with therapy. Tell patient of potential need for long-term therapy.
• Warn patient taking Fansidar to stop drug and notify doctor at first sign of rash.
• Tell patient to take first prophylactic dose 1 to 2 days before traveling.

---

*Liquid contains alcohol.    **May contain tartrazine.    †Canada    ‡Australia    §U.K.    ◇OTC

clofazimine
cycloserine
dapsone
ethambutol hydrochloride
isoniazid
pyrazinamide
rifabutin
rifampin
rifapentine
streptomycin sulfate
(See Chapter 11, AMINOGLYCOSIDES.)

## COMBINATION PRODUCTS
RIFAMATE: isoniazid 150 mg and rifampin 300 mg.
RIFATER: isoniazid 50 mg, rifampin 120 mg, and pyrazinamide 300 mg.
RIMACTANE/INH DUAL PACK: 30 300-mg isoniazid tablets and 60 300-mg rifampin capsules.

---

## clofazimine
Lamprene

*Pregnancy Risk Category C*

## HOW SUPPLIED
*Capsules:* 50 mg

## ACTION
Unknown. Thought to inhibit mycobacterial growth by binding preferentially to mycobacterial DNA. Also has anti-inflammatory effects that suppress skin reactions of erythema nodosum leprosum.

| Route | Onset | Peak | Duration |
|-------|-------|------|----------|
| P.O. | Unknown | 1-6 hr | Unknown |

## INDICATIONS & DOSAGE
*Dapsone-resistant leprosy (Hansen's disease)—*
**Adults:** 100 mg P.O. daily with other antileprotics for 3 years. Then, clofazimine *alone,* 100 mg daily.
*Erythema nodosum leprosum—*
**Adults:** 100 to 200 mg P.O. daily for up to 3 months; when prolonged, concomi-

tant corticosteroid therapy is necessary. Dose is tapered to 100 mg daily as soon as possible. Doses above 200 mg daily are not recommended.

## ADVERSE REACTIONS
**EENT:** *conjunctival and corneal pigmentation, dryness, burning, itching, irritation.*
**GI:** *epigastric pain, diarrhea, nausea, vomiting, GI intolerance, **bowel obstruction, bleeding.***
**Hematologic:** eosinophilia.
**Hepatic:** elevated albumin, serum bilirubin, and AST.
**Metabolic:** hypokalemia, elevated blood glucose level.
**Skin:** *pink to brownish black pigmentation, ichthyosis and dryness,* rash, pruritus.
**Other:** ***splenic infarction,*** discolored body fluids and excrement.

## INTERACTIONS
**Drug-drug.** *Dapsone:* impaired anti-inflammatory effects of clofazimine. No intervention appears necessary.
*Isoniazid:* may decrease level of drug in the skin and increase serum and urine levels of clofazimine. Monitor for decreased effectiveness.
*Rifampin:* decreased rifampin bioavailability. Monitor for decreased effectiveness.

## EFFECTS ON DIAGNOSTIC TESTS
None reported.

## CONTRAINDICATIONS
No known contraindications.

## NURSING CONSIDERATIONS
• Use cautiously in patients with GI dysfunction, such as abdominal pain and diarrhea.
• Give doses exceeding 100 mg daily for as short a period as possible and only under close medical supervision.
• If patient complains of colic, burning abdominal pain, or other GI symptoms, notify doctor, who may reduce dose or increase interval between doses.

---

Reactions may be *common,* uncommon, ***life-threatening,*** or COMMON AND LIFE-THREATENING.

**✓Patient teaching**
* Advise patient to take drug with meals or milk.
* Warn patient that clofazimine may discolor skin, body fluids, and excrement. The color ranges from pink to brownish black. Reassure patient that the unsightly skin discoloration is reversible but may not disappear until several months or years after drug treatment ends.
* Tell patient to apply skin oil or cream to help reverse skin dryness or ichthyosis.

---

## cycloserine
Seromycin

*Pregnancy Risk Category C*

### HOW SUPPLIED
*Capsules:* 250 mg

### ACTION
Inhibits cell-wall biosynthesis by interfering with the bacterial use of amino acids. Action may be bacteriostatic or bactericidal, depending on the concentration of drug attained at the site of infection and the susceptibility of the infecting organism.

| Route | Onset | Peak | Duration |
|-------|-------|------|----------|
| P.O. | Unknown | 4-8 hr | Unknown |

### INDICATIONS & DOSAGE
*Adjunctive treatment in pulmonary or extrapulmonary tuberculosis—*
**Adults:** initially, 250 mg P.O. q 12 hours for 2 weeks; then, if blood levels are below 25 to 30 mcg/ml and no toxicity has developed, dose is increased to 250 mg q 8 hours for 2 weeks. If optimum blood levels are still not achieved and no toxicity has developed, then dose is increased to 250 mg q 6 hours. Maximum dose is 1 g/day. If CNS toxicity occurs, drug is discontinued for 1 week, then resumed at 250 mg daily for 2 weeks. If no serious toxic effects occur, dose is increased by 250-mg increments q 10 days until blood level of 25 to 30 mcg/ml is obtained.
**Children:** 10 to 20 mg/kg/day P.O. in two divided doses (maximum of 0.75 to 1 g).

*Acute urinary tract infections—*
**Adults:** 250 mg P.O. q 12 hours for 2 weeks.

### ADVERSE REACTIONS
**CNS:** *seizures,* drowsiness, somnolence, headache, tremor, dysarthria, vertigo, confusion, loss of memory, *possible suicidal tendencies,* psychosis, hyperirritability, paresthesia, paresis, hyperreflexia, *coma.*
**CV:** *sudden heart failure.*
**Hepatic:** elevated transaminase level.
**Other:** hypersensitivity reactions (allergic dermatitis).

### INTERACTIONS
**Drug-drug.** *Ethionamide:* increased risk of CNS toxicity (seizures). Monitor patient closely.
*Isoniazid:* CNS toxicity (dizziness or drowsiness). Monitor patient closely.
**Drug-lifestyle.** *Alcohol use:* increased risk of CNS toxicity (seizures). Monitor patient closely.

### EFFECTS ON DIAGNOSTIC TESTS
None reported.

### CONTRAINDICATIONS
Contraindicated in patients hypersensitive to drug and in those with seizure disorders, depression or severe anxiety, psychosis, and severe renal insufficiency. Also contraindicated in patients who use alcohol excessively.

### NURSING CONSIDERATIONS
* Use cautiously in patients with impaired renal function; reduced dose is required.
* Obtain specimen for culture and sensitivity tests before therapy begins and periodically thereafter to detect possible resistance.
* Cycloserine is considered a "second-line" drug in the treatment of tuberculosis and should always be administered with other antituberculotics to prevent the development of resistant organisms.
* Monitor serum cycloserine levels periodically as ordered, especially in patients receiving high doses (over 500 mg daily) because toxic reactions may occur with blood levels above 30 mcg/ml.

- Monitor results of hematologic tests and renal and liver function studies.
- Observe patient for psychotic symptoms, hallucinations, and possible suicidal tendencies.
- Administer pyridoxine, anticonvulsant, tranquilizer, or sedative, as ordered, to relieve adverse reactions.

☑ **Patient teaching**
- Warn patient to avoid alcohol, which may cause serious neurologic reactions.
- Advise patient not to perform hazardous activities if drowsiness occurs.
- Tell patient to report adverse reactions promptly because dosage adjustment may be necessary or other medications may be prescribed to relieve adverse reactions.

## dapsone
Avlosulfon†, Dapsone 100‡

*Pregnancy Risk Category C*

### HOW SUPPLIED
*Tablets:* 25 mg, 100 mg

### ACTION
Unknown. May inhibit folic acid biosynthesis in susceptible organisms.

| Route | Onset | Peak | Duration |
|-------|-------|------|----------|
| P.O. | Unknown | 4-8 hr | Unknown |

### INDICATIONS & DOSAGE
*All forms of leprosy (Hansen's disease)—*
**Adults:** 100 mg P.O. daily, indefinitely; give with rifampin 600 mg P.O. monthly for 6 months.
**Children:** 1 to 2 mg/kg P.O. daily for minimum of 3 years.
*Dermatitis herpetiformis—*
**Adults:** 50 mg P.O. daily; increased to 300 mg daily, p.r.n.

### ADVERSE REACTIONS
**CNS:** insomnia, psychosis, headache, paresthesia, peripheral neuropathy, vertigo.
**CV:** tachycardia.
**EENT:** tinnitus, blurred vision.
**GI:** anorexia, abdominal pain, nausea, vomiting, pancreatitis.

**GU:** albuminuria, nephrotic syndrome, renal papillary necrosis, male infertility.
**Hematologic:** *hemolytic anemia, agranulocytosis, aplastic anemia.*
**Respiratory:** pulmonary eosinophilia.
**Skin:** lupus erythematosus, phototoxicity, *exfoliative dermatitis, toxic erythema, erythema multiforme, toxic epidermal necrolysis,* morbilliform and scarlatiniform reactions, urticaria, *erythema nodosum.*
**Other:** fever, infectious mononucleosis–like syndrome, *sulfone syndrome.*

### INTERACTIONS
**Drug-drug.** *Activated charcoal:* may decrease dapsone's GI absorption and enterohepatic recycling. Monitor closely.
*Didanosine:* possible therapeutic failure of dapsone, leading to an increase in infection. Avoid concomitant use.
*Folic acid antagonists (such as methotrexate):* increased risk of adverse hematologic reactions. Avoid concomitant use.
*PABA:* may antagonize the effect of dapsone by interfering with the primary mechanism of action. Monitor for lack of efficacy.
*Probenecid:* reduces urinary excretion of dapsone metabolites, increasing plasma concentrations. Monitor closely.
*Rifampin:* increased hepatic metabolism of dapsone. Monitor for lack of efficacy.
*Trimethoprim:* increased serum levels of both drugs may occur, possibly increasing the pharmacologic and toxic effects of each drug. Monitor closely.
**Drug-lifestyle.** *Sun exposure:* may cause photosensitivity. Tell patient to avoid prolonged exposure to sunlight or sunlamps.

### EFFECTS ON DIAGNOSTIC TESTS
None reported.

### CONTRAINDICATIONS
Contraindicated in patients with hypersensitivity to drug. Also contraindicated in breast-feeding women because of risk of tumorigenicity.

### NURSING CONSIDERATIONS
- Use cautiously in patients with chronic renal, hepatic, or CV disease; refractory types of anemia; and G6PD deficiency.

---

Reactions may be *common,* uncommon, *life-threatening,* or COMMON AND LIFE-THREATENING.

• Obtain baseline CBC as ordered. Monitor CBC weekly for the first month, monthly for 6 months, and semiannually thereafter.

• Be prepared to reduce or temporarily discontinue dapsone if hemoglobin falls below 9 g/dl, WBC count falls below 5,000/mm$^3$, or RBC count falls below 2.5 million/mm$^3$ or remains low.

• If generalized, diffuse dermatitis occurs, notify doctor and prepare to interrupt therapy.

• Administer antihistamines, as ordered, to combat allergic dermatitis.

• Monitor patient for signs and symptoms of erythema nodosum reaction (malaise, fever, painful inflammatory induration in the skin and mucosa, iritis, and neuritis), which may occur during therapy as a result of *Mycobacterium leprae* bacilli. In severe cases, therapy should be stopped and glucocorticoids given cautiously.

• Watch for and report signs and symptoms of sulfone syndrome, including fever, malaise, jaundice (with hepatic necrosis), lymphadenopathy, methemoglobinemia, and hemolytic anemia.

☑ **Patient teaching**

• *Alert:* Because of the risk of tumorigenicity, breast-feeding should be discontinued during therapy. Instruct breast-feeding woman to immediately notify doctor if cyanosis occurs in infant.

• Inform patient of need for long-term therapy. Stress importance of compliance with drug therapy.

• Advise patient to avoid unprotected exposure to sunlight or sunlamps.

---

## ethambutol hydrochloride
Etibi†, Myambutol

*Pregnancy Risk Category C*

### HOW SUPPLIED
*Tablets:* 100 mg, 400 mg

### ACTION
Unknown. Appears to interfere with the synthesis of one or more metabolites of susceptible bacteria, altering cellular metabolism during cell division (bacteriostatic).

| Route | Onset | Peak | Duration |
|-------|-------|------|----------|
| P.O. | Unknown | 2-4 hr | Unknown |

### INDICATIONS & DOSAGE
*Adjunctive treatment in pulmonary tuberculosis—*
**Adults and children over age 13:** in patients who have not received previous antitubercular therapy, 15 mg/kg P.O. as a single daily dose.

Retreatment: 25 mg/kg P.O. daily as a single dose for 60 days (or until bacteriologic smears and cultures become negative) with at least one other antituberculotic; then decreased to 15 mg/kg/day as a single dose.

### ADVERSE REACTIONS
**CNS:** headache, dizziness, mental confusion, possible hallucinations, malaise, peripheral neuritis.
**CV:** *thrombocytopenia.*
**EENT:** optic neuritis, bloody sputum.
**GI:** anorexia, nausea, vomiting, abdominal pain, GI upset.
**Hepatic:** abnormal liver function test results.
**Musculoskeletal:** joint pain.
**Skin:** dermatitis, pruritus, *toxic epidermal necrolysis.*
**Other:** *anaphylactoid reactions,* fever, elevated uric acid level, precipitation of acute gout.

### INTERACTIONS
**Drug-drug.** *Aluminum salts:* may delay and reduce absorption of ethambutol. Separate administration times by several hours.

### EFFECTS ON DIAGNOSTIC TESTS
None reported.

### CONTRAINDICATIONS
Contraindicated in patients with optic neuritis or hypersensitivity to drug and in children under age 13.

### NURSING CONSIDERATIONS
• Use cautiously in patients with impaired renal function, cataracts, recurrent eye in-

---

flammations, gout, and diabetic retinopathy.
• Perform visual acuity and color discrimination tests before and during therapy.
• Obtain AST and ALT levels before therapy, and monitor these levels every 3 to 4 weeks, as ordered.
• Anticipate dosage reduction in patients with impaired renal function.
• Always administer ethambutol with other antituberculotics to prevent the development of resistant organisms.
• Monitor serum uric acid level as ordered; observe patient for signs of gout.

☑ **Patient teaching**
• Reassure patient that visual disturbances will generally disappear several weeks to months after drug is stopped. Optic neuritis is related to dose and duration of treatment.
• Inform patient that drug is administered concurrently with other antituberculotics.
• Stress importance of compliance with drug therapy.

## isoniazid (isonicotinic acid hydrazide, INH)
Isotamine†, Laniazid, Nydrazid**, PMS-Isoniazid†

*Pregnancy Risk Category C*

### HOW SUPPLIED
*Tablets:* 100 mg, 300 mg
*Oral solution:* 50 mg/5 ml
*Injection:* 100 mg/ml

### ACTION
Unknown. Appears to inhibit cell-wall biosynthesis by interfering with lipid and DNA synthesis (bactericidal).

| Route | Onset | Peak | Duration |
|---|---|---|---|
| P.O., I.M. | Unknown | 1-2 hr | Unknown |

### INDICATIONS & DOSAGE
*Actively growing tubercle bacilli—*
**Adults:** 5 mg/kg P.O. or I.M. daily in a single dose, up to 300 mg/day, continued for 6 months to 2 years.
**Infants and children:** 10 to 20 mg/kg P.O. or I.M. daily in a single dose, up to

300 mg/day, continued long enough to prevent relapse. Coadministration of at least one other antituberculotic is recommended.
*Prevention of tubercle bacilli in those exposed to tuberculosis or those with positive skin test whose chest X-rays and bacteriologic studies are consistent with nonprogressive tuberculosis—*
**Adults:** 300 mg P.O. daily in a single dose, continued for 6 months to 1 year.
**Infants and children:** 10 mg/kg P.O. daily in a single dose, up to 300 mg/day, continued for 1 year.

### ADVERSE REACTIONS
**CNS:** *peripheral neuropathy, seizures,* toxic encephalopathy, memory impairment, toxic psychosis.
**EENT:** optic neuritis and atrophy.
**GI:** nausea, vomiting, epigastric distress.
**GU:** gynecomastia.
**Hematologic:** *agranulocytosis,* hemolytic anemia, *aplastic anemia,* eosinophilia, *thrombocytopenia,* sideroblastic anemia.
**Hepatic:** *hepatitis,* jaundice, *elevated serum transaminase levels,* bilirubinemia.
**Metabolic:** hyperglycemia, metabolic acidosis, hypocalcemia, hypophosphatemia.
**Skin:** irritation at I.M. injection site.
**Other:** rheumatic and lupus-like syndromes, *hypersensitivity reactions,* pyridoxine deficiency.

### INTERACTIONS
**Drug-drug.** *Aluminum-containing antacids and laxatives:* may decrease the rate and amount of isoniazid absorbed. Give isoniazid at least 1 hour before antacid or laxative.
*Benzodiazepines:* isoniazid may inhibit the metabolic clearance of benzodiazepines that undergo oxidative metabolism (diazepam, triazolam), possibly increasing the activity of the benzodiazepine. Monitor closely.
*Carbamazepine, halothane:* increased risk of isoniazid hepatotoxicity. Use together cautiously.
*Carbamazepine, phenytoin:* increased plasma levels of these anticonvulsants. Monitor closely.
*Cycloserine, meperidine:* may increase CNS adverse reactions and hypotension

(meperidine only). Institute safety precautions.

*Disulfiram:* may cause neurologic symptoms, including changes in behavior and coordination. Avoid concomitant use.

*Enflurane:* in rapid acetylators of isoniazid, high-output renal failure may occur because of nephrotoxic levels of inorganic fluoride. Monitor renal function.

*Ketoconazole:* serum concentrations of ketoconazole may be decreased. Monitor for lack of efficacy.

*Oral anticoagulants:* anticoagulant activity may be enhanced. Monitor patient closely.

**Drug-food.** *Foods containing tyramine:* may cause hypertensive crisis. Tell patient to avoid such foods or eat in small quantities.

**Drug-lifestyle.** *Alcohol use:* may be associated with increased incidence of isoniazid-related hepatitis. Avoid concomitant use.

**EFFECTS ON DIAGNOSTIC TESTS**
Isoniazid alters results of urine glucose tests that use cupric sulfate method (Benedict's reagent or Diastix).

**CONTRAINDICATIONS**
Contraindicated in patients with acute hepatic disease or isoniazid-associated liver damage.

**NURSING CONSIDERATIONS**
• Use cautiously in patients with chronic non-isoniazid-associated liver disease, seizure disorders (especially in those taking phenytoin), severe renal impairment, and chronic alcoholism and in elderly patients.
• Always administer isoniazid with other antituberculotics to prevent the development of resistant organisms.
• Keep in mind that isoniazid pharmacokinetics may vary among patients because drug is metabolized in the liver by genetically controlled acetylation. Fast acetylators metabolize the drug up to five times as fast as slow acetylators. About 50% of blacks and whites are slow acetylators; over 80% of Chinese, Japanese, and Inuits are fast acetylators.

• Peripheral neuropathy is more common in patients who are slow acetylators or who are malnourished, alcoholic, or diabetic.
• Monitor hepatic function closely for changes. Elevated liver function study results occur in about 15% of patients; most abnormalities are mild and transient, but some may persist throughout treatment.
• Administer pyridoxine, as ordered, to prevent peripheral neuropathy, especially in malnourished patients.

☑ **Patient teaching**
• Instruct patient to take drug exactly as prescribed; warn against discontinuing drug without doctor's consent.
• Advise patient to take drug with food if GI irritation occurs.
• Tell patient to notify doctor immediately if signs and symptoms of liver impairment occur (anorexia, fatigue, malaise, jaundice, dark urine).
• Advise patient to avoid alcoholic beverages while taking drug. Also tell him to avoid certain foods (fish, such as skipjack and tuna, and tyramine-containing products, such as aged cheese, beer, and chocolate) because drug has some MAO inhibitor activity.
• Encourage patient to comply fully with treatment, which may take months or years.

---

## pyrazinamide
pms-Pyrazinamide†, Tebrazid†, Zinamide‡

*Pregnancy Risk Category C*

**HOW SUPPLIED**
*Tablets:* 500 mg

**ACTION**
Unknown.

| Route | Onset | Peak | Duration |
|-------|---------|--------|----------|
| P.O. | Unknown | 1-2 hr | Unknown |

**INDICATIONS & DOSAGE**
*Adjunctive treatment of tuberculosis (when primary and secondary antituberculotics can't be used or have failed)—*
**Adults:** 15 to 30 mg/kg P.O. once daily. Maximum dose is 3 g daily. Or, when

compliance is a problem, 50 to 70 mg/kg (based on lean body mass) P.O. twice weekly.

**ADVERSE REACTIONS**
**CNS:** malaise.
**GI:** anorexia, nausea, vomiting.
**GU:** dysuria, interstitial nephritis.
**Hematologic:** sideroblastic anemia, ***thrombocytopenia.***
**Hepatic:** *hepatotoxicity, hepatitis.*
**Metabolic:** hyperuricemia, gout.
**Musculoskeletal:** *arthralgia, myalgia.*
**Skin:** rash, urticaria, pruritus, photosensitivity.
**Other:** fever, porphyria.

**INTERACTIONS**
None significant.

**EFFECTS ON DIAGNOSTIC TESTS**
Pyrazinamide may interfere with urine ketone determinations. Drug's systemic effects may temporarily decrease 17-ketosteroid levels. Drug may increase protein-bound iodine and urate levels.

**CONTRAINDICATIONS**
Contraindicated in patients with severe hepatic disease, acute gout, or hypersensitivity to drug.

**NURSING CONSIDERATIONS**
• Use cautiously in patients with diabetes mellitus, renal failure, or gout.
• Always administer pyrazinamide with other antituberculotics to prevent the development of resistant organisms.
• Drug is administered for the initial 2 months of a 6-month or longer treatment regimen for drug-susceptible patients. Patients with HIV infection may require longer courses of therapy.
• A reduced dosage is needed in patients with renal impairment because nearly 100% of the drug is excreted in urine.
• Question doses that exceed 35 mg/kg because they may cause liver damage.
• Monitor hematopoietic studies and serum uric acid levels, as ordered.
• Monitor liver function studies; assess for jaundice and liver tenderness or enlargement before and frequently during therapy.

• Notify doctor at once if signs and symptoms of gout and liver impairment (anorexia, fatigue, malaise, jaundice, dark urine, and liver tenderness) occur.
• When used with surgical management of tuberculosis, start pyrazinamide 1 to 2 weeks before surgery and continue for 4 to 6 weeks postoperatively.

☑ **Patient teaching**
• Inform patient that other antituberculotics will be required concomitantly.
• Instruct patient to report adverse reactions promptly.
• Stress importance of compliance with drug therapy. If daily therapy poses a problem, tell patient to ask doctor about twice-weekly dosing.

## rifabutin
Mycobutin

*Pregnancy Risk Category B*

**HOW SUPPLIED**
*Capsules:* 150 mg

**ACTION**
Inhibits DNA-dependent RNA polymerase in susceptible bacteria, blocking bacterial protein synthesis.

| Route | Onset | Peak | Duration |
|-------|-------|------|----------|
| P.O. | Unknown | 2-4 hr | Unknown |

**INDICATIONS & DOSAGE**
*Prevention of disseminated* Mycobacterium avium *complex in patients with advanced HIV infection—*
**Adults:** 300 mg P.O. daily as a single dose or divided b.i.d.

**ADVERSE REACTIONS**
**CNS:** headache.
**GI:** dyspepsia, eructation, flatulence, diarrhea, nausea, vomiting, abdominal pain, anorexia, taste perversion.
**GU:** discolored urine.
**Hematologic:** NEUTROPENIA, LEUKOPENIA, ***thrombocytopenia,*** eosinophilia.
**Hepatic:** increased aminotransferases.
**Musculoskeletal:** myalgia.
**Skin:** *rash.*

---

Reactions may be *common,* uncommon, *life-threatening,* or COMMON AND LIFE-THREATENING.

**Other:** fever.

## INTERACTIONS
**Drug-drug.** *Drugs metabolized by the liver, zidovudine:* may alter serum levels of these drugs. Dosage adjustments may be necessary.
*Oral contraceptives:* decreased effectiveness. Instruct patient to use nonhormonal forms of birth control.
**Drug-food.** *High-fat foods:* reduced rate but not extent of absorption. Avoid concurrent administration.

## EFFECTS ON DIAGNOSTIC TESTS
None reported.

## CONTRAINDICATIONS
Contraindicated in patients with hypersensitivity to drug or other rifamycin derivatives (such as rifampin). Also contraindicated in patients with active tuberculosis because single-agent therapy with rifabutin increases the risk of inducing bacterial resistance to both rifabutin and rifampin.

## NURSING CONSIDERATIONS
• Use cautiously in patients with preexisting neutropenia and thrombocytopenia. Perform baseline hematologic studies and repeat periodically.
• Mix drug with soft foods such as applesauce for patients who have difficulty swallowing.
• Dose may be divided twice daily to decrease GI adverse effects.
• *Alert:* Don't confuse rifabutin, rifampin, and rifapentine.

### ☑ Patient teaching
• Instruct patient to take drug for as long as prescribed, exactly as directed, even after feeling better.
• Tell patient that drug or its metabolites may color urine, feces, sputum, saliva, tears, and skin brownish orange. Tell him to avoid wearing soft contact lenses because they may be permanently stained.
• Instruct patient to report photophobia, excessive lacrimation, or eye pain immediately; drug may cause uveitis (rare).

## rifampin (rifampicin)
Rifadin, Rifadin IV, Rimactane, Rimycin‡, Rofact†

*Pregnancy Risk Category C*

### HOW SUPPLIED
*Capsules:* 150 mg, 300 mg
*Injection:* 600 mg

### ACTION
Inhibits DNA-dependent RNA polymerase, thus impairing RNA synthesis (bactericidal).

| Route | Onset | Peak | Duration |
|-------|-------|------|----------|
| P.O. | Unknown | 2-4 hr | Unknown |
| I.V. | Unknown | Unknown | Unknown |

### INDICATIONS & DOSAGE
*Pulmonary tuberculosis—*
**Adults:** 600 mg P.O. or I.V. daily in single dose 1 hour before or 2 hours after meals.
**Children over age 5:** 10 to 20 mg/kg P.O. or I.V. daily in single dose 1 hour before or 2 hours after meals. Maximum daily dose is 600 mg. Administration with other antituberculotics is recommended.
*Meningococcal carriers—*
**Adults:** 600 mg P.O. or I.V. q 12 hours for 2 days; or 600 mg P.O. or I.V. once daily for 4 days.
**Children ages 1 month to 12 years:** 10 mg/kg P.O. or I.V. q 12 hours for 2 days, not to exceed 600 mg/day; or 20 mg/kg once daily for 4 days.
**Neonates:** 5 mg/kg P.O. or I.V. q 12 hours for 2 days.

### ADVERSE REACTIONS
**CNS:** headache, fatigue, drowsiness, behavioral changes, dizziness, mental confusion, generalized numbness, ataxia.
**CV:** *shock.*
**EENT:** visual disturbances, exudative conjunctivitis.
**GI:** epigastric distress, anorexia, nausea, vomiting, abdominal pain, diarrhea, flatulence, sore mouth and tongue, pseudomembranous colitis, pancreatitis.
**GU:** hemoglobinuria, hematuria, *acute renal failure,* menstrual disturbances.

---

**Hematologic:** eosinophilia, ***thrombocytopenia,*** transient leukopenia, hemolytic anemia.
**Hepatic:** ***hepatotoxicity,*** transient abnormalities in liver function tests.
**Musculoskeletal:** osteomalacia.
**Respiratory:** shortness of breath, wheezing.
**Skin:** pruritus, urticaria, rash.
**Other:** flulike syndrome, discoloration of body fluids, hyperuricemia, porphyria exacerbation.

## INTERACTIONS
**Drug-drug.** *Acetaminophen, analgesics, anticoagulants, anticonvulsants, barbiturates, beta blockers, cardiac glycosides, clofibrate, chloramphenicol, corticosteroids, cyclosporine, dapsone, diazepam, disopyramide, methadone, mexiletine, narcotics, oral contraceptives, progestins, quinidine, sulfonylureas, theophylline, verapamil:* reduced effectiveness of these drugs. Monitor closely.
*Halothane:* may increase risk of hepatotoxicity of both drugs. Monitor liver function closely.
*Ketoconazole, para-aminosalicylate sodium:* may interfere with absorption of rifampin. Give these drugs 8 to 12 hours apart.
*Probenecid:* may increase rifampin levels. Use cautiously.
**Drug-lifestyle.** *Alcohol use:* may increase risk of hepatotoxicity. Avoid use of alcohol during therapy.

## EFFECTS ON DIAGNOSTIC TESTS
Rifampin alters standard serum folate and vitamin $B_{12}$ assays. Rifampin may cause temporary retention of sulfobromophthalein in the liver excretion test. It may also interfere with contrast material in gallbladder studies and urinalysis based on spectrophotometry.

## CONTRAINDICATIONS
Contraindicated in patients with hypersensitivity to rifampin or related drugs.

## NURSING CONSIDERATIONS
• Use cautiously in patients with liver disease.

• Treatment with at least one other antituberculotic is recommended.
• Give 1 hour before or 2 hours after meals for optimal absorption; however, if GI irritation occurs, patient may take rifampin with meals.
• Monitor hepatic function, hematopoietic studies, and serum uric acid levels, as ordered. Drug's systemic effects may cause asymptomatic elevation of liver function tests (14%) and serum uric acid.
• Watch for and report to doctor signs of hepatic impairment.
• Drug may cause hemorrhage in neonates of rifampin-treated mothers.
• *Alert:* Don't confuse rifabutin, rifampin, and rifapentine.

### I.V. administration
• Reconstitute drug with 10 ml of sterile water for injection to make a solution containing 60 mg/ml. Add to 100 ml of $D_5W$ and infuse over 30 minutes, or add to 500 ml of $D_5W$ and infuse over 3 hours. Prepare and use the solution within a 4-hour period. When dextrose is contraindicated, drug may be diluted with normal saline for injection. Don't use other I.V. solutions.

### Patient teaching
• Instruct patient who develops drug-induced GI upset to take drug with meals.
• Warn patient about drowsiness and possible red-orange discoloration of urine, feces, saliva, sweat, sputum, and tears. Soft contact lenses may be permanently stained.
• Advise patient to avoid alcoholic beverages during drug therapy.

## rifapentine
Priftin

*Pregnancy Risk Category C*

### HOW SUPPLIED
*Tablets (film-coated):* 150 mg

### ACTION
Inhibits DNA-dependent RNA polymerase in susceptible strains of *Mycobacterium tuberculosis.* Drug demonstrates

---

Reactions may be *common,* uncommon, ***life-threatening,*** or COMMON AND LIFE-THREATENING.

bactericidal activity against the organism both intra- and extracellularly.

| Route | Onset | Peak | Duration |
|-------|-------|------|----------|
| P.O. | Unknown | 5-6 hr | Unknown |

## INDICATIONS & DOSAGE
*Pulmonary tuberculosis, with at least one other antituberculotic to which the isolate is susceptible—*
**Adults:** during the intensive phase of short-course therapy, 600 mg P.O. twice weekly for 2 months, with an interval between doses of not less than 3 days (72 hours).

During the continuation phase of short-course therapy, 600 mg P.O. once weekly for 4 months with isoniazid or another agent to which the isolate is susceptible.

## ADVERSE REACTIONS
**CNS:** headache, dizziness, pain.
**CV:** hypertension.
**GI:** anorexia, nausea, vomiting, dyspepsia, diarrhea.
**GU:** pyuria, proteinuria, hematuria, urinary casts.
**Hematologic:** *neutropenia,* lymphopenia, anemia, *leukopenia,* thrombocytosis.
**Hepatic:** elevated AST and ALT.
**Musculoskeletal:** arthralgia.
**Respiratory:** hemoptysis.
**Skin:** rash, pruritus, acne, maculopapular rash.
**Other:** *hyperuricemia.*

## INTERACTIONS
**Drug-drug.** *Antiarrhythmics (disopyramide, mexiletine, quinidine, tocainide), antibiotics (chloramphenicol, clarithromycin, dapsone, doxycycline, fluoroquinolones), anticonvulsants (phenytoin), antifungals (fluconazole, itraconazole, ketoconazole), barbiturates, benzodiazepines (diazepam), beta blockers, calcium channel blockers (diltiazem, nifedipine, verapamil), cardiac glycosides, clofibrate, corticosteroids, haloperidol, HIV protease inhibitors (indinavir, nelfinavir, ritonavir, saquinavir), immunosuppressants (cyclosporine, tacrolimus), levothyroxine, narcotic analgesics (methadone), oral anticoagulants (warfarin), oral hypoglycemics (sulfonylureas), oral or other systemic hormonal contraceptives progestins, quinine, reverse transcriptase inhibitors (delavirdine, zidovudine), sildenafil, theophylline, tricyclic antidepressants (amitriptyline, nortriptyline):* rifapentine induces metabolism of the hepatic cytochrome P-450 enzyme system, decreasing the activity of these drugs. Dosage adjustments may be needed

## EFFECTS ON DIAGNOSTIC TESTS
May alter serum assays for folate and vitamin $B_{12}$.

## CONTRAINDICATIONS
Contraindicated in patients with history of hypersensitivity to a rifamycin (rifapentine, rifampin, or rifabutin).

## NURSING CONSIDERATIONS
• Use drug cautiously and with frequent monitoring in patients with liver disease.
• Rifamycin antibiotics have been associated with hepatotoxicity. Monitor liver function test results before beginning drug therapy.
• Drug therapy may affect liver function test results, CBC, and platelet counts; monitor carefully.
• Coadministration of pyridoxine (vitamin $B_6$) is recommended in malnourished patients, in those predisposed to neuropathy (alcoholics, diabetics), and in adolescents.
• *Alert:* Give drug with appropriate daily companion drugs. Compliance with all medications, especially with daily companion drugs on the days when rifapentine isn't given, is crucial for early sputum conversion and protection from relapse of tuberculosis.
• Administration of drug during the last 2 weeks of pregnancy may lead to postnatal hemorrhage in the mother or infant. Monitor clotting parameters closely if drug is given.
• Rifapentine can turn body tissues and fluids red-orange and can permanently stain contact lenses.
• Notify doctor of persistent or severe diarrhea.
• *Alert:* Don't confuse rifabutin, rifampin, and rifapentine.

## ☑ Patient teaching

• Stress importance of strict compliance with drug and daily companion medications as well as necessary follow-up visits and laboratory tests.
• Advise patient to use nonhormonal methods of birth control.
• Tell patient to take drug with food if nausea, vomiting, or GI upset occurs.
• Instruct patient to notify doctor if the following occur: fever, loss of appetite, malaise, nausea, vomiting, darkened urine, yellowish discoloration of the skin and eyes, pain or swelling of the joints, or excessive loose stools or diarrhea.
• Instruct patient to protect pills from excessive heat.
• Tell patient that rifapentine can turn body fluids red-orange. If patient wears contact lenses, these can become permanently stained.

amikacin sulfate
gentamicin sulfate
neomycin sulfate
streptomycin sulfate
tobramycin sulfate

## COMBINATION PRODUCTS
NEOSPORIN G.U. IRRIGANT: 40 mg
neomycin sulfate and 200,000 U
polymyxin B sulfate/ml.

## amikacin sulfate
Amikin

*Pregnancy Risk Category D*

### HOW SUPPLIED
*Injection:* 50 mg/ml, 250 mg/ml

### ACTION
Inhibits protein synthesis by binding directly to the 30S ribosomal subunit. Generally bactericidal.

| Route | Onset | Peak | Duration |
|-------|-------|------|----------|
| I.V. | Immediate | Immediate | 8-12 hr |
| I.M. | Unknown | 1 hr | 8-12 hr |

### INDICATIONS & DOSAGE
*Serious infections due to sensitive strains of* Pseudomonas aeruginosa, Escherichia coli, Proteus, Klebsiella, Serratia, Enterobacter, Acinetobacter, Providencia, Citrobacter, *or* Staphylococcus—
**Adults and children:** 15 mg/kg/day divided q 8 to 12 hours I.M. or I.V. infusion.
**Neonates:** initially, loading dose of 10 mg/kg I.V.; then 7.5 mg/kg q 12 hours.
*Uncomplicated urinary tract infection—*
**Adults:** 250 mg I.M. or I.V. b.i.d.
*Adjust-a-dose:* For adult patients with impaired renal function, initially, 7.5 mg/kg. Subsequent doses and frequency determined by blood amikacin levels and renal function studies.

### ADVERSE REACTIONS
**CNS:** *neuromuscular blockade.*

**EENT:** *ototoxicity.*
**GU:** *azotemia, nephrotoxicity;* possible elevation in BUN, nonprotein nitrogen, or serum creatinine levels; possible increase in urinary excretion of casts.
**Musculoskeletal:** arthralgia.
**Respiratory:** *apnea.*

### INTERACTIONS
**Drug-drug.** *Acyclovir, amphotericin B, cisplatin, methoxyflurane, vancomycin, other aminoglycosides:* increased nephrotoxicity. Use together cautiously.
*Cephalosporins:* increased nephrotoxicity. Use together cautiously.
*Dimenhydrinate:* may mask symptoms of ototoxicity. Use with caution.
*General anesthetics, neuromuscular blockers:* may potentiate neuromuscular blockade. Monitor closely.
*Indomethacin:* may increase serum trough and peak levels of amikacin. Monitor serum amikacin level closely.
*I.V. loop diuretics (such as furosemide):* increased ototoxicity. Use cautiously.
*Parenteral penicillins (such as ticarcillin):* amikacin inactivation in vitro. Don't mix together.

### EFFECTS ON DIAGNOSTIC TESTS
None reported.

### CONTRAINDICATIONS
Contraindicated in patients with hypersensitivity to drug or other aminoglycosides.

### NURSING CONSIDERATIONS
• Use cautiously in patients with impaired renal function or neuromuscular disorders, in neonates and infants, and in elderly patients.
• Obtain specimen for culture and sensitivity tests before giving first dose. Therapy may begin pending results.
• Evaluate patient's hearing before and during therapy. Notify doctor if patient complains of tinnitus, vertigo, or hearing loss.

---

\*Liquid contains alcohol.   \*\*May contain tartrazine.   †Canada   ‡Australia   §U.K.   ◊OTC

- Weigh patient and review renal function studies before therapy begins.
- Obtain blood for peak amikacin level 1 hour after I.M. injection and 30 minutes to 1 hour after I.V. infusion ends; for trough levels, draw blood just before next dose. Don't collect blood in a heparinized tube; heparin is incompatible with aminoglycosides.
- Peak blood levels over 35 mcg/ml and trough levels over 10 mcg/ml may be associated with higher incidence of toxicity.
- Monitor renal function (output, specific gravity, urinalysis, BUN and creatinine levels, and creatinine clearance). Report decreasing renal function.
- Watch for superinfection (continued fever and other signs and symptoms of new infection, especially of upper respiratory tract).
- Therapy is usually continued for 7 to 10 days. If no response occurs after 3 to 5 days, therapy may be stopped and new specimens obtained for culture and sensitivity testing.
- *Alert:* Don't confuse Amikin with Amicar.

**I.V. administration**
- Dilute I.V. drug in 100 to 200 ml of $D_5W$ or normal saline solution and infuse over 30 to 60 minutes.
- After I.V. infusion, flush line with normal saline solution or $D_5W$.

**Patient teaching**
- Instruct patient to report adverse reactions promptly.
- Encourage patient to maintain adequate fluid intake.

---

## gentamicin sulfate
Cidomycin†, Garamycin, Gentamicin Sulfate ADD-Vantage, Genticin§, Jenamicin

*Pregnancy Risk Category D*

### HOW SUPPLIED
*Injection:* 40 mg/ml (adult), 10 mg/ml (pediatric)

*I.V. infusion (premixed):* 40 mg, 60 mg, 70 mg, 80 mg, 90 mg, 100 mg, 120 mg in normal saline solution

### ACTION
Inhibits protein synthesis by binding directly to the 30S ribosomal subunit. Usually bactericidal.

| Route | Onset | Peak | Duration |
|-------|-------|------|----------|
| I.V. | Immediate | 30-90 min | Unknown |
| I.M. | Unknown | 30-90 min | Unknown |

### INDICATIONS & DOSAGE
*Serious infections due to sensitive strains of* Pseudomonas aeruginosa, Escherichia coli, Proteus, Klebsiella, Serratia, Enterobacter, Citrobacter, *or* Staphylococcus—
**Adults:** 3 mg/kg daily in divided doses I.M. or I.V. infusion q 8 hours. For life-threatening infections, patient may receive up to 5 mg/kg daily in three to four divided doses; dose should be reduced to 3 mg/kg daily as soon as clinically indicated.
**Children:** 2 to 2.5 mg/kg q 8 hours I.M. or by I.V. infusion.
**Neonates over age 1 week or infants:** 2.5 mg/kg q 8 hours I.M. or by I.V. infusion.
**Neonates under age 1 week and preterm infants:** 2.5 mg/kg q 12 hours I.M. or by I.V. infusion.
*Meningitis—*
**Adults:** systemic therapy as above.
**Children:** systemic therapy as above.
*Endocarditis prophylaxis for GI or GU procedure or surgery—*
**Adults:** 1.5 mg/kg I.M. or I.V. 30 minutes before procedure or surgery. Maximum dose is 80 mg. Given with ampicillin (vancomycin in penicillin-allergic patients).
**Children:** 2 mg/kg I.M. or I.V. 30 minutes before procedure or surgery. Maximum dose is 80 mg. Given with ampicillin (vancomycin in penicillin-allergic patients).
*After hemodialysis to maintain therapeutic blood levels—*
**Adults:** 1 to 1.7 mg/kg I.M. or by I.V. infusion after each dialysis.
**Children:** 2 to 2.5 mg/kg I.M. or by I.V. infusion after each dialysis.

*Adjust-a-dose:* For adult patients with impaired renal function, doses and frequency are determined by serum gentamicin levels and renal function.

## ADVERSE REACTIONS
**CNS:** headache, lethargy, encephalopathy, confusion, dizziness, *seizures,* numbness, peripheral neuropathy, vertigo, ataxia, tingling.
**CV:** hypotension.
**EENT:** *ototoxicity,* blurred vision, tinnitus.
**GI:** vomiting, nausea.
**GU:** *nephrotoxicity;* possible elevation in BUN, nonprotein nitrogen, or serum creatinine levels; possible increase in urinary excretion of casts.
**Hematologic:** anemia, eosinophilia, *leukopenia, thrombocytopenia, agranulocytosis.*
**Hepatic:** increased ALT, AST, bilirubin, LD.
**Musculoskeletal:** muscle twitching, myasthenia gravis–like syndrome.
**Respiratory:** *apnea.*
**Skin:** rash, urticaria, pruritus.
**Other:** fever, *anaphylaxis;* injection site pain.

## INTERACTIONS
**Drug-drug.** *Acyclovir, amphotericin B, cisplatin, methoxyflurane, vancomycin, other aminoglycosides:* increased ototoxicity and nephrotoxicity. Use together cautiously.
*Cephalosporins:* increased nephrotoxicity. Use together cautiously.
*Dimenhydrinate:* may mask symptoms of ototoxicity. Use with caution.
*General anesthetics, neuromuscular blockers:* may potentiate neuromuscular blockade. Monitor closely.
*Indomethacin:* may increase serum peak and trough levels of gentamicin. Monitor serum gentamicin levels closely.
*I.V. loop diuretics (such as furosemide):* increased ototoxicity. Use cautiously.
*Parenteral penicillins (such as ampicillin and ticarcillin):* gentamicin inactivation in vitro. Don't mix together.

## EFFECTS ON DIAGNOSTIC TESTS
None reported.

## CONTRAINDICATIONS
Contraindicated in hypersensitivity to drug or other aminoglycosides.

## NURSING CONSIDERATIONS
• Use cautiously in neonates, infants, elderly patients, and patients with impaired renal function or neuromuscular disorders.
• Obtain specimen for culture and sensitivity tests before giving first dose.
• Evaluate patient's hearing before and during therapy. Notify doctor if patient complains of tinnitus, vertigo, or hearing loss.
• Weigh patient and review renal function studies before therapy begins.
• *Alert:* Use preservative-free formulations of gentamicin when intrathecal route is ordered.
• Obtain blood for peak gentamicin level 1 hour after I.M. injection or 30 minutes after I.V. infusion finishes; for trough levels, draw blood just before next dose. Don't collect blood in a heparinized tube; heparin is incompatible with aminoglycosides.
• Peak blood levels over 10 mcg/ml and trough levels over 2 mcg/ml may be associated with higher incidence of toxicity.
• Monitor urine output, specific gravity, urinalysis, BUN and creatinine levels, and creatinine clearance. Notify doctor of signs of decreasing renal function.
• Hemodialysis for 8 hours removes up to 50% of drug from blood.
• Watch for superinfection (continued fever and other signs and symptoms of new infection, especially of upper respiratory tract).
• Therapy usually continues for 7 to 10 days. If no response occurs in 3 to 5 days, therapy may be stopped and new specimens obtained for culture and sensitivity testing.

### I.V. administration
• When giving by intermittent I.V. infusion, dilute with 50 to 200 ml of D₅W or normal saline injection and infuse over 30 minutes to 2 hours. After completing I.V. infusion, flush the line with normal saline solution or D₅W.

---

*Liquid contains alcohol.  **May contain tartrazine.  †Canada  ‡Australia  §U.K.  ◊OTC

☑ **Patient teaching**
- Instruct patient to report adverse reactions promptly.
- Encourage patient to maintain adequate fluid intake.
- Caution patient not to perform hazardous activities if adverse CNS reactions occur.

---

## neomycin sulfate
Mycifradin†, Neo-fradin, Neosulf‡, Neo-Tabs, Nivemycin§

*Pregnancy Risk Category D*

---

### HOW SUPPLIED
*Tablets:* 500 mg
*Oral solution:* 125 mg/5 ml

### ACTION
Inhibits protein synthesis by binding directly to the 30S ribosomal subunit. Generally bactericidal.

| Route | Onset | Peak | Duration |
|---|---|---|---|
| P.O. | Unknown | 1-4 hr | 8 hr |

### INDICATIONS & DOSAGE
*Infectious diarrhea due to enteropathogenic Escherichia coli—*
**Adults:** 50 mg/kg daily P.O. in four divided doses for 2 to 3 days; maximum of 3 g daily is usually adequate.
**Children:** 50 to 100 mg/kg daily P.O. divided q 4 to 6 hours for 2 to 3 days.
*Suppression of intestinal bacteria preoperatively—*
**Adults:** 1 g P.O. q hour for four doses; then 1 g q 4 hours for the balance of the 24 hours. A saline cathartic should precede therapy.
**Children:** 40 to 100 mg/kg daily P.O. divided q 4 to 6 hours. First dose should follow saline cathartic.
*Adjunct treatment in hepatic coma—*
**Adults:** 1 to 3 g P.O. q.i.d. for 5 to 6 days; or 200 ml of 1% solution or 100 ml of 2% solution as enema retained for 20 to 60 minutes q 6 hours. In patients with chronic hepatic insufficiency, 4 g/day indefinitely may be needed.
**Children:** 50 to 100 mg/kg/day P.O. in divided doses for 5 to 6 days.

### ADVERSE REACTIONS
**EENT:** *ototoxicity.*
**GI:** nausea, vomiting, diarrhea, malabsorption syndrome, *Clostridium difficile*–associated colitis.
**GU:** *nephrotoxicity;* possible elevation in BUN, nonprotein nitrogen, or serum creatinine levels; possible increase in urinary excretion of casts.

### INTERACTIONS
**Drug-drug.** *Acyclovir, amphotericin B, cisplatin, methoxyflurane, vancomycin, other aminoglycosides:* increased nephrotoxicity. Use together cautiously.
*Cephalosporins:* increased nephrotoxicity. Use together cautiously.
*Digoxin:* decreased digoxin absorption. Monitor closely.
*Dimenhydrinate:* may mask symptoms of ototoxicity. Use with caution.
*I.V. loop diuretics (such as furosemide):* increased ototoxicity. Use cautiously.
*Oral anticoagulants:* inhibited vitamin K–producing bacteria; may potentiate anticoagulant effect. Monitor PT and INR.

### EFFECTS ON DIAGNOSTIC TESTS
None reported.

### CONTRAINDICATIONS
Contraindicated in patients hypersensitive to other aminoglycosides and in those with intestinal obstruction.

### NURSING CONSIDERATIONS
- Use cautiously in patients with impaired renal function, neuromuscular disorders, or ulcerative bowel lesions and in elderly patients. Never administer drug parenterally.
- Monitor renal function (output, specific gravity, urinalysis, BUN and creatinine levels, and creatinine clearance). Notify doctor of signs and symptoms of decreasing renal function.
- Evaluate patient's hearing before and during prolonged therapy. Notify doctor if patient complains of tinnitus, vertigo, or hearing loss. Onset of deafness may occur several weeks after drug is stopped.
- Watch for superinfection (fever or other signs and symptoms of new infection).

---

Reactions may be *common*, uncommon, *life-threatening*, or COMMON AND LIFE-THREATENING.

• In adjunctive treatment of hepatic coma, decrease the patient's dietary protein, and assess neurologic status frequently during therapy.

• For preoperative disinfection, provide a low-residue diet and a cathartic immediately before oral administration of neomycin, as ordered.

• The ototoxic and nephrotoxic properties of neomycin limit its usefulness.

• Neomycin is nonabsorbable at the recommended dosage. However, more than 4 g/day may be systemically absorbed and lead to nephrotoxicity.

• Drug is available with polymyxin B as a urinary bladder irrigant.

☑ **Patient teaching**
• Instruct patient to report adverse reactions promptly.

• Encourage patient to maintain adequate fluid intake.

## streptomycin sulfate

*Pregnancy Risk Category D*

### HOW SUPPLIED
*Injection:* 1 g/2.5-ml ampules

### ACTION
Inhibits protein synthesis by binding directly to the 30S ribosomal subunit. Generally bactericidal.

| Route | Onset | Peak | Duration |
|-------|---------|--------|----------|
| I.M. | Unknown | 1-2 hr | Unknown |

### INDICATIONS & DOSAGE
*Streptococcal endocarditis—*
**Adults:** 1 g q 12 hours I.M. for 1 week; then 500 mg I.M. q 12 hours for 1 week, given with penicillin.
**Elderly:** 500 mg I.M. q 12 hours for entire 2 weeks, given with penicillin.
*Primary and adjunctive treatment in tuberculosis—*
**Adults:** 15 mg/kg (maximum of 1 g) I.M. daily for 2 to 3 months; then 1 g I.M. two or three times weekly.
**Children:** 20 to 40 mg/kg (maximum of 1 g) I.M. daily in divided doses injected deeply into large muscle mass. Given

with other antituberculotics, but *not* with capreomycin; continued until sputum specimen becomes negative.
**Elderly:** 10 mg/kg I.M. daily.
*Enterococcal endocarditis—*
**Adults:** 1 g I.M. q 12 hours for 2 weeks; then 500 mg I.M. q 12 hours for 4 weeks, given with penicillin.
*Tularemia—*
**Adults:** 1 to 2 g I.M. daily in divided doses injected deeply into upper outer quadrant of buttocks; continued for 7 to 14 days or until patient is afebrile for 5 to 7 days.

### ADVERSE REACTIONS
**CNS:** *neuromuscular blockade,* vertigo, paresthesia of the face.
**EENT:** *ototoxicity.*
**GI:** vomiting, nausea.
**GU:** some nephrotoxicity (not as frequently as with other aminoglycosides); possible elevation in BUN, nonprotein nitrogen, or serum creatinine levels; possible increase in urinary excretion of casts.
**Hematologic:** eosinophilia, *leukopenia, thrombocytopenia, hemolytic anemia.*
**Respiratory:** *apnea.*
**Skin:** *exfoliative dermatitis.*
**Other:** hypersensitivity reactions, *anaphylaxis.*

### INTERACTIONS
**Drug-drug.** *Acyclovir, amphotericin B, cisplatin, methoxyflurane, vancomycin, other aminoglycosides:* increased nephrotoxicity. Use together cautiously.
*Cephalosporins:* increased nephrotoxicity. Use together cautiously.
*Dimenhydrinate:* may mask symptoms of streptomycin-induced ototoxicity. Use together cautiously.
*General anesthetics, neuromuscular blockers:* may potentiate neuromuscular blockade. Monitor closely.
*I.V. loop diuretics (such as furosemide):* increased ototoxicity. Use together cautiously.

### EFFECTS ON DIAGNOSTIC TESTS
Streptomycin may cause a false-positive reaction in copper sulfate tests for urine glucose (Benedict's reagent or Diastix).

---

## CONTRAINDICATIONS

Contraindicated in patients with hypersensitivity to drug or other aminoglycosides.

## NURSING CONSIDERATIONS

• Use cautiously in patients with impaired renal function or neuromuscular disorders and in elderly patients.
• Obtain specimen for culture and sensitivity tests before giving first dose except when treating tuberculosis. Therapy may begin pending results.
• Evaluate patient's hearing before therapy and for 6 months afterward. Notify doctor if patient complains of hearing loss, roaring noises, or fullness in ears.
• *Alert:* Never administer streptomycin I.V.
• Protect hands when preparing because drug is irritating.
• For I.M. administration, inject deeply into upper outer quadrant of buttocks. Rotate injection sites.
• Obtain blood for peak streptomycin level 1 to 2 hours after I.M. injection; for trough levels, draw blood just before next dose. Don't use a heparinized tube because heparin is incompatible with aminoglycosides.
• Watch for signs and symptoms of superinfection (continued fever and other signs of new infection).
• In primary treatment of tuberculosis, streptomycin is discontinued when sputum becomes negative.

### ☑ Patient teaching

• Instruct patient to report adverse reactions promptly.
• Encourage patient to maintain adequate fluid intake.
• Emphasize need for blood tests to monitor streptomycin levels and determine the effectiveness of therapy.

---

## tobramycin sulfate
Nebcin, TOBI

*Pregnancy Risk Category D*

## HOW SUPPLIED

*Multidose vials:* 80 mg/2 ml, 20 mg/2 ml (pediatric)

*Powder for injection:* 1.2 g
*Premixed parenteral injection for I.V. infusion:* 60 mg or 80 mg in normal saline solution
*Nebulizer solution (for inhalation):* 300 mg/5 ml

## ACTION

Inhibits protein synthesis by binding directly to the 30S ribosomal subunit. Generally bactericidal.

| Route | Onset | Peak | Duration |
|-------|-------|------|----------|
| I.V. | Immediate | Immediate | 8 hr |
| I.M. | Unknown | 30-90 min | 8 hr |
| Inhalation | Unknown | Unknown | Unknown |

## INDICATIONS & DOSAGE

*Serious infections due to sensitive strains of* Escherichia coli, Proteus, Klebsiella, Enterobacter, Serratia, Morganella morganii, Staphylococcus aureus, Pseudomonas, Citrobacter, *or* Providencia—
**Adults:** 3 mg/kg I.M. or I.V. daily in divided doses. Up to 5 mg/kg daily divided q 6 to 8 hours for life-threatening infections; dose should be reduced to 3 mg/kg daily as soon as clinically indicated.
**Children:** 6 to 7.5 mg/kg I.M. or I.V. daily in three or four divided doses.
**Neonates under age 1 week or premature infants:** up to 4 mg/kg/day I.V. or I.M. in two equal doses q 12 hours.
*Adjust-a-dose:* For patients with renal impairment, loading dose is 1 mg/kg; then decreased doses at 8-hour intervals or same dose at prolonged intervals.
*Management of cystic fibrosis patients with* Pseudomonas aeruginosa—
**Adults and children ages 6 and older:** 300 mg via nebulizer q 12 hours for 28 days (cycle of 28 days on drug and 28 days off).

## ADVERSE REACTIONS

**CNS:** headache, lethargy, confusion, disorientation, *seizures.*
**EENT:** *ototoxicity, hoarseness, pharyngitis.*
**GI:** vomiting, nausea, diarrhea.
**GU:** *nephrotoxicity;* possible elevation in BUN, nonprotein nitrogen, or serum crea-

---

tinine levels; possible increase in urinary excretion of casts.

**Hematologic:** anemia, eosinophilia, *leukopenia, thrombocytopenia, agranulocytosis.*

**Musculoskeletal:** muscle twitching.

**Respiratory:** bronchospasm.

**Skin:** rash, urticaria, pruritus.

**Other:** electrolyte imbalances, fever.

## INTERACTIONS

**Drug-drug.** *Acyclovir, amphotericin B, cisplatin, methoxyflurane, vancomycin, other aminoglycosides:* increased nephrotoxicity. Use together cautiously.

*Cephalosporins:* increased nephrotoxicity. Use together cautiously.

*Dimenhydrinate:* may mask symptoms of ototoxicity. Use with caution.

*General anesthetics, neuromuscular blockers:* may potentiate neuromuscular blockade. Monitor closely.

*I.V. loop diuretics (such as furosemide):* increased ototoxicity. Use together cautiously.

*Parenteral penicillins (such as ticarcillin):* tobramycin inactivation in vitro. Don't mix together.

## EFFECTS ON DIAGNOSTIC TESTS

None reported.

## CONTRAINDICATIONS

Contraindicated in patients with hypersensitivity to drug or other aminoglycosides.

## NURSING CONSIDERATIONS

• Use cautiously in patients with impaired renal function or neuromuscular disorders and in elderly patients.

• Obtain specimen for culture and sensitivity tests before giving first dose. Therapy may begin pending results.

• Weigh patient and review renal function studies before therapy.

• Evaluate patient's hearing before and during therapy. Notify doctor if patient complains of tinnitus, vertigo, or hearing loss.

• Administer nebulizer solution over 10 to 15 minutes using hand-held Pari LC Plus reusable nebulizer with DeVilbiss Pulmo-Aide compressor.

• Don't dilute or mix TOBI with dornase alpha in the nebulizer.

• Obtain blood for peak level 1 hour after I.M. injection or ½ hour after the infusion stops; draw blood for trough level just before next dose. Don't collect blood in a heparinized tube; heparin is incompatible with aminoglycosides.

• *Alert:* Peak blood levels over 12 mcg/ml and trough levels over 2 mcg/ml may be associated with increased toxicity.

• Monitor renal function (output, specific gravity, urinalysis, creatinine clearance, and BUN and creatinine levels). Notify doctor of signs and symptoms of decreasing renal function.

• Watch for signs and symptoms of superinfection (continued fever and other signs of new infection).

• If no response occurs in 3 to 5 days, therapy may be stopped and new specimens obtained for culture and sensitivity testing.

• *Alert:* Don't confuse tobramycin with Trobicin.

### I.V. administration

• For adults, dilute in 50 to 100 ml of normal saline solution or $D_5W$; use a smaller volume for children. Infuse over 20 to 60 minutes. After I.V. infusion, flush line with normal saline solution or $D_5W$.

### Patient teaching

• Instruct patient to report adverse reactions promptly.

• Caution patient not to perform hazardous activities if adverse CNS reactions occur.

• Encourage patient to maintain adequate fluid intake.

• Instruct patient on how to use and maintain nebulizer.

• Tell patient on multiple inhaled therapies to use TOBI last.

• Instruct patient not to use TOBI if it's cloudy, if there are particles in the solution, or if it has been stored at room temperature for more than 28 days.

---

amoxicillin/clavulanate potassium
amoxicillin trihydrate
ampicillin
ampicillin sodium
ampicillin trihydrate
ampicillin sodium/sulbactam
   sodium
cloxacillin sodium
dicloxacillin sodium
mezlocillin sodium
nafcillin sodium
oxacillin sodium
penicillin G benzathine
penicillin G potassium
penicillin G procaine
penicillin G sodium
penicillin V potassium
piperacillin sodium
piperacillin sodium/tazobactam
   sodium
ticarcillin disodium
ticarcillin disodium/clavulanate
   potassium

**COMBINATION PRODUCTS**
None.

---

## amoxicillin/clavulanate potassium (amoxycillin/clavulanate potassium)
Augmentin, Clavulin†

*Pregnancy Risk Category B*

---

### HOW SUPPLIED
*Tablets (chewable):* 125 mg amoxicillin trihydrate, 31.25 mg clavulanic acid; 200 mg amoxicillin trihydrate, 28.5 mg clavulanic acid; 250 mg amoxicillin trihydrate, 62.5 mg clavulanic acid
*Tablets (film-coated):* 250 mg amoxicillin trihydrate, 125 mg clavulanic acid; 500 mg amoxicillin trihydrate, 125 mg clavulanic acid; 875 mg amoxicillin trihydrate, 125 mg clavulanic acid
*Oral suspension:* 125 mg amoxicillin trihydrate and 31.25 mg clavulanic acid/5 ml (after reconstitution); 200 mg amoxicillin trihydrate and 28.5 mg clavulanic acid/5 ml (after reconstitution); 250 mg amoxicillin trihydrate and 62.5 mg clavulanic acid/5 ml (after reconstitution); 400 mg amoxicillin trihydrate and 57 mg clavulanic acid/5 ml (after reconstitution)

### ACTION
An aminopenicillin that prevents bacterial cell-wall synthesis during replication. Clavulanic acid increases amoxicillin effectiveness by inactivating beta-lactamases, which destroy amoxicillin.

| Route | Onset | Peak | Duration |
|-------|-------|------|----------|
| P.O. | Unknown | 1-2.5 hr | 6-8 hr |

### INDICATIONS & DOSAGE
*Lower respiratory infections, otitis media, sinusitis, skin and skin-structure infections, and urinary tract infections due to susceptible strains of gram-positive and gram-negative organisms—*
**Adults and children weighing 40 kg (88 lb) or over:** 250 mg (based on the amoxicillin component) P.O. q 8 hours; or 500 mg q 12 hours. For more severe infections, 500 mg q 8 hours or 875 mg P.O. q 12 hours.
**Children ages 3 months and older and weighing under 40 kg:** 20 to 45 mg/kg (based on the amoxicillin component and severity of infection) P.O. daily in divided doses q 8 to 12 hours.
**Children under age 3 months:** 30 mg/kg/day P.O. divided q 12 hours based on the amoxicillin component. The 125 mg/5-ml oral suspension is recommended.
***Adjust-a-dose:*** Don't give the 875-mg tablet to patients with renal impairment and creatinine clearance under 30 ml/minute. If creatinine clearance is 10 to 30 ml/minute, dosage is 250 to 500 mg P.O. q 12 hours. If creatinine clearance is under 10 ml/minute, dosage is 250 to 500 mg P.O. q 24 hours. Give hemodialysis patients 250 to 500 mg P.O. q 24 hours

with an additional dose both during and at the end of dialysis.

## ADVERSE REACTIONS
**CNS:** agitation, anxiety, insomnia, confusion, behavioral changes, dizziness.
**GI:** *nausea,* vomiting, *diarrhea,* indigestion, gastritis, stomatitis, glossitis, black "hairy" tongue, enterocolitis, pseudomembranous colitis.
**GU:** vaginitis.
**Hematologic:** anemia, *thrombocytopenia,* thrombocytopenic purpura, eosinophilia, *leukopenia, agranulocytosis.*
**Other:** *hypersensitivity reactions, anaphylaxis,* overgrowth of nonsusceptible organisms.

## INTERACTIONS
**Drug-drug.** *Allopurinol:* increased incidence of rash. Monitor patient.
*Oral contraceptives:* efficacy of oral contraceptives may be decreased. Recommend additional form of contraception during penicillin therapy.
*Probenecid:* increased blood levels of amoxicillin and other penicillins. Probenecid may be used for this purpose.

## EFFECTS ON DIAGNOSTIC TESTS
Amoxicillin/clavulanate potassium alters results of urine glucose tests that use cupric sulfate (Benedict's reagent or Clinitest). Make urine glucose determinations with glucose oxidase methods (Chemstrip uG). Positive Coombs' tests have occurred with other clavulanate combinations.

## CONTRAINDICATIONS
Contraindicated in patients with hypersensitivity to drug or other penicillins and in those with a previous history of amoxicillin-associated cholestatic jaundice or hepatic dysfunction.

## NURSING CONSIDERATIONS
• Use cautiously in patients with other drug allergies, especially to cephalosporins (possible cross-sensitivity), and in those with mononucleosis (high incidence of maculopapular rash).
• Before giving drug, ask patient about allergic reactions to penicillin. However, a negative history of penicillin allergy is no guarantee against an allergic reaction.
• Obtain specimen for culture and sensitivity tests before giving first dose. Therapy may begin pending results.
• Give drug at least 1 hour before a bacteriostatic antibiotic.
• Observe patient closely. With large doses and prolonged therapy, bacterial or fungal superinfection may occur, especially in elderly, debilitated, or immunosuppressed patients.
• Avoid use of 250-mg tablet in children under 40 kg. Use chewable form instead.
• *Alert:* Both 250-mg and 500-mg film-coated tablets contain the same amount of clavulanic acid (125 mg). Therefore, two 250-mg tablets are not equivalent to one 500-mg tablet.
• This drug combination is particularly useful in clinical settings with a high prevalence of amoxicillin-resistant organisms.
• After reconstitution, refrigerate the oral suspension; discard after 10 days.
• *Alert:* Don't confuse amoxicillin with amoxapine.

### ☑ Patient teaching
• Tell patient to take entire quantity of drug exactly as prescribed, even after feeling better.
• Instruct patient to take drug with food to prevent GI upset. If he is taking the oral suspension, tell him to keep drug refrigerated, to shake it well before administration, and to discard remaining drug after 10 days.
• Tell patient to call doctor if a rash occurs because rash is a sign of an allergic reaction.

## amoxicillin trihydrate (amoxycillin trihydrate)
Alphamox‡, Amoxil, Apo-Amoxi†, Cilamox‡, Moxacin‡, Novamoxin†, Nu-Amoxi†, Trimox, Wymox

*Pregnancy Risk Category B*

## HOW SUPPLIED
*Tablets (chewable):* 125 mg, 250 mg
*Capsules:* 250 mg, 500 mg

*Oral suspension:* 50 mg/ml (pediatric drops), 125 mg/5 ml, 250 mg/5 ml (after reconstitution)

## ACTION
An aminopenicillin that inhibits cell-wall synthesis during bacterial multiplication. Bacteria resist amoxicillin by producing penicillinases—enzymes that hydrolyze amoxicillin.

| Route | Onset | Peak | Duration |
|-------|-------|------|----------|
| P.O. | Unknown | 1-2 hr | 6-8 hr |

## INDICATIONS & DOSAGE
*Systemic infections, acute and chronic urinary tract infections due to susceptible strains of gram-positive and gram-negative organisms—*
**Adults and children weighing 20 kg (44 lb) or over:** 250 to 500 mg P.O. q 8 hours.
**Children weighing under 20 kg:** 20 mg/kg P.O. daily in divided doses q 8 hours; in severe infection, 40 mg/kg P.O. daily in divided doses q 8 hours or 500 mg to 1 g/m² P.O. in divided doses q 8 hours.
*Uncomplicated gonorrhea—*
**Adults and children weighing over 45 kg (99 lb):** 3 g P.O. with 1 g probenecid given as a single dose.
**Children ages 2 and older weighing under 45 kg:** 50 mg/kg (maximum of 3 g) P.O. with 25 mg/kg (up to 1 g) of probenecid as a single dose. Don't give probenecid to children under age 2.
*Endocarditis prophylaxis for dental and GI/GU procedures—*
**Adults:** 2 g P.O. 1 hour before procedure.
**Children:** 50 mg/kg P.O. 1 hour before procedure.

## ADVERSE REACTIONS
**CNS:** lethargy, hallucinations, *seizures,* anxiety, confusion, agitation, depression, dizziness, fatigue.
**GI:** *nausea,* vomiting, *diarrhea,* glossitis, stomatitis, gastritis, abdominal pain, enterocolitis, pseudomembranous colitis, black "hairy" tongue.
**GU:** interstitial nephritis, nephropathy, vaginitis.
**Hematologic:** anemia, *thrombocytopenia,* thrombocytopenic purpura, eosinophilia, *leukopenia,* hemolytic anemia, *agranulocytosis.*
**Other:** *hypersensitivity reactions, anaphylaxis,* overgrowth of nonsusceptible organisms.

## INTERACTIONS
**Drug-drug.** *Allopurinol:* increased incidence of rash. Monitor patient.
*Oral contraceptives:* efficacy of oral contraceptives may be decreased. Recommend additional form of contraception during penicillin therapy.
*Probenecid:* increased blood levels of amoxicillin and other penicillins. Probenecid may be used for this purpose.

## EFFECTS ON DIAGNOSTIC TESTS
Amoxicillin may alter results of urine glucose tests that use cupric sulfate (Benedict's reagent or Clinitest). Make urine glucose determinations with glucose oxidase methods (Diastix or Chemstrip uG). Amoxicillin may falsely cause a positive Coombs' test.

## CONTRAINDICATIONS
Contraindicated in patients with hypersensitivity to drug or other penicillins.

## NURSING CONSIDERATIONS
• Use cautiously in patients with other drug allergies, especially to cephalosporins (possible cross-sensitivity), and in those with mononucleosis (high incidence of maculopapular rash).
• Before giving, ask patient about allergic reactions to penicillin. A negative history of penicillin allergy is no guarantee against allergic reaction.
• Obtain specimen for culture and sensitivity tests before giving first dose. Therapy may begin pending results.
• Give amoxicillin at least 1 hour before a bacteriostatic antibiotic.
• Observe patient closely. With large doses and prolonged therapy, superinfection may occur, especially in elderly, debilitated, or immunosuppressed patients.
• Store Trimox oral suspension at room temperature for up to 2 weeks. Be sure to check individual product labels for storage information.

---

Reactions may be *common,* uncommon, *life-threatening,* or COMMON AND LIFE-THREATENING.

- Amoxicillin generally causes fewer cases of diarrhea than does ampicillin.
- *Alert:* Don't confuse amoxicillin with amoxapine.

☑ **Patient teaching**
- Tell patient to take entire quantity exactly as prescribed, even after he feels better.
- Instruct patient to take drug with food.
- Tell patient to notify doctor if rash, fever, or chills develop. A rash is the most common allergic reaction, especially if allopurinol is also being taken.
- Tell parent to place pediatric drops directly on child's tongue for swallowing or add to formula, milk, fruit juice, water, ginger ale, or a cold drink; patient should take immediately and consume entirely.

---

**ampicillin**
Apo-Ampi†, Novo Ampicillin†, Nu-Ampi†, Omnipen-N

**ampicillin sodium**
Ampicin†, Ampicyn‡, Omnipen-N, Penbritin†, Totacillin-N

**ampicillin trihydrate**
Omnipen, Penbritin†, Principen, Totacillin

*Pregnancy Risk Category B*

## HOW SUPPLIED
*Capsules:* 250 mg, 500 mg
*Oral suspension:* 125 mg/5 ml, 250 mg/5 ml
*Injection:* 125 mg, 250 mg, 500 mg, 1 g, 2 g

## ACTION
An aminopenicillin that inhibits cell-wall synthesis during microorganism multiplication. Bacteria resist ampicillin by producing penicillinases—enzymes that hydrolyze ampicillin.

| Route | Onset | Peak | Duration |
|-------|-------|------|----------|
| P.O. | Unknown | 2 hr | 6-8 hr |
| I.V. | Immediate | Immediate | Unknown |
| I.M. | Unknown | 1 hr | Unknown |

## INDICATIONS & DOSAGE
*Systemic infections and acute and chronic urinary tract infections due to susceptible strains of gram-positive and gram-negative organisms—*
**Adults and children weighing 40 kg (88 lb) or more:** 250 to 500 mg P.O. q 6 hours; or 1 to 12 g I.M. or I.V. daily in divided doses q 4 to 6 hours.
**Children weighing under 40 kg:** 25 to 100 mg/kg/day P.O. in equally divided doses q 6 hours; or 25 to 50 mg/kg/day I.M. or I.V. in divided doses q 6 to 8 hours. Pediatric dosages shouldn't exceed recommended adult dosages.
*Meningitis—*
**Adults:** 150 to 200 mg/kg/day I.V. in divided doses q 3 to 4 hours. May be given I.M. after 3 days of I.V. therapy.
**Children:** 100 to 200 mg/kg I.V. daily in divided doses q 3 to 4 hours. Give I.V. for 3 days; then give I.M.
*Uncomplicated gonorrhea—*
**Adults and children weighing over 45 kg (99 lb):** 3.5 g P.O. with 1 g probenecid given as a single dose.
*Endocarditis prophylaxis for dental and GI/GU procedures—*
**Adults:** 2 g I.M. or I.V. within 30 minutes before procedure.
**Children:** 50 mg/kg I.M. or I.V. within 30 minutes before procedure.
*Note:* Give drug with gentamicin in high-risk procedures.

## ADVERSE REACTIONS
**CNS:** lethargy, hallucinations, *seizures,* anxiety, confusion, agitation, depression, dizziness, fatigue.
**CV:** vein irritation, thrombophlebitis.
**GI:** *nausea,* vomiting, *diarrhea,* glossitis, stomatitis, gastritis, abdominal pain, enterocolitis, pseudomembranous colitis, black "hairy" tongue.
**GU:** interstitial nephritis, nephropathy, vaginitis.
**Hematologic:** anemia, *thrombocytopenia,* thrombocytopenic purpura, eosinophilia, *leukopenia,* hemolytic anemia, *agranulocytosis.*
**Other:** *hypersensitivity reactions (erythematous maculopapular rash, urticaria, anaphylaxis),* overgrowth of non-

---

susceptible organisms, pain at injection site.

## INTERACTIONS
**Drug-drug.** *Allopurinol:* increased incidence of rash. Monitor patient.
*Oral contraceptives:* efficacy of oral contraceptives may be decreased. Recommend additional form of contraception during penicillin therapy.
*Probenecid:* increased blood levels of ampicillin and other penicillins. Probenecid may be used for this purpose.

## EFFECTS ON DIAGNOSTIC TESTS
Drug alters results of urine glucose tests that use cupric sulfate (Benedict's reagent or Clinitest). Make urine glucose determinations with glucose oxidase methods (Diastix or Chemstrip uG). Ampicillin may falsely decrease serum aminoglycoside levels.

## CONTRAINDICATIONS
Contraindicated in patients with hypersensitivity to drug or other penicillins.

## NURSING CONSIDERATIONS
• Use cautiously in patients with other drug allergies, especially to cephalosporins (possible cross-sensitivity), and in those with mononucleosis (high incidence of maculopapular rash).
• Before giving drug, ask patient about allergic reactions to penicillin. A negative history of penicillin allergy is no guarantee against a future allergic reaction.
• Obtain specimen for culture and sensitivity tests before giving first dose. Therapy may begin pending results.
• Give drug I.M. or I.V. only if prescribed and the infection is severe or if patient can't take oral dose.
• Administer drug 1 to 2 hours before or 2 to 3 hours after meals. When given orally, drug may cause GI disturbances. Food may interfere with absorption.
• Give ampicillin at least 1 hour before a bacteriostatic antibiotic.
• Observe patient closely. With large doses or prolonged therapy, bacterial or fungal superinfection may occur, especially in elderly, debilitated, or immunosuppressed patients.

• Dosage should be decreased in patients with impaired renal function.
• In pediatric meningitis, ampicillin may be given with parenteral chloramphenicol for 24 hours pending cultures.

## I.V. administration
• For I.V. injection, reconstitute with bacteriostatic water for injection. Use 5 ml for the 125-mg, 250-mg, or 500-mg vials; 7.4 ml for the 1-g vials; or 14.8 ml for the 2-g vials. Give direct I.V. injections over 3 to 5 minutes for doses of 500 mg or less; over 10 to 15 minutes for larger doses. Don't exceed a rate of 100 mg/minute. Or, dilute in 50 to 100 ml of normal saline for injection and give by intermittent infusion over 15 to 30 minutes.
• *Alert:* Don't mix with solutions containing dextrose or fructose because these substances promote rapid breakdown of ampicillin.
• Use initial dilution within 1 hour. Follow manufacturer's directions for stability data when ampicillin is further diluted for I.V. infusion.
• Give I.V. intermittently to prevent vein irritation. Change site every 48 hours.

## Patient teaching
• Tell patient to take entire quantity of medication exactly as prescribed, even after he feels better.
• Instruct patient to take oral form on an empty stomach 1 hour before or 2 hours after meals.
• Inform patient to notify doctor if rash, fever, or chills develop. A rash is the most common allergic reaction, especially if allopurinol is also being taken.
• Advise patient to report discomfort at I.V. injection site.

## ampicillin sodium/sulbactam sodium
Unasyn

*Pregnancy Risk Category B*

## HOW SUPPLIED
*Injection:* vials and piggyback vials containing 1.5 g (1 g ampicillin sodium with 0.5 g sulbactam sodium), 3 g (2 g ampi-

cillin sodium with 1 g sulbactam sodium), and 10 g (10 g ampicillin sodium with 5 g sulbactam sodium)

## ACTION

An aminopenicillin that inhibits cell-wall synthesis during microorganism multiplication. Sulbactam inactivates bacterial beta-lactamase, which inactivates ampicillin, causing bacterial resistance to it.

| Route | Peak | Onset | Duration |
|-------|------|-------|----------|
| I.V. | 15 min | Immediate | Unknown |
| I.M. | Unknown | Unknown | Unknown |

## INDICATIONS & DOSAGE

*Intra-abdominal, gynecologic, and skin-structure infections due to susceptible strains—*

**Adults and children weighing over 40 kg (88 lb):** dosage expressed as total drug (each 1.5-g vial contains 1 g ampicillin sodium and 0.5 g sulbactam sodium)— 1.5 to 3 g I.M. or I.V. q 6 hours. Maximum daily dose is 4 g sulbactam and 8 g ampicillin (12 g of combined drugs).
**Children ages 1 and older weighing below 40 kg:** 300 mg/kg/day (200 mg ampicillin/100 mg sulbactam) I.V. in divided doses q 6 hours. Don't exceed 4 g daily.
*Adjust-a-dose:* For renally impaired patients with creatinine clearance of 15 to 29 ml/minute, give 1.5 to 3 g q 12 hours; if creatinine clearance is 5 to 14 ml/minute, give 1.5 to 3 g q 24 hours.

## ADVERSE REACTIONS

**CV:** vein irritation, thrombophlebitis.
**GI:** *nausea,* vomiting, *diarrhea,* glossitis, stomatitis, gastritis, black "hairy" tongue, enterocolitis, pseudomembranous colitis.
**GU:** increased BUN, creatinine.
**Hematologic:** anemia, ***thrombocytopenia,*** thrombocytopenic purpura, eosinophilia, *leukopenia, agranulocytosis.*
**Hepatic:** increased liver function tests.
**Other:** *hypersensitivity reactions, anaphylaxis, overgrowth of nonsusceptible organisms,* pain at injection site.

## INTERACTIONS

**Drug-drug.** *Allopurinol:* increased incidence of rash. Monitor patient.

*Oral contraceptives:* efficacy of oral contraceptives may be decreased. Recommend additional form of contraception during penicillin therapy.
*Probenecid:* increased levels of ampicillin. Probenecid may be used for this purpose.

## EFFECTS ON DIAGNOSTIC TESTS

Ampicillin alters results of urine glucose tests that use cupric sulfate (Benedict's reagent or Clinitest). Make urine glucose determinations with glucose oxidase methods (Diastix). In pregnant women, transient decreases in serum estradiol, conjugated estrone, conjugated estriol, and estriol glucuronide levels may occur.

## CONTRAINDICATIONS

Contraindicated in patients with hypersensitivity to drug or other penicillins.

## NURSING CONSIDERATIONS

• Use cautiously in patients with other drug allergies, especially to cephalosporins (possible cross-sensitivity), and in those with mononucleosis (high incidence of maculopapular rash).
• Before giving drug, ask patient about allergic reactions to penicillin. However, a negative history of penicillin allergy is no guarantee against a future allergic reaction.
• Obtain specimen for culture and sensitivity tests before giving first dose. Therapy may begin pending results.
• Monitor liver function tests during therapy, especially in patients with impaired liver function.
• Don't use I.M. route in children.
• For I.M. injection, reconstitute with sterile water for injection or 0.5% or 2% lidocaine hydrochloride injection. Add 3.2 ml to a 1.5-g vial (or 6.4 ml to a 3-g vial) to yield a concentration of 375 mg/ml. Administer deeply.
• Observe patient closely. With large doses and prolonged therapy, bacterial or fungal superinfection may occur, especially in elderly, debilitated, or immunosuppressed patients.
• Dosage should be decreased in patients with impaired renal function.

## I.V. administration

• When preparing I.V. injection, reconstitute powder with one of the following diluents: normal saline solution, sterile water for injection, $D_5W$, lactated Ringer's injection, 1/6 M sodium lactate, dextrose 5% or half-normal saline for injection, and 10% invert sugar. Stability varies with diluent, temperature, and concentration of solution.

• After reconstitution, allow vials to stand for a few minutes to allow foam to dissipate. This will permit visual inspection of contents for particles.

• When giving I.V., don't add or mix with other drugs because they might prove incompatible.

• Give drug at least 1 hour before a bacteriostatic antibiotic.

• *Alert:* Give I.V. dose by slow injection (over 10 to 15 minutes) or dilute in 50 to 100 ml of a compatible diluent, and infuse over 15 to 30 minutes. If permitted, give intermittently to prevent vein irritation. Change site every 48 hours.

## ✓ Patient teaching

• Tell patient to report a rash, fever, or chills. A rash is the most common allergic reaction.

• Advise patient to report discomfort at I.V. insertion site.

• Warn patient that I.M. injection may cause pain at injection site.

---

## cloxacillin sodium
Apo-Cloxi†, Cloxapen,
Novo-Cloxin†, Nu-Cloxi†,
Orbenin†

*Pregnancy Risk Category B*

## HOW SUPPLIED
*Capsules:* 250 mg, 500 mg
*Oral solution:* 125 mg/5 ml (after reconstitution)

## ACTION
A penicillinase-resistant penicillin that inhibits cell-wall synthesis during microorganism multiplication. Bacteria resist penicillins by producing penicillinases—enzymes that convert penicillins to inactive penicillic acid. Cloxacillin resists these enzymes.

| Route | Onset | Peak | Duration |
|-------|-------|------|----------|
| P.O. | Unknown | 2 hr | 6 hr |

## INDICATIONS & DOSAGE
*Systemic infections due to penicillinase-producing staphylococci—*
**Adults and children weighing over 20 kg (44 lb):** 250 to 500 mg P.O. q 6 hours.
**Children weighing 20 kg or less:** 50 to 100 mg/kg P.O. daily, in divided doses q 6 hours (maximum of 4 g daily).

## ADVERSE REACTIONS
**CNS:** lethargy, hallucinations, *seizures,* anxiety, confusion, agitation, depression, dizziness, fatigue.
**GI:** *nausea,* vomiting, *epigastric distress, diarrhea,* enterocolitis, pseudomembranous colitis, black "hairy" tongue, abdominal pain.
**GU:** interstitial nephritis, nephropathy.
**Hematologic:** eosinophilia, anemia, *thrombocytopenia, leukopenia,* hemolytic anemia, *agranulocytosis,* transient reductions in RBC, WBC, and platelet counts.
**Hepatic:** transient elevations in liver function tests.
**Other:** *hypersensitivity reactions, anaphylaxis,* overgrowth of nonsusceptible organisms.

## INTERACTIONS
**Drug-drug.** *Oral contraceptives:* efficacy of oral contraceptives may be decreased. Recommend additional form of contraception during penicillin therapy.
*Probenecid:* increased blood levels of cloxacillin and other penicillins. Probenecid may be used for this purpose.
**Drug-food.** *Any food:* may interfere with absorption. Give 1 to 2 hours before or 2 to 3 hours after meals.
*Carbonated beverages, fruit juice:* inactivates drug. Don't give together.

## EFFECTS ON DIAGNOSTIC TESTS
Drug alters test results for urine and serum proteins; it produces false-positive or elevated results in turbidimetric urine and serum protein tests using sulfosali-

---

Reactions may be *common,* uncommon, *life-threatening,* or COMMON AND LIFE-THREATENING.

cylic acid or trichloroacetic acid; it also reportedly produces false results on the Bradshaw screening test for Bence Jones protein.

**CONTRAINDICATIONS**
Contraindicated in patients with hypersensitivity to drug or other penicillins.

**NURSING CONSIDERATIONS**
• Use cautiously in patients with other drug allergies, especially to cephalosporins (possible cross-sensitivity), and in those with mononucleosis (high incidence of maculopapular rash).
• Before giving drug, ask patient about allergic reactions to penicillin. However, a negative history of penicillin allergy is no guarantee against a future allergic reaction.
• Obtain specimen for culture and sensitivity tests before giving first dose. Therapy may begin pending results.
• Give drug 1 to 2 hours before or 2 to 3 hours after meals. Drug may cause GI disturbances. Food may interfere with its absorption.
• Give cloxacillin at least 1 hour before a bacteriostatic antibiotic.
• As ordered, periodically assess renal, hepatic, and hematopoietic function in patients receiving long-term therapy.
• Elevated liver function test results may indicate drug-induced cholestasis or hepatitis.
• Observe patient closely. With large doses and prolonged therapy, bacterial or fungal superinfection may occur, especially in elderly, debilitated, or immunosuppressed patients.

✅**Patient teaching**
• Tell patient to take entire quantity of drug exactly as prescribed, even after he feels better.
• Instruct patient to take drug on an empty stomach.
• *Alert:* Instruct patient to take each dose with a full glass of water, not with fruit juice or carbonated beverage, because their acid will inactivate the drug.
• Advise patient to notify doctor if rash, fever, or chills develop. A rash is the most common allergic reaction.

## diclanxacillin sodium
Diclocil‡, Dycill, Dynapen, Pathocil

*Pregnancy Risk Category B*

**HOW SUPPLIED**
*Capsules:* 125 mg, 250 mg, 500 mg
*Oral suspension:* 62.5 mg/5 ml (after reconstitution)

**ACTION**
A penicillinase-resistant penicillin that inhibits cell-wall synthesis during microorganism multiplication. Bacteria resist penicillins by producing penicillinases—enzymes that convert penicillins to inactive penicillic acid. Dicloxacillin resists these enzymes.

| Route | Onset | Peak | Duration |
|-------|-------|------|----------|
| P.O. | Unknown | 2 hr | 6 hr |

**INDICATIONS & DOSAGE**
*Systemic infections due to penicillinase-producing staphylococci—*
**Adults and children weighing over 40 kg (88 lb):** 125 to 250 mg P.O. q 6 hours.
**Children weighing 40 kg or less:** 12.5 to 25 mg/kg P.O. daily, in divided doses q 6 hours depending on severity.

**ADVERSE REACTIONS**
**CNS:** neuromuscular irritability, *seizures,* lethargy, hallucinations, anxiety, confusion, agitation, depression, dizziness, fatigue.
**GI:** *nausea,* vomiting, *epigastric distress,* flatulence, *diarrhea,* enterocolitis, pseudomembranous colitis, black "hairy" tongue, abdominal pain.
**GU:** interstitial nephritis, nephropathy.
**Hematologic:** anemia, *thrombocytopenia,* eosinophilia, *leukopenia,* hemolytic anemia, *agranulocytosis.*
**Hepatic:** transient elevations in liver function test results.
**Other:** *hypersensitivity reactions (pruritus, urticaria, rash, anaphylaxis),* overgrowth of nonsusceptible organisms.

**INTERACTIONS**
**Drug-drug.** *Oral contraceptives:* efficacy of oral contraceptives may be decreased.

---

Recommend additional form of contraception during penicillin therapy.
*Probenecid:* increased blood levels of dicloxacillin and other penicillins. Probenecid may be used for this purpose.

## EFFECTS ON DIAGNOSTIC TESTS
Drug produces false-positive or elevated results in turbidimetric urine and serum protein tests using sulfosalicylic acid or trichloroacetic acid; it also reportedly produces false results on the Bradshaw screening test for Bence Jones protein.

## CONTRAINDICATIONS
Contraindicated in patients with hypersensitivity to drug or other penicillins. It is not recommended for use in newborns.

## NURSING CONSIDERATIONS
• Use cautiously in patients with other drug allergies, especially to cephalosporins (possible cross-sensitivity), and in those with mononucleosis (high incidence of maculopapular rash).
• Before giving drug, ask patient about allergic reactions to penicillin. However, a negative history of penicillin allergy is no guarantee against a future allergic reaction.
• Obtain specimen for culture and sensitivity tests before giving first dose. Therapy may begin pending results.
• Give drug 1 to 2 hours before or 2 to 3 hours after meals. Drug may cause GI disturbances. Food may interfere with absorption.
• Give dicloxacillin at least 1 hour before a bacteriostatic antibiotic.
• As ordered, periodically assess renal, hepatic, and hematopoietic function in patients receiving long-term therapy.
• Elevated liver function test results may indicate drug-induced cholestasis or hepatitis.
• Observe patient closely. With large doses and prolonged therapy, bacterial or fungal superinfection may occur, especially in elderly, debilitated, or immunosuppressed patients.

✓ **Patient teaching**
• Tell patient to take entire quantity of drug exactly as prescribed, even after he feels better.

• Instruct patient to take drug on an empty stomach.
• Advise patient to notify doctor if rash, fever, or chills develop. A rash is the most common allergic reaction.

---

## mezlocillin sodium
Mezlin

*Pregnancy Risk Category B*

### HOW SUPPLIED
*Injection:* 1 g, 2 g, 3 g, 4 g, 20 g

### ACTION
An extended-spectrum penicillin that inhibits cell-wall synthesis during microorganism multiplication. Bacteria resist mezlocillin by producing penicillinases—enzymes that hydrolyze mezlocillin.

| Route | Onset | Peak | Duration |
|-------|-------|------|----------|
| I.V. | Immediate | Immediate | Unknown |
| I.M. | Unknown | 45-90 min | Unknown |

### INDICATIONS & DOSAGE
*Systemic infections due to susceptible strains of gram-positive and especially gram-negative organisms (including* Proteus *and* Pseudomonas aeruginosa*)—*
**Adults:** 100 to 300 mg/kg daily I.V. or I.M. in four to six divided doses. Usual dose is 3 g q 4 hours or 4 g q 6 hours. For serious infections, up to 24 g daily may be administered.
**Children ages 1 month to 12 years:** 50 mg/kg q 4 hours I.V. or I.M.
*Adjust-a-dose:* For renally impaired patients with creatinine clearance of 10 to 30 ml/minute, 1.5 g q 6 hours for urinary tract infection or 3 g q 8 hours for serious infection; for creatinine clearance below 10 ml/minute, 1.5 g q 8 hours for urinary tract infection or 2 g q 8 hours for serious infection.

### ADVERSE REACTIONS
**CNS:** neuromuscular irritability, *seizures.*
**CV:** vein irritation, phlebitis.
**GI:** nausea, diarrhea, vomiting, abnormal taste sensation, pseudomembranous colitis.
**GU:** interstitial nephritis.

---

Reactions may be *common,* uncommon, *life-threatening,* or COMMON AND LIFE-THREATENING.

Hematologic: *bleeding, neutropenia, thrombocytopenia,* eosinophilia, *leukopenia, hemolytic anemia.* Hepatic: transient elevations in liver function test results.
Metabolic: *hypokalemia.*
Other: *hypersensitivity reactions, anaphylaxis,* overgrowth of nonsusceptible organisms, pain at injection site.

## INTERACTIONS

Drug-drug. *Aminoglycoside antibiotics (such as amikacin, gentamicin, tobramycin):* chemically incompatible. Don't mix together in I.V. solution. Give 1 hour apart, especially in patients with renal impairment.
*Oral contraceptives:* efficacy of oral contraceptives may be decreased. Recommend additional form of contraception during penicillin therapy.
*Probenecid:* increased blood levels of mezlocillin. Probenecid may be used for this purpose.
*Vecuronium:* prolonged neuromuscular blockade. Use with caution.

## EFFECTS ON DIAGNOSTIC TESTS

Drug alters tests for urine or serum proteins; it interferes with turbidimetric methods that use sulfosalicylic acid, trichloroacetic acid, acetic acid, or nitric acid. Mezlocillin does not interfere with tests using bromphenol blue (Albustix, Albutest, Multistix). Positive Coombs' tests have been reported in patients taking mezlocillin.

## CONTRAINDICATIONS

Contraindicated in patients with hypersensitivity to drug or other penicillins.

## NURSING CONSIDERATIONS

• Use cautiously in patients with other drug allergies, especially to cephalosporins (possible cross-sensitivity), and in those with bleeding tendencies, uremia, or hypokalemia.
• Before giving drug, ask patient about allergic reactions to penicillin. A negative history of penicillin allergy, however, is no guarantee against future allergic reaction.
• Obtain specimen for culture and sensitivity tests before giving first dose. Therapy may begin pending results.

• When administering I.M., don't give more than 2 g per injection. Inject deeply and slowly (12 to 15 seconds) into the body of a large muscle.
• Check CBC and platelet counts frequently, as ordered. Drug may cause thrombocytopenia.
• Monitor serum potassium level.
• **Alert:** Institute seizure precautions. Patients with high serum levels of drug may have seizures.
• Observe patient closely. With large doses and prolonged therapy, bacterial or fungal superinfection may occur, especially in elderly, debilitated, or immunosuppressed patients.
• Dosage should be altered in patients with impaired renal function.
• Drug is almost always used with another antibiotic such as gentamicin.
• **Alert:** Don't confuse methicillin with mezlocillin.

### I.V. administration

• Reconstitute drug with at least 10 ml/g of drug using sterile water for injection, $D_5W$, or normal saline for injection. Solutions with a concentration not exceeding 10% may be given by direct injection over 3 to 5 minutes. Or, dilute in about 50 to 100 ml of suitable I.V. solution, and give by intermittent infusion over 30 minutes.
• Give I.V. intermittently to prevent vein irritation. Change site every 48 hours.
• Give drug at least 1 hour before bacteriostatic antibiotics.

### ✓ Patient teaching

• Instruct patient to report adverse reactions promptly.
• Tell patient to alert nurse if discomfort occurs at I.V. site.
• Caution patient to limit salt intake during mezlocillin therapy because of drug's high sodium content.

## nafcillin sodium
Nallpen, Unipen

*Pregnancy Risk Category B*

## HOW SUPPLIED
*Capsules:* 250 mg

*Injection:* 500 mg, 1 g, 2 g, 10 g
*I.V. infusion piggyback:* 1 g, 2 g

## ACTION
A penicillinase-resistant penicillin that inhibits cell-wall synthesis during microorganism multiplication. Bacteria resist penicillins by producing penicillinases—enzymes that hydrolyze penicillins. Nafcillin resists these enzymes.

| Route | Onset | Peak | Duration |
|-------|-------|------|----------|
| P.O. | Unknown | 0.5-2 hr | Unknown |
| I.V. | Immediate | Immediate | Unknown |
| I.M. | Unknown | 0.5-1 hr | Unknown |

## INDICATIONS & DOSAGE
*Systemic infections due to penicillinase-producing staphylococci—*
**Adults:** 250 to 500 mg P.O. q 4 to 6 hours (more severe infections may be treated with 1 g P.O. q 4 to 6 hours); or 500 mg I.M. q 4 to 6 hours or I.V. q 4 hours, or (for more severe infections) 1 g I.M. or I.V. q 4 hours.
**Children over age 1 month and weighing under 40 kg (88 lb):** 25 to 50 mg/kg P.O. daily, in divided doses q 6 hours; or 25 mg/kg I.M. b.i.d. or 100 to 200 mg/kg I.M. or I.V. daily in divided doses q 4 to 6 hours.
**Neonates:** 10 mg/kg I.M. b.i.d. or 10 mg/kg P.O. t.i.d. or q.i.d.

## ADVERSE REACTIONS
**CV:** vein irritation, thrombophlebitis.
**GI:** *nausea,* vomiting, diarrhea.
**Hematologic:** *neutropenia, agranulocytosis, thrombocytopenia.*
**Other:** *hypersensitivity reactions, anaphylaxis.*

## INTERACTIONS
**Drug-drug.** *Aminoglycosides:* synergistic effect; monitor closely. Chemical and physical incompatibility. Don't mix together in same I.V. solution.
*Oral contraceptives:* efficacy of oral contraceptives may be decreased. Recommend additional form of contraception during penicillin therapy.
*Probenecid:* increased blood levels of nafcillin. Probenecid may be used for this purpose.

*Rifampin:* dose-dependent antagonism. Monitor closely.
*Warfarin:* increased risk of bleeding when used with I.V. nafcillin. Monitor PT and INR closely.

## EFFECTS ON DIAGNOSTIC TESTS
Turbidimetric urine and serum proteins are falsely positive or elevated in tests using sulfosalicylic acid or trichloroacetic acid.

## CONTRAINDICATIONS
Contraindicated in patients with hypersensitivity to drug or other penicillins.

## NURSING CONSIDERATIONS
• Use cautiously in patients with other drug allergies, especially to cephalosporins (possible cross-sensitivity), and in those with GI distress.
• Before giving drug, ask patient about allergic reactions to penicillin. However, a negative history of penicillin allergy is no guarantee against a future allergic reaction.
• Obtain specimen for culture and sensitivity tests before giving first dose. Therapy may begin pending results.
• Give drug 1 to 2 hours before or 2 to 3 hours after meals. When given orally, drug may cause GI disturbances. Food may interfere with absorption.
• Give drug at least 1 hour before a bacteriostatic antibiotic.
• Observe patient closely. With large doses and prolonged therapy, bacterial or fungal superinfection may occur, especially in elderly, debilitated, or immunosuppressed patients.
• Monitor serum sodium because each gram of nafcillin contains 2.9 mEq of sodium.
• An abnormal urinalysis result may indicate drug-induced interstitial nephritis.

### ⬧ I.V. administration
• Reconstitute piggyback containers according to manufacturer's instructions. Reconstitute 500-mg, 1-g, and 2-g vials with sterile water for injection, $D_5W$, or normal saline for injection. Add 1.7 ml for each 500 mg of drug. Reconstituted drug may be given I.M. Or, dilute with 15

to 30 ml of sterile water for injection or half-normal or normal saline for injection, and give by direct injection into a vein or into the tubing of a free-flowing I.V. solution over 5 to 10 minutes. Or dilute drug to a concentration of 2 to 40 mg/ml, and give by intermittent I.V. infusion over 30 to 60 minutes.

• Avoid continuous I.V. infusions to prevent vein irritation. Change site every 48 hours.

☑ **Patient teaching**
• Tell patient to take entire quantity of medication exactly as prescribed, even after he feels better.
• Instruct patient to take oral form of drug on an empty stomach.
• Advise patient to notify doctor if rash, fever, or chills develop. A rash is the most common allergic reaction.

## oxacillin sodium
Bactocill

*Pregnancy Risk Category B*

### HOW SUPPLIED
*Capsules:* 250 mg, 500 mg
*Oral solution:* 250 mg/5 ml (after reconstitution)
*Injection:* 250 mg, 500 mg, 1 g, 2 g, 4 g
*I.V. infusion:* 1 g, 2 g

### ACTION
A penicillinase-resistant penicillin that inhibits cell-wall synthesis during microorganism multiplication. Bacteria resist penicillins by producing penicillinases—enzymes that convert penicillins to inactive penicillic acid. Oxacillin resists these enzymes.

| Route | Onset | Peak | Duration |
|-------|-------|------|----------|
| P.O. | Unknown | 0.5-2 hr | Unknown |
| I.V. | Immediate | Immediate | Unknown |
| I.M. | Unknown | 0.5 hr | Unknown |

### INDICATIONS & DOSAGE
*Systemic infections due to penicillinase-producing staphylococci—*
**Adults and children weighing over 40 kg (88 lb):** 500 mg to 1 g P.O. q 4 to 6 hours; or 250 mg to 1 g I.M. or I.V. q 4 to 6 hours.
**Children over age 1 month weighing 40 kg or less:** 50 to 100 mg/kg P.O. daily, in divided doses q 6 hours; or 50 to 200 mg/kg I.M. or I.V. daily in divided doses q 4 to 6 hours, depending on severity.
**Premature infants and neonates:** 25 mg/kg/day I.M. or I.V. in equally divided doses q 6 to 12 hours.

### ADVERSE REACTIONS
**CNS:** neuropathy, neuromuscular irritability, *seizures,* lethargy, hallucinations, anxiety, confusion, agitation, depression, dizziness, fatigue.
**CV:** *thrombophlebitis.*
**GI:** oral lesions, nausea, vomiting, diarrhea, enterocolitis, pseudomembranous colitis.
**GU:** interstitial nephritis, nephropathy.
**Hematologic:** *thrombocytopenia,* eosinophilia, *hemolytic anemia, neutropenia,* anemia, *agranulocytosis.*
**Hepatic:** elevated liver enzymes.
**Other:** *hypersensitivity reactions, anaphylaxis,* overgrowth of nonsusceptible organisms.

### INTERACTIONS
**Drug-drug.** *Aminoglycosides:* possible synergistic effect. Monitor closely. Chemical and physical incompatibility. Don't mix together in same I.V. solution.
*Oral contraceptives:* efficacy of oral contraceptives may be decreased. Recommend additional form of contraception during penicillin therapy.
*Probenecid:* increased blood levels of oxacillin and other penicillins. Probenecid may be used for this purpose.
*Rifampin:* possible antagonism. Monitor closely.

### EFFECTS ON DIAGNOSTIC TESTS
Turbidimetric urine and serum proteins are falsely positive or elevated in tests using sulfosalicylic acid or trichloroacetic acid.

### CONTRAINDICATIONS
Contraindicated in patients with hypersensitivity to drug or other penicillins.

## NURSING CONSIDERATIONS

• Use cautiously in patients with other drug allergies, especially to cephalosporins (possible cross-sensitivity), and in neonates and infants.
• Before giving drug, ask patient about allergic reactions to penicillin. However, a negative history of penicillin allergy is no guarantee against a future allergic reaction.
• Obtain specimen for culture and sensitivity tests before giving first dose. Therapy may begin pending results.
• Give drug I.M. or I.V. only if ordered and the infection is severe or if the patient can't take oral dose.
• Give drug 1 to 2 hours before or 2 to 3 hours after meals. When given orally, drug may cause GI disturbances. Food may interfere with absorption.
• Administer drug at least 1 hour before a bacteriostatic antibiotic.
• Monitor periodic liver function studies; watch for elevated AST and ALT levels. Elevations in liver function test results may indicate drug-induced hepatitis or cholestasis.
• Abnormal urinalysis results may indicate drug-induced interstitial nephritis.
• Observe patient closely. With large doses and prolonged therapy, bacterial or fungal superinfection may occur, especially in elderly, debilitated, or immunosuppressed patients.

### I.V. administration

• For direct I.V. injection, reconstitute drug with sterile water for injection or normal saline for injection. Use 5 ml of diluent for a 250- or 500-mg vial, 10 ml of diluent for a 1-g vial, 20 ml of diluent for a 2-g vial, or 40 ml of diluent for a 4-g vial. When the solution is clear, withdraw the ordered dose and inject over 10 minutes. When giving by piggyback injection, reconstitute 1-g piggyback vial with 20 to 100 ml of diluent; reconstitute 2-g vial with 19 to 99 ml of diluent. For intermittent infusion, further dilute drug to a concentration of 5 to 40 mg/ml.
• To prevent vein irritation, avoid continuous infusions. Change site every 48 hours.

### ☑ Patient teaching

• Tell patient to take entire quantity of drug exactly as prescribed, even after he feels better.
• Instruct patient to take drug on an empty stomach.
• Advise patient to notify doctor if rash, fever, or chills develop. A rash is the most common allergic reaction.

---

## penicillin G benzathine (benzylpenicillin benzathine)
Bicillin L-A, Permapen

*Pregnancy Risk Category B*

### HOW SUPPLIED
*Injection:* 300,000 U/ml, 600,000 U/ml, 1,200,000 U/2 ml, 2,400,000 U/4 ml

### ACTION
A natural penicillin that inhibits cell-wall synthesis during microorganism multiplication. Bacteria resist penicillins by producing penicillinases—enzymes that convert penicillins to inactive penicillic acid.

| Route | Onset | Peak | Duration |
|-------|-------|------|----------|
| I.M. | Unknown | 13-24 hr | 1-4 wk |

### INDICATIONS & DOSAGE
*Congenital syphilis—*
**Children under age 2:** 50,000 U/kg I.M. as a single dose.
*Group A streptococcal upper respiratory infections—*
**Adults:** 1.2 million U I.M. as a single injection.
**Children weighing 27 kg (60 lb) or more:** 900,000 U I.M. as a single injection.
**Children weighing less than 27 kg:** 300,000 to 600,000 U I.M. as a single injection.
*Prophylaxis of poststreptococcal rheumatic fever—*
**Adults and children:** 1.2 million U I.M. once monthly.
*Syphilis of less than 1 year's duration—*
**Adults:** 2.4 million U I.M. as a single dose.
**Children:** 50,000 U/kg (up to the adult dosage) I.M as a single dose.

---

*Syphilis of more than 1 year's duration—*
**Adults:** 2.4 million U I.M. weekly for 3 successive weeks.
**Children:** 50,000 U/kg I.M. weekly for 3 successive weeks.

## ADVERSE REACTIONS
**CNS:** neuropathy, *seizures,* lethargy, hallucinations, anxiety, confusion, agitation, depression, dizziness, fatigue.
**GI:** nausea, vomiting, enterocolitis, pseudomembranous colitis.
**GU:** interstitial nephritis, nephropathy.
**Hematologic:** eosinophilia, hemolytic anemia, *thrombocytopenia, leukopenia,* anemia, *agranulocytosis.*
**Other:** *hypersensitivity reactions, maculopapular and exfoliative dermatitis, anaphylaxis,* pain, sterile abscess at injection site.

## INTERACTIONS
**Drug-drug.** *Aminoglycosides:* physical and chemical incompatibility. Administer separately.
*Colestipol:* decreased serum concentrations of penicillin G benzathine. Administer penicillin G benzathine 1 hour before or 4 hours after colestipol.
*Oral contraceptives:* efficacy of oral contraceptives may be decreased. Recommend additional form of contraception during penicillin therapy.
*Probenecid:* increased blood levels of penicillin. Probenecid may be used for this purpose.
*Tetracycline:* may antagonize the effects. Avoid concurrent use.

## EFFECTS ON DIAGNOSTIC TESTS
Penicillin G interferes with turbidimetric methods using sulfosalicylic acid, trichloracetic acid, acetic acid, and nitric acid. Drug does not interfere with tests using bromphenol blue (Albustix, Albutest, Multistix). It alters urine glucose testing using cupric sulfate (Benedict's reagent); use Diastix or Chemstrip uG instead. Penicillin G may cause falsely elevated results of urine specific gravity tests in patients with low urine output and dehydration and falsely elevated Norymberski and Zimmerman tests results for 17-ketogenic steroids. It causes false-positive CSF protein test results (Folin-Ciocalteau method) and may cause positive Coombs' test results. Drug may falsely decrease serum aminoglycoside levels. Adding beta-lactamase to the sample inactivates the penicillin, rendering the assay more accurate. Or, the sample can be spun down and frozen immediately after collection.

## CONTRAINDICATIONS
Contraindicated in patients with hypersensitivity to drug or other penicillins.

## NURSING CONSIDERATIONS
● Use cautiously in patients with other drug allergies, especially to cephalosporins (possible cross-sensitivity).
● Before giving drug, ask patient about allergic reactions to penicillin. However, a negative history of penicillin allergy is no guarantee against a future allergic reaction.
● Obtain specimen for culture and sensitivity tests before giving first dose. Therapy may begin pending results.
● Shake medication well before injection.
● *Alert:* Never give I.V. Inadvertent I.V. administration has caused cardiac arrest and death.
● Inject deeply into upper outer quadrant of buttocks in adults; in midlateral thigh in infants and small children. Avoid injection into or near major nerves or blood vessels to prevent permanent neurovascular damage.
● Give drug at least 1 hour before a bacteriostatic antibiotic.
● Drug's extremely slow absorption time makes allergic reactions difficult to treat.
● Observe patient closely. With large doses and prolonged therapy, bacterial or fungal superinfection may occur, especially in elderly, debilitated, or immunosuppressed patients.
● *Alert:* Don't confuse drug with polycillin, penicillamine, or the various types of penicillin.

### ✓ Patient teaching
● Tell patient to report adverse reactions promptly.
● Inform patient that fever and eosinophilia are the most common reactions.

• Warn patient that I.M. injection may be painful but that ice applied to the site may ease discomfort.

---

## penicillin G potassium
## (benzylpenicillin potassium)
Megacillin†, Pfizerpen

*Pregnancy Risk Category B*

### HOW SUPPLIED
*Tablets:* 500,000 U†
*Oral suspension:* 250,000 U†, 500,000 U†
*Injection:* 1 million U, 5 million U, 10 million U, 20 million U
*Premixed injection:* 1 million U/50 ml, 2 million U/50 ml, 3 million U/50 ml

### ACTION
A natural penicillin that inhibits cell-wall synthesis during microorganism multiplication. Bacteria resist penicillins by producing penicillinases—enzymes that convert penicillins to inactive penicillic acid.

| Route | Onset | Peak | Duration |
|-------|-------|------|----------|
| P.O. | Unknown | 30-60 min | Unknown |
| I.V. | Immediate | Immediate | Unknown |
| I.M. | Unknown | 15-30 min | Unknown |

### INDICATIONS & DOSAGE
*Moderate to severe systemic infection—*
**Adults and children ages 12 and older:** highly individualized; 1.6 to 3.2 million U P.O. daily in divided doses q 6 hours; 1.2 to 24 million U I.M. or I.V. daily in divided doses q 4 to 6 hours.
**Children under age 12:** 25,000 to 100,000 U/kg P.O. daily in divided doses q 6 hours; or 25,000 to 400,000 U/kg I.M. or I.V. daily in divided doses q 4 to 6 hours.

### ADVERSE REACTIONS
**CNS:** neuropathy, *seizures,* lethargy, hallucinations, anxiety, confusion, agitation, depression, dizziness, fatigue.
**CV:** thrombophlebitis.
**GI:** nausea, vomiting, enterocolitis, pseudomembranous colitis.
**GU:** interstitial nephritis, nephropathy.
**Hematologic:** hemolytic anemia, *leukopenia, thrombocytopenia,* anemia, eosinophilia, *agranulocytosis.*

**Metabolic:** *possible severe potassium poisoning.*
**Other:** *hypersensitivity reactions, maculopapular eruptions, exfoliative dermatitis, anaphylaxis,* overgrowth of nonsusceptible organisms, pain at injection site.

### INTERACTIONS
**Drug-drug.** *Aminoglycosides:* physical and chemical incompatibility. Administer separately.
*Colestipol:* decreased serum levels of penicillin G potassium. Administer penicillin G potassium 1 hour before or 4 hours after colestipol.
*Oral contraceptives:* efficacy of oral contraceptives may be decreased. Recommend additional form of contraception during penicillin therapy.
*Potassium-sparing diuretics:* possible increased risk of hyperkalemia. Don't use together.
*Probenecid:* increased blood levels of penicillin. Probenecid may be used for this purpose.

### EFFECTS ON DIAGNOSTIC TESTS
Penicillin G interferes with turbidimetric methods using sulfosalicylic acid, trichloroacetic acid, acetic acid, and nitric acid. It does not interfere with tests using bromphenol blue (Albustix, Albutest, Multistix). Drug alters urine glucose testing using cupric sulfate (Benedict's reagent); use Diastix or Chemstrip uG instead. Penicillin G may cause falsely elevated results of urine specific gravity tests in patients with low urine output and dehydration and falsely elevated Norymberski and Zimmerman tests results for 17-ketogenic steroids. It causes false-positive CSF protein test results (Folin-Ciocalteau method) and may cause positive Coombs' test results. Drug may falsely decrease serum aminoglycoside levels. Adding beta-lactamase to the sample inactivates the penicillin, rendering the assay more accurate. Or, the sample can be spun down and frozen immediately after collection.

### CONTRAINDICATIONS
Contraindicated in patients with hypersensitivity to drug or other penicillins.

---

Reactions may be *common,* uncommon, *life-threatening,* or COMMON AND LIFE-THREATENING.

## NURSING CONSIDERATIONS
• Use cautiously in patients with other drug allergies, especially to cephalosporins (possible cross-sensitivity).
• Before giving drug, ask patient about allergic reactions to penicillin. However, a negative history of penicillin allergy is no guarantee against a future allergic reaction.
• Obtain specimen for culture and sensitivity tests before giving first dose. Therapy may begin pending results.
• For I.M. injection, administer deeply into large muscle; may be extremely painful.
• Give drug 1 to 2 hours before or 2 to 3 hours after meals. When given orally, drug may cause GI disturbances. Food may interfere with absorption.
• Give penicillin G potassium at least 1 hour before a bacteriostatic antibiotic.
• Monitor renal function closely. Patients with poor renal function are predisposed to high blood levels of drug.
• Monitor serum potassium and sodium levels closely in patients receiving more than 10 million U I.V. daily.
• Observe patient closely. With large doses and prolonged therapy, bacterial or fungal superinfection may occur, especially in elderly, debilitated, or immunosuppressed patients.
• *Alert:* Institute seizure precautions. Patients with high blood levels of drug may develop seizures.
• *Alert:* Don't confuse drug with polycillin, penicillamine, or the various types of penicillin.

**I.V. administration**
• Reconstitute drug with sterile water for injection, $D_5W$, or normal saline for injection. Volume of diluent varies with manufacturer.
• Give drug via intermittent I.V. infusion over 30 minutes to 2 hours.

**Patient teaching**
• Tell patient taking oral form to take entire amount exactly as prescribed, even after he feels better.
• Instruct patient to take oral drug on empty stomach.
• Tell patient to notify doctor if rash, fever, or chills develop. A rash is the most common allergic reaction.

• Warn patient that I.M. injection may be painful but that ice applied to the site may help alleviate discomfort.

---

## penicillin G procaine (benzylpenicillin procaine)
Ayercillin†, Wycillin

*Pregnancy Risk Category B*

### HOW SUPPLIED
*Injection:* 600,000 U/ml, 1,200,000 U/ml, 2,400,000 U/ml

### ACTION
A natural penicillin that inhibits cell-wall synthesis during microorganism multiplication. Bacteria resist penicillins by producing penicillinases—enzymes that convert penicillins to inactive penicillic acid.

| Route | Onset | Peak | Duration |
|-------|---------|--------|----------|
| I.M. | Unknown | 1-4 hr | 1-5 days |

### INDICATIONS & DOSAGE
*Moderate to severe systemic infection—*
**Adults:** 600,000 to 1.2 million U I.M. daily in a single dose.
**Children over age 1 month:** 25,000 to 50,000 U/kg I.M. daily in a single dose.
*Uncomplicated gonorrhea—*
**Adults and children weighing 45 kg (99 lb):** 1 g probenecid P.O.; after 30 minutes, 4.8 million U of penicillin G procaine I.M., divided between two injection sites as a single dose.
*Pneumococcal pneumonia—*
**Adults and children over age 12:** 600,000 to 1 million U I.M. daily for 7 to 10 days.

### ADVERSE REACTIONS
**CNS:** *seizures,* lethargy, hallucinations, anxiety, confusion, agitation, depression, dizziness, fatigue.
**GI:** nausea, vomiting, enterocolitis, pseudomembranous colitis.
**GU:** interstitial nephritis, nephropathy.
**Hematologic:** *thrombocytopenia, hemolytic anemia, leukopenia,* anemia, eosinophilia, *agranulocytosis.*
**Musculoskeletal:** arthralgia.

---

**Other:**, *hypersensitivity reactions, anaphylaxis,* overgrowth of nonsusceptible organisms.

## INTERACTIONS
**Drug-drug.** *Aminoglycosides:* physical and chemical incompatibility. Administer separately.
*Colestipol:* decreased serum concentrations of penicillin G procaine. Administer penicillin G procaine 1 hour before or 4 hours after colestipol.
*Oral contraceptives:* efficacy of oral contraceptives may be decreased. Recommend additional form of contraception during penicillin therapy.
*Probenecid:* increased blood levels of penicillin. Probenecid may be used for this purpose.

## EFFECTS ON DIAGNOSTIC TESTS
Penicillin G interferes with turbidimetric methods using sulfosalicylic acid, trichloroacetic acid, acetic acid, and nitric acid. Drug does not interfere with tests using bromphenol blue (Albustix, Albutest, Multistix). Penicillin G alters urine glucose testing using cupric sulfate (Benedict's reagent); use Diastix instead. Penicillin G may cause falsely elevated results of urine specific gravity tests in patients with low urine output and dehydration and falsely elevated Norymberski and Zimmerman tests results for 17-ketogenic steroids. It causes false-positive CSF protein test results (Folin-Ciocalteau method) and may cause positive Coombs' test results. Drug may falsely decrease serum aminoglycoside levels. Adding beta-lactamase to the sample inactivates the penicillin, rendering the assay more accurate. Or, the sample can be spun down and frozen immediately after collection.

## CONTRAINDICATIONS
Contraindicated in patients with hypersensitivity to drug or other penicillins.

## NURSING CONSIDERATIONS
• Use cautiously in patients with other drug allergies, especially to cephalosporins (possible cross-sensitivity). Some formulations contain sulfites, which may cause allergic reactions in sensitive persons.
• Before giving drug, ask patient about allergic reactions to penicillin. However, a negative history of penicillin allergy is no guarantee against a future allergic reaction.
• Obtain specimen for culture and sensitivity tests before giving first dose. Therapy may begin pending results.
• Give deep I.M. in upper outer quadrant of buttocks in adults; in midlateral thigh in small children. Don't give S.C. Don't massage injection site. Avoid injection near major nerves or blood vessels to prevent permanent neurovascular damage.
• *Alert:* Never give I.V. Inadvertent I.V. administration has resulted in death due to CNS toxicity due to penicillin G procaine.
• Give drug at least 1 hour before a bacteriostatic antibiotic.
• Allergic reactions are hard to treat because of drug's slow absorption rate.
• Monitor renal and hematopoietic function periodically, as ordered.
• Observe patient closely. With large doses and prolonged therapy, bacterial or fungal superinfection may occur, especially in elderly, debilitated, or immunosuppressed patients.
• *Alert:* Don't confuse drug with polycillin, penicillamine, or the various types of penicillin.

☑ **Patient teaching**
• Tell patient to report adverse reactions promptly. A rash is the most common allergic reaction.
• Warn patient that I.M. injection may be painful but that ice applied to the site may help alleviate discomfort.

---

**penicillin G sodium (benzylpenicillin sodium)**
Crystapen†

*Pregnancy Risk Category B*

## HOW SUPPLIED
*Injection:* 5 million-U vial

---

## ACTION
A natural penicillin that inhibits cell-wall synthesis during active multiplication. Bacteria resist penicillins by producing penicillinases—enzymes that convert penicillins to inactive penicillic acid.

| Route | Onset | Peak | Duration |
|-------|-------|------|----------|
| I.V. | Immediate | Immediate | Unknown |
| I.M. | Unknown | 15-30 min | Unknown |

## INDICATIONS & DOSAGE
*Moderate to severe systemic infection—*
**Adults and children ages 12 and older:** 1.2 to 24 million U daily I.M. or I.V. in divided doses q 4 to 6 hours.
**Children under age 12:** 25,000 to 400,000 U/kg daily I.M. or I.V. in divided doses q 4 to 6 hours.

## ADVERSE REACTIONS
**CNS:** neuropathy, *seizures,* lethargy, hallucinations, anxiety, confusion, agitation, depression, dizziness, fatigue.
**CV:** *heart failure,* thrombophlebitis, vein irritation.
**GI:** nausea, vomiting, enterocolitis, pseudomembranous colitis.
**GU:** interstitial colitis, nephropathy.
**Hematologic:** hemolytic anemia, *leukopenia, thrombocytopenia, agranulocytosis,* anemia, eosinophilia.
**Musculoskeletal:** arthralgia.
**Other:** *hypersensitivity reactions, anaphylaxis,* overgrowth of nonsusceptible organisms, pain at injection site.

## INTERACTIONS
**Drug-drug.** *Aminoglycosides:* physical and chemical incompatibility. Administer separately.
*Colestipol:* decreased serum levels of penicillin G sodium. Administer penicillin G sodium 1 hour before or 4 hours after colestipol.
*Oral contraceptives:* efficacy of oral contraceptives may be decreased. Recommend additional form of contraception during penicillin therapy.
*Probenecid:* increased blood levels of penicillin. Probenecid may be used for this purpose.

## EFFECTS ON DIAGNOSTIC TESTS
Drug interferes with turbidimetric methods using sulfosalicylic acid, trichloroacetic acid, acetic acid, and nitric acid. Penicillin G does not interfere with tests using bromphenol blue (Albustix, Albutest, Multistix). Penicillin G alters urine glucose testing using cupric sulfate (Benedict's reagent); use Diastix instead. It may cause falsely elevated results of urine specific gravity tests in patients with low urine output and dehydration and falsely elevated Norymberski and Zimmerman tests results for 17-ketogenic steroids. It causes false-positive CSF protein test results (Folin-Ciocalteau method) and may cause positive Coombs' test results. Drug may falsely decrease serum aminoglycoside levels. Adding beta-lactamase to the sample inactivates the penicillin, rendering the assay more accurate. Or, the sample can be spun down and frozen immediately after collection.

## CONTRAINDICATIONS
Contraindicated in patients with hypersensitivity to drug or other penicillins and in those on sodium-restricted diets.

## NURSING CONSIDERATIONS
• Use cautiously in patients with other drug allergies, especially to cephalosporins (possible cross-allergenicity).
• Before giving drug, ask patient about allergic reactions to penicillin. However, a negative history of penicillin allergy is no guarantee against a future allergic reaction.
• Obtain specimen for culture and sensitivity tests before giving first dose. Therapy may begin pending results.
• Give penicillin G sodium at least 1 hour before a bacteriostatic antibiotic.
• Observe patient closely. With large doses and prolonged therapy, bacterial or fungal superinfection may occur, especially in elderly, debilitated, or immunosuppressed patients.
• *Alert:* Institute seizure precautions. Patients with high blood levels of drug may develop seizures.
• *Alert:* Don't confuse drug with polycillin, penicillamine, or the various types of penicillin.

## I.V. administration
• Reconstitute drug with sterile water for injection, normal saline for injection, or D$_5$W. Check manufacturer's instructions for volume of diluent necessary to produce desired drug level.
• Give by intermittent I.V. infusion: Dilute drug in 50 to 100 ml, and give over 30 minutes to 2 hours q 4 to 6 hours.
• In neonates and children, give divided doses over 15 to 30 minutes.

## ✓ Patient teaching
• Tell patient to report adverse reactions promptly.
• Instruct patient to alert nurse if discomfort occurs at I.V. site.
• Warn patient receiving I.M. injection that the injection may be painful but that ice applied to site may help alleviate discomfort.

---

## penicillin V potassium (phenoxymethylpenicillin potassium)
Abbocillin VK‡, Apo-Pen VK†, Beepen-VK, Cilicaine VK‡, Nadopen-V-200†, Nadopen-V-400†, Novo-Pen-VK†, Nu-Pen-VK†, Pen Vee†, Pen• Vee K, PVF K†, PVK‡, V-Cillin K, Veetids**

*Pregnancy Risk Category B*

### HOW SUPPLIED
*Tablets:* 250 mg, 500 mg
*Tablets (film-coated):* 250 mg, 500 mg
*Capsules:* 250 mg‡
*Oral suspension:* 125 mg/5 ml, 250 mg/5 ml (after reconstitution)

### ACTION
A natural penicillin that inhibits cell-wall synthesis during microorganism multiplication. Bacteria resist penicillins by producing penicillinases—enzymes that convert penicillins to inactive penicillic acid.

| Route | Onset | Peak | Duration |
|-------|-------|------|----------|
| P.O. | Unknown | 0.5-1 hr | Unknown |

### INDICATIONS & DOSAGE
*Mild to moderate systemic infections—*
**Adults and children ages 12 and older:** 125 to 500 mg (400,000 to 800,000 U) P.O. q 6 hours.
**Children under age 12:** 15 to 62.5 mg/kg (25,000 to 100,000 U/kg) P.O. daily in divided doses q 6 to 8 hours.

### ADVERSE REACTIONS
**CNS:** neuropathy.
**GI:** *epigastric distress,* vomiting, diarrhea, *nausea,* black "hairy" tongue.
**GU:** nephropathy.
**Hematologic:** eosinophilia, hemolytic anemia, *leukopenia, thrombocytopenia.*
**Other:** *hypersensitivity reactions, anaphylaxis,* overgrowth of nonsusceptible organisms.

### INTERACTIONS
**Drug-drug.** *Oral contraceptives:* efficacy of oral contraceptives may be decreased. Recommend additional form of contraception during penicillin therapy.
*Probenecid:* increased blood levels of penicillin. Probenecid may be used for this purpose.

### EFFECTS ON DIAGNOSTIC TESTS
Drug interferes with turbidimetric methods using sulfosalicylic acid, trichloroacetic acid, acetic acid, and nitric acid. It does not interfere with tests using bromphenol blue (Albustix, Albutest, Multistix).

### CONTRAINDICATIONS
Contraindicated in patients with hypersensitivity to drug or other penicillins.

### NURSING CONSIDERATIONS
• Use cautiously in patients with other drug allergies, especially to cephalosporins (possible cross-sensitivity), and in those with GI disturbances.
• Before giving drug, ask patient about allergic reactions to penicillins. However, a negative history of penicillin allergy is no guarantee against a future allergic reaction.
• Obtain specimen for culture and sensitivity tests before giving first dose. Therapy may begin pending results.

---

Reactions may be *common,* uncommon, **life-threatening,** or COMMON AND LIFE-THREATENING.

- Give drug at least 1 hour before a bacteriostatic antibiotic.
- As ordered, periodically assess renal and hematopoietic function in patients receiving long-term therapy.
- Observe patient closely. With large doses and prolonged therapy, bacterial or fungal superinfection may occur, especially in elderly, debilitated, or immunosuppressed patients.
- The American Heart Association considers amoxicillin the preferred agent for endocarditis prophylaxis because GI absorption is better and serum levels are sustained longer. Penicillin V is considered an alternative agent.
- *Alert:* Don't confuse drug with polycillin, penicillamine, or the various types of penicillin.

### ☑ Patient teaching

- Instruct patient to take entire quantity of drug exactly as prescribed, even after he feels better.
- Tell patient to take drug with food if stomach upset occurs.
- Advise patient to notify doctor if rash, fever, or chills develop. A rash is the most common allergic reaction.

---

## piperacillin sodium
Pipracil, Pipril‡

*Pregnancy Risk Category B*

### HOW SUPPLIED
*Injection:* 2 g, 3 g, 4 g, 40 g

### ACTION
Extended-spectrum penicillin that inhibits cell-wall synthesis during microorganism multiplication. Bacteria resist penicillins by producing penicillinases—enzymes that convert penicillins to inactive penicillic acid.

| Route | Onset | Peak | Duration |
|-------|-------|------|----------|
| I.V. | Immediate | Immediate | Unknown |
| I.M. | Unknown | 30-50 min | Unknown |

### INDICATIONS & DOSAGE
*Systemic infections due to susceptible strains of gram-positive and especially gram-negative organisms (including* Proteus *and* Pseudomonas aeruginosa)—
**Adults and children over age 12:** 100 to 300 mg/kg (may go up to 600 mg/kg/day in cystic fibrosis patients) I.V. or I.M. daily in divided doses q 4 to 6 hours, not to exceed 24 g daily.
*Prophylaxis of surgical infections—*
**Adults:** 2 g I.V., given 30 to 60 minutes before surgery. Dose may be repeated during surgery and once or twice more after surgery.
*Adjust-a-dose:* For patients with creatinine clearance of 20 to 40 ml/minute, 3 to 4 g I.V. q 8 hours; if creatinine clearance is below 20 ml/minute, 3 to 4 g I.V. q 12 hours depending on severity of infection.

### ADVERSE REACTIONS
**CNS:** *seizures,* headache, dizziness, fatigue.
**CV:** vein irritation, phlebitis.
**GI:** nausea, diarrhea, vomiting, pseudomembranous colitis.
**GU:** interstitial nephritis.
**Hematologic:** *bleeding, neutropenia,* eosinophilia, *leukopenia, thrombocytopenia.*
**Hepatic:** transient elevations in liver function tests.
**Metabolic:** *hypokalemia,* hypernatremia.
**Musculoskeletal:** *prolonged muscle relaxation.*
**Other:** *hypersensitivity reactions, anaphylaxis,* overgrowth of nonsusceptible organisms, pain at injection site.

### INTERACTIONS
**Drug-drug.** *Oral contraceptives:* efficacy of oral contraceptives may be decreased. Recommend additional form of contraception during penicillin therapy.
*Probenecid:* increased blood levels of piperacillin. Probenecid may be used for this purpose.
*Vecuronium:* prolonged neuromuscular blockade: Don't use together.

### EFFECTS ON DIAGNOSTIC TESTS
Drug may falsely decrease serum aminoglycoside levels and may cause positive Coombs' tests.

---

## CONTRAINDICATIONS

Contraindicated in patients with hypersensitivity to drug or other penicillins.

## NURSING CONSIDERATIONS

• Use cautiously in patients with other drug allergies, especially to cephalosporins (possible cross-sensitivity), and in those with bleeding tendencies, uremia, and hypokalemia.
• Before giving drug, ask patient about allergic reactions to penicillin. However, a negative history of penicillin allergy is no guarantee against a future allergic reaction.
• Obtain specimen for culture and sensitivity tests before giving first dose. Therapy may begin pending results.
• Give piperacillin at least 1 hour before a bacteriostatic antibiotic.
• For I.M. injection, reconstitute with sterile or bacteriostatic water for injection, normal saline for injection (with or without preservative), or 0.5% to 1% lidocaine hydrochloride. Add 2 ml of diluent for each gram of drug. Final solution will contain 1 g/2.5 ml.
• Check CBC and platelet counts frequently, as ordered. Drug may cause thrombocytopenia.
• Monitor serum potassium and sodium levels.
• Monitor INR in patients receiving warfarin therapy because drug may prolong PT.
• *Alert:* Institute seizure precautions. Patients with high serum levels of drug may have seizures.
• Observe patient closely. With large doses and prolonged therapy, bacterial or fungal superinfection may occur, especially in elderly, debilitated, or immunosuppressed patients.
• Patients with cystic fibrosis tend to be most susceptible to fever or rash.
• Drug may be better suited for patients on sodium-free diets than ticarcillin (piperacillin contains 1.85 mEq of sodium/g).
• Keep in mind that piperacillin is typically used with another antibiotic such as gentamicin.

## I.V. administration

• Reconstitute each gram of drug with 5 ml of diluent, such as sterile or bacteriostatic water for injection, normal saline for injection (with or without preservative), $D_5W$, or dextrose 5% in normal saline for injection. Shake until dissolved. Inject reconstituted solution directly into a vein or into the tubing of a free-flowing I.V. solution over 3 to 5 minutes. Or, dilute with at least 50 ml of a compatible I.V. solution, and give by intermittent infusion over 30 minutes.
• Avoid continuous infusions to prevent vein irritation. Change site every 48 hours.
• Aminoglycoside antibiotics, such as gentamicin and tobramycin, are chemically incompatible with piperacillin. Don't mix in the same I.V. container.

## Patient teaching

• Tell patient to report adverse reactions promptly.
• Instruct patient receiving drug I.V. to report discomfort at I.V. site.
• Advise patient to limit salt intake during therapy because drug contains 1.85 mEq of sodium/g.

---

## piperacillin sodium/ tazobactam sodium
Zosyn

*Pregnancy Risk Category B*

### HOW SUPPLIED

*Powder for injection:* 2 g piperacillin and 0.25 g tazobactam per vial, 3 g piperacillin and 0.375 g tazobactam per vial, 4 g piperacillin and 0.5 g tazobactam per vial

### ACTION

Piperacillin is an extended-spectrum penicillin that inhibits cell-wall synthesis during microorganism multiplication. Tazobactam increases piperacillin's effectiveness by inactivating beta-lactamases, which destroy penicillins.

| Route | Onset | Peak | Duration |
|-------|-------|------|----------|
| I.V. | Immediate | Immediate | Unknown |

## INDICATIONS & DOSAGE

*Appendicitis (complicated by rupture or abscess) and peritonitis due to* Escherichia coli, Bacteroides fragilis, B. ovatus, B. thetaiotaomicron, *or* B. vulgatus; *skin and skin-structure infections due to* Staphylococcus aureus; *postpartum endometritis or pelvic inflammatory disease due to* E. coli; *moderately severe community-acquired pneumonia due to* Haemophilus influenzae—

**Adults:** 3 g piperacillin and 0.375 g tazobactam I.V. q 6 hours.

*Adjust-a-dose:* For renally impaired adults with creatinine clearance of 20 to 40 ml/minute, dosage is 2 g piperacillin and 0.25 g tazobactam I.V. q 6 hours; if it is below 20 ml/minute, 2 g piperacillin and 0.25 g tazobactam I.V. q 8 hours.

*Nosocomial pneumonia (moderate to severe) due to piperacillin-resistant, beta-lactamase-producing strains of* S. aureus—

**Adults:** initially, 3.375 g I.V. over 30 minutes q 4 hours. Administer with an aminoglycoside.

## ADVERSE REACTIONS

**CNS:** *headache, insomnia,* agitation, dizziness, anxiety.

**CV:** hypertension, tachycardia, chest pain, edema; inflammation, phlebitis at I.V. site.

**EENT:** rhinitis.

**GI:** *diarrhea, nausea, constipation,* vomiting, dyspepsia, stool changes, abdominal pain.

**GU:** interstitial nephritis, candidiasis.

**Hematologic:** *leukopenia,* anemia, eosinophilia, *thrombocytopenia.*

**Respiratory:** dyspnea.

**Skin:** rash, pruritus.

**Other:** fever; pain, *anaphylaxis.*

## INTERACTIONS

**Drug-drug.** *Oral anticoagulants:* prolonged effectiveness. Monitor PT and INR closely.

*Oral contraceptives:* efficacy of oral contraceptives may be decreased. Recommend additional form of contraception during penicillin therapy.

*Probenecid:* increased blood levels of piperacillin. Probenecid may be used for this purpose.

*Vecuronium:* prolonged neuromuscular blockade. Monitor closely.

## EFFECTS ON DIAGNOSTIC TESTS

As with other penicillins, piperacillin/ tazobactam may result in a false-positive reaction for urine glucose using a copper reduction method (such as Clinitest). Glucose tests based on enzymatic glucose oxidase reactions (such as Diastix) are recommended.

## CONTRAINDICATIONS

Contraindicated in patients with hypersensitivity to drug or other penicillins.

## NURSING CONSIDERATIONS

● Use cautiously in patients with other drug allergies, especially to cephalosporins (possible cross-sensitivity), and in those with bleeding tendencies, uremia, and hypokalemia.

● Obtain specimen for culture and sensitivity tests before giving first dose. Therapy may begin pending results.

● Because hemodialysis removes 6% of the piperacillin dose and 21% of the tazobactam dose, supplemental doses may be needed after hemodialysis.

● Observe patient closely. With large doses and prolonged therapy, bacterial and fungal superinfection may occur, especially in elderly, debilitated, or immunosuppressed patients.

● Drug contains 2.35 mEq sodium/g; monitor patient's sodium intake.

● There appears to be an increase of fever and rash in patients with cystic fibrosis. Monitor closely.

### I.V. administration

● Reconstitute each gram of piperacillin with 5 ml of diluent, such as sterile or bacteriostatic water for injection, normal saline for injection, bacteriostatic normal saline for injection, $D_5W$, dextrose 5% in normal saline for injection, or dextran 6% in normal saline for injection. Don't use lactated Ringer's injection. Shake until dissolved. Further dilute to a final volume of 50 ml before infusion.

• Infuse over at least 30 minutes. Discontinue any primary infusion during administration if possible. Don't mix with other drugs. Aminoglycoside antibiotics (such as amikacin, gentamicin, and tobramycin) are chemically incompatible with this drug. Don't mix in the same I.V. container.
• Use drug immediately after reconstitution. Discard unused drug after 24 hours if stored at room temperature or 48 hours if refrigerated. Once diluted, drug is stable in I.V. bags for 24 hours at room temperature or 1 week if refrigerated.
• Change I.V. site every 48 hours.

✓ **Patient teaching**
• Tell patient to report adverse reactions promptly.
• Instruct patient to alert nurse if discomfort occurs at I.V. site.

## ticarcillin disodium
Ticar

*Pregnancy Risk Category B*

### HOW SUPPLIED
*Injection:* 1 g, 3 g, 6 g
*I.V. infusion:* 3 g

### ACTION
An extended-spectrum penicillin that inhibits cell-wall synthesis during microorganism multiplication. Bacteria resist penicillins by producing penicillinases—enzymes that convert penicillins to inactive penicillic acid.

| Route | Onset | Peak | Duration |
|-------|-------|------|----------|
| I.V. | Immediate | Immediate | Unknown |
| I.M. | Unknown | 30-75 min | Unknown |

### INDICATIONS & DOSAGE
*Severe systemic infections due to susceptible strains of gram-positive and especially gram-negative organisms (including* Pseudomonas *and* Proteus)—
**Adults:** 200 to 300 mg/kg I.V. daily in divided doses q 4 to 6 hours.
**Children:** 50 to 300 mg/kg I.V. daily in divided doses q 4 to 6 hours.
*Adjust-a-dose:* For patients with renal failure, if creatinine clearance is 30 to 60 ml/minute, dosage is 2 g I.V. q 4 hours; if clearance is 10 to 29 ml/minute, 2 g I.V. q 8 hours; and if it is below 10 ml/minute, 2 g I.V. q 12 hours or 1 g I.M. q 6 hours.

### ADVERSE REACTIONS
**CNS:** *seizures,* neuromuscular excitability.
**CV:** vein irritation, phlebitis.
**GI:** nausea, diarrhea, vomiting, pseudomembranous colitis.
**Hematologic:** *leukopenia, neutropenia,* eosinophilia, *thrombocytopenia,* hemolytic anemia.
**Hepatic:** transient elevations in liver function studies.
**Metabolic:** hypokalemia, hypernatremia.
**Other:** *hypersensitivity reactions, anaphylaxis,* overgrowth of nonsusceptible organisms, pain at injection site.

### INTERACTIONS
**Drug-drug.** *Lithium:* altered renal elimination of lithium. Monitor serum lithium levels closely.
*Oral contraceptives:* efficacy of oral contraceptives may be decreased. Recommend additional form of contraception during penicillin therapy.
*Probenecid:* increased blood levels of ticarcillin and other penicillins. Probenecid may be used for this purpose.

### EFFECTS ON DIAGNOSTIC TESTS
Ticarcillin interferes with turbidimetric methods that use sulfosalicylic acid, trichloroacetic acid, acetic acid, or nitric acid. Ticarcillin does not interfere with tests using bromphenol blue (Albustix, Albutest, Multistix). Ticarcillin may falsely decrease serum aminoglycoside concentrations. Systemic effects of ticarcillin may cause positive Coombs' test.

### CONTRAINDICATIONS
Contraindicated in patients with hypersensitivity to drug or other penicillins.

### NURSING CONSIDERATIONS
• Use cautiously in patients with other drug allergies, especially to cephalosporins (possible cross-sensitivity), and in those with impaired renal function, hemorrhagic conditions, hypokalemia, or

---

Reactions may be *common,* uncommon, *life-threatening,* or COMMON AND LIFE-THREATENING.

sodium restrictions (drug contains 5.2 to 6.5 mEq sodium/g).

• Before giving drug, ask patient about allergic reactions to penicillin. However, a negative history of penicillin allergy is no guarantee against a future allergic reaction.

• Obtain specimen for culture and sensitivity tests before giving first dose. Therapy may begin pending results.

• Give ticarcillin at least 1 hour before a bacteriostatic antibiotic.

• For I.M. injection, reconstitute drug using sterile water for injection, normal saline for injection, or lidocaine 1% (without epinephrine). Use 2 ml diluent for each gram of drug. Give deeply I.M. into large muscle. Don't exceed 2 g per injection.

• Monitor serum potassium and sodium levels.

• Check CBC and platelet counts frequently, as ordered. Drug may cause thrombocytopenia.

• *Alert:* Institute seizure precautions. Patients with high blood levels of ticarcillin may develop seizures.

• Ticarcillin is typically used with another antibiotic such as gentamicin.

• Observe patient closely. With large doses and prolonged therapy, bacterial or fungal superinfection may occur, especially in elderly, debilitated, or immunosuppressed patients.

• Monitor INR in patients receiving warfarin therapy because drug may prolong PT.

**◖ I.V. administration**
• Reconstitute drug using D5W, normal saline injection, sterile water for injection, or other compatible solution. Add 4 ml of diluent for each gram of drug. Further dilute to a maximum concentration of 50 mg/ml, and inject slowly directly into a vein or into the tubing of a free-flowing I.V. solution. Or, dilute to a concentration of 10 to 100 mg/ml, and give by intermittent infusion over 30 to 120 minutes in adults or 10 to 20 minutes in neonates.

• Aminoglycoside antibiotics (such as amikacin, gentamicin, and tobramycin) are chemically incompatible with this drug. Don't mix in the same I.V. container.

• Avoid continuous infusion to prevent vein irritation. Change site every 48 hours.

**☑ Patient teaching**
• Tell patient to report adverse reactions promptly.
• Instruct patient to alert nurse if discomfort occurs at I.V. insertion site.

---

## ticarcillin disodium/ clavulanate potassium
Timentin

*Pregnancy Risk Category B*

### HOW SUPPLIED
*Injection:* 3 g ticarcillin and 100 mg clavulanic acid in 3.1-g and 31-g vials
*Premixed:* 3.1 g/100 ml

### ACTION
Ticarcillin is an extended-spectrum penicillin that inhibits cell-wall synthesis during microorganism replication. Clavulanic acid increases ticarcillin's effectiveness by inactivating beta-lactamases, which destroy ticarcillin.

| Route | Onset | Peak | Duration |
|-------|-------|------|----------|
| I.V. | Immediate | Immediate | Unknown |

### INDICATIONS & DOSAGE
*Lower respiratory tract, urinary tract, bone and joint, and skin and skin-structure infections and septicemia when due to beta-lactamase-producing strains of bacteria or by ticarcillin-susceptible organisms—*
**Adults:** 3.1 g (3 g ticarcillin and 100 mg clavulanic acid) administered by I.V. infusion q 4 to 6 hours.
*Adjust-a-dose:* For patients with renal failure, if creatinine clearance is 30 to 60 ml/minute, dosage is 2 g I.V. q 4 hours; if it is 10 to 29 ml/minute, 2 g I.V. q 8 hours; and if it is below 10 ml/minute, 2 g I.V. q 12 hours (with hepatic dysfunction, q 24 hours).

### ADVERSE REACTIONS
**CNS:** *seizures,* neuromuscular excitability, headache, giddiness.

---

**CV:** vein irritation, phlebitis.
**GI:** nausea, diarrhea, stomatitis, vomiting, epigastric pain, flatulence, pseudomembranous colitis, taste and smell disturbances.
**Hematologic:** *leukopenia, neutropenia,* eosinophilia, *thrombocytopenia,* hemolytic anemia, anemia.
**Hepatic:** transient elevations in liver function studies.
**Metabolic:** hypokalemia, hypernatremia.
**Other:** *hypersensitivity reactions, anaphylaxis,* overgrowth of nonsusceptible organisms, pain at injection site.

## INTERACTIONS
**Drug-drug.** *Oral contraceptives:* efficacy of oral contraceptives may be decreased. Recommend additional form of contraception during penicillin therapy.
*Probenecid:* increased blood levels of ticarcillin. Probenecid may be used for this purpose.

## EFFECTS ON DIAGNOSTIC TESTS
Drug interferes with turbidimetric methods that use sulfosalicylic acid, trichloroacetic acid, acetic acid, or nitric acid. Drug does not interfere with tests using bromphenol blue (Albustix, Albutest, Multistix). Systemic effects of drug may cause positive Coombs' test.

## CONTRAINDICATIONS
Contraindicated in patients with hypersensitivity to drug or other penicillins.

## NURSING CONSIDERATIONS
• Use cautiously in patients with other drug allergies, especially to cephalosporins (possible cross-sensitivity), and in those with impaired renal function, hemorrhagic conditions, hypokalemia, or sodium restrictions (drug contains 4.5 mEq sodium/g).
• Before giving drug, ask patient about allergic reactions to penicillin. However, a negative history of penicillin allergy is no guarantee against a future allergic reaction.
• Obtain specimen for culture and sensitivity tests before giving first dose. Therapy may begin pending results.

• Give drug at least 1 hour before a bacteriostatic antibiotic.
• Check CBC and platelet counts frequently, as ordered. Drug may cause thrombocytopenia.
• Monitor serum potassium.
• Observe patient closely. With large doses and prolonged therapy, bacterial or fungal superinfection may occur, especially in elderly, debilitated, or immunosuppressed patients.

### I.V. administration
• Reconstitute drug with 13 ml of sterile water for injection or normal saline for injection. Further dilute to a maximum of 10 to 100 mg/ml (based on ticarcillin component), and administer by I.V. infusion over 30 minutes. In fluid restricted patients, dilute to a maximum of 48 mg/ml if using $D_5W$, 43 mg/ml if using normal saline for injection, or 86 mg/ml if using sterile water for injection.
• Drug is chemically incompatible with aminoglycoside antibiotics (amikacin, gentamicin, tobramycin). Don't mix in the same I.V. container.

### Patient teaching
• Tell patient to report adverse reactions promptly.
• Instruct patient to alert nurse if discomfort occurs at I.V. site.
• Advise patient to limit salt intake during drug therapy because of high sodium content.

---

Reactions may be *common*, uncommon, *life-threatening*, or COMMON AND LIFE-THREATENING.

cefaclor
cefadroxil
cefazolin sodium
cefdinir
cefepime hydrochloride
cefixime
cefmetazole sodium
cefonicid sodium
cefoperazone sodium
cefotaxime sodium
cefotetan disodium
cefoxitin sodium
cefpodoxime proxetil
cefprozil
ceftazidime
ceftibuten
ceftizoxime sodium
ceftriaxone sodium
cefuroxime axetil
cefuroxime sodium
cephalexin hydrochloride
cephalexin monohydrate
cephradine
loracarbef

**COMBINATION PRODUCTS**
None.

---

cefaclor
Ceclor, Distaclor§, Distaclor MR§

*Pregnancy Risk Category B*

**HOW SUPPLIED**
*Capsules*: 250 mg, 500 mg
*Tablets (extended-release):* 375 mg, 500 mg
*Oral suspension:* 125 mg/5 ml, 187 mg/ 5 ml, 250 mg/5 ml, 375 mg/5 ml

**ACTION**
A second-generation cephalosporin that inhibits cell-wall synthesis, promoting osmotic instability; usually bactericidal.

| Route | Onset | Peak | Duration |
|-------|-------|------|----------|
| P.O. | Unknown | 0.5-1 hr | Unknown |
| P.O. (extended) | Unknown | 1.5-2.5 hr | Unknown |

**INDICATIONS & DOSAGE**
*Respiratory or urinary tract, skin, and soft-tissue infections and otitis media due to* Haemophilus influenzae, Streptococcus pneumoniae, S. pyogenes, Escherichia coli, Proteus mirabilis, Klebsiella *species, and staphylococci—*
**Adults:** 250 to 500 mg P.O. q 8 hours. For pharyngitis or otitis media, daily dose may be given in two equally divided doses q 12 hours. For extended-release forms, 500 mg P.O. q 12 hours for 7 days for bronchitis; for pharyngitis or skin and skin-structure infections, 375 mg P.O. q 12 hours for 10 days and 7 to 10 days, respectively.
**Children:** 20 mg/kg daily P.O. in divided doses q 8 hours. For pharyngitis or otitis media, daily dose may be given in two equally divided doses q 12 hours. In more serious infections, 40 mg/kg daily are recommended, not to exceed 1 g daily.

**ADVERSE REACTIONS**
**CNS:** dizziness, headache, somnolence, malaise.
**GI:** *nausea,* vomiting, *diarrhea,* anorexia, dyspepsia, abdominal cramps, pseudomembranous colitis, oral candidiasis.
**GU:** vaginal candidiasis, vaginitis.
**Hematologic:** *transient leukopenia,* anemia, eosinophilia, *thrombocytopenia,* lymphocytosis.
**Hepatic:** transient increases in liver enzymes.
**Skin:** *maculopapular rash,* dermatitis, pruritus.
**Other***: hypersensitivity reactions (serum sickness, anaphylaxis),* fever.

**INTERACTIONS**
**Drug-drug.** *Antacids:* absorption of extended-release cefaclor is decreased if

---

\*Liquid contains alcohol.    \*\*May contain tartrazine.    †Canada    ‡Australia    §U.K.    ◊OTC

taken within 1 hour. Separate administration by 1 hour.
*Chloramphenicol:* antagonistic effect. Don't use together.
*Probenecid:* may inhibit excretion and increase blood levels of cefaclor. Monitor patient.

## EFFECTS ON DIAGNOSTIC TESTS
Cefaclor may cause false-positive Coombs' test results and false-positive results in urine glucose tests using cupric sulfate (Benedict's reagent or Clinitest); use glucose oxidase tests (Diastix or Chemstrip uG) instead. Drug also causes false elevations in serum or urine creatinine levels in tests using Jaffé's reaction.

## CONTRAINDICATIONS
Contraindicated in patients with hypersensitivity to drug or other cephalosporins.

## NURSING CONSIDERATIONS
• Use cautiously in patients with impaired renal function or a history of sensitivity to penicillin and in breast-feeding women.
• Obtain specimen for culture and sensitivity tests before giving first dose. Therapy may begin pending results.
• With large doses or prolonged therapy, monitor for superinfection, especially in high-risk patients.
• Store reconstituted suspension in refrigerator. Suspension is stable for 14 days if refrigerated. Shake well before use.
• *Alert:* Don't confuse drug with other cephalosporins that sound alike.

☑**Patient teaching**
• Tell patient to take entire amount of drug exactly as prescribed, even after he feels better.
• Tell patient that drug may be taken with meals. If suspension is used, instruct him to shake container well before measuring dose and to keep the drug refrigerated.
• Advise patient to notify doctor if rash develops or signs and symptoms of superinfection appear.
• Inform patient not to crush, cut, or chew extended-release tablets.

# cefadroxil
Duricef

*Pregnancy Risk Category B*

## HOW SUPPLIED
*Tablets:* 1 g
*Capsules:* 500 mg
*Oral suspension:* 125 mg/5 ml, 250 mg/5 ml, 500 mg/5 ml

## ACTION
A first-generation cephalosporin that inhibits cell-wall synthesis, promoting osmotic instability; usually bactericidal.

| Route | Onset | Peak | Duration |
|-------|-------|------|----------|
| P.O. | Unknown | 1-2 hr | Unknown |

## INDICATIONS & DOSAGE
*Urinary tract infections due to* Escherichia coli, Proteus mirabilis, *and* Klebsiella *species; skin and soft-tissue infections due to staphylococci and streptococci; pharyngitis or tonsillitis due to group A beta-hemolytic streptococci—*
**Adults:** 1 to 2 g P.O. daily, depending on infection being treated. Usually given once daily or b.i.d.
**Children:** 30 mg/kg P.O. daily in two divided doses q 12 hours.
*Adjust-a-dose:* For renally impaired patients with creatinine clearance of 25 to 50 ml/minute, 1 g P.O. followed by 500 mg q 12 hours; if clearance is between 10 and 24 ml/minute, 500 mg q 24 hours; and if it is below 10 ml/minute, 500 mg q 36 hours.

## ADVERSE REACTIONS
**CNS:** *seizures.*
**GI:** pseudomembranous colitis, *nausea,* vomiting, *diarrhea,* glossitis, abdominal cramps, oral candidiasis.
**GU:** genital pruritus, candidiasis, vaginitis, renal dysfunction.
**Hematologic:** *transient neutropenia,* eosinophilia, *leukopenia,* anemia, *agranulocytosis, thrombocytopenia.*
**Hepatic:** transient increases in liver enzymes.
**Respiratory:** dyspnea.

---

Reactions may be *common,* uncommon, *life-threatening,* or COMMON AND LIFE-THREATENING.

**Skin:** *maculopapular and erythematous rashes,* urticaria.
**Other:** *hypersensitivity reactions, anaphylaxis, angioedema,* fever.

## INTERACTIONS
**Drug-drug.** *Probenecid:* may inhibit excretion and increase blood levels of cefadroxil. Use together cautiously.

## EFFECTS ON DIAGNOSTIC TESTS
Cefadroxil causes false-positive results in urine glucose tests using cupric sulfate (Benedict's reagent or Clinitest); use glucose oxidase test (Diastix or Chemstrip uG) instead. Drug causes false elevations in serum or urine creatinine levels in tests using Jaffé's reaction. Positive Coombs' test results occur in about 3% of patients taking cephalosporins.

## CONTRAINDICATIONS
Contraindicated in patients with hypersensitivity to drug or other cephalosporins.

## NURSING CONSIDERATIONS
• Use cautiously in patients with a history of sensitivity to penicillin and in breast-feeding women. Also use cautiously in patients with impaired renal function; dosage adjustments may be necessary.
• Obtain specimen for culture and sensitivity tests before giving first dose. Therapy may begin pending results.
• If creatinine clearance is below 50 ml/minute, dosage interval should be lengthened so drug doesn't accumulate. Monitor renal function in patients with renal dysfunction.
• With large doses or prolonged therapy, monitor for superinfection, especially in high-risk patients.
• **Alert:** Don't confuse drug with other cephalosporins that sound alike.

☑ **Patient teaching**
• Instruct patient to take drug with food or milk to lessen GI discomfort.
• Tell patient to take entire amount of drug exactly as prescribed, even after he feels better.
• Advise patient to notify doctor if rash develops or if signs and symptoms of su-

perinfection, such as recurring fever, chills, and malaise appear.

---

### cefazolin sodium
Ancef, Kefzol, Zolicef

*Pregnancy Risk Category B*

## HOW SUPPLIED
*Injection (parenteral):* 250 mg, 500 mg, 1 g, 5 g, 10 g, 20 g
*Infusion:* 500 mg/50-ml vial, 1 g/50-ml vial

## ACTION
A first-generation cephalosporin that inhibits cell-wall synthesis, promoting osmotic instability; usually bactericidal.

| Route | Onset | Peak | Duration |
|-------|-------|------|----------|
| I.V. | Immediate | Immediate | Unknown |
| I.M. | Unknown | 1-2 hr | Unknown |

## INDICATIONS & DOSAGE
*Perioperative prophylaxis in contaminated surgery—*
**Adults:** 1 g I.M. or I.V. 30 to 60 minutes before surgery; then 0.5 to 1 g I.M. or I.V. q 6 to 8 hours for 24 hours. In long operations (over 2 hours), another 0.5- to 1-g I.M. or I.V. dose may be administered intraoperatively.
   *Note:* In cases in which infection would be devastating, prophylaxis may be continued for 3 to 5 days.
*Serious infections of respiratory, biliary, and GU tracts; skin, soft-tissue, bone, and joint infections; septicemia; endocarditis due to* Escherichia coli, Enterobacteriaceae, *gonococci,* Haemophilus influenzae, Klebsiella, Proteus mirabilis, Staphylococcus aureus, Streptococcus pneumoniae, *and group A beta-hemolytic streptococci—*
**Adults:** 250 mg I.M. or I.V. q 8 hours to 1.5 g I.M. or I.V. q 6 hours. Maximum 12 g/day in life-threatening situations.
**Children over age 1 month:** 25 to 50 mg/kg/day I.M. or I.V. in three or four divided doses. In severe infections, dose may be increased to 100 mg/kg/day.
*Adjust-a-dose:* For patients with renal failure with creatinine clearance of 35 to

---

*Liquid contains alcohol.   **May contain tartrazine.   †Canada   ‡Australia   §U.K.   ◊OTC

54 ml/minute, give full dose q 8 hours; if clearance is 11 to 34 ml/minute, give 50% usual dose q 12 hours; if clearance is below 10 ml/minute, give 50% of usual dose q 18 to 24 hours.

## ADVERSE REACTIONS
**CV:** *phlebitis, thrombophlebitis with I.V. injection.*
**GI:** pseudomembranous colitis, nausea, anorexia, vomiting, *diarrhea*, glossitis, dyspepsia, abdominal cramps, anal pruritus, oral candidiasis.
**GU:** genital pruritus, candidiasis, vaginitis.
**Hematologic:** *neutropenia, leukopenia,* eosinophilia, *thrombocytopenia.*
**Hepatic:** transient increases in liver enzymes.
**Skin:** *maculopapular and erythematous rashes, urticaria, pruritus, pain, induration, sterile abscesses, tissue sloughing at injection site,* **Stevens-Johnson syndrome.**
**Other:** *hypersensitivity reactions, serum sickness, anaphylaxis.*

## INTERACTIONS
**Drug-drug.** *Probenecid:* may inhibit excretion and increase blood levels of cefazolin. Use cautiously.

## EFFECTS ON DIAGNOSTIC TESTS
Cephalosporins cause false-positive results in urine glucose tests using cupric sulfate (Benedict's reagent or Clinitest); use glucose oxidase tests (Diastix or Chemstrip uG) instead. Drug causes false elevations in serum or urine creatinine levels in tests using Jaffé's reaction. Drug also causes positive Coombs' test results.

## CONTRAINDICATIONS
Contraindicated in patients with hypersensitivity to drug or other cephalosporins.

## NURSING CONSIDERATIONS
• Use cautiously in patients with a history of sensitivity to penicillin and in breast-feeding women. Also use cautiously and with dosage adjustments in patients with renal failure.

• Obtain specimen for culture and sensitivity tests before giving first dose. Therapy may begin pending results.
• Dose and dosing interval will be adjusted if creatinine clearance is below 55 ml/minute.
• After reconstitution, inject drug I.M. without further dilution (this drug is not as painful as other cephalosporins). Administer injection deeply into a large muscle mass, such as the gluteus maximus or lateral aspect of the thigh.
• With large doses or prolonged therapy, monitor for superinfection, especially in high-risk patients.
• *Alert:* Don't confuse drug with other cephalosporins that sound alike.

### I.V. administration
• Reconstitute drug with sterile water, bacteriostatic water, or normal saline solution as follows: 2 ml to 500-mg vial; 2.5 ml to 1-g vial. Shake well until dissolved. Resultant concentration: 225 mg/ml or 330 mg/ml, respectively.
• Reconstituted cefazolin is stable for 24 hours at room temperature or 96 hours under refrigeration.
• For direct injection, further dilute Ancef with 5 ml, or Kefzol with 10 ml, of sterile water for injection. Inject into a large vein or into the tubing of a free-flowing I.V. solution over 3 to 5 minutes. For intermittent infusion, add reconstituted drug to 50 to 100 ml of compatible solution or use premixed solution. Commercially available frozen solutions of cefazolin in $D_5W$ should be given only by intermittent or continuous I.V. infusion.
• Alternate injection sites if I.V. therapy lasts longer than 3 days. Use of small I.V. needles in larger available veins may be preferable.

### Patient teaching
• Instruct patient to report adverse reactions promptly.
• Tell patient to alert nurse if discomfort occurs at I.V. injection site.

---

Reactions may be *common,* uncommon, **life-threatening,** or COMMON AND LIFE-THREATENING.

## cefdinir
Omnicef

*Pregnancy Risk Category B*

### HOW SUPPLIED
*Capsules:* 300 mg
*Suspension:* 125 mg/5 ml

### ACTION
A third-generation cephalosporin whose bactericidal activity results from inhibition of cell-wall synthesis. Drug is stable in the presence of some beta-lactamase enzymes, causing some microorganisms resistant to penicillins and cephalosporins to be susceptible to cefdinir. Excluding *Pseudomonas, Enterobacter, Enterococcus,* and methicillin-resistant *Staphylococcus* species, cefdinir's spectrum of activity includes a broad range of gram-positive and gram-negative aerobic microorganisms.

| Route | Onset | Peak | Duration |
|-------|-------|------|----------|
| P.O. | Unknown | 2-4 hr | Unknown |

### INDICATIONS & DOSAGE
*Mild to moderate infections due to susceptible strains of microorganisms for conditions of community-acquired pneumonia, acute exacerbations of chronic bronchitis, acute maxillary sinusitis, acute bacterial otitis media, and uncomplicated skin and skin-structure infections—*
**Adults and children ages 13 and older:** 300 mg P.O. q 12 hours; or 600 mg P.O. q 24 hours for 10 days. (Use q 12-hour dosages for pneumonia and skin infections.)
**Children ages 6 months to 12 years:** 7 mg/kg P.O. q 12 hours or 14 mg/kg P.O. q 24 hours for 10 days, up to maximum dose of 600 mg daily. (Use q 12-hour dosages for skin infections.)
*Pharyngitis, tonsillitis—*
**Adults and children ages 13 and older:** 300 mg P.O. q 12 hours for 5 to 10 days; or 600 mg P.O. q 24 hours for 10 days.
**Children ages 6 months to 12 years:** 7 mg/kg P.O. q 12 hours for 5 to 10 days; or 14 mg/kg P.O. q 24 hours for 10 days.

*Adjust-a-dose:* If creatinine clearance is below 30 ml/minute, dosage is reduced to 300 mg P.O. once daily for adults and 7 mg/kg (up to 300 mg) P.O. once daily for children. In patients receiving chronic hemodialysis, dosage is 300 mg or 7 mg/kg P.O. at end of each dialysis session and subsequently every other day.

### ADVERSE REACTIONS
**CNS:** headache.
**GI:** abdominal pain, *diarrhea,* nausea, vomiting.
**GU:** vaginal candidiasis, vaginitis, increased urine proteins and RBCs.
**Hepatic:** elevated GGT and alkaline phosphatase.
**Skin:** rash, cutaneous candidiasis.

### INTERACTIONS
**Drug-drug.** *Antacids (magnesium- and aluminum-containing), iron supplements, multivitamins containing iron:* decrease cefdinir's rate of absorption and bioavailability; administer such preparations 2 hours before or after cefdinir dose.
*Probenecid:* inhibits the renal excretion of cefdinir. Monitor patient.

### EFFECTS ON DIAGNOSTIC TESTS
False positive reaction for ketones (tests using nitroprusside only) and glucose (Clinitest, Benedict's or Fehling's solution) in urine may occur. Cephalosporins may occasionally induce a positive direct Coombs' test.

### CONTRAINDICATIONS
Contraindicated in patients with known allergy to cephalosporins.

### NURSING CONSIDERATIONS
• Use cautiously in patients with known hypersensitivity to penicillin because of the possibility of cross-sensitivity with other beta-lactam antibiotics. Also use with caution in patients with history of colitis and renal insufficiency.
• Prolonged drug treatment may result in possible emergence and overgrowth of resistant organisms. Monitor for signs and symptoms of superinfection.
• Pseudomembranous colitis has been reported with cefdinir and should be con-

sidered in patients with diarrhea subsequent to antibiotic therapy or in those with history of colitis.

• *Alert:* Don't confuse drug with other cephalosporins that sound alike.

### ☑ Patient teaching
• Instruct patient to take antacids and iron supplements 2 hours before or after a dose of cefdinir.
• Inform diabetic patient that each teaspoon of suspension contains 2.86 g of sucrose.
• Tell patient that drug may be taken without regard to meals.
• Advise patient to report severe diarrhea or diarrhea accompanied by abdominal pain.
• Tell patient to report adverse reactions or signs and symptoms of superinfection promptly.

---

## cefepime hydrochloride
Maxipime

*Pregnancy Risk Category B*

### HOW SUPPLIED
*Injection:* 500 mg/vial, 1 g/100-ml piggyback bottle, 1 g/ADD-Vantage vial, 1 g/15-ml vial, 2 g/100-ml piggyback bottle, 2 g/vial

### ACTION
A fourth-generation cephalosporin that inhibits bacterial cell-wall synthesis, promotes osmotic instability, and destroys bacteria.

| Route | Onset | Peak | Duration |
|-------|-------|------|----------|
| I.V., I.M. | 0.5 hr | 1-2 hr | Unknown |

### INDICATIONS & DOSAGE
*Mild to moderate urinary tract infections due to* Escherichia coli, Klebsiella pneumoniae, *or* Proteus mirabilis, *including cases associated with concurrent bacteremia with these microorganisms*—
**Adults and children ages 12 and older:** 0.5 to 1 g I.M. (I.M. route used only for infections due to *E. coli*); or I.V. infused over 30 minutes q 12 hours for 7 to 10 days.

*Severe urinary tract infections, including pyelonephritis, due to* E. coli *or* K. pneumoniae—
**Adults and children ages 12 and older:** 2 g I.V. infused over 30 minutes q 12 hours for 10 days.
*Moderate to severe pneumonia due to* Streptococcus pneumoniae, Pseudomonas aeruginosa, K. pneumoniae, *or* Enterobacter *species*—
**Adults and children ages 12 and older:** 1 to 2 g I.V. infused over 30 minutes q 12 hours for 10 days.
*Moderate to severe skin infections, uncomplicated skin infections, and skin-structure infections due to* Staphylococcus aureus *(methicillin-susceptible strains only) or* S. pyogenes—
**Adults and children ages 12 and older:** 2 g I.V. infused over 30 minutes q 12 hours for 10 days.
*Complicated intra-abdominal infections (used with metronidazole) due to* E. coli, viridans group streptococci, P. aeruginosa, K. pneumoniae, Enterobacter *species, or* B. fragilis—
**Adults:** 2 g I.V. infused over 30 minutes q 12 hours for 7 to 10 days.
❋ *NEW INDICATION: Uncomplicated and complicated urinary tract infections (including pyelonephritis), uncomplicated skin and skin-structure infections, and pneumonia; as empiric therapy for febrile neutropenic children*—
**Children ages 2 months to 16 years weighing up to 40 kg (88 lb):** 50 mg/kg/dose I.V. infused over 30 minutes q 12 hours (q 8 hours for febrile neutropenia) for 7 to 10 days; dosage shouldn't exceed the recommended adult dosage (2 g/dose).
*Adjust-a-dose:* For renally impaired patients with creatinine clearance of 30 to 60 ml/minute, give full dose q 24 hours; if clearance is 11 to 29 ml/minute, give 50% usual dose q 24 hours; and if clearance is below 11 ml/minute, give 25% of usual dose q 24 hours.

### ADVERSE REACTIONS
**CNS:** headache.
**CV:** phlebitis.
**GI:** colitis, diarrhea, nausea, vomiting, oral candidiasis.

---

Reactions may be *common*, uncommon, *life-threatening*, or COMMON AND LIFE-THREATENING.

**GU:** vaginitis.
**Skin:** rash, pruritus, urticaria.
**Other:** pain, inflammation, fever.

## INTERACTIONS
**Drug-drug.** *Aminoglycosides:* may increase risk of nephrotoxicity. Monitor renal function closely.
*Potent diuretics (such as furosemide):* may increase risk of nephrotoxicity. Monitor renal function closely.

## EFFECTS ON DIAGNOSTIC TESTS
Cefepime may cause a false-positive reaction for glucose in the urine when using Clinitest tablets. Glucose tests based on enzymatic glucose oxidase reactions (such as Diastix or Chemstrip uG) should be used instead. A positive direct Coombs' test may occur during treatment with drug.

## CONTRAINDICATIONS
Contraindicated in patients with hypersensitivity to drug, other cephalosporins or beta-lactam antibiotics, or penicillins.

## NURSING CONSIDERATIONS
• Use cautiously in patients with renal impairment, poor nutrition, or history of GI disease (particularly colitis); in those receiving a protracted course of antimicrobial therapy; and in breast-feeding women.
• Safety of drug in children under age 12 has not been established.
• Obtain culture and sensitivity tests before giving first dose, if appropriate. Therapy may begin pending results.
• Dosage adjustment is necessary in patients with impaired renal function. Monitor renal function.
• For I.M. administration, constitute drug using sterile water for injection, normal saline for injection, 5% dextrose injection, 0.5% or 1% lidocaine hydrochloride, or bacteriostatic water for injection with parabens or benzyl alcohol. Follow manufacturer's guidelines for quantity of diluent to use.
• Inspect solution for particulate matter before use. The powder and its solutions tend to darken, depending on storage conditions. Product potency is not adversely affected when stored as recommended.
• Monitor patient for superinfection. Drug may cause overgrowth of nonsusceptible bacteria or fungi.
• Many cephalosporins can reduce PT activity. Patients at risk include those with renal or hepatic impairment or poor nutrition and those receiving prolonged cefepime therapy. Monitor PT and INR in these patients as ordered. Administer exogenous vitamin K as indicated and ordered.
• *Alert:* Don't confuse drug with other cephalosporins that sound alike.

## I.V. administration
• Follow manufacturer's guidelines closely when reconstituting drug. Variations occur in constituting drug for administration, depending on concentration of drug ordered and how drug is packaged (piggyback vial, ADD-Vantage vial, or regular vial). Also be aware that the type of diluent used for constitution varies, depending on the product used. Use only solutions recommended by the manufacturer. The resulting solution should be administered over about 30 minutes.
• Intermittent I.V. infusion with a Y-type administration set can be accomplished with compatible solutions. However, during infusion of a solution containing cefepime, discontinuing the other solution is recommended.

## Patient teaching
• Warn patient receiving drug I.M. that pain may occur at injection site.
• Instruct patient to report signs and symptoms of superinfection or GI disturbance.

---

**cefixime**
Suprax

*Pregnancy Risk Category B*

## HOW SUPPLIED
*Tablets:* 200 mg, 400 mg
*Oral suspension:* 100 mg/5 ml (after reconstitution)

---

## ACTION
A third-generation cephalosporin that inhibits cell-wall synthesis, promoting osmotic instability; usually bactericidal.

| Route | Onset | Peak | Duration |
|-------|-------|------|----------|
| P.O. | Unknown | 3.1-4.4 hr | Unknown |

## INDICATIONS & DOSAGE
*Uncomplicated urinary tract infections due to* Escherichia coli *and* Proteus mirabilis; *otitis media due to* Haemophilus influenzae *(beta-lactamase positive and negative strains),* Moraxella (Branhamella) catarrhalis, *and* Streptococcus pyogenes; *pharyngitis and tonsillitis due to* S. pyogenes; *acute bronchitis and acute exacerbations of chronic bronchitis due to* S. pneumoniae *and* H. influenzae *(beta-lactamase positive and negative strains)*—

**Adults and children over age 12 or weighing over 50 kg (110 lb):** 400 mg/day P.O. as a single 400-mg tablet or 200 mg q 12 hours.

**Children ages 12 and less or weighing 50 kg or less:** 8 mg/kg/day suspension P.O. as a single daily dose or 4 mg/kg q 12 hours.

*Uncomplicated gonorrhea due to* Neisseria gonorrhoeae—

**Adults:** 400 mg P.O. as a single dose.

*Adjust-a-dose:* For patients with renal failure, if creatinine clearance is 21 to 60 ml/minute or patient undergoes hemodialysis, give 75% of dose at usual intervals; if less than 20 ml/minute, give 50% of usual dose at usual intervals.

## ADVERSE REACTIONS
**CNS:** headache, dizziness.
**GI:** *diarrhea,* loose stools, abdominal pain, nausea, vomiting, dyspepsia, flatulence, pseudomembranous colitis.
**GU:** genital pruritus, vaginitis, genital candidiasis, transient increases in BUN and serum creatinine levels.
**Hematologic:** *thrombocytopenia, leukopenia,* eosinophilia.
**Hepatic:** transient increases in liver enzyme levels.
**Skin:** pruritus, rash, urticaria, *erythema multiforme, Stevens-Johnson syndrome.*

**Other:** drug fever, *hypersensitivity reactions, serum sickness, anaphylaxis.*

## INTERACTIONS
**Drug-drug.** *Carbamazepine:* elevated carbamazepine levels reported when administered together. Avoid concomitant use.
*Probenecid:* may inhibit excretion and increase blood levels of cefixime. Use together cautiously.
*Salicylates:* may displace cefixime from plasma protein-binding sites. Clinical significance is unknown.

## EFFECTS ON DIAGNOSTIC TESTS
Cefixime may cause false-positive results in urine glucose tests using cupric sulfate (Benedict's reagent or Clinitest); use glucose oxidase tests (Diastix or Chemstrip uG) instead. Drug may cause false-positive results in tests for urine ketones that utilize nitroprusside (but not nitroferricyanide). Positive direct Coombs' test results have been seen with other cephalosporins.

## CONTRAINDICATIONS
Contraindicated in patients with hypersensitivity to drug or other cephalosporins.

## NURSING CONSIDERATIONS
• *Alert:* Use cautiously and with reduced dosage in patients with renal dysfunction. Monitor renal function.
• Use cautiously in patients with a history of sensitivity to penicillin and in breast-feeding women.
• Obtain specimen for culture and sensitivity tests before giving first dose. Therapy may begin pending results.
• To prepare oral suspension, add required amount of water to powder in two portions. Shake well after each addition. After mixing, suspension is stable for 14 days. No need to refrigerate, but keep tightly closed. Shake well before use.
• With large doses or prolonged therapy, monitor for superinfection, especially in high-risk patients.
• *Alert:* Don't confuse drug with other cephalosporins that sound alike.

---

Reactions may be *common,* uncommon, *life-threatening,* or COMMON AND LIFE-THREATENING.

☑**Patient teaching**
- Tell patient to take all of the drug prescribed, even after he feels better.
- Instruct patient using oral suspension to shake container before measuring dose. Tell him that suspension does not need to be refrigerated.
- Advise patient to notify doctor if rash or signs and symptoms of superinfection develop.

---

## cefmetazole sodium
Zefazone

*Pregnancy Risk Category B*

### HOW SUPPLIED
*Injection:* 1-g vial, 2-g vial, 1 g/50 ml, 2 g/50 ml premixed solution

### ACTION
A semisynthetic cephamycin antibiotic pharmacologically similar to second-generation cephalosporins that inhibit cell-wall synthesis, promoting osmotic instability; usually bactericidal.

| Route | Onset | Peak | Duration |
|-------|-------|------|----------|
| I.V. | Unknown | Immediate | Unknown |

### INDICATIONS & DOSAGE
*Lower respiratory tract infections due to* Streptococcus pneumoniae, Staphylococcus aureus *(penicillinase- and non-penicillinase-producing strains),* Escherichia coli, *and* Haemophilus influenzae *(non-penicillinase-producing strains); intra-abdominal infections due to* E. coli *or* Bacteroides fragilis; *skin and skin-structure infections due to* S. aureus *(penicillinase- and non-penicillinase-producing strains),* S. epidermidis, Streptococcus pyogenes, S. agalactiae, E. coli, Proteus mirabilis, Klebsiella pneumoniae, *and* B. fragilis—
**Adults:** 2 g I.V. q 6 to 12 hours for 5 to 14 days.
*Urinary tract infections due to* E. coli—
**Adults:** 2 g I.V. q 12 hours.
*Prophylaxis in patients undergoing vaginal hysterectomy—*
**Adults:** 2 g I.V. 30 to 90 minutes before surgery as a single dose; or 1 g I.V. 30 to 90 minutes before surgery, repeated in 8 and 16 hours.
*Prophylaxis in patients undergoing abdominal hysterectomy—*
**Adults:** 1 g I.V. 30 to 90 minutes before surgery, repeated in 8 and 16 hours.
*Prophylaxis in patients undergoing cesarean section—*
**Adults:** 2 g I.V. as a single dose after clamping cord; or 1 g I.V. after clamping cord, repeated in 8 and 16 hours.
*Prophylaxis in patients undergoing colorectal surgery—*
**Adults:** 2 g I.V. as a single dose 30 to 90 minutes before surgery. May follow with additional 2-g doses in 8 and 16 hours.
*Prophylaxis in high-risk patients undergoing cholecystectomy—*
**Adults:** 1 g I.V. 30 to 90 minutes before surgery, repeated in 8 and 16 hours.
*Adjust-a-dose:* For patients with renal failure, if creatinine clearance is 50 to 90 ml/minute, give 1 to 2 g q 12 hours; if clearance is 30 to 49 ml/minute, give 1 to 2 g q 16 hours; if clearance is 10 to 29 ml/minute, give 1 to 2 g q 24 hours; if clearance is less than 10 ml/minute, give 1 to 2 g q 48 hours (administered after hemodialysis).

### ADVERSE REACTIONS
**CNS:** headache.
**CV:** *shock,* hypotension, phlebitis, thrombophlebitis.
**EENT:** epistaxis, altered color perception.
**GI:** nausea, vomiting, *diarrhea,* epigastric pain, pseudomembranous colitis, candidiasis, bleeding.
**GU:** vaginitis, hot flashes.
**Hepatic:** elevated liver function test results.
**Musculoskeletal:** joint pain and inflammation.
**Respiratory:** pleural effusion, dyspnea, respiratory distress.
**Skin:** rash, pruritus, generalized erythema.
**Other:** fever, bacterial or fungal superinfection, *hypersensitivity reactions, serum sickness, anaphylaxis,* pain at injection site.

---

*\*Liquid contains alcohol.   \*\*May contain tartrazine.   †Canada   ‡Australia   §U.K.   ◇OTC*

## INTERACTIONS
**Drug-drug.** *Aminoglycosides:* potential increased risk of nephrotoxicity. Monitor closely.
*Probenecid:* may inhibit excretion and increase blood levels of cefmetazole. May be used for this effect.
**Drug-lifestyle.** *Alcohol use:* possible disulfiram-like reaction. Avoid for 24 hours before and after administration of cefmetazole.

## EFFECTS ON DIAGNOSTIC TESTS
Drug causes false-positive results of urine glucose tests that use cupric sulfate (Benedict's reagent or Clinitest); use glucose oxidase tests (Diastix or Chemstrip uG) instead. Cefmetazole may cause positive Coombs' test results.

## CONTRAINDICATIONS
Contraindicated in patients with hypersensitivity to drug or other cephalosporins.

## NURSING CONSIDERATIONS
• Use cautiously in patients with a history of sensitivity to penicillin and in breast-feeding women.
• Obtain specimen for culture and sensitivity tests before giving first dose. Therapy may begin pending results.
• Monitor patient for bacterial and fungal superinfections. Prolonged use may result in overgrowth of nonsusceptible organisms.
• Monitor INR in patients at risk (from renal or hepatic impairment, malnutrition, or prolonged therapy), as ordered. Drug's chemical structure includes the methylthiotetrazole side chain that has been associated with bleeding disorders. However, such bleeding has not been reported with drug.
• In patients undergoing hemodialysis, give dose at end of hemodialysis session.
• Monitor renal function.
• *Alert:* Don't confuse drug with other cephalosporins that sound alike.

## I.V. administration
• Reconstitute drug with bacteriostatic water for injection, sterile water for injection, or normal saline for injection. After reconstitution, drug may be further diluted to concentrations ranging from 1 to 20 mg/ml by adding it to normal saline injection, $D_5W$, or lactated Ringer's injection. Reconstituted or dilute solutions are stable for 24 hours at room temperature (77° F [25° C]) or 1 week if refrigerated at 46° F (8° C).

### ✓ Patient teaching
• Tell patient to report adverse reactions promptly.
• Instruct patient to alert nurse if discomfort occurs at I.V. insertion site.

---

## cefonicid sodium
Monocid

*Pregnancy Risk Category B*

## HOW SUPPLIED
*Injection:* 1 g
*Infusion:* 1 g/100 ml

## ACTION
A second-generation cephalosporin that inhibits cell-wall synthesis, promoting osmotic instability; usually bactericidal.

| Route | Onset | Peak | Duration |
|-------|-------|------|----------|
| I.V. | Immediate | Immediate | Unknown |
| I.M. | Unknown | 1-2 hr | Unknown |

## INDICATIONS & DOSAGE
*Perioperative prophylaxis in contaminated surgery—*
**Adults:** 1 g I.M. or I.V. 30 to 60 minutes before surgery; then 1 g I.M. or I.V. daily for 2 days after surgery. If used for prophylaxis in cesarean section, 1 g I.M. or I.V. after umbilical cord is clamped.
*Serious infections of the lower respiratory and urinary tracts; skin and skin-structure infections; septicemia; bone and joint infections; preoperative prophylaxis. Susceptible microorganisms include* Streptococcus pneumoniae, Klebsiella pneumoniae, Escherichia coli, Haemophilus influenzae, Proteus mirabilis, Staphylococcus aureus, S. epidermidis, *and* Streptococcus pyogenes—
**Adults:** usual dosage is 1 g I.V. or I.M. q 24 hours; in life-threatening infections, 2 g q 24 hours.

---

*Adjust-a-dose:* For patients with renal failure, if creatinine clearance is 60 to 79 ml/minute, give 10 to 25 mg/kg q 24 hours; if clearance is 40 to 59 ml/minute, give 8 to 20 mg/kg q 24 hours; if clearance is 20 to 39 ml/minute, give 4 to 15 mg/kg q 24 hours; if clearance is 10 to 19 ml/minute, give 4 to 15 mg/kg q 48 hours; if clearance is 5 to 9 ml/minute, give 4 to 15 mg/kg q 3 to 5 days; if clearance is below 5 ml/minute, give 3 to 4 mg/kg q 3 to 5 days.

## ADVERSE REACTIONS
**CNS:** dizziness, headache, malaise, paresthesia.
**CV:** *phlebitis, thrombophlebitis.*
**GI:** pseudomembranous colitis, diarrhea.
**GU:** *acute renal failure,* interstitial nephritis.
**Hematologic:** *neutropenia, leukopenia,* eosinophilia, anemia, thrombocytosis, *thrombocytopenia,* prolonged PT and INR.
**Hepatic:** elevated liver function test results.
**Musculoskeletal:** myalgia.
**Skin:** *maculopapular and erythematous rashes, urticaria, pain, induration, sterile abscesses, tissue sloughing at injection site.*
**Other:** *hypersensitivity reactions, serum sickness, anaphylaxis,* fever.

## INTERACTIONS
**Drug-drug.** *Probenecid:* may inhibit excretion and increase blood levels of cefonicid. Use together cautiously.

## EFFECTS ON DIAGNOSTIC TESTS
Cefonicid causes positive Coombs' test results and false-positive results in urine glucose tests using cupric sulfate (Benedict's reagent or Clinitest); use glucose oxidase tests (Diastix or Chemstrip uG) instead. Drug causes false elevations in serum or urine creatinine levels in tests using Jaffé's reaction.

## CONTRAINDICATIONS
Contraindicated in patients with hypersensitivity to drug or other cephalosporins.

## NURSING CONSIDERATIONS
• Use cautiously in patients with a history of sensitivity to penicillin and in breast-feeding women. Also use cautiously and with dosage adjustments in patients with renal failure. Monitor renal function.
• Obtain specimen for culture and sensitivity tests before giving first dose. Therapy may begin pending results.
• Dosing interval will be adjusted for patients with renal impairment.
• For I.M. use, when administering 2-g I.M. doses once daily, divide the dose equally and inject deeply into large muscle masses, such as the gluteus maximus or the lateral aspect of the thigh.
• With large doses or prolonged therapy, monitor for superinfection, especially in high-risk patients.
• The chemical structure of drug includes the methylthiotetrazole side chain that has been associated with bleeding disorders. However, such bleeding has not been reported with drug.
• *Alert:* Don't confuse drug with other cephalosporins that sound alike.

## I.V. administration
• Reconstitute drug in 1-g vial with 2.5 ml of sterile water for injection (yields a concentration of 325 mg/ml). Shake well. Reconstitute drug in piggyback vials with 50 to 100 ml of sterile water for injection, bacteriostatic water for injection, or normal saline solution.
• Infuse over 20 to 30 minutes.

## Patient teaching
• Tell patient to report adverse reactions or signs and symptoms of superinfection promptly.
• Instruct patient to alert nurse if discomfort is felt at I.V. insertion site.

## cefoperazone sodium
Cefobid

*Pregnancy Risk Category B*

## HOW SUPPLIED
*Infusion:* 1 g, 2 g piggyback
*Parenteral:* 1-g, 2-g vials; 1 g, 2 g premixed

## ACTION
A third-generation cephalosporin that inhibits cell-wall synthesis, promoting osmotic instability; usually bactericidal.

| Route | Onset | Peak | Duration |
|-------|-------|------|----------|
| I.V. | Immediate | Immediate | Unknown |
| I.M. | Unknown | 1-2 hr | Unknown |

## INDICATIONS & DOSAGE
*Serious infections of the respiratory tract; intra-abdominal, gynecologic, and skin infections; bacteremia; septicemia due to susceptible microorganisms* (Streptococcus pneumoniae *and* S. pyogenes; Staphylococcus aureus *[penicillinase- and non-penicillinase-producing] and* S. epidermidis; enterococci; Escherichia coli; Klebsiella; Haemophilus influenzae; Enterobacter; Citrobacter; Proteus; *some* Pseudomonas, *including* P. aeruginosa; *and* Bacteroides fragilis)—
**Adults:** usual dosage is 1 to 2 g q 12 hours I.M. or I.V. In severe infections or in infections due to less sensitive organisms, total daily dose (or frequency) may be increased to 16 g/day.
*Adjust-a-dose:* For patients with hepatic or biliary obstruction, total daily dose shouldn't exceed 4 g/day. In patients with hepatic and substantial renal impairment, total daily dose shouldn't exceed 2 g/day.

## ADVERSE REACTIONS
**CV:** *phlebitis, thrombophlebitis.*
**GI:** pseudomembranous colitis, nausea, vomiting, *diarrhea.*
**Hematologic:** *transient neutropenia, eosinophilia,* anemia, hypoprothrombinemia, bleeding, elevated INR.
**Hepatic:** mildly elevated liver enzymes.
**Skin:** *maculopapular and erythematous rashes, urticaria, pain, induration, sterile abscesses, temperature elevation, tissue sloughing at I.M. injection site.*
**Other:** *hypersensitivity reactions, serum sickness, anaphylaxis,* fever.

## INTERACTIONS
**Drug-drug.** *Probenecid:* may inhibit excretion and increase blood levels of cefoperazone. Use together cautiously.
**Drug-lifestyle.** *Alcohol use:* possible disulfiram-like reaction. Warn patient not to drink alcohol for several days after discontinuing cefoperazone.

## EFFECTS ON DIAGNOSTIC TESTS
Cephalosporins cause false-positive results in urine glucose tests using cupric sulfate (Benedict's reagent or Clinitest); use glucose oxidase (Diastix or Chemstrip uG) instead. Cefoperazone may cause positive Coombs' test results.

## CONTRAINDICATIONS
Contraindicated in patients with hypersensitivity to drug or other cephalosporins.

## NURSING CONSIDERATIONS
• Use cautiously in patients with impaired renal function or with a history of sensitivity to penicillin. Also use cautiously in breast-feeding women.
• Doses of 4 g/day should be given cautiously to patients with hepatic disease or biliary obstruction. Higher dosages require monitoring of serum levels.
• Periodically monitor liver and renal function and compare to baseline.
• Obtain specimen for culture and sensitivity tests before giving first dose. Therapy may begin pending results.
• To prepare drug for I.M. injection: using the 1-g vial, dissolve drug with 2 ml of sterile water for injection; then add 0.6 ml of 2% lidocaine hydrochloride for a final concentration of 333 mg/ml. Or, dissolve drug with 2.8 ml of sterile water for injection; then add 1 ml of 2% lidocaine hydrochloride for a final concentration of 250 mg/ml. When using the 2-g vial, dissolve drug with 3.8 ml of sterile water for injection; then add 1.2 ml of 2% lidocaine hydrochloride for final concentration of 333 mg/ml. Or, dissolve drug with 5.4 ml of sterile water for injection; then add 1.8 ml of 2% lidocaine hydrochloride for concentration of 250 mg/ml.
• For I.M. administration, inject deeply into a large muscle mass, such as the gluteus maximus or the lateral aspect of the thigh.
• With large doses or prolonged therapy, monitor for superinfection, especially in high-risk patients.
• Monitor INR regularly. The drug's chemical structure includes the methyl-

thiotetrazole side chain that has been associated with bleeding disorders. Vitamin K promptly reverses bleeding if it occurs.
• *Alert:* Don't confuse drug with other cephalosporins that sound alike.

### I.V. administration
• Reconstitute drug in 1- or 2-g vial with a minimum of 2.8 ml of compatible I.V. solution; the manufacturer recommends using 5 ml/g. Give by direct injection into a large vein or into the tubing of a free-flowing I.V. solution over 3 to 5 minutes. When giving by intermittent infusion, add reconstituted drug to 20 to 40 ml of a compatible I.V. solution and infuse over 15 to 30 minutes.

### Patient teaching
• Tell patient to report adverse reactions and signs and symptoms of superinfection promptly.
• Instruct patient to alert nurse if discomfort occurs at I.V. insertion site.

---

## cefotaxime sodium
Claforan

*Pregnancy Risk Category B*

### HOW SUPPLIED
*Injection:* 500 mg, 1 g, 2-g vials, 10-g bottle
*Infusion:* 1-g, 2-g premixed package

### ACTION
A third-generation cephalosporin that inhibits cell-wall synthesis, promoting osmotic instability; usually bactericidal.

| Route | Onset | Peak | Duration |
|-------|-------|------|----------|
| I.V. | Immediate | Immediate | Unknown |
| I.M. | Unknown | 30 min | Unknown |

### INDICATIONS & DOSAGE
*Perioperative prophylaxis in contaminated surgery—*
**Adults:** 1 g I.M. or I.V. 30 to 60 minutes before surgery. Patients undergoing bowel surgery should receive preoperative mechanical bowel cleansing and a nonabsorbable anti-infective agent such as neomycin. Patients undergoing cesarean

section should receive 1 g I.M. or I.V. as soon as the umbilical cord is clamped; then 1 g I.M. or I.V. 6 and 12 hours later.
*Uncomplicated gonorrhea due to penicillinase-producing strains of* Neisseria gonorrhoeae *or non-penicillinase-producing strains of the organism—*
**Adults and adolescents:** 500 mg I.M. as a single dose.
*Serious infections of the lower respiratory and urinary tracts, CNS, skin, bone, and joints; gynecologic and intra-abdominal infections; bacteremia; septicemia due to susceptible microorganisms, such as streptococci (including* Streptococcus pneumoniae *and* S. pyogenes), *Staphylococcus aureus (penicillinase- and non-penicillinase-producing) and* S. epidermidis, Escherichia coli, Klebsiella, Haemophilus influenzae, Serratia marcescens, Pseudomonas *species (including* P. aeruginosa), Enterobacter, Proteus, *and* Peptostreptococcus—
**Adults:** usual dose is 1 g I.V. or I.M. q 6 to 8 hours. Up to 12 g daily can be given in life-threatening infections.
**Children weighing 50 kg (110 lb) or more:** the usual adult dose, but dosage shouldn't exceed 12 g daily.
**Children ages 1 month to 12 years weighing less than 50 kg:** 50 to 180 mg/kg/day I.M. or I.V. in four to six divided doses.
**Neonates ages 1 to 4 weeks:** 50 mg/kg I.V. q 8 hours.
**Neonates to age 1 week:** 50 mg/kg I.V. q 12 hours.
*Adjust-a-dose:* For patients with renal failure, if creatinine clearance is below 20 ml/minute, give half usual dose at usual interval.

### ADVERSE REACTIONS
**CNS:** headache.
**CV:** *phlebitis, thrombophlebitis.*
**GI:** pseudomembranous colitis, nausea, vomiting, *diarrhea.*
**GU:** vaginitis, candidiasis, interstitial nephritis.
**Hematologic:** *transient neutropenia,* eosinophilia, hemolytic anemia, *thrombocytopenia, agranulocytosis.*
**Hepatic:** elevated liver function test results.

---

**Skin:** *maculopapular and erythematous rashes, urticaria, pain, induration, sterile abscesses, temperature elevation, tissue sloughing at I.M. injection site.*
**Other:** *hypersensitivity reactions, serum sickness, anaphylaxis,* elevated temperature.

## INTERACTIONS

**Drug-drug.** *Aminoglycosides:* may increase risk of nephrotoxicity. Monitor closely.
*Probenecid:* may inhibit excretion and increase blood levels of cefotaxime. Use together cautiously.

## EFFECTS ON DIAGNOSTIC TESTS

Cefotaxime may cause positive Coombs' test results.

## CONTRAINDICATIONS

Contraindicated in patients with hypersensitivity to drug or other cephalosporins.

## NURSING CONSIDERATIONS

• Use cautiously in patients with a history of sensitivity to penicillin and in breast-feeding women. Also use cautiously and with dosage adjustments in patients with renal failure. Monitor renal function.
• Obtain specimen for culture and sensitivity tests before giving first dose. Therapy may begin pending results.
• For I.M. administration, inject deeply into a large muscle mass, such as the gluteus maximus or the lateral aspect of the thigh.
• With large doses or prolonged therapy, monitor for superinfection, especially in high-risk patients.
• *Alert:* Don't confuse drug with other cephalosporins that sound alike.

## I.V. administration

• For direct injection, reconstitute drug in 500-mg, 1-g, or 2-g vials with 10 ml of sterile water for injection. Solutions containing 1 g/14 ml are isotonic. Inject drug into a large vein or into the tubing of a free-flowing I.V. solution over 3 to 5 minutes.
• For I.V. infusion, reconstitute drug in infusion vials with 50 to 100 ml of $D_5W$ or

normal saline solution. Infuse drug over 20 to 30 minutes. Interrupt flow of primary I.V. solution during infusion.

## Patient teaching

• Tell patient to report adverse reactions and signs and symptoms of superinfection promptly.
• Instruct patient to alert nurse if discomfort occurs at I.V. insertion site.

---

## cefotetan disodium
Cefotan

*Pregnancy Risk Category B*

## HOW SUPPLIED

*Injection:* 1 g, 2 g, 10 g
*Infusion:* 1 g, 2 g piggyback and premixed

## ACTION

A second-generation cephalosporin that inhibits cell-wall synthesis, promoting osmotic instability; usually bactericidal.

| Route | Onset | Peak | Duration |
|-------|-------|------|----------|
| I.V. | Immediate | Immediate | Unknown |
| I.M. | Unknown | 1.5-3 hr | Unknown |

## INDICATIONS & DOSAGE

*Serious urinary tract and lower respiratory tract infections and gynecologic, skin and skin-structure, intra-abdominal, and bone and joint infections due to susceptible streptococci,* Staphylococcus aureus *(penicillinase- and non-penicillinase-producing) and* S. epidermidis, Escherichia coli, Klebsiella, Enterobacter, Proteus, Haemophilus influenzae, Neisseria gonorrhoeae, *and* Bacteroides, *including* B. fragilis—
**Adults:** 1 to 2 g I.V. or I.M. q 12 hours for 5 to 10 days. Up to 6 g daily in life-threatening infections.
*Perioperative prophylaxis—*
**Adults:** 1 to 2 g I.V. given once 30 to 60 minutes before surgery. In cesarean section, dose should be administered as soon as umbilical cord is clamped.
*Adjust-a-dose:* For patients with renal failure, if creatinine clearance is 10 to 30 ml/minute, give usual dose q 24 hours;

if clearance is below 10 ml/minute, give usual dose q 48 hours.

**ADVERSE REACTIONS**
**CV:** *phlebitis, thrombophlebitis.*
**GI:** pseudomembranous colitis, nausea, *diarrhea.*
**GU:** *nephrotoxicity.*
**Hematologic:** *transient neutropenia,* eosinophilia, hemolytic anemia, hypoprothrombinemia, bleeding, thrombocytosis, *agranulocytosis, thrombocytopenia,* prolonged PT and INR.
**Hepatic:** elevated liver function test results.
**Skin:** *maculopapular and erythematous rashes, urticaria, pain, induration, sterile abscesses, tissue sloughing at injection site.*
**Other:** *hypersensitivity reactions, serum sickness, anaphylaxis,* elevated temperature.

**INTERACTIONS**
**Drug-drug.** *Aminoglycosides:* possible synergistic effect and possible increased risk of nephrotoxicity. Use with caution.
*Probenecid:* may inhibit excretion and increase blood levels of cefotetan. Sometimes used for this effect.
**Drug-lifestyle.** *Alcohol use:* possible disulfiram-like reaction. Warn patient not to drink alcohol for several days after discontinuing cefotetan.

**EFFECTS ON DIAGNOSTIC TESTS**
Cefotetan causes false-positive results in urine glucose tests using cupric sulfate (Benedict's reagent or Clinitest); use glucose oxidase tests (Diastix or Chemstrip uG) instead. Drug causes false elevations in serum or urine creatinine levels in tests using Jaffé's reaction and may cause positive Coombs' test results.

**CONTRAINDICATIONS**
Contraindicated in patients with hypersensitivity to drug or other cephalosporins.

**NURSING CONSIDERATIONS**
• Use cautiously in patients with history of sensitivity to penicillin and in breast-feeding women. Also use cautiously and with dosage adjustments in patients with renal failure. Monitor renal function.
• Obtain specimen for culture and sensitivity tests before giving first dose. Therapy may begin pending results.
• Reconstitute for I.M. injection with sterile water or bacteriostatic water for injection, normal saline for injection, or 0.5% or 1% lidocaine hydrochloride. Shake to dissolve and let stand until clear.
• Reconstituted solution is stable for 24 hours at room temperature or 96 hours if refrigerated.
• With large doses or prolonged therapy, monitor for superinfection, especially in high-risk patients.
• Drug's chemical structure includes the methylthiotetrazole side chain that has been associated with bleeding disorders. However, such bleeding has not been reported with this drug. Monitor PT and INR.
• *Alert:* Don't confuse drug with other cephalosporins that sound alike.

**I.V. administration**
• Reconstitute drug with sterile water for injection. Drug may then be mixed with 50 to 100 ml of $D_5W$ or normal saline solution. Interrupt flow of primary I.V. solution during cefotetan infusion.
• Infuse over 20 to 60 minutes.

**Patient teaching**
• Tell patient to report adverse reactions and signs and symptoms of superinfection promptly.
• Instruct patient to alert nurse if discomfort occurs at I.V. site.
• Tell patient to notify doctor if loose stools or diarrhea occurs.

**cefoxitin sodium**
Mefoxin

*Pregnancy Risk Category B*

**HOW SUPPLIED**
*Injection:* 1 g, 2 g, 10 g
*Infusion:* 1 g, 2 g in 50-ml or 100-ml container

---

## ACTION
A second-generation cephalosporin that inhibits cell-wall synthesis, promoting osmotic instability; usually bactericidal.

| Route | Onset | Peak | Duration |
|-------|-------|------|----------|
| I.V. | Immediate | Immediate | Unknown |
| I.M. | Unknown | 20-30 min | Unknown |

## INDICATIONS & DOSAGE
*Serious infections of respiratory and GU tracts; skin; soft-tissue, bone, and joint infections; bloodstream and intra-abdominal infections due to susceptible organisms (such as* Escherichia coli *and other coliform bacteria,* Staphylococcus aureus *[penicillinase- and nonpenicillinase-producing] and* S. epidermidis, streptococci, Klebsiella, Haemophilus influenzae, *and* Bacteroides, *including* B. fragilis); *perioperative prophylaxis—*
**Adults:** 1 to 2 g I.V. or I.M. q 6 to 8 hours for uncomplicated infections. Up to 12 g daily in life-threatening infections.
**Children over age 3 months:** 80 to 160 mg/kg daily I.V. or I.M., given in four to six equally divided doses. Maximum daily dose is 12 g.
*Prophylaxis in surgery—*
**Adults:** 2 g I.M. or I.V. 30 to 60 minutes before surgery, then 2 g I.M. or I.V. q 6 hours for 24 hours (72 hours after prosthetic arthroplasty).
**Children ages 3 months and older:** 30 to 40 mg/kg I.M. or I.V. 30 to 60 minutes before surgery, then 30 to 40 mg/kg q 6 hours for 24 hours (72 hours after prosthetic arthroplasty).
*Adjust-a-dose:* For patients with renal failure, if creatinine clearance is 30 to 50 ml/minute, give 1 to 2 g q 8 to 12 hours; if clearance is 10 to 29 ml/minute, give 1 to 2 g q 12 to 24 hours; and if clearance is below 10 ml/minute, give 500 mg q 24 to 48 hours.

## ADVERSE REACTIONS
**CV:** hypotension; *phlebitis, thrombophlebitis.*
**GI:** pseudomembranous colitis, nausea, vomiting, *diarrhea.*
**GU:** *acute renal failure.*

**Hematologic:** *transient neutropenia,* eosinophilia, hemolytic anemia, anemia, *thrombocytopenia.*
**Hepatic:** transient increases in liver enzyme levels.
**Respiratory:** dyspnea.
**Skin:** *maculopapular and erythematous rashes, urticaria, exfoliative dermatitis, pain, induration, sterile abscesses, tissue sloughing at injection site.*
**Other:** *hypersensitivity reactions, serum sickness, anaphylaxis,* elevated temperature.

## INTERACTIONS
**Drug-drug.** *Nephrotoxic drugs:* possible increased risk of nephrotoxicity. Monitor closely.
*Probenecid:* may inhibit excretion and increase blood levels of cefoxitin. Sometimes used for this effect.

## EFFECTS ON DIAGNOSTIC TESTS
Cefoxitin causes false-positive results in urine glucose tests using cupric sulfate (Benedict's reagent or Clinitest); use glucose oxidase tests (Diastix or Chemstrip uG) instead. Drug causes false elevations in serum or urine creatinine levels in tests using Jaffé's reaction and may cause positive Coombs' test results.

## CONTRAINDICATIONS
Contraindicated in patients with hypersensitivity to drug or other cephalosporins.

## NURSING CONSIDERATIONS
• Use cautiously in patients with a history of sensitivity to penicillin and in breast-feeding women. Also use cautiously and with dosage adjustments in patients with renal failure. Monitor renal function.
• Obtain specimen for culture and sensitivity tests before giving first dose. Therapy may begin pending results.
• For I.M. use, reconstitute each 1 g of drug with 2 ml of sterile water for injection or 0.5% or 1% lidocaine hydrochloride (without epinephrine) to minimize pain. Inject deeply into a large muscle mass, such as the gluteus maximus or the lateral aspect of the thigh.

• After reconstitution, store for 24 hours at room temperature or 1 week under refrigeration.
• With large doses or prolonged therapy, monitor for superinfection, especially in high-risk patients.
• *Alert:* Don't confuse drug with other cephalosporins that sound alike.

### I.V. administration
• Reconstitute 1 g with at least 10 ml of sterile water for injection and 2 g with 10 to 20 ml of sterile water for injection. Solutions of $D_5W$ and normal saline for injection can also be used. For direct injection, inject drug into a large vein or into the tubing of a free-flowing I.V. solution over 3 to 5 minutes. For intermittent infusion, add reconstituted drug to 50 or 100 ml of $D_5W$ or $D_{10}W$ or normal saline for injection. Interrupt flow of primary I.V. solution during infusion.
• Assess I.V. site frequently. Such use has been linked to development of thrombophlebitis.

### ☑ Patient teaching
• Tell patient to report adverse reactions and signs and symptoms of superinfection promptly.
• Instruct patient to alert nurse if discomfort is felt at I.V. site.
• Instruct patient to notify doctor if loose stools or diarrhea occurs.

---

## cefpodoxime proxetil
Vantin

*Pregnancy Risk Category B*

### HOW SUPPLIED
*Tablets (film-coated):* 100 mg, 200 mg
*Oral suspension:* 50 mg/5 ml, 100 mg/5 ml in 100-ml bottles

### ACTION
A third-generation cephalosporin that inhibits cell-wall synthesis, promoting osmotic instability; usually bactericidal.

| Route | Onset | Peak | Duration |
|-------|-------|------|----------|
| P.O. | Unknown | 2-3 hr | Unknown |

### INDICATIONS & DOSAGE
*Acute, community-acquired pneumonia due to non-beta-lactamase-producing strains of* Haemophilus influenzae *or* Streptococcus pneumoniae—
**Adults and children ages 13 and older:** 200 mg P.O. q 12 hours for 14 days.
*Acute bacterial exacerbation of chronic bronchitis due to* S. pneumoniae, H. influenzae *(non-beta-lactamase-producing strains only), or* Moraxella (Branhamella) catarrhalis—
**Adults and children ages 13 and older:** 200 mg P.O. q 12 hours for 10 days.
*Uncomplicated gonorrhea in men and women; rectal gonococcal infections in women—*
**Adults and children ages 13 and older:** 200 mg P.O. as a single dose. Follow with doxycycline 100 mg P.O. b.i.d. for 7 days.
*Uncomplicated skin and skin-structure infections due to* Staphylococcus aureus *or* S. pyogenes—
**Adults and children ages 13 and older:** 400 mg P.O. q 12 hours for 7 to 14 days.
*Acute otitis media due to* S. pneumoniae, H. influenzae, *or* M. catarrhalis—
**Children ages 6 months and older:** 5 mg/kg (not to exceed 200 mg) P.O. q 12 hours or 10 mg/kg P.O. daily for 10 days.
*Pharyngitis or tonsillitis due to* S. pyogenes—
**Adults:** 100 mg P.O. q 12 hours for 10 days.
**Children ages 6 months and older:** 5 mg/kg (not to exceed 100 mg) P.O. q 12 hours for 10 days.
*Uncomplicated urinary tract infections due to* Escherichia coli, Klebsiella pneumoniae, Proteus mirabilis, *or* S. saprophyticus—
**Adults:** 100 mg P.O. q 12 hours for 7 days.
✻ *NEW INDICATION: Mild to moderate acute maxillary sinusitis due to* H. influenzae, S. pneumoniae, *or* M. catarrhalis—
**Adults and adolescents ages 12 and older:** 200 mg P.O. q 12 hours for 10 days.
**Children ages 2 months to 11 years:** 5 mg/kg P.O. q 12 hours for 10 days; maximum is 200 mg/dose.
*Adjust-a-dose:* For patients with renal failure, if creatinine clearance is below

---

30 ml/minute, dosage interval should be increased to q 24 hours. Dialysis patients should receive drug three times weekly after dialysis.

## ADVERSE REACTIONS
**CNS:** headache.
**GI:** *diarrhea,* nausea, vomiting, abdominal pain.
**GU:** vaginal fungal infections.
**Skin:** rash.
**Other:** *hypersensitivity reactions, anaphylaxis.*

## INTERACTIONS
**Drug-drug.** *Antacids, H2-antagonists:* decreased absorption of cefpodoxime. Avoid concomitant use.
*Probenecid:* decreased excretion of cefpodoxime. Monitor for toxicity.
**Drug-food.** *Any food:* increased absorption. Give drug with food.

## EFFECTS ON DIAGNOSTIC TESTS
Drug may induce a positive direct Coombs' test. Urine glucose determinations may be false-positive with copper sulfate tests (Clinitest); glucose enzymatic tests (Diastix or Chemstrip uG) are not affected.

## CONTRAINDICATIONS
Contraindicated in patients with hypersensitivity to drug or other cephalosporins.

## NURSING CONSIDERATIONS
• Use cautiously in patients with a history of penicillin hypersensitivity because of risk of cross-sensitivity and in patients receiving nephrotoxic drugs because other cephalosporins have been shown to have nephrotoxic potential. Because drug appears in breast milk, use cautiously in breast-feeding women.
• Monitor renal function and compare to baseline.
• Obtain specimen for culture and sensitivity tests before giving first dose. Therapy may begin pending results.
• Administer drug with food to enhance absorption. Shake suspension well before using.

• Store suspension in the refrigerator (36° to 46° F [2° to 8° C]). Discard unused portion after 14 days.
• Monitor for superinfection. Drug may cause overgrowth of nonsusceptible bacteria or fungi.
• *Alert:* Don't confuse drug with other cephalosporins that sound alike.

## ☑ Patient teaching
• Tell patient to take all of the drug as prescribed, even after he feels better.
• Instruct patient to take drug with food. If patient is using suspension, tell him to shake container before measuring dose and to keep container refrigerated.
• Tell patient to call doctor if rash or signs and symptoms of superinfection develop.
• Instruct patient to notify doctor if loose stools or diarrhea occurs.

---

## cefprozil
Cefzil

*Pregnancy Risk Category B*

## HOW SUPPLIED
*Tablets:* 250 mg, 500 mg
*Oral suspension:* 125 mg/5 ml, 250 mg/5 ml

## ACTION
A second-generation cephalosporin that interferes with cell-wall synthesis during microorganism replication, leading to osmotic instability and cell lysis (bactericidal).

| Route | Onset | Peak | Duration |
|-------|-------|------|----------|
| P.O. | Unknown | 1.5 hr | Unknown |

## INDICATIONS & DOSAGE
*Pharyngitis or tonsillitis due to* Streptococcus pyogenes—
**Adults and children ages 13 and older:** 500 mg P.O. daily for at least 10 days.
*Otitis media due to* S. pneumoniae, Haemophilus influenzae, *and* Moraxella (Branhamella) catarrhalis—
**Infants and children ages 6 months to 12 years:** 15 mg/kg P.O. q 12 hours for 10 days.
*Secondary bacterial infections of acute bronchitis and acute bacterial exacerba-*

*tion of chronic bronchitis due to* S. pneumoniae, H. influenzae, *and* M. catarrhalis—

**Adults and children ages 13 and older:**
500 mg P.O. q 12 hours for 10 days.

*Uncomplicated skin and skin-structure infections due to* Staphylococcus aureus *and* S. pyogenes—

**Adults and children ages 13 and older:**
250 or 500 mg P.O. q 12 hours or 500 mg daily.

*Acute sinusitis due to* S. pneumoniae, H. influenzae *(beta-lactamase positive and negative strains), and* M. catarrhalis *(including beta-lactamase-producing strains)—*

**Adults and children ages 13 and older:**
250 mg P.O. q 12 hours for 10 days; for moderate to severe infection, 500 mg P.O. q 12 hours for 10 days.

**Children ages 6 months to 12 years:**
7.5 mg/kg P.O. q 12 hours for 10 days; for moderate to severe infections, 15 mg/kg P.O. q 12 hours for 10 days.

*Adjust-a-dose:* For patients with renal failure, if creatinine clearance is below 30 ml/minute, give 50% of usual dose.

## ADVERSE REACTIONS
**CNS:** dizziness, hyperactivity, headache, nervousness, insomnia, confusion, somnolence.
**GI:** *diarrhea, nausea,* vomiting, abdominal pain.
**GU:** elevated BUN level, elevated serum creatinine level, genital pruritus, vaginitis.
**Hematologic:** decreased leukocyte count, eosinophilia.
**Hepatic:** elevated liver enzymes, cholestatic jaundice (rare).
**Skin:** rash, urticaria, diaper rash.
**Other:** superinfection, *hypersensitivity reactions, serum sickness, anaphylaxis.*

## INTERACTIONS
**Drug-drug.** *Aminoglycosides:* potential increased risk of nephrotoxicity. Monitor closely.
*Probenecid:* may inhibit excretion and increase blood levels of cefprozil. Use together cautiously.

## EFFECTS ON DIAGNOSTIC TESTS
Cephalosporins may produce a false-positive result for urine glucose tests that use copper reduction method (Benedict's reagent, Fehling's solution, or Clinitest tablets); use enzymatic glucose oxidase methods instead. A false-negative reaction may occur in the ferricyanide test for blood glucose.

## CONTRAINDICATIONS
Contraindicated in patients with hypersensitivity to drug or other cephalosporins.

## NURSING CONSIDERATIONS
• Use cautiously in patients with history of sensitivity to penicillin and in breast-feeding women. Also use cautiously in patients with impaired hepatic or renal function.
• Monitor renal function and liver function test results.
• Obtain specimen for culture and sensitivity tests before giving first dose. Therapy may begin pending results.
• Administer after hemodialysis treatment is completed; drug is removed by hemodialysis.
• Monitor for superinfection. May cause overgrowth of nonsusceptible bacteria or fungi.
• *Alert:* Don't confuse drug with other cephalosporins that sound alike.

### ☑ Patient teaching
• Advise patient to take drug as prescribed, even after he feels better.
• Tell patient to shake suspension well before measuring dose.
• Inform patient that oral suspensions contain the drug in a bubble-gum-flavored form to improve palatability and promote compliance in children. Tell him to refrigerate reconstituted suspension and to discard unused drug after 14 days.
• Instruct patient to notify doctor if rash or signs and symptoms of superinfection occur.

## ceftazidime
Ceptaz, Fortaz, Fortum§,
Kefadim§, Tazicef, Tazidime

*Pregnancy Risk Category B*

### HOW SUPPLIED
*Injection (with sodium carbonate):*
500 mg, 1 g, 2 g, 6 g (pharmacy bulk
package)
*Injection (with arginine):* 1 g, 2 g, 6 g,
10 g (pharmacy bulk package)
*Infusion:* 1 g, 2 g in 50-ml and 100-ml
vials (premixed)

### ACTION
A third-generation cephalosporin that inhibits cell-wall synthesis, promoting osmotic instability; usually bactericidal.

| Route | Onset | Peak | Duration |
|-------|-------|------|----------|
| I.V. | Immediate | Immediate | Unknown |
| I.M. | Unknown | 1 hr | Unknown |

### INDICATIONS & DOSAGE
*Serious infections of the lower respiratory
and urinary tracts; gynecologic, intra-
abdominal, CNS, and skin infections;
bacteremia; and septicemia due to susceptible microorganisms, such as streptococci (including* Streptococcus pneumoniae *and* S. pyogenes), Staphylococcus
aureus *(penicillinase- and non-
penicillinase-producing),* Escherichia
coli, Klebsiella, Proteus, Enterobacter,
Haemophilus influenzae, Pseudomonas,
*and some strains of* Bacteroides—
**Adults and children ages 12 and older:**
1 g I.V. or I.M. q 8 to 12 hours; up to 6 g
daily in life-threatening infections.
**Children ages 1 month to 11 years:** 25
to 50 mg/kg I.V. q 8 hours (sodium carbonate formulation).
**Neonates up to age 4 weeks:** 30 mg/kg
I.V. q 12 hours (sodium carbonate formulation).
*Uncomplicated urinary tract infections—*
**Adults:** 250 mg I.V. or I.M. q 12 hours.
*Complicated urinary tract infections—*
**Adults and children ages 12 and older:**
500 mg to 1 g I.V. or I.M. q 8 to 12 hours.
*Adjust-a-dose:* For patients with renal
failure, if creatinine clearance is 31 to
50 ml/minute, give 1 g q 12 hours; if
clearance is 16 to 30 ml/minute, give 1 g
q 24 hours; if clearance is 6 to 15 ml/
minute, give 500 mg q 24 hours; if clearance is below 5 ml/minute, give 500 mg q
48 hours.

### ADVERSE REACTIONS
**CNS:** headache, dizziness, paresthesia,
*seizures.*
**CV:** *phlebitis, thrombophlebitis.*
**GI:** pseudomembranous colitis, nausea,
vomiting, diarrhea, abdominal cramps.
**GU:** vaginitis, candidiasis.
**Hematologic:** eosinophilia; thrombocytosis, *leukopenia,* hemolytic anemia,
*agranulocytosis, thrombocytopenia.*
**Hepatic:** transient elevation in liver enzyme levels.
**Skin:** *maculopapular and erythematous
rashes, urticaria, pain, induration, sterile abscesses, tissue sloughing at injection site.*
**Other:** *hypersensitivity reactions, serum
sickness, anaphylaxis.*

### INTERACTIONS
**Drug-drug.** *Aminoglycosides:* additive or
synergistic effect against some strains of
*Pseudomonas aeruginosa* and Enterobac-
teriaceae. Monitor for effects.
*Chloramphenicol:* antagonistic effect.
Avoid concomitant use.
*Probenecid:* may inhibit excretion and in-
crease drug levels. May be used as a ther-
apeutic effect.

### EFFECTS ON DIAGNOSTIC TESTS
Drug causes false-positive results in urine
glucose tests using cupric sulfate (Benedict's reagent or Clinitest); use glucose
oxidase (Diastix or Chemstrip uG) instead. Ceftazidime may cause positive
Coombs' test results.

### CONTRAINDICATIONS
Contraindicated in patients with hypersensitivity to drug or other cephalosporins.

### NURSING CONSIDERATIONS
• Use cautiously in patients with a history
of sensitivity to penicillin and in breast-
feeding women. Also use cautiously and

with dosage adjustments in patients with renal failure. Monitor renal function.

• Obtain specimen for culture and sensitivity tests before giving first dose. Therapy may begin pending results.

• For I.M. administration, inject deeply into a large muscle mass, such as the gluteus maximus or the lateral aspect of the thigh.

• With large doses or prolonged therapy, monitor for superinfection, especially in high-risk patients.

• *Alert:* Commercially available preparations contain either sodium carbonate (Fortaz, Magnacef, Tazicef, Tazidime) or arginine (Ceptaz, Pentacef) to facilitate dissolution of drug. Safety and efficacy of arginine-containing solutions in children younger than age 12 have not been established.

• Ceftazidime is removed by hemodialysis; a supplemental dose of drug is indicated after each dialysis period, as ordered.

• *Alert:* Don't confuse drug with other cephalosporins that sound alike.

## ▢ I.V. administration

• Reconstitute solutions containing sodium carbonate with sterile water for injection. Add 5 ml to a 500-mg vial; 10 ml to a 1-g or 2-g vial. Shake well to dissolve drug. Carbon dioxide is released during dissolution, and positive pressure will develop in the vial. Reconstitute arginine-containing solutions with 10 ml of sterile water for injection. This formulation won't release gas bubbles. Each brand of ceftazidime includes specific instructions for reconstitution. Read them carefully.

• Infuse over 15 to 30 minutes.

## ✅ Patient teaching

• Tell patient to report adverse reactions or signs and symptoms of superinfection promptly.

• Instruct patient to alert nurse if discomfort is felt at I.V. insertion site.

• Advise patient to notify doctor if loose stools or diarrhea occurs.

# ceftibuten
Cedax

*Pregnancy Risk Category B*

## HOW SUPPLIED
*Capsules:* 400 mg
*Oral suspension:* 90 mg/5 ml, 180 mg/5 ml

## ACTION
A third-generation cephalosporin that exerts its bacterial action by binding to essential target proteins of the bacterial cell wall, which leads to inhibition of cell-wall synthesis.

| Route | Onset | Peak | Duration |
|-------|---------|--------|----------|
| P.O. | Unknown | 2-4 hr | Unknown |

## INDICATIONS & DOSAGE
*Acute bacterial exacerbation of chronic bronchitis due to* Haemophilus influenzae, Moraxella catarrhalis, *or penicillin-susceptible strains of* Streptococcus pneumoniae—
**Adults and children weighing over 45 kg (99 lb):** 400 mg P.O. daily for 10 days.
*Pharyngitis and tonsillitis due to* S. pyogenes; *acute bacterial otitis media due to* H. influenzae, M. catarrhalis, *or* S. pyogenes—
**Adults and children weighing over 45 kg:** 400 mg P.O. daily for 10 days.
**Children under 45 kg:** 9 mg/kg P.O. daily for 10 days.
*Adjust-a-dose:* For adult patients with renal impairment, if creatinine clearance is 30 to 49 ml/minute, give 4.5 mg/kg or 200 mg P.O. q 24 hours; if clearance is 5 to 29 ml/minute, give 2.25 mg/kg or 100 mg P.O. q 24 hours. In patients undergoing hemodialysis two or three times weekly, give single dose of 400 mg (capsule) or 9 mg/kg (suspension) P.O. after each hemodialysis session. Maximum dose is 400 mg.

## ADVERSE REACTIONS
**CNS:** headache, dizziness, aphasia, psychosis.

**GI:** nausea, vomiting, diarrhea, dyspepsia, abdominal pain, loose stools, pseudomembranous colitis.
**GU:** elevated BUN levels, toxic nephropathy, renal dysfunction.
**Hematologic:** elevated eosinophil levels, decreased hemoglobin levels, altered platelet count, *aplastic anemia,* hemolytic anemia, *hemorrhage, neutropenia, agranulocytosis, pancytopenia.*
**Hepatic:** hepatic cholestasis, elevated liver enzymes and bilirubin.
**Skin:** *Stevens-Johnson syndrome.*
**Other:** allergic reaction, *anaphylaxis,* drug fever.

## INTERACTIONS
**Drug-food.** *Any food:* decreased bioavailability of drug, which slows its absorption. Administer drug 2 hours before or 1 hour after a meal.

## EFFECTS ON DIAGNOSTIC TESTS
Although drug isn't known to affect the direct Coombs' test, other cephalosporins have caused a false-positive direct Coombs' test. Some cephalosporins may cause a false-positive test for urinary glucose.

## CONTRAINDICATIONS
Contraindicated in patients with hypersensitivity to cephalosporins.

## NURSING CONSIDERATIONS
• Use cautiously in patients with history of hypersensitivity to penicillin.
• Use cautiously in patients with impaired renal failure or GI disease, especially colitis. Monitor renal function.
• Use cautiously in elderly patients.
• Safety and effectiveness in infants under age 6 months have not been established.
• Drug should be used in pregnancy only if clearly needed. Not known if drug appears in breast milk; use cautiously in breast-feeding women.
• Obtain specimen for culture and sensitivity tests before giving first dose. Therapy may begin pending test results.
• When preparing oral suspension, first tap the bottle to loosen powder. Follow chart supplied by manufacturer for amount of water to add to powder when mixing oral suspension form. Add water in two portions; shake well after each step. After mixing, suspension is stable for 14 days if refrigerated.
• Shake oral suspension well before administering.
• *Alert:* If allergic reaction is suspected, drug should be discontinued. Emergency treatment may be required.
• Drug may cause overgrowth of nonsusceptible bacteria or fungi. Monitor patient for superinfection.
• Pseudomembranous colitis has been reported with nearly all antibacterial agents. Consider this diagnosis in patients who develop diarrhea secondary to therapy. Obtain specimens for *Clostridium difficile,* as ordered.
• *Alert:* Don't confuse drug with other cephalosporins that sound alike.

### ☑ Patient teaching
• Instruct patient to take all of the drug prescribed, even if he feels better.
• Tell patient using oral suspension to take it at least 2 hours before or 1 hour after a meal, and to shake bottle well before measuring.
• Inform patient to store oral suspension in the refrigerator, with lid tightly closed, and to discard unused drug after 14 days.
• Caution breast-feeding woman that it's unknown if drug appears in breast milk.
• Tell diabetic patient that suspension contains 1 g sucrose/teaspoon.
• Instruct patient to report adverse reactions or signs and symptoms of superinfection.
• Tell patient to notify doctor if loose stools or diarrhea occurs.

## ceftizoxime sodium
Cefizox

*Pregnancy Risk Category B*

### HOW SUPPLIED
*Injection:* 500 mg, 1 g, 2 g, 10g
*Infusion:* 1 g, 2 g in 100-ml vials or in 50 ml of $D_5W$

## ACTION
A third-generation cephalosporin that inhibits cell-wall synthesis, promoting osmotic instability; usually bactericidal.

| Route | Onset | Peak | Duration |
|-------|-------|------|----------|
| I.V. | Immediate | Immediate | Unknown |
| I.M. | Unknown | 0.5-1.5 hr | Unknown |

## INDICATIONS & DOSAGE
*Serious infections of the lower respiratory and urinary tracts, gynecologic infections, bacteremia, septicemia, meningitis, intra-abdominal infections, bone and joint infections, and skin infections due to susceptible microorganisms, such as streptococci (including* Streptococcus pneumoniae *and* S. pyogenes), Staphylococcus aureus *and* S. epidermidis, Escherichia coli, Klebsiella, Haemophilus influenzae, Enterobacter, Proteus, *some* Pseudomonas, *and* Peptostreptococcus—
**Adults:** usual dosage is 1 to 2 g I.V. or I.M. q 8 to 12 hours. In life-threatening infections, up to 2 g q 4 hours.
**Children over age 6 months:** 50 mg/kg I.V. q 6 to 8 hours. For serious infections, up to 200 mg/kg/day in divided doses may be used. Don't exceed 12 g/day.
*Adjust-a-dose:* For patients with renal failure, if creatinine clearance is 50 to 79 ml/minute, give 500 mg to 1.5 g q 8 hours; if clearance is 5 to 49 ml/minute, give 250 mg to 1 g q 12 hours; if clearance is below 5 ml/minute or patient undergoes hemodialysis, give 500 mg to 1 g q 48 hours, or 250 to 500 mg q 24 hours.

## ADVERSE REACTIONS
**CV:** *phlebitis, thrombophlebitis.*
**GI:** pseudomembranous colitis, nausea, anorexia, vomiting, *diarrhea.*
**GU:** vaginitis.
**Hematologic: transient neutropenia,** eosinophilia, hemolytic anemia, thrombocytosis, anemia, *thrombocytopenia.*
**Hepatic:** transient elevation in liver enzymes.
**Respiratory:** dyspnea.
**Skin:** *maculopapular and erythematous rashes, urticaria,. pain, induration, sterile abscesses, tissue sloughing at injection site.*

**Other:** *hypersensitivity reactions, serum sickness, anaphylaxis,* elevated temperature.

## INTERACTIONS
**Drug-drug.** *Aminoglycosides:* potential increase in nephrotoxicity. Avoid use.
*Probenecid:* may inhibit excretion and increase blood levels of ceftizoxime. May be used for this effect.

## EFFECTS ON DIAGNOSTIC TESTS
Ceftizoxime causes false-positive results in urine glucose tests using cupric sulfate (Benedict's reagent or Clinitest); use glucose oxidase (Diastix or Chemstrip uG) instead. Drug also causes false elevations in urine creatinine levels using Jaffé's reaction and may cause positive Coombs' test results.

## CONTRAINDICATIONS
Contraindicated in patients with hypersensitivity to drug or other cephalosporins.

## NURSING CONSIDERATIONS
• Use cautiously in patients with history of sensitivity to penicillin and in breastfeeding women. Also use cautiously and with dosage adjustments in patients with renal failure. Monitor renal function.
• Obtain specimen for culture and sensitivity tests before giving first dose. Therapy may begin pending results.
• To prepare I.M. injection, mix 1.5 ml of diluent per 500 mg of drug. For I.M. administration, inject deeply into a large muscle mass, such as the gluteus maximus or the lateral aspect of the thigh. Larger doses (2 g) should be divided and administered at two separate sites.
• With large doses or prolonged therapy, monitor for superinfection, especially in high-risk patients.
• *Alert:* Don't confuse drug with other cephalosporins that sound alike.

## I.V. administration
• To reconstitute powder, add 5 ml of sterile water to a 500-mg vial, 10 ml to a 1-g vial, or 20 ml to a 2-g vial.

• Inject directly into vein over 3 to 5 minutes or slowly into I.V. tubing with free-flowing compatible solution.
• Reconstitute drug in piggyback vials with 50 to 100 ml of normal saline solution or D₅W. Shake well.
• Infuse over 15 to 30 minutes.

☑ **Patient teaching**
• Tell patient to report adverse reactions and signs and symptoms of superinfection promptly.
• Instruct patient to alert nurse if discomfort is felt at I.V. site.
• Tell patient to notify doctor if loose stools or diarrhea occurs.

---

**ceftriaxone sodium**
Rocephin

*Pregnancy Risk Category B*

## HOW SUPPLIED
*Injection:* 250 mg, 500 mg, 1 g, 2 g, 10 g
*Infusion:* 1 g, 2 g piggyback; 1 g, 2 g/50 ml premixed

## ACTION
A third-generation cephalosporin that inhibits cell-wall synthesis, promoting osmotic instability; usually bactericidal.

| Route | Onset | Peak | Duration |
|-------|-------|------|----------|
| I.V. | Immediate | Immediate | Unknown |
| I.M. | Unknown | 1.5-4 hr | Unknown |

## INDICATIONS & DOSAGE
*Uncomplicated gonococcal vulvovaginitis—*
**Adults:** 125 mg I.M. as a single dose, plus azithromycin 1 g P.O. as a single dose or doxycycline 100 mg P.O. b.i.d. for 7 days. Alternatively, give ceftriaxone 250 mg I.M. as a single dose.
*Most infections due to susceptible organisms; serious infections of the lower respiratory and urinary tracts; gynecologic, bone and joint, intra-abdominal, and skin infections; bacteremia; septicemia; and Lyme disease due to such susceptible microorganisms as streptococci (including* Streptococcus pneumoniae *and* S. pyogenes); *Staphylococcus aureus (penicilli-*

nase- and non-penicillinase-producing) *and* S. epidermidis, Escherichia coli, Klebsiella, Haemophilus influenzae, Neisseria meningitidis, N. gonorrhoeae, Enterobacter, Proteus, Peptostreptococcus, Pseudomonas, *and* Serratia marcescens—
**Adults and children over age 12:** 1 to 2 g I.M. or I.V. daily or in equally divided doses q 12 hours. Total daily dosage shouldn't exceed 4 g.
**Children ages 12 and younger:** 50 to 75 mg/kg I.M. or I.V., not to exceed 2 g/day, given in divided doses q 12 hours.
*Meningitis—*
**Adults and children:** initially, 100 mg/kg I.M. or I.V. (not to exceed 4 g); thereafter, 100 mg/kg I.M. or I.V., given once daily or in divided doses q 12 hours, not to exceed 4 g, for 7 to 14 days.
*Perioperative prophylaxis—*
**Adults:** 1 g I.V. as a single dose 30 minutes to 2 hours before surgery.
*Acute bacterial otitis media—*
**Children:** 50 mg/kg (not to exceed 1 g) I.M. as a single dose.

## ADVERSE REACTIONS
**CNS:** headache, dizziness.
**CV:** phlebitis.
**GI:** pseudomembranous colitis, nausea, vomiting, diarrhea.
**GU:** genital pruritus, candidiasis, elevated BUN levels.
**Hematologic:** eosinophilia, thrombocytosis, *leukopenia.*
**Hepatic:** elevated liver function test results.
**Skin:** pain, induration, tenderness at injection site, *rash;* pruritus.
**Other:** *hypersensitivity reactions, serum sickness, anaphylaxis,* elevated temperature, chills.

## INTERACTIONS
**Drug-drug.** *Aminoglycosides:* additive or synergistic effect against some strains of *P. aeruginosa* and Enterobacteriaceae. Monitor patient.
*Probenecid:* high doses (1 or 2 g/day) may enhance hepatic clearance of ceftriaxone and shorten its half-life. Avoid concomitant use.

---

Reactions may be *common,* uncommon, *life-threatening,* or COMMON AND LIFE-THREATENING.

## EFFECTS ON DIAGNOSTIC TESTS
Ceftriaxone causes false-positive results in urine glucose tests using cupric sulfate (Benedict's reagent or Clinitest); instead use glucose oxidase (Diastix or Chemstrip uG). Drug also causes false elevations in urine creatinine levels in tests using Jaffé's reaction, and may cause positive Coombs' test results.

## CONTRAINDICATIONS
Contraindicated in patients with hypersensitivity to drug or other cephalosporins.

## NURSING CONSIDERATIONS
• Use cautiously in patients with a history of sensitivity to penicillin and in breast-feeding women.
• Obtain specimen for culture and sensitivity tests before giving first dose. Therapy may begin pending results.
• A commercially available intramuscular kit containing 1% lidocaine as a diluent is available from the manufacturer.
• For I.M. administration, inject deeply into a large muscle mass, such as the gluteus maximus or the lateral aspect of the thigh.
• With large doses or prolonged therapy, monitor for superinfection, especially in high-risk patients.
• Drug is commonly used in home antibiotic programs for outpatient treatment of serious infections such as osteomyelitis.
• *Alert:* Don't confuse drug with other cephalosporins that sound alike.

### I.V. administration
• Reconstitute drug with sterile water for injection, normal saline injection, $D_5W$ or $D_{10}W$ injection, or a combination of NaCl and dextrose injection and other compatible solutions. Reconstitute by adding 2.4 ml of diluent to the 250-mg vial, 4.8 ml to the 500-mg vial, 9.6 ml to the 1-g vial, and 19.2 ml to the 2-g vial. All reconstituted solutions yield a concentration that averages 100 mg/ml. After reconstitution, dilute further for intermittent infusion to desired concentration. I.V. dilutions are stable for 24 hours at room temperature.

### ✓ Patient teaching
• Tell patient to report adverse reactions promptly.
• Instruct patient to alert nurse if discomfort occurs at I.V. insertion site.
• Teach home care patient and family how to prepare and administer drug.
• If home care patient is a diabetic who is testing his urine for glucose, tell him drug may affect results of cupric sulfate tests; he should use an enzymatic test instead.
• Tell patient to notify doctor if loose stools or diarrhea occurs.

---

## cefuroxime axetil
Ceftin, Zinnat§

## cefuroxime sodium
Kefurox, Zinacef

*Pregnancy Risk Category B*

## HOW SUPPLIED
**cefuroxime axetil**
*Tablets:* 125 mg, 250 mg, 500 mg
*Suspension:* 125 mg/5 ml, 250 mg/5 ml
**cefuroxime sodium**
*Injection:* 750 mg, 1.5 g, 7.5 g
*Infusion:* 750 mg, 1.5-g premixed, frozen solution

## ACTION
A second-generation cephalosporin that inhibits cell-wall synthesis, promoting osmotic instability; usually bactericidal.

| Route | Onset | Peak | Duration |
|-------|-------|------|----------|
| P.O. | Unknown | 15-60 min | Unknown |
| I.V. | Immediate | Immediate | Unknown |
| I.M. | Unknown | 2 hr | Unknown |

## INDICATIONS & DOSAGE
Injectable form: *Serious infections of the lower respiratory and urinary tracts; skin and skin-structure infections; bone and joint infections; septicemia; meningitis; and gonorrhea; and for perioperative prophylaxis.* Oral form: *Otitis media, pharyngitis, tonsillitis, infections of the urinary and lower respiratory tracts, and skin and skin-structure infections. Among susceptible organisms are* Streptococcus pneumoniae *and* S. pyogenes, Haemoph-

ilus influenzae, Klebsiella, Staphylococcus aureus, Escherichia coli, Moraxella (Branhamella) catarrhalis *(including beta-lactamase-producing strains),* Enterobacter, *and* Neisseria gonorrhoeae—

**Adults and children ages 12 and older:** usual dosage of cefuroxime sodium is 750 mg to 1.5 g I.M. or I.V. q 8 hours for 5 to 10 days. For life-threatening infections and infections due to less susceptible organisms, 1.5 g I.M. or I.V. q 6 hours; for bacterial meningitis, up to 3 g I.V. q 8 hours.

Or, administer 250 mg of cefuroxime axetil P.O. q 12 hours. For severe infections, dosage may be increased to 500 mg q 12 hours.

**Children and infants over age 3 months:** 50 to 100 mg/kg/day of cefuroxime sodium I.M. or I.V. in equally divided doses q 6 to 8 hours. Higher dosage of 100 mg/kg/day (not to exceed maximum adult dosage) should be used for more severe or serious infections. For bacterial meningitis, 200 to 240 mg/kg I.V. in divided doses q 6 to 8 hours. For other infections, 125 to 250 mg of cefuroxime axetil P.O. q 12 hours for a child who can swallow pills.

*Uncomplicated urinary tract infections—*

**Adults:** 125 to 250 mg P.O. q 12 hours.

*Otitis media—*

**Children ages 2 and older:** 250 mg P.O. q 12 hours.

**Children under age 2:** 125 mg P.O. q 12 hours.

*Perioperative prophylaxis—*

**Adults:** 1.5 g I.V. 30 to 60 minutes before surgery; in lengthy operations, 750 mg I.V. or I.M. q 8 hours. For open-heart surgery, 1.5 g I.V. at induction of anesthesia and then q 12 hours for a total dosage of 6 g.

*Early Lyme disease (erythema migrans) due to* Borrelia burgdorferi—

**Adults and children ages 13 and older:** 500 mg P.O. b.i.d. for 20 days.

*Secondary bacterial infection of acute bronchitis—*

**Adults:** 250 to 500 mg P.O. (tablets) b.i.d. for 5 to 10 days.

*Adjust-a-dose:* For parenteral administration in patients with renal failure, if creatinine clearance is 10 to 20 ml/minute, give 750 mg I.M. or I.V. q 12 hours; if clearance is below 10 ml/minute, give 750 mg I.M. or I.V. q 24 hours.

**ADVERSE REACTIONS**
**CV:** *phlebitis, thrombophlebitis.*
**GI:** pseudomembranous colitis, nausea, anorexia, vomiting, *diarrhea.*
**Hematologic:** *transient neutropenia,* eosinophilia, *hemolytic anemia,* **thrombocytopenia,** decreased hematocrit and hemoglobin levels.
**Hepatic:** transient increases in liver enzymes.
**Skin:** *maculopapular and erythematous rashes, urticaria, pain, induration, sterile abscesses, temperature elevation, tissue sloughing at I.M. injection site.*
**Other***:* **hypersensitivity reactions, serum sickness, anaphylaxis.**

**INTERACTIONS**
**Drug-drug.** *Aminoglycosides:* synergistic activity against some organisms; potential for increased nephrotoxicity. Monitor closely.
*Diuretics:* increased risk of adverse renal reactions. Monitor closely.
*Probenecid:* may inhibit excretion and increase blood levels of cefuroxime. Sometimes used for this effect.
**Drug-food.** *Any food:* increased absorption. Give drug with food.

**EFFECTS ON DIAGNOSTIC TESTS**
Cefuroxime causes false-positive results in urine glucose tests using cupric sulfate (Benedict's reagent or Clinitest); use glucose oxidase tests (Diastix or Chemstrip uG) instead. Drug also causes false elevations in serum or urine creatinine levels in tests using Jaffé's reaction, and may cause positive Coombs' test results.

**CONTRAINDICATIONS**
Contraindicated in patients with hypersensitivity to drug or other cephalosporins.

**NURSING CONSIDERATIONS**
• Use cautiously in patients with history of sensitivity to penicillin and in breastfeeding women. Also use cautiously and

---

with reduced dosage in patients with impaired renal function. Monitor renal function.

• Obtain specimen for culture and sensitivity tests before giving first dose. Therapy may begin pending results.

• For I.M. administration, inject deeply into a large muscle mass, such as the gluteus maximus or the lateral aspect of the thigh.

• Absorption of cefuroxime axetil is enhanced by food.

• Keep in mind that cefuroxime axetil tablets may be crushed for patients who cannot swallow tablets. Tablets may be dissolved in small amounts of apple, orange, or grape juice or chocolate milk. However, the drug has a bitter taste that is difficult to mask, even with food.

• *Alert:* Cefuroxime axetil film-coated tablet and oral suspension aren't bioequivalent. Don't substitute on a mg/mg basis.

• With large doses or prolonged therapy, monitor for superinfection, especially in high-risk patients.

• *Alert:* Don't confuse drug with other cephalosporins that sound alike.

### I.V. administration
• For each 750-mg vial of Kefurox, reconstitute with 9 ml of sterile water for injection. Withdraw 8 ml from the vial for the proper dose. For each 1.5-g vial of Kefurox, reconstitute with 16 ml of sterile water for injection; withdraw entire contents of vial for a dose. For each 750-mg vial of Zinacef, reconstitute with 8 ml of sterile water for injection; for each 1.5-g vial, reconstitute with 16 ml. In each case, withdraw entire contents of vial for a dose.

• To give by direct injection, inject into a large vein or into the tubing of a free-flowing I.V. solution over 3 to 5 minutes.

• For intermittent infusion, add reconstituted drug to 100 ml $D_5W$, normal saline for injection, or other compatible I.V. solution. Infuse over 15 to 60 minutes.

### ☑ Patient teaching
• Tell patient to take all of the drug as prescribed, even after he feels better.

• Instruct patient to take oral form with food. If patient has difficulty swallowing tablets, tell him how to dissolve or crush tablets but warn him that the bitter taste that results is hard to mask, even with food. If suspension is being used, tell patient to shake container well before measuring dose.

• Tell patient to notify doctor if rash or signs and symptoms of superinfection occur.

• Inform patient receiving drug I.V. to alert nurse if discomfort occurs at I.V. insertion site.

• Tell patient to notify doctor if loose stools or diarrhea occurs.

---

## cephalexin hydrochloride
Keftab

## cephalexin monohydrate
Apo-Cephalex†, Biocef, Keflex, Novo-Lexin†, Nu-Cephalex†

*Pregnancy Risk Category B*

### HOW SUPPLIED
**cephalexin hydrochloride**
*Tablets:* 500 mg
**cephalexin monohydrate**
*Tablets:* 250 mg, 500 mg, 1 g
*Capsules:* 250 mg, 500 mg
*Oral suspension:* 125 mg/5 ml, 250 mg/5 ml

### ACTION
A first-generation cephalosporin that inhibits cell-wall synthesis, promoting osmotic instability; usually bactericidal.

| Route | Onset | Peak | Duration |
|-------|-------|------|----------|
| P.O. | Unknown | 1 hr | Unknown |

### INDICATIONS & DOSAGE
*Respiratory tract, GI tract, skin, soft-tissue, bone, and joint infections and otitis media due to* Escherichia coli *and other coliform bacteria,* group A beta-hemolytic streptococci, Klebsiella, Proteus mirabilis, Streptococcus pneumoniae, *and* staphylococci—
**Adults:** 250 mg to 1 g P.O. q 6 hours or 500 mg q 12 hours. Maximum 4 g daily.

**Children:** 6 to 12 mg/kg P.O. q 6 hours (monohydrate only). Maximum 25 mg/kg q 6 hours.
*Adjust-a-dose:* For adults with impaired renal function, initial dose is the same. Recommended subsequent dosing for creatinine clearance below 5 ml/minute, 250 mg P.O. q 12 to 24 hours; for creatinine clearance of 5 to 10 ml/minute, 250 mg P.O. q 12 hours; and for creatinine clearance of 11 to 40 ml/minute, 500 mg P.O. q 8 to 12 hours.

## ADVERSE REACTIONS
**CNS:** dizziness, headache, fatigue, agitation, confusion, hallucinations.
**GI:** pseudomembranous colitis, *nausea, anorexia,* vomiting, *diarrhea,* gastritis, glossitis, dyspepsia, abdominal pain, anal pruritus, tenesmus, oral candidiasis.
**GU:** genital pruritus, candidiasis, vaginitis, interstitial nephritis.
**Hematologic:** *neutropenia,* eosinophilia, anemia, *thrombocytopenia.*
**Hepatic:** transient increases in liver enzymes.
**Musculoskeletal:** arthritis, arthralgia, joint pain.
**Skin:** *maculopapular and erythematous rashes, urticaria.*
**Other:** *hypersensitivity reactions, serum sickness, anaphylaxis.*

## INTERACTIONS
**Drug-drug.** *Probenecid:* may increase blood levels of cephalosporins. May be used for this effect.

## EFFECTS ON DIAGNOSTIC TESTS
Cephalexin causes false-positive results in urine glucose tests using cupric sulfate (Benedict's reagent or Clinitest); use glucose oxidase tests (Diastix or Chemstrip uG) instead. Drug also causes false elevations in serum or urine creatinine levels in tests using Jaffé's reaction. Positive Coombs' test results occur in about 3% of patients taking cephalexin.

## CONTRAINDICATIONS
Contraindicated in patients with hypersensitivity to cephalosporins.

## NURSING CONSIDERATIONS
• Use cautiously in breast-feeding women and in patients with impaired renal function or history of sensitivity to penicillin. Monitor renal function.
• Ask patient about past reaction to cephalosporin or penicillin therapy before giving first dose.
• Obtain specimen for culture and sensitivity tests before giving first dose. Therapy may begin pending results.
• To prepare oral suspension: Add required amount of water to powder in two portions. Shake well after each addition. After mixing, store in refrigerator. The mixture will remain stable for 14 days without significant loss of potency. Keep tightly closed and shake well before using.
• With large doses or prolonged therapy, monitor for superinfection, especially in high-risk patients.
• Group A beta-hemolytic streptococcal infections should be treated for a minimum of 10 days.
• *Alert:* Don't confuse drug with other cephalosporins that sound alike.

☑ **Patient teaching**
• Tell patient to take all of the drug exactly as prescribed, even after he feels better.
• Instruct patient to take drug with food or milk to lessen GI discomfort. If patient is taking suspension form, instruct him to shake container well before measuring dose and to store in refrigerator.
• Tell patient to notify doctor if rash or signs and symptoms of superinfection develop.

## cephradine
Velosef**

*Pregnancy Risk Category B*

## HOW SUPPLIED
*Capsules:* 250 mg, 500 mg
*Oral suspension:* 125 mg/5 ml, 250 mg/5 ml

## ACTION
First-generation cephalosporin that inhibits cell-wall synthesis, promoting osmotic instability; usually bactericidal.

| Route | Onset | Peak | Duration |
|-------|-------|------|----------|
| P.O. | Unknown | 1 hr | Unknown |

## INDICATIONS & DOSAGE
*Serious infections of respiratory, GU, or GI tract; skin and soft-tissue infections; bone and joint infections; septicemia; endocarditis; and otitis media due to such susceptible organisms as* Escherichia coli *and other coliform bacteria, group A beta-hemolytic streptococci,* Klebsiella, Proteus mirabilis, Staphylococcus aureus, Streptococcus pneumoniae, S. viridans, *and staphylococci; perioperative prophylaxis—*
**Adults:** 250 to 500 mg P.O. q 6 hours or 500 mg to 1 g P.O. q 12 hours.
**Children over age 9 months:** 25 to 50 mg/kg P.O. daily in divided doses q 6 to 12 hours.
*Otitis media—*
**Children:** 75 to 100 mg/kg P.O. daily in equally divided doses q 6 to 12 hours. Don't exceed 4 g daily.

All patients, regardless of age and weight, may be given larger doses (up to 1 g q.i.d.) for severe or chronic infections.

## ADVERSE REACTIONS
**CNS:** dizziness, headache, malaise, paresthesia.
**GI:** pseudomembranous colitis, *nausea, anorexia,* vomiting, heartburn, abdominal cramps, *diarrhea,* oral candidiasis.
**GU:** genital pruritus, candidiasis, vaginitis.
**Hematologic:** *transient neutropenia,* eosinophilia, ***thrombocytopenia.***
**Hepatic:** transient increases in liver enzymes.
**Skin:** *maculopapular and erythematous rashes, urticaria.*
**Other:** *hypersensitivity reactions, serum sickness, anaphylaxis.*

## INTERACTIONS
**Drug-drug.** *Probenecid:* may increase blood levels of cephalosporins. Sometimes used for this effect.

## EFFECTS ON DIAGNOSTIC TESTS
Cephradine causes false-positive results in urine glucose tests using cupric sulfate (Benedict's reagent or Clinitest); instead use glucose oxidase tests (Diastix or Chemstrip uG). Drug also causes false elevations in serum or urine creatinine levels in tests using Jaffé's reaction, and may cause positive Coombs' test results.

## CONTRAINDICATIONS
Contraindicated in patients with hypersensitivity to drug and to other cephalosporins.

## NURSING CONSIDERATIONS
• Use cautiously in patients with impaired renal function or with a history of sensitivity to penicillin. Also use cautiously in breast-feeding women.
• Monitor renal function.
• Obtain specimen for culture and sensitivity tests before giving first dose. Therapy may begin pending results.
• Group A beta-hemolytic streptococcal infections should be treated for a minimum of 10 days.
• With large doses or prolonged therapy, monitor for superinfection, especially in high-risk patients.
• *Alert:* Don't confuse drug with other cephalosporins that sound alike.

### ☑ Patient teaching
• Instruct patient to take all of the drug as prescribed, even after he feels better.
• Inform patient to take drug with food or milk to lessen GI discomfort. If patient is taking suspension form, tell him to shake it well before measuring dose.
• Tell patient to notify doctor if rash or signs and symptoms of superinfection occur.
• Instruct patient to notify doctor if loose stools or diarrhea occurs.

---

## loracarbef
Lorabid

*Pregnancy Risk Category B*

---

## HOW SUPPLIED
*Pulvules:* 200 mg, 400 mg

---

*Powder for oral suspension:* 100 mg/ 5 ml, 200 mg/5 ml in 50-ml, 75-ml and 100-ml bottles

## ACTION
A synthetic beta-lactam antibiotic of the carbacephem class with actions similar to second-generation cephalosporins. Inhibits cell-wall synthesis, promoting osmotic instability; usually bactericidal.

| Route | Onset | Peak | Duration |
|-------|-------|------|----------|
| P.O. | Unknown | 0.5-1 hr | Unknown |

## INDICATIONS & DOSAGE
*Secondary bacterial infections of acute bronchitis—*
**Adults:** 200 to 400 mg P.O. q 12 hours for 7 days.
*Acute bacterial exacerbations of chronic bronchitis—*
**Adults:** 400 mg P.O. q 12 hours for 7 days.
*Pneumonia—*
**Adults:** 400 mg P.O. q 12 hours for 14 days.
*Pharyngitis, sinusitis, tonsillitis—*
**Adults:** 200 to 400 mg P.O. q 12 hours for 10 days.
**Children ages 6 months to 12 years:** 15 mg/kg P.O. daily in divided doses q 12 hours for 10 days.
*Acute otitis media—*
**Children ages 6 months to 12 years:** 30 mg/kg (oral suspension) P.O. daily in divided doses q 12 hours for 10 days.
*Uncomplicated skin and skin-structure infections—*
**Adults:** 200 mg P.O. q 12 hours for 7 days.
*Impetigo—*
**Children ages 6 months to 12 years:** 15 mg/kg P.O. daily in divided doses q 12 hours for 7 days.
*Uncomplicated cystitis—*
**Adults:** 200 mg P.O. daily for 7 days.
*Uncomplicated pyelonephritis—*
**Adults:** 400 mg P.O. q 12 hours for 14 days.
*Adjust-a-dose:* Patients with creatinine clearance of 50 ml/minute or more don't require dose and interval changes. If creatinine clearance is 10 to 49 ml/minute, give half of usual dose at same interval; if

it is below 10 ml/minute, give usual dose q 3 to 5 days. Hemodialysis patients require an additional dose after dialysis.

## ADVERSE REACTIONS
**CNS:** headache, somnolence, nervousness, insomnia, dizziness.
**CV:** vasodilation.
**GI:** diarrhea, nausea, vomiting, abdominal pain, anorexia, pseudomembranous colitis.
**GU:** vaginal candidiasis, transient increases in BUN and creatinine levels.
**Hematologic:** *transient thrombocytopenia, leukopenia,* eosinophilia, increased PT and INR, pancytopenia, *neutropenia.*
**Hepatic:** transient elevations in AST, ALT, and alkaline phosphatase levels.
**Skin:** rash, urticaria, pruritus, *erythema multiforme.*
**Other:** *hypersensitivity reactions, anaphylaxis.*

## INTERACTIONS
**Drug-drug.** *Probenecid:* decreased excretion of loracarbef, causing increased plasma levels. Monitor for toxicity.
**Drug-food.** *Any food:* decreased absorption. Have patent take drug on empty stomach at least 1 hour before or 2 hours after a meal.

## EFFECTS ON DIAGNOSTIC TESTS
Drug can cause positive direct Coombs' test results.

## CONTRAINDICATIONS
Contraindicated in patients with hypersensitivity to drug or other cephalosporins and in patients with diarrhea due to pseudomembranous colitis.

## NURSING CONSIDERATIONS
• Use cautiously in pregnant or breast-feeding women. Safety and efficacy of drug have not been established in infants under age 6 months.
• Obtain specimen for culture and sensitivity tests before giving first dose. Therapy may begin pending results.
• To reconstitute powder for oral suspension, add 30 ml of water in two portions to the 50-ml bottle or 60 ml of water in

two portions to the 100-ml bottle; shake
after each addition.
• After reconstitution, store oral suspension for 14 days at room temperature (59°
to 86° F [15° to 30° C]).
• Monitor for superinfection. May cause
overgrowth of nonsusceptible bacteria or
fungi.
• Monitor renal function.
• *Alert:* Monitor patient for seizures.
Beta-lactam antibiotics may trigger
seizures in susceptible patients, especially
when given without dosage modification
to those with renal impairment. If
seizures occur, discontinue drug and notify doctor. Administer anticonvulsants as
ordered.
• For otitis media, remember that the
more rapidly absorbed oral suspension
produces higher peak plasma levels than
do the capsules.
• *Alert:* Don't confuse Lorabid with
Lortab.

**☑ Patient teaching**
• Instruct patient to take all of the drug
prescribed, even after he feels better.
• Tell patient to take drug on an empty
stomach, at least 1 hour before or 2 hours
after meals. Tell him to shake container of
suspension well before measuring dose.
• Advise patient to discard unused portion
after 14 days.
• Instruct patient to notify doctor if rash
or signs and symptoms of superinfection
appear.
• Instruct patient to notify doctor if loose
stools or diarrhea occurs.

**demeclocycline hydrochloride**
**doxycycline calcium**
**doxycycline hyclate**
**doxycycline hydrochloride**
**doxycycline monohydrate**
**minocycline hydrochloride**
**tetracycline hydrochloride**

## COMBINATION PRODUCTS
UROBIOTIC-250: oxytetracycline hydrochloride 250 mg, sulfamethizole 250 mg, and phenazopyridine hydrochloride 50 mg.
HELIDAC: tetracycline 500 mg, bismuth salicylate 262.4 mg, and metronidazole 250 mg.

---

**demeclocycline hydrochloride**
Declomycin, Ledermycin‡

*Pregnancy Risk Category D*

## HOW SUPPLIED
*Tablets (film-coated):* 150 mg, 300 mg
*Capsules:* 150 mg

## ACTION
Unknown. Thought to exert bacteriostatic effect by binding to the 30S and possibly 50S ribosomal subunits of microorganisms, thus inhibiting protein synthesis. May also alter the cytoplasmic membrane of susceptible microorganisms.

| Route | Onset | Peak | Duration |
|-------|-------|------|----------|
| P.O. | Unknown | 3-4 hr | Unknown |

## INDICATIONS & DOSAGE
*Infections due to susceptible gram-positive and gram-negative organisms (including* Haemophilus ducreyi, Yersinia pestis, *and* Campylobacter fetus), *Rickettsiae, Mycoplasma pneumoniae, Chlamydia trachomatis; psittacosis; granuloma inguinale—*
**Adults:** 150 mg P.O. q 6 hours or 300 mg P.O. q 12 hours.

**Children over age 8:** 6.6 to 13.2 mg/kg P.O. daily, in divided doses q 6 to 12 hours.
*Gonorrhea—*
**Adults:** initially, 600 mg P.O.; then 300 mg P.O. q 12 hours for 4 days (for total of 3 g).

## ADVERSE REACTIONS
**CNS:** *intracranial hypertension,* dizziness.
**CV:** pericarditis.
**EENT:** dysphagia, tinnitus, visual disturbances.
**GI:** anorexia, *nausea, vomiting, diarrhea,* enterocolitis, glossitis, anogenital inflammation, pancreatitis.
**GU:** elevated serum BUN levels.
**Hematologic:** *neutropenia,* eosinophilia, *thrombocytopenia, hemolytic anemia.*
**Hepatic:** elevated liver enzymes.
**Metabolic:** diabetes insipidus syndrome.
**Skin:** *maculopapular and erythematous rashes, photosensitivity, increased pigmentation,* urticaria.
**Other:** *hypersensitivity reactions, anaphylaxis,* permanent tooth discoloration, bone growth retardation if used in children under age 9.

## INTERACTIONS
**Drug-drug.** *Antacids (including sodium bicarbonate) and laxatives containing aluminum, magnesium, or calcium; antidiarrheals:* decreased antibiotic absorption. Give antibiotic 1 hour before or 2 hours after any of these drugs.
*Ferrous sulfate and other iron products, zinc:* decreased antibiotic absorption. Give antibiotic 2 hours before or 3 hours after iron administration.
*Methoxyflurane:* may cause nephrotoxicity with tetracyclines. Avoid concurrent use.
*Oral anticoagulants:* increased anticoagulant effect. Monitor PT and INR, and adjust dosage as ordered.
*Oral contraceptives:* decreased contraceptive effectiveness and increased risk of

---

Reactions may be *common,* uncommon, *life-threatening,* or COMMON AND LIFE-THREATENING.

breakthrough bleeding. Use a nonhormonal birth control method.
*Penicillins:* may interfere with bactericidal action of penicillins. Avoid use together.
**Drug-food.** *Milk, dairy products, other foods:* decreased antibiotic absorption. Give antibiotic 1 hour before or 2 hours after any of the above.
**Drug-lifestyle.** *Sun exposure:* photosensitivity reactions may occur. Take precautions.

**EFFECTS ON DIAGNOSTIC TESTS**
Demeclocycline causes false-negative results in urine glucose tests using glucose oxidase reagent (Diastix or Chemstrip uG). Drug also causes false elevations in fluorometric tests for urine catecholamines.

**CONTRAINDICATIONS**
Contraindicated in patients with hypersensitivity to drug or other tetracyclines.

**NURSING CONSIDERATIONS**
• Use cautiously in patients with impaired renal or hepatic function. Use of these drugs during last half of pregnancy and in children under age 9 may cause permanent discoloration of teeth, enamel defects, and bone growth retardation.
• Be alert for signs and symptoms of diabetes insipidus syndrome, including polyuria, polydipsia, and weakness.
• Monitor renal and liver function test results.
• Monitor fluid balance and daily weights in patients with impaired kidney and liver function.
• Obtain specimen for culture and sensitivity tests before giving first dose. Therapy may begin pending test results.
• *Alert:* Check expiration date. Outdated or deteriorated tetracyclines have been associated with reversible nephrotoxicity (Fanconi's syndrome).
• Don't expose drug to light or heat; store in tightly capped container.
• With large doses or prolonged therapy, monitor for superinfection, especially in high-risk patients.
• Check patient's tongue for signs of candidal infection. Stress good oral hygiene.

☑ **Patient teaching**
• Instruct patient to take entire amount of drug, exactly as prescribed, even after he feels better.
• Explain that drug's effectiveness is reduced when taken with milk or other dairy products, food, antacids, or iron products. Tell patient to take each dose with a full glass of water on an empty stomach, at least 1 hour before or 2 hours after meals. Also tell him to take drug at least 1 hour before bedtime to prevent esophageal irritation or ulceration.
• Warn patient to avoid direct sunlight and ultraviolet light, wear protective clothing, and use sunscreen. Photosensitivity reactions may occur within a few minutes to several hours after sun exposure. Photosensitivity persists for some time after discontinuation of drug.
• Instruct patient to report signs and symptoms of superinfection.

---

**doxycycline calcium**
Vibramycin

**doxycycline hyclate**
Apo-Doxy†, Doryx, Doxy Caps, Doxy 100, Doxy 200, Doxycin†, Novo-Doxylin†, Vibramycin, Vibra-Tabs

**doxycycline hydrochloride**
Doryx‡, Doxylin‡, Vibramycin‡

**doxycycline monohydrate**
Monodox, Vibramycin

*Pregnancy Risk Category D*

**HOW SUPPLIED**
**doxycycline calcium**
*Oral suspension:* 50 mg/5 ml
**doxycycline hyclate**
*Tablets (film-coated):* 100 mg
*Capsules:* 50 mg, 100 mg
*Capsules (enteric-coated pellets):* 100 mg
*Injection:* 100 mg, 200 mg
**doxycycline hydrochloride**
*Tablets:* 50 mg‡, 100 mg‡
*Capsules:* 50 mg‡, 100 mg‡
**doxycycline monohydrate**
*Capsules:* 50 mg, 100 mg

---

*Oral suspension:* 25 mg/5 ml

## ACTION
Unknown. Thought to exert bacteriostatic effect by binding to the 30S and possibly 50S ribosomal subunits of microorganisms, thus inhibiting protein synthesis. May also alter the cytoplasmic membrane of susceptible microorganisms.

| Route | Onset | Peak | Duration |
|-------|-------|------|----------|
| P.O. | Unknown | 1.5-4 hr | Unknown |
| I.V. | Immediate | Unknown | Unknown |

## INDICATIONS & DOSAGE
*Infections due to susceptible gram-positive and gram-negative organisms (including* Haemophilus ducreyi, Yersinia pestis, *and* Campylobacter fetus), Rickettsiae, Mycoplasma pneumoniae, Chlamydia trachomatis, *and* Borrelia burgdorferi *(Lyme disease); psittacosis; granuloma inguinale—*
**Adults and children over age 8 weighing at least 45 kg (99 lb):** 100 mg P.O. q 12 hours on first day; then 100 mg P.O. daily. Or, 200 mg I.V. on first day in one or two infusions; then 100 to 200 mg I.V. daily.
**Children over age 8 and under 45 kg:** 4.4 mg/kg P.O. or I.V. daily, in divided doses q 12 hours on first day; then 2.2 to 4.4 mg/kg daily in one or two divided doses.
    Give I.V. infusion slowly (minimum 1 hour). Infusion must be completed within 12 hours (within 6 hours in lactated Ringer's solution or dextrose 5% in lactated Ringer's solution).
*Gonorrhea in patients allergic to penicillin—*
**Adults:** 100 mg P.O. b.i.d. for 7 days (10 days for epididymitis).
*Primary or secondary syphilis in patients allergic to penicillin—*
**Adults:** 300 mg P.O. daily in divided doses for at least 10 days.
*Uncomplicated urethral, endocervical, or rectal infections due to* C. trachomatis *or* Ureaplasma urealyticum—
**Adults:** 100 mg P.O. b.i.d. for at least 7 days (10 days for epididymitis).
*Prophylaxis of malaria—*
**Adults:** 100 mg P.O. daily.

**Children over age 8:** 2 mg/kg P.O. once daily. Dose shouldn't exceed that of adults.
    *Note:* Prophylaxis should begin 1 to 2 days before travel to endemic area and continued until 4 weeks after travel.
*Pelvic inflammatory disease—*
**Adults:** 100 mg I.V. q 12 hours with cefoxitin or cefotetan and continued for at least 2 days after symptomatic improvement; thereafter, 100 mg P.O. q 12 hours for a total course of 14 days.

## ADVERSE REACTIONS
**CNS:** *intracranial hypertension.*
**CV:** pericarditis, thrombophlebitis.
**EENT:** glossitis, dysphagia.
**GI:** anorexia, *epigastric distress, nausea, vomiting, diarrhea,* oral candidiasis, enterocolitis, anogenital inflammation.
**Hematologic:** *neutropenia,* eosinophilia, *thrombocytopenia,* hemolytic anemia.
**Hepatic:** elevated liver enzymes.
**Musculoskeletal:** bone growth retardation in children under age 9.
**Skin:** *maculopapular and erythematous rashes, photosensitivity, increased pigmentation,* urticaria.
**Other:** *hypersensitivity reactions, anaphylaxis,* superinfection; permanent discoloration of teeth, enamel defects.

## INTERACTIONS
**Drug-drug.** *Antacids (including sodium bicarbonate) and laxatives containing aluminum, magnesium, or calcium; antidiarrheals:* decreased antibiotic absorption. Give antibiotic 1 hour before or 2 hours after any of these drugs.
*Carbamazepine, phenobarbital:* decreased antibiotic effect. Avoid if possible.
*Ferrous sulfate and other iron products, zinc:* decreased antibiotic absorption. Give drug 2 hours before or 3 hours after iron administration.
*Methoxyflurane:* may cause nephrotoxicity with tetracyclines. Monitor carefully.
*Oral anticoagulants:* increased anticoagulant effect. Monitor PT and INR, and adjust dosage as ordered.
*Oral contraceptives:* decreased contraceptive effectiveness and increased risk of breakthrough bleeding. Use a nonhormonal form of birth control.

---

Reactions may be *common*, uncommon, *life-threatening*, or COMMON AND LIFE-THREATENING.

*Penicillins:* may interfere with bactericidal action of penicillins. Avoid use together.
**Drug-lifestyle.** *Alcohol use:* decreased antibiotic effect. Avoid use together.
*Sun exposure:* photosensitivity reactions may occur. Take precautions.

**EFFECTS ON DIAGNOSTIC TESTS**
Drug causes false-negative results in urine glucose tests using glucose oxidase reagent (Diastix or Chemstrip uG). Parenteral dosage form may cause false-positive Clinitest results. Drug also causes false elevations in fluorometric tests for urine catecholamines.

**CONTRAINDICATIONS**
Contraindicated in patients with hypersensitivity to drug or other tetracyclines.

**NURSING CONSIDERATIONS**
● Use cautiously in patients with impaired renal or hepatic function. Use of these drugs during last half of pregnancy and in children under age 9 may cause permanent discoloration of teeth, enamel defects, and bone growth retardation.
● Obtain specimen for culture and sensitivity tests before giving first dose. Therapy may begin pending test results.
● *Alert:* Check expiration date. Outdated or deteriorated tetracyclines have been associated with reversible nephrotoxicity (Fanconi's syndrome).
● Administer drug with milk or food if adverse GI reactions develop.
● Reconstituted injectable solution is stable for 72 hours if refrigerated and protected from light.
● With large doses or prolonged therapy, monitor for superinfection, especially in high-risk patients.
● Check patient's tongue for signs of fungal infection. Stress good oral hygiene.
● Drug isn't indicated for the treatment of neurosyphilis.
● *Alert:* Don't confuse doxycycline, doxylamine, and dicyclomine.

**I.V. administration**
● Reconstitute powder for injection with sterile water for injection. Use 10 ml in 100-mg vial and 20 ml in 200-mg vial.

Dilute solution to 100 to 1,000 ml for I.V. infusion. Avoid extravasation. Don't infuse solutions that are more concentrated than 1 mg/ml. Infusion time varies with dose, but usually ranges from 1 to 4 hours. Monitor I.V. infusion site for signs of thrombophlebitis, which may occur with I.V. administration.
● Don't expose drug to light or heat. Protect it from sunlight during infusion.

**Patient teaching**
● Tell patient to take entire amount of drug exactly as prescribed, even after he feels better.
● Instruct patient to report adverse reactions promptly. If drug is being administered I.V., tell patient to alert nurse if discomfort occurs at I.V site.
● Advise patient to take oral form of drug with food or milk if stomach upset occurs. Also advise patient not to take oral tablets or capsules within 1 hour of bedtime because of possible esophageal irritation or ulceration.
● Warn patient to avoid direct sunlight and ultraviolet light, wear protective clothing, and use sunscreen. Photosensitivity reactions may occur within a few minutes to several hours after exposure. Photosensitivity persists for some time after therapy ends.
● Tell patient to report signs and symptoms of superinfection to the doctor.

**minocycline hydrochloride**
Apo-Minocycline†, Dynacin, Minocin*, Minomycin‡, Vectrin

*Pregnancy Risk Category D*

**HOW SUPPLIED**
*Tablets (film-coated):* 50 mg, 100 mg
*Capsules (pellet-filled):* 50 mg, 100 mg
*Oral suspension:* 50 mg/5 ml
*Injection:* 100 mg

**ACTION**
Unknown. Thought to exert bacteriostatic effect by binding to the 30S and possibly 50S ribosomal subunits of microorganisms, thus inhibiting protein synthesis.

May also alter the cytoplasmic membrane of susceptible microorganisms.

| Route | Onset | Peak | Duration |
|-------|-------|------|----------|
| P.O. | Unknown | 1-4 hr | Unknown |
| I.V. | Immediate | Immediate | Unknown |

## INDICATIONS & DOSAGE

*Infections due to susceptible gram-negative and gram-positive organisms (including* Haemophilus ducreyi, Yersinia pestis, *and* Campylobacter fetus), *Rickettsiae,* Mycoplasma pneumoniae, *and* Chlamydia trachomatis; *psittacosis; granuloma inguinale—*
**Adults:** initially, 200 mg I.V.; then 100 mg I.V. q 12 hours. Don't exceed 400 mg/day. Or, 200 mg P.O. initially; then 100 mg P.O. q 12 hours. May use 100 or 200 mg P.O. initially; then 50 mg q.i.d.
**Children over age 8:** initially, 4 mg/kg P.O. or I.V.; then 2 mg/kg q 12 hours.
    Give I.V. in 500- to 1,000-ml solution without calcium and administer over 6 hours.
*Gonorrhea in patients allergic to penicillin—*
**Adults:** initially, 200 mg P.O.; then 100 mg q 12 hours for at least 4 days.
*Syphilis in patients allergic to penicillin—*
**Adults:** initially, 200 mg P.O.; then 100 mg q 12 hours for 10 to 15 days.
*Meningococcal carrier state—*
**Adults:** 100 mg P.O. q 12 hours for 5 days.
*Uncomplicated urethral, endocervical, or rectal infection due to* C. trachomatis *or* Ureaplasma urealyticum—
**Adults:** 100 mg P.O. b.i.d. for at least 7 days.
*Uncomplicated gonococcal urethritis in men—*
**Adults:** 100 mg P.O. b.i.d. for 5 days.

## ADVERSE REACTIONS

**CNS:** headache, *intracranial hypertension,* light-headedness, dizziness, vertigo.
**CV:** pericarditis, *thrombophlebitis.*
**EENT:** dysphagia, glossitis.
**GI:** *anorexia,* epigastric distress, oral candidiasis, *nausea,* vomiting, *diarrhea,* enterocolitis, inflammatory lesions in anogenital region.

**GU:** elevated BUN.
**Hematologic:** *neutropenia,* eosinophilia, *thrombocytopenia,* hemolytic anemia.
**Hepatic:** elevated liver enzymes.
**Musculoskeletal:** bone growth retardation in children under age 9.
**Skin:** *maculopapular and erythematous rashes, photosensitivity, increased pigmentation, urticaria.*
**Other:** *hypersensitivity reactions, anaphylaxis,* superinfection; permanent discoloration of teeth, enamel defects.

## INTERACTIONS

**Drug-drug.** *Antacids (including sodium bicarbonate) and laxatives containing aluminum, magnesium, or calcium; antidiarrheals:* decreased antibiotic absorption. Give antibiotic 1 hour before or 2 hours after any of these drugs.
*Ferrous sulfate and other iron products, zinc:* decreased antibiotic absorption. Give drug 2 hours before or 3 hours after iron administration.
*Methoxyflurane:* may cause nephrotoxicity when given with tetracyclines. Monitor carefully.
*Oral anticoagulants:* increased anticoagulant effect. Monitor PT and INR, and adjust dosage as ordered.
*Oral contraceptives:* decreased contraceptive effectiveness and increased risk of breakthrough bleeding. Use a nonhormonal form of birth control.
*Penicillins:* may interfere with bactericidal action of penicillins. Avoid use together.
**Drug-lifestyle.** *Sun exposure:* photosensitivity reactions may occur. Take precautions.

## EFFECTS ON DIAGNOSTIC TESTS

Minocycline causes false-negative results in urine glucose tests using glucose oxidase reagent (Diastix or Chemstrip uG). Drug also causes false elevations in fluorometric tests for urine catecholamines. Parenteral form may cause false-positive reading of copper sulfate tests (Clinitest).

## CONTRAINDICATIONS

Contraindicated in patients with hypersensitivity to drug or other tetracyclines.

---

Reactions may be *common,* uncommon, **life-threatening**, or COMMON AND LIFE-THREATENING.

## NURSING CONSIDERATIONS
• Use cautiously in patients with impaired renal or hepatic function. Use of these drugs during last half of pregnancy and in children under age 9 may cause permanent discoloration of teeth, enamel defects, and bone growth retardation.
• Monitor renal and liver function test results.
• Obtain specimen for culture and sensitivity tests before first dose. Therapy may begin pending test results.
• *Alert:* Check expiration date. Outdated or deteriorated tetracyclines have been associated with reversible nephrotoxicity (Fanconi's syndrome).
• Don't expose drug to light or heat. Keep cap tightly closed.
• With large doses or prolonged therapy, monitor for superinfection, especially in high-risk patients.
• Check patient's tongue for signs of candidal infection. Stress good oral hygiene.
• Drug may cause tooth discoloration in young adults. Observe for brown pigmentation, and notify doctor if it occurs.
• Drug is not indicated for the treatment of neurosyphilis.
• *Alert:* Don't confuse minocin, niacin, and mithracin.

🖒 **I.V. administration**
• Reconstitute 100 mg of powder with 5 ml of sterile water for injection, with further dilution to 500 to 1,000 ml for I.V. infusion. Although reconstituted solution is stable for 24 hours at room temperature, use as soon as possible. Infusions are usually given over 6 hours.
• Patient may develop thrombophlebitis with I.V. administration. Avoid extravasation. Switch to oral therapy as soon as possible.

☑ **Patient teaching**
• Tell patient to take entire amount of drug exactly as prescribed, even after he feels better.
• Instruct patient to take oral form of drug with a full glass of water. Drug may be taken with food. Tell patient not to take within 1 hour of bedtime to avoid esophageal irritation or ulceration.

• Warn patient to avoid driving or other hazardous tasks because of possible adverse CNS effects.
• Caution patient to avoid direct sunlight and ultraviolet light, wear protective clothing, and use sunscreen. Photosensitivity reactions may occur within a few minutes to several hours after exposure. Photosensitivity persists for some time after discontinuation of therapy.

---

## tetracycline hydrochloride
Achromycin V, Apo-Tetra†, Novo-Tetra†, Nu-Tetra†, Panmycin**, Sumycin, Sustamycin§, Tetrachel§

*Pregnancy Risk Category D*

### HOW SUPPLIED
*Tablets:* 250 mg, 500 mg
*Capsules:* 100 mg, 250 mg, 500 mg
*Oral suspension:* 125 mg/5 ml

### ACTION
Unknown. Thought to exert bacteriostatic effect by binding to the 30S and possibly 50S ribosomal subunits of microorganisms, thus inhibiting protein synthesis. May also alter the cytoplasmic membrane of susceptible microorganisms.

| Route | Onset | Peak | Duration |
|-------|-------|------|----------|
| P.O. | Unknown | 1-4 hr | Unknown |

### INDICATIONS & DOSAGE
*Infections due to susceptible gram-negative and gram-positive organisms (including* Haemophilus ducreyi, Yersinia pestis, *and* Campylobacter fetus), *Rickettsia,* Mycoplasma pneumoniae, *and* Chlamydia trachomatis; *psittacosis; granuloma inguinale—*
**Adults:** 250 to 500 mg P.O. q 6 hours.
**Children over age 8:** 25 to 50 mg/kg P.O. daily, in divided doses q 6 hours.
*Uncomplicated urethral, endocervical, or rectal infections due to* C. trachomatis—
**Adults:** 500 mg P.O. q.i.d. for at least 7 days, 10 days for epididymitis, and 21 days for lymphogranuloma venereum.

---

*Brucellosis—*
**Adults:** 500 mg P.O. q 6 hours for 3 weeks with 1 g of streptomycin I.M. q 12 hours for first week; once daily for second week.
*Gonorrhea in patients allergic to penicillin—*
**Adults:** initially, 1.5 g P.O.; then 500 mg q 6 hours for total dose of 9 g; for epididymitis, 500 mg P.O. q 6 hours for 7 days.
*Syphilis in patients allergic to penicillin—*
**Adults:** total of 30 to 40 g P.O. in equally divided doses over 10 to 15 days.
*Acne—*
**Adults and adolescents:** initially, 250 mg P.O. q 6 hours; then 125 to 500 mg daily or every other day.
*Helicobacter pylori infection—*
**Adults:** 500 mg P.O. q 6 hours for 10 to 14 days with other agents, such as metronidazole, bismuth subsalicylate, amoxicillin, or omeprazole.
*Cholera—*
**Adults:** 500 mg P.O. q 6 hours for 48 to 72 hours.
*Malaria due to* Plasmodium falciparum—
**Adults:** 250 to 500 mg P.O. daily for 7 days with quinine sulfate 650 mg P.O. q 8 hours for 3 to 7 days.

## ADVERSE REACTIONS
**CNS:** dizziness, headache, *intracranial hypertension.*
**CV:** pericarditis.
**EENT:** sore throat, glossitis, dysphagia.
**GI:** anorexia, *epigastric distress, nausea, vomiting, diarrhea,* esophagitis, oral candidiasis, stomatitis, enterocolitis, inflammatory lesions in anogenital region.
**GU:** increased BUN.
**Hematologic:** *neutropenia,* eosinophilia, *thrombocytopenia.*
**Hepatic:** elevated liver enzymes.
**Musculoskeletal:** *bone growth retardation* in children under age 9.
**Skin:** *candidal superinfection, maculopapular and erythematous rash, urticaria, photosensitivity, increased pigmentation.*
**Other:** hypersensitivity reactions; *permanent discoloration of teeth, enamel defects.*

## INTERACTIONS
**Drug-drug.** *Antacids (including sodium bicarbonate) and laxatives containing aluminum, magnesium, or calcium; antidiarrheals containing kaolin, pectin, or bismuth subsalicylate:* decreased antibiotic absorption. Give antibiotic 1 hour before or 2 hours after any of these drugs.
*Ferrous sulfate and other iron products, zinc:* decreased antibiotic absorption. Give tetracyclines 2 hours before or 3 hours after iron administration.
*Lithium carbonate:* may alter serum lithium levels. Monitor levels.
*Methoxyflurane:* may cause severe nephrotoxicity with tetracyclines. Monitor carefully.
*Oral anticoagulants:* potentiated anticoagulant effects. Monitor PT and INR, and adjust anticoagulant dosage as ordered.
*Oral contraceptives:* decreased contraceptive effectiveness and increased risk of breakthrough bleeding. Use a nonhormonal form of birth control.
*Penicillins:* may interfere with bactericidal action of penicillins. Avoid use together.
**Drug-food.** *Milk, dairy products, other foods:* decreased antibiotic absorption. Give antibiotic 1 hour before or 2 hours after any of the above.
**Drug-lifestyle.** *Sun exposure:* photosensitivity reactions may occur. Take precautions.

## EFFECTS ON DIAGNOSTIC TESTS
Tetracycline causes false-negative results in urine glucose tests using glucose oxidase reagent (Diastix or Chemstrip uG) and false elevations in fluorometric tests for urine catecholamines.

## CONTRAINDICATIONS
Contraindicated in patients with hypersensitivity to drug or other tetracyclines.

## NURSING CONSIDERATIONS
• Use with extreme caution in patients with impaired renal or hepatic function. Monitor renal and liver function test results. Also use with extreme caution (if at all) during last half of pregnancy and in children under age 9 because drug may cause permanent discoloration of teeth,

---

Reactions may be *common,* uncommon, *life-threatening,* or COMMON AND LIFE-THREATENING.

enamel defects, and bone growth retardation.
• Obtain specimen for culture and sensitivity tests before giving first dose. Therapy may begin pending test results.
• *Alert:* Check expiration date. Outdated or deteriorated tetracyclines have been associated with reversible nephrotoxicity (Fanconi's syndrome).
• Don't expose drug to light or heat.
• With large doses or prolonged therapy, monitor for superinfection, especially in high-risk patients.
• Check patient's tongue for signs of candidal infection. Stress good oral hygiene.
• Drug is not indicated for the treatment of neurosyphilis.

### ☑ Patient teaching
• Tell patient to take drug exactly as prescribed, even after he feels better, and to take entire amount prescribed.
• Explain that effectiveness is reduced when taken with milk or other dairy products, food, antacids, or iron products. Tell patient to take each dose with a full glass of water on an empty stomach, at least 1 hour before or 2 hours after meals. Also tell him to take it at least 1 hour before bedtime to prevent esophageal irritation or ulceration.
• Warn patient to avoid direct sunlight and ultraviolet light, wear protective clothing, and use sunscreen. Photosensitivity reactions may occur within a few minutes to several hours after sun exposure. Photosensitivity persists after discontinuation of drug.

co-trimoxazole
sulfadiazine
sulfamethoxazole
sulfisoxazole
sulfisoxazole acetyl

## COMBINATION PRODUCTS

AZO-SULFAMETHOXAZOLE† tablets (film-coated): sulfamethoxazole 500 mg and phenazopyridine hydrochloride 100 mg.
AZO-SULFISOXAZOLE tablets (film-coated): sulfisoxazole 500 mg and phenazopyridine hydrochloride 50 mg.
ERYZOLE, PEDIAZOLE, SULFIMYCIN suspension: sulfisoxazole 600 mg and erythromycin ethylsuccinate 200 mg/5 ml.

## co-trimoxazole (sulfamethoxazole-trimethoprim)

Apo-Sulfatrim†, Apo-Sulfatrim DS†, Bactrim*, Bactrim DS, Bactrim I.V., Novo-Trimel†, Novo-Trimel D.S.†, Nu-Cotrimox†, Resprim‡, Roubac†, Septra*, Septra DS, Septra I.V., Septrin‡, SMZ-TMP, Sulfatrim

*Pregnancy Risk Category C (contraindicated at term)*

## HOW SUPPLIED

*Tablets (single-strength):* trimethoprim 80 mg and sulfamethoxazole 400 mg
*Tablets (double-strength):* trimethoprim 160 mg and sulfamethoxazole 800 mg
*Oral suspension:* trimethoprim 40 mg and sulfamethoxazole 200 mg/5 ml
*Injection:* trimethoprim 16 mg/ml and sulfamethoxazole 80 mg/ml in 5-ml, 10-ml, 20-ml, and 30-ml vials

## ACTION

Sulfamethoxazole inhibits formation of dihydrofolic acid from PABA; trimethoprim inhibits dihydrofolate reductase for-

mation. Both decrease bacterial folic acid synthesis; bactericidal.

| Route | Onset | Peak | Duration |
|-------|-------|------|----------|
| P.O. | Unknown | 1-4 hr | Unknown |
| I.V. | Immediate | Immediate | Unknown |

## INDICATIONS & DOSAGE

*Shigellosis or urinary tract infections (UTIs) due to susceptible strains of* Escherichia coli, Proteus *(indole positive or negative),* Klebsiella, *or* Enterobacter—
**Adults:** 160 mg trimethoprim/800 mg sulfamethoxazole (double-strength tablet) P.O. q 12 hours for 10 to 14 days in UTIs and for 5 days in shigellosis. If indicated, I.V. infusion is given: 8 to 10 mg/kg/day (based on trimethoprim component) in two to four divided doses q 6, 8, or 12 hours for up to 14 days for severe UTIs. Maximum daily dose is 960 mg trimethoprim.
**Children ages 2 months and older:** 8 mg/kg/day (based on trimethoprim component) P.O., in two divided doses q 12 hours (10 days for UTIs; 5 days for shigellosis). If indicated, I.V. infusion is given: 8 to 10 mg/kg/day (based on trimethoprim component) in two to four divided doses q 6, 8, or 12 hours. Adult dose shouldn't be exceeded.
*Otitis media in patients with penicillin allergy or penicillin-resistant infections—*
**Children ages 2 months and older:** 8 mg/kg/day (based on trimethoprim component) P.O., in two divided doses q 12 hours for 10 to 14 days.
*Chronic bronchitis, upper respiratory tract infections—*
**Adults:** 160 mg trimethoprim/800 mg sulfamethoxazole P.O. q 12 hours for 10 to 14 days.
*Traveler's diarrhea—*
**Adults:** 160 mg trimethoprim/800 mg sulfamethoxazole P.O. b.i.d. for 3 to 5 days. Some patients may require 2 days or less of therapy.

*UTIs in men with prostatitis—*
**Adults:** 160 mg trimethoprim/800 mg sulfamethoxazole P.O. b.i.d. for 3 to 6 months.
*Prophylaxis for chronic UTIs—*
**Adults:** 40 mg trimethoprim/200 mg sulfamethoxazole (½ tablet) or 80 mg trimethoprim/400 mg sulfamethoxazole P.O. daily or three times weekly for 3 to 6 months.
*Prophylaxis for* Pneumocystis carinii *pneumonia—*
**Adults:** 160 mg of trimethoprim/800 mg sulfamethoxazole P.O. daily.
**Children ages 2 months and older:**
150 mg/m$^2$ trimethoprim/750 mg/m$^2$ sulfamethoxazole P.O daily in two divided doses on 3 consecutive days each week.
*P. carinii pneumonia—*
**Adults and children over age 2 months:**
15 to 20 mg/kg/day (based on trimethoprim) I.V. or P.O. in three or four divided doses for 14 days.
*Adjust-a-dose:* For patients with renal failure with creatinine clearance of 15 to 30 ml/minute, daily dose should be reduced by 50%. Drug isn't recommended for patients with creatinine clearance below 15 ml/minute.

## ADVERSE REACTIONS
**CNS:** headache, mental depression, aseptic meningitis, tinnitus, apathy, *seizures,* hallucinations, ataxia, nervousness, fatigue, vertigo, insomnia.
**CV:** thrombophlebitis.
**GI:** *nausea, vomiting, diarrhea,* abdominal pain, anorexia, stomatitis, pancreatitis, pseudomembranous colitis.
**GU:** *toxic nephrosis with oliguria and anuria,* crystalluria, hematuria, interstitial nephritis, increased BUN and serum creatinine levels.
**Hematologic:** *agranulocytosis, aplastic anemia,* megaloblastic anemia, *thrombocytopenia, leukopenia, hemolytic anemia.*
**Hepatic:** jaundice, *hepatic necrosis,* elevated liver function test results.
**Musculoskeletal:** arthralgia, myalgia, muscle weakness.
**Respiratory:** pulmonary infiltrates.
**Skin:** *erythema multiforme, Stevens-Johnson syndrome, generalized skin* eruption, *epidermal necrolysis, exfoliative dermatitis,* photosensitivity, urticaria, pruritus.
**Other:** *hypersensitivity reactions, serum sickness, drug fever, anaphylaxis.*

## INTERACTIONS
**Drug-drug.** *Cyclosporine:* may decrease cyclosporine levels and increase nephrotoxicity risk. Avoid concomitant use.
*Methotrexate:* may increase methotrexate concentrations. Use together cautiously.
*Oral anticoagulants:* increased anticoagulant effect. Monitor for bleeding.
*Oral antidiabetics:* increased hypoglycemic effect. Monitor blood glucose levels.
*Oral contraceptives:* decreased contraceptive effectiveness and increased risk of breakthrough bleeding. Suggest a nonhormonal contraceptive.
*Phenytoin:* may inhibit hepatic metabolism of phenytoin. Monitor closely.
**Drug-lifestyle.** *Sun exposure:* photosensitivity reactions may occur. Take precautions.

## EFFECTS ON DIAGNOSTIC TESTS
Trimethoprim can interfere with serum methotrexate assay as determined by the competitive binding protein technique. No interference occurs if radioimmunoassay is used.

## CONTRAINDICATIONS
Contraindicated in patients with severe renal impairment (creatinine clearance below 15 ml/minute), porphyria, megaloblastic anemia due to folate deficiency, or hypersensitivity to trimethoprim or sulfonamides. Also contraindicated in pregnant women at term, in breast-feeding women, and in infants under age 2 months.

## NURSING CONSIDERATIONS
• Use cautiously and in reduced dosages in patients with impaired hepatic or renal function (creatinine clearance 15 to 30 ml/minute), severe allergy or bronchial asthma, G6PD deficiency, and blood dyscrasia.
• Monitor renal and liver function test results.

---

*Liquid contains alcohol.    **May contain tartrazine.    †Canada    ‡Australia    §U.K.    ◊OTC

• Obtain specimen for culture and sensitivity tests before first dose. Therapy may begin pending results.
• *Alert:* Double-check dosage, which may be written as trimethoprim component.
• *Alert:* Note that the "DS" product means "double strength."
• Never administer drug I.M.
• Promptly report complaints of rash, sore throat, fever, cough, mouth sores, or iris lesions—early signs and symptoms of erythema multiforme, which may progress to the sometimes fatal condition, Stevens-Johnson syndrome. These symptoms may also represent early signs of blood dyscrasias.
• Watch for superinfection (fever or other signs or symptoms of new infection).
• *Alert:* Adverse reactions, especially hypersensitivity reactions, rash, and fever, occur much more frequently in patients with AIDS.

**I.V. administration**
• Dilute each 5 ml of concentrate for I.V. infusion in 75 to 125 ml of $D_5W$ before administration. Don't mix with other drugs or solutions. Infuse slowly over 60 to 90 minutes. Don't give by rapid infusion or bolus injection. Don't refrigerate; use within 6 hours.

**Patient teaching**
• Tell patient to take drug as prescribed, even if he feels better.
• Encourage patient to maintain adequate fluid intake.
• Tell patient to report adverse reactions promptly.
• Instruct patient receiving drug I.V. to alert nurse if discomfort occurs at I.V. insertion site.
• Advise patient to avoid prolonged sun exposure, wear protective clothing, and use sunscreen.
• Instruct patient to take oral medication with 8 oz (240 ml) of water on an empty stomach.

# sulfadiazine
Coptin†

*Pregnancy Risk Category C
(contraindicated at term)*

## HOW SUPPLIED
*Tablets:* 500 mg

## ACTION
Inhibits formation of dihydrofolic acid from PABA, decreasing bacterial folic acid synthesis; bacteriostatic.

| Route | Onset | Peak | Duration |
|-------|-------|------|----------|
| P.O. | Unknown | 4-6 hr | Unknown |

## INDICATIONS & DOSAGE
*Asymptomatic meningococcal carriers—*
**Adults:** 1 g P.O. q 12 hours for 2 days.
**Children ages 1 to 12:** 500 mg P.O. q 12 hours for 2 days.
**Children ages 2 to 12 months:** 500 mg P.O. daily for 2 days.
*Rheumatic fever prophylaxis, as an alternative to penicillin—*
**Children weighing over 30 kg (66 lb):** 1 g P.O. daily.
**Children under 30 kg:** 500 mg P.O. daily.
*Adjunct treatment in toxoplasmosis—*
**Adults:** 2 to 8 g P.O. daily divided q 6 hours for 6 to 8 weeks or until improvement occurs. Usually given with pyrimethamine.
**Children:** 100 to 200 mg/kg P.O. daily divided q 6 hours (maximum 6 g daily) for 6 to 8 weeks or until improvement occurs. Usually given with pyrimethamine.
*Malaria, treatment of chloroquine-resistant* Plasmodium falciparum—
**Adults:** 500 mg P.O. q.i.d. for 5 days with quinine sulfate and pyrimethamine.
**Children:** 25 to 50 mg/kg P.O. q.i.d. (maximum 2 g daily) for 5 days with quinine sulfate and pyrimethamine.
*Nocardiosis—*
**Adults:** 4 to 8 g P.O. daily given in divided doses for a minimum of 6 weeks.

## ADVERSE REACTIONS
**CNS:** headache, mental depression, *seizures,* hallucinations.

---

Reactions may be *common,* uncommon, *life-threatening,* or COMMON AND LIFE-THREATENING.

**GI:** *nausea, vomiting, diarrhea,* abdominal pain, anorexia, stomatitis.
**GU:** *toxic nephrosis with oliguria and anuria,* crystalluria, hematuria, elevated serum creatinine level.
**Hematologic:** *agranulocytosis, aplastic anemia,* megaloblastic anemia, *thrombocytopenia, leukopenia, hemolytic anemia.*
**Hepatic:** elevated liver function test results, jaundice.
**Skin:** *erythema multiforme, Stevens-Johnson syndrome, generalized skin eruption, epidermal necrolysis, exfoliative dermatitis,* photosensitivity, urticaria, pruritus.
**Other:** *hypersensitivity reactions, serum sickness, drug fever, anaphylaxis,* local irritation, extravasation.

## INTERACTIONS
**Drug-drug.** *Methotrexate:* may increase methotrexate levels. Use together cautiously.
*Oral anticoagulants:* increased anticoagulant effect. Monitor for bleeding.
*Oral antidiabetics:* increased hypoglycemic effect. Monitor blood glucose levels.
*Oral contraceptives:* decreased contraceptive effectiveness and increased risk of breakthrough bleeding. Suggest a nonhormonal contraceptive.
*PABA-containing drugs:* inhibited antibacterial action. Don't use together.
**Drug-lifestyle.** *Sun exposure:* photosensitivity reactions may occur. Take precautions.

## EFFECTS ON DIAGNOSTIC TESTS
Drug alters urine glucose tests using cupric sulfate (Benedict's reagent or Clinitest).

## CONTRAINDICATIONS
Contraindicated in patients with hypersensitivity to sulfonamides, in those with porphyria, in infants under age 2 months (except in congenital toxoplasmosis), in pregnant women at term, and in breast-feeding women.

## NURSING CONSIDERATIONS
• Use cautiously and in reduced doses in patients with impaired hepatic or renal function, bronchial asthma, history of multiple allergies, G6PD deficiency, and blood dyscrasia.
• Give drug on schedule to maintain constant blood level.
• Monitor for signs of blood dyscrasia (purpura, ecchymoses, sore throat, fever, and pallor). Report them immediately.
• Promptly report complaints of rash, sore throat, fever, cough, mouth sores, or iris lesions—early signs and symptoms of erythema multiforme, which may progress to the sometimes fatal Stevens-Johnson syndrome.
• Monitor urine cultures, CBCs, and urinalyses before and during therapy, as ordered.
• Monitor renal and liver function test results.
• Watch for superinfection (fever or other signs or symptoms of new infection).
• Folic or folinic acid may be used during rest periods in toxoplasmosis therapy to reverse hematopoietic depression or anemia associated with pyrimethamine and sulfadiazine.
• Monitor fluid intake and output. Maintain intake between 3,000 and 4,000 ml daily for adults to produce output of 1,500 ml daily. If fluid intake is not adequate to prevent crystalluria, sodium bicarbonate may be administered to alkalinize urine, as ordered. Monitor urine pH daily.
• *Alert:* Don't confuse sulfadiazine with sulfasalazine. Don't confuse sulfonamide drugs.

☑ **Patient teaching**
• Tell patient to take drug as prescribed, even if he feels better.
• Inform patient to drink a glass of water with each dose and plenty of water each day to prevent crystalluria.
• Instruct patient to report adverse reactions promptly.
• Warn patient to avoid prolonged exposure to sunlight, wear protective clothing, and use sunscreen.

## sulfamethoxazole
## (sulphamethoxazole)
Apo-Sulfamethoxazole†, Gantanol

*Pregnancy Risk Category C
(contraindicated at term)*

### HOW SUPPLIED
*Tablets:* 500 mg

### ACTION
Inhibits formation of dihydrofolic acid from PABA, decreasing bacterial folic acid synthesis; bacteriostatic.

| Route | Onset | Peak | Duration |
|-------|-------|------|----------|
| P.O. | Unknown | 2 hr | Unknown |

### INDICATIONS & DOSAGE
*Urinary tract and systemic infections—*
**Adults:** initially, 2 g P.O.; then 1 g P.O. b.i.d. up to t.i.d. for severe infections.
*Chlamydia trachomatis (lymphogranuloma venereum)—*
**Adults:** 1 g P.O. b.i.d. for 21 days.
**Children and infants over age 2 months:** initially, 50 to 60 mg/kg P.O.; then 25 to 30 mg/kg b.i.d. Maximum daily dose shouldn't exceed 75 mg/kg.

### ADVERSE REACTIONS
**CNS:** headache, mental depression, *seizures,* hallucinations, aseptic meningitis, tinnitus, apathy.
**GI:** *nausea, vomiting, diarrhea,* abdominal pain, anorexia, stomatitis, pancreatitis, pseudomembranous colitis.
**GU:** *toxic nephrosis with oliguria and anuria,* crystalluria, hematuria, interstitial nephritis.
**Hematologic:** *agranulocytosis, aplastic anemia,* megaloblastic anemia, *thrombocytopenia, leukopenia, hemolytic anemia.*
**Hepatic:** elevated liver function test results, jaundice.
**Skin:** *erythema multiforme, Stevens-Johnson syndrome, generalized skin eruption, epidermal necrolysis, exfoliative dermatitis,* photosensitivity, urticaria, pruritus.
**Other:** *hypersensitivity reactions, serum sickness, drug fever, anaphylaxis.*

### INTERACTIONS
**Drug-drug.** *Methotrexate:* may increase methotrexate levels. Use together cautiously.
*Oral anticoagulants:* increased anticoagulant effect. Monitor for bleeding.
*Oral antidiabetics:* increased hypoglycemic effect. Monitor blood glucose levels.
*Oral contraceptives:* decreased contraceptive effectiveness and increased risk of breakthrough bleeding. Suggest a nonhormonal contraceptive.
*Phenytoin:* may increase phenytoin effect. Monitor closely.
**Drug-lifestyle.** *Sun exposure:* may cause photosensitivity reactions. Use precautions.

### EFFECTS ON DIAGNOSTIC TESTS
Drug alters results of urine glucose tests using cupric sulfate (Benedict's reagent or Clinitest).

### CONTRAINDICATIONS
Contraindicated in patients with hypersensitivity to sulfonamides, in those with porphyria, in infants under age 2 months (except in congenital toxoplasmosis), in pregnant women at term, and in breast-feeding women.

### NURSING CONSIDERATIONS
• Use cautiously and in reduced dosages in patients with impaired hepatic or renal function, severe allergy or bronchial asthma, G6PD deficiency, and blood dyscrasia.
• Monitor renal and liver function test results.
• Obtain specimen for culture and sensitivity tests before first dose. Therapy may begin pending results.
• Monitor urine cultures, CBCs, and urinalyses before and during therapy, as ordered.
• Watch for superinfection (fever or other signs or symptoms of new infection).
• Monitor fluid intake and output. Maintain intake between 3,000 and 4,000 ml daily for adults to produce output of 1,500 ml daily. If fluid intake is not adequate to prevent crystalluria, sodium bicarbonate may be administered to alkalinize urine, as ordered. Monitor urine pH daily.

---

Reactions may be *common*, uncommon, *life-threatening*, or COMMON AND LIFE-THREATENING.

• *Alert:* Don't confuse sulfamethoxazole with sulfamethizole. Don't confuse the combination products (such as Gantanol) with sulfamethoxazole alone.

### ☑ Patient teaching
• Tell patient to take drug as prescribed, even if he feels better.
• Instruct patient to drink a glass of water with each dose and plenty of water each day to prevent crystalluria.
• *Alert:* Tell patient to notify doctor of early signs and symptoms of blood dyscrasia (sore throat, fever, and pallor). Also tell patient to be alert for flulike symptoms, cough, and lesions of the iris, skin, and mucous membranes—early signs of erythema multiforme, which can progress to the sometimes fatal Stevens-Johnson syndrome.
• Warn patient to avoid prolonged exposure to sunlight, to wear protective clothing, and to use sunscreen.

---

## sulfisoxazole (sulfafurazole, sulphafurazole)
Novo-Soxazole†

## sulfisoxazole acetyl
Gantrisin Pediatric

*Pregnancy Risk Category C (contraindicated at term)*

### HOW SUPPLIED
**sulfisoxazole**
*Tablets:* 500 mg
**sulfisoxazole acetyl**
*Liquid:* 500 mg/5 ml

### ACTION
Inhibits formation of dihydrofolic acid from PABA, decreasing bacterial folic acid synthesis; bacteriostatic.

| Route | Onset | Peak | Duration |
|-------|-------|------|----------|
| P.O. | Unknown | 1-4 hr | Unknown |

### INDICATIONS & DOSAGE
*Urinary tract and systemic infections—*
**Adults:** initially, 2 to 4 g P.O.; then 4 to 8 g daily divided in four to six doses.

**Children over age 2 months:** initially, 75 mg/kg P.O. daily or 2 g/m² P.O.; then 150 mg/kg or 4 g/m² P.O. daily in divided doses q 6 hours. Total daily dose shouldn't exceed 6 g.
*Chlamydia trachomatis (lymphogranuloma venereum)—*
**Adults:** 500 mg to 1 g P.O. q.i.d. for 21 days.
*Uncomplicated urethral, endocervical, or rectal infections due to* C. trachomatis—
**Adults:** 500 mg P.O. q.i.d. for 10 days.
*Adjust-a-dose:* For patients with renal failure, use normal dose at longer intervals. If creatinine clearance is 10 to 50 ml/min ute, give q 8 to12 hours; if clearance is less than 10 ml/minute, give q 12 to 24 hours.

### ADVERSE REACTIONS
**CNS:** headache, mental depression, *seizures,* hallucinations.
**CV:** tachycardia, palpitations, syncope, cyanosis.
**GI:** *nausea, vomiting, diarrhea,* abdominal pain, anorexia, stomatitis, pseudomembranous colitis.
**GU:** *toxic nephrosis with oliguria and anuria,* crystalluria, hematuria, *acute renal failure.*
**Hematologic:** *agranulocytosis, aplastic anemia,* megaloblastic anemia, *thrombocytopenia, leukopenia, hemolytic anemia.*
**Hepatic:** jaundice, elevated liver function test results, *hepatitis.*
**Skin:** *erythema multiforme, generalized skin eruption, epidermal necrolysis, exfoliative dermatitis,* photosensitivity, urticaria, pruritus.
**Other:** *hypersensitivity reactions, serum sickness, drug fever, anaphylaxis.*

### INTERACTIONS
**Drug-drug.** *Methotrexate:* may increase methotrexate levels. Use together cautiously.
*Oral anticoagulants:* increased anticoagulant effect. Monitor for bleeding.
*Oral antidiabetics:* increased hypoglycemic effect. Monitor blood glucose levels.
*Oral contraceptives:* decreased contraceptive effectiveness, increased risk of break-

---

through bleeding. Suggest a nonhormonal contraceptive.
**Drug-lifestyle.** *Sun exposure:* photosensitivity reactions may occur. Use precautions.

## EFFECTS ON DIAGNOSTIC TESTS
Drug alters results of urine glucose tests using cupric sulfate (Benedict's reagent or Clinitest).

## CONTRAINDICATIONS
Contraindicated in patients with hypersensitivity to sulfonamides, in infants under age 2 months (except in congenital toxoplasmosis), in pregnant women at term, and in breast-feeding women.

## NURSING CONSIDERATIONS
• Use cautiously in patients with impaired hepatic or renal function, severe allergy or bronchial asthma, and G6PD deficiency.
• Monitor renal and liver function test results.
• Obtain specimen for culture and sensitivity tests before giving first dose. Therapy may begin pending results.
• Monitor urine cultures, CBCs, PT, and urinalyses before and during therapy, as ordered.
• Report moderate to severe diarrhea to doctor.
• Watch for superinfection (fever or other signs or symptoms of new infection).
• Monitor fluid intake and output. Maintain intake between 3,000 and 4,000 ml daily for adults to produce output of 1,500 ml daily. If fluid intake is not adequate to prevent crystalluria, sodium bicarbonate may be administered to alkalinize urine, as ordered. Monitor urine pH daily.
• *Alert:* Don't confuse sulfisoxazole with sulfasalazine. Don't confuse the combination products (such as Gantrisin) with sulfamethoxazole alone.

### ☑ Patient teaching
• Tell patient to take drug as prescribed, even if he feels better.
• Instruct patient to drink a glass of water with each dose and plenty of water each day to prevent crystalluria.

• *Alert:* Tell patient to notify doctor if early signs of blood dyscrasia (sore throat, fever, and pallor) and moderate to severe diarrhea occur.
• Warn patient to avoid sunlight, wear protective clothing, and use sunscreen.

---

Reactions may be *common*, uncommon, ***life-threatening***, or COMMON AND LIFE-THREATENING.

alatrofloxacin mesylate
ciprofloxacin
enoxacin
levofloxacin
lomefloxacin hydrochloride
nalidixic acid
norfloxacin
ofloxacin
sparfloxacin
trovafloxacin mesylate

**COMBINATION PRODUCTS**
None.

---

### ciprofloxacin
Cipro, Cipro I.V., Ciproxin‡

*Pregnancy Risk Category C*

#### HOW SUPPLIED
*Tablets (film-coated):*100 mg, 250 mg, 500 mg, 750 mg
*Infusion (premixed):* 200 mg in 100 ml D₅W, 400 mg in 200 ml D₅W
*Injection:* 200 mg, 400 mg

#### ACTION
Inhibits bacterial DNA synthesis, mainly by blocking DNA gyrase; bactericidal.

| Route | Onset | Peak | Duration |
|-------|-------|------|----------|
| P.O. | Unknown | 0.5-2.3 hr | Unknown |
| I.V. | Unknown | Immediate | Unknown |

#### INDICATIONS & DOSAGE
*Mild to moderate urinary tract infections (UTIs) due to* Escherichia coli, Klebsiella pneumoniae, Enterobacter cloacae, Serratia marcescens, Proteus mirabilis, Providencia rettgeri, Morganella morganii, Citrobacter diversus, C. freundii, Pseudomonas aeruginosa, Staphylococcus epidermidis, *and* Enterococcus faecalis—
**Adults:** 250 mg P.O. or 200 mg I.V. q 12 hours.
*Severe or complicated UTIs; mild to moderate bone and joint infections due to* E. cloacae, P. aeruginosa, *and* S. marcescens;

*mild to moderate respiratory infections due to* E. coli, K. pneumoniae, E. cloacae, P. mirabilis, P. aeruginosa, Haemophilus influenzae, *and* H. parainfluenzae; *mild to moderate skin and skin-structure infections due to* E. coli, K. pneumoniae, E. cloacae, P. mirabilis, P. vulgaris, Providencia stuartii, M. morganii, C. freundii, Streptococcus pyogenes, P. aeruginosa, Staphylococcus aureus, *and* S. epidermidis; *infectious diarrhea due to* E. coli, Campylobacter jejuni, Shigella flexneri, *and* S. sonnei; *typhoid fever—*
**Adults:** 500 mg P.O. or 400 mg I.V. q 12 hours.
*Severe or complicated bone or joint infections, severe respiratory tract infections, severe skin and skin-structure infections—*
**Adults:** 750 mg P.O. q 12 hours.
*Chronic bacterial prostatitis due to* E. coli *or* P. mirabilis—
**Adults:** 500 mg P.O. q 12 hours for 28 days.
*Complicated intra-abdominal infections (used with metronidazole) due to* E. coli, P. aeruginosa, P. mirabilis, K. pneumoniae, *or* Bacteroides fragilis—
**Adults:** 500 mg P.O. or 400 mg I.V. q 12 hours for 7 to 14 days.
*Acute uncomplicated cystitis—*
**Adults:** 100 mg P.O. q 12 hours for 3 days.
*Mild to moderate acute sinusitis—*
**Adults:** 500 mg P.O. q 12 hours for 10 days.
✳ *NEW INDICATION:* Mild to moderate acute sinusitis due to H. influenzae, Streptococcus pneumoniae, *or* Moraxella catarrhalis; *mild to moderate chronic bacterial prostatitis due to* Escherichia coli *or* P. mirabilis—
**Adults:** 400 mg I.V. infusion given over 60 minutes q 12 hours.
*Adjust-a-dose:* For patients with renal failure, if creatinine clearance is 30 to 50 ml/minute, give 250 to 500 mg P.O. q 12 hours or the usual I.V. dose; if clearance is 5 to 29 ml/minute, give 250 to 500 mg P.O. q 18 hours or 200 to 400 mg

---

I.V. q 18 to 24 hours. If patient is on hemodialysis, give 250 to 500 mg P.O. q 24 hours (after dialysis)

## ADVERSE REACTIONS
**CNS:** headache, restlessness, tremor, dizziness, fatigue, drowsiness, insomnia, depression, light-headedness, confusion, hallucinations, *seizures,* paresthesia.
**GI:** *nausea, diarrhea,* vomiting, abdominal pain or discomfort, oral candidiasis, pseudomembranous colitis, dyspepsia, flatulence, constipation.
**GU:** crystalluria, increased serum creatinine and BUN levels, interstitial nephritis.
**Hematologic:** eosinophilia, *leukopenia, neutropenia, thrombocytopenia.*
**Hepatic:** elevated liver enzymes.
**Musculoskeletal:** arthralgia, arthropathy, joint or back pain, joint inflammation, joint stiffness, tendon rupture, aching, neck or chest pain.
**Skin:** *rash,* photosensitivity, *Stevens-Johnson syndrome, toxic epidermal necrolysis, exfoliative dermatitis.*
**Other:** hypersensitivity; thrombophlebitis, burning, pruritus, erythema, edema.

## INTERACTIONS
**Drug-drug.** *Antacids containing aluminum hydroxide or magnesium hydroxide, iron supplements, iron- or zinc-containing multivitamins, sucralfate:* decreased ciprofloxacin absorption. Separate administration by at least 2 hours.
*Probenecid:* may elevate serum level of ciprofloxacin. Monitor for toxicity.
*Theophylline:* increased plasma theophylline levels and prolonged theophylline half-life. Monitor blood levels of theophylline and observe for adverse effects.
**Drug-herb.** *Yerba maté:* may decrease clearance of yerba maté's methylxanthines and cause toxicity. Use together cautiously.
**Drug-food.** *Caffeine:* increased effect of caffeine. Monitor closely.
*Dairy products, other foods:* delayed peak serum levels. Give drug on an empty stomach.
**Drug-lifestyle.** *Sun exposure:* photosensitivity reactions may occur. Take precautions.

## EFFECTS ON DIAGNOSTIC TESTS
None reported.

## CONTRAINDICATIONS
Contraindicated in patients sensitive to fluoroquinolone antibiotics.

## NURSING CONSIDERATIONS
• Use cautiously in patients with CNS disorders, such as severe cerebral arteriosclerosis or seizure disorders, and in those at increased risk for seizures. Drug may cause CNS stimulation.
• Obtain specimen for culture and sensitivity tests before giving first dose. Therapy may begin pending results.
• Administer oral form 2 hours after a meal or 2 hours before or after taking antacids, sucralfate, or products that contain iron (such as vitamins with mineral supplements). Food does not affect absorption but may delay peak serum levels.
• Long-term therapy may result in overgrowth of organisms resistant to ciprofloxacin.
• Safety in children under age 18 has not been established. Drug may cause cartilage erosion.
• Monitor patient's intake and output and observe for signs of crystalluria.
• Tendon rupture has been reported in patients receiving quinolones. Discontinue if pain, inflammation, or rupture of a tendon occurs.

### 🔲 I.V. administration
• Dilute drug using $D_5W$ or normal saline for injection to a final concentration of 1 to 2 mg/ml before use. Infuse slowly (over 1 hour) into a large vein to minimize discomfort and reduce the risk of venous irritation.
• If administering drug through a Y-type set, discontinue the other I.V. solution during ciprofloxacin infusion.

### ☑ Patient teaching
• Tell patient to take drug as prescribed, even after he feels better.
• Advise patient to drink plenty of fluids to reduce risk of crystalluria.
• Warn patient to avoid hazardous tasks that require alertness, such as driving, until CNS effects of drug are known.

• Instruct patient to avoid caffeine while taking drug because of potential for cumulative caffeine effects.
• Advise patient that hypersensitivity reactions may occur even after first dose. If a rash or other allergic reaction appears, tell him to stop drug immediately and notify doctor.
• Tell patient to avoid excessive sunlight or artificial ultraviolet light during therapy and to stop drug and call doctor if phototoxicity occurs.
• Because drug appears in breast milk, inform female patient to discontinue breast-feeding during treatment or to ask to be treated with another drug.
• Tell patient to take drug on an empty stomach, 2 hours after a meal.

---

### enoxacin
Penetrex

*Pregnancy Risk Category C*

#### HOW SUPPLIED
*Tablets (film-coated):* 200 mg, 400 mg

#### ACTION
Inhibits bacterial DNA synthesis, mainly by blocking DNA gyrase; bactericidal.

| Route | Onset | Peak | Duration |
|-------|-------|------|----------|
| P.O. | Unknown | 1-3 hr | Unknown |

#### INDICATIONS & DOSAGE
*Uncomplicated urinary tract infections (UTIs) due to susceptible strains of* Escherichia coli, Staphylococcus epidermidis, *and* S. saprophyticus—
**Adults ages 18 and older:** 200 mg P.O. q 12 hours for 7 days.
*Severe or complicated UTIs due to susceptible strains of* E. coli, Proteus mirabilis, Pseudomonas aeruginosa, S. epidermidis, *and* Enterobacter cloacae—
**Adults ages 18 and older:** 400 mg P.O. q 12 hours for 14 days.
*Uncomplicated urethral or endocervical gonorrhea—*
**Adults:** 400 mg P.O. as a single dose.
    Doxycycline therapy may follow to treat possible coexisting chlamydial infection.

*Adjust-a-dose:* For patients with renal failure, if creatinine clearance is 30 ml/minute or less, therapy is started with usual initial dose. Subsequent doses are decreased by 50%.

#### ADVERSE REACTIONS
**CNS:** headache, restlessness, tremor, light-headedness, confusion, hallucinations, *seizures.*
**GI:** *nausea, diarrhea,* vomiting, abdominal pain or discomfort, oral candidiasis.
**GU:** crystalluria.
**Hematologic:** eosinophilia.
**Hepatic:** elevated liver enzymes.
**Respiratory:** dyspnea, cough.
**Skin:** *rash,* photosensitivity, pruritus.
**Other:** hypersensitivity.

#### INTERACTIONS
**Drug-drug.** *Aminophylline, cyclosporine, theophylline:* increased levels of these drugs because of decreased metabolism. Use together cautiously.
*Antacids containing aluminum hydroxide or magnesium hydroxide, oral iron supplements, sucralfate:* decreased enoxacin absorption. Separate administration times by at least 2 hours.
*Bismuth subsalicylate:* bioavailability of enoxacin is decreased when given within 60 minutes of bismuth subsalicylate. Avoid concomitant use.
*Digoxin:* may increase digoxin serum levels. Monitor closely for toxicity.
*Oral anticoagulants:* increased anticoagulant effect. Use together cautiously.
**Drug-food.** *Any food:* affects absorption. Give drug on empty stomach.
*Caffeine:* increased effect of caffeine. Monitor closely.

#### EFFECTS ON DIAGNOSTIC TESTS
None reported.

#### CONTRAINDICATIONS
Contraindicated in patients with hypersensitivity to drug or other fluoroquinolone antibiotics.

#### NURSING CONSIDERATIONS
• Use cautiously in patients with CNS disorders, such as severe cerebral arteriosclerosis or seizure disorders, and in those at

---

*Liquid contains alcohol.    **May contain tartrazine.    †Canada    ‡Australia    §U.K.    ◊OTC

increased risk for seizures. Drug may cause CNS stimulation.
• Use cautiously and with dosage adjustments in patients with impaired renal or hepatic function. Monitor renal function and liver function tests.
• Obtain specimen for culture and sensitivity tests before giving first dose. Therapy may begin pending results.
• **Alert:** Before treatment for gonorrhea begins, patient should have an initial serologic test for syphilis. Drug hasn't been effective in treating syphilis and may mask signs and symptoms of infection. Have the serologic test repeated in 1 to 3 months.
• Administer 2 hours after a meal or 2 hours before or after antacids containing magnesium hydroxide or aluminum hydroxide, sucralfate, or products that contain iron (such as vitamins with mineral supplements).
• Monitor closely for superinfection.
• Safety in children under age 18 has not been established. Drug has caused cartilage erosion.
• Tendon rupture has been reported in patients receiving quinolones. Discontinue if pain, inflammation, or rupture of a tendon occurs.

☑ **Patient teaching**
• Tell patient to take drug as prescribed, even after he feels better.
• Instruct patient to take drug on an empty stomach.
• Advise patient to drink plenty of fluids to reduce risk of crystalluria.
• Warn patient to avoid hazardous tasks until adverse CNS effects of drug are known.
• Warn patient not to drink beverages containing caffeine. Enoxacin inhibits the metabolism of caffeine and can result in toxicity.
• Advise patient to avoid overexposure to direct sunlight, use a sunblock, and wear protective clothing while outdoors.
• Instruct patient to stop taking drug at first signs of an allergic reaction and to notify doctor.

## levofloxacin
Levaquin

*Pregnancy Risk Category C*

### HOW SUPPLIED
*Tablets:* 250 mg, 500 mg
*Single-use vials:* 500 mg
*Infusion (premixed):* 250 mg in 50 ml $D_5W$, 500 mg in 100 ml $D_5W$

### ACTION
Inhibits bacterial DNA gyrase and prevents DNA replication, transcription, repair, and recombination in susceptible bacteria.

| Route | Onset | Peak | Duration |
|-------|-------|------|----------|
| P.O., I.V. | Unknown | 1-2 hr | Unknown |

### INDICATIONS & DOSAGE
*Note:* Indicated for treatment of mild, moderate, and severe infections due to susceptible microorganisms in adults ages 18 and older.
*Acute maxillary sinusitis due to susceptible strains of* Streptococcus pneumoniae, Moraxella catarrhalis, *or* Haemophilus influenzae—
**Adults:** 500 mg P.O. or I.V. daily for 10 to 14 days. (See *Adjust-a-dose,* p. 147.)
*Acute bacterial exacerbation of chronic bronchitis due to* Staphylococcus aureus, S. pneumoniae, M. catarrhalis, H. influenzae, *or* H. parainfluenzae—
**Adults:** 500 mg P.O. or I.V. daily for 7 days. (See *Adjust-a-dose,* p. 147.)
*Community-acquired pneumonia due to* S. aureus, S. pneumoniae, M. catarrhalis, H. influenzae, H. parainfluenzae, Klebsiella pneumoniae, Chlamydia pneumoniae, Legionella pneumophila, *or* Mycoplasma pneumoniae—
**Adults:** 500 mg P.O. or I.V. daily for 7 to 14 days. (See *Adjust-a-dose,* p. 147.)
*Mild to moderate skin and skin-structure infections due to* S. aureus *or* S. pyogenes—
**Adults:** 500 mg P.O. or I.V. daily for 7 to 10 days. (See *Adjust-a-dose,* p. 147.)
✷ *NEW INDICATION: Mild to moderate uncomplicated urinary tract infection due to*

Escherichia coli, K. pneumoniae, *or* S. saprophyticus—
**Adults:** 250 mg P.O. daily for 3 days.
*Adjust-a-dose:* If creatinine clearance is 20 to 49 ml/minute, subsequent dosages are half the initial dose. If 10 to 19 ml/minute, subsequent dosages are half initial dose and the interval is increased to q 48 hours for above indications.
*Urinary tract infections (mild to moderate) due to* Enterococcus faecalis, Enterobacter cloacae, E. coli, K. pneumoniae, Proteus mirabilis, *or* Pseudomonas aeruginosa—
**Adults:** 250 mg P.O. or I.V. daily for 10 days. (See *Adjust-a-dose* below.)
*Acute pyelonephritis (mild to moderate) due to* E. coli—
**Adults:** 250 mg P.O. or I.V. daily for 10 days. (See *Adjust-a-dose* below.)
*Adjust-a-dose:* If creatinine clearance is 10 to 19 ml/minute, dosage interval is increased to q 48 hours.

## ADVERSE REACTIONS
**CNS:** headache, insomnia, dizziness, encephalopathy, paresthesia, *seizures.*
**CV:** chest pain, palpitations, vasodilation.
**GI:** nausea, diarrhea, constipation, vomiting, abdominal pain, dyspepsia, flatulence, *pseudomembranous colitis.*
**GU:** vaginitis.
**Hematologic:** eosinophilia, hemolytic anemia, lymphopenia.
**Metabolic:** hypoglycemia.
**Musculoskeletal:** back pain, tendon rupture.
**Respiratory:** allergic pneumonitis.
**Skin:** rash, photosensitivity, pruritus, erythema multiforme, *Stevens-Johnson syndrome.*
**Other:** pain, hypersensitivity reactions, *anaphylaxis, multisystem organ failure.*

## INTERACTIONS
**Drug-drug.** *Antacids containing aluminum or magnesium, iron salts, products containing zinc, sucralfate:* may interfere with GI absorption of levofloxacin. Administer at least 2 hours apart.
*Antidiabetics:* may alter blood glucose levels. Monitor blood glucose levels closely.
*NSAIDs:* may increase CNS stimulation. Monitor for seizure activity.

*Theophylline:* decreased clearance of theophylline with some fluoroquinolones. Monitor theophylline levels.
*Warfarin and derivatives:* increased effect of oral anticoagulant with some fluoroquinolones. Monitor PT and INR.
**Drug-lifestyle.** *Sun exposure:* photosensitivity reactions may occur. Take precautions.

## EFFECTS ON DIAGNOSTIC TESTS
Drug may cause an abnormal ECG.

## CONTRAINDICATIONS
Contraindicated in patients with hypersensitivity to drug, its components, or other fluoroquinolones.

## NURSING CONSIDERATIONS
• Safety and efficacy of drug in children under age 18 and in pregnant and breast-feeding women have not been established.
• Use cautiously in patients with history of seizure disorders or other CNS diseases, such as cerebral arteriosclerosis. If patient experiences symptoms of excessive CNS stimulation (restlessness, tremor, confusion, hallucinations), discontinue medication and notify doctor. Institute seizure precautions.
• Use cautiously and with dosage adjustment, as ordered, in patients with renal impairment.
• Acute hypersensitivity reactions may require treatment with epinephrine, oxygen, I.V. fluids, antihistamines, corticosteroids, pressor amines, and airway management.
• Most antibacterial drugs can cause pseudomembranous colitis. Notify doctor if diarrhea occurs. Drug may be discontinued.
• Obtain specimen for culture and sensitivity before starting therapy and as needed to determine if bacterial resistance has occurred.
• Monitor blood glucose and renal, hepatic, and hematopoietic blood studies, as ordered.

**◖ I.V. administration**
• Levofloxacin injection should be administered only by I.V. infusion. Dilute drug in single-use vials, according to manufacturer's instructions, with $D_5W$ or normal

saline for injection to a final concentration of 5 mg/ml. Reconstituted solution should be clear, slightly yellow, and free of particulate matter. Reconstituted drug is stable for 72 hours at room temperature, for 14 days when refrigerated in plastic containers, and for 6 months when frozen. Thaw at room temperature or in refrigerator only. Don't mix with other drugs. Infuse over 60 minutes.

### ☑ Patient teaching
• Tell patient to take drug as prescribed, even if symptoms disappear.
• Advise patient to take drug with plenty of fluids and to avoid antacids, sucralfate, and products containing iron or zinc for at least 2 hours before and after each dose.
• Warn patient to avoid hazardous tasks until adverse CNS effects of drug are known.
• Advise patient to avoid excessive sunlight, use sunblock, and wear protective clothing when outdoors.
• Instruct patient to stop drug and notify doctor if rash or other signs or symptoms of hypersensitivity develop.
• Tell patient to notify doctor if he experiences pain or inflammation; tendon rupture can occur with drug.
• Instruct diabetic patient to monitor blood glucose levels and notify doctor if a hypoglycemic reaction occurs.
• Instruct patient to notify doctor if loose stools or diarrhea occurs.

## lomefloxacin hydrochloride
Maxaquin

*Pregnancy Risk Category C*

### HOW SUPPLIED
*Tablets (film-coated):* 400 mg

### ACTION
Inhibits bacterial DNA gyrase, an enzyme necessary for bacterial replication; bactericidal.

| Route | Onset | Peak | Duration |
|-------|-------|------|----------|
| P.O. | Unknown | 1.5 hr | Unknown |

### INDICATIONS & DOSAGE
*Acute bacterial exacerbations of chronic bronchitis due to* Haemophilus influenzae *or* Moraxella (Branhamella) catarrhalis—
**Adults:** 400 mg P.O. daily for 10 days.
*Uncomplicated urinary tract infections (cystitis) due to* Escherichia coli, Klebsiella pneumoniae, Proteus mirabilis, *or* Staphylococcus saprophyticus—
**Adults:** 400 mg P.O. daily for 10 days.
*Complicated urinary tract infections due to* E. coli, K. pneumoniae, P. mirabilis, *or* Pseudomonas aeruginosa; *possibly effective against infections due to* Citrobacter diversus *or* Enterobacter cloacae—
**Adults:** 400 mg P.O. daily for 14 days.
*Adjust-a-dose:* For patients with creatinine clearance of 10 to 40 ml/minute, give loading dose of 400 mg P.O. on first day; then 200 mg daily for duration of therapy. Hemodialysis removes negligible amounts of drug.
*Prophylaxis of infections after transurethral surgical procedures—*
**Adults:** 400 mg P.O. as a single dose 2 to 6 hours before surgery.
*Prophylaxis of urinary tract infections after transrectal prostate biopsy—*
**Adults:** 400 mg P.O. as a single dose 1 to 6 hours before procedure.

### ADVERSE REACTIONS
**CNS:** *dizziness, headache,* abnormal dreams, fatigue, malaise, asthenia, agitation, anorexia, anxiety, confusion, depersonalization, depression, insomnia, nervousness, somnolence, *seizures, coma,* hyperkinesis, tremor, vertigo, paresthesia.
**CV:** flushing, hypotension, hypertension, edema, syncope, arrhythmia, tachycardia, bradycardia, extrasystoles, cyanosis, angina pectoris, *MI, cardiac failure, pulmonary embolism,* cerebrovascular disorder, cardiomyopathy, phlebitis.
**EENT:** epistaxis, abnormal vision, conjunctivitis, eye pain, earache, tinnitus, tongue discoloration, taste perversion, thirst.
**GI:** *diarrhea, nausea,* dry mouth, increased appetite, pseudomembranous colitis, abdominal pain, dyspepsia, vomiting, flatulence, constipation, inflammation, dysphagia, bleeding.

---

Reactions may be *common,* uncommon, *life-threatening,* or COMMON AND LIFE-THREATENING.

**GU:** dysuria, hematuria, anuria, epididymitis, orchitis, vaginitis, vaginal candidiasis, intermenstrual bleeding, perineal pain.
**Hematologic:** thrombocythemia, *thrombocytopenia.*
**Hepatic:** elevated liver enzymes.
**Metabolic:** hypoglycemia.
**Musculoskeletal:** leg cramps, arthralgia, myalgia, chest or back pain.
**Respiratory:** dyspnea, *bronchospasm,* respiratory disorder or infection, increased sputum, stridor.
**Skin:** pruritus, skin disorder, skin exfoliation, eczema, rash, urticaria, *photosensitivity.*
**Other:** *anaphylaxis,* increased diaphoresis, lymphadenopathy, chills, allergic reaction, facial edema, flulike syndrome, decreased heat tolerance, gout.

**INTERACTIONS**
**Drug-drug.** *Antacids, sucralfate:* impaired absorption after binding with lomefloxacin in GI tract. Give no less than 4 hours before or 2 hours after a dose.
*Cimetidine:* increased half-life of other fluoroquinolones when administered to patients taking cimetidine; lomefloxacin has not been tested. Monitor for toxicity.
*Cyclosporine, warfarin:* increased effects on serum levels when combined with other fluoroquinolones; lomefloxacin has not been tested. Monitor for toxicity.
*NSAIDs:* possibility of increased CNS stimulation and seizures. Use cautiously.
*Probenecid:* decreased excretion of lomefloxacin. Monitor for toxicity.
**Drug-lifestyle.** *Sun exposure:* photosensitivity reactions may occur. Take precautions.

**EFFECTS ON DIAGNOSTIC TESTS**
None reported.

**CONTRAINDICATIONS**
Contraindicated in patients with hypersensitivity to drug or other fluoroquinolones.

**NURSING CONSIDERATIONS**
• Use cautiously in patients with known or suspected CNS disorders, such as seizure disorder or cerebral arteriosclerosis, that may predispose the patient to seizures.

• Obtain culture and sensitivity tests before giving first dose. Therapy may begin pending results.
• Although most fluoroquinolones exhibit photosensitizing effects, it appears that photosensitization and phototoxicity are more common with lomefloxacin.
• Prolonged use may result in overgrowth of organisms resistant to lomefloxacin.
• Safety in children under age 18 hasn't been established. Drug has caused cartilage erosion.
• Tendon rupture has been reported in patients receiving quinolones. Discontinue if pain, inflammation, or rupture of a tendon occurs.

✅ **Patient teaching**
• Tell patient to take drug as prescribed, even after he feels better.
• Advise patient that hypersensitivity reactions may occur even after first dose. If rash or other allergic reaction appears, patient should stop taking drug and notify doctor.
• Warn patient to avoid hazardous tasks until CNS effects of drug are known.
• Advise patient to wear protective clothing, use a sunscreen, and avoid prolonged exposure to sunlight during treatment and for a few days after therapy ends. If sunburn occurs, tell him to call doctor promptly.
• Tell patient that drug may be taken with or without food.
• Instruct patient to notify doctor if loose stools or diarrhea occurs.

---

**nalidixic acid**
NegGram

*Pregnancy Risk Category B (safe use in first trimester unknown)*

**HOW SUPPLIED**
*Caplets:* 250 mg, 500 mg, 1 g
*Oral suspension:* 250 mg/5 ml

**ACTION**
Inhibits microbial DNA synthesis.

| Route | Onset | Peak | Duration |
|-------|-------|------|----------|
| P.O. | Unknown | 1-2 hr | Unknown |

## INDICATIONS & DOSAGE
*Acute and chronic urinary tract infections due to susceptible gram-negative organisms* (Proteus, Klebsiella, Enterobacter, *and* Escherichia coli)—
**Adults:** 1 g P.O. q.i.d. for 7 to 14 days; 2 g daily for long-term use.
**Children over age 3 months:** 55 mg/kg P.O. daily divided q.i.d. for 7 to 14 days; 33 mg/kg daily for long-term use.

## ADVERSE REACTIONS
**CNS:** drowsiness, weakness, headache, dizziness, vertigo, *seizures,* malaise, confusion, hallucinations, psychosis, *increased intracranial pressure and bulging fontanelles in infants and children.*
**EENT:** sensitivity to light, change in color perception, diplopia, blurred vision.
**GI:** *abdominal pain, nausea, vomiting,* diarrhea.
**Hematologic:** eosinophilia, *leukopenia, thrombocytopenia,* hemolytic anemia.
**Musculoskeletal:** arthralgia, joint stiffness.
**Skin:** pruritus, photosensitivity, urticaria, rash.
**Other:** *angioedema, anaphylactoid reaction.*

## INTERACTIONS
**Drug-drug.** *Nitrofurantoin:* antagonizes effects of nalidixic acid. Monitor closely.
*Oral anticoagulants:* increased anticoagulant effect. Monitor for bleeding.
**Drug-lifestyle.** *Sun exposure:* photosensitivity reactions may occur. Take precautions.

## EFFECTS ON DIAGNOSTIC TESTS
Drug may cause false-positive results in urine glucose tests using cupric sulfate (such as Benedict's reagent, Fehling's solution, and Clinitest). Urine 17-ketosteroid and urine 17-ketogenic steroid levels may be falsely elevated because nalidixic acid interacts with *M*-dinitrobenzene, used to measure these urine metabolites. Urine vanillylmandelic acid levels may also be falsely elevated.

## CONTRAINDICATIONS
Contraindicated in patients with hypersensitivity to drug, in those with seizure disorders, and in infants under age 3 months.

## NURSING CONSIDERATIONS
• Use with extreme caution in prepubertal children; drug has caused cartilage erosion.
• Use cautiously in patients with impaired hepatic or renal function or with severe cerebral arteriosclerosis. Monitor renal and liver function test results.
• Obtain specimen for culture and sensitivity tests before starting therapy and repeat as needed. Therapy may begin pending results.
• Monitor CBC and renal and liver function studies during long-term therapy, as ordered.
• Resistant bacteria may emerge in the first 48 hours of therapy.

☑ **Patient teaching**
• Tell patient to take drug as prescribed, even after he feels better.
• Instruct patient to take drug with food to prevent GI upset.
• Tell patient to avoid exposure to sunlight, to wear protective clothing, and to use sunscreen.
• Tell patient to report visual disturbances or CNS symptoms immediately.

---

## norfloxacin
Noroxin, Utinor§

*Pregnancy Risk Category C*

## HOW SUPPLIED
*Tablets (film-coated):* 400 mg

## ACTION
Inhibits bacterial DNA synthesis, mainly by blocking DNA gyrase; bactericidal.

| Route | Onset | Peak | Duration |
|-------|-------|------|----------|
| P.O. | Unknown | 0.5-2 hr | Unknown |

## INDICATIONS & DOSAGE
*Complicated or uncomplicated urinary tract infections due to susceptible strains*

*of* Enterococcus faecalis, Escherichia coli, Klebsiella pneumoniae, Enterobacter aerogenes, E. cloacae, Proteus mirabilis, P. vulgaris, Pseudomonas aeruginosa, Citrobacter freundii, Staphylococcus agalactiae, S. aureus, S. epidermidis, S. saprophyticus, *and* Serratia marcescens—
**Adults:** for uncomplicated infections, 400 mg P.O. q 12 hours for 7 to 10 days. For complicated infections, 400 mg P.O. q 12 hours for 10 to 21 days. (See *Adjust-a Dose* below.)
*Cystitis due to* E. coli, K. pneumoniae, *or* P. mirabilis—
**Adults:** 400 mg P.O. q 12 hours for 3 days. (See *Adjust-a-dose* below.)
*Acute, uncomplicated urethral and cervical gonorrhea—*
**Adults:** 800 mg P.O. as a single dose, followed by doxycycline therapy to treat any coexisting chlamydial infection.
*Adjust-a-dose:* For adult patients with creatinine clearance of 30 ml/minute or less, 400 mg once daily for above indications.

## ADVERSE REACTIONS
**CNS:** fatigue, somnolence, headache, dizziness, *seizures,* depression, insomnia.
**GI:** nausea, constipation, flatulence, heartburn, dry mouth, abdominal pain, diarrhea, vomiting, anorexia.
**GU:** increased serum creatinine and BUN levels, crystalluria.
**Hematologic:** eosinophilia, hematocrit may decrease, *neutropenia.*
**Hepatic:** ALT, AST, and alkaline phosphatase levels may increase.
**Musculoskeletal:** back pain.
**Skin:** rash, photosensitivity.
**Other:** *hypersensitivity reactions, anaphylaxis,* fever, hyperhidrosis.

## INTERACTIONS
**Drug-drug.** *Antacids, iron products, sucralfate:* may hinder absorption. Separate administration times by 2 hours.
*Cyclosporine:* increased serum concentrations of cyclosporine. Monitor serum levels.
*Nitrofurantoin*: antagonizes effects of norfloxacin. Monitor closely.
*Oral anticoagulants:* increased anticoagulant effect. Monitor closely.

*Probenecid:* may increase serum levels of norfloxacin by decreasing its excretion. Monitor for toxicity.
*Theophylline:* possibly impaired theophylline metabolism, resulting in increased plasma levels and risk of toxicity. Monitor closely.

## EFFECTS ON DIAGNOSTIC TESTS
None reported.

## CONTRAINDICATIONS
Contraindicated in patients with hypersensitivity to drug or other fluoroquinolones.

## NURSING CONSIDERATIONS
• Use cautiously in patients with conditions such as cerebral arteriosclerosis that may predispose them to seizure disorders. Also use cautiously in those with renal impairment. Monitor renal function.
• Safety in children under age 18 has not been established. Drug has caused cartilage erosion.
• Obtain culture and sensitivity before starting therapy.
• Tendon rupture has been reported in patients receiving quinolones. Discontinue if pain, inflammation, or rupture of a tendon occurs.

### ☑ Patient teaching
• Tell patient to take drug as prescribed, even after he feels better.
• Advise patient to take drug 1 hour before or 2 hours after meals because food, antacids, iron products, and sucralfate may hinder absorption.
• Warn patient not to exceed the recommended dosages and to drink several glasses of water throughout the day to maintain hydration and adequate urine output.
• Warn patient to avoid hazardous tasks that require alertness until CNS effects of drug are known.
• Instruct patient to avoid exposure to sunlight, to wear protective clothing, and to use sunscreen while outdoors.

## ofloxacin
Floxin, Floxin I.V., Tarivid§

*Pregnancy Risk Category C*

### HOW SUPPLIED
*Tablets (film-coated):* 200 mg, 300 mg, 400 mg
*Injection:* 20 mg/ml, 40 mg/ml; 200 mg, 400 mg premixed in $D_5W$

### ACTION
Inhibits bacterial DNA synthesis by blocking DNA gyrase; bactericidal.

| Route | Onset | Peak | Duration |
|-------|-------|------|----------|
| P.O. | Unknown | 0.5-2 hr | Unknown |
| I.V. | Unknown | Immediate | Unknown |

### INDICATIONS & DOSAGE
*Lower respiratory tract infections due to susceptible strains of* Haemophilus influenzae *or* Streptococcus pneumoniae—
**Adults:** 400 mg I.V. or P.O. q 12 hours for 10 days.
*Cervicitis or urethritis due to* Chlamydia trachomatis *or* Neisseria gonorrhoeae—
**Adults:** 300 mg I.V. or P.O. q 12 hours for 7 days.
*Acute, uncomplicated gonorrhea—*
**Adults:** 400 mg I.V. or P.O. as a single dose with doxycycline.
*Mild to moderate skin and skin-structure infections due to susceptible strains of* Staphylococcus aureus, S. pyogenes, *or* Proteus mirabilis—
**Adults:** 400 mg I.V. or P.O. q 12 hours for 10 days.
*Cystitis due to* Escherichia coli *or* Klebsiella pneumoniae—
**Adults:** 200 mg I.V. or P.O. q 12 hours for 3 days.
*Urinary tract infections due to susceptible strains of* Citrobacter diversus, Enterobacter aerogenes, E. coli, P. mirabilis, *or* Pseudomonas aeruginosa—
**Adults:** 200 mg I.V. or P.O. q 12 hours for 7 days. Complicated infections may require therapy for 10 days.
*Prostatitis due to* E. coli—
**Adults:** 300 mg I.V. or P.O. q 12 hours for 6 weeks.

*Epididymitis—*
**Adults:** 300 mg P.O. q 12 hours for 10 days.
*Pelvic inflammatory disease (outpatient)—*
**Adults:** 400 mg P.O. q 12 hours for 14 days with metronidazole.
*Adjust-a-dose:* For renally impaired patients with creatinine clearance of 10 to 50 ml/minute, reduce dosing interval to once q 24 hours. If creatinine clearance is below 20 ml/minute, give half the recommended dose q 24 hours.

### ADVERSE REACTIONS
**CNS:** headache, dizziness, fatigue, lethargy, malaise, drowsiness, sleep disorders, nervousness, insomnia, *seizures.*
**CV:** chest pain, phlebitis.
**EENT:** visual disturbances.
**GI:** *nausea,* anorexia, abdominal pain or discomfort, diarrhea, vomiting, constipation, dry mouth, flatulence, dysgeusia.
**GU:** vaginitis, vaginal discharge, genital pruritus.
**Hepatic:** elevated liver enzymes.
**Metabolic:** hyperglycemia.
**Musculoskeletal:** trunk pain.
**Skin:** rash, pruritus, photosensitivity.
**Other:** *hypersensitivity reactions, anaphylaxis,* fever.

### INTERACTIONS
**Drug-drug.** *Antacids containing magnesium or aluminum hydroxide, iron salts, sucralfate, products containing zinc:* may interfere with GI absorption of ofloxacin. Separate administration by at least 2 hours.
*Antidiabetics:* may cause alterations in blood glucose levels. Monitor levels closely.
*NSAIDs:* risk of increased CNS stimulation and seizures. Use cautiously.
*Oral anticoagulants:* increased effect. Monitor for bleeding and altered PT.
*Theophylline:* decreased clearance of theophylline with some fluoroquinolones. Monitor theophylline levels.
**Drug-food.** *Any food:* decreased absorption. Give drug on an empty stomach.
**Drug-lifestyle.** *Sun exposure:* photosensitivity reactions may occur. Take precautions.

---

Reactions may be *common,* uncommon, *life-threatening,* or COMMON AND LIFE-THREATENING.

**EFFECTS ON DIAGNOSTIC TESTS**
None reported.

**CONTRAINDICATIONS**
Contraindicated in patients with hypersensitivity to drug or other fluoroquinolones.

**NURSING CONSIDERATIONS**
• Use cautiously in patients with a history of seizure disorders or other CNS diseases such as cerebral arteriosclerosis.
• Use cautiously and with dosage adjustment in patients with renal failure, as prescribed, because drug is mainly eliminated by renal excretion.
• Obtain culture and sensitivity before first dose.
• Monitor regular blood studies and hepatic and renal function tests during prolonged therapy, as ordered.
• *Alert:* Patients treated for gonorrhea should have a serologic test for syphilis. Drug is not effective against syphilis, and treatment of gonorrhea may mask or delay symptoms of syphilis.
• Safety in children under age 18 has not been established. Drug has caused cartilage erosion.
• Tendon rupture has been reported in patients receiving quinolones. Discontinue if pain, inflammation, or rupture of a tendon occurs.

**◨ I.V. administration**
• Dilute concentrate for injection before use. Single-use vials containing 20 or 40 mg/ml must be diluted to a maximum concentration of 4 mg/ml with a compatible I.V. solution, such as $D_5W$, normal saline for injection, $D_5W$ in normal saline for injection, or sterile water for injection. Infuse over at least 60 minutes.
• Because compatibility with other drugs is not known, don't mix ofloxacin with other drugs. If giving infusion at a Y-site, discontinue the flow of the other solution.

**☑ Patient teaching**
• Tell patient to take drug as prescribed, even after he feels better.
• Advise patient to take drug with plenty of fluids, but not with meals, and to avoid antacids, sucralfate, and products containing iron or zinc for at least 2 hours before and after each dose.
• Warn patient to avoid hazardous tasks until adverse CNS effects of drug are known.
• Inform patient to use sunscreen and wear protective clothing while outdoors.
• Tell patient to stop drug and notify doctor if rash or other signs of hypersensitivity develop.

---

**sparfloxacin**
Zagam

*Pregnancy Risk Category C*

---

**HOW SUPPLIED**
*Tablets:* 200 mg

**ACTION**
Inhibits bacterial DNA gyrase and prevents DNA replication, transcription, repair, and deactivation in susceptible bacteria.

| Route | Onset | Peak | Duration |
|-------|-------|------|----------|
| P.O. | Unknown | 3-6 hr | Unknown |

**INDICATIONS & DOSAGE**
*Acute bacterial exacerbation of chronic bronchitis due to* Staphylococcus aureus, Streptococcus pneumoniae, Chlamydia pneumoniae, Enterobacter cloacae, Klebsiella pneumoniae, Moraxella catarrhalis, Haemophilus influenzae, *or* H. parainfluenzae—
**Adults over age 18:** 400 mg P.O. on first day as a loading dose; then 200 mg daily for total of 10 days of therapy.
*Community-acquired pneumonia due to* S. pneumoniae, M. catarrhalis, H. influenzae, H. parainfluenzae, C. pneumoniae, *or* Mycoplasma pneumoniae—
**Adults over age 18:** 400 mg P.O. on first day as a loading dose; then 200 mg daily for total of 10 days of therapy.
*Adjust-a-dose:* For renally impaired patients with creatinine clearance below 50 ml/minute, give a loading dose of 400 mg P.O.; then, 200 mg P.O. q 48 hours for total of 9 days of therapy.

---

## ADVERSE REACTIONS

**CNS:** headache, dizziness, insomnia, asthenia, somnolence, *seizures.*
**CV:** prolonged QT interval, vasodilatation.
**EENT:** dry mouth, taste perversion.
**GI:** nausea, diarrhea, vomiting, abdominal pain, dyspepsia, flatulence, *pseudomembranous colitis.*
**GU:** vaginal candidiasis.
**Hematologic:** elevated WBC counts.
**Hepatic:** elevated ALT and AST levels.
**Musculoskeletal:** tendon rupture.
**Skin:** rash, photosensitivity, pruritus.
**Other:** hypersensitivity reactions, *anaphylaxis.*

## INTERACTIONS

**Drug-drug.** *Antacids containing aluminum or magnesium, iron salts, sucralfate, zinc:* may interfere with GI absorption of levofloxacin. Administer at least 4 hours apart.
*Drugs that prolong the QT interval or cause torsades de pointes (including amiodarone, bepridil, cisapride, class IA antiarrhythmics [such as procainamide and quinidine], class III drugs [such as sotalol], disopyramide, erythromycin, pentamidine, phenothiazines, tricyclic antidepressants):* may cause torsades de pointes. Sparfloxacin is contraindicated in these patients.
**Drug-lifestyle.** *Sun exposure:* photosensitivity reactions may occur. Take precautions.

## EFFECTS ON DIAGNOSTIC TESTS

Drug may produce false-negative culture results for *Mycobacterium tuberculosis.*

## CONTRAINDICATIONS

Contraindicated in patients with a history of hypersensitivity or photosensitivity reactions to drug and in those who cannot avoid the sun. Avoid administration with drugs known to prolong the QT interval or cause torsades de pointes. Drug isn't recommended for patients with heart conditions that predispose them to arrhythmias.

## NURSING CONSIDERATIONS

• Safety and efficacy of levofloxacin in pregnant and breast-feeding women and in patients under age 18 have not been established.
• Use cautiously in patients with history of seizure disorder or other CNS diseases such as cerebral arteriosclerosis. If patient experiences symptoms of excessive CNS stimulation (restlessness, tremor, confusion, hallucinations), discontinue drug and notify doctor. Then institute seizure precautions.
• Use cautiously and with dosage adjustment in patients with renal impairment. Monitor renal function.
• Acute hypersensitivity reactions may require treatment with epinephrine, oxygen, I.V. fluids, antihistamines, corticosteroids, and pressor amines, and airway management.
• Obtain specimen for culture and sensitivity before starting therapy and as needed and ordered to determine if bacterial resistance has occurred.

### ☑ Patient teaching

• Tell patient that drug may be taken with food, milk, or products that contain caffeine.
• Tell patient to take drug as prescribed, even if symptoms disappear.
• Advise patient to take drug with plenty of fluids and to avoid antacids, sucralfate, and products containing iron or zinc for at least 4 hours after each dose.
• Warn patient to avoid hazardous tasks until adverse CNS effects of drug are known.
• *Alert:* Advise patient to avoid direct, indirect, and artificial ultraviolet light, even with sunscreen on, during treatment and for 5 days after treatment. Patient should stop taking drug and notify doctor if signs or symptoms of phototoxicity (skin burning, redness, swelling, blisters, rash, itching) occur.
• Tell patient to stop drug and notify doctor if rash or other signs of hypersensitivity develop.
• Instruct patient to discontinue drug and notify doctor of pain or inflammation; tendon rupture can occur with drug use. He should rest and refrain from exercise until diagnosis is made.
• Instruct patient to notify doctor if loose stools or diarrhea occurs.

---

Reactions may be *common*, uncommon, *life-threatening*, or COMMON AND LIFE-THREATENING.

## trovafloxacin mesylate
Trovan Tablets

## alatrofloxacin mesylate
Trovan I.V.

*Pregnancy Risk Category C*

### HOW SUPPLIED
*Tablets:* 100 mg, 200 mg
*Injection:* 5 mg/ml in 40-ml (200 mg) and 60-ml (300 mg) vials

### ACTION
Trovafloxacin is related to the fluoro-quinolones with in vitro activity against a wide range of gram-positive and gram-negative aerobic and anaerobic microorganisms. Bactericidal action results from inhibition of DNA gyrase and topoisomerase IV, two enzymes involved in bacterial replication.

| Route | Onset | Peak | Duration |
|-------|-------|------|----------|
| P.O., I.V. | Unknown | 1 hr | Unknown |

### INDICATIONS & DOSAGE
*Nosocomial pneumonia due to* Escherichia coli, Pseudomonas aeruginosa, Haemophilus influenzae, *or* Staphylococcus aureus; *gynecologic and pelvic infections due to* E. coli, Bacteroides fragilis, *viridans group streptococci,* Enterococcus faecalis, Streptococcus agalactiae, Peptostreptococcus *species,* Prevotella *species, or* Gardnerella vaginalis; *complicated intra-abdominal infections including postsurgical infections due to* E. coli, B. fragilis, *viridans group streptococci,* P. aeruginosa, Klebsiella pneumoniae, Peptostreptococcus *species, or* Prevotella *species—*
**Adults:** 300 mg I.V. daily; then 200 mg P.O. daily for 7 to 14 days (10 to 14 days for pneumonia).
*Community-acquired pneumonia due to* S. pneumoniae, H. influenzae, K. pneumoniae, S. aureus, Mycoplasma pneumoniae, Moraxella catarrhalis, Legionella pneumophila, *or* Chlamydia pneumoniae; *complicated skin and skin-structure infections including diabetic foot infections due to* S. aureus, S. agalactiae, P. aeruginosa, E. fae-

calis, E. coli, *or* Proteus mirabilis *(not for treatment of osteomyelitis)—*
**Adults:** 200 mg P.O. or I.V. daily; then 200 mg P.O. daily for 7 to 14 days (10 to 14 days for complicated skin and skin-structure infections).
*Prophylaxis of infection associated with elective colorectal surgery or vaginal and abdominal hysterectomy—*
**Adults:** 200 mg P.O. or I.V as a single dose 30 minutes to 4 hours before surgery.
*Acute sinusitis due to* H. influenzae, M. catarrhalis, *or* S. pneumoniae; *chronic prostatitis due to* E. coli, E. faecalis, *or* S. epidermis; *cervicitis due to* C. trachomatis; *and pelvic inflammatory disease (mild to moderate) due to* Neisseria gonorrhoeae *or* C. trachomatis—
**Adults:** 200 mg P.O. daily for 5 days (cervicitis), 10 days (acute sinusitis), 14 days (pelvic inflammatory disease), or 28 days (chronic prostatitis).
*Uncomplicated urinary tract infections due to* E. coli; *uncomplicated skin and skin-structure infections due to* S. aureus, S. pyogenes, *or* S. agalactiae; *acute bacterial exacerbation of chronic bronchitis due to* H. influenzae, M. catarrhalis, S. pneumoniae, S. aureus, *or* Haemophilus parainfluenzae; *and uncomplicated gonorrhea due to* N. gonorrhoeae—
**Adults:** 100 mg P.O. daily for 3 days (urinary tract infections), 7 to 10 days (skin and skin-structure infections, bronchitis) or single dose for treatment of gonorrhea.
***Adjust-a-dose:*** For patients with mild to moderate cirrhosis (Child-Pugh Class A and B), reduce 300-mg I.V. dose to 200-mg I.V. and 200-mg I.V. or P.O. dose to 100-mg I.V. or P.O.; no reduction is needed for 100-mg P.O. dose.

### ADVERSE REACTIONS
**CNS:** *dizziness,* light-headedness, headache, *seizures,* psychosis.
**GI:** diarrhea, nausea, vomiting, abdominal pain, pseudomembranous colitis.
**GU:** vaginitis, increased BUN and creatinine levels.
**Hematologic:** bone marrow aplasia *(anemia, thrombocytopenia, leukopenia),* decreased hemoglobin and hematocrit, increased platelets.

---

**Hepatic:** increased ALT and AST.
**Musculoskeletal:** arthralgia, arthropathy, myalgia.
**Skin:** pruritus, rash, injection-site reaction, photosensitivity.

## INTERACTIONS
**Drug-drug.** *Antacids containing aluminum, magnesium, or citric acid buffered with sodium citrate (Bicitra), iron-containing preparations, I.V. morphine, sucralfate:* bioavailability of trovafloxacin is significantly reduced following use with these agents. Give these agents 2 hours before or 2 hours after trovafloxacin. Avoid morphine I.V. for 4 hours if trovafloxacin is taken with food.
**Drug-lifestyle.** *Sun exposure:* photosensitivity reactions may occur. Take precautions.

## EFFECTS ON DIAGNOSTIC TESTS
None reported.

## CONTRAINDICATIONS
Contraindicated in patients with hypersensitivity to drug, alatrofloxacin, or other quinolone antimicrobials or any other components of these products.

## NURSING CONSIDERATIONS
• Use cautiously in patients with CNS disorders (such as cerebral atherosclerosis or epilepsy) and in those at increased risk for seizures. As with other quinolones, drug may cause neurologic complications such as seizures, psychosis, or increased intracranial pressure. Monitor patient with preexisting condition closely.
• Perform periodic assessment of liver function because of potential for increases in ALT, AST, and alkaline phosphatase levels.
• *Alert:* Using drug for more than 2 weeks greatly increases the risk of serious liver injury. Liver injury has also been reported following reexposure to drug. Therefore, drug should be limited to patients with life- or limb-threatening infections who received their initial treatment as an inpatient in a hospital or a long-term care nursing facility. Drug shouldn't be used if effective and safer alternative antimicrobial therapy is available.

• Drug can be given as a single daily dose without regard to food.
• Moderate to severe phototoxicity reactions have occurred in patients exposed to direct sunlight.
• No dosage adjustment is necessary when switching from I.V. to oral form.
• If *P. aeruginosa* is the known or presumed pathogen, treatment with an aminoglycoside or aztreonam may be indicated.

### ◑ I.V. administration
• Alatrofloxacin mesylate is supplied in single-use vials that must be further diluted with an appropriate solution ($D_5W$, half-normal saline) before administration. Don't dilute drug with normal saline or lactated Ringer's solution. Follow package insert for specific instructions regarding preparation of desired dosage.
• After dilution, administer alatrofloxacin mesylate by I.V. infusion over 60 minutes. Avoid rapid bolus or infusion. Don't administer drug and solutions containing multivalent cations (such as magnesium) through same I.V. line.

### ☑ Patient teaching
• Inform patient that drug may be taken without regard to meals; however, tell him to take products containing iron, aluminum, magnesium (vitamins, minerals, antacids), or sucralfate at least 2 hours before or 2 hours after trovafloxacin dose.
• Advise patient to take drug with meals or at bedtime if light-headedness or dizziness occurs.
• Warn patient to avoid excessive sunlight or artificial ultraviolet light and to use an effective sunscreen to prevent sunburn.
• Instruct patient to discontinue treatment, refrain from exercise, and seek medical advice if pain, inflammation, or rupture of a tendon occurs.
• Advise patient to discontinue drug at first sign of rash, hives, difficulty swallowing or breathing, or other symptoms suggesting an allergic reaction and to seek medical help immediately.
• Instruct patient to notify doctor if severe diarrhea occurs; this may indicate pseudomembranous colitis.

---

Reactions may be *common*, uncommon, *life-threatening*, or COMMON AND LIFE-THREATENING.

abacavir sulfate
acyclovir sodium
amantadine hydrochloride
amprenavir
cidofovir
delavirdine mesylate
didanosine
efavirenz
famciclovir
fomivirsen sodium
foscarnet sodium
ganciclovir
indinavir sulfate
lamivudine
lamivudine/zidovudine
nelfinavir mesylate
nevirapine
oseltamivir phosphate
ribavirin
rimantadine hydrochloride
ritonavir
saquinavir
saquinavir mesylate
stavudine
valacyclovir hydrochloride
zalcitabine
zanamivir
zidovudine

**COMBINATION PRODUCTS**
None.

**✳ NEW DRUG**

## abacavir sulfate
Ziagen

*Pregnancy Risk Category C*

**HOW SUPPLIED**
*Tablets:* 300 mg
*Oral solution:* 20 mg/ml

**ACTION**
Converted intracellularly to the active metabolite carbovir triphosphate, which inhibits the activity of HIV-1 reverse transcriptase, thereby terminating viral DNA growth.

| Route | Onset | Peak | Duration |
|-------|-------|------|----------|
| P.O. | Unknown | Unknown | Unknown |

**INDICATIONS & DOSAGE**
*HIV-1 infection—*
**Adults:** 300 mg P.O. b.i.d. with other antiretrovirals.
**Children ages 3 months to 16 years:** 8 mg/kg P.O. b.i.d. (up to maximum of 300 mg P.O. b.i.d.) with other antiretrovirals.

**ADVERSE REACTIONS**
**CNS:** insomnia and sleep disorders, headache.
**GI:** *nausea, vomiting,* diarrhea, loss of appetite, anorexia.
**Metabolic:** *elevated triglyceride levels.*
**Skin:** rash.
**Other:** *hypersensitivity reaction,* fever.

**INTERACTIONS**
**Drug-lifestyle.** *Alcohol use:* decreased elimination of abacavir, increasing overall exposure to drug. Monitor alcohol consumption. Use together cautiously.

**EFFECTS ON DIAGNOSTIC TESTS**
None reported.

**CONTRAINDICATIONS**
Contraindicated in patients with previous hypersensitivity to drug or its components.

**NURSING CONSIDERATIONS**
• Use cautiously when administering drug to patients with known risk factors for liver disease. Lactic acidosis and severe hepatomegaly with steatosis, including fatal cases, have been reported with the use of nucleoside analogues alone or in combination, including abacavir and other antiretrovirals.
• Women are more likely than men to experience lactic acidosis and severe hepatomegaly with steatosis. Obesity and prolonged nucleoside exposure may be risk factors.

---

*Liquid contains alcohol.   **May contain tartrazine.   †Canada   ‡Australia   §U.K.   ◇OTC

• Discontinue treatment, as ordered, in patients who develop signs or symptoms of lactic acidosis or pronounced hepatotoxicity, which may include hepatomegaly and steatosis even in absence of elevated transaminase levels.

• Use cautiously in pregnant women because no adequate studies of the effects of abacavir on pregnancy exist. Use during pregnancy only if the potential benefits outweigh the risk. Register pregnant women taking abacavir with the Antiretroviral Pregnancy Registry at 1-800-258-4263.

• *Alert:* Don't restart drug after a hypersensitivity reaction because severe signs and symptoms will recur within hours and may include life-threatening hypotension and death. To facilitate reporting of hypersensitivity reactions, register patients with the Abacavir Hypersensitivity Registry at 1-800-270-0425.

• *Alert:* Abacavir can cause fatal hypersensitivity reactions; as soon as patient develops signs or symptoms of hypersensitivity (such as fever, rash, fatigue, nausea, vomiting, diarrhea, or abdominal pain), discontinue drug and seek medical attention immediately.

• Always give drug with other antiretrovirals and never alone.

• Drug may cause mildly elevated blood glucose levels.

☑ **Patient teaching**

• Inform patient that abacavir can cause a life-threatening hypersensitivity reaction. Warn patient that, if he develops signs or symptoms of hypersensitivity (such as fever, rash, severe tiredness, achiness, a generally ill feeling, nausea, vomiting, diarrhea, or stomach pain), to stop taking drug and notify his doctor immediately.

• Include information leaflet about drug with each new prescription and refill. Patient should also receive, and be instructed to carry, a warning card summarizing signs and symptoms of abacavir hypersensitivity reaction.

• Inform patient that this drug isn't a cure for HIV infection. Tell patient that drug hasn't been shown to reduce the risk of transmission of HIV to others through sexual contact or blood contamination and that its long-term effects are unknown.

• Tell patient to take drug exactly as prescribed.

• Inform patient that drug can be taken with or without food.

---

## acyclovir sodium
Avirax†, Zovirax

*Pregnancy Risk Category C*

---

### HOW SUPPLIED
*Capsules:* 200 mg
*Tablets:* 400 mg, 800 mg
*Suspension:* 200 mg/5 ml
*Injection:* 500 mg/vial, 1 g/vial

### ACTION
Interferes with DNA synthesis and inhibits viral multiplication.

| Route | Onset | Peak | Duration |
|-------|-------|------|----------|
| P.O. | Unknown | 2.5 hr | Unknown |
| I.V. | Immediate | Immediate | Unknown |

### INDICATIONS & DOSAGE
*Initial and recurrent episodes of mucocutaneous herpes simplex virus (HSV-1 and HSV-2) infections in immunocompromised patients; severe initial episodes of genital herpes in patients who are not immunocompromised—*
**Adults and children ages 12 and older:** 5 mg/kg given I.V. at a constant rate over 1 hour q 8 hours for 7 to 14 days (5 to 7 days for severe initial episode of genital herpes).
**Children under age 12:** 250 mg/m$^2$ given I.V. at a constant rate over 1 hour q 8 hours for 7 days.
*Initial genital herpes—*
**Adults:** 200 mg P.O. q 4 hours while awake (total of five capsules daily); or 400 mg P.O. q 8 hours. Continue for 7 to 10 days for treatment of initial genital herpes episodes.
*Intermittent therapy for recurrent genital herpes—*
**Adults:** 200 mg P.O. q 4 hours while awake (total of five capsules daily). Treat-

---

Reactions may be *common*, uncommon, *life-threatening*, or COMMON AND LIFE-THREATENING.

ment should continue for 5 days. Initiate therapy at first sign of recurrence.

*Long-term suppressive therapy for recurrent genital herpes—*

**Adults:** 400 mg P.O. b.i.d. for up to 12 months. Or, 200 mg P.O. three to five times daily for up to 12 months.

*Varicella (chickenpox) infections in immunocompromised patients—*

**Adults and children ages 12 and older:** 10 mg/kg I.V. infused at a constant rate over 1 hour q 8 hours for 7 days. Dosage for obese patients is 10 mg/kg (based on ideal body weight) q 8 hours for 7 days. Don't exceed maximum dosage equivalent of 500 mg/m$^2$ q 8 hours.

**Children under age 12:** 500 mg/m$^2$ I.V. infused at a constant rate over 1 hour q 8 hours for 7 to 10 days.

*Varicella infection in immunocompetent patients—*

**Adults and children ages 2 and older:** 20 mg/kg (maximum 800 mg/dose) P.O. q.i.d. for 5 days. Start therapy as soon as symptoms appear to achieve maximum efficacy.

Or, in adults and children weighing over 40 kg (88 lb), 800 mg P.O. q.i.d. for 5 days. In children ages 2 and older weighing 40 kg or less, 20 mg/kg P.O. q.i.d. for 5 days.

*Acute herpes zoster infection in immunocompetent patients—*

**Adults and children ages 12 and older:** 800 mg P.O. q 4 hours five times daily for 7 to 10 days.

*Herpes simplex encephalitis—*

**Adults and children over age 6 months:** 10 mg/kg I.V. infused at a constant rate over 1 hour q 8 hours for 10 days.

Or, in children ages 6 months to 12 years, 500 mg/m$^2$ I.V. infused at a constant rate over 1 hour q 8 hours for 10 days.

*Adjust-a-dose:* For patients with renal failure, if creatinine clearance is over 50 ml/minute, I.V. dose is 100% of dose q 8 hours; if clearance is 25 to 50 ml/minute, 100% of dose q 12 hours; if clearance is 10 to 24 ml/minute, 100% of dose q 24 hours; if clearance is below 10 ml/minute, 50% of dose q 24 hours.

P.O. dosage: If normal dose is 200 mg q 4 hours five times daily and creatinine clearance is below 10 ml/minute, 200 mg P.O. q 12 hours. If normal dose is 400 mg q 12 hours and creatinine clearance is below 10 ml/minute, 200 mg q 12 hours. If normal dose is 800 mg q 4 hours five times daily and creatinine clearance is below 10 ml/minute, 800 mg q 12 hours; and if creatinine clearance is 10 to 25 ml/minute, 800 mg q 8 hours.

## ADVERSE REACTIONS

**CNS:** *malaise, headache,* **encephalopathic changes,** including **lethargy, obtundation, tremor, confusion, hallucinations, agitation, seizures, coma.**

**GI:** *nausea, vomiting,* diarrhea.

**GU:** *transient elevations of serum creatinine and BUN levels,* hematuria, **acute renal failure.**

**Hematologic:** **thrombocytopenia, leukopenia,** thrombocytosis.

**Skin:** rash, itching, urticaria.

**Other:** *inflammation, phlebitis at injection site.*

## INTERACTIONS

**Drug-drug.** *Interferon:* may have synergistic effect. Monitor closely.

*Probenecid:* increased acyclovir blood levels. Monitor for possible toxicity.

*Zidovudine:* may cause drowsiness or lethargy. Use together cautiously.

## EFFECTS ON DIAGNOSTIC TESTS

None reported.

## CONTRAINDICATIONS

Contraindicated in patients with hypersensitivity to drug.

## NURSING CONSIDERATIONS

• Use cautiously in patients with underlying neurologic problems, renal disease, or dehydration and in those receiving other nephrotoxic drugs. Monitor renal function.

• *Alert:* Don't administer I.M. or S.C.

• Encephalopathic changes are more likely to occur in patients with neurologic disorders or in those who have had neurologic reactions to cytotoxic drugs.

• Because there are no adequate studies in pregnant women, acyclovir should be used during pregnancy only if potential benefits outweigh risks to fetus.

### 🜂 I.V. administration

• Administer I.V. infusion over at least 1 hour to prevent renal tubular damage. Don't give by bolus injection. Bolus injection, dehydration (decreased urine output), preexisting renal disease, and concomitant use of other nephrotoxic drugs increase the risk of renal toxicity.

• Concentrated solutions (7 mg/ml or more) may be associated with a higher incidence of phlebitis.

• Encourage fluid intake because patient must be adequately hydrated during acyclovir infusion. Monitor intake and output especially within the first 2 hours after I.V. administration.

### ✅ Patient teaching

• Tell patient to take drug as prescribed, even after he feels better.

• Instruct patient that drug is effective in managing herpes infection but does not eliminate or cure it. Warn patient that acyclovir will not prevent spread of infection to others.

• Instruct patient about early symptoms of herpes infection (such as tingling, itching, or pain). Tell him to notify doctor and get a prescription for acyclovir before the infection fully develops. Treatment started early is most effective.

---

### amantadine hydrochloride
Symmetrel

*Pregnancy Risk Category C*

### HOW SUPPLIED
*Capsules:* 100 mg
*Syrup:* 50 mg/5 ml
*Tablets:* 100 mg

### ACTION
Unknown. Possibly inhibits the uncoating of the virus.

| Route | Onset | Peak | Duration |
|-------|-------|------|----------|
| P.O. | Unknown | 1-4 hr | Unknown |

### INDICATIONS & DOSAGE
*Prophylaxis or symptomatic treatment of influenza type A virus, respiratory tract illnesses—*
**Adults up to age 65 with normal renal function:** 200 mg P.O. daily in a single dose.
**Children ages 9 to 12:** 100 mg P.O. b.i.d.
**Children ages 1 to 9 or weighing less than 45 kg (99 lb):** 4.4 to 8.8 mg/kg P.O. as a total daily dose given once daily or divided equally b.i.d. Maximum daily dose is 150 mg.
**Elderly:** 100 mg P.O. once daily in patients over age 65 with normal renal function.

Begin treatment within 24 to 48 hours after symptoms appear and continue for 24 to 48 hours after symptoms disappear (usually 2 to 7 days of therapy). Start prophylaxis as soon as possible after initial exposure and continue for at least 10 days after exposure. May continue prophylactic treatment up to 90 days for repeated or suspected exposures if influenza vaccine is unavailable. If used with influenza vaccine, continue dose for 2 to 3 weeks until antibody response to vaccine has developed.

*Adjust-a-dose:* For patients with renal failure, if creatinine clearance is 30 to 50 ml/minute, give 200 mg the first day and 100 mg thereafter; if clearance is 15 to 29 ml/minute, give 200 mg the first day, then 100 mg on alternate days; if clearance is below 15 ml/minute, give 200 mg q 7 days.

### ADVERSE REACTIONS
**CNS:** depression, fatigue, confusion, *dizziness,* hallucinations, anxiety, *irritability,* ataxia, *insomnia,* headache, *lightheadedness.*
**CV:** peripheral edema, orthostatic hypotension, **heart failure.**
**GI:** anorexia, *nausea,* constipation, vomiting, dry mouth.
**Skin:** *livedo reticularis.*

### INTERACTIONS
**Drug-drug.** *Anticholinergics:* increased anticholinergic effects. Use together cautiously. Dosage of anticholinergic agent

---

Reactions may be *common,* uncommon, **life-threatening,** or COMMON AND LIFE-THREATENING.

may be reduced before initiation of amantadine.
*CNS stimulants:* additive CNS stimulation. Use together cautiously.
**Drug-herb.** *Jimsonweed:* may adversely
affect CV function. Avoid concomitant
use.

**EFFECTS ON DIAGNOSTIC TESTS**
None reported.

**CONTRAINDICATIONS**
Contraindicated in patients with hypersensitivity to drug.

**NURSING CONSIDERATIONS**
● Use cautiously in patients with seizure
disorders, heart failure, peripheral edema,
hepatic disease, mental illness, eczema-
toid rash, renal impairment, orthostatic
hypotension, and CV disease and in elderly patients. Monitor renal and liver function tests.
● *Alert:* Elderly patients are more susceptible to adverse neurologic effects. Monitor for mental status changes.
● *Alert:* Don't confuse amantadine with rimantadine.

☑**Patient teaching**
● If insomnia occurs, tell patient to take
drug several hours before bedtime.
● If orthostatic hypotension occurs, instruct patient not to stand or change positions too quickly.
● Instruct patient to notify doctor of adverse reactions, especially dizziness, depression, anxiety, nausea, and urine retention.

✳ *NEW DRUG*

## amprenavir
Agenerase

*Pregnancy Risk Category C*

**HOW SUPPLIED**
*Capsules:* 50 mg, 150 mg
*Oral solution:* 15 mg/ml

**ACTION**
Inhibits HIV-1 protease by binding to the
active site of HIV-1 protease, which caus-

es immature noninfectious viral particles
to form.

| Route | Onset | Peak | Duration |
|-------|-------|------|----------|
| P.O. | Unknown | 1-2 hr | Unknown |

**INDICATIONS & DOSAGE**
*HIV-1 infection (with other antiretrovi-
rals)—*
**Adults and adolescents ages 13 to 16
weighing over 50 kg (110 lb):** 1,200 mg
(eight 150-mg capsules) P.O. b.i.d. with
other antiretrovirals.
**Children ages 4 to 12 and adolescents
ages 13 to 16 weighing less than 50 kg:**
*Capsules—*20 mg/kg P.O. b.i.d. or 15 mg/
kg P.O. t.i.d. (to maximum daily dose of
2,400 mg) with other antiretrovirals. *Oral
solution—*22.5 mg/kg (1.5 ml/kg) P.O.
b.i.d. or 17 mg/kg (1.1ml/kg) P.O. t.i.d. (to
maximum daily dose of 2,800 mg) with
other antiretrovirals.
*Adjust-a-dose:* For patients with liver impairment and a Child-Pugh score from 5
to 8, dose for capsules should be reduced
to 450 mg P.O. b.i.d. In patients with a
Child-Pugh score from 9 to 12, dose for
capsules should be reduced to 300 mg
P.O. b.i.d.

**ADVERSE REACTIONS**
**CNS:** *paresthesia,* depressive or mood
disorders.
**GI:** *nausea, vomiting, diarrhea or loose
stools,* taste disorders.
**Metabolic:** *hyperglycemia, hypertriglyc-
eridemia,* hypercholesterolemia.
**Skin:** *rash,* **Stevens-Johnson syndrome.**

**INTERACTIONS**
**Drug-drug.** *Amiodarone, lidocaine,
quinidine, tricyclic antidepressants:* inhibited metabolism of these drugs. Monitor drug levels closely.
*Antacids, didanosine:* decreased absorption. Separate administration by at least 1
hour.
*Anticonvulsants, such as carbamazepine,
phenobarbital, and phenytoin:* potentially
decreased amprenavir levels. Monitor patient closely and adjust dosage as needed.
*Bepridil, cisapride, dihydroergotamine,
ergotamine, midazolam, triazolam:* inhibited metabolism of these drugs, which

may cause serious or life-threatening adverse reactions. Don't use together.

*Rifabutin:* decreased amprenavir levels and increased rifabutin levels. Reduce rifabutin dosage to at least half the recommended dosage. Monitor CBC weekly for neutropenia.

*Rifampin:* 90% reduced plasma amprenavir levels. Don't use together.

*Sildenafil:* increased sildenafil levels, which may increase the frequency of sildenafil-associated adverse reactions, such as hypotension, visual changes, and priapism. Use together cautiously.

*Warfarin:* inhibited metabolism of warfarin, which may cause serious or life-threatening adverse reactions. Monitor INR closely.

**Drug-food.** *High-fat foods:* decreased absorption of drug. Avoid taking drug with high-fat foods.

## EFFECTS ON DIAGNOSTIC TESTS
None reported.

## CONTRAINDICATIONS
Contraindicated in patients with hypersensitivity to drug or its components. Drug can cause severe or life-threatening rash, including Stevens-Johnson syndrome. Therapy should be discontinued if patient develops a severe or life-threatening rash or a moderate rash accompanied by systemic signs and symptoms.

## NURSING CONSIDERATIONS
• Use cautiously in patients with moderate or severe hepatic impairment, diabetes mellitus, a known sulfonamide allergy, or hemophilia A or B.

• Use cautiously in pregnant women because no adequate studies exist regarding the effects of amprenavir when administered during pregnancy. Use during pregnancy only if the potential benefits outweigh the risks. Register pregnant woman taking amprenavir with the Antiretroviral Pregnancy Registry by calling 1-800-258-4263.

• *Alert:* Because amprenavir may interact with many drugs, obtain patient's complete drug history. Ask patient to show you the drugs he's taking.

• Patient shouldn't be given high-fat foods because they may decrease absorption of amprenavir.

• Monitor patient for adverse reactions. A patient taking a protease inhibitor may experience a redistribution of body fat, including central obesity, dorsocervical fat enlargement (buffalo hump), peripheral wasting, breast enlargement, and cushingoid appearance. The mechanism and long-term consequences of these effects are unknown.

• Drug provides high daily doses of vitamin E. Advise patient taking drug not to take supplemental vitamin E because high vitamin levels may exacerbate the blood coagulation defect of vitamin K deficiency that anticoagulant therapy or malabsorption causes.

• Protease inhibitors have caused spontaneous bleeding in some patients with hemophilia A or B. In some patients, additional factor VIII was required. In many of the reported cases, treatment with protease inhibitors was continued or restarted.

• Amprenavir capsules aren't interchangeable with amprenavir oral solution on a milligram-per-milligram basis.

### ☑ Patient teaching
• Advise patient that drug isn't a cure for HIV infection; patient may continue to develop opportunistic infections and other complications from the disease. Also, tell patient that drug doesn't reduce risk of HIV transmission through sexual contact.

• Tell patient that, although drug can be taken without regard to food, he shouldn't take it with a high-fat meal because of decreased drug absorption.

• Tell patient to report adverse reactions, especially rash.

• Advise patient to take drug daily, as prescribed, with other antiretrovirals. Dosage mustn't be altered or discontinued without doctor's approval.

• Inform patient to take an antacid or didanosine 1 hour before or after amprenavir to prevent a decrease in amprenavir absorption.

• If a dose is missed by more than 4 hours, advise patient to wait and take the next dose at the regularly scheduled time.

---

Reactions may be *common*, uncommon, *life-threatening*, or COMMON AND LIFE-THREATENING.

If a dose is missed by less than 4 hours, advise him to take the dose as soon as possible and then take the next dose at the regularly scheduled time. If a dose is skipped, patient shouldn't double-dose.
• Advise patient using hormonal contraception to use another contraceptive measure during drug therapy.
• Advise patient to notify doctor if pregnancy occurs during therapy.
• Advise patient not to take supplemental vitamin E because drug contains a significant amount of the vitamin.

---

## cidofovir
Vistide

*Pregnancy Risk Category C*

### HOW SUPPLIED
*Injection:* 75 mg/ml in 5-ml vial

### ACTION
Suppresses CMV replication by selective inhibition of viral DNA synthesis.

| Route | Onset | Peak | Duration |
|-------|-------|------|----------|
| I.V. | Unknown | Unknown | Unknown |

### INDICATIONS & DOSAGE
*CMV retinitis in patients with AIDS—*
**Adults:** initially, 5 mg/kg I.V. infused over 1 hour once weekly for 2 consecutive weeks; then maintenance dose of 5 mg/kg I.V. infused over 1 hour once q 2 weeks. Administer probenecid and prehydration with normal saline solution I.V. concomitantly; may reduce potential for nephrotoxicity.
*Adjust-a-dose:* For patients with renal failure, if serum creatinine increases 0.3 to 0.4 mg/dl above baseline, dose is reduced to 3 mg/kg at same rate and frequency. If serum creatinine increases 0.5 mg/dl or more above baseline, drug is discontinued.

### ADVERSE REACTIONS
**CNS:** *asthenia, headache,* amnesia, anxiety, confusion, **seizures,** depression, dizziness, abnormal gait, hallucinations, insomnia, neuropathy, paresthesia, somnolence, malaise.

**CV:** hypotension, orthostatic hypotension, pallor, syncope, tachycardia, vasodilation.
**EENT:** amblyopia, conjunctivitis, eye disorders, *ocular hypotony,* iritis, retinal detachment, uveitis, abnormal vision, taste perversion.
**GI:** *nausea, vomiting, diarrhea, anorexia, abdominal pain,* dry mouth, colitis, constipation, tongue discoloration, dyspepsia, dysphagia, flatulence, gastritis, melena, oral candidiasis, rectal disorders, stomatitis, aphthous stomatitis, mouth ulcerations, weight loss.
**GU:** *elevated creatinine levels,* **nephrotoxicity,** *proteinuria,* decreased creatinine clearance levels, glycosuria, hematuria, urinary incontinence, urinary tract infection.
**Hematologic:** NEUTROPENIA, *anemia,* **thrombocytopenia.**
**Hepatic:** hepatomegaly, abnormal liver function test results, increased alkaline phosphatase levels.
**Metabolic:** fluid imbalance, hyperglycemia, hyperlipemia, hypocalcemia, hypokalemia, decreased serum bicarbonate level.
**Musculoskeletal:** arthralgia, myasthenia, myalgia, pain in back, chest, or neck.
**Respiratory:** asthma, bronchitis, coughing, *dyspnea,* hiccups, increased sputum, lung disorders, pharyngitis, pneumonia, rhinitis, sinusitis.
**Skin:** *rash, alopecia,* acne, skin discoloration, dry skin, herpes simplex, pruritus, sweating, urticaria.
**Other:** *fever, infections, chills,* allergic reactions, facial edema, **sarcoma, sepsis.**

### INTERACTIONS
**Drug-drug.** *Nephrotoxic agents (such as aminoglycosides, amphotericin B, foscarnet, I.V. pentamidine):* may increase nephrotoxicity. Avoid concomitant use.
*Probenecid:* known to interact with the metabolism or renal tubular excretion of many drugs. Monitor closely.

### EFFECTS ON DIAGNOSTIC TESTS
None reported.

### CONTRAINDICATIONS
Contraindicated in patients with hypersensitivity to drug or history of clinically

---

severe hypersensitivity to probenecid or other sulfur-containing drugs. Also contraindicated in patients receiving agents with nephrotoxic potential and in those with serum creatinine exceeding 1.5 mg/dl, a calculated creatinine clearance of 55 ml/minute or less, or a urine protein of 100 mg/dl or more (equivalent to 2+ proteinuria or more). Don't administer as a direct intraocular injection because it may be associated with significant decreases in intraocular pressure and vision impairment. Don't administer drug to breast-feeding women.

## NURSING CONSIDERATIONS

• Use cautiously in patients with impaired renal function. Monitor renal function tests and patient's fluid balance.
• Administer 1 L normal saline as ordered, usually over 1- to 2-hour period immediately before each cidofovir infusion.
• Administer probenecid, as ordered, with cidofovir.
• Monitor renal function (serum creatinine and urine protein) before each dose. Dosage may be modified by a doctor if changes in renal function occur.
• Drug shouldn't be used in patients with baseline serum creatinine level exceeding 1.5 mg/dl or calculated creatinine clearance of 55 ml/minute or less unless potential benefits outweigh potential risks.
• Fanconi's syndrome and decreased serum bicarbonate levels associated with renal tubular damage have been reported in patients receiving cidofovir. Monitor patient closely.
• Monitor WBC counts with differential before each dose.
• Granulocytopenia has been observed with drug treatment. Monitor neutrophil counts during therapy.
• Intraocular pressure, visual acuity, and ocular symptoms should be monitored periodically.
• Cidofovir is indicated only for the treatment of CMV retinitis in patients with AIDS. Safety and efficacy of drug have not been established for treating other CMV infections, congenital or neonatal CMV disease, or CMV disease in patients not infected with HIV.

• Cidofovir has been known to be carcinogenic and teratogenic and has caused hypospermia.
• Discontinue zidovudine therapy or reduce dosage by 50%, as ordered, on the days cidofovir is administered; probenecid reduces metabolic clearance of zidovudine.
• Dosage adjustment may be necessary in elderly patients with renal impairment.
• Safety and effectiveness in children have not been established.
• It's unknown if cidofovir appears in breast milk.

### 🛑 I.V. administration
• Because of the potential for increased nephrotoxicity, don't exceed recommended dosages or frequency or rate of administration.
• To prepare cidofovir for infusion, extract the appropriate amount of cidofovir from the vial using a syringe and transfer the dose to an infusion bag containing 100 ml of normal saline solution. Infuse the entire volume I.V. at a constant rate over a 1-hour period. Use a standard infusion pump for administration.
• Because of the mutagenic properties of cidofovir, drug should be prepared in a class II laminar flow biological safety cabinet. Personnel preparing drug should wear surgical gloves and a closed front surgical gown with knit cuffs.
• If drug contacts the skin, wash membranes and flush thoroughly with water. Excess drug and all other materials used in the admixture preparation and administration should be placed in a leakproof, puncture-proof container. Recommended method of disposal is high temperature incineration.
• Cidofovir infusion admixtures should be administered within 24 hours of preparation; refrigerator or freezer storage shouldn't be used to extend this 24-hour period. If admixtures are not used immediately, they may be refrigerated at 36° to 46° F (2° to 8° C) for no more than 24 hours. Allow cidofovir to reach room temperature before use.
• Don't add other drugs or supplements to admixture for concurrent administration.

---

Reactions may be *common*, uncommon, *life-threatening*, or COMMON AND LIFE-THREATENING.

• Compatibility with Ringer's solution, lactated Ringer's solution, or bacteriostatic infusion fluids has not been evaluated.

☑**Patient teaching**
• Inform patient that drug is not a cure for CMV retinitis and that regular ophthalmologic follow-up examinations are necessary.
• Alert patient on zidovudine therapy that he'll need to obtain dosage guidelines on days cidofovir is administered.
• Tell patient that close monitoring of renal function will be needed and that abnormalities may require a change in cidofovir therapy.
• Stress importance of completing a full course of probenecid with each cidofovir dose. Tell patient to take probenecid after a meal to decrease nausea.
• Advise woman of childbearing age to use effective contraception during and for 1 month following treatment with cidofovir.
• Advise man to practice barrier contraception during and for 3 months after treatment with drug.
• Advise breast-feeding woman that it's unknown if cidofovir appears in breast milk.

---

**delavirdine mesylate**
Rescriptor

*Pregnancy Risk Category C*

**HOW SUPPLIED**
*Tablets:* 100 mg

**ACTION**
A nonnucleoside reverse-transcriptase inhibitor of HIV-1. Drug binds directly to reverse transcriptase and blocks RNA- and DNA-dependent DNA polymerase activities.

| Route | Onset | Peak | Duration |
|-------|-------|------|----------|
| P.O. | Unknown | 1 hr | Unknown |

**INDICATIONS & DOSAGE**
*HIV-1 infection when therapy is warranted—*
**Adults:** 400 mg P.O. t.i.d. with other appropriate antiretroviral agents.

**ADVERSE REACTIONS**
**CNS:** abnormal coordination, agitation, amnesia, anxiety, change in dreams, cognitive impairment, confusion, depression, disorientation, dizziness, emotional lability, fatigue, hallucinations, headache, hyperesthesia, hyperreflexia, hypoesthesia, impaired concentration, lethargy, malaise, insomnia, manic symptoms, migraine, nervousness, neuropathy, nightmares, pallor, paralysis, paranoid symptoms, paresthesia, restlessness, somnolence, tingling, tremor, vertigo, weakness.
**CV:** bradycardia, chest pain, edema, orthostatic hypotension, palpitation, syncope, tachycardia, vasodilation.
**EENT:** blepharitis, conjunctivitis, diplopia, dry eyes, ear pain, epistaxis, nystagmus, pharyngitis, photophobia, rhinitis, sinusitis, taste perversion, tinnitus.
**GI:** anorexia, aphthous stomatitis, bloody stools, colitis, constipation, decreased appetite, diarrhea, diverticulitis, duodenitis, dry mouth, dyspepsia, dysphagia, enteritis, esophagitis, fecal incontinence, flatulence, gagging, gastritis, gastroesophageal reflux, GI bleeding, gingivitis, gum hemorrhage, increased thirst and appetite, increased saliva, mouth ulcer, *nausea*, nonspecific hepatitis, pancreatitis, rectal disorder, sialadenitis, stomatitis, tongue edema or ulceration, vomiting, abdominal cramps, distention, or pain, weight gain or loss.
**GU:** epididymitis, hematuria, hemospermia, impotence, renal calculi, renal pain, metrorrhagia, nocturia, polyuria, proteinuria, vaginal candidiasis.
**Hematologic:** anemia, ecchymosis, eosinophilia, granulocytosis, *neutropenia, pancytopenia,* petechiae, prolonged PTT, purpura, spleen disorder, *thrombocytopenia.*
**Hepatic:** increased ALT and AST levels.
**Metabolic:** alcohol intolerance; bilirubinemia; hyperkalemia; hyperuricemia; hypocalcemia; hyponatremia; hypophosphatemia; peripheral edema; increased gamma glutamyl transpeptidase, lipase, serum alkaline phosphatase, serum amylase, serum CK, and serum creatinine levels.
**Musculoskeletal:** bone disorder, arthralgia or arthritis of single and multiple

---

joints, asthenia, bone pain, back pain, flank pain, leg cramps, muscle cramps, muscular weakness, myalgia, neck rigidity, tendon disorder, tenosynovitis.
**Respiratory:** chest congestion, bronchitis, dyspnea, laryngismus, cough, upper respiratory tract infection.
**Skin:** alopecia, angioedema, dermal leukocytoblastic vasculitis, dermatitis, desquamation, diaphoresis, dry skin, epidermal cyst, erythema, erythema multiforme, folliculitis, fungal dermatitis, maculopapular rash, nail disorder, petechial rash, pruritus, *rash*, sebaceous cyst, seborrhea, skin nodule, **Stevens-Johnson syndrome**, urticaria, vesiculobullous rash.
**Other:** allergic reaction, breast enlargement, chills, decreased libido, fever, flu-like syndrome, lip edema, pain, trauma, tetany.

## INTERACTIONS
**Drug-drug.** *Amphetamines, benzodiazepines, calcium channel blockers, cisapride, ergot alkaloid preparations, quinidine:* may result in potentially serious or life-threatening adverse effects. Avoid concomitant use.
*Antacids:* reduced absorption of delavirdine. Separate doses by at least 1 hour.
*Carbamazepine, phenobarbital, phenytoin, rifampin:* substantially decreased plasma delavirdine levels. Avoid coadministration.
*Clarithromycin:* increased concentrations of both drugs. Monitor carefully.
*Dapsone, warfarin:* delavirdine increases plasma concentrations of these drugs. Monitor carefully.
*Didanosine:* coadministration with delavirdine results in a 20% decrease in absorption of both drugs. Separate administration by at least 1 hour.
*Fluoxetine, ketoconazole:* increased delavirdine trough levels. Monitor patient.
*H$_2$-receptor antagonists:* may reduce absorption of delavirdine. Chronic use of these drugs with delavirdine isn't recommended.
*Indinavir:* increased plasma levels of indinavir. A lower dosage of indinavir should be considered.

*Rifabutin:* decreased delavirdine levels and increased rifabutin levels. Use together cautiously.
*Saquinavir:* fivefold increase in systemic levels of saquinavir. Monitor AST and ALT levels frequently when used together.

## EFFECTS ON DIAGNOSTIC TESTS
None reported.

## CONTRAINDICATIONS
Contraindicated in patients with hypersensitivity to drug's formulation.

## NURSING CONSIDERATIONS
• Use cautiously in patients with impaired hepatic function.
• Drug-induced rash is more common in patients with lower CD4+ cell counts and usually occurs within first 3 weeks of treatment. It's typically diffuse, maculopapular, erythematous, and often pruritic. It occurs commonly and its incidence doesn't appear to be significantly reduced by adjusted drug doses.
• Rash occurs mainly on the upper body and proximal arms. Using diphenhydramine, hydroxyzine, or topical corticosteroids may relieve symptoms.
• Because drug's effects in patients with hepatic or renal impairment have not been studied, monitor renal and liver function test results carefully.
• Drug has not been shown to reduce risk of transmission of HIV-1.
• Because resistance develops rapidly when used as monotherapy, always use drug with appropriate antiretroviral therapy.
• Monitor patient's fluid balance and weight.

### ✓ Patient teaching
• Tell patient to discontinue drug and call doctor if severe rash or such symptoms as fever, blistering, oral lesions, conjunctivitis, swelling, or muscle or joint aches occur.
• Inform patient that drug is not a cure for HIV-1 infection and that they may continue to acquire illnesses associated with HIV-1 infection, including opportunistic infections. Therapy has not been shown to reduce the incidence or frequency of such

illnesses. Drug has not been shown to reduce transmission of HIV.
- Advise patient to remain under medical supervision when taking drug because the long-term effects are not known.
- Tell patient to take drug as prescribed and not to alter doses without doctor's approval. If a dose is missed, tell patient to take the next dose as soon as possible; he shouldn't double the next dose.
- Inform patient that drug may be dispersed in water before ingestion. Add tablets to at least 5 oz (148 ml) of water, allow to stand for a few minutes, and stir until a uniform dispersion occurs. Tell patient to drink dispersion promptly, rinse glass, and swallow the rinse to ensure that entire dose is consumed.
- Tell patient that drug may be taken without regard to food.
- Instruct patient with achlorhydria to take drug with an acidic beverage, such as orange or cranberry juice.
- Instruct patient to take drug and antacids at least 1 hour apart.
- Advise patient to report use of other prescription or OTC medications.

## didanosine (ddl)
Videx

*Pregnancy Risk Category B*

### HOW SUPPLIED
*Tablets (buffered, chewable):* 25 mg, 50 mg, 100 mg, 150 mg
*Powder for oral solution (buffered):* 100 mg/packet, 167 mg/packet, 250 mg/packet,
*Powder for oral solution (pediatric):* 4-oz, 8-oz glass bottles containing 2 g and 4 g of Videx, respectively

### ACTION
Inhibits the enzyme HIV-RNA-dependent DNA polymerase (reverse transcriptase) and terminates DNA chain growth.

| Route | Onset | Peak | Duration |
|-------|-------|------|----------|
| P.O. | Unknown | 0.5-1 hr | Unknown |

### INDICATIONS & DOSAGE
*HIV infection when antiretroviral therapy is warranted—*
**Adults weighing 60 kg (132 lb) and over:** 200 mg (tablets) P.O. q 12 hours; or 250 mg buffered powder P.O. q 12 hours.
**Adults under 60 kg:** 125 mg (tablets) P.O. q 12 hours; or 167 mg buffered powder P.O. q 12 hours.
**Children:** 90 to 150 mg/m² P.O. q 12 hours.
*Adjust-a-dose:* Dialysis patients should receive 25% of usual dose.

### ADVERSE REACTIONS
**CNS:** *headache, seizures,* confusion, anxiety, nervousness, abnormal thinking, twitching, depression, *peripheral neuropathy, dizziness,* asthenia, insomnia.
**CV:** hypertension, edema, **heart failure.**
**EENT:** retinal changes, optic neuritis.
**GI:** *diarrhea, nausea, vomiting, abdominal pain, pancreatitis,* dry mouth, anorexia.
**Hematologic:** *leukopenia,* granulocytosis, **thrombocytopenia,** anemia.
**Hepatic:** *hepatic failure,* elevated liver enzymes.
**Respiratory:** dyspnea, pneumonia.
**Skin:** rash, pruritus, alopecia.
**Other:** pain, infection, sarcoma, allergic reactions, myopathy, increased serum uric acid levels, *chills, fever.*

### INTERACTIONS
**Drug-drug.** *Antacids containing magnesium or aluminum hydroxides:* enhanced adverse effects of the antacid component (including diarrhea or constipation) when administered with didanosine tablets or pediatric suspension. Avoid concomitant use.
*Dapsone, drugs that require gastric acid for adequate absorption, ketoconazole:* decreased absorption from buffering action. Administer these drugs 2 hours before didanosine.
*Fluoroquinolones, tetracyclines:* decreased absorption from buffering agents in didanosine tablets or antacids in pediatric suspension. Avoid concomitant use.
*Itraconazole:* decreased serum levels of itraconazole. Avoid concomitant use.
**Drug-food.** *Any food:* decreased rate of absorption. Give drug on an empty stomach at least 30 minutes before a meal.

---

*Liquid contains alcohol.   **May contain tartrazine.   †Canada   ‡Australia   §U.K.   ◇OTC

## EFFECTS ON DIAGNOSTIC TESTS
None reported.

## CONTRAINDICATIONS
Contraindicated in patients with history of hypersensitivity to any component of the formulation.

## NURSING CONSIDERATIONS
• Use cautiously in patients with history of pancreatitis; fatalities have occurred. Also use cautiously in patients with peripheral neuropathy, renal or hepatic impairment, or hyperuricemia. Monitor liver and renal function tests.
• Administer didanosine on an empty stomach, regardless of the dosage form used; administering drug with meals can decrease absorption by 50%.
• To administer single-dose packets containing buffered powder for oral solution, pour contents into 4 oz (120 ml) of water. Don't use fruit juice or other beverages that may be acidic. Stir for 2 or 3 minutes until the powder dissolves completely. Administer immediately.
• The powder for oral solution has been associated with a high incidence of diarrhea. The manufacturer suggests switching to the tablet formulation if diarrhea is a problem.
• *Alert:* The pediatric powder for oral solution must be prepared by a pharmacist before dispensing. It must be constituted with purified USP water and then diluted with an antacid (either Mylanta Double Strength Liquid or Maalox TC Suspension) to a final concentration of 10 mg/ml. The admixture is stable for 30 days if refrigerated (at 36° to 46° F [2° to 8° C]). Shake the solution well before measuring the dose.
• *Alert:* Don't confuse drug with other antivirals that use abbreviations for identification.

☑ **Patient teaching**
• Instruct patient to take drug on an empty stomach.
• Because the tablets contain buffers that raise stomach pH to levels that prevent degradation of the active drug, instruct patient to chew tablets thoroughly before swallowing and drink at least 1 oz (30 ml) of water with each dose. Teach patient how to prepare crushed tablets or buffered powder form for ingestion, if appropriate.
• Inform patient receiving a sodium-restricted diet that each two-tablet dose of didanosine contains 529 mg of sodium; each single packet of buffered powder for oral solution contains 1.38 g of sodium.
• Tell patient to report symptoms of pancreatitis, such as abdominal pain, nausea, vomiting, diarrhea.

---

## efavirenz
Sustiva

*Pregnancy Risk Category C*

## HOW SUPPLIED
*Capsules:* 50 mg, 100 mg, 200 mg

## ACTION
A nonnucleoside, reverse transcriptase inhibitor (NNRTI) that inhibits the transcription of HIV-1 RNA to DNA, a critical step in the viral replication process. Therefore, drug lowers the amount of HIV in the blood (the viral load) and increases CD4 lymphocytes.

| Route | Onset | Peak | Duration |
|-------|-------|------|----------|
| P.O. | Unknown | 3-5 hr | Unknown |

## INDICATIONS & DOSAGE
*HIV-1 infection—*
**Adults:** 600 mg P.O. once daily.
**Children ages 3 and older weighing 40 kg (88 lb) or more:** 600 mg P.O. once.
**Children ages 3 and older weighing 10 to under 40 kg (22 to under 88 lb):**
Children 10 to under 15 kg (22 to under 33 lb): 200 mg P.O. once daily.
Children 15 to under 20 kg (33 to under 44 lb): 250 mg P.O. once daily.
Children 20 to under 25 kg (44 to under 55 lb): 300 mg P.O. once daily.
Children 25 to under 32.5 kg (55 to under 72 lb): 350 mg P.O. once daily.
Children 32.5 to under 40 kg (72 to under 88 lb): 400 mg P.O. once daily.
  *Note:* Give all above doses with a protease inhibitor or nucleoside analogue reverse transcriptase inhibitors.

---

## ADVERSE REACTIONS

**CNS:** abnormal dreams or thinking, agitation, amnesia, confusion, depersonalization, depression, *dizziness,* euphoria, fatigue, hallucinations, headache, hypoesthesia, impaired concentration, insomnia, somnolence, nervousness.
**GI:** abdominal pain, anorexia, *diarrhea,* dyspepsia, flatulence, *nausea,* vomiting.
**GU:** hematuria, kidney stones.
**Hepatic:** increased AST, ALT, and total cholesterol levels.
**Skin:** increased sweating, *erythema multiforme, Stevens-Johnson syndrome, toxic epidermal necrolysis, rash,* pruritus.
**Other:** fever.

## INTERACTIONS

**Drug-drug.** *Cisapride, ergot derivatives, midazolam, triazolam:* competition for cytochrome P-450 enzyme system may result in inhibition of the metabolism of these drugs and cause serious or life-threatening adverse effects (such as arrhythmias, prolonged sedation, or respiratory depression). Avoid concomitant use.
*Clarithromycin, indinavir:* decreased plasma levels. Consider alternative therapy or dosage adjustment.
*Drugs that induce the cytochrome P-450 enzyme system (phenobarbital, rifampin, rifabutin):* increased clearance of efavirenz resulting in lowered plasma levels. Avoid concomitant use.
*Estrogens, ritonavir:* increased plasma levels. Monitor patient.
*Oral contraceptives:* potential interaction of efavirenz with oral contraceptives has not been determined. Suggest use of a reliable method of barrier contraception in addition to oral contraceptives.
*Psychoactive drugs:* additive CNS effects. Avoid concomitant use.
*Saquinavir:* plasma levels of saquinavir decreased significantly. Don't use with saquinavir as sole protease inhibitor.
*Warfarin:* plasma levels and effects potentially increased or decreased. Monitor INR.
**Drug-food.** *High-fat meals:* increased absorption of drug. Instruct patient to maintain a proper low-fat diet.
**Drug-lifestyle.** *Alcohol:* enhanced CNS effects. Avoid concomitant use.

## EFFECTS ON DIAGNOSTIC TESTS

Drug therapy may cause false-positive urine cannabinoid test results.

## CONTRAINDICATIONS

Contraindicated in patients with hypersensitivity to drug or its components.

## NURSING CONSIDERATIONS

• Use cautiously in patients with hepatic impairment or in those concurrently receiving hepatotoxic drugs. Monitor liver function test results in patients with history of hepatitis B or C and in those also taking ritonavir.
• Monitor cholesterol levels.
• *Alert:* Drug should be used with other antiretroviral drugs because resistant viruses emerge rapidly when used alone. Drug shouldn't be used as monotherapy, or added on as a single agent to a failing regimen.
• Using drug with ritonavir is associated with a higher frequency of adverse effects (such as dizziness, nausea, paresthesia) and laboratory abnormalities (elevated liver enzymes).
• Administer drug at bedtime to decrease noticeable CNS adverse effects.
• Pregnancy must be ruled out before starting therapy in women of childbearing age.
• Children may be more prone to adverse reactions, especially diarrhea, nausea, vomiting, and rash.

### ☑ Patient teaching

• Instruct patient to take drug with water, juice, milk, or soda. It may be taken without regard to meals.
• Inform patient about need for scheduled blood tests to monitor liver function and cholesterol levels.
• Tell patient to use a reliable method of barrier contraception in addition to oral contraceptives and to notify doctor immediately if pregnancy is suspected.
• Inform patient that drug is not a cure for HIV infection and that it will not affect the development of opportunistic infections and other complications associated with HIV infection or transmission of HIV to others through sexual contact or blood contamination.

---

*Liquid contains alcohol.   **May contain tartrazine.   †Canada   ‡Australia   §U.K.   ◇OTC

• Instruct patient to take drug at the same time daily and always with other antiretroviral drugs.
• Tell patient to take drug exactly as prescribed and not to discontinue it without medical approval. Also instruct patient to report adverse reactions if they occur.
• Inform patient that rash is the most common adverse effect. Tell patient to report rash immediately because it may be serious (in rare cases).
• Advise patient to report use of other drugs.
• Advise patient that dizziness, difficulty sleeping or concentrating, drowsiness, or unusual dreams may occur the first few days of therapy. Reassure him that these symptoms generally resolve after 2 to 4 weeks and may be less problematic if drug is taken at bedtime.
• Tell patient to avoid alcoholic beverages, driving, or operating machinery until the drug's effects are known.

## famciclovir
Famvir

*Pregnancy Risk Category B*

### HOW SUPPLIED
*Tablets:* 125 mg, 250 mg, 500 mg

### ACTION
A guanosine nucleoside that's converted to penciclovir, which enters viral cells and inhibits DNA polymerase and viral DNA synthesis.

| Route | Onset | Peak | Duration |
|-------|-------|------|----------|
| P.O. | Unknown | 1 hr | Unknown |

### INDICATIONS & DOSAGE
*Acute herpes zoster infection (shingles)—*
**Adults:** 500 mg P.O. q 8 hours for 7 days.
*Adjust-a-dose:* For patients with reduced renal function, if creatinine clearance is 60 ml/minute or more, 500 mg P.O. q 8 hours; if clearance is 40 to 59 ml/minute, 500 mg P.O. q 12 hours; if 20 to 39 ml/minute, 500 mg P.O. q 24 hours; and if below 20 ml/minute, 250 mg P.O. q 24 hours.

For hemodialysis patients, 250 mg P.O. after each hemodialysis session.
*Recurrent episodes of genital herpes—*
**Adults:** 125 mg P.O. b.i.d. for 5 days. Therapy begins as soon as symptoms occur.
*Adjust-a-dose:* For patients with reduced renal function, if creatinine clearance is 40 ml/minute or more, 125 mg P.O. q 12 hours; if 20 to 39 ml/minute, 125 mg P.O. q 24 hours; if below 20 ml/minute, 125 mg P.O. q 24 hours.

For hemodialysis patients, 125 mg P.O. after each hemodialysis session.
*Recurrent mucocutaneous herpes simplex infections in HIV-infected patients—*
**Adults:** 500 mg P.O. b.i.d. for 7 days.
*Adjust-a-dose:* For patients with reduced renal function, if creatinine clearance is 40 ml/minute or more, 500 mg P.O. q 12 hours; if 20 to 39 ml/minute, 500 mg P.O. q 24 hours; and if below 20 ml/minute, 250 mg P.O. q 24 hours.

For hemodialysis patients, 250 mg P.O. after each hemodialysis session.

### ADVERSE REACTIONS
**CNS:** *headache,* fatigue, dizziness, paresthesia, somnolence.
**EENT:** pharyngitis, sinusitis.
**GI:** diarrhea, *nausea,* vomiting, constipation, anorexia, abdominal pain.
**Musculoskeletal:** back pain, arthralgia.
**Skin:** pruritus; zoster-related signs, symptoms, and complications.
**Other:** fever.

### INTERACTIONS
**Drug-drug.** *Probenecid:* may increase plasma levels of famciclovir. Monitor patient for increased adverse effects.

### EFFECTS ON DIAGNOSTIC TESTS
None reported.

### CONTRAINDICATIONS
Contraindicated in patients with hypersensitivity to drug.

### NURSING CONSIDERATIONS
• Use cautiously in patients with renal or hepatic impairment. Dosage adjustment may be needed. Monitor renal and liver function tests.

---

Reactions may be *common,* uncommon, *life-threatening,* or COMMON AND LIFE-THREATENING.

• Drug may be taken without regard to meals.

### ✓ Patient teaching
• Inform patient that drug is not a cure for genital herpes but can decrease the length and severity of symptoms.
• Teach patient how to prevent spread of infection to others.
• Urge patient to recognize the early symptoms of herpes infection, such as tingling, itching, and pain, and to report them. Treatment is more effective if therapy is started within 48 hours of rash onset.

---

## fomivirsen sodium
Vitravene

*Pregnancy Risk Category C*

### HOW SUPPLIED
*Intravitreal injection:* preservative-free, 0.25-ml, single-use vials containing 6.6 mg/ml

### ACTION
A phosphorothioate oligonucleotide that inhibits human CMV replication by binding to the target mRNA and subsequently inhibiting virus replication.

| Route | Onset | Peak | Duration |
|-------|-------|------|----------|
| Intravitreal | Unknown | Unknown | Unknown |

### INDICATIONS & DOSAGE
*Local treatment of CMV retinitis in patients with AIDS, who are intolerant of or have a contraindication to other treatments or who were insufficiently responsive to previous treatment—*
**Adults:** induction dose is 330 mcg (0.05 ml) by intravitreal injection every other week for two doses. Subsequent maintenance dose is 330 mcg (0.05 ml) by intravitreal injection once q 4 weeks after induction.

### ADVERSE REACTIONS
**CNS:** asthenia, headache, abnormal thinking, depression, dizziness, neuropathy, pain.
**CV:** chest pain.

**EENT:** abnormal or blurred vision, anterior chamber inflammation, cataract, conjunctival hemorrhage, decreased visual acuity, desaturation of color vision, eye pain, floaters, increased intraocular pressure, photophobia, retinal detachment, retinal edema, retinal hemorrhage, retinal pigment changes, *uveitis, vitreitis,* application site reaction, conjunctival hyperemia, conjunctivitis, corneal edema, decreased peripheral vision, eye irritation, hypotony, keratic precipitates, optic neuritis, photopsia, retinal vascular disease, visual field defect, vitreous hemorrhage, vitreous opacity, sinusitis.
**GI:** abdominal pain, anorexia, diarrhea, nausea, vomiting, decreased weight, oral candidiasis, *pancreatitis.*
**GU:** catheter infection, *kidney failure.*
**Hematologic:** anemia, lymphoma-like reaction, *neutropenia, thrombocytopenia.*
**Hepatic:** abnormal liver function tests, increased GGT.
**Metabolic:** dehydration.
**Musculoskeletal:** back pain.
**Respiratory:** bronchitis, dyspnea, increased cough, pneumonia.
**Skin:** rash, sweating.
**Other:** allergic reactions, cachexia, fever, flulike syndrome, infection, *sepsis,* systemic CMV.

### INTERACTIONS
None significant.

### EFFECTS ON DIAGNOSTIC TESTS
None reported.

### CONTRAINDICATIONS
Contraindicated in patients with hypersensitivity to drug or its components or in those who have recently (within 2 to 4 weeks) been treated with either I.V. or intravitreal cidofovir because of an increased risk of exaggerated ocular inflammation.

### NURSING CONSIDERATIONS
• *Alert:* Drug is for ophthalmic use by intravitreal injection only.
• Drug provides localized therapy limited to the treated eye, and does not provide treatment for systemic CMV disease.

---

*Liquid contains alcohol.  **May contain tartrazine.  †Canada  ‡Australia  §U.K.  ◊OTC

Monitor patient for extraocular CMV disease or disease in the contralateral eye.
• Ocular inflammation (uveitis) is more common during induction dosing.
• Monitor light perception and optic nerve head perfusion postinjection.
• Watch for intraocular pressure. This is usually transient and returns to normal without treatment or with temporary use of topical medications.

☑ **Patient teaching**
• Inform patient that drug is not a cure for CMV retinitis, and that some patients continue to experience progression of retinitis during and following treatment.
• Tell patient that drug treats only the eye in which it has been injected, and that CMV may also exist in the body. Stress importance of follow-up visits to monitor progress and to check for additional infections.
• Instruct patient to also have regular ophthalmologic follow-up examinations.
• Advise HIV-infected patient to continue taking antiretroviral therapy as indicated.

## foscarnet sodium (phosphonoformic acid)
Foscavir

*Pregnancy Risk Category C*

### HOW SUPPLIED
*Injection:* 24 mg/ml in 250- and 500-ml bottles

### ACTION
Inhibits all known herpesviruses in vitro by blocking the pyrophosphate binding site on DNA polymerases and reverse transcriptases.

| Route | Onset | Peak | Duration |
|-------|-------|------|----------|
| I.V. | Unknown | Immediate | Unknown |

### INDICATIONS & DOSAGE
*CMV retinitis in patients with AIDS—*
**Adults:** initially, 60 mg/kg I.V. as an induction treatment in patients with normal renal function. Administer q 8 hours for 2 to 3 weeks, depending on clinical response. Follow with a maintenance infusion of 90 to 120 mg/kg daily. Or, 90 mg/kg IV q 12 hours is used for induction.
*Acyclovir-resistant HSV infections-*
**Adults:** 40 mg/kg I.V. over 1 hour q 8 to 12 hours for 2 to 3 weeks or until healed.
**Adjust-a-dose:** Refer to package insert for very specific dose adjustments. Dosage must be adjusted when creatinine clearance is below 1.5 ml/minute/kg. If creatinine clearance falls below 0.4 ml/minute/kg, discontinue drug.

### ADVERSE REACTIONS
**CNS:** *headache,* **seizures,** *fatigue, malaise, asthenia, paresthesia, dizziness, hypoesthesia, neuropathy,* tremor, ataxia, generalized spasms, dementia, stupor, sensory disturbances, meningitis, aphasia, abnormal coordination, EEG abnormalities, depression, confusion, anxiety, insomnia, somnolence, nervousness, amnesia, agitation, aggressive reaction, hallucinations.
**CV:** *hypertension, palpitations, ECG abnormalities, sinus tachycardia,* cerebrovascular disorder, *first-degree AV block, hypotension, flushing,* edema.
**EENT:** visual disturbances, taste perversion, eye pain, conjunctivitis, sinusitis, pharyngitis, rhinitis.
**GI:** *nausea, diarrhea, vomiting, abdominal pain, anorexia,* constipation, dysphagia, rectal hemorrhage, dry mouth, dyspepsia, melena, flatulence, ulcerative stomatitis, **pancreatitis.**
**GU:** *abnormal renal function, decreased creatinine clearance and increased serum creatinine levels, albuminuria, dysuria, polyuria, urethral disorder, urine retention, urinary tract infections,* **acute renal failure,** candidiasis.
**Hematologic:** *anemia, granulocytopenia,* **leukopenia, bone marrow suppression, thrombocytopenia,** platelet abnormalities, thrombocytosis, WBC count abnormalities, lymphadenopathy.
**Hepatic:** increased liver enzymes; increased serum bilirubin, alkaline phosphatase, ALT, and AST levels; abnormal hepatic function.
**Metabolic:** hypokalemia, hypomagnesemia, hypophosphatemia or hyperphosphatemia, hypocalcemia, hyponatremia.

Reactions may be *common*, uncommon, *life-threatening*, or COMMON AND LIFE-THREATENING.

**Musculoskeletal:** leg cramps, arthralgia, myalgia, back or chest pain.
**Respiratory:** *cough, dyspnea,* pneumonitis, respiratory insufficiency, pulmonary infiltration, stridor, pneumothorax, *bronchospasm,* hemoptysis, flulike symptoms.
**Skin:** *rash, diaphoresis,* pruritus, skin ulceration, erythematous rash, seborrhea, skin discoloration, facial edema.
**Other:** ***death,*** *fever,* pain, sepsis, rigors, inflammation and pain at infusion site, lymphoma-like disorder, sarcoma, bacterial or fungal infections, abscess.

### INTERACTIONS
**Drug-drug.** *Nephrotoxic drugs (such as aminoglycosides, amphotericin B):* increased risk of nephrotoxicity. Avoid concomitant use.
*Pentamidine:* increased risk of nephrotoxicity; severe hypocalcemia has also been reported. Avoid concomitant use.
*Zidovudine:* possible increased incidence or severity of anemia. Monitor blood counts.

### EFFECTS ON DIAGNOSTIC TESTS
None reported.

### CONTRAINDICATIONS
Contraindicated in patients with hypersensitivity to drug.

### NURSING CONSIDERATIONS
• Use cautiously and with reduced dosage in patients with abnormal renal function, as ordered. Because drug is nephrotoxic, it can worsen renal impairment. Some degree of nephrotoxicity occurs in most patients treated with drug.
• Because drug is highly toxic and toxicity is probably dose-related, always use the lowest effective maintenance dose during therapy.
• Monitor creatinine clearance frequently during therapy because of drug's adverse effects on renal function. A baseline 24-hour creatinine clearance is recommended, followed by regular determinations two to three times weekly during induction and at least once every 1 to 2 weeks during maintenance.
• Because drug can alter serum electrolytes, monitor levels using a schedule

similar to that established for creatinine clearance. Assess patient for tetany and seizures associated with abnormal electrolyte levels.
• Monitor patient's hemoglobin and hematocrit levels. Anemia is common (in up to 33% of patients treated with drug). It may be severe enough to require transfusions.
• Keep in mind that drug administration is associated with a dose-related transient decrease in ionized serum calcium, which may not always be reflected in patient's laboratory values.

### I.V. administration
• Use an infusion pump to administer foscarnet. To minimize renal toxicity, make sure patient is adequately hydrated before and during the infusion.
• Administer induction treatment over 1 hour; maintenance infusions over 2 hours.
• *Alert:* Don't exceed the recommended dosage, infusion rate, or frequency of administration. All doses must be individualized according to patient's renal function.

### Patient teaching
• Explain the importance of adequate hydration throughout therapy.
• Advise patient to report perioral tingling, numbness in the extremities, and paresthesia.
• Instruct patient to alert nurse if discomfort occurs at I.V. insertion site.

# ganciclovir
Cymevene§, Cytovene

*Pregnancy Risk Category C*

### HOW SUPPLIED
*Capsules:* 250 mg
*Injection:* 500 mg/vial

### ACTION
Inhibits binding of deoxyguanosine triphosphate to DNA polymerase, resulting in inhibition of DNA synthesis.

| Route | Onset | Peak | Duration |
|-------|-------|------|----------|
| P.O. | Unknown | 1.8-3 hr | Unknown |
| I.V. | Unknown | Immediate | Unknown |

## INDICATIONS & DOSAGE

*CMV retinitis in immunocompromised individuals, including patients with AIDS and normal renal function—*
**Adults and children over age 3 months:** induction treatment is 5 mg/kg I.V. q 12 hours for 14 to 21 days. Maintenance treatment is 5 mg/kg I.V. daily for 7 days weekly, or 6 mg/kg daily for 5 days weekly. Or, 1,000 mg P.O. t.i.d. with food.
*Adjust-a-dose:* Refer to package insert for very specific dose adjustments. Dosage is adjusted for patients with impaired renal function and is based on creatinine clearance levels.

Dosage adjustment is necessary in patients with creatinine clearance below 70 ml/minute.
*Prevention of CMV disease in patients with advanced HIV infection and normal renal function—*
**Adults:** 1,000 mg P.O. t.i.d. with food.
*Prevention of CMV disease in transplant recipients with normal renal function—*
**Adults:** 5 mg/kg I.V. (given at a constant rate over 1 hour) q 12 hours for 7 to 14 days; then 5 mg/kg daily for 7 days weekly, or 6 mg/kg daily for 5 days weekly. Duration of therapy depends on degree of immunosuppression.

## ADVERSE REACTIONS

**CNS:** altered dreams, confusion, ataxia, headache, *seizures, coma,* dizziness, somnolence, tremor, abnormal thinking, agitation, amnesia, anxiety, neuropathy, paresthesia, asthenia.
**EENT:** retinal detachment in CMV retinitis patients.
**GI:** *nausea, vomiting, diarrhea, anorexia, abdominal pain,* flatulence, dyspepsia, dry mouth.
**GU:** *increased serum creatinine levels.*
**Hematologic:** *agranulocytosis, thrombocytopenia, leukopenia, anemia.*
**Hepatic:** abnormal liver function test results.
**Respiratory:** pneumonia.
**Skin:** *rash, sweating,* pruritus.
**Other:** *fever,* infection, chills, sepsis, and inflammation, pain, and phlebitis at injection site.

## INTERACTIONS

**Drug-drug.** *Cytotoxic drugs:* increased toxic effects, especially hematologic effects and stomatitis. Monitor closely.
*Didanosine:* increased plasma levels of didanosine when used concomitantly. Monitor closely.
*Imipenem/cilastatin:* heightened seizure activity with concomitant use. Monitor closely.
*Immunosuppressants (such as azathioprine, corticosteroids, cyclosporine):* enhanced immune and bone marrow suppression. Use together cautiously.
*Probenecid:* increased ganciclovir blood levels. Monitor closely.
*Zidovudine:* increased incidence of agranulocytosis with concurrent use. Monitor closely.

## EFFECTS ON DIAGNOSTIC TESTS
None reported.

## CONTRAINDICATIONS
Contraindicated in patients with hypersensitivity to drug or acyclovir and in those with an absolute neutrophil count below 500 mm$^3$ or a platelet count below 25,000 mm$^3$.

## NURSING CONSIDERATIONS
• Use cautiously and in reduced dosage in patients with renal dysfunction. Monitor renal function tests.
• Use caution when preparing ganciclovir solution, which is alkaline.
• *Alert:* Don't administer S.C. or I.M.
• Because of the frequency of agranulocytosis and thrombocytopenia, obtain neutrophil and platelet counts every 2 days during twice-daily ganciclovir dosing and at least weekly thereafter.

### I.V. administration
• Administer infusion over at least 1 hour. Too-rapid infusions will result in increased toxicity. Use an infusion pump. Don't administer as an I.V. bolus.

### Patient teaching
• Explain importance of adequate hydration during therapy.
• Instruct patient to report adverse reactions promptly.

---

Reactions may be *common,* uncommon, *life-threatening,* or COMMON AND LIFE-THREATENING.

• Tell patient to notify nurse if discomfort occurs at I.V. insertion site.
• Advise patient that drug causes birth defects. Instruct women to use effective birth control methods during treatment; men should use barrier contraception during, and for at least 90 days following, treatment with ganciclovir.

## indinavir sulfate
Crixivan

*Pregnancy Risk Category C*

### HOW SUPPLIED
*Capsules:* 200 mg, 400 mg

### ACTION
Inhibits HIV protease, enzyme required for the proteolytic cleavage of viral polyprotein precursors into individual functional proteins found in infectious HIV. Indinavir binds to the protease active site and inhibits activity of the enzyme, preventing cleavage of the viral polyproteins and resulting in formation of immature noninfectious viral particles.

| Route | Onset | Peak | Duration |
|-------|-------|------|----------|
| P.O. | Unknown | < 1 hr | Unknown |

### INDICATIONS & DOSAGE
*HIV infection when antiretroviral therapy is warranted—*
**Adults:** 800 mg P.O. q 8 hours.
*Adjust-a-dose:* For patients with mild to moderate hepatic insufficiency due to cirrhosis, reduce dosage to 600 mg P.O. q 8 hours.

### ADVERSE REACTIONS
**CNS:** headache, insomnia, dizziness, somnolence, asthenia, malaise, fatigue.
**CV:** chest pain, palpitations.
**EENT:** blurred vision, eye pain or swelling.
**GI:** abdominal pain, *nausea,* diarrhea, vomiting, acid regurgitation, anorexia, dry mouth, taste perversion.
**GU:** nephrolithiasis, hematuria.
**Hematologic:** decreased hemoglobin, platelet, or neutrophil count.

**Hepatic:** elevation in ALT, AST, and serum amylase levels.
**Metabolic:** *hyperbilirubinemia,* hyperglycemia.
**Musculoskeletal:** back pain.
**Other:** flank pain.

### INTERACTIONS
**Drug-drug.** *Cisapride, midazolam, triazolam:* possible inhibition of the metabolism of these drugs because of competition for CYP3A4 by indinavir, creating potential for serious or life-threatening events, such as arrhythmias or prolonged sedation. Don't administer concurrently.
*Clarithromycin:* increased serum levels of both drugs. Monitor closely.
*Didanosine:* possible degradation of didanosine, formulated with buffering agents to increase pH. If administered with indinavir, administer at least 1 hour apart on an empty stomach. Normal gastric pH (acidic) may be necessary for optimum absorption of indinavir but rapidly degrades didanosine.
*Ketoconazole:* increased plasma level of indinavir. Consider dosage reduction of indinavir to 600 mg P.O. q 8 hours when coadministered.
*Rifabutin:* increased plasma levels. Reduce dosage of rifabutin by 50% if administered with indinavir.
*Rifampin:* markedly diminished plasma levels of indinavir. Avoid concomitant administration of indinavir and rifampin.
*Ritonavir:* increased indinavir levels. Monitor closely.
**Drug-food.** *Any food:* substantially decreased absorption of oral indinavir. Don't give together.

### EFFECTS ON DIAGNOSTIC TESTS
None reported.

### CONTRAINDICATIONS
Contraindicated in patients with hypersensitivity to any component of drug.

### NURSING CONSIDERATIONS
• Use cautiously in patients with hepatic insufficiency due to cirrhosis.
• Drug must be taken at 8-hour intervals.
• Drug may cause nephrolithiasis. If signs and symptoms of nephrolithiasis occur,

---

*Liquid contains alcohol.   **May contain tartrazine.   †Canada   ‡Australia   §U.K.   ◇OTC

doctor may stop drug for 1 to 3 days during acute phases.
• To prevent nephrolithiasis, patient should maintain adequate hydration (at least 48 oz or 1.5 L of fluids q 24 hours while on indinavir).
• Safety and effectiveness in children have not been established.

### ☑ Patient teaching
• Tell patient that drug is not a cure for HIV infection and that he may continue to develop opportunistic infections and other complications associated with HIV infection. Drug has not been shown to reduce the risk of HIV transmission.
• Instruct patient on use of barrier protection during sexual activity.
• Caution patient not to adjust dosage or discontinue indinavir therapy without first consulting his doctor.
• Advise patient that if a dose of indinavir is missed, he should take the next dose at the regularly scheduled time and shouldn't double the dose.
• Instruct patient to take drug on an empty stomach with water 1 hour before or 2 hours after a meal. Or, he may take it with other liquids (such as skim milk, juice, coffee, or tea) or a light meal. Inform patient that a meal high in fat, calories, and protein reduces absorption of drug.
• Instruct patient to store and use capsules in the original container and to keep desiccant in the bottle; capsules are sensitive to moisture.
• Tell patient to drink at least 48 oz (1.5 L) of fluid daily.
• Advise woman to avoid breast-feeding because indinavir may appear in breast milk. Also, in order to prevent transmitting the virus to the infant, an HIV-positive woman shouldn't breast-feed

---

### lamivudine
Epivir, Epivir-HBV

*Pregnancy Risk Category C*

### HOW SUPPLIED
*Tablets:* 100 mg, 150 mg
*Oral solution:* 5 mg/ml, 10 mg/ml

### ACTION
A synthetic nucleoside analogue that inhibits HIV reverse transcription via viral DNA chain termination. RNA- and DNA-dependent DNA polymerase activities are also inhibited.

| Route | Onset | Peak | Duration |
|-------|-------|------|----------|
| P.O. | Unknown | 1-3 hr | Unknown |

### INDICATIONS & DOSAGE
*HIV infection concomitantly with zidovudine—*
**Adults weighing 50 kg (110 lb) or more and children ages 12 and older:** 150 mg P.O. b.i.d.
**Adults under 50 kg:** 2 mg/kg P.O. b.i.d.
**Children ages 3 months to 12 years:** 4 mg/kg P.O. b.i.d. Maximum dose is 150 mg b.i.d.
*Adjust-a-dose:* For patients with renal impairment, if creatinine clearance is 30 to 49 ml/minute, 150 mg P.O. daily. If clearance is 15 to 29 ml/minute, 150 mg P.O. on day 1, then 100 mg daily; if 5 to 14 ml/minute, 150 mg on day 1, then 50 mg daily; if less than 5 ml/minute, 50 mg on day 1, then 25 mg daily.
✳ *NEW INDICATION: Chronic hepatitis B associated with evidence of hepatitis B viral replication and active liver inflammation—*
**Adults:** 100 mg P.O. once daily (Epivir-HBV).
*Adjust-a-dose:* For patients with renal impairment, if creatinine clearance is 30 to 49 ml/minute, 100 mg first dose; then 50 mg P.O. once daily. If clearance is 15 to 29 ml/minute, 100 mg first dose; then 25 mg P.O. once daily. If creatinine clearance is 5 to 14 ml/minute, 35 mg first dose; then 15 mg P.O. once daily. If less than 5 ml/minute, 35 mg first dose; then 10 mg P.O. once daily.

### ADVERSE REACTIONS
Adverse reactions pertain to the combination therapy of lamivudine and zidovudine.
**CNS:** *headache, fatigue, neuropathy, malaise, dizziness, insomnia and other sleep disorders,* depressive disorders.
**GI:** *nausea, diarrhea, vomiting, anorexia,* abdominal pain, abdominal cramps, dyspepsia, pancreatitis.

---

Reactions may be *common*, uncommon, *life-threatening*, or COMMON AND LIFE-THREATENING.

**EENT:** *nasal symptoms.*
**Hematologic:** *neutropenia,* anemia, *thrombocytopenia.*
**Hepatic:** elevated liver enzymes and bilirubin.
**Musculoskeletal:** *musculoskeletal pain,* myalgia, arthralgia.
**Respiratory:** *cough.*
**Skin:** rash.
**Other:** *fever, chills.*

**INTERACTIONS**
**Drug-drug.** *Trimethoprim/sulfamethoxazole:* may cause increased blood level of lamivudine because of decreased clearance of lamivudine. Monitor patient closely.
*Zidovudine:* increased serum zidovudine level. Monitor patient closely.

**EFFECTS ON DIAGNOSTIC TESTS**
None reported.

**CONTRAINDICATIONS**
Contraindicated in patients with hypersensitivity to drug.

**NURSING CONSIDERATIONS**
• *Alert:* Use drug with extreme caution, if at all, in children with history of pancreatitis or other significant risk factors for development of pancreatitis. Stop lamivudine treatment immediately and notify doctor if clinical signs, symptoms, or laboratory abnormalities suggest pancreatitis. Monitor serum amylase level.
• Use cautiously in patients with renal impairment.
• Breast-feeding should be discontinued if lamivudine is prescribed.
• Administer drug with zidovudine. It's not currently indicated for use alone unless for chronic hepatitis B virus infection.
• Safety and effectiveness of treatment with Epivir-HBV beyond 1 year have not been established; optimum duration of treatment isn't known. Patients should be tested for HIV before initiating treatment and during therapy because formulation and dosage of lamivudine in Epivir-HBV aren't appropriate for those dually infected with hepatitis B virus and HIV. If lamivudine is administered to patients

with hepatitis B virus and HIV, the higher dosage indicated for HIV therapy should be used as part of an appropriate combination regimen.
• Monitor patient's CBC, platelet count, renal and liver function studies, as ordered. Report abnormalities.
• An Antiretroviral Pregnancy Registry has been established to monitor maternal-fetal outcomes of pregnant women exposed to lamivudine. To register a pregnant patient, the doctor can call 1-800-258-4263.

☑ **Patient teaching**
• Inform patient that long-term effects of lamivudine are unknown.
• Stress importance of taking lamivudine exactly as prescribed.
• Teach parents the signs and symptoms of pancreatitis. Advise them to report signs and symptoms immediately.

---

**lamivudine/zidovudine**
Combivir

*Pregnancy Risk Category C*

**HOW SUPPLIED**
*Tablets:* 150 mg lamivudine and 300 mg zidovudine

**ACTION**
Inhibit reverse transcriptase via DNA chain termination. Both drugs are also weak inhibitors of DNA polymerase. Together, they have synergistic antiretroviral activity. Combination therapy with lamivudine and zidovudine is targeted at suppressing or delaying the emergence of resistant strains that can occur with retroviral monotherapy because dual resistance requires multiple mutations.

| Route | Onset | Peak | Duration |
|-------|-------|------|----------|
| P.O. | Unknown | Unknown | Unknown |

**INDICATIONS & DOSAGE**
*HIV infection—*
**Adults and children ages 12 and older weighing over 50 kg (110 lb):** one tablet P.O. b.i.d.

**ADVERSE REACTIONS**
**CNS:** *headache, malaise, fatigue, insomnia, dizziness, neuropathy,* depression.
**EENT:** *nasal signs and symptoms.*
**GI:** *nausea, diarrhea, vomiting, anorexia,* abdominal pain, abdominal cramps, dyspepsia.
**Hematologic:** *neutropenia,* anemia.
**Hepatic:** increased ALT, AST, amylase.
**Musculoskeletal:** *musculoskeletal pain,* myalgia, arthralgia.
**Respiratory:** *cough.*
**Skin:** rash.
**Other:** *fever, chills.*

**INTERACTIONS**
**Drug-drug.** *Ganciclovir, interferon-alpha, other bone marrow suppressive or cytotoxic agents:* may increase zidovudine's hematologic toxicity. Monitor patient.

**EFFECTS ON DIAGNOSTIC TESTS**
None reported.

**CONTRAINDICATIONS**
Contraindicated in patients with known hypersensitivity to drug's components and in those requiring dosage adjustments, such as children under age 12, those weighing under 50 kg, and those with creatinine clearance below 50 ml/minute. Also contraindicated in patients experiencing dose-limiting adverse effects.

**NURSING CONSIDERATIONS**
• Use combination cautiously in patients with bone marrow suppression as evidenced by granulocyte count below 1,000 cells/mm$^3$ or hemoglobin level below 9.5 g/dl.
• Lactic acidosis and severe hepatomegaly with steatosis have been reported in patients receiving lamivudine and zidovudine alone and in combination. Notify doctor if signs of lactic acidosis or hepatotoxicity develop (abdominal pain, jaundice).
• Monitor for bone marrow toxicity with frequent blood counts, particularly in patients with advanced HIV infection. Monitor patients for signs and symptoms of lactic acidosis and hepatotoxicity.

• Assess patient's fine motor skills and peripheral sensation for evidence of peripheral neuropathies.
• An Antiretroviral Pregnancy Registry has been established to monitor maternal-fetal outcomes of pregnant women exposed to Combivir. To register a pregnant patient, doctor can call 1-800-258-4263.

☑ **Patient teaching**
• Advise patient that the lamivudine/zidovudine combination drug therapy is not a cure for HIV infection, and that he may continue to experience illness including opportunistic infections.
• Warn patient that HIV transmission can still occur with drug therapy.
• Educate patient about using protection when engaging in sexual activities to prevent disease transmission.
• Teach patient signs and symptoms of neutropenia and anemia (fever, chills, infection, fatigue) and instruct him to report such occurrences.
• Tell patient to have blood counts followed closely while on drug, especially if he has advanced disease.
• Advise patient to consult doctor or pharmacist before taking other drugs.
• Warn patient to report abdominal pain immediately.
• Instruct patient to report signs and symptoms of myopathy or myositis (muscle inflammation, pain, weakness, decrease in muscle size).
• Stress importance of taking combination drug therapy exactly as prescribed to reduce the development of resistance.
• Tell patient he may take combination with or without food.
• Inform woman that breast-feeding is contraindicated in HIV infection and during drug therapy.

---

**nelfinavir mesylate**
Viracept

*Pregnancy Risk Category B*

**HOW SUPPLIED**
*Tablets:* 250 mg
*Powder:* 50 mg/g powder in 144-g bottle

## ACTION
An HIV-1 protease inhibitor, thereby preventing cleavage of the viral polyprotein, resulting in the production of immature, noninfectious virus.

| Route | Onset | Peak | Duration |
|-------|-------|------|----------|
| P.O. | Unknown | 2-4 hr | Unknown |

## INDICATIONS & DOSAGE
*HIV infection when antiretroviral therapy is warranted—*
**Adults:** 1,250 mg b.i.d. or 750 mg P.O. t.i.d. with meals or light snack.
**Children ages 2 to 13:** 20 to 30 mg/kg/dose P.O. t.i.d. with meals or light snack; don't exceed 750 mg t.i.d.

Recommended children's dose given t.i.d. is shown below.

| Body weight (kg) | Level 1-g scoops | Level teaspoons | Tablets |
|------------------|------------------|-----------------|---------|
| 7 to < 8.5 | 4 | 1 | - |
| 8.5 to < 10.5 | 5 | 1.25 | - |
| 10.5 to < 12 | 6 | 1.5 | - |
| 12 to < 14 | 7 | 1.75 | - |
| 14 to < 16 | 8 | 2 | - |
| 16 to < 18 | 9 | 2.25 | - |
| 18 to < 23 | 10 | 2.5 | 2 |
| 23 | 15 | 3.75 | 3 |

## ADVERSE REACTIONS
**CNS:** anxiety, depression, dizziness, emotional lability, hyperkinesia, insomnia, migraine, headache, paresthesia, *seizures,* sleep disorders, malaise, somnolence, *suicidal ideation.*
**EENT:** iritis, eye disorder, pharyngitis, rhinitis, sinusitis.
**GI:** nausea, *diarrhea,* flatulence, anorexia, dyspepsia, epigastric pain, GI bleeding, pancreatitis, mouth ulceration, vomiting.
**GU:** sexual dysfunction, renal calculus, urine abnormality.
**Hematologic:** anemia, *leukopenia, thrombocytopenia.*
**Hepatic:** *hepatitis,* elevated liver function test results, jaundice, bilirubinemia.
**Metabolic:** dehydration, hyperglycemia, hyperlipidemia, hyperuricemia, hypoglycemia, increased amylase and creatinine phosphokinase levels, metabolic acidosis.
**Musculoskeletal:** back pain, arthralgia, arthritis, cramps, myalgia, myasthenia, myopathy.
**Respiratory:** dyspnea.
**Skin:** rash, dermatitis, folliculitis, fungal dermatitis, pruritus, sweating, urticaria.
**Other:** allergic reactions, fever, hypersensitivity reactions, including *bronchospasm,* moderate to severe rash, edema.

## INTERACTIONS
**Drug-drug.** *Amiodarone, cisapride, ergot derivatives, midazolam, quinidine, triazolam:* nelfinavir may produce large increases in plasma levels of these drugs, which may increase risk for serious or life-threatening adverse effects. Don't administer concurrently.
*Carbamazepine, phenobarbital, phenytoin:* may reduce the effectiveness of nelfinavir by decreasing nelfinavir plasma levels. Monitor closely.
*HIV protease inhibitors (indinavir, ritonavir):* may increase nelfinavir plasma levels. Use together cautiously.
*Oral contraceptives (ethinyl estradiol, norethindrone):* nelfinavir may decrease plasma levels. Suggest alternative or additional contraceptive measures during nelfinavir therapy.
*Rifabutin:* nelfinavir dramatically increases rifabutin plasma levels. Therefore, reduce dose of rifabutin to one-half the usual dose.
*Rifampin:* decreased nelfinavir plasma levels. Don't use together.

## EFFECTS ON DIAGNOSTIC TESTS
None reported.

## CONTRAINDICATIONS
Contraindicated in patients with hypersensitivity to drug or its components.

## NURSING CONSIDERATIONS
• Use cautiously in patients with hepatic dysfunction or hemophilia types A and B. Monitor liver function test results.
• Drug dosage is the same whether used alone or with other antiretroviral drugs.
• Twice-daily dosing hasn't been established in pediatric patients.

*Liquid contains alcohol.   **May contain tartrazine.   †Canada   ‡Australia   §U.K.   ◊OTC

• Administer oral powder in children unable to take tablets. May mix oral powder with small amount of water, milk, formula, soy formula, soy milk, or dietary supplements. Tell patient to consume entire contents.

• Don't reconstitute with water in its original container.

• Use reconstituted powder within 6 hours.

• Mixing with acidic foods or juice is not recommended because of bitter taste.

• It's not known if drug appears in breast milk. Because safety has not been established, HIV-infected women should be advised not to breast-feed to avoid transmitting the virus to the infant.

• *Alert:* Don't confuse nelfinavir with nevirapine.

**☑ Patient teaching**

• Advise patient to take drug with food.

• Inform patient that drug is not a cure for HIV infection.

• Tell patient that long-term effects of drug are currently unknown and that there are no supporting data that nelfinavir reduces risk of transmission of HIV.

• Advise patient to take drug daily as prescribed and not to alter dose or discontinue drug without medical approval.

• If patient misses a dose, tell him to take the dose as soon as possible and then return to his normal schedule. If a dose is skipped, advise patient not to double-dose.

• Tell patient that diarrhea is the most common adverse effect and that it can be controlled with loperamide if necessary.

• Instruct patient taking oral contraceptives to use alternative or additional contraceptive measures while on nelfinavir therapy.

• Warn patient with phenylketonuria that powder contains 11.2 mg phenylalanine per gram.

• Advise patient to report use of other prescribed or OTC drugs because of possible drug interactions.

## nevirapine
Viramune

*Pregnancy Risk Category C*

### HOW SUPPLIED
*Tablets:* 200 mg
*Oral suspension:* 50 mg/5 ml

### ACTION
Binds directly to reverse transcriptase and blocks RNA-dependent and DNA-dependent DNA polymerase activities by causing a disruption of the enzyme's catalytic site.

| Route | Onset | Peak | Duration |
|-------|-------|------|----------|
| P.O. | Unknown | 4 hr | Unknown |

### INDICATIONS & DOSAGE
*Adjunct treatment in patients with HIV-1 infection who have experienced clinical or immunologic deterioration—*
**Adults:** 200 mg P.O. daily for the first 14 days, followed by 200 mg P.O. b.i.d. Used with nucleoside analogue antiretroviral agents.
❋ *NEW INDICATION: Adjunct treatment in children infected with HIV-1—*
**Children ages 2 months to 8 years:** 4 mg/kg P.O. once daily for first 14 days, followed by 7 mg/kg P.O. b.i.d. thereafter. Maximum daily dose is 400 mg.
**Children ages 8 and older:** 4 mg/kg P.O. once daily for first 14 days; then 4 mg/kg P.O. b.i.d. thereafter. Maximum daily dose is 400 mg.

### ADVERSE REACTIONS
**CNS:** headache, paresthesia.
**GI:** *nausea,* diarrhea, abdominal pain, ulcerative stomatitis.
**Hematologic:** *neutropenia,* decreased hemoglobin.
**Hepatic:** hepatitis, increased ALT, AST, gamma-glutamyl transpeptidase, and total bilirubin levels.
**Musculoskeletal:** myalgia.
**Skin:** *rash, blistering, **Stevens-Johnson syndrome.***
**Other:** *fever.*

---

Reactions may be *common,* uncommon, *life-threatening*, or COMMON AND LIFE-THREATENING.

## INTERACTIONS

**Drug-drug.** *Drugs extensively metabolized by P-450 CYP3A:* may lower plasma levels of these drugs, requiring dosage adjustment. Monitor closely.

*Protease inhibitors, oral contraceptives, other hormonal contraceptives:* may decrease plasma levels of these drugs. Don't administer concomitantly.

*Rifabutin, rifampin:* more data needed to assess whether dosage adjustments are necessary. When administering with nevirapine, monitor closely.

## EFFECTS ON DIAGNOSTIC TESTS

None reported.

## CONTRAINDICATIONS

Contraindicated in patients with hypersensitivity to drug.

## NURSING CONSIDERATIONS

• Use cautiously in patients with impaired renal and hepatic function; pharmacokinetics have not been evaluated in those patients.

• Clinical chemistry tests, including renal and liver function tests, should be performed before initiating drug therapy and regularly throughout therapy.

• Drug should be used with at least one additional antiretroviral drug.

• **Alert:** Monitor patient for blistering, oral lesions, conjunctivitis, muscle or joint aches, or general malaise. Be especially alert for a severe rash or rash accompanied by fever. Report such signs and symptoms to doctor. Patients who experience a rash during the initial 14 days of therapy shouldn't have the dosage increased until the rash has resolved. Most rashes occur within the first 6 weeks of therapy.

• Moderate and severe liver function test abnormalities may warrant temporary discontinuance of therapy; drug may be restarted at half the previous dose level as ordered.

• Patients who have nevirapine therapy interrupted for more than 7 days should restart therapy as if receiving drug for the first time.

• Antiretroviral therapy may be changed if disease progresses while patient is receiving nevirapine.

• Safety and effectiveness in children have not been established.

• Nevirapine appears in breast milk.

• **Alert:** Don't confuse nevirapine with nelfinavir.

### ☑ Patient teaching

• Inform patient that nevirapine is not a cure for HIV and that illnesses associated with advanced HIV-1 infection may still occur. Explain that drug does not reduce risk of HIV-1 transmission.

• Instruct patient to report rash immediately and to discontinue drug until told to resume.

• Stress importance of taking drug exactly as prescribed. If a dose is missed, tell patient to take the next dose as soon as possible. If a dose is skipped, patient shouldn't double next dose.

• Tell patient not to use other drugs unless approved by a doctor.

• Advise woman of childbearing age that oral contraceptives and other hormonal methods of birth control shouldn't be used with nevirapine.

• Advise woman to avoid breast-feeding during drug therapy to reduce risk of postnatal HIV transmission.

✳ *NEW DRUG*

## oseltamivir phosphate
Tamiflu

*Pregnancy Risk Category C*

## HOW SUPPLIED

*Capsules:* 75 mg

## ACTION

Inhibits influenza virus enzyme neuraminidase, which is thought to play a role in viral particle aggregation and release from the host cell. Neuraminidase inhibition, therefore, appears to interfere with viral replication.

| Route | Onset | Peak | Duration |
|-------|-------|------|----------|
| P.O. | Unknown | Unknown | Unknown |

## INDICATIONS & DOSAGE
*Uncomplicated, acute illness due to influenza infection in patients who have been symptomatic for 2 days or less—*
**Adults:** 75 mg P.O. b.i.d. for 5 days.
*Adjust-A-Dose:* For patients with creatinine clearance less than 30 ml/minute, reduce dose to 75 mg P.O. once daily for 5 days.

## ADVERSE REACTIONS
**CNS:** dizziness, insomnia, headache, vertigo, fatigue.
**GI:** abdominal pain, diarrhea, nausea, vomiting.
**Respiratory:** bronchitis, cough.

## INTERACTIONS
None significant.

## EFFECTS ON DIAGNOSTIC TESTS
None reported.

## CONTRAINDICATIONS
Contraindicated in patients with hypersensitivity to drug or its components.

## NURSING CONSIDERATIONS
• Use cautiously in patients with chronic cardiac or respiratory diseases, or any medical condition that may require imminent hospitalization. Also use cautiously in patients with renal failure, especially those with creatinine clearance less than 10 ml/minute.
• There is no evidence supporting drug use in treatment of viral infections other than influenza virus types A and B.
• Drug must be given within 2 days of onset of symptoms.
• Drug is used to treat flu symptoms, not to prevent influenza.
• Drug isn't a replacement for the annual influenza vaccination. Patients for whom vaccine is indicated should continue to receive the vaccine each fall.
• Safety and efficacy of repeated treatment courses have not been established.
• Drug may be given with meals to decrease GI adverse effects.
• It's unknown if drug or its active metabolite appear in breast milk. Use only if potential benefits outweigh potential risks to infant.

• Store at controlled room temperature (59° to 86° F [15° to 30° C]).

## PATIENT TEACHING
• Instruct patient to begin treatment as soon as possible after appearance of flu symptoms.
• Inform patient that drug may be taken with or without meals. If nausea or vomiting occurs, he can take drug with food or milk.
• Tell patient that, if a dose is missed, it should be taken as soon as possible. He should skip missed dose, however, if next dose is due within 2 hours, and take the next dose on schedule.
• Advise patient to complete the full 5 days of treatment, even if symptoms are resolved.
• Alert patient that drug is not a replacement for the annual influenza vaccination. Patients for whom vaccine is indicated should continue to receive the vaccine each fall.

# ribavirin
Virazole

*Pregnancy Risk Category X*

## HOW SUPPLIED
*Powder to be reconstituted for inhalation:* 6 g in 100-ml glass vial

## ACTION
Inhibits viral activity by an unknown mechanism, possibly by inhibiting RNA and DNA synthesis by depleting intracellular nucleotide pools.

| Route | Onset | Peak | Duration |
|-------|-------|------|----------|
| Inhalation | Unknown | Unknown | Unknown |

## INDICATIONS & DOSAGE
*Hospitalized infants and young children infected by respiratory syncytial virus (RSV)—*
**Infants and young children:** solution in concentration of 20 mg/ml delivered via the Viratek Small Particle Aerosol Generator (SPAG-2) and mechanical ventilator or oxygen hood, face mask, or oxygen tent at a rate of about 12.5 L of mist per

minute. Treatment is carried out for 12 to 18 hours/day for at least 3 days, and no more than 7 days.

## ADVERSE REACTIONS
**CV:** *cardiac arrest,* hypotension, *brady-cardia.*
**EENT:** conjunctivitis.
**Hematologic:** anemia, reticulocytosis.
**Hepatic:** elevated bilirubin, AS, and ALT levels.
**Respiratory:** worsening respiratory state, *apnea,* bacterial pneumonia, pneumothorax.
**Other:** rash or erythema of eyelids.

## INTERACTIONS
None significant.

## EFFECTS ON DIAGNOSTIC TESTS
None reported.

## CONTRAINDICATIONS
Contraindicated in patients with hypersensitivity to drug. Although drug is used in children, manufacturer states that it's contraindicated in women who are or may become pregnant during treatment.

## NURSING CONSIDERATIONS
• Administer ribavirin aerosol by the Viratek Small Particle Aerosol Generator (SPAG-2) only. Don't use any other aerosol-generating device.
• Use sterile USP water for injection, not bacteriostatic water. Water used to reconstitute this drug mustn't contain any antimicrobial agent.
• Discard solutions placed in the SPAG-2 unit at least every 24 hours before adding newly reconstituted solution.
• The most frequent adverse effects reported in health care personnel exposed to aerosolized ribavirin include eye irritation and headache. Pregnant personnel should be advised of these effects.
• *Alert:* Monitor ventilator function frequently. Ribavirin may precipitate in ventilator apparatus, causing equipment malfunction with serious consequences.
• Store reconstituted solutions at room temperature for 24 hours.
• Ribavirin aerosol is indicated only for severe lower respiratory tract infection caused by RSV. Although treatment may begin while awaiting diagnostic test results, existence of RSV infection must eventually be documented.
• Most infants and children with RSV infection don't require treatment because the disease is commonly mild and self-limiting. Infants with underlying conditions, such as prematurity or cardiopulmonary disease, experience RSV in its severest form and benefit most from treatment with ribavirin aerosol.

### ✅ Patient teaching
• Inform parents of need for drug and answer any questions.
• Encourage parents to report any subtle change in child immediately to nurse.

---

## rimantadine hydrochloride
Flumadine

*Pregnancy Risk Category C*

## HOW SUPPLIED
*Tablets (film-coated):* 100 mg
*Syrup:* 50 mg/5 ml

## ACTION
Unknown. Appears to prevent viral uncoating, an early step in virus reproductive cycle.

| Route | Onset | Peak | Duration |
|-------|-------|------|----------|
| P.O. | Unknown | 6 hr | Unknown |

## INDICATIONS & DOSAGE
*Prophylaxis of influenza A—*
**Adults and children over age 10:**
100 mg P.O. b.i.d.
**Children ages 1 to 9 years:** 5 mg/kg (not to exceed 150 mg) P.O. once daily.
**Elderly:** 100 mg P.O. daily.
*Adjust-a-dose:* For patients with severe hepatic or renal dysfunction or those experiencing adverse effects with normal dosage, 100 mg P.O. daily.
Prophylaxis should begin as soon as possible after initial exposure and should be continued through course of influenza A outbreak. Safety of prolonged therapy over 6 weeks has not been established. Can be used for prophylaxis in children

up to 6 weeks after first dose of influenza vaccine or until 2 weeks after second dose of vaccine.
*Influenza A—*
**Adults:** 100 mg P.O. b.i.d. initiated within 24 to 48 hours after onset of symptoms and continued for 48 hours after symptoms disappear (usually 7-day total course).

### ADVERSE REACTIONS
**CNS:** insomnia, headache, dizziness, nervousness, fatigue, asthenia.
**GI:** nausea, vomiting, anorexia, dry mouth, abdominal pain.

### INTERACTIONS
**Drug-drug.** *Acetaminophen, aspirin:* reduced level of rimantadine. Monitor for decreased effectiveness of rimantadine.
*Cimetidine:* may decrease clearance of rimantadine. Monitor for adverse reactions.

### EFFECTS ON DIAGNOSTIC TESTS
None reported.

### CONTRAINDICATIONS
Contraindicated in patients with hypersensitivity to drug or amantadine.

### NURSING CONSIDERATIONS
• Use cautiously in patients with renal or hepatic impairment and in patients with a history of seizures. Pregnant patients should consider the risks compared with the benefits before taking drug.
• Consider the risk to contacts of treated patients who may be subject to morbidity from influenza A. Influenza A–resistant strains can emerge during therapy. Patients taking drug may still be able to spread the disease.
• *Alert:* Don't confuse rimantadine with amantadine.

### ☑ Patient teaching
• Instruct patient to take drug several hours before bedtime to prevent insomnia.
• Inform patient that he may still be able to infect others with influenza A and to take infection-control precautions.

## ritonavir
Norvir

*Pregnancy Risk Category B*

### HOW SUPPLIED
*Capsules:* 100 mg
*Oral solution:* 80 mg/ml

### ACTION
An HIV protease inhibitor with activity against HIV-1 and HIV-2 proteases. HIV protease is an enzyme required for the proteolytic cleavage of viral polyprotein precursors into the individual functional proteins in infectious HIV. Ritonavir binds to the protease active site and inhibits activity of the enzyme, preventing cleavage of the viral polyproteins and resulting in the formation of immature, noninfectious viral particles.

| Route | Onset | Peak | Duration |
|-------|-------|------|----------|
| P.O. | Unknown | 2-4 hr | Unknown |

### INDICATIONS & DOSAGE
*HIV infection with nucleoside analogues or as monotherapy when antiretroviral therapy is warranted—*
**Adults:** 600 mg P.O. b.i.d with meals. If nausea occurs, gradually increasing dose may provide some relief: 300 mg b.i.d. for 1 day, 400 mg b.i.d. for 2 days, 500 mg b.i.d. for 1 day, and then 600 mg b.i.d. thereafter.

### ADVERSE REACTIONS
**CNS:** *asthenia,* headache, malaise, circumoral paresthesia, dizziness, insomnia, paresthesia, peripheral paresthesia, somnolence, thinking abnormality, migraine headache.
**CV:** vasodilation.
**EENT:** local throat irritation, blepharitis, diplopia, pharyngitis, photophobia, *taste perversion.*
**GI:** abdominal pain, anorexia, constipation, *diarrhea, nausea, vomiting,* dyspepsia, flatulence, cramping, jaundice.
**GU:** dysuria, hematuria, nocturia, polyuria, pyelonephritis, urethritis, hyperuricemia.

---

Reactions may be *common,* uncommon, *life-threatening,* or COMMON AND LIFE-THREATENING.

**Hematologic:** decreased hemoglobin and hematocrit levels, *leukopenia, thrombocytopenia,* decreased neutrophil and eosinophil levels.

**Hepatic:** elevated triglycerides, AST, ALT, GGT, alkaline phosphatase, total bilirubin, altered PT and INR.

**Metabolic:** hyperlipidemia, hyperglycemia, hyperkalemia.

**Musculoskeletal:** increased CK level, myalgia.

**Skin:** rash, sweating, urticaria.

**Other:** fever.

## INTERACTIONS

**Drug-drug.** *Agents that increase CYP3A activity (such as carbamazepine, dexamethasone, phenobarbital, phenytoin, rifabutin, rifampin):* may increase clearance of ritonavir, resulting in decreased ritonavir plasma levels. Monitor patient closely.

*Alprazolam, clorazepate, diazepam, dihydroergotamine, ergotamine, estazolam, flurazepam, midazolam, triazolam, zolpidem:* significantly increased levels of these drugs. Because of risk of extreme sedation and respiratory depression, don't give these drugs with ritonavir.

*Amiodarone, bupropion, cisapride, clozapine, encainide, flecainide, meperidine, piroxicam, propafenone, propoxyphene, quinidine, rifabutin:* significantly increased plasma levels of these drugs, which increases patient's risk of arrhythmias, hematologic abnormalities, seizures, or other potentially serious adverse effects. Avoid concomitant use.

*Clarithromycin:* reduced creatinine clearance. Patients with impaired renal function receiving drug with ritonavir require a 50% reduction in clarithromycin dose if creatinine clearance is 30 to 60 ml/minute and a 75% reduction if it is below 30 ml/minute.

*Desipramine:* increased overall serum levels of desipramine. Concomitant administration may require a dosage adjustment when administered with ritonavir. Monitor patient.

*Directly glucuronidated drugs:* ritonavir may increase activity of glucoronosyl transferases with loss of therapeutic effects from these drugs; may signify need for dosage alteration of these drugs. Concomitant use should be accompanied by therapeutic drug level monitoring and increased monitoring of therapeutic and adverse effects, especially for drugs with narrow therapeutic margins, such as oral anticoagulants and immunosuppressants. Dosage reduction greater than 50% may be required for drugs extensively metabolized by CYP3A.

*Disulfiram or other drugs that produce disulfiram-like reactions such as metronidazole:* increased risk of disulfiram-like reactions. Ritonavir formulations contain alcohol that can produce reactions when co-administered. Monitor patient.

*Oral contraceptives containing ethinyl estradiol:* decreased overall serum levels of the contraceptive. Advise patient that concomitant therapy may require a dosage increase in the oral contraceptive or use of other contraceptive measures.

*Saquinavir:* inhibited metabolism of saquinavir, resulting in greatly increased plasma levels. Safety of this combination has not been established.

*Theophylline:* decreased overall serum levels of theophylline. Increased dosage may be required when coadministered with ritonavir. Monitor level.

**Drug-food.** *Any food:* increased absorption. Give drug with food.

**Drug-lifestyle.** *Smoking:* decreased overall serum levels of ritonavir. Avoid use.

## EFFECTS ON DIAGNOSTIC TESTS
None reported.

## CONTRAINDICATIONS
Contraindicated in patients with hypersensitivity to drug or its components.

## NURSING CONSIDERATIONS
• Use cautiously in patients with hepatic insufficiency.

• Drug may be administered alone or with nucleoside analogues.

• Patients beginning combination regimens with ritonavir and nucleosides may improve GI tolerance by starting ritonavir alone and subsequently adding nucleosides before completing 2 weeks of ritonavir.

• Safety and effectiveness in children under age 12 have not been established.

• It's unknown whether ritonavir appears in breast milk.

## ✅ Patient teaching

• Inform patient that drug is not a cure for HIV infection. He may continue to develop opportunistic infections and other complications associated with HIV infection. Drug has not been shown to reduce the risk of transmitting HIV to others through sexual contact or blood contamination.

• Caution patient to take drug as prescribed and not to adjust dosage or discontinue therapy without first consulting the doctor.

• Tell patient he may improve the taste of ritonavir oral solution by mixing it with chocolate milk, Ensure, or Advera within 1 hour of the scheduled dose.

• Instruct patient to take drug with a meal to improve absorption.

• Tell patient that if a dose is missed, he should take the next dose as soon as possible. If a dose is skipped, he shouldn't double the next dose.

• Advise patient to report use of other drugs, including OTC drugs; ritonavir interacts with some drugs when taken together.

• Advise woman not to breast-feed to prevent transmission of infection.

---

## saquinavir
Fortovase

## saquinavir mesylate
Invirase

*Pregnancy Risk Category B*

## HOW SUPPLIED
**saquinavir**
*Capsules (soft gelatin):* 200 mg
**saquinavir mesylate**
*Capsules (hard gelatin):* 200 mg

## ACTION
Inhibits the activity of HIV protease and prevents the cleavage of HIV polyproteins, which are essential for HIV maturation.

| Route | Onset | Peak | Duration |
|-------|-------|------|----------|
| P.O. | Unknown | Unknown | Unknown |

## INDICATIONS & DOSAGE
*Adjunct treatment of advanced HIV infection in selected patients—*
**Adults:** 600 mg (Invirase) or 1,200 mg (Fortovase) P.O. t.i.d. taken within 2 hours after a full meal and with a nucleoside analogue such as zalcitabine at a dose of 0.75 mg P.O. t.i.d. or zidovudine at a dose of 200 mg P.O. t.i.d.

## ADVERSE REACTIONS
**CNS:** paresthesia, headache, dizziness, asthenia, numbness.
**CV:** chest pain.
**GI:** diarrhea, ulcerated buccal mucosa, abdominal pain, nausea, dyspepsia, pancreatitis.
**Hematologic:** *pancytopenia, thrombocytopenia.*
**Musculoskeletal:** musculoskeletal pain.
**Respiratory:** bronchitis, cough.
**Skin:** rash.

## INTERACTIONS
**Drug-drug.** *Cisapride:* increased serum level of this drug, increased risk of arrhythmias, and sudden death. Avoid concomitant use.
*Ketoconazole, ritonavir:* increased serum saquinavir levels. Monitor patient closely.
*Phenobarbital, phenytoin, rifabutin, rifampin:* reduced steady-state level of saquinavir. Use together cautiously.
**Drug-food.** *Any food:* increased absorption. Give drug with food.

## EFFECTS ON DIAGNOSTIC TESTS
None reported.

## CONTRAINDICATIONS
Contraindicated in patients with hypersensitivity to drug or to any component contained in the capsule.

## NURSING CONSIDERATIONS
• Safety of drug is not established in pregnant or breast-feeding women or in children under age 16.
• *Alert:* Don't confuse the two forms of this drug because dosages are different.
• CBC, platelets, electrolytes, uric acid, liver enzymes, and bilirubin should be evaluated before therapy begins and at ap-

---

Reactions may be *common,* uncommon, **life-threatening**, or COMMON AND LIFE-THREATENING.

propriate intervals throughout therapy, as ordered.
• If serious toxicity occurs during treatment, drug should be discontinued until cause is identified or the toxicity resolves. Drug may be resumed with no dosage modifications.
• Monitor patient's hydration if adverse GI reactions occur.
• Notify doctor if adverse reactions occur. Obtain order for a mild analgesic if drug causes headache, an antiemetic if drug causes nausea, or an antidiarrheal if drug causes diarrhea.
• Be alert for adverse reactions associated with adjunct therapy (zidovudine or zalcitabine).

☑ **Patient teaching**
• Advise patient to take drug within 2 hours after a full meal.
• Inform patient that drug is usually administered with other AIDS-related antivirals.
• Instruct patient to take drug around the clock, not missing any doses, to decrease the risk of developing HIV resistance.
• Inform patient that change from Invirase to Fortovase capsules should be made only under doctor's supervision.
• Tell patient to store Fortovase capsules in the refrigerator; Invirase capsules can be kept at room temperature.

---

**stavudine (2,3 didehydro-3-deoxythymidine, d4T)**
Zerit

*Pregnancy Risk Category C*

**HOW SUPPLIED**
*Capsules:* 15 mg, 20 mg, 30 mg, 40 mg
*Oral solution:* 1 mg/ml

**ACTION**
A thymidine nucleoside analogue that prevents replication of retroviruses, including HIV, by inhibiting the enzyme reverse transcriptase and causing termination of DNA chain growth.

| Route | Onset | Peak | Duration |
|-------|-------|------|----------|
| P.O. | Unknown | 1 hr | Unknown |

**INDICATIONS & DOSAGE**
*HIV-infected patients who have received prolonged prior zidovudine therapy—*
**Adults weighing 60 kg (132 lb) or more:** 40 mg P.O. q 12 hours.
**Adults under 60 kg:** 30 mg P.O. q 12 hours.
**Children:** 2 mg/kg/day P.O. in divided doses q 12 hours for children under 30 kg (66 lb); adult dose should be used for children 30 kg or more.
*Adjust-a-dose:* For patients with renal impairment, if creatinine clearance is 26 to 50 ml/minute, 20 mg (if weight exceeds 60 kg) or 15 mg (if weight is below 60 kg) P.O. q 12 hours; if creatinine clearance is 10 to 25 ml/minute, 20 mg (if weight exceeds 60 kg) or 15 mg (if weight is below 60 kg) P.O. q 24 hours.

**ADVERSE REACTIONS**
**CNS:** peripheral neuropathy, headache, malaise, insomnia, anxiety, *asthenia,* depression, nervousness, dizziness.
**CV:** chest pain.
**EENT:** conjunctivitis.
**GI:** *abdominal pain, diarrhea, nausea, vomiting, anorexia,* dyspepsia, constipation, weight loss, pancreatitis.
**Hematologic:** *neutropenia, thrombocytopenia,* anemia, increased AST and ALT levels.
**Hepatic:** *hepatotoxicity.*
**Musculoskeletal:** *arthralgia, myalgia, back pain.*
**Respiratory:** *dyspnea.*
**Skin:** *rash, diaphoresis, pruritus,* maculopapular rash.
**Other:** *chills, fever*

**INTERACTIONS**
None significant.

**EFFECTS ON DIAGNOSTIC TESTS**
None reported.

**CONTRAINDICATIONS**
Contraindicated in patients with hypersensitivity to drug.

**NURSING CONSIDERATIONS**
• Use cautiously in patients with renal impairment or history of peripheral neuropathy. Dosage adjustment is necessary for

---

*Liquid contains alcohol.    **May contain tartrazine.    †Canada    ‡Australia    §U.K.    ◇OTC

creatinine clearance below 50 ml/minute; dosage adjustment or discontinuation is necessary in onset of peripheral neuropathy. Also use cautiously in pregnant women.
• *Alert:* Peripheral neuropathy appears to be the major dose-limiting adverse effect of stavudine. It may or may not resolve after drug is discontinued.
• Monitor CBC and serum levels of creatinine, AST, ALT, and alkaline phosphatase, as ordered.
• *Alert:* Don't confuse drug with other antivirals that may use initials for identification.

☑ **Patient teaching**
• Tell patient that drug may be taken without regard to meals.
• Warn patient not to take other drugs for HIV or AIDS unless the doctor has approved them.
• Teach patient signs and symptoms of peripheral neuropathy (pain, burning, aching, weakness, or pins and needles in the extremities) and tell him to report these immediately.
• Tell patient to monitor weight patterns and report weight loss or gain.

## valacyclovir hydrochloride
Valtrex

*Pregnancy Risk Category B*

### HOW SUPPLIED
*Tablets:* 500 mg, 1 g

### ACTION
Rapidly converts to acyclovir, which in turn becomes incorporated into viral DNA, thereby terminating growth of the DNA chain; inhibits viral DNA polymerase, causing inhibition of viral replication.

| Route | Onset | Peak | Duration |
|-------|-------|------|----------|
| P.O. | 30 min | Unknown | Unknown |

### INDICATIONS & DOSAGE
*Herpes zoster infection (shingles)—*
**Adults:** 1 g P.O. t.i.d. for 7 days.
*Adjust-a-dose:* For renally impaired patients with creatinine clearance of 50 ml/

minute or more, use regular dose; if 30 to 49 ml/minute, 1 g P.O. q 12 hours; if 10 to 29 ml/minute, 1 g P.O. q 24 hours; if below 10 ml/minute, 500 mg P.O. q 24 hours.
For hemodialysis patients, 1 g P.O. after hemodialysis.
*Initial episode of genital herpes—*
**Adults:** 1 g P.O. b.i.d. for 10 days.
*Adjust-a-dose:* For renally impaired patients with creatinine clearance of 30 ml/minute or more, dosage is 1 g P.O. q 12 hours; if 10 to 29 ml/minute, 1 g P.O. q 24 hours; if below 10 ml/minute, 500 mg P.O. q 24 hours.
For hemodialysis patients, 1 g P.O. after hemodialysis.
*Recurrent genital herpes—*
**Adults:** 500 mg P.O. b.i.d. for 5 days, given at the first sign or symptom of an episode.
*Adjust-a-dose:* For renally impaired patients with creatinine clearance of 30 ml/minute or more, dosage is 500 mg P.O. q 12 hours; if 29 ml/minute or less, 500 mg P.O. q 24 hours.
For hemodialysis patients, 500 mg P.O. after hemodialysis.

### ADVERSE REACTIONS
**CNS:** *headache,* asthenia, dizziness.
**GI:** *nausea,* vomiting, diarrhea, constipation, abdominal pain, anorexia.

### INTERACTIONS
**Drug-drug.** *Cimetidine, probenecid:* reduced rate but not extent of conversion of valacyclovir to acyclovir and reduced renal clearance of acyclovir, thus increasing acyclovir blood levels. Monitor for possible toxicity.

### EFFECTS ON DIAGNOSTIC TESTS
None reported.

### CONTRAINDICATIONS
Contraindicated in patients with hypersensitivity or intolerance to valacyclovir, acyclovir, or components of the formulation.

### NURSING CONSIDERATIONS
• Valacyclovir isn't recommended for use in patients with HIV infection or in bone

marrow or renal transplant recipients due to the occurrence of thrombotic thrombocytopenic purpura and hemolytic uremic syndrome in these patient populations in clinical trials of valacyclovir at doses of 8 g/day.

• Use cautiously in elderly patients, those with renal impairment, and those receiving other nephrotoxic drugs. Monitor renal function test results.

• Safety and efficacy in children have not been established.

• Use during pregnancy should be considered only if the benefits outweigh the risks.

• Alert doctor if patient is breast-feeding; drug may need to be discontinued.

• Although there have been no reports of overdosage, precipitation of acyclovir in renal tubules may occur when solubility (2.5 mg/ml) is exceeded in the intratubular fluid. With acute renal failure and anuria, the patient may benefit from hemodialysis until renal function is restored.

**☑ Patient teaching**

• Inform patient that valacyclovir may be taken without regard to meals.

• Teach patient the signs and symptoms of herpes infection (rash, tingling, itching, and pain), and advise him to notify doctor immediately if they occur. Treatment should be initiated as soon as possible after symptoms appear, preferably within 48 hours of the onset of zoster rash.

• Tell patient that valacyclovir is not a cure for herpes but may decrease the length and severity of symptoms.

## zalcitabine
## (dideoxycytidine, ddC)
Hivid

*Pregnancy Risk Category C*

### HOW SUPPLIED
*Tablets:* 0.375 mg, 0.75 mg

### ACTION
Inhibits replication of HIV by blocking viral DNA synthesis.

| Route | Onset | Peak | Duration |
|-------|-------|------|----------|
| P.O. | Unknown | 1-2 hr | Unknown |

### INDICATIONS & DOSAGE
*Monotherapy for treatment of advanced HIV disease in patients who either can't tolerate zidovudine or who have disease progression while receiving zidovudine—*
**Adults and children ages 13 and older:** 0.75 mg P.O. q 8 hours.
*Therapy with zidovudine for treatment of advanced HIV disease (CD4+ cell count 300/mm³ or less)—*
**Adults and children ages 13 and older:** 0.75 mg P.O. q 8 hours given with zidovudine 200 mg P.O. q 8 hours.
*Adjust-a-dose:* For renally impaired patients with creatinine clearance of 10 to 40 ml/minute, dosage is 0.75 mg P.O. q 12 hours; if clearance is below 10 ml/minute, 0.75 mg P.O. q 24 hours.

If patient experiences moderate discomfort with signs and symptoms of peripheral neuropathy, discontinue drug temporarily. If symptoms improve after discontinuation, drug may be reintroduced at 0.375 mg P.O. q 8 hours.

### ADVERSE REACTIONS
**CNS:** *peripheral neuropathy, headache, fatigue,* dizziness, confusion, **seizures,** impaired concentration, amnesia, insomnia, mental depression, tremor, hypertonia, anxiety.
**CV:** cardiomyopathy, **heart failure,** chest pain.
**EENT:** pharyngitis, ocular pain, abnormal vision, ototoxicity, nasal discharge.
**GI:** nausea, vomiting, diarrhea, abdominal pain, anorexia, constipation, stomatitis, esophageal ulcer, glossitis, pancreatitis.
**Hematologic:** anemia, **neutropenia, leukopenia, thrombocytopenia.**
**Hepatic:** increased AST, ALT and alkaline phosphatase.
**Metabolic:** hypoglycemia.
**Musculoskeletal:** myalgia, arthralgia.
**Respiratory:** cough.
**Skin:** pruritus; night sweats; *erythematous, maculopapular, or follicular rash;* urticaria.
**Other:** *fever.*

### INTERACTIONS
**Drug-drug.** *Aminoglycosides, amphotericin B, foscarnet, other drugs that may*

*impair renal function:* increased risk of nephrotoxicity. Avoid concomitant use when possible.

*Antacids containing aluminum or magnesium:* decreased bioavailability of zalcitabine. Don't use together.

*Chloramphenicol, cisplatin, dapsone, didanosine, disulfiram, ethionamide, glutethimide, gold salts, hydralazine, iodoquinol, isoniazid, metronidazole, nitrofurantoin, other drugs that can cause peripheral neuropathy, phenytoin, ribavirin, stavudine, vincristine:* increased risk of peripheral neuropathy. Avoid concomitant use.

*Cimetidine, probenecid:* increased serum zalcitabine levels. Monitor patient carefully.

*Pentamidine:* increased risk of pancreatitis. Avoid concomitant use when possible.

**Drug-food.** *Any food:* decreased rate of absorption. Give drug on an empty stomach.

**EFFECTS ON DIAGNOSTIC TESTS**
None reported.

**CONTRAINDICATIONS**
Contraindicated in patients with hypersensitivity to drug or its components.

**NURSING CONSIDERATIONS**
• Use with extreme caution in patients with preexisting peripheral neuropathy.
• Use cautiously in patients with hepatic failure, history of pancreatitis or heart failure, or baseline cardiomyopathy. Monitor liver function test results and pancreatic enzymes.
• Toxic effects of drug may cause abnormalities in several laboratory tests, including CBC, hemoglobin, leukocyte, reticulocyte, granulocyte, and platelet counts; and AST, ALT, and alkaline phosphatase levels.
• Don't administer drug with food because it decreases the rate and extent of absorption.
• Assess for signs and symptoms of peripheral neuropathy, characterized by numbness and burning in the extremities, the drug's major toxic effects. If drug isn't withdrawn, peripheral neuropathy can progress to sharp shooting pain or severe continuous burning pain requiring opioid analgesics. The pain may or may not be reversible.
• **Alert:** Don't confuse drug with other antivirals that may use initials for identification.

✓ **Patient teaching**
• Instruct patient to take drug on an empty stomach.
• Make sure patient understands that the drug doesn't cure HIV infection and that opportunistic infections may still occur despite continued use. Review safe sex practices with patient.
• Inform patient that peripheral neuropathy is the major toxic condition associated with drug and that pancreatitis is the major life-threatening toxic reaction. Review the signs and symptoms of these adverse reactions, and instruct patient to call doctor promptly if any appear.
• Instruct patient of childbearing age to use an effective contraceptive while taking drug.

☀ *NEW DRUG*

## zanamivir
Relenza

*Pregnancy Risk Category B*

**HOW SUPPLIED**
*Powder for inhalation:* 5 mg/blister

**ACTION**
Likely exerts its antiviral action by inhibiting neuraminidase on the surface of the influenza virus, potentially altering virus particle aggregation and release.

| Route | Onset | Peak | Duration |
|-------|-------|------|----------|
| Inhalation | Unknown | 1-2 hr | Unknown |

**INDICATIONS & DOSAGE**
*Uncomplicated acute illness due to influenza virus in patients who have been symptomatic for no more than 2 days—*
**Adults and adolescents ages 12 and older:** 2 oral inhalations (one 5-mg blister per inhalation for total dose of 10 mg) b.i.d. using the Diskhaler inhalation device for 5 days. Two doses should be tak-

en on first day of treatment provided there is at least 2 hours between doses. Subsequent doses should be about 12 hours apart (in the morning and evening) at about the same time each day.

**ADVERSE REACTIONS**
**CNS:** headache, dizziness.
**EENT:** nasal signs and symptoms; sinusitis; ear, nose, and throat infections.
**GI:** diarrhea, nausea, vomiting.
**Respiratory:** bronchitis, cough.

**INTERACTIONS**
None significant.

**EFFECTS ON DIAGNOSTIC TESTS**
None reported.

**CONTRAINDICATIONS**
Contraindicated in patients with known hypersensitivity to drug or its components.

**NURSING CONSIDERATIONS**
• Use cautiously in patients with severe or decompensated chronic obstructive pulmonary disease, asthma, or other underlying respiratory disease.
• Keep in mind that patients with underlying respiratory disease should have a fast-acting bronchodilator available in case of wheezing while taking zanamivir. Patients scheduled to use an inhaled bronchodilator for asthma should use their bronchodilator before taking zanamivir.
• No data are available to support safety and efficacy of zanamivir in patients who begin treatment after 48 hours of symptoms.
• Safety and efficacy of drug haven't been established for influenza prophylaxis. Use of drug shouldn't affect evaluation of patient for annual influenza vaccination.
• Lymphopenia, neutropenia, and a rise in liver enzyme and CK levels have been reported during zanamivir treatment.
• Monitor patient for bronchospasm and decline in lung function. Stop drug, as ordered, in such situations.

☑ **Patient teaching**
• Tell patient to carefully read the instructions regarding how to use the Diskhaler

inhalation device properly to administer drug.
• Advise patient to keep the Diskhaler level when loading and inhaling zanamivir. Tell him to always check inside the mouthpiece of the Diskhaler before each use to make sure it's free of foreign objects.
• Tell patient to exhale fully before putting the mouthpiece in his mouth; then, keeping the Diskhaler level, to close his lips around the mouthpiece and breathe in steadily and deeply. Advise patient to hold his breath for a few seconds after inhaling to help drug stay in the lungs.
• Advise patient with underlying respiratory disease who is scheduled to use an inhaled bronchodilator to do so before taking zanamivir. Tell patient to have a fast-acting bronchodilator available in case of wheezing while taking zanamivir.
• Advise patient that it's important to finish the entire 5-day course of treatment even if he starts to feel better and symptoms improve before the fifth day.
• Advise patient that the use of zanamivir has not been shown to reduce the risk of transmission of influenza virus to others.

---

**zidovudine
(azidothymidine, AZT)**
Apo-Zidovudine†, Novo-AZT†,
Retrovir

*Pregnancy Risk Category C*

**HOW SUPPLIED**
*Capsules:* 100 mg
*Tablets:* 300 mg
*Syrup:* 50 mg/5 ml
*Injection:* 10 mg/ml

**ACTION**
Inhibits replication of HIV by blocking DNA synthesis.

| Route | Onset | Peak | Duration |
|-------|-------|------|----------|
| P.O., I.V. | Unknown | 0.5-1.5 hr | Unknown |

---

## INDICATIONS & DOSAGE

*Symptomatic HIV infection, including AIDS—*

**Adults and children ages 12 and older:** 100 mg P.O. q 4 hours around the clock, 300 mg (1 tablet) P.O. q 12 hours, 200 mg P.O. q 8 hours, or 1 mg/kg I.V. q 4 hours six times daily.

**Children ages 3 months to 12 years:** 180 mg/m² P.O. q 6 hours (720 mg/m²/day), not to exceed 200 mg q 6 hours.

*Asymptomatic HIV infection—*

**Adults and children ages 12 and older:** 100 mg P.O. q 4 hours while awake (500 mg daily). Or, 1 mg/kg I.V. q 4 hours while awake (5 mg/kg/day).

**Children ages 3 months to 12 years:** 180 mg/m² P.O. q 6 hours (720 mg/m²/day), not to exceed 200 mg q 6 hours.

*To reduce risk of transmission of HIV from infected mother with a baseline CD4+ lymphocyte count exceeding 200 cells/mm³ to the newborn—*

**Adults:** 100 mg P.O. five times daily given initially between 14 and 34 weeks' gestation and continued throughout pregnancy. During labor, administer loading dose of 2 mg/kg I.V. over 1 hour followed by continuous I.V. infusion of 1 mg/kg/hour until umbilical cord is clamped.

**Neonates:** 2 mg/kg P.O. (syrup) q 6 hours for 6 weeks, beginning within 12 hours after birth. Or, 1.5 mg/kg I.V. q 6 hours.

*Therapy with zalcitabine or other antiretroviral agents for treatment of advanced HIV disease—*

**Adults and children ages 13 and older:** 200 mg P.O. q 8 hours or 300 mg (1 tablet) P.O. q 12 hours given with zalcitabine 0.75 mg P.O. q 8 hours or other antiretroviral agents.

*Adjust-a-dose:* For patient with end-stage renal disease or patient receiving hemodialysis or peritoneal dialysis, 100 mg P.O. or 1 mg/kg I.V. q 6 to 8 hours.

## ADVERSE REACTIONS

**CNS:** *headache,* **seizures,** paresthesia, *malaise,* insomnia, *asthenia, dizziness,* somnolence.

**GI:** nausea, anorexia, abdominal pain, vomiting, constipation, diarrhea, taste perversion, dyspepsia, pancreatitis.

**Hematologic:** *severe bone marrow suppression, anemia, agranulocytosis, thrombocytopenia.*

**Hepatic:** increased liver enzyme levels.

**Musculoskeletal:** myalgia.

**Skin:** *rash.*

**Other:** diaphoresis, *fever,* lactic acidosis.

## INTERACTIONS

**Drug-drug:** *Acetaminophen, aspirin, indomethacin:* may impair hepatic metabolism of zidovudine, increasing drug's toxicity. Monitor closely.

*Acyclovir:* possible seizures, lethargy, and fatigue. Use together cautiously.

*Amphotericin B, dapsone, flucytosine, pentamidine:* increased risk of nephrotoxicity and bone marrow suppression. Monitor closely.

*Fluconazole, methadone, valproic acid:* increased zidovudine level. Monitor for toxicity.

*Ganciclovir, interferon-alpha:* increased risk of hematologic toxicity. Monitor closely.

*Other cytotoxic drugs:* additive adverse effects on the bone marrow. Avoid concomitant use.

*Probenecid:* may decrease the renal clearance of zidovudine. Avoid concomitant use.

*Ribavirin:* antagonized antiviral activity of zidovudine against HIV. Avoid concomitant use.

## EFFECTS ON DIAGNOSTIC TESTS

Drug may cause depression of formed elements (erythrocytes, leukocytes, and platelets) in peripheral blood.

## CONTRAINDICATIONS

Contraindicated in patients with hypersensitivity to drug.

## NURSING CONSIDERATIONS

• Use cautiously and with close monitoring in patients with advanced symptomatic HIV infection and in patients with severe bone marrow depression.

• Use with caution in patients with hepatomegaly, hepatitis, or other known risk factors for liver disease and in those with renal insufficiency. Monitor renal and liver function tests.

---

Reactions may be *common,* uncommon, *life-threatening,* or COMMON AND LIFE-THREATENING.

• Monitor blood studies every 2 weeks, as ordered, to detect anemia or agranulocytosis. Patients may require dosage reduction or temporary discontinuation of drug.
• Drug may temporarily decrease morbidity and mortality in certain patients with AIDS.

### ☐ I.V. administration
• Dilute drug before administration. Remove the calculated dose from the vial; add to $D_5W$ to achieve a concentration that doesn't exceed 4 mg/ml. Infuse drug over 1 hour at a constant rate. Avoid rapid infusion or bolus injection. Adding mixture to biological or colloidal fluids (for example, blood products, protein solutions) isn't recommended. Protect undiluted vials from light.

### ☑ Patient teaching
• Tell patient to take drug exactly as directed and not to share it with others.
• Instruct patient to take drug on an empty stomach. To avoid esophageal irritation, tell patient to take drug while sitting upright and with adequate amount of fluids.
• Remind patient that he must comply with the dosage schedule. Suggest ways to avoid missing doses, perhaps by using an alarm clock.
• Advise patient that blood transfusions may be needed during treatment. Zidovudine frequently causes a low RBC count.
• Warn patient not to take other drugs for AIDS unless doctor has approved them.
• Advise pregnant, HIV-infected patient that drug therapy only reduces the risk of HIV transmission to her newborn. Long-term risks to infants are unknown.
• Advise patient that monotherapy is no longer recommended, and to discuss any questions with doctor.
• Advise health care worker considering zidovudine prophylaxis after occupational exposure (following needle-stick injury, for example) that drug's safety or efficacy has not yet been proved.

---

*Liquid contains alcohol.    **May contain tartrazine.    †Canada    ‡Australia    §U.K.    ◊OTC

**azithromycin**
**clarithromycin**
**dirithromycin**
**erythromycin base**
**erythromycin estolate**
**erythromycin ethylsuccinate**
**erythromycin lactobionate**
**erythromycin stearate**

**COMBINATION PRODUCTS**
ERYZOLE, PEDIAZOLE, SULFIMYCIN: erythromycin (200 mg) and sulfisoxazole (600 mg)/5 ml.

---

**azithromycin**
Zithromax

*Pregnancy Risk Category B*

### HOW SUPPLIED
*Capsules:* 250 mg; Z-pak (contains 5 days of therapy)
*Injection:* 500 mg
*Oral suspension:* 100 mg/5 ml,
200 mg/5 ml
*Single-dose powder for oral suspension:* 1 g
*Tablets:* 250 mg, 600 mg

### ACTION
Binds to the 50S subunit of bacterial ribosomes, blocking protein synthesis; bacteriostatic or bactericidal, depending on concentration.

| Route | Onset | Peak | Duration |
|-------|-------|------|----------|
| P.O. | Unknown | 2.5-4.4 hr | Unknown |
| I.V. | Unknown | Unknown | Unknown |

### INDICATIONS & DOSAGE
*Acute bacterial exacerbations of COPD due to* Haemophilus influenzae, Moraxella (Branhamella) catarrhalis, *or* Streptococcus pneumoniae; *uncomplicated skin and skin-structure infections due to* Staphylococcus aureus, Streptococcus pyogenes, *or* S. agalactiae; *second-line*

*therapy of pharyngitis or tonsillitis due to* S. pyogenes—
**Adults and adolescents ages 16 and older:** 500 mg P.O. as a single dose on day 1; then 250 mg daily on days 2 through 5. Total dose is 1.5 g.
*Community-acquired pneumonia due to* Chlamydia pneumoniae, H. influenzae, Mycoplasma pneumoniae, S. pneumoniae; *I.V. form can also be used for* Legionella pneumophila, M. catarrhalis, *and* S. aureus—
**Adults and adolescents ages 16 and older:** 500 mg P.O. as a single dose on day 1; then 250 mg P.O. daily on days 2 through 5. Total dose is 1.5 g. For patients requiring initial I.V. therapy, 500 mg I.V. as a single daily dose for 2 days; then 500 mg P.O. as a single daily dose to complete a 7-to 10-day course of therapy. Switch from I.V. to P.O. therapy should be done at the doctor's discretion and based on patient's clinical response.
*Nongonococcal urethritis or cervicitis due to* C. trachomatis—
**Adults and adolescents ages 16 and older:** 1 g P.O. as a single dose.
*Prevention of disseminated* Mycobacterium avium *complex disease in patients with advanced HIV infection*—
**Adults:** 1,200 mg P.O. once weekly, as indicated.
*Urethritis and cervicitis due to* Neisseria gonorrhoeae—
**Adults:** 2 g P.O. as a single dose.
*Pelvic inflammatory disease due to* C. trachomatis, N. gonorrhoeae, *or* M. hominis *in patients who require initial I.V. therapy*—
**Adults:** 500 mg I.V. as a single daily dose for 1 to 2 days; then 250 mg P.O. daily to complete a 7-day course of therapy. Switch from I.V. to P.O. therapy should be at doctor's discretion and based on patient's clinical response.
*Genital ulcer disease in men caused by* H. ducreyi *(chancroid)*—
**Adults:** 1 g P.O. as a single dose.

---

Reactions may be *common*, uncommon, *life-threatening*, or COMMON AND LIFE-THREATENING.

*Otitis media—*
**Children over age 6 months:** 10 mg/kg (maximum 500 mg) P.O. on day 1; then 5 mg/kg (maximum 250 mg) on days 2 to 5.
*Pharyngitis, tonsillitis—*
**Children over age 2:** 12 mg/kg (maximum 500 mg) P.O. daily for 5 days.
*Dental prophylaxis in patients allergic to penicillin—*
**Adults:** 500 mg P.O. 1 hour before procedure.
**Children:** 15 mg/kg P.O. 1 hour before procedure.

## ADVERSE REACTIONS
**CNS:** dizziness, vertigo, headache, fatigue, somnolence.
**CV:** palpitations, chest pain.
**GI:** *nausea, vomiting, diarrhea, abdominal pain,* dyspepsia, flatulence, melena, cholestatic jaundice, pseudomembranous colitis.
**GU:** candidiasis, vaginitis, nephritis.
**Skin:** rash, photosensitivity.
**Other:** *angioedema.*

## INTERACTIONS
**Drug-drug.** *Aluminum- and magnesium-containing antacids:* lowered peak plasma levels of azithromycin. Separate administration times by at least 2 hours.
*Carbamazepine, cyclosporine, phenytoin:* may increase levels of these drugs. Monitor closely.
*Digoxin:* may cause elevated digoxin levels. Monitor closely.
*Ergotamine:* acute ergotamine toxicity has occurred. Monitor closely.
*Pimozide:* prolongation of QT interval and ventricular tachycardia have been associated with other macrolide anti-infectives. Monitor patient closely.
*Theophylline:* may increase plasma theophylline levels with other macrolides; effect of azithromycin is unknown. Monitor theophylline levels carefully.
*Triazolam:* may decrease clearance of triazolam. Monitor closely.
*Warfarin:* may increase INR with other macrolides; effect of azithromycin is unknown. Monitor INR carefully.
**Drug-food.** *Any food:* decreased absorption of capsules and multidose oral suspension formulation. Take the preparations on an empty stomach.
**Drug-lifestyle.** *Sun exposure:* photosensitivity reactions may occur. Take precautions.

## EFFECTS ON DIAGNOSTIC TESTS
None reported.

## CONTRAINDICATIONS
Contraindicated in patients with hypersensitivity to erythromycin or other macrolides.

## NURSING CONSIDERATIONS
• Use cautiously in patients with impaired hepatic function.
• Obtain specimen for culture and sensitivity tests before giving first dose. Therapy may begin pending results.
• Administer capsules and multidose oral suspension 1 hour before or 2 hours after meals; don't administer with antacids. Tablets and single-dose packets for oral suspension can be taken with or without food.
• Monitor for superinfection. May cause overgrowth of nonsusceptible bacteria or fungi.
• Single-dose, 1-g packets for suspension should be reconstituted with 2 oz (60 ml) of water, mixed, and administered to patient. Patient should rinse glass with additional 2 oz of water and drink to ensure he has consumed entire dose. Packets are not for pediatric use.

### I.V. administration
• Reconstitute drug in 500-mg vial with 4.8 ml of sterile water for injection and shake well until all the drug is dissolved (yields a concentration of 100 mg/ml). Dilute solution further in at least 250 ml of normal saline, half-normal saline, $D_5W$, or lactated Ringer's solution to yield a concentration range of 1 to 2 mg/ml.
• *Alert:* Infuse a 500-mg dose of azithromycin I.V. over 1 hour or more. Never give it as a bolus or an I.M. injection.

### Patient teaching
• Tell patient to take drug as prescribed, even after he feels better.

## clarithromycin
Biaxin, Klaricid§

*Pregnancy Risk Category C*

### HOW SUPPLIED
*Tablets (film-coated):* 250 mg, 500 mg
*Suspension:* 125 mg/5 ml, 250 mg/5 ml

### ACTION
Binds to the 50S subunit of bacterial ribosomes, blocking protein synthesis; bacteriostatic or bactericidal, depending on concentration.

| Route | Onset | Peak | Duration |
|-------|-------|------|----------|
| P.O. | Unknown | 2-4 hr | Unknown |

### INDICATIONS & DOSAGE
*Pharyngitis or tonsillitis due to* Streptococcus pyogenes—
**Adults:** 250 mg P.O. q 12 hours for 10 days.
**Children:** 15 mg/kg/day P.O. in divided doses q 12 hours for 10 days.
*Acute maxillary sinusitis due to* S. pneumoniae, Haemophilus influenzae, *or* Moraxella (Branhamella) catarrhalis—
**Adults:** 500 mg P.O. q 12 hours for 14 days.
**Children:** 15 mg/kg/day P.O. in divided doses q 12 hours for 10 days.
*Acute exacerbations of chronic bronchitis due to* M. catarrhalis *or* S. pneumoniae; *pneumonia due to* S. pneumoniae, Chlamydia pneumoniae, *or* Mycoplasma pneumoniae—
**Adults:** 250 mg P.O. q 12 hours for 7 to 14 days.
*Acute exacerbations of chronic bronchitis due to* H. influenzae—
**Adults:** 500 mg P.O. q 12 hours for 7 to 14 days.
*Uncomplicated skin and skin-structure infections due to* Staphylococcus aureus *or* S. pyogenes—
**Adults:** 250 mg P.O. q 12 hours for 7 to 14 days.
**Children:** 15 mg/kg/day P.O. in divided doses q 12 hours for 10 days.
*Acute otitis media caused by* H. influenzae, M. catarrhalis, *or* S. pneumoniae—

**Children:** 7.5 mg/kg P.O. q 12 hours for 10 days.
*Mycobacterium avium complex (MAC) disease in patients with HIV infection—*
**Adults:** 500 mg P.O. q 12 hours, with other antimycobacterial drugs, for life.
**Children:** 7.5 mg/kg P.O. (maximum of 500 mg) q 12 hours, with other antimycobacterial drugs, for life.
*Prophylaxis against MAC disease in patients with advanced HIV infection—*
**Adults:** 500 mg P.O. q 12 hours.
**Children:** 7.5 mg/kg P.O. (maximum of 500 mg) q 12 hours.
*Active duodenal ulcer associated with* Helicobacter pylori *infection—*
**Adults:** 500 mg P.O. t.i.d. for 14 days with omeprazole 40 mg P.O. each morning. Omeprazole therapy should continue at a dose of 20 mg P.O. each morning for days 15 to 28. Or, 500 mg P.O. t.i.d. for 14 days with ranitidine bismuth citrate 400 mg P.O. b.i.d. Ranitidine bismuth citrate therapy continues for days 15 to 28. Or, 500 mg P.O. b.i.d. plus lansoprazole 30 mg P.O. b.i.d. and amoxicillin 1 g P.O. b.i.d. for 14 days.
*Dental prophylaxis in patients allergic to penicillin—*
**Adults:** 500 mg P.O. 1 hour before procedure.
**Children:** 15 mg/kg P.O. 1 hour before procedure.

### ADVERSE REACTIONS
**CNS:** headache.
**CV:** *ventricular arrhythmias.*
**GI:** *diarrhea, nausea, abnormal taste, dyspepsia, abdominal pain or discomfort, pseudomembranous colitis.*
**GU:** *increased BUN.*
**Hematologic:** *increased INR, **leukopenia, thrombocytopenia.***
**Hepatic:** elevated liver studies.
**Skin:** rash, **Stevens-Johnson syndrome,** urticaria.

### INTERACTIONS
**Drug-drug.** *Cisapride, pimozide:* altered metabolism of these drugs, with prolongation of QT interval and ventricular tachycardia. Don't use these drugs with clarithromycin.

---

Reactions may be *common*, uncommon, ***life-threatening**,* or COMMON AND LIFE-THREATENING.

*Carbamazepine:* may increase serum levels of carbamazepine. Monitor blood levels.
*Digoxin:* may increase serum digoxin levels. Monitor for digitalis toxicity.
*Fluconazole:* increased clarithromycin levels. Monitor closely.
*Theophylline:* increased plasma theophylline levels possible with other macrolides; effect of clarithromycin is unknown. Monitor theophylline levels carefully.
*Warfarin:* increased INR possible with other macrolides; effect of clarithromycin is unknown. Monitor INR carefully.
*Zidovudine:* decreased zidovudine levels. Monitor effectiveness of zidovudine closely.

**EFFECTS ON DIAGNOSTIC TESTS**
None reported.

**CONTRAINDICATIONS**
Contraindicated in patients with hypersensitivity to erythromycin or other macrolides and in those receiving cisapride, and pimozide.

**NURSING CONSIDERATIONS**
• Use cautiously in patients with hepatic or renal impairment.
• Obtain specimen for culture and sensitivity tests before giving first dose. Therapy may begin pending results.
• Monitor patient for superinfection. Drug may cause overgrowth of nonsusceptible bacteria or fungi.

☑ **Patient teaching**
• Tell patient to take drug as prescribed, even after he feels better.
• Instruct patient to report persistent adverse reactions.
• Inform patient that drug may be taken with or without food. He shouldn't refrigerate the suspension form. Discard unused portion after 10 days.

---

**dirithromycin**
Dynabac

*Pregnancy Risk Category C*

**HOW SUPPLIED**
*Tablets (enteric-coated):* 250 mg

**ACTION**
Inhibits bacterial RNA-dependent protein synthesis by binding to the 50S subunit of the ribosome.

| Route | Onset | Peak | Duration |
|-------|-------|------|----------|
| P.O. | Unknown | 4 hr | Unknown |

**INDICATIONS & DOSAGE**
*Acute bacterial exacerbations of chronic bronchitis due to* Moraxella (Branhamella) catarrhalis, Streptococcus pneumoniae, *or* Haemophilus influenzae; *secondary bacterial infection of acute bronchitis due to* M. catarrhalis *or* S. pneumoniae; *uncomplicated skin and skin-structure infections due to* Staphylococcus aureus *(methicillin-susceptible strains) or* S. pyogenes—
**Adults and children ages 12 and older:** 500 mg P.O. daily with food (or within 1 hour after eating) for 5 to 7 days.
*Community-acquired pneumonia due to* Legionella pneumophila, Mycoplasma pneumoniae, *or* S. pneumoniae—
**Adults and children ages 12 and older:** 500 mg P.O. daily with food (or within 1 hour after eating) for 14 days.
*Pharyngitis or tonsillitis due to* S. pyogenes—
**Adults and children ages 12 and older:** 500 mg P.O. daily with food (or within 1 hour after eating) for 10 days.

**ADVERSE REACTIONS**
**CNS:** headache, dizziness, vertigo, asthenia, insomnia.
**GI:** abdominal pain, nausea, diarrhea, vomiting, dyspepsia, flatulence.
**Hepatic:** increased liver enzyme levels.
**Hematologic:** increased platelet, eosinophil, and neutrophil counts.
**Metabolic:** hyperkalemia.
**Respiratory:** increased cough, dyspnea.
**Skin:** rash, pruritus, urticaria.
**Other:** pain, decreased bicarbonate levels, increased CK level.

**INTERACTIONS**
**Drug-drug.** *Antacids, H$_2$-antagonists:* may slightly increase the absorption of dirithromycin when it is administered immediately after these drugs. Do not give together.

---

*Liquid contains alcohol.   **May contain tartrazine.   †Canada   ‡Australia   §U.K.   ◇OTC

*Theophylline:* may alter steady-state plasma levels of theophylline. Monitor theophylline plasma levels. Dosage adjustments may be needed.

   *Note:* Alfentanil, oral anticoagulants, bromocriptine, carbamazepine, cyclosporine, digoxin, disopyramide, ergotamine, hexobarbital, lovastatin, phenytoin, triazolam, and valproate have been reported to interact with erythromycin products. It's unknown whether these same drugs interact with dirithromycin. Until further data are available, use caution during coadministration.

**Drug-food.** *Any food:* increased absorption. Administer drug with food.

**EFFECTS ON DIAGNOSTIC TESTS**
None reported.

**CONTRAINDICATIONS**
Contraindicated in patients with hypersensitivity to drug, erythromycin, or other macrolide antibiotics.

**NURSING CONSIDERATIONS**
• Use cautiously in patients with hepatic insufficiency and in breast-feeding women. Monitor liver function test results.
• Safety of drug in children under age 12 hasn't been established.
• Obtain culture and sensitivity results to ensure organism is sensitive to dirithromycin. Drug isn't recommended for empiric use.
• Drug shouldn't be used in patients with known, suspected, or potential bacteremias because serum levels are inadequate to provide antibacterial coverage of organisms within the bloodstream.
• Administer drug with food or within 1 hour of food intake.
• Monitor patient for superinfection. Drug may cause overgrowth of nonsusceptible bacteria or fungi.

☑ **Patient teaching**
• Tell patient to take drug as prescribed, even after he feels better.
• Instruct patient to take drug with food or within 1 hour after eating and not to cut, chew, or crush the tablet.

## erythromycin base
Apo-Erythro Base†, EMU-V Tablets‡, E-Base, E-Mycin, Erybid†, Eryc, Ery-Tab, Erythromid†, Erythromycin Base Filmtab, Erythromycin Delayed-Release, Novo-Rythro Encap†, PCE Dispertab

## erythromycin estolate
Ilosone, Ilosone Pulvules, Novo-Rythro†

## erythromycin ethylsuccinate
Apo-Erythro-ES†, E.E.S., EES-400‡, EES granules‡, Erymin§, EryPed, EryPed 200, EryPed 400, Erythroped§, Erythroped A§, Novo-Rythro†

## erythromycin lactobionate
Erythrocin, Erythromycin Lactobionate

## erythromycin stearate
Apo-Erythro-S†, Erythrocin Stearate, Novo-Rythro†

*Pregnancy Risk Category B*

**HOW SUPPLIED**
**erythromycin base**
*Tablets (enteric-coated):* 250 mg, 333 mg, 500 mg
*Tablets (filmtabs):* 250 mg, 500 mg
*Capsules (delayed-release):* 250 mg
**erythromycin estolate**
*Tablets:* 500 mg
*Capsules:* 250 mg
*Oral suspension:* 125 mg/5 ml, 250 mg/5 ml
**erythromycin ethylsuccinate**
*Tablets (film-coated):* 400 mg
*Tablets (chewable):* 200 mg
*Oral suspension:* 200 mg/5 ml, 400 mg/5 ml, 100 mg/2.5 ml
**erythromycin lactobionate**
*Injection:* 500-mg, 1-g vials
**erythromycin stearate**
*Tablets (film-coated):* 250 mg, 500 mg

---

Reactions may be *common*, uncommon, ***life-threatening***, or COMMON AND LIFE-THREATENING.

## ACTION

Inhibits bacterial protein synthesis by binding to the 50S subunit of the ribosome. Bacteriostatic or bactericidal, depending on concentration.

| Route | Onset | Peak | Duration |
|-------|-------|------|----------|
| P.O. | Unknown | 1-4 hr | Unknown |
| I.V. | Unknown | Immediate | Unknown |

## INDICATIONS & DOSAGE

*Acute pelvic inflammatory disease due to* Neisseria gonorrhoeae—
**Adults:** 500 mg I.V. (lactobionate) q 6 hours for 3 days; then 250 mg (base, estolate, stearate) or 400 mg (ethylsuccinate) P.O. q 6 hours for 7 days.
**Children:** initially, 20 mg/kg (base, ethylsuccinate, stearate) P.O. 1½ to 2 hours before procedure; then half the initial dose 6 hours later.
*Intestinal amebiasis due to* Entamoeba histolytica—
**Adults:** 400 mg P.O. (ethylsuccinate) q.i.d. for 10 to 14 days. I.V. therapy not effective.
**Children:** 30 to 50 mg/kg (ethylsuccinate) P.O. daily, in divided doses, for 10 to 14 days. I.V. therapy not effective.
*Erythrasma—*
**Adults:** 250 mg P.O. (base, estolate, stearate) t.i.d. for 21 days.
*Rheumatic fever prophylaxis—*
**Adults:** 250 mg (base, estolate, stearate) P.O. q 12 hours.
*Mild to moderately severe respiratory tract, skin, and soft-tissue infections due to sensitive group A beta-hemolytic streptococci,* Streptococcus pneumoniae, Mycoplasma pneumoniae, Corynebacterium diphtheriae, *or* Bordetella pertussis—
**Adults:** 250 to 500 mg (base, estolate, stearate) P.O. q 6 hours; or 400 to 800 mg (ethylsuccinate) P.O. q 6 hours; or 15 to 20 mg/kg I.V. daily, as continuous infusion or in divided doses q 6 hours for 10 days (3 weeks for *Mycoplasma* infection).
**Children:** 30 to 50 mg/kg (oral erythromycin salts) P.O. daily, in divided doses q 6 hours; or 15 to 20 mg/kg I.V. daily, in divided doses q 4 to 6 hours for 10 days (3 weeks for *Mycoplasma* infection).

Listeria monocytogenes *infection—*
**Adults:** 250 mg (base, estolate, stearate) P.O. q 6 hours or 500 mg P.O. q 12 hours.
*Nongonococcal urethritis due to* Ureaplasma urealyticum—
**Adults:** 500 mg (base, estolate, stearate) P.O. q 6 hours for at least 7 days.
*Syphilis in patients allergic to penicillin—*
**Adults:** 500 mg (base, estolate, stearate) P.O. q.i.d. for 2 weeks.
*Legionnaires' disease—*
**Adults:** 500 mg to 1 g I.V. or P.O. (base, estolate, stearate) or 800 to 1,600 mg (ethylsuccinate) q 6 hours for 10 to 14 days.
*Uncomplicated urethral, endocervical, or rectal infections due to* Chlamydia trachomatis *when tetracyclines are contraindicated—*
**Adults:** 500 mg (base, estolate, stearate) or 800 mg (ethylsuccinate) P.O. q.i.d. for 14 days.
*Urogenital* C. trachomatis *infections during pregnancy—*
**Adults:** 500 mg (base, estolate, stearate) P.O. q.i.d. for at least 7 days or 250 mg (base, estolate, stearate) or 400 mg (ethylsuccinate) P.O. q.i.d. for at least 14 days.
*Conjunctivitis due to* C. trachomatis *in neonates—*
**Neonates:** 50 mg/kg (base, estolate, stearate) P.O. daily in four divided doses for 14 days.
*Pneumonia in infants caused by* C. trachomatis—
**Infants:** 50 mg/kg/day (base, estolate, stearate) P.O. in four divided doses for 21 days or 15 to 20 mg/kg/day (lactobionate) I.V. as a continuous infusion or in four divided doses.

## ADVERSE REACTIONS

**CV:** *ventricular arrhythmias.*
**EENT:** hearing loss (with high I.V. doses).
**GI:** *abdominal pain and cramping, nausea, vomiting, diarrhea.*
**Hepatic:** cholestatic jaundice (with erythromycin estolate).
**Skin:** urticaria, rash, eczema.
**Other:** overgrowth of nonsusceptible bacteria or fungi; *anaphylaxis;* fever; *vein irritation, thrombophlebitis after I.V. injection.*

---

*Liquid contains alcohol.  **May contain tartrazine.  †Canada  ‡Australia  §U.K.  ◇OTC

## INTERACTIONS

**Drug-drug.** *Carbamazepine:* increased carbamazepine blood levels and increased risk of toxicity. Monitor closely.
*Cisapride:* may increase cisapride levels, leading to toxicity including arrhythmias.
*Clindamycin, lincomycin:* may be antagonistic. Don't use together.
*Cyclosporine:* increased levels of cyclosporine. Monitor closely.
*Digoxin:* increased serum digoxin levels. Monitor for digoxin toxicity.
*Disopyramide:* increased disopyramide plasma levels resulting, in some cases, in arrhythmias and prolonged QT intervals. Monitor ECG.
*Midazolam, triazolam:* increased effects of these drugs. Monitor closely.
*Oral anticoagulants:* increased anticoagulant effect. Monitor PT and INR closely.
*Theophylline:* decreased erythromycin blood level and increased theophylline toxicity. Use together cautiously.
**Drug-herb.** *Pill-bearing spurge:* may inhibit CYP3A enzymes, affecting drug metabolism. Use together cautiously.

## EFFECTS ON DIAGNOSTIC TESTS

Erythromycin may interfere with fluorometric determination of urine catecholamines. AST and ALT may become falsely elevated during erythromycin therapy (rare).

## CONTRAINDICATIONS

Contraindicated in patients with hypersensitivity to drug or other macrolides. Erythromycin estolate is contraindicated in patients with hepatic disease.

## NURSING CONSIDERATIONS

• Use erythromycin salts cautiously in patients with impaired hepatic function. Monitor liver function test results.
• Erythromycin estolate isn't recommended during pregnancy because of the potential adverse effects on the mother and fetus.
• Obtain urine specimen for culture and sensitivity tests before giving first dose. Therapy may begin pending results.
• When administering suspension, be sure to note the concentration.

• Monitor patient for superinfection. Drug may cause overgrowth of nonsusceptible bacteria or fungi.
• Monitor hepatic function (increased serum levels of alkaline phosphatase, ALT, AST, and bilirubin may occur). Erythromycin estolate may cause serious hepatotoxicity in adults (reversible cholestatic jaundice). Other erythromycin salts cause hepatotoxicity to a lesser degree.
• Drug may falsely elevate levels of urinary 17-hydroxycorticosteroids and 17-ketosteroids.
• Drug may interfere with colorimetric assays, resulting in falsely elevated AST and ALT levels.
• Keep in mind that coated tablets or encapsulated pellets have caused fewer instances of GI upset; they may be better tolerated by patients who cannot tolerate erythromycin.
• Drug isn't indicated for the treatment of neurosyphilis.

### ◖ I.V. administration

• Reconstitute drug according to manufacturer's directions and dilute each 250 mg in at least 100 ml of normal saline solution. Infuse over 1 hour.
• *Alert:* Don't administer erythromycin lactobionate with other drugs.

### ☑ Patient teaching

• Tell patient to take drug as prescribed, even after he feels better.
• Instruct patient to take oral form of drug with full glass of water 1 hour before or 2 hours after meals for best absorption. Drug may be taken with food if GI upset occurs. Coated tablets may be taken with meals. Tell patient not to drink fruit juice with drug. Chewable erythromycin tablets shouldn't be swallowed whole.
• Instruct patient to report adverse reactions, especially nausea, abdominal pain, and fever.

---

Reactions may be *common*, uncommon, *life-threatening*, or COMMON AND LIFE-THREATENING.

## Miscellaneous anti-infectives

aztreonam
bacitracin
chloramphenicol sodium
  succinate
clindamycin hydrochloride
clindamycin palmitate
  hydrochloride
clindamycin phosphate
imipenem and cilastatin sodium
meropenem
nitrofurantoin macrocrystals
nitrofurantoin microcrystals
quinupristin/dalfopristin
spectinomycin hydrochloride
trimethoprim
vancomycin hydrochloride

**COMBINATION PRODUCTS**
MACROBID: nitrofurantoin macrocrystals
25 mg and nitrofurantoin monohydrate
75 mg.

---

aztreonam
Azactam

*Pregnancy Risk Category B*

**HOW SUPPLIED**
*Injection:* 500-mg vials, 1-g vials, 2-g
vials

**ACTION**
Inhibits bacterial cell-wall synthesis, ultimately causing cell-wall destruction; bactericidal.

| Route | Onset | Peak | Duration |
|-------|-------|------|----------|
| I.V. | Unknown | Immediate | Unknown |
| I.M. | Unknown | < 1 hr | Unknown |

**INDICATIONS & DOSAGE**
*Urinary tract infections, lower respiratory
tract infections, septicemia, skin and skin-
structure infections, intra-abdominal infections, surgical infections, and gynecologic infections due to susceptible strains
of the following gram-negative aerobic
organisms:* Escherichia coli, Klebsiella

pneumoniae, Proteus mirabilis,
Pseudomonas aeruginosa, Enterobacter
cloacae, Klebsiella oxytoca, *and* Citrobacter *species,* Serratia marcescens;
*respiratory infections due to* Haemophilus
influenzae—
**Adults:** 500 mg to 2 g I.V. or I.M. q 8 to
12 hours. For severe systemic or life-
threatening infections, 2 g q 6 to 8 hours
may be given. Maximum dose is 8 g daily.
**Children ages 9 months to 15 years:**
30 mg/kg q 6 to 8 hours I.V. Maximum
dose is 120 mg/kg/day.
*Adjust-a-dose:* For adults with renal impairment, if creatinine clearance is 10 to
30 ml/minute, dose is 1 to 2 g; then 50%
usual dose at the usual interval. If clearance is less than 10 ml/minute, 500 mg to
2 g; then 25% usual dose at usual interval.
For adults with alcoholic cirrhosis, decrease dose by 20% to 25%.

**ADVERSE REACTIONS**
**CNS:** *seizures,* headache, insomnia, confusion.
**CV:** hypotension.
**GI:** diarrhea, nausea, vomiting,
pseudomembranous colitis.
**GU:** increased BUN and serum creatinine
levels.
**Hematologic:** *neutropenia,* anemia, *pancytopenia, thrombocytopenia,* leukocytosis, thrombocytosis, prolonged PT, INR,
and PTT.
**Hepatic:** transient elevation of ALT and
AST.
**Other:** *hypersensitivity reactions (rash,
anaphylaxis),* thrombophlebitis, discomfort and swelling at I.M. injection site, increased LD.

**INTERACTIONS**
**Drug-drug.** *Aminoglycosides, beta-lactam
antibiotics, other anti-infectives:* synergistic effectiveness. Avoid concomitant use.
*Cefoxitin, imipenem:* possible antagonistic effect. Avoid concomitant use.
*Probenecid:* increased serum aztreonam
levels. Avoid concomitant use.

---

*Liquid contains alcohol.   **May contain tartrazine.   †Canada   ‡Australia   §U.K.   ◇OTC

## EFFECTS ON DIAGNOSTIC TESTS
Drug therapy alters urine glucose determinations using cupric sulfate (Clinitest or Benedict's reagent). Coombs' test results may become positive during therapy.

## CONTRAINDICATIONS
Contraindicated in patients with hypersensitivity to drug.

## NURSING CONSIDERATIONS
• Use cautiously in elderly patients and in those with impaired renal function. Dosage adjustment may be necessary. Monitor renal function tests.
• Obtain culture and sensitivity tests before giving first dose. Therapy may begin pending results.
• Administer I.M. injections deep into a large muscle mass, such as the upper outer quadrant of the gluteus maximus or the lateral aspect of the thigh. Doses exceeding 1 g should be given I.V.
• Don't give I.M. injection to children.
• Observe patient for signs of superinfection.
• Because drug is ineffective against gram-positive and anaerobic organisms, anticipate using it with other antibiotics for immediate treatment of life-threatening illnesses. Aztreonam is a narrow-spectrum antibiotic, effective only against gram-negative organisms.
• Patients who are allergic to penicillins or cephalosporins may not be allergic to aztreonam. However, close monitoring of those who have had an immediate hypersensitivity reaction to these antibiotics is recommended.

## I.V. administration
• To administer a bolus of aztreonam, inject drug slowly (over 3 to 5 minutes) directly into a vein or I.V. tubing. Give infusions over 20 minutes to 1 hour.

## Patient teaching
• Warn patient receiving I.M. drug that pain and swelling at the injection site may occur.
• Tell patient to alert nurse if discomfort occurs at I.V. insertion site.
• Instruct patient to report adverse reactions and signs of superinfection promptly.

# bacitracin
BACI-IM, Bacitin†

*Pregnancy Risk Category C*

## HOW SUPPLIED
*Injection:* 50,000-U vials

## ACTION
Hinders bacterial cell-wall synthesis, damaging the bacterial plasma membrane and making the cell more vulnerable to osmotic pressure.

| Route | Onset | Peak | Duration |
|-------|---------|--------|----------|
| I.M. | Unknown | 1-2 hr | Unknown |

## INDICATIONS & DOSAGE
*Pneumonia or empyema due to susceptible staphylococci—*
**Infants weighing over 2.5 kg (5.5 lb):** 1,000 U/kg I.M. daily, divided q 8 to 12 hours for up to 12 days.
**Infants under 2.5 kg:** 900 U/kg I.M. daily, divided q 8 to 12 hours for up to 12 days.

## ADVERSE REACTIONS
**EENT:** ototoxicity.
**GI:** nausea, vomiting.
**GU:** *nephrotoxicity (albuminuria, cylindruria, oliguria, anuria, tubular and glomerular necrosis),* increased BUN and serum creatinine.
**Skin:** urticaria, rash.
**Other:** injection site pain.

## INTERACTIONS
**Drug-drug.** *Inhalation anesthetics, neuromuscular blockers:* prolonged muscle weakness. Monitor patient for excessive muscle weakness or respiratory distress. *Nephrotoxic drugs (such as aminoglycosides):* increased nephrotoxicity. Use together cautiously.

## EFFECTS ON DIAGNOSTIC TESTS
Urinary sediment tests may show increased protein and cast excretion.

## CONTRAINDICATIONS
Contraindicated in patients with impaired renal function or hypersensitivity to drug.

Because of significant risk of neurotoxicity, limit I.M. use to infants with staphylococcal pneumonia.

## NURSING CONSIDERATIONS
• Use cautiously in patients with myasthenia gravis and neuromuscular disease.
• Obtain culture and sensitivity tests before giving first dose.
• Assess baseline renal function studies before and during therapy.
• Administer by deep I.M. injection only.
• Concentration of bacitracin should be between 5,000 and 10,000 U/ml. Reconstitute 50,000-U vial with 9.8 ml of diluent. Store in refrigerator. Drug is inactivated if stored at room temperature.
• Maintain adequate fluid intake, and monitor urine output closely.
• Provide measures to keep urine pH above 6 to reduce risk of nephrotoxicity.
• Prolonged therapy may result in overgrowth of nonsusceptible organisms, especially *Candida albicans*.

### ☑ Patient teaching
• Warn patient that injection may be painful.
• Instruct patient to report adverse reactions promptly.

---

## chloramphenicol sodium succinate
Chloromycetin Sodium Succinate, Kemicetine§, Pentamycetin†

*Pregnancy Risk Category C*

### HOW SUPPLIED
*Injection:* 1-g vial; 1 g, 2 g premixed (frozen)

### ACTION
Inhibits bacterial protein synthesis by binding to the 50S subunit of the ribosome; bacteriostatic.

| Route | Onset | Peak | Duration |
|-------|-------|------|----------|
| I.V. | Unknown | 1-3 hr | Unknown |

### INDICATIONS & DOSAGE
Haemophilus influenzae *meningitis, acute* Salmonella typhi *infection, and meningitis, bacteremia, or other severe infections due to sensitive* Salmonella *species,* Rickettsia, *lymphogranuloma, psittacosis, or various sensitive gram-negative organisms—*
**Adults:** 50 to 100 mg/kg I.V. daily, divided q 6 hours. Maximum dose is 100 mg/kg daily.
**Full-term infants over age 2 weeks with normal metabolic processes:** up to 50 mg/kg I.V. daily, divided q 6 hours.
**Premature infants, neonates ages 2 weeks or less, and children and infants with immature metabolic processes:** 25 mg/kg I.V. once daily. I.V. route must be used to treat meningitis.

### ADVERSE REACTIONS
**CNS:** headache, mild depression, confusion, delirium, peripheral neuropathy with prolonged therapy.
**EENT:** optic neuritis (in patients with cystic fibrosis), decreased visual acuity.
**GI:** nausea, vomiting, stomatitis, diarrhea, enterocolitis, glossitis.
**Hepatic:** jaundice.
**Hematologic:** *aplastic anemia, hypoplastic anemia, granulocytopenia, thrombocytopenia.*
**Other:** *hypersensitivity reactions, anaphylaxis, gray syndrome in neonates.*

### INTERACTIONS
**Drug-drug.** *Anticoagulants, barbiturates, hydantoins, iron salts, sulfonylureas:* increased blood levels of these drugs possible. Monitor for toxicity.
*Penicillins:* synergistic effects may develop in the treatment of certain microorganisms, but antagonism may also occur. Monitor effectiveness closely.
*Rifampin:* may reduce chloramphenicol levels. Monitor for changes in effectiveness.
*Vitamin $B_{12}$:* may decrease response of vitamin B in patients with pernicious anemia. Monitor closely.

### EFFECTS ON DIAGNOSTIC TESTS
False elevation of urine PABA levels result if chloramphenicol is administered during a bentiromide test for pancreatic function. Treatment with chloramphenicol causes false-positive results on tests for

urine glucose using cupric sulfate (Clinitest).

**CONTRAINDICATIONS**
Contraindicated in patients with hypersensitivity to drug.

**NURSING CONSIDERATIONS**
• Use cautiously in patients with impaired hepatic or renal function, acute intermittent porphyria, and G6PD deficiency and with other drugs that cause bone marrow suppression or blood disorders.
• *Alert:* Use with caution in premature infants and newborns because potentially fatal gray syndrome may occur. Symptoms include abdominal distention, gray cyanosis, vasomotor collapse, respiratory distress, and death within a few hours of symptom onset.
• Obtain specimen for culture and sensitivity tests before giving first dose. Therapy may begin pending results.
• Obtain plasma levels. Therapeutic plasma levels are as follows: peak, 10 to 20 mcg/ml; trough, 5 to 10 mcg/ml.
• Monitor CBC, platelets, serum iron, and reticulocytes before and every 2 days during therapy, as ordered. Stop drug immediately if anemia, reticulocytopenia, leukopenia, or thrombocytopenia develops, and notify doctor.
• Monitor for evidence of superinfection.

🔲 **I.V. administration**
• Give I.V. slowly over at least 1 minute. Check injection site daily for phlebitis and irritation.
• Reconstitute 1-g vial of powder for injection with 10 ml of sterile water for injection. Concentration will be 100 mg/ml. Stable for 30 days at room temperature, but refrigeration recommended. Don't use cloudy solutions.

✅ **Patient teaching**
• Instruct patient to notify doctor if adverse reactions occur, especially nausea, vomiting, diarrhea, fever, confusion, sore throat, or mouth sores.
• Tell patient receiving drug I.V. to alert nurse if discomfort occurs at I.V. insertion site.

• Instruct patient to report symptoms of superinfection.

---

**clindamycin hydrochloride**
Cleocin HCl, Dalacin C†‡

**clindamycin palmitate hydrochloride**
Cleocin Pediatric, Dalacin C Flavored Granules†

**clindamycin phosphate**
Cleocin Phosphate, Dalacin C†‡, Dalacin C Phosphate†‡

*Pregnancy Risk Category B*

---

**HOW SUPPLIED**
**clindamycin hydrochloride**
*Capsules:* 75 mg, 150 mg, 300 mg
**clindamycin palmitate hydrochloride**
*Granules for oral solution:* 75 mg/5 ml
**clindamycin phosphate**
*Injection:* 150-mg base/ml, 300-mg base/2 ml, 600-mg base/4 ml, 900-mg base/6 ml, 9,000-mg base/60 ml
*Injectable infusion (in 5% dextrose):* 300 mg (50 ml), 600 mg (50 ml), 900 mg (50 ml)

**ACTION**
Inhibits bacterial protein synthesis by binding to the 50S subunit of the ribosome.

| Route | Onset | Peak | Duration |
|-------|-------|------|----------|
| P.O. | Unknown | 45-60 min | Unknown |
| I.V. | Unknown | Immediate | Unknown |
| I.M. | Unknown | 3 hr | Unknown |

**INDICATIONS & DOSAGE**
*Infections due to sensitive staphylococci, streptococci, pneumococci,* Bacteroides, Fusobacterium, Clostridium perfringens, *and other sensitive aerobic and anaerobic organisms—*
**Adults:** 150 to 450 mg P.O. q 6 hours; or 300 to 600 mg I.M. or I.V. q 6, 8, or 12 hours.
**Children over age 1 month:** 8 to 20 mg/kg P.O. daily, in divided doses q 6 to 8 hours; or 15 to 40 mg/kg I.M. or I.V. daily, in divided doses q 6 or 8 hours.

*Pelvic inflammatory disease—*
**Adults:** 900 mg I.V. q 8 hours with gentamicin. Continue at least 48 hours after improvement in symptoms; then switch to oral clindamycin 450 mg 4 times daily for a total course of 10 to 14 days or doxycycline 100 mg P.O. q 12 hours for total of 10 to 14 days.
*Pneumocystis carinii pneumonia—*
**Adults:** 600 mg I.V. q 6 hours (or, 900 mg IV q 8 hours) or 300 to 450 mg P.O. q 6 hours with primaquine.

## ADVERSE REACTIONS
**CV:** thrombophlebitis.
**GI:** *nausea,* vomiting, abdominal pain, *diarrhea, pseudomembranous colitis.*
**Hematologic:** *transient leukopenia,* eosinophilia, *thrombocytopenia.*
**Hepatic:** jaundice; transient increases in serum bilirubin, alkaline phosphatase, and AST.
**Skin:** maculopapular rash, urticaria.
**Other:** *anaphylaxis.*

## INTERACTIONS
**Drug-drug.** *Erythromycin:* may block access of clindamycin to its site of action. Avoid concomitant use.
*Kaolin:* decreased absorption of oral clindamycin. Separate administration times.
*Neuromuscular blockers:* potentiated neuromuscular blockade possible. Monitor closely.
**Drug-food.** *Diet foods with sodium cyclamate:* decreased serum level of drug. Don't use together.

## EFFECTS ON DIAGNOSTIC TESTS
None reported.

## CONTRAINDICATIONS
Contraindicated in patients with hypersensitivity to drug or lincomycin.

## NURSING CONSIDERATIONS
• Use cautiously in neonates and patients with renal or hepatic disease, asthma, history of GI disease, or significant allergies.
• Drug does not penetrate blood-brain barrier.
• Obtain culture and sensitivity tests before giving first dose. Therapy may begin pending results.

• For I.M. administration, inject deeply. Rotate sites. Doses over 600 mg per injection are not recommended.
• I.M. injection may raise CK in response to muscle irritation.
• Don't refrigerate reconstituted oral solution because it will thicken. Drug is stable for 2 weeks at room temperature.
• Monitor renal, hepatic, and hematopoietic functions during prolonged therapy, as ordered.
• Observe patient for signs of superinfection.
• *Alert:* Don't give opioid antidiarrheals to treat drug-induced diarrhea; they may prolong and worsen diarrhea.

### I.V. administration
• When giving I.V., check site daily for phlebitis and irritation. For I.V. infusion, dilute each 300 mg in 50-ml solution, and give no faster than 30 mg/minute (over 10 to 60 minutes). Never give undiluted as a bolus.

### Patient teaching
• Advise patient taking the capsule form to take it with a full glass of water to prevent esophageal irritation.
• Warn patient that I.M. injection may be painful.
• Tell patient to alert nurse if discomfort occurs at I.V. insertion site.
• Instruct patient to notify doctor if adverse reactions, especially diarrhea, occur. Warn him not to treat such diarrhea himself.

# imipenem and cilastatin sodium
Primaxin IM, Primaxin IV

*Pregnancy Risk Category C*

## HOW SUPPLIED
*Powder for injection:* 250 mg, 500 mg, 750 mg

## ACTION
Imipenem is bactericidal and inhibits bacterial cell-wall synthesis. Cilastatin inhibits the enzymatic breakdown of imipenem in the kidneys, thereby achiev-

ing adequate antibacterial levels of imipenem in the urine.

| Route | Onset | Peak | Duration |
|-------|-------|------|----------|
| I.V. | Unknown | Immediate | Unknown |
| I.M. | Unknown | 1-2 hr | Unknown |

## INDICATIONS & DOSAGE

*Serious infections of the lower respiratory and urinary tracts, intra-abdominal and gynecologic infections, bacterial septicemia, bone and joint infections, skin and soft-tissue infections, and endocarditis. Most known microorganisms are susceptible:* Acinetobacter, Enterococcus, Staphylococcus, Streptococcus, Escherichia coli, Haemophilus, Klebsiella, Morganella, Proteus, Enterobacter, Pseudomonas aeruginosa, *and* Bacteroides, *including* B. fragilis—
**Adults weighing over 70 kg (154 lb):** 250 mg to 1 g by I.V. infusion q 6 to 8 hours. Maximum daily dose is 50 mg/kg/day or 4 g/day, whichever is less. Or, 500 to 750 mg I.M. q 12 hours. Maximum daily dose is 1,500 mg.
*Adjust-a-dose:* For children over age 12, patients under 70 kg, and those who are renally impaired, refer to package insert for dosage adjustments based on weight, creatinine clearance, and severity of infection.

## ADVERSE REACTIONS

**CNS:** *seizures,* dizziness, somnolence.
**CV:** hypotension.
**GI:** nausea, vomiting, diarrhea, *pseudomembranous colitis.*
**GU:** increased BUN or serum creatinine levels.
**Hematologic:** eosinophilia, *thrombocytopenia, leukopenia.*
**Hepatic:** transient increases in AST, ALT, alkaline phosphatase, and bilirubin.
**Skin:** rash, urticaria, pruritus.
**Other:** *hypersensitivity reactions, anaphylaxis,* fever; increased LD; thrombophlebitis, injection site pain.

## INTERACTIONS

**Drug-drug.** *Aminoglycosides:* synergistic effect. Monitor closely.
*Beta-lactam antibiotics:* possible in vitro antagonism. Avoid concomitant use.

*Ganciclovir:* may cause seizures. Avoid concomitant use.
*Probenecid:* increased serum levels of cilastatin. Avoid concomitant use.

## EFFECTS ON DIAGNOSTIC TESTS

Drug may interfere with glucose determination by Benedict's solution or Clinitest.

## CONTRAINDICATIONS

Contraindicated in patients with hypersensitivity to drug.

## NURSING CONSIDERATIONS

• Use cautiously in patients allergic to penicillins or cephalosporins because drug has similar properties.
• Also use cautiously in patients with history of seizure disorders, especially if they also have compromised renal function.
• Use with caution in children under age 3 months.
• Obtain culture and sensitivity tests before giving first dose. Therapy may begin pending results.
• Adjust dosage for patients with a creatinine clearance below 70 ml/minute. Monitor renal function tests.
• *Alert:* If seizures develop and persist despite anticonvulsant therapy, notify doctor; drug should then be discontinued.
• Monitor patient for bacterial or fungal superinfections and resistant infections during and after therapy.

### I.V. administration

• Don't administer by direct I.V. bolus injection. Each 250- or 500-mg dose should be given by I.V. infusion over 20 to 30 minutes. Each 1-g dose should be infused over 40 to 60 minutes. If nausea occurs, the infusion may be slowed.
• When reconstituting powder, shake until the solution is clear. Solutions may range from colorless to yellow; variations of color within this range don't affect drug's potency. After reconstitution, solution is stable for 10 hours at room temperature and for 48 hours when refrigerated.

### Patient teaching

• Instruct patient to report adverse reactions promptly.

• Tell patient to alert nurse if discomfort occurs at I.V. insertion site.
• Inform patient to notify doctor if loose stools or diarrhea occurs.

---

## meropenem
Meronem§, Merrem I.V.

*Pregnancy Risk Category B*

### HOW SUPPLIED
*Powder for injection:* 500 mg, 1 g

### ACTION
Inhibits cell-wall synthesis in bacteria. It readily penetrates cell wall of most gram-positive and gram-negative bacteria to reach penicillin-binding-protein targets.

| Route | Onset | Peak | Duration |
|-------|-------|------|----------|
| I.V. | Unknown | 1 hr | Unknown |

### INDICATIONS & DOSAGE
*Complicated appendicitis and peritonitis due to viridans group streptococci,* Escherichia coli, Klebsiella pneumoniae, Pseudomonas aeruginosa, Bacteroides fragilis, Bacteroides thetaiotaomicron, *and* Peptostreptococcus *species; bacterial meningitis (pediatric patients only) due to* Streptococcus pneumoniae, Haemophilus influenzae, *and* Neisseria meningitidis—
**Adults:** 1 g I.V. q 8 hours over 15 to 30 minutes as I.V. infusion or over 3 to 5 minutes as I.V. bolus injection (5 to 20 ml).
**Children ages 3 months and older weighing below 50 kg (110 lb):**
20 mg/kg (intra-abdominal infection) or 40 mg/kg (bacterial meningitis) q 8 hours over 15 to 30 minutes as I.V. infusion or over 3 to 5 minutes as I.V. bolus injection (5 to 20 ml). Maximum dosage is 2 g I.V. q 8 hours.
**Children 50 kg and over:** 1 g I.V. q 8 hours for intra-abdominal infections and 2 g I.V. q 8 hours for meningitis.
*Adjust-a-dose:* For patients with renal insufficiency or renal failure and creatinine clearance of 26 to 50 ml/minute, usual dose q 12 hours; if clearance is 10 to 25 ml/minute, half the usual dose q 12 hours; and if it is below 10 ml/minute, half the usual dose q 24 hours.

### ADVERSE REACTIONS
**CNS:** *seizures,* headache.
**GI:** diarrhea, nausea, vomiting, constipation, pseudomembranous colitis, oral candidiasis, glossitis.
**GU:** increased creatinine or BUN levels, presence of RBCs in urine.
**Hematologic:** increased or decreased platelet count, increased eosinophil count, positive direct or indirect Coombs' test, decreased hemoglobin level or hematocrit, decreased WBC count, prolonged or shortened PT, INR, or PTT.
**Hepatic:** increased levels of ALT, AST, alkaline phosphatase, LD, and bilirubin.
**Respiratory:** *apnea,* dyspnea.
**Skin:** rash, pruritus.
**Other:** *hypersensitivity, anaphylactic reaction;* inflammation, phlebitis, thrombophlebitis (at injection site).

### INTERACTIONS
**Drug-drug.** *Probenecid:* inhibited renal excretion of meropenem. Drug competes with meropenem for active tubular secretion, which significantly increases elimination half-life of drug and the extent of systemic exposure. Administration of probenecid with meropenem is not recommended.

### EFFECTS ON DIAGNOSTIC TESTS
Drug may cause a positive direct or indirect Coombs' test.

### CONTRAINDICATIONS
Contraindicated in patients with hypersensitivity to components of drug or other drugs in same class and in those who have demonstrated anaphylactic reactions to beta-lactams.

### NURSING CONSIDERATIONS
• Use cautiously in elderly patients and in those with a history of seizure disorders or impaired renal function.
• Safety and effectiveness of drug have not been established for patients under age 3 months.

---

• It's unknown whether meropenem appears in breast milk. Use drug cautiously in breast-feeding women.

• Drug is not used to treat methicillin-resistant staphylococci.

• Obtain specimen for culture and sensitivity test before giving first dose. Therapy may begin pending test results.

• *Alert:* Serious and occasionally fatal hypersensitivity reactions have been reported in patients receiving therapy with beta-lactams. Before therapy is initiated, determine whether previous hypersensitivity reactions to penicillins, cephalosporins, other beta-lactams, or other allergens have occurred.

• Discontinue drug and notify doctor if an allergic reaction occurs. Serious anaphylactic reactions require immediate emergency treatment.

• Seizures and other CNS adverse reactions associated with meropenem therapy can occur in patients with CNS disorders, bacterial meningitis, and compromised renal function.

• If seizures occur during drug therapy, discontinue infusion and notify doctor. Dosage adjustment may be ordered.

• Monitor patient for signs and symptoms of superinfection. Drug may cause overgrowth of nonsusceptible bacteria or fungi.

• Periodic assessment of organ system functions, including renal, hepatic, and hematopoietic function, is recommended during prolonged therapy.

• Monitor patient's fluid balance and weight carefully.

**I.V. administration**
• For I.V. bolus administration, add 10 ml of sterile water for injection to 500 mg/20-ml vial or 20 ml to 1 g/30-ml vial. Shake to dissolve, and let stand until clear.
• For I.V. infusion, infusion vials (500 mg/100 ml and 1 g/100 ml) may be directly reconstituted with a compatible infusion fluid. Or, an injection vial may be reconstituted, then the resulting solution added to an I.V. container and further diluted with an appropriate infusion fluid. Don't use ADD-Vantage vials for this purpose. For ADD-Vantage vials, constitute only with half-normal saline injec-

tion, normal saline injection, or 5% dextrose injection in 50-, 100-, or 250-ml Abbott ADD-Vantage flexible diluent containers. Follow manufacturer's guidelines closely when using ADD-Vantage vials.
• Don't mix or add meropenem to solutions containing other drugs.
• Use freshly prepared solutions of drug immediately whenever possible. Stability of drug varies with type of drug used (injection vial, infusion vial, or ADD-Vantage container). Consult manufacturer's literature for details.

**✓ Patient teaching**
• Advise breast-feeding woman of risk of transmitting drug to infant through breast milk.
• Instruct patient to report adverse reactions or signs and symptoms of superinfection.

## nitrofurantoin macrocrystals
Macrobid, Macrodantin

## nitrofurantoin microcrystals
Apo-Nitrofurantoin†, Furadantin, Furalan, Macrodantin, Novo-Furantoin†

*Pregnancy Risk Category B*

### HOW SUPPLIED
**nitrofurantoin macrocrystals**
*Capsules:* 25 mg, 50 mg, 100 mg
**nitrofurantoin microcrystals**
*Oral suspension:* 25 mg/5 ml

### ACTION
Unknown. Appears to interfere with bacterial enzyme systems and possibly with bacterial cell-wall formation.

| Route | Onset | Peak | Duration |
|-------|-------|------|----------|
| P.O. | Unknown | Unknown | Unknown |

### INDICATIONS & DOSAGE
*Urinary tract infections due to susceptible* Escherichia coli, Staphylococcus aureus, *enterococci; or certain strains of* Klebsiella *and* Enterobacter—
**Adults and children over age 12:** 50 to 100 mg P.O. q.i.d. with meals and h.s.

**Children ages 1 month to 12 years:** 5 to 7 mg/kg P.O. daily, divided q.i.d.
*Long-term suppression therapy—*
**Adults:** 50 to 100 mg P.O. daily h.s.
**Children:** 1 mg/kg P.O. daily in a single dose h.s. or divided into two doses given q 12 hours.

## ADVERSE REACTIONS
**CNS:** *peripheral neuropathy,* headache, dizziness, drowsiness, *ascending polyneuropathy with high doses or renal impairment.*
**GI:** *anorexia, nausea, vomiting,* abdominal pain, *diarrhea.*
**Hematologic:** *hemolysis in patients with G6PD deficiency, agranulocytosis, thrombocytopenia.*
**Hepatic:** *hepatitis, hepatic necrosis,* elevated bilirubin and alkaline phosphatase.
**Metabolic:** hypoglycemia.
**Respiratory:** *pulmonary sensitivity reactions, asthmatic attacks.*
**Skin:** maculopapular, erythematous, or eczematous eruption; transient alopecia; pruritus; urticaria; *exfoliative dermatitis; Stevens-Johnson syndrome.*
**Other:** *hypersensitivity reactions, anaphylaxis,* drug fever, overgrowth of nonsusceptible organisms in urinary tract.

## INTERACTIONS
**Drug-drug.** *Magnesium-containing antacids:* decreased nitrofurantoin absorption. Separate administration times by 1 hour.
*Probenecid, sulfinpyrazone:* increased blood levels and decreased urine levels. May result in increased toxicity and lack of therapeutic effect. Don't use together.
**Drug-food.** *Any food:* increased absorption. Give drug with food.

## EFFECTS ON DIAGNOSTIC TESTS
Nitrofurantoin may cause false-positive results in urine glucose tests using cupric sulfate (such as Benedict's reagent, Fehling's solution, or Clinitest) because it reacts with these agents.

## CONTRAINDICATIONS
Contraindicated in infants ages 1 month and under and in patients with moderate to severe renal impairment, anuria, oli-guria, or creatinine clearance under 60 ml/minute. Contraindicated in pregnancy at term (38 to 42 weeks) and during labor and delivery.

## NURSING CONSIDERATIONS
• Use cautiously in patients with renal impairment, anemia, diabetes mellitus, electrolyte abnormalities, vitamin B deficiency, debilitating disease, and G6PD deficiency. Drug may precipitate an asthma attack in patients with a history of asthma.
• Obtain urine specimen for culture and sensitivity tests before starting therapy and repeat as needed. Therapy may begin pending results.
• Give drug with food or milk to minimize GI distress and improve absorption.
• Monitor fluid intake and output carefully. May turn urine brown or darker.
• Monitor CBC and pulmonary status regularly.
• Monitor the patient for signs of superinfection. Use of nitrofurantoin may result in growth of nonsusceptible organisms, especially Pseudomonas.
• Monitor patient for pulmonary sensitivity reactions including cough, chest pain, fever, chills, dyspnea, pulmonary infiltration with consolidation or effusions.
• *Alert:* Hypersensitivity may develop when used for long-term therapy.
• Some patients may experience fewer adverse GI effects with nitrofurantoin macrocrystals.
• Dual-release capsules (25 mg nitrofurantoin macrocrystals combined with 75 mg nitrofurantoin monohydrate) enable patients to take drug only twice daily.
• Continue treatment for 3 days after sterile urine specimens have been obtained.
• Store drug in amber container. Keep away from metals other than stainless steel or aluminum to avoid precipitate formation.

☑ **Patient teaching**
• Instruct patient to take drug for as long as prescribed, exactly as directed, even after he feels better.
• Tell patient to take drug with food or milk to minimize stomach upset.

- Instruct patient to report adverse reactions.
- Alert patient that drug may turn urine a harmless dark yellow or brown color.
- Warn patient not to store drug in container made of metal other than stainless steel or aluminum.

✳ *NEW DRUG*

## quinupristin/dalfopristin
Synercid

*Pregnancy Risk Category B*

### HOW SUPPLIED
*Injection:* 500 mg/10 ml (150 mg quinupristin and 350 mg dalfopristin)

### ACTION
The two antibiotics work synergistically to inhibit or destroy susceptible bacteria through combined inhibition on protein synthesis in bacterial cells. Without the ability to manufacture new proteins, the bacterial cells are inactivated or die.

| Route | Onset | Peak | Duration |
|-------|-------|------|----------|
| I.V. | Unknown | Unknown | Unknown |

### INDICATIONS & DOSAGE
*Serious or life-threatening infections associated with vancomycin-resistant* Enterococcus faecium *(VREF) bacteremia—*
**Adults and adolescents ages 16 and older:** 7.5 mg/kg I.V. infusion over 1 hour every 8 hours. Treatment duration should be determined by site and severity of infection.
*Complicated skin and skin structure infections due to* Staphylococcus aureus *(methicillin susceptible) or* Streptococcus pyogenes—
**Adults and adolescents ages 16 and older:** 7.5 mg/kg by I.V. infusion over 1 hour every 12 hours for at least 7 days.

### ADVERSE REACTIONS
**CNS:** headache, pain.
**CV:** thrombophlebitis.
**GI:** nausea, diarrhea, vomiting.
**Hepatic:** *elevated total and conjugated bilirubin levels,* altered liver function studies.

**Musculoskeletal:** arthralgia, myalgia.
**Skin:** rash, pruritus.
**Other:** *inflammation, pain, edema at infusion site; infusion site reaction.*

### INTERACTIONS
**Drug-drug.** *Cyclosporine:* metabolism is reduced and levels may be increased. Monitor cyclosporine levels.
*Drugs metabolized by cytochrome P-450 3A4 (carbamazepine, delavirdine, diazepam, diltiazem, disopyramide, docetaxel, indinavir, lidocaine, lovastatin, methylprednisolone, midazolam, nevirapine, nifedipine, paclitaxel, ritonavir, tacrolimus, verapamil, vinblastine, and others):* increased plasma levels of these drugs that could increase their therapeutic effects and adverse reactions. Use together cautiously.
*Drugs metabolized by cytochrome P-450 3A4 that may prolong the QT$_c$ interval (such as cisapride, quinidine):* decreased metabolism of these drugs, resulting in prolongation of QT$_c$ interval. Avoid concomitant use.

### EFFECTS ON DIAGNOSTIC TESTS
None reported.

### CONTRAINDICATIONS
Contraindicated in patients with hypersensitivity to drug or other streptogramin antibiotics.

### NURSING CONSIDERATIONS
- Quinupristin/dalfopristin isn't active against *Enterococcus faecalis.* Appropriate blood cultures are needed to avoid misidentifying *E. faecalis* as *E. faecium.*
- Because mild to life-threatening pseudomembranous colitis has been reported with use of quinupristin/dalfopristin, consider this diagnosis in patients who develop diarrhea during or following therapy with drug.
- Adverse reactions, such as arthralgia and myalgia, may be reduced by decreasing dosage interval to every 12 hours, as ordered.
- Because overgrowth of nonsusceptible organisms may occur, monitor patient closely for signs and symptoms of superinfection.

---

Reactions may be *common,* uncommon, **life-threatening**, or COMMON AND LIFE-THREATENING.

• Monitor liver function tests during therapy, as ordered.

### ◖ I.V. administration
• Reconstitute powder for injection by adding 5 ml of either sterile water for injection or $D_5W$ and gently swirling the vial by manual rotation to ensure dissolution; avoid shaking to limit foaming. Reconstituted solutions must be further diluted within 30 minutes.
• The appropriate dose, according to patient's weight, of reconstituted solution should be added to 250 ml of $D_5W$ to make a final concentration of no more than 2 mg/ml. This diluted solution is stable for 5 hours at room temperature or 54 hours if refrigerated.
• Fluid restricted patients with a central venous catheter may receive dose in 100 ml of $D_5W$. This concentration isn't recommended for peripheral venous administration.
• If moderate to severe peripheral venous irritation occurs, consider increasing infusion volume to 500 or 750 ml, changing injection site, or infusing by a central venous catheter.
• Administer all doses by I.V. infusion over 1 hour. An infusion pump or device may be used to control rate of infusion.
• *Alert:* Quinupristin/dalfopristin is incompatible with saline and heparin solutions. Don't dilute drug with solutions containing saline or infuse into lines that contain saline or heparin. Flush line with $D_5W$ before and after each dose.

### ☑ Patient teaching
• Advise patient to immediately report irritation at I.V. site, pain in joints or muscles, and diarrhea.
• Tell patient about importance of reporting persistent or worsening signs and symptoms of infection, such as pain or erythema.

# spectinomycin hydrochloride
Trobicin

*Pregnancy Risk Category B*

## HOW SUPPLIED
*Powder for injection:* 2 g

## ACTION
Inhibits protein synthesis by binding to the 30S subunit of the ribosome.

| Route | Onset | Peak | Duration |
|-------|-------|------|----------|
| I.M. | Unknown | 1-2 hr | Unknown |

## INDICATIONS & DOSAGE
*Acute gonococcal urethritis and proctitis in men and cervicitis and proctitis in women; alternative therapy for patient allergic to beta-lactam antibiotics—*
**Adults:** 2 g I.M. single dose injected deeply into the upper outer quadrant of the buttock.
*Disseminated gonococcal infection—*
**Adults:** 2 g I.M. q 12 hours for 24 to 48 hours; then switch to cefixime, ciprofloxacin, or ofloxacin.

## ADVERSE REACTIONS
**CNS:** insomnia, dizziness.
**GI:** nausea.
**GU:** decreased urine output and creatinine clearance, increased BUN.
**Hematologic:** decreased hemoglobin levels and hematocrit.
**Hepatic:** increased AST, serum alkaline phosphatase.
**Skin:** urticaria.
**Other:** *anaphylaxis,* fever, chills, injection site pain.

## INTERACTIONS
None significant.

## EFFECTS ON DIAGNOSTIC TESTS
None reported.

## CONTRAINDICATIONS
Contraindicated in patients with hypersensitivity to drug.

---

*Liquid contains alcohol.    **May contain tartrazine.    †Canada    ‡Australia    §U.K.    ◇OTC

## NURSING CONSIDERATIONS
• Spectinomycin isn't effective for pharyngeal gonorrhea.
• Know that fever and chills may mask or delay the symptoms of incubating syphilis.
• Shake vial vigorously after reconstitution and before withdrawing dose. Store at room temperature after reconstitution and use within 24 hours.
• Use 20G needle to administer drug.

☑ **Patient teaching**
• Inform patient that drug is not effective in the treatment of syphilis. Tell him that serologic test for syphilis should be performed before therapy begins and for 3 months afterward.
• Tell patient to report adverse reactions promptly.
• Instruct patient to have all infection sites cultured 7 days after treatment to confirm eradication of organism.

---

## trimethoprim
Ipral§, Monotrim§, Proloprim, Trimopan§, Trimpex, Triprim‡

*Pregnancy Risk Category C*

---

## HOW SUPPLIED
*Tablets:* 100 mg, 200 mg

## ACTION
Interferes with the action of dihydrofolate reductase, inhibiting bacterial synthesis of folic acid.

| Route | Onset | Peak | Duration |
|-------|-------|------|----------|
| P.O. | Unknown | 1-4 hr | Unknown |

## INDICATIONS & DOSAGE
*Uncomplicated urinary tract infections due to susceptible strains of* Escherichia coli, Proteus mirabilis, Klebsiella pneumoniae, Enterobacter *species, and coagulase-negative* Staphylococcus, *including* S. saprophyticus—
**Adults:** 200 mg P.O. daily as a single dose or in divided doses q 12 hours for 10 days.
*Note:* Drug is not recommended for children under age 12.

*Adjust-a-dose:* For patients with creatinine clearance of 15 to 30 ml/minute, 50 mg P.O. q 12 hours; if clearance is below 15 ml/minute, don't use drug.

## ADVERSE REACTIONS
**GI:** *epigastric distress, nausea, vomiting, glossitis.*
**GU:** increased BUN and serum creatinine.
**Hematologic:** *thrombocytopenia, leukopenia,* megaloblastic anemia, methemoglobinemia.
**Hepatic:** elevated liver function test results.
**Skin:** *rash, pruritus, exfoliative dermatitis.*
**Other:** fever.

## INTERACTIONS
**Drug-drug.** *Phenytoin:* may decrease phenytoin metabolism and increase its serum levels. Monitor for toxicity.

## EFFECTS ON DIAGNOSTIC TESTS
Drug interferes with serum methotrexate assays.

## CONTRAINDICATIONS
Contraindicated in patients with hypersensitivity to drug and in those with documented megaloblastic anemia due to folate deficiency.

## NURSING CONSIDERATIONS
• Use cautiously in patients with impaired hepatic or renal function. Dosage should be decreased in patients with severely impaired renal function. Also use cautiously in patients with possible folate deficiency. Monitor renal and liver function test results.
• Obtain urine specimen for culture and sensitivity tests before giving first dose. Therapy may begin pending results.
• Monitor CBC routinely. Clinical signs and symptoms, such as sore throat, fever, pallor, or purpura, may be early indications of serious blood disorders.
• Monitor patient's fluid balance.
• *Alert:* Prolonged use of trimethoprim at high doses may cause bone marrow suppression.

---

Reactions may be *common*, uncommon, *life-threatening*, or COMMON AND LIFE-THREATENING.

• Because resistance to trimethoprim develops rapidly when administered alone, it's usually given with other drugs.
• *Alert:* Trimethoprim is also used with sulfamethoxazole; don't confuse the two products.

### ☑ Patient teaching
• Instruct patient to take entire amount of drug, as prescribed, even after he feels better.
• Tell patient to report adverse reactions promptly, especially signs of infection or unusual bruising.
• Inform patient of the need for adequate hydration during therapy.

## vancomycin hydrochloride
Vancocin, Vancoled

*Pregnancy Risk Category C*

### HOW SUPPLIED
*Capsules:* 125 mg, 250 mg
*Powder for oral solution:* 1-g bottles, 10-g bottles
*Powder for injection:* 500-mg vials, 1-g vials, 5 g, 10 g

### ACTION
Hinders bacterial cell-wall synthesis, damaging the bacterial plasma membrane and making the cell more vulnerable to osmotic pressure. Also interferes with RNA synthesis.

| Route | Onset | Peak | Duration |
|-------|-------|------|----------|
| P.O. | Unknown | Unknown | Unknown |
| I.V. | Unknown | Immediate | Unknown |

### INDICATIONS & DOSAGE
*Serious or severe infections when other antibiotics are ineffective or contraindicated, including those caused by methicillin-resistant* Staphylococcus aureus, Staphylococcus epidermidis, *or diphtheroid organisms—*
**Adults:** 1 to 1.5 g I.V. q 12 hours (dose based on weight and renal function; longer dosing intervals necessary in renal dysfunction).
**Children:** 10 mg/kg I.V. q 6 hours.

**Neonates and young infants:** 15 mg/kg I.V. loading dose, followed by 10 mg/kg I.V. q 12 hours if child is under age 1 week or 10 mg/kg I.V. q 8 hours if age is over 1 week but under 1 month.
*Antibiotic-associated pseudomembranous* (Clostridium difficile) *and staphylococcal enterocolitis—*
**Adults:** 125 to 500 mg P.O. q 6 hours for 7 to 10 days.
**Children:** 40 mg/kg P.O. daily, in divided doses q 6 hours for 7 to 10 days. Maximum daily dose is 2 g.
*Endocarditis prophylaxis for dental procedures—*
**Adults:** 1 g I.V. slowly over 1 hour, starting 1 hour before procedure.
**Children:** 20 mg/kg I.V. over 1 hour, starting 1 hour before procedure.

### ADVERSE REACTIONS
**CV:** hypotension.
**EENT:** tinnitus, ototoxicity.
**GI:** nausea, pseudomembranous colitis.
**GU:** *nephrotoxicity,* increased BUN and serum creatinine levels.
**Hematologic:** *neutropenia, leukopenia,* eosinophilia.
**Respiratory:** wheezing, dyspnea.
**Skin:** "red-neck" syndrome with rapid I.V. infusion.
**Other:** chills, fever, *anaphylaxis,* superinfection, pain, thrombophlebitis at injection site.

### INTERACTIONS
**Drug-drug.** *Aminoglycosides, amphotericin B, cisplatin, pentamidine:* increased risk of nephrotoxicity and ototoxicity. Monitor closely.

### EFFECTS ON DIAGNOSTIC TESTS
None reported.

### CONTRAINDICATIONS
Contraindicated in patients with hypersensitivity to drug.

### NURSING CONSIDERATIONS
• Use cautiously in patients receiving other neurotoxic, nephrotoxic, or ototoxic drugs; in patients over age 60; and in those with impaired hepatic or renal function, preexisting hearing loss, or allergies

to other antibiotics. Patients with renal dysfunction require dosage adjustment. Serum levels should be monitored to adjust I.V. dosage. Normal therapeutic levels of vancomycin are as follows: peak, 30 to 40 mg/L (drawn 1 hour after infusion ends); trough, 5 to 10 mg/L (drawn just before next dose is given).

• Monitor patient's fluid balance and observe for oliguria and cloudy urine.

• Obtain culture and sensitivity tests before giving first dose. Therapy may begin pending results.

• Obtain hearing evaluation and renal function studies before therapy.

• Monitor patient carefully for "red-neck" syndrome, which can occur if drug is infused too rapidly. Signs and symptoms include maculopapular rash on face, neck, trunk, and extremities, pruritis and hypotension associated with histamine release. If this reaction occurs, stop infusion and notify the doctor.

• Don't give drug I.M.

• *Alert:* Oral administration is ineffective for systemic infections, and I.V. administration is ineffective for pseudomembranous (*C. difficile*) diarrhea.

• Keep in mind that the oral preparation is stable for 2 weeks if refrigerated.

• Monitor renal function (BUN, serum creatinine, urinalysis, creatinine clearance, and urine output) during therapy. Also monitor for signs and symptoms of superinfection.

• Have patient's hearing evaluated during prolonged therapy.

• When drug is used to treat staphylococcal endocarditis, it will be given for at least 4 weeks.

## I.V. administration

• For I.V. infusion, dilute in 200 ml normal saline for injection or $D_5W$, and infuse over 60 minutes; if dose is greater than 1 g, infuse over 90 minutes. Check site daily for phlebitis and irritation. Report pain at infusion site. Avoid extravasation; severe irritation and necrosis can result.

• Refrigerate I.V. solution after reconstitution and use within 14 days.

## Patient teaching

• Tell patient to take entire amount of drug exactly as directed, even after he feels better.

• Instruct patient receiving drug I.V. to alert nurse if discomfort occurs at I.V. insertion site.

**amrinone lactate**
**digoxin**
**milrinone lactate**

**COMBINATION PRODUCTS**
None.

---

## amrinone lactate
Inocor

*Pregnancy Risk Category C*

### HOW SUPPLIED
*Injection:* 5 mg/ml in 20-ml ampules

### ACTION
Unknown. Thought to produce inotropic action by increasing cellular levels of cAMP. Produces vasodilation through a direct relaxant effect on vascular smooth muscle.

| Route | Onset | Peak | Duration |
|-------|-------|------|----------|
| I.V. | 2-5 min | 10 min | 0.5-2 hr |

### INDICATIONS & DOSAGE
*Short-term management of heart failure—*
**Adults:** initially, 0.75 mg/kg I.V. bolus over 2 to 3 minutes. Then begin maintenance infusion of 5 to 10 mcg/kg/minute. May give additional bolus of 0.75 mg/kg 30 minutes after starting therapy. Don't exceed total daily dose of 10 mg/kg.

### ADVERSE REACTIONS
**CV:** *arrhythmias,* hypotension, chest pain.
**GI:** nausea, vomiting, anorexia, abdominal pain.
**Hematologic:** *thrombocytopenia.*
**Hepatic:** elevated enzymes.
**Other:** burning at injection site, *hypersensitivity reactions (pericarditis, ascites, myositis vasculitis, pleuritis),* fever.

### INTERACTIONS
**Drug-drug.** *Cardiac glycosides:* enhanced inotropic effect. Beneficial drug interaction.

*Disopyramide:* excessive hypotension. Monitor patient.

### EFFECTS ON DIAGNOSTIC TESTS
Drug may decrease serum potassium or increase serum hepatic enzymes.

### CONTRAINDICATIONS
Contraindicated in patients with hypersensitivity to amrinone or bisulfites.

### NURSING CONSIDERATIONS
• Drug shouldn't be used in patients with severe aortic or pulmonic valvular disease in place of surgical correction of the obstruction or during acute phase of MI.
• Use cautiously in patients with hypertrophic cardiomyopathy.
• Amrinone is primarily prescribed for patients who have not responded to cardiac glycosides, diuretics, and vasodilators.
• Dosage depends on clinical response, including assessment of pulmonary artery wedge pressure and cardiac output.
• Anticipate that drug may be added to cardiac glycoside therapy in patients with atrial fibrillation and flutter because it slightly enhances AV conduction and increases ventricular response rate.
• Monitor platelet count. If it falls below 150,000/mm$^3$, decrease dosage as ordered.
• Patients with end-stage cardiac disease may receive home treatment with an amrinone drip while awaiting heart transplantation.
• *Alert:* Don't confuse amrinone (an inotrope) with amiodarone (an antiarrhythmic with negative chronotropic effects). Be alert to drug that patient should be receiving and the reason for its use.

### ☐ I.V. administration
• Administer drug with an infusion pump and use as supplied, or dilute in half-normal saline or normal saline solution to a concentration of 1 to 3 mg/ml. Use diluted solution within 24 hours.
• Don't dilute with solutions containing dextrose because a slow chemical reaction

---

*Liquid contains alcohol.   **May contain tartrazine.   †Canada   ‡Australia   §U.K.   ◇OTC

occurs over 24 hours. Amrinone can be injected into free-flowing dextrose infusions through a Y-connector or directly into tubing.

*Alert:* Don't administer furosemide and amrinone through the same I.V. line because precipitation occurs.

• Monitor blood pressure and heart rate throughout the infusion. If patient's blood pressure falls, slow or stop infusion and notify doctor.

*Alert:* Don't confuse amrinone with amiodarone.

☑ **Patient teaching**
• Warn patient that burning may occur at the site of injection.
• Instruct home care patient and family on administration; tell them to report adverse reactions promptly.

---

## digoxin
Digoxin, Lanoxicaps, Lanoxin*, Novodigoxin†

*Pregnancy Risk Category C*

### HOW SUPPLIED
*Tablets:* 0.125 mg, 0.25 mg
*Capsules:* 0.05 mg, 0.1 mg, 0.2 mg
*Elixir:* 0.05 mg/ml
*Injection:* 0.05 mg/ml†, 0.1 mg/ml (pediatric), 0.25 mg/ml

### ACTION
Inhibits sodium potassium–activated adenosine triphosphatase, thereby promoting movement of calcium from extracellular to intracellular cytoplasm and strengthening myocardial contraction. Also acts on CNS to enhance vagal tone, slowing conduction through the SA and AV nodes and providing an antiarrhythmic effect.

| Route | Onset | Peak | Duration |
|-------|-------|------|----------|
| P.O. | 1.5-2 hr | 2-6 hr | 3-4 days |
| I.V. | 5-30 min | 1-4 hr | 3-4 days |

### INDICATIONS & DOSAGE
*Heart failure, paroxysmal supraventricular tachycardia, atrial fibrillation and flutter—*

**Adults:** loading dose is 0.5 to 1 mg I.V. or P.O. in divided doses over 24 hours; maintenance dose is 0.125 to 0.5 mg I.V. or P.O. daily (average is 0.25 mg). Depending on response, larger doses may be needed for arrhythmias.
**Elderly:** for patients over age 65, 0.125 mg P.O. daily as maintenance dose. Frail or underweight elderly patients may require only 0.0625 mg daily or 0.125 mg every other day.
**Premature neonates:** loading dose is 0.015 to 0.025 mg/kg I.V. in three divided doses over 24 hours; maintenance dose is 0.01 mg/kg daily, divided q 12 hours.
**Neonates:** loading dose is 0.025 to 0.035 mg/kg P.O., divided q 8 hours over 24 hours; I.V. loading dose is 0.02 to 0.03 mg/kg; maintenance dose is 0.01 mg/kg P.O. daily, divided q 12 hours.
**Children ages 1 month to 2 years:** loading dose is 0.035 to 0.06 mg/kg P.O. in three divided doses over 24 hours; I.V. loading dose is 0.03 to 0.05 mg/kg; maintenance dose is 0.01 to 0.02 mg/kg P.O. daily, divided q 12 hours.
**Children over age 2:** loading dose is 0.02 to 0.04 mg/kg P.O. daily, divided q 8 hours over 24 hours; I.V. loading dose is 0.025 to 0.035 mg/kg; maintenance dose is 0.012 mg/kg P.O. daily, divided q 12 hours.
*Adjust-a-dose:* Smaller loading and maintenance doses are given to patients with impaired renal function.

### ADVERSE REACTIONS
**CNS:** *fatigue, generalized muscle weakness, agitation, hallucinations,* headache, malaise, dizziness, vertigo, stupor, paresthesia.
**CV:** *arrhythmias (most commonly, conduction disturbances with or without AV block, PVCs, and supraventricular arrhythmias);* arrhythmias may lead to increased severity of heart failure and hypotension.
**EENT:** yellow-green halos around visual images, blurred vision, light flashes, photophobia, diplopia.
**GI:** *anorexia, nausea,* vomiting, diarrhea.

---

Reactions may be *common*, uncommon, **life-threatening**, or COMMON AND LIFE-THREATENING.

## INTERACTIONS

**Drug-drug.** *Amiloride:* inhibited digoxin effect and increased digoxin excretion. Monitor for altered digoxin effect.

*Amiodarone, diltiazem, nifedipine, quinidine, verapamil:* increased digoxin blood levels. Monitor for toxicity.

*Amphotericin B, carbenicillin, corticosteroids, diuretics (including loop diuretics, chlorthalidone, metolazone, thiazides), ticarcillin:* hypokalemia predisposing patient to digitalis toxicity. Monitor serum potassium levels.

*Antacids, kaolin-pectin:* decreased absorption of oral digoxin. Schedule doses as far as possible from oral digoxin administration.

*Anticholinergics:* may increase digoxin absorption of oral digoxin tablets. Monitor blood levels and observe for toxicity.

*Cholestyramine, colestipol, metoclopramide:* decreased absorption of oral digoxin. Monitor for decreased digitoxin effect and low blood levels. Space doses by giving digoxin 1½ hours before or 2 hours after other drugs.

*Parenteral calcium, thiazides:* hypercalcemia and hypomagnesemia predisposing patient to digitalis toxicity. Monitor serum calcium and serum magnesium levels.

**Drug-herb.** *Betel palm, fumitory, lily of the valley, goldenseal, motherwort, rue, shepherd's purse:* possible enhanced cardiac effects. Avoid concomitant use.

*Licorice, oleander, Siberian ginseng, squill:* possible enhanced toxicity. Monitor patient closely.

## EFFECTS ON DIAGNOSTIC TESTS
None reported.

## CONTRAINDICATIONS

Contraindicated in patients with digitalis-induced toxicity, ventricular fibrillation, ventricular tachycardia unless caused by heart failure, or hypersensitivity to drug.

## NURSING CONSIDERATIONS

• Use with extreme caution in elderly patients and in those with acute MI, incomplete AV block, sinus bradycardia, PVCs, chronic constrictive pericarditis, hypertrophic cardiomyopathy, renal insufficiency, severe pulmonary disease, or hypothyroidism.

• Patients with hypothyroidism are extremely sensitive to cardiac glycosides and may need larger doses.

• Before administering loading dose, obtain baseline data (heart rate and rhythm, blood pressure, and electrolytes) and question patient about use of cardiac glycosides within the previous 2 to 3 weeks.

• Loading dose is divided over the first 24 hours unless the situation indicates otherwise.

• Before giving drug, take apical-radial pulse for 1 minute. Record and notify doctor of significant changes (sudden increase or decrease in pulse rate, pulse deficit, irregular beats and, particularly, regularization of a previously irregular rhythm). If these occur, check blood pressure and obtain a 12-lead ECG.

• Toxic effects on the heart may be life-threatening and require immediate attention.

• Absorption of digoxin from liquid-filled capsules is superior to absorption from tablets or elixir. Expect dosage reduction of 20% to 25% when changing from tablets or elixir to liquid-filled capsules or parenteral therapy.

• Monitor serum digoxin levels. Therapeutic levels range from 0.5 to 2 ng/ml. Obtain blood for digoxin levels 8 hours after last oral dose.

• *Alert:* Excessive slowing of the pulse rate (60 beats/minute or less) may be a sign of digitalis toxicity. Withhold drug and notify doctor.

• Monitor serum potassium levels carefully. Take corrective action before hypokalemia occurs.

• Withhold drug for 1 to 2 days before elective cardioversion. Adjust dose after cardioversion.

• *Alert:* Don't confuse digoxin with doxepin, Desoxyn, or digitoxin.

**I.V. administration**
• Infuse drug slowly over at least 5 minutes.

**Patient teaching**
• Instruct patient and a responsible family member about drug action, dosage regi-

men, how to take pulse, reportable signs, and follow-up care.
• Encourage patient to eat potassium-rich foods.
• Tell patient not to substitute one brand of digoxin for another.

---

## milrinone lactate
Primacor

*Pregnancy Risk Category C*

### HOW SUPPLIED
*Injection:* 1 mg/ml
*Injection (premixed):* 200 mcg/ml in $D_5W$

### ACTION
Produces inotropic action by increasing cellular levels of cAMP. Produces vasodilation by directly relaxing vascular smooth muscle.

| Route | Onset | Peak | Duration |
|-------|-------|------|----------|
| I.V. | 5-15 min | 1-2 hr | 3-6 hr |

### INDICATIONS & DOSAGE
*Short-term treatment of heart failure—*
**Adults:** initial loading dose is 50 mcg/kg I.V., administered slowly over 10 minutes; then continuous I.V. infusion of 0.375 to 0.75 mcg/kg/minute. Titrate infusion dose based on clinical and hemodynamic responses, as ordered.
*Adjust-a-dose:* For patients with renal failure, if creatinine clearance is 50 ml/minute or less, titrate dosage to maximum clinical effect; don't exceed 1.13 mg/kg/day.

### ADVERSE REACTIONS
**CNS:** headache.
**CV:** VENTRICULAR ARRHYTHMIAS, *ventricular ectopic activity,* nonsustained ventricular tachycardia, *sustained ventricular tachycardia, ventricular fibrillation.*

### INTERACTIONS
None significant.

### EFFECTS ON DIAGNOSTIC TESTS
None reported.

### CONTRAINDICATIONS
Contraindicated in patients with hypersensitivity to drug.

### NURSING CONSIDERATIONS
• Drug shouldn't be used in patients with severe aortic or pulmonic valvular disease in place of surgical correction of the obstruction or during acute phase of MI.
• Use cautiously in patients with atrial flutter or fibrillation because drug slightly shortens AV node conduction time and may increase ventricular response rate. Administer a cardiac glycoside, if ordered, before beginning milrinone therapy.
• Drug is typically given with digoxin and diuretics.
• Inotropics may aggravate outflow tract obstruction in hypertrophic subaortic stenosis.
• Improved cardiac output may enhance urine output. Expect dosage reduction in patient's diuretic therapy as heart failure improves. Potassium loss may predispose patient to digitalis toxicity.
• Monitor fluid and electrolyte status, blood pressure, heart rate, and renal function during therapy. Excessive decrease in blood pressure requires discontinuing or slowing rate of infusion.

### I.V. administration
• Prepare I.V. infusion solution using half-normal saline or normal saline or $D_5W$. Prepare the 100-mcg/ml solution by adding 180 ml of diluent per 20-mg (20-ml) vial, the 150-mcg/ml solution by adding 113 ml of diluent per 20-mg (20-ml) vial, and the 200-mcg/ml solution by adding 80 ml of diluent per 20-mg (20-ml) vial.
• *Alert:* Administering furosemide into an I.V. line containing milrinone causes formation of a precipitate.

### Patient teaching
• Instruct patient to report adverse reactions promptly.
• Tell patient to alert nurse if discomfort occurs at I.V. insertion site.

---

adenosine
amiodarone hydrochloride
atropine sulfate
bretylium tosylate
diltiazem hydrochloride
(See Chapter 22, ANTIANGINALS.)
disopyramide
disopyramide phosphate
esmolol hydrochloride
flecainide acetate
ibutilide fumarate
lidocaine hydrochloride
mexiletine hydrochloride
moricizine hydrochloride
phenytoin
(See Chapter 30, ANTICONVULSANTS.)
phenytoin sodium
(See Chapter 30, ANTICONVULSANTS.)
procainamide hydrochloride
propafenone hydrochloride
propranolol hydrochloride
(See Chapter 22, ANTIANGINALS.)
quinidine bisulfate
quinidine gluconate
quinidine polygalacturonate
quinidine sulfate
sotalol
tocainide hydrochloride
verapamil hydrochloride
(See Chapter 22, ANTIANGINALS.)

**COMBINATION PRODUCTS**
None.

---

## adenosine
Adenocard, Adenocor§

*Pregnancy Risk Category C*

---

**HOW SUPPLIED**
*Injection:* 3 mg/ml in 2-ml and 5-ml vials

**ACTION**
A naturally occurring nucleoside that acts on the AV node to slow conduction and inhibit reentry pathways. Adenosine is also useful in treating paroxysmal supraventricular tachycardia (PSVT) as-

sociated with accessory bypass tracts (Wolff-Parkinson-White syndrome).

| Route | Onset | Peak | Duration |
|-------|-------|------|----------|
| I.V. | Immediate | Immediate | Unknown |

**INDICATIONS & DOSAGE**
*Conversion of PSVT to sinus rhythm—*
**Adults:** 6 mg I.V. by rapid bolus injection over 1 to 2 seconds. If PSVT isn't eliminated in 1 to 2 minutes, 12 mg by rapid I.V. push may be given and repeated if needed. Single doses over 12 mg aren't recommended.

**ADVERSE REACTIONS**
**CNS:** dizziness, light-headedness, numbness, tingling in arms, headache.
**CV:** *facial flushing.*
**GI:** nausea.
**Respiratory:** chest pressure, *dyspnea, shortness of breath.*

**INTERACTIONS**
**Drug-drug.** *Carbamazepine:* higher degrees of heart block may occur. Use with caution.
*Digoxin, verapamil:* potential for ventricular fibrillation. Monitor closely.
*Dipyridamole:* may potentiate adenosine's effects. Smaller doses may be needed.
*Methylxanthines:* antagonism of adenosine's effects. Patients receiving theophylline may require higher doses or may not respond to adenosine therapy.
**Drug-herb.** *Guarana:* may decrease response. Monitor patient.
**Drug-food.** *Caffeine:* may antagonize adenosine's effects. Patient may require higher doses or not respond to adenosine therapy.

**EFFECTS ON DIAGNOSTIC TESTS**
None reported.

**CONTRAINDICATIONS**
Contraindicated in patients with hypersensitivity to drug and in those with second- or third-degree heart block or sinus

---

\*Liquid contains alcohol.    \*\*May contain tartrazine.    †Canada    ‡Australia    §U.K.    ◇OTC

node disease (such as sick sinus syndrome or symptomatic bradycardia) unless an artificial pacemaker is present; adenosine decreases conduction through the AV node and may produce first-, second-, or third-degree heart block. Patients who develop high level heart block after a single dose of adenosine shouldn't receive additional doses.

## NURSING CONSIDERATIONS
• *Alert:* Because of the potential for new arrhythmias, including heart block or transient asystole, monitor cardiac rhythm and be prepared to administer appropriate therapy.
• Use cautiously in patients with asthma because bronchoconstriction may occur.
• Crystals may form if solution is cold. If crystals are visible, gently warm solution to room temperature. Don't use solutions that aren't clear.
• Discard unused drug; adenosine lacks preservatives.

### I.V. administration
• Rapid I.V. injection is needed to ensure drug action. Administer directly into a vein if possible; when giving through an I.V. line, use the port closest to the patient, and flush immediately and rapidly with normal saline solution to ensure that drug quickly reaches the systemic circulation.

### ☑ Patient teaching
• Instruct patient to report adverse reactions promptly.
• Tell patient to alert nurse if discomfort occurs at I.V. site.

---

## amiodarone hydrochloride
Aratac‡, Cordarone,
Cordarone X‡

*Pregnancy Risk Category D*

## HOW SUPPLIED
*Tablets:* 100 mg‡, 200 mg
*Injection:* 50 mg/ml

## ACTION
Unknown. Thought to prolong the refractory period and action potential duration.

| Route | Onset | Peak | Duration |
|-------|-------|------|----------|
| P.O. | Variable | Unknown | Variable |
| I.V. | Unknown | Unknown | Variable |

## INDICATIONS & DOSAGE
*Recurrent ventricular fibrillation or recurrent hemodynamically unstable ventricular tachycardia nonresponsive to adequate doses of other antiarrhythmics or when alternative agents can't be tolerated—*
**Adults:** loading dose is 800 to 1,600 mg P.O. daily divided b.i.d. for 1 to 3 weeks until initial therapeutic response occurs; then 600 to 800 mg P.O. daily for 1 month, followed by 200 to 600 mg P.O. daily for maintenance.
 Or, give loading dose of 150 mg I.V. over 10 minutes (15 mg/minute); then 360 mg I.V. over next 6 hours (1 mg/minute), followed by 540 mg I.V. over next 18 hours (0.5 mg/minute). After first 24 hours, continue with maintenance I.V. infusion of 720 mg/24 hours (0.5 mg/minute).

## ADVERSE REACTIONS
**CNS:** peripheral neuropathy, ataxia, paresthesia, *tremor,* insomnia, sleep disturbances, headache, *malaise, fatigue.*
**CV:** bradycardia, hypotension, ***arrhythmias, heart failure, heart block, sinus arrest,*** edema.
**EENT:** *asymptomatic corneal microdeposits,* optic neuropathy or neuritis resulting in visual impairment, abnormal taste and smell, *visual disturbances.*
**GI:** anorexia, *nausea, vomiting,* constipation, abdominal pain.
**Hepatic:** *elevated liver enzymes,* hepatic dysfunction, ***hepatic failure.***
**Respiratory:** ***adult respiratory distress syndrome,*** SEVERE PULMONARY TOXICITY.
**Skin:** *photosensitivity,* solar dermatitis.
**Other:** *hypothyroidism,* hyperthyroidism, ***coagulation abnormalities.***

## INTERACTIONS
**Drug-drug.** *Antiarrhythmics:* amiodarone may reduce hepatic or renal clearance of certain antiarrhythmics (especially fle-

---

Reactions may be *common,* uncommon, *life-threatening,* or COMMON AND LIFE-THREATENING.

cainide, procainamide, quinidine). Use of amiodarone with other antiarrhythmics (especially mexiletine, propafenone, quinidine, disopyramide, procainamide) may induce torsades de pointes. Avoid concomitant use.

*Antihypertensives:* increased hypotensive effect. Use together cautiously.

*Beta blockers, calcium channel blockers:* increased cardiac depressant effects; may potentiate slowing of SA node and AV conduction. Use together cautiously.

*Cyclosporine:* increased serum creatinine levels. Serum creatinine level can remain elevated even after cyclosporine dose is reduced. Monitor closely.

*Digoxin:* increased serum digoxin levels (average of 70% to 100%). Monitor digoxin levels closely and adjust dosage as ordered. Digoxin dosage should be reduced by half or discontinued.

*Phenytoin:* may decrease phenytoin metabolism. Monitor serum phenytoin levels and adjust dosage as ordered.

*Theophylline:* increased theophylline levels with toxicity may occur. Monitor serum theophylline levels.

*Warfarin:* potentiation of anticoagulant response with the potential for serious or fatal bleeding. Decrease warfarin dosage 33% to 50% when amiodarone is initiated. Monitor patient closely.

**Drug-herb.** *Pennyroyal:* may change the rate of formation of toxic metabolites of pennyroyal. Avoid concurrent use.

**Drug-lifestyle.** *Sun exposure:* photosensitivity reaction may occur. Take precautions.

**EFFECTS ON DIAGNOSTIC TESTS**
None reported.

**CONTRAINDICATIONS**
Contraindicated in patients with hypersensitivity to drug. Also contraindicated in those with cardiogenic shock, second- or third-degree AV block, severe SA node disease resulting in preexisting bradycardia unless an artificial pacemaker is present, and in those in whom bradycardia has caused syncope.

**NURSING CONSIDERATIONS**
● Use with extreme caution in patients receiving other antiarrhythmics.
● Use cautiously in patients with pulmonary, hepatic, or thyroid disease.
● Be aware of the high incidence of adverse reactions.
● Obtain baseline pulmonary, liver, and thyroid function tests.
● Administer loading doses in a hospital setting and with continuous ECG monitoring because of the slow onset of antiarrhythmic effect and the risk of life-threatening arrhythmias.
● Divide oral loading dose into two equal doses and give with meals to decrease GI intolerance. Maintenance dose may be given once daily, but may be divided into two doses taken with meals if GI intolerance occurs.
● *Alert:* Drug poses major and potentially life-threatening management problems in patients at risk for sudden death and should be used only in patients with documented, life-threatening, recurrent ventricular arrhythmias nonresponsive to documented adequate doses of other antiarrhythmics or when alternative agents can't be tolerated. Amiodarone can cause fatal toxicities, including hepatic and pulmonary toxicity.
● Monitor carefully for pulmonary toxicity. Incidence increases in patients receiving doses over 400 mg/day.
● Monitor for symptoms of pneumonitis—exertional dyspnea, nonproductive cough, and pleuritic chest pain. Monitor pulmonary function tests and chest X-ray.
● Monitor liver and thyroid function tests and serum electrolytes, particularly potassium and magnesium levels.
● Instillation of methylcellulose ophthalmic solution is recommended during amiodarone therapy to minimize corneal microdeposits. Within 1 to 4 months after beginning amiodarone therapy, most patients show corneal microdeposits upon slit-lamp ophthalmic examination. However, only 2% to 3% have actual vision disturbances.
● Monitor blood pressure and heart rate and rhythm frequently. Perform continuous ECG monitoring during initiation and

---

alteration of dosage. Notify doctor of significant change.
• **Alert:** Don't confuse amiodarone with amiloride or amrinone.

### I.V. administration
• Drug may be given I.V. only in facilities where continuous ECG monitoring and electrophysiologic techniques are available. Mix initial dose of 150 mg in 100 ml of $D_5W$ solution. Mix infusions planned for administration over 30 minutes or more in glass bottles. Administer repeat doses through a central venous catheter.
• Administer I.V. amiodarone whenever possible via a central line dedicated to that purpose.
• Use an in-line filter with I.V. administration.
• Continuously monitor cardiac status of patient receiving drug I.V.

### Patient teaching
• Advise patient to use a sunscreen or protective clothing to prevent photosensitivity reaction. Monitor for burning or tingling skin followed by erythema and possible skin blistering. A blue-gray discoloration of the exposed skin may occur.
• Tell patient to take oral drug with food if GI reactions occur.
• Inform patient that adverse effects of drug are more prevalent at high doses and become more frequent with treatment lasting over 6 months but are generally reversible when drug is stopped. Resolution of adverse reactions may take up to 4 months.

## atropine sulfate

*Pregnancy Risk Category C*

### HOW SUPPLIED
*Tablets:* 0.4 mg
*Injection:* 0.05 mg/ml, 0.1 mg/ml, 0.3 mg/ml, 0.4 mg/ml, 0.5 mg/ml, 0.8 mg/ml, 1 mg/ml

### ACTION
An anticholinergic that inhibits acetylcholine at the parasympathetic neuroeffector junction, blocking vagal effects on the SA and AV nodes, thereby enhancing conduction through the AV node and increasing the heart rate.

| Route | Onset | Peak | Duration |
|-------|-------|------|----------|
| P.O. | 0.5-2 hr | 1-2 hr | 4 hr |
| I.V. | Immediate | 2-4 min | 4 hr |
| I.M. | 5-40 min | 20-60 min | 4 hr |
| S.C. | Unknown | Unknown | Unknown |

### INDICATIONS & DOSAGE
*Symptomatic bradycardia, bradyarrhythmia (junctional or escape rhythm)—*
**Adults:** usually 0.5 to 1 mg I.V. push, repeated q 3 to 5 minutes to maximum of 2 mg p.r.n. Lower doses (below 0.5 mg) can cause bradycardia.
**Children:** 0.01 mg/kg I.V.; may repeat q 4 to 6 hours; maximum dose is 0.4 mg or $0.3 mg/m^2$.
*Antidote for anticholinesterase insecticide poisoning—*
**Adults:** 2 to 3 mg I.V. repeated q 5 to 10 minutes until muscarinic symptoms disappear or signs of atropine toxicity appear. Severe poisoning may require up to 6 mg hourly.
**Children:** 0.05 mg/kg I.M. or I.V. repeated q 10 to 30 minutes until muscarinic signs and symptoms subside (may be repeated if they reappear) or until atropine toxicity occurs.
*Preoperatively to diminish secretions and block cardiac vagal reflexes—*
**Adults and children weighing 20 kg (44 lb) or more:** 0.4 to 0.6 mg I.M. or S.C. 30 to 60 minutes before anesthesia.
**Children under 20 kg:** 0.01 mg/kg I.M. or S.C. up to maximum dose of 0.4 mg 30 to 60 minutes before anesthesia.
*Adjunct treatment of peptic ulcer disease, treatment of functional GI disorders such as irritable bowel syndrome—*
**Adults:** 0.4 to 0.6 mg P.O. q 4 to 6 hours.
**Children:** 0.01 mg/kg or $0.3 mg/m^2$ P.O. (not to exceed 0.4 mg) q 4 to 6 hours.

### ADVERSE REACTIONS
**CNS:** *headache, restlessness,* ataxia, disorientation, hallucinations, delirium, *insomnia, dizziness,* excitement, agitation, confusion.

**CV:** palpitations, bradycardia, tachycardia.
**EENT:** photophobia, *blurred vision, mydriasis,* cycloplegia, increased intraocular pressure.
**GI:** *dry mouth,* thirst, *constipation,* nausea, vomiting.
**GU:** urine retention, impotence.
**Other:** severe allergic reactions, ***anaphylaxis, urticaria.***

## INTERACTIONS
**Drug-drug.** *Antacids:* decreased absorption of anticholinergics. Separate administration times by at least 1 hour.
*Anticholinergics, drugs with anticholinergic effects (such as amantadine, antiarrhythmics, antiparkinsonians, glutethimide, meperidine, phenothiazines, tricyclic antidepressants):* additive anticholinergic effects. Use together cautiously.
*Ketoconazole, levodopa:* decreased absorption. Avoid concomitant use.
*Methotrimeprazine:* may produce extrapyramidal symptoms. Monitor patient carefully.
*Potassium chloride wax-matrix tablets:* increased risk of mucosal lesions. Use cautiously.
**Drug-herb.** *Jaborandi tree, pill-bearing spurge:* decreased effectiveness of drug. Avoid concomitant use.
*Jimsonweed:* may adversely affect CV function. Avoid concomitant use.
*Squaw vine:* tannic acid may decrease metabolic breakdown. Monitor patient.

## EFFECTS ON DIAGNOSTIC TESTS
None reported.

## CONTRAINDICATIONS
Contraindicated in patients with hypersensitivity to drug and in those with acute angle-closure glaucoma, obstructive uropathy, obstructive disease of GI tract, paralytic ileus, toxic megacolon, intestinal atony, unstable CV status in acute hemorrhage, tachycardia, myocardial ischemia, asthma, myasthenia gravis.

## NURSING CONSIDERATIONS
• Use cautiously in patients with Down syndrome because they may be more sensitive to drug.

• Many adverse reactions (such as dry mouth and constipation) vary with the dose.
• Monitor patients for paradoxical initial bradycardia, especially those receiving small doses (0.4 to 0.6 mg). This usually disappears within 2 minutes.
• *Alert:* Watch for tachycardia in cardiac patients because it may precipitate ventricular fibrillation.
• Monitor fluid intake and urine output. Drug causes urine retention and urinary hesitancy.

### ◖ I.V. administration
• Administer via direct I.V. into a large vein or I.V. tubing over at least 1 minute.
• Slow I.V. administration may cause paradoxical slowing of the heart rate.

### ☑ Patient teaching
• Teach patient receiving oral form of drug how to handle distressing anticholinergic effects.
• Instruct patient to report serious or persistent adverse reactions promptly.
• Tell patient about potential for photophobia and suggest use of sunglasses.

# bretylium tosylate
Bretylate†

*Pregnancy Risk Category C*

## HOW SUPPLIED
*Injection:* 50 mg/ml in 10-ml ampules, vials, and syringes and in 20-ml vials

## ACTION
Unknown. Considered a class III antiarrhythmic that initially exerts transient adrenergic stimulation through release of norepinephrine. Subsequent depletion of norepinephrine causes adrenergic blocking actions to predominate, prolonging repolarization and increasing duration of action potential and an effective refractory period.

| Route | Onset | Peak | Duration |
|-------|-------|------|----------|
| I.V. | Immediate | Immediate | 6-24 hr |
| I.M. | 5-40 min | 1 hr | 6-24 hr |

### INDICATIONS & DOSAGE
*Ventricular fibrillation or hemodynamically unstable ventricular tachycardia unresponsive to other antiarrhythmics—*
**Adults:** 5 mg/kg by I.V. push over 1 minute. If needed, dose increased to 10 mg/kg and repeated q 15 to 30 minutes until 30 to 35 mg/kg have been given. For continuous suppression, diluted solution administered at 1 to 2 mg/minute continuously or 5 to 10 mg/kg diluted over more than 8 minutes q 6 hours.

### ADVERSE REACTIONS
**CNS:** *vertigo, dizziness, light-headedness, syncope.*
**CV:** severe hypotension, bradycardia, anginal pain, *transient arrhythmias,* transient hypertension, increased PVC.
**GI:** severe nausea, vomiting.

### INTERACTIONS
**Drug-drug.** *All antihypertensives:* may potentiate hypotension. Monitor blood pressure.
*Other antiarrhythmics:* additive or antagonistic antiarrhythmic effects. Monitor for additive toxicity.
*Sympathomimetics:* bretylium may potentiate effects of drugs given to correct hypotension. Monitor for effects.

### EFFECTS ON DIAGNOSTIC TESTS
None reported.

### CONTRAINDICATIONS
Contraindicated in digitalized patients unless arrhythmia is life-threatening and not caused by cardiac glycosides, and in those unresponsive to other antiarrhythmics.

### NURSING CONSIDERATIONS
• Use with extreme caution in patients with fixed cardiac output (aortic stenosis and pulmonary hypertension) to avoid severe and sudden drop in blood pressure.
• Keep patient supine until tolerance to hypotension develops.
• Monitor patient closely. The initial release of norepinephrine caused by bretylium may induce transient hypertension and arrhythmias.
• Monitor blood pressure and heart rate and rhythm continuously. Immediately report significant change. If supine systolic blood pressure falls below 75 mm Hg, the doctor may order norepinephrine, dopamine, or volume expanders.
• Observe for increased anginal pain in susceptible patients.

### I.V. administration
• When used for maintenance therapy, dilute using dextrose or normal saline for injection before administration. Follow manufacturer's guidelines for specific dilution method (varies according to dosage). When administering as direct I.V. injection, use a 20G to 22G needle and inject over 1 minute into a vein or I.V. line containing a free-flowing, compatible solution.
• For intermittent I.V. administration, dilute and give over a period of 8 minutes or more to minimize nausea and vomiting.

### ☑ Patient teaching
• Instruct patient to report adverse reactions immediately.
• Tell patient to alert nurse if discomfort occurs at I.V. insertion site.
• Inform patient to avoid sudden postural changes.

---

## disopyramide
Dirythmin SA§, Rythmodan†‡

## disopyramide phosphate
Norpace, Norpace CR, Rythmodan Injection‡, Rythmodan-LA†

*Pregnancy Risk Category C*

### HOW SUPPLIED
**disopyramide**
*Capsules:* 100 mg†, 150 mg†
**disopyramide phosphate**
*Tablets (sustained-release):* 250 mg†
*Capsules:* 100 mg, 150 mg
*Capsules (controlled-release):* 100 mg, 150 mg
*Injection:* 10 mg/ml†‡§

### ACTION
Unknown. Considered a class IA antiarrhythmic that depresses phase O and pro-

longs the action potential. All class I drugs have membrane-stabilizing effects.

| Route | Onset | Peak | Duration |
|-------|-------|------|----------|
| P.O. | 0.5-3.5 hr | 2-2.5 hr | 1.5-8.5 hr |
| I.V. | Unknown | Unknown | Unknown |

## INDICATIONS & DOSAGE

*Ventricular tachycardia and ventricular arrhythmias believed to be life-threatening—*
P.O.—
**Adults weighing over 50 kg (110 lb):** 150 mg q 6 hours with conventional capsules or 300 mg q 12 hours with extended-release preparations.
**Adults 50 kg or less:** highly individualized.
**Children under age 1:** 10 to 30 mg/kg P.O. daily, divided into four doses (q 6 hours).
**Children ages 1 to 4:** 10 to 20 mg/kg P.O. daily, divided into four doses (q 6 hours).
**Children ages 4 to 12:** 10 to 15 mg/kg P.O. daily, divided into four doses (q 6 hours).
**Children ages 12 to 18:** 6 to 15 mg/kg P.O. daily, divided into four doses (q 6 hours).
*Adjust-a-dose:* For patients with advanced renal insufficiency, if creatinine clearance is 30 to 40 ml/minute, 100 mg q 8 hours; between 15 and 30 ml/minute, 100 mg q 12 hours; if it is below 15 ml/minute, 100 mg q 24 hours.
I.V.—
**Adults:** for parenteral use, initially give 2 mg/kg I.V. slowly (over not less than 15 minutes). Administer until arrhythmias are eliminated or patient has received 150 mg. Repeat dosage if conversion is successful but arrhythmias return. Total I.V. dosage shouldn't exceed 300 mg in first hour. Follow with I.V. infusion of 0.4 mg/kg/hour (usually 20 to 30 mg/hour) to maximum of 800 mg/day.

## ADVERSE REACTIONS

**CNS:** dizziness, agitation, depression, fatigue, headache, nervousness, acute psychosis, syncope.
**CV:** *hypotension, heart failure, heart block,* edema, *arrhythmias,* shortness of breath, chest pain.
**EENT:** blurred vision, dry eyes or nose, *dry mouth.*
**GI:** nausea, vomiting, anorexia, bloating, gas, weight gain, abdominal pain, *constipation, diarrhea.*
**GU:** *urinary hesitancy.*
**Hepatic:** cholestatic jaundice.
**Musculoskeletal:** muscle weakness.
**Skin:** rash, pruritus, dermatosis.
**Other:** aches, pain.

## INTERACTIONS

**Drug-drug.** *Antiarrhythmics:* possible additive or antagonized antiarrhythmic effects. Monitor closely.
*Erythromycin:* increased disopyramide levels may occur. Monitor closely.
*Phenytoin:* increased metabolism of disopyramide. Monitor for decreased antiarrhythmic effect.
*Rifampin:* may decrease disopyramide levels. Monitor closely.
**Drug-herb.** *Jimsonweed:* may adversely affect CV function. Avoid concomitant use.

## EFFECTS ON DIAGNOSTIC TESTS
None reported.

## CONTRAINDICATIONS
Contraindicated in patients with hypersensitivity to drug and in those with sick sinus syndrome, cardiogenic shock, or second- or third-degree heart block in the absence of an artificial pacemaker.

## NURSING CONSIDERATIONS
• Use with extreme caution and avoid, if possible, in patients with heart failure. Use cautiously in patients with underlying conduction abnormalities, urinary tract diseases (especially prostatic hyperplasia), hepatic or renal impairment, myasthenia gravis, or acute angle-closure glaucoma.
• Correct electrolyte abnormalities before therapy begins, as ordered.
• Check apical pulse before administering drug. Notify doctor if pulse rate is slower than 60 beats/minute or faster than 120 beats/minute.
• Don't use sustained-release or controlled-release preparations for control of ventricular arrhythmias when therapeu-

tic blood levels must be rapidly attained, in patients with cardiomyopathy or possible cardiac decompensation, or in those with severe renal impairment.

• For use in young children, pharmacist may prepare disopyramide suspension, using 100-mg capsules and cherry syrup. Suspension should be dispensed in amber glass bottles and protected from light.

• Watch for recurrence of arrhythmias and check for adverse reactions; notify doctor if any occur.

• Discontinue drug if heart block develops, if QRS complex widens by more than 25%, or if QT interval lengthens by more than 25% above baseline.

• When transferring patient from immediate-release to sustained-release capsules, advise him to take the first sustained-release capsule 6 hours after taking the last immediate-release capsule.

• *Alert:* Don't confuse disopyramide with desipramine or dipyridamole.

### 🔵 I.V. administration

• Add 200 mg to 200 to 500 ml of a compatible solution, such as normal saline or D₅W. Administer slowly, over at least 15 minutes. Don't mix with other drugs; switch to oral therapy as soon as possible.

### ☑ Patient teaching

• Teach patient importance of taking drug on time and exactly as prescribed. This may require use of an alarm clock for overnight doses.

• If not contraindicated, advise patient to chew gum or hard candy to relieve dry mouth and to increase fiber and fluid intake to relieve constipation.

---

## esmolol hydrochloride
Brevibloc

*Pregnancy Risk Category C*

### HOW SUPPLIED
*Injection:* 10 mg/ml in 10-ml vials, 250 mg/ml in 10-ml ampules

### ACTION
A class II antiarrhythmic and ultrashort-acting selective beta blocker that decreas-

es heart rate, contractility, and blood pressure.

| Route | Onset | Peak | Duration |
|-------|-------|------|----------|
| I.V. | Immediate | 30 min | 30 min after infusion |

### INDICATIONS & DOSAGE
*Supraventricular tachycardia; to control ventricular rate in patients with atrial fibrillation or flutter in perioperative, postoperative, or other emergent circumstances; noncompensatory sinus tachycardia when heart rate requires specific interventions—*
**Adults:** loading dose is 500 mcg/kg/minute by I.V. infusion over 1 minute; then 4-minute maintenance infusion of 50 mcg/kg/minute. If adequate response doesn't occur within 5 minutes, loading dose is repeated and followed by maintenance infusion of 100 mcg/kg/minute for 4 minutes. Loading dose is repeated and maintenance infusion is increased by 50-mcg/kg/minute increments. Maximum maintenance infusion for tachycardia is 200 mcg/kg/minute.
*Perioperative and postoperative tachycardia or hypertension—*
**Adults:** for perioperative treatment of tachycardia or hypertension, 80 mg (about 1 mg/kg) I.V. bolus over 30 seconds; then 150 mcg/kg/minute I.V. infusion, if needed. Titrate infusion rate, p.r.n., to maximum of 300 mcg/kg/minute. Dosage for postoperative treatment of tachycardia and hypertension is same as for supraventricular tachycardia.

### ADVERSE REACTIONS
**CNS:** anxiety, depression, dizziness, somnolence, headache, agitation, fatigue, confusion.
**CV:** HYPOTENSION (SOMETIMES WITH DIAPHORESIS), peripheral ischemia.
**GI:** *nausea,* vomiting.
**Other:** inflammation, induration (at infusion site).

### INTERACTIONS
**Drug-drug.** *Digoxin:* serum digoxin levels may be increased by 10% to 20%. Monitor serum digoxin levels.
*Morphine:* may increase esmolol blood levels. Titrate esmolol carefully.

---

Reactions may be *common*, uncommon, *life-threatening*, or COMMON AND LIFE-THREATENING.

*Reserpine and other catecholamine-depleting drugs:* may cause additive bradycardia and hypotension. Titrate esmolol carefully.
*Succinylcholine:* esmolol may prolong neuromuscular blockade. Monitor closely.

**EFFECTS ON DIAGNOSTIC TESTS**
None reported.

**CONTRAINDICATIONS**
Contraindicated in patients with sinus bradycardia, heart block greater than first-degree, cardiogenic shock, or overt heart failure.

**NURSING CONSIDERATIONS**
• Use cautiously in patients with impaired renal function, diabetes, or bronchospasm.
• Esmolol solutions are incompatible with diazepam, furosemide, sodium bicarbonate, and thiopental sodium.
• *Alert:* Monitor ECG and blood pressure continuously during infusion. Up to 50% of all patients treated with esmolol develop hypotension. Monitor closely, especially if patient's pretreatment blood pressure was low.
• Hypotension can usually be reversed within 30 minutes by decreasing the dose or, if needed, by stopping the infusion. Notify doctor if this becomes necessary.
• If a local reaction develops at the infusion site, change to another site. Avoid using butterfly needles.
• Esmolol is recommended only for short-term use, no longer than 48 hours.
• When patient's heart rate becomes stable, esmolol will be replaced by alternative (longer-acting) antiarrhythmics, such as propranolol, digoxin, or verapamil. A half-hour after the first dose of the alternative agent is administered, reduce infusion rate by 50%. Monitor patient response and, if heart rate is controlled for 1 hour after administration of the second dose of the alternative drug, discontinue esmolol infusion.

**⚡ I.V. administration**
• Don't give esmolol by I.V. push; use an infusion control device. The 10-mg/ml single-dose vials may be used without diluting, but the injection concentrate (250 mg/ml) must be diluted to maximum level of 10 mg/ml before infusion. Remove 20 ml from 500 ml of D₅W, lactated Ringer's solution, half-normal or normal saline solution and add two ampules of esmolol (final level 10 mg/ml). Don't mix in sodium bicarbonate.

**✅ Patient teaching**
• Instruct patient to report adverse reactions promptly.
• Tell patient to alert nurse if discomfort occurs at I.V. site.

---

**flecainide acetate**
Tambocor

*Pregnancy Risk Category C*

**HOW SUPPLIED**
*Tablets:* 50 mg, 100 mg, 150 mg
*Injection:* 10 mg/ml‡

**ACTION**
A class IC antiarrhythmic that decreases excitability, conduction velocity, and automaticity as a result of slowed atrial, AV node, His-Purkinje system, and intraventricular conduction; causes a slight but significant prolongation of refractory periods in these tissues.

| Route | Onset | Peak | Duration |
|-------|-------|------|----------|
| P.O. | Unknown | 2-3 hr | Unknown |
| I.V. | Immediate | Immediate | Unknown |

**INDICATIONS & DOSAGE**
*Paroxysmal supraventricular tachycardia, paroxysmal atrial fibrillation or flutter in patients without structural heart disease; life-threatening ventricular arrhythmias such as sustained ventricular tachycardia—*
**Adults:** for paroxysmal supraventricular tachycardia, 50 mg P.O. q 12 hours. Increased in increments of 50 mg b.i.d. q 4 days. Maximum dose is 300 mg/day.
*Adjust-a-dose:* For patients with renal impairment, if creatinine clearance is 35 ml/minute or less, initial dose is 100 mg once daily or 50 mg b.i.d.

---

For life-threatening ventricular arrhythmias, 100 mg P.O. q 12 hours. Increase in increments of 50 mg b.i.d. q 4 days until efficacy is achieved. Maximum dose is 400 mg daily for most patients.

Initial dosage for patients with heart failure is 50 mg P.O. q 12 hours.

*Note:* Where available, flecainide may be given by I.V. injection‡—

**Adults:** 2 mg/kg I.V. push over not less than 10 minutes to maximum dose of 150 mg; or dilute dose and administer as an infusion.

## ADVERSE REACTIONS
**CNS:** *dizziness, headache,* fatigue, tremor, anxiety, insomnia, depression, malaise, paresthesia, ataxia, vertigo, *lightheadedness, syncope,* asthenia.
**CV:** *new or worsened arrhythmias,* chest pain, *heart failure, cardiac arrest,* palpitations, edema, flushing.
**EENT:** eye pain, eye irritation, *blurred vision and other visual disturbances.*
**GI:** nausea, constipation, abdominal pain, dyspepsia, vomiting, diarrhea, anorexia.
**Respiratory:** *dyspnea.*
**Skin:** rash.
**Other:** fever.

## INTERACTIONS
**Drug-drug.** *Amiodarone, cimetidine:* altered pharmacokinetics. Monitor for toxicity.
*Digoxin:* flecainide may increase plasma digoxin levels by 15% to 25%. Monitor serum digoxin levels.
*Disopyramide, verapamil:* negative inotropic properties may be additive with flecainide. Avoid concurrent administration.
*Propranolol, other beta blockers:* both flecainide and propranolol plasma levels increase by 20% to 30%. Monitor for propranolol and flecainide toxicity.
*Urine acidifying and alkalinizing drugs:* extremes of urine pH may substantially alter excretion of flecainide. Monitor for flecainide toxicity or decreased effectiveness.
**Drug-lifestyle.** *Smoking:* lowered flecainide serum levels. Monitor closely.

## EFFECTS ON DIAGNOSTIC TESTS
None reported.

## CONTRAINDICATIONS
Contraindicated in patients with hypersensitivity to drug and in those with pre-existing second- or third-degree AV block or right bundle-branch block when associated with a left hemiblock (in the absence of an artificial pacemaker), recent MI, or cardiogenic shock.

## NURSING CONSIDERATIONS
• Use cautiously in patients with preexisting heart failure, cardiomyopathy, severe renal or hepatic disease, prolonged QT interval, sick sinus syndrome, or blood dyscrasia.
• When used to prevent ventricular arrhythmias, drug should be reserved for patients with documented life-threatening arrhythmias.
• Check that pacing threshold was determined 1 week before and after initiating therapy in patients with pacemakers because flecainide can alter endocardial pacing thresholds.
• Correct hypokalemia or hyperkalemia as ordered before giving flecainide because these electrolyte disturbances may alter drug's effect.
• Most patients can be adequately maintained on an every-12-hour dosing schedule, but some need to receive flecainide every 8 hours.
• Dosage adjustments should be made only once every 3 to 4 days.
• Monitor serum flecainide levels, especially in patients with renal failure or heart failure. Therapeutic serum levels of flecainide range from 0.2 to 1 mcg/ml. Incidence of adverse effects increases when trough blood levels exceed 1 mcg/ml.

### I.V. administration
• When administering by I.V. push, give over at least 10 minutes. For I.V. infusion, mix only with $D_5W$.
• Because of drug's long half-life, its full therapeutic effect may take 3 to 5 days. Administer concomitant I.V. lidocaine, as ordered, for first several days.

### Patient teaching
• Stress importance of taking drug exactly as prescribed.

---

Reactions may be *common,* uncommon, ***life-threatening,*** or COMMON AND LIFE-THREATENING.

• Instruct patient to report adverse reactions promptly and to limit fluid and sodium intake to minimize fluid retention.
• Tell patient receiving drug I.V. to alert nurse if discomfort occurs at insertion site.

---

## ibutilide fumarate
Corvert

*Pregnancy Risk Category C*

### HOW SUPPLIED
*Injection:* 0.1 mg/ml in 10-ml vials

### ACTION
Prolongs action potential in isolated cardiac myocyte and increases atrial and ventricular refractoriness, namely class III electrophysiologic effects.

| Route | Onset | Peak | Duration |
|-------|-------|------|----------|
| I.V. | Unknown | Unknown | Unknown |

### INDICATIONS & DOSAGE
*Rapid conversion of atrial fibrillation or atrial flutter of recent onset to sinus rhythm—*
**Adults weighing 60 kg (132 lb) or more:** 1 mg I.V. over 10 minutes.
**Adults under 60 kg:** 0.01 mg/kg I.V. over 10 minutes.

### ADVERSE REACTIONS
**CNS:** headache.
**CV:** ventricular extrasystoles, nonsustained VT, hypotension, bundle-branch block, *sustained polymorphic VT,* AV block, *heart failure,* hypertension, prolonged QT interval, bradycardia, palpitation, tachycardia.
**GI:** nausea.

### INTERACTIONS
**Drug-drug.** *Class IA antiarrhythmics (disopyramide, procainamide, quinidine), other class III drugs (amiodarone, sotalol):* increased potential for prolonged refractoriness. Don't give these drugs for at least 5 half-lives before and 4 hours after ibutilide dose.
*Digoxin:* supraventricular arrhythmias may mask cardiotoxicity associated with excessive digoxin levels. Use cautiously.

*H₁-receptor antagonist antihistamines, phenothiazines, tetracyclic antidepressants, tricyclic antidepressants, other drugs that prolong QT interval:* increased risk for proarrhythmia. Monitor closely.

### EFFECTS ON DIAGNOSTIC TESTS
None reported.

### CONTRAINDICATIONS
Contraindicated in patients with hypersensitivity to drug or its components.

### NURSING CONSIDERATIONS
• Drug isn't recommended in patients with history of polymorphic VT and in breast-feeding women.
• Use cautiously in patients with hepatic or renal dysfunction.
• Safety of drug hasn't been established in children.
• Drug should be given only by skilled personnel. Cardiac monitor, intracardiac pacing, cardioverter or defibrillator, and medication for sustained VT must be available.
• Before therapy, hypokalemia and hypomagnesemia should be corrected to reduce the potential for proarrhythmia. Patients with atrial fibrillation of more than 2 to 3 days' duration must be adequately anticoagulated, generally over at least 2 weeks.
• Monitor ECG continuously during administration and for at least 4 hours afterward or until QTc interval returns to baseline; drug can induce or worsen ventricular arrhythmias. Longer monitoring is required if ECG shows arrhythmia.

### ◖ I.V. administration
• Drug may be given undiluted or diluted in 50 ml of diluent, and may be added to normal saline for injection or 5% dextrose injection before infusion. Contents of 10-ml vial (0.1 mg/ml) may be added to 50-ml infusion bag to form admixture of about 0.017 mg/ml ibutilide. Use aseptic technique. Drug can be used with polyvinyl chloride plastic bags or polyolefin bags.
• Administer drug over 10 minutes.
• *Alert:* Infusion should be stopped if arrhythmia is terminated or patient develops ventricular tachycardia (VT) or marked prolongation of QT or QTc interval. If ar-

---

rhythmia isn't terminated 10 minutes after infusion ends, may give a second 10-minute infusion of equal strength.
• Admixtures with approved diluents are stable for 24 hours at room temperature; 48 hours if refrigerated.
• Don't infuse parenteral products that contain particulate matter or are discolored.

☑ **Patient teaching**
• Tell patient to report adverse reactions promptly.
• Instruct patient to alert nurse of discomfort at injection site.

---

**lidocaine hydrochloride (lignocaine hydrochloride)**
LidoPen Auto-Injector, Xylocaine, Xylocard†‡

*Pregnancy Risk Category B*

## HOW SUPPLIED
*Injection (for I.M. use):* 300 mg/3 ml automatic injection device
*Injection (for direct I.V. use):* 1% (10 mg/ml), 2% (20 mg/ml)
*Injection (for I.V. admixtures):* 4% (40 mg/ml), 10% (100 mg/ml), 20% (200 mg/ml)
*Infusion (premixed):* 0.2% (2 mg/ml), 0.4% (4 mg/ml), 0.8% (8 mg/ml)

## ACTION
A class IB antiarrhythmic that decreases the depolarization, automaticity, and excitability in the ventricles during the diastolic phase by direct action on the tissues, especially the Purkinje network.

| Route | Onset | Peak | Duration |
|-------|-------|------|----------|
| I.V. | Immediate | Immediate | 10-20 min |
| I.M. | 5-15 min | 10 min | 2 hr |

## INDICATIONS & DOSAGE
*Ventricular arrhythmias due to MI, cardiac manipulation, or cardiac glycosides—*
**Adults:** 50 to 100 mg (1 to 1.5 mg/kg) by I.V. bolus at 25 to 50 mg/minute. Bolus dose is repeated q 3 to 5 minutes until arrhythmias subside or adverse reactions develop. Don't exceed 300-mg total bolus

during a 1-hour period. Simultaneously, constant infusion of 20 to 50 mcg/kg/minute (1 to 4 mg/minute) is begun. If single bolus has been given, smaller bolus dose may be repeated 15 to 20 minutes after start of infusion to maintain therapeutic serum level. Or, 200 to 300 mg I.M.; then second I.M. dose 60 to 90 minutes later, if needed.
**Children:** 0.5 to 1 mg/kg by I.V. bolus; then infusion of 10 to 50 mcg/kg/minute.
**Elderly:** reduce dosage and rate of infusion by 50%.
*Adjust-a-dose:* For patients with heart failure, renal or liver disease, or those weighing under 50 kg (110 lb), use reduced dosage.

## ADVERSE REACTIONS
**CNS:** *confusion, tremor,* lethargy, somnolence, *stupor, restlessness,* anxiety, hallucinations, nervousness, *light-headedness,* paresthesia, muscle twitching, *seizures.*
**CV:** hypotension, bradycardia, *new or worsened arrhythmias, cardiac arrest.*
**EENT:** *tinnitus, blurred or double vision.*
**GI:** vomiting.
**Respiratory:** *respiratory depression and arrest.*
**Other:** *anaphylaxis,* soreness at injection site, sensation of cold.

## INTERACTIONS
**Drug-drug.** *Beta blockers, cimetidine:* decreased metabolism of lidocaine. Monitor for toxicity.
*Mexiletine, tocainide:* additive pharmacologic effects. Avoid concomitant use.
*Phenytoin, procainamide, propranolol, quinidine:* additive cardiac depressant effects. Monitor carefully.
**Drug-herb.** *Pareira:* may add to or potentiate the effects of neuromuscular blockade. Avoid concomitant use.
**Drug-lifestyle.** *Smoking:* may increase metabolism of lidocaine. Monitor closely.

## EFFECTS ON DIAGNOSTIC TESTS
Because I.M. lidocaine therapy may increase CK levels, isoenzyme tests should be performed for differential diagnosis of acute MI.

---

Reactions may be *common,* uncommon, *life-threatening,* or COMMON AND LIFE-THREATENING.

## CONTRAINDICATIONS
Contraindicated in patients with hypersensitivity to the amide-type local anesthetics, Adams-Stokes syndrome, Wolff-Parkinson-White syndrome, and severe degrees of SA, AV, or intraventricular block in absence of artificial pacemaker.

## NURSING CONSIDERATIONS
• Use cautiously and in reduced dosages in patients with complete or second-degree heart block or sinus bradycardia, in elderly patients, in those with heart failure or renal or hepatic disease, and in those weighing under 110 lb (50 kg).
• Give I.M. injections in the deltoid muscle only.
• Monitor isoenzymes when using I.M. drug for suspected MI. A patient who has received I.M. lidocaine will show a sevenfold increase in serum CK level. Such an increase originates in the skeletal muscle, not the heart.
• Monitor serum levels as ordered. Therapeutic levels are 2 to 5 mcg/ml.
• *Alert:* Monitor patient for toxicity. In many severely ill patients, seizures may be the first sign of toxicity. However, severe reactions are usually preceded by somnolence, confusion, and paresthesia.
• If signs of toxicity such as dizziness occur, stop drug at once and notify doctor. Continuing could lead to seizures and coma. Give oxygen via nasal cannula if not contraindicated. Keep oxygen and cardiopulmonary resuscitation equipment available.
• Monitor patient's response, especially blood pressure and serum electrolytes, BUN, and creatinine levels, as ordered. Notify doctor promptly if abnormalities develop.
• Discontinue infusion and notify doctor if arrhythmias worsen or ECG changes, such as widening QRS complex or substantially prolonged PR interval, are evident.

**I.V. administration**
• Lidocaine injections containing 40, 100, or 200 mg/ml are for the preparation of I.V. infusion solutions only and must be diluted before use.
• Prepare I.V. infusion by adding 1 g of lidocaine hydrochloride (using 25 ml of 4% or 5 ml of 20% injection) to 1 L of 5% dextrose injection to provide a solution containing 1 mg/ml.
• A more concentrated solution of up to 8 mg/ml may be used if patient is fluid restricted.
• Patients receiving infusions must be on a cardiac monitor and must be attended at all times. Use an infusion control device for administering infusion precisely. Don't exceed rate of 4 mg/minute; faster rate greatly increases risk of toxicity.
• Injections containing preservatives shouldn't be given I.V.

☑ **Patient teaching**
• Inform patient receiving lidocaine I.M. that drug may cause soreness at injection site. Instruct patient receiving drug I.V. to alert nurse if discomfort occurs at the insertion site.
• Tell patient to report adverse reactions promptly because toxicity can occur.

## mexiletine hydrochloride
Mexitil

*Pregnancy Risk Category C*

### HOW SUPPLIED
*Capsules:* 50 mg‡, 100 mg†, 150 mg, 200 mg, 250 mg
*Injection:* 250 mg/10 ml‡

### ACTION
A class IB antiarrhythmic that blocks the fast sodium channel in cardiac tissues, especially the Purkinje network, without involving the autonomic nervous system. Drug reduces the rate of rise and amplitude of the action potential and decreases automaticity in the Purkinje fibers. It also shortens the duration of the action potential and, to a lesser extent, decreases the effective refractory period in the Purkinje fibers.

| Route | Onset | Peak | Duration |
|-------|-------|------|----------|
| P.O. | 0.5-2 hr | 2-3 hr | Unknown |
| I.V. | Immediate | Immediate | Unknown |

## INDICATIONS & DOSAGE

*Refractory life-threatening ventricular arrhythmias, including ventricular tachycardia and PVC—*
**Adults:** 200 to 400 mg P.O.; then 200 mg q 8 hours. Dose increased q 2 to 3 days to 400 mg q 8 hours if satisfactory control isn't obtained. Patients who respond well to a q-12-hour schedule may be given up to 450 mg q 12 hours.
*Note:* Where available, mexiletine may be given I.V.‡—
**Adults:** loading dose is 100 to 250 mg I.V. at a rate of 25 mg/minute. Then prepare an infusion solution of 250 mg mexiletine in 500 ml of $D_5W$, and administer the first 120 ml (60 mg) over 1 hour. If clinical response is inadequate, give another bolus of 200 mg over 10 to 20 minutes. Maintenance dose is 0.5 mg/minute (1 ml/minute of prepared solution).

## ADVERSE REACTIONS

**CNS:** *tremor, dizziness,* blurred vision, diplopia, confusion, *light-headedness, incoordination,* changes in sleep habits, paresthesia, weakness, fatigue, speech difficulties, tinnitus, depression, *nervousness,* headache.
**CV:** NEW OR WORSENED ARRHYTHMIAS, palpitations, chest pain, nonspecific edema, angina.
**GI:** *nausea, vomiting, upper GI distress, heartburn,* diarrhea, constipation, dry mouth, changes in appetite, abdominal pain.
**Hepatic:** transient alterations in liver function tests.
**Skin:** rash.

## INTERACTIONS

**Drug-drug.** *Antacids, atropine, narcotics:* slowed mexiletine absorption. Monitor patient.
*Cimetidine:* increased or decreased mexiletine blood levels. Monitor carefully.
*Methylxanthines (such as caffeine, theophylline):* reduced clearance of methylxanthines, possibly resulting in toxicity. Monitor carefully.
*Metoclopramide:* mexiletine absorption may be accelerated. Monitor for toxicity.

*Phenobarbital, phenytoin, rifampin, urine acidifiers:* decreased mexiletine blood levels. Monitor carefully.
*Urine alkalinizers:* increased mexiletine blood levels. Monitor carefully.

## EFFECTS ON DIAGNOSTIC TESTS

None reported.

## CONTRAINDICATIONS

Contraindicated in patients with cardiogenic shock or preexisting second- or third-degree AV block in the absence of an artificial pacemaker.

## NURSING CONSIDERATIONS

• Use cautiously in patients with preexisting first-degree heart block, a ventricular pacemaker, preexisting sinus node dysfunction, intraventricular conduction disturbances, hypotension, severe heart failure, or seizure disorder.
• When changing from lidocaine to mexiletine, stop the lidocaine infusion when the first mexiletine dose is given. Keep the infusion line open, however, until the arrhythmia is satisfactorily controlled.
• Administer oral dose with meals or antacids to lessen GI distress.
• If patient may be a good candidate for q-12-hour therapy, notify doctor. Twice-daily dosage enhances compliance.
• Monitor therapeutic levels, as ordered. Levels range from 0.5 to 2 mcg/ml.
• An early sign of mexiletine toxicity is tremor, usually a fine tremor of the hands, progressing to dizziness and then to ataxia and nystagmus as drug level in the blood increases. Monitor for and question patients about these symptoms.
• Monitor blood pressure and heart rate and rhythm frequently. Notify doctor of significant change.

### 🔃 I.V. administration

• Mexiletine injection is compatible with normal saline, $D_5W$, 5% sodium bicarbonate, 1/6 M sodium lactate, and 10% fructose (levulose) solutions.
• Administer I.V. dose during continuous ECG monitoring.

---

Reactions may be *common,* uncommon, *life-threatening,* or COMMON AND LIFE-THREATENING.

✓ **Patient teaching**
• Tell patient to take drug exactly as prescribed and to take with food or antacids if GI reactions occur.
• Instruct patient to report adverse reactions promptly.
• Tell patient receiving drug I.V. to report discomfort at insertion site.

---

**moricizine hydrochloride**
Ethmozine

*Pregnancy Risk Category B*

**HOW SUPPLIED**
*Tablets:* 200 mg, 250 mg, 300 mg

**ACTION**
A class I antiarrhythmic that reduces the fast inward current carried by sodium ions across myocardial cell membranes. Drug has potent local anesthetic activity and membrane-stabilizing effect.

| Route | Onset | Peak | Duration |
|-------|-------|------|----------|
| P.O. | Unknown | 0.5-2 hr | 10-24 hr |

**INDICATIONS & DOSAGE**
*Life-threatening ventricular arrhythmias—*
**Adults:** individualized dosage is based on clinical response and patient tolerance. Therapy should begin in the hospital. Most patients respond to 600 to 900 mg P.O. daily in divided doses q 8 hours. Daily dose increased q 3 days by 150 mg until desired effect is seen.
*Adjust-a-dose:* For patients with hepatic or renal impairment, 600 mg or less P.O. daily.

**ADVERSE REACTIONS**
**CNS:** *dizziness,* headache, fatigue, hyperesthesia, anxiety, asthenia, depression, nervousness, paresthesia, sleep disorders.
**CV:** *ventricular tachycardia, PVC, supraventricular arrhythmias, ECG abnormalities including conduction defects, sinus pause, junctional rhythm, and AV block, heart failure,* palpitations, thrombophlebitis, chest pain, *cardiac death,* hypotension, hypertension, vasodilation, cerebrovascular events.

**EENT:** blurred vision.
**GI:** nausea, vomiting, abdominal pain, dyspepsia, diarrhea, dry mouth.
**GU:** urine retention, urinary frequency, dysuria.
**Hepatic:** elevated liver function test results.
**Musculoskeletal:** musculoskeletal pain.
**Respiratory:** dyspnea.
**Skin:** rash, diaphoresis.
**Other:** drug-induced fever.

**INTERACTIONS**
**Drug-drug.** *Cimetidine:* increased plasma levels and decreased clearance of moricizine. Begin moricizine therapy at low dosage (not more than 600 mg daily), and monitor plasma levels and therapeutic effect closely.
*Digoxin, propranolol:* additive prolongation of PR interval. Monitor closely.
*Theophylline:* increased clearance and reduced plasma levels of theophylline. Monitor plasma levels and therapeutic response; adjust theophylline dosage as needed.

**EFFECTS ON DIAGNOSTIC TESTS**
None reported.

**CONTRAINDICATIONS**
Contraindicated in patients with hypersensitivity to drug, cardiogenic shock, or preexisting second- or third-degree AV block or right bundle-branch block when associated with left hemiblock (bifascicular block) unless an artificial pacemaker is present.

**NURSING CONSIDERATIONS**
• Because drug appears in breast milk, a decision should be made to discontinue breast-feeding or drug, depending on potential benefit of therapy to mother.
• Use with extreme caution in patients with sick sinus syndrome because drug may cause sinus bradycardia or sinus arrest. Also use with extreme caution in patients with coronary artery disease and left ventricular dysfunction because these patients may be at risk for sudden death when treated with the drug.
• Patients with hepatic or renal dysfunction will have decreased moricizine clear-

---

ance. Administer drug cautiously and monitor effects closely.

• When substituting moricizine for another antiarrhythmic, previous drug should be withdrawn for one to two of the drug's half-lives before moricizine is started. Patients who have shown a tendency to develop life-threatening arrhythmias after withdrawal of previous antiarrhythmic drug therapy should be hospitalized during withdrawal and adjustment to moricizine. Guidelines used for when to start moricizine therapy are

–disopyramide, 6 to 12 hours after the last dose.

–flecainide, 12 to 24 hours after last dose.

–mexiletine, 8 to 12 hours after last dose.

–procainamide, 3 to 6 hours after last dose.

–propafenone, 8 to 12 hours after last dose.

–quinidine, 6 to 12 hours after last dose.

–tocainide, 8 to 12 hours after last dose.

• Determine electrolyte status and correct imbalances before therapy, as ordered. Hypokalemia, hyperkalemia, and hypomagnesemia may alter the effects of drug.

• *Alert:* Don't confuse Ethmozine with Erythrocin.

☑ **Patient teaching**

• Instruct patient to take drug exactly as prescribed and not to abruptly discontinue use.

• Tell patient to avoid hazardous activities if adverse CNS reactions or blurred vision occurs.

• Instruct patient to report persistent or serious adverse reactions promptly.

---

**procainamide hydrochloride**
Procanbid, Promine, Pronestyl**,
Pronestyl-SR

*Pregnancy Risk Category C*

**HOW SUPPLIED**
*Tablets:* 250 mg, 375 mg, 500 mg
*Tablets (extended-release):* 250 mg, 500 mg, 750 mg, 1,000 mg
*Capsules:* 250 mg, 375 mg, 500 mg
*Injection:* 100 mg/ml, 500 mg/ml

**ACTION**
A class IA antiarrhythmic that decreases excitability, conduction velocity, automaticity, and membrane responsiveness with prolonged refractory period. Larger than usual doses may induce AV block.

| Route | Onset | Peak | Duration |
|-------|-------|------|----------|
| P.O. | Unknown | 0.75-2.5 hr | Unknown |
| I.V. | Immediate | Immediate | Unknown |
| I.M. | 10-30 min | 15-60 min | Unknown |

**INDICATIONS & DOSAGE**
*Life-threatening ventricular arrhythmias—*
**Adults:** 50 to 100 mg by slow I.V. push q 5 minutes, no faster than 25 to 50 mg/minute until arrhythmias disappear, adverse reactions develop, or 500 mg has been given. Or, give a loading dose I.V. infusion of 500 to 600 mg over 25 to 30 minutes. Usual effective dose is 500 to 600 mg. When arrhythmias disappear, give continuous infusion of 1 to 6 mg/minute. If arrhythmias recur, repeat bolus as above and increase infusion rate. Or, give 50 mg/kg I.M. in divided doses q 3 to 6 hours until oral therapy begins.

For P.O. administration, give 50 mg/kg daily in divided doses q 3 hours (average is 250 to 500 mg q 3 hours); for extended-release tablets, give 50 mg/kg daily in divided doses q 6 hours. For Procanbid extended-release tablets, give 50 mg/kg daily in equally divided doses q 12 hours.
*Adjust-a-dose:* For patients with renal or hepatic dysfunction, decreased dosages or longer dosing intervals may be needed.

**ADVERSE REACTIONS**
**CNS:** hallucinations, confusion, *seizures,* depression, dizziness.
**CV:** *hypotension,* bradycardia, AV block, *ventricular fibrillation, ventricular asystole.*
**GI:** abdominal pain, nausea, vomiting, anorexia, diarrhea, bitter taste.
**Hepatic:** increased bilirubin, alkaline phosphatase, ALT, and AST levels.
**Skin:** *maculopapular rash, urticaria, pruritus, flushing, angioneurotic edema.*
**Other:** *fever, lupus-like syndrome,* elevated LD.

---

Reactions may be *common,* uncommon, *life-threatening,* or COMMON AND LIFE-THREATENING.

## INTERACTIONS
**Drug-drug.** *Amiodarone:* increased procainamide levels and toxicity; additive effects on QT interval and QRS complex. Avoid concomitant use.
*Anticholinergics:* additive antivagal effects. Monitor closely.
*Anticholinesterases:* may decrease effect of anticholinesterases. Anticholinesterase dosage may need to be increased.
*Beta blockers, cimetidine, ranitidine, trimethoprim:* may increase procainamide blood levels. Monitor for toxicity.
*Neuromuscular blockers:* increased skeletal muscle relaxant effects. Monitor patient closely.
**Drug-herb.** *Jimsonweed:* may adversely affect CV function. Avoid concomitant use.
*Licorice:* may prolong QT interval and be additive. Use cautiously.
**Drug-lifestyle.** *Alcohol use:* reduced drug levels. Avoid use.

## EFFECTS ON DIAGNOSTIC TESTS
Drug will invalidate bentiromide test results; discontinue at least 3 days before bentiromide test. Procainamide may alter edrophonium test results, and may cause positive antinuclear antibody (ANA) titers, positive direct antiglobulin (Coombs') tests, and ECG changes.

## CONTRAINDICATIONS
Contraindicated in patients with hypersensitivity to procaine and related drugs and in those with complete, second-, or third-degree heart block in the absence of an artificial pacemaker. Also contraindicated in those with myasthenia gravis; systemic lupus erythematosus; or atypical ventricular tachycardia (torsades de pointes) because procainamide may aggravate this condition.

## NURSING CONSIDERATIONS
• Use with extreme caution when treating patients with ventricular tachycardia during coronary occlusion.
• Use cautiously in patients with heart failure or conduction disturbances, such as bundle-branch heart block, sinus bradycardia, or digitalis intoxication, and in those with hepatic or renal insufficien-cy. Also use cautiously in patients with preexisting blood dyscrasias or bone marrow suppression.
• Monitor plasma levels of procainamide and its active metabolite NAPA. To suppress ventricular arrhythmias, therapeutic serum levels of procainamide are 4 to 8 mcg/ml; therapeutic levels of NAPA are 10 to 30 mcg/ml.
• Monitor QT interval closely in patients with renal failure.
• Hypokalemia predisposes patient to arrhythmias; therefore, monitor serum electrolytes, especially potassium level.
• Elderly patients may be more likely to develop hypotension. Monitor blood pressure carefully.
• Monitor CBC frequently during first 3 months of therapy.
• Positive ANA titer is common in about 60% of patients who don't have symptoms of lupus-like syndrome. This response seems to be related to prolonged use, not dosage. May progress to systemic lupus erythematosus if drug isn't discontinued.
• **Alert:** Don't confuse procainamide with probenecid.

## 🔲 I.V. administration
• **Alert:** Monitor blood pressure and ECG continuously during I.V. administration. Watch for prolonged QT intervals and QRS complexes, heart block, or increased arrhythmias. If they occur, withhold drug, obtain rhythm strip, and notify doctor immediately.
• Dilute with compatible I.V. solution such as 5% dextrose injection and administer with the patient in supine position at a rate not exceeding 25 to 50 mg/minute.
• Attend patient receiving infusions at all times. Use an infusion control device to administer infusion precisely.
• Note that the vials for I.V. injection contain 1 g of drug: 100 mg/ml (10 ml) or 500 mg/ml (2 ml).
• Keep patient in supine position during I.V. administration. If drug is given too rapidly, hypotension can occur. Watch closely for adverse reactions during infusion, and notify doctor if they occur.

---

*Liquid contains alcohol.   **May contain tartrazine.   †Canada   ‡Australia   §U.K.   ◇OTC

☑ **Patient teaching**

• Stress importance of taking drug exactly as prescribed. This may require use of an alarm clock for nighttime doses.

• Instruct patient to report fever, rash, muscle pain, diarrhea, bleeding, bruises, or pleuritic chest pain.

• Tell patient not to crush or break extended-release tablets.

• Reassure patient who is taking the extended-release form that a wax-matrix "ghost" from the tablet may be passed in stools. Drug is completely absorbed before this occurs.

## propafenone hydrochloride
Arythmol§, Rythmol

*Pregnancy Risk Category C*

### HOW SUPPLIED
*Tablets:* 150 mg, 225 mg, 300 mg

### ACTION
A class IC antiarrhythmic that reduces inward sodium current in Purkinje and myocardial cells. Drug decreases excitability, conduction velocity, and automaticity in AV nodal, His-Purkinje, and intraventricular tissue and causes slight but significant prolongation of refractory period in AV nodal tissue.

| Route | Onset | Peak | Duration |
|-------|-------|------|----------|
| P.O. | Unknown | 3.5 hr | Unknown |

### INDICATIONS & DOSAGE
*Suppression of life-threatening ventricular arrhythmias such as sustained ventricular tachycardia—*
**Adults:** initially, 150 mg P.O. q 8 hours. May increase dosage at 3- to 4-day intervals to 225 mg q 8 hours; if needed, increase dosage to 300 mg q 8 hours. Maximum daily dose is 900 mg.

### ADVERSE REACTIONS
**CNS:** anxiety, ataxia, *dizziness,* drowsiness, fatigue, headache, insomnia, syncope, tremor.
**CV:** atrial fibrillation, bradycardia, bundle-branch block, *heart failure,* angina, chest pain, edema, first-degree AV block, hypotension, increased QRS complex, intraventricular conduction delay, palpitations, ***proarrhythmic events, including ventricular tachycardia, PVC, ventricular fibrillation.***
**EENT:** blurred vision.
**GI:** abdominal pain or cramps, constipation, diarrhea, dyspepsia, anorexia, flatulence, *nausea, vomiting,* dry mouth, unusual taste.
**Musculoskeletal:** joint pain.
**Respiratory:** dyspnea.
**Skin:** rash, diaphoresis.

### INTERACTIONS
**Drug-drug.** *Antiarrhythmics:* increased risk of heart failure. Monitor closely.
*Cardiac glycosides, cyclosporine, oral anticoagulants:* propafenone may increase serum levels of these agents by 35% to 85%, resulting in toxicity. Monitor closely.
*Cimetidine:* decreased metabolism of propafenone. Monitor closely.
*Desipramine:* decreased metabolism of desipramine. Monitor closely.
*Local anesthetics:* increased risk of CNS toxicity. Monitor closely.
*Metoprolol, propranolol:* propafenone slows the metabolism of these agents. Adjust dosage as ordered.
*Quinidine:* slowed metabolism of propafenone. Avoid concomitant use.
*Rifampin:* increased clearance of propafenone. Monitor closely.
*Theophylline:* decreased metabolism of theophylline. Monitor closely.

### EFFECTS ON DIAGNOSTIC TESTS
Drug may cause positive antinuclear antibody (ANA) titers.

### CONTRAINDICATIONS
Contraindicated in patients with hypersensitivity to drug and in those with severe or uncontrolled heart failure; cardiogenic shock; SA, AV, or intraventricular disorders of impulse conduction in the absence of a pacemaker; bradycardia; marked hypotension; bronchospastic disorders; or electrolyte imbalance.

---

## NURSING CONSIDERATIONS

• Use cautiously in patients with heart failure because propafenone can exert a negative inotropic effect on the heart. Also use cautiously in patients taking other cardiac depressant drugs and in those with hepatic or renal failure.

• To minimize adverse GI reactions, administer drug with food.

• Continuous cardiac monitoring is recommended during initiation of therapy and during dosage adjustments. If PR interval or QRS complex increases by more than 25%, a reduction in dosage may be needed.

• During use with digoxin, frequently monitor ECG and serum digoxin levels.

☑ **Patient teaching**

• Stress importance of taking drug exactly as prescribed.

• Tell patient to report adverse reactions promptly.

---

### quinidine bisulfate
(66.4% quinidine base), Kinidin Durules‡

### quinidine gluconate
(62% quinidine base) Quinaglute Dura-Tabs, Quinate†

### quinidine polygalacturonate
(60.5% quinidine base) Cardioquin

### quinidine sulfate
(83% quinidine base) Apo-Quinidine†, Cin-Quin, Novoquinidin†, Quinidex Extentabs, Quinora

*Pregnancy Risk Category C*

## HOW SUPPLIED
**quinidine bisulfate**
*Tablets (extended-release):* 250 mg†‡
**quinidine gluconate**
*Tablets (extended-release):* 324 mg, 325 mg†, 330 mg
*Injection:* 80 mg/ml
**quinidine polygalacturonate**
*Tablets:* 275 mg

**quinidine sulfate**
*Tablets:* 200 mg, 300 mg
*Tablets (extended-release):* 300 mg
*Capsules:* 200 mg, 300 mg
*Injection:* 200 mg/ml†

## ACTION
A class IA antiarrhythmic that has both direct and indirect (anticholinergic) effects on cardiac tissue. Drug decreases automaticity, conduction velocity, and membrane responsiveness. The effective refractory period is prolonged, and the anticholinergic action reduces vagal tone.

| Route | Onset | Peak | Duration |
|-------|-------|------|----------|
| P.O. | 1-3 hr | 1-6 hr | 6-8 hr |
| I.V. | Immediate | Immediate | Unknown |
| I.M. | 0.5-1.5 min | Unknown | Unknown |

## INDICATIONS & DOSAGE
*Atrial flutter or fibrillation—*
**Adults:** 300 to 400 mg quinidine sulfate or equivalent base P.O. q 6 hours. Or, 200 mg P.O. q 2 to 3 hours for 5 to 8 doses, increased daily until sinus rhythm is restored or toxic effects develop. Administer quinidine only after AV node has been blocked with a beta blocker, digoxin, or a calcium channel blocker to avoid increasing AV conduction. Maximum dose is 3 to 4 g daily.
*Paroxysmal supraventricular tachycardia—*
**Adults:** 400 to 600 mg P.O. gluconate q 2 to 3 hours until toxic adverse reactions develop or arrhythmia subsides.
*Premature atrial and ventricular contractions, paroxysmal AV junctional rhythm, paroxysmal atrial tachycardia, paroxysmal ventricular tachycardia, maintenance after cardioversion of atrial fibrillation or flutter—*
**Adults:** test dose is 200 mg P.O. or I.M. Quinidine sulfate or equivalent base 200 to 400 mg P.O. q 4 to 6 hours or 600 mg quinidine sulfate extended-release every 8 to 12 hours; or quinidine gluconate 800 mg (10 ml of commercially available solution) added to 40 ml of $D_5W$, infused I.V. at 2.5 mg/kg/minute.
**Children:** 30 mg/kg/24 hours or 900 mg/ $m^2$/24 hours P.O. in five divided doses.

---

*Severe* Plasmodium falciparum *malaria—*
**Adults:** 10 mg/kg gluconate I.V. diluted in 250 ml of normal saline solution and infused over 1 to 2 hours; then a continuous maintenance infusion of 0.02 mg/kg/minute for 72 hours or until parasitemia is reduced to less than 1%.
*Adjust-a-dose:* Use reduced dosage for patients with impaired hepatic function or heart failure.

## ADVERSE REACTIONS
**CNS:** *vertigo, headache, light-headedness,* confusion, ataxia, depression, dementia.
**CV:** *PVC; ventricular tachycardia; atypical ventricular tachycardia (torsades de pointes); hypotension; complete AV block,* tachycardia; *aggravated heart failure; ECG changes (particularly widening of QRS complex, widened QT and PR intervals).*
**EENT:** *tinnitus,* excessive salivation, blurred vision, diplopia, photophobia.
**GI:** *diarrhea, nausea, vomiting,* anorexia, abdominal pain.
**Hematologic:** *hemolytic anemia, thrombocytopenia, agranulocytosis.*
**Hepatic:** *hepatotoxicity.*
**Respiratory:** acute asthmatic attack, *respiratory arrest.*
**Skin:** rash, petechial hemorrhage of buccal mucosa, pruritus, urticaria, lupus erythematosus, photosensitivity.
**Other:** *angioedema, fever, cinchonism.*

## INTERACTIONS
**Drug-drug.** *Acetazolamide, antacids, sodium bicarbonate, thiazide diuretics:* may increase quinidine blood levels because of alkaline urine. Monitor for increased effect.
*Amiodarone, cimetidine:* increased serum quinidine levels. Monitor for increased effect.
*Barbiturates, phenytoin, rifampin:* may lower blood levels of quinidine. Monitor for decreased effect.
*Digoxin:* increased serum digoxin levels after initiating quinidine therapy. Monitor closely.
*Fluvoxamine, nefazodone, tricyclic antidepressants:* increased blood levels with increased effect. Monitor closely.

*Nifedipine:* may decrease quinidine blood levels. Monitor carefully.
*Other antiarrhythmics (such as lidocaine, procainamide, propranolol):* increased risk of toxicity. Use together cautiously.
*Verapamil:* may result in hypotension, bradycardia, or AV block. Monitor blood pressure and heart rate.
*Warfarin:* increased anticoagulant effect. Monitor closely.
**Drug-herb.** *Jimsonweed:* may adversely affect CV function. Avoid concomitant use.
*Licorice:* may prolong the QT interval and be additive. Use together cautiously.

## EFFECTS ON DIAGNOSTIC TESTS
None reported.

## CONTRAINDICATIONS
Contraindicated in patients with idiosyncrasy or hypersensitivity to quinidine or related cinchona derivatives and in those with myasthenia gravis, intraventricular conduction defects, digitalis toxicity when AV conduction is grossly impaired, abnormal rhythms due to escape mechanisms, and history of prolonged QT syndrome. Also contraindicated in patients who developed thrombocytopenia with prior exposure to quinidine or quinine.

## NURSING CONSIDERATIONS
• Use cautiously in patients with asthma, muscle weakness, or infection accompanied by fever because hypersensitivity reactions to drug may be masked.
• Also use cautiously in patients with hepatic or renal impairment because systemic accumulation may occur.
• Check apical pulse rate and blood pressure before therapy. If extremes in pulse rate are detected, withhold drug and notify doctor at once.
• Anticoagulant therapy is commonly advised before quinidine therapy in long-standing atrial fibrillation because restoration of normal sinus rhythm may result in thromboembolism caused by dislodgment of thrombi from atrial wall.
• *Alert:* When changing route of administration or oral salt form, be aware that dosage needs to be altered to compensate for variations in quinidine base content.

• Never use discolored (brownish) quinidine solution.

• Don't crush extended-release tablets.

• Quinidine gluconate I.M. is no longer recommended for treatment of arrhythmias because of erratic absorption.

• *Alert:* Patients with severe malaria should be hospitalized in an intensive-care setting. Continuous monitoring is needed. Decrease infusion rate if plasma quinidine level exceeds 6 mcg/ml, uncorrected QT interval exceeds 0.6 second, or QRS complex widening exceeds 25% of baseline.

• Monitor liver function test results during first 4 to 8 weeks of therapy.

• Monitor serum quinidine levels as ordered. Therapeutic plasma levels for antiarrhythmic effects are 2 to 5 mcg/ml.

• Monitor patient response carefully. If adverse GI reactions occur, especially diarrhea, notify doctor. Check quinidine blood levels, which are toxic when greater than 8 mcg/ml. GI symptoms may be decreased by giving drug with meals or aluminum hydroxide antacids.

• Store drug away from heat and direct light.

• *Alert:* Don't confuse quinidine with quinine or clonidine.

### 🔲 I.V. administration

• For quinidine gluconate infusion to treat atrial fibrillation/flutter in adults, dilute 800 mg (10 ml of injection) with 40 ml 5% dextrose injection and infuse at a rate of up to 0.25 mg/kg/minute.

• During infusion, continuously monitor patient's blood pressure and ECG.

• Titrate rate so that the arrhythmia is corrected without disturbing the normal mechanism of the heart beat.

• For quinidine gluconate infusion to treat malaria, dilute in 5 ml/kg (usually 250 ml) normal saline and infuse over 1 to 2 hours, followed by a continuous maintenance infusion.

### ✅ Patient teaching

• Stress importance of taking drug exactly as prescribed and taking it with food if adverse GI reactions occur.

• Tell patient not to crush or chew extended-release tablets.

• Tell patient to report persistent or serious adverse reactions promptly, especially signs and symptoms of quinidine toxicity.

---

## sotalol
Beta-Cardone§, Betapace, Sotacor†‡

*Pregnancy Risk Category B*

### HOW SUPPLIED
*Tablets:* 80 mg, 120 mg, 160 mg, 240 mg

### ACTION
A nonselective beta blocker that depresses sinus heart rate, slows AV conduction, decreases cardiac output, and lowers systolic and diastolic blood pressure.

| Route | Onset | Peak | Duration |
|-------|-------|------|----------|
| P.O. | Unknown | 2.5-4 hr | Unknown |

### INDICATIONS & DOSAGE
*Documented, life-threatening ventricular arrhythmias—*
**Adults:** initially, 80 mg P.O. b.i.d. Dosage is increased q 2 to 3 days as needed and tolerated; most patients respond to daily dose of 160 to 320 mg. A few patients with refractory arrhythmias have received as much as 640 mg daily.

*Adjust-a-dose:* For patients with renal failure, if creatinine clearance is above 60 ml/minute, no adjustment in dosage interval is needed. If creatinine clearance is 30 to 60 ml/minute, dosage interval is increased to q 24 hours; if clearance is between 10 and 30 ml/minute, q 36 to 48 hours; and if it's below 10 ml/minute, dosage must be individualized.

### ADVERSE REACTIONS
**CNS:** *asthenia, headache, dizziness, weakness, fatigue,* sleep problems, *lightheadedness.*
**CV:** *bradycardia, **arrhythmias, heart failure, AV block, proarrhythmic events, including polymorphic ventricular tachycardia, PVC, ventricular fibrillation,** edema, palpitations, chest pain,* ECG abnormalities, hypotension.
**GI:** *nausea, vomiting,* diarrhea, dyspepsia.

**Hepatic:** increased liver enzyme levels.
**Metabolic:** hyperglycemia
**Respiratory:** *dyspnea, bronchospasm.*

## INTERACTIONS
**Drug-drug.** *Antiarrhythmics:* additive effects. Avoid concomitant use.
*Antihypertensives, catecholamine-depleting drugs (such as guanethidine, reserpine):* enhanced hypotensive effects. Monitor closely.
*Calcium channel blockers:* enhanced myocardial depression. Avoid concomitant use.
*Clonidine:* beta blockers may enhance rebound effect after withdrawal of clonidine. Discontinue sotalol several days before withdrawing clonidine.
*General anesthetics:* may cause additional myocardial depression. Monitor closely.
*Insulin, oral antidiabetics:* may cause hyperglycemia. Adjust dosage. May mask symptoms of hypoglycemia.
**Drug-food.** *Any food:* decreased absorption by 20%. Give drug on empty stomach.

## EFFECTS ON DIAGNOSTIC TESTS
Drug may cause a false-positive catecholamine level.

## CONTRAINDICATIONS
Contraindicated in patients with hypersensitivity to drug and in those with severe sinus node dysfunction, sinus bradycardia, second- and third-degree AV block in the absence of an artificial pacemaker, congenital or acquired long QT syndrome, cardiogenic shock, uncontrolled heart failure, and bronchial asthma.

## NURSING CONSIDERATIONS
• Use cautiously in patients with renal impairment or diabetes mellitus. Beta blockers may mask signs and symptoms of hypoglycemia.
• Because proarrhythmic events may occur at start of therapy and during dosage adjustments, patient should be hospitalized. Facilities and personnel should be available for cardiac rhythm monitoring and interpretation of ECG.
• Although patients receiving I.V. lidocaine have started sotalol therapy without

ill effect, other antiarrhythmics should be withdrawn before therapy with sotalol. Sotalol therapy typically is delayed until two or three half-lives of the withdrawn drug have elapsed. After withdrawal of amiodarone, sotalol shouldn't be administered until the QT interval normalizes.
• Dosage should be adjusted slowly, allowing 2 to 3 days between dosage increments for adequate monitoring of QT intervals and for plasma levels of drug to reach a steady-state level.
• Monitor serum electrolytes regularly, especially if patient is receiving diuretics. Electrolyte imbalances, such as hypokalemia or hypomagnesemia, may enhance QT-interval prolongation and increase the risk of serious arrhythmias such as torsades de pointes.
• ***Alert:*** Don't confuse sotalol with Statrol or Stadol.

✓ **Patient teaching**
• Explain importance of taking drug as prescribed, even when the patient is feeling well. Caution against suddenly discontinuing drug.
• Caution against taking OTC drugs and decongestants while taking drug.
• Because food can interfere with absorption, tell patient to take drug on an empty stomach, 1 hour before or 2 hours after meals.

## tocainide hydrochloride
Tonocard

*Pregnancy Risk Category C*

### HOW SUPPLIED
*Tablets:* 400 mg, 600 mg

### ACTION
A class IB antiarrhythmic that blocks the fast sodium channel in cardiac tissues, especially the Purkinje network, without involvement of the autonomic nervous system. It reduces the rate of rise and amplitude of the action potential and decreases automaticity in the Purkinje fibers. It shortens the duration of action potential and, to a lesser extent, decreases the effec-

tive refractory period in the Purkinje fibers.

| Route | Onset | Peak | Duration |
|-------|-------|------|----------|
| P.O. | Unknown | 0.5-2 hr | 8 hr |

## INDICATIONS & DOSAGE
*Suppression of symptomatic life-threatening ventricular arrhythmias—*
**Adults:** initially, 400 mg P.O. q 8 hours. Usual dose is between 1,200 and 1,800 mg daily in three divided doses.
*Adjust-a-dose:* For patients with renal or hepatic impairment, dose less than 1,200 mg daily may be adequate.

## ADVERSE REACTIONS
**CNS:** ataxia, *light-headedness, tremor,* paresthesia, *dizziness, vertigo,* drowsiness, fatigue, confusion, headache.
**CV:** hypotension, ***new or worsened arrhythmias, heart failure,*** bradycardia, palpitations.
**EENT:** blurred vision, tinnitus.
**GI:** *nausea, vomiting,* diarrhea, anorexia.
**Hepatic:** hepatitis, abnormal liver function test results.
**Skin:** rash, diaphoresis.

## INTERACTIONS
**Drug-drug.** *Beta blockers:* decreased myocardial contractility; increased CNS toxicity. Monitor closely.
*Disopyramide, lidocaine, mexiletine, phenytoin, procainamide, quinidine:* additive pharmacologic effect and CV and CNS toxicity. Monitor patient.
*Rifampin:* increased clearance of tocainide. Monitor efficacy of tocainide.

## EFFECTS ON DIAGNOSTIC TESTS
None reported.

## CONTRAINDICATIONS
Contraindicated in patients with hypersensitivity to lidocaine or other amide-type local anesthetics and in those with second- or third-degree AV block in the absence of an artificial pacemaker.

## NURSING CONSIDERATIONS
• Use cautiously in patients with heart failure or diminished cardiac reserve and in those with hepatic or renal impairment.

These patients often may be treated effectively with a lower dose.
• Drug may ease transition from I.V. lidocaine to oral antiarrhythmic. Monitor patient carefully.
• Correct potassium deficits, as ordered; drug may be ineffective in hypokalemia.
• Monitor patient for tremor, which may indicate that maximum dosage has been reached.

### ☑ Patient teaching
• Instruct patient to report immediately unusual bruising or bleeding or signs of infection. Agranulocytosis and bone marrow suppression have been reported in patients taking usual doses of drug, typically within first 12 weeks of therapy.
• Advise patient to report sudden onset of pulmonary symptoms, such as coughing, wheezing, or exertional dyspnea. Drug has been associated with serious pulmonary toxicity.
• Tell elderly patient to take safety precautions because dizziness and falling may occur.

amlodipine besylate
amyl nitrite
bepridil hydrochloride
diltiazem hydrochloride
isosorbide dinitrate
isosorbide mononitrate
nadolol
nicardipine hydrochloride
nifedipine
nitroglycerin
propranolol hydrochloride
verapamil
verapamil hydrochloride

**COMBINATION PRODUCTS**
LOTREL: amlodipine 2.5 mg and benazepril hydrochloride 10 mg, amlodipine 5 mg and benazepril hydrochloride 10 mg, amlodipine 5 mg and benazepril hydrochloride 20 mg.

---

**amlodipine besylate**
Istin§, Norvasc

*Pregnancy Risk Category C*

**HOW SUPPLIED**
*Tablets:* 2.5 mg, 5 mg, 10 mg

**ACTION**
Inhibits calcium ion influx across cardiac and smooth-muscle cells, thus decreasing myocardial contractility and oxygen demand; also dilates coronary arteries and arterioles.

| Route | Onset | Peak | Duration |
|-------|-------|------|----------|
| P.O. | Unknown | 6-12 hr | 24 hr |

**INDICATIONS & DOSAGE**
*Chronic stable angina, vasospastic angina (Prinzmetal's or variant angina)—*
**Adults:** initially, 5 to 10 mg P.O. daily. Most patients require 10 mg daily.
**Elderly:** initially, 5 mg P.O. daily.
***Adjust-a-dose:*** For small, frail patients or those with hepatic insufficiency, initially 5 mg P.O. daily.

*Hypertension—*
**Adults:** initially, 2.5 to 5 mg P.O. daily. Dosage adjusted according to patient response and tolerance. Maximum daily dose is 10 mg.
**Elderly:** initially, 2.5 mg P.O. daily.
***Adjust-a-dose:*** For small, frail, patients; those currently receiving other antihypertensives; or those with hepatic insufficiency, initially 2.5 mg P.O. daily.

**ADVERSE REACTIONS**
**CNS:** *headache,* somnolence, fatigue, dizziness, light-headedness, paresthesia.
**CV:** *edema,* flushing, palpitations.
**GI:** nausea, abdominal pain.
**Musculoskeletal:** muscle pain.
**Respiratory:** dyspnea.
**Skin:** rash, pruritus.

**INTERACTIONS**
None significant.

**EFFECTS ON DIAGNOSTIC TESTS**
None reported.

**CONTRAINDICATIONS**
Contraindicated in patients with hypersensitivity to drug.

**NURSING CONSIDERATIONS**
• Use cautiously in patients receiving other peripheral vasodilators, especially those with severe aortic stenosis, and in those with heart failure. Because drug is metabolized by the liver, use cautiously and in reduced dosage in patients with severe hepatic disease.
• *Alert:* Monitor patient carefully. Some patients, especially those with severe obstructive coronary artery disease, have developed increased frequency, duration, or severity of angina or acute MI after initiation of calcium channel blocker therapy or at time of dosage increase.
• Monitor blood pressure frequently during initiation of therapy. Because drug-induced vasodilation has a gradual onset, acute hypotension is rare.

---

Reactions may be *common,* uncommon, *life-threatening,* or COMMON AND LIFE-THREATENING.

• Notify doctor if signs of heart failure occur, such as swelling of hands and feet or shortness of breath.
• **Alert:** Don't confuse amlodipine with amiloride.

### ☑ Patient teaching
• Caution patient to continue taking drug, even when feeling better.
• Tell patient S.L. nitroglycerin may be taken as needed when angina symptoms are acute. If patient continues nitrate therapy during adjustment of amlodipine dosage, urge continued compliance.

---

## amyl nitrite

*Pregnancy Risk Category X*

### HOW SUPPLIED
*Ampules (crushable):* 0.3 ml

### ACTION
Unknown. Drug's effect is thought to be the result of dilation of both arterial and venous beds. The net effect is a reduction in myocardial oxygen demand, improving perfusion to the ischemic myocardium. Drug converts hemoglobin to methemoglobin (which binds cyanide) to treat cyanide poisoning.

| Route | Onset | Peak | Duration |
|-------|-------|------|----------|
| Inhalation | 30 sec | Unknown | 3-5 min |

### INDICATIONS & DOSAGE
*Relief of angina pectoris—*
**Adults and children:** 0.3 ml by inhalation (one glass ampule), p.r.n.
*Antidote for cyanide poisoning—*
**Adults and children:** 0.3 ml by inhalation for 15 to 60 seconds q 5 minutes until sodium nitrite infusion is available.

### ADVERSE REACTIONS
**CNS:** *headache, sometimes with throbbing;* dizziness; weakness, syncope.
**CV:** *orthostatic hypotension, tachycardia,* flushing, palpitations.
**GI:** nausea, vomiting.
**Hematologic:** methemoglobinemia.
**Skin:** cutaneous vasodilation, rash.
**Other:** *hypersensitivity reactions.*

### INTERACTIONS
**Drug-drug.** *Calcium channel blockers:* increased risk of symptomatic orthostatic hypotension. Monitor closely.
**Drug-lifestyle.** *Alcohol use:* severe hypotension and CV collapse may occur. Monitor patient.

### EFFECTS ON DIAGNOSTIC TESTS
Drug alters the Zlatkis-Zak color reaction, causing a false decrease in serum cholesterol levels.

### CONTRAINDICATIONS
Contraindicated in patients with hypersensitivity to nitrates; also contraindicated in those with severe anemia, angle-closure glaucoma, orthostatic hypotension, early MI, and increased intracranial pressure, and during pregnancy.

### NURSING CONSIDERATIONS
• Use cautiously in patients with glaucoma (except angle-closure type, which is a contraindication), volume depletion, or hypotension.
• Extinguish all cigarettes before administering because ampule may ignite.
• Wrap ampule in cloth and crush. Hold near patient's nose and mouth so vapor is inhaled.
• Watch for orthostatic hypotension.
• Store away from light.
• Drug is claimed to have aphrodisiac benefits and is often abused. Street name is "Amy."

### ☑ Patient teaching
• Show patient how to administer drug. Stress importance of extinguishing all cigarettes before use.
• Tell patient to sit and avoid position changes while inhaling drug to prevent orthostatic hypotension.
• Advise patient to take a mild analgesic for drug-induced headache.

---

## bepridil hydrochloride
Vascor

*Pregnancy Risk Category C*

### HOW SUPPLIED
*Tablets:* 200 mg, 300 mg, 400 mg

### ACTION
A calcium channel blocker that inhibits calcium ion influx across cardiac and smooth-muscle cells, thereby dilating coronary arteries and peripheral arteries and arterioles. Drug may reduce heart rate, decrease myocardial contractility, and slow AV node conduction.

| Route | Onset | Peak | Duration |
|-------|-------|------|----------|
| P.O. | 1 hr | 2-3 hr | 24 hr |

### INDICATIONS & DOSAGE
*Chronic stable angina in patients who can't tolerate or who fail to respond to other agents—*
**Adults:** initially, 200 mg P.O. daily. After 10 days, dosage increased based on response. Maintenance daily dose in most patients is 300 mg; maximum daily dose is 400 mg.

### ADVERSE REACTIONS
**CNS:** *dizziness,* drowsiness, *nervousness, headache,* insomnia, paresthesia, *asthenia,* tremor.
**CV:** edema, flushing, palpitations, tachycardia, ***ventricular arrhythmias, including torsades de pointes, ventricular tachycardia, ventricular fibrillation.***
**EENT:** tinnitus.
**GI:** *nausea, diarrhea,* constipation, abdominal discomfort, dry mouth, anorexia.
**Hepatic:** increased ALT levels, abnormal liver function test results.
**Respiratory:** dyspnea, shortness of breath.
**Skin:** rash.
**Other:** flulike syndrome.

### INTERACTIONS
**Drug-drug.** *Antiarrhythmics, cardiac glycosides, drugs that increase QT interval:* may exaggerate prolongation of the QT interval or depression of AV node with bepridil. Monitor closely.
*Digoxin:* serum digoxin levels may be increased. Monitor combined use.
*Fentanyl:* may cause severe hypotension. Monitor patient.

### EFFECTS ON DIAGNOSTIC TESTS
None reported.

### CONTRAINDICATIONS
Contraindicated in patients with hypersensitivity to drug; also contraindicated in those with uncompensated cardiac insufficiency, sick sinus syndrome second- or third-degree AV block unless pacemaker is present, hypotension (below 90 mm Hg systolic), congenital QT-interval prolongation, or history of serious ventricular arrhythmias. Don't use in those receiving other drugs that prolong the QT interval.

### NURSING CONSIDERATIONS
• Use cautiously in patients with left bundle-branch block, sinus bradycardia, impaired renal or hepatic function, or heart failure.
• Monitor patient for adverse reactions. Bepridil has been associated with severe ventricular arrhythmias, including torsades de pointes.
• Dosage shouldn't be adjusted more frequently than every 10 to 14 days because of bepridil's long half-life and the time it takes to reach steady-state blood levels.
• *Alert:* Don't confuse bepridil with Prepidil.

### ☑ Patient teaching
• Instruct patient to take drug exactly as directed.
• Tell patient to protect drug from light.

# diltiazem hydrochloride
Adizem-60§, Adizem-SR§,
Adizem-XL Plus§, Angitil SR§,
Apo-Diltiaz†, Calcicard CR§,
Cardizem, Cardizem CD,
Cardizem SR, Dilacor XR,
Dilzem SR§, Dilzem XL§,
Slozem§, Tiazac, Tildiem§,
Tildiem LA§, Tildiem Retard§,
Viazem XL§, Zemtard 300XL§

*Pregnancy Risk Category C*

## HOW SUPPLIED
*Tablets:* 30 mg, 60 mg, 90 mg, 120 mg
*Capsules (extended-release; Cardizem CD, Dilacor XR, Tiazac):* 120 mg, 180 mg, 240 mg, 300 mg, 360 mg (Tiazac)
*Capsules (sustained-release; Cardizem SR):* 60 mg, 90 mg, 120 mg, 180 mg, 240 mg
*Injection:* 5 mg/ml

## ACTION
A calcium channel blocker that inhibits calcium ion influx across cardiac and smooth-muscle cells, decreasing myocardial contractility and oxygen demand. Also dilates coronary arteries and arterioles.

| Route | Onset | Peak | Duration |
|---|---|---|---|
| P.O. | 0.5-1 hr | 2-3 hr | 6-8 hr |
| P.O. (extended, sustained) | 2-3 hr | 10-14 hr | 12-24 hr |
| I.V. | Within 3 min | 2-7 min | 1-10 hr |

## INDICATIONS & DOSAGE
*Vasospastic angina (Prinzmetal's or variant angina), classic chronic stable angina pectoris—*
**Adults:** 30 mg P.O. t.i.d. or q.i.d. before meals and h.s., increased gradually to maximum of 360 mg daily in divided doses. Or, 120 or 180 mg (extended-release). Adjusted as needed and tolerated to maximum of 480 mg daily.
*Hypertension—*
**Adults:** 60 to 120 mg P.O. b.i.d. (sustained-release). Adjusted to effect. Maximum dose is 360 mg daily. Or, initially 180 to 240 mg daily (extended-release). Dosage adjusted, p.r.n.
*Atrial fibrillation or flutter, paroxysmal supraventricular tachycardia—*
**Adults:** 0.25 mg/kg as an I.V. bolus injection over 2 minutes. If response is inadequate, 0.35 mg/kg I.V. after 15 minutes followed by a continuous infusion of 10 mg/hour. Some patients respond well to a rate of 5 mg/hour; maximum dose is 15 mg/hour.

## ADVERSE REACTIONS
**CNS:** *headache,* dizziness, asthenia, somnolence.
**CV:** *edema,* **arrhythmias,** flushing, bradycardia, hypotension, conduction abnormalities, **heart failure,** AV block, abnormal ECG.
**GI:** *nausea, constipation,* abdominal discomfort.
**Hepatic:** acute hepatic injury.
**Skin:** *rash.*

## INTERACTIONS
**Drug-drug.** *Anesthetics:* effects may be potentiated. Monitor patient.
*Carbamazepine:* increased levels of carbamazepine. Monitor carbamazepine levels and watch for signs and symptoms of toxicity.
*Cimetidine:* may inhibit diltiazem metabolism. Monitor for toxicity, additive AV node conduction slowing.
*Cyclosporine:* diltiazem may increase serum cyclosporine levels, possibly by decreasing its metabolism, leading to increased risk of cyclosporine toxicity. If used concurrently, monitor cyclosporine levels.
*Digoxin:* diltiazem may increase serum levels of digoxin. Monitor for toxicity.
*Furosemide:* forms a precipitate when mixed with diltiazem injection. Administer through separate I.V. lines.
*Propranolol, other beta blockers:* may precipitate heart failure or prolong conduction time. Use together cautiously.

## EFFECTS ON DIAGNOSTIC TESTS
None reported.

---

*Liquid contains alcohol.    **May contain tartrazine.    †Canada    ‡Australia    §U.K.    ◊OTC

## CONTRAINDICATIONS

Contraindicated in patients with hypersensitivity to drug, sick sinus syndrome or second- or third-degree AV block in the absence of an artificial pacemaker, systolic blood pressure below 90 mm Hg, acute MI, or pulmonary congestion (documented by X-ray).

## NURSING CONSIDERATIONS

• Use cautiously in elderly patients and in those with heart failure or impaired hepatic or renal function.
• Monitor blood pressure and heart rate during initiation of therapy and during dosage adjustments.
• If systolic blood pressure is below 90 mm Hg or heart rate is below 60 beats/minute, withhold dose and notify doctor.
• *Alert:* Don't confuse Cardizem SR with Cardene SR.

🔲 **I.V. administration**
• For direct I.V. injection, no dilution of 5 mg/ml injection is necessary.
• For continuous I.V. infusion, 5 mg/ml injection should be added to 100, 200 or 500 ml of normal saline, 5% dextrose, or 5% dextrose and half-normal saline to produce a final concentration of 1, 0.83, or 0.45 mg/ml.
• Drug in monovials labeled as containing 100 mg should be reconstituted according to manufacturer's directions.
• For direct injection or continuous infusion, give slowly under continuous ECG and blood pressure monitoring.
• Infusions lasting longer than 24 hours aren't recommended.

☑ **Patient teaching**
• Advise patient to avoid hazardous activities during initiation of therapy.
• If nitrate therapy is prescribed during adjustment of diltiazem dosage, urge patient compliance. Tell patient that S.L. nitroglycerin especially may be taken concomitantly as needed when angina symptoms are acute.
• Tell patient to swallow Dilacor XR whole, and not to open, crush, or chew it.

## isosorbide dinitrate
Apo-ISDN†, Cedocard Retard§, Cedocard SR†, Dilatrate-SR, Ismo Retard§, Isonate, Isorbid, Isordil, Isordil Tembids, Isordil Titradose, Isotrate, Novosorbide†, Sorbid SA§, Sorbichew§, Sorbitrate

## isosorbide mononitrate
Elantan§, Imdur, Isib 60XL§, ISMO, Isotrate§, Modisal XL§, Monit§, Mono-Cedocard§, Monoket, Monosorb XL 60§

*Pregnancy Risk Category C*

## HOW SUPPLIED
**isosorbide dinitrate**
*Tablets:* 5 mg, 10 mg, 20 mg, 30 mg, 40 mg
*Tablets (S.L.):* 2.5 mg, 5 mg, 10 mg
*Tablets (chewable):* 5 mg, 10 mg
*Tablets (sustained-release):* 40 mg
*Capsules:* 40 mg
*Capsules (sustained-release):* 40 mg
**isosorbide mononitrate**
*Tablets:* 10 mg, 20 mg
*Tablets (extended-release):* 30 mg, 60 mg, 120 mg

## ACTION
Not completely known. Thought to reduce cardiac oxygen demand by decreasing preload and afterload. Drug also may increase blood flow through the collateral coronary vessels.

| Route | Onset | Peak | Duration |
|---|---|---|---|
| P.O. | 15-40 min | Unknown | 4-6 hr |
| P.O. (S.L.) | 2-5 min | Unknown | 1.5 hr |
| P.O. (chewable) | 2-5 min | Unknown | 2-2.5 hr |
| P.O. (extended) | 0.5-4 hr | Unknown | 12 hr |

## INDICATIONS & DOSAGE
*Acute angina attacks (S.L. and chewable tablets of isosorbide dinitrate only), prophylaxis in situations likely to cause angina attacks—*
**Adults:** *S.L. form*—2.5 to 5 mg S.L. for prompt relief of angina pain, repeated q 5 to 10 minutes (maximum of three doses

for each 30-minute period). For prophylaxis, 2.5 to 10 mg q 2 to 3 hours.
*Chewable form*—5 to 10 mg, p.r.n., for acute attack or q 2 to 3 hours for prophylaxis, but only after initial test dose of 5 mg to determine risk of severe hypotension.
*Oral form (isosorbide dinitrate)*—5 to 30 mg P.O. t.i.d. or q.i.d. for prophylaxis only (use smallest effective dose); 20 to 40 mg P.O. (sustained-release) q 6 to 12 hours.
*Oral form (isosorbide mononitrate using Imdur)*—30 to 60 mg P.O. once daily upon arising; increased to 120 mg once daily after several days, if needed.
*Oral form (isosorbide mononitrate using ISMO or Monoket)*—20 mg b.i.d. with the two doses given 7 hours apart.

## ADVERSE REACTIONS
**CNS:** *headache;* dizziness; weakness.
**CV:** *orthostatic hypotension, tachycardia, palpitations, ankle edema, fainting, flushing.*
**GI:** nausea, vomiting.
**Skin:** cutaneous vasodilation, rash.
**Other:** sublingual burning.

## INTERACTIONS
**Drug-drug.** *Antihypertensives:* may increase hypotensive effects. Monitor closely during initial therapy.
*Sildenafil:* may increase hypotensive effects. Avoid concomitant use.
**Drug-lifestyle.** *Alcohol use:* may increase hypotension. Avoid concomitant use.

## EFFECTS ON DIAGNOSTIC TESTS
May interfere with serum cholesterol determination tests using the Zlatkis-Zak color reaction, causing a falsely decreased value.

## CONTRAINDICATIONS
Contraindicated in patients with hypersensitivity or idiosyncrasy to nitrates, severe hypotension, angle-closure glaucoma, increased intracranial pressure, shock, or acute MI with low left ventricular filling pressure.

## NURSING CONSIDERATIONS
• Use cautiously in patients with blood volume depletion (such as from diuretic therapy) or mild hypotension.
• To prevent development of tolerance, a nitrate-free interval of 8 to 12 hours/day has been recommended. The regimen for isosorbide mononitrate (one tablet upon awakening with the second dose in 7 hours, or one extended-release tablet daily) is intended to minimize nitrate tolerance by providing a substantial nitrate-free interval.
• Monitor blood pressure and intensity and duration of drug response.
• Drug may cause headaches, especially at beginning of therapy. Dosage may be reduced temporarily, but tolerance usually develops. Treat headache with aspirin or acetaminophen.
• **Alert:** Don't confuse Isordil with Isuprel or Inderal.

### ☑ Patient teaching
• Caution patient to take medication regularly, as prescribed, and to keep it accessible at all times.
• **Alert:** Advise patient that abrupt discontinuation of drug may cause coronary vasospasm with increased angina symptoms and potential risk of MI.
• Tell patient to take S.L. tablet at first sign of attack. The tablet should be wet with saliva and placed under the tongue until absorbed; the patient should sit down and rest. Dose may be repeated every 10 to 15 minutes for a maximum of three doses. If drug doesn't provide relief, tell patient to seek medical help promptly.
• Advise patient who complains of tingling sensation with S.L. drug to try holding tablet in buccal pouch.
• Warn patient not to confuse S.L. with P.O. form.
• Advise patient taking P.O. form of isosorbide dinitrate to take oral tablet on an empty stomach either 30 minutes before or 1 to 2 hours after meals, to swallow oral tablets whole, and to chew chewable tablets thoroughly before swallowing.
• Tell patient to minimize orthostatic hypotension by changing to upright position slowly. Advise him to go up and down stairs carefully and to lie down at first sign of dizziness.

---

*Liquid contains alcohol.   **May contain tartrazine.   †Canada   ‡Australia   §U.K.   ◇OTC

• Inform patient to store drug in a cool place, in a tightly closed container, and away from light.

## nadolol
Corgard

*Pregnancy Risk Category C*

### HOW SUPPLIED
*Tablets:* 20 mg, 40 mg, 80 mg, 120 mg, 160 mg

### ACTION
A beta blocker that reduces cardiac oxygen demand by blocking catecholamine-induced increases in heart rate, blood pressure, and force of myocardial contraction. Depresses renin secretion.

| Route | Onset | Peak | Duration |
|-------|-------|------|----------|
| P.O. | Unknown | 2-4 hr | Unknown |

### INDICATIONS & DOSAGE
*Angina pectoris—*
**Adults:** 40 mg P.O. once daily. Dosage increased in 40- to 80-mg increments at 3- to 7-day intervals until optimum response occurs. Usual maintenance dose is 40 to 80 mg once daily; up to 240 mg once daily may be needed.
*Hypertension—*
**Adults:** 20 to 40 mg P.O. once daily. Dosage increased in 40- to 80-mg increments until optimum response occurs. Usual maintenance dose is 40 to 80 mg once daily. Doses of 320 mg may be needed.
*Adjust-a-dose:* For patients with renal failure, dosage interval should be adjusted based on creatinine clearance. For creatinine clearance of over 50 ml/minute, give dose q 24 hours; for clearance of 31 to 50 ml/minute, give dose q 24 to 36 hours; for clearance of 10 to 30 ml/minute, give dose q 24 to 48 hours; and for clearance below 10 ml/minute, give dose q 40 to 60 hours.

### ADVERSE REACTIONS
**CNS:** fatigue, dizziness.
**CV:** *bradycardia, hypotension, **heart failure,*** peripheral vascular disease, rhythm and conduction disturbances.
**GI:** nausea, vomiting, diarrhea, abdominal pain, constipation, anorexia.
**Respiratory:** *increased airway resistance.*
**Skin:** rash.
**Other:** fever.

### INTERACTIONS
**Drug-drug.** *Antihypertensives:* enhanced antihypertensive effect. Monitor closely.
*Cardiac glycosides:* excessive bradycardia and additive effects on AV conduction. Use together cautiously.
*Epinephrine:* severe vasoconstriction and reflex bradycardia. Monitor blood pressure carefully.
*Insulin, oral antidiabetics:* can alter dosage requirements in previously stabilized diabetic patients. Observe patient carefully.
*Phenothiazines:* can result in additive hypotensive effects. Monitor closely.
*NSAIDs:* decreased antihypertensive effect. Monitor blood pressure and adjust dosage.

### EFFECTS ON DIAGNOSTIC TESTS
None reported.

### CONTRAINDICATIONS
Contraindicated in patients with bronchial asthma, sinus bradycardia and greater than first-degree heart block, and cardiogenic shock.

### NURSING CONSIDERATIONS
• Use cautiously in patients with heart failure, chronic bronchitis, emphysema, or renal or hepatic impairment and in patients undergoing major surgery involving general anesthesia. Also use cautiously in diabetic patients because beta blockers may mask certain signs and symptoms of hypoglycemia.
• Check apical pulse before giving drug. If slower than 60 beats/minute, withhold drug and call doctor.
• Monitor blood pressure frequently. If patient develops severe hypotension, administer a vasopressor, as prescribed.
• *Alert:* Abrupt discontinuation can exacerbate angina and precipitate MI. Dosage should be reduced gradually over 1 to 2 weeks.

---

Reactions may be *common,* uncommon, *life-threatening,* or COMMON AND LIFE-THREATENING.

• Nadolol masks signs and symptoms of shock and hyperthyroidism.

☑ **Patient teaching**
• Explain importance of taking drug as prescribed, even when patient is feeling well.
• Teach patient how to check pulse rate and to do so before each dose. If pulse rate is below 60 beats/minute, tell patient to notify doctor.
• Caution patient not to discontinue drug suddenly.

---

## nicardipine hydrochloride
Cardene, Cardene IV,
Cardene SR

*Pregnancy Risk Category C*

### HOW SUPPLIED
*Capsules (immediate-release):* 20 mg, 30 mg
*Capsules (sustained-release):* 30 mg, 45 mg, 60 mg
*Injection:* 2.5 mg/ml

### ACTION
A calcium channel blocker that inhibits calcium ion influx across cardiac and smooth-muscle cells, decreasing myocardial contractility and oxygen demand. Also dilates coronary arteries and arterioles.

| Route | Onset | Peak | Duration |
|---|---|---|---|
| P.O. (immediate) | 0.5-1.5 min | Unknown | Unknown |
| P.O. (sustained) | 20 min | 1-4 hr | 12 hr |
| I.V. | Immediate | Immediate | Unknown |

### INDICATIONS & DOSAGE
*Chronic stable angina (used alone or with other antianginals)—*
**Adults:** initially, 20 mg P.O. t.i.d. (immediate-release only). Dosage adjusted based on patient response q 3 days. Usual dosage range is 20 to 40 mg t.i.d.
*Hypertension—*
**Adults:** initially, 20 mg P.O. t.i.d. (immediate-release); range, 20 to 40 mg t.i.d. Or, 30 mg b.i.d. (sustained-release);

range, 30 to 60 mg b.i.d. Dosage increased based on patient response. Or, for patients unable to take oral nicardipine, 50 ml/hour (5 mg/hour) I.V. infusion initially; then increased by 25 ml/hour (2.5 mg/hour) q 15 minutes up to maximum of 150 ml/hour (15 mg/hour).

### ADVERSE REACTIONS
**CNS:** *dizziness, light-headedness, headache, asthenia.*
**CV:** *peripheral edema, palpitations,* angina, tachycardia, *flushing.*
**GI:** nausea, abdominal discomfort, dry mouth.
**Skin:** rash.

### INTERACTIONS
**Drug-drug.** *Antihypertensives:* enhanced antihypertensive effect. Monitor closely.
*Beta blockers:* may increase cardiac depressant effects. Monitor closely.
*Cimetidine:* may decrease metabolism of calcium channel blockers. Monitor for increased pharmacologic effect.
*Cyclosporine:* nicardipine may increase plasma levels of cyclosporine. Monitor for toxicity.
*Theophylline:* pharmacologic effects of theophylline may be enhanced. Monitor for toxicity.

### EFFECTS ON DIAGNOSTIC TESTS
None reported.

### CONTRAINDICATIONS
Contraindicated in patients with hypersensitivity to drug or advanced aortic stenosis.

### NURSING CONSIDERATIONS
• Use cautiously in patients with hypotension, heart failure, or impaired hepatic and renal function.
• Measure blood pressure frequently during initial therapy. Maximum blood pressure response occurs about 1 hour after dosing with the immediate-release form and 2 to 4 hours with the sustained-release form. Check for potential orthostatic hypotension. Because large swings in blood pressure may occur based on blood level of drug, assess adequacy of antihypertensive effect 8 hours after dosing.

---

• Extended-release form is preferred because of improved medication adherence, fewer fluctuations in blood pressure, and increased risk in mortality with short-acting agents.
• *Alert:* Don't confuse Cardene with Cardura or codeine. Don't confuse Cardene SR with Cardizem SR.

### I.V. administration
• Dilute with compatible I.V. solution before administration.
• Administer by slow I.V. infusion in a concentration of 0.1mg/ml.
• Closely monitor blood pressure during and after completion of infusion.
• Titrate infusion rate, as ordered, if hypotension or tachycardia occurs.
• Change peripheral infusion site every 12 hours to minimize risk of venous irritation.
• When switching to oral therapy other than nicardipine, initiate therapy upon discontinuation of the infusion. If oral nicardipine is to be used, administer first dose of t.i.d. regimen 1 hour before discontinuing infusion.

### ☑ Patient teaching
• Tell patient to take oral form of drug exactly as prescribed.
• Advise patient to report chest pain immediately. Some patients may experience increased frequency, severity, or duration of chest pain at beginning of therapy or during dosage adjustments.

## nifedipine
Adalat, Adalat CC, Adalat XL†, Adalat PA†, Adipine MR§, Apo-Nifed†, Cardilate MR§, Coracten§, Hypolar Retard 20§, Nifedotard 20 MR§, Nifelease§, Nifensar XL§, Novo-Nifedin†, Nu-Nifed†, Procardia, Procardia XL, Tensipine MR§, Unipine XL§

*Pregnancy Risk Category C*

## HOW SUPPLIED
*Tablets (extended-release):* 30 mg, 60 mg, 90 mg
*Capsules:* 10 mg, 20 mg

## ACTION
Unknown. Thought to inhibit calcium ion influx across cardiac and smooth-muscle cells, decreasing contractility and oxygen demand. Also may dilate coronary arteries and arterioles.

| Route | Onset | Peak | Duration |
|-------|-------|------|----------|
| P.O. | 20 min | 0.5-1 hr | 4-8 hr |
| P.O. (extended) | 20 min | 6 hr | 24 hr |

## INDICATIONS & DOSAGE
*Vasospastic angina (Prinzmetal's or variant angina), classic chronic stable angina pectoris—*
**Adults:** initially 10 mg P.O. t.i.d. Usual effective dosage range is 10 to 20 mg t.i.d. Some patients may require up to 30 mg q.i.d. Maximum daily dose is 180 mg.
*Hypertension—*
**Adults:** 30 or 60 mg P.O. (extended-release form) once daily. Adjusted over 7 to 14 days. Doses larger than 90 mg (for Adalat CC) and 120 mg (for Procardia XL) aren't recommended.

## ADVERSE REACTIONS
**CNS:** *dizziness, light-headedness, headache, weakness,* syncope, nervousness.
**CV:** *peripheral edema,* hypotension, palpitations, **heart failure, MI,** pulmonary edema, *flushing.*
**EENT:** nasal congestion.
**GI:** *nausea,* diarrhea, constipation, abdominal discomfort.
**Hepatic:** increased serum levels of alkaline phosphate, LD, AST, and ALT.
**Metabolic:** hypokalemia.
**Musculoskeletal:** muscle cramps.
**Respiratory:** dyspnea, cough.
**Skin:** rash, pruritus.

## INTERACTIONS
**Drug-drug.** *Cimetidine, ranitidine:* decreased nifedipine metabolism. Dosage may be adjusted.
*Digoxin:* may cause elevated digoxin levels. Monitor closely.
*Fentanyl:* severe hypotension may occur. Monitor closely.

Reactions may be *common,* uncommon, *life-threatening*, or COMMON AND LIFE-THREATENING.

*Propranolol, other beta blockers,:* may cause hypotension and heart failure. Use together cautiously.
*Phenytoin:* may reduce phenytoin metabolism. Monitor closely.
**Drug-food.** *Grapefruit juice:* increased bioavailability of nifedipine. Avoid concomitant use. Monitor patient closely if given together.

**EFFECTS ON DIAGNOSTIC TESTS**
None reported.

**CONTRAINDICATIONS**
Contraindicated in patients with hypersensitivity to drug.

**NURSING CONSIDERATIONS**
• Use cautiously in patients with heart failure or hypotension and in elderly patients. Use extended-release tablets cautiously in patients with severe GI narrowing.
• When a rapid response to drug is desired, have patient bite and swallow the capsule. If he can't chew capsules, the liquid can be withdrawn by puncturing the capsule with a needle and squeezing the contents into the mouth. When these methods are used, continuous blood pressure and ECG monitoring is recommended. These methods aren't recommended for the treatment of hypertension.
• Despite widespread S.L. use of nifedipine capsules, this route of administration should be avoided. Peak serum levels are lower and take longer to occur than when capsules are bitten and swallowed.
• Monitor blood pressure regularly, especially in patients who are taking beta blockers or antihypertensives.
• Although rebound effect hasn't been observed when drug is stopped, dosage should be reduced slowly under doctor's supervision.
• *Alert:* Don't confuse nifedipine with nimodipine or nicardipine.

☑ **Patient teaching**
• If patient is kept on nitrate therapy while nifedipine dosage is being adjusted, urge continued compliance. S.L. nitroglycerin especially may be taken as needed when angina symptoms are acute.

• Tell patient he may briefly develop angina exacerbation when beginning drug therapy or when dosage is increased.
• Instruct patient to swallow extended-release tablets without breaking, crushing, or chewing.
• Instruct patient to avoid taking drug with grapefruit juice.
• Reassure patient who is taking the extended-release form that a wax-matrix "ghost" from the tablet may be passed in the stools. Drug is completely absorbed before this occurs.
• Warn patient not to switch brands. Procardia XL and Adalat CC aren't therapeutically equivalent because of major differences in their pharmacokinetics.
• Tell patient to protect capsules from direct light and moisture and to store at room temperature.

---

## nitroglycerin (glyceryl trinitrate)
Anginine‡, Deponit, Minitran, Nitradisc‡, Nitro-Bid, Nitro-Bid IV, Nitrocine, Nitrodisc, Nitro-Dur, Nitrogard, Nitrogard SR†, Nitroglyn, Nitrol, Nitrolingual, Nitrong, Nitrostat, Nitro-Time, NTS, Transderm-Nitro, Transderm-Nitro‡, Tridil

*Pregnancy Risk Category C*

---

**HOW SUPPLIED**
*Tablets (buccal):* 1 mg, 2 mg, 3 mg
*Tablets (S.L.):* 0.15 mg (¹⁄₄₀₀ gr), 0.3 mg (¹⁄₂₀₀ gr), 0.4 mg (¹⁄₁₅₀ gr), 0.6 mg (¹⁄₁₀₀ gr)
*Tablets (sustained-release):* 2.6 mg, 6.5 mg, 9 mg, 13 mg
*Capsules (sustained-release):* 2.5 mg, 6.5 mg, 9 mg, 13 mg
*Aerosol (translingual):* 0.4 mg metered spray
*Topical:* 2% ointment
*Transdermal:* 0.1 mg, 0.2 mg, 0.3 mg, 0.4 mg, 0.6 mg, 0.8 mg per hour release rate
*Injection:* 0.5 mg/ml, 5 mg/ml

---

## ACTION
A nitrate that reduces cardiac oxygen demand by decreasing left ventricular end-diastolic pressure (preload) and, to a lesser extent, systemic vascular resistance (afterload). Also increases blood flow through the collateral coronary vessels.

| Route | Onset | Peak | Duration |
|---|---|---|---|
| P.O. | 20-45 min | Unknown | 3-8 hr |
| P.O. (buccal) | 3 min | Unknown | 3-5 hr |
| P.O. (S.L.) | 1-3 min | Unknown | 0.5-1 hr |
| I.V. | Immediate | Immediate | 3-5 min |
| Trans-lingual | 2-4 min | Unknown | 0.5-1 hr |
| Topical | 30 min | Unknown | 2-12 hr |
| Trans-dermal | 30 min | Unknown | 24 hr |

## INDICATIONS & DOSAGE
*Prophylaxis against chronic anginal attacks—*
**Adults:** 2.5 or 2.6 mg sustained-release capsule or tablet q 8 to 12 hours, adjusted upward to an effective dose in 2.5- or 2.6-mg increments b.i.d. to q.i.d. Or, use 2% ointment: Start dosage with ½-inch ointment, increasing by ½-inch increments until desired results are achieved. Range of dosage with ointment is ½ to 5 inches. Usual dose is 1 to 2 inches. Or, transdermal disc or pad (Nitrodisc, Nitro-Dur, or Transderm-Nitro) 0.2 to 0.4 mg/hour once daily.
*Acute angina pectoris, prophylaxis to prevent or minimize anginal attacks before stressful events—*
**Adults:** 1 S.L. tablet (gr ¹⁄₄₀₀, ¹⁄₂₀₀, ¹⁄₁₅₀, ¹⁄₁₀₀) dissolved under the tongue or in the buccal pouch as soon as angina begins. Repeat q 5 minutes, if needed, for 15 minutes. Or, using Nitrolingual spray, one or two sprays into mouth, preferably onto or under the tongue. Repeat q 3 to 5 minutes, if needed, to a maximum of three doses within a 15-minute period. Or, 1 to 3 mg transmucosally q 3 to 5 hours during waking hours.
*Hypertension associated with surgery, heart failure associated with MI, angina pectoris in acute situations, to produce controlled hypotension during surgery (by I.V. infusion)—*
**Adults:** initial infusion rate is 5 mcg/minute, increased p.r.n. by 5 mcg/minute q 3 to 5 minutes until response occurs. If a 20 mcg/minute rate doesn't produce a response, may increase dosage by as much as 20 mcg/minute q 3 to 5 minutes. Up to 100 mcg/minute may be needed.

## ADVERSE REACTIONS
**CNS:** *headache, dizziness,* weakness.
**CV:** *orthostatic hypotension, tachycardia, flushing, palpitations,* fainting.
**GI:** nausea, vomiting.
**Skin:** cutaneous vasodilation, contact dermatitis (patch), rash.
**Other:** *hypersensitivity reactions,* sublingual burning.

## INTERACTIONS
**Drug-drug.** *Antihypertensives:* possible enhanced hypotensive effect. Monitor closely.
*Heparin:* I.V. nitroglycerin interferes with anticoagulant effect of heparin in some patients. Monitor PTT.
*Sildenafil:* may increase risk of hypotension. Avoid concomitant use.
**Drug-lifestyle.** *Alcohol use:* possible increased hypotension. Avoid alcohol intake.

## EFFECTS ON DIAGNOSTIC TESTS
Nitroglycerin may interfere with serum cholesterol determination tests using the Zlatkis-Zak color reaction, resulting in falsely decreased values.

## CONTRAINDICATIONS
Contraindicated in patients with early MI, severe anemia, increased intracranial pressure, angle-closure glaucoma, orthostatic hypotension, allergy to adhesives (transdermal), or hypersensitivity to nitrates. I.V. nitroglycerin is contraindicated in patients with hypersensitivity to I.V. form, cardiac tamponade, restrictive cardiomyopathy, or constrictive pericarditis.

## NURSING CONSIDERATIONS
• Use cautiously in patients with hypotension or volume depletion.
• Closely monitor vital signs during infusion. Be particularly aware of blood pressure, especially in a patient with an MI. Excessive hypotension may worsen the MI.

• To apply ointment, measure the prescribed amount on the application paper; then place the paper on any nonhairy area. Don't rub in. Cover with plastic film to aid absorption and to protect clothing. Remove all excess ointment from previous site before applying the next dose. Avoid getting ointment on fingers.

• Transdermal dosage forms can be applied to any nonhairy part of the skin except distal parts of the arms or legs (absorption won't be maximal at distal sites).

• Remove transdermal patch before defibrillation. Because of the aluminum backing on the patch, the electric current may cause arcing that can result in damage to paddles and burns to the patient.

• When stopping transdermal treatment of angina, gradually reduce the dose and frequency of application over 4 to 6 weeks, as ordered.

• Monitor blood pressure and intensity and duration of drug response.

• Drug may cause headaches, especially at beginning of therapy. Dosage may be reduced temporarily, but tolerance usually develops. Treat headache with aspirin or acetaminophen.

• Tolerance to drug can be minimized with a 10- to 12-hour nitrate-free interval. To achieve this, remove the transdermal system in the early evening and apply a new system the next morning or omit the last daily dose of a buccal, sustained-release, or ointment form. Check with the doctor for alterations in dosage regimen if tolerance is suspected.

• *Alert:* Don't confuse Nitro-Bid with Nicobid or nitroglycerin with nitroprusside.

### ◻ I.V. administration
• Dilute with $D_5W$ or normal saline for injection. Concentration shouldn't exceed 400 mcg/ml. Always administer with an infusion control device and titrate to desired response. Also, always mix in glass bottles and avoid use of I.V. filters because drug binds to plastic. Regular polyvinyl chloride tubing can bind up to 80% of drug, making it necessary to infuse higher dosages. A special nonabsorbent polyvinyl chloride tubing is available from the manufacturer; patients receive more drug when these infusion sets are used. Always use the same type of infusion set when changing I.V. lines.

• When changing the concentration of infusion, flush the I.V. administration set with 15 to 20 ml of the new concentration before use. This will clear the line of the old drug solution.

### ☑ Patient teaching
• Caution patient to take nitroglycerin regularly, as prescribed, and to have it accessible at all times.

• *Alert:* Advise patient that abrupt discontinuation of drug causes coronary vasospasms.

• Teach patient how to administer the prescribed form of nitroglycerin.

• Tell patient to take S.L. tablet at first sign of attack. The tablet should be wet with saliva and placed under the tongue until absorbed, and the patient should sit down and rest. Dose may be repeated every 5 minutes for a maximum of three doses. If drug doesn't provide relief, medical help should be obtained promptly.

• Advise patient who complains of a tingling sensation with S.L. drug to try holding tablet in buccal pouch.

• Tell patient to take oral tablets on an empty stomach either 30 minutes before or 1 to 2 hours after meals, to swallow oral tablets whole, and not to chew tablets.

• Remind patient using translingual aerosol form that he shouldn't inhale the spray, but should release it onto or under the tongue. Also tell him to wait about 10 seconds or so before swallowing.

• Tell patient to place the buccal tablet between the lip and gum above the incisors or between the cheek and gum. Tablets shouldn't be swallowed or chewed.

• Tell patient to take an additional dose before anticipated stress or at bedtime if angina is nocturnal.

• Instruct patient wearing transdermal patch to use caution when near a microwave oven. Leaking radiation may heat patch's metallic backing and cause burns.

• Advise patient to avoid alcohol.

• To minimize orthostatic hypotension, tell patient to change to upright position slowly. Advise him to go up and down stairs carefully and to lie down at the first sign of dizziness.

• Tell patient to store drug in cool, dark place in a tightly closed container. Remove cotton from container because it absorbs drug.

• Tell patient to store S.L. tablets in original container or other container specifically approved for this use and to carry the container in a jacket pocket or purse, not in a pocket close to the body.

---

## propranolol hydrochloride
Apo-Propranolol†, Deralin‡, Inderal, Inderal LA, Novopranol†, pms Propranolol†

*Pregnancy Risk Category C*

### HOW SUPPLIED
*Tablets:* 10 mg, 20 mg, 40 mg, 60 mg, 80 mg, 90 mg
*Capsules (extended-release):* 60 mg, 80 mg, 120 mg, 160 mg
*Oral solution:* 4 mg/ml, 8 mg/ml, 80 mg/ml (concentrate)
*Injection:* 1 mg/ml

### ACTION
A nonselective beta blocker that reduces cardiac oxygen demand by blocking catecholamine-induced increases in heart rate, blood pressure, and force of myocardial contraction. Depresses renin secretion and prevents vasodilation of cerebral arteries.

| Route | Onset | Peak | Duration |
|-------|-------|------|----------|
| P.O. | 30 min | 1-1.5 hr | 12 hr |
| I.V. | Immediate | 1 min | 5 min |

### INDICATIONS & DOSAGE
*Angina pectoris—*
**Adults:** total daily doses of 80 to 320 mg P.O. when given b.i.d., t.i.d., or q.i.d. Or, one 80-mg extended-release capsule daily. Dosage increased at 3- to 7-day intervals.
*Mortality reduction after MI—*
**Adults:** 180 to 240 mg P.O. daily in divided doses beginning 5 to 21 days after MI has occurred. Usually administered t.i.d. or q.i.d.
*Supraventricular, ventricular, and atrial arrhythmias; tachyarrhythmias caused by*
*excessive catecholamine action during anesthesia, hyperthyroidism, or pheochromocytoma—*
**Adults:** 0.5 to 3 mg by slow I.V. push, not to exceed 1 mg/minute. After 3 mg have been given, another dose may be given in 2 minutes; subsequent doses, no sooner than q 4 hours. May be diluted and infused slowly. Usual maintenance dose is 10 to 30 mg P.O. t.i.d. or q.i.d.
*Hypertension—*
**Adults:** initially, 80 mg P.O. daily in two to four divided doses or extended-release form once daily. Increased at 3- to 7-day intervals to maximum daily dose of 640 mg. Usual maintenance dose is 160 to 480 mg daily.
*Prevention of frequent, severe, uncontrollable, or disabling migraine or vascular headache—*
**Adults:** initially, 80 mg P.O. daily in divided doses or one extended-release capsule daily. Usual maintenance dose is 160 to 240 mg daily, t.i.d. or q.i.d.
*Essential tremor—*
**Adults:** 40 mg (tablets, oral solution) P.O. b.i.d. Usual maintenance dose is 120 to 320 mg daily in three divided doses.
*Hypertrophic subaortic stenosis—*
**Adults:** 20 to 40 mg P.O. t.i.d. or q.i.d.; or 80 to 160 mg extended-release capsules once daily.
*Adjunct therapy in pheochromocytoma—*
**Adults:** 60 mg P.O. daily in divided doses with an alpha blocker 3 days before surgery.

### ADVERSE REACTIONS
**CNS:** *fatigue, lethargy,* vivid dreams, hallucinations, mental depression, lightheadedness, insomnia.
**CV:** *bradycardia, hypotension,* **heart failure,** intermittent claudication, intensification of AV block.
**GI:** abdominal cramping, constipation, diarrhea, nausea, vomiting.
**GU:** elevated BUN levels.
**Hematologic:** *agranulocytosis.*
**Hepatic:** elevated serum transaminase, alkaline phosphatase, and LDH levels.
**Respiratory:** *bronchospasm.*
**Skin:** rash.
**Other:** fever.

---

Reactions may be *common*, uncommon, *life-threatening*, or COMMON AND LIFE-THREATENING.

## INTERACTIONS

**Drug-drug.** *Aminophylline:* antagonized beta-blocking effects of propranolol. Use together cautiously.

*Cardiac glycosides, diltiazem, verapamil:* hypotension, bradycardia, and increased depressant effect on myocardium. Use together cautiously.

*Cimetidine:* inhibited metabolism of propranolol. Monitor for increased beta-blocking effect.

*Epinephrine:* severe vasoconstriction. Monitor blood pressure and observe patient carefully.

*Glucagon, isoproterenol:* antagonized propranolol effect. May be used therapeutically and in emergencies.

*Haloperidol:* cardiac arrest has occurred with concomitant therapy. Avoid use together.

*Insulin, oral antidiabetics:* can alter requirements for these drugs in previously stabilized diabetics. Monitor for hypoglycemia.

*Phenothiazines, reserpine:* additive effect. Use cautiously.

**Drug-herb.** *Betel palm:* decreased temperature-elevating effects and enhanced CNS effects. Avoid concomitant use.

**Drug-lifestyle.** *Cocaine use:* increased angina-inducing potential of cocaine. Monitor patient carefully.

## EFFECTS ON DIAGNOSTIC TESTS
None reported.

## CONTRAINDICATIONS
Contraindicated in patients with bronchial asthma, sinus bradycardia and heart block greater than first-degree, cardiogenic shock, and heart failure (unless failure is secondary to a tachyarrhythmia that can be treated with propranolol).

## NURSING CONSIDERATIONS
• Use cautiously in patients with renal impairment, nonallergic bronchospastic diseases, or hepatic disease and in those taking other antihypertensives. Because drug blocks some symptoms of hypoglycemia, use with caution in patients with diabetes mellitus. Also use cautiously in patients with thyrotoxicosis because drug may mask some signs and symptoms of that disorder. Elderly patients may experience enhanced adverse reactions and may need dosage adjustment.

• Always check patient's apical pulse before giving drug. If extremes in pulse rates occur, withhold drug and notify doctor immediately.

• Give drug consistently with meals. Food may increase absorption of propranolol.

• Drug masks common signs and symptoms of shock and hypoglycemia.

• **Alert:** Don't discontinue drug before surgery for pheochromocytoma. Before any surgical procedure, tell anesthesiologist that patient is receiving propranolol.

• Compliance may be improved by administering drug twice daily or as extended-release capsule. Check with doctor.

• **Alert:** Don't confuse propranolol with Pravachol. Don't confuse Inderal with Inderide, Isordil, Adderall, or Imuran.

### I.V. administration

• Give by direct injection into a large vessel or into the tubing of a free-flowing, compatible I.V. solution; continuous I.V. infusion generally isn't recommended. Or, dilute drug with normal saline and give by intermittent infusion over 10 to 15 minutes in 0.1- to 0.2-mg increments. Drug is compatible with $D_5W$ and half-normal and normal saline and lactated Ringer's solutions.

• Infusion rate shouldn't exceed 1 mg/minute.

• Double-check dose and route. I.V. doses are much smaller than oral doses.

• Monitor blood pressure, ECG, central venous pressure, and heart rate and rhythm frequently, especially during I.V. administration. If patient develops severe hypotension, notify doctor; a vasopressor may be prescribed.

• For overdose, give I.V. isoproterenol, I.V. atropine, or glucagon; refractory cases may require a pacemaker.

### Patient teaching

• Caution patient to continue taking this drug as prescribed, even when he is feeling well.

• Instruct patient to take drug with food.

• **Alert:** Tell patient not to discontinue drug suddenly because this can exacerbate angina and precipitate MI.

# verapamil
Apo-Verap†, Calan, Isoptin, Novo-Veramil†, Nu-Verap†

# verapamil hydrochloride
Anpec‡, Calan, Calan SR, Cordilox‡, Cordilox SR‡, Half-Securon SR§, Isoptin, Isoptin SR, Novo-Veramil†, Securon§, Securon SR§, Univer§, Veracaps SR‡, Verapress MR§, Verelan

*Pregnancy Risk Category C*

## HOW SUPPLIED
**verapamil**
*Tablets:* 40 mg, 80 mg, 120 mg
**verapamil hydrochloride**
*Tablets:* 40 mg, 80 mg, 120 mg, 160 mg‡
*Tablets (extended-release):* 120 mg, 180 mg, 240 mg, 360 mg
*Capsules (extended-release):* 120 mg, 160 mg‡, 180 mg, 240 mg, 360 mg
*Injection:* 2.5 mg/ml

## ACTION
Not clearly defined. A calcium channel blocker that inhibits calcium ion influx across cardiac and smooth-muscle cells, thus decreasing myocardial contractility and oxygen demand; it also dilates coronary arteries and arterioles.

| Route | Onset | Peak | Duration |
|-------|-------|------|----------|
| P.O. | 0.5 hr | 1-2 hr | 8-10 hr |
| P.O. (extended) | 0.5 hr | 5-9 hr | 24 hr |
| I.V. | Immediate | 1-5 min | 1-6 hr |

## INDICATIONS & DOSAGE
*Vasospastic angina (Prinzmetal's or variant angina); classic chronic, stable angina pectoris; chronic atrial fibrillation—*
**Adults:** starting dose is 80 to 120 mg P.O. t.i.d. Dosage increased at weekly intervals, p.r.n. Some patients may require up to 480 mg daily.
*Supraventricular arrhythmias—*
**Adults:** 0.075 to 0.15 mg/kg (5 to 10 mg) by I.V. push over 2 minutes with ECG and blood pressure monitoring. Repeat dose in 30 minutes if no response occurs.

**Children under age 1:** 0.1 to 0.2 mg/kg as I.V. bolus over 2 minutes with continuous ECG monitoring. Repeat dose in 30 minutes if no response occurs.
**Children ages 1 to 15:** 0.1 to 0.3 mg/kg as I.V. bolus over 2 minutes; not to exceed 5 mg.
*Hypertension—*
**Adults:** 240 mg extended-release tablet P.O. once daily in the morning. If response isn't adequate, give an additional 120 mg in the evening or 240 mg q 12 hours or an 80-mg immediate-release tablet t.i.d.

## ADVERSE REACTIONS
**CNS:** dizziness, headache, asthenia.
**CV:** *transient hypotension,* **heart failure,** pulmonary edema, bradycardia, AV block, ***ventricular asystole, ventricular fibrillation,*** peripheral edema.
**GI:** *constipation,* nausea.
**Hepatic:** elevated liver enzymes.
**Skin:** rash.

## INTERACTIONS
**Drug-drug.** *Antihypertensives, quinidine:* may result in hypotension. Monitor blood pressure.
*Carbamazepine, cardiac glycosides:* may increase serum levels of these drugs. Monitor for toxicity.
*Cyclosporine:* may increase cyclosporine serum levels. Monitor cyclosporine levels.
*Disopyramide, flecainide, propranolol, other beta blockers (including ophthalmic timolol):* may cause heart failure. Use together cautiously.
*Lithium:* may decrease or increase serum lithium levels. Monitor closely.
*Rifampin:* may decrease oral bioavailability of verapamil. Monitor patient for lack of effect.
**Drug-herb.** *Black catechu:* additive effects. Avoid concomitant use.
*Yerba maté:* may decrease clearance of yerba maté methylxanthines and cause toxicity. Use together cautiously.
**Drug-food.** *Any food:* increased absorption. Take drug with food.
**Drug-lifestyle.** *Alcohol use:* verapamil may enhance the effects of alcohol. Avoid use.

---

Reactions may be *common,* uncommon, *life-threatening*, or COMMON AND LIFE-THREATENING.

**EFFECTS ON DIAGNOSTIC TESTS**
None reported.

**CONTRAINDICATIONS**
Contraindicated in patients with hypersensitivity to drug, severe left ventricular dysfunction, cardiogenic shock, second- or third-degree AV block or sick sinus syndrome except in presence of functioning pacemaker, atrial flutter or fibrillation and accessory bypass tract syndrome, severe heart failure (unless secondary to verapamil therapy), and severe hypotension. I.V. verapamil is contraindicated in patients receiving I.V. beta blockers and in those with ventricular tachycardia.

**NURSING CONSIDERATIONS**
• Use cautiously in elderly patients and in patients with increased intracranial pressure or hepatic or renal disease.
• Although drug should be taken with food, taking extended-release tablets with food may decrease rate and extent of absorption but allows smaller fluctuations of peak and trough blood levels.
• Patients with severely compromised cardiac function or those receiving beta blockers should receive lower doses of verapamil. Monitor these patients closely.
• If verapamil is being used to terminate supraventricular tachycardia, doctor may have the patient perform vagal maneuvers after receiving drug.
• Monitor blood pressure at the start of therapy and during dosage adjustments. Assist patient with ambulation because dizziness may occur.
• Notify doctor if signs and symptoms of heart failure, such as swelling of hands and feet and shortness of breath, occur.
• Monitor liver function during prolonged treatment, as ordered.
• *Alert:* Don't confuse Isoptin with Intropin, or Verelan with Vivarin, Voltaren, Ferralyn, or Virilon.

**I.V. administration**
• Give drug by direct injection into a vein or into the tubing of a free-flowing, compatible I.V. solution. Compatible solutions include $D_5W$ and half-normal saline, normal saline, Ringer's, and lactated Ringer's solutions. Administer I.V. doses over at least 2 minutes to minimize risk of adverse reactions, or 3 minutes in elderly patients.
• Monitor ECG and blood pressure continuously in patient receiving I.V. verapamil.

**☑ Patient teaching**
• Instruct patient to take oral form of drug exactly as prescribed.
• Tell patient to take drug with food.
• Caution patient against abruptly discontinuing drug.
• If patient is kept on nitrate therapy during adjustment of oral verapamil dosage, urge continued compliance. S.L. nitroglycerin especially may be taken as needed when angina symptoms are acute.
• Encourage patient to increase fluid and fiber intake to combat constipation. Administer a stool softener, as ordered.

# 23

## Antihypertensives

acebutolol hydrochloride
amlodipine besylate
(See Chapter 22, ANTIANGINALS.)
atenolol
benazepril hydrochloride
betaxolol hydrochloride
bisoprolol fumarate
candesartan cilexetil
captopril
carteolol hydrochloride
carvedilol
clonidine
clonidine hydrochloride
diazoxide
diltiazem hydrochloride
(See Chapter 22, ANTIANGINALS.)
doxazosin mesylate
enalaprilat
enalapril maleate
eprosartan mesylate
felodipine
fenoldopam mesylate
fosinopril sodium
guanabenz acetate
guanadrel sulfate
guanfacine hydrochloride
hydralazine hydrochloride
irbesartan
isradipine
labetalol hydrochloride
lisinopril
losartan potassium
methyldopa
methyldopate hydrochloride
metoprolol succinate
metoprolol tartrate
minoxidil
moexipril hydrochloride
nadolol
(See Chapter 22, ANTIANGINALS.)
nicardipine hydrochloride
(See Chapter 22, ANTIANGINALS.)
nifedipine
(See Chapter 22, ANTIANGINALS.)
nisoldipine
nitroprusside sodium
penbutolol sulfate
perindopril erbumine
phentolamine mesylate

pindolol
prazosin hydrochloride
propranolol hydrochloride
(See Chapter 22, ANTIANGINALS.)
quinapril hydrochloride
ramipril
telmisartan
terazosin hydrochloride
timolol maleate
trandolapril
valsartan
verapamil hydrochloride
(See Chapter 22, ANTIANGINALS.)

## COMBINATION PRODUCTS

ALDOCLOR-150: chlorothiazide 150 mg
and methyldopa 250 mg.
ALDOCLOR-250: chlorothiazide 250 mg
and methyldopa 250 mg.
ALDORIL-15: hydrochlorothiazide 15 mg
and methyldopa 250 mg.
ALDORIL-25: hydrochlorothiazide 25 mg
and methyldopa 250 mg.
ALDORIL D30: hydrochlorothiazide 30 mg
and methyldopa 500 mg.
ALDORIL D50: hydrochlorothiazide 50 mg
and methyldopa 500 mg.
APRESAZIDE 25/25: hydrochlorothiazide
25 mg and hydralazine hydrochloride
25 mg.
APRESAZIDE 50/50: hydrochlorothiazide
50 mg and hydralazine hydrochloride
50 mg.
APRESAZIDE 100/50: hydrochlorothiazide
50 mg and hydralazine hydrochloride
100 mg.
APRESOLINE-ESIDRIX: hydrochlorothiazide
15 mg and hydralazine hydrochloride
25 mg.
CAM-AP-ES: hydrochlorothiazide 15 mg,
hydralazine hydrochloride 25 mg, and reserpine 0.1 mg.
CAPOZIDE 25/15: hydrochlorothiazide
15 mg and captopril 25 mg.
CAPOZIDE 25/25: hydrochlorothiazide
25 mg and captopril 25 mg.
CAPOZIDE 50/15: hydrochlorothiazide
15 mg and captopril 50 mg.

---

Reactions may be *common*, uncommon, *life-threatening*, or COMMON AND LIFE-THREATENING.

CAPOZIDE 50/25: hydrochlorothiazide 25 mg and captopril 50 mg.

CHERAPAS: hydrochlorothiazide 15 mg, hydralazine hydrochloride 25 mg, and reserpine 0.1 mg.

COMBIPRES 0.1: chlorthalidone 15 mg and clonidine hydrochloride 0.1 mg.

COMBIPRES 0.2: chlorthalidone 15 mg and clonidine hydrochloride 0.2 mg.

COMBIPRES 0.3: chlorthalidone 15 mg and clonidine hydrochloride 0.3 mg.

CORZIDE: nadolol 40 mg or 80 mg and bendroflumethiazide 5 mg.

DEMI-REGROTON: chlorthalidone 25 mg and reserpine 0.125 mg.

DIURESE-R: trichlormethiazide 4 mg and reserpine 0.1 mg.

DIURIGEN WITH RESERPINE: chlorothiazide 250 mg and reserpine 0.125 mg.

DIUTENSEN-R: methyclothiazide 2.5 mg and reserpine 0.1 mg.

ENDURONYL: methyclothiazide 5.0 mg and deserpidine 0.25 mg.

ENDURONYL FORTE: methyclothiazide 5.0 mg and deserpidine 0.5 mg.

ESIMIL: hydrochlorothiazide 25 mg and guanethidine monosulfate 10 mg.

HYDROPINE: hydroflumethiazide 25 mg and reserpine 0.125 mg.

HYDROPINE H.P: hydroflumethiazide 50 mg and reserpine 0.125 mg.

HYDROPRES-50: hydrochlorothiazide 50 mg and reserpine 0.125 mg.

HYDRO-SERP: hydrochlorothiazide 25 or 50 mg and reserpine 0.125 mg.

HYDROSERPINE: hydrochlorothiazide 25 or 50 mg and reserpine 0.125 mg.

HYDROTENSIN tablets: hydrochlorothiazide 25 mg and reserpine 0.125 mg.

HYZAAR: losartan 50 mg and hydrochlorothiazide 12.5 mg.

INDERIDE 40/25: propranolol hydrochloride 40 mg and hydrochlorothiazide 25 mg.

INDERIDE 80/25: propranolol hydrochloride 80 mg and hydrochlorothiazide 25 mg.

INDERIDE LA 80/50: propranolol hydrochloride 80 mg and hydrochlorothiazide 50 mg.

INDERIDE LA 120/50: propranolol hydrochloride 120 mg and hydrochlorothiazide 50 mg.

INDERIDE LA 160/50: propranolol hydrochloride 160 mg and hydrochlorothiazide 50 mg.

LEXXEL: enalapril maleate 5 mg and felodipine 5 mg.

LOPRESSOR HCT 50/25: metoprolol tartrate 50 mg and hydrochlorothiazide 25 mg.

LOPRESSOR HCT 100/25: metoprolol tartrate 100 mg and hydrochlorothiazide 25 mg.

LOPRESSOR HCT 100/50: metoprolol tartrate 100 mg and hydrochlorothiazide 50 mg.

LOTREL 2.5/10: amlodipine besylate 2.5 mg and benazepril hydrochloride 10 mg.

LOTREL 5/10: amlodipine besylate 5 mg and benazepril hydrochloride 10 mg.

LOTREL 5/20: amlodipine besylate 5 mg and benazepril hydrochloride 20 mg.

MAXZIDE: triamterene 75 mg and hydrochlorothiazide 50 mg.

MINIZIDE 1: polythiazide 0.5 mg and prazosin hydrochloride 1 mg.

MINIZIDE 2: polythiazide 0.5 mg and prazosin hydrochloride 2 mg.

MINIZIDE 5: polythiazide 0.5 mg and prazosin hydrochloride 5 mg.

NAQUIVAL: trichlormethiazide 4 mg and reserpine 0.1 mg.

PRINZIDE 12.5: lisinopril 20 mg and hydrochlorothiazide 12.5 mg.

PRINZIDE 25: lisinopril 20 mg and hydrochlorothiazide 25 mg.

RAUZIDE**: bendroflumethiazide 4 mg and powdered rauwolfia serpentina 50 mg.

REGROTON: chlorthalidone 50 mg and reserpine 0.25 mg.

RENESE-R: polythiazide 2 mg and reserpine 0.25 mg.

SALUTENSIN TABLETS: hydroflumethiazide 50 mg and reserpine 0.125 mg.

SALUTENSIN-DEMI: hydroflumethiazide 25 mg and reserpine 0.125 mg.

SER-A-GEN: hydrochlorothiazide 15 mg, hydralazine hydrochloride 25 mg, and reserpine 0.1 mg.

SERALAZIDE: hydrochlorothiazide 15 mg, hydralazine hydrochloride 25 mg, and reserpine 0.1 mg.

SER-AP-ES: hydrochlorothiazide 15 mg, reserpine 0.1 mg, and hydralazine hydrochloride 25 mg.

SERPAZIDE: hydrochlorothiazide 15 mg, hydralazine hydrochloride 25 mg, and reserpine 0.1 mg.
TENORETIC 50: atenolol 50 mg and chlorthalidone 25 mg.
TENORETIC 100: atenolol 100 mg and chlorthalidone 25 mg.
TIMOLIDE 10-25: timolol maleate 10 mg and hydrochlorothiazide 25 mg.
TRI-HYDROSERPINE: hydrochlorothiazide 15 mg, hydralazine hydrochloride 25 mg, and reserpine 0.1 mg.
VASERETIC 10-25: enalapril maleate 10 mg and hydrochlorothiazide 25 mg.
ZESTORETIC: lisinopril 20 mg and hydrochlorothiazide 12.5 mg.
ZESTORETIC: lisinopril 20 mg and hydrochlorothiazide 25 mg.
ZIAC TABLETS: bisoprolol fumarate 2.5 mg, 5 mg, or 10 mg and hydrochlorothiazide 6.5 mg.

---

## acebutolol hydrochloride
Monitan†, Sectral

*Pregnancy Risk Category B*

---

### HOW SUPPLIED
*Capsules:* 200 mg, 400 mg
*Tablets:* 100 mg†, 200 mg, 400 mg

### ACTION
Unknown. Possible mechanisms include reduced cardiac output, decreased sympathetic outflow to peripheral vasculature, and inhibition of renin release. Drug decreases myocardial contractility and heart rate and has mild intrinsic sympathomimetic activity.

| Route | Onset | Peak | Duration |
|-------|-------|------|----------|
| P.O. | 1-1.5 hr | 2.5 hr | 24 hr |

### INDICATIONS & DOSAGE
*Hypertension—*
**Adults:** 400 mg P.O. either as a single daily dose or in divided doses b.i.d. Maximum daily dose is 1,200 mg.
*Ventricular arrhythmias—*
**Adults:** 400 mg P.O. daily divided b.i.d. Dosage increased to provide an adequate clinical response. Usual dose is 600 to 1,200 mg daily.

**Elderly:** may need lower dosage; dose should not exceed 800 mg daily.
*Adjust-a-dose:* For renally impaired patients with creatinine clearance of 25 to 50 ml/minute, reduce dosage by 50%; if clearance is below 25 ml/minute, reduce dosage by 75%.

### ADVERSE REACTIONS
**CNS:** *fatigue,* headache, dizziness, insomnia, depression.
**CV:** chest pain, edema, bradycardia, **heart failure,** *hypotension.*
**GI:** nausea, constipation, diarrhea, dyspepsia, flatulence, vomiting.
**GU:** dysuria, impotence, nocturia, urinary frequency.
**Musculoskeletal:** arthralgia, myalgia.
**Respiratory:** dyspnea, **bronchospasm,** cough.
**Skin:** rash.

### INTERACTIONS
**Drug-drug.** *Cardiac glycosides, diltiazem, verapamil:* excessive bradycardia and increased depressant effect on myocardium. Use together cautiously.
*Catecholamine-depleting drugs such as reserpine:* effects may be additive. Monitor closely.
*Diuretics, other antihypertensives:* increased hypotensive effect. Use together cautiously.
*Insulin, oral antidiabetics:* can alter dosage requirements in previously stabilized diabetic patients. Observe patient carefully.
*NSAIDs:* decreased antihypertensive effect. Monitor blood pressure and adjust dosage.
*Sympathomimetics:* effects antagonized by acebutolol. Greater than usual dosages of beta-adrenergic agonist bronchodilators may be needed.

### EFFECTS ON DIAGNOSTIC TESTS
Drug may cause positive antinuclear antibody titers.

### CONTRAINDICATIONS
Contraindicated in patients with persistent severe bradycardia, second- and third-degree heart block, overt cardiac failure, and cardiogenic shock.

---

## NURSING CONSIDERATIONS
• Use cautiously in those with cardiac failure, peripheral vascular disease, bronchospastic disease, and diabetes.
• Check apical pulse before giving drug; if slower than 60 beats/minute, withhold drug and call doctor. Also monitor blood pressure.
• Before surgery, tell anesthesiologist that patient is taking drug.
• Acebutolol may mask signs and symptoms of hyperthyroidism.
• Drug loses its selectivity for the beta$_1$ receptor at higher doses. Monitor for peripheral effects.
• *Alert:* Discontinue drug gradually over 2 weeks.
• Keep in mind that drug can mask signs and symptoms of hypoglycemia in diabetic patients.
• *Alert:* Don't confuse Sectral with Factrel or Septra.

☑ **Patient teaching**
• Instruct patient to take drug exactly as prescribed.
• Tell patient to avoid taking OTC oral cold preparations or topical nasal decongestants because of risk of severe hypertensive reaction.
• Warn patient not to discontinue drug suddenly, and to notify doctor promptly of unpleasant adverse reactions.
• Teach patient how to take his pulse and instruct him to withhold the dose and notify doctor if pulse rate is below 60 beats/minute.

---

## atenolol
Anselol‡, Apo-Atenol†, Noten‡, Nu-Atenol†, Tenormin, Tensig‡

*Pregnancy Risk Category D*

## HOW SUPPLIED
*Tablets:* 25 mg, 50 mg, 100 mg
*Injection:* 5 mg/10 ml

## ACTION
A beta blocker that selectively blocks beta$_1$-adrenergic receptors; decreases cardiac output, peripheral resistance, and cardiac oxygen consumption; and depresses renin secretion.

| Route | Onset | Peak | Duration |
|-------|-------|-------|----------|
| P.O. | 1 hr | 2-4 hr | 24 hr |
| I.V. | 5 min | 5 min | 12 hr |

## INDICATIONS & DOSAGE
*Hypertension—*
**Adults:** initially, 50 mg P.O. daily as a single dose, increased to 100 mg once daily after 7 to 14 days. Dosages over 100 mg are unlikely to produce further benefit.
*Angina pectoris—*
**Adults:** 50 mg P.O. once daily, increased, p.r.n., to 100 mg daily after 7 days for optimal effect. Maximum dose is 200 mg daily.
*To reduce CV mortality and risk of re-infarction in patients with acute MI—*
**Adults:** 5 mg I.V. over 5 minutes; then another 5 mg after 10 minutes. After an additional 10 minutes, 50 mg P.O.; then 50 mg P.O. in 12 hours. Thereafter, 100 mg P.O. daily (as a single dose or 50 mg b.i.d.) for at least 7 days.
*Adjust-a-dose:* For renally impaired patients with creatinine clearance of 15 to 35 ml/minute, maximum dose is 50 mg/day; if it is below 15 ml/minute, maximum dose is 25 mg/day.
    Hemodialysis patients need 25 to 50 mg after each dialysis session; monitor closely because of risk of hypotension.

## ADVERSE REACTIONS
**CNS:** *fatigue,* lethargy, vertigo, drowsiness, *dizziness.*
**CV:** *bradycardia, hypotension,* **heart failure,** intermittent claudication.
**GI:** nausea, diarrhea.
**GU:** elevated BUN and creatinine.
**Hematologic:** elevated platelet count.
**Hepatic:** elevated transaminase, alkaline phosphatase, LD levels.
**Metabolic:** elevated serum levels of potassium, uric acid; increased or decreased serum glucose levels in diabetic patients.
**Respiratory:** dyspnea, ***bronchospasm.***
**Skin:** rash.
**Other:** fever, leg pain.

---

## INTERACTIONS
**Drug-drug.** *Antihypertensives:* enhanced hypotensive effect. Use together cautiously. *Cardiac glycosides, diltiazem, verapamil:* excessive bradycardia and increased depressant effect on myocardium. Use together cautiously.
*Insulin, oral antidiabetics:* can alter dosage requirements in previously stabilized diabetic patient. Observe patient carefully.
*Reserpine:* may cause hypotension. Use with caution.

## EFFECTS ON DIAGNOSTIC TESTS
Drug may cause changes in exercise tolerance and ECG.

## CONTRAINDICATIONS
Contraindicated in patients with sinus bradycardia, greater than first-degree heart block, overt cardiac failure, or cardiogenic shock.

## NURSING CONSIDERATIONS
• Use cautiously in patients at risk for heart failure and in patients with bronchospastic disease, diabetes, hyperthyroidism, and impaired renal or hepatic function.
• Check apical pulse before giving drug; if slower than 60 beats/minute, withhold drug and call doctor.
• Monitor patient's blood pressure.
• Beta blockers may mask tachycardia associated with hyperthyroidism. In patients with suspected thyrotoxicosis, withdraw beta blocker gradually, as ordered, to avoid thyroid storm.
• Drug may mask signs and symptoms of hypoglycemia in diabetic patients.
• *Alert:* Withdraw drug gradually over 2 weeks to avoid serious adverse reactions.
• *Alert:* Don't confuse atenolol with timolol or albuterol.

## I.V. administration
• Give by slow I.V. injection, not exceeding 1 mg/minute. I.V. doses may be mixed with $D_5W$, normal saline, or dextrose and saline solutions. Solution is stable for 48 hours after mixing.

## ☑ Patient teaching
• Instruct patient to take drug exactly as prescribed, at the same time every day.
• Caution patient not to stop drug suddenly, but to call doctor if unpleasant adverse reactions occur.
• Teach patient how to take his pulse. Tell him to withhold drug and call doctor if pulse rate is below 60 beats/minute.
• Tell woman to notify doctor if pregnancy occurs. Drug will need to be discontinued.

---

## benazepril hydrochloride
Lotensin

*Pregnancy Risk Category C (D in second and third trimesters)*

## HOW SUPPLIED
*Tablets:* 5 mg, 10 mg, 20 mg, 40 mg

## ACTION
Drug and its active metabolite, benazeprilat, inhibit ACE, preventing conversion of angiotensin I to angiotensin II, a potent vasoconstrictor. Reduced formation of angiotensin II decreases peripheral arterial resistance, thus decreasing aldosterone secretion, which in turn reduces sodium and water retention and lowers blood pressure. Drug also exhibits antihypertensive activity in patients with low-renin hypertension.

| Route | Onset | Peak | Duration |
|-------|-------|------|----------|
| P.O. | 1 hr | 2-4 hr | 24 hr |

## INDICATIONS & DOSAGE
*Hypertension—*
**Adults:** for patients not receiving a diuretic, 10 mg P.O. daily initially. Dosage adjusted as needed and tolerated; most patients take 20 to 40 mg daily in one or two divided doses. For patients receiving a diuretic, 5 mg P.O. daily.
*Adjust-a-dose:* For renally impaired patients with creatinine clearance below 30 ml/minute, 5 mg P.O. daily. Dose may be adjusted up to 40 mg/day.

## ADVERSE REACTIONS
**CNS:** headache, dizziness, drowsiness, fatigue, somnolence.

---

Reactions may be *common*, uncommon, *life-threatening*, or COMMON AND LIFE-THREATENING.

**CV:** symptomatic hypotension.
**GI:** nausea.
**GU:** impotence, increased serum creatinine and BUN levels.
**Metabolic:** hyperkalemia.
**Musculoskeletal:** arthralgia, arthritis, myalgia.
**Respiratory:** dry, persistent, nonproductive cough.
**Skin:** hypersensitivity reactions, increased diaphoresis.

## INTERACTIONS
**Drug-drug.** *Diuretics, other antihypertensives:* risk of excessive hypotension. Discontinue diuretic or lower dose of benazepril as needed.
*Lithium:* increased serum lithium levels and lithium toxicity. Coadminister with caution; monitor serum lithium levels.
*Potassium-sparing diuretics, potassium supplements:* risk of hyperkalemia. Monitor closely.
**Drug-food.** *Salt substitutes containing potassium:* risk of hyperkalemia. Monitor closely.

## EFFECTS ON DIAGNOSTIC TESTS
None reported.

## CONTRAINDICATIONS
Contraindicated in patients with hypersensitivity to ACE inhibitors.

## NURSING CONSIDERATIONS
• Use cautiously in patients with impaired hepatic or renal function.
• Safety and efficacy of dosages over 80 mg/day have not been established.
• Monitor for hypotension. Excessive hypotension can occur when drug is given with diuretics. If possible, diuretic therapy should be discontinued 2 to 3 days before starting benazepril to decrease potential for excessive hypotensive response. If drug does not adequately control blood pressure, diuretic may be reinstituted with care.
• Measure blood pressure when drug levels are at peak (2 to 6 hours after administration) and at trough (just before a dose) to verify adequate blood pressure control.
• Assess renal and hepatic function before and periodically throughout therapy.

Monitor serum potassium levels, as ordered.
• *Alert:* Don't confuse benazepril with Benadryl or Lotensin with Loniten or lovastatin.

☑ **Patient teaching**
• Instruct patient to avoid salt substitutes; these products may contain potassium, which can cause hyperkalemia in patients taking drug.
• Inform patient that light-headedness can occur, especially during first few days of therapy. Tell him to rise slowly to minimize this effect and to report dizziness to doctor. If syncope occurs, he should stop drug and call doctor immediately.
• Warn patient to use caution in hot weather and during exercise. Inadequate fluid intake, vomiting, diarrhea, and excessive perspiration can lead to light-headedness and syncope.
• Advise patient to report signs of infection, such as fever and sore throat. Tell him to call doctor if the following signs or symptoms occur: easy bruising or bleeding; swelling of tongue, lips, face, eyes, mucous membranes, or extremities; difficulty swallowing or breathing; or hoarseness.
• Tell woman to notify doctor if pregnancy occurs. Drug will need to be discontinued.

---

## betaxolol hydrochloride
Kerlone

*Pregnancy Risk Category C*

### HOW SUPPLIED
*Tablets:* 10 mg, 20 mg

### ACTION
Unknown. A selective beta blocker that decreases blood pressure, possibly by slowing heart rate and decreasing cardiac output.

| Route | Onset | Peak | Duration |
|-------|-------|------|----------|
| P.O. | 3 hr | 2-4 hr | 24-48 hr |

## INDICATIONS & DOSAGE
*Hypertension (used alone or with other antihypertensives)—*
**Adults:** initially, 10 mg P.O. once daily; if needed, 20 mg P.O. once daily if desired response is not achieved in 7 to 14 days. Maximum daily dose 40 mg.

## ADVERSE REACTIONS
**CNS:** dizziness, fatigue, headache, insomnia, lethargy, anxiety.
**CV:** bradycardia, chest pain, *heart failure*, edema.
**EENT:** pharyngitis.
**GI:** nausea, diarrhea, dyspepsia.
**GU:** impotence.
**Musculoskeletal:** arthralgia.
**Respiratory:** dyspnea, *bronchospasm.*
**Skin:** rash.

## INTERACTIONS
**Drug-drug.** *Calcium channel blockers:* increased risk of hypotension, left-sided heart failure, and AV conduction disturbances. Use I.V. calcium channel blockers with caution.
*Catecholamine-depleting drugs, reserpine:* may have an additive effect. Monitor closely.
*General anesthetics:* increased hypotensive effects. Observe carefully for excessive hypotension or bradycardia or orthostatic hypotension.
*Lidocaine:* may increase lidocaine's effects. Monitor patient.

## EFFECTS ON DIAGNOSTIC TESTS
Oral beta blockers have been reported to decrease serum glucose levels as a result of blockage of normal glycogen release after hypoglycemia. Oral beta blockers may alter the results of glucose tolerance tests.

## CONTRAINDICATIONS
Contraindicated in patients with hypersensitivity to drug; also contraindicated in those with severe bradycardia, greater than first-degree heart block, cardiogenic shock, or uncontrolled heart failure.

## NURSING CONSIDERATIONS
• Use cautiously in patients with heart failure controlled by cardiac glycosides and diuretics because these patients may exhibit signs of cardiac decompensation with beta-blocker therapy.
• When discontinuing drug, withdraw over 2 weeks.
• Monitor blood pressure closely.
• Monitor blood glucose levels regularly in patients with diabetes. Beta blockade may inhibit glycogenolysis as well as the signs and symptoms of hypoglycemia (such as tachycardia and blood pressure changes).
• Withdrawal of beta-blocker therapy before surgery is controversial. Withdrawal is sometimes advocated to prevent impairment of cardiac responsiveness to reflex stimuli and decreased responsiveness to administration of catecholamines. Advise anesthesiologist that patient is receiving a beta blocker so that isoproterenol or dobutamine can be readily available for reversal of drug's cardiac effects.
• Beta blockers may mask tachycardia associated with hyperthyroidism. In patients with suspected thyrotoxicosis, withdraw beta blocker gradually, as ordered, to avoid thyroid storm.

☑ **Patient teaching**
• Instruct patient to take drug exactly as prescribed.
• *Alert:* Advise patient that abrupt discontinuation may precipitate angina pectoris in patients with unrecognized coronary artery disease.
• Emphasize importance of promptly reporting signs and symptoms of heart failure, including shortness of breath or difficulty breathing, unusually fast heartbeat, cough, and fatigue with exertion.

---

**bisoprolol fumarate**
Emcor§, Monocor§, Zebeta

*Pregnancy Risk Category C*

## HOW SUPPLIED
*Tablets:* 5 mg, 10 mg

## ACTION
Not completely defined. A beta blocker that decreases myocardial contractility, heart rate, and cardiac output; it lowers

blood pressure and reduces myocardial oxygen consumption.

| Route | Onset | Peak | Duration |
|-------|-------|------|----------|
| P.O. | Unknown | 1-4 hr | 24 hr |

## INDICATIONS & DOSAGE
*Hypertension (used alone or with other antihypertensives)—*
**Adults:** initially, 5 mg P.O. once daily. If response is inadequate, increase to 10 mg once daily or to 20 mg P.O. daily if needed. Maximum recommended dose is 20 mg daily.
*Adjust-a-dose:* For patients with renal or hepatic impairment, 2.5 mg P.O. daily initially. Adjust subsequent dosage cautiously.

## ADVERSE REACTIONS
**CNS:** asthenia, fatigue, dizziness, *headache,* hypoesthesia, vivid dreams, depression, insomnia.
**CV:** bradycardia, peripheral edema, chest pain, *heart failure.*
**EENT:** pharyngitis, rhinitis, sinusitis.
**GI:** nausea, vomiting, diarrhea, dry mouth.
**Musculoskeletal:** arthralgia.
**Respiratory:** cough, dyspnea.

## INTERACTIONS
**Drug-drug:** *Calcium channel blockers:* can cause myocardial depression and AV conduction inhibition. Monitor closely.
*Guanethidine, reserpine:* can cause hypotension. Monitor closely.
*NSAIDs:* decreased antihypertensive effect. Monitor blood pressure and adjust dosage.

## EFFECTS ON DIAGNOSTIC TESTS
Drug may produce hypoglycemia and interfere with glucose or insulin tolerance tests.

## CONTRAINDICATIONS
Contraindicated in patients with hypersensitivity to drug, cardiogenic shock, overt cardiac failure, marked sinus bradycardia, or second- or third-degree AV block.

## NURSING CONSIDERATIONS
• Use cautiously in patients with bronchospastic disease. In general, these patients should avoid beta blockers because blockade of pulmonary beta$_2$ receptors may result in worsening of symptoms. For patients who can't tolerate or don't respond to other antihypertensives, bisoprolol is given in low doses, starting with 2.5 mg P.O. daily. Bisoprolol blocks beta$_2$ receptors in higher doses (20 mg daily or more).
• Also use cautiously in patients with diabetes, peripheral vascular disease, or thyroid disease and in those with a history of heart failure.
• Monitor blood pressure frequently.
• Closely monitor blood glucose levels in diabetic patients. Beta blockers may mask some signs and symptoms of hypoglycemia, such as tachycardia.
• Drug must be withdrawn gradually over 1 to 2 weeks.
• Beta blockers may mask tachycardia associated with hyperthyroidism. In patients with suspected thyrotoxicosis, withdraw beta blocker gradually, as ordered, to avoid thyroid storm.
• *Alert:* Don't confuse Zebeta with Dia-Beta.

☑ **Patient teaching**
• Explain to patient importance of taking drug as prescribed, even when he is feeling well.
• Advise patient not to stop drug suddenly but to call doctor if unpleasant adverse reactions occur.
• Tell patient to check with doctor or pharmacist before taking OTC medications.

## candesartan cilexetil
Atacand

*Pregnancy Risk Category C (D in second and third trimesters)*

## HOW SUPPLIED
*Tablets:* 4 mg, 8 mg, 16 mg, 32 mg

## ACTION
Inhibits vasoconstrictive action of angiotensin II by blocking angiotensin II recep-

tor on the surface of vascular smooth muscle and other tissue cells.

| Route | Onset | Peak | Duration |
|-------|-------|------|----------|
| P.O. | Unknown | 3-4 hr | 24 hr |

## INDICATIONS & DOSAGE
*Hypertension (used alone or with other antihypertensives)—*
**Adults:** initially, 16 mg P.O. once daily when used as monotherapy; usual range is 8 to 32 mg P.O. daily as a single dose or divided b.i.d.

## ADVERSE REACTIONS
**CNS:** dizziness, fatigue, headache.
**CV:** chest pain, peripheral edema.
**EENT:** pharyngitis, rhinitis, sinusitis.
**GI:** abdominal pain, diarrhea, nausea, vomiting.
**GU:** albuminuria.
**Musculoskeletal:** arthralgia, back pain.
**Respiratory:** coughing, bronchitis, upper respiratory tract infection.

## INTERACTIONS
**Drug-drug.** *Potassium-sparing diuretics, potassium supplements:* risk of hyperkalemia. Monitor closely.
**Drug-food.** *Salt substitutes containing potassium:* risk of hyperkalemia. Monitor closely.

## EFFECTS ON DIAGNOSTIC TESTS
None reported.

## CONTRAINDICATIONS
Contraindicated in patients with hypersensitivity to drug or its ingredients.

## NURSING CONSIDERATIONS
• Use cautiously in patients whose renal function depends on the renin-angiotensin-aldosterone system (such as patients with heart failure) because of risk of oliguria and progressive azotemia with acute renal failure or death.
• Use cautiously in patients who are volume- or salt-depleted because of potential for symptomatic hypotension. Start therapy with a lower dosage range, as ordered, and monitor blood pressure carefully.
• Drugs such as candesartan that act directly on the renin-angiotensin system can cause fetal and neonatal morbidity and death when given to pregnant women. These problems have not been detected when exposure has been limited to first trimester. If pregnancy is suspected, notify doctor because drug should be discontinued.
• If hypotension occurs after a dose of candesartan, place patient in the supine position and, if needed, give an I.V. infusion of normal saline, as ordered.
• Most of drug's antihypertensive effect is present within 2 weeks. Maximal antihypertensive effect is obtained within 4 to 6 weeks. Diuretic may be added if blood pressure is not controlled by drug alone.
• Carefully monitor therapeutic response and the occurrence of adverse reactions in elderly patients and in those with renal disease.

### ✔Patient teaching
• Inform woman of childbearing age of the consequences of second and third trimester exposure to drug. Advise her to notify doctor immediately if pregnancy is suspected.
• Advise breast-feeding woman of the risk of adverse effects on the infant and the need to either stop breast-feeding or discontinue drug.
• Instruct patient to store drug at room temperature and to keep container tightly sealed.
• Inform patient to report adverse reactions without delay.
• Tell patient that drug may be taken without regard to meals.

## captopril
Acenorm‡, Capoten, Enzace‡, Novo-Captoril†

*Pregnancy Risk Category C (D in second and third trimesters)*

## HOW SUPPLIED
*Tablets:* 12.5 mg, 25 mg, 50 mg, 100 mg

## ACTION
Not clearly defined. Thought to inhibit ACE, preventing conversion of angiotensin I to angiotensin II, a potent vaso-

constrictor. Reduced formation of angiotensin II decreases peripheral arterial resistance, thus decreasing aldosterone secretion, thereby reducing sodium and water retention and lowering blood pressure.

| Route | Onset | Peak | Duration |
|-------|-------|------|----------|
| P.O. | 0.25-1 hr | 1-1.5 hr | 6-12 hr |

## INDICATIONS & DOSAGE
*Hypertension—*
**Adults:** 25 mg P.O. b.i.d. or t.i.d. initially. If blood pressure isn't satisfactorily controlled in 1 to 2 weeks, increase dosage to 50 mg b.i.d. or t.i.d. If not satisfactorily controlled after another 1 to 2 weeks, expect a diuretic to be added. If further blood pressure reduction is needed, dosage may be raised to 150 mg t.i.d. while continuing diuretic. Maximum daily dose is 450 mg.
*Heart failure, to reduce risk of death and to slow development of heart failure after MI—*
**Adults:** initially, 6.25 to 12.5 mg P.O. t.i.d. Gradually increased to 50 mg t.i.d., p.r.n. Maximum daily dose is 450 mg.
*Diabetic nephropathy—*
**Adults:** 25 mg P.O. t.i.d.

## ADVERSE REACTIONS
**CNS:** dizziness, fainting, headache, malaise, fatigue.
**CV:** *tachycardia, hypotension,* angina pectoris.
**GI:** abdominal pain, anorexia, constipation, diarrhea, dry mouth, dysgeusia, nausea, vomiting.
**Hematologic:** *leukopenia, agranulocytosis, pancytopenia,* anemia, *thrombocytopenia.*
**Hepatic:** transient increase in hepatic enzymes.
**Metabolic:** hyperkalemia.
**Respiratory:** dyspnea, *dry, persistent, nonproductive cough..*
**Skin:** *urticarial rash, maculopapular rash,* pruritus, alopecia.
**Other:** fever, *angioedema of face and extremities.*

## INTERACTIONS
**Drug-drug.** *Antacids:* decreased captopril effect. Separate administration times.
*Digoxin:* may increase serum digoxin level by 15% to 30%. Monitor closely.
*Diuretics, other antihypertensives:* risk of excessive hypotension. Diuretic may need to be discontinued or captopril dosage lowered.
*Insulin, oral antidiabetics:* risk of hypoglycemia when captopril therapy is initiated. Monitor closely.
*Lithium:* increased lithium levels and symptoms of toxicity possible. Monitor patient closely.
*NSAIDs:* may reduce antihypertensive effect. Monitor blood pressure.
*Potassium-sparing diuretics, potassium supplements:* increased risk of hyperkalemia. Avoid these drugs unless hypokalemic blood levels are confirmed.
**Drug-herb.** *Black catechu:* additional hypotensive effect. Avoid concomitant use.
**Drug-food.** *Salt substitutes containing potassium:* risk of hyperkalemia. Monitor closely.

## EFFECTS ON DIAGNOSTIC TESTS
Drug may cause false-positive results for urinary acetone.

## CONTRAINDICATIONS
Contraindicated in patients with hypersensitivity to drug or other ACE inhibitors.

## NURSING CONSIDERATIONS
• Use cautiously in patients with impaired renal function or serious autoimmune disease, especially systemic lupus erythematosus, and in those who have been exposed to other drugs known to affect WBC counts or immune response.
• Monitor patient's blood pressure and pulse rate frequently.
• *Alert:* Elderly patients may be more sensitive to drug's hypotensive effects.
• Drug is associated with the most frequent occurrence of cough compared with other ACE inhibitors.
• In patients with impaired renal function or collagen vascular disease, monitor WBC and differential counts before starting treatment, every 2 weeks for the first 3 months of therapy, and periodically thereafter.
• *Alert:* Don't confuse captopril with Capitol.

---

*Liquid contains alcohol.   **May contain tartrazine.   †Canada   ‡Australia   §U.K.   ◊OTC

☑ **Patient teaching**
• Instruct patient to take drug 1 hour before meals; food in the GI tract may reduce absorption.
• Inform patient that light-headedness is possible, especially during first few days of therapy. Tell him to rise slowly to minimize this effect and to report occurrence to doctor. If syncope occurs, he should stop drug and call doctor immediately.
• Tell patient to use caution in hot weather and during exercise. Inadequate fluid intake, vomiting, diarrhea, and excessive perspiration can lead to light-headedness and syncope.
• Advise patient to report signs and symptoms of infection, such as fever and sore throat.
• Tell woman to notify doctor if pregnancy occurs. Drug will need to be discontinued.

---

## carteolol hydrochloride
Cartrol

*Pregnancy Risk Category C*

### HOW SUPPLIED
*Tablets:* 2.5 mg, 5 mg

### ACTION
Unknown. A nonselective beta blocker with intrinsic sympathomimetic activity. Its antihypertensive effects are probably caused by decreased sympathetic outflow from the brain and decreased cardiac output. Drug doesn't have a consistent effect on renin output.

| Route | Onset | Peak | Duration |
|-------|---------|--------|----------|
| P.O. | Unknown | 1-3 hr | 24 hr |

### INDICATIONS & DOSAGE
*Hypertension—*
**Adults:** initially, 2.5 mg P.O. as a single daily dose; gradually increased to 5 or 10 mg as a single daily dose, p.r.n. Doses that exceed 10 mg daily don't produce a greater response and may actually decrease it.
*Adjust-a-dose:* For patients with substantial renal failure, if creatinine clearance is over 60 ml/minute, dosage interval is 24 hours; if between 20 and 60 ml/minute, dosage interval is 48 hours; if below 20 ml/minute, dosage interval is 72 hours.

### ADVERSE REACTIONS
**CNS:** lassitude, fatigue, somnolence, *asthenia,* paresthesia.
**CV:** conduction disturbances, bradycardia.
**EENT:** nasal congestion.
**GI:** diarrhea, nausea, abdominal pain.
**Musculoskeletal:** *muscle cramps,* arthralgia.
**Skin:** sweating, rash.

### INTERACTIONS
**Drug-drug.** *Calcium channel blockers:* increased risk of hypotension, left-sided heart failure, and AV conduction disturbances. Use I.V. calcium channel blockers with caution.
*Cardiac glycosides:* may produce additive effects on slowing AV node conduction. Avoid concomitant use.
*Catecholamine-depleting drugs, reserpine:* may have an additive effect. Monitor closely.
*General anesthetics:* increased hypotensive effects. Observe carefully for excessive hypotension or bradycardia or orthostatic hypotension.
*Insulin, oral antidiabetics:* may alter hypoglycemic response. Adjust dosage as needed.

### EFFECTS ON DIAGNOSTIC TESTS
None reported.

### CONTRAINDICATIONS
Contraindicated in patients with bronchial asthma, severe bradycardia, greater than first-degree heart block, cardiogenic shock, or uncontrolled heart failure.

### NURSING CONSIDERATIONS
• Use cautiously in patients with heart failure controlled by cardiac glycosides and diuretics because these patients may exhibit signs of cardiac decompensation with beta-blocker therapy.
• Monitor blood pressure frequently.
• Beta blockade may inhibit glycogenolysis and the signs and symptoms of hypoglycemia (such as tachycardia and blood

pressure changes). It may also attenuate insulin release. Monitor blood glucose levels frequently.

• Withdrawal of beta-blocker therapy before surgery is controversial. Withdrawal may be advocated to prevent impairment of cardiac responsiveness to reflex stimuli and decreased responsiveness to administration of catecholamines. However, the beta-blocking effects of carteolol may persist for weeks, and discontinuing drug before surgery may be impractical. Advise anesthesiologist that patient is receiving a beta blocker so that isoproterenol or dobutamine can be readily available for reversal of drug's cardiac effects.

• Beta blockers may mask tachycardia associated with hyperthyroidism. In patients with suspected thyrotoxicosis, gradually withdraw beta-blocker therapy, as ordered, to avoid thyroid storm.

• **Alert:** Patients with unrecognized coronary artery disease may exhibit signs of angina pectoris on withdrawal of drug. Monitor closely.

☑ **Patient teaching**
• Instruct patient to take drug exactly as prescribed.
• Tell patient not to stop drug suddenly but to call doctor and discuss unpleasant adverse reactions.
• Emphasize importance of reporting signs and symptoms of heart failure, including shortness of breath or difficulty breathing, unusually fast heartbeat, cough, or fatigue with exertion.

---

## carvedilol
Coreg, Eucardic§

*Pregnancy Risk Category C*

### HOW SUPPLIED
*Tablets:* 3.125 mg, 6.25 mg, 12.5 mg, 25 mg

### ACTION
Nonselective beta blocker with alpha$_1$-blocking activity.

| Route | Onset | Peak | Duration |
|-------|-------|------|----------|
| P.O. | Unknown | 1-2 hr | 7-10 hr |

### INDICATIONS & DOSAGE
*Hypertension—*
**Adults:** dosage highly individualized. Initially, 6.25 mg P.O. b.i.d. Obtain a standing blood pressure 1 hour after initial dose. If tolerated, continue dosage for 7 to 14 days. May increase to 12.5 mg P.O. b.i.d. for 7 to 14 days, following blood pressure monitoring protocol noted above. Maximum dose is 25 mg P.O. b.i.d. as tolerated.
*Heart failure—*
**Adults:** dosage highly individualized. Initially, 3.125 mg P.O. b.i.d. for 2 weeks; if tolerated, can increase to 6.25 mg P.O. b.i.d. Dosage may be doubled q 2 weeks as tolerated. Maximum dose for patients under 85 kg (187 lb) is 25 mg P.O. b.i.d.; for those over 85 kg, dose is 50 mg P.O. b.i.d.
*Adjust-a-dose:* If patient experiences bradycardia with pulse rate below 55 beats/minute, use reduced dosage.

### ADVERSE REACTIONS
**CNS:** *dizziness, fatigue,* headache, hypoesthesia, insomnia, pain, paresthesia, somnolence, vertigo, syncope, malaise.
**CV:** aggravated angina pectoris, *AV block, bradycardia, chest pain,* fluid overload, hypertension, hypotension, orthostatic hypotension, edema.
**EENT:** abnormal vision, pharyngitis, rhinitis, sinusitis.
**GI:** abdominal pain, *diarrhea,* melena, nausea, periodontitis, vomiting.
**GU:** abnormal renal function, albuminuria, hematuria, impotence, urinary tract infection, elevated BUN levels.
**Hematologic:** purpura, *thrombocytopenia, decreased PT and INR.*
**Hepatic:** increased serum alkaline phosphatase, ALT, and AST levels.
**Metabolic:** dehydration, glycosuria, gout, hypercholesterolemia, *hyperglycemia,* hypertriglyceridemia, hypervolemia, hypovolemia, hyperuricemia, hypoglycemia, hyponatremia, weight gain.
**Musculoskeletal:** arthralgia, back pain, myalgia,
**Respiratory:** bronchitis, dyspnea, *upper respiratory tract infection.*
**Other:** allergy, fever, peripheral edema, *sudden death,* viral infection.

---

## INTERACTIONS

**Drug-drug.** *Calcium channel blockers:* can cause isolated conduction disturbances. Monitor patient's heart rhythm and blood pressure.

*Catecholamine-depleting drugs, such as MAO inhibitors, reserpine:* may cause bradycardia or severe hypotension. Monitor patient closely.

*Cimetidine:* increased bioavailability of carvedilol. Monitor vital signs carefully.

*Clonidine:* may potentiate blood pressure and heart rate–lowering effects. Monitor vital signs closely.

*Digoxin:* increased levels of digoxin by about 15% when given concurrently. Monitor digoxin levels.

*Fluoxetine, quinidine, paroxetine, propafenone:* increased blood levels of carvedilol by inhibiting metabolism. Monitor vital signs closely.

*Insulin, oral antidiabetics:* concomitant use may enhance hypoglycemic properties. Monitor blood glucose levels.

*Rifampin:* reduced plasma levels of carvedilol by 70%. Monitor vital signs closely.

**Drug-food.** *Any food:* delayed rate of absorption of carvedilol but does not alter extent of bioavailability. Advise patient to take drug with food to minimize orthostatic effects.

## EFFECTS ON DIAGNOSTIC TESTS
None reported.

## CONTRAINDICATIONS
Contraindicated in patients with hypersensitivity to drug and in those with New York Heart Association class IV decompensated cardiac failure requiring I.V. inotropic therapy. Also contraindicated in those with bronchial asthma or related bronchospastic conditions, second- or third-degree AV block, sick sinus syndrome (unless a permanent pacemaker is in place), cardiogenic shock, severe bradycardia, or symptomatic hepatic impairment.

## NURSING CONSIDERATIONS
• Use cautiously in hypertensive patients with left-sided heart failure, perioperative patients who receive anesthetics that depress myocardial function (such as ether, cyclopropane, and trichloroethylene), diabetic patients receiving insulin or oral antidiabetics, and in those subject to spontaneous hypoglycemia. Also use with caution in patients with thyroid disease (may mask hyperthyroidism; withdrawal may precipitate thyroid storm or exacerbation of hyperthyroidism), pheochromocytoma, Prinzmetal's or variant angina, bronchospastic disease, or peripheral vascular disease (may precipitate or aggravate symptoms of arterial insufficiency). Also use cautiously in breast-feeding women.

• ***Alert:*** Patients receiving beta-blocker therapy with a history of severe anaphylactic reaction to several allergens may be more reactive to repeated challenge (accidental, diagnostic, or therapeutic). They may be unresponsive to dosages of epinephrine typically used to treat allergic reactions.

• Mild hepatocellular injury may occur during therapy. At first sign of hepatic dysfunction, perform tests for hepatic injury or jaundice; if present, stop drug.

• If drug must be stopped, discontinue it gradually over 1 to 2 weeks.

• Monitor patient with heart failure for worsened condition, renal dysfunction, or fluid retention; diuretics may need to be increased.

• Monitor diabetic patient closely; drug may mask signs of hypoglycemia, or hyperglycemia may be worsened.

• Observe patient for dizziness or lightheadedness for 1 hour after administration of each new dosage.

• Before initiation of carvedilol, dosages of digoxin, diuretics, and ACE inhibitors should be stabilized.

• Safety and efficacy in patients under age 18 haven't been established.

• Monitor elderly patients carefully; plasma levels are about 50% higher in elderly patients compared with younger ones.

### ✅ Patient teaching
• Tell patient not to interrupt or discontinue drug without medical approval.
• Inform patient that improvement of heart failure symptoms might take several weeks of drug therapy.

---

Reactions may be *common*, uncommon, ***life-threatening***, or COMMON AND LIFE-THREATENING.

• Advise patient with heart failure to call doctor if weight gain or shortness of breath occurs.
• Inform patient that he may experience low blood pressure when standing. If dizziness or fainting (rare) occur, advise him to sit or lie down. Notify doctor if symptoms persist.
• Caution patient against performing hazardous tasks during initiation of therapy.
• Advise diabetic patient to promptly report changes in blood glucose level.
• Inform patient who wears contact lenses that decreased lacrimation may occur.

## clonidine
Catapres-TTS

## clonidine hydrochloride
Catapres, Dixarit†‡

*Pregnancy Risk Category C*

### HOW SUPPLIED
**clonidine**
*Transdermal:* TTS-1 (releases 0.1 mg/24 hours), TTS-2 (releases 0.2 mg/24 hours), TTS-3 (releases 0.3 mg/24 hours)
**clonidine hydrochloride**
*Tablets:* 0.025 mg†‡, 0.1 mg, 0.2 mg, 0.3 mg

### ACTION
Unknown. Thought to stimulate alpha$_2$-adrenergic receptors centrally and inhibit the central vasomotor centers, thereby decreasing sympathetic outflow to the heart, kidneys, and peripheral vasculature, resulting in decreased peripheral vascular resistance, systolic and diastolic blood pressure, and heart rate.

| Route | Onset | Peak | Duration |
|---|---|---|---|
| P.O. | 0.5-1 hr | 2-4 hr | 12-24 hr |
| Transdermal | 2-3 days | 2-3 days | 7-8 days |

### INDICATIONS & DOSAGE
*Essential and renal hypertension—*
**Adults:** initially, 0.1 mg P.O. b.i.d.; then increased by 0.1 to 0.2 mg daily on a weekly basis. Usual range is 0.2 to 0.6 mg daily in divided doses; infrequently, dosages as high as 2.4 mg daily are used.

Or, a transdermal patch is applied to a nonhairy area of intact skin on upper arm or torso once q 7 days, starting with 0.1-mg system and adjusted with another 0.1-mg system or larger system.
**Children:** 50 to 400 mcg P.O. b.i.d.

### ADVERSE REACTIONS
**CNS:** *drowsiness, dizziness,* fatigue, *sedation, weakness,* malaise, agitation, depression.
**CV:** orthostatic hypotension, bradycardia, *severe rebound hypertension.*
**GI:** *constipation, dry mouth,* nausea, vomiting, anorexia.
**GU:** urine retention, impotence, loss of libido.
**Metabolic:** weight gain.
**Skin:** *pruritus, dermatitis* with transdermal patch, rash.

### INTERACTIONS
**Drug-drug.** *CNS depressants:* enhanced CNS depression. Use together cautiously.
*Diuretics, other antihypertensives:* increased hypotensive effect. Monitor closely.
*Levodopa:* may reduce effectiveness of levodopa. Monitor patient.
*MAO inhibitors, prazosin, tricyclic antidepressants:* may decrease antihypertensive effect. Use together cautiously.
*Propranolol, other beta blockers,:* paradoxical hypertensive response. Monitor carefully.
*Verapamil:* may cause AV block and severe hypotension. Monitor carefully.
**Drug-herb.** *Capsicum:* may reduce antihypertensive effectiveness. Avoid concomitant use.

### EFFECTS ON DIAGNOSTIC TESTS
Clonidine may decrease urinary excretion of vanillylmandelic acid and catecholamines, and may cause a weakly positive Coombs' test.

### CONTRAINDICATIONS
Contraindicated in patients with hypersensitivity to drug. Transdermal form is contraindicated in patients with hypersensitivity to any component of the adhesive layer of transdermal system.

## NURSING CONSIDERATIONS
• Use cautiously in patients with severe coronary insufficiency, recent MI, cerebrovascular disease, chronic renal failure, or impaired liver function.
• Drug may be given to rapidly lower blood pressure in some hypertensive emergencies.
• Monitor blood pressure and pulse rate frequently. Dosage is usually adjusted to patient's blood pressure and tolerance.
• Elderly patients may be more sensitive than younger ones to drug's hypotensive effects.
• Observe patient for tolerance to drug's therapeutic effects, which may require increased dosage.
• Noticeable antihypertensive effects of transdermal clonidine may take 2 to 3 days. Oral antihypertensive therapy may have to be continued in the interim.
• *Alert:* Remove transdermal patch before defibrillation to prevent arcing.
• When stopping therapy in patients receiving both clonidine and a beta blocker, gradually withdraw the beta blocker first to minimize adverse reactions, as ordered.
• Discontinuation of drug before surgery is not recommended.
• *Alert:* Don't confuse clonidine with quinidine or clomiphene; or Catapres with Cetapred or Combipres.

☑ **Patient teaching**
• Instruct patient to take drug exactly as prescribed.
• Advise patient that abrupt discontinuation of drug may cause severe rebound hypertension. Tell him dosage must be reduced gradually over 2 to 4 days as instructed by doctor.
• Tell patient to take the last dose immediately before retiring.
• Reassure patient that the transdermal patch usually adheres despite showering and other routine daily activities. Instruct him on the use of the adhesive overlay to provide additional skin adherence if needed. Also tell him to place patch at a different site each week.
• Caution patient that drug may cause drowsiness but that this adverse effect will usually diminish over 4 to 6 weeks.

• Inform patient that orthostatic hypotension can be minimized by rising slowly and avoiding sudden position changes.

---

### diazoxide
Eudemine§, Hyperstat IV

*Pregnancy Risk Category C*

## HOW SUPPLIED
*Injection:* 300 mg/20 ml, 15 mg/ml

## ACTION
Unknown. Directly relaxes arteriolar smooth muscle and decreases peripheral vascular resistance.

| Route | Onset | Peak | Duration |
|-------|-------|------|----------|
| I.V. | 1 min | 2-5 min | 2-12 hr |

## INDICATIONS & DOSAGE
*Hypertensive crisis—*
**Adults and children:** 1 to 3 mg/kg by I.V. bolus (to maximum of 150 mg) q 5 to 15 minutes until adequate response is seen. Repeat at 4- to 24-hour intervals, p.r.n.

## ADVERSE REACTIONS
**CNS:** *headache,* dizziness, lightheadedness, weakness, *seizures, paralysis,* euphoria, *cerebral ischemia.*
**CV:** *sodium and water retention,* orthostatic hypotension, flushing, warmth, angina, myocardial ischemia, *arrhythmias,* ECG changes, *shock, MI.*
**EENT:** optic nerve infarction.
**GI:** *nausea, vomiting,* abdominal discomfort, dry mouth, constipation, diarrhea.
**Metabolic:** *hyperglycemia,* hyperuricemia.
**Skin:** inflammation and pain resulting from extravasation, diaphoresis.

## INTERACTIONS
**Drug-drug.** *Antihypertensives such as hydralazine, beta blockers, methyldopa, minoxidil, nitrites, prazosin, reserpine:* risk of severe hypotension. Don't administer within 6 hours of each other.
*Hydantoins:* may decrease levels of hydantoins, resulting in decreased anticonvulsant action. Monitor closely.

---

Reactions may be *common,* uncommon, *life-threatening,* or COMMON AND LIFE-THREATENING.

*Sulfonylureas:* may cause hyperglycemia. Monitor serum glucose levels.
*Thiazide diuretics:* may increase diazoxide's effects. Use together cautiously.

**EFFECTS ON DIAGNOSTIC TESTS**
Drug inhibits glucose-stimulated insulin release and may cause false-negative insulin response to glucagon. Drug may increase renin secretion and IgG, and decrease cortisol levels.

**CONTRAINDICATIONS**
Contraindicated in patients with hypersensitivity to drug, other thiazides, or other sulfonamide-derived drugs. Also contraindicated in those with compensatory hypertension (such as that associated with coarctation of the aorta or arteriovenous shunt).

**NURSING CONSIDERATIONS**
• Use cautiously in patients with impaired cerebral or cardiac function or uremia.
• Check patient's standing blood pressure before discontinuing close monitoring for hypotension.
• Monitor patient's fluid intake and output carefully. If fluid or sodium retention develops, doctor may order diuretics.
• Weigh patient daily and notify doctor of weight increase.
• Diazoxide may alter requirements for insulin, diet, or oral antidiabetics in patients with previously controlled diabetes. Monitor blood glucose level daily; watch for signs and symptoms of severe hyperglycemia or hyperosmolar hyperosmotic nonketotic syndrome. Insulin may be needed.
• Check uric acid levels frequently and report abnormalities to doctor.
• *Alert:* Don't confuse diazoxide with Dyazide or diazepam, or Hyperstat with Nitrostat, Hyper-Tet, or HyperHep.

🖐 **I.V. administration**
• Protect I.V. solutions from light. Darkened I.V. solutions of diazoxide are subpotent and shouldn't be used.
• Administer drug through peripheral vein only.
• Take care to avoid extravasation.

• Monitor blood pressure and ECG continuously. Place patient in supine position or in Trendelenburg's position during and for 1 hour after infusion. Notify doctor immediately if severe hypotension develops. Keep norepinephrine available.

☑ **Patient teaching**
• Inform patient that orthostatic hypotension can be minimized by rising slowly and avoiding sudden position changes. Tell patient to remain in supine position for 60 minutes after injection.
• Tell patient to alert nurse if discomfort occurs at I.V. insertion site.

---

**doxazosin mesylate**
Cardura, Carduran‡

*Pregnancy Risk Category C*

**HOW SUPPLIED**
*Tablets:* 1 mg, 2 mg, 4 mg, 8 mg

**ACTION**
An alpha$_1$ blocker that acts on the peripheral vasculature to reduce peripheral vascular resistance and produce vasodilation.

| Route | Onset | Peak | Duration |
|-------|-------|------|----------|
| P.O. | 1-2 hr | 2-3 hr | 24 hr |

**INDICATIONS & DOSAGE**
*Essential hypertension—*
**Adults:** initially, 1 mg P.O. daily; determine effect on standing and supine blood pressure at 2 to 6 hours and 24 hours after dosing. If needed, dosage is increased to 2 mg daily. To minimize adverse reactions, dosage is adjusted slowly (dosage typically increased only q 2 weeks). If needed, dosage increased to 4 mg daily; then 8 mg. Maximum daily dose is 16 mg; however, dosages over 4 mg daily are associated with a greater incidence of adverse reactions.
*BPH—*
**Adults:** initially, 1 mg P.O. once daily in the morning or evening; may be increased to 2 mg and, thereafter, 4 mg and 8 mg once daily, p.r.n. Recommended adjustment interval is 1 to 2 weeks.

---

## ADVERSE REACTIONS

**CNS:** *dizziness,* vertigo, somnolence, drowsiness, *asthenia, headache.*
**CV:** *orthostatic hypotension,* hypotension, edema, palpitations, ***arrhythmias,*** tachycardia.
**EENT:** rhinitis, pharyngitis, abnormal vision.
**GI:** nausea, vomiting, diarrhea, constipation.
**Hematologic:** *leukopenia, neutropenia.*
**Musculoskeletal:** arthralgia, myalgia.
**Respiratory:** dyspnea.
**Skin:** rash, pruritus.
**Other:** pain.

## INTERACTIONS

**Drug-herb.** *Butcher's broom:* possible diminished effect of doxazosin. Avoid concomitant use.

## EFFECTS ON DIAGNOSTIC TESTS

None reported.

## CONTRAINDICATIONS

Contraindicated in patients with hypersensitivity to drug and quinazoline derivatives (including prazosin and terazosin).

## NURSING CONSIDERATIONS

• Use cautiously in patients with impaired hepatic function.
• Monitor blood pressure closely.
• If syncope occurs, place patient in a recumbent position and treat supportively. A transient hypotensive response isn't considered a contraindication to continued therapy.
• *Alert:* Don't confuse doxazosin with doxapram, doxorubicin, or doxepin; or Cardura with Coumadin, K-Dur, Cardene, or Cordarone.

☑ **Patient teaching**
• Instruct patient to take drug exactly as prescribed.
• *Alert:* Advise patient that he is susceptible to a first-dose effect—consisting of marked orthostatic hypotension with dizziness or syncope—similar to that produced by other alpha blockers. Orthostatic hypotension is most common after first dose but also can occur during dosage adjustment or interruption of therapy. Warn

patient that dizziness or fainting may occur. Advise him to avoid driving and other hazardous activities until drug's CNS effects are known.

---

## enalaprilat
Innovace§, Vasotec I.V.

## enalapril maleate
Amprace‡, Renitec‡, Vasotec

*Pregnancy Risk Category C (D in second and third trimesters)*

---

## HOW SUPPLIED
**enalaprilat**
*Injection:* 1.25 mg/ml
**enalapril maleate**
*Tablets:* 2.5 mg, 5 mg, 10 mg, 20 mg

## ACTION

Unknown. Inhibits ACE, preventing conversion of angiotensin I to angiotensin II, a potent vasoconstrictor. Reduced formation of angiotensin II decreases peripheral arterial resistance, thus decreasing aldosterone secretion.

| Route | Onset | Peak | Duration |
|-------|-------|------|----------|
| P.O. | 1 hr | 4-6 hr | 24 hr |
| I.V. | 15 min | 1-4 hr | 6 hr |

## INDICATIONS & DOSAGE

*Hypertension—*
**Adults:** in patients not receiving diuretics, initially 5 mg P.O. once daily; then adjusted based on response. Usual dosage range is 10 to 40 mg daily as a single dose or two divided doses. Or, 1.25 mg I.V. infusion over 5 minutes q 6 hours.
*Adjust-a-dose:* For patients on diuretics, initially 2.5 mg P.O. once daily. Or, 0.625 mg I.V. over 5 minutes, repeated in 1 hour if needed; then 1.25 mg I.V. q 6 hours.
*To convert from I.V. therapy to oral therapy—*
**Adults:** initially, 2.5 mg P.O. once daily; if patient was receiving 0.625 mg I.V. q 6 hours, then 2.5 mg P.O once daily. Dosage is adjusted based on response.

---

Reactions may be *common,* uncommon, ***life-threatening,*** or COMMON AND LIFE-THREATENING.

*To convert from oral therapy to I.V. therapy—*
**Adults:** 1.25 mg I.V. over 5 minutes q 6 hours. Higher dosages haven't shown greater efficacy.
*Adjust-a-dose:* For patients with renal impairment or hyponatremia, if serum creatinine level is over 1.6 mg/dl or serum sodium level is below 130 mEq/L, dosage is initiated at 2.5 mg P.O. daily and adjusted slowly.
*Management of symptomatic heart failure—*
**Adults:** initially, 2.5 mg P.O. daily or b.i.d. increased gradually over several weeks. Maintenance is 5 to 20 mg daily, given in two divided doses. Maximum daily dose is 40 mg given in two divided doses.

## ADVERSE REACTIONS
**CNS:** headache, dizziness, fatigue, vertigo, asthenia, syncope.
**CV:** *hypotension,* chest pain, angina.
**GI:** diarrhea, nausea, abdominal pain, vomiting.
**GU:** decreased renal function in patients with bilateral renal artery stenosis or heart failure, increased BUN and creatinine levels.
**Hematologic:** decreased hemoglobin level and hematocrit, bone marrow depression.
**Hepatic:** increased liver function test results, decreased bilirubin level.
**Respiratory:** dyspnea; *dry, persistent, tickling, nonproductive cough.*
**Skin:** rash.
**Other:** *angioedema.*

## INTERACTIONS
**Drug-drug.** *Diuretics:* excessive reduction of blood pressure. Use together cautiously.
*Insulin, oral antidiabetics:* risk of hypoglycemia, especially at initiation of enalapril therapy. Monitor closely.
*Lithium:* lithium toxicity can occur. Monitor lithium levels.
*NSAIDs:* may reduce antihypertensive effect. Monitor blood pressure.
*Potassium-sparing diuretics, potassium supplements:* increased risk of hyper-

kalemia. Avoid these drugs unless hypokalemic blood levels are confirmed.
**Drug-food.** *Salt substitutes containing potassium:* risk of hyperkalemia. Monitor closely.

## EFFECTS ON DIAGNOSTIC TESTS
None reported.

## CONTRAINDICATIONS
Contraindicated in patients with hypersensitivity to drug or history of angioedema related to previous treatment with an ACE inhibitor.

## NURSING CONSIDERATIONS
• Use cautiously in renally impaired patients.
• Monitor blood pressure response to drug closely.
• Monitor CBC with differential counts before and during therapy.
• Diabetic patients, those with impaired renal function or heart failure, and those receiving drugs that can increase serum potassium level may develop hyperkalemia. Monitor potassium intake and serum potassium level.
• *Alert:* Don't confuse enalapril with Anafranil or Eldepryl.

 **I.V. administration**
• Inject drug slowly over at least 5 minutes, or dilute in 50 ml of a compatible solution and infuse over 15 minutes. Compatible solutions include $D_5W$, normal saline for injection, dextrose 5% in lactated Ringer's injection, dextrose 5% in normal saline for injection and Isolyte E.

 **Patient teaching**
• Instruct patient to report breathing difficulty or swelling of face, eyes, lips, or tongue. Angioedema (including laryngeal edema) may occur, especially after first dose.
• Advise patient to report signs of infection, such as fever and sore throat.
• Inform patient that light-headedness can occur, especially during first few days of therapy. Tell him to rise slowly to minimize this effect and to notify doctor if symptoms develop. If syncope occurs, he

should stop taking drug and call doctor immediately.
• Tell patient to use caution in hot weather and during exercise. Inadequate fluid intake, vomiting, diarrhea, and excessive perspiration can lead to light-headedness and syncope.
• Advise patient to avoid salt substitutes; these products may contain potassium, which can cause hyperkalemia in patients taking this drug.
• Tell woman to notify doctor if pregnancy occurs. Drug will need to be discontinued.

✳ *NEW DRUG*

## eprosartan mesylate
Teveten

*Pregnancy Risk Category C (D in second and third trimesters)*

### HOW SUPPLIED
*Tablets:* 400 mg, 600 mg

### ACTION
An angiotensin II receptor antagonist that reduces blood pressure by blocking the vasostrictor and aldosterone-secreting effects of angiotensin II. Eprosartan selectively blocks the binding of angiotensin II to its receptor sites found in many tissues, such as vascular smooth muscle and the adrenal gland.

| Route | Onset | Peak | Duration |
|-------|-------|------|----------|
| P.O. | 1-2 hr | 1-3 hr | 24 hr |

### INDICATIONS & DOSAGE
*Hypertension (alone or with other antihypertensives)—*
**Adults:** initially, 600 mg P.O. daily. Dose ranges from 400 to 800 mg daily, given as single daily dose or two divided doses.

### ADVERSE REACTIONS
**CNS:** depression, fatigue, headache, dizziness.
**CV:** chest pain.
**EENT:** pharyngitis, rhinitis, sinusitis.
**GI:** abdominal pain, dyspepsia, diarrhea.
**GU:** urinary tract infection, increased BUN levels.

**Hematologic:** *neutropenia.*
**Metabolic:** hypertriglyceridemia.
**Musculoskeletal:** arthralgia, myalgia.
**Respiratory:** cough, upper respiratory tract infection, bronchitis.
**Other:** injury, viral infection, dependent edema.

### INTERACTIONS
None significant.

### EFFECTS ON DIAGNOSTIC TESTS
None known.

### CONTRAINDICATIONS
Contraindicated in patients with hypersensitivity to eprosartan or its components.

### NURSING CONSIDERATIONS
• Use cautiously in patients with an activated renin-angiotensin system, such as volume- or salt-depleted patients, and in patients whose renal function may depend on the activity of the renin-angiotensin-aldosterone system, such as patients with severe heart failure. Also use cautiously in patients with renal artery stenosis.
• Correct hypovolemia and hyponatremia before initiating therapy, as ordered, to reduce the risk of symptomatic hypotension.
• Monitor blood pressure closely for 2 hours during initiation of treatment. If hypotension occurs, place patient in a supine position and, if needed, give an intravenous infusion of normal saline, as ordered.
• A transient episode of hypotension isn't a contraindication to continued treatment. Drug may be restarted once patient's blood pressure has stabilized.
• Drug may be used alone or with other antihypertensives, such as diuretics and calcium channel blockers. Maximal blood pressure response may take 2 to 3 weeks.
• Monitor patient for facial or lip swelling because angioedema has occurred with other angiotensin II antagonists.
• Closely observe infants exposed to eprosartan in utero for hypotension, oliguria, and hyperkalemia.
• Safety and effectiveness in pediatric patients haven't been established.

Reactions may be *common*, uncommon, *life-threatening*, or COMMON AND LIFE-THREATENING.

### ☑ Patient teaching
• Advise woman of childbearing age to use a reliable form of contraception and to notify her doctor immediately if pregnancy is suspected. Treatment may need to be discontinued under medical supervision.
• Advise patient to report facial or lip swelling and signs and symptoms of infection, such as fever and sore throat.
• Tell patient to notify doctor before taking OTC medication to treat a dry cough.
• Inform patient that drug may be taken without regard to meals.
• Advise breast feeding woman of potential for serious adverse reactions in breast-fed infants. A decision should be made to either discontinue drug or stop breast-feeding.
• Tell patient to store drug at a controlled room temperature of 68° to 77° F (20° to 25° C).

## felodipine
Agon SR‡, Plendil, Plendil ER‡, Renedil†

*Pregnancy Risk Category C*

### HOW SUPPLIED
*Tablets (extended-release):* 2.5 mg, 5 mg, 10 mg

### ACTION
Unknown. A dihydropyridine-derivative calcium channel blocker that prevents entry of calcium ions into vascular smooth-muscle and cardiac cells; shows some selectivity for smooth muscle as compared with cardiac muscle.

| Route | Onset | Peak | Duration |
|-------|-------|------|----------|
| P.O. | 2-5 hr | 2.5-5 hr | 24 hr |

### INDICATIONS & DOSAGE
*Hypertension—*
**Adults:** initially, 5 mg P.O. daily. Dosage is adjusted based on patient response, generally at intervals not less than 2 weeks. Usual dose is 2.5 to 10 mg daily; maximum recommended dose is 10 mg daily.

**Elderly:** 2.5 mg P.O. daily; dosage is adjusted as for adults. Maximum recommended dose is 10 mg daily.
*Adjust-a-dose:* For patients with impaired hepatic function, 2.5 mg P.O. daily; dosage adjusted as for adults. Maximum recommended dose is 10 mg daily.

### ADVERSE REACTIONS
**CNS:** *headache,* dizziness, paresthesia, asthenia.
**CV:** *peripheral edema,* chest pain, palpitations, flushing.
**EENT:** rhinorrhea, pharyngitis.
**GI:** abdominal pain, nausea, constipation, diarrhea.
**Musculoskeletal:** muscle cramps, back pain.
**Respiratory:** upper respiratory tract infection, cough.
**Skin:** rash.

### INTERACTIONS
**Drug-drug.** *Anticonvulsants:* decreased plasma level of felodipine. Avoid concomitant use.
*Cimetidine:* decreased clearance of felodipine. Use lower doses of felodipine.
*Metoprolol:* may alter pharmacokinetics of metoprolol. No dosage adjustment appears needed; monitor for adverse effects.
*Theophylline:* may slightly decrease theophylline levels. Monitor patient's response closely.
**Drug-food.** *Grapefruit juice:* increased bioavailability and effect when taken together. Monitor closely.

### EFFECTS ON DIAGNOSTIC TESTS
None reported.

### CONTRAINDICATIONS
Contraindicated in patients with hypersensitivity to drug.

### NURSING CONSIDERATIONS
• Use cautiously in patients with heart failure, particularly those receiving beta blockers, and in patients with impaired hepatic function.
• Monitor blood pressure for response.
• Monitor patient for peripheral edema, which appears to be both dose- and age-related. It's more common in patients tak-

ing higher doses, especially those over age 60.
- *Alert:* Don't confuse Plendil with pindolol.

☑ **Patient teaching**
- Tell patient to swallow tablets whole and not to crush or chew them.
- Advise patient not to take drug with grapefruit juice.
- Advise patient to continue taking drug even when he feels better, to watch his diet, and to check with doctor or pharmacist before taking other drugs, including OTC drugs.
- Advise patient to observe good oral hygiene and to see a dentist regularly; use of drug has been associated with mild gingival hyperplasia.

---

## fenoldopam mesylate
Corlopam

*Pregnancy Risk Category B*

### HOW SUPPLIED
*Ampules:* 10 mg/ml in single-dose ampules of 5 ml

### ACTION
Rapid-acting vasodilator. Drug is an agonist for $D_1$-like dopamine receptors and binds with moderate affinity to $alpha_2$ adrenoceptors.

| Route | Onset | Peak | Duration |
|-------|-------|------|----------|
| I.V. | 15 min | 20 min | Unknown |

### INDICATIONS & DOSAGE
*Short-term (up to 48 hours) hospital management of severe hypertension when rapid but quickly reversible reduction of blood pressure is indicated, including malignant hypertension with deteriorating end-organ function—*
**Adults:** administer by continuous I.V. infusion. Initiate infusion rates at 0.025 to 0.3 mcg/kg/minute and titrate upward or downward no more frequently than q 15 minutes to achieve desired blood pressure. Recommended increments for titration are 0.05 to 0.1 mcg/kg/minute.

### ADVERSE REACTIONS
**CNS:** dizziness, headache, insomnia.
**CV:** hypotension, palpitations, bradycardia, tachycardia, angina, *MI,* T-wave inversion, flushing, nonspecific chest pain.
**EENT:** nasal congestion.
**GI:** nausea, vomiting, abdominal pain, constipation, diarrhea.
**GU:** oliguria.
**Hematologic:** leukocytosis, bleeding.
**Hepatic:** increased LD and transaminase levels.
**Metabolic:** hypokalemia, increased BUN and glucose levels.
**Musculoskeletal:** limb cramp, back pain.
**Respiratory:** dyspnea.
**Other:** pyrexia.

### INTERACTIONS
**Drug-drug.** *Beta blockers:* may cause hypotension. Avoid concurrent use.

### EFFECTS ON DIAGNOSTIC TESTS
None reported.

### CONTRAINDICATIONS
No known contraindications.

### NURSING CONSIDERATIONS
- Use with caution in patients with glaucoma or ocular hypertension because drug can cause dose-dependent increases in intraocular pressure. Drug may cause symptomatic hypotension; use particular caution when administering to patients who have sustained an acute cerebral infarction or hemorrhage. Use during pregnancy only if clearly needed. Drug may appear in breast milk; use caution in administering to breast-feeding women.
- Safety and effectiveness in children have not been established.
- Drug causes a dose-related tachycardia that diminishes over time but remains substantial at higher doses.
- *Alert:* Drug contains sodium metabisulfite, which may cause allergy-type reactions (including anaphylactic symptoms and severe asthmatic episodes in susceptible individuals). Sulfite sensitivity is more frequent in asthmatics than in nonasthmatics.
- Monitor serum electrolyte levels and watch for hypokalemia.

---

Reactions may be *common,* uncommon, *life-threatening,* or COMMON AND LIFE-THREATENING.

## I.V. administration
• Follow manufacturer's instructions for diluting drug. Diluted solution is stable at room temperature for at least 24 hours.
• Infuse drug with a calibrated mechanical infusion pump.
• Don't use a bolus dose.
• Infusion may be abruptly discontinued or gradually tapered. Oral antihypertensives can be added once blood pressure is stable during infusion or after infusion discontinuation.
• Monitor blood pressure frequently during infusions. Check blood pressure and heart rate every 15 minutes until patient is stable.

## ☑ Patient teaching
• Tell patient that drug causes dose-related decreases in blood pressure and increases in heart rate. Advise patient to change positions slowly to avoid orthostatic symptoms.
• Encourage patient to report adverse reactions promptly.

---

## fosinopril sodium
Monopril, Staril§

*Pregnancy Risk Category C (D in second and third trimesters)*

### HOW SUPPLIED
*Tablets:* 10 mg, 20 mg, 40 mg

### ACTION
Antihypertensive action not clearly defined. Inhibits ACE, preventing conversion of angiotensin I to angiotensin II, a potent vasoconstrictor. Reduced formation of angiotensin II decreases peripheral arterial resistance, thus decreasing aldosterone secretion.

| Route | Onset | Peak | Duration |
|-------|-------|------|----------|
| P.O. | 1 hr | 3 hr | 24 hr |

### INDICATIONS & DOSAGE
*Hypertension—*
**Adults:** initially, 10 mg P.O. daily. Dosage is adjusted based on blood pressure response at peak and trough levels. Usual

dose is 20 to 40 mg; maximum is 80 mg daily. Dosage is divided if needed.
*Heart failure—*
**Adults:** initially, 10 mg P.O. once daily. Dosage increased over several weeks to a maximum of 40 mg P.O. daily, if needed.
*Adjust-a-dose:* For patients with moderate to severe renal failure or vigorous diuresis, initially, 5 mg P.O. once daily.

### ADVERSE REACTIONS
**CNS:** *CVA,* headache, dizziness, fatigue, syncope, paresthesia, sleep disturbance.
**CV:** chest pain, angina, *MI,* rhythm disturbances, palpitations, hypotension, orthostatic hypotension.
**EENT:** tinnitus, sinusitis.
**GI:** nausea, vomiting, diarrhea, *pancreatitis,* dry mouth, abdominal distention, abdominal pain, constipation.
**GU:** sexual dysfunction, decreased libido, renal insufficiency, elevated BUN and serum creatinine levels.
**Hematologic:** decreased hemoglobin level and hematocrit.
**Hepatic:** *hepatitis,* elevated liver function test results.
**Metabolic:** hyperkalemia.
**Musculoskeletal:** arthralgia, musculoskeletal pain, myalgia.
**Respiratory:** *bronchospasm; dry, persistent, tickling, nonproductive cough.*
**Skin:** urticaria, rash, photosensitivity, pruritus.
**Other:** *angioedema,* gout.

### INTERACTIONS
**Drug-drug.** *Antacids:* may impair absorption. Separate administration times by at least 2 hours.
*Diuretics, other antihypertensives:* risk of excessive hypotension. Diuretic may need to be discontinued or fosinopril dosage lowered.
*Lithium:* increased serum lithium levels and lithium toxicity. Monitor serum lithium levels.
*Potassium-sparing diuretics, potassium supplements:* risk of hyperkalemia. Monitor closely during concomitant use.
**Drug-food.** *Salt substitutes containing potassium:* risk of hyperkalemia. Monitor closely during concomitant use.

---

## EFFECTS ON DIAGNOSTIC TESTS
False low measurements of digoxin levels may result with the Digi-Tab radio-immunoassay kit for digoxin; other kits may be used.

## CONTRAINDICATIONS
Contraindicated in patients with hypersensitivity to drug or other ACE inhibitors and in breast-feeding women.

## NURSING CONSIDERATIONS
• Use cautiously in patients with impaired renal or hepatic function.
• Monitor blood pressure for effect.
• Monitor potassium intake and serum potassium level. Diabetic patients, those with impaired renal function, and those receiving drugs that can increase serum potassium level may develop hyperkalemia.
• Other ACE inhibitors have been associated with agranulocytosis and neutropenia. Monitor CBC with differential counts, as ordered, before therapy and periodically thereafter.
• Assess renal and hepatic function before and periodically throughout therapy.
• *Alert:* Don't confuse fosinopril with lisinopril or Monopril with Monurol.

☑ **Patient teaching**
• Tell patient to avoid salt substitutes; these products may contain potassium that can cause hyperkalemia in patients taking drug.
• Advise patient to report signs of infection, such as fever and sore throat.
• Instruct patient to call doctor if the following signs or symptoms occur: easy bruising or bleeding; swelling of tongue, lips, face, eyes, mucous membranes, or extremities; difficulty swallowing or breathing; and hoarseness.
• Tell patient to use caution in hot weather and during exercise. Inadequate fluid intake, vomiting, diarrhea, and excessive perspiration can lead to light-headedness and syncope.
• Tell woman to notify doctor if pregnancy occurs. Drug will need to be discontinued.

# guanabenz acetate
Wytensin

*Pregnancy Risk Category C*

## HOW SUPPLIED
*Tablets:* 4 mg, 8 mg

## ACTION
Unknown. A centrally acting antihypertensive whose action is thought to be due to central alpha-adrenergic stimulation, which results in decreased sympathetic outflow to the heart, kidneys, and peripheral vasculature.

| Route | Onset | Peak | Duration |
|-------|-------|------|----------|
| P.O. | 1 hr | 2-5 hr | 12 hr |

## INDICATIONS & DOSAGE
*Hypertension—*
**Adults:** initially, 2 to 4 mg P.O. b.i.d. Dosage increased in increments of 4 to 8 mg/day q 1 to 2 weeks. Maximum daily dose is 32 mg b.i.d. To ensure adequate overnight blood pressure control, give last dose h.s.

## ADVERSE REACTIONS
**CNS:** *drowsiness, sedation, dizziness, weakness,* headache.
**CV:** *rebound hypertension.*
**GI:** *dry mouth.*
**Hepatic:** elevated liver enzyme levels.
**Other:** reduced serum cholesterol and total triglyceride levels.

## INTERACTIONS
**Drug-drug.** *CNS depressants:* may cause increased sedation. Use together cautiously.
*Diuretics, other antihypertensives:* increased risk of excessive hypotension. Dosage adjustment may be needed.
*MAO inhibitors, tricyclic antidepressants:* may decrease antihypertensive effect. Monitor closely.

## EFFECTS ON DIAGNOSTIC TESTS
None reported.

---

Reactions may be *common*, uncommon, *life-threatening*, or COMMON AND LIFE-THREATENING.

**CONTRAINDICATIONS**
Contraindicated in patients with hypersensitivity to drug.

**NURSING CONSIDERATIONS**
• Use cautiously in the elderly and in patients with severe coronary insufficiency, recent MI, cerebrovascular disease, or severe hepatic or renal failure.
• Monitor blood pressure. Elderly patients may be more sensitive than younger ones to drug's hypotensive effects.
• Chronic use of guanabenz decreases plasma levels of norepinephrine, dopamine, and beta-hydroxylase, and plasma renin activity.
• Store drug in light-resistant container.
• *Alert:* Don't confuse guanabenz with guanadrel or guanfacine.

☑ **Patient teaching**
• Caution patient that abrupt discontinuation of drug may cause rebound hypertension.
• Advise patient to avoid hazardous tasks that require alertness until drug's CNS effects are known.
• Inform patient that orthostatic hypotension can be minimized by rising slowly and avoiding sudden position changes. Dry mouth can be relieved by chewing gum or sucking on sour hard candy or ice chips.
• Warn patient that tolerance to alcohol or other CNS depressants may be diminished.

---

**guanadrel sulfate**
Hylorel

*Pregnancy Risk Category B*

---

**HOW SUPPLIED**
*Tablets:* 10 mg, 25 mg

**ACTION**
Acts peripherally, inhibiting norepinephrine release and depleting norepinephrine stores in adrenergic nerve endings.

| Route | Onset | Peak | Duration |
|-------|-------|------|----------|
| P.O. | 2 hr | 4-6 hr | 4-14 hr |

**INDICATIONS & DOSAGE**
*Hypertension—*
**Adults:** initially, 5 mg P.O. b.i.d. Dosage adjusted until blood pressure is controlled. Most patients need dosages of 20 to 75 mg/day, usually given in divided doses. b.i.d.; however, tolerance to hypotensive effect may necessitate upward adjustment to 100 to 400 mg daily in three to four divided doses.
*Adjust-a-dose:* For patients with renal impairment, if creatinine clearance is 30 to 60 ml/minute, dosage is reduced to 5 mg P.O. once daily; if clearance is below 30 ml/minute, dosage interval is increased to 48 hours. Dosage is adjusted q 7 to 14 days.

**ADVERSE REACTIONS**
**CNS:** depression, *fatigue, drowsiness, faintness, headache, confusion, paresthesia.*
**CV:** *palpitations, chest pain, peripheral edema, orthostatic hypotension.*
**EENT:** *visual disturbances.*
**GI:** *diarrhea,* dry mouth, *indigestion, constipation, anorexia,* nausea, vomiting, abdominal pain, glossitis.
**GU:** impotence, *ejaculation disturbances, nocturia, urination frequency.*
**Metabolic:** *weight gain.*
**Musculoskeletal:** *aching limbs, leg cramps.*
**Respiratory:** *shortness of breath, cough.*

**INTERACTIONS**
**Drug-drug.** *Amphetamines, ephedrine, methylphenidate, norepinephrine, phenothiazines, tricyclic antidepressants:* may inhibit guanadrel's antihypertensive effect. Adjust dose accordingly.
*Diuretics, other antihypertensives:* hypotensive effect of guanadrel increased. Monitor blood pressure closely.
*MAO inhibitors:* antagonized hypotensive effects of guanadrel. Don't give guanadrel concurrently or within 1 week of MAO inhibitor therapy.

**EFFECTS ON DIAGNOSTIC TESTS**
None reported.

---

## CONTRAINDICATIONS

Contraindicated in patients with hypersensitivity to drug, known or suspected pheochromocytoma, or frank heart failure. Avoid use with or within 1 week of MAO inhibitor therapy.

## NURSING CONSIDERATIONS

• Use cautiously in patients with regional vascular disease, bronchial asthma, or history of peptic ulcer disease.
• Monitor both supine and standing blood pressure, especially during dosage adjustment periods.
• Elderly patients may be more sensitive to drug's hypotensive effects.
• Drug should be discontinued 48 to 72 hours before surgery to minimize risk of vascular collapse during anesthesia.
• *Alert:* Don't confuse guanadrel with gonadorelin or guanabenz.

☑️**Patient teaching**
• Inform patient that orthostatic hypotension can be minimized by rising slowly from a supine position and by avoiding sudden position changes. Dry mouth can be relieved by chewing gum or sucking on sour hard candy or ice chips.
• Warn patient to avoid strenuous exercise and hot showers, which may cause a hypotensive reaction. An ambient temperature that is too hot or alcohol ingestion also may potentiate drug's hypotensive effects.
• Tell patient to check with doctor or pharmacist before taking cold, cough, or allergy preparations.

---

## guanfacine hydrochloride
Tenex

*Pregnancy Risk Category B*

### HOW SUPPLIED
*Tablets:* 1 mg, 2 mg

### ACTION
Unknown. Possibly inhibits the central vasomotor center, thereby decreasing sympathetic outflow to the heart, kidneys, and peripheral vasculature, and decreasing blood pressure.

| Route | Onset | Peak | Duration |
|-------|-------|------|----------|
| P.O. | Unknown | 1-4 hr | 24 hr |

### INDICATIONS & DOSAGE
*Hypertension—*
**Adults:** initially, 1 mg P.O. daily h.s. Dosage may be increased to 2 mg P.O. h.s. after 3 to 4 weeks, p.r.n. Dosage may be further increased to 3 mg P.O. h.s. after an additional 3 to 4 weeks, p.r.n. Average dose is 1 to 3 mg daily.

### ADVERSE REACTIONS
**CNS:** *dizziness,* fatigue, headache, insomnia, *somnolence,* asthenia.
**CV:** bradycardia.
**GI:** *constipation,* diarrhea, nausea, *dry mouth.*
**Skin:** dermatitis, pruritus.

### INTERACTIONS
**Drug-drug.** *CNS depressants:* may potentially increase sedation. Use together cautiously.
*Tricyclic antidepressants:* may inhibit antihypertensive effects. Avoid concurrent use.

### EFFECTS ON DIAGNOSTIC TESTS
Drug alters urinary catecholamine levels and urinary vanillylmandelic acid excretion (may be decreased during therapy but may increase on abrupt withdrawal). Plasma growth hormone levels may be increased after a single dose; long-term elevation does not follow long-term use.

### CONTRAINDICATIONS
Contraindicated in patients with hypersensitivity to drug.

### NURSING CONSIDERATIONS
• Use cautiously in patients with severe coronary insufficiency, recent MI, cerebrovascular disease, or chronic renal or hepatic insufficiency.
• Monitor blood pressure frequently.
• Incidence and severity of adverse reactions increase with higher dosages.
• Drug may be used alone or with a diuretic.

---

Reactions may be *common,* uncommon, ***life-threatening**,* or **COMMON AND LIFE-THREATENING.**

• **Alert:** Don't confuse guanfacine with guanidine, guaifenesin, or guanabenz; or Tenex with Xanax, Entex, or Ten-K.

☑ **Patient teaching**
• Tell patient not to discontinue therapy abruptly. Rebound hypertension is less common than with similar drugs but may occur.
• Advise patient to avoid activities that require alertness until response to drug is established; drowsiness may occur.

---

## hydralazine hydrochloride
Alphapress‡, Apresoline**,
Novo-Hylazin†, Suprest†

*Pregnancy Risk Category C*

### HOW SUPPLIED
*Tablets:* 10 mg, 25 mg, 50 mg, 100 mg
*Injection:* 20 mg/ml

### ACTION
Unknown. A direct-acting vasodilator that primarily relaxes arteriolar smooth muscle.

| Route | Onset | Peak | Duration |
|-------|-------|------|----------|
| P.O. | 20-30 min | 1-2 hr | 2-4 hr |
| I.V. | 5-20 min | 10-80 min | 2-6 hr |
| I.M. | 10-30 min | 1 hr | 2-6 hr |

### INDICATIONS & DOSAGE
*Essential hypertension (orally, alone or with other antihypertensives), severe essential hypertension (parenterally, to lower blood pressure quickly)—*
**Adults:** *P.O.*—initially, 10 mg P.O. q.i.d.; gradually increased to 50 mg q.i.d., p.r.n. Maximum recommended dose is 200 mg daily, but some patients may need 300 to 400 mg daily.
*I.V.*—10 to 20 mg given slowly and repeated as needed, switching to oral antihypertensives as soon as possible.
*I.M.*—10 to 50 mg, repeated as needed, switching to oral form as soon as possible.
**Children:** *P.O.*—initially, 0.75 mg/kg/day P.O. divided into four doses; gradually increased over 3 to 4 weeks to maximum of

7.5 mg/kg or 200 mg daily. Maximum initial P.O. dose is 25 mg.
*I.V.*—0.1 to 0.2 mg/kg I.V. q 4 to 6 hours, p.r.n. Maximum initial parenteral dose is 20 mg.

### ADVERSE REACTIONS
**CNS:** peripheral neuritis, *headache, dizziness.*
**CV:** orthostatic hypotension, *tachycardia,* edema, *angina, palpitations.*
**EENT:** nasal congestion.
**GI:** *nausea, vomiting, diarrhea, anorexia,* constipation.
**Hematologic:** *neutropenia, leukopenia, agranulocytopenia, agranulocytosis, thrombocytopenia with or without purpura;* decreased hemoglobin level and RBC count.
**Skin:** rash.
**Other:** *lupus-like syndrome.*

### INTERACTIONS
**Drug-drug.** *Diazoxide, MAO inhibitors:* may cause severe hypotension. Use together cautiously.
*Diuretics, other hypotensive drugs:* increased risk of excessive hypotension. Dosage adjustment may be needed.
*Indomethacin:* may decrease effects of hydralazine. Monitor blood pressure.

### EFFECTS ON DIAGNOSTIC TESTS
Drug may cause positive antinuclear antibody titer and positive lupus erythematosus cell preparation.

### CONTRAINDICATIONS
Contraindicated in patients with hypersensitivity to drug, coronary artery disease, or mitral valvular rheumatic heart disease.

### NURSING CONSIDERATIONS
• Use cautiously in patients with suspected cardiac disease, CVA, or severe renal impairment and in those taking other antihypertensives.
• Monitor patient's blood pressure, pulse rate, and body weight frequently. Hydralazine may be given with diuretics and beta blockers to decrease sodium retention and tachycardia and to prevent angina attacks.

---

• Elderly patients may be more sensitive than younger ones to drug's hypotensive effects.

• Monitor CBC, lupus erythematosus cell preparation, and antinuclear antibody titer determination before therapy and periodically during long-term therapy, as ordered.

• *Alert:* Watch patient closely for signs and symptoms of lupus-like syndrome (sore throat, fever, muscle and joint aches, rash). Notify doctor immediately if these develop.

• Compliance may be improved by administering drug b.i.d. Check with doctor.

• *Alert:* Don't confuse hydralazine with hydroxyzine or Apresoline with Apresazide.

**I.V. administration**

• Give drug slowly and repeat as needed, generally q 4 to 6 hours.

• Hydralazine will undergo color changes in most infusion solutions; these color changes don't indicate loss of potency.

• Drug is compatible with normal saline, Ringer's, and lactated Ringer's solutions, and several other common I.V. solutions. Drug may undergo a reaction with dextrose. The manufacturer doesn't recommend mixing drug in infusion solutions. Check with pharmacist for additional compatibility information.

• Oral therapy should replace parenteral therapy as soon as possible.

**Patient teaching**

• Instruct patient to take oral form with meals to increase absorption.

• Inform patient that orthostatic hypotension can be minimized by rising slowly and avoiding sudden position changes.

• Tell woman to notify doctor if she suspects pregnancy; drug should be stopped.

## irbesartan
Aprovel§, Avapro

*Pregnancy Risk Category C (D in second and third trimesters)*

### HOW SUPPLIED
*Tablets:* 75 mg, 150 mg, 300 mg

### ACTION
Produces antihypertensive effect by competitive antagonist activity at the angiotensin II receptor.

| Route | Onset | Peak | Duration |
|-------|-------|------|----------|
| P.O. | Unknown | 1.5-2 hr | 24 hr |

### INDICATIONS & DOSAGE
*Hypertension–*
**Adults:** initially 150 mg P.O. daily, increased to maximum of 300 mg daily if needed.
*Adjust-a-dose:* For volume- and salt-depleted patients, initially 75 mg P.O. daily.

### ADVERSE REACTIONS
**CNS:** fatigue, anxiety, dizziness, headache.
**CV:** chest pain, edema, tachycardia.
**EENT:** pharyngitis, rhinitis, sinus abnormality.
**GI:** diarrhea, dyspepsia, abdominal pain, nausea, vomiting.
**GU:** urinary tract infection.
**Musculoskeletal:** musculoskeletal trauma or pain.
**Respiratory:** upper respiratory tract infection.
**Skin:** rash.

### INTERACTIONS
None significant.

### EFFECTS ON DIAGNOSTIC TESTS
None reported.

### CONTRAINDICATIONS
Contraindicated in patients with hypersensitivity to drug or its ingredients.

### NURSING CONSIDERATIONS
• Use during pregnancy can cause injury and death to the developing fetus. When pregnancy is detected, discontinue drug as soon as possible.

• Use with caution in patients with impaired renal function, heart failure, and renal artery stenosis and in breast-feeding women.

• Drug may be administered with a diuretic or other antihypertensive, if needed, for control of hypertension.

---

Reactions may be *common,* uncommon, *life-threatening,* or COMMON AND LIFE-THREATENING.

• Symptomatic hypotension may occur in volume- or salt-depleted patients (vigorous diuretic use or dialysis). The cause of volume depletion should be corrected before administration or before a lower dose is used.

• If hypotension occurs, place patient in a supine position and give an I.V. infusion of normal saline solution if needed. Once blood pressure has stabilized after a transient hypotensive episode, drug may be continued without problems.

☑ **Patient teaching**
• Warn woman of childbearing age of consequences of drug exposure to fetus. Tell her to call doctor immediately if pregnancy is suspected.
• Tell patient that drug may be taken once daily without regard to food.

---

## isradipine
DynaCirc, Prescal§

*Pregnancy Risk Category C*

---

### HOW SUPPLIED
*Capsules:* 2.5 mg, 5 mg

### ACTION
Unknown. A calcium channel blocker that inhibits calcium ion influx across cardiac and smooth-muscle cells and is thought to decrease arteriolar resistance and blood pressure.

| Route | Onset | Peak | Duration |
|-------|-------|------|----------|
| P.O. | 2 hr | 1.5 hr | 12 hr |

### INDICATIONS & DOSAGE
*Essential hypertension—*
**Adults:** initially, 1.25 to 2.5 mg P.O. b.i.d., alone or with a thiazide diuretic. To increase dosage, adjust gradually. If response is inadequate after first 2 to 4 weeks, dose increased by 5-mg daily increments q 2 to 4 weeks to maximum of 20 mg daily.

### ADVERSE REACTIONS
**CNS:** dizziness, *headache,* fatigue, syncope.

**CV:** edema, flushing, angina, tachycardia.
**GI:** nausea, diarrhea, abdominal discomfort, vomiting.
**Respiratory:** dyspnea.
**Skin:** rash.

### INTERACTIONS
**Drug-drug.** *Cimetidine:* increases levels of isradipine. Monitor for increased effects.
*Fentanyl anesthesia:* severe hypotension has been reported with use of a beta blocker and a calcium channel blocker. Avoid concomitant use.
*Rifampin:* reduced isradipine effects. Monitor closely.

### EFFECTS ON DIAGNOSTIC TESTS
None reported.

### CONTRAINDICATIONS
Contraindicated in patients with hypersensitivity to drug.

### NURSING CONSIDERATIONS
• Use cautiously in patients with heart failure, especially if given with a beta blocker.
• Monitor patient for adverse reactions. Like other calcium channel blockers, isradipine is known to cause symptomatic hypotension. Most adverse reactions are mild and transient and are related to vasodilation (dizziness, edema, flushing, palpitations, and tachycardia).
• Monitor blood pressure closely.
• Before surgery, inform anesthesiologist that patient is taking a calcium channel blocker.
• *Alert:* Don't confuse DynaCirc with Dynacin.

☑ **Patient teaching**
• Tell patient that drug has some diuretic activity. He may note an increased need to void.
• Advise patient to avoid hazardous tasks if adverse CNS reactions occur.

---

## labetalol hydrochloride
Normodyne, Presolol‡, Trandate

*Pregnancy Risk Category C*

### HOW SUPPLIED
*Tablets:* 100 mg, 200 mg, 300 mg
*Injection:* 5 mg/ml

### ACTION
Unknown. Possibly related to reduced peripheral vascular resistance mainly as a result of alpha and beta blockade.

| Route | Onset | Peak | Duration |
|-------|-------|------|----------|
| P.O. | 20 min | 2-4 hr | 8-12 hr |
| I.V. | 2-5 min | 5 min | 2-4 hr |

### INDICATIONS & DOSAGE
*Hypertension—*
**Adults:** 100 mg P.O. b.i.d. with or without a diuretic. If needed, dosage is increased to 200 mg b.i.d. after 2 days. Further increases may be made q 2 to 3 days until optimum response is reached. Usual maintenance dose is 200 to 400 mg b.i.d.
*Severe hypertension, hypertensive emergencies—*
**Adults:** 200 mg diluted in 160 ml of $D_5W$, infused at 2 mg/minute until satisfactory response is obtained; then infusion is stopped. May be repeated q 6 to 12 hours.
   Or, administered by repeated I.V. injection: initially, 20 mg I.V. slowly over 2 minutes. Repeat injections of 40 to 80 mg q 10 minutes until maximum dose of 300 mg is reached, p.r.n.

### ADVERSE REACTIONS
**CNS:** vivid dreams, fatigue, headache, paresthesia, syncope, transient scalp tingling, *dizziness.*
**CV:** *orthostatic hypotension, ventricular arrhythmias.*
**EENT:** nasal stuffiness.
**GI:** nausea, vomiting.
**GU:** sexual dysfunction, urine retention.
**Respiratory:** dyspnea, *bronchospasm.*
**Skin:** rash.

### INTERACTIONS
**Drug-drug.** *Beta-adrenergic agonists:* may blunt bronchodilator effect of these drugs in patients with bronchospasm. Therefore, greater than normal doses of these drugs may be needed.
*Cimetidine:* may enhance labetalol's effect. Give together cautiously.
*Halothane:* additive hypotensive effect. Monitor blood pressure closely.
*Insulin, oral antidiabetics:* can alter dosage requirements in previously stabilized diabetic patient. Observe patient carefully.

### EFFECTS ON DIAGNOSTIC TESTS
Drug may cause a false-positive increase of urine free and total catecholamine levels when measured by a nonspecific trihydroxindole fluorometric method. Drug causes increases in serum transaminases and blood urea levels.

### CONTRAINDICATIONS
Contraindicated in patients with hypersensitivity to drug; also contraindicated in those with bronchial asthma, overt cardiac failure, greater than first-degree heart block, cardiogenic shock, severe bradycardia, or other conditions associated with severe and prolonged hypotension.

### NURSING CONSIDERATIONS
• Use cautiously in patients with heart failure, hepatic failure, chronic bronchitis, emphysema, preexisting peripheral vascular disease, and pheochromocytoma.
• Monitor blood pressure frequently. Know that drug masks common signs and symptoms of shock.
• If dizziness occurs, ask doctor if patient may take a dose at bedtime or take smaller doses t.i.d. to help minimize this adverse reaction.
• Monitor blood glucose levels in diabetic patients closely because beta blockers may mask certain signs and symptoms of hypoglycemia.
• *Alert:* Don't confuse Trandate with Trental or Tridrate.

### ◖I.V. administration
• Drug may be given by slow, direct I.V. injection over 2 minutes at 10-minutes intervals.

---

Reactions may be *common,* uncommon, *life-threatening,* or COMMON AND LIFE-THREATENING.

• For I.V. infusion, prepare by diluting with 5% dextrose or normal saline solutions, e.g., 200 mg of drug to 160 ml 5% dextrose solution to yield a concentration of 1 mg/ml.
• Administer labetalol injection with an infusion control device. Monitor blood pressure closely: every 5 minutes for 30 minutes, then every 30 minutes for 2 hours, then hourly for 6 hours. Patient should remain in a supine position for 3 hours after infusion.
• When administered I.V. for hypertensive emergencies, drug produces a rapid, predictable fall in blood pressure within 5 to 10 minutes.
• *Alert:* Sodium bicarbonate injection is incompatible with I.V. labetalol.

☑ **Patient teaching**
• Tell patient that abrupt discontinuation of therapy can exacerbate angina and precipitate MI.
• Advise patient that dizziness is the most troublesome adverse reaction and tends to occur in the early stages of treatment, in patients also receiving diuretics, and in those receiving higher dosages. Inform patient that dizziness can be minimized by rising slowly and avoiding sudden position changes.
• Warn patient that transient scalp tingling may occur, especially at beginning of therapy, but is harmless.

---

## lisinopril
Carace§, Prinivil, Zestril

*Pregnancy Risk Category C (D in second and third trimesters)*

### HOW SUPPLIED
*Tablets:* 2.5 mg, 5 mg, 10 mg, 20 mg, 40 mg

### ACTION
Unknown. Thought to result primarily from suppression of the renin-angiotensin-aldosterone system.

| Route | Onset | Peak | Duration |
|-------|-------|------|----------|
| P.O. | 1 hr | 7 hr | 24 hr |

### INDICATIONS & DOSAGE
*Hypertension—*
**Adults:** initially, 10 mg P.O. daily for patients not receiving a diuretic. Most patients are well controlled on 20 to 40 mg daily as a single dose.
*Adjust-a-dose:* For patients receiving a diuretic, 5 mg P.O. daily. For patients with renal impairment, dosage is based on creatinine clearance: if clearance is 10 to 30 ml/minute, 5 mg P.O. daily; if clearance is below 10 ml/minute, 2.5 mg P.O. daily.
*Treatment adjunct in heart failure (with diuretics and cardiac glycosides)—*
**Adults:** initially, 5 mg P.O. daily; increased as needed to maximum of 20 mg P.O. daily.
*Adjust-a-dose:* For patients with serum sodium level less than 130 mEq/L or creatinine clearance below 30 ml/minute, initiate dose at 2.5 mg daily.
*Hemodynamically stable patients within 24 hours of acute MI to improve survival—*
**Adults:** initially 5 mg P.O.; then 5 mg after 24 hours, 10 mg after 48 hours, followed by 10 mg once daily for 6 weeks.
*Adjust-a-dose:* For patients with low systolic blood pressure (120 mm Hg or less) when treatment is started or during first 3 days after an infarct, dose should be decreased to 2.5 mg P.O. If hypotension occurs (systolic blood pressure 100 mm Hg or less), daily maintenance dose of 5 mg may be reduced to 2.5 mg if needed. If prolonged hypotension occurs (systolic blood pressure below 90 mm Hg for over 1 hour), drug should be withdrawn.

### ADVERSE REACTIONS
**CNS:** *dizziness,* headache, fatigue, paresthesia.
**CV:** hypotension, *orthostatic hypotension,* chest pain.
**EENT:** *nasal congestion.*
**GI:** *diarrhea,* nausea, dyspepsia.
**GU:** impaired renal function, impotence, increased BUN and creatinine levels.
**Hepatic:** increased liver enzymes and serum bilirubin levels.
**Metabolic:** hyperkalemia.
**Respiratory:** dyspnea; dry, persistent, tickling, nonproductive cough.
**Skin:** rash.

---

## INTERACTIONS

**Drug-drug.** *Allopurinol:* increased risk of hypersensitivity reaction. Use with caution.

*Capsaicin:* may increase risk of ACE inhibitor–induced cough. Monitor patient.

*Diuretics, thiazide diuretics:* excessive hypotension with diuretics. Monitor closely.

*Indomethacin, phenothiazines:* attenuated hypotensive effect. Monitor closely.

*Insulin, oral antidiabetics:* risk of hypoglycemia, especially at initiation of lisinopril therapy. Monitor closely.

*Potassium-sparing diuretics, potassium supplements:* possible hyperkalemia. Monitor closely.

**Drug-food.** *Potassium-containing salt substitutes:* possible hyperkalemia. Monitor closely.

## EFFECTS ON DIAGNOSTIC TESTS
None reported.

## CONTRAINDICATIONS
Contraindicated in patients with hypersensitivity to ACE inhibitors or history of angioedema related to previous treatment with ACE inhibitor.

## NURSING CONSIDERATIONS
• Use cautiously in patients with impaired renal function; dosage adjustment is needed. Also use cautiously in patients at risk for hyperkalemia.

• When used in acute MI, patient should receive, as appropriate, the standard recommended treatment, such as thrombolytics, aspirin, and beta blockers.

• Monitor blood pressure frequently. If drug does not adequately control blood pressure, diuretics may be added.

• Monitor WBC with differential counts before therapy, every 2 weeks for first 3 months of therapy, and periodically thereafter.

• *Alert:* Don't confuse lisinopril with fosinopril or Lioresal; Zestril with Zostrix; or Prinivil with Proventil or Prilosec.

### ✓ Patient teaching
• *Alert:* Rarely, angioedema (including laryngeal edema) may occur, especially after first dose. Advise patient to report signs or symptoms, such as swelling of face, eyes, lips, or tongue; or breathing difficulty.

• Inform patient that light-headedness can occur, especially during first few days of therapy. Tell him to rise slowly to minimize this effect and to report symptoms to doctor. If syncope occurs, he should stop taking drug and call doctor immediately.

• Tell patient not to discontinue drug suddenly but to call doctor if unpleasant adverse reactions occur.

• Advise patient to report signs and symptoms of infection, such as fever and sore throat.

• Tell woman to notify doctor if pregnancy occurs. Drug will need to be discontinued.

• Instruct patient not to use salt substitutes that contain potassium without first consulting doctor.

---

## losartan potassium
Cozaar

*Pregnancy Risk Category C (D in second and third trimesters)*

## HOW SUPPLIED
*Tablets:* 25 mg, 50 mg

## ACTION
An angiotensin II receptor antagonist that inhibits the vasoconstricting and aldosterone-secreting effects of angiotensin II by selectively blocking the binding of angiotensin II to its receptor sites that are found in many tissues, including vascular smooth muscle and adrenal glands.

| Route | Onset | Peak | Duration |
|-------|--------|------|----------|
| P.O. | Unknown | 1 hr | Unknown |

## INDICATIONS & DOSAGE
*Hypertension—*
**Adults:** initially, 25 to 50 mg P.O. daily. Maximum daily dose is 100 mg in one or two divided doses.

*Adjust-a-dose:* For patients with impaired hepatic function and in those who are intravascularly volume-depleted (such as those receiving diuretics), use lowest dosage (25 mg) initially.

---

Reactions may be *common,* uncommon, *life-threatening,* or COMMON AND LIFE-THREATENING.

## ADVERSE REACTIONS
**CNS:** dizziness, insomnia.
**EENT:** nasal congestion, sinusitis.
**GI:** diarrhea, dyspepsia.
**Musculoskeletal:** muscle cramps, myalgia, back or leg pain.
**Respiratory:** cough, upper respiratory tract infection.

## INTERACTIONS
**Drug-drug.** *Potassium-sparing diuretics, potassium supplements:* possible hyperkalemia. Monitor closely.
**Drug-food.** *Salt substitutes containing potassium:* risk of hyperkalemia. Monitor closely.

## EFFECTS ON DIAGNOSTIC TESTS
None reported.

## CONTRAINDICATIONS
Contraindicated in patients with hypersensitivity to drug.

## NURSING CONSIDERATIONS
• Breast-feeding isn't recommended during losartan therapy.
• Use cautiously in patients with impaired renal or hepatic function.
• Drugs that act directly on the renin-angiotensin system (such as losartan) can cause fetal and neonatal morbidity and death when given to pregnant women. These problems have not been detected when exposure has been limited to the first trimester. If pregnancy is suspected, notify doctor because drug should be discontinued.
• Drug can be used alone or with other antihypertensives.
• If antihypertensive effect measured by the serum trough level of drug, using once-daily dosing, is inadequate, a b.i.d. regimen using the same total daily dose or an increase in dose may give a more satisfactory response.
• Monitor patient's blood pressure closely to evaluate effectiveness of therapy. When losartan is used alone, the effect on blood pressure is notably less in black patients than in patients of other races.
• Monitor patients who are also taking diuretics for symptomatic hypotension.

• Regularly assess the patient's renal function (via serum creatinine and BUN levels), as ordered.
• Patients with severe heart failure whose renal function depends on the angiotensin-aldosterone system have experienced acute renal failure during ACE inhibitor therapy. Manufacturer of losartan states that drug would be expected to have the same effect. Closely monitor patient, especially during first few weeks of therapy.
• *Alert:* Don't confuse Cozaar with Zocor.

☑ **Patient teaching**
• Tell patient to avoid salt substitutes; these products may contain potassium, which can cause hyperkalemia in patients taking losartan.
• Inform woman of childbearing age about consequences of second- and third-trimester exposure to drug; instruct her to notify doctor immediately if pregnancy is suspected.

# methyldopa
Aldomet, Apo-Methyldopa†, Aldopren‡, Dopamet†, Hydopa‡, Novo-Medopa†, Nu-Medopa†

# methyldopate hydrochloride
Aldomet

*Pregnancy Risk Category B (P.O.); C (I.V.)*

## HOW SUPPLIED
**methyldopa**
*Tablets:* 125 mg, 250 mg, 500 mg
*Oral suspension:* 250 mg/5 ml
**methyldopate hydrochloride**
*Injection:* 250 mg/5 ml

## ACTION
Unknown. Thought to inhibit the central vasomotor centers, thereby decreasing sympathetic outflow to the heart, kidneys, and peripheral vasculature.

| Route | Onset | Peak | Duration |
|---|---|---|---|
| P.O. | Unknown | 4-6 hr | 12-48 hr |
| I.V. | Unknown | 4-6 hr | 10-16 hr |

## INDICATIONS & DOSAGE

*Hypertension, hypertensive crisis—*
**Adults:** *P.O.*—initially, 250 mg P.O. b.i.d. to t.i.d. in first 48 hours. Then increased, p.r.n., q 2 days. May give entire daily dose in evening or h.s. Adjust dosages if other antihypertensives are added to or deleted from therapy. Maintenance dose is 500 mg to 2 g daily in two to four divided doses. Maximum recommended daily dose is 3 g.
*I.V.*—250 to 500 mg q 6 hours. Maximum dosage is 1 g q 6 hours. Switch to oral antihypertensives as soon as possible.
**Children:** initially, 10 mg/kg P.O. daily in two to four divided doses; or, 20 to 40 mg/kg I.V. daily in four divided doses. Increase dose daily until desired response occurs. Maximum daily dose is 65 mg/kg or 3 g, whichever is less.

## ADVERSE REACTIONS

**CNS:** *sedation,* headache, weakness, dizziness, *decreased mental acuity,* paresthesia, parkinsonism, involuntary choreoathetoid movements, psychic disturbances, depression, nightmares.
**CV:** bradycardia, *orthostatic hypotension,* aggravated angina, ***myocarditis,*** *edema.*
**EENT:** *nasal congestion.*
**GI:** nausea, vomiting, diarrhea, ***pancreatitis,*** *dry mouth,* constipation.
**GU:** gynecomastia, altered serum creatinine levels.
**Hematologic:** ***hemolytic anemia, thrombocytopenia, leukopenia, bone marrow depression.***
**Hepatic:** ***hepatic necrosis,*** abnormal liver function tests, ***hepatitis.***
**Musculoskeletal:** arthralgia.
**Skin:** rash.
**Other:** galactorrhea, drug-induced fever.

## INTERACTIONS

**Drug-drug.** *Amphetamines, nonselective beta blockers, norepinephrine, phenothiazines, tricyclic antidepressants:* possible hypertensive effects. Monitor carefully.
*Anesthetics:* may need lower doses of anesthetics while on methyldopa. Use together cautiously.
*Barbiturates:* may decrease actions of methyldopa. Monitor closely.

*Haloperidol:* adverse mental symptoms and increased sedation when used with methyldopa. Use together cautiously.
*Levodopa:* additive hypotensive effects may increase adverse CNS reactions. Monitor closely.
*Lithium:* may increase lithium levels. Monitor for increased lithium levels.
*Tolbutamide:* Metabolism of tolbutamide may be impaired. Monitor for hypoglycemic effect.
**Drug-herb.** *Capsicum:* may reduce antihypertensive effectiveness. Avoid concomitant use.

## EFFECTS ON DIAGNOSTIC TESTS

Drug may cause falsely high levels of urine catecholamines, interfering with the diagnosis of pheochromocytoma. A positive direct antiglobulin (Coombs') test may also occur.

## CONTRAINDICATIONS

Contraindicated in patients with hypersensitivity to drug, active hepatic disease (such as acute hepatitis), or active cirrhosis. Also contraindicated if previous methyldopa therapy has been associated with liver disorders.

## NURSING CONSIDERATIONS

• Use cautiously in patients with history of impaired hepatic function or sulfite sensitivity and in breast-feeding women.
• Monitor patient's blood pressure regularly. Elderly patients are more likely than younger ones to experience hypotension and sedation.
• After dialysis, monitor patient for hypertension and notify doctor if needed. Patient may need an extra dose of methyldopa.
• Monitor CBC with differential counts before therapy and periodically thereafter.
• Patients who need blood transfusions should have direct and indirect Coombs' tests to prevent crossmatching problems.
• Monitor patient's Coombs' test results. In patients who have received drug for several months, positive reaction to direct Coombs' test indicates hemolytic anemia.

---

- Observe for and report involuntary choreoathetoid movements. Drug may have to be discontinued.
- *Alert:* Don't confuse Aldomet with Aldoril or Anzemet.

### ☐ I.V. administration
- Dilute appropriate dose in 100 ml D₅W and infuse slowly over 30 to 60 minutes.

### ☑ Patient teaching
- Tell patient not to suddenly stop taking drug, but to notify doctor if unpleasant adverse reactions occur.
- Instruct patient to report signs and symptoms of infection.
- Tell patient to check his weight daily and to notify doctor of weight gain over 5 lb. Sodium and water retention may occur but can be relieved with diuretics.
- Warn patient that drug may impair ability to perform tasks that require mental alertness, particularly at start of therapy. A once-daily dose at bedtime will minimize daytime drowsiness.
- Inform patient that orthostatic hypotension can be minimized by rising slowly and avoiding sudden position changes. Dry mouth can be relieved by chewing gum or sucking on sour hard candy or ice chips.
- Tell patient that urine may turn dark if left standing in toilet bowl or if toilet bowl has been treated with bleach.

---

### metoprolol succinate
Toprol XL

### metoprolol tartrate
Apo-Metoprolol†, Apo-Metoprolol (Type L)†, Betaloc†‡, Betaloc Durules†, Lopresor†, Lopresor SR†, Lopressor, Minax‡, Novo-Metoprol†, Nu-Metop†

*Pregnancy Risk Category C*

---

### HOW SUPPLIED
**metoprolol succinate**
*Tablets (extended-release):* 50 mg, 100 mg, 200 mg
**metoprolol tartrate**
*Tablets:* 50 mg, 100 mg

*Tablets (extended-release):* 100 mg†, 200 mg†
*Injection:* 1 mg/ml in 5-ml ampules

### ACTION
Unknown. A beta blocker that decreases myocardial contractility, heart rate, cardiac output, and blood pressure and reduces myocardial oxygen use. Also depresses renin secretion.

| Route | Onset | Peak | Duration |
|---|---|---|---|
| P.O. | 15 min | 1 hr | 6-12 hr |
| P.O. (extended) | 15 min | 6-12 hr | 24 hr |
| I.V. | 5 min | 20 min | 5-8 hr |

### INDICATIONS & DOSAGE
*Hypertension—*
**Adults:** initially, 50 mg P.O. b.i.d. or 100 mg P.O. once daily; then up to 100 to 450 mg daily in two or three divided doses. Or, 50 to 100 mg of extended-release tablets (tartrate equivalent) once daily. Dosage is adjusted as needed and tolerated at intervals of not less than 1 week to maximum of 400 mg daily.
*Early intervention in acute MI (metoprolol tartrate)—*
**Adults:** three 5-mg I.V. boluses q 2 minutes. Then, beginning 15 minutes after last dose, 25 to 50 mg P.O. q 6 hours for 48 hours. Maintenance dose is 100 mg P.O. b.i.d. for 3 months to 3 years.
*Angina pectoris—*
**Adults:** initially, 100 mg P.O. daily as a single dose or in two equally divided doses; increased at weekly intervals until an adequate response or a pronounced decrease in heart rate is seen. Effects of daily dose beyond 400 mg are not known. Or, give 100 mg of extended-release tablets (tartrate equivalent) once daily. Dose adjusted as needed and tolerated at intervals of not less than 1 week to maximum of 400 mg daily.

### ADVERSE REACTIONS
**CNS:** *fatigue, dizziness,* depression.
**CV:** *bradycardia,* hypotension, *heart failure, AV block.*
**GI:** nausea, diarrhea.
**Hepatic:** elevated serum transaminase, alkaline phosphatase, and LD levels.

---

**Metabolic:** elevated uric acid levels.
**Respiratory:** dyspnea.
**Skin:** rash.

## INTERACTIONS
**Drug-drug.** *Barbiturates, rifampin:* increased metabolism of metoprolol. Monitor for decreased effect.
*Cardiac glycosides, diltiazem, verapamil:* excessive bradycardia and increased depressant effect on myocardium. Use together cautiously.
*Catecholamine-depleting drugs such as reserpine, $H_2$ antagonists, MAO inhibitors:* may have additive effect when given with beta blockers. Monitor for hypotension and bradycardia.
*Chlorpromazine, cimetidine, verapamil:* decreased hepatic clearance. Monitor for greater beta-blocking effect.
*Indomethacin:* decreased antihypertensive effect. Monitor blood pressure and adjust dosage.
*Insulin, oral antidiabetics:* can alter dosage requirements in previously stabilized diabetic patients. Observe patient carefully.
*Propafenone:* may increase metoprolol serum levels. Monitor vital signs.
*Terbutaline:* may antagonize bronchodilatory effects of terbutaline. Monitor patient.
**Drug-food.** *Any food:* may increase absorption. Give drug with food.

## EFFECTS ON DIAGNOSTIC TESTS
None reported.

## CONTRAINDICATIONS
Contraindicated in patients with hypersensitivity to drug or other beta blockers. Also contraindicated in patients with sinus bradycardia, heart block greater than first-degree, cardiogenic shock, or overt cardiac failure when used to treat hypertension or angina. When used to treat MI, drug is contraindicated in patients with heart rate less than 45 beats/minute, second- or third-degree heart block, PR interval of 0.24 seconds or longer with first-degree heart block, systolic blood pressure below 100 mm Hg, or moderate to severe cardiac failure.

## NURSING CONSIDERATIONS
• Use cautiously in patients with heart failure, diabetes, or respiratory or hepatic disease.
• Always check patient's apical pulse rate before giving drug. If it's slower than 60 beats/minute, withhold drug and call doctor immediately.
• Monitor blood glucose levels closely in diabetic patients because drug masks common signs of hypoglycemia.
• Monitor blood pressure frequently; metoprolol masks common signs and symptoms of shock.
• Beta blockers may mask tachycardia associated with hyperthyroidism. In patients with suspected thyrotoxicosis, withdraw beta blocker gradually, as ordered, to avoid thyroid storm.
• Store drug at room temperature and protect from light. Discard solution if it's discolored or contains particles.
• $Beta_1$ selectivity is lost at higher doses. Monitor for peripheral side effects.
• *Alert:* Don't confuse metoprolol with metaproterenol or metolazone.

### I.V. administration
• Give drug undiluted by direct injection. Although mixing with other drugs should be avoided, metoprolol is compatible when mixed with meperidine hydrochloride or morphine sulfate or when administered with alteplase infusion at a Y-site connection.

### Patient teaching
• Instruct patient to take drug exactly as prescribed and to take it with meals.
• Tell patient not to stop drug suddenly but to notify doctor about unpleasant adverse reactions. Inform him that drug must be withdrawn gradually over 1 to 2 weeks.

---

**minoxidil**
Loniten

*Pregnancy Risk Category C*

## HOW SUPPLIED
*Tablets:* 2.5 mg, 10 mg

---

## ACTION

Unknown. Drug's predominant effect produces direct arteriolar vasodilation.

| Route | Onset | Peak | Duration |
|-------|-------|------|----------|
| P.O. | 0.5 hr | 2-3 hr | 2-5 days |

## INDICATIONS & DOSAGE

*Severe hypertension—*
**Adults:** initially, 2.5 to 5 mg P.O. as a single dose. Effective dosage range is usually 10 to 40 mg daily. Maximum dose is
100 mg daily.
**Children under age 12:** 0.2 mg/kg P.O.
(maximum 5 mg) as a single daily dose.
Effective dosage range is usually 0.25 to
1 mg/kg daily. Maximum dose is 50 mg.

## ADVERSE REACTIONS

**CV:** *edema, tachycardia, pericardial effusion and tamponade,* **heart failure,** ECG
changes, rebound hypertension.
**GI:** nausea, vomiting.
**GU:** elevated BUN and serum creatinine
levels.
**Hematologic:** transiently decreased hemoglobin levels and hematocrit.
**Hepatic:** elevated serum alkaline phosphatase level.
**Metabolic:** weight gain.
**Skin:** rash, ***Stevens-Johnson syndrome.***
**Other:** *hypertrichosis* (elongation, thickening, and enhanced pigmentation of fine
body hair), breast tenderness.

## INTERACTIONS

**Drug-drug.** *Antihypertensives:* severe orthostatic hypotension. Advise patient to
stand up slowly.

## EFFECTS ON DIAGNOSTIC TESTS

Minoxidil may alter direction and magni-
tude of T waves on ECG and elevate antinuclear antibody titers.

## CONTRAINDICATIONS

Contraindicated in patients with hypersensitivity to drug; also contraindicated in
those with pheochromocytoma.

## NURSING CONSIDERATIONS

• Use cautiously in those with impaired
renal function and after acute MI.

• Closely monitor blood pressure and
pulse rate at beginning of therapy.
• Elderly patients may be more sensitive
than younger ones to drug's hypotensive
effects.
• Drug is removed by hemodialysis. Be
sure to administer dose after dialysis.
• Monitor fluid intake and urine output.
Check for weight gain and edema.
• *Alert:* Don't confuse Loniten with
Lotensin.

☑ **Patient teaching**
• Make sure patient receives and reads
manufacturer's package insert that describes the drug and its adverse reactions.
Also provide an oral explanation.
• Tell patient not to suddenly stop taking
drug, but to call doctor if unpleasant adverse effects occur.
• Make sure patient understands importance of compliance with total treatment
regimen. Drug is usually prescribed with
a beta blocker to control tachycardia and a
diuretic to counteract fluid retention.
• Teach patient how to take his own pulse
and to notify doctor of increases over 20
beats/minute.
• Tell patient to weigh himself at least
weekly and to report weight gain of more
than 5 lb (2.2 kg).
• About 8 of 10 patients will experience
hypertrichosis within 3 to 6 weeks of beginning treatment. Unwanted hair can be
controlled with a depilatory or shaving.
Assure patient that extra hair will disappear within 1 to 6 months of stopping minoxidil. Advise patient, however, not to
discontinue drug without doctor's approval.

## moexipril hydrochloride
Perdix§, Univasc

*Pregnancy Risk Category C (D in
second and third trimesters)*

## HOW SUPPLIED

*Tablets:* 7.5 mg, 15 mg

## ACTION
Unknown. Drug's effect is thought to result primarily from suppression of renin-angiotensin-aldosterone system.

| Route | Onset | Peak | Duration |
|-------|-------|------|----------|
| P.O. | 1 hr | 1.5 hr | 24 hr |

## INDICATIONS & DOSAGE
*Hypertension—*
**Adults:** initially, 7.5 mg (3.75 mg if patient is receiving a diuretic) P.O. once daily 1 hour before meal. If control is inadequate, dosage may be increased or dose divided. Recommended maintenance dose is 7.5 to 30 mg daily, in one or two divided doses 1 hour before meal. Subsequent dosage depends on response.
*Adjust-a-dose:* For renally impaired patients with creatinine clearance less than 40 ml/minute, initial dose is 3.75 mg/day; adjust to maximum of 15 mg/day.

## ADVERSE REACTIONS
**CNS:** dizziness, headache, fatigue.
**CV:** peripheral edema, hypotension, orthostatic hypotension, chest pain, flushing.
**EENT:** pharyngitis, rhinitis, sinusitis.
**GI:** diarrhea, dyspepsia, nausea.
**GU:** urinary frequency, elevated creatinine and BUN levels.
**Hepatic:** elevated liver enzymes.
**Metabolic:** hyperkalemia.
**Musculoskeletal:** myalgia.
**Respiratory:** upper respiratory tract infection; persistent, nonproductive cough.
**Skin:** rash.
**Other:** *anaphylactoid reactions,* flulike syndrome, pain.

## INTERACTIONS
**Drug-drug.** *Diuretics:* risk of excessive hypotension. Expect diuretic to be discontinued or moexipril dose lowered.
*Lithium:* increased serum lithium level and lithium toxicity. Use together cautiously and monitor serum lithium levels frequently.
*Potassium-sparing diuretics, potassium supplements:* risk of hyperkalemia. Monitor serum potassium level closely.
**Drug-food.** *Salt substitutes containing potassium:* risk of hyperkalemia. Monitor serum potassium level closely.

## EFFECTS ON DIAGNOSTIC TESTS
None reported.

## CONTRAINDICATIONS
Contraindicated in patients with hypersensitivity to drug or history of angioedema related to treatment with ACE inhibitor.

## NURSING CONSIDERATIONS
• Safety of drug has not been established in children.
• Use cautiously in patients with impaired renal function, heart failure, or renal artery stenosis and in breast-feeding women.
• Monitor for excessive hypotension.
• Measure blood pressure at trough (just before dose) to verify blood pressure control.
• Assess renal function before and during therapy. Monitor serum potassium level, as ordered.
• Other ACE inhibitors have been associated with agranulocytosis and neutropenia. Monitor CBC with differential before therapy, especially in patients who have collagen-vascular disease with impaired renal function.
• Because angioedema associated with the tongue, glottis, or larynx can cause a fatal airway obstruction, have appropriate therapy ready, such as S.C. epinephrine 1:1,000 (0.3 to 0.5 ml) and equipment to ensure a patent airway.

### ☑ Patient teaching
• Tell patient to take drug on an empty stomach at least 1 hour before a meal to avoid impaired absorption.
• Advise patient to avoid salt substitutes with potassium, which can cause hyperkalemia in patients taking drug.
• Tell patient to use caution in hot weather and during exercise. Inadequate fluid intake, vomiting, diarrhea, and excessive perspiration can lead to light-headedness and syncope.
• Urge patient to rise slowly to minimize light-headedness. Tell him to stop taking drug and to notify doctor immediately if syncope occurs.
• Advise patient to report fever; sore throat; easy bruising or bleeding; swelling of tongue, lips, face, eyes, mucous mem-

branes, or extremities; difficulty swallowing or breathing; or hoarseness.
• Tell woman to notify doctor if pregnancy occurs. Drug must be discontinued.

## nisoldipine
Sular, Syscor MR§

*Pregnancy Risk Category C*

### HOW SUPPLIED
*Tablets (extended-release):* 10 mg, 20 mg, 30 mg, 40 mg

### ACTION
Prevents calcium ions from entering vascular smooth-muscle cells, thereby causing dilation of arterioles, which in turn decreases peripheral vascular resistance.

| Route | Onset | Peak | Duration |
|-------|-------|------|----------|
| P.O. | Unknown | 6-12 hr | 24 hr |

### INDICATIONS & DOSAGE
*Hypertension—*
**Adults:** initially, 20 mg P.O. once daily; increased by 10 mg/week or at longer intervals, p.r.n. Usual maintenance dose is 20 to 40 mg/day. Dosages over 60 mg/day are not recommended.
**Elderly:** initially, 10 mg P.O. once daily; dosage is adjusted as for adults.
*Adjust-a-dose:* For patients with impaired liver function, initially 10 mg P.O. once daily; dosage is adjusted as for adults.

### ADVERSE REACTIONS
**CNS:** *headache,* dizziness.
**CV:** vasodilation, palpitation, chest pain.
**EENT:** sinusitis, pharyngitis.
**GI:** nausea.
**Skin:** rash.
**Other:** *peripheral edema.*

### INTERACTIONS
**Drug-drug.** *Cimetidine:* increased bioavailability and peak levels of nisoldipine. Monitor blood pressure closely.
*Quinidine:* decreased bioavailability of nisoldipine. Adjust dosage accordingly.
**Drug-food.** *Grapefruit juice:* increased bioavailability and level of drug. Monitor blood pressure closely.

*High-fat meal:* increased peak drug level. Monitor blood pressure closely.

### EFFECTS ON DIAGNOSTIC TESTS
None reported.

### CONTRAINDICATIONS
Contraindicated in patients with hypersensitivity to dihydropyridine calcium channel blockers. Drug should not be used in breast-feeding women.

### NURSING CONSIDERATIONS
• Use cautiously in patients with heart failure or compromised ventricular function, particularly those receiving beta blockers and patients with severe hepatic dysfunction.
• Monitor patient carefully. Some patients, especially those with severe obstructive coronary artery disease, have developed increased frequency, duration, or severity of angina or even acute MI after starting calcium channel blocker therapy or at time of dosage increase.
• Monitor blood pressure regularly, especially during initial administration and during dosage adjustment.

### ✔ Patient teaching
• Tell patient to take drug as prescribed, even if he feels better.
• Advise patient to swallow tablet whole and not to chew, divide, or crush it.
• Remind patient not to take drug with a high-fat meal or with grapefruit juice. Both may increase drug level in the body beyond the intended amount.

## nitroprusside sodium
Nipride†, Nitropress

*Pregnancy Risk Category C*

### HOW SUPPLIED
*Injection:* 50 mg/vial in 2-ml, 5-ml vials

### ACTION
Relaxes both arteriolar and venous smooth muscle.

| Route | Onset | Peak | Duration |
|-------|-------|------|----------|
| I.V. | Immediate | 1-2 min | 10 min |

## INDICATIONS & DOSAGE

*To lower blood pressure quickly in hypertensive emergencies, to produce controlled hypotension during anesthesia, to reduce preload and afterload in cardiac pump failure or cardiogenic shock (may be used with or without dopamine)—*

**Adults and children:** 50-mg vial diluted with 2 to 3 ml of $D_5W$ and then added to 250, 500, or 1,000 ml of $D_5W$; begin infusion at 0.25 to 0.3 mcg/kg/minute I.V. and gradually titrate q few minutes to a maximum infusion rate of 10 mcg/ kg/minute.

***Adjust-a-dose:*** Patients taking other antihypertensives with nitroprusside are extremely sensitive to nitroprusside. Titrate dosage accordingly. Use with caution in patients with renal failure; reduce dosage as much as possible.

## ADVERSE REACTIONS

**CNS:** *headache, dizziness,* loss of consciousness, apprehension, ***increased intracranial pressure,*** restlessness.
**CV:** bradycardia, hypotension, tachycardia, palpitations, ECG changes, flushing.
**GI:** *nausea, abdominal pain,* ileus.
**GU:** increased serum creatinine levels.
**Metabolic:** acidosis, hypothyroidism.
**Musculoskeletal:** *muscle twitching.*
**Skin:** pink color, rash, *diaphoresis.*
**Other:** ***thiocyanate toxicity, methemoglobinemia, cyanide toxicity,*** venous streaking, irritation at infusion site.

## INTERACTIONS

**Drug-drug.** *Antihypertensives:* may cause sensitivity to nitroprusside. Adjust dosage as ordered.
*Ganglionic blocking drugs, general anesthetics, negative inotropic agents, other antihypertensives:* additive effects. Monitor blood pressure closely.

## EFFECTS ON DIAGNOSTIC TESTS

None reported.

## CONTRAINDICATIONS

Contraindicated in patients with hypersensitivity to drug; also contraindicated in those with compensatory hypertension (such as in arteriovenous shunt or coarctation of the aorta), inadequate cerebral circulation, acute heart failure associated with reduced peripheral vascular resistance, congenital optic atrophy, or tobacco-induced amblyopia.

## NURSING CONSIDERATIONS

● Use with extreme caution in patients with increased intracranial pressure. Use cautiously in patients with hypothyroidism, hepatic or renal disease, hyponatremia, or low vitamin $B_{12}$ level.
● Obtain baseline vital signs before giving drug; find out what parameters doctor wants to achieve.
● Keep patient in the supine position when initiating or titrating drug therapy.
● ***Alert:*** Don't confuse nitroprusside with nitroglycerin.

### 🔲 I.V. administration

● Don't use bacteriostatic water for injection or sterile saline solution for reconstitution.
● Prepare solution by dissolving 50 mg in 2 to 3 ml of 5% dextrose injection or according to manufacturer's instructions.
● Further dilute concentration in 250, 500 or 1,000 ml of 5% dextrose to provide solutions containing 200, 100 or 50 mcg/ml, respectively.
● Reconstitute ADD-Vantage vials labeled as containing 50 mg of drug according to manufacturer's directions.
● Because drug is sensitive to light, wrap I.V. solution in foil; it's not necessary to wrap the tubing. Fresh solution should have faint brownish tint. Discard after 24 hours.
● Infuse with an infusion pump. Drug is best given via piggyback through a peripheral line with no other drug. Don't titrate rate of main I.V. line while drug is being infused. Even a small bolus of nitroprusside can cause severe hypotension.
● Check blood pressure every 5 minutes at start of infusion and every 15 minutes thereafter. If severe hypotension occurs, discontinue nitroprusside infusion—effects of drug quickly reverse. Notify doctor. If possible, start an arterial pressure line. Regulate drug flow to specified level.
● ***Alert:*** Excessive doses or rapid infusion greater than 10 mcg/kg/minute can cause cyanide toxicity. If these factors are present, check serum thiocyanate levels q 72

hours. Levels above 100 mcg/ml are associated with toxicity. If profound hypotension, metabolic acidosis, dyspnea, headache, loss of consciousness, ataxia, and vomiting occur, discontinue drug immediately and notify doctor.

☑ **Patient teaching**
• Instruct patient to report adverse reactions promptly.
• Tell patient to alert nurse if discomfort occurs at I.V. insertion site.

---

**penbutolol sulfate**
Levatol

*Pregnancy Risk Category C*

**HOW SUPPLIED**
*Tablets:* 20 mg

**ACTION**
Unknown.

| Route | Onset | Peak | Duration |
|-------|-------|------|----------|
| P.O. | 1 hr | 1.5-3 hr | 24 hr |

**INDICATIONS & DOSAGE**
*Mild to moderate hypertension—*
**Adults:** 20 mg P.O. once daily. Usually given with other antihypertensives such as thiazide diuretics. Maximum dose is 80 mg/day.

**ADVERSE REACTIONS**
**CNS:** *dizziness,* headache, fatigue, insomnia, asthenia.
**CV:** chest pain, *heart failure.*
**GI:** nausea, diarrhea, dyspepsia.
**GU:** impotence.
**Respiratory:** cough, dyspnea, upper respiratory tract infection.
**Skin:** excessive diaphoresis.

**INTERACTIONS**
**Drug-drug.** *Clonidine:* may cause paradoxical hypertension. Also, beta blockers may enhance rebound hypertension when clonidine is withdrawn. Monitor closely.
*Digoxin, diltiazem, verapamil:* may produce additive depressant effects on AV node conduction. Monitor closely.

*Insulin, oral antidiabetics:* hypoglycemic response to these drugs may be altered. Monitor patient closely.
*Lidocaine:* volume of distribution affected. May need higher loading doses of lidocaine.
*NSAIDs:* may decrease antihypertensive effects. Monitor closely.
*Prazosin, terazosin:* first-dose orthostatic hypotension seen with these drugs may be enhanced. Use together cautiously.
*Sympathomimetics, including dobutamine, dopamine, isoproterenol, norepinephrine:* decreased hypotensive response. Monitor closely.
*Theophylline:* may decrease bronchodilator effect. Monitor patient closely.

**EFFECTS ON DIAGNOSTIC TESTS**
Drug may interfere with glucose or insulin tolerance tests.

**CONTRAINDICATIONS**
Contraindicated in patients with hypersensitivity to drug or other beta blockers and in those with sinus bradycardia, cardiogenic shock, overt cardiac failure, greater than first-degree heart block, or bronchial asthma.

**NURSING CONSIDERATIONS**
• Use cautiously in patients with heart failure controlled by drug therapy and in those with a history of bronchospastic disease. Also use cautiously in diabetic patients because beta-blockers may mask certain signs and symptoms of hypoglycemia.
• Always check patient's apical pulse before giving drug. If you detect extremes in pulse rates, withhold drug and call doctor immediately.
• Monitor blood pressure, ECG, and heart rate and rhythm frequently.
• *Alert:* Don't confuse Levatol with Lipitor.

☑ **Patient teaching**
• Instruct patient to take drug exactly as prescribed.
• Tell patient not to stop drug suddenly but to notify doctor if unpleasant adverse reactions occur.

---

• Teach patient signs and symptoms of heart failure (edema and pulmonary congestion). Advise him to notify doctor if these occur.

✳ NEW DRUG

## perindopril erbumine
Aceon

*Pregnancy Risk Category C (D in second and third trimesters)*

### HOW SUPPLIED
*Tablets:* 2 mg, 4 mg, 8 mg

### ACTION
A prodrug that's converted by the liver to the active metabolite perindoprilat, which inhibits ACE activity, thereby preventing conversion of angiotensin I to angiotensin II, a potent vasoconstrictor. Inhibition of ACE results in decreased vasoconstriction and decreased aldosterone activity, thus reducing sodium and water retention and lowering blood pressure.

| Route | Onset | Peak | Duration |
|-------|-------|------|----------|
| P.O. | Unknown | 1 hr | Unknown |

### INDICATIONS & DOSAGE
*Essential hypertension—*
**Adults:** initially, 4 mg P.O. once daily. Increase dosage until blood pressure is controlled or to maximum of 16 mg/day; usual maintenance dose is 4 to 8 mg once daily; may be given in two divided doses.
**Elderly:** initially, 4 mg P.O. daily as one dose or in two divided doses. Dosage increases exceeding 8 mg/day should only occur under close medical supervision.
*Adjust-a-dose:* For renally impaired patients, initially, 2 mg P.O. daily. Maximum maintenance dose is 8 mg/day. In patients taking diuretics, initially, 2 to 4 mg P.O. daily as one dose or in two divided doses with close medical supervision for several hours and until blood pressure has stabilized. Adjust dose based on patient's blood pressure response.

### ADVERSE REACTIONS
**CNS:** dizziness, asthenia, sleep disorder, paresthesia, depression, somnolence, nervousness, *headache.*
**CV:** palpitation, edema, chest pain, abnormal ECG.
**EENT:** rhinitis, sinusitis, ear infection, pharyngitis, tinnitus.
**GI:** dyspepsia, diarrhea, abdominal pain, nausea, vomiting, flatulence.
**GU:** proteinuria, urinary tract infection, male sexual dysfunction, menstrual disorder.
**Hepatic:** increased ALT level.
**Metabolic:** triglyceride increase.
**Musculoskeletal:** back pain, hypertonia, neck pain, joint pain, myalgia, arthritis, low or upper extremity pain.
**Respiratory:** *cough,* upper respiratory tract infection.
**Skin:** rash.
**Other:** viral infection, fever, injury, seasonal allergy.

### INTERACTIONS
**Drug-drug.** *Diuretics:* additive hypotensive effect. Monitor patient closely.
*Potassium-sparing diuretics (amiloride, spironolactone, triamterene), potassium supplements, other drugs capable of increasing serum potassium level(cyclosporine, heparin, indomethacin):* additive hyperkalemic effect. Use together cautiously and monitor serum potassium level frequently.
*Lithium:* increased serum lithium level and signs and symptoms of lithium toxicity can occur. Use together cautiously and monitor serum lithium level. Use of a diuretic may further increase risk of lithium toxicity.
**Drug-food.** *Salt substitutes containing potassium:* may increase risk of hyperkalemia. Use together cautiously.

### EFFECTS ON DIAGNOSTIC TESTS
None reported.

### CONTRAINDICATIONS
Contraindicated in patients with hypersensitivity to drug or other ACE inhibitors and in those with a history of angioedema secondary to ACE inhibitors. Also contraindicated in pregnant women.

---

Reactions may be *common,* uncommon, *life-threatening,* or COMMON AND LIFE-THREATENING.

## NURSING CONSIDERATIONS

• Use cautiously in patients with a history of angioedema unrelated to ACE inhibitor therapy. Also use cautiously in patients with impaired renal function, heart failure, ischemic heart disease, cerebrovascular disease or renal artery stenosis, and in patients with collagen vascular disease, such as systemic lupus erythematosus or scleroderma.

• *Alert:* Angioedema involving the face, extremities, lips, tongue, glottis, and larynx has been reported in patients treated with perindopril. Discontinue drug and observe patient until swelling disappears. If swelling is confined to face and lips, it will probably resolve without treatment, but antihistamines may be useful in relieving symptoms. Angioedema associated with involvement of the tongue, glottis, or larynx may be fatal because of airway obstruction. Appropriate therapy, such as subcutaneous epinephrine solution, should be promptly administered, as ordered.

• Patients with a history of angioedema unrelated to ACE inhibitor therapy may be at increased risk for angioedema while receiving an ACE inhibitor.

• Other ACE inhibitors have been associated with agranulocytosis and neutropenia. Monitor CBC with differential before therapy, especially in renally impaired patients with systemic lupus erythematosus or scleroderma.

• Excessive hypotension can occur when drug is given with diuretics. If possible, diuretic should be discontinued 2 to 3 days before starting perindopril to decrease potential for excessive hypotensive response. If it isn't possible to discontinue the diuretic, consider starting perindopril with a lower dosage or decreasing dosage of diuretic.

• Monitor patient at risk for hypotension closely during initiation of therapy, for first 2 weeks of treatment, and whenever dosage of perindopril or concomitant diuretic is increased. If severe hypotension occurs, place patient in supine position and treat symptomatically.

• Hypotension can occur when initiating therapy or adjusting dosage in patient who is volume- or salt-depleted as a result of prolonged diuretic therapy, dietary salt restriction, dialysis, diarrhea, or vomiting. Volume and salt depletion should be corrected before starting drug.

• ACE inhibitors have rarely been associated with a syndrome of cholestatic jaundice, fulminant hepatic necrosis, and death. Discontinue drug in patient who develops jaundice or marked elevations of hepatic enzymes during therapy.

• Monitor renal function before and periodically throughout therapy. Drug shouldn't be used in patient with a creatinine clearance less than 30 ml/minute.

• Monitor serum potassium levels closely.

### ✓ Patient teaching

• Inform patient that angioedema, including laryngeal edema, can occur during therapy, especially with the first dose. Advise patient to stop taking drug and immediately report any signs or symptoms suggestive of angioedema (swelling of face, extremities, eyes, lips, tongue, hoarseness or difficulty in swallowing or breathing).

• Advise patient to report promptly any sign of infection (sore throat, fever) or jaundice (yellowing of eyes or skin).

• Advise patient to avoid salt substitutes containing potassium unless instructed otherwise by doctor.

• Caution patient that light-headedness may occur, especially during first few days of therapy. Advise patient to report light-headedness and, if fainting occurs, to discontinue drug and consult doctor promptly.

• Caution patient that inadequate fluid intake or excessive perspiration, diarrhea, or vomiting can lead to an excessive drop in blood pressure.

• Advise woman of childbearing age of the consequences of second and third trimester exposure to drug. Advise her to notify doctor immediately if pregnancy is suspected.

---

## phentolamine mesylate
Regitine, Rogitine†

*Pregnancy Risk Category C*

### HOW SUPPLIED
*Injection:* 5 mg/ml in 1-ml vials, 10 mg/ml‡

---

## ACTION
An alpha blocker that competitively blocks the effects of catecholamines on alpha-adrenergic receptors.

| Route | Onset | Peak | Duration |
|-------|-------|------|----------|
| I.V. | Immediate | Within 2 minutes | 15-30 minutes |
| I.M. | Unknown | Within 20 minutes | 30-45 minutes |

## INDICATIONS & DOSAGE
*To aid in diagnosis of pheochromocytoma, to control or prevent hypertension before or during pheochromocytomectomy—*
**Adults:** I.V. diagnostic dose is 2.5 mg with close monitoring of blood pressure. Before surgical removal of tumor, 5 mg I.M. or I.V. During surgery, patient may need 5 mg I.V.
**Children:** I.V. diagnostic dose is 1 mg with close monitoring of blood pressure. Before surgical removal of tumor, 1 mg I.V. or I.M. During surgery, patient may need 1 mg I.V.
*Dermal necrosis and sloughing after I.V. extravasation of norepinephrine—*
**Adults and children:** infiltrate area with 5 to 10 mg phentolamine in 10 ml of normal saline solution, or give half the dose through the infiltrated I.V. and the other half around the site. Must be done within 12 hours.

## ADVERSE REACTIONS
**CNS:** *dizziness, weakness, flushing, **cerebrovascular occlusion,** cerebrovascular spasm.*
**CV:** *hypotension, **shock, arrhythmias,** tachycardia, **MI.***
**EENT:** *nasal congestion.*
**GI:** *diarrhea, nausea, vomiting.*

## INTERACTIONS
**Drug-drug.** *Ephedrine, epinephrine:* excessive hypotension. Don't use together.

## EFFECTS ON DIAGNOSTIC TESTS
None reported.

## CONTRAINDICATIONS
Contraindicated in patients with hypersensitivity to drug and in those with angina, coronary artery disease, or MI or history of MI.

## NURSING CONSIDERATIONS
• Use cautiously in patients with gastritis or peptic ulcer.
• When drug is given as a diagnostic test for pheochromocytoma, take patient's blood pressure first; monitor blood pressure frequently during administration.
• *Alert:* Don't administer epinephrine to treat phentolamine-induced hypotension because it may cause additional fall in blood pressure ("epinephrine reversal"). Use norepinephrine instead, as ordered.
• *Alert:* Don't confuse phentolamine with phentermine.

### I.V. administration
• Reconstitute drug by adding 1 ml of sterile water for injection to vial containing 5 mg of drug; resulting solution contains 5 mg of phentolamine per ml.
• Delay injection until effect of venipuncture on blood pressure has passed. Then, rapidly inject drug.
• For pheochromocytoma diagnosis, inject drug rapidly. Test is positive if severe hypotension results.

### Patient teaching
• Explain use and administration of drug.
• Tell patient to report adverse reactions promptly.

---

## pindolol
Apo-Pindol†, Barbloc‡, Novo-Pindol†, Syn-Pindol†, Visken

*Pregnancy Risk Category B*

## HOW SUPPLIED
*Tablets:* 5 mg, 10 mg, 15 mg‡

## ACTION
Unknown. A nonselective beta blocker that has intrinsic sympathomimetic activity. Possible mechanisms include reduced cardiac output, decreased sympathetic

---

Reactions may be *common,* uncommon, *life-threatening,* or COMMON AND LIFE-THREATENING.

outflow to peripheral vasculature, and inhibition of renin release by the kidneys.

| Route | Onset | Peak | Duration |
|-------|---------|--------|----------|
| P.O. | Unknown | 1-2 hr | 24 hr |

## INDICATIONS & DOSAGE
*Hypertension—*
**Adults:** initially, 5 mg P.O. b.i.d. Dose increased as needed and tolerated to maximum of 60 mg daily.

## ADVERSE REACTIONS
**CNS:** *insomnia, fatigue, dizziness, nervousness,* vivid dreams, weakness, paresthesia.
**CV:** *edema,* bradycardia, **heart failure,** chest pain.
**GI:** *nausea,* abdominal discomfort.
**Hepatic:** elevated serum transaminase, alkaline phosphatase, and LD levels.
**Metabolic:** elevated uric acid levels.
**Musculoskeletal:** *muscle pain, joint pain.*
**Respiratory:** *increased airway resistance,* dyspnea.
**Skin:** rash, pruritus.

## INTERACTIONS
**Drug-drug.** *Cardiac glycosides, diltiazem, verapamil:* excessive bradycardia and additive depression of AV node. Use together cautiously.
*Catecholamine-depleting drugs such as reserpine:* may have additive effects. Monitor for hypotension and bradycardia.
*Epinephrine:* severe vasoconstriction. Monitor blood pressure and observe patient carefully.
*Indomethacin:* decreased antihypertensive effect. Monitor blood pressure and adjust dosage.
*Insulin, oral antidiabetics:* can alter requirements for these drugs in previously stabilized diabetic patients. Monitor patient for hypoglycemia.

## EFFECTS ON DIAGNOSTIC TESTS
None reported.

## CONTRAINDICATIONS
Contraindicated in patients with hypersensitivity to drug and in those with bronchial asthma, severe bradycardia, heart block greater than first degree, cardiogenic shock, or overt cardiac failure.

## NURSING CONSIDERATIONS
• Use cautiously in patients with heart failure, nonallergic bronchospastic disease, diabetes, hyperthyroidism, and impaired renal or hepatic function.
• Always check patient's apical pulse rate before giving drug. If extremes in pulse rate are detected, withhold drug and call doctor immediately.
• Monitor blood pressure frequently and notify doctor if severe hypotension occurs. A vasopressor may be needed.
• Withdraw drug over 1 to 2 weeks after long-term therapy, as ordered.
• Monitor blood glucose levels in diabetic patients closely because drug masks certain signs and symptoms of hypoglycemia.
• Beta blockers may mask tachycardia associated with hyperthyroidism. In patients with suspected thyrotoxicosis, withdraw beta blocker gradually, as ordered, to avoid thyroid storm.
• **Alert:** Don't confuse pindolol with Parlodel, Panadol, or Plendil; or Visken with Visine.

☑**Patient teaching**
• Tell patient to take drug exactly as prescribed.
• Tell patient not to stop drug suddenly but to call doctor to discuss unpleasant adverse drug reactions.

---

**prazosin hydrochloride**
Hypovase§, Minipress

*Pregnancy Risk Category C*

## HOW SUPPLIED
*Capsules:* 1 mg, 2 mg, 5 mg

## ACTION
Unknown. Drug's alpha-adrenergic blocking activity is thought to account primarily for its effects.

| Route | Onset | Peak | Duration |
|-------|-----------|--------|----------|
| P.O. | 0.5-1.5 hr | 2-4 hr | 7-10 hr |

## INDICATIONS & DOSAGE
*Mild to moderate hypertension, alone or with a diuretic or other antihypertensive—*
**Adults:** oral test dose is 1 mg h.s. to prevent "first-dose syncope." Initial dose is 1 mg P.O. b.i.d. or t.i.d. Dosage increased slowly. Maximum daily dose is 20 mg. Maintenance dose is 6 to 15 mg daily in three divided doses. Some patients need larger dosages (up to 40 mg daily). If other antihypertensives or diuretics are added to drug, prazosin is decreased to 1 to 2 mg t.i.d. and readjusted.

## ADVERSE REACTIONS
**CNS:** *dizziness,* headache, drowsiness, nervousness, paresthesia, weakness, *first-dose syncope,* depression.
**CV:** orthostatic hypotension, *palpitations,* edema.
**EENT:** blurred vision, tinnitus, conjunctivitis, epistaxis, nasal congestion.
**GI:** vomiting, diarrhea, abdominal cramps, *nausea,* elevated serum uric acid.
**GU:** priapism, impotence, urinary frequency, incontinence, elevated BUN.
**Hepatic:** liver function test abnormalities.
**Musculoskeletal:** arthralgia, myalgia.
**Respiratory:** dyspnea.
**Skin:** pruritus.
**Other:** fever.

## INTERACTIONS
**Drug-drug.** *Propranolol, other beta blockers:* increased frequency of syncope with loss of consciousness. Advise patient to sit or lie down if dizziness occurs.
*Verapamil:* increased serum prazosin levels. Monitor closely.
**Drug-herb.** *Butcher's broom:* possible diminished effect. Avoid concomitant use.

## EFFECTS ON DIAGNOSTIC TESTS
Drug alters results of screening tests for pheochromocytoma and causes increases in levels of the urinary metabolite of norepinephrine and vanillylmandelic acid; it may cause positive antinuclear antibody titer.

## CONTRAINDICATIONS
Contraindicated in patients with hypersensitivity to drug or other alpha₁ blockers.

## NURSING CONSIDERATIONS
• Use cautiously in patients receiving other antihypertensives.
• Monitor patient's blood pressure and pulse rate frequently.
• Elderly patients may be more sensitive to drug's hypotensive effects.
• Compliance might be improved with twice-daily dosing. Suggest this dosing change with doctor if problems with compliance is suspected.
• *Alert:* If initial dose is greater than 1 mg, severe syncope with loss of consciousness may occur (first-dose syncope).

### ✅ Patient teaching
• Warn patient that dizziness may occur with first dose. If he experiences dizziness, tell him to sit or lie down. Reassure him that this effect disappears with continued dosing.
• Tell patient not to suddenly stop taking drug but to call doctor if unpleasant adverse reactions occur.
• Advise patient to minimize orthostatic hypotension by rising slowly and avoiding sudden position changes. Dry mouth can be relieved by chewing gum or sucking on sour hard candy or ice chips.

---

## quinapril hydrochloride
Accupril, Accupro§, Asig‡

*Pregnancy Risk Category C (D in second and third trimesters)*

## HOW SUPPLIED
*Tablets:* 5 mg, 10 mg, 20 mg, 40 mg

## ACTION
Unknown. Thought to be involved with inhibiting conversion of angiotensin I to angiotensin II, a potent vasoconstrictor. Reduced formation of angiotensin II decreases peripheral arterial resistance, thus decreasing aldosterone secretion.

| Route | Onset | Peak | Duration |
|-------|-------|------|----------|
| P.O. | 1 hr | 2-6 hr | 24 hr |

## INDICATIONS & DOSAGE
*Hypertension—*
**Adults:** initially, 10 to 20 mg P.O. daily.

---

Reactions may be *common,* uncommon, **life-threatening,** or COMMON AND LIFE-THREATENING.

Dosage adjusted based on patient response at intervals of about 2 weeks. Most patients are controlled at 20, 40, or 80 mg daily as a single dose or in two divided doses. If patient is taking a diuretic, initiate therapy with 5 mg daily.

**Elderly:** for patients over age 65, initiate therapy at 10 mg P.O. daily.

*Heart failure—*

**Adults:** initially, 5 mg P.O. b.i.d. if patient is receiving a diuretic and 10 to 20 mg P.O. b.i.d. if patient isn't receiving a diuretic. Dosage increased at weekly intervals. Usual effective dose is 20 to 40 mg b.i.d. in equally divided doses.

*Adjust-a-dose:* For renally impaired patients with creatinine clearance over 60 ml/minute, give 10 mg daily; if clearance is 30 to 60 ml/minute, give 5 mg daily; and if clearance is 10 to 30 ml/minute, give 2.5 mg daily.

## ADVERSE REACTIONS

**CNS:** somnolence, vertigo, nervousness, headache, dizziness, fatigue, depression.
**CV:** palpitations, tachycardia, angina, hypertensive crisis, orthostatic hypotension, rhythm disturbances.
**GI:** dry mouth, abdominal pain, constipation, vomiting, nausea, hemorrhage.
**Hepatic:** elevated liver enzyme levels.
**Metabolic:** hyperkalemia.
**Respiratory:** dry, persistent, tickling, nonproductive cough.
**Skin:** pruritus, photosensitivity, diaphoresis.

## INTERACTIONS

**Drug-drug.** *Diuretics, other antihypertensives:* risk of excessive hypotension. Discontinue diuretic or lower dose of quinapril as needed.
*Lithium:* increased serum lithium levels and lithium toxicity. Monitor serum lithium levels.
*Potassium-sparing diuretics, potassium supplements:* risk of hyperkalemia. Monitor closely during concomitant use.
*Tetracycline:* absorption decreased with administration of quinapril. Avoid concomitant use.
**Drug-food.** *Salt substitutes containing potassium:* risk of hyperkalemia. Monitor closely during concomitant use.

## EFFECTS ON DIAGNOSTIC TESTS
None reported.

## CONTRAINDICATIONS
Contraindicated in patients with hypersensitivity to ACE inhibitors or history of angioedema related to treatment with an ACE inhibitor.

## NURSING CONSIDERATIONS
• Use cautiously in patients with impaired renal function.
• Assess renal and hepatic function before and periodically throughout therapy.
• Monitor blood pressure for effectiveness of therapy.
• Monitor serum potassium levels as ordered. Risk factors for the development of hyperkalemia include renal insufficiency, diabetes, and concomitant use of drugs that raise potassium level.
• Other ACE inhibitors have been associated with agranulocytosis and neutropenia. Monitor CBC with differential counts before therapy and periodically thereafter, as ordered.

☑**Patient teaching**
• Advise patient to report signs of infection, such as fever and sore throat.
• *Alert:* Angioedema (including laryngeal edema) may occur, especially after first dose. Advise patient to report signs or symptoms of angioedema, such as breathing difficulty or swelling of face, eyes, lips, or tongue.
• Light-headedness can occur, especially during first few days of therapy. Tell patient to rise slowly to minimize effect and to report symptoms to doctor. If syncope occurs, he should stop taking drug and call doctor immediately.
• Inform patient that inadequate fluid intake, vomiting, diarrhea, and excessive perspiration can lead to light-headedness and syncope. Tell him to use caution in hot weather and during exercise.
• Tell patient to avoid salt substitutes. These products may contain potassium, which can cause hyperkalemia in patients taking quinapril.
• Tell woman to notify doctor if pregnancy occurs. Drug will need to be discontinued.

---

# ramipril
Altace, Ramace‡, Tritace‡

*Pregnancy Risk Category C (D in second and third trimesters)*

## HOW SUPPLIED
*Capsules:* 1.25 mg, 2.5 mg, 5 mg, 10 mg

## ACTION
Unknown. Thought to be involved with inhibiting conversion of angiotensin I to angiotensin II, a potent vasoconstrictor. Reduced formation of angiotensin II decreases peripheral arterial resistance, thus decreasing aldosterone secretion.

| Route | Onset | Peak | Duration |
|-------|-------|------|----------|
| P.O. | 1-2 hr | 1-3 hr | 24 hr |

## INDICATIONS & DOSAGE
*Hypertension—*
**Adults:** initially, 2.5 mg P.O. once daily for patients not receiving a diuretic, and 1.25 mg P.O. once daily for patients receiving a diuretic. Dosage increased as needed, based on patient response. Maintenance dose is 2.5 to 20 mg daily as a single dose or in divided doses.
*Adjust-a-dose:* For renally impaired patients with creatinine clearance below 40 ml/minute, give 1.25 mg P.O. daily. Dosage is adjusted gradually based on response. Maximum daily dose is 5 mg.
*Heart failure—*
**Adults:** initially, 2.5 mg P.O. b.i.d. If hypotension occurs, dosage decreased to 1.25 mg P.O. b.i.d. Dosage may be gradually increased to maximum of 5 mg P.O. b.i.d., p.r.n.
*Adjust-a-dose:* For renally impaired patients with creatinine clearance below 40 ml/minute, give 1.25 mg P.O. daily. Dosage is adjusted gradually based on response. Maximum daily dose is 2.5 mg b.i.d.

## ADVERSE REACTIONS
**CNS:** headache, dizziness, fatigue, asthenia, malaise, light-headedness, anxiety, amnesia, depression, insomnia, nervousness, neuralgia, neuropathy, paresthesia, somnolence, tremor, vertigo, syncope.
**CV:** *heart failure,* orthostatic hypotension, angina, chest pain, palpitations, *MI,* edema.
**EENT:** epistaxis, tinnitus.
**GI:** nausea, vomiting, abdominal pain, anorexia, constipation, diarrhea, dyspepsia, dry mouth, gastroenteritis.
**GU:** impotence, elevated BUN and creatinine levels.
**Hematologic:** decreased hemoglobin and hematocrit level.
**Hepatic:** elevated liver enzyme and bilirubin levels.
**Metabolic:** hyperglycemia, hyperkalemia, weight gain.
**Musculoskeletal:** arthralgia, arthritis, myalgia.
**Respiratory:** dyspnea; dry, persistent, tickling, nonproductive cough.
**Skin:** hypersensitivity reactions, rash, dermatitis, pruritus, photosensitivity, increased diaphoresis.
**Other:** elevated uric acid levels.

## INTERACTIONS
**Drug-drug.** *Diuretics:* excessive hypotension, especially at start of therapy. Discontinue diuretic at least 3 days before therapy begins, increase sodium intake, or reduce starting dose of ramipril.
*Insulin, oral antidiabetics:* risk of hypoglycemia, especially at start of ramipril therapy. Monitor closely.
*Lithium:* increased serum lithium levels. Use together cautiously and monitor serum lithium levels.
*Potassium-sparing diuretics, potassium supplements:* increased risk of hyperkalemia because ramipril attenuates potassium loss. Monitor plasma potassium levels closely.
**Drug-food.** *Salt substitutes containing potassium:* increased risk of hyperkalemia because ramipril attenuates potassium loss. Monitor plasma potassium levels closely.

## EFFECTS ON DIAGNOSTIC TESTS
None reported.

## CONTRAINDICATIONS
Contraindicated in patients with hypersensitivity to ACE inhibitors or history of angioedema related to treatment with an ACE inhibitor.

## NURSING CONSIDERATIONS
• Use cautiously in patients with renal impairment.
• Monitor blood pressure regularly for drug effectiveness.
• Closely assess renal function in patients during first few weeks of therapy. Regular assessment of renal function (serum creatinine and BUN levels) is advisable. Patients with severe heart failure whose renal function depends on the renin-angiotensin-aldosterone system have experienced acute renal failure during ACE inhibitor therapy. Hypertensive patients with renal artery stenosis also may show signs of worsening renal function during first few days of therapy.
• Monitor CBC with differential counts before therapy and periodically thereafter. Decreased blood counts may occur especially in patients with impaired renal function or collagen vascular diseases (systemic lupus erythematosus or scleroderma).
• Monitor serum potassium levels. Risk factors for the development of hyperkalemia include renal insufficiency, diabetes, and concomitant use of agents that raise potassium levels.

☑ **Patient teaching**
• Tell patient to call doctor to discuss adverse reactions. Dosage adjustment or discontinuation of drug may be needed.
• *Alert:* Rarely, angioedema (including laryngeal edema) may occur, especially after first dose. Advise patient to report signs or symptoms of angioedema, such as breathing difficulty or swelling of face, eyes, lips, or tongue.
• Inform patient that light-headedness can occur, especially during the first few days of therapy. Tell him to rise slowly to minimize this effect and to report symptoms to doctor. If syncope occurs, patient should stop taking drug and call doctor immediately.
• Tell patient that, if he has difficulty swallowing capsules, he can open drug and sprinkle contents on a small amount of applesauce.
• Advise patient to report signs and symptoms of infection, such as fever and sore throat.

• Tell patient to avoid salt substitutes. These products may contain potassium, which can cause hyperkalemia in patients taking ramipril.
• Tell woman to notify doctor if pregnancy occurs. Drug will need to be discontinued.

---

## telmisartan
Micardis

*Pregnancy Risk Category C (D in second and third trimesters)*

### HOW SUPPLIED
*Tablets:* 40 mg, 80 mg

### ACTION
Blocks the vasoconstricting and aldosterone-secreting effects of angiotensin II by selectively blocking the binding of angiotensin II to the $AT_1$ receptor in many tissues, such as vascular smooth muscle and the adrenal gland.

| Route | Onset | Peak | Duration |
|-------|-------|------|----------|
| P.O. | Unknown | 0.5-1 hr | 24 hr |

### INDICATIONS & DOSAGE
*Hypertension (used alone or with other antihypertensives)—*
**Adults:** 40 mg P.O. daily. Blood pressure response is dose related over a range of 20 to 80 mg daily.

### ADVERSE REACTIONS
**CNS:** dizziness, pain, fatigue, headache.
**CV:** chest pain, hypertension, peripheral edema.
**EENT:** pharyngitis, sinusitis.
**GI:** abdominal pain, diarrhea, dyspepsia, nausea.
**GU:** urinary tract infection.
**Hepatic:** elevated liver enzyme levels.
**Musculoskeletal:** back pain, myalgia.
**Respiratory:** cough, upper respiratory tract infection.
**Other:** flulike symptoms.

### INTERACTIONS
**Drug-drug.** *Digoxin:* increased digoxin plasma levels. Monitor digoxin levels closely.

*Warfarin:* slightly decreased plasma warfarin levels. Monitor INR.

**Drug-food.** *Salt substitutes containing potassium:* risk of hyperkalemia. Monitor closely.

**EFFECTS ON DIAGNOSTIC TESTS**
None reported.

**CONTRAINDICATIONS**
Contraindicated in patients with hypersensitivity to drug or its components.

**NURSING CONSIDERATIONS**
• Use cautiously in patients with biliary obstruction disorders or renal and hepatic insufficiency and in those with an activated renin-angiotensin system, such as volume- or salt-depleted patients (for example, those being treated with high doses of diuretics).
• Drugs such as telmisartan that act on the renin-angiotensin system can cause fetal and neonatal morbidity and death when administered to pregnant women. These problems have not been detected when exposure has been limited to the first trimester. If pregnancy is suspected, notify doctor because drug should be discontinued.
• Monitor for hypotension following initiation of drug. Place patient in supine position if hypotension occurs and administer I.V. normal saline if needed, as ordered.
• Most of the antihypertensive effect occurs within 2 weeks. Maximal blood pressure reduction is generally reached after 4 weeks. Diuretic may be added if blood pressure is not controlled by drug alone.
• In patients whose renal function may depend on the activity of the renin-angiotensin-aldosterone system (such as those with severe heart failure), treatment with ACE inhibitors and angiotensin receptor antagonists has been associated with oliguria or progressive azotemia and (rarely) with acute renal failure or death.
• Drug is not removed by hemodialysis. Patients undergoing dialysis may develop orthostatic hypotension. Closely monitor blood pressure.

☑ **Patient teaching**
• Instruct patient to report suspected pregnancy to doctor immediately.
• Inform woman of childbearing age of the consequences of second and third trimester exposure to drug.
• Advise breast-feeding woman about risk of adverse drug effects in infant and the need to discontinue drug or breast-feeding.
• Tell patient that, if transient hypotension occurs, he should lie down if feeling dizzy, rise slowly from a lying to standing position, and climb stairs slowly.
• Tell patient that drug may be taken without regard to meals.
• Tell patient that drug shouldn't be removed from blister-sealed packet until immediately before use.

---

**terazosin hydrochloride**
Hytrin

*Pregnancy Risk Category C*

**HOW SUPPLIED**
*Tablets:* 1 mg, 2 mg, 5 mg, 10 mg
*Capsules:* 1 mg, 2 mg, 5 mg, 10 mg

**ACTION**
Decreases blood pressure by vasodilation produced in response to blockade of alpha$_1$-adrenergic receptors. It improves urine flow in patients with BPH by blocking alpha$_1$-adrenergic receptors in the smooth muscle of the bladder neck and prostate, thus relieving urethral pressure and reestablishing urine flow.

| Route | Onset | Peak | Duration |
|-------|-------|------|----------|
| P.O. | 15 min | 2-3 hr | 24 hr |

**INDICATIONS & DOSAGE**
*Hypertension—*
**Adults:** initially, 1 mg P.O. h.s. Dosage increased gradually based on response. Usual dosage range is 1 to 5 mg daily. Maximum recommended dose is 20 mg daily.
*Symptomatic BPH—*
**Adults:** initially, 1 mg P.O. h.s. Dosage increased in a stepwise fashion to 2, 5, or 10 mg once daily to achieve optimal response. Most patients need 10 mg daily for optimal response.

## ADVERSE REACTIONS
**CNS:** asthenia, dizziness, headache, nervousness, paresthesia, somnolence.
**CV:** palpitations, orthostatic hypotension, tachycardia, *peripheral edema.*
**EENT:** *nasal congestion,* sinusitis, blurred vision.
**GI:** nausea.
**GU:** impotence.
**Hematologic:** decreases in hematocrit, WBC, and hemoglobin, total protein, and albumin levels.
**Musculoskeletal:** back pain, muscle pain.
**Respiratory:** dyspnea.

## INTERACTIONS
**Drug-drug.** *Antihypertensives:* excessive hypotension. Use together cautiously.
*Clonidine:* clonidine's antihypertensive effect may be decreased. Monitor patient.
**Drug-herb.** *Butcher's broom:* possible diminished effect. Avoid concomitant use.

## EFFECTS ON DIAGNOSTIC TESTS
None reported.

## CONTRAINDICATIONS
Contraindicated in patients with hypersensitivity to drug.

## NURSING CONSIDERATIONS
• Monitor blood pressure frequently.
• *Alert:* If terazosin is discontinued for several days, dosage will need to be readjusted using initial dosing regimen (1 mg P.O. h.s.).

### ☑ Patient teaching
• Tell patient not to discontinue drug suddenly, but to call doctor if adverse reactions occur.
• Warn patient to avoid hazardous activities that require mental alertness, such as driving or operating heavy machinery, for 12 hours after first dose.

## timolol maleate
Apo-Timol†, Betim§, Blocadren

*Pregnancy Risk Category C*

## HOW SUPPLIED
*Tablets:* 5 mg, 10 mg, 20 mg

## ACTION
Unknown. In MI, drug may decrease myocardial oxygen requirements. For migraine headache prophylaxis, drug prevents arterial dilation through beta blockade.

| Route | Onset | Peak | Duration |
|-------|-------|------|----------|
| P.O. | 15-30 min | 1-2 hr | 6-12 hr |

## INDICATIONS & DOSAGE
*Hypertension—*
**Adults:** initially, 10 mg P.O. b.i.d. Usual daily maintenance dose is 20 to 40 mg. Maximum daily dose is 60 mg. Allow at least 7 days between increases in dosage.
*MI (long-term prophylaxis in patients who have survived acute phase)—*
**Adults:** 10 mg P.O. b.i.d.
*Migraine headache prophylaxis—*
**Adults:** initially, 10 mg P.O. b.i.d. Increase dosage as needed and tolerated to maximum of 30 mg daily as a divided dose. Discontinue treatment if no response occurs after 6 to 8 weeks at maximum dose.

## ADVERSE REACTIONS
**CNS:** fatigue, lethargy, dizziness.
**CV:** *bradycardia, hypotension, heart failure,* peripheral vascular disease, *arrhythmias.*
**GI:** nausea, vomiting, diarrhea.
**GU:** slightly increased BUN levels.
**Hematologic:** decreased hemoglobin and hematocrit level.
**Metabolic:** hyperkalemia, hyperglycemia.
**Respiratory:** dyspnea, *bronchospasm, increased airway resistance,* pulmonary edema.
**Skin:** pruritus.
**Other:** increased uric acid levels.

## INTERACTIONS
**Drug-drug.** *Cardiac glycosides, diltiazem, verapamil:* excessive bradycardia and increased depressant effect on myocardium. Use together cautiously.
*Catecholamine-depleting drugs such as reserpine:* may have additive effect when given with beta blockers. Monitor for hypotension and bradycardia.

*Indomethacin:* decreased antihypertensive effect. Monitor blood pressure and adjust dosage.

*Insulin, oral antidiabetics:* can alter requirements for these drugs in previously stabilized diabetic patients. Monitor patient for hypoglycemia.

**EFFECTS ON DIAGNOSTIC TESTS**
None reported.

**CONTRAINDICATIONS**
Contraindicated in patients with hypersensitivity to drug and in those with bronchial asthma, severe COPD, sinus bradycardia and heart block greater than first-degree, cardiogenic shock, or heart failure.

**NURSING CONSIDERATIONS**
• Use cautiously in patients with heart failure; hepatic, renal, or respiratory disease; diabetes; and hyperthyroidism.
• Check patient's apical pulse rate before giving drug. If extremes in pulse rates are detected, withhold drug and call doctor immediately.
• Monitor blood pressure frequently.
• Monitor blood glucose levels in diabetic patients; drug can mask signs and symptoms of hypoglycemia.
• *Alert:* Don't confuse timolol with atenolol.

☑ **Patient teaching**
• Tell patient to take drug exactly as prescribed.
• Instruct patient not to discontinue drug suddenly but to call doctor to discuss unpleasant adverse reactions. Tell him dosage should be reduced gradually over 1 to 2 weeks.

---

**trandolapril**
Gopten§, Odrik§, Mavik

*Pregnancy Risk Category C (D in second and third trimesters)*

**HOW SUPPLIED**
*Tablets:* 1 mg, 2 mg, 4 mg

**ACTION**
Unknown. Thought to result primarily from inhibition of circulating and tissue ACE activity, thereby reducing angiotensin II formation, decreasing vasoconstriction and aldosterone secretion, and increasing plasma renin. Decreased aldosterone secretion leads to diuresis, natriuresis, and a small increase in serum potassium. Drug is converted in the liver to the prodrug, trandolaprilat.

| Route | Onset | Peak | Duration |
|-------|-------|------|----------|
| P.O. | Unknown | 1-10 hr | 24 hr |

**INDICATIONS & DOSAGE**
*Hypertension—*
**Adults:** for patients not receiving a diuretic, initially 1 mg for a nonblack patient and 2 mg for a black patient P.O. once daily. If control isn't adequate, dosage can be increased at intervals of at least 1 week. Maintenance doses for most patients range from 2 to 4 mg daily. Some patients receiving once-daily doses of 4 mg may need b.i.d. doses. For a patient receiving a diuretic concurrently, initial dose of trandolapril should be 0.5 mg P.O. once daily. Subsequent dosage adjustment based on blood pressure response.
*Heart failure or ventricular dysfunction following an MI—*
**Adults:** initially 1 mg P.O. daily, adjusted to 4 mg P.O. daily. If patient can't tolerate 4 mg, continue at highest tolerated dose.
*Adjust-a-dose:* For patients with hepatic disease or renal failure, if creatinine clearance is below 30 ml/minute, initial dose is 0.5 mg daily.

**ADVERSE REACTIONS**
**CNS:** dizziness, headache, fatigue, drowsiness, insomnia, paresthesia, vertigo, anxiety.
**CV:** chest pain, first-degree AV block, *bradycardia,* edema, flushing, hypotension, palpitations.
**EENT:** epistaxis, throat irritation.
**GI:** diarrhea, dyspepsia, abdominal distention, abdominal pain or cramps, constipation, vomiting, *pancreatitis.*
**GU:** elevated BUN and creatinine levels, urinary frequency, impotence, decreased libido.

---

Reactions may be *common,* uncommon, *life-threatening,* or COMMON AND LIFE-THREATENING.

**Hematologic:** *neutropenia, leukopenia.*
**Hepatic:** elevated liver enzyme levels.
**Metabolic:** hyperkalemia, hyponatremia.
**Respiratory:** dyspnea; persistent, non-productive cough; upper respiratory tract infection.
**Skin:** rash, pruritus, pemphigus.

## INTERACTIONS
**Drug-drug.** *Diuretics:* increased risk of excessive hypotension. Diuretic may be discontinued or treatment initiated with a lower dose of trandolapril, as ordered.
*Lithium:* increased serum lithium levels and lithium toxicity. Avoid concomitant use. Monitor serum lithium levels.
*Potassium-sparing diuretics, potassium supplements:* increased risk of hyperkalemia. Monitor serum potassium level closely.
**Drug-food.** *Salt substitutes containing potassium:* increased risk of hyperkalemia. Monitor serum potassium level closely.

## EFFECTS ON DIAGNOSTIC TESTS
None reported.

## CONTRAINDICATIONS
Contraindicated in patients with hypersensitivity to drug or a history of angioedema related to previous treatment with an ACE inhibitor. Drug isn't recommended for use during pregnancy.

## NURSING CONSIDERATIONS
● Use cautiously in patients with impaired renal function, heart failure, or renal artery stenosis.
● Monitor serum potassium levels closely.
● Monitor for hypotension. Excessive hypotension can occur when drug is given with diuretics. If possible, diuretic therapy should be discontinued 2 to 3 days before starting trandolapril to decrease potential for excessive hypotension response. If drug doesn't adequately control blood pressure, diuretic therapy may be reinstituted cautiously, as ordered.
● Assess patient's renal function before and periodically throughout therapy.
● Other ACE inhibitors have been associated with agranulocytosis and neutropenia. Monitor CBC with differential before

therapy, especially in patients with collagen vascular disease with impaired renal function.
● *Alert:* Angioedema with involvement of the tongue, glottis, or larynx may be fatal because of airway obstruction. Appropriate therapy should be ordered, including epinephrine 1:1,000 (0.3 to 0.5 ml) S.C.; have resuscitation equipment for maintaining a patent airway readily available.
● If patient develops jaundice, discontinue drug under doctor's advice because, although rare, ACE inhibitors have been associated with a syndrome of cholestatic jaundice, fulminant hepatic necrosis, and death.
● Safety and effectiveness of drug in children haven't been established.
● It's unknown if drug appears in breast milk. Drug shouldn't be given to breast-feeding women.

## ☑ Patient teaching
● Instruct patient to report jaundice.
● Advise patient to report fever and sore throat (signs of infection), easy bruising or bleeding; swelling of the tongue, lips, face, eyes, mucous membranes, or extremities; difficulty swallowing or breathing; hoarseness; and nonproductive, persistent cough.
● Tell patient to avoid salt substitutes during drug therapy. These products may contain potassium, which can cause hyperkalemia.
● Tell patient that light-headedness can occur, especially during first few days of therapy. Advise him to rise slowly to minimize this effect and to report it immediately.
● Advise patient to use caution in hot weather and during exercise. Inadequate fluid intake, vomiting, diarrhea, and excessive perspiration can lead to light-headedness and syncope.
● Tell woman to report suspected pregnancy immediately. Drug will need to be discontinued.
● Advise patient planning to undergo surgery or receive anesthesia to inform doctor that he is taking this drug.

## valsartan
Diovan

*Pregnancy Risk Category C (D in second and third trimesters)*

### HOW SUPPLIED
*Capsules:* 80 mg, 160 mg

### ACTION
Blocks the binding of angiotensin II to receptor sites in vascular smooth muscle and the adrenal gland, which inhibits the pressor effects of the renin-angiotensin-aldosterone system.

| Route | Onset | Peak | Duration |
|-------|-------|------|----------|
| P.O. | 2 hr | 2-4 hr | 24 hr |

### INDICATIONS & DOSAGE
*Hypertension (used alone or with other antihypertensives)—*
**Adults:** initially, 80 mg P.O. once daily. Expect to see a reduction in blood pressure in 2 to 4 weeks. If additional antihypertensive effect is needed, dosage may be increased to 160 or 320 mg daily, or a diuretic may be added. (Addition of a diuretic has a greater effect than dosage increases beyond 80 mg.) Usual dosage range is 80 to 320 mg daily.

### ADVERSE REACTIONS
**CNS:** dizziness, headache, insomnia, fatigue.
**CV:** edema.
**EENT:** rhinitis, sinusitis, pharyngitis.
**GI:** abdominal pain, diarrhea, nausea.
**Hematologic:** *neutropenia.*
**Metabolic:** hyperkalemia.
**Musculoskeletal:** arthralgia.
**Respiratory:** upper respiratory tract infection, cough.
**Other:** viral infection.

### INTERACTIONS
**Drug-drug.** *Diuretics:* risk of excessive hypotension. Assess fluid status before starting concomitant therapy. Monitor closely.
*Potassium-sparing diuretics, potassium:* increased risk of hyperkalemia. Monitor serum potassium level closely.

**Drug-food.** *Any food:* decreased peak levels. Give drug on an empty stomach.

### EFFECTS ON DIAGNOSTIC TESTS
None reported.

### CONTRAINDICATIONS
Contraindicated in patients with hypersensitivity to drug.

### NURSING CONSIDERATIONS
• Use cautiously in patients with renal or hepatic disease.
• Drug can cause fetal or neonatal morbidity and death if administered to a pregnant woman in the second or third trimester. Breast-feeding women shouldn't take drug.
• Safety and effectiveness of drug in children haven't been established.
• Monitor for hypotension. Excessive hypotension can occur when drug is given with high doses of diuretics. Correct volume and salt depletions, as ordered, before starting drug.

### ☑ Patient teaching
• Tell woman to notify doctor if pregnancy occurs. Drug will need to be discontinued.
• Tell patient that drug may be taken without regard to food.

---

Reactions may be *common*, uncommon, *__life-threatening__*, or COMMON AND LIFE-THREATENING.

**atorvastatin calcium**
**cerivastatin sodium**
**cholestyramine**
**colestipol hydrochloride**
**fenofibrate (micronized)**
**fluvastatin sodium**
**gemfibrozil**
**lovastatin**
**niacin**
(See Chapter 90, VITAMINS AND MINER-
ALS.)
**pravastatin sodium**
**simvastatin**

**COMBINATION PRODUCTS**
None.

---

## atorvastatin calcium
Lipitor

*Pregnancy Risk Category X*

---

### HOW SUPPLIED
*Tablets:* 10 mg, 20 mg, 40 mg

### ACTION
Inhibits 3-hydroxy-3-methylglutaryl-
coenzyme A reductase, an early (and rate-
limiting) step in cholesterol biosynthesis.

| Route | Onset | Peak | Duration |
|-------|-------|------|----------|
| P.O. | Unknown | 1-2 hr | Unknown |

### INDICATIONS & DOSAGE
*Adjunct to diet to reduce low-density
lipoprotein (LDL), total cholesterol, apo
B, and triglyceride levels in patients with
primary hypercholesterolemia and mixed
dyslipidemia (Fredrickson types IIa and
IIb); primary dysbetalipoproteinemia
(Fredrickson type III) that doesn't respond adequately to diet; adjunctive therapy to diet for elevated serum triglyceride
levels (Fredrickson type IV)—*
**Adults:** initially, 10 mg P.O. once daily.
Dosage increased, p.r.n., to maximum single dose of 80 mg daily. Dosage based on

blood lipid levels drawn within 2 to 4
weeks after starting therapy.
*Alone or as an adjunct to lipid-lowering
treatments such as LDL apheresis in patients with homozygous familial hypercholesterolemia—*
**Adults:** 10 to 80 mg P.O. once daily.

### ADVERSE REACTIONS
**CNS:** *headache,* asthenia, insomnia.
**EENT:** rhinitis, pharyngitis, sinusitis.
**GI:** abdominal pain, dyspepsia, flatu-
lence, nausea, constipation, diarrhea.
**GU:** urinary tract infection.
**Hepatic:** increased liver function test re-
sults.
**Musculoskeletal:** arthritis, arthralgia,
myalgia.
**Respiratory:** bronchitis.
**Skin:** rash.
**Other:** infection, flulike syndrome, aller-
gic reaction, peripheral edema.

### INTERACTIONS
**Drug-drug.** *Antacids:* may decrease plasma levels of drug. Monitor patient.
*Azole antifungals, cyclosporine, ery-
thromycin, fibric acid derivatives, niacin:*
possible risk of rhabdomyolysis. Avoid
concomitant use.
*Colestipol:* may decrease plasma levels of
drug. Monitor patient.
*Digoxin:* may increase plasma digoxin
levels. Monitor serum digoxin levels.
*Erythromycin:* will increase plasma level
of drug. Monitor patient.
*Oral contraceptives:* increased levels of
hormones. Consider when selecting an
oral contraceptive.

### EFFECTS ON DIAGNOSTIC TESTS
None reported.

### CONTRAINDICATIONS
Contraindicated in patients hypersensitive
to drug and in those with active liver disease or conditions associated with unexplained persistent elevations of serum
transaminase levels. Also contraindicated

---

in pregnant and breast-feeding women and in women of childbearing age (except those not at risk for becoming pregnant).

## NURSING CONSIDERATIONS
• Use cautiously in patients with history of liver disease or heavy alcohol use.
• Drug should be withheld or discontinued in patients at risk for renal failure secondary to rhabdomyolysis due to trauma; in serious, acute conditions that suggest myopathy; and in major surgery; severe acute infection; hypotension; uncontrolled seizures; or severe metabolic, endocrine, and electrolyte disorders.
• Use of atorvastatin in children has been limited to those over age 9 with homozygous familial hypercholesterolemia.
• Initiate drug therapy only after diet and other nonpharmacologic treatments prove ineffective. Patient should follow a standard low-cholesterol diet before and during therapy.
• Before initiating treatment, secondary causes for hypercholesterolemia should be excluded and a baseline lipid profile done. Obtain periodic liver function test results and lipid levels, as ordered, before starting treatment and at 6 and 12 weeks after initiation, or after an increase in dosage and periodically thereafter.
• Drug may be given as a single dose at any time of day, with or without food.
• Watch for signs of myositis.
• *Alert:* Don't confuse Lipitor with Levatol.

☑ **Patient teaching**
• Teach patient about proper dietary management, weight control, and exercise. Explain their importance in controlling elevated serum lipid levels.
• Warn patient to avoid alcohol.
• Tell patient to inform doctor of adverse reactions, such as muscle pain, malaise, and fever.
• Advise patient that drug can be taken at any time of day and without regard to meals.
• *Alert:* Inform woman that drug is contraindicated during pregnancy because of potential of danger to the fetus. Advise her to notify doctor immediately if pregnancy occurs or is suspected.

## cerivastatin sodium
Baycol, Lipobay§

*Pregnancy Risk Category X*

### HOW SUPPLIED
*Tablets*: 0.2 mg, 0.3 mg

### ACTION
Competitively inhibits 3-hydroxy-3-methylglutaryl-coenzyme A (HMG-CoA) reductase, which is responsible for the conversion of HMG-CoA, a precursor of cholesterol. The result is a reduction in the plasma cholesterol level.

| Route | Onset | Peak | Duration |
|-------|-------|------|----------|
| P.O. | 1 wk | 4 wk | Unknown |

### INDICATIONS & DOSAGE
*Adjunct to diet to reduce total and low-density cholesterol levels in patients with primary hypercholesterolemia or mixed dyslipidemia (Fredrickson types IIa and IIb) when diet and other nonpharmacologic measures have been inadequate—*
**Adults:** 0.4 mg P.O. daily in the evening.
*Adjust-a-dose:* For patients with moderate or severe renal dysfunction (creatinine clearance 60 ml/minute or less), starting dose is 0.2 mg P.O. daily.
✱ *NEW INDICATION: Adjunct to diet for treatment of elevated triglycerides and apolipoprotein B levels in patients with primary hypercholesterolemia and mixed dyslipidemia (Fredrickson types IIa and IIb) when diet and other nonpharmacologic measures has been inadequate—*
**Adults:** 0.4 mg P.O. daily in the evening.

### ADVERSE REACTIONS
**CNS:** dizziness, *headache*, insomnia, asthenia.
**CV:** chest pain, peripheral edema.
**EENT:** *pharyngitis, rhinitis,* sinusitis.
**GI:** constipation, diarrhea, dyspepsia, flatulence, nausea, abdominal pain.
**GU:** urinary tract infection.
**Hepatic:** elevated transaminase, CK, alkaline phosphatase, GGT, and bilirubin levels.
**Metabolic:** altered thyroid function.

---

Reactions may be *common*, uncommon, *life-threatening*, or COMMON AND LIFE-THREATENING.

**Musculoskeletal:** arthralgia, back or leg pain, myalgia.
**Respiratory:** increased cough.
**Skin:** rash.
**Other:** flulike syndrome.

## INTERACTIONS
**Drug-drug.** *Azole antifungals, cyclosporine, erythromycin, fibric acid derivatives, immunosuppressants, niacin:* may increase the incidence of myopathy. Use together cautiously.
*Cholestyramine:* decreased absorption and decreased peak plasma levels of cerivastatin when given within 4 hours of drug. Use together cautiously.
*Erythromycin:* may decrease hepatic metabolism of drug and has resulted in increases of cerivastatin of up to 50%. Use together cautiously.

## EFFECTS ON DIAGNOSTIC TESTS
None reported.

## CONTRAINDICATIONS
Contraindicated in patients with hypersensitivity to drug and in those with active liver disease or unexplained persistent elevations of serum transaminase levels; also contraindicated in pregnant or breastfeeding women.

## NURSING CONSIDERATIONS
• Use cautiously in patients with history of liver disease or heavy alcohol use.
• Safety and efficacy of drug in children haven't been established.
• Drug should be given to women of childbearing age only if conception is highly unlikely and they have been warned of potential risks to fetus.
• Therapy with lipid-lowering drugs should be started after appropriate diet, exercise, and weight reduction programs have proved unsuccessful in controlling cholesterol levels.
• Perform liver function tests before starting treatment, at 6 and 12 weeks after initiation of therapy, and periodically thereafter.
• Withhold drug temporarily in patients experiencing an acute or serious condition predisposing them to renal failure secondary to rhabdomyolysis. Rare cases of

rhabdomyolysis have been reported with other HMG-CoA reductase inhibitors.

☑ **Patient teaching**
• Tell patient to take drug in the early evening at least 1 hour before or 4 hours after cholestyramine or colestipol.
• Inform patient that drug can be taken without regard to meals.
• Advise patient that it may take up to 4 weeks for full therapeutic effect to occur.
• Caution woman to stop drug if pregnancy occurs or is suspected.
• Tell patient to notify doctor if an unexplained muscle pain, tenderness, or weakness (particularly if accompanied by fever or malaise) occurs.

---

## cholestyramine
LoCholest, Prevalite, Questran**,
Questran Light, Questran Lite‡

*Pregnancy Risk Category C*

### HOW SUPPLIED
*Powder:* 378-g cans, 9-g single-dose packets. Each scoop of powder or single-dose packet contains 4 g of cholestyramine resin.
*Tablets:* 1 g

### ACTION
A bile-acid sequestrant that combines with bile acid to form an insoluble compound that is excreted. The liver must synthesize new bile acid from cholesterol, which reduces low-density-lipoprotein cholesterol levels.

| Route | Onset | Peak | Duration |
|-------|-------|------|----------|
| P.O. | Unknown | Unknown | 2-4 wk |

### INDICATIONS & DOSAGE
*Primary hyperlipidemia or pruritus due to partial bile obstruction, adjunct for reduction of elevated serum cholesterol in patients with primary hypercholesterolemia—*
**Adults:** 4 g once or twice daily. Maintenance dose is 8 to 16 g daily divided into two doses. Maximum daily dose is 24 g.

---

## ADVERSE REACTIONS

**CNS:** headache, anxiety, vertigo, dizziness, insomnia, fatigue, syncope, tinnitus.
**GI:** *constipation, fecal impaction,* hemorrhoids, *abdominal discomfort,* flatulence, *nausea,* vomiting, steatorrhea, GI bleeding, diarrhea, anorexia.
**GU:** hematuria, dysuria.
**Hematologic:** anemia, bleeding tendencies, ecchymoses.
**Hepatic:** increased serum alkaline phosphatase levels.
**Metabolic:** hyperchloremic acidosis (with long-term use or very high doses).
**Musculoskeletal:** backache, muscle and joint pains, osteoporosis.
**Skin:** *rash;* irritation of skin, tongue, and perianal area.
**Other:** *vitamin A, D, E, and K deficiencies from decreased absorption.*

## INTERACTIONS

**Drug-drug.** *Acetaminophen, beta blockers, cardiac glycosides, corticosteroids, estrogens, fat-soluble vitamins (A, D, E, and K), iron preparations, niacin, penicillin G, phenobarbital, progestins, tetracycline, thiazide diuretics, thyroid hormones, warfarin and other coumarin derivatives:* absorption may be substantially decreased by cholestyramine. Administer other drugs 1 hour before or 4 to 6 hours after cholestyramine.

## EFFECTS ON DIAGNOSTIC TESTS

Cholecystography using iopanoic acid will yield abnormal results because iopanoic acid is also bound by cholestyramine.

## CONTRAINDICATIONS

Contraindicated in patients with hypersensitivity to bile-acid sequestering resins or in those with complete biliary obstruction.

## NURSING CONSIDERATIONS

• Use cautiously in patients predisposed to constipation and in those with conditions aggravated by constipation, such as severe, symptomatic coronary artery disease.
• Monitor serum cholesterol and triglyceride levels regularly during therapy.
• Monitor serum levels of cardiac glycosides in patients receiving cardiac glycosides and cholestyramine concurrently. If cholestyramine therapy is discontinued, adjust dosage of cardiac glycosides as ordered to avoid toxicity.
• Monitor bowel habits. Encourage a diet high in fiber and fluids. If severe constipation develops, decrease dosage, add a stool softener, or discontinue drug, as ordered.
• Long-term use may be associated with deficiencies of vitamins A, D, E, and K and folic acid.
• *Alert:* Don't confuse Questran with Quarzan.

### ☑ Patient teaching

• *Alert:* Tell patient never to take drug in its dry form; esophageal irritation or severe constipation may result.
• To prepare, instruct patient to use a large glass containing water, milk, or juice (especially pulpy fruit juice). He should sprinkle the powder on the surface of the preferred beverage, let the mixture stand for a few minutes, and then stir thoroughly. Mixing with carbonated beverages may result in excessive foaming. After drinking preparation, patient should swirl a small additional amount of liquid in the same glass and then drink again to ensure ingestion of the entire dose.
• Advise patient to take all other drugs at least 1 hour before or 4 to 6 hours after cholestyramine to avoid blocking their absorption.
• Teach patient about proper dietary management of serum lipids. When appropriate, recommend weight-control, exercise, and smoking-cessation programs.

---

## colestipol hydrochloride
Colestid

*Pregnancy Risk Category NR*

---

## HOW SUPPLIED

*Granules:* 300-g and 500-g bottles, 5-g packets
*Tablets:* 1 g

---

## ACTION
Combines with bile acid to form an insoluble compound that is excreted in feces. The liver must synthesize new bile acid from cholesterol; this leads to reduced low-density-lipoprotein cholesterol levels.

| Route | Onset | Peak | Duration |
|-------|-------|------|----------|
| P.O. | 1 mo | Unknown | 1 mo |

## INDICATIONS & DOSAGE
*Primary hypercholesterolemia—*
**Adults:** initially, 5g P.O. daily or b.i.d., increased in 5-mg increments q 1 to 2 months, p.r.n. Usual dose is 5 to 30 g (granules) P.O. once daily or in divided doses. Or, 2 to 16 g (tablets) P.O. daily given once or in divided doses.

## ADVERSE REACTIONS
**CNS:** headache, dizziness, anxiety, vertigo, insomnia, fatigue, syncope, tinnitus.
**CV:** angina, chest pain.
**GI:** *constipation, fecal impaction,* hemorrhoids, abdominal discomfort, flatulence, nausea, vomiting, steatorrhea, GI bleeding, diarrhea, anorexia.
**GU:** dysuria, hematuria.
**Hematologic:** anemia, ecchymoses, bleeding tendencies.
**Hepatic:** increased serum alkaline phosphatase, ALT, and AST levels.
**Metabolic:** hyperchloremic acidosis.
**Musculoskeletal:** backache, muscle and joint pain, osteoporosis.
**Skin:** rash, irritation of tongue and perianal area.
**Other:** vitamin A, D, E, and K deficiencies from decreased absorption.

## INTERACTIONS
**Drug-drug.** *Chlorothiazide, furosemide, penicillin G, tetracycline:* colestipol may decrease absorption. Separate administration times; give other drugs at least 1 hour before or 4 hours after colestipol.
*Oral antidiabetics:* may antagonize response to colestipol. Monitor serum lipids.

## EFFECTS ON DIAGNOSTIC TESTS
None reported.

## CONTRAINDICATIONS
Contraindicated in patients with hypersensitivity reactions to bile-acid sequestering resins.

## NURSING CONSIDERATIONS
• Use cautiously in patients predisposed to constipation and in those with conditions aggravated by constipation, such as severe, symptomatic coronary artery disease.
• Monitor serum cholesterol and triglyceride levels regularly during therapy.
• Monitor bowel habits; if severe constipation develops, decrease dosage or add stool softener, as ordered. Encourage a diet high in fiber and fluids.
• Monitor serum levels of cardiac glycosides in patients concurrently receiving cardiac glycosides and colestipol. If colestipol therapy is discontinued, adjust dosage of cardiac glycosides to avoid toxicity, as ordered.

### ☑ Patient teaching
• *Alert:* Tell patient never to take drug in its dry form; esophageal irritation or severe constipation may result.
• To prepare, instruct patient to use a large glass containing water, milk, or juice (especially pulpy fruit juice). He should sprinkle the powder on the surface of the preferred beverage, let the mixture stand a few minutes, and then stir thoroughly to obtain a uniform suspension. After drinking this preparation, patient should swirl a small additional amount of liquid in the same glass and then drink it to ensure ingestion of the entire dose.
• To enhance palatability, tell patient to mix and refrigerate the next daily dose the previous evening.
• Instruct patient taking tablet form to swallow tablets whole and not to crush, cut, or chew them.
• Advise patient to take all other drugs at least 1 hour before or 4 to 6 hours after colestipol to avoid blocking their absorption.
• Teach patient about proper dietary management of serum lipids. When appropriate, recommend weight-control, exercise, and smoking-cessation programs.

---

*Liquid contains alcohol.    **May contain tartrazine.    †Canada    ‡Australia    §U.K.    ◇OTC

• Inform patient that long-term use may be associated with deficiencies of vitamins A, D, E, and K and folic acid. Instruct patient to report any unusual signs or symptoms.

---

## fenofibrate (micronized)
Tricor

*Pregnancy Risk Category C*

### HOW SUPPLIED
*Capsules:* 67 mg

### ACTION
Unknown. Thought to lower triglyceride levels by inhibiting triglyceride synthesis, resulting in a decrease in the amount of very-low-density lipoproteins (VLDL) released into the circulation. Drug may stimulate breakdown of triglyceride-rich protein.

| Route | Onset | Peak | Duration |
|-------|-------|------|----------|
| P.O. | Unknown | 6-8 hr | Unknown |

### INDICATIONS & DOSAGE
*Adjunct to diet for treatment of patients with very high serum triglyceride levels (types IV and V hyperlipidemia) who are at risk for pancreatitis and who don't respond adequately to a determined dietary effort—*
**Adults:** initially, 67 mg P.O. daily. Dosage may be increased following repeat serum triglyceride estimations at 4- to 8-week intervals to maximum dose of three capsules daily (201 mg).
*Adjust-a-dose:* Minimize dose for patients with severe renal impairment. Initiate therapy with dose of 67 mg/day and increase only after effects on renal function and triglyceride levels have been evaluated at initial dose. No modification is needed for patients with moderate renal impairment.

### ADVERSE REACTIONS
**CNS:** dizziness, localized pain, asthenia, fatigue, paresthesia, insomnia, increased appetite, headache.
**CV:** *arrhythmias.*

**EENT:** eye irritation, eye floaters, earache, conjunctivitis, blurred vision, rhinitis, sinusitis.
**GI:** dyspepsia, eructation, flatulence, nausea, vomiting, abdominal pain, constipation, diarrhea.
**GU:** increased BUN and creatinine levels, polyuria, vaginitis.
**Hematologic:** decreased hemoglobin level.
**Hepatic:** increased ALT, AST levels.
**Musculoskeletal:** arthralgia.
**Respiratory:** cough.
**Skin:** pruritus, rash.
**Other:** decreased uric acid levels, hypersensitivity reaction, *infection,* flulike syndrome, decreased libido.

### INTERACTIONS
**Drug-drug.** *Bile-acid sequestrants:* may bind and inhibit absorption of fenofibrate. Give drug 1 hour before or 4 to 6 hours after bile-acid sequestrants.
*Coumarin-type anticoagulants:* potentiation of anticoagulant effect, prolonged PT and INR. Monitor PT and INR closely. Dosage of anticoagulant may need to be reduced.
*Cyclosporine, immunosuppressants, nephrotoxic drugs:* induced renal dysfunction may compromise the elimination of fenofibrate. Use together cautiously.
*3-Hydroxy-3-methylglutaryl coenzyme A (HMG-CoA) reductase inhibitors:* no data are available on concomitant use with fenofibrate. Because of risk of myopathy, rhabdomyolysis, and acute renal failure reported with concomitant use of HMG-CoA reductase inhibitors and gemfibrozil (another fibrate derivative), don't give these drugs together.
**Drug-food.** *Any food:* absorption of fenofibrate is increased when administered with food. Give drug with meals.
**Drug-lifestyle.** *Alcohol use:* may elevate triglyceride levels. Avoid concomitant use.

### EFFECTS ON DIAGNOSTIC TESTS
None reported.

### CONTRAINDICATIONS
Contraindicated in patients with hypersensitivity to drug and in those with pre-

---

existing gallbladder disease, hepatic dysfunction, primary biliary cirrhosis, severe renal dysfunction, or unexplained persistent liver function abnormalities.

## NURSING CONSIDERATIONS
• Use cautiously in patients with a history of pancreatitis.
• Obtain baseline lipid levels and liver function tests before starting therapy. Perform periodic monitoring of liver function for duration of drug therapy. Discontinue drug if enzyme levels persist above three times normal limit.
• Monitor for signs and symptoms of pancreatitis, myositis, rhabdomyolysis, cholelithiasis, and renal failure. Be alert to occurrence of myalgia, muscle tenderness, or weakness, especially in the presence of malaise or fever.
• If an adequate response hasn't been obtained after 2 months of treatment with maximum daily dose, therapy must be discontinued.
• Drug lowers serum uric acid levels in patients with or without hyperuricemia by increasing uric acid excretion.
• Beta blockers, estrogens, and thiazide diuretics may increase plasma triglyceride levels; the continued use of these drugs should be evaluated.
• Mild to moderate decreases in hemoglobin level, hematocrit, and WBC count may occur on initiation of therapy but stabilize on long-term administration.

☑ **Patient teaching**
• Inform patient that drug therapy doesn't reduce the importance of adhering to triglyceride-lowering diet.
• Advise patient to promptly report unexplained muscle weakness, pain, or tenderness, especially if accompanied by malaise or fever.
• Inform patient to take drug with meals to optimize drug absorption.
• Advise patient to continue weight-control measures, including diet and exercise, and to reduce alcohol intake before starting drug therapy.
• Instruct patient who is also taking bile-acid resins to take fenofibrate 1 hour before or 4 to 6 hours after taking bile-acid resin.

• Advise woman about potential for tumor growth.
• Tell woman that a decision must be made to discontinue either breast-feeding or drug therapy.

## fluvastatin sodium
Lescol

*Pregnancy Risk Category X*

### HOW SUPPLIED
*Capsules:* 20 mg, 40 mg

### ACTION
Inhibits 3-hydroxy-3-methylglutaryl coenzyme A reductase, which is an early (and rate-limiting) step in the synthetic pathway of cholesterol.

| Route | Onset | Peak | Duration |
|-------|-------|------|----------|
| P.O. | Unknown | 1 hr | Unknown |

### INDICATIONS & DOSAGE
*Reduction of low-density lipoprotein and total cholesterol levels in patients with primary hypercholesterolemia (types IIa and IIb)—*
**Adults:** initially, 20 to 40 mg P.O. h.s., increased p.r.n. to maximum of 80 mg daily (in divided doses).
*To slow progression of coronary atherosclerosis in patients with coronary artery disease—*
**Adults:** initially, 20 to 40 mg P.O. h.s., increased p.r.n. to maximum of 80 mg daily (in divided doses).
✱ *NEW INDICATION: Elevated triglycerides and apolipoprotein B levels in patients with primary hypercholesterolemia and mixed dyslipidemia whose response to dietary restriction and other nonpharmacologic measures has been inadequate—*
**Adults:** initially, 20 to 40 mg P.O. h.s., increased p.r.n. to maximum of 80 mg daily (in divided doses).

### ADVERSE REACTIONS
**CNS:** headache, fatigue, dizziness, insomnia.
**EENT:** sinusitis, rhinitis, pharyngitis.
**GI:** dyspepsia, diarrhea, nausea, vomiting, abdominal pain, constipation, flatulence.

---

**Hematologic:** *thrombocytopenia, hemolytic anemia, leukopenia.*
**Hepatic:** increased liver enzymes, elevated CK levels.
**Metabolic:** abnormal thyroid function tests.
**Musculoskeletal:** arthralgia, back pain, myalgia.
**Respiratory:** *upper respiratory infection,* cough, bronchitis.
**Other:** hypersensitivity reactions.

## INTERACTIONS
**Drug-drug.** *Cholestyramine, colestipol:* may bind with fluvastatin in the GI tract and decrease absorption. Separate administration times by at least 4 hours.
*Cimetidine, omeprazole, ranitidine:* decreased fluvastatin metabolism. Monitor for enhanced effects.
*Cyclosporine and other immunosuppressants, erythromycin, gemfibrozil, niacin:* possible increased risk of polymyositis and rhabdomyolysis. Avoid concomitant use.
*Digoxin:* may alter digoxin pharmacokinetics. Monitor serum digoxin levels carefully.
*Rifampin:* enhanced fluvastatin metabolism and decreased plasma levels. Monitor for lack of effect.
*Warfarin:* increased anticoagulant effect with bleeding. Monitor patient.
**Drug-lifestyle.** *Alcohol use:* increased risk of hepatotoxicity. Avoid concomitant use.

## EFFECTS ON DIAGNOSTIC TESTS
None reported.

## CONTRAINDICATIONS
Contraindicated in patients with hypersensitivity to drug and in those with active liver disease or conditions associated with unexplained persistent elevations of serum transaminase levels; also contraindicated in pregnant and breast-feeding women and in women of childbearing age unless there is no risk of pregnancy.

## NURSING CONSIDERATIONS
• Use cautiously in patients with severe renal impairment and history of liver disease or heavy alcohol use.

• Drug should be initiated only after diet and other nonpharmacologic therapies have proved ineffective. Patient should be on a standard low-cholesterol diet during therapy.
• Liver function tests should be performed at the start of therapy and periodically thereafter.
• Watch for signs of myositis.
• *Alert:* Don't confuse fluvastatin with fluoxetine.

☑ **Patient teaching**
• Tell patient that drug may be taken without regard to meals; however, efficacy is enhanced if drug is taken in the evening.
• Teach patient about proper dietary management, weight control, and exercise. Explain their importance in controlling elevated serum lipid levels.
• Warn patient to avoid alcohol.
• Tell patient to notify doctor of adverse reactions, particularly muscle aches and pains.
• *Alert:* Inform woman that drug is contraindicated during pregnancy. Advise her to notify doctor immediately if pregnancy occurs.

## gemfibrozil
Apo-Gemfibrozil†, Lopid

*Pregnancy Risk Category C*

### HOW SUPPLIED
*Tablets:* 600 mg
*Capsules:* 300 mg

### ACTION
Inhibits peripheral lipolysis and reduces triglyceride synthesis in the liver. It lowers serum triglyceride levels and increases high-density-lipoprotein cholesterol levels.

| Route | Onset | Peak | Duration |
|-------|-------|------|----------|
| P.O. | 2-5 days | 4 wk | Unknown |

### INDICATIONS & DOSAGE
*Types IV and V hyperlipidemia unresponsive to diet and other drugs, reduction of risk of coronary heart disease in patients with type IIb hyperlipidemia who cannot*

*tolerate or who are refractory to treatment with bile-acid sequestrants or niacin—*
**Adults:** 1,200 mg P.O. daily in two divided doses, 30 minutes before morning and evening meals.

## ADVERSE REACTIONS
**CNS:** headache, fatigue, vertigo.
**CV:** atrial fibrillation.
**GI:** *abdominal and epigastric pain,* diarrhea, nausea, vomiting, *dyspepsia,* constipation, acute appendicitis.
**Hematologic:** *anemia, leukopenia,* eosinophilia, *thrombocytopenia.*
**Hepatic:** bile duct obstruction, elevated liver enzymes.
**Metabolic:** hypokalemia.
**Skin:** rash, dermatitis, pruritus, eczema.

## INTERACTIONS
**Drug-drug.** *Lovastatin:* myopathy with rhabdomyolysis has been reported. Don't use together.
*Oral anticoagulants:* gemfibrozil may enhance the clinical effects of oral anticoagulants. Monitor closely.

## EFFECTS ON DIAGNOSTIC TESTS
None reported.

## CONTRAINDICATIONS
Contraindicated in patients with hypersensitivity to drug and in those with hepatic or severe renal dysfunction (including primary biliary cirrhosis) or preexisting gallbladder disease.

## NURSING CONSIDERATIONS
• Periodic CBCs and liver function tests should be performed during the first 12 months of therapy.
• If drug has no beneficial effects after 3 months of therapy, expect doctor to discontinue it.

### ✔Patient teaching
• Instruct patient to take drug 30 minutes before breakfast and dinner.
• Teach patient about proper dietary management of serum lipids. When appropriate, recommend weight-control, exercise, and smoking-cessation programs.

• Because of possible dizziness and blurred vision, advise patient to avoid driving or other potentially hazardous activities until CNS effects of drug are known.
• Tell patient to observe bowel movements and to report evidence of steatorrhea or other signs of bile duct obstruction.

# lovastatin (mevinolin)
Mevacor

*Pregnancy Risk Category X*

## HOW SUPPLIED
*Tablets:* 10 mg, 20 mg, 40 mg

## ACTION
Inhibits 3-hydroxy-3-methylglutaryl coenzyme A reductase, which is an early (and rate-limiting) step in the synthetic pathway of cholesterol.

| Route | Onset | Peak | Duration |
|-------|-------|------|----------|
| P.O. | Unknown | 2 hr | Unknown |

## INDICATIONS & DOSAGE
*Reduction of low-density lipoprotein and total cholesterol levels in patients with primary hypercholesterolemia (types IIa and IIb), to slow the progression of coronary atherosclerosis associated with coronary artery disease—*
**Adults:** initially, 20 mg P.O. once daily with evening meal. Recommended dosage range is 10 to 80 mg daily in one or two divided doses.
*Adjust-a-dose:* For patients receiving immunosuppressants, initially 10 mg P.O. daily. Maximum daily dose is 20 mg.
✷ *NEW INDICATION: Primary prevention of coronary heart disease in patients without symptomatic cardiovascular disease, average to moderately elevated total cholesterol and low-density lipoprotein cholesterol, and below average high-density lipoprotein cholesterol—*
**Adults:** initially, 20 mg P.O. once daily with evening meal. Recommended dosage range is 10 to 80 mg daily in one or two divided doses.

## ADVERSE REACTIONS

**CNS:** headache, dizziness, peripheral neuropathy, insomnia.
**CV:** chest pain.
**EENT:** blurred vision.
**GI:** constipation, diarrhea, dyspepsia, flatulence, abdominal pain or cramps, heartburn, nausea, vomiting.
**Hepatic:** elevated serum CK or serum transaminase levels.
**Musculoskeletal:** muscle cramps, myalgia, myositis, *rhabdomyolysis.*
**Skin:** rash, pruritus, alopecia.

## INTERACTIONS

**Drug-drug.** *Azole antifungals, clarithromycin, cyclosporine or other immunosuppressants, erythromycin, gemfibrozil, nefazodone, niacin:* possible increased risk of polymyositis and rhabdomyolysis (maximum recommended lovastatin dose is 20 mg daily); monitor patient closely.
*Oral anticoagulants:* lovastatin may enhance the clinical effects of oral anticoagulants. Monitor patient closely.
**Drug-lifestyle.** *Alcohol use:* increased risk of hepatotoxicity. Avoid concomitant use.

## EFFECTS ON DIAGNOSTIC TESTS

None reported.

## CONTRAINDICATIONS

Contraindicated in patients with hypersensitivity to drug and in those with active liver disease or conditions associated with unexplained persistent elevations of serum transaminase levels; also contraindicated in pregnant and breast-feeding women, in women of childbearing age unless there is no risk of pregnancy, and in patients taking mibefradil.

## NURSING CONSIDERATIONS

• Use cautiously in patients who consume substantial quantities of alcohol or have a past history of liver disease.
• Drug should be initiated only after diet and other nonpharmacologic therapies have proved ineffective. Patient should be on a standard low-cholesterol diet during therapy.

• Liver function tests should be performed at the start of therapy and periodically thereafter.
• **Alert:** Don't confuse lovastatin with Lotensin; or Leustatin, or Livostin; or Mevacor with Mivacron.

☑ **Patient teaching**
• Instruct patient to take drug with the evening meal, when absorption is enhanced and cholesterol biosynthesis is greater.
• Teach patient about proper dietary management of serum lipids. When appropriate, recommend weight-control, exercise, and smoking-cessation programs.
• Advise patient to have periodic eye examinations; related compounds have been shown to cause cataracts.
• Inform patient to store tablets at room temperature in a light-resistant container.
• Advise patient to promptly report unexplained muscle pain, tenderness or weakness, particularly when accompanied by malaise or fever.
• **Alert:** Inform female patient that drug is contraindicated during pregnancy. Advise her to notify doctor immediately if pregnancy occurs.

---

## pravastatin sodium (eptastatin)
Lipostat§, Pravachol

*Pregnancy Risk Category X*

## HOW SUPPLIED

*Tablets:* 10 mg, 20 mg, 40 mg

## ACTION

Inhibits 3-hydroxy-3-methylglutaryl coenzyme A reductase, which is an early (and rate-limiting) step in the synthetic pathway of cholesterol.

| Route | Onset | Peak | Duration |
|-------|-------|------|----------|
| P.O. | Unknown | 1-1.5 hr | Unknown |

## INDICATIONS & DOSAGE

*Adjunct to diet to reduce low-density lipoprotein, total cholesterol, and triglyceride levels in patients with primary hypercholesterolemia and mixed dyslipi-*

demia (Fredrickson types IIa and IIb); primary prevention of coronary events in hypercholesterolemic patients without clinical evidence of heart disease—

**Adults:** initially, 10 or 20 mg P.O. h.s. Dosage adjusted q 4 weeks based on patient tolerance and response; maximum daily dose is 40 mg.

**Elderly:** initially, 10 mg P.O. h.s. Most patients respond to daily dose of 20 mg or less.

Reduction of risk of acute coronary events or slowing progression of coronary atherosclerosis in hypercholesterolemic patients with clinical evidence of coronary artery disease, including prior MI; reduction of risk of undergoing myocardial revascularization procedure; reduction of risk of recurrent MI, stroke, or transient ischemic attacks in post-MI patients with normal cholesterol levels—

**Adults:** initially, 10 or 20 mg P.O. h.s. Dosage adjusted q 4 weeks based on patient tolerance and response; maximum daily dose is 40 mg.

**Elderly:** initially, 10 mg P.O. h.s. Most patients respond to daily dose of 20 mg or less.

*Adjust-a-dose:* Patients taking immunosuppressants should be initiated at 10 mg P.O. daily. Maximum dose is 20 mg P.O. daily.

## ADVERSE REACTIONS

**CNS:** headache, dizziness, fatigue.
**CV:** chest pain.
**EENT:** rhinitis.
**GI:** vomiting, diarrhea, heartburn, abdominal pain, constipation, flatulence, nausea.
**GU:** renal failure secondary to myoglobinuria, urinary abnormality.
**Hepatic:** increased serum ALT, AST, CK, alkaline phosphatase, and bilirubin levels.
**Metabolic:** abnormal thyroid function tests.
**Musculoskeletal:** myositis, myopathy, *localized muscle pain,* myalgia.
**Respiratory:** cough, influenza, common cold.
**Skin:** rash.
**Other:** flulike symptoms, *rhabdomyolysis.*

## INTERACTIONS

**Drug-drug.** *Cholestyramine, colestipol:* concomitant administration decreases plasma levels of pravastatin. Administer pravastatin 1 hour before or 4 hours after these drugs.

*Drugs that decrease levels or activity of endogenous steroids (such as cimetidine, ketoconazole, spironolactone):* may increase risk of developing endocrine dysfunction. No intervention appears needed; take complete drug history in patients who develop endocrine dysfunction.

*Erythromycin, fibric acid derivatives (such as clofibrate, gemfibrozil), immunosuppressants (such as cyclosporine), high doses (1 g or more daily) of niacin (nicotinic acid):* may increase the risk of rhabdomyolysis. Monitor patient closely if concomitant use cannot be avoided.

*Gemfibrozil:* decreases protein-binding and urinary clearance of pravastatin. Avoid concomitant use.

*Hepatotoxic drugs:* increased risk of hepatotoxicity. Avoid concomitant use.

**Drug-lifestyle.** *Alcohol use:* increased risk of hepatotoxicity. Avoid concomitant use.

## EFFECTS ON DIAGNOSTIC TESTS

None reported.

## CONTRAINDICATIONS

Contraindicated in patients with hypersensitivity to drug and in those with active liver disease or conditions that cause unexplained, persistent elevations of serum transaminase levels; also contraindicated in pregnant and breast-feeding women and in women of childbearing age unless there is no risk of pregnancy.

## NURSING CONSIDERATIONS

• Use cautiously in patients who consume large quantities of alcohol or have history of liver disease.
• Drug should be initiated only after diet and other nonpharmacologic therapies prove ineffective. Patients should be on a standard low-cholesterol diet during therapy.
• Liver function tests should be performed at start of therapy and periodically thereafter. A liver biopsy may be per-

---

formed if elevated liver enzyme levels persist.
• *Alert:* Don't confuse Pravachol with Prevacid or propranolol.

### ☑ Patient teaching
• Instruct patient to take the recommended dose in the evening, preferably at bedtime.
• Teach patient about proper dietary management of serum lipids. When appropriate, recommend weight-control, exercise, and smoking-cessation programs.
• *Alert:* Inform woman that drug is contraindicated during pregnancy. Advise her to notify doctor immediately if pregnancy occurs.

---

## simvastatin (synvinolin)
Lipex‡, Zocor

*Pregnancy Risk Category X*

### HOW SUPPLIED
*Tablets:* 5 mg, 10 mg, 20 mg, 40 mg

### ACTION
Inhibits 3-hydroxy-3-methylglutaryl coenzyme A reductase, which is an early (and rate-limiting) step in the synthetic pathway of cholesterol.

| Route | Onset | Peak | Duration |
|-------|-------|------|----------|
| P.O. | Unknown | 1.3-2.4 hr | Unknown |

### INDICATIONS & DOSAGE
*Adjunct to diet for reduction of low-density lipoprotein (LDL) and total cholesterol levels in patients with primary hypercholesterolemia (types IIa and IIb) and mixed dyslipidemia and in patients with coronary heart disease and hypercholesterolemia to reduce the risk of coronary death, nonfatal MI, stroke, transient ischemic attack, and undergoing myocardial revascularization procedures—*
**Adults:** initially, 20 mg P.O. daily in the evening. Dosage adjusted q 4 weeks based on patient tolerance and response; maximum daily dose is 80 mg.
**Elderly:** initially, 5 mg P.O. daily in the evening. Maximum daily dose is 20 mg.

*Reduction of total cholesterol and LDL in patients with homozygous familial hypercholesterolemia—*
**Adults:** 40 mg daily in the evening or 80 mg daily given in three divided doses of 20 mg, 20 mg, and 40 mg in the evening.

### ADVERSE REACTIONS
**CNS:** headache, asthenia.
**GI:** abdominal pain, constipation, diarrhea, dyspepsia, flatulence, nausea, vomiting.
**Hepatic:** elevated liver enzyme levels.
**Respiratory:** upper respiratory tract infection.

### INTERACTIONS
**Drug-drug.** *Antifungals, clarithromycin, erythromycin, fibric acid derivatives (such as clofibrate, gemfibrozil), immunosuppressants (such as cyclosporine), nefazodone, high doses (1 g or more daily) of niacin (nicotinic acid):* may increase risk of rhabdomyolysis. Monitor patient closely if concomitant use cannot be avoided. Limit daily dose of simvastatin to 10 mg if the patient must take cyclosporine.
*Digoxin:* simvastatin may slightly elevate digoxin levels. Closely monitor plasma digoxin levels at initiation of simvastatin therapy.
*Drugs that decrease levels or activity of endogenous steroids (such as cimetidine, ketoconazole, spironolactone):* may increase risk of developing endocrine dysfunction. No intervention appears needed; take complete drug history in patients who develop endocrine dysfunction.
*Hepatotoxic drugs:* increased risk of hepatotoxicity. Avoid concomitant use.
*Warfarin:* anticoagulant effect may be slightly enhanced. Monitor INR at start of therapy and during dosage adjustments.
**Drug-lifestyle.** *Alcohol use:* increased risk of hepatotoxicity. Avoid concomitant use.

### EFFECTS ON DIAGNOSTIC TESTS
None reported.

### CONTRAINDICATIONS
Contraindicated in patients with hypersensitivity to drug and in those with active liver disease or conditions that cause un-

---

*Reactions may be* common, *uncommon,* **life-threatening**, *or* COMMON AND LIFE-THREATENING.

explained persistent elevations of serum transaminase levels; also contraindicated in pregnant and breast-feeding women and in women of childbearing age unless there is no risk of pregnancy.

## NURSING CONSIDERATIONS
• Use cautiously in patients who consume substantial quantities of alcohol or have a history of liver disease.
• Drug is initiated only after diet and other nonpharmacologic therapies prove ineffective. Patient should be on a standard low-cholesterol diet during therapy.
• Liver function tests should be performed at start of therapy and periodically thereafter. A liver biopsy may be performed if enzyme elevations persist.
• *Alert:* Don't confuse Zocor with Cozaar or Zorac.

### ☑ Patient teaching
• Instruct patient to take drug with the evening meal; absorption is enhanced and cholesterol biosynthesis is greater.
• Teach patient about proper dietary management of serum lipids. When appropriate, recommend weight-control, exercise, and smoking-cessation programs.
• Tell patient to inform doctor if adverse reactions occur, particularly muscle aches and pains.
• *Alert:* Inform woman that drug is contraindicated during pregnancy. Advise her to notify doctor immediately if pregnancy occurs.

abciximab
alprostadil
arbutamine hydrochloride
cilostazol
clopidogrel bisulfate
dipyridamole
eptifibatide
midodrine hydrochloride
pentoxifylline
ticlopidine hydrochloride
tirofiban hydrochloride

**COMBINATION PRODUCTS**
None.

---

abciximab
ReoPro

*Pregnancy Risk Category C*

**HOW SUPPLIED**
*Injection:* 2 mg/ml

**ACTION**
Binds to the glycoprotein IIb/IIIa
(GPIIb/IIIa) receptor of human platelets
and inhibits platelet aggregation.

| Route | Onset | Peak | Duration |
|-------|-------|------|----------|
| I.V. | Immediate | Immediate | 48 hr |

**INDICATIONS & DOSAGE**
*Adjunct to percutaneous transluminal
coronary angioplasty (PTCA) or atherectomy for the prevention of acute cardiac
ischemic complications in patients at high
risk for abrupt closure of treated coronary
vessel—*
**Adults:** 0.25 mg/kg as an I.V. bolus administered 10 to 60 minutes before start
of PTCA or atherectomy; then a continuous I.V. infusion of 10 mcg/minute for 12
hours.
*Patients with unstable angina not re-
sponding to conventional medical therapy
who are to undergo percutaneous coronary intervention within 24 hours—*
**Adults:** 0.25 mg/kg as an I.V. bolus; then

an 18- to 24-hour infusion of 10 mcg/
minute, concluding 1 hour after percutaneous coronary intervention.

**ADVERSE REACTIONS**
**CNS:** hyperesthesia, hypoesthesia, confu-
sion, headache.
**CV:** *hypotension,* bradycardia, peripheral
edema.
**EENT:** abnormal vision.
**GI:** *nausea,* vomiting, abdominal pain.
**Hematologic:** *bleeding, **thrombocytope-
nia,*** anemia, leukocytosis.
**Respiratory:** pleural effusion, pleurisy,
pneumonia.
**Other:** pain.

**INTERACTIONS**
**Drug-drug.** *Antiplatelet drugs, dipyridamole, heparin, NSAIDs, other anticoagulants, thrombolytics, ticlopidine:* increased risk of bleeding. Monitor patient
closely.

**EFFECTS ON DIAGNOSTIC TESTS**
None reported.

**CONTRAINDICATIONS**
Contraindicated in patients with hypersensitivity to drug, its ingredients, or
murine proteins. Also contraindicated in
those with active internal bleeding, recent
(within 6 weeks) GI or GU bleeding of
clinical significance, CVA within past 2
years or with significant residual neurologic deficit, bleeding diathesis, thrombocytopenia (under 100,000/mm³), recent
(within 6 weeks) major surgery or trauma,
intracranial neoplasm, intracranial arteriovenous malformation, intracranial
aneurysm, severe uncontrolled hypertension, or history of vasculitis. Drug is contraindicated when oral anticoagulants
have been administered within past 7 days
unless PT is 1.2 times control or less or
when I.V. dextran is used before PTCA or
is intended to be used during PTCA.

---

## NURSING CONSIDERATIONS

• Use with caution in patients at increased risk for bleeding, including those under 165 lb (75 kg) or over age 65, those who have a history of GI disease, and those who are receiving thrombolytics. Conditions that increase patient's risk of bleeding include PTCA within 12 hours of onset of symptoms for acute MI, prolonged PTCA (lasting more than 70 minutes), or failed PTCA. Heparin used with drug also may contribute to the risk of bleeding.

• Patients undergoing PTCA and who have one or more of the following conditions should be considered as candidates for drug therapy: unstable angina or a non-Q-wave MI, acute Q-wave MI within 12 hours of onset of symptoms, presence of two type B lesions in the artery to be dilated, presence of one type B lesion in the artery to be dilated in women over age 65 or in diabetic patients, presence of one type C lesion in the artery to be dilated, or angioplasty of an infarct-related lesion within 7 days of MI.

• Review and monitor concomitant drugs; drug is intended for use with aspirin and heparin.

• *Alert:* Keep epinephrine, dopamine, theophylline, antihistamines, and corticosteroids readily available in case of anaphylaxis.

• Monitor patient closely for bleeding. Bleeding associated with therapy is categorized as follows: bleeding observed at the arterial access site used for cardiac catheterization and internal bleeding involving the GI or GU tract or retroperitoneal sites.

• Institute bleeding precautions. Maintain patient on bed rest for 6 to 8 hours following sheath removal or discontinuation of drug infusion, whichever is later. Minimize or avoid, if possible, arterial and venous punctures; I.M. injections; use of urinary catheters, nasogastric tubes, or automatic blood pressure cuffs; and nasotracheal intubation.

• *Alert:* Don't confuse abciximab with arcitumomab.

### I.V. administration

• Inspect solution for particulate matter before administration. If visibly opaque particles occur, discard solution and obtain new vial. Withdraw needed amount of drug for I.V. bolus injection through a sterile, nonpyrogenic, low-protein-binding, 0.2- or 0.22-micron filter into a syringe. Administer I.V. bolus 10 to 60 minutes before procedure.

• Withdraw 4.5 ml of drug for continuous I.V. infusion through a sterile, nonpyrogenic, low-protein-binding, 0.2- or 0.22-micron filter into a syringe. Inject into 250 ml of sterile normal saline solution or $D_5W$, and infuse at a rate of 10 mcg/minute for 12 hours via a continuous infusion pump equipped with an in-line filter. Discard unused portion at end of 12-hour infusion.

• Administer drug in a separate I.V. line; no other drug should be added to the infusion solution.

### ✓ Patient teaching

• Explain use and administration of drug to patient and family.

• Instruct patient to report adverse reactions immediately.

---

## alprostadil
### Prostin VR Pediatric

*Pregnancy Risk Category NR*

### HOW SUPPLIED
*Injection:* 500 mcg/ml

### ACTION
A prostaglandin derivative that relaxes the smooth muscle of the ductus arteriosus.

| Route | Onset | Peak | Duration |
|-------|-------|------|----------|
| I.V. | 20 min | 1-2 hr | Length of infusion |

### INDICATIONS & DOSAGE
*Palliative therapy for temporary maintenance of patency of ductus arteriosus until surgery can be performed—*
**Infants:** 0.05 to 0.1 mcg/kg/minute by I.V. infusion. When therapeutic response is achieved, infusion rate reduced to lowest dose that will maintain response. Maximum dose is 0.4 mcg/kg/minute. Or, drug can be administered through umbili-

cal artery catheter placed at ductal opening.

## ADVERSE REACTIONS
**CNS:** *seizures.*
**CV:** *bradycardia,* hypotension, tachycardia, *cardiac arrest,* edema, *flushing.*
**GI:** diarrhea.
**Hematologic:** disseminated intravascular coagulation.
**Metabolic:** hypokalemia.
**Respiratory:** APNEA.
**Other:** *fever, sepsis.*

## INTERACTIONS
None significant.

## EFFECTS ON DIAGNOSTIC TESTS
None reported.

## CONTRAINDICATIONS
No known contraindications.

## NURSING CONSIDERATIONS
• A differential diagnosis should be made between respiratory distress syndrome and cyanotic heart disease before drug is administered. Drug shouldn't be used in neonates with respiratory distress syndrome.
• Use cautiously in neonates with bleeding tendencies because drug inhibits platelet aggregation.
• Keep respiratory support available.
• In infants with restricted pulmonary blood flow, measure drug's effectiveness by monitoring blood oxygenation. In infants with restricted systemic blood flow, measure drug's effectiveness by monitoring systemic blood pressure and blood pH.
• Monitor arterial pressure by umbilical artery catheter, auscultation, or Doppler transducer. Slow rate of infusion if arterial pressure falls significantly.
• *Alert:* Apnea and bradycardia may reflect drug overdose; if either occurs, stop infusion immediately.
• Keep in mind that CV and CNS adverse reactions are more frequent in infants weighing under 4.5 lb (2 kg) and in those receiving infusions for longer than 48 hours.
• *Alert:* Don't confuse alprostadil with alprazolam.

## ▣ I.V. administration
• Dilute drug before administering. Prepare fresh solution daily; discard solution after 24 hours.
• For infusion, 1 ml of concentrate labeled as containing 500 mcg is diluted in normal saline or dextrose 5% injection to provide a solution containing 2 to 20 mcg/ml.
• When using a device with a volumetric infusion chamber, add appropriate volume of diluent to the chamber; then add 1 ml of alprostadil concentrate.
• During dilution, avoid direct contact between concentrate and wall of plastic volumetric infusion chamber because solution may become hazy. If this occurs, discard solution.
• Don't use diluents that contain benzyl alcohol. Fatal toxic syndrome may occur.
• Reduce infusion rate if fever or significant hypotension occurs.
• Drug isn't recommended for direct injection or intermittent infusion. Administer by continuous infusion using a constant-rate pump. Infuse through a large peripheral or central vein or through an umbilical artery catheter placed at the level of the ductus arteriosus. If flushing from peripheral vasodilation occurs, reposition catheter.

## ☑ Patient teaching
• Inform parents of the need for drug and explain its use.
• Encourage parents to ask questions and express concerns.

---

## arbutamine hydrochloride
GenESA

*Pregnancy Risk Category B*

## HOW SUPPLIED
*Injection:* 20-ml prefilled syringe containing 1 mg (0.05 mg/ml)

## ACTION
A sympathomimetic that increases cardiac workload through both positive inotropic and chronotropic actions.

| Route | Onset | Peak | Duration |
|-------|-------|------|----------|
| I.V. | 1 min | Unknown | Variable |

---

Reactions may be *common,* uncommon, *life-threatening,* or COMMON AND LIFE-THREATENING.

## INDICATIONS & DOSAGE
*Single-dose diagnostic aid in patients with suspected coronary artery disease who can't exercise adequately—*
**Adults:** 0.1 mcg/kg/minute for 1 minute via GenESA I.V. infusion system. The device adjusts dose until maximal heart rate limit (set by user) or maximal infusion rate of 0.8 mcg/kg/minute (maximum total dose, 10 mcg/kg) is achieved.

## ADVERSE REACTIONS
**CNS:** anxiety, dizziness, fatigue, headache, hypoesthesia, paresthesia, *tremor.*
**CV:** *angina pectoris,* ARRHYTHMIAS, chest pain, flushing, hypotension, hot flashes, palpitation, vasodilation.
**EENT:** dry mouth, taste perversion.
**GI:** nausea.
**Respiratory:** dyspnea.
**Skin:** increased sweating.
**Other:** pain.

## INTERACTIONS
**Drug-drug.** *Beta blockers:* may attenuate arbutamine's effects. Discontinue drug at least 48 hours before administration of arbutamine.

## EFFECTS ON DIAGNOSTIC TESTS
None reported.

## CONTRAINDICATIONS
Contraindicated in patients with known hypersensitivity to drug and in those with idiopathic hypertrophic subaortic stenosis, a history of recurrent sustained ventricular tachycardia, or heart failure (New York Heart Association class III or IV). Also contraindicated in patients who have an implanted cardiac pacemaker or automated cardioverter or defibrillator and in those receiving digoxin, atropine, other anticholinergic drugs, or tricyclic antidepressants.

## NURSING CONSIDERATIONS
• Use cautiously in patients with a known sulfite allergy. Arbutamine contains sodium metabisulfite, which may produce an allergic response in susceptible patients.
• Avoid use in patients with unstable angina, mechanical left ventricular outflow obstruction (such as severe valvular aortic stenosis), uncontrolled systemic hypertension, cardiac transplantation, history of cerebrovascular disease, peripheral vascular disorder resulting in cerebral or aortic aneurysm, narrow-angle glaucoma, supraventricular tachyarrhythmias or ventricular arrhythmias, or uncontrolled hyperthyroidism. Don't use in patients receiving class I antiarrhythmics, such as quinidine, lidocaine, or flecainide.
• Safety and efficacy of drug in patients with recent history (within 30 days) of MI haven't been evaluated; don't use in these patients.
• Don't administer atropine to enhance drug-induced chronotropic response; coadministration may lead to tachyarrhythmias.
• *Alert:* Before using the GenESA system, read and understand the manufacturer's directions.
• Monitor blood pressure, heart rate, and a diagnostic quality ECG continuously throughout drug infusion.
• A crash cart should be available by the bedside during drug administration.
• Transient prolongation of the corrected QT interval, as measured from a surface ECG, occurs with administration.
• Transient reductions in serum potassium levels may occur but rarely to hypokalemic levels.

### I.V. administration
• Drug is manufactured with a prefilled glass syringe and plunger rod.
• *Alert:* Don't dilute drug before use. Drug should only be administered via the prefilled syringe using the GenESA system (a closed-loop, computer-controlled, I.V. infusion device). Before administration, syringe should be inspected for evidence of particulate matter or discoloration.

### Patient teaching
• Instruct patient on need to discontinue beta blockers at least 48 hours before undergoing cardiac stress testing with arbutamine as ordered by doctor.
• Inform patient that drug will temporarily increase heart rate, but that he will be closely monitored.

- Inform patient of potential adverse events.

✳ *NEW DRUG*

## cilostazol
Pletal

*Pregnancy Risk Category C*

### HOW SUPPLIED
*Tablets:* 50 mg, 100 mg

### ACTION
A quinolinone derivative thought to inhibit the enzyme phosphodiesterase III, thus inhibiting platelet aggregation and causing vasodilation.

| Route | Onset | Peak | Duration |
|-------|-------|------|----------|
| P.O. | Unknown | 2-4 hr | Unknown |

### INDICATIONS & DOSAGE
*Reduction of symptoms of intermittent claudication—*
**Adults:** 100 mg P.O. b.i.d., at least 30 minutes before or 2 hours after breakfast and dinner.
*Adjust-a-dose:* Decrease dose to 50 mg P.O. b.i.d. during coadministration with drugs that may interact to cause an increase in serum cilostazol levels.

### ADVERSE REACTIONS
**CNS:** *headache, dizziness,* vertigo.
**CV:** *palpitation,* tachycardia.
**EENT:** *pharyngitis, rhinitis.*
**GI:** *abnormal stools, diarrhea,* dyspepsia, abdominal pain, flatulence, nausea.
**Musculoskeletal:** back pain, myalgia.
**Respiratory:** increased cough.
**Other:** *infection,* peripheral edema.

### INTERACTIONS
**Drug-drug.** *Diltiazem:* increased plasma cilostazol levels. Reduce cilostazol dose to 50 mg b.i.d. during coadministration.
*Erythromycin, other macrolides:* increased serum cilostazol levels and serum levels of one of the metabolites. Reduce cilostazol dose to 50 mg b.i.d. during coadministration.
*Omeprazole:* increased serum levels of active cilostazol metabolite. Reduce

cilostazol dose to 50 mg b.i.d. during coadministration.
*Strong inhibitors of CYP3A4 (such as fluconazole, fluoxetine, fluvoxamine, itraconazole, ketoconazole, miconazole, nefazodone, sertraline):* possible increased levels of cilostazol and its metabolites. Reduce cilostazol dose to 50 mg b.i.d. during coadministration.
**Drug-food.** *Grapefruit juice:* increased drug levels. Avoid grapefruit juice during therapy.
**Drug-lifestyle.** *Smoking:* may decrease drug exposure. Monitor patient closely.

### EFFECTS ON DIAGNOSTIC TESTS
None reported.

### CONTRAINDICATIONS
Contraindicated in patients with known or suspected hypersensitivity to drug or its components and in those with heart failure of any severity.

### NURSING CONSIDERATIONS
- Use cautiously in patients with severe underlying heart disease; also use cautiously with other drugs having antiplatelet activity.
- *Alert:* Cilostazol and similar drugs that inhibit the enzyme phosphodiesterase decrease the likelihood of survival in patients with class III and IV heart failure.
- *Alert:* CV risk is unknown in patients who use drug on long-term basis and in those with severe underlying heart disease.
- Drug should be given at least 30 minutes before or 2 hours after breakfast and dinner.
- Beneficial effects of drug may not be apparent for up to 12 weeks following initiation of therapy.
- Dosage can be reduced or discontinued without such rebound effects as platelet hyperaggregation.
- Drug may cause reduced triglyceride levels and increased high-density lipoprotein cholesterol level.

### ✓ Patient teaching
- Instruct patient that drug should be taken on an empty stomach, at least 30 min-

---

utes before or 2 hours after breakfast and dinner.
• Tell patient that beneficial effect of drug on intermittent claudication isn't likely to be noticed for 2 to 4 weeks and that it may take as long as 12 weeks.
• Instruct patient to avoid consuming grapefruit juice during drug therapy.
• Inform patient that CV risk is unknown in patients who use drug on a long-term basis and in those with have severe underlying heart disease.
• Tell patient that drug may cause dizziness. Caution patient not to drive or perform other activities that require alertness until response to drug is known.

## clopidogrel bisulfate
Plavix

*Pregnancy Risk Category B*

### HOW SUPPLIED
*Tablets*: 75 mg

### ACTION
Inhibits platelet aggregation by inhibiting the binding of adenosine diphosphate (ADP) to its platelet receptor inhibiting ADP-mediated activation and subsequent platelet aggregation. Because clopidogrel acts by irreversibly modifying the platelet ADP receptor, platelets exposed to the drug are affected for their life span.

| Route | Onset | Peak | Duration |
|-------|-------|------|----------|
| P.O. | 2 hr | Unknown | 5 days |

### INDICATIONS & DOSAGE
*To reduce atherosclerotic events in patients with atherosclerosis documented by recent CVA, MI, or peripheral arterial disease—*
**Adults:** 75 mg P.O. daily.

### ADVERSE REACTIONS
**CNS:** headache, dizziness, fatigue, depression.
**CV:** edema, hypertension.
**EENT:** rhinitis, epistaxis.
**GI:** *hemorrhage,* abdominal pain, dyspepsia, gastritis, constipation, diarrhea, ulcers.

**GU:** urinary tract infection.
**Hematologic:** purpura.
**Musculoskeletal:** arthralgia.
**Respiratory:** bronchitis, coughing, dyspnea, upper respiratory tract infection.
**Skin:** *rash,* pruritus.
**Other:** flulike syndrome, pain.

### INTERACTIONS
**Drug-drug.** *Aspirin, NSAIDs:* may increase risk of GI bleeding. Use cautiously.
*Heparin, warfarin:* safety hasn't been established. Use together cautiously.
**Drug-herb.** *Red clover:* possible increased risk of bleeding. Use together cautiously.

### EFFECTS ON DIAGNOSTIC TESTS
None reported.

### CONTRAINDICATIONS
Contraindicated in patients with hypersensitivity to drug or its components and in those with pathologic bleeding (such as peptic ulcer or intracranial hemorrhage).

### NURSING CONSIDERATIONS
• Use with caution in patients at risk for increased bleeding from trauma, surgery, or other pathologic conditions and in those with hepatic impairment.
• Platelet aggregation won't return to normal for at least 5 days after drug has been discontinued.
• Drug is usually used in patients hypersensitive or intolerant to aspirin or after stent placement.

### ☑ Patient teaching
• Inform patient it may take longer than usual to stop bleeding. Tell him to refrain from activities in which trauma and bleeding may occur and encourage him to wear a seat belt when in a car.
• Instruct patient to notify doctor if unusual bleeding or bruising occurs.
• Tell patient to inform doctor or dentist that he is taking drug before having surgery or starting new drug therapy.
• Inform patient that drug may be taken without regard to meals.

---

## dipyridamole
Apo-Dipyridamole FC†,
Persantine IV, Novo-Dipiradol†,
Persantin‡, Persantine**

*Pregnancy Risk Category B*

### HOW SUPPLIED
*Tablets:* 25 mg, 50 mg, 75 mg
*Injection:* 10 mg/2 ml

### ACTION
Unknown. Possibly involves drug's ability to increase adenosine, which is a coronary vasodilator and platelet aggregation inhibitor.

| Route | Onset | Peak | Duration |
|-------|-------|------|----------|
| P.O. | Unknown | 75 min | Unknown |
| I.V. | Unknown | 2 min | Unknown |

### INDICATIONS & DOSAGE
*Inhibition of platelet adhesion in prosthetic heart valves (with warfarin or aspirin)—*
**Adults:** 75 to 100 mg P.O. q.i.d.
*Alternative to exercise in evaluation of coronary artery disease during thallium myocardial perfusion scintigraphy—*
**Adults:** 0.57 mg/kg as an I.V. infusion at a constant rate over 4 minutes (0.142 mg/kg/minute).

### ADVERSE REACTIONS
**CNS:** *headache, dizziness,* syncope.
**CV:** flushing, hypotension; angina, chest pain, *ECG abnormalities,* blood pressure lability, hypertension.
**GI:** *nausea,* vomiting, diarrhea, abdominal distress.
**Skin:** rash, irritation, pruritus.

### INTERACTIONS
**Drug-drug.** *Heparin:* may increase risk of bleeding. Monitor closely.
*Theophylline:* may prevent the coronary vasodilation by I.V. dipyridamole; could lead to a false-negative thallium-imaging result. Avoid concomitant use.

### EFFECTS ON DIAGNOSTIC TESTS
None reported.

### CONTRAINDICATIONS
Contraindicated in patients with hypersensitivity to drug.

### NURSING CONSIDERATIONS
• Use cautiously in patients with hypotension.
• If patient develops GI distress, administer drug 1 hour before meals or with meals.
• Observe for adverse reactions, especially with large doses. Monitor blood pressure.
• Observe for signs and symptoms of bleeding; note prolonged bleeding time (especially with large doses or long-term therapy).
• Dipyridamole's value as part of an antithrombotic regimen is controversial; its use may not provide significantly better results than aspirin alone.
• *Alert:* Don't confuse dipyridamole with disopyramide or Persantine with Periactin.

### ⬛ I.V. administration
• If administering as a diagnostic agent, dilute in half-normal or normal saline or $D_5W$ in at least a 1:2 ratio for a total volume of 20 to 50 ml. Inject [201]Tl within 5 minutes after completing the 4-minute dipyridamole infusion.

### ☑ Patient teaching
• Instruct patient to take drug exactly as prescribed.
• Tell patient to report adverse reactions promptly.
• Tell patient receiving drug I.V. to alert nurse if discomfort occurs at insertion site.

## eptifibatide
Integrilin

*Pregnancy Risk Category B*

### HOW SUPPLIED
*Injection:* 10-ml (2 mg/ml), 100-ml (0.75 mg/ml) vials

---

Reactions may be *common*, uncommon, *life-threatening*, or COMMON AND LIFE-THREATENING.

## ACTION
Reversibly binds to the glycoprotein IIb/IIIa (GP IIb/IIIa) receptor on human platelets and inhibits platelet aggregation.

| Route | Onset | Peak | Duration |
|-------|-------|------|----------|
| I.V. | Immediate | Immediate | 4-6 hr after end of infusion |

## INDICATIONS & DOSAGE
*Patients with acute coronary syndrome (unstable angina or non-Q-wave MI), including patients who are to be managed medically and those undergoing percutaneous coronary intervention—*
**Adults:** I.V. bolus of 180 mcg/kg (maximum dose of 22.6 mg) as soon as possible following diagnosis; then a continuous I.V. infusion of 2 mcg/kg/minute (maximum infusion rate of 15 mg/hour) for up to 72 hours. Infusion rate may be decreased to 0.5 mcg/kg/minute during percutaneous coronary intervention. Infusion should then be continued for an additional 20 to 24 hours after procedure for up to 96 hours.
*Patients not presenting with an acute coronary syndrome who are undergoing percutaneous coronary intervention—*
**Adults:** I.V. bolus of 135 mcg/kg administered immediately before procedure; then continuous infusion of 0.5 mcg/kg/minute for 20 to 24 hours.

## ADVERSE REACTIONS
**CV:** hypotension.
**GU:** hematuria.
**Hematologic:** *bleeding, **thrombocytopenia.***
**Other:** bleeding at femoral artery access site.

## INTERACTIONS
**Drug-drug.** *Clopidogrel, dipyridamole, NSAIDs, oral anticoagulants (warfarin), thrombolytics, ticlopidine:* increased risk of bleeding. Monitor patient closely.
*Other inhibitors of platelet receptor IIb/IIIa:* potential for serious bleeding. Don't administer together.

## EFFECTS ON DIAGNOSTIC TESTS
None reported.

## CONTRAINDICATIONS
Contraindicated in patients with known hypersensitivity to drug or its ingredients and in those with history of bleeding diathesis or evidence of active abnormal bleeding within previous 30 days, severe hypertension (systolic blood pressure over 200 mm Hg or diastolic blood pressure over 110 mm Hg) not adequately controlled with antihypertensives, major surgery within previous 6 weeks, history of stroke within 30 days or history of hemorrhagic stroke, current or planned use of another parenteral GP IIb/IIIa inhibitor, or platelet count below 100,000/mm[3]; also contraindicated in patients whose serum creatinine is 2 mg/dl or higher (for the 180 mcg/kg bolus and 2 mcg/kg/minute infusion) or 4 mg/dl or higher (for the 135 mcg/kg bolus and 0.5 mcg/kg/minute infusion) and in patients who are dependent on renal dialysis.

## NURSING CONSIDERATIONS
• Use cautiously in patients at increased risk for bleeding and in patients over 315 lb (143 kg).
• Drug is intended for use with heparin and aspirin.
• Discontinue eptifibatide and heparin and achieve sheath hemostasis by standard compressive techniques at least 4 hours before hospital discharge.
• If patient is to undergo coronary artery bypass graft surgery, infusion should be stopped before surgery.
• Minimize use of arterial and venous punctures, I.M. injections, urinary catheters, and nasotracheal and nasogastric tubes.
• When obtaining I.V. access, avoid use of noncompressible sites (such as subclavian or jugular veins).
• Monitor patient for bleeding.
• If patient's platelet count is below 100,000/mm[3], discontinue eptifibatide and heparin.
• Perform baseline laboratory tests before start of drug therapy; also determine hematocrit, PT, INR, APTT, platelet count, and hemoglobin and serum creatinine levels.

• Store vials in refrigerator at 36° to 46° F (2° to 8° C). Protect from light until administration.

### ▮ I.V. administration
• Withdraw bolus dose from 10-ml vial into a syringe and administer by I.V. push over 1 to 2 minutes. Administer I.V. infusion undiluted directly from 100-ml vial using an infusion pump.
• Inspect solution for particulate matter before use. If particles are visible, the sterility is suspect; discard solution.
• Drug may be administered in same I.V. line as alteplase, atropine, dobutamine, heparin, lidocaine, meperidine, metoprolol, midazolam, morphine, nitroglycerin, or verapamil.
• Don't administer drug in same I.V. line as furosemide.
• Drug may be administered in same I.V. line with normal saline or normal saline and 5% dextrose; main infusion may also contain up to 60 mEq/L of potassium chloride.

### ☑ Patient teaching
• Explain that drug is a blood thinner used to prevent chest pain and heart attack.
• Explain that the risk of serious bleeding is far outweighed by the benefits of drug.
• Instruct patient to report chest discomfort or other adverse events immediately.

---

## midodrine hydrochloride
ProAmatine

*Pregnancy Risk Category C*

### HOW SUPPLIED
*Tablets:* 2.5 mg, 5 mg

### ACTION
Forms an active metabolite, desglymidodrine, which is an alpha$_1$-agonist. It increases blood pressure by activating alpha-adrenergic receptors in arteriolar and venous vasculature.

| Route | Onset | Peak | Duration |
|-------|-------|------|----------|
| P.O. | Unknown | 1-2 hr | Unknown |

### INDICATIONS & DOSAGE
*Symptomatic orthostatic hypotension unresponsive to standard clinical care—*
**Adults:** 10 mg P.O. t.i.d. Suggested dosing schedule: Dose 1 shortly before or upon arising in the morning; dose 2 at midday; and dose 3 in late afternoon but no later than 6 p.m.
*Adjust-a-dose:* For patients with abnormal renal function, initial dose of 2.5 mg is recommended.

### ADVERSE REACTIONS
**CNS:** *paresthesia,* headache, confusion, anxiety.
**CV:** ***supine hypertension, vasodilation.***
**GI:** dry mouth.
**GU:** urine retention, frequency, and urgency; *dysuria.*
**Skin:** *piloerection, pruritus,* rash.
**Other:** pain, chills.

### INTERACTIONS
**Drug-drug.** *Alpha-adrenergic agonists:* enhanced vasopressor effects. Monitor blood pressure closely.
*Alpha blockers:* may antagonize drug effects. Avoid concomitant use.
*Beta blockers, cardiac glycosides, psychopharmacologic agents:* may enhance or cause bradycardia, AV block, or arrhythmias. Avoid concomitant use.
*Fludrocortisone:* may increase risk of supine hypertension. May also lead to increased intraocular pressure and worsened glaucoma. Monitor closely.

### EFFECTS ON DIAGNOSTIC TESTS
None reported.

### CONTRAINDICATIONS
Contraindicated in patients with severe organic heart disease, persistent and excessive supine hypertension, acute renal disease, urine retention, pheochromocytoma, or thyrotoxicosis.

### NURSING CONSIDERATIONS
• Use cautiously in patients with history of urine retention, visual problems, diabetes, or renal or hepatic impairment and in breast-feeding women.

---

Reactions may be *common*, uncommon, ***life-threatening***, or COMMON AND LIFE-THREATENING.

• Drug should be used in pregnancy only if benefit justifies potential risk to the fetus.

• Safety and effectiveness of drug in children haven't been established.

• Monitor supine and sitting blood pressures closely, and notify doctor if supine blood pressure increases excessively.

• Drug should be taken during the day when patient can be upright and performing activities of daily living. Space doses at least 3 hours apart. Midodrine shouldn't be given after the evening meal or within 4 hours of bedtime, to reduce potential for supine hypertension during sleep.

• Drug should be continued only if patient experiences symptomatic improvement during initial therapy.

• Perform renal and hepatic tests before and during drug therapy as ordered.

• *Alert:* Don't confuse ProAmatine with protamine.

☑ **Patient teaching**

• Instruct patient about proper dosing intervals; tell him to take last dose of the day 4 hours before bedtime.

• Tell patient to report symptoms of supine hypertension (cardiac awareness, pounding in ears, headache, blurred vision) immediately to doctor and to stop drug.

• Tell patient to consult doctor before taking OTC drugs.

## pentoxifylline
Trental

*Pregnancy Risk Category C*

### HOW SUPPLIED
*Tablets (extended-release):* 400 mg

### ACTION
Unknown. Improves capillary blood flow, probably by increasing RBC flexibility and lowering blood viscosity.

| Route | Onset | Peak | Duration |
|-------|-------|------|----------|
| P.O. | Unknown | 1 hr | Unknown |

### INDICATIONS & DOSAGE
*Intermittent claudication due to chronic occlusive vascular disease—*
**Adults:** 400 mg P.O. t.i.d. with meals. May decrease to 400 mg b.i.d. if GI and CNS adverse effects occur.

### ADVERSE REACTIONS
**CNS:** headache, dizziness.
**GI:** dyspepsia, nausea, vomiting.

### INTERACTIONS
**Drug-drug.** *Anticoagulants:* increased anticoagulant effect. Adjust anticoagulant dosage as ordered.
*Antihypertensives:* increased hypotensive effect. Dosage adjustments may be needed.
*Theophylline:* may cause increase of theophylline level. Monitor closely.
**Drug-lifestyle.** *Smoking:* vasoconstriction may result. Advise patient to avoid smoking; it may worsen his condition.

### EFFECTS ON DIAGNOSTIC TESTS
None reported.

### CONTRAINDICATIONS
Contraindicated in patients intolerant to methylxanthines, such as caffeine, theophylline, and theobromine, and in those with recent cerebral or retinal hemorrhage.

### NURSING CONSIDERATIONS
• Drug is useful in patients who aren't good surgical candidates.

• Elderly patients may be more sensitive to drug's effects.

• *Alert:* Don't confuse Trental with Trendar or Trandate.

☑ **Patient teaching**

• Advise patient to take with meals to minimize GI upset.

• Instruct patient to swallow tablet whole, without breaking, crushing, or chewing.

• Tell patient to report GI or CNS adverse reactions; doctor may reduce dosage.

• Inform patient not to discontinue drug during the first 8 weeks of therapy unless directed by doctor.

---

*Liquid contains alcohol.  **May contain tartrazine.  †Canada  ‡Australia  §U.K.  ◊ OTC

## ticlopidine hydrochloride
Ticlid

*Pregnancy Risk Category B*

### HOW SUPPLIED
*Tablets:* 250 mg

### ACTION
Unknown. An antiplatelet that probably blocks adenosine diphosphate–induced platelet-to-fibrinogen and platelet-to-platelet binding.

| Route | Onset | Peak | Duration |
|-------|-------|------|----------|
| P.O. | Unknown | 2 hr | Unknown |

### INDICATIONS & DOSAGE
*To reduce risk of thrombotic stroke in patients with history of stroke or who have experienced stroke precursors—*
**Adults:** 250 mg P.O. b.i.d. with meals.

### ADVERSE REACTIONS
**CNS:** dizziness, peripheral neuropathy.
**CV:** vasculitis.
**EENT:** conjunctival hemorrhage.
**GI:** *diarrhea,* nausea, dyspepsia, abdominal pain, anorexia, vomiting, flatulence, bleeding.
**GU:** hematuria, dark-colored urine.
**Hematologic:** *neutropenia, pancytopenia, agranulocytosis, immune thrombocytopenia.*
**Hepatic:** abnormal liver function tests.
**Musculoskeletal:** arthropathy, myositis.
**Respiratory:** *allergic pneumonitis.*
**Skin:** rash, pruritus, ecchymoses, maculopapular rash, urticaria, *thrombocytopenic purpura.*
**Other:** hypersensitivity reactions, postoperative bleeding.

### INTERACTIONS
**Drug-drug.** *Antacids:* decreased plasma ticlopidine levels. Separate administration times by at least 2 hours.
*Aspirin:* effects of aspirin on platelets potentiated. Avoid concomitant use.
*Cimetidine:* decreased clearance of ticlopidine and increased risk of toxicity. Avoid concomitant use.

*Digoxin:* slight decrease in serum digoxin levels. Monitor serum digoxin levels.
*Phenytoin:* possible elevation in serum phenytoin level. Monitor closely.
*Theophylline:* decreased theophylline clearance and risk of toxicity. Monitor closely and adjust theophylline dosage as ordered.
**Drug-herb.** *Red clover:* possible increased risk of bleeding. Use together cautiously.

### EFFECTS ON DIAGNOSTIC TESTS
A positive antinuclear antibody titer has been reported rarely.

### CONTRAINDICATIONS
Contraindicated in patients with hypersensitivity to drug and in those with severe hepatic impairment, hematopoietic disorders, active pathologic bleeding from peptic ulceration, or active intracranial bleeding.

### NURSING CONSIDERATIONS
• Use cautiously and with close monitoring of CBC and WBC differentials. Moderate to severe neutropenia and agranulocytosis have occurred in patients taking ticlopidine.
• Because of life-threatening adverse reactions, use drug only in patients who are allergic to, can't tolerate, or have failed aspirin therapy.
• Monitor baseline liver function tests before therapy.
• Determine CBC and WBC differentials at second week of therapy and repeat every 2 weeks until end of third month, as ordered.
• Monitor liver function tests and repeat if dysfunction is suspected.
• Thrombocytopenia has occurred rarely. Discontinue drug in patients with platelet count of 80,000/mm³ or less. If needed, give methylprednisolone 20 mg I.V. to normalize bleeding time within 2 hours, as ordered.
• When used preoperatively, drug may decrease incidence of graft occlusion in patients receiving coronary artery bypass grafts and reduce severity of drop in platelet count in patients receiving extra-

---

Reactions may be *common*, uncommon, *life-threatening*, or COMMON AND LIFE-THREATENING.

corporeal hemoperfusion during open heart surgery.

### ✅ Patient teaching
• Tell patient to take drug with meals.
• Warn patient to avoid aspirin and aspirin-containing products and to check with doctor or pharmacist before taking OTC drugs.
• Explain that drug will prolong bleeding time and that unusual or prolonged bleeding should be reported. Advise patient to tell dentists and other doctors that he is taking ticlopidine.
• Stress importance of regular blood tests. Because neutropenia can result from increased risk of infection, tell patient to immediately report signs and symptoms of infection, such as fever, chills, or sore throat.
• If drug is being substituted for a fibrinolytic or anticoagulant, tell patient to discontinue those drugs before starting ticlopidine therapy, as ordered.
• Advise patient to discontinue drug 10 to 14 days before undergoing elective surgery, as ordered. Also tell patient to immediately report yellow skin or sclera, severe or persistent diarrhea, rashes, S.C. bleeding, light-colored stools, or dark urine.

---

## tirofiban hydrochloride
Aggrastat

*Pregnancy Risk Category B*

### HOW SUPPLIED
*Injection:* 50-ml vials (250 mcg/ml), 500-ml premixed vials (50 mcg/ml)

### ACTION
Reversibly binds to the glycoprotein IIb/IIIa (GP IIb/IIIa) receptor on human platelets and inhibits platelet aggregation.

| Route | Onset | Peak | Duration |
|-------|-------|------|----------|
| I.V. | Immediate | Immediate | 4-6 hr after end of infusion |

### INDICATIONS & DOSAGE
*Acute coronary syndrome, with heparin and/or aspirin, including patients who are* to be managed medically and those undergoing percutaneous transluminal coronary angioplasty (PTCA) or atherectomy—
**Adults:** I.V. loading dose of 0.4 mcg/kg/minute for 30 minutes; then continuous I.V. infusion of 0.1 mcg/kg/minute. Continue infusion through angiography and for 12 to 24 hours after angioplasty or atherectomy.
*Adjust-a-dose:* For patients with renal insufficiency (creatinine clearance below 30 ml/minute), use a loading dose of 0.2 mcg/kg/minute for 30 minutes; then continuous infusion of 0.05 mcg/kg/minute. Continue infusion through angiography and for 12 to 24 hours after angioplasty or atherectomy.

### ADVERSE REACTIONS
**CNS:** dizziness, headache.
**CV:** *bradycardia, coronary artery dissection,* edema.
**GI:** nausea, *occult bleeding.*
**Hematologic:** *bleeding, thrombocytopenia,* decreased hemoglobin level and hematocrit.
**Musculoskeletal:** leg pain.
**Skin:** sweating.
**Other:** fever, bleeding at arterial access site, pelvic pain, vasovagal reaction.

### INTERACTIONS
**Drug-drug.** *Clopidogrel, dipyridamole, NSAIDs, oral anticoagulants such as warfarin, thrombolytics, ticlopidine:* increased risk of bleeding. Monitor patient closely.
*Levothyroxine, omeprazole:* increased renal clearance of tirofiban. Monitor patient.

### EFFECTS ON DIAGNOSTIC TESTS
None reported.

### CONTRAINDICATIONS
Contraindicated in patients with known hypersensitivity to drug or its ingredients and in those with active internal bleeding or history of bleeding diathesis within the previous 30 days and in those with history of intracranial hemorrhage, intracranial neoplasm, arteriovenous malformation, aneurysm, thrombocytopenia following

---

*Liquid contains alcohol.    **May contain tartrazine.    †Canada    ‡Australia    §U.K.    ◊OTC

prior exposure to tirofiban, stroke within 30 days, or hemorrhagic stroke

Drug is also contraindicated in those with history, symptoms, or findings suggestive of aortic dissection; severe hypertension (systolic blood pressure over 180 mm Hg or diastolic blood pressure over 110 mm Hg); acute pericarditis; major surgical procedure or severe physical trauma within previous month; or concomitant use of another parenteral GP IIb/IIIa inhibitor.

## NURSING CONSIDERATIONS
• Use cautiously in patients with increased risk of bleeding, including those with hemorrhagic retinopathy or platelet count below 150,000/mm$^3$.
• Monitor hemoglobin level and hematocrit and platelet counts before starting therapy, 6 hours following loading dose, and at least daily during therapy.
• Monitor patient for bleeding.
• Minimize injection and avoid noncompatible I.V. sites.
• Administer drug with concomitant aspirin and heparin.
• Safety and effectiveness of drug haven't been studied in patients under age 18.
• Notify doctor if thrombocytopenia occurs.
• The most common adverse effect is bleeding at the arterial access site for cardiac catheterization.
• Store drug at room temperature. Protect from light.

## I.V. administration
• Dilute 50-ml injection vials (250 mcg/ml) to same strength as 500-ml premixed vials (50 mcg/ml) as follows: withdraw and discard 100 ml from a 500-ml bag of sterile normal saline or $D_5W$ and replace this volume with 100 ml of tirofiban injection (from two 50-ml vials) or withdraw 50 ml from a 250-ml bag of sterile normal saline or $D_5W$ and replace this volume with 50 ml of tirofiban injection, to achieve a concentration of 50 mcg/ml.
• Inspect solution for particulate matter before administration, and check for leaks by squeezing the inner bag firmly. If particles are visible or if leaks occur, discard solution.

• Discard unused solution 24 hours following the start of infusion.
• Heparin and tirofiban can be administered through same I.V. catheter.

## Patient teaching
• Explain that drug is a blood thinner that is used to prevent chest pain and heart attack.
• Explain that risk of serious bleeding is far outweighed by the benefits of drug.
• Instruct patient to report chest discomfort or other adverse events immediately.
• Inform patient that frequent blood sampling may be needed to evaluate therapy.

---

Reactions may be *common*, uncommon, *life-threatening*, or COMMON AND LIFE-THREATENING.

**acetaminophen**
**aspirin**
**choline magnesium trisalicylate**
**diflunisal**
**magnesium salicylate**

## COMBINATION PRODUCTS

ALLEREST NO-DROWSINESS ◊, COLDRINE ◊, ORNEX NO DROWSINESS CAPLETS ◊, SINUS-RELIEF, SINUTAB NO DROWSINESS ◊: acetaminophen 325 mg and pseudoephedrine hydrochloride 30 mg.

AMAPHEN, ANOQUAN, BUTACE, ENDOLOR, ESGIC, FEMCET, FIORICET, ISOPAP, MEDIGESIC, REPAN, TENCET, TRIAD, TWO-DYNE: acetaminophen 325 mg, caffeine 40 mg, and butalbital 50 mg.

ASCRIPTIN, MAGNAPRIN: aspirin 325 mg, magnesium hydroxide 50 mg, aluminum hydroxide 50 mg, and calcium carbonate 50 mg ◊.

ASCRIPTIN A/D, MAGNAPRIN ARTHRITIS STRENGTH: aspirin 325 mg, magnesium hydroxide 75 mg, aluminum hydroxide 75 mg, and calcium carbonate 75 mg ◊.

BUFFERIN AF NITE TIME ◊, EXCEDRIN P.M. ◊: acetaminophen 500 mg and diphenhydramine citrate 38 mg.

CAMA ARTHRITIS PAIN RELIEVER: aspirin 500 mg, magnesium oxide 150 mg, and aluminum hydroxide 150 mg.

DOAN'S P.M. EXTRA STRENGTH ◊: magnesium salicylate 500 mg and diphenhydramine 25 mg.

EXCEDRIN EXTRA STRENGTH ◊: aspirin 250 mg, acetaminophen 250 mg, and caffeine 65 mg.

EXCEDRIN MIGRAINE: acetaminophen 250 mg, aspirin 250 mg, and caffeine 65 mg.

FIORGEN, FIORINAL, ISOLLYL, LANORINAL, MARNAL: aspirin 325 mg, caffeine 40 mg, and butalbital 50 mg.

MIDRIN: isometheptene mucate 65 mg, dichloralphenazone 100 mg, and acetaminophen 325 mg.

P-A-C ANALGESIC ◊: aspirin 400 mg and caffeine 32 mg.

PHRENILIN: acetaminophen 325 mg and butalbital 50 mg.

PHRENILIN FORTE: acetaminophen 650 mg and butalbital 50 mg.

SINUS EXCEDRIN EXTRA STRENGTH ◊: acetaminophen 500 mg and pseudoephedrine hydrochloride 30 mg.

SINUTAB ◊: acetaminophen 325 mg, chlorpheniramine 2 mg, and pseudoephedrine hydrochloride 30 mg.

SINUTAB MAXIMUM STRENGTH WITHOUT DROWSINESS ◊: acetaminophen 500 mg, pseudoephedrine hydrochloride 30 mg.

TECNAL†: aspirin 330 mg, caffeine 40 mg, and butalbital 50 mg.

VANQUISH ◊: aspirin 227 mg, acetaminophen 194 mg, caffeine 33 mg, aluminum hydroxide 25 mg, and magnesium hydroxide 50 mg.

---

## acetaminophen (APAP, paracetamol)

Abenol† ◊; Aceta Elixir* ◊; Acetaminophen Uniserts ◊; Aceta Tablets ◊; Actamin ◊; Actamin Extra† ◊; Actimol† ◊; Aminofen ◊; Aminofen Max ◊; Anacin-3 ◊; Anacin-3 Extra Strength ◊; Apacet Capsules ◊; Apacet Elixir* ◊; Apacet Extra Strength Caplets ◊; Apacet Extra Strength Tablets ◊; Apacet, Infants' ◊; Apacet Regular Strength Tablets ◊; Apo-Acetaminophen† ◊; Arthritis Pain Formula Aspirin Free ◊; Atasol Caplets† ◊; Atasol Drops† ◊; Atasol Forte Caplets† ◊; Atasol Forte Tablets† ◊; Atasol Tablets† ◊; Banesin ◊; Dapa ◊; Dapa X-S ◊; Datril Extra-Strength; Dymadon‡ ◊; Dymadon P‡ ◊; Exdol† ◊; Exdol Strong† ◊; Feverall, Children's; Feverall Junior Strength; Feverall Sprinkle Caps, Children's; Feverall Sprinkle Caps Junior Strength; Genapap Children's Elixir ◊; Genapap Children's Tablets ◊; Genapap Extra Strength Caplets ◊;

---

Genapap Extra Strength Tablets ◇;
Genapap, Infants' ◇; Genapap
Regular Strength Tablets ◇;
Genebs Extra Strength Caplets ◇;
Genebs Regular Strength
Tablets ◇; Genebs X-Tra ◇;
Halenol Children's* ◇; Liquiprin
Infants' Drops ◇; Mapap,
Children's* ◇; Mapap Infant
Drops ◇; Meda Cap ◇; Neopap ◇;
Oraphen-PD ◇; Panadol ◇;
Panadol, Children's ◇; Panadol
Extra Strength ◇; Panadol,
Infants' ◇; Panadol Junior Strength
Caplets ◇; Panadol Maximum
Strength Caplets ◇; Panadol
Maximum Strength Tablets ◇;
Panamax‡ ◇; Paralgin‡ ◇;
Redutemp ◇; Robigesic† ◇;
Rounox† ◇; Snaplets-FR ◇; St.
Joseph Aspirin-Free Fever Reducer
for Children ◇; Suppap-120 ◇;
Suppap-325 ◇; Suppap-650 ◇;
Tapanol Extra Strength Caplets ◇;
Tapanol Extra Strength Tablets ◇;
Tempra ◇; Tempra Caplets ◇;
Tempra Chewable Tablets ◇;
Tempra Drops ◇; Tempra D.S. ◇;
Tempra, Infants' ◇; Tempra
Syrup ◇; Tylenol Caplets ◇; Tylenol
Children's Chewable Tablets ◇;
Tylenol Children's Elixir ◇; Tylenol
Children's Tablets ◇; Tylenol
Drops ◇; Tylenol Elixir* ◇; Tylenol
Extended Relief ◇; Tylenol Extra
Strength Adult Liquid Pain
Reliever ◇; Tylenol Extra Strength
Caplets ◇; Tylenol Extra Strength
Gelcaps ◇; Tylenol Extra Strength
Tablets ◇; Tylenol, Infants' Drops;
Tylenol Infants' Suspension
Drops ◇; Tylenol Junior Strength
Caplets ◇; Tylenol Junior Strength
Tablets ◇; Tylenol Regular Strength
Caplets ◇; Tylenol Regular
Strength Tablets ◇; Tylenol
Tablets ◇; Valorin ◇; Valorin Extra ◇

*Pregnancy Risk Category B*

## HOW SUPPLIED
*Tablets:* 160 mg ◇, 325 mg ◇, 500 mg ◇,
650 mg ◇
*Tablets (chewable):* 80 mg ◇

*Caplets:* 160 mg, 500 mg ◇
*Caplets (extended-release):* 650 mg
*Capsules:* 500 mg ◇, 325 mg ◇
*Gelcaps:* 500 mg ◇
*Oral liquid:* 160 mg/5 ml ◇, 500 mg/
15 ml ◇
*Oral solution:* 48 mg/ml ◇, 100 mg/ml ◇
*Oral suspension:* 80 mg/ml, 120 mg/
5 ml‡, 160 mg/5 ml ◇
*Oral syrup:* 16 mg/ml ◇
*Elixir:* 80 mg/5 ml, 120 mg/5 ml,
160 mg/5 ml* ◇, 325 mg/5 ml* ◇
*Sprinkles:* 80 mg/capsule, 160 mg/capsule
*Suppositories:* 80 mg ◇, 120 mg ◇, 125
mg ◇, 300 mg ◇, 325 mg ◇, 650 mg ◇

## ACTION
Unknown. Thought to produce analgesia
by blocking generation of pain impulses,
probably by inhibiting prostaglandin synthesis in the CNS or the synthesis or action of other substances that sensitize pain
receptors to mechanical or chemical stimulation. It is thought to relieve fever by
central action in the hypothalamic heat-
regulating center.

| Route | Onset | Peak | Duration |
|-------|-------|------|----------|
| P.O., P.R. | Unknown | 1-3 hr | 3-4 hr |

## INDICATIONS & DOSAGE
*Mild pain or fever—*
**Adults:** 325 to 650 mg P.O. q 4 to 6
hours; or 1 g P.O. t.i.d. or q.i.d., p.r.n. Or,
two extended-release caplets P.O. q 8
hours. Or, 650 mg P.R. q 4 to 6 hours,
p.r.n. Maximum dose shouldn't exceed
4 g daily. Dose for long-term therapy
shouldn't exceed 2.6 g daily.
*P.O.—*
**Children over age 14:** 650 mg P.O. q 4 to
6 hours.
**Children ages 12 to 14:** 640 mg P.O. q 4
to 6 hours.
**Children age 11:** 480 mg P.O. q 4 to 6
hours.
**Children ages 9 to 10:** 400 mg P.O. q 4 to
6 hours.
**Children ages 6 to 8:** 320 mg P.O. q 4 to
6 hours.
**Children ages 4 to 5:** 240 mg P.O. q 4 to
6 hours.
**Children ages 2 to 3:** 160 mg P.O. q 4 to
6 hours.

Reactions may be *common*, uncommon, **life-threatening**, or COMMON AND LIFE-THREATENING.

**Children ages 12 to 23 months:** 120 mg P.O. q 4 to 6 hours.
**Children ages 4 to 11 months:** 80 mg P.O. q 4 to 6 hours.
**Children up to age 3 months:** 40 mg P.O. q 4 to 6 hours.
*P.R.—*
**Children ages 6 to 12:** 325 mg P.R. q 4 to 6 hours.
**Children ages 3 to 6:** 120 to 125 mg P.R. q 4 to 6 hours.
**Children ages 1 to 3:** 80 mg P.R. q 4 to 6 hours.
**Children ages 3 to 11 months:** 80 mg P.R. q 6 hours.

## ADVERSE REACTIONS
**Hematologic:** hemolytic anemia, *neutropenia, leukopenia, pancytopenia.*
**Hepatic:** *severe liver damage,* jaundice.
**Metabolic:** hypoglycemia.
**Skin:** rash, urticaria.

## INTERACTIONS
**Drug-drug.** *Barbiturates, carbamazepine, hydantoins, rifampin, sulfinpyrazone:* high doses or long-term use of these drugs may reduce therapeutic effects and enhance hepatotoxic effects of acetaminophen. Avoid concomitant use.
*Warfarin:* may increase hypoprothrombinemic effects with long-term use with high doses of acetaminophen. Monitor INR closely.
*Zidovudine:* may increase incidence of bone marrow suppression because of impaired zidovudine metabolism. Monitor patient closely.
**Drug-herb.** *Watercress:* may inhibit oxidative metabolism of acetaminophen. Avoid concomitant use.
**Drug-food.** *Caffeine:* may enhance analgesic effects of acetaminophen. Avoid concomitant use.
**Drug-lifestyle.** *Alcohol use:* increased risk of hepatic damage. Avoid concomitant use.

## EFFECTS ON DIAGNOSTIC TESTS
Drug may cause a false-positive test result for urinary 5-hydroxyindoleacetic acid or interfere with home glucose testing.

## CONTRAINDICATIONS
Contraindicated in patients with hypersensitivity to drug.

## NURSING CONSIDERATIONS
• Use cautiously in patients with history of chronic alcohol use because hepatotoxicity has occurred after therapeutic doses.
• Many OTC products contain acetaminophen; be aware of this when calculating total daily dose.
• Use liquid form for children and patients who have difficulty swallowing.
• Acetaminophen may produce false-positive decreases in blood glucose levels in home monitoring systems.

☑ **Patient teaching**
• Tell parents to consult doctor before giving drug to children under age 2.
• Tell patient that drug is only for short-term use and to consult doctor if administering to children for more than 5 days or adults for more than 10 days.
• Tell patient not to use for self-medication of marked fever (over 103.1° F [39.5° C]), fever persisting longer than 3 days, or recurrent fever unless directed by doctor.
• *Alert:* Warn patient that high doses or unsupervised long-term use can cause hepatic damage. Excessive ingestion of alcohol may increase the risk of hepatotoxicity.
• Tell breast-feeding woman that acetaminophen appears in breast milk in low levels (less than 1% of dose). Drug may be used safely if therapy is short-term and doesn't exceed recommended doses.

---

**aspirin (acetylsalicylic acid)**
Artria S.R. ◇ , ASA ◇ , Aspergum ◇ , Aspro‡ , Bayer Aspirin ◇ , Bex‡ , Coryphen† ◇ , Easprin ◇ , Ecotrin ◇ , Empirin ◇ , Entrophen† ◇ , Halfprin , Norwich Extra Strength ◇ , Novasen† ◇ , Solprin‡ , Vincent's Powders‡ , ZORprin ◇

*Pregnancy Risk Category C (D in third trimester)*

## HOW SUPPLIED
*Tablets:* 325 mg ◇ , 500 mg ◇

---

*Tablets (chewable):* 81 mg ◇
*Tablets (enteric-coated):* 165 mg,
325 mg ◇, 500 mg ◇, 650 mg ◇, 975 mg
*Tablets (controlled-release):* 800 mg
*Tablets (timed-release):* 650 mg ◇
*Chewing gum:* 227.5 mg ◇
*Suppositories:* 120 mg ◇, 200 mg ◇,
300 mg ◇, 600 mg ◇

## ACTION
Produces analgesia by blocking prostaglandin synthesis (peripheral action). Aspirin and other salicylates may prevent the lowering of the pain threshold that occurs when prostaglandins sensitize pain receptors to mechanical and chemical stimulation. Exerts its anti-inflammatory effect by inhibiting prostaglandin synthesis; also may inhibit the synthesis or action of other mediators of the inflammatory response. Drug relieves fever by acting on the hypothalamic heat-regulating center to cause peripheral vasodilation, thus increasing peripheral blood supply and promoting sweating, which leads to heat loss and to cooling by evaporation. In low doses, aspirin also appears to impede clotting by blocking prostaglandin synthesis, which prevents formation of the platelet-aggregating substance thromboxane $A_2$.

| Route | Onset | Peak | Duration |
|---|---|---|---|
| P.O. (tablet) | 5-30 min | 25-40 min | 1-4 hr |
| P.O. (buffered) | 5-30 min | 1-2 hr | 1-4 hr |
| P.O. (extended) | 5-30 min | 1-4 hr | 1-4 hr |
| P.O. (enteric-coated) | 5-30 min | Variable | 1-4 hr |
| P.O. (solution) | 5-30 min | 15-40 min | 1-4 hr |
| P.R. | Unknown | 3-4 hr | Unknown |

## INDICATIONS & DOSAGE
*Rheumatoid arthritis, osteoarthritis, or other polyarthritic or inflammatory conditions—*
**Adults:** initially, 2.4 to 3.6 g P.O. daily in divided doses. Maintenance dosage is 3.2 to 6 g P.O. daily in divided doses.
*Juvenile rheumatoid arthritis—*
**Children:** 60 to 110 mg/kg/day P.O. divided q 6 to 8 hours.

*Mild pain or fever—*
**Adults and children over age 11:** 325 to 650 mg P.O. or P.R. q 4 hours, p.r.n.
**Children ages 2 to 11:** 10 to 15 mg/kg/dose P.O. or P.R. q 4 hours up to 80 mg/kg/day.
*Prevention of thrombosis—*
**Adults:** 1.3 g P.O. daily in two to four divided doses.
*Reduction of risk of heart attack in patients with previous MI or unstable angina—*
**Adults:** 160 to 325 mg P.O. daily.
*Kawasaki syndrome (mucocutaneous lymph node syndrome)—*
**Adults:** 80 to 180 mg/kg P.O. daily in four divided doses during febrile phase. When fever subsides, dose decreased to 10 mg/kg once daily, adjusted according to serum salicylate level.
*Acute rheumatic fever—*
**Adults:** 5 to 8 g P.O. daily.
**Children:** 100 mg/kg/day P.O. for 2 weeks; then 75 mg/kg/day P.O. for 4 to 6 weeks.

## ADVERSE REACTIONS
**EENT:** *tinnitus, hearing loss.*
**GI:** *nausea,* GI distress, occult bleeding, dyspepsia, ***GI bleeding.***
**Hematologic:** *leukopenia, thrombocytopenia, prolonged bleeding time.*
**Hepatic:** abnormal liver function tests, ***hepatitis.***
**Skin:** *rash,* bruising, urticaria.
**Other:** *angioedema, **hypersensitivity reactions (anaphylaxis, asthma), Reye's syndrome.***

## INTERACTIONS
**Drug-drug.** *ACE inhibitors:* may decrease antihypertensive effects. Monitor blood pressure closely.
*Ammonium chloride, other urine acidifiers:* increased blood levels of aspirin products. Monitor for aspirin toxicity.
*Antacids in high doses, other urine alkalinizers:* decreased levels of aspirin products. Monitor for decreased aspirin effect.
*Anticoagulants:* increased risk of bleeding. Avoid using together if possible.
*Beta blockers:* decreased antihypertensive effect. Avoid long-term aspirin use if patient is taking antihypertensives.

---

Reactions may be *common*, uncommon, ***life-threatening***, or COMMON AND LIFE-THREATENING.

*Corticosteroids:* enhanced salicylate elimination. Monitor for decreased salicylate effect.

*Methotrexate:* increased risk of methotrexate toxicity. Avoid concomitant use.

*Nizatidine:* may increase risk of salicylate toxicity in patients receiving high doses of aspirin. Monitor closely.

*NSAIDs, including diflunisal, fenoprofen, ibuprofen, indomethacin, meclofenamate, naproxen, piroxicam:* altered pharmacokinetics of these agents, leading to lowered serum levels and decreased effectiveness. Avoid concomitant use.

*NSAIDs, corticosteroids:* increased risk of GI bleeding. Avoid concomitant use.

*Oral antidiabetics:* increased hypoglycemic effect. Monitor closely.

*Probenecid, sulfinpyrazone:* decreased uricosuric effect. Avoid aspirin during therapy with these drugs.

*Valproic acid:* may increase serum valproic acid levels. Avoid concomitant use.

**Drug-herb.** *Horse chestnut, kelpware, red clover:* increased risk of bleeding. Monitor patient closely for increased effects.

**Drug-food.** *Caffeine:* may increase the absorption of aspirin. Monitor for increased effects.

**Drug-lifestyle.** *Alcohol use:* increased risk of GI bleeding. Avoid concomitant use.

## EFFECTS ON DIAGNOSTIC TESTS

Aspirin interferes with urinary glucose analysis performed with Diastix, Chemstrip uG, Clinitest, and Benedict's solution, and with urinary 5-hydroxyindoleacetic acid and vanillylmandelic acid tests. Aspirin may also interfere with the Gerhardt's test for urine acetoacetic acid.

## CONTRAINDICATIONS

Contraindicated in patients with hypersensitivity to drug and in those with NSAID-induced sensitivity reactions, G6PD deficiency, or bleeding disorders, such as hemophilia, von Willebrand's disease, or telangiectasia.

## NURSING CONSIDERATIONS

• Use cautiously in patients with GI lesions, impaired renal function, hypoprothrombinemia, vitamin K deficiency, thrombocytopenia, thrombotic thrombocytopenic purpura, or severe hepatic impairment.

• *Alert:* Because of epidemiologic association with Reye's syndrome, the Centers for Disease Control and Prevention recommends not giving salicylates to children or teenagers with chickenpox or flu-like illness.

• For inflammatory conditions, rheumatic fever, and thrombosis, aspirin is administered on a scheduled, rather than p.r.n., basis.

• Because enteric-coated and sustained-release tablets are slowly absorbed, they aren't suitable for rapid relief of acute pain, fever, or inflammation. They do cause less GI bleeding and may be better suited for long-term therapy, such as treatment of arthritis.

• For patient with swallowing difficulties, crush nonenteric-coated aspirin and dissolve in soft food or liquid. Administer liquid immediately after mixing because drug will break down rapidly.

• For patients who can't tolerate oral drugs, ask doctor about possibility of using aspirin rectal suppositories. Watch for rectal mucosal irritation or bleeding.

• Febrile, dehydrated children can develop toxicity rapidly.

• Monitor elderly patients closely because they may be more susceptible to aspirin's toxic effects.

• Monitor blood salicylate levels as indicated and ordered. Therapeutic blood salicylate level in arthritis is 10 to 30 mg/100 ml. Tinnitus may occur at plasma levels of 30 mg/100 ml and above, but this isn't a reliable indicator of toxicity, especially in very young patients and those over age 60. With long-term therapy, mild toxicity may occur at plasma levels of 20 mg/100 ml.

• During prolonged therapy, hematocrit, hemoglobin level, PT, INR, and renal function should be assessed periodically as ordered.

• Aspirin irreversibly inhibits platelet aggregation. It should be discontinued 5 to 7 days before elective surgery, as ordered, to allow time for the production and release of new platelets.

• *Alert:* Don't confuse aspirin with
Asendin or Afrin.

☑ **Patient teaching**
• Tell patient who is allergic to tartrazine
dye to avoid aspirin.
• Advise patient on sodium-restricted diet
that 1 tablet of buffered aspirin contains
553 mg of sodium.
• Advise patient to take with food, milk,
antacid, or large glass of water to reduce
adverse GI reactions.
• Tell patient that sustained-release or enteric-coated preparations shouldn't be
crushed or chewed but should be swallowed whole.
• Instruct patient to discard aspirin tablets
with a strong vinegar-like odor.
• Tell patient to consult doctor if administering to children for more than 5 days or
adults for more than 10 days.
• Advise patient receiving prolonged
treatment with large doses of aspirin to
watch for petechiae, bleeding gums, and
signs of GI bleeding, and to maintain adequate fluid intake. Encourage use of a
soft-bristled toothbrush.
• Because of many possible drug interactions involving aspirin, warn patient taking prescription drugs to check with doctor or pharmacist before taking aspirin or
OTC products containing aspirin.
• Inform pregnant woman to avoid aspirin
during last trimester of pregnancy unless
specifically directed by doctor.
• Caution parents to keep out of reach of
children because aspirin is a leading
cause of poisoning in children. Encourage
use of child-resistant containers.

---

**choline magnesium
trisalicylate (choline salicylate
and magnesium salicylate)**
Trilisate

*Pregnancy Risk Category C*

**HOW SUPPLIED**
*Tablets:* 500 mg, 750 mg, 1,000 mg of
salicylate
*Solution:* 500 mg of salicylate/5 ml

**ACTION**
Produces analgesia and anti-inflammatory
effects by blocking prostaglandin synthesis (peripheral action). Salicylates may
prevent the lowering of the pain threshold
that occurs when prostaglandins sensitize
pain receptors to stimulation. Salicylates
relieve fever by acting on the hypothalamic heat-regulating center to produce peripheral vasodilation.

| Route | Onset | Peak | Duration |
|-------|-------|------|----------|
| P.O. | Unknown | 1-2 hr | Unknown |

**INDICATIONS & DOSAGE**
*Rheumatoid arthritis and osteoarthritis or
other polyarthritic or inflammatory conditions—*
**Adults:** initially, 1.5 to 2.5 g P.O. daily as
a single dose or in two or three divided
doses. Dosage is adjusted according to
patient response. Maintenance dose range
is 1 to 4.5 g daily.
**Elderly:** 750 mg P.O. t.i.d.
*Mild to moderate pain and fever—*
**Adults:** 2 to 3 g P.O. daily in divided doses q 4 to 6 hours.
**Children:** for those weighing 37 kg (82
lb) or less, 50 mg/kg/day P.O. in divided
doses b.i.d.; for those over 37 kg,
2,250 mg/day.

**ADVERSE REACTIONS**
**EENT:** tinnitus, hearing loss.
**GI:** GI distress, nausea, vomiting.
**Skin:** rash.
**Other:** *hypersensitivity reactions, ana-
phylaxis, Reye's syndrome.*

**INTERACTIONS**
**Drug-drug.** *ACE inhibitors, beta blockers, diuretics:* effects of these agents may
be decreased. Monitor patient closely.
*Ammonium chloride, other urine acidi-
fiers:* increased blood levels of salicylates. Monitor for salicylate toxicity.
*Antacids in high doses, other urine alka-
linizers:* decreased levels of salicylates.
Monitor for decreased salicylate effect.
*Corticosteroids:* enhanced salicylate elimination. Monitor for decreased salicylate
effect.
*Methotrexate:* increased risk of methotrexate toxicity. Avoid concomitant use.

---

*NSAIDs, corticosteroids:* enhanced risk of adverse GI effects. Avoid concomitant use.
*Oral anticoagulants:* increased risk of bleeding. Use together cautiously.
*Oral hypoglycemics:* increased effect of sulfonylureas. Monitor for symptoms of hypoglycemia.
*Uricosurics:* decreased uricosuric effect. Avoid concomitant use.
**Drug-lifestyle.** *Alcohol use:* enhanced risk of adverse GI effects. Avoid concomitant use.

### EFFECTS ON DIAGNOSTIC TESTS
Choline salicylates may interfere with urinary glucose analysis performed via Diastix, Chemstrip uG, Clinitest, and Benedict's solution. These drugs also interfere with urinary 5-hydroxyindoleacetic acid and vanillylmandelic acid.

### CONTRAINDICATIONS
Contraindicated in patients with hypersensitivity to drug and in those with hemophilia, bleeding ulcers, or hemorrhagic states.

### NURSING CONSIDERATIONS
• Use cautiously in patients with renal insufficiency, hepatic impairment, peptic ulcer disease, and gastritis.
• *Alert:* Because of epidemiologic association with Reye's syndrome, the Centers for Disease Control and Prevention recommends not giving salicylates to children or teenagers with chickenpox or flu-like illness.
• Febrile, dehydrated children can develop toxicity rapidly.
• Monitor serum salicylate levels in long-term therapy. Therapeutic blood salicylate level in arthritis is 15 to 30 mg/100 ml and 5 to 15 mg/100 ml for pain and fever relief. Tinnitus may occur at plasma levels of 30 mg/100 ml and above, but this isn't a reliable indicator of toxicity, especially in the very young and in those over age 60. In long-term therapy, mild toxicity may occur at plasma levels of 20 mg/100 ml.
• Periodically monitor hemoglobin level, PT, and INR in patients receiving long-term treatment with large doses.

• Drug causes less GI distress than aspirin. If an antacid is needed, give antacid 2 hours after meals and choline magnesium trisalicylate before meals.

### ☑ Patient teaching
• Tell patient to take tablets with food and to take solution with a full glass of water. Solution may be mixed with fruit juice, but not antacids.
• Warn patient not to take drug longer than prescribed or to increase dosage without consulting doctor.

---

# diflunisal
## Dolobid

*Pregnancy Risk Category C*

---

### HOW SUPPLIED
*Tablets:* 250 mg, 500 mg

### ACTION
Unknown. Probably related to inhibition of prostaglandin synthesis.

| Route | Onset | Peak | Duration |
| --- | --- | --- | --- |
| P.O. | 1 hr | 2-3 hr | 8-12 hr |

### INDICATIONS & DOSAGE
*Osteoarthritis, rheumatoid arthritis—*
**Adults:** 500 to 1,000 mg P.O. daily in two divided doses, usually q 12 hours. Maximum dose is 1,500 mg daily.
**Elderly:** in patients over age 65, one-half usual adult dose.
*Mild to moderate pain—*
**Adults:** 1 g P.O.; then 500 mg q 8 to 12 hours. A lower dose of 500 mg P.O. followed by 250 mg q 8 to 12 hours may be appropriate.

### ADVERSE REACTIONS
**CNS:** dizziness, somnolence, insomnia, headache, fatigue.
**EENT:** tinnitus.
**GI:** nausea, dyspepsia, GI pain, diarrhea, vomiting, constipation, flatulence, stomatitis.
**GU:** renal impairment, hematuria, *interstitial nephritis.*
**Skin:** rash, pruritus, sweating, erythema multiforme, *Stevens-Johnson syndrome.*

---

## INTERACTIONS
**Drug-drug.** *Acetaminophen, hydrochlorothiazide, indomethacin:* diflunisal may substantially increase blood levels, increasing risk of toxicity. Avoid concomitant use.
*Antacids, aspirin:* decreased diflunisal blood levels. Monitor for possible decreased therapeutic effect.
*Anticoagulants, thrombolytics:* diflunisal may enhance pharmacologic effects of these drugs. Use together cautiously.
*Cyclosporine:* diflunisal may enhance the nephrotoxicity of cyclosporine. Avoid concomitant use.
*Methotrexate:* diflunisal may enhance the toxicity of methotrexate. Avoid concomitant use.
*Sulindac:* diflunisal decreases blood levels of sulindac's active metabolite. Monitor for reduced effect.

## EFFECTS ON DIAGNOSTIC TESTS
Physiologic effects of the drug may prolong bleeding time; increase serum BUN, creatinine, and potassium levels; decrease serum uric acid level; and increase liver function test results.

## CONTRAINDICATIONS
Contraindicated in patients with hypersensitivity to drug and in those for whom acute asthmatic attacks, urticaria, or rhinitis are precipitated by aspirin or other NSAIDs.

## NURSING CONSIDERATIONS
• Use cautiously in GI bleeding, history of peptic ulcer disease, renal impairment, compromised cardiac function, hypertension, or other conditions predisposing patient to fluid retention.
• *Alert:* Because of the epidemiologic association with Reye's syndrome, the Centers for Disease Control and Prevention recommends not giving salicylates to children and teenagers with chickenpox or flulike illness.

☑ **Patient teaching**
• Advise patient to take with water, milk, or meals.
• Tell patient that tablets must be swallowed whole.

• Instruct patient to avoid aspirin or acetaminophen while using diflunisal unless ordered.
• Inform breast-feeding woman that drug appears in breast milk and that a decision should be made to discontinue either breast-feeding or drug.

---

**magnesium salicylate**
Doan's, Doan's P.M. Extra-Strength† ◊, Magan ◊, Mobidin ◊

*Pregnancy Risk Category C*

---

## HOW SUPPLIED
*Tablets:* 545 mg, 600 mg
*Caplets:* 325 mg ◊, 500 mg ◊

## ACTION
Produces analgesia and anti-inflammatory effect by blocking prostaglandin synthesis (peripheral action). Salicylates may prevent the lowering of the pain threshold that occurs when prostaglandins sensitize pain receptors to stimulation; salicylates relieve fever by acting on the hypothalamic heat-regulating center to produce peripheral vasodilation.

| Route | Onset | Peak | Duration |
|-------|-------|------|----------|
| P.O. | Unknown | 1.5-2 hr | Unknown |

## INDICATIONS & DOSAGE
*Arthritis—*
**Adults:** 545 mg to 1.2 g P.O. t.i.d. or q.i.d.
*Mild pain or fever—*
**Adults and children over age 11:** 300 to 600 mg P.O. q 4 hours, not to exceed 3.5 g daily.

## ADVERSE REACTIONS
**EENT:** tinnitus, hearing loss.
**GI:** nausea, vomiting, *GI distress.*
**Hepatic:** abnormal liver function tests, *hepatitis.*
**Skin:** rash, bruising.
**Other:** *hypersensitivity reactions (anaphylaxis, asthma), Reye's syndrome.*

## INTERACTIONS
**Drug-drug.** *ACE inhibitors, beta blockers, diuretics, uricosurics:* effects of these

---

drugs may be decreased. Monitor patient closely.

*Ammonium chloride, other urine acidifiers:* increased blood levels of salicylates. Monitor for salicylate toxicity.
*Antacids in high doses, other urine alkalinizers:* decreased levels of salicylates. Monitor for decreased salicylate effect.
*Anticoagulants:* increased risk of bleeding. Avoid using together.
*Corticosteroids:* enhanced salicylate elimination. Monitor for decreased salicylate effect.
*Methotrexate:* increased risk of methotrexate toxicity. Avoid concomitant use.
*Other NSAIDs, corticosteroids:* increased risk of GI bleeding. Avoid concomitant use.
**Drug-lifestyle.** *Alcohol use:* increased risk of GI bleeding. Avoid concomitant use.

**EFFECTS ON DIAGNOSTIC TESTS**
In high doses, drug may cause false-positive urine glucose test results using copper sulfate method; it may cause false-negative urine glucose test results using glucose enzymatic method. False increases or decreases in urine vanillylmandelic acid tests and false increases in serum uric acid have been seen. Magnesium salicylate may interfere with the Gerhardt's test for urine acetoacetic acid.

**CONTRAINDICATIONS**
Contraindicated in patients with hypersensitivity to drug and in those with aspirin bleeding disorders or severe chronic renal insufficiency because of risk of magnesium toxicity.

**NURSING CONSIDERATIONS**
• Use cautiously in patients with hypoprothrombinemia and vitamin K deficiency.
• *Alert:* Because of epidemiologic association with Reye's syndrome, the Centers for Disease Control and Prevention recommends not giving salicylates to children or teenagers with chickenpox or flu-like illness.
• Febrile, dehydrated children can develop toxicity rapidly.
• Monitor serum salicylate levels in long-term use, as ordered. Therapeutic blood salicylate level in arthritis is 10 to 30 mg/100 ml. Tinnitus may occur at plasma levels of 30 mg/100 ml and above, but this isn't a reliable indicator of toxicity, especially in very young patients and those over age 60. With long-term therapy, mild toxicity may occur at plasma levels of 20 mg/100 ml.
• Monitor hemoglobin level, PT, and INR in long-term treatment with large doses.

**✓ Patient teaching**
• Advise patient that risk of GI irritation can be reduced by taking drug with food, milk, antacid, or a large glass of water.
• Instruct patient not to crush or cut tablets and caplets.

---

## Nonsteroidal anti-inflammatory drugs

celecoxib
diclofenac potassium
diclofenac sodium
etodolac
fenoprofen calcium
flurbiprofen
ibuprofen
indomethacin
indomethacin sodium
   trihydrate
ketoprofen
ketorolac tromethamine
nabumetone
naproxen
naproxen sodium
oxaprozin
piroxicam
rofecoxib
sulindac

## COMBINATION PRODUCTS

ADVIL COLD AND SINUS CAPLETS ◊,
DIMETAPP SINUS CAPLETS, DRISTAN
SINUS CAPLETS ◊, MOTRIN IB SINUS,
SINE-AID IB CAPLETS: pseudoephedrine
hydrochloride 30 mg and ibuprofen
200 mg.
ARTHROTEC: diclofenac 50 mg and miso-
prostol 200 mcg.
ARTHROTEC: diclofenac 75 mg and miso-
prostol 200 mcg.

✳ *NEW DRUG*

## celecoxib
Celebrex

*Pregnancy Risk Category C*

## HOW SUPPLIED
*Capsules:* 100 mg, 200 mg

## ACTION
A selective NSAID that is thought to inhibit prostaglandin synthesis, primarily
via inhibition of cyclooxygenase-2 (COX-
2). Its anti-inflammatory effects and analgesic and antipyretic properties are

thought to be related to a decrease in
prostaglandin synthesis.

| Route | Onset | Peak | Duration |
|-------|-------|------|----------|
| P.O. | Unknown | 3 hr | Unknown |

## INDICATIONS & DOSAGE
*Relief of signs and symptoms of osteo-
arthritis—*
**Adults:** 200 mg P.O. daily as a single
dose or divided equally b.i.d.
*Relief of signs and symptoms of rheuma-
toid arthritis—*
**Adults:** 100 to 200 mg P.O. b.i.d.
*Adjust-a-dose:* For patients weighing less
than 50 kg (110 lb), start at lowest recommended dosage. For patients with moderate hepatic impairment (Child-Pugh Class
II), start therapy with reduced dosage.

## ADVERSE REACTIONS
**CNS:** dizziness, *headache,* insomnia.
**EENT:** pharyngitis, rhinitis, sinusitis.
**GI:** abdominal pain, diarrhea, dyspepsia,
flatulence, nausea.
**GU:** elevated BUN level.
**Hepatic:** elevated liver enzyme levels.
**Metabolic:** hyperchloremia, hypophos-
phatemia.
**Musculoskeletal:** back pain.
**Respiratory:** upper respiratory tract in-
fection.
**Skin:** rash.
**Other:** peripheral edema, accidental in-
jury.

## INTERACTIONS
**Drug-drug.** *ACE inhibitors:* diminished
antihypertensive effects. Monitor patient's
blood pressure.
*Aluminum- and magnesium-containing
antacids:* reduced celecoxib levels. Separate administration times.
*Aspirin:* increased risk of ulcers; low aspirin dosages can be used safely to prevent CV events. Monitor patient for signs
and symptoms of GI bleeding.

---

*Fluconazole:* increased celecoxib levels. Reduce dosage of celecoxib to minimal effective dose.

*Furosemide:* NSAIDs can reduce sodium excretion associated with diuretics, leading to sodium retention. Monitor patient for swelling and increased blood pressure.

*Lithium:* increased lithium level. Monitor plasma lithium levels closely during treatment.

*Warfarin:* increased PT and bleeding complications. Monitor PT and INR, and check for signs and symptoms of bleeding.

**Drug-lifestyle.** *Long-term alcohol use, smoking:* increased risk of GI irritation or bleeding. Check for signs and symptoms of bleeding.

**EFFECTS ON DIAGNOSTIC TESTS**
None reported.

**CONTRAINDICATIONS**
Contraindicated in patients with hypersensitivity to drug, sulfonamides, aspirin, or other NSAIDs, and in those with severe hepatic impairment; also contraindicated in pregnant women in third trimester.

**NURSING CONSIDERATIONS**
• Use cautiously in patients with history of ulcers or GI bleeding, advanced renal disease, dehydration, anemia, symptomatic liver disease, hypertension, edema, heart failure, or asthma and in those with known or suspected history as poor P-4502C9 metabolizers. Also use cautiously in elderly or debilitated patients.

• *Alert:* Patients may be allergic to drug if they are allergic and have had anaphylactic reactions to sulfonamides, aspirin, or other NSAIDs.

• Patient with history of ulcers or GI bleeding is at higher risk for GI bleeding while taking NSAIDs such as celecoxib. Other risk factors for GI bleeding include treatment with corticosteroids or anticoagulants, longer duration of NSAID treatment, smoking, alcoholism, older age, and poor overall health.

• Although drug may be used with low aspirin dosages, the combination may increase risk of GI bleeding.

• Monitor for signs and symptoms of overt and occult bleeding.

• NSAIDs such as celecoxib can cause fluid retention; closely monitor patients with hypertension, edema, or heart failure.

• Drug may be hepatotoxic; monitor for signs and symptoms of liver toxicity.

• Before starting drug therapy, rehydrate patient who is dehydrated.

• Although drug can be given without regard to meals, food may decrease GI upset.

• *Alert:* Don't confuse Celebrex with Cerebyx or Celexa.

**☑ Patient teaching**
• Tell patient to report history of allergic reactions to sulfonamides, aspirin, or other NSAIDs before starting therapy.

• Instruct patient to promptly report signs of GI bleeding, such as bloody vomitus, blood in urine or stool, and black, tarry stools.

• Advise patient to report rash, unexplained weight gain, or edema immediately.

• Tell woman to notify doctor if she becomes pregnant or is planning to become pregnant during drug therapy.

• Instruct patient to take drug with food if stomach upset occurs.

• Teach patient that all NSAIDs, including celecoxib, may adversely affect the liver. Signs and symptoms of liver toxicity include nausea, fatigue, lethargy, itching, jaundice, right upper quadrant tenderness, and flulike syndrome. Advise patient to stop therapy and seek immediate medical advice if he experiences these signs or symptoms.

• Inform patient that it may take several days before he feels consistent pain relief.

---

**diclofenac potassium**
Cataflam

**diclofenac sodium**
Diclomax Retard§, Fenac‡, Voltaren, Voltaren XR, Voltaren Rapide†, Voltaren SR†, Voltarol§

*Pregnancy Risk Category B*

**HOW SUPPLIED**
*Tablets:* 50 mg
*Tablets (enteric-coated):* 25 mg, 50 mg, 75 mg

*Tablets (extended-release):* 100 mg
*Suppositories:* 50 mg†, 100 mg†

## ACTION

Unknown. Produces anti-inflammatory, analgesic, and antipyretic effects, possibly by inhibiting prostaglandin synthesis.

| Route | Onset | Peak | Duration |
|-------|-------|------|----------|
| P.O., P.R. | 10 min | 1 hr | 8 hr |
| P.O. (enteric) | 30 min | 2-3 hr | 8 hr |

## INDICATIONS & DOSAGE

*Ankylosing spondylitis—*
**Adults:** 25 mg P.O. q.i.d. (and h.s., p.r.n.)
*Osteoarthritis—*
**Adults:** 50 mg P.O. b.i.d. or t.i.d., or 75 mg P.O. b.i.d. Maintenance dose is 100 mg P.O. daily (extended-release diclofenac sodium only).
*Rheumatoid arthritis—*
**Adults:** 50 mg P.O. t.i.d. or q.i.d. Or, 75 mg P.O. b.i.d. (diclofenac sodium only), 100 mg P.O. daily (extended-release form), or 50 to 100 mg P.R. (where available) h.s. as substitute for last oral dose of the day. Not to exceed 225 mg daily.
*Analgesia, primary dysmenorrhea—*
**Adults:** 50 mg P.O. t.i.d. (diclofenac potassium only).

## ADVERSE REACTIONS

**CNS:** anxiety, depression, dizziness, drowsiness, insomnia, irritability, headache, *aseptic meningitis.*
**CV:** *heart failure,* hypertension, edema, fluid retention.
**EENT:** tinnitus, *laryngeal edema,* swelling of the lips and tongue, blurred vision, eye pain, night blindness, epistaxis, taste disorder, reversible hearing loss.
**GI:** abdominal pain or cramps, constipation, diarrhea, indigestion, nausea, abdominal distention, flatulence, peptic ulceration, *bleeding,* melena, bloody diarrhea, appetite change, colitis.
**GU:** proteinuria, *acute renal failure,* oliguria, interstitial nephritis, papillary necrosis, *nephrotic syndrome,* fluid retention.
**Hepatic:** elevated liver enzyme levels, jaundice, *hepatitis, hepatotoxicity.*
**Metabolic:** hypoglycemia; hyperglycemia.
**Musculoskeletal:** back, leg, or joint pain.
**Respiratory:** asthma.
**Skin:** rash, pruritus, urticaria, eczema, dermatitis, alopecia, photosensitivity, bullous eruption, *Stevens-Johnson syndrome* (rare), allergic purpura.
**Other:** *anaphylaxis, anaphylactoid reactions, angioedema.*

## INTERACTIONS

**Drug-drug.** *Anticoagulants, including warfarin:* possible increased incidence of bleeding. Monitor patient closely.
*Aspirin:* may decrease effectiveness of diclofenac and increase GI toxicity. Concomitant use not recommended by manufacturer.
*Beta blockers:* antihypertensive effects may be blunted. Monitor closely.
*Cyclosporine, digoxin, lithium, methotrexate:* diclofenac may reduce renal clearance of these drugs and increase risk of toxicity. Monitor patient closely.
*Diuretics:* decreased effectiveness of diuretics. Avoid concomitant use.
*Insulin, oral antidiabetics:* diclofenac may alter requirements for antidiabetics. Monitor patient closely.
*Phenytoin:* increased serum levels. Monitor for toxicity.
*Potassium-sparing diuretics:* enhanced potassium retention and increased serum potassium levels. Monitor serum potassium level.
**Drug-lifestyle.** *Sun exposure:* may cause photosensitivity reactions. Take precautions.

## EFFECTS ON DIAGNOSTIC TESTS

None reported.

## CONTRAINDICATIONS

Contraindicated in patients with hypersensitivity to drug and in those with hepatic porphyria or history of asthma, urticaria, or other allergic reactions after taking aspirin or other NSAIDs. Drug isn't recommended for use during late pregnancy or breast-feeding.

---

Reactions may be *common,* uncommon, *life-threatening,* or **COMMON AND LIFE-THREATENING.**

## NURSING CONSIDERATIONS
• Use cautiously in patients with history of peptic ulcer disease, hepatic dysfunction, cardiac disease, hypertension, conditions associated with fluid retention, or impaired renal function.
• Because NSAIDs impair the synthesis of renal prostaglandins, they can decrease renal blood flow and lead to reversible renal impairment, especially in patients with preexisting renal failure, liver dysfunction, or heart failure; in elderly patients; and in those taking diuretics. Monitor these patients closely.
• Elevations of liver test results may occur during therapy. Monitor serum transaminase, especially ALT levels, periodically in patients undergoing long-term therapy, as ordered. The first serum transaminase measurement should be no later than 8 weeks after therapy is begun.
• Because of their antipyretic and anti-inflammatory actions, NSAIDs may mask the signs and symptoms of infection.
• *Alert:* Don't confuse diclofenac with Diflucan or Duphalac.

### ☑ Patient teaching
• Tell patient to take drug with milk or meals to minimize GI distress.
• Instruct patient not to crush, break, or chew enteric-coated tablets.
• Serious GI toxicity, including peptic ulceration and bleeding, can occur in patients taking NSAIDs despite absence of GI symptoms. Teach patient signs and symptoms of GI bleeding, and tell him to contact doctor immediately if these occur.
• Teach patient the signs and symptoms of hepatotoxicity, including nausea, fatigue, lethargy, pruritus, jaundice, right upper quadrant tenderness, and flulike symptoms. Tell him to contact doctor immediately if these symptoms occur.
• Advise patient to avoid consumption of alcohol or aspirin during drug therapy.
• Tell patient to wear sunscreen or protective clothing because drug may cause photosensitivity reactions.
• Warn patient to avoid hazardous activities that require alertness until adverse CNS effects of drug are known.
• Tell pregnant woman to avoid use of drug during last trimester.

## etodolac
Lodine, Lodine XL

*Pregnancy Risk Category C*

### HOW SUPPLIED
*Capsules:* 200 mg, 300 mg
*Tablets:* 400 mg, 500 mg
*Tablets (extended-release):* 400 mg, 500 mg, 600 mg

### ACTION
Unknown. Possibly related to inhibition of prostaglandin biosynthesis.

| Route | Onset | Peak | Duration |
|-------|-------|------|----------|
| P.O. | 30 min | 1-2 hr | 4-12 hr |
| P.O. (extended) | Unknown | 3-12 hr | 6-12 hr |

### INDICATIONS & DOSAGE
*Acute pain—*
**Adults:** 200 to 400 mg P.O. q 6 to 8 hours, p.r.n., not to exceed 1,200 mg daily. In patients weighing 60 kg (132 lb) or less, don't exceed total daily dose of 20 mg/kg.
*Acute and chronic management of osteoarthritis and rheumatoid arthritis—*
**Adults:** 600 to 1,000 mg P.O. daily, divided into two or three doses. Maximum dose is 1,200 mg/day. For extended-release product, 400 to 1,000 mg P.O. daily. Maximum dose is 1,000 mg/day.

### ADVERSE REACTIONS
**CNS:** asthenia, malaise, dizziness, depression, drowsiness, nervousness, insomnia, syncope.
**CV:** hypertension, *heart failure,* flushing, palpitations, edema, fluid retention.
**EENT:** blurred vision, tinnitus, photophobia.
**GI:** *dyspepsia,* flatulence, abdominal pain, diarrhea, nausea, constipation, gastritis, melena, vomiting, anorexia, *peptic ulceration with or without GI bleeding or perforation,* ulcerative stomatitis, thirst, dry mouth.
**GU:** dysuria, urinary frequency, *renal failure.*

**Hematologic:** anemia (rare), *leukopenia,* hemolytic anemia.
**Hepatic:** *hepatitis.*
**Metabolic:** weight gain.
**Respiratory:** asthma.
**Skin:** pruritus, rash, *Stevens-Johnson syndrome.*
**Other:** chills, fever.

## INTERACTIONS
**Drug-drug.** *Antacids:* may decrease peak levels of drug. Monitor for decreased effect of etodolac.
*Aspirin:* reduced protein-binding of etodolac without altering its clearance. Clinical significance unknown. May increase GI toxicity. Avoid concomitant use.
*Beta blockers, diuretics:* effects may be blunted. Monitor closely.
*Cyclosporine:* impaired elimination and increased risk of nephrotoxicity. Avoid concomitant use.
*Digoxin, lithium, methotrexate:* etodolac may impair elimination of these drugs, resulting in increased levels and risk of toxicity. Monitor blood levels.
*Phenytoin:* increased serum levels of phenytoin. Monitor for toxicity.
*Warfarin:* etodolac decreases the protein-binding of warfarin but doesn't change its clearance. Although no dosage adjustment is needed, monitor INR closely and watch for bleeding.
**Drug-lifestyle.** *Alcohol use:* increased chance of adverse effects. Avoid use.
*Sun exposure:* photosensitivity reactions may occur; take precautions.

## EFFECTS ON DIAGNOSTIC TESTS
A false-positive test for urinary bilirubin may be caused by phenolic metabolites.

## CONTRAINDICATIONS
Contraindicated in patients with hypersensitivity to drug and in those with history of aspirin- or NSAID-induced asthma, rhinitis, urticaria, or other allergic reactions.

## NURSING CONSIDERATIONS
• Use cautiously in patients with history of renal or hepatic impairment or GI bleeding, ulceration, and perforation.

• Because NSAIDs impair the synthesis of renal prostaglandins, they can decrease renal blood flow and lead to reversible renal impairment, especially in patients with preexisting renal failure, liver dysfunction, or heart failure; in elderly patients; and in those taking diuretics. Monitor these patients closely.
• *Alert:* Drug appears to cause fewer GI problems than most NSAIDs. Minimal GI blood loss has been reported at dosages up to 1,200 mg daily.
• *Alert:* Don't confuse Lodine with codeine, iodine, or Iopidine.

## ☑ Patient teaching
• Tell patient to take drug with milk or meals to minimize GI discomfort.
• Serious GI toxicity, including peptic ulceration and bleeding, can occur in patients taking NSAIDs despite absence of GI symptoms. Teach patient signs and symptoms of GI bleeding, and tell him to contact doctor immediately if they occur.
• Advise patient to avoid consumption of alcohol or aspirin while taking drug.
• Warn patient to avoid hazardous activities that require alertness until adverse CNS effects of drug are known.
• Because of possibility of photosensitivity reactions, advise patient to use a sunblock, wear protective clothing, and avoid prolonged exposure to sunlight.
• Tell pregnant woman to avoid use of drug during last trimester.

# fenoprofen calcium
Fenopron§, Nalfon

*Pregnancy Risk Category NR*

## HOW SUPPLIED
*Tablets:* 600 mg
*Capsules:* 200 mg, 300 mg

## ACTION
Unknown. Produces anti-inflammatory, analgesic, and antipyretic effects, possibly by inhibiting prostaglandin synthesis.

| Route | Onset | Peak | Duration |
|-------|-------|------|----------|
| P.O. | 15-30 min | 2 hr | 4-6 hr |

---

Reactions may be *common,* uncommon, **life-threatening,** or **COMMON AND LIFE-THREATENING.**

## INDICATIONS & DOSAGE
*Rheumatoid arthritis, osteoarthritis—*
**Adults:** 300 to 600 mg P.O. t.i.d. or q.i.d. Maximum dose is 3.2 g daily.
*Mild to moderate pain—*
**Adults:** 200 mg P.O. q 4 to 6 hours, p.r.n.

## ADVERSE REACTIONS
**CNS:** *headache,* dizziness, *somnolence,* fatigue, nervousness, asthenia, tremor, confusion.
**CV:** peripheral edema, palpitations.
**EENT:** tinnitus, blurred vision, decreased hearing, nasopharyngitis.
**GI:** epigastric distress, nausea, *GI bleeding,* vomiting, occult blood loss, peptic ulceration, constipation, anorexia, dyspepsia, flatulence.
**GU:** oliguria, interstitial nephritis, proteinuria, cystitis, hematuria, elevated BUN and creatinine.
**Hematologic:** prolonged bleeding time, anemia, bruising, hemolytic anemia.
**Hepatic:** elevated liver enzyme levels, *hepatitis.*
**Metabolic:** hyperkalemia.
**Respiratory:** dyspnea, upper respiratory tract infections.
**Skin:** pruritus, rash, urticaria, increased diaphoresis.
**Other:** *angioedema.*

## INTERACTIONS
**Drug-drug.** *Aspirin:* decreased fenoprofen half-life; may increase GI toxicity. Avoid concomitant use.
*Corticosteroids:* increased risk of adverse GI reactions. Avoid concomitant use.
*Diuretics:* decreased diuretic effectiveness. Monitor patient closely.
*Oral anticoagulants, sulfonylureas:* fenoprofen enhances pharmacologic effects of these drugs. Use together cautiously.
*Phenobarbital:* enhanced metabolism of fenoprofen. Monitor for lack of fenoprofen effectiveness.
**Drug-lifestyle.** *Alcohol use:* increased risk of adverse GI reactions. Avoid concomitant use.

## EFFECTS ON DIAGNOSTIC TESTS
Drug or its metabolite may cross-react with the antibody used in the Amerlex-M assay. Limited data suggest that drug may alter free and total $T_3$ levels determined by the Corning method.

## CONTRAINDICATIONS
Contraindicated in patients with hypersensitivity to drug and in those with history of aspirin- or NSAID-induced asthma, urticaria or rhinitis, or significantly impaired renal function; also contraindicated during pregnancy.

## NURSING CONSIDERATIONS
● Use cautiously in elderly patients and in those with history of serious GI events or peptic ulcer disease, compromised cardiac function, or hypertension.
● Safety of drug hasn't been established in pregnant women. Use during pregnancy isn't recommended.
● Because NSAIDs impair the synthesis of renal prostaglandins, they can decrease renal blood flow and lead to reversible renal impairment, especially in patients with preexisting renal failure, liver dysfunction, or heart failure; in elderly patients; and in those taking diuretics. Monitor these patients closely during therapy.
● Because of their antipyretic and anti-inflammatory actions, NSAIDs may mask the signs and symptoms of infection.
● Renal, hepatic, ocular, and auditory function should be checked periodically in long-term therapy. Drug should be stopped if abnormalities occur.
● Drug isn't recommended for use in children.
● *Alert:* Don't confuse Nalfon with Naldecon.

### ☑ Patient teaching
● Tell patient that full therapeutic effect for arthritis may be delayed for 2 to 3 weeks.
● Inform patient to take drug 30 minutes before or 2 hours after meals. If adverse GI reactions occur, tell him that drug may be taken with milk or meals.
● Serious GI toxicity, including peptic ulceration and bleeding, can occur in patients taking NSAIDs despite the absence of GI symptoms. Teach patient the signs and symptoms of GI bleeding, and tell him to contact doctor immediately if they occur.

• Advise patient to avoid consumption of alcohol or aspirin while taking drug.
• Warn patient to avoid hazardous activities that require alertness until adverse CNS effects of drug are known.

---

## flurbiprofen
Ansaid, Apo-Flurbiprofen†, Froben†, Froben SR†, Ocufen Ophthalmic

*Pregnancy Risk Category C*

### HOW SUPPLIED
*Tablets:* 50 mg, 100 mg
*Capsules (extended-release):* 200 mg†
*Ophthalmic solution:* 0.03%

### ACTION
Unknown. Possibly inhibits prostaglandin synthesis.

| Route | Onset | Peak | Duration |
|---|---|---|---|
| P.O. | Unknown | 1.5 hr | Unknown |
| Ophthalmic | Unknown | Unknown | Unknown |

### INDICATIONS & DOSAGE
*Rheumatoid arthritis, osteoarthritis—*
**Adults:** 200 to 300 mg P.O. daily, divided b.i.d. to q.i.d. Patients maintained on 200 mg daily may switch to one 200-mg extended-release capsule (where available) P. O. daily taken in the evening after food. Doses over 300 mg/day aren't recommended.
**Elderly:** may require lower dosage. Monitor closely.
*Adjust-a-dose:* For debilitated patients and those with hepatic or renal dysfunction, reduced dosage may be needed. Monitor closely.
*Inhibition of intraoperative miosis—*
**Adults:** 1 drop in the eye(s) undergoing surgery beginning 2 hours before surgery and repeated at 30-minute intervals for total of 4 drops per affected eye.

### ADVERSE REACTIONS
**CNS:** headache, anxiety, insomnia, dizziness, increased reflexes, tremors, amnesia, asthenia, drowsiness, malaise, depression.
**CV:** edema, *heart failure,* hypertension, vasodilation.
**EENT:** rhinitis, tinnitus, visual changes, epistaxis (oral form); ocular stinging or burning, ocular discomfort, itching, foreign body sensation, tearing, dry eyes, dull eye pain, photophobia (ophthalmic form)
**GI:** dyspepsia, diarrhea, abdominal pain, nausea, constipation, *bleeding,* flatulence, vomiting.
**GU:** symptoms suggesting urinary tract infection, hematuria, interstitial nephritis, *renal failure.*
**Hematologic:** *thrombocytopenia, neutropenia,* anemia, *aplastic anemia.*
**Hepatic:** elevated liver enzymes, jaundice.
**Metabolic:** weight changes.
**Respiratory:** asthma.
**Skin:** rash, photosensitivity, urticaria.
**Other:** *angioedema.*

### INTERACTIONS
**Drug-drug.** *Anticoagulants:* increased risk of bleeding. Monitor patient closely.
*Aspirin:* decreased flurbiprofen levels. May increase GI toxicity. Avoid concomitant use.
*Beta blockers:* antihypertensive effect of beta blockers may be impaired. Monitor blood pressure.
*Cyclosporine:* increased risk of nephrotoxicity. Avoid concomitant use.
*Diuretics:* possible decreased diuretic effect. Monitor patient closely.
*Lithium:* serum lithium levels may be increased. Avoid use together.
*Methotrexate:* increased risk of methotrexate toxicity. Monitor patient closely.
**Drug-lifestyle.** *Alcohol use:* increased risk of adverse GI reactions. Avoid concomitant use.
*Sun exposure:* photosensitivity reactions may occur. Take precautions.

### EFFECTS ON DIAGNOSTIC TESTS
None reported.

### CONTRAINDICATIONS
Contraindicated in patients with hypersensitivity to drug and history of aspirin- or NSAID-induced asthma, urticaria, or other allergic-type reactions. Ophthalmic

---

Reactions may be *common*, uncommon, **life-threatening**, or COMMON AND LIFE-THREATENING.

form should be used cautiously in patients with history of herpes simplex keratitis.

## NURSING CONSIDERATIONS
• Use cautiously in patients with history of peptic ulcer disease, hepatic dysfunction, cardiac disease, or other conditions associated with fluid retention or impaired renal function.
• Safety and effectiveness of drug use in children haven't been established.
• Drug use isn't recommended during last trimester of pregnancy.
• Elderly or debilitated patients and those patients with hepatic or renal dysfunction may be at risk for renal toxicity, jaundice, or toxic hepatitis. Periodically monitor renal and hepatic function, as ordered.
• Because NSAIDs impair the synthesis of renal prostaglandins, they can decrease renal blood flow and lead to reversible renal impairment, especially in patients with preexisting renal failure, liver dysfunction, or heart failure; in elderly patients; and in those taking diuretics. Monitor these patients closely during therapy.
• Patients receiving long-term therapy should have periodic liver function studies, eye examinations, and hematocrit determinations.
• Ophthalmic solution may be absorbed systemically, causing systemic adverse reactions. Monitor patient closely.

### ☑ Patient teaching
• Instruct patient to take drug with food, milk, or antacid if GI upset occurs.
• Tell patient taking extended-release capsules to swallow them whole and not to crush, chew, or break open the capsules.
• Serious GI toxicity, including peptic ulceration and bleeding, can occur in patients taking NSAIDs despite absence of GI symptoms. Teach patient the signs and symptoms of GI bleeding, and tell him to notify doctor immediately if they occur.
• Advise patient to avoid consumption of alcohol or aspirin while taking drug.
• Warn patient to avoid hazardous activities that require mental alertness until CNS effects are known.

# ibuprofen
ACT-3‡, Actiprofen‡, Advil◇, Apo-Ibuprofen†, Bayer Select Pain Relief Formula, Brufen‡, Children's Advil, Children's Motrin◇, Excedrin IB◇, Excedrin IB Caplets◇, Genpril Caplets◇, Genpril Tablets◇, Haltran◇, Ibuprin◇, Ibuprohm◇, Ibuprohm Caplets◇, Ibu-Tab◇, Junifen Sugar Free§, Medipren◇, Medipren Caplets◇, Menadol, Midol IB, Motrin, Motrin-IB Caplets◇, Motrin-IB Tablets◇, Novo-Profen†, Nuprin◇, Nuprin Caplets◇, Nurofen‡, Nurofen Junior‡, Pamprin-IB, Pedia Profen, Rafen‡, Rufen, Saleto-200, Saleto-400, Saleto-600, Saleto-800, Trendar◇

*Pregnancy Risk Category NR*

## HOW SUPPLIED
*Tablets:* 100 mg, 200 mg◇, 300 mg, 400 mg, 600 mg, 800 mg
*Tablets (chewable):* 50 mg, 100 mg
*Oral suspension:* 100 mg/5 ml
*Oral drops:* 40 mg/ml

## ACTION
Unknown. Produces anti-inflammatory, analgesic, and antipyretic effects, possibly by inhibiting prostaglandin synthesis.

| Route | Onset | Peak | Duration |
|-------|-------|------|----------|
| P.O. | Variable | 1-2 hr | 4-6 hr |

## INDICATIONS & DOSAGE
*Rheumatoid arthritis, osteoarthritis, arthritis—*
**Adults:** 300 to 800 mg P.O. t.i.d. or q.i.d. not to exceed 3.2 g daily.
*Mild to moderate pain, dysmenorrhea—*
**Adults:** 400 mg P.O. q 4 to 6 hours, p.r.n.
*Fever—*
**Adults:** 200 to 400 mg P.O. q 4 to 6 hours. Don't exceed 1.2 g daily or give longer than 3 days.
**Children ages 6 months to 12 years:** if fever is below 102.5° F (39.2° C), the recommended dose is 5 mg/kg P.O. q 6 to 8 hours. Treat higher fevers with 10 mg/kg

q 6 to 8 hours. Don't exceed 40 mg/kg daily.

*Juvenile arthritis—*
**Children:** 30 to 70 mg/kg/day P.O. in three or four divided doses.

## ADVERSE REACTIONS
**CNS:** headache, dizziness, nervousness, *aseptic meningitis.*
**CV:** peripheral edema, fluid retention, edema.
**EENT:** tinnitus.
**GI:** epigastric distress, nausea, occult blood loss, peptic ulceration, diarrhea, constipation, dyspepsia, flatulence, heartburn, decreased appetite.
**GU:** acute renal failure, azotemia, cystitis, hematuria, increased BUN and creatinine.
**Hematologic:** prolonged bleeding time, anemia, *neutropenia, pancytopenia, thrombocytopenia, aplastic anemia, leukopenia, agranulocytosis.*
**Hepatic:** elevated liver enzyme levels.
**Metabolic:** hypoglycemia, hyperkalemia.
**Respiratory:** *bronchospasm.*
**Skin:** pruritus, rash, urticaria, *Stevens-Johnson syndrome.*
**Other:** decreased serum uric acid levels.

## INTERACTIONS
**Drug-drug.** *Antihypertensives, furosemide, thiazide diuretics:* ibuprofen may decrease the effectiveness of diuretics or antihypertensives. Monitor patient closely.
*Aspirin:* may decrease serum levels of ibuprofen. Avoid concomitant use.
*Aspirin, corticosteroids:* increased risk of adverse GI reactions. Avoid concomitant use.
*Cyclosporine:* nephrotoxicity of both drugs may be increased. Avoid concomitant use.
*Digoxin, lithium, oral anticoagulants:* ibuprofen may increase plasma levels or effects of these drugs. Monitor for toxicity.
*Methotrexate:* decreased methotrexate clearance and increased toxicity. Use together cautiously.
**Drug-lifestyle.** *Alcohol use:* increased risk of adverse GI reactions. Avoid concomitant use.
*Sun exposure:* may cause photosensitivity reactions. Take precautions.

## EFFECTS ON DIAGNOSTIC TESTS
None reported.

## CONTRAINDICATIONS
Contraindicated in patients with hypersensitivity to drug and in those with angioedema, syndrome of nasal polyps, or bronchospastic reaction to aspirin or other NSAIDs.

## NURSING CONSIDERATIONS
• Use cautiously in patients with GI disorders, history of peptic ulcer disease, hepatic or renal disease, cardiac decompensation, hypertension, or known intrinsic coagulation defects.
• Use of drug in pregnant women isn't recommended.
• Check renal and hepatic function periodically in patients on long-term therapy. Stop drug if abnormalities occur and notify doctor.
• Because of their antipyretic and anti-inflammatory actions, NSAIDs may mask the signs and symptoms of infection.
• Blurred or diminished vision and changes in color vision have occurred.
• It may take 1 to 2 weeks before full anti-inflammatory effects occur.
• *Alert:* Don't confuse Trendar with Trandate.

### ☑ Patient teaching
• Tell patient to take with meals or milk to reduce adverse GI reactions.
• *Alert:* Drug is available OTC in several brands (200 mg). Instruct patient not to exceed 1.2 g daily, give to children under age 12, or self-medicate for extended periods without consulting doctor.
• Tell patient that full therapeutic effect for arthritis may be delayed for 2 to 4 weeks. Although analgesic effect occurs at low dosage levels, anti-inflammatory effect doesn't occur at dosages below 400 mg q.i.d.
• Caution patient that use with aspirin, alcohol, or corticosteroids may increase risk of GI adverse reactions.
• Serious GI toxicity, including peptic ulceration and bleeding, can occur in patients taking NSAIDs despite absence of GI symptoms. Teach patient signs and

symptoms of GI bleeding, and tell him to notify doctor immediately if they occur.
• Warn patient to avoid hazardous activities that require mental alertness until CNS effects are known.
• Advise patient to wear sunscreen to avoid photosensitivity reactions.

## indomethacin
Apo-Indomethacin†, Arthrexin‡, Indochron E-R, Indocid†‡, Indocid SR†, Indocin, Indocin SR, Novo-Methacin†

## indomethacin sodium trihydrate
Apo-Indomethacin†, Indocid PDA, Indocin I.V., Novo-Methacin†

*Pregnancy Risk Category NR*

## HOW SUPPLIED
**indomethacin**
*Capsules:* 25 mg, 50 mg
*Capsules (sustained-release):* 75 mg
*Oral suspension:* 25 mg/5 ml
*Suppositories:* 50 mg
**indomethacin sodium trihydrate**
*Injection:* 1-mg vials

## ACTION
Unknown. Produces anti-inflammatory, analgesic, and antipyretic effects, possibly by inhibiting prostaglandin synthesis.

| Route | Onset | Peak | Duration |
|-------|-------|------|----------|
| P.O. | 0.5 hr | 1-4 hr | 4-6 hr |
| I.V. | Immediate | Immediate | 4-6 hr |
| P.R. | Unknown | Unknown | 4-6 hr |

## INDICATIONS & DOSAGE
*Moderate to severe rheumatoid arthritis or osteoarthritis, ankylosing spondylitis—*
**Adults:** 25 mg P.O. or P.R. b.i.d. or t.i.d. with food or antacids; increase daily dose by 25 or 50 mg q 7 days, up to 200 mg daily. Or, sustained-release capsules (75 mg): 75 mg P.O. to start, in morning or h.s., followed, if needed, by 75 mg b.i.d.
*Acute gouty arthritis—*
**Adults:** 50 mg P.O. t.i.d. Dose reduced as soon as possible; then discontinued.

Sustained-release capsules shouldn't be used for this condition.
*Acute painful shoulders (bursitis or tendinitis)—*
**Adults:** 75 to 150 mg P.O. daily in divided doses t.i.d. or q.i.d. for 7 to 14 days.
*To close a hemodynamically significant patent ductus arteriosus in premature neonates (I.V. form only)—*
**Neonates under age 48 hours:** 0.2 mg/kg I.V.; then two doses of 0.1 mg/kg at 12- to 24-hour intervals.
**Neonates ages 2 to 7 days:** 0.2 mg/kg I.V.; then two doses of 0.2 mg/kg at 12- to 24-hour intervals.
**Neonates over age 7 days:** 0.2 mg/kg I.V.; then two doses of 0.25 mg/kg at 12- to 24-hour intervals.

## ADVERSE REACTIONS
*P.O. and P.R.—*
**CNS:** *headache,* dizziness, depression, drowsiness, confusion, somnolence, fatigue, peripheral neuropathy, psychic disturbances, syncope, *vertigo.*
**CV:** hypertension, edema.
**EENT:** blurred vision, corneal and retinal damage, hearing loss, tinnitus.
**GI:** nausea, anorexia, diarrhea, peptic ulceration, *GI bleeding,* constipation, dyspepsia, *pancreatitis.*
**GU:** hematuria.
**Hematologic:** iron deficiency anemia.
**Metabolic:** hyperkalemia.
**Skin:** pruritus, urticaria, *Stevens-Johnson syndrome.*
**Other:** *hypersensitivity reactions (rash, respiratory distress).*
*I.V.—*
**GU:** hematuria, proteinuria, interstitial nephritis.

## INTERACTIONS
**Drug-drug.** *Aminoglycosides, cyclosporine, methotrexate:* indomethacin may enhance the toxicity of these drugs. Avoid concomitant use.
*Anticoagulants:* increased risk of bleeding. Monitor patient closely.
*Antihypertensives:* reduced antihypertensive effect. Monitor patient closely. *Antihypertensives, furosemide, thiazide diuretics:* impaired response to both drugs. Avoid using together if possible.

*Aspirin:* decreased blood levels of indomethacin. Avoid concomitant use.

*Aspirin, corticosteroids:* increased risk of GI toxicity. Don't use together.

*Diflunisal, probenecid:* decreased indomethacin excretion. Watch for increased incidence of indomethacin adverse reactions.

*Digoxin:* indomethacin may prolong half-life of digoxin. Use together cautiously.

*Dipyridamole:* enhanced fluid retention. Avoid concomitant use.

*Lithium:* increased plasma lithium levels. Monitor for toxicity.

*Penicillamine:* may increase bioavailability of penicillamine. Monitor closely.

*Phenytoin:* increased serum phenytoin levels may occur. Monitor closely.

*Triamterene:* possible nephrotoxicity. Monitor patient closely.

**Drug-herb.** *Senna:* blocked diarrheal effects. Avoid concomitant use.

**Drug-lifestyle.** *Alcohol use:* increased risk of GI toxicity. Don't use together.

## EFFECTS ON DIAGNOSTIC TESTS
Drug may interfere with results of dexamethasone suppression test. It may also interfere with urinary 5-hydroxyindoleacetic acid determinations.

## CONTRAINDICATIONS
Contraindicated in patients with hypersensitivity to drug or history of aspirin- or NSAID-induced asthma, rhinitis, or urticaria. Also contraindicated in pregnant or breast-feeding women and in infants with untreated infection, active bleeding, coagulation defects or thrombocytopenia, congenital heart disease in whom patency of the ductus arteriosus is needed, necrotizing enterocolitis, or impaired renal function. Suppositories are contraindicated in patients with history of proctitis or recent rectal bleeding.

## NURSING CONSIDERATIONS
• Use cautiously in patients with epilepsy, parkinsonism, hepatic or renal disease, CV disease, infection, and mental illness or depression. Also use cautiously in elderly patients and patients with history of GI disease.

• Because of its high incidence of adverse effects during chronic use, indomethacin shouldn't be used routinely as an analgesic or antipyretic.

• Use of drug in pregnant women isn't recommended.

• Administer oral dose with food, milk, or antacid to prevent GI upset.

• If ductus arteriosus reopens, a second course of one to three doses may be given. If ineffective, surgery may be needed.

• Monitor for bleeding in patients receiving anticoagulants, patients with coagulation defects, and neonates.

• Because NSAIDs impair the synthesis of renal prostaglandins, they can decrease renal blood flow and lead to reversible renal impairment, especially in patients with preexisting renal failure, liver dysfunction, or heart failure; in elderly patients; and in those taking diuretics. Monitor these patients closely during therapy.

• Drug causes sodium retention; monitor for weight gain (especially in elderly patients) and increased blood pressure in patients with hypertension.

• Because of their antipyretic and anti-inflammatory actions, NSAIDs may mask signs and symptoms of infection.

## I.V. administration
• Reconstitute powder for injection with sterile water or normal saline for injection or normal saline. For each 1-mg vial, add 1 ml of diluent for a solution containing 1 mg/ml.

• *Alert:* Use only preservative-free sterile NaCl or sterile water to prepare I.V. injection. Never use diluents containing benzyl alcohol because it has been associated with toxicity in newborns. Because the injection contains no preservatives, reconstitute drug immediately before administration, and discard unused solution.

• Withhold administration of second or third scheduled I.V. dose if anuria or marked oliguria is evident; notify doctor.

• Monitor carefully for bleeding and for reduced urine output with I.V. administration.

## Patient teaching
• Tell patient to take oral drug with food, milk, or antacid to prevent GI upset.

---

Reactions may be *common*, uncommon, *life-threatening*, or COMMON AND LIFE-THREATENING.

- Alert patient that use of oral form with aspirin, alcohol, or corticosteroids may increase risk of adverse GI reactions.
- Serious GI toxicity, including peptic ulceration and bleeding, can occur in patients taking oral NSAIDs despite absence of GI symptoms. Teach patient signs and symptoms of GI bleeding, and tell him to notify doctor immediately if they occur.
- Warn patient to avoid hazardous activities that require mental alertness until CNS effects are known.
- Tell patient to notify doctor immediately if visual or hearing changes occur. Patient on long-term oral therapy should have regular eye examinations, hearing tests, CBC, and renal function tests to monitor for toxicity.

## ketoprofen
Actron, Apo-Keto†, Apo-Keto-E†, Novo-Keto-EC†, Orudis, Orudis E†, Orudis KT, Orudis SR†‡, Oruvail, Rhodis†, Rhodis-EC†

*Pregnancy Risk Category B*

## HOW SUPPLIED
*Tablets:* 12.5 mg ◊
*Tablets (extended-release):* 200 mg†
*Tablets (enteric-coated):* 50 mg†, 100 mg†
*Capsules (extended-release):* 100 mg, 150 mg, 200 mg
*Capsules:* 25 mg, 50 mg, 75 mg
*Suppositories:* 100 mg†

## ACTION
Unknown. Produces anti-inflammatory, analgesic, and antipyretic effects, possibly by inhibiting prostaglandin synthesis.

| Route | Onset | Peak | Duration |
| --- | --- | --- | --- |
| P.O., P.R. | 1-2 hr | 0.5-2 hr | 3-4 hr |

## INDICATIONS & DOSAGE
*Rheumatoid arthritis, osteoarthritis—*
**Adults:** 75 mg t.i.d. or 50 mg q.i.d. or 200 mg as an extended-release tablet once daily. Maximum dose is 300 mg daily or 200mg daily for extended-release capsules. Or, where suppository is available,
100 mg P.R. b.i.d.; or 1 suppository h.s. (with oral ketoprofen during the day).
**Elderly:** reduce initial dose to between one-third and one-half of normal initial dose.
*Mild to moderate pain, dysmenorrhea—*
**Adults:** 25 to 50 mg P.O. q 6 to 8 hours, p.r.n.
**Elderly:** reduce initial dose to between one-third and one-half of normal initial dose.
*Minor aches and pain or fever—*
**Adults:** 12.5 mg q 4 to 6 hours. Don't exceed 25 mg in a 4- to 6-hour period or 75 mg in 24 hours.
**Elderly:** reduce initial dose to between one-third and one-half of normal initial dose.
***Adjust-a-dose:*** For patients with impaired renal function, reduce initial dose to between one-third and one-half of normal initial dose.

## ADVERSE REACTIONS
**CNS:** headache, dizziness, CNS excitation or depression.
**EENT:** tinnitus, visual disturbances.
**GI:** nausea, abdominal pain, diarrhea, constipation, flatulence, *peptic ulceration, dyspepsia,* anorexia, vomiting, stomatitis.
**GU:** *nephrotoxicity,* elevated BUN.
**Hematologic:** prolonged bleeding time.
**Hepatic:** elevated liver enzymes.
**Respiratory:** dyspnea.
**Skin:** rash, photosensitivity.
**Other:** peripheral edema.

## INTERACTIONS
**Drug-drug.** *Aspirin, corticosteroids:* increased risk of adverse GI reactions. Avoid concomitant use.
*Aspirin, probenecid:* increased plasma levels of ketoprofen. Avoid concomitant use.
*Cyclosporine:* increased nephrotoxicity. Avoid use together.
*Hydrochlorothiazide, other diuretics:* decreased diuretic effectiveness. Monitor for lack of effect.
*Lithium, methotrexate, phenytoin:* increased levels of these drugs, leading to toxicity. Monitor patient closely.
*Warfarin:* increased risk of bleeding. Monitor patient closely.

---

*Liquid contains alcohol.   **May contain tartrazine.   †Canada   ‡Australia   §U.K.   ◊OTC

**Drug-lifestyle.** *Alcohol use:* increased risk of GI toxicity. Don't use together.
*Sun exposure:* may cause photosensitivity reactions. Take precautions.

## EFFECTS ON DIAGNOSTIC TESTS

In vitro interactions with glucose determinations have been reported with glucose oxidase and peroxidase methods. Drug may interfere with serum iron determinations (false increases or decreases depending on method used) and produce false increases in serum bilirubin levels. These interactions were reported with drug levels above those seen clinically (60 mg/ml).

## CONTRAINDICATIONS

Contraindicated in patients with hypersensitivity to drug and in those with history of aspirin- or NSAID-induced asthma, urticaria, or other allergy-type reactions.

## NURSING CONSIDERATIONS

• Use cautiously in patients with history of peptic ulcer disease, renal dysfunction, hypertension, heart failure, or fluid retention.
• Avoid use during last trimester of pregnancy.
• Sustained-release form isn't recommended for patients in acute pain.
• Because NSAIDs impair synthesis of renal prostaglandins, they can decrease renal blood flow and lead to reversible renal impairment, especially in patients with preexisting renal failure, liver dysfunction, or heart failure; in elderly patients; and in those taking diuretics. Monitor these patients closely during therapy.
• Check renal and hepatic function every 6 months or as indicated.
• NSAIDs may mask signs and symptoms of infection because of their antipyretic and anti-inflammatory actions.
• Drug isn't recommended for use in children.

☑ **Patient teaching**
• *Alert:* Drug is available OTC. Instruct patient not to exceed dosage of 75 mg/day.
• Tell patient to take drug 30 minutes before or 2 hours after meals. If adverse GI reactions occur, patient may take drug with milk or meals.

• Tell patient that full therapeutic effect may be delayed for 2 to 4 weeks.
• Serious GI toxicity, including peptic ulceration and bleeding, can occur in patient taking NSAIDs despite absence of GI symptoms. Teach patient signs and symptoms of GI bleeding, and tell him to notify doctor immediately if they occur.
• Alert patient that use with aspirin, alcohol, or corticosteroids may increase risk of adverse GI reactions.
• Warn patient to avoid hazardous activities that require mental alertness until CNS effects are known.
• Because drug has been associated with photosensitivity reactions, advise patient to use a sunblock, wear protective clothing, and avoid prolonged exposure to sunlight.
• Instruct patient to report visual or auditory adverse reactions immediately.

---

## ketorolac tromethamine
Toradol

*Pregnancy Risk Category C*

## HOW SUPPLIED
*Tablets:* 10 mg
*Injection:* 15 mg/ml, 30 mg/ml

## ACTION
Unknown. Thought to inhibit prostaglandin synthesis.

| Route | Onset | Peak | Duration |
|-------|-------|------|----------|
| P.O. | 0.5-1 hr | 0.5-1 hr | 6-8 hr |
| I.V. | Immediate | Immediate | 6-8 hr |
| I.M. | 10 min | 0.5-1 hr | 6-8 hr |

## INDICATIONS & DOSAGE
*Short-term management of moderately severe, acute pain for single-dose treatment—*
**Adults:** in patients under age 65, 60 mg I.M. or 30 mg I.V.
**Elderly:** in patients ages 65 and older, 30 mg I.M. or 15 mg I.V.
*Adjust-a-dose:* For renally impaired patients or those weighing below 50 kg (110 lb), 30 mg I.M. or 15 mg I.V.

---

Reactions may be **common**, uncommon, *life-threatening*, or COMMON AND LIFE-THREATENING.

*Short-term management of moderately severe, acute pain for multiple-dose treatment—*
**Adults:** for patients under age 65, 30 mg I.M. or I.V. q 6 hours. Maximum daily dose is 120 mg.
**Elderly:** for patients ages 65 and older, 15 mg I.M. or I.V. q 6 hours. Maximum daily dose is 60 mg.
*Adjust-a-dose:* For renally impaired patients or those weighing below 50 kg (110 lb), 15 mg I.M. or I.V. q 6 hours. Maximum daily dose is 60 mg.
*Short-term management of moderately severe, acute pain when switching from parenteral to oral administration (oral therapy is indicated only as continuation of parenterally administered drug and should never be given without patient first having received parenteral therapy)—*
**Adults:** for patients under age 65, 20 mg P.O. as single dose; then 10 mg P.O. q 4 to 6 hours. Maximum daily dose is 40 mg.
**Elderly:** for patients ages 65 and older, 10 mg P.O. as single dose; then 10 mg P.O. q 4 to 6 hours. Maximum daily dose is 40 mg.
*Adjust-a-dose:* For renally impaired patients or those weighing below 50 kg (110 lb), 10 mg P.O. as single dose; then 10 mg P.O. q 4 to 6 hours. Maximum daily dose is 40 mg.

## ADVERSE REACTIONS
**CNS:** drowsiness, sedation, dizziness, headache.
**CV:** edema, hypertension, palpitations, ***arrhythmias.***
**GI:** *nausea, dyspepsia, GI pain,* diarrhea, ***peptic ulceration,*** vomiting, constipation, flatulence, stomatitis.
**Hematologic:** decreased platelet adhesion, purpura, prolonged bleeding time.
**Hepatic:** elevated liver function tests.
**Skin:** pruritus, rash, diaphoresis.
**Other:** pain at injection site.

## INTERACTIONS
**Drug-drug.** *ACE inhibitors:* may increase risk of renal impairment, particularly in volume-depleted patients. Don't use together in volume-depleted patients.
*Anticoagulants, salicylates:* ketorolac may increase levels of free (unbound) sal-

icylates or anticoagulants in the blood. Use with extreme caution and monitor patient closely.
*Antihypertensives, diuretics:* decreased effectiveness. Monitor patient closely.
*Lithium:* increased lithium levels. Monitor patient closely.
*Methotrexate:* decreased methotrexate clearance and increased toxicity. Don't use together.

## EFFECTS ON DIAGNOSTIC TESTS
None reported.

## CONTRAINDICATIONS
Contraindicated in patients with hypersensitivity to drug and in those with active peptic ulcer disease, recent GI bleeding or perforation, advanced renal impairment, risk for renal impairment due to volume depletion, suspected or confirmed cerebrovascular bleeding, hemorrhagic diathesis, incomplete hemostasis, or high risk of bleeding. Also contraindicated in patients with history of peptic ulcer disease or GI bleeding, past allergic manifestations to aspirin or other NSAIDs, and during labor and delivery or breast-feeding. Also contraindicated as prophylactic analgesic before major surgery or intraoperatively when hemostasis is critical; and in patients currently receiving aspirin, an NSAID, or probenecid. Don't administer drug epidurally or intrathecally because of alcohol content.

## NURSING CONSIDERATIONS
● Use of ketorolac isn't recommended in children.
● Use cautiously in patients with hepatic or renal impairment.
● *Alert:* The maximum combined duration of therapy (parenteral and oral) must be limited to 5 days.
● I.M. administration may cause pain at the injection site. Holding pressure over the site for 15 to 30 seconds after the injection may minimize local effects. Give deep I.M.
● Carefully observe patients with coagulopathies and those taking anticoagulants. Ketorolac inhibits platelet aggregation and can prolong bleeding time. This effect will disappear within 48 hours of discon-

tinuing drug. It won't alter platelet count, INR, PTT, or PT.
• NSAIDs may mask signs and symptoms of infection because of their antipyretic and anti-inflammatory actions.
• *Alert:* Don't confuse Toradol with Tegretol.

## I.V. administration
• Don't mix with morphine sulfate, meperidine hydrochloride, promethazine hydrochloride, or hydroxyzine hydrochloride. Ketorolac will precipitate out in solution.
• Dilute with normal saline, 5% dextrose, 5% dextrose and normal saline, Ringer's, lactated Ringer's, or Plasma-Lyte A.
• Give I.V. injection in no less than 15 seconds.

## Patient teaching
• Warn patient receiving drug I.M. that pain may occur at injection site.
• Serious GI toxicity, including peptic ulceration and bleeding, can occur in patient taking NSAIDs despite absence of GI symptoms. Teach patient signs and symptoms of GI bleeding, and tell him to notify doctor immediately if they occur.

---

## nabumetone
Relafen, Relifex§

*Pregnancy Risk Category C*

## HOW SUPPLIED
*Tablets:* 500 mg, 750 mg

## ACTION
Unknown. Probably acts by inhibiting prostaglandin synthesis.

| Route | Onset | Peak | Duration |
|-------|---------|--------|----------|
| P.O. | Unknown | 2-4 hr | Unknown |

## INDICATIONS & DOSAGE
*Rheumatoid arthritis, osteoarthritis—*
**Adults:** initially, 1,000 mg P.O. daily as a single dose or in divided doses b.i.d. Maximum daily dose is 2,000 mg.

## ADVERSE REACTIONS
**CNS:** dizziness, headache, fatigue, insomnia, nervousness, somnolence.
**CV:** vasculitis, edema.
**EENT:** tinnitus.
**GI:** *diarrhea, dyspepsia, abdominal pain,* constipation, flatulence, nausea, dry mouth, gastritis, stomatitis, anorexia, vomiting, ***bleeding,*** ulceration.
**Respiratory:** dyspnea, pneumonitis.
**Skin:** pruritus, rash, increased diaphoresis.

## INTERACTIONS
**Drug-drug.** *Diuretics:* NSAIDs may decrease diuretic effectiveness. Monitor patients closely during therapy.
*Warfarin, other highly protein-bound drugs,:* increased risk of adverse effects from displacement of drugs by nabumetone. Use together cautiously.
**Drug-food.** *Any food:* increased absorption. Give drug with food.
**Drug-lifestyle.** *Alcohol use:* associated with an increased risk of additive GI toxicity. Avoid concomitant use.

## EFFECTS ON DIAGNOSTIC TESTS
None reported.

## CONTRAINDICATIONS
Contraindicated in patients with hypersensitivity reactions and history of aspirin- or NSAID-induced asthma, urticaria, or other allergic-type reactions.

## NURSING CONSIDERATIONS
• Use cautiously in patients with renal or hepatic impairment; heart failure, hypertension, or other conditions that may predispose patient to fluid retention; and in patients with history of peptic ulcer disease.
• Use of drug isn't recommended during third trimester of pregnancy.
• Because NSAIDs impair the synthesis of renal prostaglandins, they can decrease renal blood flow and lead to reversible renal impairment, especially in patients with preexisting renal failure, liver dysfunction, or heart failure; in elderly patients; and in those taking diuretics. Monitor these patients closely during therapy.

---

Reactions may be *common*, uncommon, ***life-threatening***, OR **COMMON AND LIFE-THREATENING**.

• During long-term therapy, periodically monitor renal and liver function, CBC, and hematocrit as ordered; assess patients for signs and symptoms of GI bleeding.
• Drug isn't recommended for use in children.

✓ **Patient teaching**
• Instruct patient to take drug with food, milk, or antacids. Drug is absorbed more rapidly when taken with food or milk.
• Advise patient to limit alcohol intake because of additive GI toxicity risk.
• Serious GI toxicity, including peptic ulceration and bleeding, can occur in patient taking NSAIDs despite absence of GI symptoms. Teach patient signs and symptoms of GI bleeding and tell him to notify doctor immediately if they occur.
• Warn patient against hazardous activities that require mental alertness until CNS effects are known.

---

## naproxen

Apo-Naproxen†, EC-Naprosyn, Naprosyn, Naprosyn-E†, Naprosyn-SR, Naxen†, Novo-Naprox†, Nu-Naprox†, Nycopren§

## naproxen sodium

Aleve ◇, Anaprox, Anaprox DS, Apo-Napro-Na†, Naprelan, Naprogesic‡, Novo-Naprox Sodium†, Synflex†

*Pregnancy Risk Category B*

### HOW SUPPLIED
**naproxen**
*Tablets:* 250 mg, 375 mg, 500 mg
*Tablets (delayed-release):* 375 mg, 500 mg
*Tablets (extended-release):* 750 mg, 1,000 mg
*Oral suspension:* 125 mg/5 ml
*Suppositories:* 500 mg‡
**naproxen sodium**
*Tablets (controlled-release):* 421.5 mg, 550 mg
*Tablets (film-coated):* 220 mg ◇, 275 mg, 550 mg
*Note:* 275 mg of naproxen sodium contains 250 mg of naproxen.

### ACTION
Unknown. Produces anti-inflammatory, analgesic, and antipyretic effects, possibly by inhibiting prostaglandin synthesis.

| Route | Onset | Peak | Duration |
|-------|-------|------|----------|
| P.O. | 1 hr | 2-4 hr | 7 hr |
| P.R. | Unknown | Unknown | Unknown |

### INDICATIONS & DOSAGE
*Rheumatoid arthritis, osteoarthritis, ankylosing spondylitis, pain, dysmenorrhea, tendinitis, bursitis—*
**Adults:** 250 to 500 mg (naproxen) b.i.d.; maximum is 1.5 g daily for a limited time. Or, 375 to 500 mg delayed-release (EC-Naprosyn) b.i.d.; or 750 to 1,000 mg controlled-release (Naprelan) daily; or 275 to 550 mg naproxen sodium b.i.d.
*Juvenile arthritis*
**Children:** 10 mg/kg P.O. in two divided doses.
*Acute gout—*
**Adults:** 750 mg (naproxen) P.O.; then 250 mg q 8 hours until attack subsides. Or, 825 mg naproxen sodium; then 275 mg q 8 hours until attack subsides. Or, 1,000 to 1,500 mg/day controlled-release (Naprelan) on first day; then 1,000 mg daily until attack subsides.
*Mild to moderate pain, primary dysmenorrhea—*
**Adults:** 500 mg (naproxen) P.O.; then 250 mg q 6 to 8 hours up to 1.25 g/day. Or, 550 mg naproxen sodium; then 275 mg q 6 to 8 hours up to 1,375 mg/day. Or, 1,000 mg controlled-release (Naprelan) once daily.
**Elderly:** for patients over age 65, don't exceed 400 mg/day.

### ADVERSE REACTIONS
**CNS:** headache, drowsiness, dizziness, vertigo.
**CV:** edema, palpitations.
**EENT:** visual disturbances, *tinnitus,* auditory disturbances.
**GI:** epigastric distress, occult blood loss, nausea, *peptic ulceration,* constipation, dyspepsia, heartburn, diarrhea, stomatitis, thirst.
**GU:** elevated BUN and creatinine levels.
**Hematologic:** increased bleeding time.
**Hepatic:** elevated liver enzyme levels.

---

*Liquid contains alcohol. **May contain tartrazine. †Canada ‡Australia §U.K. ◇OTC

**Metabolic:** hyperkalemia.
**Respiratory:** dyspnea.
**Skin:** pruritus, rash, urticaria, ecchymosis, diaphoresis, purpura.

## INTERACTIONS
**Drug-drug:** *ACE inhibitors:* may increase risk of renal impairment. Use together cautiously.
*Antihypertensives, diuretics:* decreased effect of these drugs. Monitor patient closely.
*Aspirin, corticosteroids:* increased risk of adverse GI reactions. Avoid concomitant use.
*Methotrexate:* increased risk of toxicity. Monitor patient closely.
*Oral anticoagulants, other sulfonylureas, highly protein-bound drugs:* increased risk of toxicity. Monitor patient closely.
*Probenecid:* decreased elimination of naproxen. Monitor for toxicity.
**Drug-lifestyle.** *Alcohol use:* increased risk of adverse GI reactions. Avoid concomitant use.

## EFFECTS ON DIAGNOSTIC TESTS
Drug and its metabolite may interfere with urinary 5-hydroxyindoleacetic acid and 17-hydroxycorticosteroid determinations.

## CONTRAINDICATIONS
Contraindicated in patients with hypersensitivity to drug and in those with the syndrome of asthma, rhinitis, and nasal polyps.

## NURSING CONSIDERATIONS
• Use cautiously in elderly patients and in patients with renal disease, CV disease, GI disorders, hepatic disease, or a history of peptic ulcer disease.
• Drug should be avoided during last trimester of pregnancy.
• Because NSAIDs impair synthesis of renal prostaglandins, they can decrease renal blood flow and lead to reversible renal impairment, especially in patients with preexisting renal failure, liver dysfunction, or heart failure; in elderly patients; and in those taking diuretics. Monitor these patients closely during therapy.

• Monitor CBC and renal and hepatic function every 4 to 6 months or as indicated and ordered during long-term therapy.
• Because of their antipyretic and anti-inflammatory actions, NSAIDs may mask signs and symptoms of infection.

☑ **Patient teaching**
• *Alert:* Drug is available OTC (naproxen sodium, 200 mg). Instruct patient not to exceed 600 mg in 24 hours. Dosage in patient over age 65 shouldn't exceed 400 mg/day.
• Advise patient to take drug with food or milk to minimize GI upset. A full glass of water or other liquid should be taken with each dose.
• Tell patient taking prescription doses of naproxen for arthritis that full therapeutic effect may be delayed 2 to 4 weeks.
• Warn patient against taking both naproxen and naproxen sodium at the same time because both circulate in the blood as the naproxen anion.
• Serious GI toxicity, including peptic ulceration and bleeding, can occur in patient taking NSAIDs despite absence of GI symptoms. Teach patient signs and symptoms of GI bleeding and tell him to notify doctor immediately if they occur.
• Caution patient that use with aspirin, alcohol, or corticosteroids may increase risk of adverse GI reactions.
• Warn patient against hazardous activities that require mental alertness until CNS effects are known.

---

**oxaprozin**
Daypro

*Pregnancy Risk Category C*

## HOW SUPPLIED
*Caplets:* 600 mg

## ACTION
Unknown. Produces anti-inflammatory, analgesic, and antipyretic effects, possibly by inhibiting prostaglandin synthesis.

| Route | Onset | Peak | Duration |
|-------|-------|------|----------|
| P.O. | Unknown | 3-5 hr | Unknown |

## INDICATIONS & DOSAGE
*Osteoarthritis, rheumatoid arthritis—*
**Adults:** initially, 1,200 mg P.O. daily.
Then, individualized to smallest effective
dose to minimize adverse reactions.
Smaller patients or those with mild symptoms may need only 600 mg daily. Maximum is 1,800 mg or 26 mg/kg, whichever
is lower, in divided doses.

## ADVERSE REACTIONS
**CNS:** depression, sedation, somnolence,
confusion, sleep disturbances.
**EENT:** tinnitus, blurred vision.
**GI:** nausea, dyspepsia, diarrhea, constipation, abdominal pain or distress, anorexia,
flatulence, vomiting, ***hemorrhage,*** stomatitis.
**GU:** dysuria, urinary frequency.
**Hematologic:** prolonged bleeding time,
anemia.
**Hepatic:** elevated liver function test results with long-term use; severe hepatic
dysfunction (rare).
**Skin:** *rash,* photosensitivity.

## INTERACTIONS
**Drug-drug.** *Antihypertensives, diuretics:*
decreased effect. Monitor patient closely
and adjust dosage, as ordered.
*Aspirin:* oxaprozin displaces salicylates
from plasma protein-binding sites, increasing risk of salicylate toxicity. Avoid
concomitant use.
*Aspirin, corticosteroids:* increased risk of
adverse GI reactions. Avoid concomitant
use.
*Cyclosporine:* nephrotoxicity may be increased. Avoid use together.
*Lithium, phenytoin:* serum levels of these
drugs may be increased. Avoid concomitant use.
*Methotrexate:* increased risk of methotrexate toxicity. Avoid concomitant use.
*Oral anticoagulants:* although problems
haven't been reported, there is an increased risk of bleeding. Use together
cautiously.
**Drug-lifestyle.** *Alcohol use:* increased
risk of adverse GI reactions. Avoid concomitant use.
*Sun exposure:* photosensitivity reactions
may occur. Take precautions.

## EFFECTS ON DIAGNOSTIC TESTS
None reported.

## CONTRAINDICATIONS
Contraindicated in patients with hypersensitivity to drug and in those with the
syndrome of nasal polyps, angioedema,
and bronchospastic reaction to aspirin or
other NSAIDs.

## NURSING CONSIDERATIONS
• Use cautiously in patients with history
of peptic ulcer disease, hepatic or renal
dysfunction, hypertension, CV disease, or
conditions predisposing patient to fluid
retention.
• Because renal prostaglandins play a role
in the maintenance of renal perfusion, patients with preexisting conditions leading
to a reduction in renal blood flow may experience renal toxicity with NSAID therapy. Patients at greatest risk are the elderly,
those taking diuretics, and those with impaired renal, hepatic, or cardiac function.
Closely monitor renal function in these
patients, and discontinue NSAID therapy
if problems develop.
• Elevations of liver function test results
can occur after long-term use. These abnormal findings may persist, worsen, or
resolve with continued therapy. Rarely,
patients may progress to severe hepatic
dysfunction. Periodically monitor liver
function tests in patients receiving longterm therapy, and closely monitor patients
with abnormal test results.
• Because of their antipyretic and antiinflammatory actions, NSAIDs may mask
signs and symptoms of infection.
• *Alert:* Don't confuse oxaprozin with oxazepam.

### ✓ Patient teaching
• Tell patient to take drug 30 minutes before or 2 hours after meals. If adverse GI
reactions occur, drug may be taken with
milk or meals.
• Inform patient that full therapeutic effects may be delayed for 2 to 4 weeks.
• Serious GI toxicity, including peptic ulceration and bleeding, can occur in patient taking NSAIDs despite absence of
GI symptoms. Teach patient signs and

---

symptoms of GI bleeding and tell him to notify doctor immediately if they occur.
• Tell patient to report adverse visual or auditory reactions immediately.
• Warn patient against hazardous activities that require mental alertness until CNS effects are known.
• Because drug has been associated with photosensitivity reactions, advise patient to use a sunblock, wear protective clothing, and avoid prolonged exposure to sunlight.

## piroxicam
Apo-Piroxicam†, Feldene, Novo-Pirocam†, Pirox‡

*Pregnancy Risk Category B (D in third trimester or near delivery)*

### HOW SUPPLIED
*Capsules:* 10 mg, 20 mg

### ACTION
Unknown. Produces anti-inflammatory, analgesic, and antipyretic effects, possibly by inhibiting prostaglandin synthesis.

| Route | Onset | Peak | Duration |
|-------|-------|------|----------|
| P.O. | 1 hr | 3-5 hr | 48-72 hr |

### INDICATIONS & DOSAGE
*Osteoarthritis, rheumatoid arthritis—*
**Adults:** 20 mg P.O. daily. If desired, dose may be divided b.i.d.

### ADVERSE REACTIONS
**CNS:** headache, drowsiness, dizziness, somnolence, vertigo.
**CV:** peripheral edema.
**EENT:** auditory disturbances.
**GI:** epigastric distress, nausea, occult blood loss, *peptic ulceration, severe GI bleeding,* diarrhea, constipation, abdominal pain, dyspepsia, flatulence, anorexia, stomatitis.
**GU:** *nephrotoxicity,* elevated BUN and creatinine levels.
**Hematologic:** prolonged bleeding time, anemia, *leukopenia, agranulocytosis,* eosinophilia.
**Hepatic:** elevated liver enzymes.
**Metabolic:** hyperkalemia, hypoglycemia in diabetic patients.

**Respiratory:** *bronchospasm.*
**Skin:** pruritus, rash, urticaria, *photosensitivity.*

### INTERACTIONS
**Drug-drug.** *Antihypertensives, diuretics:* decreased effects. Avoid use together.
*Aspirin, corticosteroids:* increased risk of GI toxicity. Decreased plasma levels of piroxicam. Avoid concomitant use.
*Cyclosporine, methotrexate:* increased toxicity. Monitor patient closely.
*Lithium:* increased plasma lithium levels. Monitor for toxicity.
*Oral anticoagulants, other highly protein-bound drugs:* increased risk of toxicity. Monitor patient closely.
*Oral antidiabetics:* enhanced antidiabetic effects. Monitor patient closely.
**Drug-lifestyle.** *Alcohol use:* increased risk of GI toxicity. Decreased plasma levels of piroxicam. Avoid concomitant use.
*Sun exposure:* photosensitivity reactions may occur. Take precautions.

### EFFECTS ON DIAGNOSTIC TESTS
None reported.

### CONTRAINDICATIONS
Contraindicated in patients with hypersensitivity to drug and in those with bronchospasm or angioedema precipitated by aspirin or NSAIDs. Also contraindicated in pregnant or breast-feeding women.

### NURSING CONSIDERATIONS
• Use cautiously in elderly patients and in patients with GI disorders, history of renal or peptic ulcer disease, cardiac disease, hypertension, or conditions predisposing to fluid retention.
• Because NSAIDs impair the synthesis of renal prostaglandins, they can decrease renal blood flow and lead to reversible renal impairment, especially in the elderly; patients with preexisting renal failure, liver dysfunction, or heart failure; and in those taking diuretics. Monitor closely.
• Check renal, hepatic, and auditory function and CBC periodically during prolonged therapy. Discontinue drug if abnormalities occur and notify doctor.

• NSAIDs may mask signs and symptoms of infection because of their antipyretic and anti-inflammatory actions.

☑ **Patient teaching**
• Tell patient to take drug with milk, antacids, or meals if GI adverse reactions occur.
• Inform patient that full therapeutic effects may be delayed for 2 to 4 weeks.
• Serious GI toxicity, including peptic ulceration and bleeding, can occur in patient taking NSAIDs despite absence of GI symptoms. Teach patient signs and symptoms of GI bleeding and tell him when to report them to doctor.
• Warn patient against hazardous activities that require mental alertness until CNS effects are known.
• Because drug causes adverse skin reactions more often than other drugs in its class, advise patient to use a sunblock, wear protective clothing, and avoid prolonged exposure to sunlight. Photosensitivity reactions are the most common.

✳ *NEW DRUG*

## rofecoxib
Vioxx

*Pregnancy Risk Category C*

### HOW SUPPLIED
*Tablets:* 12.5 mg, 25 mg
*Oral suspension:* 12.5 mg/5 ml, 25 mg/5 ml

### ACTION
Unknown. Produces anti-inflammatory, analgesic, and antipyretic effects, possibly by inhibiting prostaglandin synthesis.

| Route | Onset | Peak | Duration |
|-------|-------|------|----------|
| P.O. | Unknown | 2-3 hr | Unknown |

### INDICATIONS & DOSAGE
*Relief of signs and symptoms of osteoarthritis—*
**Adults:** initially, 12.5 mg P.O. once daily, increased, p.r.n., to maximum of 25 mg P.O. once daily.

*Management of acute pain, treatment of primary dysmenorrhea—*
**Adults:** 50 mg P.O. once daily, p.r.n., for up to 5 days.

### ADVERSE REACTIONS
**CNS:** headache, asthenia, fatigue, dizziness.
**CV:** hypertension, lower-extremity edema.
**EENT:** sinusitis.
**GI:** diarrhea, dyspepsia, epigastric discomfort, heartburn, nausea, abdominal pain.
**GU:** urinary tract infection.
**Musculoskeletal:** back pain.
**Respiratory:** bronchitis, upper respiratory tract infection.
**Other:** flulike syndrome.

### INTERACTIONS
**Drug-drug.** *ACE inhibitors:* decreased antihypertensive effects of ACE inhibitors. Monitor patient closely.
*Aspirin:* increased rate of GI ulceration and other complications. Don't use together, if possible. If used together, monitor patient closely for GI bleeding.
*Furosemide, thiazide diuretics:* potentially reduced efficacy of these drugs. Monitor patient closely.
*Lithium:* increased plasma lithium levels and decreased lithium clearance. Monitor patient closely for toxic reaction to lithium.
*Methotrexate:* increased plasma methotrexate levels. Monitor patient closely for toxic reaction to methotrexate.
*Rifampin:* decreased rofecoxib levels by about 50%. Initiate therapy with a higher dosage of rofecoxib.
*Warfarin:* increased effects of warfarin. Monitor INR more frequently in the first few days after therapy is initiated or dosage is changed.
**Drug-lifestyle.** *Long-term alcohol use, smoking:* increased risk of GI bleeding. Monitor patient closely for such bleeding.

### EFFECTS ON DIAGNOSTIC TESTS
None reported.

### CONTRAINDICATIONS
Contraindicated in patients with hypersensitivity to drug or its components and

in those who have experienced asthma, urticaria, or allergy-type reactions after taking aspirin or other NSAIDs. Also contraindicated in patients with advanced kidney disease or moderate or severe hepatic insufficiency, and in pregnant women because drug may cause ductus arteriosus to close prematurely.

## NURSING CONSIDERATIONS
• *Alert:* NSAIDs may cause serious GI toxicity. Signs and symptoms include bleeding, ulceration, and perforation of the stomach, small intestine, and large intestine. Such toxicity can occur any time, with or without warning. To minimize risk of an adverse GI event, use lowest effective dosage for the shortest possible duration. Monitor patient closely for GI bleeding.
• Use cautiously in patients with history of ulcer disease or GI bleeding and in those taking such drugs as oral corticosteroids and anticoagulants. Also use cautiously in patients with conditions, such as older age, alcoholism, poor general health status, and addiction to smoking, that may increase risk of GI bleeding.
• Use cautiously in patients who are considerably dehydrated. Rehydration is recommended before therapy begins.
• In patients with fluid retention, hypertension, or heart failure, use cautiously and initiate therapy at the lowest recommended dosage. Monitor blood pressure and check patient for fluid retention or worsening heart failure.
• In patients over age 65, initiate therapy at the lowest recommended dosage.
• Patient may be allergic to drug if he has an allergy to aspirin or other NSAIDs.
• Drug may be hepatotoxic. Monitor patient for signs and symptoms of liver toxicity. Drug should be discontinued, as ordered, if signs and symptoms consistent with liver disease develop.
• Oral suspension should be shaken well before it's administered.
• Patients undergoing long-term treatment should have their hemoglobin level and hematocrit checked if they experience signs or symptoms of anemia or blood loss.

☑ **Patient teaching**
• Warn patient that he may experience signs and symptoms of GI bleeding, including bloody vomitus, blood in urine and stool, and black, tarry stools. Advise patient to call doctor if he experiences these signs or symptoms.
• Advise patient to report rash, unexplained weight gain, or edema.
• Tell patient to avoid aspirin and aspirin-containing products unless doctor has instructed him otherwise.
• Inform patient to avoid OTC anti-inflammatories such as ibuprofen (Advil) unless doctor has instructed him otherwise.
• Tell patient that all NSAIDs, including rofecoxib, may adversely affect the liver. Signs and symptoms of liver toxicity include nausea, fatigue, lethargy, itching, jaundice, right upper quadrant tenderness, and flulike syndrome. Advise him to stop therapy and call doctor immediately if he experiences these signs or symptoms.
• Instruct woman to inform doctor if she becomes pregnant or is planning to become pregnant while taking drug.
• Tell patient that drug may be taken without regard to food, although taking it with food may decrease GI upset.
• Tell patient that the most common adverse effects of drug are dyspepsia, epigastric discomfort, heartburn, and nausea. Tell him that taking drug with food may help minimize these effects.

## sulindac
Aclin‡, Apo-Sulin†, Clinoril, Novo-Sundac†, Saldac‡

*Pregnancy Risk Category NR*

## HOW SUPPLIED
*Tablets:* 100 mg‡, 150 mg, 200 mg

## ACTION
Produces anti-inflammatory, analgesic, and antipyretic effects, possibly by inhibiting prostaglandin synthesis.

| Route | Onset | Peak | Duration |
|-------|-------|------|----------|
| P.O. | Unknown | 2-4 hr | Unknown |

## INDICATIONS & DOSAGE
*Osteoarthritis, rheumatoid arthritis, ankylosing spondylitis—*
**Adults:** initially, 150 mg P.O. b.i.d.; increased to 200 mg b.i.d., p.r.n. Maximum dose is 400 mg daily.
*Acute subacromial bursitis or supraspinatus tendinitis, acute gouty arthritis—*
**Adults:** 200 mg P.O. b.i.d. for 7 to 14 days. Dosage reduced as symptoms subside. Maximum dose is 400 mg daily.

## ADVERSE REACTIONS
**CNS:** dizziness, headache, nervousness, psychosis.
**CV:** hypertension, *heart failure,* palpitations, edema.
**EENT:** tinnitus, transient visual disturbances.
**GI:** *epigastric distress, peptic ulceration,* occult blood loss, nausea, constipation, dyspepsia, flatulence, anorexia, *GI bleeding.*
**GU:** interstitial nephritis, increased BUN and serum creatinine levels.
**Hematologic:** prolonged bleeding time.
**Hepatic:** increased serum alkaline phosphatase and transaminase levels.
**Metabolic:** hyperkalemia.
**Skin:** rash, pruritus.
**Other:** drug fever, *anaphylaxis, angioedema, hypersensitivity syndrome.*

## INTERACTIONS
**Drug-drug.** *Anticoagulants:* increased risk of bleeding. Monitor PT and INR closely.
*Aspirin:* decreased sulindac plasma level and increased risk of GI adverse reactions. Don't use together.
*Cyclosporine:* increased nephrotoxicity of cyclosporine. Avoid concomitant use.
*Diflunisal, dimethyl sulfoxide:* decreased metabolism of sulindac to its active metabolite, reducing its effectiveness. Don't use together.
*Methotrexate:* increased methotrexate toxicity. Avoid concomitant use.
*Sulfonamides, sulfonylureas, other highly protein-bound drugs:* possible displacement of these drugs from plasma protein-binding sites, leading to increased toxicity. Monitor closely.

*Probenecid:* increased plasma levels of sulindac and its active metabolite. Monitor for toxicity.

## EFFECTS ON DIAGNOSTIC TESTS
None reported.

## CONTRAINDICATIONS
Contraindicated in patients with hypersensitivity to drug and in those in whom acute asthmatic attacks, urticaria, or rhinitis is precipitated by aspirin or NSAIDs.

## NURSING CONSIDERATIONS
● Use cautiously in patients with a history of ulcers and GI bleeding, renal dysfunction, compromised cardiac function, hypertension, or conditions predisposing to fluid retention.
● Use of drug in pregnant women isn't recommended.
● Periodically monitor hepatic and renal function and CBC in patients receiving long-term therapy, as ordered.
● NSAIDs may mask signs and symptoms of infection.

### ✓ Patient teaching
● Tell patient to take drug with food, milk, or antacids.
● Serious GI toxicity, including peptic ulceration and bleeding, can occur in patient taking NSAIDs despite the absence of GI symptoms. Teach patient signs and symptoms of GI bleeding, including fatigue, weakness, black tarry stool, coffee ground emesis, and tell him to contact doctor immediately if they occur.
● *Alert:* Tell patient to notify doctor immediately if easy bruising or prolonged bleeding occurs.
● Advise patient to avoid hazardous activities that require mental alertness until CNS effects are known.
● Instruct patient to report edema and have blood pressure checked monthly. Drug causes sodium retention but is thought to have less effect on the kidneys than do other NSAIDs.
● Advise patient to notify doctor and have complete eye examination if visual disturbances occur.

---

*Liquid contains alcohol.    **May contain tartrazine.    †Canada    ‡Australia    §U.K.    ◊OTC

alfentanil hydrochloride
buprenorphine hydrochloride
butorphanol tartrate
codeine phosphate
codeine sulfate
fentanyl citrate
fentanyl transdermal system
fentanyl transmucosal
hydromorphone hydrochloride
meperidine hydrochloride
methadone hydrochloride
morphine hydrochloride
morphine sulfate
morphine tartrate
nalbuphine hydrochloride
oxycodone hydrochloride
oxycodone pectinate
oxymorphone hydrochloride
pentazocine hydrochloride
pentazocine hydrochloride and
    naloxone hydrochloride
pentazocine lactate
propoxyphene hydrochloride
propoxyphene napsylate
remifentanil hydrochloride
sufentanil citrate
tramadol hydrochloride

## COMBINATION PRODUCTS

222†: aspirin 375 mg, codeine phosphate 8 mg, and caffeine citrate 30 mg.

282 MEP†: aspirin 375 mg, codeine phosphate 15 mg, and caffeine citrate 30 mg.

292†: aspirin 375 mg, codeine phosphate 30 mg, and caffeine citrate 30 mg.

293†: aspirin 375 mg, codeine phosphate 30 mg, codeine phosphate (slow-release) 30 mg, and caffeine citrate 30 mg.

692†: aspirin 375 mg, propoxyphene hydrochloride 65 mg, and caffeine 30 mg.

A.C. & C.†: aspirin 375 mg, codeine phosphate 8 mg, and caffeine 30 mg.

ACETA WITH CODEINE, EMPRACET-30†, EMTEC-30†: acetaminophen 300 mg and codeine phosphate 30 mg.

ANACIN WITH CODEINE†: aspirin 325 mg, codeine phosphate 8 mg, and caffeine 32 mg.

ANCASAL 8†, C2 WITH CODEINE†: aspirin 375 mg, codeine phosphate 8 mg, and caffeine 15 mg.

ANEXSIA 5/500: hydrocodone bitartrate 5 mg, acetaminophen 500 mg.

CAPITAL WITH CODEINE, TYLENOL WITH CODEINE ELIXIR*: acetaminophen 120 mg and codeine phosphate 12 mg/5 ml.

DARVOCET-N 50: acetaminophen 325 mg and propoxyphene napsylate 50 mg.

DARVOCET-N 100, PROPACET 100: acetaminophen 650 mg and propoxyphene napsylate 100 mg.

DARVON COMPOUND-65†: aspirin 389 mg, propoxyphene hydrochloride 65 mg, and caffeine 32.4 mg.

DARVON-N COMPOUND†: aspirin 375 mg, propoxyphene napsylate 100 mg, and caffeine 30 mg.

DARVON-N WITH A.S.A.†: aspirin 325 mg and propoxyphene napsylate 100 mg.

DARVON WITH A.S.A.†: aspirin 325 mg and propoxyphene hydrochloride 65 mg.

E-LOR, WYGESIC: acetaminophen 650 mg and propoxyphene hydrochloride 65 mg.

EMPIRIN WITH CODEINE NO. 3, PHENAPHEN WITH CODEINE NO. 3: aspirin 325 mg and codeine phosphate 30 mg.

EMPIRIN WITH CODEINE NO. 4, PHENAPHEN WITH CODEINE NO. 4: aspirin 325 mg and codeine phosphate 60 mg.

EMPRACET-60†: acetaminophen 300 mg and codeine phosphate 60 mg.

ENDOCET, OXYCOCET†, PERCOCET, ROXICET: acetaminophen 325 mg and oxycodone hydrochloride 5 mg.

ENDODAN†, OXYCODAN†, PERCODAN†: aspirin 325 mg and oxycodone hydrochloride 5 mg.

FIORICET WITH CODEINE: acetaminophen 325 mg, butalbital 50 mg, caffeine 40 mg, and codeine phosphate 30 mg.

FIORINAL WITH CODEINE: aspirin 325 mg, butalbital 50 mg, caffeine 40 mg, and codeine 30 mg.

INNOVAR: droperidol 2.5 mg and fentanyl citrate 0.05 mg/ml.

LENOLTEC WITH CODEINE NO. 1†, LORCET 10/650: acetaminophen 650 mg and hydrocodone bitartrate 10 mg.
LORCET PLUS: acetaminophen 650 mg, hydrocodone bitartrate 7.5 mg
LORTAB 2.5/500: acetaminophen 500 mg and hydrocodone bitartrate 2.5 mg.
LORTAB 5/500: acetaminophen 500 mg and hydrocodone bitartrate 5 mg.
LORTAB 7.5/500: acetaminophen 500 mg and hydrocodone bitartrate 7.5 mg.
NOVO-GESIC C8†: acetaminophen 300 mg, codeine phosphate 8 mg, and caffeine 15 mg.
PERCODAN-DEMI: aspirin 325 mg, oxycodone hydrochloride 2.25 mg, and oxycodone terephthalate 0.19 mg.
PERCODAN-DEMI†: aspirin 325 mg and oxycodone hydrochloride 2.5 mg.
PERCODAN, ROXIPRIN: aspirin 325 mg, oxycodone hydrochloride 4.5 mg, and oxycodone terephthalate 0.38 mg.
ROUNOX AND CODEINE 15†: acetaminophen 325 mg and codeine phosphate 15 mg.
ROUNOX AND CODEINE 30†: acetaminophen 325 mg and codeine phosphate 30 mg.
ROUNOX AND CODEINE 60†: acetaminophen 325 mg and codeine phosphate 60 mg.
ROXICET 5/500, TYLOX: acetaminophen 500 mg and oxycodone hydrochloride 5 mg.
ROXICET ORAL SOLUTION*: acetaminophen 325 mg and oxycodone hydrochloride 5 mg/5 ml.
TALACEN: acetaminophen 650 mg and pentazocine hydrochloride 25 mg.
TALWIN COMPOUND: aspirin 325 mg and pentazocine hydrochloride 12.5 mg.
TYLENOL WITH CODEINE NO. 1: acetaminophen 300 mg and codeine phosphate 7.5 mg.
TYLENOL WITH CODEINE NO. 2: acetaminophen 300 mg and codeine phosphate 15 mg.
TYLENOL WITH CODEINE NO. 3: acetaminophen 300 mg and codeine phosphate 30 mg.
TYLENOL WITH CODEINE NO. 4: acetaminophen 300 mg and codeine phosphate 60 mg.
VICODIN: acetaminophen 500 mg and hydrocodone bitartrate 5 mg.
VICODIN ES: acetaminophen 750 mg and hydrocodone bitartrate 7.5 mg.

# alfentanil hydrochloride
Alfenta, CD Rapifen§

*Controlled Substance Schedule II*
*Pregnancy Risk Category C*

## HOW SUPPLIED
*Injection:* 500 mcg/ml

## ACTION
Binds with opiate receptors in the CNS, altering both perception of and emotional response to pain through an unknown mechanism.

| Route | Onset | Peak | Duration |
|-------|-------|------|----------|
| I.V. | 1 min | 1.5-2 min | 5-10 min |

## INDICATIONS & DOSAGE
*Adjunct to general anesthetic—*
**Adults:** initially, 8 to 50 mcg/kg I.V.; then increments of 3 to 15 mcg/kg I.V. q 5 to 20 minutes.
*As a primary anesthetic—*
**Adults:** initially, 130 to 245 mcg/kg I.V.; then 0.5 to 1.5 mcg/kg/minute I.V.
*Monitored anesthesia care—*
**Adults:** initially, 3 to 8 mcg/kg I.V.; then 3 to 5 mcg/kg I.V. q 5 to 20 minutes or 0.25 to 1 mcg/kg/minute I.V. Total dose is 3 to 40 mcg/kg I.V.
**Elderly:** Clearance reduced by about 30% in patients ages 65 and older, leading to a prolonged half-life. Dosage should be reduced.
*Adjust-a-dose:* For debilitated patients, dosage should be reduced. In obese patients, dosage is based on lean body weight.

## ADVERSE REACTIONS
**CNS:** anxiety, headache, confusion, dizziness, sleepiness, sedation.
**CV:** *hypotension, hypertension,* BRADYCARDIA, *tachycardia,* ARRHYTHMIAS.
**EENT:** blurred vision.
**GI:** *nausea, vomiting.*
**Musculoskeletal:** skeletal muscle movements.
**Respiratory:** *chest wall rigidity, bronchospasm, respiratory depression,* hypercapnia, *respiratory arrest,* laryngospasm.
**Skin:** pruritus, urticaria.

---

*Liquid contains alcohol.    **May contain tartrazine.    †Canada    ‡Australia    §U.K.    ◊OTC

**Other:** increased amylase and lipase plasma levels.

## INTERACTIONS
**Drug-drug.** *Cimetidine:* CNS toxicity. Monitor closely.
*CNS depressants:* additive effects. Use together cautiously.
*Diazepam:* CV depression and decreased blood pressure with high doses of alfentanil. Monitor closely.
**Drug-lifestyle.** *Alcohol use:* additive effects. Use together cautiously.

## EFFECTS ON DIAGNOSTIC TESTS
None reported.

## CONTRAINDICATIONS
Contraindicated in patients with hypersensitivity to drug.

## NURSING CONSIDERATIONS
• Use cautiously in patients with head injury, pulmonary disease, decreased respiratory reserve, or hepatic or renal impairment.
• *Alert:* To administer small volumes of alfentanil accurately, use a tuberculin syringe.
• Accidental skin contact should be treated by rinsing the area with water.
• Periodically monitor postoperative vital signs and bladder function. Because drug decreases both rate and depth of respirations, monitoring of arterial oxygen saturation may aid in assessing respiratory depression.
• *Alert:* Don't confuse alfentanil with Anafranil, fentanyl, or sufentanil; or Alfenta with Sufenta.

## I.V. administration
• Drug is compatible with $D_5W$, $D_5W$ in lactated Ringer's solution, and normal saline solution. Infusions containing 25 to 80 mcg/ml are used most frequently.
• Discontinue infusion at least 10 to 15 minutes before end of surgery.
• Drug should be administered only by persons specifically trained in use of I.V. anesthetics.
• Keep narcotic antagonist (naloxone) and resuscitation equipment available when giving drug I.V.

## ☑Patient teaching
• Explain anesthetic effect of drug and preoperative and postoperative care measures.
• Inform patient that another analgesic will be available to relieve pain after effects of drug have worn off.

---

**buprenorphine hydrochloride**
Buprenex, Temgesic‡

*Controlled Substance Schedule V*
*Pregnancy Risk Category C*

## HOW SUPPLIED
*Injection:* 0.324 mg (equivalent to 0.3 mg base/ml)

## ACTION
Binds with opiate receptors in the CNS, altering both perception of and emotional response to pain through an unknown mechanism.

| Route | Onset | Peak | Duration |
|-------|-------|------|----------|
| I.V. | Immediate | 2 min | 6 hr |
| I.M. | 15 min | 1 hr | 6 hr |

## INDICATIONS & DOSAGE
*Moderate to severe pain—*
**Adults and children ages 13 and older:** 0.3 mg I.M. or slow I.V. q 6 hours, p.r.n. or around the clock; dose repeated (up to 0.3 mg), if needed, 30 to 60 minutes after initial dose.
**Children ages 2 to 12:** 2 to 6 mcg/kg I.M. or I.V. q 4 to 6 hours.
**Elderly:** reduce dose by one-half.
*Adjust-a-dose:* Reduce dose by one-half in high-risk patients, such as debilitated patients.

## ADVERSE REACTIONS
**CNS:** *dizziness, sedation,* headache, confusion, nervousness, euphoria, *vertigo, increased intracranial pressure.*
**CV:** hypotension, bradycardia, tachycardia, hypertension.
**EENT:** *miosis,* blurred vision.
**GI:** *nausea,* vomiting, constipation, dry mouth.
**GU:** urine retention.
**Respiratory:** *respiratory depression,* hypoventilation, dyspnea.

---

Reactions may be *common,* uncommon, *life-threatening,* or COMMON AND LIFE-THREATENING.

**Skin:** pruritus, diaphoresis.

## INTERACTIONS
**Drug-drug.** *CNS depressants, MAO inhibitors:* additive effects. Use together cautiously.
**Drug-lifestyle.** *Alcohol use:* additive effects. Use together cautiously.

## EFFECTS ON DIAGNOSTIC TESTS
None reported.

## CONTRAINDICATIONS
Contraindicated in patients with hypersensitivity to drug.

## NURSING CONSIDERATIONS
• Use cautiously in elderly or debilitated patients or in those with head injury, intracranial lesions, and increased intracranial pressure; severe respiratory, liver, or kidney impairment; CNS depression or coma; thyroid irregularities; adrenal insufficiency; and prostatic hyperplasia, urethral stricture, acute alcoholism, delirium tremens, or kyphoscoliosis.
• S.C. administration isn't recommended.
• Buprenorphine 0.3 mg is equal to 10 mg of morphine and 75 mg of meperidine in analgesic potency. It has longer duration of action than morphine or meperidine.
• *Alert:* Naloxone won't completely reverse the respiratory depression caused by buprenorphine overdose; an overdose may necessitate mechanical ventilation. Larger than customary doses of naloxone (more than 0.4 mg) and doxapram also may be ordered.
• Accidental skin exposure should be treated by removing exposed clothing and rinsing skin with water.
• Drug's narcotic antagonist properties may precipitate withdrawal syndrome in narcotic-dependent patients.
• If dependence occurs, withdrawal symptoms may appear up to 14 days after drug is stopped.
• *Alert:* Don't confuse Buprenex with Bumex.

## I.V. administration
• Give drug by direct I.V. injection, slowly into a vein or through tubing of a free-flowing, compatible I.V. solution over not less than 2 minutes.
• When mixed in a 1:1 volume ratio, drug is compatible with atropine sulfate, diphenhydramine hydrochloride, droperidol, glycopyrrolate, haloperidol lactate, hydroxyzine hydrochloride, promethazine hydrochloride, scopolamine hydrochloride, 5% dextrose, 5% dextrose and normal saline, NaCl, lactated Ringer's, and normal saline injections.

### ✓ Patient teaching
• Caution ambulatory patient about getting out of bed or walking.
• When drug is used postoperatively, encourage patient to turn, cough, and breathe deeply to prevent atelectasis.

---

## butorphanol tartrate
Stadol, Stadol NS

*Controlled Substance Schedule IV*
*Pregnancy Risk Category C*

## HOW SUPPLIED
*Injection:* 1 mg/ml, 2 mg/ml
*Nasal spray:* 10 mg/ml

## ACTION
Binds with opiate receptors in the CNS, altering both perception of and emotional response to pain through an unknown mechanism.

| Route | Onset | Peak | Duration |
|-------|-------|------|----------|
| I.V. | 2-3 min | 30-60 min | 3-4 hr |
| I.M. | 10-15 min | 30-60 min | 3-4 hr |
| Nasal | 15 min | 1-2 hr | 4-5 hr |

## INDICATIONS & DOSAGE
*Moderate to severe pain—*
**Adults:** 1 to 4 mg I.M. q 3 to 4 hours, p.r.n. or around the clock; or 0.5 to 2 mg I.V. q 3 to 4 hours, p.r.n. or around the clock. Not to exceed 4 mg per dose. Or, 1 mg by nasal spray q 3 to 4 hours (1 spray in one nostril); repeated in 60 to 90 minutes if pain relief is inadequate. For severe pain, 2 mg (1 spray in each nostril) q 3 to 4 hours.
**Elderly:** use one-half of usual dose at twice the interval for I.V. use; for nasal

use, allow 1.5 to 2 hours to elapse before repeating dose.
*Labor for patients at full term and in early labor—*
**Adults:** 1 to 2 mg I.V. or I.M.; repeated after 4 hours, p.r.n.
*Preoperative anesthesia or preanesthesia—*
**Adults:** 2 mg. I.M. 60 to 90 minutes before surgery.
*Adjunct to balanced anesthesia—*
**Adults:** 2 mg I.V. shortly before induction, or 0.5 to 1.0 mg I.V. in increments during anesthesia.
**Elderly:** one-half of usual dose at twice the interval for I.V. use.
*Adjust-a-dose:* For patients with renal or hepatic impairment, increase dosage interval to 6 to 8 hours.

## ADVERSE REACTIONS
**CNS:** confusion, nervousness, lethargy, headache, *somnolence, dizziness, insomnia,* anxiety, paresthesia, euphoria, hallucinations, flushing, increased intracranial pressure.
**CV:** palpitations, vasodilation, hypotension.
**EENT:** blurred vision, *nasal congestion (with nasal spray),* tinnitus, unpleasant taste.
**GI:** *nausea, vomiting,* constipation, anorexia.
**Respiratory:** *respiratory depression.*
**Skin:** rash, hives, clamminess, excessive diaphoresis.
**Other:** sensation of heat.

## INTERACTIONS
**Drug-drug.** *CNS depressants:* additive effects. Use together cautiously.
**Drug-lifestyle.** *Alcohol use:* additive effects. Use together cautiously.

## EFFECTS ON DIAGNOSTIC TESTS
None reported.

## CONTRAINDICATIONS
Contraindicated in patients with hypersensitivity to drug or to preservative, benzethonium chloride and in those with narcotic addiction; may precipitate withdrawal syndrome.

## NURSING CONSIDERATIONS
• Use cautiously in patients with head injury, increased intracranial pressure, acute MI, ventricular dysfunction, coronary insufficiency, respiratory disease or depression, and renal or hepatic dysfunction. Also administer cautiously to patients who have recently received repeated doses of narcotic analgesic medication.
• S.C. route isn't recommended.
• Respiratory depression apparently doesn't increase with larger dosage.
• Psychological and physical addiction may occur.
• Periodically monitor postoperative vital signs and bladder function. Because drug decreases both rate and depth of respirations, monitoring of arterial oxygen saturation may aid in assessing respiratory depression.
• *Alert:* Don't confuse Stadol with sotalol.

### I.V. administration
• Give by direct injection into a vein or into the tubing of a free-flowing I.V. solution. Compatible solutions include $D_5W$ and normal saline.

### Patient teaching
• Caution ambulatory patient about getting out of bed or walking. Warn outpatient to avoid driving and other potentially hazardous activities that require mental alertness until drug's CNS effects are known.
• Inform patient about administration technique for and storage of nasal spray, if applicable.
• Instruct patient to avoid alcohol during therapy.

---

**codeine phosphate**
Paveral†

**codeine sulfate**

*Controlled Substance Schedule II*
*Pregnancy Risk Category C*

---

## HOW SUPPLIED
**codeine phosphate**
*Oral solution:* 15 mg/5 ml, 10 mg/ml†
*Tablets (soluble):* 30 mg, 60 mg
*Injection:* 30 mg/ml, 60 mg/ml

---

## codeine sulfate
*Tablets:* 15 mg, 30 mg, 60 mg
*Tablets (soluble):* 15 mg, 30 mg, 60 mg

## ACTION
Binds with opiate receptors in the CNS, altering both perception of and emotional response to pain through an unknown mechanism. Drug also suppresses the cough reflex by direct action on the cough center in the medulla.

| Route | Onset | Peak | Duration |
|-------|-------|------|----------|
| P.O. | 30-45 min | 1-2 hr | 4-6 hr |
| I.V. | Immediate | Immediate | 4-6 hr |
| I.M. | 10-30 min | 0.5-1 hr | 4-6 hr |
| S.C. | 10-30 min | Unknown | 4-6 hr |

## INDICATIONS & DOSAGE
*Mild to moderate pain—*
**Adults:** 15 to 60 mg P.O. or 15 to 60 mg (phosphate) S.C., I.M., or I.V. q 4 to 6 hours, p.r.n. Maximum dose is 360 mg/day.
**Children over age 1:** 0.5 mg/kg P.O., S.C., or I.M. q 4 hours, p.r.n. *Don't use I.V. in children.*
*Nonproductive cough—*
**Adults:** 10 to 20 mg P.O. q 4 to 6 hours. Maximum dose is 120 mg/day.
**Children ages 6 to 12:** 5 to 10 mg P.O. q 4 to 6 hours. Maximum dose is 60 mg/day.
**Children ages 2 to 6:** 2.5 to 5 mg P.O. q 4 to 6 hours. Don't exceed 30 mg/day.

## ADVERSE REACTIONS
**CNS:** *sedation, clouded sensorium,* euphoria, dizziness, light-headedness.
**CV:** hypotension, bradycardia, flushing.
**GI:** nausea, vomiting, *constipation,* dry mouth, ileus.
**GU:** urine retention.
**Respiratory:** *respiratory depression.*
**Skin:** pruritus, *diaphoresis.*
**Other:** physical dependence, increased plasma amylase and lipase levels.

## INTERACTIONS
**Drug-drug.** *CNS depressants, general anesthetics, hypnotics, MAO inhibitors, other narcotic analgesics, sedatives, tranquilizers, tricyclic antidepressants:* additive effects. Use together with extreme caution. Monitor patient response.

**Drug-lifestyle.** *Alcohol use:* additive effects. Use together cautiously.

## EFFECTS ON DIAGNOSTIC TESTS
Codeine may delay gastric emptying, increase biliary tract pressure resulting from contraction of the sphincter of Oddi, and interfere with hepatobiliary imaging studies.

## CONTRAINDICATIONS
Contraindicated in patients with hypersensitivity to drug.

## NURSING CONSIDERATIONS
• Use with extreme caution in patients with head injury, increased intracranial pressure, increased CSF pressure, hepatic or renal disease, hypothyroidism, Addison's disease, acute alcoholism, seizures, severe CNS depression, bronchial asthma, COPD, respiratory depression, and shock. Also use with extreme caution in elderly or debilitated patients.
• *Alert:* Don't mix with other solutions because codeine phosphate is incompatible with many drugs.
• Don't administer discolored solution.
• Codeine and aspirin or acetaminophen are often prescribed together to provide enhanced pain relief.
• For full analgesic effect, administer drug before patient has intense pain.
• Drug is an antitussive and shouldn't be used when cough is a valuable diagnostic sign or is beneficial (as after thoracic surgery).
• Monitor cough type and frequency.
• Monitor respiratory and circulatory status.
• Opiates may cause constipation. Assess bowel function and need for stool softeners or laxatives.
• *Alert:* Don't confuse codeine with Cardene, Lodine, or Cordran.

### I.V. administration
• Give drug by direct injection into a large vein. Administer very slowly.

### Patient teaching
• Advise patient that GI distress caused by oral administration can be minimized by taking with milk or meals.

• Instruct patient to ask for or to take drug before pain is intense.

• Caution ambulatory patient about getting out of bed or walking. Warn outpatient to avoid driving and other potentially hazardous activities that require mental alertness until drug's CNS effects are known.

• Advise patient to avoid alcohol during therapy.

## fentanyl citrate
Sublimaze

## fentanyl transdermal system
Duragesic-25, Duragesic-50, Duragesic-75, Duragesic-100

## fentanyl transmucosal
Fentanyl Oralet

*Controlled Substance Schedule II*
*Pregnancy Risk Category C*

## HOW SUPPLIED
*Injection:* 50 mcg/ml
*Transdermal system:* patches designed to release 25 mcg, 50 mcg, 75 mcg, or 100 mcg of fentanyl per hour
*Transmucosal:* 100 mcg, 200 mcg, 300 mcg, 400 mcg

## ACTION
Binds with opiate receptors in the CNS, altering both perception of and emotional response to pain through an unknown mechanism.

| Route | Onset | Peak | Duration |
|---|---|---|---|
| I.V. | 1-2 min | 3-5 min | 0.5-1 hr |
| I.M. | 7-15 min | 20-30 min | 1-2 hr |
| Trans-dermal | 12-24 hr | 1-3 days | Variable |
| Trans-mucosal | 5-15 min | 20-30 min | Unknown |

## INDICATIONS & DOSAGE
*Adjunct to general anesthetic—*
**Adults:** for low-dose therapy, 2 mcg/kg I.V. For moderate-dose therapy, 2 to 20 mcg/kg I.V.; then 25 to 100 mcg I.V., p.r.n. For high-dose therapy, 20 to 50 mcg/kg I.V.; then 25 mcg to one-half initial loading dose I.V., p.r.n.
*Adjunct to regional anesthesia—*
**Adults:** 50 to 100 mcg I.M. or slowly I.V. over 1 to 2 minutes, p.r.n.
*Induction and maintenance of anesthesia—*
**Children ages 2 to 12:** 2 to 3 mcg/kg I.V.
*Postoperatively—*
**Adults:** 50 to 100 mcg I.M. q 1 to 2 hours, p.r.n.
*Preoperatively—*
**Adults:** 50 to 100 mcg I.M. 30 to 60 minutes before surgery. Or, 5 mcg/kg dispensed as oralet unit, 20 to 40 minutes before need of desired effects.
*Management of chronic pain—*
**Adults:** one transdermal system applied to a portion of the upper torso on an area of skin that isn't irritated and hasn't been irradiated. Therapy initiated with the 25-mcg/hour system; dosage adjusted as needed and tolerated. Each system may be worn for 72 hours, although some patients may require systems to be applied q 48 hours. Upward adjustment may be done q 3 days after initial dose; then 6 days thereafter.

## ADVERSE REACTIONS
**CNS:** *sedation, somnolence, clouded sensorium, euphoria,* dizziness, headache, *confusion, asthenia,* nervousness, hallucinations, anxiety, depression, **seizures.**
**CV:** hypotension, hypertension, **arrhythmias,** chest pain.
**GI:** nausea, vomiting, constipation, ileus, abdominal pain, dry mouth, anorexia, diarrhea, dyspepsia.
**GU:** urine retention.
**Respiratory:** *respiratory depression,* hypoventilation, dyspnea, **apnea.**
**Skin:** reaction at application site, *pruritus, diaphoresis.*
**Other:** physical dependence, increased plasma amylase and lipase levels.

## INTERACTIONS
**Drug-drug.** *CNS depressants, general anesthetics, hypnotics, MAO inhibitors, other narcotic analgesics, sedatives, tricyclic antidepressants:* additive effects. Use together with extreme caution. Fentanyl dose should be reduced by one-

quarter to one-third. Also give above drugs in reduced dosages.

*Diazepam:* CV depression when given with high doses of fentanyl. Monitor closely.

*Droperidol:* hypotension and decreased pulmonary arterial pressure. Use together cautiously.

**Drug-lifestyle.** *Alcohol use:* additive effects. Use together cautiously.

## EFFECTS ON DIAGNOSTIC TESTS
None reported.

## CONTRAINDICATIONS
Contraindicated in patients with known intolerance of drug. Fentanyl patch is contraindicated for pain management following surgery, mild or intermittent pain that can be managed with nonnarcotic agents, or in doses exceeding 25 mcg/hour initially.

## NURSING CONSIDERATIONS
• Use with caution in patients with head injury, increased CSF pressure, COPD, decreased respiratory reserve, potentially compromised respirations, hepatic or renal disease, and cardiac bradyarrhythmias. Also use with caution in elderly or debilitated patients.

• For better analgesic effect, administer drug before patient has intense pain.

• *Alert:* High doses can produce muscle rigidity, which can be reversed with neuromuscular blockers; however, patient must be artificially ventilated.

• Monitor circulatory and respiratory status and urinary function carefully. Drug may cause respiratory depression, hypotension, urine retention, nausea, vomiting, ileus, or altered level of consciousness without regard to route of administration.

• Periodically monitor postoperative vital signs and bladder function. Because drug decreases both rate and depth of respirations, monitoring of arterial oxygen saturation (Sao₂) may help assess respiratory depression. Immediately report respiratory rate below 12 breaths/minute, decreased respiratory volume, or decreased Sao₂.

*Transdermal form*

• Transdermal fentanyl isn't recommended for postoperative pain.

• Don't give transdermal fentanyl to patients under age 12 or patients under age 18 weighing less than 110 lb (50 kg).

• Dosage equivalent charts are available to calculate the fentanyl transdermal dose based on the daily morphine intake—for example, for every 90 mg of oral morphine or 15 mg of I.M. morphine per 24 hours, 25 mcg/hour of transdermal fentanyl is needed.

• Dosage adjustments in patients using the transdermal system should be made gradually. Reaching steady-state levels of a new dosage may take up to 6 days; delay dosage adjustment until after at least two applications.

• Monitor patients who develop adverse reactions to the transdermal system for at least 12 hours after removal. Serum levels of fentanyl drop gradually and may take as long as 17 hours to decline by 50%.

• Most patients experience good control of pain for 3 days while wearing the transdermal system, but a few may need a new application after 48 hours.

• Because serum fentanyl level rises for the first 24 hours after application, analgesic effect can't be evaluated on the first day. Be sure patient has adequate supplemental analgesic to prevent breakthrough pain.

• When reducing opiate therapy or switching to a different analgesic, the transdermal system should be withdrawn gradually. Because fentanyl's serum level drops gradually after removal, give half of the equianalgesic dose of the new analgesic 12 to 18 hours after removal, as ordered.

*Transmucosal form*

• Remove foil overwrap of fentanyl oralet just before administration.

• Have patient place the fentanyl oralet in mouth and suck (not chew or swallow) it.

• Remove fentanyl oralet unit, using the handle, after it has been consumed, patient shows adequate effect, or patient shows signs of respiratory depression. Place any remaining portion in the plastic overwrap provided, and dispose accordingly for Schedule II drugs.

• *Alert:* Don't confuse fentanyl with alfentanil.

## I.V. administration
• Only staff trained in administration of I.V. anesthetics and management of their potential adverse effects should administer I.V. fentanyl.
• Drug is often used I.V. with droperidol to produce neuroleptanalgesia.
• Keep narcotic antagonist (naloxone) and resuscitation equipment available when giving drug I.V.

## Patient teaching
• When used for pain control, instruct patient to ask for drug before pain becomes intense.
• When drug is used postoperatively, encourage patient to turn, cough, and breathe deeply to prevent atelectasis.
• Instruct patient to avoid performing hazardous activities until CNS effects subside.
• Tell home care patient to avoid drinking alcohol or taking other CNS-type drugs while receiving fentanyl because additive effects can occur.
• Teach patient about the proper application of the prescribed transdermal patch. Tell patient to clip hair at application site, but not to use a razor, which may irritate the skin. Wash area with clear water if necessary, but not with soaps, oils, lotions, alcohol, or other substances that may irritate the skin or prevent adhesion. Dry area completely before application.
• Tell patient to remove transdermal system from package just before applying, hold in place for 30 seconds, and be sure the edges of patch adhere to skin.
• Teach patient to dispose of the transdermal patch by folding so the adhesive side adheres to itself and then flushing it down the toilet.
• Tell patient that, if another patch is needed after 48 to 72 hours, to apply it to a new site.
• Inform patient that heat from fever or environment, such as from heating pads, electric blankets, heat lamps, hot tubs, or water beds, may increase transdermal delivery and cause toxicity requiring dosage adjustment. Instruct patient to notify doctor if fever occurs or if he'll be spending time in a hot climate.

# hydromorphone hydrochloride (dihydromorphinone hydrochloride)
CD Palladone§,
CD Palladone SR§, Dilaudid,
Dilaudid-5, Dilaudid-HP

*Controlled Substance Schedule II*
*Pregnancy Risk Category C*

## HOW SUPPLIED
*Tablets:* 1 mg, 2 mg, 3 mg, 4 mg, 8 mg
*Injection:* 1 mg/ml, 2 mg/ml, 3 mg/ml, 4 mg/ml, 10 mg/ml
*Suppositories:* 3 mg
*Syrup:* 1 mg/5 ml**
*Liquid:* 5 mg/5 ml

## ACTION
Binds with opiate receptors in the CNS, altering both perception of and emotional response to pain through an unknown mechanism. It also suppresses the cough reflex by direct action on the cough center in the medulla.

| Route | Onset | Peak | Duration |
|-------|-------|------|----------|
| P.O. | 30 min | 1.5-2 hr | 4 hr |
| I.V. | 10-15 min | 15-30 min | 2-3 hr |
| I.M. | 15 min | 0.5-1 hr | 4-5 hr |
| S.C. | 15 min | 0.5-1.5 hr | 4 hr |
| P.R. | Unknown | Unknown | 4 hr |

## INDICATIONS & DOSAGE
*Moderate to severe pain—*
**Adults:** 2 to 4 mg P.O. q 4 to 6 hours, p.r.n.; or 1 to 4 mg I.M., S.C., or I.V. (slowly over at least 2 to 5 minutes) q 4 to 6 hours, p.r.n.; or 3 mg P.R. suppository q 6 to 8 hours, p.r.n.
*Cough—*
**Adults and children over age 12:** 1 teaspoon (5 ml) P.O. q 3 to 4 hours, p.r.n.

## ADVERSE REACTIONS
**CNS:** *sedation, somnolence, clouded sensorium,* dizziness, *euphoria.*
**CV:** hypotension, bradycardia.
**EENT:** blurred vision, diplopia, nystagmus.
**GI:** nausea, vomiting, constipation, ileus.
**GU:** urine retention.

---

Reactions may be *common,* uncommon, **life-threatening**, or COMMON AND LIFE-THREATENING.

**Respiratory:** *respiratory depression, bronchospasm.*
**Other:** induration with repeated S.C. injections, physical dependence, increased plasma amylase and lipase levels.

## INTERACTIONS
**Drug-drug.** *CNS depressants, general anesthetics, hypnotics, MAO inhibitors, other narcotic analgesics, sedatives, tranquilizers, tricyclic antidepressants:* additive effects. Use together with extreme caution. Reduce hydromorphone dose and monitor patient response.
**Drug-lifestyle.** *Alcohol use:* additive effects. Use together cautiously.

## EFFECTS ON DIAGNOSTIC TESTS
Drug may delay gastric emptying; increased biliary tract pressure resulting from contraction of the sphincter of Oddi may interfere with hepatobiliary imaging studies.

## CONTRAINDICATIONS
Contraindicated in patients with hypersensitivity to drug and in those with intracranial lesions associated with increased intracranial pressure; also contraindicated whenever ventilator function is depressed, such as in status asthmaticus, COPD, cor pulmonale, emphysema, and kyphoscoliosis.

## NURSING CONSIDERATIONS
• Use with extreme caution in patients with hepatic or renal disease, hypothyroidism, Addison's disease, prostatic hyperplasia, or urethral stricture. Also use with caution in elderly or debilitated patients.
• For better analgesic effect, give drug before patient has intense pain.
• Dilaudid-HP, a highly concentrated form (10 mg/ml), may be administered in smaller volumes to prevent the discomfort associated with large-volume I.M. or S.C. injections. Check dosage carefully.
• Rotate injection sites to avoid induration with S.C. injection.
• Monitor respiratory and circulatory status and bowel function.
• Keep narcotic antagonist (naloxone) available.

• Drug may worsen or mask gallbladder pain.
• Drug is a commonly abused narcotic.
• *Alert:* Don't confuse hydromorphone with morphine or Dilaudid with Dilantin.

### I.V. administration
• Give by direct injection over no less than 2 minutes. For infusion, drug may be mixed in $D_5W$, normal saline, dextrose 5% in normal saline, dextrose 5% in half-normal saline, or Ringer's or lactated Ringer's solutions.
• Respiratory depression and hypotension can occur with I.V. administration. Give very slowly and monitor patient constantly. Keep resuscitation equipment available.

### Patient teaching
• Instruct patient to ask for or take drug before pain becomes intense.
• Tell patient to store suppositories in refrigerator.
• Tell patient to take drug with food if GI upset occurs.
• When drug is used postoperatively, encourage patient to turn, cough, and deep-breath to avoid atelectasis.
• Caution ambulatory patient about getting out of bed or walking. Warn outpatient to avoid hazardous activities that require mental alertness until drug's CNS effects are known.
• Advise patient to avoid alcohol during therapy.

---

**meperidine hydrochloride (pethidine hydrochloride)**
CD Pamergan-P100§,
CD Pethidine§, Demerol

*Controlled Substance Schedule II*
*Pregnancy Risk Category B (D if used for prolonged periods or in high doses at term)*

## HOW SUPPLIED
*Tablets:* 50 mg, 100 mg
*Syrup:* 50 mg/5 ml
*Injection:* 10 mg/ml, 25 mg/ml, 50 mg/ml, 75 mg/ml, 100 mg/ml

---

*Liquid contains alcohol.   **May contain tartrazine.   †Canada   ‡Australia   §U.K.   ◊OTC

## ACTION
Binds with opiate receptors in the CNS, altering both perception of and emotional response to pain through an unknown mechanism.

| Route | Onset | Peak | Duration |
|-------|-------|------|----------|
| P.O. | 15 min | 1-1.5 hr | 2-4 hr |
| I.V. | 1 min | 5-7 min | 2-4 hr |
| I.M. | 10-15 min | 30-50 min | 2-4 hr |
| S.C. | 10-15 min | 40-60 min | 2-4 hr |

## INDICATIONS & DOSAGE
*Moderate to severe pain—*
**Adults:** 50 to 150 mg P.O., I.M., or S.C. q 3 to 4 hours, p.r.n.
**Children:** 1.1 to 1.8 mg/kg P.O., I.M., or S.C. q 3 to 4 hours. Maximum dose is 100 mg q 4 hours, p.r.n.
*Preoperatively—*
**Adults:** 50 to 100 mg I.M. or S.C. 30 to 90 minutes before surgery.
**Children:** 1 to 2 mg/kg I.M. or S.C. up to the adult dose 30 to 90 minutes before surgery.
*Adjunct to anesthesia—*
**Adults:** repeated slow I.V. injections of fractional doses (10 mg/ml); or, continuous I.V. infusion of a more dilute solution (1 mg/ml) titrated to patient's needs.
*Obstetric analgesia—*
**Adults:** 50 to 100 mg I.M. or S.C. when pain becomes regular; repeated at 1- to 3-hour intervals.

## ADVERSE REACTIONS
**CNS:** *sedation, somnolence, clouded sensorium, euphoria,* paradoxical excitement, tremor, *dizziness,* **seizures,** headache, hallucinations, syncope, *light-headedness.*
**CV:** hypotension, bradycardia, tachycardia, **cardiac arrest, shock.**
**GI:** constipation, ileus, dry mouth, *nausea, vomiting,* biliary tract spasms.
**GU:** urine retention.
**Musculoskeletal:** muscle twitching.
**Respiratory:** **respiratory depression,** respiratory arrest.
**Skin:** pruritus, urticaria, *diaphoresis.*
**Other:** physical dependence, phlebitis after I.V. delivery, pain at injection site, local tissue irritation, induration (after S.C. injection), increased plasma amylase and lipase levels.

## INTERACTIONS
**Drug-drug.** *Aminophylline, barbiturates, heparin, methicillin, morphine sulfate, phenytoin, sodium bicarbonate, sulfonamides:* incompatible when mixed in the same I.V. container. Don't use together.
*CNS depressants, general anesthetics, hypnotics, other narcotic analgesics, phenothiazines, sedatives, tricyclic antidepressants:* possible respiratory depression, hypotension, profound sedation, or coma. Use together with extreme caution. Reduce meperidine dosage.
*MAO inhibitors:* increased CNS excitation or depression that can be severe or fatal. Don't use together.
*Phenytoin:* decreased blood levels of meperidine. Monitor for decreased analgesia.
**Drug-herb.** *Parsley:* may promote or produce serotonin syndrome. Avoid concomitant use.
**Drug-lifestyle.** *Alcohol use:* additive effects. Use together cautiously.

## EFFECTS ON DIAGNOSTIC TESTS
None reported.

## CONTRAINDICATIONS
Contraindicated in patients with hypersensitivity to drug and in those who have received MAO inhibitors within past 14 days.

## NURSING CONSIDERATIONS
• Use with extreme caution in patients with increased intracranial pressure, head injury, asthma, and other respiratory conditions; supraventricular tachycardias, seizures, acute abdominal conditions, hepatic or renal disease, hypothyroidism, Addison's disease, urethral stricture, and prostatic hyperplasia; and in elderly or debilitated patients.
• Drug may be used in some patients allergic to morphine.
• S.C. injection isn't recommended because it's very painful. However, it may be suitable for occasional use.
• **Alert:** Oral dose is less than half as effective as parenteral dose. Give I.M. if possible. When changing from parenteral to oral route, dosage should be increased.

---

• Syrup has local anesthetic effect. Give with full glass of water.
• Drug and its active metabolite normeperidine accumulate in the body. Monitor for increased toxic effect, especially in patients with impaired renal function.
• Because drug toxicity frequently appears after several days of treatment, drug isn't recommended for treatment of chronic pain.
• Monitor respirations of neonates exposed to drug during labor. Have resuscitation equipment and naloxone available.
• Monitor respiratory and CV status carefully. Don't give if respirations are below 12 breaths/minute, if respiratory rate or depth is decreased, or if change in pupils is noted.
• Watch for withdrawal symptoms if drug is discontinued abruptly after long-term use.
• Monitor bladder function in postoperative patients.
• Monitor bowel function. Patient may need a laxative or stool softener.
• *Alert:* Don't confuse Demerol with Demulen, Dymelor, or Temaril.

### I.V. administration
• Give drug slowly by direct I.V. injection. Meperidine also may be given by slow continuous I.V. infusion. Drug is compatible with most I.V. solutions, including $D_5W$, normal saline, and Ringer's or lactated Ringer's solutions.
• Keep narcotic antagonist (naloxone) available when giving this drug I.V.

### ✓ Patient teaching
• When drug is used postoperatively, encourage patient to turn, cough, and deep-breath and to use an incentive spirometer to prevent atelectasis.
• Caution ambulatory patient about getting out of bed or walking. Warn outpatient to avoid driving and other potentially hazardous activities that require mental alertness until drug's CNS effects are known.
• Advise patient to avoid alcohol during therapy.

## methadone hydrochloride
Dolophine, Methadose, Physeptone‡

*Controlled Substance Schedule II*
*Pregnancy Risk Category C*

### HOW SUPPLIED
*Tablets:* 5 mg, 10 mg
*Dispersible tablets (for methadone maintenance therapy):* 40 mg
*Oral solution:* 5 mg/5 ml, 10 mg/5 ml, 10 mg/10 ml, 10 mg/ml (concentrate)
*Injection:* 10 mg/ml

### ACTION
Binds with opiate receptors at many sites in the CNS (brain, brain stem, and spinal cord), altering both perception of and emotional response to pain through an unknown mechanism.

| Route | Onset | Peak | Duration |
|---|---|---|---|
| P.O. | 0.5-1 hr | 1.5-2 hr | 4-6 hr |
| I.M., S.C. | 10-20 min | 1-2 hr | 4-5 hr |

### INDICATIONS & DOSAGE
*Severe pain—*
**Adults:** 2.5 to 10 mg P.O., I.M., or S.C. q 3 to 4 hours, p.r.n.
*Narcotic withdrawal syndrome—*
**Adults:** 15 to 40 mg P.O. daily (highly individualized). Maintenance dose is 20 to 120 mg P.O. daily. Dosage adjusted, p.r.n. Daily doses over 120 mg require special state and federal approval.

### ADVERSE REACTIONS
**CNS:** *sedation, somnolence, clouded sensorium,* euphoria, *dizziness,* choreic movements, **seizures,** headache, insomnia, agitation, *light-headedness,* syncope.
**CV:** hypotension, bradycardia, **shock, cardiac arrest,** palpitations, edema.
**EENT:** visual disturbances.
**GI:** *nausea, vomiting,* constipation, ileus, dry mouth, anorexia, biliary tract spasm.
**GU:** urine retention.
**Respiratory:** *respiratory depression, respiratory arrest.*
**Skin:** diaphoresis, pruritus, urticaria.
**Other:** physical dependence, pain at injection site, tissue irritation, induration

(following S.C. injection), decreased libido, increased plasma amylase levels.

## INTERACTIONS
**Drug-drug.** *Ammonium chloride, other urine acidifiers, phenytoin:* may reduce methadone effect. Monitor for decreased pain control.
*CNS depressants, general anesthetics, hypnotics, MAO inhibitors, sedatives, tranquilizers, tricyclic antidepressants:* possible respiratory depression, hypotension, profound sedation, or coma. Use together with extreme caution. Monitor patient response.
*Rifampin:* withdrawal symptoms; reduced blood levels of methadone. Use together cautiously.
**Drug-lifestyle.** *Alcohol use:* additive effects. Use together cautiously.

## EFFECTS ON DIAGNOSTIC TESTS
None reported.

## CONTRAINDICATIONS
Contraindicated in patients with hypersensitivity to drug.

## NURSING CONSIDERATIONS
• Use with extreme caution in patients with acute abdominal conditions, severe hepatic or renal impairment, hypothyroidism, Addison's disease, prostatic hyperplasia, urethral stricture, head injury, increased intracranial pressure, asthma, and other respiratory conditions. Also use with caution in elderly or debilitated patients.
• Oral liquid form legally required in maintenance programs. Completely dissolve tablets in one-half cup of orange juice or powdered citrus drink.
• For parenteral use, I.M. injection is preferred. Rotate injection sites.
• Oral dose is half as potent as injected dose.
• An around-the-clock regimen is needed to manage severe, chronic pain.
• Patient treated for narcotic withdrawal syndrome usually will require an additional analgesic if pain control is needed.
• Monitor patient closely because drug has cumulative effect; marked sedation can occur after repeated doses.

• Monitor circulatory and respiratory status and bladder and bowel function. Patient may need a laxative.
• When used as an adjunct in the treatment of narcotic addiction (maintenance), withdrawal usually will be delayed and mild.

### ☑ Patient teaching
• Caution ambulatory patient about getting out of bed or walking. Warn outpatient to avoid hazardous activities that require mental alertness until drug's CNS effects are known.
• Instruct patient to increase fluid and fiber in diet, if not contraindicated, to combat constipation.
• Advise patient to avoid alcohol during therapy.

## morphine hydrochloride
Morphitec†, M.O.S.†, M.O.S.-S.R.†

## morphine sulfate
Anamorph‡, Astramorph PF, CD Morcap SR§, CD MST Continus§, CD Sevredol§, CD Zomorph§, Duramorph, Epimorph†, Infumorph 200, Infumorph 500, Morphine H.P.†, MS Contin, MSIR, MS/L, OMS Concentrate, Oramorph SR, RMS Uniserts, Roxanol, Roxanol 100, Roxanol Rescudose, Roxanol UD, Statex

## morphine tartrate‡

*Controlled Substance Schedule II*
*Pregnancy Risk Category C*

## HOW SUPPLIED
**morphine hydrochloride**
*Tablets:* 10 mg†, 20 mg†, 40 mg†, 60 mg†
*Tablets (extended-release):* 30 mg†, 60 mg†
*Oral solution:* 1 mg/ml†, 5 mg/ml†, 10 mg/ml†, 50 mg/ml†
*Syrup:* 1 mg/ml†, 5 mg/ml†, 10 mg/ml†, 20 mg/ml†, 50 mg/ml†
*Suppositories:* 10 mg†, 20 mg†, 30 mg†

---

Reactions may be *common*, uncommon, *life-threatening*, or COMMON AND LIFE-THREATENING.

### morphine sulfate
*Tablets:* 15 mg, 30 mg
*Tablets (extended-release):* 15 mg, 30 mg,
60 mg, 100 mg, 200 mg
*Soluble tablets:* 10 mg, 15 mg, 30 mg
*Oral solution:* 10 mg/5 ml, 20 mg/5 ml,
20 mg/ml (concentrate), 100 mg/5 ml
*Syrup:* 1 mg/ml, 5 mg/ml
*Injection (with preservative):* 0.5 mg/ml,
1 mg/ml, 2 mg/ml, 3 mg/ml, 4 mg/ml,
5 mg/ml, 8 mg/ml, 10 mg/ml, 15 mg/ml,
25 mg/ml, 50 mg/ml
*Injection (without preservative):*
0.5 mg/ml, 1 mg/ml, 10 mg/ml, 25 mg/ml
*Suppositories:* 5 mg, 10 mg, 20 mg,
30 mg
### morphine tartrate
*Injection:* 80 mg/ml‡

## ACTION
Binds with opiate receptors in the CNS,
altering both perception of and emotional
response to pain through an unknown
mechanism.

| Route | Onset | Peak | Duration |
|---|---|---|---|
| P.O. | 1 hr | 1-2 hr | 4-12 hr |
| I.V. | 5 min | 20 min | 4-5 hr |
| I.M. | 10-30 min | 30-60 min | 4-5 hr |
| S.C. | 10-30 min | 50-90 min | 4-5 hr |
| P.R. | 20-30 min | 20-60 min | 4-5 hr |
| Epidural | 15-60 min | 15-60 min | 24 hr |
| Intrathecal | 15-60 min | 30-60 min | 24 hr |

## INDICATIONS & DOSAGE
*Severe pain—*
**Adults:** 5 to 20 mg S.C. or I.M. or 2.5 to
15 mg I.V. q 4 hours, p.r.n. Or, 10 to
30 mg P.O. or 10 to 20 mg P.R. q 4 hours,
p.r.n. When given by continuous I.V. infusion, a loading dose of 15 mg I.V. may
be followed by a continuous infusion of
0.8 to 10 mg/hour. Fifteen to 30 mg
extended-release tablets P.O. q 8 to 12
hours may also be given. As an epidural
injection, 5 mg by epidural catheter; then,
if adequate pain relief not obtained within
1 hour, additional doses of 1 to 2 mg giv-
en at intervals sufficient to assess efficacy. Maximum total epidural dose should-
n't exceed 10 mg/24 hours. As an intrathecal injection, a single dose of 0.2 to
1 mg may provide pain relief for 24 hours

(only in the lumbar area). Repeat injections not recommended.
**Children:** 0.1 to 0.2 mg/kg S.C. or I.M. q
4 hours. Maximum single dose is 15 mg.

## ADVERSE REACTIONS
**CNS:** *sedation, somnolence, clouded sensorium, euphoria, seizures, dizziness,
nightmares (with long-acting oral forms),
light-headedness,* hallucinations, nervousness, depression, syncope.
**CV:** hypotension, *bradycardia, shock,
cardiac arrest,* tachycardia, hypertension.
**GI:** *nausea, vomiting, constipation,* ileus,
dry mouth, biliary tract spasms, anorexia.
**GU:** urine retention.
**Hematologic:** *thrombocytopenia.*
**Respiratory:** *respiratory depression, apnea, respiratory arrest.*
**Skin:** pruritus and skin flushing (with
epidural administration), diaphoresis, edema.
**Other:** physical dependence, decreased
libido, increased plasma amylase levels.

## INTERACTIONS
**Drug-drug.** *CNS depressants, general
anesthetics, hypnotics, MAO inhibitors,
other narcotic analgesics, sedatives, tranquilizers, tricyclic antidepressants:* possible respiratory depression, hypotension,
profound sedation, or coma. Use together
with extreme caution. Reduce morphine
dose and monitor patient response.
**Drug-lifestyle.** *Alcohol use:* additive effects. Use together cautiously.

## EFFECTS ON DIAGNOSTIC TESTS
None reported.

## CONTRAINDICATIONS
Contraindicated in patients with hypersensitivity to drug or conditions that
would preclude administration of opioids
by I.V. route (acute bronchial asthma or
upper airway obstruction).

## NURSING CONSIDERATIONS
• Use with extreme caution in patients
with head injury, increased intracranial
pressure, seizures, chronic pulmonary disease, prostatic hyperplasia, severe hepatic
or renal disease, acute abdominal conditions, hypothyroidism, Addison's disease,

and urethral stricture. Also use with extreme caution in elderly or debilitated patients.
• Keep narcotic antagonist (naloxone) and resuscitation equipment available.
• Oral solutions of various concentrations and an intensified oral solution (20 mg/ml) are available. Carefully note the strength administered.
• Don't crush, break, or chew extended-release tablets.
• Oral capsules may be carefully opened and the entire beaded contents poured into cool, soft foods, such as water, orange juice, applesauce, or pudding; mixture should be consumed immediately.
• S.L. administration may be ordered. Measure oral solution with tuberculin syringe. Administer dose a few drops at a time to allow maximal S.L. absorption and minimize swallowing.
• Refrigeration of rectal suppository isn't necessary. In some patients, rectal and oral absorption may not be equivalent.
• Preservative-free preparations are available for epidural and intrathecal administration.
• When given epidurally, monitor closely for respiratory depression up to 24 hours after the injection. Check respiratory rate and depth every 30 to 60 minutes for 24 hours.
• Morphine is the drug of choice in relieving MI pain; may cause transient decrease in blood pressure.
• An around-the-clock regimen best manages severe, chronic pain.
• Morphine may worsen or mask gallbladder pain.
• Monitor circulatory, respiratory, bladder, and bowel functions carefully. Drug may cause respiratory depression, hypotension, urine retention, nausea, vomiting, ileus, or altered level of consciousness regardless of the route used. Withhold dose and notify doctor if respirations are below 12 breaths/minute.
• Constipation is frequently severe with maintenance dose. Ensure that stool softener or other laxative is ordered.
• **Alert:** Don't confuse morphine with hydromorphone.

### I.V. administration
• When given by direct injection, 2.5 to 15 mg may be diluted in 4 or 5 ml of sterile water for injection and given over 4 to 5 minutes. Or, drug may be mixed with $D_5W$ to a concentration of 0.1 to 1 mg/ml and administered by a continuous infusion device. Morphine sulfate is compatible with most common I.V. solutions.

### Patient teaching
• When drug is used postoperatively, encourage patient to turn, cough, and breathe deeply and to use incentive spirometer to prevent atelectasis.
• Caution ambulatory patient about getting out of bed or walking. Warn outpatient to avoid driving and other potentially hazardous activities that require mental alertness until drug's adverse CNS effects are known.
• Advise patient to avoid alcohol during therapy.

## nalbuphine hydrochloride
Nubain

*Pregnancy Risk Category B*

### HOW SUPPLIED
*Injection:* 10 mg/ml, 20 mg/ml

### ACTION
Binds with opiate receptors in the CNS, altering both perception of and emotional response to pain through an unknown mechanism.

| Route | Onset | Peak | Duration |
|-------|-------|------|----------|
| I.V. | 2-3 min | 30 min | 3-6 hr |
| I.M. | 15 min | 1 hr | 3-6 hr |
| S.C. | 15 min | Unknown | 3-6 hr |

### INDICATIONS & DOSAGE
*Moderate to severe pain—*
**Adults:** for an average (70-kg [154-lb]) person, 10 to 20 mg S.C., I.M., or I.V. q 3 to 6 hours, p.r.n. Maximum daily dose is 160 mg.
*Adjunct to balanced anesthesia—*
**Adults:** 0.3 mg/kg to 3.0 mg/kg I.V. over 10 to 15 minutes; then maintenance doses

of 0.25 to 0.50 mg/kg in single I.V. dose,
p.r.n.

## ADVERSE REACTIONS

**CNS:** *headache, sedation, dizziness, vertigo,* nervousness, depression, restlessness, crying, euphoria, hostility, unusual dreams, confusion, hallucinations, speech difficulty, delusions.
**CV:** hypertension, hypotension, tachycardia, *bradycardia.*
**EENT:** blurred vision, dry mouth.
**GI:** cramps, dyspepsia, bitter taste, nausea, vomiting, constipation, biliary tract spasms.
**GU:** urinary urgency.
**Respiratory:** *respiratory depression,* dyspnea, asthma, *pulmonary edema.*
**Skin:** pruritus, burning, urticaria, clamminess.

## INTERACTIONS

**Drug-drug.** *CNS depressants, general anesthetics, hypnotics, MAO inhibitors, sedatives, tranquilizers, tricyclic antidepressants:* possible respiratory depression, hypertension, profound sedation, or coma. Use together with extreme caution. Monitor patient response.
*Narcotic analgesics:* possible decreased analgesic effect. Avoid concomitant use.
**Drug-lifestyle.** *Alcohol use:* additive effects. Use together cautiously.

## EFFECTS ON DIAGNOSTIC TESTS
None reported.

## CONTRAINDICATIONS
Contraindicated in patients with hypersensitivity to drug.

## NURSING CONSIDERATIONS
• Use cautiously in patients with history of drug abuse or in patients with emotional instability, head injury, increased intracranial pressure, impaired ventilation, MI accompanied by nausea and vomiting, upcoming biliary surgery, and hepatic or renal disease.
• Drug acts as a narcotic antagonist; may precipitate withdrawal syndrome. For patients who have received opiates longterm, administer 25% of the usual dose initially, as ordered. Observe for signs of withdrawal.

• *Alert:* Drug causes respiratory depression, which at 10 mg is equal to the respiratory depression produced by 10 mg of morphine.
• Monitor circulatory and respiratory status and bladder and bowel function. Withhold dose and notify doctor if respirations are shallow or rate is below 12 breaths/minute.
• Constipation is often severe with maintenance therapy. Make sure stool softener or other laxative is ordered.
• Psychological and physical dependence may occur with prolonged use.
• *Alert:* Don't confuse Nubain with Navane.

**I.V. administration**
• Inject slowly over at least 2 to 3 minutes into a vein or into an I.V. line containing a compatible, free-flowing I.V. solution, such as $D_5W$, normal saline, or lactated Ringer's solution.
• Respiratory depression can be reversed with naloxone. Keep resuscitation equipment available, particularly when administering I.V.

**Patient teaching**
• Caution ambulatory patient about getting out of bed or walking. Warn outpatient to avoid driving and other potentially hazardous activities that require mental alertness until drug's CNS effects are known.
• Instruct patient on how to manage troublesome adverse effects such as constipation.

---

**oxycodone hydrochloride**
Endone‡, OxyContin, Oxy IR,
Roxicodone, Roxicodone Intensol,
Supeudol†

**oxycodone pectinate**
Proladone‡

*Controlled Substance Schedule II*
*Pregnancy Risk Category C*

## HOW SUPPLIED
**oxycodone hydrochloride**
*Capsules:* 5 mg
*Tablets:* 5 mg

*Tablets (controlled-release):* 10 mg,
20 mg, 40 mg, 80 mg
*Oral solution:* 5 mg/5 ml, 20 mg/ml (concentrate)
*Suppositories:* 10 mg†, 20 mg†
**oxycodone pectinate**
*Suppositories:* 30 mg‡

## ACTION
Binds with opiate receptors in the CNS,
altering both perception of and emotional
response to pain through an unknown
mechanism.

| Route | Onset | Peak | Duration |
|-------|-------|------|----------|
| P.O. | 10-15 min | 1 hr | 3-6 hr |
| P.R. | Unknown | Unknown | Unknown |

## INDICATIONS & DOSAGE
*Moderate to severe pain—*
**Adults:** 5 mg P.O. q 6 hours, p.r.n. Or, 1
to 3 suppositories P.R. daily, p.r.n., or 10
mg (controlled-release tablets) P.O. q 12
hours, p.r.n., for patients not currently receiving opiates.

## ADVERSE REACTIONS
**CNS:** *sedation, somnolence, clouded sensorium, euphoria, dizziness, lightheadedness.*
**CV:** *hypotension,* **bradycardia.**
**GI:** *nausea, vomiting,* constipation, ileus.
**GU:** urine retention.
**Hepatic:** increased liver enzymes.
**Respiratory:** *respiratory depression.*
**Skin:** diaphoresis, pruritus.
**Other:** physical dependence, increased
plasma amylase and lipase levels.

## INTERACTIONS
**Drug-drug.** *Anticoagulants:* oxycodone
hydrochloride products containing aspirin
may increase anticoagulant effect. Monitor clotting times. Use together cautiously.
*CNS depressants, general anesthetics,
hypnotics, MAO inhibitors, other narcotic
analgesics, sedatives, tranquilizers, tricyclic antidepressants:* additive effects.
Use together with extreme caution. Reduce oxycodone dose and monitor patient
response.
**Drug-lifestyle.** *Alcohol use:* additive effects. Use together cautiously.

## EFFECTS ON DIAGNOSTIC TESTS
None reported.

## CONTRAINDICATIONS
Contraindicated in patients with hypersensitivity to drug and in those suspected
of having paralytic ileus.

## NURSING CONSIDERATIONS
• Use with extreme caution in patients
with head injury, increased intracranial
pressure, seizures, asthma, COPD, prostatic hyperplasia, severe hepatic or renal
disease, acute abdominal conditions, urethral stricture, hypothyroidism, Addison's
disease, and arrhythmias. Also use with
extreme caution in elderly or debilitated
patients.
• For full analgesic effect, administer
drug before patient has intense pain.
• To minimize GI upset, administer drug
after meals or with milk.
• Single-drug oxycodone solution or
tablets are especially useful for patients
who shouldn't take aspirin or acetaminophen.
• Monitor circulatory and respiratory status. Withhold dose and notify doctor if
respirations are shallow or if respiratory
rate falls below 12 breaths/minute.
• Monitor patient's bladder and bowel patterns. Patient may require a laxative because drug has a constipating effect.
• The 80-mg controlled-release tablet
should be reserved for opioid-dependent
patients who are taking daily doses of 160
mg or more.
• In patients who are taking more than 60
mg daily, dosing should be tapered when
discontinued to prevent withdrawal.

☑ **Patient teaching**
• Instruct patient to ask for drug before
pain is intense.
• Tell patient to take drug with milk or after eating.
• Advise patient to swallow extended-release tablets whole.
• Caution ambulatory patient about getting out of bed or walking. Warn outpatient to avoid driving and other potentially
hazardous activities that require mental
alertness until drug's CNS effects are
known.

---

Reactions may be *common,* uncommon, *__life-threatening,__* or COMMON AND LIFE-THREATENING.

• Advise patient to avoid alcohol during therapy.
• Advise patient that drug shouldn't be discontinued abruptly.

---

## oxymorphone hydrochloride
Numorphan, Numorphan H.P.

*Controlled Substance Schedule II*
*Pregnancy Risk Category C (D if used for prolonged periods or high doses at term)*

### HOW SUPPLIED
*Injection:* 1 mg/ml, 1.5 mg/ml
*Suppositories:* 5 mg

### ACTION
Binds with opiate receptors in the CNS, altering both perception of and emotional response to pain through an unknown mechanism.

| Route | Onset | Peak | Duration |
|-------|-------|------|----------|
| I.V. | 5-10 min | 15-30 min | 3-4 hr |
| I.M. | 10-15 min | 0.5-1.5 hr | 3-6 hr |
| S.C. | 10-20 min | 1-1.5 hr | 3-6 hr |
| P.R. | 15-30 min | 2 hr | 3-6 hr |

### INDICATIONS & DOSAGE
*Moderate to severe pain—*
**Adults:** 1 to 1.5 mg I.M. or S.C. q 4 to 6 hours, p.r.n.; or 0.5 mg I.V. q 4 to 6 hours, p.r.n.; or 5 mg P.R. q 4 to 6 hours, p.r.n.
*Analgesia during labor—*
**Adults:** 0.5 to 1 mg I.M.

### ADVERSE REACTIONS
**CNS:** *sedation, somnolence, clouded sensorium, euphoria,* dizziness, **seizures** (with large doses), light-headedness, headache.
**CV:** *hypotension,* **bradycardia.**
**GI:** *nausea, vomiting, constipation,* ileus.
**GU:** *urine retention.*
**Respiratory:** *respiratory depression.*
**Skin:** pruritus.
**Other:** physical dependence, increased plasma amylase levels.

### INTERACTIONS
**Drug-drug.** *CNS depressants, general anesthetics, MAO inhibitors, phenothi-*
*azines, sedative hypnotics, tricyclic antidepressants:* additive effects. Use together with extreme caution.
**Drug-lifestyle.** *Alcohol use:* additive effects. Use together cautiously.

### EFFECTS ON DIAGNOSTIC TESTS
None reported.

### CONTRAINDICATIONS
Contraindicated in patients with hypersensitivity to drug and in those with acute asthma attacks, severe respiratory depression, upper airway obstruction, or paralytic ileus. Don't use to treat pulmonary edema caused by a respiratory irritant.

### NURSING CONSIDERATIONS
• Use with extreme caution in patients with head injury, increased intracranial pressure, seizures, asthma, COPD, acute abdominal conditions, prostatic hyperplasia, severe hepatic or renal disease, urethral stricture, respiratory depression, hypothyroidism, Addison's disease, and arrhythmias. Also use with extreme caution in elderly or debilitated patients.
• Keep narcotic antagonist (naloxone) and resuscitation equipment available.
• Drug isn't for mild pain. May worsen gallbladder pain.
• For better effect, administer drug before patient has intense pain.
• Monitor CV and respiratory status. Withhold dose and notify doctor if respirations decrease or rate is below 12 breaths/minute.
• Monitor patient's bladder and bowel function. Patient may need laxative.
• *Alert:* Don't confuse oxymorphone with oxymetholone.

### I.V. administration
• Give drug by direct I.V. injection. If necessary, drug may be diluted in normal saline solution.

### Patient teaching
• Instruct patient to ask for drug before pain is intense.
• When drug is used postoperatively, encourage patient to turn, cough, and breathe deeply and to use incentive spirometer to avoid atelectasis.

---

*Liquid contains alcohol.  **May contain tartrazine.  †Canada  ‡Australia  §U.K.  ◇OTC

• Caution ambulatory patient about getting out of bed or walking. Warn outpatient to avoid driving and other potentially hazardous activities that require mental alertness until drug's CNS effects are known.
• Instruct patient to store suppositories in refrigerator.
• Advise patient to avoid alcohol during therapy.

---

**pentazocine hydrochloride**
Fortral†‡, Talwin†

**pentazocine hydrochloride and naloxone hydrochloride**
Talwin NX

**pentazocine lactate**
Fortral‡, Talwin

*Controlled Substance Schedule IV*
*Pregnancy Risk Category C*

## HOW SUPPLIED
**pentazocine hydrochloride**
*Tablets:* 25 mg‡, 50 mg†‡
**pentazocine hydrochloride and naloxone hydrochloride**
*Tablets:* 50 mg pentazocine hydrochloride and 500 mcg naloxone hydrochloride
**pentazocine lactate**
*Injection:* 30 mg/ml

## ACTION
Drug binds with opiate receptors at many sites in the CNS, altering both perception of and emotional response to pain through an unknown mechanism.

| Route | Onset | Peak | Duration |
|---|---|---|---|
| P.O. | 15-30 min | 1-3 hr | 2-3 hr |
| I.V. | 2-3 min | 15-30 min | 2-3 hr |
| I.M., S.C. | 10-20 min | 30-60 min | 2-3 hr |

## INDICATIONS & DOSAGE
*Moderate to severe pain—*
**Adults:** 50 to 100 mg P.O. q 3 to 4 hours, p.r.n. Maximum oral dose is 600 mg/day. Or, 30 mg I.M., I.V., or S.C. q 3 to 4 hours, p.r.n. Maximum parenteral dose is 360 mg/day. Single doses above 30 mg

I.V. or 60 mg I.M. or S.C. aren't recommended.
*Labor—*
**Adults:** 30 mg I.M. or 20 mg I.V. q 2 to 3 hours when contractions become regular.

## ADVERSE REACTIONS
**CNS:** *sedation,* visual disturbances, hallucinations, drowsiness, *dizziness, lightheadedness,* confusion, *euphoria,* headache, psychotomimetic effects.
**CV:** circulatory depression, **shock,** hypertension.
**EENT:** dry mouth.
**GI:** *nausea, vomiting,* constipation.
**GU:** urine retention.
**Respiratory:** *respiratory depression,* dyspnea, **apnea.**
**Skin:** induration, nodules, sloughing, sclerosis at injection site; diaphoresis; pruritus.
**Other:** *hypersensitivity reactions, anaphylaxis,* physical and psychological dependence.

## INTERACTIONS
**Drug-drug.** *CNS depressants:* additive effects. Use together cautiously.
*Fluoxetine:* additive effects resulting in serotonin syndrome. Use together cautiously.
*Narcotic analgesics:* possible decreased analgesic effect. Avoid concomitant use.
**Drug-lifestyle.** *Alcohol use:* additive effects. Use together cautiously.
*Smoking:* may increase requirements for pentazocine. Monitor drug's effectiveness.

## EFFECTS ON DIAGNOSTIC TESTS
Drug may interfere with certain laboratory tests for urinary 17-hydroxycorticosteroids.

## CONTRAINDICATIONS
Contraindicated in patients with hypersensitivity to drug or its components. It isn't recommended for children under age 12.

## NURSING CONSIDERATIONS
• Use cautiously in patients with hepatic or renal disease, acute MI, head injury, increased intracranial pressure, and respiratory depression.

---

• Have naloxone readily available. Respiratory depression can be reversed with naloxone.

• *Alert:* When giving by S.C. or I.M. injection, rotate injection sites to minimize tissue irritation. If possible, avoid giving by S.C. route.

• Drug has narcotic antagonist properties. May precipitate withdrawal syndrome in narcotic-dependent patients.

• Psychological and physical dependence may occur with prolonged use.

### I.V. administration
• Give drug by direct I.V. injection slowly. Don't mix in syringe with aminophylline, barbiturates, or other alkaline substances.

• Talwin Nx, the oral pentazocine available in the United States, contains the narcotic antagonist naloxone. This prevents illicit I.V. use.

### ✓ Patient teaching
• Instruct patient to ask for drug before pain is intense.

• Caution ambulatory patient about getting out of bed or walking. Warn outpatient to avoid driving and other potentially hazardous activities that require mental alertness until drug's CNS effects are known.

• Advise patient to avoid alcohol during therapy.

• Instruct patient or family to report skin rash, disorientation, or confusion to doctor.

---

## propoxyphene hydrochloride
(dextropropoxyphene hydrochloride)
Darvon, Dolene, Novo-Propoxyn†, 642†

## propoxyphene napsylate
(dextropropoxyphene napsylate)
Darvon-N, Doloxene‡

*Controlled Substance Schedule IV*
*Pregnancy Risk Category C*

### HOW SUPPLIED
**propoxyphene hydrochloride**
*Capsules:* 32 mg, 65 mg

**propoxyphene napsylate**
*Tablets:* 100 mg
*Oral suspension:* 10 mg/ml

### ACTION
Binds with opiate receptors in the CNS, altering both perception of and emotional response to pain through an unknown mechanism.

| Route | Onset | Peak | Duration |
|-------|-------|------|----------|
| P.O. | 15-60 min | 2-2.5 hr | 4-6 hr |

### INDICATIONS & DOSAGE
*Mild to moderate pain—*
**Adults:** 65 mg (hydrochloride) P.O. q 4 hours, p.r.n. Maximum dose is 390 mg/day.
*Mild to moderate pain—*
**Adults:** 100 mg (napsylate) P.O. q 4 hours, p.r.n. Maximum dose is 600 mg/day.
*Adjust-a-dose:* For patients with hepatic or renal dysfunction, reduce dose.

### ADVERSE REACTIONS
**CNS:** *dizziness,* headache, *sedation,* euphoria, light-headedness, weakness, hallucinations.
**GI:** *nausea, vomiting,* constipation, abdominal pain.
**Hepatic:** abnormal liver function tests.
**Respiratory:** *respiratory depression.*
**Other:** psychological and physical dependence.

### INTERACTIONS
**Drug-drug.** *Carbamazepine:* may increase carbamazepine levels. Monitor closely.
*CNS depressants:* additive effects. Use together cautiously.
*Warfarin:* may increase anticoagulant effect. Monitor PT and INR.
**Drug-lifestyle.** *Alcohol use:* additive effects. Use together cautiously.
*Smoking:* increased metabolism of propoxyphene. Monitor closely.

### EFFECTS ON DIAGNOSTIC TESTS
Drug may cause false decreases in tests for urinary steroid excretion.

### CONTRAINDICATIONS
Contraindicated in patients with hypersensitivity to drug.

---

*Liquid contains alcohol.  **May contain tartrazine.  †Canada  ‡Australia  §U.K.  ◇OTC

## NURSING CONSIDERATIONS
- Use cautiously in hepatic or renal disease, emotional instability, or history of drug or alcohol abuse.
- Remember that 65 mg of propoxyphene hydrochloride equals 100 mg of propoxyphene napsylate.
- Drug is considered a mild narcotic analgesic, but pain relief is equivalent to that provided by aspirin. Tolerance and physical dependence may occur. Drug is used with aspirin or acetaminophen to maximize analgesia.
- Smokers may need increased dosage because smoking may induce liver enzymes responsible for the metabolism of the drug, thereby decreasing its efficacy.

☑ **Patient teaching**
- Advise patient to take drug with food or milk to minimize GI upset.
- Warn patient not to exceed recommended dosage. Respiratory depression, hypotension, profound sedation, and coma may result if used in excessive doses or with other CNS depressants. Advise patient to avoid alcohol intake or use of other CNS-type drugs when taking propoxyphene.
- Caution ambulatory patient about getting out of bed or walking. Warn outpatient to avoid driving and other hazardous activities that require mental alertness until drug's CNS effects are known.

---

## remifentanil hydrochloride
Ultiva

*Controlled Substance Schedule II*
*Pregnancy Risk Category C*

---

### HOW SUPPLIED
*Injection (vials):* 1 mg/3 ml, 2 mg/5 ml, 5 mg/10 ml

### ACTION
Binds with μ-opiate receptors throughout CNS, resulting in analgesia and anesthesia.

| Route | Onset | Peak | Duration |
|-------|-------|------|----------|
| I.V. | Immediate | Unknown | 5-10 min |

### INDICATIONS & DOSAGE
*Induction of anesthesia through intubation—*
**Adults:** 0.5 to 1 mcg/kg/minute with hypnotic or volatile agent; may load with 1 mcg/kg over 30 to 60 seconds if endotracheal intubation is to occur less than 8 minutes after start of drug infusion.
*Maintenance of anesthesia—*
**Adults:** 0.25 to 0.4 mcg/kg/minute, dependent on concurrent anesthetic therapy (nitrous oxide, isoflurane, propofol). Increase doses by 25% to 100% and decrease by 25% to 50% q 2 to 5 minutes, p.r.n. If rate exceeds 1 mcg/kg/minute, consider increases in concomitant anesthetics. May supplement with 1 mcg/kg boluses over 30 to 60 seconds q 2 to 5 minutes, p.r.n.
*Continuation as analgesic immediately postoperatively—*
**Adults:** initially, 0.1 mcg/kg/minute. Adjust rate by 0.025-mcg/kg/minute increments q 5 minutes, p.r.n. Rates over 0.2 mcg/kg/minute are associated with respiratory depression (under 8 breaths/minute).
*Monitored anesthesia care—*
**Adults:** as single I.V. dose: 0.5 to 1 mcg/kg over 30 to 60 seconds starting 90 seconds before placement of local or regional anesthetic. As continuous I.V. infusion: 0.1 mcg/kg/minute beginning 5 minutes before giving local anesthetic; after placement of local anesthetic, titrate rate to 0.05 mcg/kg/minute. Titrate rate by 0.025 mcg/kg/minute q 5 minutes, p.r.n. Rates over 0.2 mcg/kg/minute are associated with respiratory depression (less than 8 breaths/minute). Decrease dose by 50% if given with 2 mg midazolam. Bolus doses administered simultaneously with continuously infusing remifentanil to spontaneously breathing patients aren't recommended.
**Elderly:** decrease initial dose by 50%.
*Adjust-a-dose:* For obese patients (more than 30% over ideal body weight), base starting dose on ideal body weight.

### ADVERSE REACTIONS
**CNS:** agitation, dizziness, headache.
**CV:** *bradycardia,* hypertension, *hypotension,* tachycardia.

---

Reactions may be *common,* uncommon, *life-threatening,* or COMMON AND LIFE-THREATENING.

**EENT:** visual disturbances.
**GI:** *nausea, vomiting.*
**Musculoskeletal:** *muscle rigidity.*
**Respiratory: *apnea, hypoxia, respiratory depression.***
**Skin:** flushing, pain at injection site, pruritus, sweating.
**Other:** chills, fever, postoperative pain, shivering, warm sensation.

## INTERACTIONS
**Drug-drug.** *Benzodiazepine, hypnotics, inhaled anesthetics:* produce a synergistic effect. Monitor patient closely.

## EFFECTS ON DIAGNOSTIC TESTS
None reported.

## CONTRAINDICATIONS
Contraindicated in patients with hypersensitivity to fentanyl analogues. Don't use via epidural or intrathecal routes because of presence of glycine in preparation.

## NURSING CONSIDERATIONS
• Use cautiously in breast-feeding women because fentanyl analogues appear in breast milk.
• Monitor vital signs and oxygenation continually throughout drug administration.
• Don't use as a single agent in general anesthesia.
• Manage respiratory depression in spontaneously breathing patients by decreasing infusion rate by 50% or by temporarily discontinuing infusion.
• Skeletal muscle rigidity may occur. To treat, either stop or decrease the rate of infusion in spontaneously breathing patients.
• Effects of long-term (over 16 hours) use in intensive care settings aren't known.
• Bradycardia has been reported and responds to ephedrine, atropine, and glycopyrrolate.
• Interruption of drug infusion results in rapid reversal (no residual opioid effects within 5 to 10 minutes of infusion discontinuation) of effects; adequate postoperative anesthesia should first be established.
• Drug shouldn't be used outside the monitored anesthesia care setting. Keep

narcotic antagonist (naloxone) and resuscitation equipment available. Naloxone may be used to manage severe respiratory depression.
• Drug is incompatible with blood products.
• Obtain history from patient regarding previous adverse anesthesia reactions in patient or patient's family.

### ◖I.V. administration
• To reconstitute solution, add 1 ml of diluent per mg of drug. Shake well to dissolve. Reconstituted solution contains 1 mg/ml and should be clear and colorless. Further dilute to concentration of 25, 50, or 250 mcg/ml before administration. Drug is stable at room temperature for 24 hours when in final concentration in $D_5W$, $D_5W$ in normal saline, normal saline, half-normal saline, or $D_5W$ in lactated Ringer's solution. Drug is stable for 4 hours when mixed in lactated Ringer's solution. Continuous infusion of drug must be administered by infusion device. Upon discontinuation of drug, I.V. tubing should be cleared to avoid inadvertent administration of drug at a later time.
• Hypotension may occur and can be treated by decreasing rate of infusion or administering I.V. fluids or catecholamine.
• I.V. bolus administration should be used only during maintenance of general anesthesia. In nonintubated patients, single doses should be administered over 30 to 60 seconds.

### ✔Patient teaching
• Reassure patient that appropriate monitoring will occur during anesthesia administration.

## sufentanil citrate
Sufenta

*Controlled Substance Schedule II*
*Pregnancy Risk Category C*

## HOW SUPPLIED
*Injection:* 50 mcg/ml

## ACTION

Binds with opiate receptors in the CNS, altering both perception of and emotional response to pain through an unknown mechanism.

| Route | Onset | Peak | Duration |
|-------|-------|------|----------|
| I.V. | 1 min | 1 min | 5 min |

## INDICATIONS & DOSAGE

*Adjunct to general anesthetic—*
**Adults:** 1 to 8 mcg/kg I.V. administered with nitrous oxide and oxygen; additional 10 to 25 mcg I.V. may be given, p.r.n., when movement or changes in vital signs indicate surgical stress or lightening of analgesia.
*As primary anesthetic—*
**Adults:** 8 to 30 mcg/kg I.V. administered with 100% oxygen and a muscle relaxant; additional 25 to 50 mcg I.V. may be given, p.r.n., when movement or changes in vital signs indicate surgical stress or lightening of analgesia.
**Children under age 12 undergoing CV surgery:** 10 to 25 mcg/kg I.V. administered with 100% oxygen and a muscle relaxant. Additional doses up to 50 mcg may be given, p.r.n.
**Elderly:** reduced dosage is needed.
***Adjust-a-dose:*** Use reduced dosage in debilitated patients. For obese patients who exceed 20% of their ideal body weight, base dosage calculations on an estimate of ideal weight.

## ADVERSE REACTIONS

**CNS:** chills, somnolence.
**CV:** *hypotension,* hypertension, ***arrhythmias, bradycardia,*** tachycardia.
**GI:** nausea, vomiting.
**Respiratory:** *chest wall rigidity, apnea, bronchospasm.*
**Skin:** *pruritus,* erythema.
**Other:** intraoperative muscle movement; increased plasma amylase, lipase, and serum prolactin levels.

## INTERACTIONS

**Drug-drug.** *CNS depressants:* additive effects. Use together cautiously.
**Drug-lifestyle.** *Alcohol use:* additive effects. Use together cautiously.

## EFFECTS ON DIAGNOSTIC TESTS

None reported.

## CONTRAINDICATIONS

Contraindicated in patients with hypersensitivity to drug.

## NURSING CONSIDERATIONS

• Use with extreme caution in head injury; in pulmonary, hepatic, or renal disease; in decreased respiratory reserve; and in elderly or debilitated patients.
• When used at doses over 8 mcg/kg, postoperative mechanical ventilation and observation are essential because of prolonged respiratory depression.
• Keep narcotic antagonist (naloxone) and resuscitation equipment available.
• Because drug decreases both rate and depth of respirations, monitoring of arterial oxygen saturation may aid in assessing respiratory depression. Notify doctor if respirations decrease or rate falls below 12 breaths/minute.
• Monitor respirations of neonates exposed to drug during labor.
• *Alert:* High doses can produce muscle rigidity reversible by neuromuscular blockers; however, patient must be artificially ventilated.
• Monitor postoperative vital signs frequently, including circulatory and respiratory status and urinary function. Drug may cause respiratory depression, hypotension, urine retention, nausea, vomiting, ileus, or altered level of consciousness.
• *Alert:* Don't confuse sufentanil with alfentanil, or Sufenta with Survanta.

### 🔲 I.V. administration

• Drug should be administered only by persons trained in the use of I.V. anesthetics.
• Give drug by direct I.V. injection. Drug has been given by intermittent I.V. infusion, but drug compatibility and stability in I.V. solutions isn't fully known.

### ✅ Patient teaching

• Inform patient and family of need for drug and answer any questions.

---

Reactions may be *common,* uncommon, *life-threatening,* or COMMON AND LIFE-THREATENING.

• Encourage turning, coughing, and deep breathing postoperatively to prevent atelectasis.

---

## tramadol hydrochloride
Ultram, Zamadol§, Zydol§

*Pregnancy Risk Category C*

### HOW SUPPLIED
*Tablets:* 50 mg

### ACTION
Unknown. A centrally acting synthetic analgesic compound not chemically related to opiates. Drug is thought to bind to opioid receptors and inhibit reuptake of norepinephrine and serotonin.

| Route | Onset | Peak | Duration |
|-------|-------|------|----------|
| P.O. | Unknown | 2 hr | Unknown |

### INDICATIONS & DOSAGE
*Moderate to moderately severe pain—*
**Adults:** 50 to 100 mg P.O. q 4 to 6 hours, p.r.n. Maximum dose is 400 mg daily.
**Elderly:** for patients over age 75, maximum dose is 300 mg/day in divided doses.
*Adjust-a-dose:* For renally impaired patients with creatinine clearance below 30 ml/minute, increase dose interval to q 12 hours; maximum daily dose is 200 mg. In patients with cirrhosis, give 50 mg q 12 hours.

### ADVERSE REACTIONS
**CNS:** *dizziness, vertigo, headache, somnolence,* CNS stimulation, asthenia, anxiety, confusion, coordination disturbance, euphoria, nervousness, sleep disorder, *seizures,* malaise.
**CV:** vasodilation.
**EENT:** visual disturbances.
**GI:** *nausea, constipation, vomiting,* dyspepsia, dry mouth, diarrhea, abdominal pain, anorexia, flatulence.
**GU:** urine retention, urinary frequency, menopausal symptoms, proteinuria, increased creatinine clearance.
**Hematologic:** decreased hemoglobin levels.

**Hepatic:** increased liver enzyme levels.
**Musculoskeletal:** hypertonia.
**Respiratory:** *respiratory depression.*
**Skin:** pruritus, diaphoresis, rash.

### INTERACTIONS
**Drug-drug.** *Carbamazepine:* increased tramadol metabolism. Patients receiving chronic carbamazepine therapy at a dose of up to 800 mg daily may need up to twice the recommended dose of tramadol.
*CNS depressants:* additive effects. Use together with caution. Dosage of tramadol may need to be reduced.
*Cyclobenzaprine, MAO inhibitors, neuroleptics, selective serotonin reuptake inhibitors, tricyclic antidepressants:* increased risk of seizures. Monitor patient closely.
*Quinidine:* increased levels of tramadol. Monitor patient closely.

### EFFECTS ON DIAGNOSTIC TESTS
None reported.

### CONTRAINDICATIONS
Contraindicated in patients with hypersensitivity to drug and in those with acute intoxication from alcohol, hypnotics, centrally acting analgesics, opioids, or psychotropic drugs.

### NURSING CONSIDERATIONS
• Use cautiously in patients at risk for seizures or respiratory depression; in increased intracranial pressure or head injury, acute abdominal conditions, and in renal or hepatic impairment; and in physical dependence on opioids.
• Monitor CV and respiratory status. Withhold dose and notify doctor if respirations decrease or rate is below 12 breaths/minute.
• Monitor bowel and bladder function. Anticipate need for laxative.
• For better analgesic effect, give drug before onset of intense pain.
• Monitor patients at risk for seizures. Drug may reduce seizure threshold.
• Monitor patient for drug dependence. Drug can produce dependence similar to

---

that of codeine or dextropropoxyphene and thus has potential for abuse.

### ✓ Patient teaching
• Tell patient to take drug as prescribed and not to increase dose or dosage interval unless ordered by doctor.
• Caution ambulatory patient to be careful when rising and walking. Warn outpatient to avoid driving and other potentially hazardous activities that require mental alertness until drug's CNS effects are known.
• Advise patient to check with doctor before taking OTC drugs; drug interactions can occur.

**chloral hydrate**
**estazolam**
**flurazepam hydrochloride**
**pentobarbital**
**pentobarbital sodium**
**phenobarbital sodium**
(See Chapter 30, ANTICONVULSANTS.)
**secobarbital sodium**
**temazepam**
**triazolam**
**zaleplon**
**zolpidem tartrate**

## COMBINATION PRODUCTS
TUINAL 100 mg PULVULES: amobarbital
sodium 50 mg and secobarbital sodium
50 mg.
TUINAL 200 mg PULVULES: amobarbital
sodium 100 mg and secobarbital sodium
100 mg.

## chloral hydrate
Aquachloral Supprettes, Noctec,
Novo-Chlorhydrate†

*Controlled Substance Schedule IV*
*Pregnancy Risk Category C*

## HOW SUPPLIED
*Capsules:* 250 mg, 500 mg
*Syrup:* 250 mg/5 ml, 500 mg/5 ml
*Suppositories:* 324 mg, 500 mg, 648 mg

## ACTION
Unknown. Sedative effects may be caused
by its primary metabolite, trichloro-
ethanol.

| Route | Onset | Peak | Duration |
|-------|-------|------|----------|
| P.O. | 0.5 hr | Unknown | 4-8 hr |
| P.R. | Unknown | Unknown | 4-8 hr |

## INDICATIONS & DOSAGE
*Sedation—*
**Adults:** 250 mg P.O. or P.R. t.i.d. after
meals.

**Children:** 25 mg/kg/day P.O. or P.R.
Maximum daily dose is 500 mg per single
dose; doses may be divided.
*Insomnia—*
**Adults:** 500 mg to 1 g P.O. or P.R. 15 to
30 minutes before bedtime.
**Children:** 50 mg/kg P.O. or P.R. 15 to 30
minutes before bedtime. Maximum single
dose is 1 g.
*Preoperatively—*
**Adults:** 500 mg to 1 g P.O. or P.R. 30
minutes before surgery.
*Premedication for EEG—*
**Children:** 20 to 25 mg/kg P.O. or P.R.

## ADVERSE REACTIONS
**CNS:** drowsiness, nightmares, dizziness,
ataxia, paradoxical excitement, hangover,
somnolence, disorientation, delirium,
light-headedness, hallucinations, confusion, vertigo, malaise.
**GI:** *nausea, vomiting, diarrhea,* flatulence.
**Hematologic:** eosinophilia, *leukopenia.*
**Skin:** hypersensitivity reactions.
**Other:** physical and psychological dependence.

## INTERACTIONS
**Drug-drug.** *CNS depressants, including
narcotic analgesics:* excessive CNS depression or vasodilation reaction. Use together cautiously.
*Furosemide I.V.:* causes sweating, flushes,
variable blood pressure, nausea, and un-
easiness. Use together cautiously or use a
different hypnotic drug.
*Oral anticoagulants:* increased risk of
bleeding. Monitor patient closely.
*Phenytoin:* decreased phenytoin levels.
Monitor closely.
**Drug-lifestyle.** *Alcohol use:* excessive
CNS and respiratory depression. Use together cautiously.

## EFFECTS ON DIAGNOSTIC TESTS
Drug therapy may produce false-positive
results for urine glucose with tests using
cupric sulfate, such as Benedict's reagent.

---

*Liquid contains alcohol.    **May contain tartrazine.    †Canada    ‡Australia    §U.K.    ◊OTC

It doesn't interfere with Diastix or Chemstrip uG results. It will interfere with fluorometric tests for urine catecholamines; don't use drug for 48 hours before the test. Drug may interfere with Reddy-Jenkins-Thorn test for urinary 17-hydroxycorticosteroids. It may also cause a false-positive phentolamine test.

## CONTRAINDICATIONS
Contraindicated in patients with hypersensitivity to drug and in those with hepatic or renal impairment, or severe cardiac disease. Oral administration contraindicated in patients with gastric disorders.

## NURSING CONSIDERATIONS
• Use with extreme caution in patients with severe cardiac disease. Use cautiously in patients with mental depression, suicidal tendencies, or history of drug abuse.
• *Alert:* Note two strengths of oral liquid form. Double-check dose, especially when administering to children. Fatal overdoses have occurred.
• To minimize unpleasant taste and stomach irritation, dilute or administer with liquid. Drug should be taken after meals.
• Take precautions to prevent hoarding or self-overdosing by patients who are depressed, suicidal, or drug-dependent or who have history of drug abuse.
• Long-term use isn't recommended; drug loses its efficacy in promoting sleep after 14 days of continued use. Long-term use may cause drug dependence, and patient may experience withdrawal symptoms if drug is suddenly stopped.
• Don't administer drug for 48 hours before fluorometric test, as ordered.
• Monitor BUN levels as ordered; large doses may raise BUN levels.

### ✓ Patient teaching
• Instruct patient to take capsule with a full glass of water or juice and to swallow capsule whole.
• Tell patient to avoid alcohol during therapy.
• Caution patient about performing activities that require mental alertness or physical coordination.
• Advise patient to store drug in dark container; store suppositories in refrigerator.

## estazolam
ProSom

*Controlled Substance Schedule IV*
*Pregnancy Risk Category X*

### HOW SUPPLIED
*Tablets:* 1 mg, 2 mg

### ACTION
Unknown. Thought to act on the limbic system and thalamus of the CNS by binding to specific benzodiazepine receptors.

| Route | Onset | Peak | Duration |
|-------|-------|------|----------|
| P.O. | Unknown | 1-3 hr | Unknown |

### INDICATIONS & DOSAGE
*Insomnia—*
**Adults:** 1 mg P.O. h.s. Some patients may need 2 mg.
**Elderly:** 1 mg P.O. h.s. Use higher doses with extreme care. Frail elderly or debilitated patients may take 0.5 mg, but this low dose may be only marginally effective.

### ADVERSE REACTIONS
**CNS:** fatigue, dizziness, daytime drowsiness, *somnolence, asthenia,* hypokinesia, abnormal thinking.
**GI:** dyspepsia, abdominal pain.
**Hepatic:** increased AST levels.
**Musculoskeletal:** back pain, stiffness.

### INTERACTIONS
**Drug-drug.** *Cimetidine, disulfiram, isoniazid, oral contraceptives:* may impair metabolism and clearance of benzodiazepines and prolong their plasma half-life. Monitor for increased CNS depression.
*CNS depressants, including antihistamines, opiate analgesics, and other benzodiazepines:* increased CNS depression. Avoid concomitant use.
*Digoxin:* Digoxin serum levels may increase, resulting in toxicity. Monitor closely.
*Phenytoin:* possible increase in phenytoin levels, resulting in toxicity. Monitor closely.
*Rifampin:* may increase metabolism and clearance and decrease plasma half-life. Monitor for decreased effectiveness.

---

Reactions may be *common,* uncommon, *life-threatening,* or COMMON AND LIFE-THREATENING.

*Theophylline:* pharmacologic antagonism. Monitor for decreased effectiveness of estazolam.

**Drug-lifestyle.** *Alcohol use:* excessive CNS and respiratory depression. Use together cautiously.

*Smoking:* may increase metabolism and clearance and decrease plasma half-life. Monitor for decreased effectiveness.

**EFFECTS ON DIAGNOSTIC TESTS**
None reported.

**CONTRAINDICATIONS**
Contraindicated in patients with hypersensitivity to drug and during pregnancy.

**NURSING CONSIDERATIONS**
• Use cautiously in patients with depression, suicidal tendencies, or hepatic, renal, or pulmonary disease.
• Liver and renal function and CBC should be checked before and periodically during long-term therapy, as ordered.
• Take precautions to prevent hoarding by depressed, suicidal, or drug-dependent patients or those with history of drug abuse.
• Patients who receive prolonged treatment with benzodiazepines may experience withdrawal symptoms if drug is suddenly discontinued (possibly after 6 weeks of continuous therapy).
• *Alert:* Don't confuse ProSom with Proscar, Prozac, or Psorcon.

☑ **Patient teaching**
• Advise patient to inform doctor if pregnancy is suspected or is being planned during therapy.
• Tell patient not to increase dosage but to inform doctor if he thinks that drug is no longer effective.
• Caution patient about performing activities that require mental alertness or physical coordination.
• Warn patient that additive depressant effects can occur if alcohol is consumed while taking drug or within 24 hours after taking drug.
• Warn patient not to abruptly discontinue use after taking for 1 month or more.

## flurazepam hydrochloride
Apo-Flurazepam†, Dalmane, Novo-Flupam†

*Controlled Substance Schedule IV*
*Pregnancy Risk Category NR*

**HOW SUPPLIED**
*Capsules:* 15 mg, 30 mg

**ACTION**
Unknown. A benzodiazepine that probably acts on the limbic system, thalamus, and hypothalamus of the CNS to produce hypnotic effects.

| Route | Onset | Peak | Duration |
|-------|-------|------|----------|
| P.O. | Unknown | 0.5-1 hr | Unknown |

**INDICATIONS & DOSAGE**
*Insomnia—*
**Adults:** 15 to 30 mg P.O. h.s. Dose repeated once, p.r.n.
**Elderly:** initiate with 15-mg dose until response determined.

**ADVERSE REACTIONS**
**CNS:** *daytime sedation, dizziness, drowsiness, disturbed coordination,* lethargy, confusion, *headache,* lightheadedness, nervousness, hallucinations, staggering, ataxia, disorientation, *coma.*
**GI:** nausea, vomiting, heartburn, diarrhea, abdominal pain.
**Hepatic:** elevated liver enzyme levels.
**Other:** physical or psychological dependence.

**INTERACTIONS**
**Drug-drug.** *Cimetidine:* increased sedation. Monitor carefully.
*CNS depressants, including narcotic analgesics:* excessive CNS depression. Use together cautiously.
*Digoxin:* Digoxin serum levels may increase, resulting in toxicity. Monitor closely.
*Disulfiram, isoniazid, oral contraceptives:* decreased metabolism of benzodiazepines, leading to toxicity. Monitor closely.
*Phenytoin:* increased phenytoin levels. Monitor for toxicity.

---

*Liquid contains alcohol.    **May contain tartrazine.    †Canada    ‡Australia    §U.K.    ◊OTC

*Rifampin:* enhanced metabolism of benzodiazepines. Monitor for decreased effectiveness.
*Theophylline:* antagonist with flurazepam. Monitor for decreased effectiveness.
**Drug-lifestyle.** *Alcohol use:* excessive CNS and respiratory depression. Use together cautiously.
*Smoking:* may increase metabolism and clearance and decrease plasma half-life. Monitor for decreased effectiveness.

### EFFECTS ON DIAGNOSTIC TESTS
Minor changes in EEG patterns (usually low-voltage, fast activity) may occur during and after flurazepam therapy.

### CONTRAINDICATIONS
Contraindicated in patients with hypersensitivity to drug and during pregnancy.

### NURSING CONSIDERATIONS
• Use cautiously in patients with impaired hepatic or renal function, chronic pulmonary insufficiency, mental depression, suicidal tendencies, or history of drug abuse.
• Check hepatic and renal function and CBC before and periodically during long-term therapy. Drug may cause elevations in certain liver function tests (AST, ALT, total and direct bilirubin, and alkaline phosphatase).
• Assess mental status before initiating therapy. Elderly patients are more sensitive to drug's adverse CNS reactions.
• Take precautions to prevent hoarding or self-overdosing by patients who are depressed, suicidal, or drug-dependent or who have history of drug abuse.
• Physical and psychological dependence is possible with long-term use.
• *Alert:* Don't confuse Dalmane with Dialume or Demulen.

☑ **Patient teaching**
• Inform patient that drug is more effective on second, third, and fourth nights because active metabolite accumulates.
• Warn patient not to abruptly discontinue use after taking for 1 month or more.
• Tell patient to avoid alcohol while taking drug.

• Caution patient about performing activities that require mental alertness or physical coordination.

## pentobarbital
Nembutal*†**

## pentobarbital sodium
Nembutal Sodium*, Nova Rectal†, NovoPentobarb†

*Controlled Substance Schedule II (III for suppositories)*
*Pregnancy Risk Category D*

### HOW SUPPLIED
**pentobarbital**
*Elixir:* 18.2 mg/5 ml
**pentobarbital sodium**
*Capsules:* 50 mg, 100 mg
*Injection:* 50 mg/ml
*Suppositories:* 30 mg, 60 mg, 120 mg, 200 mg

### ACTION
Unknown. Probably interferes with transmission of impulses from the thalamus to the cortex of the brain. A barbiturate.

| Route | Onset | Peak | Duration |
|-------|-------|------|----------|
| P.O. | 20 min | 0.5-1 hr | 1-4 hr |
| I.V. | Immediate | Immediate | 15 min |
| I.M. | 10-25 min | Unknown | Unknown |
| P.R. | 20 min | Unknown | 1-4 hr |

### INDICATIONS & DOSAGE
*Sedation—*
**Adults:** 20 mg P.O. t.i.d. or q.i.d.
**Children:** 2 to 6 mg/kg P.O. daily in three divided doses. Maximum daily dose is 100 mg.
*Insomnia—*
**Adults:** 100 to 200 mg P.O. h.s. or 150 to 200 mg deep I.M.; 100 mg initially I.V., then additional small doses up to a total of 500 mg; 120 or 200 mg P.R.
**Children:** 2 to 6 mg/kg or 125 mg/m$^2$ I.M. Maximum dose is 100 mg. P.R. dose for children ages 2 months to 1 year is 30 mg; ages 1 to 4, 30 or 60 mg; ages 5 to 11, 60 mg; ages 12 to 14, 60 or 120 mg.
*Preoperative sedation—*
**Adults:** 150 to 200 mg I.M.

Reactions may be *common*, uncommon, *life-threatening*, or COMMON AND LIFE-THREATENING.

**Children:** 5 mg/kg P.O. or I.M. if child is age 10 or older; 5 mg/kg I.M. or P.R. if child is under age 10.

## ADVERSE REACTIONS
**CNS:** *drowsiness, lethargy, hangover,* paradoxical excitement in elderly patients, somnolence.
**GI:** nausea, vomiting.
**Hematologic:** exacerbation of porphyria.
**Respiratory:** *respiratory depression.*
**Skin:** rash, urticaria, *Stevens-Johnson syndrome.*
**Other:** *angioedema,* physical and psychological dependence.

## INTERACTIONS
**Drug-drug.** *CNS depressants, including narcotic analgesics:* excessive CNS and respiratory depression. Use together cautiously.
*Corticosteroids, digitoxin, doxycycline, estrogens and oral contraceptives, oral anticoagulants, theophylline, verapamil:* pentobarbital may enhance the metabolism of these drugs. Monitor for decreased effect.
*Griseofulvin:* decreased absorption of griseofulvin. Monitor effectiveness of griseofulvin.
*MAO inhibitors:* inhibited metabolism of barbiturates; may cause prolonged CNS depression. Reduce barbiturate dosage.
*Rifampin:* may decrease barbiturate levels. Monitor for decreased effect.
**Drug-herb.** *Kava:* may cause additive effects. Avoid concomitant use.
**Drug-lifestyle.** *Alcohol use:* excessive CNS and respiratory depression. Use together cautiously.

## EFFECTS ON DIAGNOSTIC TESTS
Drug may cause a false-positive phentolamine test. The physiologic effects of drug may impair the absorption of cyanocobalamin $^{57}$Co. Drug may decrease serum bilirubin levels in neonates, epileptic patients, and patients with congenital, nonhemolytic, unconjugated hyperbilirubinemia. EEG patterns show a change in low-voltage, fast activity; changes persist for a time after discontinuation of therapy.

## CONTRAINDICATIONS
Contraindicated in patients with hypersensitivity to barbiturates and in those with porphyria.

## NURSING CONSIDERATIONS
• Use cautiously in patients with acute or chronic pain, mental depression, suicidal tendencies, history of drug abuse, or hepatic impairment. Also administer cautiously to elderly or debilitated patients.
• Assess mental status before initiating therapy and use reduced doses, as ordered. Elderly patients are more sensitive to drug's adverse CNS effects.
• *Alert:* Administer I.M. injection deeply. Superficial injection may cause pain, sterile abscess, and sloughing.
• To ensure accurate dosage, don't divide suppositories.
• Take precautions to prevent hoarding or self-overdosing by patients who are depressed, suicidal, or drug-dependent or who have a history of drug abuse.
• Watch for signs of barbiturate toxicity: coma, pupillary constriction, cyanosis, clammy skin, and hypotension. Overdose can be fatal.
• Inspect patient's skin. Skin eruptions may precede potentially fatal reactions to barbiturate therapy. Discontinue drug when skin reactions occur and call doctor. In some patients, high fever, stomatitis, headache, or rhinitis may precede skin reactions.
• Drug has no analgesic effect and may cause restlessness or delirium in patients with pain.
• Long-term use isn't recommended; drug loses its efficacy in promoting sleep after 14 days of continued use. Long-term high dosage may cause drug dependence, and patient may experience withdrawal symptoms if drug is suddenly discontinued. Withdraw barbiturates gradually.
• *Alert:* Don't confuse pentobarbital with phenobarbital.

### ◖ I.V. administration
• I.V. administration of barbiturates may cause severe respiratory depression, laryngospasm, or hypotension. Have emergency resuscitation equipment available.

• To minimize deterioration, use I.V. injection solution within 30 minutes after opening container. Don't use cloudy solution.
• Reserve I.V. injection for emergency treatment, which should be given under close supervision. Administer slowly at a rate not exceeding 50 mg/minute.
• Parenteral solution is alkaline. Local tissue reactions and injection site pain have followed I.V. use. Avoid extravasation. Assess patency of I.V. site before and during administration.
• Don't mix in syringe or in I.V. solutions or lines with other drugs.

☑ **Patient teaching**
• Inform patient that morning hangover is common after hypnotic dose, which suppresses REM sleep. Patient may experience increased dreaming after drug is discontinued.
• Caution patient about performing activities that require mental alertness or physical coordination.
• Tell patient to avoid alcohol while taking drug.
• Instruct patient using oral contraceptives to consider alternative birth control methods because drug may decrease oral contraceptive's effect.

---

## secobarbital sodium
Novo-Secobarb†, Seconal Sodium

*Controlled Substance Schedule II*
*Pregnancy Risk Category D*

### HOW SUPPLIED
*Capsules:* 100 mg
*Injection:* 50 mg/ml

### ACTION
Unknown. Probably interferes with transmission of impulses from the thalamus to the cortex of the brain.

| Route | Onset | Peak | Duration |
|-------|-------|------|----------|
| P.O. | 15 min | 15-30 min | 1-4 hr |
| I.V. | Immediate | 1-3 min | 15 min |
| I.M. | Unknown | 7-10 min | Unknown |

### INDICATIONS & DOSAGE
*Preoperative sedation—*
**Adults:** 200 to 300 mg P.O. 1 to 2 hours before surgery; or 1 mg/kg I.M. 10 to 15 minutes before surgery.
**Children:** 2 to 6 mg/kg P.O. 1 to 2 hours before surgery. Maximum single dose is 100 mg P.O., or 4 to 5 mg/kg I.M. as a single dose.
*Insomnia—*
**Adults:** 100 to 200 mg P.O. or I.M. or 50 to 250 mg I.V.
**Children:** 3 to 5 mg/kg I.M. or 125 mg/m$^2$, not to exceed 100 mg, with no more than 5 ml injected in any one site.
*Acute tetanus seizure—*
**Adults and children:** 5.5 mg/kg I.M. or slow I.V., repeated q 3 to 4 hours, if needed; I.V. injection rate not to exceed 50 mg/15 seconds.
*Status epilepticus—*
**Children:** 15 to 20 mg/kg I.V. over 15 minutes.

### ADVERSE REACTIONS
**CNS:** *drowsiness, lethargy, hangover,* paradoxical excitement (in elderly patients), somnolence.
**CV:** hypotension with I.V. use.
**GI:** nausea, vomiting.
**Hematologic:** exacerbation of porphyria.
**Respiratory:** *respiratory depression.*
**Skin:** rash, urticaria, ***Stevens-Johnson syndrome,*** tissue reactions, injection-site pain.
**Other:** *angioedema,* physical and psychological dependence.

### INTERACTIONS
**Drug-drug.** *Chloramphenicol, MAO inhibitors, valproic acid:* inhibited metabolism of barbiturates; may cause prolonged CNS depression. Reduce barbiturate dosage.
*CNS depressants, including narcotic analgesics:* excessive CNS and respiratory depression. Use together cautiously.
*Corticosteroids, digitoxin, doxycycline, estrogens and oral contraceptives, oral anticoagulants, theophylline, tricyclic antidepressants, verapamil:* secobarbital may enhance the metabolism of these drugs. Monitor for decreased effect.

---

Reactions may be *common*, uncommon, *life-threatening*, or COMMON AND LIFE-THREATENING.

*Griseofulvin:* decreased absorption of griseofulvin. Monitor effectiveness of griseofulvin.

*Rifampin:* may decrease barbiturate levels. Monitor for decreased effect.

**Drug-lifestyle.** *Alcohol use:* excessive CNS and respiratory depression. Use together cautiously.

## EFFECTS ON DIAGNOSTIC TESTS

Drug may cause a false-positive phentolamine test. The physiologic effects of drug may impair the absorption of cyanocobalamin $^{57}$Co. Drug may decrease serum bilirubin levels in neonates, epileptic patients, and patients with congenital, nonhemolytic, unconjugated hyperbilirubinemia. EEG patterns are altered, with a change in low-voltage, fast activity; changes persist for a time after discontinuation of therapy.

## CONTRAINDICATIONS

Contraindicated in patients with hypersensitivity to barbiturates and in those with marked liver impairment, respiratory disease in which dyspnea or obstruction is evident, or porphyria.

## NURSING CONSIDERATIONS

• Use cautiously in patients with acute or chronic pain, depression, suicidal tendencies, history of drug abuse, or hepatic or renal impairment. Also use cautiously in elderly or debilitated patients.

• Assess mental status before initiating therapy. Elderly patients are more sensitive to the drug's adverse CNS effects.

• Secobarbital sodium injection isn't compatible with lactated Ringer's solution, but is compatible with Ringer's solution, sterile water for injection, and normal saline. Don't mix with acidic solutions.

• Use injection solution within 30 minutes after opening container to minimize deterioration. Don't use cloudy solution.

• *Alert:* Give I.M. injection deeply. Superficial injection may cause pain, sterile abscess, and sloughing.

• Take precautions to prevent hoarding or self-overdosing by patients who are depressed, suicidal, or drug-dependent or who have a history of drug abuse.

• Watch for signs of barbiturate toxicity: coma, pupillary constriction, cyanosis, clammy skin, and hypotension. Overdose can be fatal.

• Inspect patient's skin. Skin eruptions may precede potentially fatal reactions to barbiturate therapy. Discontinue drug when skin reactions occur and notify doctor. In some patients, high fever, stomatitis, headache, or rhinitis may precede skin reactions.

• Long-term use isn't recommended; drug loses its efficacy in promoting sleep after 14 days of continued use.

## I.V. administration

• I.V. injection is reserved for emergency treatment; it should be given under close supervision by direct injection and administered slowly at a rate not exceeding 50 mg/15 seconds. May be administered as supplied or diluted with sterile water for injection, normal saline, or Ringer's injection. Don't use lactated Ringer's injection.

• Don't add to acidic solutions because precipitate will form.

• Local tissue reactions and injection-site pain have been noted with I.V. use. Assess patency of I.V. site before and during administration.

• I.V. administration of barbiturates may cause severe respiratory depression, laryngospasm, or hypotension. Have emergency resuscitation equipment readily available.

## Patient teaching

• Tell patient that morning hangover is common after hypnotic dose, which suppresses REM sleep. Patient may experience increased dreaming after drug is discontinued.

• Tell patient to avoid alcohol while taking drug.

• Caution patient about performing activities that require mental alertness or physical coordination.

• Instruct patient using oral contraceptives to consider alternative birth control methods.

## temazepam
Euhypnos 10‡, Euhypnos 20‡,
Nomapam‡, Normison‡, Restoril,
Temaze‡, Temtabs‡

*Controlled Substance Schedule IV
Pregnancy Risk Category X*

### HOW SUPPLIED
*Capsules:* 10 mg‡, 15 mg, 20 mg‡, 30 mg

### ACTION
Unknown. A benzodiazepine that probably acts on the limbic system, thalamus,
and hypothalamus of the CNS to produce
hypnotic effects.

| Route | Onset | Peak | Duration |
|-------|-------|------|----------|
| P.O. | Unknown | 1-2 hr | Unknown |

### INDICATIONS & DOSAGE
*Insomnia—*
**Adults:** 15 to 30 mg P.O. h.s.
**Elderly:** in patients over age 65, 15 mg
P.O. h.s.

### ADVERSE REACTIONS
**CNS:** drowsiness, dizziness, lethargy, disturbed coordination, daytime sedation,
confusion, nightmares, vertigo, euphoria,
weakness, headache, fatigue, nervousness, anxiety, depression.
**EENT:** blurred vision.
**GI:** diarrhea, nausea, dry mouth.
**Hepatic:** increased liver function test results.
**Other:** physical and psychological dependence.

### INTERACTIONS
**Drug-drug.** *CNS depressants:* increased
CNS depression. Use together cautiously.
**Drug-lifestyle.** *Alcohol use:* increased
CNS depression. Use together cautiously.

### EFFECTS ON DIAGNOSTIC TESTS
Minor changes in EEG patterns (usually
low-voltage, fast activity) may occur during and after therapy.

### CONTRAINDICATIONS
Contraindicated in patients with hypersensitivity to drug or other benzodiazepines and during pregnancy.

### NURSING CONSIDERATIONS
• Use cautiously in patients with chronic
pulmonary insufficiency, impaired hepatic or renal function, severe or latent mental depression, suicidal tendencies, and
history of drug abuse.
• Assess mental status before initiating
therapy. Elderly patients are more sensitive to drug's adverse CNS effects.
• Take precautions to prevent hoarding or
self-overdosing by patients who are depressed, suicidal, or drug-dependent or
who have history of drug abuse.
• *Alert:* Don't confuse Restoril with Vistaril.

☑ **Patient teaching**
• Tell patient to avoid alcohol during therapy.
• Caution patient about performing activities that require mental alertness or physical coordination.
• Warn patient not to discontinue drug
abruptly if taken for 1 month or longer.
• Tell patient that onset of drug's effects
may take as long as 2 to 2½ hours.

## triazolam
Apo-Triazo†, Halcion,
Novo-Triolam†

*Controlled Substance Schedule IV
Pregnancy Risk Category X*

### HOW SUPPLIED
*Tablets:* 0.125 mg, 0.25 mg

### ACTION
Unknown. A benzodiazepine that probably acts on the limbic system, thalamus,
and hypothalamus of the CNS to produce
hypnotic effects.

| Route | Onset | Peak | Duration |
|-------|-------|------|----------|
| P.O. | Unknown | 1-2 hr | Unknown |

## INDICATIONS & DOSAGE
*Insomnia—*
**Adults:** 0.125 to 0.5 mg P.O. h.s.
**Elderly:** 0.125 mg P.O. h.s.; increased, p.r.n., to 0.25 mg P.O. h.s.

## ADVERSE REACTIONS
**CNS:** *drowsiness,* dizziness, headache, rebound insomnia, amnesia, lack of coordination, mental confusion, depression, nervousness, ataxia.
**GI:** nausea, vomiting.
**Hepatic:** increased liver function test results.
**Other:** physical or psychological dependence.

## INTERACTIONS
**Drug-drug.** *Cimetidine, erythromycin:* may cause prolonged triazolam blood levels. Monitor for increased sedation.
*CNS depressants:* excessive CNS depression. Use together cautiously.
**Drug-lifestyle.** *Alcohol use:* excessive CNS depression. Use together cautiously.

## EFFECTS ON DIAGNOSTIC TESTS
Minor changes in EEG patterns (usually low-voltage, fast activity) may occur during and after therapy.

## CONTRAINDICATIONS
Contraindicated in patients with hypersensitivity to benzodiazepines and during pregnancy.

## NURSING CONSIDERATIONS
• Use cautiously in patients with impaired hepatic or renal function, chronic pulmonary insufficiency, sleep apnea, mental depression, suicidal tendencies, or history of drug abuse. Also use cautiously in breast-feeding women.
• Assess mental status before initiating therapy. Elderly patients are more sensitive to drug's CNS effects.
• Take precautions to prevent hoarding or self-overdosing by patients who are depressed, suicidal, or drug-dependent or who have history of drug abuse.
• *Alert:* Don't confuse Halcion with Haldol, Healon, or halcinonide.

## ☑ Patient teaching
• Warn patient not to take more than the prescribed amount; overdose can occur at total daily dose of 2 mg (or four times highest recommended amount).
• Tell patient to avoid alcohol while taking drug.
• Warn patient not to discontinue drug abruptly if taken for 2 weeks or longer.
• Caution patient about performing activities that require mental alertness or physical coordination.
• Inform patient that drug tends not to cause morning drowsiness.
• Tell patient that rebound insomnia may develop for 1 or 2 nights after stopping therapy.

❋ *NEW DRUG*

## zaleplon
## Sonata

*Controlled Substance Schedule IV*
*Pregnancy Risk Category C*

## HOW SUPPLIED
*Capsules:* 5 mg, 10 mg

## ACTION
A hypnotic with chemical structure unrelated to benzodiazepines that interacts with the gamma-aminobutyric acid BZ receptor complex in the CNS. Modulation of this complex is thought to be responsible for sedative, anxiolytic, muscle relaxant, and anticonvulsant effects of benzodiazepines.

| Route | Onset | Peak | Duration |
|-------|-------|------|----------|
| P.O. | 1 hr | 1 hr | 3-4 hr |

## INDICATIONS & DOSAGE
*Short-term treatment for insomnia—*
**Adults:** 10 mg P.O. daily immediately before bedtime; may increase dose to 20 mg if needed. Low-weight adults may respond to 5-mg dose.
**Elderly:** initially, 5 mg P.O. daily immediately before bedtime; doses over 10 mg aren't recommended.
*Adjust-a-dose:* For debilitated patients, initially, 5 mg P.O. daily immediately be-

fore bedtime; doses over 10 mg aren't recommended.

For patients with mild to moderate hepatic failure or those receiving cimetidine concomitantly, 5 mg P.O. daily immediately before bedtime.

## ADVERSE REACTIONS
**CNS:** *headache,* amnesia, dizziness, somnolence, depression, hypertonia, nervousness, depersonalization, hallucinations, vertigo, difficulty concentrating, anxiety, paresthesia, hypoesthesia, tremor, asthenia, migraine, malaise.
**CV:** chest pain, peripheral edema.
**EENT:** abnormal vision, conjunctivitis, eye pain, ear pain, hyperacusis, epistaxis, smell alteration.
**GI:** constipation, dry mouth, anorexia, dyspepsia, nausea, abdominal pain, colitis.
**GU:** dysmenorrhea.
**Musculoskeletal:** arthritis, myalgia, back pain.
**Respiratory:** bronchitis.
**Skin:** pruritus, rash, photosensitivity reaction.
**Other:** fever.

## INTERACTIONS
**Drug-drug.** *Carbamazepine, phenobarbital, phenytoin, rifampin, other CYP3A4:* may reduce bioavailability and peak levels of zaleplon by about 80%. Consider an alternative hypnotic.
*Cimetidine:* increases zaleplon bioavailability and peak levels by 85%. For patient taking cimetidine, use an initial zaleplon dose of 5 mg.
*CNS depressants (imipramine, thioridazine):* may produce additive CNS effects. Use cautiously together.
**Drug-food.** *High-fat foods, heavy meals:* prolong absorption, delaying peak zaleplon levels by about 2 hours; sleep onset may be delayed. Separate administration from meals.
**Drug-lifestyle.** *Alcohol use:* concurrent use may increase CNS effects. Avoid concomitant use.

## EFFECTS ON DIAGNOSTIC TESTS
None reported.

## CONTRAINDICATIONS
Contraindicated in patients with severe hepatic impairment.

## NURSING CONSIDERATIONS
• Use cautiously in elderly and debilitated patients, in those with compromised respiratory function, and in those with signs and symptoms of depression.
• Because drug works rapidly, it should only be given immediately before bedtime or after patient has gone to bed and has experienced difficulty falling asleep.
• Don't administer drug with or following a high-fat or heavy meal.
• Closely monitor patients with compromised respiratory function due to preexisting illness, and elderly or debilitated patients since they are more sensitive to respiration depression.
• Limit hypnotics use to 7 to 10 days. Reevaluate patient if hypnotics are to be taken for more than 2 to 3 weeks.
• Initiate treatment only after careful evaluation of patient because sleep disturbances may be a symptom of an underlying physical or psychiatric disorder.
• Adverse reactions are usually dose-related. Notify doctor about a dose reduction if adverse reactions are bothersome to patient.

☑**Patient teaching**
• Advise patient that drug works rapidly and should only be taken immediately before bedtime or after he has gone to bed and has experienced difficulty falling asleep.
• Advise patient to take drug only if he will be able to sleep for at least 4 undisturbed hours.
• Caution patient that drowsiness, dizziness, light-headedness, and difficulty with coordination most frequently occur within 1 hour after taking drug.
• Advise patient to avoid performing activities that require mental alertness until CNS effects of drug are known.
• Advise patient to avoid alcohol while taking drug and to notify doctor before taking other prescription or OTC drugs.
• Tell patient not to take drug after a high fat or heavy meal.

---

Reactions may be *common*, uncommon, *life-threatening*, or COMMON AND LIFE-THREATENING.

• Advise patient to report continued sleep problems despite use of drug.

• Notify patient that dependence can occur, and that drug is recommended for short-term use only.

• Warn patient not to abruptly discontinue drug because withdrawal symptoms, including unpleasant feelings, stomach and muscle cramps, vomiting, sweating, shakiness, and seizures, may occur.

• Notify patient that insomnia may recur for a few nights after stopping drug, but should resolve on its own.

• Advise patient that drug may cause changes in behavior and thinking, including outgoing or aggressive behavior, loss of personal identity, confusion, strange behavior, agitation, hallucinations, worsening of depression, or suicidal thoughts. Tell patient to notify doctor immediately if these symptoms occur.

---

## zolpidem tartrate
Ambien, Stilnoct§

*Controlled Substance Schedule IV*
*Pregnancy Risk Category B*

### HOW SUPPLIED
*Tablets:* 5 mg, 10 mg

### ACTION
Although drug interacts with one of three identified gamma-aminobutyric acid-benzodiazepine receptor complexes, it isn't a benzodiazepine. It exhibits hypnotic activity but no muscle relaxant or anticonvulsant properties.

| Route | Onset | Peak | Duration |
|-------|-------|------|----------|
| P.O. | Rapid | 0.5-2 hr | Unknown |

### INDICATIONS & DOSAGE
*Short-term management of insomnia—*
**Adults:** 10 mg P.O. immediately before bedtime.
**Elderly:** 5 mg P.O. immediately before bedtime. Maximum daily dose is 10 mg.
*Adjust-a-dose:* For debilitated patients and for those with hepatic insufficiency, 5 mg P.O. immediately before bedtime. Maximum daily dose is 10 mg.

### ADVERSE REACTIONS
**CNS:** daytime drowsiness, lightheadedness, abnormal dreams, amnesia, dizziness, *headache,* hangover, sleep disorder, lethargy, depression.
**CV:** palpitations.
**EENT:** sinusitis, pharyngitis, dry mouth.
**GI:** nausea, vomiting, diarrhea, dyspepsia, constipation, abdominal pain.
**Musculoskeletal:** myalgia, arthralgia.
**Skin:** rash.
**Other:** back or chest pain, flulike syndrome, hypersensitivity reactions.

### INTERACTIONS
**Drug-drug.** *CNS depressants:* excessive CNS depression. Use together cautiously.
**Drug-lifestyle**. *Alcohol use:* excessive CNS depression. Use together cautiously.

### EFFECTS ON DIAGNOSTIC TESTS
None reported.

### CONTRAINDICATIONS
No known contraindications.

### NURSING CONSIDERATIONS
• Use cautiously in patients with compromised respiratory status.

• Hypnotics should be used only for short-term management of insomnia, usually 7 to 10 days.

• The smallest effective dose should be used in all patients.

• Take precautions to prevent hoarding or self-overdosing by patients who are depressed, suicidal, or drug-dependent or who have history of drug abuse.

• *Alert:* Don't confuse Ambien with Amen.

### ✓ Patient teaching
• For rapid sleep onset, instruct patient not to take drug with or immediately after meals.

• Tell patient to avoid alcohol during drug therapy.

• Caution patient about performing activities that require mental alertness or physical coordination.

---

acetazolamide sodium
   (See Chapter 62, DIURETICS.)
carbamazepine
clonazepam
clorazepate dipotassium
   (See Chapter 32, ANTIANXIETY DRUGS.)
diazepam
   (See Chapter 32, ANTIANXIETY DRUGS.)
divalproex sodium
ethosuximide
fosphenytoin sodium
gabapentin
lamotrigine
magnesium sulfate
phenobarbital
phenobarbital sodium
phenytoin
phenytoin sodium
phenytoin sodium (extended)
primidone
tiagabine hydrochloride
topiramate
valproate sodium
valproic acid

**COMBINATION PRODUCTS**
None.

---

carbamazepine
Apo-Carbamazepine†, Atretol,
Carbatrol, Epitol, Novo-
Carbamaz†, Tegretol, Tegretol
CR†, Tegretol-XR, Teril‡

*Pregnancy Risk Category C*

**HOW SUPPLIED**
*Tablets:* 200 mg
*Tablets (chewable):* 100 mg
*Tablets (extended-release)†:* 100 mg,
200 mg, 400 mg
*Capsules (extended-release):* 200 mg,
300 mg
*Oral suspension:* 100 mg/5 ml

**ACTION**
Unknown. Thought to stabilize neuronal
membranes and limit seizure activity by
either increasing efflux or decreasing influx of sodium ions across cell membranes in the motor cortex during generation of nerve impulses.

| Route | Onset | Peak | Duration |
|-------|-------|------|----------|
| P.O. | Unknown | 1.5-12 hr | Unknown |

**INDICATIONS & DOSAGE**
*Generalized tonic-clonic and complex
partial seizures, mixed seizure patterns—*
**Adults and children over age 12:** initially, 200 mg P.O. b.i.d. for tablets, or 1 teaspoon of suspension P.O. q.i.d. with
meals. May be increased at weekly intervals by 200 mg P.O. daily in divided doses
at 6- to 8-hour intervals. Adjusted to minimum effective level. Maximum daily
dose is 1 g/day in children ages 12 to 15,
and 1.2 g/day in patients over age 15.
Usual maintenance dose is 800 to 1,200
mg/day.
**Children ages 6 to 12:** initially, 100 mg
P.O. b.i.d. or ½ teaspoon of suspension
P.O. q.i.d. with meals, increased at weekly
intervals by 100 mg P.O. daily. Maximum
daily dose is 1 g/day. Usual maintenance
dose is 400 to 800 mg/day.
*Trigeminal neuralgia—*
**Adults:** initially, 100 mg P.O. b.i.d. or ½
teaspoon of suspension q.i.d. with meals,
increased by 100 mg q 12 hours for
tablets or ½ teaspoon of suspension q.i.d.
until pain is relieved. Maximum daily
dose is 1.2 g/day. Maintenance dose is
200 to 400 mg P.O. b.i.d.

**ADVERSE REACTIONS**
**CNS:** *dizziness, vertigo, drowsiness,* fatigue, *ataxia,* **worsening of seizures** (usually in patients with mixed seizure disorders, including atypical absence seizures),
confusion, headache, syncope.
**CV:** *heart failure,* hypertension, hypotension, aggravation of coronary artery disease, ***arrhythmias, AV block.***
**EENT:** conjunctivitis, dry mouth and
pharynx, blurred vision, diplopia, nystagmus.

**GI:** *nausea, vomiting,* abdominal pain, diarrhea, anorexia, stomatitis, glossitis.
**GU:** urinary frequency, urine retention, impotence, albuminuria, glycosuria, elevated BUN levels.
**Hematologic:** *aplastic anemia, agranulocytosis,* eosinophilia, leukocytosis, *thrombocytopenia.*
**Hepatic:** elevated liver function test results, *hepatitis.*
**Metabolic:** SIADH, decreased thyroid function test results.
**Respiratory:** pulmonary hypersensitivity.
**Skin:** rash, urticaria, erythema multiforme, *Stevens-Johnson syndrome,* excessive diaphoresis.
**Other:** fever, chills.

## INTERACTIONS
**Drug-drug.** *Cimetidine, danazol, diltiazem, fluoxetine, fluvoxamine, isoniazid, macrolides such as erythromycin, propoxyphene, valproic acid, verapamil:* may increase carbamazepine blood levels. Use cautiously.
*Doxycycline, felbamate, haloperidol, oral contraceptives, phenytoin, theophylline, warfarin:* carbamazepine may decrease blood levels of these drugs. Monitor for decreased effect.
*Lithium:* increased CNS toxicity of lithium. Avoid concomitant use.
*MAO inhibitors:* increased depressant and anticholinergic effects. Don't use together.
*Phenobarbital, phenytoin, primidone:* may decrease carbamazepine levels. Monitor for decreased effect.
**Drug-herb.** *Plantains:* psyllium seed has been reported to inhibit GI absorption. Avoid concomitant use.

## EFFECTS ON DIAGNOSTIC TESTS
Drug may interfere with some pregnancy tests.

## CONTRAINDICATIONS
Contraindicated in patients with hypersensitivity to carbamazepine or tricyclic antidepressants or history of previous bone marrow suppression; also contraindicated in those who have taken an MAO inhibitor within 14 days of therapy.

## NURSING CONSIDERATIONS
• Use cautiously in patients with mixed seizure disorders because they may experience an increased incidence of seizures.
• Obtain baseline determinations of urinalysis, BUN level, liver function, CBC, platelet and reticulocyte counts, and serum iron level, as ordered. Monitor periodically thereafter.
• Shake oral suspension well before measuring dose.
• When administering by nasogastric tube, mix dose with an equal volume of water, normal saline solution, or $D_5W$. Flush tube with 100 ml of diluent after administering dose.
• Never discontinue drug suddenly when treating seizures. Notify doctor immediately if adverse reactions occur.
• Adverse reactions may be minimized by gradually increasing dosage.
• Therapeutic carbamazepine blood level is 4 to 12 mcg/ml. Monitor blood levels and effects closely. Ask patient when last dose was taken to better evaluate blood levels.
• When managing seizures, institute appropriate precautions.
• *Alert:* Observe for signs of anorexia or subtle appetite changes, which may indicate excessive blood levels
• *Alert:* Don't confuse Tegretol with Toradol or Tegopen.

☑ **Patient teaching**
• Instruct patient to take drug with food to minimize GI distress. Tell patient taking suspension form to shake container well before measuring dose.
• Tell patient not to chew or crush extended release form and that broken or chipped tablets shouldn't be taken. Tegretol-XR tablet coating may appear in the stool because it isn't absorbed.
• Advise patient to keep tablets in the original container and to keep the container tightly closed and away from moisture. Some formulations may harden when exposed to excessive moisture, resulting in decreased bioavailability and loss of seizure control.
• Inform patient that, when drug is used for trigeminal neuralgia, an attempt to de-

crease dosage or withdraw drug is usually done every 3 months.
• Advise patient to notify doctor immediately if fever, sore throat, mouth ulcers, or easy bruising or bleeding occurs.
• Tell patient that drug may cause mild to moderate dizziness and drowsiness when first taken. Advise him to avoid hazardous activities until effects disappear, usually within 3 to 4 days.
• Advise patient that periodic eye examinations are recommended.

## clonazepam
Klonopin, Paxam‡, Rivotril†

*Controlled Substance Schedule IV*
*Pregnancy Risk Category D*

### HOW SUPPLIED
*Tablets:* 0.5 mg, 1 mg, 2 mg
*Drops:* 2.5 mg/ml‡
*Injection:* 1 mg/ml‡

### ACTION
Unknown. A benzodiazepine that probably acts by facilitating the effects of the inhibitory neurotransmitter gamma-aminobutyric acid.

| Route | Onset | Peak | Duration |
|-------|-------|------|----------|
| P.O. | Unknown | 1-2 hr | Unknown |
| I.V. | Unknown | Unknown | Unknown |

### INDICATIONS & DOSAGE
*Lennox-Gastaut syndrome, atypical absence seizures, akinetic and myoclonic seizures—*
**Adults:** initially, not to exceed 1.5 mg P.O. daily in three divided doses. May be increased by 0.5 to 1 mg q 3 days until seizures are controlled. If given in unequal doses, largest dose given h.s. Maximum recommended daily dose is 20 mg.
**Children up to age 10 or 30 kg (66 lb):** initially, 0.01 to 0.03 mg/kg P.O. daily (not to exceed 0.05 mg/kg daily) in two or three divided doses. Increased by 0.25 to 0.5 mg q third day to maximum maintenance dose of 0.1 to 0.2 mg/kg daily, p.r.n.
*Status epilepticus (where parenteral form is available)—*
**Adults:** 1 mg by slow I.V. infusion.

**Children:** 0.5 mg by slow I.V. infusion.
*Panic disorder—*
**Adults:** initially, 0.25 mg P.O. b.i.d.; increase to target dose of 1 mg/day after 3 days. Some patients may benefit from doses up to maximum of 4 mg/day. To achieve 4 mg/day, dosage increased in increments of 0.125 to 0.25 mg b.i.d. q 3 days as tolerated until panic disorder is controlled. Discontinue drug gradually with decrease of 0.125 mg b.i.d. q 3 days until drug is stopped.

### ADVERSE REACTIONS
**CNS:** *drowsiness,* ataxia, behavioral disturbances (especially in children), slurred speech, tremor, confusion, agitation, depression.
**CV:** palpitations.
**EENT:** nystagmus, abnormal eye movements, sore gums.
**GI:** constipation, gastritis, change in appetite, nausea, anorexia, diarrhea.
**GU:** dysuria, enuresis, nocturia, urine retention.
**Hematologic:** *leukopenia, thrombocytopenia,* eosinophilia.
**Hepatic:** elevated liver function test results.
**Respiratory:** *respiratory depression,* chest congestion, shortness of breath.
**Skin:** rash.

### INTERACTIONS
**Drug-drug.** *Carbamazepine, phenobarbital, phenytoin:* lowered plasma clonazepam levels. Monitor closely.
*CNS depressants:* increased CNS depression. Avoid concomitant use.
**Drug-lifestyle.** *Alcohol use:* increased CNS depression. Avoid concomitant use.

### EFFECTS ON DIAGNOSTIC TESTS
None reported.

### CONTRAINDICATIONS
Contraindicated in patients with hypersensitivity to benzodiazepines and in those with significant hepatic disease or acute angle-closure glaucoma.

### NURSING CONSIDERATIONS
• Use cautiously in patients with mixed type of seizure because drug may precipi-

tate generalized tonic-clonic seizures. Also use cautiously in children and in patients with chronic respiratory disease or open-angle glaucoma.
• Never withdraw suddenly because seizures may worsen. Call doctor at once if adverse reactions develop.
• Assess elderly patient's response closely. Elderly patients are more sensitive to drug's CNS effects.
• Monitor patient for oversedation.
• Monitor CBCs and liver function tests, as ordered.
• Withdrawal symptoms are similar to those of barbiturates.
• To reduce inconvenience of somnolence when drug is used for panic disorder, administration of one dose at bedtime may be desirable.

**◖ I.V. administration**
• Mix solutions in glass bottles because drug binds to polyvinyl chloride plastic. If polyvinyl chloride infusion bags are used, administer immediately and infuse at a rate of 60 ml/hour or faster.
• Give slowly by direct injection or by slow I.V. infusion. Drug may be diluted with $D_5W$, dextrose 2.5% in water, or normal or half-normal saline solution.

**☑ Patient teaching**
• Advise patient to avoid driving and other potentially hazardous activities that require mental alertness until drug's CNS effects are known.
• Instruct parent to monitor child's school performance because drug may interfere with attentiveness in school.
• Instruct patient and parents never to stop drug abruptly because seizures may occur.

---

**ethosuximide**
Emeside§, Zarontin

*Pregnancy Risk Category C*

**HOW SUPPLIED**
*Capsules:* 250 mg
*Syrup:* 250 mg/5 ml

**ACTION**
Not clearly defined. A succinimide derivative that probably increases seizure threshold. Drug reduces the paroxysmal spike-and-wave pattern of absence seizures by depressing nerve transmission in the motor cortex.

| Route | Onset | Peak | Duration |
|-------|-------|------|----------|
| P.O. | Unknown | 3-7 hr | Unknown |

**INDICATIONS & DOSAGE**
*Absence seizures—*
**Adults and children ages 6 and older:** 500 mg P.O. daily. Optimal dose is 20 mg/kg/day.
**Children ages 3 to 6:** 250 mg P.O. daily. Adjust dosage until control is achieved. Optimal dose is 20 mg/kg/day.
  *Note:* Doses exceeding 1.5 g daily require administration under doctor's strict supervision.

**ADVERSE REACTIONS**
**CNS:** drowsiness, headache, fatigue, dizziness, ataxia, irritability, euphoria, lethargy, depression, psychosis.
**EENT:** myopia, tongue swelling, gingival hyperplasia.
**GI:** nausea, vomiting, diarrhea, cramps, anorexia, epigastric and abdominal pain.
**GU:** vaginal bleeding, urinary frequency, abnormal renal function tests.
**Hematologic:** *leukopenia*, eosinophilia, *agranulocytosis, pancytopenia.*
**Hepatic:** elevated liver enzyme levels.
**Metabolic:** weight loss.
**Respiratory:** hiccups.
**Skin:** urticaria, pruritic and erythematous rashes, hirsutism.

**INTERACTIONS**
**Drug-drug.** *Phenytoin:* serum phenytoin levels may be increased. Monitor levels closely.
*Valproic acid:* may increase or decrease serum levels of ethosuximide. Monitor levels closely.
**Drug-lifestyle.** *Alcohol use:* increased CNS depression. Avoid concomitant use.

**EFFECTS ON DIAGNOSTIC TESTS**
Drug may cause false-positive Coombs' test results.

---

## CONTRAINDICATIONS

Contraindicated in patients with hypersensitivity to succinimide derivatives.

## NURSING CONSIDERATIONS

• Use with extreme caution in patients with hepatic or renal disease.
• Ethosuximide is currently drug of choice for treating absence seizures.
• Never withdraw drug suddenly. Call doctor immediately if adverse reactions develop.
• Monitor blood levels. Therapeutic blood levels are 40 to 100 mcg/ml.
• Obtain CBC every 3 to 6 months, as ordered.
• *Alert:* Drug may increase frequency of generalized tonic-clonic seizures when used alone in patients who have mixed types of seizures.
• *Alert:* Don't confuse ethosuximide with methsuximide or Zarontin with Zaroxolyn.

✓ **Patient teaching**
• Advise patient to take drug with food to minimize GI distress.
• Inform patient to avoid hazardous activities that require mental alertness until drug's CNS effects are known.
• Tell patient to notify doctor if rash, joint pain, fever, sore throat, or bruising occurs.
• Warn patient and parents not to stop drug abruptly.

## fosphenytoin sodium
Cerebyx

*Pregnancy Risk Category D*

## HOW SUPPLIED

*Injection:* 2 ml (150 mg fosphenytoin sodium equivalent to 100 mg phenytoin sodium), 10 ml (750 mg fosphenytoin sodium equivalent to 500 mg phenytoin sodium)

## ACTION

Drug is a prodrug of phenytoin, so its anticonvulsant action is that of phenytoin. Phenytoin is thought to stabilize neuronal membranes and limit seizure activity by modulation of voltage-dependent sodium channels of neurons, inhibition of calcium flux across neuronal membranes, modulation of voltage-dependent calcium channels of neurons, and enhancement of sodium-potassium ATPase activity of neurons and glial cells.

| Route | Onset | Peak | Duration |
|-------|-------|------|----------|
| I.V. | Unknown | End of infusion | Unknown |
| I.M. | Unknown | 30 min | Unknown |

## INDICATIONS & DOSAGE

*Status epilepticus—*
**Adults:** 15 to 20 mg phenytoin sodium equivalent (PE)/kg I.V. at 100 to 150 mg PE/minute as loading dose; then 4 to 6 mg PE/kg/day I.V. as maintenance dose. (Phenytoin may be used instead of fosphenytoin as maintenance, using the appropriate dose.)
*Prevention and treatment of seizures during neurosurgery (nonemergent loading or maintenance dosing)—*
**Adults:** loading dose of 10 to 20 mg PE/kg I.M. or I.V. at infusion rate not exceeding 150 mg PE/minute. Maintenance dose is 4 to 6 mg PE/kg/day I.V. or I.M.
*Short-term substitution for oral phenytoin therapy—*
**Adults:** same total daily dose equivalent as oral phenytoin sodium therapy given as a single daily dose I.M. or I.V. at infusion rate not exceeding 150 mg PE/minute. Some patients may require more frequent dosing.
**Elderly:** phenytoin clearance is decreased slightly in elderly patients; lower or less frequent dosing may be required.

## ADVERSE REACTIONS

**CNS:** increased or decreased reflexes, speech disorders, asthenia, ***intracranial hypertension,*** thinking abnormalities, nervousness, hypesthesia, dysarthria, extrapyramidal syndrome, brain edema, headache, *nystagmus, dizziness, somnolence, ataxia,* stupor, incoordination, paresthesia, tremor, agitation, vertigo.
**CV:** hypertension, vasodilation, tachycardia, hypotension.
**GI:** constipation, taste perversion.

---

Reactions may be *common,* uncommon, *life-threatening,* or COMMON AND LIFE-THREATENING.

**Hepatic:** increased serum levels of alkaline phosphatase and gamma glutamyl transpeptidase.

**Metabolic:** hypokalemia, hyperglycemia, decreased serum levels of $T_4$.

**Musculoskeletal:** pelvic pain, back pain, myasthenia.

**Respiratory:** pneumonia.

**Skin:** rash, ecchymosis, *pruritus*.

**Other:** lymphadenopathy, accidental injury, injection site reaction and pain, infection, chills, decreased serum folate levels.

## INTERACTIONS

Most significant drug interactions are those commonly seen with phenytoin.

**Drug-drug.** *Amiodarone, chloramphenicol, chlordiazepoxide, cimetidine, diazepam, dicumarol, disulfiram, estrogens, ethosuximide, fluoxetine, $H_2$ antagonists, halothane, isoniazid, methylphenidate, phenothiazines, phenylbutazone, salicylates, succinimides, sulfonamides, tolbutamide, trazodone:* may increase plasma phenytoin levels and thus its therapeutic effects. Use together cautiously.

*Carbamazepine, reserpine:* may decrease plasma phenytoin levels. Monitor patient.

*Corticosteroids, coumarin, digitoxin, doxycycline, estrogens, furosemide, oral contraceptives, quinidine, rifampin, theophylline, vitamin D:* efficacy may be decreased by phenytoin as a result of increased hepatic metabolism. Monitor closely.

*Phenobarbital, valproate sodium, valproic acid:* may increase or decrease plasma phenytoin levels. Similarly, the effects of phenytoin on levels of these drugs is unpredictable. Monitor patient.

*Tricyclic antidepressants:* may lower seizure threshold and require adjustments in phenytoin dosage. Use cautiously.

**Drug-lifestyle.** *Acute alcohol use:* may increase plasma phenytoin level and thus its therapeutic effects. Use cautiously.

*Chronic alcohol use:* may decrease plasma phenytoin levels. Monitor patient.

## EFFECTS ON DIAGNOSTIC TESTS

Drug may produce artificially low results in dexamethasone or metyrapone tests.

## CONTRAINDICATIONS

Contraindicated in patients with hypersensitivity to drug or its components, phenytoin, or other hydantoins; also contraindicated in those with sinus bradycardia, SA block, second- or third-degree AV block, or Adams-Stokes syndrome.

## NURSING CONSIDERATIONS

• Use cautiously in patients with porphyria and in those with history of hypersensitivity to similarly structured drugs, such as barbiturates, oxazolidinediones, and succinimides.

• *Alert:* Fosphenytoin should always be prescribed and dispensed in phenytoin sodium equivalent units (PE). Don't make adjustments in the recommended doses when substituting fosphenytoin for phenytoin, and vice versa.

• Phosphate load provided by fosphenytoin (0.0037 mmol phosphate/mg PE fosphenytoin) must be taken into consideration when treating patients who require phosphate restriction, such as those with severe renal impairment. Monitor laboratory values.

• Discontinue drug and notify doctor if rash appears. If rash is exfoliative, purpuric, or bullous or if lupus erythematosus, Stevens-Johnson syndrome, or toxic epidermal necrolysis is suspected, drug should be discontinued and alternative therapy considered. If rash is mild (measlelike or scarlatiniform), therapy may be resumed after rash disappears. If rash recurs on reinstitution of therapy, further fosphenytoin or phenytoin administration is contraindicated. Document that patient is allergic to drug.

• Drug should be stopped in patients with acute hepatotoxicity.

• I.M. administration generates systemic phenytoin levels similar enough to oral phenytoin sodium to allow essentially interchangeable use when ordered.

• Following fosphenytoin administration, phenytoin levels shouldn't be monitored until conversion to phenytoin is essentially complete—about 2 hours after the end of an I.V. infusion or 4 hours after I.M. administration.

• Interpret total phenytoin plasma levels cautiously in patients with renal or hepatic disease or hypoalbuminemia due to an increased fraction in unbound phenytoin. Unbound phenytoin levels may be more useful in these patients. When giving drug I.V., monitor patients with renal and hepatic disease because they are at increased risk for more frequent and severe adverse reactions.

• Abrupt withdrawal of drug may precipitate status epilepticus.

• *Alert:* Don't confuse Cerebyx with Cerezyme, Celexa, or Celebrex.

### ⚠ I.V. administration

• Before I.V. infusion, dilute fosphenytoin in 5% $D_5W$ or normal saline solution for injection to a level ranging from 1.5 to 25 mg PE/ml. Don't administer at a rate exceeding 150 mg PE/minute.

• For status epilepticus, administer dose of I.V. fosphenytoin at a maximum rate of 150 mg PE/minute. Typical infusion to a 110-lb patient takes 5 to 7 minutes. (An infusion of an identical molar dose of phenytoin can't be accomplished in less than 15 to 20 minutes because of adverse CV effects that accompany direct I.V. administration of phenytoin at rates above 50 mg/minute.) Don't use fosphenytoin I.M. for status epilepticus because therapeutic phenytoin levels may not be reached as rapidly as with I.V. administration.

• Patients receiving 20 mg PE/kg of drug infused at a rate of 150 mg PE/minute are expected to experience sensory discomfort, most often in the groin. Occurrence and intensity of discomfort can be lessened by slowing or temporarily stopping infusion.

• If rapid phenytoin loading is a primary goal, I.V. administration of drug is preferred because it takes longer to achieve therapeutic plasma phenytoin levels after I.M. injection than after I.V. infusion.

• Monitor patient's ECG, blood pressure, and respiration continuously throughout period during which maximal serum phenytoin levels occur—about 10 to 20 minutes after end of fosphenytoin infusions. Severe CV complications are most commonly encountered in elderly or gravely ill patients. Reducing the rate of administration or discontinuing drug may be necessary.

### ☑ Patient teaching

• Warn patient that sensory disturbances may occur with I.V. administration.

• Instruct patient to immediately report adverse reactions, especially rash.

• Warn patient never to stop drug abruptly or adjust dosage without discussing with doctor.

• Inform woman that breast-feeding isn't recommended during therapy.

---

### gabapentin
Neurontin

*Pregnancy Risk Category C*

#### HOW SUPPLIED
*Capsules:* 100 mg, 300 mg, 400 mg

#### ACTION
Unknown. Although structurally related to gamma-aminobutyric acid (GABA), drug doesn't interact with GABA receptors and isn't converted metabolically into GABA or a GABA agonist. It doesn't inhibit GABA reuptake and doesn't prevent degradation.

| Route | Onset | Peak | Duration |
|-------|-------|------|----------|
| P.O. | Unknown | Unknown | Unknown |

#### INDICATIONS & DOSAGE
*Adjunctive treatment of partial seizures with and without secondary generalization in adults with epilepsy—*
**Adults:** initially, 300 mg P.O. h.s. on day 1; 300 mg P.O. b.i.d. on day 2; then 300 mg P.O. t.i.d. on day 3. Dosage increased as needed and tolerated to 1,800 mg daily in divided doses. Doses up to 3,600 mg daily have been well tolerated.
*Adjust-a-dose:* For patients with renal failure with creatinine clearance over 60 ml/minute, give 400 mg P.O. t.i.d.; if clearance is between 30 and 60 ml/minute, 300 mg P.O. b.i.d.; between 15 and 30 ml/minute, 300 mg P.O. daily; and if clearance is under 15 ml/minute, 300 mg P.O. every other day. Patients on dialysis should receive a loading dose of 300 to 400 mg P.O.; then 200 to 300 mg P.O. q 4 hours during hemodialysis.

---

Reactions may be *common,* uncommon, *life-threatening,* or COMMON AND LIFE-THREATENING.

## ADVERSE REACTIONS
**CNS:** *fatigue, somnolence, dizziness, ataxia,* nystagmus, tremor, nervousness, dysarthria, amnesia, depression, abnormal thinking, twitching, incoordination.
**CV:** peripheral edema, vasodilation.
**EENT:** diplopia, rhinitis, pharyngitis, dry throat, coughing, amblyopia.
**GI:** nausea, vomiting, dyspepsia, dry mouth, constipation, increased appetite, dental abnormalities.
**GU:** impotence.
**Hematologic:** *leukopenia.*
**Metabolic:** weight gain.
**Musculoskeletal:** back pain, myalgia, fractures.
**Skin:** pruritus, abrasion.

## INTERACTIONS
**Drug-drug.** *Antacids:* decreased absorption of gabapentin. Separate administration times by at least 2 hours.

## EFFECTS ON DIAGNOSTIC TESTS
Drug causes false-positive results with the Ames-N-Multistix SG dipstick test for urinary protein when added to other antiepileptic drugs. The more specific sulfosalicylic acid precipitation procedure is recommended to determine the presence of urine protein.

## CONTRAINDICATIONS
Contraindicated in patients with hypersensitivity to drug.

## NURSING CONSIDERATIONS
• First dose should be given at bedtime to minimize drowsiness, dizziness, fatigue, and ataxia.
• If drug therapy is discontinued or alternative drug is substituted, do so gradually over at least 1 week, as ordered, to minimize risk of precipitating seizures.
• *Alert:* Don't suddenly withdraw other anticonvulsants in patients starting gabapentin therapy.
• Routine monitoring of plasma drug levels isn't necessary. Drug doesn't appear to alter plasma levels of other anticonvulsants.

☑ **Patient teaching**
• Instruct patient to take first dose at bedtime to minimize adverse reactions.
• Warn patient to avoid driving and operating heavy machinery until drug's CNS effects are known.

## lamotrigine
Lamictal

*Pregnancy Risk Category C*

## HOW SUPPLIED
*Tablets:* 25 mg, 100 mg, 150 mg, 200 mg
*Tablets (chewable dispersible):* 5 mg, 25 mg

## ACTION
Unknown. May inhibit release of glutamate and aspartate (excitatory neurotransmitters) in the brain via an action at voltage-sensitive sodium channels.

| Route | Onset | Peak | Duration |
|-------|-------|------|----------|
| P.O. | Unknown | 1.4-4.8 hr | Unknown |

## INDICATIONS & DOSAGE
*Adjunct therapy in treatment of partial seizures caused by epilepsy—*
**Adults and children over age 16:** for patients taking valproic acid with other enzyme-inducing antiepileptics, 25 mg P.O. every other day for 2 weeks; then 25 mg P.O. daily for 2 weeks. Continue to increase, p.r.n., by 25 to 50 mg/day q 1 to 2 weeks, with maximum dose of 150 mg P.O. daily in two divided doses.

For patients receiving enzyme-inducing antiepileptics but not valproic acid, 50 mg P.O. daily for 2 weeks; then 100 mg P.O. daily in two divided doses for 2 weeks. Increase, p.r.n., by 100 mg/day q 1 to 2 weeks. Usual maintenance dose is 300 to 500 mg P.O. daily in two divided doses.
*Adjust-a-dose:* Use lower maintenance dose for patients with severe renal impairment.
*Adjunctive treatment of generalized seizures of Lennox-Gastaut syndrome—*
**Adults and children over age 12:** for patients on an antiepileptic drug regimen with valproic acid, 25 mg P.O. every other

day for 2 weeks; then 25 mg P.O. daily for 2 weeks. Thereafter, usual maintenance dose is 100 to 400 mg P.O. daily in one or two divided doses. For patients taking enzyme-inducing antiepileptics but not valproic acid, 50 mg P.O. daily for 2 weeks; then 100 mg P.O. daily in two divided doses for 2 weeks. Thereafter, usual maintenance dose is 300 to 500 mg P.O. daily in two divided doses.

**Children ages 2 to 12 weighing over 17 kg (37 lb):** for patients on antiepileptic drug regimen with valproic acid, 0.15 mg/kg/day P.O. in one or two divided doses (rounded down to nearest 5 mg) for 2 weeks. If calculated daily dose of lamotrigine is 2.5 to 5 mg, 5 mg of lamotrigine should be taken on alternate days; then 0.3 mg/kg/day P.O. in one or two doses rounded down to nearest 5 mg for 2 weeks. Thereafter, usual maintenance dose is 1 to 5 mg/kg/day (maximum dose is 200 mg/day in one to two divided doses). For patients on an antiepileptic drug regimen without valproic acid, 0.6 mg/kg/day P.O. in two divided doses rounded down to nearest 5 mg for 2 weeks; then 1.2 mg/kg/day P.O. in two divided doses rounded down to nearest 5 mg for 2 weeks. Thereafter, usual maintenance dose is 5 to 15 mg/kg/day (maximum dose is 400 mg/day in two divided doses).

## ADVERSE REACTIONS
**CNS:** *dizziness, headache, ataxia, somnolence,* incoordination, insomnia, tremor, depression, anxiety, *seizures,* irritability, speech disorder, decreased memory, aggravated reaction, concentration disturbance, sleep disorder, emotional lability, vertigo, mind racing, dysarthria, malaise.
**CV:** palpitations.
**EENT:** *diplopia, blurred vision,* vision abnormality, nystagmus, *rhinitis,* pharyngitis.
**GI:** *nausea, vomiting,* diarrhea, dyspepsia, abdominal pain, constipation, tooth disorder, anorexia, dry mouth.
**GU:** dysmenorrhea, vaginitis, amenorrhea.
**Musculoskeletal:** muscle spasm, neck pain.
**Respiratory:** cough, dyspnea.
**Skin:** *rash,* **Stevens-Johnson syndrome, toxic epidermal necrolysis,** pruritus, hot flashes, alopecia, acne.

**Other:** flulike syndrome, fever, infection, chills.

## INTERACTIONS
**Drug-drug.** *Acetaminophen:* may decrease therapeutic effects. Monitor patient.
*Carbamazepine, phenobarbital, phenytoin, primidone:* decrease in lamotrigine's steady-state levels. Monitor patient closely.
*Folate inhibitors, such as co-trimoxazole and methotrexate:* lamotrigine inhibits dihydrofolate reductase, an enzyme involved in folic acid synthesis. May have an additive effect. Monitor patient.
*Valproic acid:* decreased clearance of lamotrigine, which increases the drug's steady-state levels. Also decreases valproic acid levels. Monitor patient closely for toxicity.
**Drug-lifestyle.** *Sun exposure:* photosensitivity reactions may occur. Take precautions.

## EFFECTS ON DIAGNOSTIC TESTS
None reported.

## CONTRAINDICATIONS
Contraindicated in patients with hypersensitivity to drug or its ingredients.

## NURSING CONSIDERATIONS
• Use cautiously in patients with renal, hepatic, or cardiac impairment.
• Drug shouldn't be discontinued abruptly because of possibility of increased seizure frequency. Instead, drug should be tapered over at least 2 weeks.
• *Alert:* Drug should be stopped at first sign of rash unless rash isn't drug-related.
• Lamotrigine dose should be lowered if drug is added to a multidrug regimen that includes valproic acid.
• Chewable dispersible tablets may be swallowed whole, chewed, or dispersed in water or diluted fruit juice. If tablets are chewed, a small amount of water or diluted fruit juice should be given to aid in swallowing.
• Safety and efficacy of drug in children under age 16 (other than those with Lennox-Gastaut syndrome) haven't been established. Children weighing less than

37 lb (17 kg) shouldn't receive drug because therapy can't be initiated using dosing guidelines and currently available tablet strength.
• Patients should be evaluated for changes in seizure activity. Adjunct anticonvulsant's serum levels should be checked, as ordered.
• *Alert:* Don't confuse lamotrigine with lamivudine or Lamictal with Lamisil.

☑ **Patient teaching**
• Inform patient that drug may cause rash. Combination therapy of valproic acid and lamotrigine may cause a serious rash. Tell patient to report rash or signs or symptoms of hypersensitivity promptly to doctor because they may warrant drug discontinuation.
• Warn patient not to engage in hazardous activity until drug's CNS effects are known.
• Warn patient that photosensitivity reactions may occur and to take precautions until tolerance is determined.

## magnesium sulfate

*Pregnancy Risk Category A*

### HOW SUPPLIED
*Injection:* 4%, 8%, 10%, 12.5%, 25%, 50%
*Injection solution:* 1% in 5% dextrose, 2% in 5% dextrose

### ACTION
May decrease acetylcholine released by nerve impulses, but its anticonvulsant mechanism is unknown.

| Route | Onset | Peak | Duration |
|-------|-------|------|----------|
| I.V. | 1-2 min | Rapid | 30 min |
| I.M. | 1 hr | Unknown | 3-4 hr |

### INDICATIONS & DOSAGE
*Prevention or control of seizures in preeclampsia or eclampsia—*
**Women:** initially, 4 g I.V. in 250 ml $D_5W$ and 4 to 5 g deep I.M. into each buttock; then 4 to 5 g deep I.M. into alternate buttock q 4 hours, p.r.n. Or, 4 g I.V. loading dose; then 1 to 2 g hourly as I.V. infusion.

Total dose shouldn't exceed 30 to 40 g daily.
*Hypomagnesemia—*
**Adults:** for mild deficiency, 1 g I.M. q 6 hours for four doses; for severe deficiency, 5 g in 1,000 ml $D_5W$ or normal saline infused over 3 hours.
*Seizures, hypertension, and encephalopathy associated with acute nephritis in children—*
**Children:** 0.2 ml/kg of 50% solution I.M. q 4 to 6 hours, p.r.n. For severe symptoms, 100 to 200 mg/kg I.V. slowly over 1 hour with 50% of dose administered in first 15 to 20 minutes. Dosage titrated according to blood magnesium levels and seizure response.
*Management of paroxysmal atrial tachycardia—*
**Adults:** 3 to 4 g I.V. over 30 seconds.
*Management of life-threatening ventricular arrhythmias, such as sustained ventricular tachycardia or torsades de pointes—*
**Adults:** 2 to 6 g I.V. over several minutes; then continuous I.V. infusion of 3 to 20 mg/minute for 5 to 48 hours. Dosage and duration of therapy are based on patient response and serum magnesium levels.

### ADVERSE REACTIONS
**CNS:** drowsiness, *depressed reflexes,* flaccid paralysis, hypothermia.
**CV:** *hypotension, flushing,* **circulatory collapse,** depressed cardiac function.
**Metabolic:** hypocalcemia.
**Respiratory:** *respiratory paralysis.*
**Skin:** diaphoresis.

### INTERACTIONS
**Drug-drug.** *Anesthetics, CNS depressants:* may cause additive CNS depression. Use cautiously.
*Cardiac glycosides:* concomitant use may exacerbate arrhythmias. Use together cautiously.
*Neuromuscular blockers:* may cause increased neuromuscular blockade. Use cautiously.

### EFFECTS ON DIAGNOSTIC TESTS
None reported.

---

## CONTRAINDICATIONS

Parenteral administration of drug contraindicated in patients with heart block or myocardial damage. Don't give in toxemia of pregnancy during 2 hours preceding delivery.

## NURSING CONSIDERATIONS

• Use cautiously in patients with impaired renal function. Also use cautiously in women who are in labor.
• If used to treat seizures, institute appropriate seizure precautions.
• *Alert:* Watch for respiratory depression and signs and symptoms of heart block.
• Keep I.V. calcium gluconate available to reverse magnesium intoxication; however, use cautiously in patients undergoing digitalization because of danger of arrhythmias.
• Check blood magnesium levels after repeated doses. Disappearance of knee-jerk and patellar reflexes is sign of impending magnesium toxicity.
• Signs of hypermagnesemia begin to appear at blood levels of 4 mEq/L.
• Monitor fluid intake and output. Urine output should be 100 ml or more in 4-hour period before each dose.
• Observe neonates for signs of magnesium toxicity, including neuromuscular or respiratory depression, when giving I.V. form of drug to toxemic mothers within 24 hours before delivery.
• *Alert:* Don't confuse magnesium sulfate with manganese sulfate.

### 🔲 I.V. administration

• If necessary, dilute to maximum level of 20%. Infuse no faster than 150 mg/minute (1.5 ml/minute of a 10% solution or 0.75 ml/minute of a 20% solution). Drug is compatible with $D_5W$.
• Maximum infusion rate is 150 mg/minute. Too-rapid infusion will induce uncomfortable feeling of heat.
• Monitor vital signs every 15 minutes when giving drug I.V.

### ✅ Patient teaching

• Inform patient of short-term need for drug, and answer any questions and address concerns.

• Review potential adverse reactions and instruct patient to promptly report any occurrences. Reassure patient that, although adverse reactions can occur, frequent monitoring of vital signs, reflexes, and blood levels will be done to ensure safety.

---

## phenobarbital (phenobarbitone)
Barbita, Solfoton

## phenobarbital sodium
Luminal Sodium

*Controlled Substance Schedule IV*
*Pregnancy Risk Category D*

### HOW SUPPLIED

*Tablets:* 15 mg, 16 mg, 30 mg, 60 mg, 100 mg
*Capsules:* 16 mg
*Elixir\*:* 15 mg/5 ml, 20 mg/5 ml
*Injection:* 30 mg/ml, 60 mg/ml, 65 mg/ml, 130 mg/ml

### ACTION

Unknown. A barbiturate that probably depresses monosynaptic and polysynaptic transmission in CNS and increases threshold for seizure activity in motor cortex. As a sedative, drug probably interferes with transmission of impulses from thalamus to cortex of brain.

| Route | Onset | Peak | Duration |
|-------|-------|------|----------|
| P.O. | 1 hr | 8-12 hr | 10-12 hr |
| I.V. | 5 min | 30 min | 4-10 hr |
| I.M. | > 5 min | > 30 min | 4-10 hr |

### INDICATIONS & DOSAGE

*All forms of epilepsy, febrile seizures—*
**Adults:** 60 to 200 mg P.O. daily in divided doses t.i.d. or as single dose h.s.
**Children:** 3 to 6 mg/kg P.O. daily, usually divided q 12 hours. Drug can be administered once daily, usually h.s.
*Status epilepticus—*
**Adults:** 200 to 600 mg I.V.
**Children:** 100 to 400 mg I.V. Don't exceed 50 mg/minute.
*Sedation—*
**Adults:** 30 to 120 mg P.O. daily in two or three divided doses.

---

Reactions may be *common,* uncommon, *life-threatening,* or COMMON AND LIFE-THREATENING.

**Children:** 3 to 5 mg/kg P.O. daily in divided doses t.i.d.
*Insomnia—*
**Adults:** 100 to 200 mg P.O. or I.M. h.s.
*Preoperative sedation—*
**Adults:** 100 to 200 mg I.M. 60 to 90 minutes before surgery.
**Children:** 16 to 100 mg I.M. or 1 to 3 mg/kg I.V., I.M., or P.O. 60 to 90 minutes before surgery.

**ADVERSE REACTIONS**
**CNS:** *drowsiness, lethargy, hangover,* paradoxical excitement in elderly patients, somnolence.
**CV:** bradycardia, hypotension.
**GI:** nausea, vomiting.
**Hematologic:** exacerbation of porphyria.
**Respiratory:** *respiratory depression, apnea.*
**Skin:** rash, *erythema multiforme, Stevens-Johnson syndrome,* urticaria, pain, swelling, thrombophlebitis, necrosis, nerve injury at injection site.
**Other:** *angioedema,* physical and psychological dependence.

**INTERACTIONS**
**Drug-drug.** *Chloramphenicol, MAO inhibitors, valproic acid:* potentiated barbiturate effect. Monitor patient for increased CNS and respiratory depression.
*CNS depressants, including narcotic analgesics:* excessive CNS depression. Monitor closely.
*Corticosteroids, digitoxin, doxycycline, estrogens and oral contraceptives, oral anticoagulants, tricyclic antidepressants:* phenobarbital may enhance metabolism of these drugs. Monitor for decreased effect.
*Diazepam:* increased effects of both drugs. Use together cautiously.
*Griseofulvin:* decreased absorption of griseofulvin. Monitor effectiveness of griseofulvin.
*Mephobarbital, primidone:* excessive phenobarbital blood levels. Monitor closely.
*Rifampin:* may decrease barbiturate levels. Monitor for decreased effect.
*Valproic acid:* increased phenobarbital levels. Monitor for toxicity.
**Drug-lifestyle.** *Alcohol use:* excessive CNS depression. Avoid concomitant use.

**EFFECTS ON DIAGNOSTIC TESTS**
Drug may cause a false-positive phentolamine test. The physiologic effects of drug may impair the absorption of cyanocobalamin $^{57}$Co. It may decrease serum bilirubin levels in neonates, epileptics, and in patients with congenital nonhemolytic, unconjugated, hyperbilirubinemia. Barbiturates may increase sulfobromophthalein retention. EEG patterns show a change in low-voltage, fast activity. Changes persist for a time after discontinuation of therapy.

**CONTRAINDICATIONS**
Contraindicated in patients with hypersensitivity to barbiturates or history of manifest or latent porphyria; also contraindicated in those with hepatic dysfunction, respiratory disease with dyspnea or obstruction, and nephritis.

**NURSING CONSIDERATIONS**
• Use cautiously in patients with acute or chronic pain, depression, suicidal tendencies, history of drug abuse, blood pressure alterations, CV disease, shock, or uremia, and in elderly or debilitated patients.
• Don't use injectable solution if it contains a precipitate.
• Give I.M. injection deeply. Superficial injection may cause pain, sterile abscess, and tissue sloughing.
• Elderly patients are more sensitive to drug's effects.
• *Alert:* Watch for signs of barbiturate toxicity: coma, asthmatic breathing, cyanosis, clammy skin, and hypotension. Overdose can be fatal.
• Therapeutic blood levels are 15 to 40 mcg/ml.
• Don't stop drug abruptly because seizures may worsen. Call doctor immediately if adverse reactions develop.
• *Alert:* Don't confuse phenobarbital with pentobarbital.

**◖ I.V. administration**
• I.V. injection is reserved for emergency treatment. Give slowly under close supervision. Monitor respirations closely. When administering, don't give more than 60 mg/minute. Have resuscitation equipment available.

---

• Don't mix parenteral form with acidic solutions; precipitation may result.
• Dilute drug in half-normal or normal saline, 5% dextrose, lactated Ringer's, or Ringer's solution.

☑ **Patient teaching**
• Ensure that patient is aware that phenobarbital is available in different milligram strengths and sizes. Advise him to check prescription and refills closely.
• Inform patient that full therapeutic effects aren't seen for 2 to 3 weeks, except when loading dose is used.
• Advise patient to avoid driving and other potentially hazardous activities that require mental alertness until drug's CNS effects are known.
• Warn patient and parents not to discontinue drug abruptly.
• Tell patient using oral contraceptives to consider another birth control method because drug may decrease effect of contraceptive.

---

**phenytoin
(diphenylhydantoin)**
Dilantin-125, Dilantin Infatabs, Epanutin§

**phenytoin sodium**
Dilantin, Phenytex

**phenytoin sodium (extended)**
Dilantin Kapseals

*Pregnancy Risk Category D*

---

**HOW SUPPLIED**
**phenytoin**
*Tablets (chewable):* 50 mg
*Oral suspension:* 125 mg/5 ml
**phenytoin sodium**
*Capsules:* 100 mg (92-mg base)
*Injection:* 50 mg/ml (46-mg base)
**phenytoin sodium (extended)**
*Capsules:* 30 mg (27.6-mg base), 100 mg (92-mg base)

**ACTION**
Unknown. A hydantoin derivative that probably stabilizes neuronal membranes and limits seizure activity by either in-

creasing efflux or decreasing influx of sodium ions across cell membranes in the motor cortex during generation of nerve impulses.

| Route | Onset | Peak | Duration |
|-------|-------|------|----------|
| P.O. | Unknown | 1.5-12 hr | Unknown |
| I.V. | Immediate | 1-2 hr | Unknown |
| I.M. | Unknown | Unknown | Unknown |

**INDICATIONS & DOSAGE**
*Control of tonic-clonic (grand mal) and complex partial (temporal lobe) seizures—*
**Adults:** highly individualized. Initially, 100 mg P.O. t.i.d., increased in increments of 100 mg P.O. q 2 to 4 weeks until desired response is obtained. Usual range is 300 to 600 mg daily. If patient is stabilized with extended-release capsules, once-daily dosing with 300-mg extended-release capsules is possible as an alternative.
**Children:** 5 mg/kg or 250 mg/m$^2$ P.O. divided b.i.d. or t.i.d. Maximum daily dose is 300 mg.
*For patient requiring a loading dose—*
**Adults:** initially, 1 g P.O. daily divided into three doses and administered at 2-hour intervals. Or, 10 to 15 mg/kg I.V. at a rate not exceeding 50 mg/minute. Normal maintenance dose is instituted 24 hours later.
**Children:** 5 mg/kg/day P.O. in two or three equally divided doses with subsequent dose individualized to maximum of 300 mg daily.
*Prevention and treatment of seizures occurring during neurosurgery—*
**Adults:** 100 to 200 mg I.M. q 4 hours during surgery and continued during postoperative period.
*Status epilepticus—*
**Adults:** loading dose of 10 to 15 mg/kg I.V. (1 to 1.5 g may be needed) at a rate not exceeding 50 mg/minute; then maintenance doses of 100 mg P.O. or I.V. q 6 to 8 hours.
**Elderly:** may require lower dosages.
**Children:** loading dose of 15 to 20 mg/kg I.V., at a rate not exceeding 1 to 3 mg/minute; then highly individualized maintenance doses.

---

Reactions may be *common,* uncommon, ***life-threatening,*** or COMMON AND LIFE-THREATENING.

## ADVERSE REACTIONS
**CNS:** *ataxia, slurred speech,* dizziness, insomnia, nervousness, twitching, headache, *mental confusion, decreased coordination.*
**CV:** periarteritis nodosa.
**EENT:** *nystagmus, diplopia,* blurred vision, *gingival hyperplasia* (especially in children).
**GI:** *nausea, vomiting,* constipation.
**Hematologic:** *thrombocytopenia, leukopenia, agranulocytosis, pancytopenia,* macrocythemia, megaloblastic anemia.
**Hepatic:** *toxic hepatitis,* increased serum levels of alkaline phosphatase or gamma-glutamyltransferase.
**Metabolic:** hyperglycemia.
**Musculoskeletal:** osteomalacia.
**Skin:** scarlatiniform or morbilliform rash; bullous or purpuric dermatitis; *exfoliative dermatitis; Stevens-Johnson syndrome;* lupus erythematosus; *hirsutism; toxic epidermal necrolysis;* photosensitivity; pain, necrosis, inflammation at injection site; discoloration of skin (purple-glove syndrome) if given by I.V. push in back of hand; hypertrichosis.
**Other:** lymphadenopathy.

## INTERACTIONS
**Drug-drug.** *Amiodarone, antihistamines, chloramphenicol, cimetidine, cycloserine, diazepam, disulfiram, isoniazid, phenylbutazone, salicylates, sulfamethizole, valproate:* may increase phenytoin activity and toxicity. Monitor patient.
*Barbiturates, carbamazepine, dexamethasone, diazoxide, folic acid, rifampin:* decreased phenytoin activity. Monitor levels.
*Carbamazepine, cardiac glycosides, oral contraceptives, quinidine, theophylline, valproic acid:* effects may be decreased by phenytoin. Monitor patient.
**Drug-food.** *Oral tube feedings with Osmolite or Isocal:* may interfere with absorption of oral phenytoin. Stop enteral feedings for 2 hours before and 2 hours after phenytoin administration.
**Drug-lifestyle.** *Long-term alcohol use:* decreased phenytoin activity. Inform patient that heavy alcohol use may diminish drug's benefits.

## EFFECTS ON DIAGNOSTIC TESTS
Drug may cause reduced serum protein-bound iodine and free thyroxine levels without evidence of hypothyroidism; a slight decrease in urinary 17-hydroxysteroid and 17-ketosteroid levels; increased urine 6-b hydroxycortisol excretion, and decreased values for dexamethasone suppression or metyrapone tests.

## CONTRAINDICATIONS
Contraindicated in patients with hypersensitivity to hydantoin and in those with sinus bradycardia, SA block, second- or third-degree AV block, or Adams-Stokes syndrome.

## NURSING CONSIDERATIONS
• Use cautiously in patients with hepatic dysfunction, hypotension, myocardial insufficiency, diabetes, and respiratory depression; in elderly or debilitated patients; and in those receiving other hydantoin derivatives.
• Elderly patients tend to metabolize phenytoin slowly and may require lower dosages.
• Phenytoin requirements usually increase during pregnancy.
• Use only clear solution for injection. A slight yellow color is acceptable. Don't refrigerate.
• Don't give I.M. unless dosage adjustments are made; drug may precipitate at injection site, cause pain, and be absorbed erratically.
• Divided doses given with or after meals may decrease adverse GI reactions.
• Drug should be discontinued if rash appears. If rash is scarlatiniform or morbilliform, drug may be resumed after rash clears. If rash reappears, therapy should be discontinued. If rash is exfoliative, purpuric, or bullous, drug won't be resumed.
• Don't withdraw drug suddenly because seizures may worsen. Call doctor at once if adverse reactions develop.
• Monitor blood levels, as ordered. Therapeutic phenytoin blood level is 10 to 20 mcg/ml.
• Monitor CBC and serum calcium level every 6 months, and periodically monitor hepatic function, as ordered. If mega-

loblastic anemia is evident, doctor may order folic acid and vitamin $B_{12}$.

• If using to treat seizures, take appropriate safety precautions.

• Mononucleosis may decrease phenytoin levels. Monitor for increased seizure activity.

• **Alert:** Dilantin doesn't follow linear kinetics, so doubling the dose doesn't result in twice initial serum levels but may result in toxic serum levels. Consult pharmacist for specific dosing recommendations.

• **Alert:** Don't confuse phenytoin with mephenytoin or Dilantin with Dilaudid.

### I.V. administration

• Administer slowly (50 mg/minute) as I.V. bolus. If giving as an infusion, don't mix drug with $D_5W$ because it will precipitate. Clear I.V. tubing first with normal saline solution. Never use cloudy solution. May mix with normal saline solution if necessary and give as an infusion over 30 minutes to 1 hour, when possible. Infusion must begin within 1 hour after preparation and should run through an in-line filter. Discard 4 hours after preparation.

• **Alert:** Check patency of I.V. catheter before administering. Extravasation has caused severe local tissue damage.

• If possible, don't administer phenytoin by I.V. push into veins on the back of the hand to avoid discoloration (purple-glove syndrome). Inject into larger veins or central venous catheter if available.

• Check vital signs, blood pressure, and ECG during I.V. administration.

### ✓ Patient teaching

• Advise patient to avoid driving and other potentially hazardous activities that require mental alertness until drug's CNS effects are known.

• Advise patient not to change brands or dosage forms once he's stabilized on therapy.

• Dilantin capsules are the only oral form that can be given once daily. Toxic levels may result if any other brand or form is given once daily. Dilantin tablets and oral suspension should never be taken once daily.

• Warn patient and parents not to stop drug abruptly.

• Stress importance of good oral hygiene and regular dental examinations. Gingivectomy may be necessary periodically if dental hygiene is poor.

• Caution patient that drug may color urine pink, red, or reddish brown.

## primidone
Apo-Primidone†, Mysoline, PMS Primidone†, Sertan†

*Pregnancy Risk Category NR*

### HOW SUPPLIED
*Tablets:* 50 mg, 250 mg
*Oral suspension:* 250 mg/5 ml

### ACTION
Unknown. Some activity may be caused by phenylethylmalonamide and phenobarbital, which are active metabolites.

| Route | Onset | Peak | Duration |
|-------|-------|------|----------|
| P.O. | Unknown | 3-4 hr | Unknown |

### INDICATIONS & DOSAGE
*Tonic-clonic, complex partial, and simple partial seizures—*
**Adults and children ages 8 and older:** initially, 100 to 125 mg P.O. h.s. on days 1 to 3; then 100 to 125 mg P.O. b.i.d. on days 4 to 6; then 100 to 125 mg P.O. t.i.d. on days 7 to 9, followed by maintenance dose of 250 mg P.O. t.i.d. Maintenance dose may be increased to 250 mg q.i.d., if needed. Dose may be increased to maximum of 2 g daily in divided doses.
**Children under age 8:** initially, 50 mg P.O. h.s. for 3 days; then 50 mg P.O. b.i.d. for days 4 to 6; then 100 mg P.O. b.i.d. for days 7 to 9, followed by maintenance dose of 125 to 250 mg P.O. t.i.d. or 10 to 25 mg/kg/day in divided doses.

### ADVERSE REACTIONS
**CNS:** *drowsiness, ataxia,* emotional disturbances, vertigo, hyperirritability, fatigue, paranoia.
**EENT:** *diplopia,* nystagmus.
**GI:** anorexia, *nausea, vomiting.*
**GU:** impotence, polyuria.

---

Reactions may be *common,* uncommon, **life-threatening,** or COMMON AND LIFE-THREATENING.

**Hematologic:** megaloblastic anemia, *thrombocytopenia.*
**Hepatic:** abnormal liver function test results.
**Skin:** morbilliform rash.

## INTERACTIONS
**Drug-drug.** *Acetazolamide, succinimide:* may decrease primidone levels. Monitor levels.
*Carbamazepine:* increased carbamazepine levels and decreased primidone and phenobarbital levels. Observe for toxicity.
*Isoniazid:* increased primidone level. Monitor levels.
*Phenytoin:* stimulated conversion of primidone to phenobarbital. Observe for increased phenobarbital effect.

## EFFECTS ON DIAGNOSTIC TESTS
None reported.

## CONTRAINDICATIONS
Contraindicated in patients with hypersensitivity to phenobarbital and in those with porphyria.

## NURSING CONSIDERATIONS
• Shake liquid suspension well.
• Don't withdraw drug suddenly because seizures may worsen. Notify doctor immediately if adverse reactions develop.
• Therapeutic blood level of primidone is 5 to 12 mcg/ml. Therapeutic blood level of phenobarbital is 15 to 40 mcg/ml.
• Monitor CBC and routine blood chemistry every 6 months.
• Brand interchange isn't recommended because of documented bioequivalence problems for primidone products marketed by different manufacturers.
• *Alert:* Don't confuse primidone with prednisone.

### ☑ Patient teaching
• Advise patient to avoid driving and other potentially hazardous activities that require mental alertness until drug's CNS effects are known.
• Warn patient and parents not to stop drug therapy suddenly.
• Tell patient that full therapeutic response may take 2 weeks or more.

## tiagabine hydrochloride
Gabitril

*Pregnancy Risk Category C*

## HOW SUPPLIED
*Tablets:* 4 mg, 12 mg, 16 mg, 20 mg

## ACTION
Unknown. May act by enhancing the activity of gamma aminobutyric acid (GABA), the major inhibitory neurotransmitter in the CNS. Drug binds to recognition sites associated with the GABA uptake carrier and may thus permit more GABA to be available for binding to receptors on postsynaptic cells.

| Route | Onset | Peak | Duration |
|-------|-------|------|----------|
| P.O. | Rapid | 45 min | 7-9 hr |

## INDICATIONS & DOSAGE
*Adjunctive therapy in treatment of partial seizures—*
**Adults:** initially, 4 mg P.O. once daily. Total daily dose may be increased by 4 to 8 mg at weekly intervals until clinical response or up to 56 mg/day. Total daily dose should be given in divided doses b.i.d. to q.i.d.
**Children ages 12 to 18:** initially, 4 mg P.O. once daily. Total daily dose may be increased by 4 mg at beginning of week 2 and thereafter by 4 to 8 mg/week until clinical response or up to 32 mg/day. Total daily dose should be given in divided doses b.i.d. to q.i.d.
*Adjust-a-dose:* For patients with impaired liver function, reduced initial and maintenance doses or longer dosing intervals may be required.

## ADVERSE REACTIONS
**CNS:** *dizziness, asthenia, somnolence, nervousness,* tremor, difficulty with concentration and attention, insomnia, ataxia, confusion, speech disorder, difficulty with memory, paresthesia, depression, emotional lability, abnormal gait, hostility, language problems, agitation.
**CV:** vasodilation.
**EENT:** nystagmus, pharyngitis.

---

**GI:** abdominal pain, *nausea,* diarrhea, vomiting, increased appetite, mouth ulceration.
**Musculoskeletal:** generalized weakness, pain, myasthenia.
**Respiratory:** increased cough.
**Skin:** rash, pruritus.

## INTERACTIONS
**Drug-drug.** *Carbamazepine, phenobarbital, phenytoin:* increased tiagabine clearance. Monitor closely.
*CNS depressants:* enhanced CNS effects. Use cautiously.
**Drug-lifestyle.** *Alcohol use:* enhanced CNS effects. Use cautiously.

## EFFECTS ON DIAGNOSTIC TESTS
None reported.

## CONTRAINDICATIONS
Contraindicated in patients with hypersensitivity to drug or its ingredients.

## NURSING CONSIDERATIONS
• Use cautiously in breast-feeding women.
• Never withdraw drug suddenly because seizure frequency may increase. Withdraw drug gradually unless safety concerns require a more rapid withdrawal.
• *Alert:* Status epilepticus and sudden unexpected death in epilepsy have occurred in patients receiving antiepilepsy drugs, including tiagabine.
• Patients who aren't receiving at least one concomitant enzyme-inducing antiepilepsy drug at time of tiagabine initiation may require lower doses or a slower dosage adjustment.
• Moderately severe to incapacitating generalized weakness has occurred in patients receiving tiagabine. Weakness resolved after dosage reduction or discontinuation of drug.

☑ **Patient teaching**
• Advise patient to take drug only as prescribed.
• Tell patient to take drug with food.
• Warn patient that drug may cause dizziness, somnolence, and other signs and symptoms of CNS depression. Advise patient to avoid driving and other potentially hazardous activities that require mental alertness until drug's CNS effects are known.
• Tell woman to call doctor if she becomes pregnant or plans to become pregnant during therapy.
• Instruct woman to notify doctor if planning to breast-feed because drug may appear in breast milk.

---

**topiramate**
Topamax

*Pregnancy Risk Category C*

## HOW SUPPLIED
*Tablets:* 25 mg, 100 mg, 200 mg

## ACTION
Unknown. Suggestive of a sodium channel blocking action. May also potentiate the activity of gamma-aminobutyrate (GABA) and antagonize the ability of kainate to activate the kainate/alpha-amino-3-hydroxy-5-methylisoxazole-4-propionic acid subtype of excitatory amino acid (glutamate) receptor.

| Route | Onset | Peak | Duration |
|-------|-------|------|----------|
| P.O. | Unknown | 2 hr | Unknown |

## INDICATIONS & DOSAGE
*Adjunctive therapy for adults with partial onset seizures—*
**Adults:** adjust up to maximum daily dose of 400 mg P.O. in divided doses b.i.d. Adjustment schedule is as follows: Week 1: 50 mg P.O. in evening; week 2, 50 mg P.O. b.i.d.; week 3, 50 mg P.O. in morning and 100 mg P.O. in evening; week 4, 100 mg P.O. b.i.d.; week 5, 100 mg P.O. in morning and 150 mg P.O. in evening; week 6, 150 mg P.O. b.i.d.; week 7, 150 mg P.O. in morning and 200 mg P.O. in evening; week 8, 200 mg P.O. b.i.d.
*Adjust-a-dose:* For renally impaired patients with creatinine clearance below 70 ml/minute, reduce dosage by 50%. For patients on hemodialysis, supplemental doses may be required to avoid rapid drops in drug levels during prolonged dialysis treatment.

---

## ADVERSE REACTIONS

**CNS:** abnormal coordination; aggressive reaction; agitation; apathy; asthenia; *ataxia; confusion;* depression; depersonalization; difficulty with concentration, attention, or language; *difficulty with memory; dizziness;* emotional lability; euphoria; **generalized tonic-clonic seizures;** hallucination; hyperkinesia; hypertonia; hypoesthesia; hypokinesia; insomnia; mood problems; *nervousness; paresthesia;* personality disorder; *psychomotor slowing;* psychosis; *somnolence; speech disorders;* stupor; **suicide attempts;** *tremor;* vertigo, malaise, *fatigue.*

**CV:** chest pain, palpitations, vasodilation, edema.

**EENT:** *abnormal vision,* conjunctivitis, *diplopia,* eye pain, hearing problems, tinnitus, pharyngitis, sinusitis, *nystagmus.*

**GI:** abdominal pain, anorexia, constipation, diarrhea, dry mouth, dyspepsia, flatulence, gastroenteritis, gingivitis, *nausea,* vomiting, taste perversion.

**GU:** amenorrhea, dysuria, dysmenorrhea, hematuria, impotence, intermenstrual bleeding, menstrual disorder, menorrhagia, micturition frequency, renal calculus, urinary incontinence, urinary tract infection, vaginitis, leukorrhea.

**Hematologic:** anemia, epistaxis, *leukopenia.*

**Hepatic:** elevated liver enzymes.

**Metabolic:** increased or decreased weight.

**Musculoskeletal:** arthralgia, back or leg pain, muscle weakness, myalgia, rigors.

**Respiratory:** bronchitis, coughing, dyspnea, *upper respiratory tract infection.*

**Skin:** acne, alopecia, increased sweating, pruritus, rash.

**Other:** breast pain, body odor, fever, flu-like syndrome, hot flashes, decreased libido, lymphadenopathy.

## INTERACTIONS

**Drug-drug.** *Carbamazepine:* decreased topiramate levels. Monitor patient.
*Carbonic anhydrase inhibitors (acetazolamide, dichlorphenamide):* increased risk of renal calculus formation. Avoid concomitant use.
*CNS depressants:* possible topiramate-induced CNS depression as well as other adverse cognitive and neuropsychiatric events. Use with caution.
*Oral contraceptives:* decreased efficacy. Report changes in bleeding patterns.
*Phenytoin:* decreased topiramate levels and increased phenytoin levels. Monitor levels.
*Valproic acid:* decrease in valproic acid and topiramate levels. Monitor patient.

**Drug-lifestyle.** *Alcohol use:* possible topiramate-induced CNS depression as well as other adverse cognitive and neuropsychiatric events. Use with caution.

## EFFECTS ON DIAGNOSTIC TESTS
None reported.

## CONTRAINDICATIONS
Contraindicated in patients with hypersensitivity to drug or its ingredients.

## NURSING CONSIDERATIONS
• Use with caution in breast-feeding or pregnant women and in those with hepatic impairment.
• If necessary, withdraw antiepileptic drugs (including topiramate) gradually to minimize risk of increased seizure activity.
• Monitoring plasma levels of topiramate isn't necessary.
• Drug is rapidly cleared by dialysis. A prolonged period of dialysis may result in low drug levels and seizures. A supplemental dose may be required.

### ✅ Patient teaching
• Tell patient to maintain adequate fluid intake during therapy to minimize risk of forming renal calculi.
• Advise patient not to drive or operate hazardous machinery until CNS effects of drug are known because drug can cause somnolence, dizziness, confusion, and difficulty concentrating.
• Tell woman that drug may decrease effectiveness of oral contraceptives. Advise woman taking oral contraceptives to report change in her bleeding patterns.
• Tell patient to avoid crushing or breaking tablets because of bitter taste.
• Inform patient that drug can be taken without regard to food.

## valproate sodium
Depacon, Depakene, Epilim‡, Valpro‡

## valproic acid
Convulex§, Depakene

## divalproex sodium
Depakote, Depakote Sprinkle, Epival†

*Pregnancy Risk Category D*

## HOW SUPPLIED
**valproate sodium**
*Syrup:* 250 mg/5 ml
**valproic acid**
*Tablets (enteric-coated):* 200 mg‡, 500 mg‡
*Tablets (crushable):* 100 mg‡
*Capsules:* 250 mg
*Syrup:* 200 mg/5 ml‡
**divalproex sodium**
*Capsules (delayed-release):* 125 mg
*Tablets (enteric-coated):* 125 mg, 250 mg, 500 mg
*Injection:* 500-mg vial

## ACTION
Unknown. Probably increases brain levels of gamma-aminobutyric acid, which transmits inhibitory nerve impulses in the CNS.

| Route | Onset | Peak | Duration |
|-------|-------|------|----------|
| P.O. | Unknown | 15 min-4 hr | Unknown |
| I.V. | Unknown | 1 hr | Unknown |

## INDICATIONS & DOSAGE
*Simple and complex absence seizures, mixed seizure types (including absence seizures)—*
**Adults and children:** initially, 15 mg/kg P.O. or I.V. daily; then increase by 5 to 10 mg/kg daily at weekly intervals up to maximum of 60 mg/kg daily.
*Mania (divalproex sodium only)—*
**Adults and children:** initially, 750 mg daily in divided doses. Adjust dosage based on patient's response; maximum dose is 60 mg/kg/day.

*Prophylaxis for migraine headache (divalproex sodium only)—*
**Adults:** initially, 250 mg P.O. b.i.d. Some patients may require up to 1,000 mg/day.
*Complex partial seizures—*
**Adults and children ages 10 and older:** 10 to 15 mg/kg P.O. or I.V. daily; then increase by 5 to 10 mg/kg daily at weekly intervals, up to 60 mg/kg/day.
**Elderly:** reduce initial dose.

## ADVERSE REACTIONS
**CNS:** asthenia, *sedation,* emotional upset, depression, psychosis, aggressiveness, hyperactivity, behavioral deterioration, muscle weakness, tremor, ataxia, *headache, dizziness,* incoordination.
**EENT:** nystagmus, *diplopia.*
**GI:** *nausea, vomiting, indigestion, diarrhea,* abdominal cramps, constipation, increased appetite, anorexia, **pancreatitis.**
**Hematologic:** **thrombocytopenia,** increased bleeding time, petechiae, bruising, eosinophilia, **hemorrhage, leukopenia, bone marrow suppression.**
**Hepatic:** *elevated liver enzyme levels,* **toxic hepatitis.**
**Metabolic:** weight gain.
**Skin:** rash, alopecia, pruritus, photosensitivity, erythema multiforme.

## INTERACTIONS
**Drug-drug.** *Aspirin, chlorpromazine, cimetidine, erythromycin, felbamate:* may cause valproic acid toxicity. Use together cautiously and monitor blood levels. Monitor patient closely.
*Benzodiazepines, other CNS depressants:* excessive CNS depression. Avoid concomitant use.
*Lamotrigine:* increased lamotrigine levels, decreased valproate levels. Monitor levels closely.
*Phenobarbital:* increased phenobarbital levels. Monitor patient closely.
*Phenytoin:* increased or decreased phenytoin levels, decreased valproate levels. Monitor patient closely.
*Rifampin:* may decrease valproate levels. Monitor levels.
*Warfarin:* valproic acid may displace warfarin from binding sites. Monitor PT and INR.

Reactions may be *common,* uncommon, **life-threatening,** or COMMON AND LIFE-THREATENING.

**Drug-lifestyle:** *Alcohol use:* excessive CNS depression. Avoid concomitant use.

**EFFECTS ON DIAGNOSTIC TESTS**
Drug may produce false-positive results for urine ketones.

**CONTRAINDICATIONS**
Contraindicated in patients with hypersensitivity to drug and in those with hepatic disease or significant hepatic dysfunction.

**NURSING CONSIDERATIONS**
• Monitor liver function studies, platelet counts, and PT and INR before starting drug and periodically thereafter, as ordered.
• Don't administer syrup to patients who need sodium restriction. Check with doctor.
• Adverse reactions may not be caused by valproic acid alone because it's usually used in combination with other anticonvulsants.
• Divalproex sodium has a lower incidence of adverse GI reactions.
• Never withdraw drug suddenly because sudden withdrawal may worsen seizures. Call doctor at once if adverse reactions develop.
• *Alert:* Serious or fatal hepatotoxicity may follow nonspecific symptoms, such as malaise, fever, and lethargy. If these symptoms occur, notify doctor at once because drug will need to be discontinued in the presence of suspected or apparent substantial hepatic dysfunction.
• Patients at high risk for hepatotoxicity include those with congenital metabolic disorders, mental retardation, or presence of organic brain disease; those taking multiple anticonvulsants; and children under age 2.
• Notify doctor if tremors occur (a dosage reduction may be necessary).
• Monitor blood levels, as ordered. Therapeutic blood level is 50 to 100 mcg/ml.
• Use caution when converting patients from a brand to a generic product because breakthrough seizures are possible.

**◖ I.V. administration**
• I.V. use is indicated only in patients who are unable to take drug orally. Switch patient to oral form as soon as clinically feasible; use of I.V. dosage for more than 14 days hasn't been studied.
• Dilute valproate sodium injection with at least 50 ml of a compatible diluent. It's physically compatible and chemically stable in $D_5W$, normal saline, and lactated Ringer's solution for 24 hours.
• Administer drug as a 60-minute I.V. infusion (but not more than 20 mg/minute) with the same frequency as oral dosage.
• Monitoring of plasma levels and dosage adjustment may be needed.

**✓ Patient teaching**
• Tell patient to take drug with food or milk to reduce adverse GI effects.
• Advise patient not to chew capsules; irritation of mouth and throat may result.
• Tell patient and parents that syrup shouldn't be mixed with carbonated beverages; mixture may be irritating to mouth and throat.
• Tell patient and parents to keep drug out of children's reach.
• Warn patient and parents not to stop drug therapy abruptly.
• Advise patient to avoid driving and other potentially hazardous activities that require mental alertness until drug's CNS effects are known.

---

amitriptyline hydrochloride
amitriptyline pamoate
amoxapine
bupropion hydrochloride
citalopram hydrobromide
clomipramine hydrochloride
desipramine hydrochloride
doxepin hydrochloride
fluoxetine hydrochloride
imipramine hydrochloride
imipramine pamoate
mirtazapine
nefazodone hydrochloride
nortriptyline hydrochloride
paroxetine hydrochloride
phenelzine sulfate
sertraline hydrochloride
tranylcypromine sulfate
trazodone hydrochloride
trimipramine maleate
venlafaxine hydrochloride

## COMBINATION PRODUCTS
ETRAFON: perphenazine 2 mg and
amitriptyline hydrochloride 25 mg.
ETRAFON 2-10: perphenazine 2 mg and
amitriptyline hydrochloride 10 mg.
ETRAFON-A: perphenazine 4 mg and
amitriptyline hydrochloride 10 mg.
ETRAFON-FORTE: perphenazine 4 mg and
amitriptyline hydrochloride 25 mg.
LIMBITROL DS: chlordiazepoxide 10 mg
and amitriptyline hydrochloride 25 mg.
TRIAVIL 2-10, TRIAVIL 4-10, TRIAVIL 2-25,
TRIAVIL 4-25 are products identical to the
Etrafon products listed above. Triavil is
also available as TRIAVIL 4-50 (perphenazine 4 mg and amitriptyline hydrochloride 50 mg).

## amitriptyline hydrochloride
Apo-Amitriptyline†, Elavil, Endep,
Levate†, Novotriptyn†, Tryptanol‡,
Tryptine‡

## amitriptyline pamoate
Elavil†

*Pregnancy Risk Category NR*

## HOW SUPPLIED
**amitriptyline hydrochloride**
*Tablets:* 10 mg, 25 mg, 50 mg, 75 mg,
100 mg, 150 mg
*Injection:* 10 mg/ml
**amitriptyline pamoate†**
*Syrup:* 10 mg/5 ml*†

## ACTION
Unknown. A tricyclic antidepressant
(TCA) that increases amount of norepinephrine, serotonin, or both in the CNS
by blocking their reuptake by the presynaptic neurons.

| Route | Onset | Peak | Duration |
|-------|-------|------|----------|
| P.O., I.M. | Unknown | 2-12 hr | Unknown |

## INDICATIONS & DOSAGE
*Depression—*
**Adults:** initially, 50 to 100 mg P.O. h.s.,
increasing to 150 mg daily; maximum
dose is 300 mg daily, if needed. Maintenance dose is 50 to 100 mg/day. Or, 20 to
30 mg I.M. q.i.d.
**Elderly and adolescents:** 10 mg P.O.
t.i.d. and 20 mg h.s. daily.

## ADVERSE REACTIONS
**CNS:** *coma, seizures,* hallucinations,
delusions, disorientation, ataxia, tremor,
peripheral neuropathy, anxiety, insomnia,
restlessness, drowsiness, dizziness, weakness, fatigue, headache, extrapyramidal
reactions.
**CV:** *MI, stroke, arrhythmias,* heart block,
*orthostatic hypotension, tachycardia,*
ECG changes, hypertension, edema.

---

Reactions may be *common,* uncommon, *life-threatening,* or COMMON AND LIFE-THREATENING.

**EENT:** blurred vision, tinnitus, mydriasis, increased intraocular pressure.
**GI:** *dry mouth,* nausea, vomiting, anorexia, epigastric distress, diarrhea, constipation, paralytic ileus.
**GU:** urine retention.
**Hematologic:** *agranulocytosis, thrombocytopenia, leukopenia,* eosinophilia.
**Hepatic:** elevated liver function test results.
**Metabolic:** hypoglycemia, hyperglycemia.
**Skin:** rash, urticaria, photosensitivity, diaphoresis.
**Other:** *hypersensitivity reaction.*
**After abrupt withdrawal of long-term therapy:** nausea, headache, malaise (doesn't indicate addiction).

## INTERACTIONS
**Drug-drug.** *Barbiturates, CNS depressants:* enhanced CNS depression. Avoid concomitant use.
*Cimetidine, fluoxetine, fluvoxamine, oral contraceptives, paroxetine, sertraline:* increased TCA blood levels. Monitor for increased antidepressant adverse effects.
*Clonidine:* may cause hypertensive crisis. Avoid coadministration.
*Epinephrine, norepinephrine:* increased hypertensive effect. Use with caution.
*MAO inhibitors:* may cause severe excitation, hyperpyrexia, or seizures, usually with high doses. Avoid concomitant use.
**Drug-lifestyle.** *Alcohol use:* enhanced CNS depression. Avoid concomitant use.
*Smoking:* may lower plasma levels of drug. Monitor for lack of effect.
*Sun exposure:* increased risk of photosensitivity reactions. Avoid unprotected or prolonged exposure to sun.

## EFFECTS ON DIAGNOSTIC TESTS
None reported.

## CONTRAINDICATIONS
Contraindicated in patients with hypersensitivity to drug and in those who have received an MAO inhibitor within past 14 days; also contraindicated during acute recovery phase of MI.

## NURSING CONSIDERATIONS
• Use cautiously in patients with history of seizures, urine retention, angle-closure glaucoma, or increased intraocular pressure; in those with hyperthyroidism, CV disease, diabetes, or impaired liver function; and in those receiving thyroid medications.
• *Alert:* Parenteral form of drug is for I.M. administration only. Drug shouldn't be given I.V.
• Amitriptyline has strong anticholinergic effects and is one of the most sedating TCAs. Anticholinergic effects have a rapid onset even though therapeutic effect is delayed for weeks.
• If signs or symptoms of psychosis occur or increase, expect doctor to reduce dosage. Record mood changes. Monitor patient for suicidal tendencies, and allow only minimum supply of drug.
• Because hypertensive episodes have occurred during surgery in patients receiving TCAs, drug should be gradually discontinued several days before surgery.
• Don't withdraw drug abruptly.
• *Alert:* Don't confuse amitriptyline with nortriptyline or aminophylline; Elavil with Equanil or Mellaril; or Endep with Depen.

☑ **Patient teaching**
• Advise patient to take full dose at bedtime, but warn him of possible morning orthostatic hypotension.
• Tell patient to avoid alcohol during drug therapy.
• Advise patient to consult doctor before taking other medications.
• Warn patient to avoid activities that require alertness and good psychomotor coordination until CNS effects of drug are known. Drowsiness and dizziness usually subside after a few weeks.
• Inform patient that dry mouth may be relieved with sugarless hard candy or gum. Saliva substitutes may be needed.
• To prevent photosensitivity reactions, advise patient to use a sunblock, wear protective clothing, and avoid prolonged exposure to strong sunlight.
• Warn patient not to stop drug therapy abruptly.

## amoxapine
Asendin

*Pregnancy Risk Category C*

### HOW SUPPLIED
*Tablets:* 25 mg, 50 mg, 100 mg, 150 mg

### ACTION
Unknown. A tricyclic antidepressant (TCA) that increases amount of norepinephrine, serotonin, or both in the CNS by blocking their reuptake by the presynaptic neurons.

| Route | Onset | Peak | Duration |
|-------|-------|------|----------|
| P.O. | Unknown | 1.5 hr | Unknown |

### INDICATIONS & DOSAGE
*Depression—*
**Adults:** initially, 50 mg P.O. b.i.d. or t.i.d. Increased to 100 mg b.i.d. or t.i.d. by end of week 1 of therapy if tolerated. Increases above 300 mg daily are made only if 300 mg daily has been ineffective during trial period of at least 2 weeks. Maximum recommended dose for outpatients is 400 mg daily. When effective dose is established, entire dose (not to exceed 300 mg) may be given h.s.
**Elderly:** initially, 25 mg P.O. b.i.d. or t.i.d. If tolerated by end of week 1, increase to 50 mg b.i.d. or t.i.d. Carefully increase up to 300 mg daily.

### ADVERSE REACTIONS
**CNS:** *drowsiness, dizziness,* excitation, tremor, weakness, confusion, anxiety, insomnia, restlessness, nightmares, ataxia, fatigue, headache, nervousness, tardive dyskinesia, EEG changes, *seizures,* extrapyramidal reactions (rare).
**CV:** *orthostatic hypotension, tachycardia,* hypertension, palpitations, edema, ECG changes.
**EENT:** blurred vision.
**GI:** *dry mouth,* constipation, nausea, excessive appetite.
**GU:** urine retention, *acute renal failure* (with overdose).
**Hepatic:** elevated liver function test results.
**Metabolic:** hypoglycemia, hyperglycemia.

**Skin:** rash, diaphoresis.
**Other:** *neuroleptic malignant syndrome (high fever, tachycardia, tachypnea, profuse diaphoresis).*
**After abrupt withdrawal of long-term therapy:** nausea, headache, malaise (doesn't indicate addiction).

### INTERACTIONS
**Drug-drug.** *Barbiturates:* decreased TCA blood levels. Monitor for decreased antidepressant effect.
*Cimetidine, fluoxetine, fluvoxamine, paroxetine, sertraline:* may increase amoxapine serum levels. Monitor for increased adverse effects.
*Clonidine, epinephrine, norepinephrine:* increased hypertensive effect. Use with caution.
*CNS depressants:* enhanced CNS depression. Avoid concomitant use.
*MAO inhibitors:* may cause severe excitation, hyperpyrexia, or seizures, usually with high doses. Avoid concomitant use.
**Drug-lifestyle.** *Alcohol use:* enhanced CNS depression. Avoid concomitant use.
*Sun exposure:* increased risk of photosensitivity. Avoid unprotected or prolonged exposure to sun.

### EFFECTS ON DIAGNOSTIC TESTS
None reported.

### CONTRAINDICATIONS
Contraindicated in patients with hypersensitivity to drug and in those who have received an MAO inhibitor within past 14 days; also contraindicated during acute recovery phase of MI.

### NURSING CONSIDERATIONS
• Use cautiously in patients with history of urine retention, angle-closure glaucoma, or increased intraocular pressure and in patients with CV disease. Use with extreme caution in patients with history of seizure disorders.
• Safe use of drug in children under age 16 hasn't been determined.
• Don't withdraw drug abruptly.
• Because hypertensive episodes have occurred during surgery in patients receiving TCAs, drug should be gradually discontinued several days before surgery.

---

Reactions may be *common,* uncommon, *life-threatening,* or COMMON AND LIFE-THREATENING.

• Expect delay of 2 weeks or more before noticeable effect. Full effect may take 4 weeks or more. However, adverse anticholinergic effects can occur rapidly.
• If signs or symptoms of psychosis occur or increase, expect doctor to reduce dosage. Record mood changes. Monitor patient for suicidal tendencies, and allow only a minimum supply of drug.
• Monitor for signs and symptoms of tardive dyskinesia, especially in elderly women.
• Drug therapy has been associated with neuroleptic malignant syndrome, a rare but life-threatening syndrome usually seen with phenothiazines. Discontinue drug immediately and institute appropriate therapy if symptoms occur.
• Relieve dry mouth with sugarless hard candy or gum. Saliva substitutes may be needed.
• *Alert:* Don't confuse amoxapine with amoxicillin, or Asendin with aspirin.

☑ **Patient teaching**
• Whenever possible, tell patient to take full dose at bedtime.
• Caution patient not to stop drug therapy abruptly.
• Warn patient to avoid activities that require alertness and good psychomotor coordination until CNS effects of drug are known. Drowsiness and dizziness usually subside after a few weeks.
• To prevent photosensitivity reactions, advise patient to use sunblock, wear protective clothing, and avoid prolonged exposure to strong sunlight.

---

## bupropion hydrochloride
Wellbutrin, Wellbutrin SR

*Pregnancy Risk Category B*

### HOW SUPPLIED
*Tablets:* 75 mg, 100 mg
*Tablets (sustained-release):* 100 mg, 150 mg

### ACTION
Unknown. Drug isn't a tricyclic antidepressant (TCA), doesn't inhibit MAO, and is a weak inhibitor of norepinephrine, dopamine, and serotonin reuptake.

| Route | Onset | Peak | Duration |
|-------|-------|------|----------|
| P.O. | Unknown | 2 hr | Unknown |
| P.O. (sustained) | Unknown | 3 hr | Unknown |

### INDICATIONS & DOSAGE
*Depression—*
**Adults:** initially, 100 mg P.O. b.i.d., increased after 3 days to 100 mg P.O. t.i.d. if needed. If no response occurs after several weeks of therapy, dose increased to 150 mg t.i.d. No single dose should exceed 150 mg. For sustained-release tablets, initially, 150 mg P.O. q morning; increased to target dose of 150 mg P.O. b.i.d. as tolerated as early as day 4 of dosing. Maximum dose is 400 mg/day.

### ADVERSE REACTIONS
**CNS:** *headache, seizures,* anxiety, confusion, delusions, euphoria, hostility, impaired sleep quality, *insomnia, sedation, tremor;* akinesia, akathisia, *agitation, dizziness,* fatigue, syncope.
**CV:** *arrhythmias,* hypertension, hypotension, palpitations, *tachycardia.*
**EENT:** *auditory disturbances,* blurred vision.
**GI:** *dry mouth,* taste disturbance, increased appetite, *constipation,* dyspepsia, *nausea, vomiting, anorexia,* diarrhea.
**GU:** impotence, menstrual complaints, urinary frequency, urine retention.
**Metabolic:** *weight loss, weight gain.*
**Musculoskeletal:** arthritis.
**Skin:** pruritus, rash, cutaneous temperature disturbance, *excessive diaphoresis.*
**Other:** fever and chills, decreased libido.

### INTERACTIONS
**Drug-drug.** *Levodopa, phenothiazines, TCAs; recent and rapid withdrawal of benzodiazepines:* increased risk of adverse reactions, including seizures. Monitor patient closely.
*MAO inhibitors:* altered seizure threshold. Avoid concomitant use.
**Drug-lifestyle.** *Alcohol use:* altered seizure threshold. Avoid concomitant use.

---

**EFFECTS ON DIAGNOSTIC TESTS**
None reported.

**CONTRAINDICATIONS**
Contraindicated in patients with hypersensitivity to drug, in those who have taken MAO inhibitors within previous 14 days, and in those with seizure disorders or history of bulimia or anorexia nervosa because of a higher incidence of seizures. Don't use with Zyban or other drugs containing bupropion and used for smoking cessation.

**NURSING CONSIDERATIONS**
• Use cautiously in patients with recent history of MI or unstable heart disease or renal or hepatic impairment.
• Many patients experience a period of increased restlessness, especially at initiation of therapy. This may include agitation, insomnia, and anxiety.
• *Alert:* Risk of seizure may be minimized by not exceeding 450 mg/day and by administering daily dose in three to four equally divided doses. Patients who experience seizures often have predisposing factors, including history of head trauma, prior seizures, or CNS tumors, or they may be taking a drug that lowers seizure threshold.
• Closely monitor patient with history of bipolar disorders. Antidepressants can cause manic episodes during the depressed phase of bipolar disorder. This is less likely to occur with bupropion than with other antidepressants.
• *Alert:* Don't confuse bupropion with buspirone, or Wellbutrin with Wellcovorin or Wellferon.

☑ **Patient teaching**
• Advise patient to take drug as scheduled and to take each day's dose in three divided doses to minimize risk of seizures.
• Advise patient to consult doctor before taking other prescription or OTC drugs.
• Tell patient to avoid alcohol while taking drug because it may contribute to development of seizures.
• Advise patient to avoid hazardous activities that require alertness and good psychomotor coordination until CNS effects of drug are known.

---

**citalopram hydrobromide**
Celexa

*Pregnancy Risk Category C*

**HOW SUPPLIED**
*Tablets:* 20 mg, 40 mg

**ACTION**
A selective serotonin reuptake inhibitor whose action is presumed to be linked to potentiation of serotonergic activity in the CNS resulting from inhibition of neuronal reuptake of serotonin.

| Route | Onset | Peak | Duration |
|-------|-------|------|----------|
| P.O. | Unknown | 4 hr | Unknown |

**INDICATIONS & DOSAGE**
*Depression—*
**Adults:** initially, 20 mg P.O. once daily, increasing to 40 mg daily after no less than 1 week. Maximum recommended dose is 40 mg daily.
**Elderly:** 20 mg/day P.O. with adjustment to 40 mg/day only for nonresponding patients.
*Adjust-a-dose:* For patients with hepatic impairment, use 20 mg/day P.O. with adjustment to 40 mg/day only for nonresponding patients.

**ADVERSE REACTIONS**
**CNS:** tremor, *somnolence, insomnia,* anxiety, agitation, dizziness, paresthesia, migraine, impaired concentration, amnesia, depression, apathy, **suicide attempt,** confusion, fatigue.
**CV:** tachycardia, orthostatic hypotension, hypotension.
**EENT:** rhinitis, sinusitis, abnormal accommodation.
**GI:** *dry mouth, nausea,* diarrhea, anorexia, dyspepsia, vomiting, abdominal pain, taste perversion, increased saliva, flatulence, increased appetite.
**GU:** dysmenorrhea, amenorrhea, ejaculation disorder, impotence, polyuria.
**Metabolic:** decreased and increased weight.
**Musculoskeletal:** arthralgia, myalgia.
**Respiratory:** upper respiratory tract infection, coughing.

---

Reactions may be *common,* uncommon, *life-threatening,* or COMMON AND LIFE-THREATENING.

**Skin:** rash, pruritus, *increased sweating.*
**Other:** fever, yawning, decreased libido.

## INTERACTIONS
**Drug-drug.** *Carbamazepine:* may increase citalopram clearance. Monitor for effects.
*CNS drugs:* additive effects. Use together cautiously.
*Drugs that inhibit cytochrome P-450 isoenzymes 3A4 and 2C19:* decreased clearance of citalopram. Monitor closely.
*Imipramine, other tricyclic antidepressants:* level of imipramine metabolite desipramine increased by about 50%. Use together cautiously.
*MAO inhibitors:* serious, sometimes fatal, reactions may occur. Don't use drug within 14 days of MAO inhibitor use.
*Lithium:* may enhance serotonergic effect of citalopram. Use with caution, and monitor lithium levels.
*Warfarin:* prothrombin time increased by 5%. Monitor closely.
**Drug-lifestyle.** *Alcohol use:* may increase CNS effects. Avoid concomitant use.

## EFFECTS ON DIAGNOSTIC TESTS
None reported.

## CONTRAINDICATIONS
Contraindicated in patients with hypersensitivity to drug or its inactive ingredients and in those also taking MAO inhibitors; also contraindicated within 14 days of stopping MAO inhibitor therapy.

## NURSING CONSIDERATIONS
• Use cautiously in patients with history of mania, seizures, suicidal ideation, or hepatic or renal impairment.
• Safety and effectiveness of drug haven't been established in children.
• Although drug hasn't been shown to impair psychomotor performance, any psychoactive drug has the potential to impair judgment, thinking, or motor skills.
• The possibility of a suicide attempt is inherent in depression and may persist until significant remission occurs. Closely supervise high-risk patients at start of drug therapy. Reduce risk of overdose by limiting amount of drug available per refill.

• At least 14 days should elapse between MAO inhibitor therapy and citalopram therapy.
• **Alert:** Don't confuse Celexa with Celebrex or Cerebyx.

✓ **Patient teaching**
• Inform patient that, although improvement may take 1 to 4 weeks, he should continue therapy as prescribed.
• Instruct patient to exercise caution when operating hazardous machinery, including automobiles, because of the potential of psychoactive drugs to impair judgment, thinking, and motor skills.
• Advise patient to consult doctor before taking other prescription or OTC drugs.
• Advise woman to consult doctor before breast-feeding.
• Warn patient to avoid concomitant use of alcohol.
• Instruct woman of childbearing age to use birth control during drug therapy and to notify doctor immediately if pregnancy is suspected.
• Caution patient against use of MAO inhibitors while taking citalopram.
• Tell patient that drug may be taken in the morning or evening without regard to meals. If drowsiness occurs, take drug in evening.

## clomipramine hydrochloride
Anafranil, Placil‡

*Pregnancy Risk Category C*

## HOW SUPPLIED
*Capsules:* 25 mg, 50 mg, 75 mg

## ACTION
Unknown. A tricyclic antidepressant (TCA) that selectively inhibits reuptake of serotonin.

| Route | Onset | Peak | Duration |
|-------|-------|------|----------|
| P.O. | ≥ 2 wk | 2-6 hr | Unknown |

## INDICATIONS & DOSAGE
*Obsessive-compulsive disorder—*
**Adults:** initially, 25 mg P.O. daily with meals, gradually increased to 100 mg daily in divided doses during first 2 weeks.

Thereafter, increased to maximum dose of 250 mg daily in divided doses with meals, p.r.n. After adjustment, total daily dose may be given h.s.

**Children and adolescents:** initially, 25 mg P.O. daily with meals, gradually increased over first 2 weeks to daily maximum of 3 mg/kg or 100 mg P.O. in divided doses, whichever is smaller. Maximum daily dose is 3 mg/kg or 200 mg, whichever is smaller; may be given h.s. after adjustment. Periodic reassessment and adjustment are necessary.

## ADVERSE REACTIONS

**CNS:** *somnolence, tremor, dizziness, headache, insomnia, nervousness, myoclonus, fatigue,* EEG changes, **seizures.**
**CV:** *orthostatic hypotension, palpitations,* tachycardia.
**EENT:** *pharyngitis, rhinitis, visual changes.*
**GI:** *dry mouth, constipation, nausea, dyspepsia, increased appetite,* diarrhea, *anorexia, abdominal pain.*
**GU:** *urinary hesitancy,* urinary tract infection, *dysmenorrhea, ejaculation failure, impotence.*
**Hematologic:** purpura.
**Metabolic:** *weight gain.*
**Musculoskeletal:** *myalgia.*
**Skin:** *diaphoresis,* rash, pruritus, dry skin.
**Other:** *altered libido.*

## INTERACTIONS

**Drug-drug.** *Barbiturates:* decreased TCA blood levels. Monitor for decreased antidepressant effect.
*Cimetidine, fluoxetine, fluvoxamine, sertraline:* increased TCA blood levels. Monitor for enhanced antidepressant effect.
*Clonidine, epinephrine, norepinephrine:* increased hypertensive effect. Use with caution.
*CNS depressants:* enhanced CNS depression. Avoid concomitant use.
*MAO inhibitors:* may cause hyperpyretic crisis, seizures, coma, or death. Avoid concomitant use.
**Drug-lifestyle.** *Alcohol use:* enhanced CNS depression. Avoid concomitant use.

*Sun exposure:* increased risk of photosensitivity. Avoid unprotected or prolonged exposure to sun.

## EFFECTS ON DIAGNOSTIC TESTS
None reported.

## CONTRAINDICATIONS
Contraindicated in patients with hypersensitivity to drug or other TCAs, in those who have taken MAO inhibitors within previous 14 days, and in patients during acute recovery period after MI.

## NURSING CONSIDERATIONS
• Use cautiously in patients with history of seizure disorders or with brain damage of varying cause; in patients receiving other seizure threshold–lowering drugs; in patients at risk for suicide; in patients with history of urine retention or angle-closure glaucoma, increased intraocular pressure, CV disease, impaired hepatic or renal function, or hyperthyroidism; in patients with tumors of the adrenal medulla; in patients receiving thyroid medication or electroconvulsive therapy; and in those undergoing elective surgery.
• Don't withdraw drug abruptly.
• Because hypertensive episodes have occurred during surgery in patients receiving TCAs, drug should be gradually discontinued several days before surgery.
• Relieve dry mouth with sugarless candy or gum. Saliva substitutes may be necessary.
• *Alert:* Don't confuse clomipramine with chlorpromazine or clomiphene, or Anafranil with enalapril, nafarelin, or alfentanil.

## ☑ Patient teaching
• Warn patient to avoid hazardous activities requiring alertness and good psychomotor coordination, especially during adjustment. Daytime sedation and dizziness may occur.
• Tell patient to avoid alcohol during drug therapy.
• Warn patient not to stop drug suddenly.
• Advise patient to use sunblock, wear protective clothing, and avoid prolonged exposure to strong sunlight to prevent photosensitivity reactions.

---

# desipramine hydrochloride
Norpramin**, Pertofran‡,
Pertofrane†

*Pregnancy Risk Category NR*

## HOW SUPPLIED
*Tablets:* 10 mg, 25 mg, 50 mg, 75 mg,
100 mg, 150 mg
*Capsules:* 25 mg, 50 mg

## ACTION
Unknown. A tricyclic antidepressant
(TCA) that increases amount of norepinephrine, serotonin, or both in the CNS
by blocking their reuptake by the presynaptic neurons.

| Route | Onset | Peak | Duration |
|-------|-------|------|----------|
| P.O. | Unknown | 4-6 hr | Unknown |

## INDICATIONS & DOSAGE
*Depression—*
**Adults:** 100 to 200 mg P.O. daily in divided doses, increased to maximum of
300 mg daily. Or, entire dose can be given
h.s.
**Elderly and adolescents:** 25 to 100 mg
P.O. daily in divided doses, increased
gradually to maximum of 150 mg daily if
needed.

## ADVERSE REACTIONS
**CNS:** *drowsiness, dizziness,* excitation,
tremor, weakness, confusion, anxiety,
restlessness, agitation, headache, nervous-
ness, EEG changes, *seizures,* extrapyra-
midal reactions.
**CV:** orthostatic hypotension, *tachycardia,*
ECG changes, hypertension.
**EENT:** *blurred vision,* tinnitus, mydriasis.
**GI:** *dry mouth,* constipation, nausea,
vomiting, anorexia, paralytic ileus.
**GU:** urine retention.
**Hepatic:** elevated liver function tests.
**Metabolic:** hypoglycemia, hyper-
glycemia.
**Skin:** rash, urticaria, photosensitivity, di-
aphoresis.
**Other:** *hypersensitivity reaction; sudden
death in children.*

**After abrupt withdrawal of long-term
therapy:** nausea, headache, malaise
(doesn't indicate addiction).

## INTERACTIONS
**Drug-drug.** *Barbiturates, CNS depressants:* enhanced CNS depression. Avoid
concomitant use.
*Cimetidine, fluvoxamine, fluoxetine,
paroxetine, sertraline:* may increase
serum desipramine levels. Monitor for adverse reactions.
*Clonidine, epinephrine, norepinephrine:*
increased hypertensive effect. Use with
caution.
*MAO inhibitors:* may cause severe excitation, hyperpyrexia, or seizures, usually
with high doses. Avoid concomitant use.
**Drug-lifestyle.** *Alcohol use:* enhanced
CNS depression. Avoid concomitant use.
*Smoking:* may lower plasma desipramine
levels. Monitor for lack of effect.
*Sun exposure:* increased risk of photosensitivity. Avoid unprotected or prolonged
sun exposure.

## EFFECTS ON DIAGNOSTIC TESTS
None reported.

## CONTRAINDICATIONS
Contraindicated in patients with hypersensitivity to drug, in those who have taken
MAO inhibitors within previous 14 days,
and during acute recovery phase of MI.

## NURSING CONSIDERATIONS
• Use with extreme caution in patients
with CV disease or history of urine retention, glaucoma, seizure disorders, or thyroid disease and in those taking thyroid
medication.
• Don't withdraw drug abruptly.
• Because hypertensive episodes have occurred during surgery in patients receiving TCAs, drug should be gradually discontinued several days before surgery.
• If signs or symptoms of psychosis occur
or increase, expect doctor to reduce
dosage. Record mood changes. Monitor
patient for suicidal tendencies, and allow
only a minimum supply of drug.
• Because desipramine produces fewer
anticholinergic effects than other TCAs, it
is often prescribed for cardiac patients.

• Recommend use of sugarless hard candy or gum to relieve dry mouth. Saliva substitutes may be necessary.
• *Alert:* Don't confuse desipramine with disopyramide or imipramine.

☑ **Patient teaching**
• Advise patient to take full dose at bedtime.
• Warn patient to avoid hazardous activities that require alertness and good psychomotor coordination until CNS effects of drug are known. Drowsiness and dizziness usually subside after a few weeks.
• Tell patient to avoid alcohol during drug therapy because it may antagonize effects of desipramine.
• Tell patient to consult doctor before taking other prescription or OTC drugs.
• Warn patient not to stop drug therapy suddenly.
• To prevent photosensitivity reactions, advise patient to use sunblock, wear protective clothing, and avoid prolonged exposure to strong sunlight.

---

**doxepin hydrochloride**
Deptran‡, Novo-Doxepin†,
Sinequan, Triadapin†

*Pregnancy Risk Category NR*

**HOW SUPPLIED**
*Capsules:* 10 mg, 25 mg, 50 mg, 75 mg, 100 mg, 150 mg
*Oral concentrate:* 10 mg/ml

**ACTION**
Unknown. A tricyclic antidepressant (TCA) that increases amount of norepinephrine, serotonin, or both in the CNS by blocking their reuptake by the presynaptic neurons.

| Route | Onset | Peak | Duration |
|-------|-------|------|----------|
| P.O. | Unknown | 2 hr | Unknown |

**INDICATIONS & DOSAGE**
*Depression—*
**Adults:** initially, 25 to 75 mg P.O. daily in divided doses to maximum of 300 mg daily. Or, entire maintenance dose may be given once daily with maximum dose of 150 mg.

**ADVERSE REACTIONS**
**CNS:** *drowsiness, dizziness,* confusion, numbness, hallucinations, paresthesia, ataxia, weakness, headache, **seizures,** extrapyramidal reactions.
**CV:** *orthostatic hypotension, tachycardia,* ECG changes.
**EENT:** *blurred vision,* tinnitus.
**GI:** *dry mouth, constipation,* nausea, vomiting, anorexia.
**GU:** urine retention.
**Hepatic:** elevated liver function test results.
**Metabolic:** hypoglycemia, hyperglycemia.
**Skin:** rash, urticaria, photosensitivity, *diaphoresis.*
**Other:** *hypersensitivity reaction.*
**After abrupt withdrawal of long-term therapy:** nausea, headache, malaise (doesn't indicate addiction).

**INTERACTIONS**
**Drug-drug.** *Barbiturates, CNS depressants:* enhanced CNS depression. Avoid concomitant use.
*Cimetidine, fluoxetine, sertraline:* may increase serum doxepin levels. Monitor for increased adverse reactions.
*Clonidine, epinephrine, norepinephrine:* increased hypertensive effect. Use with caution.
*MAO inhibitors:* may cause severe excitation, hyperpyrexia, or seizures, usually with high dosage. Avoid concomitant use.
**Drug-lifestyle.** *Alcohol use:* enhanced CNS depression. Avoid concomitant use.
*Sun exposure*: increased risk of photosensitivity reactions. Avoid unprotected or prolonged exposure to sun.

**EFFECTS ON DIAGNOSTIC TESTS**
None reported.

**CONTRAINDICATIONS**
Contraindicated in patients with hypersensitivity to drug and in those with glaucoma or tendency to urine retention; also contraindicated in those who have received an MAO inhibitor within past 14

---

Reactions may be *common,* uncommon, *life-threatening*, or COMMON AND LIFE-THREATENING.

days and during acute recovery phase of an MI.

## NURSING CONSIDERATIONS
• Don't withdraw drug abruptly.
• *Alert:* Because hypertensive episodes may occur during surgery in patients receiving TCAs, drug should be gradually discontinued several days before surgery.
• If signs or symptoms of psychosis occur or increase, expect doctor to reduce dosage. Record mood changes. Monitor patient for suicidal tendencies, and allow only a minimum supply of drug.
• Doxepin has strong anticholinergic effects; it's one of the most sedating TCAs. Adverse anticholinergic effects can occur rapidly.
• Recommend use of sugarless hard candy or gum to relieve dry mouth.
• *Alert:* Don't confuse doxepin with doxazosin, digoxin, doxapram, or Doxidan; or Sinequan with saquinavir.

### ☑ Patient teaching
• Tell patient to dilute oral concentrate with 4 oz (120 ml) of water, milk, or juice (orange, grapefruit, tomato, prune, or pineapple, but not grape); preparation is incompatible with carbonated beverages.
• Inform patient to take full dose at bedtime but warn him of possible morning orthostatic hypotension.
• Advise patient to consult doctor before taking other prescription or OTC drugs.
• Warn patient to avoid hazardous activities that require alertness and good psychomotor coordination until CNS effects of drug are known. Drowsiness and dizziness usually subside after a few weeks.
• Tell patient to avoid alcohol during drug therapy.
• Tell patient that maximum antidepressant effect may not be evident for 2 to 3 weeks.
• Warn patient not to stop drug therapy suddenly.
• To prevent photosensitivity reactions, advise patient to use sunblock, wear protective clothing, and avoid prolonged exposure to strong sunlight.

## fluoxetine hydrochloride
Prozac, Prozac-20‡, Erocap‡, Lovan‡, Zactin‡

*Pregnancy Risk Category C*

### HOW SUPPLIED
*Tablets:* 10 mg
*Pulvules:* 10 mg, 20 mg
*Oral solution:* 20 mg/5 ml

### ACTION
Unknown. Thought to be linked to drug's inhibition of CNS neuronal uptake of serotonin.

| Route | Onset | Peak | Duration |
|-------|-------|------|----------|
| P.O. | Unknown | 6-8 hr | Unknown |

### INDICATIONS & DOSAGE
*Depression, obsessive-compulsive disorder—*
**Adults:** initially, 20 mg P.O. in the morning; dosage increased based on patient response. Maximum dose is 80 mg/day.
**Elderly:** (depression only) 20 mg P.O. daily, preferably in the morning.
*Adjust-a-dose:* For patients with renal or hepatic impairment, a lower or less frequent dosage should be used.
*Binge-eating and vomiting behavior in patients with moderate to severe bulimia nervosa—*
**Adults:** 60 mg P.O. in the morning.

### ADVERSE REACTIONS
**CNS:** *nervousness, anxiety, insomnia, headache, drowsiness,* fatigue, *tremor, dizziness, asthenia.*
**CV:** palpitations, hot flashes.
**EENT:** nasal congestion, pharyngitis, cough, sinusitis.
**GI:** *nausea, diarrhea, dry mouth, anorexia,* dyspepsia, constipation, abdominal pain, vomiting, flatulence, increased appetite.
**GU:** sexual dysfunction.
**Metabolic:** weight loss
**Musculoskeletal:** muscle pain.
**Respiratory:** upper respiratory infection, respiratory distress.
**Skin:** rash, pruritus, diaphoresis.
**Other:** flulike syndrome, fever.

## INTERACTIONS
**Drug-drug.** *Carbamazepine, flecainide, vinblastine:* increased serum levels of these drugs. Monitor serum levels and patient for adverse effects.
*Cyproheptadine:* may reverse or decrease pharmacologic effect. Monitor patient closely.
*Insulin, oral antidiabetics:* altered blood glucose levels and possible altered requirements for antidiabetic medication. Adjust dosage, as ordered.
*Lithium, tricyclic antidepressants:* risk of increased adverse CNS effects. Avoid concomitant use.
*Phenytoin:* increased plasma phenytoin levels and risk of toxicity. Monitor serum phenytoin levels and adjust dosage, as ordered.
*Tryptophan:* increased agitation, restlessness, GI problems. Use with caution.
*Warfarin, other highly protein-bound drugs:* may increase plasma levels of fluoxetine and other highly protein-bound drugs. Monitor patient closely.
**Drug-lifestyle.** *Alcohol use:* increased CNS depression. Avoid concomitant use.

## EFFECTS ON DIAGNOSTIC TESTS
None reported.

## CONTRAINDICATIONS
Contraindicated in patients with hypersensitivity to drug and in those taking MAO inhibitors within 14 days of starting therapy. MAO inhibitors shouldn't be started within 5 weeks of stopping fluoxetine therapy.

## NURSING CONSIDERATIONS
● Use cautiously in patients at high risk for suicide and in those with history of hepatic, renal, or CV disease; diabetes mellitus; or seizures.
● Use antihistamines or topical corticosteroids, as ordered, to treat rashes or pruritus.
● *Alert:* Don't confuse fluoxetine with fluvoxamine or fluvastatin, or Prozac with Proscar, Prilosec, or ProSom.

## ☑ Patient teaching
● Tell patient to avoid taking drug in the afternoon because fluoxetine commonly causes nervousness and insomnia.
● Drug may cause dizziness or drowsiness. Warn patient to avoid driving and other hazardous activities that require alertness and good psychomotor coordination until CNS effects of drug are known.
● Tell patient to consult doctor before taking other prescription or OTC drugs.
● Warn patient to avoid food high in tryptophan, including meats, poultry, fish, liver, kidney, eggs, nuts, peanut butter, broad beans, and wheat germ.

---

## imipramine hydrochloride
Apo-Imipramine†, Impril†, Melipramine‡, Norfranil, Novopramine†, Tipramine, Tofranil**

## imipramine pamoate
Tofranil-PM**

*Pregnancy Risk Category D*

## HOW SUPPLIED
**imipramine hydrochloride**
*Tablets:* 10 mg, 25 mg, 50 mg
*Injection:* 12.5 mg/ml
**imipramine pamoate**
*Capsules:* 75 mg, 100 mg, 125 mg, 150 mg

## ACTION
Unknown. A tricyclic antidepressant (TCA) that increases amount of norepinephrine, serotonin, or both in the CNS by blocking their reuptake by the presynaptic neurons.

| Route | Onset | Peak | Duration |
|-------|---------|--------|----------|
| P.O. | Unknown | 1-2 hr | Unknown |
| I.M. | Unknown | 30 min | Unknown |

## INDICATIONS & DOSAGE
*Depression—*
**Adults:** 75 to 100 mg P.O. or I.M. daily in divided doses, increased in 25- to 50-mg increments. Maximum dose for outpatients is 200 mg daily; 300 mg daily may

---

be used for hospitalized patients. Entire dose may be given h.s.

**Elderly and adolescents:** initially, 30 to 40 mg daily; it usually isn't necessary to exceed 100 mg daily.

*Childhood enuresis—*

**Children ages 5 and older:** 25 mg P.O. 1 hour before bedtime. If no response within 1 week, increased to 50 mg if child is under age 12; increased to 75 mg for children ages 12 and older. In either case, maximum dose is 2.5 mg/kg/day.

## ADVERSE REACTIONS

**CNS:** *drowsiness, dizziness,* excitation, tremor, confusion, hallucinations, anxiety, ataxia, paresthesia, nervousness, EEG changes, **seizures,** extrapyramidal reactions.

**CV:** *orthostatic hypotension, tachycardia, ECG changes,* hypertension, **MI, stroke, arrhythmias, heart block,** precipitation of heart failure.

**EENT:** *blurred vision,* tinnitus, mydriasis.

**GI:** *dry mouth, constipation,* nausea, vomiting, anorexia, paralytic ileus, abdominal cramps.

**GU:** *urine retention.*

**Hepatic:** elevated liver function tests.

**Metabolic:** hypoglycemia, hyperglycemia.

**Skin:** rash, urticaria, photosensitivity, pruritus, diaphoresis.

**Other:** *hypersensitivity reaction.*

**After abrupt withdrawal of long-term therapy:** nausea, headache, malaise (doesn't indicate addiction).

## INTERACTIONS

**Drug-drug.** *Barbiturates, CNS depressants:* enhanced CNS depression. Avoid concomitant use.

*Cimetidine, fluoxetine, sertraline:* may increase serum imipramine levels. Monitor for adverse reactions.

*Clonidine, epinephrine, norepinephrine:* increased hypertensive effect. Use with caution.

*MAO inhibitors:* may cause hyperpyretic crisis, severe seizures, and death. Avoid concomitant use.

**Drug-lifestyle.** *Alcohol use:* enhanced CNS depression. Avoid concomitant use.

*Smoking:* may lower plasma levels of imipramine. Monitor for lack of effect.

*Sun exposure:* increased risk of photosensitivity. Avoid unprotected or prolonged exposure to sun.

## EFFECTS ON DIAGNOSTIC TESTS
None reported.

## CONTRAINDICATIONS
Contraindicated in patients with hypersensitivity to drug and in those receiving MAO inhibitors; also contraindicated during acute recovery phase of MI.

## NURSING CONSIDERATIONS
• Use with extreme caution in patients at risk for suicide; in patients with history of urine retention, angle-closure glaucoma, or seizure disorders; increased intraocular pressure, CV disease, impaired hepatic function, hyperthyroidism, and impaired renal function; and in patients receiving thyroid drugs. Injectable form contains sulfites, which may cause allergic reactions in hypersensitive patients.

• Don't withdraw drug abruptly.

• Because of hypertensive episodes during surgery in patients receiving TCAs, drug should be gradually discontinued several days before surgery.

• If signs or symptoms of psychosis occur or increase, expect doctor to reduce dosage. Record mood changes. Monitor patient for suicidal tendencies, and allow only a minimum supply of drug.

• To prevent relapse in children receiving drug for enuresis, drug should be withdrawn gradually.

• Recommend use of sugarless hard candy or gum to relieve dry mouth. Saliva substitutes may be necessary.

• *Alert:* Don't confuse imipramine with desipramine.

### ☑ Patient teaching
• Advise patient to take full dose at bedtime but warn him of possible morning orthostatic hypotension.

• If child is an early night bedwetter, tell parents it may be more effective to divide dose and administer the first dose earlier in the day.

---

• Tell patient to avoid alcohol while taking this drug.
• Advise patient to consult doctor before taking other prescription or OTC drugs.
• Warn patient to avoid hazardous activities that require alertness and good psychomotor coordination until CNS effects of the drug are known. Drowsiness and dizziness usually subside after a few weeks.
• Warn patient not to stop drug suddenly.
• To prevent photosensitivity reactions, advise patient to use sunblock, wear protective clothing, and avoid prolonged exposure to strong sunlight.

---

## mirtazapine
Remeron, Zispin§

*Pregnancy Risk Category C*

### HOW SUPPLIED
*Tablets:* 15 mg, 30 mg

### ACTION
Antidepressant action is thought to be due to enhancement of central noradrenergic and serotonergic activity.

| Route | Onset | Peak | Duration |
|-------|-------|------|----------|
| P.O. | Unknown | 2 hr | Unknown |

### INDICATIONS & DOSAGE
*Depression—*
**Adults:** initially, 15 mg P.O. h.s. Maintenance dosage ranges from 15 to 45 mg daily. Dosage adjustments should be made at intervals of no less than 1 to 2 weeks.

### ADVERSE REACTIONS
**CNS:** *somnolence,* dizziness, asthenia, abnormal dreams, abnormal thinking, tremors, confusion.
**CV:** edema.
**GI:** nausea, *increased appetite, dry mouth, constipation.*
**GU:** urinary frequency.
**Hepatic:** increased ALT levels.
**Metabolic:** *weight gain.*
**Musculoskeletal:** back pain, myalgia.
**Respiratory:** dyspnea.
**Other:** flulike syndrome, peripheral edema, increased cholesterol and triglycerides.

### INTERACTIONS
**Drug-drug.** *Diazepam, other CNS depressants:* possible additive CNS effects. Avoid concomitant use.
*MAO inhibitors:* sometimes fatal reactions. Avoid concomitant use.
**Drug-lifestyle.** *Alcohol use:* possible additive CNS effects. Avoid concomitant use.

### EFFECTS ON DIAGNOSTIC TESTS
None reported.

### CONTRAINDICATIONS
Contraindicated in patients with hypersensitivity to drug. Drug shouldn't be used with MAO inhibitor or within 14 days of initiating or discontinuing therapy with MAO inhibitor. At least 14 days should elapse after stopping mirtazapine before starting an MAO inhibitor.

### NURSING CONSIDERATIONS
• Use cautiously in patients with CV or cerebrovascular disease, seizure disorders, suicidal ideations, impaired hepatic or renal function, or history of mania or hypomania.
• Use cautiously in patients with conditions that predispose them to hypotension, such as dehydration, hypovolemia, or treatment with antihypertensives.
• Although incidence of agranulocytosis is rare, discontinue drug and monitor patient closely if he develops a sore throat, fever, stomatitis, or other signs and symptoms of infection with a low WBC count.
• Monitor patient closely for signs of dependence.
• Administer drug cautiously to elderly patients; decreased clearance has occurred in the elderly.
• Lower dosages tend to be more sedating than higher dosages.

☑ **Patient teaching**
• Caution patient not to perform hazardous activities if somnolence occurs.
• Tell patient to report signs and symptoms of infection, such as fever, chills, sore throat, mucous membrane ulceration, or flulike syndrome.
• Instruct patient not to use alcohol or other CNS depressants while taking drug.

---

Reactions may be *common,* uncommon, *life-threatening*, or COMMON AND LIFE-THREATENING.

- Stress importance of compliance with therapy.
- Instruct patient not to take other medications without doctor's approval.
- Tell woman of childbearing age to report suspected pregnancy immediately and to notify doctor if she is breast-feeding.

## nefazodone hydrochloride
Dutonin§, Serzone

*Pregnancy Risk Category C*

### HOW SUPPLIED
*Tablets:* 50 mg, 100 mg, 150 mg, 300 mg

### ACTION
Unknown. Inhibits neuronal uptake of serotonin (5-HT$_2$) and norepinephrine; it also occupies serotonin and alpha$_1$-adrenergic receptors in the CNS.

| Route | Onset | Peak | Duration |
|-------|-------|------|----------|
| P.O. | Unknown | 1 hr | Unknown |

### INDICATIONS & DOSAGE
*Depression—*
**Adults:** initially, 200 mg/day P.O. in two divided doses. Dosage increased in increments of 100 to 200 mg/day at intervals of no less than 1 week, p.r.n. Usual dosage range is 300 to 600 mg/day.
**Elderly:** initially, 100 mg/day P.O. in two divided doses.
*Adjust-a-dose:* For debilitated patients, initially 100 mg/day P.O. in two divided doses.

### ADVERSE REACTIONS
**CNS:** *headache, somnolence, dizziness, asthenia, insomnia, light-headedness, confusion,* memory impairment, paresthesia, vasodilation, abnormal dreams, decreased concentration, ataxia, incoordination, psychomotor retardation, tremor, hypertonia.
**CV:** orthostatic hypotension, hypotension, peripheral edema.
**EENT:** blurred vision, abnormal vision, tinnitus, visual field defect, pharyngitis.
**GI:** *dry mouth, nausea, constipation,* taste perversion, dyspepsia, diarrhea, increased appetite, vomiting.
**GU:** urinary frequency, urinary tract infection, urine retention, vaginitis.
**Musculoskeletal:** neck rigidity, arthralgia.
**Respiratory:** cough.
**Skin:** pruritus, rash.
**Other:** infection, flulike syndrome, chills, fever, breast pain, thirst.

### INTERACTIONS
**Drug-drug.** *Alprazolam, triazolam:* administration with nefazodone potentiates effects of these drugs. Don't administer concurrently. However, if necessary, dosage of alprazolam and triazolam may need to be greatly reduced.
*CNS drugs:* may alter CNS activity. Use together cautiously.
*Digoxin:* may increase digoxin level. Use together cautiously and monitor digoxin levels.
*MAO inhibitors:* may cause severe excitation, hyperpyrexia, seizures, delirium, or coma. Avoid concomitant use.
*Other highly protein-bound drugs:* may increase incidence and severity of adverse reactions. Monitor patient closely.
**Drug-lifestyle.** *Alcohol use:* enhanced CNS depression. Avoid concomitant use.

### EFFECTS ON DIAGNOSTIC TESTS
None reported.

### CONTRAINDICATIONS
Contraindicated in patients with hypersensitivity to drug or other phenylpiperazine antidepressants; also contraindicated within 14 days of MAO inhibitor therapy.

### NURSING CONSIDERATIONS
- Use cautiously in patients with CV or cerebrovascular disease that could be exacerbated by hypotension (such as history of MI, angina, or CVA) and conditions that would predispose patients to hypotension (such as dehydration, hypovolemia, and treatment with antihypertensives). Also use cautiously in patients with a history of mania.

• At least 1 week should elapse between stopping nefazodone and starting MAO inhibitor therapy, and at least 14 days should elapse before patient begins taking nefazodone after MAO inhibitor therapy has been discontinued.
• Record mood changes. Monitor patient for suicidal tendencies, and allow only minimum supply of drug.

☑ **Patient teaching**
• Warn patient not to engage in hazardous activity until CNS effects of drug are known.
• *Alert:* Instruct men who experience prolonged or inappropriate erections to stop drug immediately and notify doctor.
• Instruct woman to notify doctor if she becomes pregnant or intends to become pregnant during therapy.
• Tell patient to notify doctor if rash, hives, or related allergic reactions occur.
• Instruct patient to avoid alcohol during therapy.
• Tell patient to notify doctor before taking OTC drugs.
• Inform patient that several weeks of therapy may be required to obtain full antidepressant effect. Once improvement occurs, advise him not to discontinue drug until directed by doctor.

---

**nortriptyline hydrochloride**
Allegron‡, Aventyl*, Pamelor*

*Pregnancy Risk Category NR*

**HOW SUPPLIED**
*Tablets:* 10 mg‡, 25 mg‡
*Capsules:* 10 mg, 25 mg, 50 mg, 75 mg
*Oral solution:* 10 mg/5 ml (4% alcohol)

**ACTION**
Unknown. A tricyclic antidepressant (TCA) that increases amount of norepinephrine, serotonin, or both in the CNS by blocking their reuptake by the presynaptic neurons.

| Route | Onset | Peak | Duration |
|-------|-------|------|----------|
| P.O. | Unknown | 7-8.5 hr | Unknown |

**INDICATIONS & DOSAGE**
*Depression—*
**Adults:** 25 mg P.O. t.i.d. or q.i.d., gradually increased to maximum of 150 mg daily. Entire dose may be given h.s. Monitor plasma levels when doses above 100 mg/day are given.
**Elderly and adolescents:** 30 to 50 mg daily given once or in divided doses.

**ADVERSE REACTIONS**
**CNS:** *drowsiness, dizziness, seizures,* tremor, weakness, confusion, headache, nervousness, EEG changes, extrapyramidal reactions, insomnia, nightmares, hallucinations, paresthesia, ataxia, agitation.
**CV:** ECG changes, *tachycardia,* hypertension, hypotension, *MI, heart block, stroke.*
**EENT:** *blurred vision,* tinnitus, mydriasis.
**GI:** dry mouth, *constipation,* nausea, vomiting, anorexia, paralytic ileus.
**GU:** *urine retention.*
**Hematologic:** bone marrow depression, *agranulocytosis,* eosinophilia, *thrombocytopenia.*
**Hepatic:** elevated liver function tests.
**Metabolic:** hypoglycemia, hyperglycemia.
**Skin:** rash, urticaria, photosensitivity, diaphoresis.
**Other:** *hypersensitivity reaction.*
**After abrupt withdrawal of long-term therapy:** nausea, headache, malaise (doesn't indicate addiction).

**INTERACTIONS**
**Drug-drug.** *Barbiturates, CNS depressants:* enhanced CNS depression. Avoid concomitant use.
*Cimetidine, fluoxetine, sertraline:* may increase nortriptyline serum levels. Monitor for adverse reactions.
*Clonidine, epinephrine, norepinephrine:* increased hypertensive effect. Use with caution.
*MAO inhibitors:* may cause severe excitation, hyperpyrexia, or seizures, usually with high doses. Avoid concomitant use.
**Drug-lifestyle.** *Alcohol use:* enhanced CNS depression. Avoid concomitant use.
*Smoking:* may lower plasma levels of nortriptyline. Monitor for lack of clinical effect.

---

Reactions may be *common*, uncommon, *life-threatening*, or COMMON AND LIFE-THREATENING.

*Sun exposure*: increased risk of photosensitivity reaction. Avoid unprotected or prolonged exposure to sun.

**EFFECTS ON DIAGNOSTIC TESTS**
None reported.

**CONTRAINDICATIONS**
Contraindicated in patients with hypersensitivity to drug and during acute recovery phase of MI; also contraindicated within 14 days of MAO therapy.

**NURSING CONSIDERATIONS**
• Use with extreme caution in patients with glaucoma, suicidal tendency, history of urine retention or seizures, CV disease, or hyperthyroidism and in those receiving thyroid medication.
• Don't withdraw drug abruptly.
• Because hypertensive episodes have occurred during surgery in patients receiving TCAs, dosage should be gradually discontinued several days before surgery.
• If signs or symptoms of psychosis occur or increase, expect doctor to reduce dosage. Record mood changes. Monitor patient for suicidal tendencies, and allow him only a minimum supply of drug.
• Recommend use of sugarless hard candy or gum to relieve dry mouth. Saliva substitutes may be necessary.
• *Alert:* Don't confuse nortriptyline with amitriptyline.

☑ **Patient teaching**
• Whenever possible, advise patient to take full dose at bedtime to reduce risk of orthostatic hypotension.
• Warn patient to avoid activities that require alertness and good psychomotor coordination until CNS effects of drug are known. Drowsiness and dizziness usually subside after a few weeks.
• Tell patient to consult doctor before taking other prescription or OTC drugs.
• Warn patient not to stop drug suddenly.
• To prevent photosensitivity reactions, advise patient to use sunblock, wear protective clothing, and avoid prolonged exposure to strong sunlight.

## paroxetine hydrochloride
Paxil, Aropax‡, Seroxat§

*Pregnancy Risk Category C*

**HOW SUPPLIED**
*Tablets:* 10 mg, 20 mg, 30 mg, 40 mg

**ACTION**
Unknown. Probably linked to drug's inhibition of CNS neuronal uptake of serotonin.

| Route | Onset | Peak | Duration |
|-------|-------|------|----------|
| P.O. | Unknown | 2-8 hr | Unknown |

**INDICATIONS & DOSAGE**
*Depression—*
**Adults:** initially, 20 mg P.O. daily, preferably in the morning as indicated. If patient doesn't respond after full antidepressant effect has occurred, dose may be increased in 10-mg/day increments at weekly intervals, to maximum of 50 mg daily.
**Elderly:** initially, 10 mg P.O. daily, preferably in the morning as indicated. If patient doesn't respond after full antidepressant effect has occurred, dose may be increased in 10-mg/day increments at weekly intervals, to maximum of 40 mg daily.
*Obsessive-compulsive disorder—*
**Adults:** initially, 20 mg P.O. daily, preferably in the morning. Dose may increased in 10-mg/day increments at weekly intervals. Recommended daily dose is 40 mg daily. Maximum dose is 60 mg/day.
*Panic disorder—*
**Adults:** initially, 10 mg P.O. daily. Dose may be increased in 10-mg increments at no less than weekly intervals, to maximum of 60 mg/day.
✴ *NEW INDICATION: Social anxiety disorder—*
**Adults:** initially, 20 mg P.O. daily, preferably in the morning. Dosage range is 20 to 60 mg/day. Adjust dosage to maintain patient on lowest effective dose.
*Adjust-a-dose:* For debilitated patients or those with renal or hepatic failure, initially, 10 mg P.O. daily, preferably in the morning. If patient doesn't respond after full antidepressant effect has occurred,

dose may be increased in 10-mg/day increments at weekly intervals, to maximum of 40 mg daily.

## ADVERSE REACTIONS
**CNS:** *somnolence, dizziness, insomnia, tremor, nervousness,* anxiety, paresthesia, confusion, *headache,* agitation, *asthenia.*
**CV:** palpitations, vasodilation, orthostatic hypotension.
**EENT:** lump or tightness in throat.
**GI:** *dry mouth, nausea, constipation, diarrhea,* flatulence, vomiting, dyspepsia, dysgeusia, increased appetite, abdominal pain.
**GU:** ejaculatory disturbances, male genital disorders (including anorgasmy, erectile difficulties, delayed ejaculation or orgasm, impotence, and sexual dysfunction), urinary frequency, other urinary disorders, female genital disorders (including anorgasmy, difficulty with orgasm).
**Musculoskeletal:** myopathy, myalgia, myasthenia.
**Skin:** rash, pruritus, *diaphoresis.*
**Other:** yawning, decreased libido.

## INTERACTIONS
**Drug-drug.** *Cimetidine:* decreased hepatic metabolism of paroxetine, leading to risk of toxicity. Dosage adjustments may be necessary.
*Digoxin:* may decrease digoxin levels. Monitor closely.
*MAO inhibitors:* may increase risk of serious, sometimes fatal, adverse reactions. Avoid concomitant use.
*Phenobarbital, phenytoin:* may alter pharmacokinetics of both drugs. Dosage adjustments may be necessary.
*Procyclidine:* may increase procyclidine levels. Monitor for excessive anticholinergic effects.
*Theophylline:* decreased clearance. Dose reductions are necessary.
*Tryptophan:* may increase incidence of adverse reactions, such as diaphoresis, headache, nausea, and dizziness. Avoid concomitant use.
*Warfarin:* increased risk of bleeding. Use concomitantly with caution.
**Drug-herb.** *St. John's wort:* may result in sedative-hypnotic intoxication. Avoid concurrent use.

**Drug-lifestyle.** *Alcohol use:* may alter psychomotor function. Limit intake.

## EFFECTS ON DIAGNOSTIC TESTS
None reported.

## CONTRAINDICATIONS
Contraindicated in patients with hypersensitivity to drug and in those taking MAO inhibitors; also contraindicated within 14 days of discontinuing MAO inhibitor therapy.

## NURSING CONSIDERATIONS
• Use cautiously in patients with history of seizure disorders or mania and in those with severe, concomitant systemic illness.
• Use cautiously in patients at risk for volume depletion, and monitor appropriately.
• If signs or symptoms of psychosis occur or increase, expect doctor to reduce dosage. Record mood changes. Monitor patient for suicidal tendencies, and allow only a minimum supply of drug.
• **Alert:** Don't confuse paroxetine with paclitaxel, or Paxil with Doxil, paclitaxel, or Taxol.

### ☑ Patient teaching
• Warn patient to avoid activities that require alertness and good psychomotor coordination until CNS effects of drug are known.
• Tell patient to avoid alcohol and to consult doctor before taking other prescription or OTC drugs.

---

## phenelzine sulfate
Nardil

*Pregnancy Risk Category C*

## HOW SUPPLIED
*Tablets:* 15 mg

## ACTION
Unknown. An MAO inhibitor that probably promotes accumulation of neurotransmitters by inhibiting their metabolism.

| Route | Onset | Peak | Duration |
|-------|-------|------|----------|
| P.O. | Unknown | 2-4 hr | ≤ 10 days |

## INDICATIONS & DOSAGE
*Depression—*
**Adults:** 15 mg P.O. t.i.d., increased rapidly to 60 mg daily. Maximum dose is 90 mg daily; dose can usually be reduced to 15 mg daily.

## ADVERSE REACTIONS
**CNS:** *dizziness, vertigo, headache,* hyperreflexia, tremor, muscle twitching, *insomnia,* drowsiness, weakness, fatigue.
**CV:** *postural hypotension,* edema.
**GI:** dry mouth, *anorexia,* nausea, *constipation.*
**Hepatic:** elevated liver function tests.
**Metabolic:** weight gain.
**Skin:** diaphoresis.

## INTERACTIONS
**Drug-drug.** *Amphetamines, antihistamines, buspirone, ephedrine, levodopa, meperidine, metaraminol, methylphenidate, phenylephrine, phenylpropanolamine, sympathomimetics:* enhanced pressor effects. Avoid concomitant use.
*Antihypertensives containing thiazide diuretics, barbiturates, dextromethorphan, methotrimeprazine, narcotics, other sedatives, serotonin reuptake inhibitors, spinal anesthetics, tricyclic antidepressants:* unpredictable interaction. Use these drugs with caution and in reduced dosage.
*Insulin, oral antidiabetics:* increased risk of hypoglycemia. Use with caution and in reduced dosages.
**Drug-herb.** *Cacao tree:* potential vasopressor effects. Avoid concomitant use.
*Ginseng:* may cause headache, tremors, or mania. Avoid concomitant use.
**Drug-food.** *Foods high in tryptophan, tyramine, caffeine:* may precipitate hypertensive crisis. Avoid concomitant use. Watch for adverse effects.
**Drug-lifestyle.** *Alcohol use:* may precipitate hypertensive crisis. Avoid concomitant use.

## EFFECTS ON DIAGNOSTIC TESTS
Drug therapy elevates urinary catecholamine levels.

## CONTRAINDICATIONS
Contraindicated in patients with hypersensitivity to drug and in those with heart failure, pheochromocytoma, hypertension, significant renal impairment, cerebrovascular defect, liver disease, and CV disease. Also contraindicated during therapy with other MAO inhibitors (isocarboxazid, tranylcypromine) or within 10 days of such therapy or within 10 days of elective surgery requiring general anesthesia, cocaine use, or local anesthesia containing sympathomimetic vasoconstrictors.

## NURSING CONSIDERATIONS
• Use cautiously with antihypertensives containing thiazide diuretics, with spinal anesthetics, and in patients at risk for suicide, diabetes, or seizure disorders.
• Obtain baseline blood pressure, heart rate, CBC, and liver function test results before therapy, and continue to monitor throughout treatment.
• Discontinue MAO inhibitors 14 days before elective surgery, as ordered, to avoid drug interactions that may occur during anesthesia.
• Monitor patient closely for suicidal tendencies, and allow only a minimum supply of drug.
• If patient develops symptoms of overdose (severe hypotension, palpitations, or frequent headaches), withhold dose and notify doctor.
• *Alert:* Have phentolamine available to combat severe hypertension.
• Continue precautions 14 days after stopping drug because it has long-lasting effects.

### ☑ Patient teaching
• Advise patient to consult doctor before taking other prescription or OTC drugs. Severe adverse effects can occur if MAO inhibitors are taken with OTC cold, hay-fever, or diet preparations.
• Warn patient about the probability of orthostatic hypotension. Supervise walking. Tell patient to get out of bed slowly, sitting up first for 1 minute.
• Because MAO inhibitors may suppress chest pain in patients with angina, warn such patients to engage in moderate activities and to avoid overexertion.
• Advise patient to avoid the following foods: pickled herring, liver, dry sausage,

broad bean pods, sauerkraut, cheese, yogurt, yeast extract, meat extract, and pickled, fermented, or smoked foods. These foods have a high tyramine content that may cause a hypertensive crisis.

---

## sertraline hydrochloride
Lustral§, Zoloft

*Pregnancy Risk Category C*

### HOW SUPPLIED
*Tablets:* 50 mg, 100 mg
*Capsules†:* 25 mg, 50 mg, 100 mg

### ACTION
Unknown. Probably linked to drug's inhibition of neuronal uptake of serotonin in the CNS.

| Route | Onset | Peak | Duration |
|-------|-------|------|----------|
| P.O. | Unknown | 4.5-8.5 hr | Unknown |

### INDICATIONS & DOSAGE
*Depression—*
**Adults:** 50 mg P.O. daily. Dosage adjusted as needed and tolerated; doses of 50 to 200 mg daily have been given. Dosage adjustments should be made at intervals of no less than 1 week.
*Obsessive-compulsive disorder—*
**Adults:** 50 mg P.O. once daily. If no response, dose may be increased to maximum of 200 mg/day. Dosage adjustments should be made at intervals of no less than 1 week.
**Children ages 6 to 17:** initially 25 mg P.O. daily in children ages 6 to 12, or 50 mg P.O. daily in children ages 13 to 17. May increase dosage, p.r.n., up to 200 mg/day at intervals of no less than 1 week.
*Panic disorder—*
**Adults:** initially, 25 mg P.O. daily. After one week, increase dose to 50 mg P.O. daily. If no response, dose may be increased to maximum of 200 mg/day. Dosage adjustments should be made at intervals of no less than 1 week.
*Adjust-a-dose:* For patients with hepatic disease, lower or less frequent doses should be used.

### ADVERSE REACTIONS
**CNS:** *headache, tremor, dizziness, insomnia, somnolence,* paresthesia, hypoesthesia, *fatigue,* nervousness, anxiety, agitation, hypertonia, twitching, confusion.
**CV:** palpitations, chest pain, hot flashes.
**GI:** *dry mouth, nausea, diarrhea, loose stools, dyspepsia,* vomiting, constipation, thirst, flatulence, anorexia, abdominal pain, increased appetite.
**GU:** *male sexual dysfunction.*
**Hepatic:** elevated serum AST and ALT levels.
**Musculoskeletal:** myalgia.
**Skin:** rash, pruritus, diaphoresis.

### INTERACTIONS
**Drug-drug.** *Benzodiazepines, tolbutamide:* decreased clearance of these drugs. Clinical significance unknown; however, monitor patients for increased drug effects.
*Cimetidine:* decreased clearance of sertraline. Monitor closely.
*MAO inhibitors:* may cause serious, sometimes fatal, reactions including myoclonus rigidity, mental status changes, hyperthermia, autonomic nervous system instability, rapid fluctuations of vital signs, delirium, coma, and death. Avoid concomitant use.
*Warfarin, other highly protein-bound drugs:* may increase plasma levels of sertraline or other highly bound drug. PT or INR may increase by 8% with concomitant use of warfarin. Monitor closely.

### EFFECTS ON DIAGNOSTIC TESTS
None reported.

### CONTRAINDICATIONS
Contraindicated in patients taking MAO inhibitors or within 14 days of discontinuing MAO inhibitor therapy.

### NURSING CONSIDERATIONS
• Use cautiously in patients at risk for suicide and in those with seizure disorders, major affective disorder, or diseases or conditions that affect metabolism or hemodynamic responses.

---

• Administer sertraline once daily, either in the morning or evening. May be given with or without food.
• Record mood changes. Monitor patient for suicidal tendencies, and allow only a minimum supply of drug.

☑ **Patient teaching**
• Advise patient to use caution when performing hazardous tasks that require alertness.
• Tell patient to avoid alcohol and to consult doctor before taking OTC drugs.

---

## tranylcypromine sulfate
Parnate

*Pregnancy Risk Category C*

### HOW SUPPLIED
*Tablets:* 10 mg

### ACTION
Unknown. An MAO inhibitor that probably promotes accumulation of neurotransmitters by inhibiting MAO.

| Route | Onset | Peak | Duration |
|-------|-------|------|----------|
| P.O. | Unknown | 1-3.5 hr | ≤ 10 days |

### INDICATIONS & DOSAGE
*Depression—*
**Adults:** 10 mg P.O. t.i.d. Increased by 10 mg P.O. daily at 1- to 3-week intervals to maximum of 60 mg daily, if necessary, after 2 weeks of therapy.

### ADVERSE REACTIONS
**CNS:** *dizziness, headache,* anxiety, agitation, paresthesia, drowsiness, weakness, numbness, tremor, jitters, confusion, *vertigo.*
**CV:** *orthostatic hypotension, tachycardia,* paradoxical hypertension, palpitations, *edema.*
**EENT:** blurred vision, tinnitus.
**GI:** dry mouth, *anorexia,* nausea, diarrhea, constipation, abdominal pain.
**GU:** impotence, urine retention, impaired ejaculation.
**Hematologic:** anemia, *leukopenia, agranulocytosis, thrombocytopenia.*

**Hepatic:** *hepatitis,* elevated liver function test results.
**Metabolic:** SIADH.
**Musculoskeletal:** muscle spasm, myoclonic jerks.
**Skin:** rash.
**Other:** chills.

### INTERACTIONS
**Drug-drug.** *Amphetamines, antihistamines, antihypertensives, diuretics, ephedrine, levodopa, meperidine, metaraminol, methylphenidate, phenylephrine, phenylpropanolamine, sympathomimetics:* enhanced pressor effects of these drugs. Avoid concomitant use.
*Antiparkinsonians, barbiturates, dextromethorphan, methotrimeprazine, narcotics, other sedatives, selective serotonin reuptake inhibitors, spinal anesthetics, tricyclic antidepressants:* enhanced adverse CNS effects. Avoid concomitant use. If necessary, use with caution and in reduced dosage.
*Buspirone:* may elevate blood pressure. Monitor patient closely.
*Insulin, oral antidiabetics:* increased risk of hypoglycemia. Use with caution and in reduced dosages.
**Drug-herb.** *Cacao tree:* potential vasopressor effects. Avoid concomitant use.
*Ginseng:* may cause headache, tremors, or mania. Monitor for effects.
**Drug-food.** *Foods high in caffeine, tyramine, tryptophan:* may cause hypertensive crisis. Avoid concomitant use.
**Drug-lifestyle.** *Alcohol use:* enhanced CNS effects. Avoid concomitant use.

### EFFECTS ON DIAGNOSTIC TESTS
Drug therapy elevates urinary catecholamine levels.

### CONTRAINDICATIONS
Contraindicated in patients receiving MAO inhibitors or dibenzazepine derivatives within 2 weeks; those with pheochromocytoma, cerebrovascular or cardiovascular disease, hypertension, or heart failure; and debilitated patients.

Also contraindicated in patients with hypersensitivity to drug and in those with confirmed or suspected cerebrovascular defect, pheochromocytoma, heart failure,

---

CV disease, hypertension, hepatic disease, significant renal impairment, or history of headache; also contraindicated in those undergoing elective surgery.

## NURSING CONSIDERATIONS
• Use cautiously in patients with renal disease, diabetes, seizure disorders, Parkinson's disease, or hyperthyroidism, and in those at risk for suicide.
• Obtain baseline blood pressure, heart rate, CBC, and liver function test results before beginning therapy, and continue to monitor throughout treatment.
• Dosage usually is reduced to maintenance level as soon as possible.
• Don't withdraw drug abruptly.
• Discontinue MAO inhibitors 14 days before elective surgery, as ordered, to avoid drug interactions that may occur during anesthesia.
• Monitor patient for suicidal tendencies, and allow only a minimum supply of drug.
• If patient develops symptoms of overdose (palpitations, severe hypotension, or frequent headaches), withhold dose and notify doctor.
• *Alert:* Have phentolamine available to combat severe hypertension.
• Continue precautions for 10 days after stopping drug because it has long-lasting effects.

### ☑ Patient teaching
• Warn patient to avoid foods high in tyramine, tryptophan, or caffeine. Tranylcypromine is the MAO inhibitor most frequently reported to cause hypertensive crisis with ingestion of tyramine-rich foods, including aged cheese, Chianti wine, beer, avocados, chicken livers, chocolate, bananas, soy sauce, meat tenderizers, salami, and bologna.
• Tell patient to avoid alcohol during therapy.
• Advise patient to consult doctor before taking other prescription or OTC drugs.
• To prevent dizziness resulting from orthostatic hypotension, tell patient to get out of bed slowly, sitting up first for 1 minute.
• Because MAO inhibitors may suppress anginal pain, warn patient to perform only moderate activities and to avoid overexertion.
• Warn patient not to stop drug suddenly.
• Advise patient to avoid the following: cheese, sour cream, pickled herring, anchovies, caviar, liver, canned figs, raisins, bananas, avocados, chocolate, soy sauce, sauerkraut, broad beans, yeast extracts, yogurt, meat extracts, meat prepared with tenderizers due to their high tyramine content.

---

## trazodone hydrochloride
Desyrel, Molipaxin§, Trazon, Trialodine

*Pregnancy Risk Category C*

### HOW SUPPLIED
*Tablets:* 50 mg, 100 mg, 150 mg, 300 mg

### ACTION
Unknown. Inhibits serotonin uptake in the brain. Not a tricyclic derivative.

| Route | Onset | Peak | Duration |
|-------|-------|------|----------|
| P.O. | Unknown | 1-2 hr | Unknown |

### INDICATIONS & DOSAGE
*Depression—*
**Adults:** initial dosage, 150 mg P.O. daily in divided doses; then increased by 50 mg daily q 3 to 4 days, p.r.n. Dosage ranges from 150 to 400 mg daily. Maximum daily dose is 600 mg for inpatients and 400 mg for outpatients.

### ADVERSE REACTIONS
**CNS:** *drowsiness, dizziness,* nervousness, fatigue, confusion, tremor, weakness, hostility, anger, nightmares, vivid dreams, headache, insomnia, syncope.
**CV:** orthostatic hypotension, tachycardia, hypertension, shortness of breath, ECG changes.
**EENT:** blurred vision, tinnitus, nasal congestion.
**GI:** dry mouth, dysgeusia, constipation, nausea, vomiting, anorexia.
**GU:** urine retention; priapism, possibly leading to impotence; hematuria.
**Hematologic:** anemia.

---

Reactions may be *common,* uncommon, *life-threatening,* or COMMON AND LIFE-THREATENING.

**Hepatic:** elevated liver function test results.
**Skin:** rash, urticaria, diaphoresis.
**Other:** decreased libido.

## INTERACTIONS
**Drug-drug.** *Antihypertensives:* increased hypotensive effect of trazodone. Antihypertensive dosage may have to be decreased.
*Clonidine, CNS depressants:* enhanced CNS depression. Avoid concomitant use.
*Digoxin, phenytoin:* may increase serum levels of these drugs. Monitor for toxicity.
*MAO inhibitors:* effects unknown. Use together with extreme caution.
**Drug-herb.** *St. John's wort:* serotonin syndrome may result. Avoid concomitant use.
**Drug-lifestyle.** *Alcohol use:* enhanced CNS depression. Avoid concomitant use.

## EFFECTS ON DIAGNOSTIC TESTS
None reported.

## CONTRAINDICATIONS
Contraindicated in patients with hypersensitivity to drug.

## NURSING CONSIDERATIONS
• Use cautiously in patients with cardiac disease, during initial recovery phase of MI, and in patients at risk for suicide.
• Administer drug after meals or a light snack for optimal absorption and to decrease incidence of dizziness.
• Record mood changes. Monitor patient for suicidal tendencies, and allow only minimum supply of drug.

☑ **Patient teaching**
• *Alert:* Priapism, a persistent, painful erection, may occur in men taking trazodone. Tell patient to report it immediately because he may need surgery.
• Warn patient to avoid activities that require alertness and good psychomotor coordination until CNS effects of drug are known. Drowsiness and dizziness usually subside after first few weeks.
• Teach caregivers how to recognize signs and symptoms of suicidal tendency or suicidal ideation.

# trimipramine maleate
Apo-Trimip†, Novo-Tripramine†, Rhotrimine†, Surmontil

*Pregnancy Risk Category C*

## HOW SUPPLIED
*Tablets:* 25 mg‡
*Capsules:* 25 mg, 50 mg, 100 mg

## ACTION
Unknown. A tricyclic antidepressant (TCA) that increases amount of norepinephrine, serotonin, or both in the CNS by blocking their reuptake by the presynaptic neurons.

| Route | Onset | Peak | Duration |
|---|---|---|---|
| P.O. | Unknown | 2 hr | Unknown |

## INDICATIONS & DOSAGE
*Depression—*
**Adults:** 75 to 100 mg P.O. daily in divided doses, increased to 200 to 300 mg daily. Doses over 300 mg daily not recommended in hospitalized patients, or over 200 mg in outpatients. Total dose requirement may be given h.s.
**Elderly and adolescents:** initially, 50 mg/day, gradually increased to 100 mg/day.

## ADVERSE REACTIONS
**CNS:** *drowsiness, dizziness,* paresthesia, ataxia, hallucinations, delusions, anxiety, agitation, insomnia, tremor, weakness, confusion, headache, EEG changes, *seizures,* extrapyramidal reactions.
**CV:** *orthostatic hypotension, tachycardia,* hypertension, *arrhythmias, heart block, MI, stroke,* ECG changes.
**EENT:** *blurred vision,* tinnitus, mydriasis.
**GI:** *dry mouth, constipation,* nausea, vomiting, anorexia, paralytic ileus.
**GU:** *urine retention.*
**Hepatic:** elevated liver function tests.
**Metabolic:** altered serum glucose levels.
**Skin:** rash, urticaria, photosensitivity, *diaphoresis.*
**Other:** *hypersensitivity reaction.*
**After abrupt withdrawal of long-term therapy:** nausea, headache, malaise (doesn't indicate addiction).

---

*Liquid contains alcohol.   **May contain tartrazine.   †Canada   ‡Australia   §U.K.   ◊OTC

## INTERACTIONS
**Drug-drug.** *Barbiturates:* decreased TCA blood levels. Monitor for decreased antidepressant effect.
*Cimetidine, fluoxetine, sertraline:* may increase serum trimipramine levels. Monitor for increased adverse reactions.
*Clonidine, epinephrine, norepinephrine:* increased hypertensive effect. Use with caution.
*CNS depressants:* enhanced CNS depression. Avoid concomitant use.
*MAO inhibitors:* may cause severe excitation, hyperpyrexia, or seizures, usually with high doses. Avoid concomitant use.
**Drug-lifestyle.** *Alcohol use:* enhanced CNS depression. Avoid concomitant use.
*Sun exposure:* increased risk of photosensitivity reactions. Avoid unprotected or prolonged sun exposure.

## EFFECTS ON DIAGNOSTIC TESTS
None reported.

## CONTRAINDICATIONS
Contraindicated in patients with hypersensitivity to drug, during acute recovery phase of MI, and in those receiving MAO inhibitor therapy within 14 days.

## NURSING CONSIDERATIONS
• Use with extreme caution in patients with CV disease, history of urine retention or angle-closure glaucoma, increased intraocular pressure, hyperthyroidism, impaired hepatic function, or history of seizures and in those receiving thyroid medications, guanethidine, or similar drugs.
• Don't withdraw drug abruptly.
• *Alert:* Because hypertensive episodes have occurred during surgery in patients receiving TCAs, dosage should be gradually discontinued several days before surgery.
• If signs or symptoms of psychosis occur or increase, expect doctor to reduce dosage. Record mood changes. Monitor patient for suicidal tendencies, and allow only a minimum supply of drug.
• Recommend use of sugarless hard candy or gum to relieve dry mouth. Saliva substitutes may be necessary.

• *Alert:* Don't confuse trimipramine with triamterene or trimeprazine.

### ☑ Patient teaching
• Tell patient to take full dose at bedtime to avoid daytime sedation. Warn him about possible morning orthostatic hypotension.
• Tell patient to avoid alcohol and to consult doctor before taking other prescription or OTC drugs.
• Warn patient to avoid hazardous activities that require alertness and good psychomotor coordination until CNS effects of drug are known. Drowsiness and dizziness usually subside after a few weeks.
• Warn patient not to stop drug suddenly.
• To prevent photosensitivity reactions, advise patient to use sunblock, wear protective clothing, and avoid prolonged exposure to strong sunlight.

# venlafaxine hydrochloride
Efexor‡, Effexor, Effexor XR

*Pregnancy Risk Category C*

## HOW SUPPLIED
*Capsules (extended-release):* 37.5 mg, 75 mg, 150 mg
*Tablets:* 25 mg, 37.5 mg, 50 mg, 75 mg, 100 mg

## ACTION
Blocks reuptake of norepinephrine and serotonin into neurons in the CNS.

| Route | Onset | Peak | Duration |
|-------|-------|------|----------|
| P.O. | Unknown | Unknown | Unknown |

## INDICATIONS & DOSAGE
*Depression—*
**Adults:** initially, 75 mg P.O. daily in two or three divided doses with food. Dosage increased as tolerated and needed in increments of 75 mg/day at intervals of no less than 4 days. For moderately depressed outpatients, usual maximum dose is 225 mg/day; in certain severely depressed patients, dose may be as high as 375 mg/day. For extended-release capsules, 75 mg P.O. daily in a single dose. For some patients it may be desirable to

start at 37.5 mg P.O. daily for 4 to 7 days before increasing to 75 mg daily. Dosage may be increased at increments of 75 mg/day q 4 days to maximum of 225 mg/day.

*Adjust-a-dose:* For renally impaired patients, reduce total daily dose by 25%. For patients undergoing hemodialysis, reduce total daily dose by 50% and withhold dose until dialysis is completed. For patients with hepatic impairment, reduce total daily dose by 50%.

## ADVERSE REACTIONS

**CNS:** *headache, somnolence, dizziness, nervousness, insomnia,* anxiety, tremor, abnormal dreams, paresthesia, agitation, *asthenia.*
**CV:** hypertension, tachycardia, vasodilation.
**EENT:** blurred vision.
**GI:** *nausea, constipation,* vomiting, *dry mouth, anorexia,* diarrhea, dyspepsia, flatulence, vomiting.
**GU:** *abnormal ejaculation,* impotence, urinary frequency, impaired urination.
**Metabolic:** weight loss.
**Skin:** *diaphoresis,* rash.
**Other:** yawning, chills, infection.

## INTERACTIONS

**Drug-drug.** *MAO inhibitors:* may precipitate a syndrome similar to neuroleptic malignant syndrome (myoclonus, hyperthermia, seizures, and death). Avoid concomitant use.
**Drug-herb.** *Yohimbe:* additive stimulation. Use together cautiously.

## EFFECTS ON DIAGNOSTIC TESTS
None reported.

## CONTRAINDICATIONS
Contraindicated in patients with hypersensitivity to drug or within 14 days of MAO inhibitor therapy.

## NURSING CONSIDERATIONS
• Use cautiously in patients with renal impairment, diseases or conditions that could affect hemodynamic responses or metabolism, and in those with history of mania or seizures.

• Carefully monitor blood pressure. Drug therapy is associated with sustained, dose-dependent increases in blood pressure. Greatest increases (averaging about 7 mm Hg above baseline) occur in patients taking 375 mg daily.

### ☑ Patient teaching
• Inform patient who has received drug for 6 weeks or more that drug should be gradually discontinued by tapering dosage over a 2-week period as instructed by doctor.
• Warn patient to avoid hazardous activities that require alertness and good psychomotor coordination until CNS effects of drug are known.
• Tell patient to avoid alcohol and to consult doctor before taking other prescription or OTC drugs.

alprazolam
buspirone hydrochloride
chlordiazepoxide
chlordiazepoxide hydrochloride
clorazepate dipotassium
diazepam
doxepin hydrochloride
(See Chapter 31, ANTIDEPRESSANTS.)
hydroxyzine embonate
hydroxyzine hydrochloride
hydroxyzine pamoate
lorazepam
meprobamate
midazolam hydrochloride
oxazepam

## COMBINATION PRODUCTS
EQUAGESIC: meprobamate 200 mg and aspirin 325 mg.
LIBRAX: chlordiazepoxide hydrochloride 5 mg and clidinium bromide 2.5 mg.
LIMBITROL DS: chlordiazepoxide 10 mg and amitriptyline hydrochloride 25 mg.

---

## alprazolam
Apo-Alpraz†, Kalma‡,
Novo-Alprazol†, Nu-Alpraz†,
Ralozam‡, Xanax

*Controlled Substance Schedule IV*
*Pregnancy Risk Category D*

### HOW SUPPLIED
*Tablets:* 0.25 mg, 0.5 mg, 1 mg, 2 mg
*Oral solution:* 0.5 mg/5 ml, 1 mg/ml (concentrate)

### ACTION
Unknown. A benzodiazepine that probably potentiates the effects of gamma-aminobutyric acid, an inhibitory neurotransmitter, and depresses the CNS at the limbic and subcortical levels of the brain.

| Route | Onset | Peak | Duration |
|-------|-------|------|----------|
| P.O. | Unknown | 1-2 hr | Unknown |

### INDICATIONS & DOSAGE
*Anxiety—*
**Adults:** usual initial dose, 0.25 to 0.5 mg P.O. t.i.d. Maximum dose is 4 mg daily in divided doses.
**Elderly:** usual initial dose, 0.25 mg P.O. b.i.d. or t.i.d. Maximum dose is 4 mg daily in divided doses.
*Panic disorders—*
**Adults:** 0.5 mg P.O. t.i.d., increased at intervals of 3 to 4 days in increments of no more than 1 mg. Maximum dose is 10 mg daily in divided doses.
*Adjust-a-dose:* For debilitated patients or those with advanced hepatic disease, usual initial dose is 0.25 mg P.O. b.i.d. or t.i.d. Maximum dose is 4 mg daily in divided doses.

### ADVERSE REACTIONS
**CNS:** *drowsiness, light-headedness,* headache, confusion, tremor, dizziness, syncope, *depression,* insomnia, memory impairment, nervousness, minor changes in EEG patterns.
**CV:** hypotension, tachycardia.
**EENT:** blurred vision, nasal congestion.
**GI:** *dry mouth,* nausea, vomiting, *diarrhea, constipation,* increased salivation.
**Hepatic:** elevated liver function tests.
**Metabolic:** weight gain or loss.
**Musculoskeletal:** muscle rigidity.
**Skin:** dermatitis.

### INTERACTIONS
**Drug-drug.** *Cimetidine:* decreased alprazolam clearance with potential for increased adverse reactions. Monitor patient carefully.
*CNS depressants:* increased CNS depression. Avoid concomitant use.
*Digoxin:* may increase serum digoxin levels, increasing toxicity. Monitor patient closely.
*Tricyclic antidepressants (TCAs):* increased plasma levels of TCAs. Monitor for toxicity.
**Drug-herb.** *Kava:* may cause coma. Avoid concomitant use.

---

Reactions may be *common,* uncommon, *life-threatening,* or COMMON AND LIFE-THREATENING.

**Drug-lifestyle.** *Alcohol use:* increased CNS depression. Avoid concomitant use. *Smoking:* decreased effectiveness of benzodiazepines. Monitor patient closely.

**EFFECTS ON DIAGNOSTIC TESTS**
None reported.

**CONTRAINDICATIONS**
Contraindicated in patients with hypersensitivity to drug or other benzodiazepines and in those with acute angle-closure glaucoma.

**NURSING CONSIDERATIONS**
• Use cautiously in patients with hepatic, renal, or pulmonary disease.
• Drug isn't for daily stress or for long-term use. Further study is needed to determine the optimum duration of therapy.
• *Alert:* Don't withdraw drug abruptly; withdrawal symptoms, including seizures, may occur. Abuse or addiction is possible.
• Monitor liver, renal, and hematopoietic function studies periodically in patients receiving repeated or prolonged therapy, as ordered.
• *Alert:* Don't confuse alprazolam with alprostadil, or Xanax with Zantac or Tenex.

☑ **Patient teaching**
• Warn patient to avoid hazardous activities that require alertness and good psychomotor coordination until CNS effects of drug are known.
• Tell patient to avoid alcohol while taking drug.
• Notify patient that smoking may decrease effectiveness of drug.
• Warn patient not to abruptly stop using drug because withdrawal symptoms or seizures may occur.

---

**buspirone hydrochloride**
BuSpar

*Pregnancy Risk Category B*

---

**HOW SUPPLIED**
*Tablets:* 5 mg, 10 mg, 15 mg

**ACTION**
Unknown. May inhibit neuronal firing and reduce serotonin turnover in cortical, amygdaloid, and septohippocampal tissue.

| Route | Onset | Peak | Duration |
|-------|-------|------|----------|
| P.O. | Unknown | 40-90 min | Unknown |

**INDICATIONS & DOSAGE**
*Anxiety disorders, short-term relief of anxiety—*
**Adults:** initially, 5 mg P.O. t.i.d. Dosage increased at 3-day intervals in 5-mg increments. Usual maintenance dose is 20 to 30 mg daily in divided doses. Don't exceed 60 mg daily.

**ADVERSE REACTIONS**
**CNS:** *dizziness, drowsiness,* nervousness, insomnia, headache, light-headedness, fatigue, numbness.
**EENT:** blurred vision.
**GI:** dry mouth, nausea, diarrhea, abdominal distress.

**INTERACTIONS**
**Drug-drug.** *CNS depressants:* increased CNS depression. Avoid concomitant use.
*MAO inhibitors:* may elevate blood pressure. Avoid concomitant use.
**Drug-lifestyle.** *Alcohol use:* increased CNS depression. Avoid concomitant use.

**EFFECTS ON DIAGNOSTIC TESTS**
None reported.

**CONTRAINDICATIONS**
Contraindicated in patients with hypersensitivity to drug; also contraindicated within 14 days of MAO inhibitor therapy.

**NURSING CONSIDERATIONS**
• Use cautiously in patients with hepatic or renal failure.
• Monitor patient closely for adverse CNS reactions. Buspirone is less sedating than other antianxiety agents. However, CNS effects in individual patients may be unpredictable.
• *Alert:* Before initiating buspirone therapy in a patient already being given benzodiazepines, warn him against stopping the benzodiazepine abruptly; withdrawal reaction may occur.

---

*Liquid contains alcohol.   **May contain tartrazine.   †Canada   ‡Australia   §U.K.   ◊OTC

• Drug has shown no potential for abuse and hasn't been classified as a controlled substance; however, it isn't recommended for relief of daily stress.
• **Alert:** Don't confuse buspirone with bupropion.

☑ **Patient teaching**
• Warn patient to avoid hazardous activities that require alertness and good psychomotor coordination until CNS effects of drug are known.
• Notify patient that drug's effects may not be seen for several weeks.
• Warn patient not to abruptly withdraw benzodiazepines because of risk of withdrawal symptoms.
• Tell patient to avoid alcohol during therapy.

---

**chlordiazepoxide**
Libritabs

**chlordiazepoxide hydrochloride**
Apo-Chlordiazepoxide†, Librium, Novo-Poxide†

*Controlled Substance Schedule IV*
*Pregnancy Risk Category NR*

## HOW SUPPLIED
**chlordiazepoxide**
*Tablets:* 10 mg, 25 mg
**chlordiazepoxide hydrochloride**
*Capsules:* 5 mg, 10 mg, 25 mg
*Powder for injection:* 100-mg ampule

## ACTION
Unknown. A benzodiazepine that may exert its anxiolytic effects by facilitating the action of the inhibitory neurotransmitter gamma-aminobutyric acid. Drug depresses the CNS at the limbic and subcortical levels of the brain and suppresses the spread of seizure activity produced by epileptogenic foci in the cortex, thalamus, and limbic structures.

| Route | Onset | Peak | Duration |
|-------|-------|------|----------|
| P.O. | Unknown | 0.5-4 hr | Unknown |
| I.V. | 1-5 min | Unknown | 15-60 min |
| I.M. | Unknown | Unknown | Unknown |

## INDICATIONS & DOSAGE
*Mild to moderate anxiety—*
**Adults:** 5 to 10 mg P.O. t.i.d. or q.i.d.
**Children over 6:** 5 mg P.O. b.i.d. to q.i.d. Maximum dose is 10 mg P.O. b.i.d. or t.i.d.
*Severe anxiety—*
**Adults:** 20 to 25 mg P.O. t.i.d. or q.i.d.
**Elderly:** 5 mg P.O. b.i.d. to q.i.d.
**Adjust-a-dose:** For debilitated patients, 5 mg P.O. b.i.d. to q.i.d.
*Withdrawal symptoms of acute alcoholism—*
**Adults:** 50 to 100 mg P.O., I.M., or I.V. Repeated in 2 to 4 hours, p.r.n. Maximum dose is 300 mg daily.
*Preoperative apprehension and anxiety—*
**Adults:** 5 to 10 mg P.O. t.i.d. or q.i.d. on day preceding surgery; or 50 to 100 mg I.M. 1 hour before surgery.
*Note:* Parenteral form isn't recommended in children under age 12.

## ADVERSE REACTIONS
**CNS:** *drowsiness, lethargy,* ataxia, confusion, extrapyramidal symptoms, minor changes in EEG patterns.
**GI:** nausea, constipation.
**GU:** menstrual irregularities.
**Hematologic:** *agranulocytosis.*
**Hepatic:** elevated liver function tests, jaundice.
**Skin:** *swelling, pain at injection site;* skin eruptions, edema.
**Other:** increased or decreased libido.

## INTERACTIONS
**Drug-drug.** *Cimetidine:* decreased chlordiazepoxide clearance, with potential for increased adverse reactions. Monitor patient carefully.
*CNS depressants:* increased CNS depression. Avoid concomitant use.
*Digoxin:* increased serum digoxin levels and risk of toxicity. Monitor patient closely.
**Drug-lifestyle.** *Alcohol use:* increased CNS depression. Avoid concomitant use.
*Smoking:* decreased effectiveness of benzodiazepines. Monitor patient closely.

## EFFECTS ON DIAGNOSTIC TESTS
Drug may cause a false-positive pregnancy test, depending on method used. It may

---

Reactions may be *common,* uncommon, *life-threatening,* or COMMON AND LIFE-THREATENING.

also alter urinary 17-ketosteroids (Zimmerman reaction), urine alkaloid determination (Frings thin-layer chromatography method), and urinary glucose determinations (with Chemstrip uG and Diastix).

## CONTRAINDICATIONS
Contraindicated in patients with hypersensitivity to drug.

## NURSING CONSIDERATIONS
• Use cautiously in patients with mental depression, porphyria, or hepatic or renal disease.
• Drug should be avoided during pregnancy, especially during first trimester.
• Drug shouldn't be prescribed regularly for daily stress.
• Injectable form (as hydrochloride) comes in two types of ampules—as diluent and as powdered drug. Read directions carefully.
• Keep powder away from light and refrigerate; mix just before use and discard remainder.
• For I.M. use, add 2 ml of diluent to powder and agitate gently until clear. Use immediately. I.M. form may be absorbed erratically.
• Monitor liver, renal, and hematopoietic function studies periodically in patients receiving repeated or prolonged therapy, as ordered.
• Possibility of abuse and addiction exists. Drug shouldn't be withdrawn abruptly after long-term administration; withdrawal symptoms may occur.
• *Alert:* Drug is slowly and erratically absorbed when given I.M.
• *Alert:* Chlordiazepoxide 5 mg and 25 mg unit-dose capsules may appear similar in color when viewed through the package. When using unit doses of this or any product, verify contents and read label carefully.

## I.V. administration
• Use 5 ml of normal saline solution or sterile water for injection as diluent to an ampule containing 100 mg of drug; don't give packaged diluent I.V. because air bubbles may form when using prepackaged diluent. Administer over 1 minute.

• When giving drug I.V., make sure equipment and personnel needed for emergency airway management are available. Monitor respirations every 5 to 15 minutes and before each repeated I.V. dose.

## ✔ Patient teaching
• Warn patient to avoid hazardous activities that require alertness and good psychomotor coordination until CNS effects of drug are known.
• Tell patient to avoid alcohol while taking drug.
• Notify patient that smoking may decrease effectiveness of drug.
• Warn patient not to abruptly stop using the drug because withdrawal symptoms may occur.
• Caution woman to avoid use during pregnancy.

---

## clorazepate dipotassium
Apo-Clorazepate†, Gen-XENE, Novo-Clopate†, Tranxene, Tranxene-SD, Tranxene T-TAB

*Controlled Substance Schedule IV*
*Pregnancy Risk Category D*

## HOW SUPPLIED
*Tablets:* 3.75 mg, 7.5 mg, 11.25 mg, 15 mg, 22.5 mg
*Capsules:* 3.75 mg, 7.5 mg, 15 mg

## ACTION
Unknown. A benzodiazepine that may exert its anxiolytic effects by facilitating the action of the inhibitory neurotransmitter gamma-aminobutyric acid. Drug depresses the CNS at the limbic and subcortical levels of the brain and suppresses the spread of seizure activity produced by epileptogenic foci in the cortex, thalamus, and limbic structures.

| Route | Onset | Peak | Duration |
|---|---|---|---|
| P.O. | Unknown | 0.5-2 hr | Unknown |

## INDICATIONS & DOSAGE
*Acute alcohol withdrawal—*
**Adults:** day 1—30 mg P.O. initially; then 30 to 60 mg P.O. in divided doses; day 2—45 to 90 mg P.O. in divided doses; day

---

3—22.5 to 45 mg P.O. in divided doses; day 4—15 to 30 mg P.O. in divided doses; then gradually reduce dosage to 7.5 to 15 mg daily. Maximum recommended daily dose is 90 mg.

*Anxiety—*
**Adults:** 15 to 60 mg P.O. daily.
**Elderly:** initially, 7.5 to 15 mg daily in divided doses or as a single dose h.s.
***Adjust-a-dose:*** For debilitated patients, initially, 7.5 to 15 mg daily in divided doses or as a single dose h.s.

*Adjunct in partial seizure disorder—*
**Adults and children over age 12:** maximum recommended initial dose is 7.5 mg P.O. t.i.d. Dosage increases shouldn't exceed 7.5 mg weekly. Maximum dose is 90 mg daily.
**Children ages 9 to 12:** maximum recommended initial dose is 7.5 mg P.O. b.i.d. Dosage increases shouldn't exceed 7.5 mg weekly. Maximum dose is 60 mg daily.

## ADVERSE REACTIONS
**CNS:** *drowsiness,* dizziness, nervousness, confusion, headache, insomnia, depression, irritability, tremor, minor changes in EEG patterns.
**CV:** hypotension.
**EENT:** blurred vision, diplopia.
**GI:** nausea, vomiting, abdominal discomfort, dry mouth.
**GU:** urine retention, incontinence.
**Hepatic:** elevated liver function tests.
**Skin:** rash.

## INTERACTIONS
**Drug-drug.** *Cimetidine:* decreased clorazepate clearance, with increased potential for adverse reactions. Monitor patient carefully.
*CNS depressants:* increased CNS depression. Avoid concomitant use.
*Digoxin:* may increase serum digoxin levels and risk of toxicity. Monitor patient closely.
**Drug-lifestyle.** *Alcohol use:* increased CNS depression. Avoid concomitant use.
*Smoking:* decreased effectiveness of benzodiazepines. Monitor patient closely.

## EFFECTS ON DIAGNOSTIC TESTS
None reported.

## CONTRAINDICATIONS
Contraindicated in patients with hypersensitivity to drug and in those with acute angle-closure glaucoma.

## NURSING CONSIDERATIONS
• Drug should be avoided during pregnancy, especially during first trimester.
• Use cautiously in patients with suicidal tendencies, renal or hepatic impairment, pulmonary disease, or history of drug abuse.
• **Alert:** Monitor liver, renal, and hematopoietic function studies periodically in patients receiving repeated or prolonged therapy, as ordered.
• The possibility of abuse and addiction exists. Don't withdraw drug abruptly after prolonged use because withdrawal symptoms may occur.
• Drug isn't recommended for use in children under age 9.
• **Alert:** Don't confuse clorazepate with clofibrate.

☑ **Patient teaching**
• Warn patient to avoid activities that require alertness and good psychomotor coordination until CNS effects of drug are known.
• Tell patient to avoid alcohol while taking drug.
• Notify patient that smoking may decrease effectiveness of drug.
• Warn patient not to abruptly stop using drug because withdrawal symptoms may occur.
• Caution woman to avoid use during pregnancy.
• Inform patient that sugarless chewing gum or hard candy can relieve dry mouth.

## diazepam
Antenex‡, Apo-Diazepam†, Diastat, Diazemuls†‡, Diazepam Intensol, Ducene‡, Novo-Dipam†, PMS-Diazepam†, Valium, Vivol†

*Controlled Substance Schedule IV*
*Pregnancy Risk Category D*

## HOW SUPPLIED
*Tablets:* 2 mg, 5 mg, 10 mg

---

Reactions may be *common,* uncommon, *life-threatening,* or COMMON AND LIFE-THREATENING.

*Capsules (extended-release):* 15 mg
*Oral solution:* 5 mg/5 ml, 5 mg/ml
*Injection:* 5 mg/ml
*Sterile emulsion for injection:* 5 mg/ml
*Rectal gel twin packs:* 2.5 mg, 5 mg, 10 mg, 15 mg, 20 mg

## ACTION

Unknown. A benzodiazepine that may exert its anxiolytic effects by facilitating the action of the inhibitory neurotransmitter gamma-aminobutyric acid. Drug depresses the CNS at the limbic and subcortical levels of the brain and suppresses the spread of seizure activity produced by epileptogenic foci in the cortex, thalamus, and limbic structures.

| Route | Onset | Peak | Duration |
|-------|-------|------|----------|
| P.O. | 0.5 hr | 2 hr | 3-8 hr |
| I.V. | 1-5 min | Immediate | 15-60 min |
| I.M. | Unknown | 2 hr | Unknown |
| P.R. | Unknown | 1.5 hr | Unknown |

## INDICATIONS & DOSAGE

*Anxiety—*
**Adults:** depending on severity, 2 to 10 mg P.O. b.i.d. to q.i.d. or 15 to 30 mg extended-release capsules P.O. once daily. Or, 2 to 10 mg I.M. or I.V. q 3 to 4 hours, p.r.n.
**Children age 6 months and older:** 1 to 2.5 mg P.O. t.i.d. or q.i.d., increased gradually, as needed and tolerated.
**Elderly:** initially, 2 to 2.5 mg once or twice daily; increased gradually.
*Acute alcohol withdrawal—*
**Adults:** 10 mg P.O. t.i.d. or q.i.d. first 24 hours; reduced to 5 mg P.O. t.i.d. or q.i.d., p.r.n. Or, initially, 10 mg I.M. or I.V.; then 5 to 10 mg I.M. or I.V. q 3 to 4 hours, p.r.n.
*Before endoscopic procedures—*
**Adults:** I.V. dose titrated to desired sedative response (up to 20 mg). Or, 5 to 10 mg I.M. 30 minutes before procedure.
*Muscle spasm—*
**Adults:** 2 to 10 mg P.O. b.i.d. to q.i.d., or 15 to 30 mg extended-release capsules once daily. Or, 5 to 10 mg I.M. or I.V. initially; then 5 to 10 mg I.M. or I.V. q 3 to 4 hours, p.r.n. For tetanus, larger doses may be needed.

**Children over age 30 days to 5 years:** 1 to 2 mg I.M. or I.V. slowly, repeated q 3 to 4 hours, p.r.n.
**Children ages 5 and older:** 5 to 10 mg I.M. or I.V. q 3 to 4 hours, p.r.n.
*Preoperative sedation—*
**Adults:** 10 mg I.M. (preferred) or I.V. before surgery.
*Cardioversion—*
**Adults:** 5 to 15 mg I.V. within 5 to 10 minutes before procedure.
*Adjunct in seizure disorders—*
**Adults:** 2 to 10 mg P.O. b.i.d. to q.i.d.
**Children ages 6 months and older:** 1 to 2.5 mg P.O. t.i.d. or q.i.d. initially; increased as needed and tolerated.
*Status epilepticus, severe recurrent seizures—*
**Adults:** 5 to 10 mg I.V. (preferred) or I.M. initially. I.M. route should only be used if I.V. access is unavailable. Repeated q 10 to 15 minutes, p.r.n., up to maximum dose of 30 mg. Repeated q 2 to 4 hours, if needed.
**Children over age 30 days to 5 years:** 0.2 to 0.5 mg I.V. slowly q 2 to 5 minutes up to maximum of 5 mg. Repeated q 2 to 4 hours, if needed.
**Children ages 5 and older:** 1 mg I.V. q 2 to 5 minutes up to maximum of 10 mg. Repeated q 2 to 4 hours, if needed.
*Patients on stable regimens of antiepileptic drugs who need intermittent use of diazepam to control bouts of increased seizure activity—*
**Adults and children ages 12 and older:** 0.2 mg/kg P.R. A second dose may be given 4 to 12 hours after first.
**Children ages 6 to 11:** 0.3 mg/kg P.R.. A second dose may be given 4 to 12 hours after first.
**Children ages 2 to 5:** 0.5 mg/kg P.R.. A second dose may be given 4 to 12 hours after first.
**Adjust-a-dose:** For elderly and debilitated patients, reduce dosage to decrease the likelihood of ataxia and oversedation.
*Note:* Use Diastat rectal gel to treat no more than five episodes per month and no more than one episode every 5 days.

## ADVERSE REACTIONS
**CNS:** *drowsiness,* dysarthria, slurred speech, tremor, transient amnesia, fatigue,

---

ataxia, headache, insomnia, paradoxical anxiety, hallucinations, minor changes in EEG patterns.
**CV:** hypotension, *CV collapse, bradycardia.*
**EENT:** diplopia, blurred vision, nystagmus.
**GI:** nausea, constipation.
**GU:** incontinence, urine retention, altered libido.
**Hematologic:** *neutropenia.*
**Hepatic:** elevated liver function test results, jaundice.
**Respiratory:** *respiratory depression.*
**Skin:** rash.
**Other:** physical or psychological dependence, *acute withdrawal syndrome (after sudden discontinuation in physically dependent persons), pain, phlebitis at injection site.*

## INTERACTIONS
**Drug-drug.** *Cimetidine:* decreased clearance of diazepam, with increased potential for adverse effects. Monitor patient carefully.
*CNS depressants:* increased CNS depression. Avoid concomitant use.
*Digoxin:* may increase serum digoxin levels and risk of toxicity. Monitor patient closely.
*Phenobarbital:* increased effects of both drugs. Use together cautiously.
**Drug-lifestyle.** *Alcohol use:* increased CNS depression. Avoid concomitant use.
*Smoking:* decreased effectiveness of benzodiazepines. Monitor patient closely.

## EFFECTS ON DIAGNOSTIC TESTS
None reported.

## CONTRAINDICATIONS
Contraindicated in patients with hypersensitivity to drug or soy protein; in patients experiencing shock, coma, or acute alcohol intoxication (parenteral form); and in children under age 6 months (oral form). Diastat rectal gel is contraindicated in patients with acute narrow-angle glaucoma.

## NURSING CONSIDERATIONS
• Drug should be avoided during pregnancy, especially during first trimester.

• Use cautiously in patients with liver or renal impairment, depression, or chronic open-angle glaucoma.
• Use cautiously in elderly and debilitated patients.
• Don't mix injectable diazepam with other drugs, and don't store parenteral solution in plastic syringes.
• When using oral concentrate solution, dilute dose just before administering.
• Parenteral emulsion—a stabilized oil-in-water emulsion—should appear milky white and uniform. Avoid mixing with any other drugs or solutions, and avoid infusion sets or containers made from polyvinyl chloride. If dilution is needed, drug may be mixed with I.V. fat emulsion. Use admixture within 6 hours.
• *Alert:* Diastat rectal gel should only be administered by caregivers who can distinguish the distinct cluster of seizures or events from the patient's ordinary seizure activity, who have been instructed and can administer the treatment competently, who understand which seizure manifestations may or may not be treated with Diastat, and who are able to monitor the clinical response and recognize when immediate professional medical evaluation is needed.
• Monitor periodic liver, renal, and hematopoietic function studies in patients receiving repeated or prolonged therapy, as ordered.
• Possibility of abuse and addiction exists. Don't withdraw drug abruptly after long-term use; withdrawal symptoms may occur.
• *Alert:* Don't confuse diazepam with diazoxide.

### I.V. administration
• I.V. route is the most reliable parenteral route; I.M. administration isn't recommended because absorption is variable and injection is painful.
• Give I.V. at rate not exceeding 5 mg/minute. When injecting, administer directly into the vein. If this is impossible, inject slowly through infusion tubing as near to the vein insertion site as possible. Watch closely for phlebitis at injection site.

---

Reactions may be *common*, uncommon, *life-threatening*, or COMMON AND LIFE-THREATENING.

• Avoid extravasation. Don't inject into small veins.
• *Alert:* Monitor respirations every 5 to 15 minutes and before each repeated I.V. dose. Have emergency resuscitation equipment and oxygen at bedside.

☑ **Patient teaching**
• Warn patient to avoid activities that require alertness and good psychomotor coordination until CNS effects of drug are known.
• Tell patient to avoid alcohol while taking drug.
• Notify patient that smoking may decrease effectiveness of drug.
• Warn patient not to abruptly stop using drug because withdrawal symptoms may occur.
• Caution woman to avoid use during pregnancy.
• Instruct patient's caregiver on the proper administration technique of Diastat rectal gel.

---

**hydroxyzine embonate‡**
Atarax

**hydroxyzine hydrochloride**
Anx, Apo-Hydroxyzine†, Atarax*, Hydroxacen, Hyzine-50, Multipax†, Novo-Hydroxyzin†, QYS, Ucerax§, Vistacon-50, Vistaject-50, Vistaril, Vistazine 50

**hydroxyzine pamoate**
Vistaril

*Pregnancy Risk Category NR*

**HOW SUPPLIED**
**hydroxyzine embonate‡**
*Capsules:* 25 mg, 50 mg
**hydroxyzine hydrochloride**
*Tablets:* 10 mg, 25 mg, 50 mg, 100 mg
*Capsules:* 10 mg†‡, 25 mg†‡, 50 mg†‡
*Syrup:* 10 mg/5 ml
*Injection:* 25 mg/ml, 50 mg/ml
**hydroxyzine pamoate**
*Capsules:* 25 mg, 50 mg, 100 mg
*Oral suspension:* 25 mg/5 ml

**ACTION**
Unknown. A piperazine antihistamine whose action may be due to a suppression of activity in certain key regions of the subcortical area of the CNS.

| Route | Onset | Peak | Duration |
|-------|-------|------|----------|
| P.O. | 15-30 min | 2 hr | 4-6 hr |
| I.M. | Unknown | Unknown | 4-6 hr |

**INDICATIONS & DOSAGE**
*Anxiety—*
**Adults:** 50 to 100 mg P.O. q.i.d.
**Children under age 6:** 50 mg P.O. daily in divided doses.
**Children ages 6 and older:** 50 to 100 mg P.O. daily in divided doses.
*Preoperative and postoperative adjunctive therapy—*
**Adults:** 25 to 100 mg I.M. q 4 to 6 hours.
**Children:** 1.1 mg/kg I.M. q 4 to 6 hours.
*Pruritus due to allergies—*
**Adults:** 25 mg P.O. t.i.d. or q.i.d.
**Children under age 6:** 50 mg P.O. daily in divided doses.
**Children ages 6 and older:** 50 to 100 mg P.O. daily in divided doses.
*Psychiatric and emotional emergencies, including acute alcoholism—*
**Adults:** 50 to 100 mg I.M. q 4 to 6 hours, p.r.n.
*Nausea and vomiting (excluding nausea and vomiting of pregnancy)—*
**Adults:** 25 to 100 mg I.M.
**Children:** 1.1 mg/kg I.M.
*Antepartum and postpartum adjunctive therapy—*
**Adults:** 25 to 100 mg I.M.

**ADVERSE REACTIONS**
**CNS:** *drowsiness,* involuntary motor activity.
**GI:** *dry mouth.*
**Other:** marked discomfort at I.M. injection site, *hypersensitivity reactions.*

**INTERACTIONS**
**Drug-drug.** *CNS depressants:* increased CNS depression. Avoid concomitant use.
**Drug-lifestyle.** *Alcohol use:* increased CNS depression. Avoid concomitant use.

---

## EFFECTS ON DIAGNOSTIC TESTS
Drug therapy causes falsely elevated urinary 17-hydroxycorticosteroid levels. It also may cause false-negative skin allergen tests by attenuating or inhibiting the cutaneous response to histamine.

## CONTRAINDICATIONS
Contraindicated in patients with hypersensitivity to drug, during early pregnancy, and in breast-feeding women.

## NURSING CONSIDERATIONS
• Parenteral form (hydroxyzine hydrochloride) is for I.M. use only; never administer I.V. or S.C. The Z-track injection method is preferred.
• Aspirate I.M. injection carefully to prevent inadvertent intravascular injection. Inject deeply into a large muscle mass.
• If patient is taking other CNS drugs, observe for oversedation.
• *Alert:* Don't confuse hydroxyzine with hydroxyurea or hydralazine.

☑ **Patient teaching**
• Warn patient to avoid hazardous activities that require alertness and good psychomotor coordination until CNS effects of drug are known.
• Tell patient to avoid alcohol while taking drug.
• Advise patient to use sugarless hard candy or gum to relieve dry mouth.
• Warn woman to avoid use during pregnancy and breast feeding.

## lorazepam
Apo-Lorazepam†, Ativan, Lorazepam Intensol, Novo-Lorazem†, Nu-Loraz†◇

*Controlled Substance Schedule IV*
*Pregnancy Risk Category D*

## HOW SUPPLIED
*Tablets:* 0.5 mg, 1 mg, 2 mg
*Tablets (S.L.):* 0.5 mg†, 1 mg†, 2 mg
*Oral solution (concentrated):* 2 mg/ml
*Injection:* 2 mg/ml, 4 mg/ml

## ACTION
Unknown. A benzodiazepine that probably potentiates the effects of gamma-aminobutyric acid, an inhibitory neurotransmitter, and depresses the CNS at the limbic and subcortical levels of the brain.

| Route | Onset | Peak | Duration |
|---|---|---|---|
| P.O. | 1 hr | 2 hr | 12-24 hr |
| I.V. | 5 min | 1-1.5 hr | 6-8 hr |
| I.M. | 15-30 min | 1-1.5 hr | 6-8 hr |

## INDICATIONS & DOSAGE
*Anxiety—*
**Adults:** 2 to 6 mg P.O. daily in divided doses. Maximum dose is 10 mg daily.
**Elderly:** initially, 1 to 2 mg daily.
*Insomnia due to anxiety—*
**Adults:** 2 to 4 mg P.O. h.s.
*Preoperative sedation—*
**Adults:** 0.05 mg/kg I.M. 2 hours before procedure. Total dose shouldn't exceed 4 mg. Or, 2 mg I.V. total or 0.044 mg/kg I.V., whichever is smaller. Larger doses up to 0.05 mg/kg I.V., to total of 4 mg, may be needed.

## ADVERSE REACTIONS
**CNS:** *drowsiness,* amnesia, insomnia, agitation, *sedation,* dizziness, weakness, unsteadiness, disorientation, depression, headache.
**CV:** hypotension.
**EENT:** visual disturbances.
**GI:** abdominal discomfort, nausea, change in appetite.
**Hepatic:** elevated liver function tests.
**Other:** *acute withdrawal syndrome following sudden discontinuation in physically dependent persons.*

## INTERACTIONS
**Drug-drug.** *CNS depressants:* increased CNS depression. Avoid concomitant use.
*Digoxin:* may increase serum digoxin levels and risk of toxicity. Monitor patient closely.
**Drug-lifestyle.** *Alcohol use:* increased CNS depression. Avoid concomitant use.
*Smoking:* decreased effectiveness of benzodiazepines. Monitor patient closely.

## EFFECTS ON DIAGNOSTIC TESTS
None reported.

Reactions may be *common,* uncommon, *life-threatening,* or COMMON AND LIFE-THREATENING.

## CONTRAINDICATIONS

Contraindicated in patients with hypersensitivity to drug, other benzodiazepines, or its vehicle (used in parenteral dosage form); also contraindicated in those with acute angle-closure glaucoma.

## NURSING CONSIDERATIONS

• Drug should be avoided during pregnancy, especially during first trimester.
• Use cautiously in patients with pulmonary, renal, or hepatic impairment. Also use cautiously in elderly, acutely ill, or debilitated patients.
• For I.M. administration, inject deeply into a muscle mass. Don't dilute.
• Refrigerate parenteral form to prolong shelf life.
• Monitor liver, renal, and hematopoietic function studies periodically in patients receiving repeated or prolonged therapy, as ordered.
• *Alert:* Possibility of abuse and addiction exists. Don't withdraw drug abruptly after long-term use because withdrawal symptoms may occur.
• *Alert:* Don't confuse lorazepam with alprazolam.

### I.V. administration

• Give slowly, at rate not exceeding 2 mg/minute. Dilute with an equal volume of sterile water for injection, normal saline for injection, or dextrose 5% injection.
• *Alert:* Monitor respirations every 5 to 15 minutes and before each repeated I.V. dose. Have emergency resuscitation equipment and oxygen available.

### Patient teaching

• As a premedication for surgery, lorazepam provides substantial preoperative amnesia. Patient teaching requires extra care to ensure adequate recall. Provide written materials or inform a family member, if possible.
• Warn patient to avoid hazardous activities that require alertness or good psychomotor coordination until CNS effects of drug are known.
• Tell patient to avoid alcohol while taking drug.

• Notify patient that smoking may decrease effectiveness of drug.
• Warn patient not to abruptly stop drug because withdrawal symptoms may occur.
• Caution woman to avoid drug during pregnancy.

## meprobamate
Apo-Meprobamate†, Equanil**, Miltown-200, Miltown-400, Miltown-600, Neuramate, Probate, Trancot

*Controlled Substance Schedule IV*
*Pregnancy Risk Category D*

### HOW SUPPLIED
*Tablets:* 200 mg, 400 mg, 600 mg

### ACTION
Unknown. Appears to act at multiple sites in the CNS.

| Route | Onset | Peak | Duration |
|-------|-------|------|----------|
| P.O. | Unknown | Unknown | Unknown |

### INDICATIONS & DOSAGE
*Anxiety—*
**Adults:** 1.2 to 1.6 g P.O. daily in three or four equally divided doses. Maximum dose is 2.4 g daily.
**Children ages 6 to 12:** 200 to 600 mg P.O. in two or three divided doses.

### ADVERSE REACTIONS
**CNS:** *drowsiness,* ataxia, dizziness, slurred speech, headache, vertigo, *seizures,* syncope.
**CV:** palpitations, tachycardia, hypotension, *arrhythmias.*
**GI:** nausea, vomiting, diarrhea.
**Hematologic:** *aplastic anemia, thrombocytopenia, agranulocytosis.*
**Skin:** pruritus, urticaria, erythematous maculopapular rash, *hypersensitivity reactions.*

### INTERACTIONS
**Drug-drug.** *CNS depressants:* increased CNS depression. Avoid concomitant use.
**Drug-lifestyle.** *Alcohol use:* increased CNS depression. Avoid concomitant use.

## EFFECTS ON DIAGNOSTIC TESTS
Drug therapy may falsely elevate urinary 17-ketosteroids, 17-ketogenic steroids (as determined by the Zimmerman reaction), and 17-hydroxycorticosteroid levels (as determined by the Glenn-Nelson technique).

## CONTRAINDICATIONS
Contraindicated in patients with hypersensitivity to drug or related compounds (such as carisoprodol, mebutamate, tybamate, and carbromal); also contraindicated in those with porphyria.

## NURSING CONSIDERATIONS
• Drug should be avoided during pregnancy, especially during first trimester.
• Use cautiously in patients with impaired hepatic or renal function, seizure disorders, or suicidal tendencies.
• Miltown-600 isn't recommended for use in children.
• Give drug with meals to reduce GI distress.
• Possibility of abuse and addiction exists with long-term use. Withdraw drug gradually over 2 weeks to avoid withdrawal symptoms.
• *Alert:* After abrupt withdrawal of long-term therapy, severe generalized tonic-clonic seizures may occur.
• Periodically monitor CBC and renal and liver function tests in patients receiving high doses, as ordered.
• *Alert:* Don't confuse Miltown with Milontin.

### ☑ Patient teaching
• Advise patient to take drug with meals and not to crush or chew sustained-release capsules but to swallow them whole.
• Warn patient to avoid hazardous activities that require alertness and good psychomotor coordination until CNS effects of drug are known.
• Tell patient to avoid alcohol while taking drug.
• Advise patient to report unusual bruising or bleeding, fever, or sore throat, which may indicate serious hematologic toxicity.

• Warn patient not to abruptly stop drug because withdrawal symptoms may occur.
• Caution woman to avoid use during pregnancy.

---

## midazolam hydrochloride
Hypnovel‡, Versed, Versed Syrup

*Controlled Substance Schedule IV*
*Pregnancy Risk Category D*

## HOW SUPPLIED
*Syrup*: 2 mg/ml
*Injection:* 1 mg/ml, 5 mg/ml

## ACTION
Unknown. May depress CNS at the limbic and subcortical levels of the brain by potentiating the effects of gamma-aminobutyric acid.

| Route | Onset | Peak | Duration |
|-------|-------|------|----------|
| P.O. | 10-20 min | 45-60 min | 2-6 hr |
| I.V. | 1.5-5 min | Rapid | 2-6 hr |
| I.M. | 15 min | 15-60 min | 2-6 hr |

## INDICATIONS & DOSAGE
*Preoperative sedation (to induce sleepiness or drowsiness and relieve apprehension)—*
**Adults:** 0.07 to 0.08 mg/kg I.M. about 1 hour before surgery.
*Conscious sedation before short diagnostic or endoscopic procedures—*
**Adults under age 60:** initially, small dose not to exceed 2.5 mg I.V. administered slowly; repeated in 2 minutes, if needed, in small increments of initial dose over at least 2 minutes to achieve desired effect. Total dose of up to 5 mg may be used. Additional doses to maintain desired level of sedation may be given by slow titration in increments of 25% of dose used to first reach the sedative endpoint.
**Elderly:** 1.5 mg or less over at least 2 minutes. If additional titration is needed, give at rate not exceeding 1 mg over 2 minutes. Total doses exceeding 3.5 mg aren't usually needed.
*To induce sleepiness and amnesia and to relieve apprehension before anesthesia or*

---

Reactions may be *common*, uncommon, ***life-threatening***, or COMMON AND LIFE-THREATENING.

*before or during procedures in pediatric patients—*

I.M.—

**Children:** 0.1 to 0.15 mg/kg I.M. Doses up to 0.5 mg/kg can be used for more anxious patients.

I.V.—

**Children ages 6 months to 5 years:** 0.05 to 0.1 mg/kg I.V. over 2 to 3 minutes. Additional doses may be given in small increments after 2 to 3 minutes. Total dose of up to 0.6 mg/kg, not to exceed 6 mg, may be used.

**Children ages 6 to 12:** 0.025 to 0.05 mg/kg I.V. over 2 to 3 minutes. Additional doses may be given in small increments after 2 to 3 minutes. Total dose up to 0.4 mg/kg, not to exceed 10 mg, may be used.

**Children ages 12 to 16:** dosage as for adults; total dose not to exceed 10 mg.

P.O.—

**Infants and children ages 6 months to 5 years and less cooperative patients:** 0.25 to 1 mg/kg P.O. as a single dose, not to exceed 20 mg.

**Children ages 6 to 16 and cooperative patients:** 0.25 to 0.5 mg/kg P.O. as a single dose, up to 20 mg.

*Adjust-a-dose:* For obese children, base dose on ideal body weight; high risk or debilitated children and children receiving other sedatives need lower doses.

*Induction of general anesthesia—*

**Adults over age 55:** 0.3 mg/kg I.V. over 20 to 30 seconds if patient hasn't received premedication, or 0.2 mg/kg I.V. over 20 to 30 seconds if patient has received sedative or narcotic premedication. Additional increments of 25% of initial dose may be needed to complete induction.

**Adults under age 55:** 0.3 to 0.35 mg/kg I.V. over 20 to 30 seconds if patient hasn't received premedication, or 0.25 mg/kg I.V. over 20 to 30 seconds if patient has received sedative or narcotic premedication. Additional increments of 25% of initial dose may be needed to complete induction.

*Adjust-a-dose:* For debilitated patients, initially, 0.2 to 0.25 mg/kg. As little as 0.15 mg/kg may be needed.

*Continuous infusion for sedation of intubated patients in the critical care setting—*

**Adults:** initially, 0.01 to 0.05 mg/kg may be given I.V. over several minutes, repeated at 10- to 15-minute intervals until adequate sedation is achieved. For maintenance of sedation, usual initial infusion rate is 0.02 to 0.10 mg/kg/hour. Higher loading dose or infusion rates may be needed in some patients. Use the lowest effective rate.

**Children:** initially, 0.05 to 0.2 mg/kg may be given I.V. over at least 2 to 3 minutes; then continuous infusion at rate of 0.06 to 0.12 mg/kg/hour. Increase or decrease infusion to maintain desired effect.

**Neonates under 32 weeks' gestational age:** initially, 0.03 mg/kg/hour. Adjust rate, p.r.n., using lowest possible rate.

**Neonates over age 32 weeks' gestational age:** initially, 0.06 mg/kg/hour. Adjust rate, p.r.n., using lowest possible rate.

**ADVERSE REACTIONS**

**CNS:** headache, oversedation, drowsiness, amnesia, involuntary movements, nystagmus, paradoxical behavior or excitement.

**CV:** variations in blood pressure and pulse rate.

**GI:** *nausea,* vomiting, *hiccups.*

**Respiratory:** *decreased respiratory rate,* APNEA.

**Other:** *pain at injection site.*

**INTERACTIONS**

**Drug-drug.** *CNS depressants:* may increase risk of apnea. Avoid concomitant use. Prepare to adjust dosage of midazolam if used with opiates or other CNS depressants.

*Erythromycin:* may alter metabolism of midazolam. Use with caution.

*Oral contraceptives:* prolonged half-life of midazolam. Use with caution.

*Theophylline:* sedative effects of midazolam may be antagonized by theophylline. Use with caution.

**Drug-lifestyle.** *Alcohol use:* may increase risk of apnea. Avoid concomitant use.

**EFFECTS ON DIAGNOSTIC TESTS**

None reported.

## CONTRAINDICATIONS
Contraindicated in patients with hypersensitivity to drug and in those with acute angle-closure glaucoma, shock, coma, or acute alcohol intoxication.

## NURSING CONSIDERATIONS
• Use cautiously in patients with uncompensated acute illness and in elderly or debilitated patients.
• *Alert:* Before administering, have oxygen and resuscitation equipment available in case of severe respiratory depression. Excessive dosage or rapid infusion has been associated with respiratory arrest. Continuously monitor patients who have received midazolam, including children who have received midazolam syrup, to detect potentially life-threatening respiratory depression.
• May be mixed in the same syringe with morphine sulfate, meperidine, atropine, or scopolamine.
• When injecting I.M., give deeply into a large muscle mass.
• Monitor blood pressure, heart rate and rhythm, respirations, airway integrity, and arterial oxygen saturation during procedure.
• *Alert:* Don't confuse Versed with VePesid.

### I.V. administration
• Administer slowly over at least 2 minutes, and wait at least 2 minutes when titrating doses to effect. When mixing infusion, use 5-mg/ml vial, dilute to a concentration of 0.5 mg/ml with $D_5W$ or normal saline.
• When administering I.V., take care to avoid extravasation.

### Patient teaching
• Because drug's beneficial amnesic effect diminishes patient's recall of perioperative events, provide written information, family member instruction, and follow-up contact to ensure that patient has adequate information.
• Warn patient to avoid hazardous activities that require alertness or good psychomotor coordination until CNS effects of drug are known.

• Tell patient to avoid alcohol while taking drug.

## oxazepam
Alepam‡, Apo-Oxazepam†, Murelax‡, Novoxapam†, Serax**, Serepax‡

*Controlled Substance Schedule IV*
*Pregnancy Risk Category D*

### HOW SUPPLIED
*Tablets, capsules:* 10 mg, 15 mg, 30 mg

### ACTION
Unknown. May stimulate gamma-aminobutyric acid receptors in the ascending reticular activating system.

| Route | Onset | Peak | Duration |
|-------|-------|------|----------|
| P.O. | Unknown | 3 hr | Unknown |

### INDICATIONS & DOSAGE
*Alcohol withdrawal, severe anxiety—*
**Adults:** 15 to 30 mg P.O. t.i.d. or q.i.d.
*Mild to moderate anxiety—*
**Adults:** 10 to 15 mg P.O. t.i.d. or q.i.d.
**Elderly:** initially, 10 mg t.i.d.; increased to 15 mg t.i.d. to q.i.d.

### ADVERSE REACTIONS
**CNS:** *drowsiness, lethargy,* dizziness, vertigo, headache, syncope, tremor, slurred speech, changes in EEG patterns.
**CV:** edema.
**GI:** nausea.
**Hepatic:** *hepatic dysfunction.*
**Skin:** rash.
**Other:** altered libido.

### INTERACTIONS
**Drug-drug.** *CNS depressants:* increased CNS depression. Avoid concomitant use.
*Digoxin:* may increase serum digoxin levels and risk of toxicity. Monitor patient closely.
**Drug-lifestyle.** *Alcohol use:* increased CNS depression. Avoid concomitant use.
*Smoking:* decreased effectiveness of benzodiazepines. Monitor patient closely.

### EFFECTS ON DIAGNOSTIC TESTS
None reported.

## CONTRAINDICATIONS
Contraindicated in patients with hypersensitivity to drug and in those with psychoses.

## NURSING CONSIDERATIONS
• Drug should be avoided during pregnancy, especially during first trimester.
• Use cautiously in elderly patients and in patients with history of drug abuse or in whom a decrease in blood pressure might lead to cardiac problems.
• Monitor liver, renal, and hematopoietic function studies periodically in patients receiving repeated or prolonged therapy, as ordered.
• *Alert:* Possibility of abuse and addiction exists. Don't stop drug abruptly because withdrawal symptoms may occur.
• *Alert:* Don't confuse oxazepam with oxaprozin.

☑ **Patient teaching**
• Warn patient to avoid hazardous activities that require alertness or good psychomotor coordination until CNS effects of drug are known.
• Tell patient to avoid alcohol while taking drug.
• Notify patient that smoking may decrease effectiveness of drug.
• Warn patient not to abruptly stop drug because withdrawal symptoms may occur.
• Caution woman to avoid use during pregnancy.

**chlorpromazine hydrochloride**
**clozapine**
**fluphenazine decanoate**
**fluphenazine enanthate**
**fluphenazine hydrochloride**
**haloperidol**
**haloperidol decanoate**
**haloperidol lactate**
**loxapine hydrochloride**
**loxapine succinate**
**mesoridazine besylate**
**molindone hydrochloride**
**olanzapine**
**perphenazine**
**pimozide**
**prochlorperazine**
(See Chapter 51, ANTIEMETICS.)
**quetiapine fumarate**
**risperidone**
**thioridazine hydrochloride**
**thiothixene**
**thiothixene hydrochloride**
**trifluoperazine hydrochloride**

## COMBINATION PRODUCTS
ETRAFON: perphenazine 2 mg and
amitriptyline hydrochloride 25 mg.
ETRAFON 2-10: perphenazine 2 mg and
amitriptyline hydrochloride 10 mg.
ETRAFON-A: perphenazine 4 mg and
amitriptyline hydrochloride 10 mg.
ETRAFON-FORTE: perphenazine 4 mg and
amitriptyline hydrochloride 25 mg.
TRIAVIL 2-10, TRIAVIL 4-10, TRIAVIL 2-25,
TRIAVIL 4-25 are identical to Etrafon
products above. Triavil also is available as
TRIAVIL 4-50 (perphenazine 4 mg and
amitriptyline hydrochloride 50 mg).

---

**chlorpromazine hydrochloride**
Chlorpromanyl-5†,
Chlorpromanyl-20†,
Chlorpromanyl-40†, Largactil†‡,
Novo-Chlorpromazine†,
Ormazine, Thorazine, Thor-Prom

*Pregnancy Risk Category C*

## HOW SUPPLIED
*Tablets:* 10 mg, 25 mg, 50 mg, 100 mg,
200 mg
*Capsules (extended-release):* 30 mg,
75 mg, 150 mg, 200 mg, 300 mg
*Oral concentrate:* 30 mg/ml, 100 mg/ml
*Syrup:* 10 mg/5 ml
*Injection:* 25 mg/ml
*Suppositories:* 25 mg, 100 mg

## ACTION
Unknown. An aliphatic phenothiazine that
probably blocks postsynaptic dopamine
and alpha receptors in the brain and inhibits the medullary chemoreceptor trigger zone.

| Route | Onset | Peak | Duration |
|-------|-------|------|----------|
| P.O. | 0.5-1 hr | Unknown | 4-6 hr |
| P.O. (extended) | 0.5-1 hr | Unknown | 10-12 hr |
| I.V. | Unknown | Unknown | Unknown |
| I.M. | Unknown | Unknown | Unknown |
| P.R. | > 1 hr | Unknown | 3-4 hr |

## INDICATIONS & DOSAGE
*Psychosis—*
**Adults:** 25 to 75 mg P.O. daily in two to
four divided doses. Dosage increased by
20 to 50 mg twice weekly until symptoms
are controlled. Up to 800 mg daily may be
needed in some patients. Or, 25 to 50 mg
I.M. q 1 to 4 hours, p.r.n. Subsequent I.M.
doses should be gradually increased over
several days to maximum of 400 mg q 4
to 6 hours. Switch to oral therapy as soon
as possible.
**Children ages 6 months and older:**
0.55 mg/kg P.O. q 4 to 6 hours or I.M. q 6
to 8 hours; or 1.1 mg/kg P.R. q 6 to 8
hours. Maximum I.M. dose in children
under age 5 or weighing less than 22.7 kg
(50 lb) is 40 mg. Maximum I.M. dose in
children ages 5 to 12 or weighing 22.7 to
45.5 kg (50 to 100 lb) is 75 mg.
*Nausea and vomiting—*
**Adults:** 10 to 25 mg P.O. q 4 to 6 hours,
p.r.n.; or 50 to 100 mg P.R. q 6 to 8 hours,
p.r.n.; or 25 mg I.M. initially. If no hy-

---

Reactions may be *common*, uncommon, *life-threatening*, or COMMON AND LIFE-THREATENING.

potension occurs, 25 to 50 mg I.M. q 3 to 4 hours may be given, p.r.n., until vomiting stops.

**Children ages 6 months and older:**
0.55 mg/kg P.O. q 4 to 6 hours or I.M. q 6 to 8 hours; or 1.1 mg/kg P.R. q 6 to 8 hours. Maximum I.M. dose in children under age 5 or weighing less than 22.7 kg is 40 mg. Maximum I.M. dose in children ages 5 to 12 or weighing 22.7 to 45.5 kg is 75 mg.

*Intractable hiccups, acute intermittent porphyria—*
**Adults:** 25 to 50 mg P.O. t.i.d. or q.i.d. If symptoms persist for 2 to 3 days, 25 to 50 mg I.M. For hiccups, if symptoms still persist, 25 to 50 mg diluted in 500 to 1,000 ml of normal saline solution and infused slowly with patient in supine position.

*Tetanus—*
**Adults:** 25 to 50 mg I.V. or I.M. t.i.d. or q.i.d.

**Children ages 6 months and older:**
0.55 mg/kg I.M. or I.V. q 6 to 8 hours. Maximum parenteral dose in children weighing less than 22.7 kg is 40 mg daily; for children weighing 22.7 to 45.5 kg, 75 mg, except in severe cases.

*Surgery—*
**Adults:** preoperatively, 25 to 50 mg P.O. 2 to 3 hours before surgery or 12.5 to 25 mg I.M. 1 to 2 hours before surgery; during surgery, 12.5 mg I.M., repeated in 30 minutes if needed, or fractional 2-mg doses I.V. at 2-minute intervals to maximum dose of 25 mg; postoperatively, 10 to 25 mg P.O. q 4 to 6 hours or 12.5 to 25 mg I.M., repeated in 1 hour, if needed.

**Children ages 6 months and older:** preoperatively, 0.55 mg/kg P.O. 2 to 3 hours before surgery or I.M. 1 to 2 hours before surgery; during surgery, 0.275 mg/kg I.M., repeated in 30 minutes if needed, or fractional 1-mg doses I.V. at 2-minute intervals to maximum of 0.275 mg/kg; may repeat fractional I.V. regimen in 30 minutes, if needed; postoperatively, 0.55 mg/kg P.O. or I.M. q 4 to 6 hours (oral dose) or 1 hour (I.M. dose), if needed and if hypotension doesn't occur.

**Elderly:** lower dosages are sufficient; dosage increments should be more gradual than in adults.

## ADVERSE REACTIONS
**CNS:** *extrapyramidal reactions,* drowsiness, *sedation,* **seizures,** *tardive dyskinesia,* pseudoparkinsonism, dizziness.
**CV:** *orthostatic hypotension,* tachycardia, quinidine-like ECG effects.
**EENT:** ocular changes, blurred vision, nasal congestion.
**GI:** *dry mouth, constipation,* nausea.
**GU:** *urine retention,* menstrual irregularities, gynecomastia, inhibited ejaculation, lactation, priapism.
**Hematologic:** **leukopenia, agranulocytosis,** eosinophilia, hemolytic anemia, **aplastic anemia, thrombocytopenia.**
**Hepatic:** jaundice, abnormal liver function test results.
**Skin:** *mild photosensitivity,* allergic reactions, *pain at I.M. injection site,* sterile abscess, skin pigmentation.
**Other:** **neuroleptic malignant syndrome. After abrupt withdrawal of long-term therapy:** gastritis, nausea, vomiting, dizziness, tremor.

## INTERACTIONS
**Drug-drug.** *Antacids:* inhibited absorption of oral phenothiazines. Separate antacid and phenothiazine doses by at least 2 hours.
*Anticholinergics including antidepressants, antiparkinsonians:* increased anticholinergic activity, aggravated parkinsonian symptoms. Use with caution.
*Anticonvulsants:* may lower seizure threshold. Monitor patient closely.
*Barbiturates, lithium:* may decrease phenothiazine effect. Observe patient.
*Centrally acting antihypertensives:* decreased antihypertensive effect. Monitor blood pressure.
*CNS depressants:* increased CNS depression. Avoid concomitant use.
*Electroconvulsive therapy, insulin:* may precipitate severe reactions. Monitor patient closely.
*Propranolol:* increased levels of both propranolol and chlorpromazine. Monitor patient closely.
*Warfarin:* decreased effect of oral anticoagulants. Monitor PT and INR.
**Drug-lifestyle.** *Alcohol use:* increased CNS depression. Avoid concomitant use.

---

*Liquid contains alcohol.   **May contain tartrazine.   †Canada   ‡Australia   §U.K.   ◇OTC

*Sun exposure:* photosensitivity reactions may occur. Take precautions.

## EFFECTS ON DIAGNOSTIC TESTS
Drug causes false-positive test results for urinary porphyrins, urobilinogen, amylase, and 5-hydroxyindoleacetic acid because of darkening of urine by metabolites; it also causes false-positive results in urine pregnancy tests using human chorionic gonadotropin.

## CONTRAINDICATIONS
Contraindicated in patients with hypersensitivity to drug and in those experiencing CNS depression, bone marrow suppression, subcortical damage, or coma.

## NURSING CONSIDERATIONS
• Use cautiously in elderly or debilitated patients and in patients with hepatic or renal disease, severe CV disease (may cause sudden decrease in blood pressure), respiratory disorders, hypocalcemia, glaucoma, or prostatic hyperplasia. Also use cautiously in those exposed to extreme heat or cold (including antipyretic therapy) or organophosphate insecticides
• Use cautiously in acutely ill or dehydrated children.
• Obtain baseline blood pressure measurements before starting therapy, and monitor regularly. Watch for orthostatic hypotension, especially with parenteral administration. Monitor blood pressure before and after I.M. administration; keep patient supine for 1 hour afterward and have him get up slowly.
• Slight yellowing of injection or concentrate is common and doesn't affect potency. Discard markedly discolored solutions.
• Give deeply I.M. only in upper outer quadrant of buttocks. Massage slowly afterward to prevent sterile abscess. Keep in mind that injection stings.
• Wear gloves when preparing solutions, and prevent any contact with skin and clothing. Oral liquid and parenteral forms can cause contact dermatitis.
• Protect liquid concentrate from light. Dilute with fruit juice, milk, or semisolid food just before administration.

• Monitor patient for tardive dyskinesia, which may occur after prolonged use. It may not appear until months or years later and may disappear spontaneously or persist for life, despite discontinuation of drug.
• *Alert:* Watch for symptoms of neuroleptic malignant syndrome (extrapyramidal effects, hyperthermia, autonomic disturbance), which is rare but commonly fatal. It isn't necessarily related to length of drug use or type of neuroleptic; however, more than 60% of affected patients are men.
• Monitor therapy with weekly bilirubin tests during first month, periodic blood tests (CBC and liver function), and ophthalmic tests (long-term use), as ordered.
• Don't withdraw drug abruptly unless necessitated by severe adverse reactions.
• Withhold dose and notify doctor if jaundice, symptoms of blood dyscrasia (fever, sore throat, infection, cellulitis, weakness), or persistent extrapyramidal reactions (longer than a few hours) develop, or if such reactions occur in children or pregnant women.
• *Alert:* Don't confuse chlorpromazine with chlorpropamide, a hypoglycemic. Make sure that any drug administered is appropriate for patient's treatment.
• *Alert:* Don't confuse chlorpromazine with clomipramine.

## I.V. administration
• For direct injection, drug may be diluted with normal saline for injection and administered into a large vein or through the tubing of a free-flowing I.V. solution. Don't exceed 1 mg/minute for adults or 0.5 mg/minute for children.
• Drug may be given as an intermittent I.V. infusion; dilute with 50 or 100 ml of a compatible solution and infuse over 30 minutes.
• Chlorpromazine is compatible with most common I.V. solutions, including $D_5W$, Ringer's injection, lactated Ringer's injection, and normal saline for injection.

## Patient teaching
• Warn patient to avoid activities that require alertness or good psychomotor coordination until CNS effects of drug are

known. Drowsiness and dizziness usually subside after first few weeks.

• Tell patient to avoid alcohol while taking drug.

• Have patient report signs of urine retention or constipation.

• Tell patient to use sunblock and to wear protective clothing to avoid photosensitivity reactions. Chlorpromazine causes higher incidence of photosensitivity than any other drug in its class.

• Tell patient to relieve dry mouth with sugarless gum or hard candy.

• Advise patient receiving drug parenterally to remain supine for 1 hour afterward and to rise slowly.

---

## clozapine
Clozaril

*Pregnancy Risk Category B*

### HOW SUPPLIED
*Tablets:* 25 mg, 100 mg

### ACTION
Unknown. Binds selectively to dopaminergic receptors (both $D_1$ and $D_2$) within the limbic system of the CNS and may interfere with adrenergic, cholinergic, histaminergic, and serotonergic receptors.

| Route | Onset | Peak | Duration |
|-------|-------|------|----------|
| P.O. | Unknown | 2.5 hr | 4-12 hr |

### INDICATIONS & DOSAGE
*Schizophrenia in severely ill patients unresponsive to other therapies—*
**Adults:** initially, 12.5 mg P.O. once daily or b.i.d., adjusted upward at 25 to 50 mg daily (if tolerated) to 300 to 450 mg daily by end of 2 weeks. Individual dosage is based on clinical response, patient tolerance, and adverse reactions. Subsequent dosage shouldn't be increased more than once or twice weekly, and shouldn't exceed 100 mg. Many patients respond to doses of 300 to 600 mg daily, but some may need as much as 900 mg daily. Don't exceed 900 mg daily.

### ADVERSE REACTIONS
**CNS:** *drowsiness, sedation,* **seizures,** *dizziness,* syncope, *vertigo,* headache, tremor, disturbed sleep or nightmares, restlessness, hypokinesia or akinesia, agitation, rigidity, akathisia, confusion, fatigue, insomnia, hyperkinesia, weakness, lethargy, ataxia, slurred speech, depression, myoclonus, anxiety.
**CV:** *tachycardia, hypotension,* hypertension, chest pain, ECG changes, orthostatic hypotension.
**EENT:** visual disturbances.
**GI:** dry mouth, *constipation,* nausea, vomiting, *excessive salivation,* heartburn, diarrhea.
**GU:** urinary abnormalities (urinary frequency or urgency, urine retention), incontinence, abnormal ejaculation.
**Hematologic:** *leukopenia,* **agranulocytosis.**
**Metabolic:** fever, weight gain.
**Musculoskeletal:** muscle pain or spasm, muscle weakness.
**Skin:** rash, diaphoresis.
**After abrupt withdrawal of long-term therapy:** possible abrupt recurrence of psychotic symptoms.

### INTERACTIONS
**Drug-drug.** *Anticholinergics:* may potentiate anticholinergic effects of clozapine. Avoid concomitant use. Monitor blood pressure.
*Antihypertensives:* may potentiate hypotensive effects. Monitor blood pressure.
*Bone marrow suppressants:* may increase bone marrow toxicity. Don't use together.
*Digoxin, warfarin, other highly protein-bound drugs:* may increase serum levels of these drugs. Monitor closely for adverse reactions.
*Psychoactive drugs:* may produce additive effects. Use together cautiously.
**Drug-herb.** *Nutmeg:* may reduce effectiveness of drug therapy. Avoid concomitant use.
**Drug-food.** *Caffeine-containing beverages:* may inhibit antipsychotic effects of clozapine. Monitor closely.
**Drug-lifestyle.** *Alcohol use:* increased CNS depression. Use cautiously.

---

## EFFECTS ON DIAGNOSTIC TESTS
None reported.

## CONTRAINDICATIONS
Contraindicated in patients with uncontrolled epilepsy, history of clozapine-induced agranulocytosis, WBC count below 3,500/mm³, severe CNS depression or coma, and myelosuppressive disorders. Also contraindicated in patients taking other drugs that suppress bone marrow function.

## NURSING CONSIDERATIONS
• Use cautiously in patients with prostatic hyperplasia or angle-closure glaucoma because drug has potent anticholinergic effects
• Use cautiously in patients with hepatic, renal, or cardiac disease or in those receiving general anesthesia.
• *Alert:* Clozapine carries significant risk of agranulocytosis. If possible, patients should receive at least two trials of drug therapy with a standard antipsychotic before clozapine therapy is initiated. Baseline WBC and differential counts are needed before therapy. Monitor WBC counts weekly for at least 4 weeks after clozapine therapy is discontinued, as ordered.
• When administering clozapine, ensure that WBC counts and blood tests are performed weekly and that no more than a 1-week supply of drug is dispensed for first 6 months of therapy. If WBC count is maintained at 3,000/mm³ or more and an absolute neutrophil count at 1,500/mm³ or more during first 6 months of continuous therapy, frequency of monitoring blood counts may be reduced to every other week.
• If WBC count drops below 3,500/mm³ after therapy is initiated or if it drops substantially from baseline, monitor patient closely for signs and symptoms of infection. If WBC count is 3,000 to 3,500/mm³ and granulocyte count is above 1,500/mm³, perform WBC and differential count twice weekly. If WBC count drops below 3,000/mm³ and granulocyte count drops below 1,500/mm³, interrupt therapy, notify doctor, and monitor patient for signs and symptoms of infec-

tion. Therapy may be restarted cautiously if WBC count returns to above 3,000/mm³ and granulocyte count returns to above 1,500/mm³. Continue monitoring WBC and differential counts twice weekly until WBC count exceeds 3,500/mm³, as ordered.
• If WBC count drops below 2,000/mm³ and granulocyte count drops below 1,000/mm³, patient may need protective isolation. If infection develops, prepare cultures according to institutional policy and administer antibiotics, as ordered. Bone marrow aspiration may be deemed necessary to assess bone marrow function. Future clozapine therapy is contraindicated in such situations.
• Seizures may occur, especially in patients receiving high doses.
• Some patients experience transient fevers (temperature above 100.4° F [38° C]), especially in the first 3 weeks of therapy. Monitor closely.
• If clozapine therapy must be discontinued, withdraw drug gradually (over 1- to 2-week period). However, changes in patient's medical condition (including development of leukopenia) may need abrupt discontinuation of drug. Monitor closely for recurrence of psychotic symptoms.
• If therapy is reinstated in patient withdrawn from drug, follow usual guidelines for dosage increase. However, reexposure of patient to drug may increase severity and risk of adverse reactions. If therapy was terminated because WBC counts were below 2,000/mm³ or granulocyte counts were below 1,000/mm³, don't expect drug to be continued.
• *Alert:* Don't confuse clozapine with Cloxapen or clofazimine.

### ☑ Patient teaching
• Tell patient about need for weekly blood tests to monitor for agranulocytosis. Advise him to report flulike symptoms, fever, sore throat, lethargy, malaise, or other signs of infection.
• Warn patient to avoid hazardous activities that require alertness and good psychomotor coordination while taking drug.
• Tell patient to check with doctor before taking alcohol or OTC drugs.

---

Reactions may be *common*, uncommon, *life-threatening*, or COMMON AND LIFE-THREATENING.

• Tell patient to rise slowly to avoid orthostatic hypotension.
• Inform patient that ice chips or sugarless candy or gum may help relieve dry mouth.

---

**fluphenazine decanoate**
Modecate†‡, Modecate Concentrate†, Prolixin Decanoate

**fluphenazine enanthate**
Moditen Enanthate†, Prolixin Enanthate

**fluphenazine hydrochloride**
Anatensol‡*, Apo-Fluphenazine†, Moditen HCl†, Moditen HCl-H.P.†, Permitil*†**, Permitil Concentrate, Prolixin*†**, Prolixin Concentrate

*Pregnancy Risk Category C*

---

## HOW SUPPLIED
**fluphenazine decanoate**
*Depot injection:* 25 mg/ml
**fluphenazine enanthate**
*Depot injection:* 25 mg/ml
**fluphenazine hydrochloride**
*Tablets:* 1 mg, 2.5 mg, 5 mg, 10 mg
*Oral concentrate:* 5 mg/ml (contains 1% alcohol)
*Elixir:* 2.5 mg/5 ml (with 14% alcohol)
*I.M. injection:* 2.5 mg/ml

## ACTION
Unknown. A piperazine phenothiazine that probably blocks postsynaptic dopamine, alpha-adrenergic, and cholinergic receptors in the brain.

| Route | Onset | Peak | Duration |
|---|---|---|---|
| P.O. | < 1 hr | 0.5 hr | 6-8 hr |
| I.M. (HCl) | < 1 hr | 1.5-2 hr | 6-8 hr |
| I.M. | 24-72 hr | Unknown | 1-6 wk |
| S.C. | Unknown | Unknown | Unknown |

## INDICATIONS & DOSAGE
*Psychotic disorders—*
**Adults:** initially, 0.5 to 10 mg fluphenazine hydrochloride P.O. daily in divided doses q 6 to 8 hours; may increase cautiously to 20 mg. Higher doses (50 to 100 mg) have been given. Mainte-

nance dose is 1 to 5 mg P.O. daily. I.M. doses are one-third to one-half of oral doses. Usual I.M. dose is 1.25 mg. Use doses above 10 mg/day with caution.
Or, 12.5 to 25 mg of long-acting esters (decanoate or enanthate) I.M. or S.C. q 1 to 6 weeks; maintenance dose is 25 to 100 mg, p.r.n.
**Elderly:** use lower dosages for elderly patients (1 to 2.5 mg daily).

## ADVERSE REACTIONS
**CNS:** *extrapyramidal reactions, tardive dyskinesia,* sedation, pseudoparkinsonism, EEG changes, drowsiness, *seizures,* dizziness.
**CV:** orthostatic hypotension, tachycardia, ECG changes.
**EENT:** ocular changes, *blurred vision,* nasal congestion.
**GI:** *dry mouth, constipation.*
**GU:** *urine retention,* dark urine, menstrual irregularities, gynecomastia, inhibited ejaculation.
**Hematologic:** *leukopenia, agranulocytosis,* eosinophilia, hemolytic anemia, *aplastic anemia, thrombocytopenia.*
**Hepatic:** cholestatic jaundice, abnormal liver function test results.
**Metabolic:** weight gain, increased appetite, elevated test results for protein-bound iodine.
**Skin:** *mild photosensitivity,* allergic reactions.
**After abrupt withdrawal of long-term therapy:** gastritis, nausea, vomiting, dizziness, tremor, feeling of warmth or cold, diaphoresis, tachycardia, headache, insomnia.

## INTERACTIONS
**Drug-drug.** *Antacids:* inhibited absorption of oral phenothiazines. Separate antacid and phenothiazine doses by at least 2 hours.
*Anticholinergics:* increased anticholinergic effects. Avoid concomitant use.
*Barbiturates, lithium:* may decrease phenothiazine effect. Observe patient.
*Centrally acting antihypertensives:* decreased antihypertensive effect. Monitor blood pressure.
*CNS depressants:* increased CNS depression. Avoid concomitant use.

---

**Drug-lifestyle.** *Alcohol use:* increased CNS depression. Avoid concomitant use. *Sun exposure:* photosensitivity reactions may occur. Take precautions.

## EFFECTS ON DIAGNOSTIC TESTS
Drug causes false-positive test results for urinary porphyrins, urobilinogen, amylase, and 5-hydroxyindoleacetic acid because of darkening of urine by metabolites; it also causes false-positive urine pregnancy test results using human chorionic gonadotropin.

## CONTRAINDICATIONS
Contraindicated in patients with hypersensitivity to drug and in those experiencing CNS depression, coma, bone marrow suppression or other blood dyscrasia, subcortical damage, or liver damage.

## NURSING CONSIDERATIONS
• Use cautiously in elderly or debilitated patients and in those with pheochromocytoma, severe CV disease (may cause sudden drop in blood pressure), peptic ulcer, respiratory disorder, hypocalcemia, seizure disorder (may lower seizure threshold), severe reactions to insulin or electroconvulsive therapy, mitral insufficiency, glaucoma, or prostatic hyperplasia. Also use cautiously in those exposed to extreme heat or cold (including antipyretic therapy) or phosphorus insecticides. Use parenteral form cautiously in asthmatic patients and in those allergic to sulfites.
• Prolixin Concentrate and Permitil Concentrate are 10 times more concentrated than Prolixin elixir (5 mg/ml versus 0.5 mg/ml). Check dosage order carefully.
• Dilute liquid concentrate with water, fruit juice, milk, or semisolid food just before administration.
• For long-acting forms (decanoate and enanthate), which are oil preparations, use a dry needle of at least 21G. Allow 24 to 96 hours for onset of action. Note and report adverse reactions in patients taking these drug forms.
• Oral liquid and parenteral forms can cause contact dermatitis. Wear gloves when preparing solutions, and prevent contact with skin and clothing.

• Protect medication from light. Slight yellowing of injection or concentrate is common and doesn't affect potency. Discard markedly discolored solutions.
• Monitor patient for tardive dyskinesia, which may occur after prolonged use. It may not appear until months or years later and disappear spontaneously or persist for life, despite discontinuation of drug.
• *Alert:* Watch for symptoms of neuroleptic malignant syndrome (extrapyramidal effects, hyperthermia, autonomic disturbance), which is rare but frequently fatal. It isn't necessarily related to length of drug use or type of neuroleptic; however, more than 60% of affected patients are men.
• Monitor therapy with weekly bilirubin tests during first month, periodic blood tests (CBC and liver function), and periodic renal function and ophthalmic tests (long-term use), as ordered.
• Don't withdraw drug abruptly unless serious adverse reactions occur.
• Withhold dose and notify doctor if symptoms of blood dyscrasia (fever, sore throat, infection, cellulitis, weakness) or persistent extrapyramidal reactions (longer than a few hours) develop, especially in children or pregnant women.

### ✓ Patient teaching
• Warn patient to avoid activities that require alertness and good psychomotor coordination until CNS effects of drug are known. Drowsiness and dizziness usually subside after first few weeks.
• Warn patient to avoid alcohol while taking drug.
• Tell patient to relieve dry mouth with sugarless gum or hard candy.
• Have patient report signs of urine retention or constipation.
• Advise patient to use sunblock and to wear protective clothing to avoid photosensitivity reactions.
• Tell patient that drug may discolor urine.

---

Reactions may be *common*, uncommon, *life-threatening*, or COMMON AND LIFE-THREATENING.

# haloperidol
Apo-Haloperidol†, Dozic§,
Haldol**, Novo-Peridol†, Peridol†,
Serenace§‡

# haloperidol decanoate
Haldol Decanoate, Haldol LA†

# haloperidol lactate
Haldol, Haldol Concentrate,
Haloperidol Injection, Haloperidol
Intensol

*Pregnancy Risk Category C*

## HOW SUPPLIED
**haloperidol**
*Tablets:* 0.5 mg, 1 mg, 2 mg, 5 mg,
10 mg, 20 mg
**haloperidol decanoate**
*Injection:* 50 mg/ml, 100 mg/ml
**haloperidol lactate**
*Oral concentrate:* 2 mg/ml
*Injection:* 5 mg/ml

## ACTION
Unknown. A butyrophenone that probably
exerts its antipsychotic effects by blocking postsynaptic dopamine receptors in
the brain.

| Route | Onset | Peak | Duration |
|-------|-------|------|----------|
| P.O. | Unknown | 3-6 hr | Unknown |
| I.M. (decanoate) | Unknown | 3-9 days | Unknown |
| I.M. (lactate) | Unknown | 10-20 min | Unknown |

## INDICATIONS & DOSAGE
*Psychotic disorders—*
**Adults and children ages 12 and older:**
dosage varies for each patient. Initial
range, 0.5 to 5 mg P.O. b.i.d. or t.i.d.; or 2
to 5 mg I.M. q 4 to 8 hours, although
hourly administration may be needed until
control obtained. Maximum dose is
100 mg P.O. daily.
**Children ages 3 to 12:** 0.05 mg/kg to
0.15 mg/kg P.O. daily. Severely disturbed
children may need higher doses.
*Chronic psychotic patients who need pro-
longed therapy—*

**Adults:** 50 to 100 mg I.M. decanoate q 4
weeks.
*Nonpsychotic behavior disorders—*
**Children ages 3 to 12:** 0.05 mg/kg P.O.
daily. Maximum daily dose is 6 mg.
*Tourette syndrome—*
**Adults:** 0.5 to 5 mg P.O. b.i.d. or t.i.d., or
p.r.n.
**Children ages 3 to 12:** 0.05 to
0.075 mg/kg P.O. daily in two or three divided doses.
**Elderly:** 0.5 to 2 mg P.O. b.i.d. or t.i.d.,
increased gradually, p.r.n.
*Adjust-a-dose:* For debilitated patients,
use 0.5 to 2 mg P.O. b.i.d. or t.i.d., increased gradually, p.r.n.

## ADVERSE REACTIONS
**CNS:** *severe extrapyramidal reactions,
tardive dyskinesia,* sedation, drowsiness,
lethargy, headache, insomnia, confusion,
vertigo, *seizures.*
**CV:** tachycardia, hypotension, hyperten-
sion, ECG changes.
**EENT:** blurred vision.
**GI:** dry mouth, anorexia, constipation, di-
arrhea, nausea, vomiting, dyspepsia.
**GU:** urine retention, menstrual irregulari-
ties, gynecomastia, priapism.
**Hematologic:** *leukopenia,* leukocytosis.
**Hepatic:** altered liver function test re-
sults, jaundice.
**Skin:** rash, other skin reactions, diaphore-
sis.
**Other:** *neuroleptic malignant syndrome.*

## INTERACTIONS
**Drug-drug.** *Anticholinergics:* increased
anticholinergic effects, glaucoma. Avoid
concomitant use.
*CNS depressants:* increased CNS depres-
sion. Avoid concomitant use.
*Lithium:* lethargy and confusion after
high doses. Monitor patient.
**Drug-herb.** *Nutmeg:* may reduce effec-
tiveness or interfere with drug therapy.
Avoid concomitant use.
**Drug-lifestyle.** *Alcohol use:* increased
CNS depression. Avoid concomitant use.

## EFFECTS ON DIAGNOSTIC TESTS
None reported.

---

*Liquid contains alcohol.   **May contain tartrazine.   †Canada   ‡Australia   §U.K.   ◇OTC

## CONTRAINDICATIONS
Contraindicated in patients with hypersensitivity to drug and in those experiencing parkinsonism, coma, or CNS depression.

## NURSING CONSIDERATIONS
• Use cautiously in elderly and debilitated patients; in patients with history of seizures or EEG abnormalities, severe CV disorders, allergies, glaucoma, or urine retention; also use cautiously with anticonvulsants, anticoagulants, antiparkinsonians, or lithium.
• *Alert:* Don't administer decanoate form I.V.
• When changing from tablets to decanoate injection, patient should be given 10 to 15 times the oral dose once a month (maximum 100 mg).
• Protect drug from light. Slight yellowing of injection or concentrate is common and doesn't affect potency. Discard markedly discolored solutions.
• Don't withdraw drug abruptly unless required by severe adverse reactions.
• Monitor patient for tardive dyskinesia, which may occur after prolonged use. It may not appear until months or years later and disappear spontaneously or persist for life, despite discontinuation of drug.
• *Alert:* Watch for symptoms of neuroleptic malignant syndrome (extrapyramidal effects, hyperthermia, autonomic disturbance), which is rare but frequently fatal. It isn't necessarily related to length of drug use or type of neuroleptic; however, more than 60% of affected patients are men.
• Dilute dose with water or a beverage, such as orange juice, apple juice, tomato juice, or cola, immediately before administration.
• *Alert:* Don't confuse Haldol with Halcion or Halog.

☑ **Patient teaching**
• Although drug is the least sedating of the antipsychotics, warn patient to avoid activities that require alertness and good psychomotor coordination until CNS effects of drug are known. Drowsiness and dizziness usually subside after a few weeks.

• Warn patient to avoid alcohol while taking drug.
• Advise patient to relieve dry mouth with sugarless gum or hard candy.

---

## loxapine hydrochloride
Loxapac†, Loxitane C, Loxitane IM

## loxapine succinate
Loxapac†, Loxitane

*Pregnancy Risk Category NR*

## HOW SUPPLIED
**loxapine hydrochloride**
*Oral concentrate:* 25 mg/ml
*Injection:* 50 mg/ml
**loxapine succinate**
*Tablets:* 5 mg†, 10 mg†, 25 mg†, 50 mg†
*Capsules:* 5 mg, 10 mg, 25 mg, 50 mg

## ACTION
Unknown. A dibenzoxazepine that probably exerts its antipsychotic effects by blocking postsynaptic dopamine receptors in the brain.

| Route | Onset | Peak | Duration |
|---|---|---|---|
| P.O., I.M. | 30 min | 1.5-3 hr | 12 hr |

## INDICATIONS & DOSAGE
*Psychotic disorders—*
**Adults:** 10 mg P.O. b.i.d. to q.i.d., rapidly increasing to 60 to 100 mg P.O. daily for most patients; dosage varies among patients. If patient is unable to take oral dose, give 12.5 to 50 mg I.M. q 4 to 6 hours or longer, dosage and interval depending on patient response. Dosages exceeding 250 mg/day aren't recommended.
**Elderly:** initially, 3 to 5 mg P.O. b.i.d.

## ADVERSE REACTIONS
**CNS:** *extrapyramidal reactions, sedation,* drowsiness, **seizures,** numbness, confusion, syncope, *tardive dyskinesia,* pseudoparkinsonism, EEG changes, dizziness.
**CV:** orthostatic hypotension, tachycardia, ECG changes, hypertension.
**EENT:** *blurred vision,* nasal congestion.

---

**GI:** *dry mouth, constipation,* nausea, vomiting, paralytic ileus.
**GU:** *urine retention,* menstrual irregularities, gynecomastia.
**Hematologic:** *leukopenia, agranulocytosis, thrombocytopenia.*
**Hepatic:** elevated test results for liver enzymes, jaundice.
**Metabolic:** elevated test results for protein-bound iodine, weight gain.
**Skin:** *mild photosensitivity,* allergic reactions, rash, pruritus.

## INTERACTIONS
**Drug-drug.** *CNS depressants:* increased CNS depression. Avoid concomitant use.
**Drug-lifestyle.** *Alcohol use:* increased CNS depression. Avoid concomitant use.

## EFFECTS ON DIAGNOSTIC TESTS
Loxapine causes false-positive test results for urinary porphyrins, urobilinogen, amylase, and 5-hydroxyindoleacetic acid because of darkening of urine by metabolites; it also causes false-positive urine pregnancy test results using human chorionic gonadotropin.

## CONTRAINDICATIONS
Contraindicated in patients with hypersensitivity to dibenzoxazepines and in those experiencing coma, severe CNS depression, or drug-induced depressed states.

## NURSING CONSIDERATIONS
• Use with extreme caution in patients with seizure disorder, CV disorder, glaucoma, or history of urine retention.
• Obtain baseline blood pressure measurements before starting therapy, and monitor regularly.
• Dilute liquid concentrate with orange or grapefruit juice just before giving.
• Monitor patient for tardive dyskinesia, which may occur after prolonged use. It may not appear until months or years later, and may disappear spontaneously or persist for life, despite discontinuation of drug.
• *Alert:* Watch for symptoms of neuroleptic malignant syndrome (extrapyramidal effects, hyperthermia, autonomic disturbance), which is rare but frequently fatal.

It isn't necessarily related to length of drug use or type of neuroleptic; however, more than 60% of affected patients are men.

☑ **Patient teaching**
• Warn patient to avoid activities that require alertness and good psychomotor coordination until CNS effects of drug are known. Drowsiness and dizziness usually subside after first few weeks.
• Advise patient to report bruising, fever, or sore throat immediately.
• Tell patient to avoid alcohol while taking drug.
• Advise patient to get up slowly to avoid orthostatic hypotension.
• Tell patient to relieve dry mouth with sugarless gum or hard candy.
• Inform patient that periodic eye examinations are recommended.

## mesoridazine besylate
Serentil*, Serentil Concentrate

*Pregnancy Risk Category NR*

## HOW SUPPLIED
*Tablets:* 10 mg, 25 mg, 50 mg, 100 mg
*Oral concentrate:* 25 mg/ml (0.6% alcohol)
*Injection:* 25 mg/ml

## ACTION
Unknown. A piperidine phenothiazine and the major sulfoxide metabolite of thioridazine that probably exerts its antipsychotic effects by blocking postsynaptic dopamine receptors in the brain.

| Route | Onset | Peak | Duration |
|-------|-------|------|----------|
| P.O., I.M. | Unknown | Unknown | Unknown |

## INDICATIONS & DOSAGE
*Alcoholism—*
**Adults and children over age 12:** 25 mg P.O. b.i.d. to maximum of 200 mg daily.
*Behavior problems associated with chronic organic mental syndrome—*
**Adults and children over age 12:** 25 mg P.O. t.i.d. to maximum of 300 mg daily.

*Psychoneurotic manifestations (anxiety)—*
**Adults and children over age 12:** 10 mg P.O. t.i.d. to maximum of 150 mg daily.
*Schizophrenia—*
**Adults and children over age 12:** initially, 50 mg P.O. t.i.d. or 25 mg I.M. repeated in 30 to 60 minutes, p.r.n. Maximum oral dose is 400 mg daily; maximum daily I.M. dose is 200 mg.

## ADVERSE REACTIONS

**CNS:** *extrapyramidal reactions, tardive dyskinesia, sedation,* drowsiness, tremor, rigidity, weakness, EEG changes, dizziness.
**CV:** *hypotension,* tachycardia, ECG changes.
**EENT:** *ocular changes, blurred vision,* retinitis pigmentosa, nasal congestion.
**GI:** *dry mouth, constipation,* nausea, vomiting.
**GU:** *urine retention,* menstrual irregularities, gynecomastia, inhibited ejaculation.
**Hematologic:** *leukopenia, agranulocytosis, aplastic anemia,* eosinophilia, *thrombocytopenia.*
**Hepatic:** jaundice, abnormal liver function test results.
**Metabolic:** weight gain, elevated test results for protein-bound iodine.
**Skin:** *mild photosensitivity,* allergic reactions, pain at I.M. injection site, sterile abscess, rash.
**After abrupt withdrawal of long-term therapy:** gastritis, nausea, vomiting, dizziness, tremor, feeling of warmth or cold, diaphoresis, tachycardia, headache, insomnia.

## INTERACTIONS

**Drug-drug.** *Antacids:* inhibited absorption of oral phenothiazines. Separate antacid and phenothiazine doses by at least 2 hours.
*Anticholinergics:* may increase anticholinergic effects. Use together cautiously.
*Barbiturates:* may decrease phenothiazine effect. Observe patient.
*CNS depressants:* increased CNS depression. Use together cautiously.
**Drug-lifestyle.** *Alcohol use:* increased CNS depression. Avoid concomitant use.

*Sun exposure:* photosensitivity reactions may occur. Take precautions.

## EFFECTS ON DIAGNOSTIC TESTS

Drug causes false-positive test results for urinary porphyrins, urobilinogen, amylase, and 5-hydroxyindoleacetic acid because of darkening of urine by metabolites; it also causes false-positive urine pregnancy test results using human chorionic gonadotropin.

## CONTRAINDICATIONS

Contraindicated in patients with hypersensitivity to drug and in those experiencing severe CNS depression or coma.

## NURSING CONSIDERATIONS

• Obtain baseline blood pressure measurements before starting therapy and monitor regularly. Watch for orthostatic hypotension, especially with parenteral administration.
• Oral liquid and parenteral forms may cause contact dermatitis. Wear gloves when preparing solutions, and prevent contact with skin and clothing.
• Give deeply I.M. only in upper outer quadrant of buttocks. Massage slowly afterward to prevent sterile abscess. Keep in mind that injection may sting.
• Protect drug from light. Slight yellowing of injection or concentrate is common and doesn't affect potency. Discard markedly discolored solutions.
• Monitor patient for tardive dyskinesia, which may occur after prolonged use. It may not appear until months or years later, and may disappear spontaneously or persist for life, despite discontinuation of drug.
• *Alert:* Watch for symptoms of neuroleptic malignant syndrome (extrapyramidal effects, hyperthermia, autonomic disturbance), which is rare but frequently fatal. It isn't necessarily related to length of drug use or type of neuroleptic; however, more than 60% of affected patients are men.
• Withhold dose and notify doctor if jaundice, symptoms of blood dyscrasia (fever, sore throat, infection, cellulitis, weakness), or persistent extrapyramidal reac-

---

Reactions may be *common,* uncommon, *life-threatening*, or COMMON AND LIFE-THREATENING.

tions (longer than a few hours) develop, especially in children or pregnant women.
• Monitor therapy with weekly bilirubin tests during first month, periodic blood tests (CBC and liver function), and ophthalmic tests (long-term use), as ordered.
• Don't withdraw drug abruptly unless required by severe adverse reactions.
• *Alert:* Don't confuse Serentil with Serevent or Aventyl.

### ☑ Patient teaching
• Warn patient to avoid activities that require alertness and good psychomotor coordination until CNS effects of drug are known. Drowsiness and dizziness usually subside after a few weeks.
• Advise patient to change position slowly.
• Warn patient to avoid alcohol while taking drug.
• Have patient report signs of urine retention or constipation.
• Tell patient that drug may discolor urine.
• Instruct patient to relieve dry mouth with sugarless gum or hard candy.
• Advise patient to use sunblock and to wear protective clothing to avoid photosensitivity reactions.

---

## molindone hydrochloride
Moban

*Pregnancy Risk Category C*

### HOW SUPPLIED
*Tablets:* 5 mg, 10 mg, 25 mg, 50 mg, 100 mg
*Oral solution:* 20 mg/ml

### ACTION
Unknown. A dihydroindolone that probably blocks postsynaptic dopamine receptors in the brain.

| Route | Onset | Peak | Duration |
|-------|-------|------|----------|
| P.O. | Unknown | 1.5 hr | 24-36 hr |

### INDICATIONS & DOSAGE
*Psychotic disorders—*
**Adults:** initially, 50 to 75 mg P.O. daily; then increased to 100 to 225 mg/day in 3

or 4 days. Maintenance dose as follows: mild severity—5 to 15 mg P.O. t.i.d. to q.i.d.; moderate severity—10 to 25 mg P.O. t.i.d. or q.i.d.; acute severity—225 mg/day P.O.

### ADVERSE REACTIONS
**CNS:** *extrapyramidal reactions, tardive dyskinesia, sedation,* drowsiness, depression, euphoria, pseudoparkinsonism, EEG changes, dizziness.
**CV:** *orthostatic hypotension,* tachycardia, ECG changes.
**EENT:** *blurred vision.*
**GI:** *dry mouth, constipation,* nausea.
**GU:** *urine retention,* elevated BUN, menstrual irregularities, gynecomastia, inhibited ejaculation.
**Hematologic:** *leukopenia*, leukocytosis.
**Hepatic:** jaundice, abnormal liver function test results.
**Metabolic:** elevated free fatty acid levels, possible increase or decrease in serum glucose levels.
**Skin:** *mild photosensitivity,* allergic reactions.

### INTERACTIONS
**Drug-drug.** *CNS depressants:* increased CNS depression. Avoid concomitant use.
**Drug-lifestyle.** *Alcohol use:* increased CNS depression. Avoid concomitant use.

### EFFECTS ON DIAGNOSTIC TESTS
Drug causes false-positive results in urine pregnancy tests using human chorionic gonadotropin and enhances potential for causing seizures with metrizamide myelography.

### CONTRAINDICATIONS
Contraindicated in patients with hypersensitivity to drug and in those experiencing coma or severe CNS depression.

### NURSING CONSIDERATIONS
• Use cautiously when increased physical activity would be harmful because drug may cause hyperactivity. Also use cautiously in patients subject to seizures (may lower seizure threshold).
• Monitor patient for tardive dyskinesia, which may occur after prolonged use. It may not appear until months or years lat-

---

er, and may disappear spontaneously or persist for life, despite discontinuation of drug.

• *Alert:* Watch for symptoms of neuroleptic malignant syndrome (extrapyramidal effects, hyperthermia, autonomic disturbance), which is rare but frequently fatal. It isn't necessarily related to length of drug use or type of neuroleptic; however, more than 60% of affected patients are men.

• *Alert:* Don't confuse Moban with Mobidin.

### ☑ Patient teaching
• Warn patient to avoid activities that require alertness or good psychomotor coordination until CNS effects of drug are known. Drowsiness and dizziness usually subside after first few weeks.

• Tell patient to avoid alcohol while taking drug.

• Advise patient to relieve dry mouth with sugarless gum or hard candy.

## olanzapine
Zyprexa

*Pregnancy Risk Category C*

### HOW SUPPLIED
*Tablets:* 5 mg, 7.5 mg, 10 mg

### ACTION
Unknown. Binds to dopamine and serotonin receptors; may antagonize adrenergic, cholinergic, and histaminergic receptors.

| Route | Onset | Peak | Duration |
|-------|-------|------|----------|
| P.O. | Unknown | 6 hr | Unknown |

### INDICATIONS & DOSAGE
*Psychotic disorders—*
**Adults:** initially, 5 to 10 mg P.O. once daily. Dosage adjustments in 5-mg daily increments should occur at intervals of not less than 1 week. Most patients respond to dosages of 10 mg/day. Don't exceed 20 mg/day.
*Adjust-a-dose:* For patients who are debilitated, predisposed to hypotension, or have an alteration in metabolism due to

smoking status, sex, or age, or who are pharmacologically sensitive to drug, 5 mg initially.

### ADVERSE REACTIONS
**CNS:** *somnolence, agitation, insomnia, headache, nervousness, hostility,* parkinsonism, *dizziness,* anxiety, personality disorder, akathisia, hypertonia, tremor, amnesia, articulation impairment, euphoria, stuttering, tardive dyskinesia.
**CV:** orthostatic hypotension, tachycardia, chest pain, hypotension, edema.
**EENT:** amblyopia, blepharitis, corneal lesion, *rhinitis,* pharyngitis.
**GI:** constipation, dry mouth, abdominal pain, increased appetite, increased salivation, nausea, vomiting, thirst.
**GU:** premenstrual syndrome, hematuria, metrorrhagia, urinary incontinence, urinary tract infection.
**Hematologic:** asymptomatic increases in eosinophil count.
**Hepatic:** asymptomatic increases in AST, ALT, and GGT levels.
**Metabolic:** weight gain or loss, fever, asymptomatic increases in CK and serum prolactin levels.
**Musculoskeletal:** joint pain, extremity pain, back pain, neck rigidity, twitching.
**Respiratory:** increased cough, dyspnea.
**Skin:** vesiculobullous rash.

### INTERACTIONS
**Drug-drug.** *Antihypertensives:* may potentiate hypotensive effects. Monitor blood pressure closely.
*Carbamazepine, omeprazole, rifampin:* increased clearance of olanzapine. Monitor patient.
*Diazepam:* increased CNS effects. Monitor closely.
*Dopamine agonists, levodopa:* antagonized activity of these drugs. Monitor patient.
**Drug-herb.** *Nutmeg:* may reduce effectiveness or interfere with drug therapy. Avoid concomitant use.
**Drug-lifestyle.** *Alcohol use:* increased CNS effects. Avoid concomitant use.

### EFFECTS ON DIAGNOSTIC TESTS
None reported.

---

Reactions may be *common,* uncommon, *life-threatening,* or COMMON AND LIFE-THREATENING.

## CONTRAINDICATIONS
Contraindicated in patients with hypersensitivity to drug.

## NURSING CONSIDERATIONS
• Use cautiously in patients with heart disease, cerebrovascular disease, conditions that predispose patient to hypotension, history of seizures or conditions that might lower the seizure threshold, and hepatic impairment. Also use cautiously in elderly patients, those with a history of paralytic ileus, and those at risk for aspiration pneumonia, prostatic hyperplasia, or angle-closure glaucoma.
• Drug should be used in pregnancy only if benefit justifies potential risk to the fetus. Women taking drug shouldn't breastfeed.
• Safety and effectiveness of drug in patients under age 18 haven't been established.
• *Alert:* Watch for symptoms of neuroleptic malignant syndrome (hyperpyrexia, muscle rigidity, altered mental status, autonomic instability), which is rare but frequently fatal. Drug should be stopped immediately and patient monitored and treated as needed.
• Monitor patient for tardive dyskinesia, which may occur after prolonged use. It may not appear until months or years later, and may disappear spontaneously or persist for life, despite discontinuation of drug.
• Obtain baseline and periodic liver function tests, as ordered.
• *Alert:* Don't confuse olanzapine with olsalazine, or Zyprexa with Zyrtec.

### ☑ Patient teaching
• Warn patient to avoid hazardous tasks until adverse CNS effects of drug are known.
• Warn patient against exposure to extreme heat; drug may impair the body's ability to reduce core temperature.
• Tell patient to avoid alcohol.
• Tell patient to rise slowly to avoid orthostatic hypotension.
• Instruct patient to relieve dry mouth with ice chips or sugarless candy or gum.
• Advise woman to notify doctor if she becomes pregnant or intends to become pregnant during drug therapy. Advise her not to breast-feed during therapy.

---

## perphenazine
Apo-Perphenazine†, Fentazin§, PMS Perphenazine†, Trilafon, Trilafon Concentrate

*Pregnancy Risk Category NR*

## HOW SUPPLIED
*Tablets:* 2 mg, 4 mg, 8 mg, 16 mg
*Oral concentrate:* 16 mg/5 ml
*Syrup:* 2 mg/5 ml†
*Injection:* 5 mg/ml

## ACTION
Unknown. Probably exerts its antipsychotic effects by blocking postsynaptic dopamine receptors in the brain; inhibits the medullary chemoreceptor trigger zone.

| Route | Onset | Peak | Duration |
|---|---|---|---|
| P.O., I.M., I.V. | Unknown | Unknown | Unknown |

## INDICATIONS & DOSAGE
*Psychosis in nonhospitalized patients—*
**Adults and children over age 12:** initially, 4 to 8 mg P.O. t.i.d., reduced as soon as possible to minimum effective dose.
*Psychosis in hospitalized patients—*
**Adults and children over age 12:** initially, 8 to 16 mg P.O. b.i.d., t.i.d., or q.i.d., increased to 64 mg daily, p.r.n. Or, 5 to 10 mg I.M. q 6 hours, p.r.n. Maximum dose is 30 mg.
*Severe nausea and vomiting—*
**Adults:** 8 to 16 mg P.O. daily in divided doses to maximum of 24 mg. Or, 5 to 10 mg I.M., p.r.n. May be given I.V., diluted to 0.5 mg/ml with saline solution. I.V. dose shouldn't exceed 5 mg.

## ADVERSE REACTIONS
**CNS:** *extrapyramidal reactions, tardive dyskinesia,* sedation, pseudoparkinsonism, dizziness, *seizures,* drowsiness.
**CV:** *orthostatic hypotension,* tachycardia, ECG changes.
**EENT:** ocular changes, *blurred vision,* nasal congestion.

---

*Liquid contains alcohol.  **May contain tartrazine.  †Canada  ‡Australia  §U.K.  ◇OTC

**GI:** *dry mouth, constipation,* nausea, vomiting, diarrhea.
**GU:** *urine retention,* dark urine, menstrual irregularities, gynecomastia, inhibited ejaculation.
**Hematologic:** *leukopenia, agranulocytosis,* eosinophilia, *hemolytic anemia, thrombocytopenia.*
**Hepatic:** elevated liver enzymes test results, jaundice.
**Metabolic:** weight gain, elevated protein-bound iodine test results.
**Skin:** *mild photosensitivity,* allergic reactions, pain at I.M. injection site, sterile abscess.
**Other:** *neuroleptic malignant syndrome.* **After abrupt withdrawal of long-term therapy:** gastritis, nausea, vomiting, dizziness, tremor, feeling of warmth or cold, diaphoresis, tachycardia, headache, insomnia.

## INTERACTIONS
**Drug-drug.** *Antacids:* inhibited absorption of oral phenothiazines. Separate antacid and phenothiazine doses by at least 2 hours.
*Barbiturates:* may decrease phenothiazine effect. Observe patient.
*CNS depressants:* increased CNS depression. Avoid concomitant use.
**Drug-lifestyle.** *Alcohol use:* increased CNS depression. Avoid concomitant use.
*Sun exposure:* photosensitivity reactions may occur. Take precautions.

## EFFECTS ON DIAGNOSTIC TESTS
Drug causes false-positive test results for urinary porphyrins, urobilinogen, amylase, and 5-hydroxyindoleacetic acid because of darkening of urine by metabolites; it also causes false-positive urine pregnancy test results using human chorionic gonadotropin.

## CONTRAINDICATIONS
Contraindicated in patients with hypersensitivity to drug and in those with CNS depression, blood dyscrasia, bone marrow depression, liver damage, or subcortical damage; also contraindicated in those experiencing coma or receiving large doses of CNS depressants.

## NURSING CONSIDERATIONS
• Use cautiously with other CNS depressants or anticholinergics, and in elderly or debilitated patients.
• Use cautiously in patients with alcohol withdrawal, psychic depression, suicidal tendency, severe adverse reactions to other phenothiazines, impaired renal function, CV disease, or respiratory disorders.
• Obtain baseline blood pressure measurements before starting therapy and monitor regularly. Watch for orthostatic hypotension, especially with parenteral administration. Keep patient supine for 1 hour after administration of drug; tell him to change positions slowly.
• Prevent contact dermatitis by keeping drug away from skin and clothes. Wear gloves when preparing liquid forms.
• Dilute liquid concentrate with fruit juice, milk, carbonated beverage, or semisolid food just before giving. Exceptions: Oral concentrate causes turbidity or precipitation in colas, black coffee, grape or apple juice, or tea. Don't mix with these liquids.
• Protect drug from light. Slight yellowing of injection or concentrate is common and doesn't affect potency. Discard markedly discolored solutions.
• Give deeply I.M. only in upper outer quadrant of buttocks. Massage slowly afterward to prevent sterile abscess. Keep in mind that injection may sting.
• Monitor patient for tardive dyskinesia, which may occur after prolonged use. It may not appear until months or years later, and may disappear spontaneously or persist for life, despite discontinuation of drug.
• *Alert:* Watch for symptoms of neuroleptic malignant syndrome (extrapyramidal effects, hyperthermia, autonomic disturbance), which is rare but frequently fatal. It isn't necessarily related to length of drug use or type of neuroleptic; however, more than 60% of affected patients are men.
• Monitor therapy with weekly bilirubin tests during first month, periodic blood tests (CBC and liver function), and ophthalmic tests (long-term use), as ordered.
• Don't withdraw drug abruptly unless required by severe adverse reactions.

---

Reactions may be *common,* uncommon, *life-threatening,* or **COMMON AND LIFE-THREATENING.**

• Withhold dose and notify doctor if jaundice, symptoms of blood dyscrasia (fever, sore throat, infection, cellulitis, weakness), or persistent extrapyramidal reactions (longer than a few hours) develop.

✓ **Patient teaching**
• Tell patient what beverages to use to dilute oral concentrate.
• Warn patient to avoid activities that require alertness or good psychomotor coordination until CNS effects of drug are known. Drowsiness and dizziness usually subside after a few weeks.
• Tell patient to avoid alcohol while taking drug.
• Advise patient to report signs of urine retention or constipation.
• Tell patient to use sunblock and to wear protective clothing to avoid photosensitivity reactions.
• Advise patient to relieve dry mouth with sugarless gum or hard candy.

---

**pimozide**
Orap

*Pregnancy Risk Category C*

**HOW SUPPLIED**
*Tablets:* 2 mg, 4 mg†, 10 mg

**ACTION**
Unknown. May block dopamine nonselectively at both the presynaptic and postsynaptic receptors on neurons in the CNS.

| Route | Onset | Peak | Duration |
|-------|-------|------|----------|
| P.O. | Unknown | 4-12 hr | Unknown |

**INDICATIONS & DOSAGE**
*Suppression of motor and phonic tics in patients with Tourette syndrome refractory to first-line therapy—*
**Adults and children over age 12:** initially, 1 to 2 mg P.O. daily in divided doses; then increased every other day, p.r.n. Maintenance dose: under 0.2 mg/kg/day or 10 mg/day, whichever is less. Maximum dose is 10 mg daily.

**ADVERSE REACTIONS**
**CNS:** *parkinsonian-like symptoms,* drowsiness, headache, insomnia, other extrapyramidal symptoms (dystonia, akathisia, hyperreflexia, opisthotonos, oculogyric crisis), *tardive dyskinesia, sedation.*
**CV:** *ECG changes (prolonged QT interval),* hypotension, hypertension, tachycardia.
**EENT:** visual disturbances.
**GI:** *dry mouth, constipation.*
**GU:** impotence, urinary frequency.
**Musculoskeletal:** muscle rigidity.
**Skin:** rash, diaphoresis.
**Other:** *neuroleptic malignant syndrome.*

**INTERACTIONS**
**Drug-drug.** *Antiarrhythmics, phenothiazines, tricyclic antidepressants:* increased risk of ECG abnormalities. Monitor patient closely.
*CNS depressants:* increased CNS depression. Avoid concomitant use.
**Drug-lifestyle.** *Alcohol use:* increased CNS depression. Avoid concomitant use.

**EFFECTS ON DIAGNOSTIC TESTS**
None reported.

**CONTRAINDICATIONS**
Contraindicated in patients with hypersensitivity to drug, in treatment of simple tics or tics other than those associated with Tourette syndrome, and in concurrent drug therapy known to cause motor and phonic tics. Also contraindicated in patients with severe toxic CNS depression or congenital long QT syndrome or history of arrhythmias, and in those experiencing coma.

**NURSING CONSIDERATIONS**
• Use cautiously in patients with hepatic or renal dysfunction, glaucoma, prostatic hyperplasia, seizure disorder, or EEG abnormalities.
• *Alert:* Perform an ECG before treatment begins and periodically thereafter, as ordered. Monitor for prolonged QT interval.
• Concurrent administration of other drugs that prolong the QT interval, such as antiarrhythmics, should be avoided.

---

• Monitor patient for tardive dyskinesia, which may occur after prolonged use. It may not appear until months or years later, and may disappear spontaneously or persist for life, despite discontinuation of drug.

• *Alert:* Watch for symptoms of neuroleptic malignant syndrome (extrapyramidal effects, hyperthermia, autonomic disturbance), which is rare but frequently fatal. It isn't necessarily related to length of drug use or type of neuroleptic; however, more than 60% of affected patients are men.

• Monitor patients who also are taking anticonvulsants for increased seizure activity. Pimozide may lower the seizure threshold.

☑ **Patient teaching**
• Warn patient not to stop taking drug abruptly and not to exceed prescribed dosage.
• Tell patient to avoid alcohol while taking drug.
• Advise patient to use sugarless hard candy, gum, and liquids to relieve dry mouth.

---

**quetiapine fumarate**
Seroquel

*Pregnancy Risk Category C*

**HOW SUPPLIED**
*Tablets:* 25 mg, 100 mg, 200 mg

**ACTION**
Unknown. A dibenzoxazepine that may block dopamine $D_2$ receptors and serotonin $5\text{-}HT_2$ receptors in the brain and $H_1$ and $alpha_1$ receptors.

| Route | Onset | Peak | Duration |
|-------|---------|--------|----------|
| P.O. | Unknown | 1.5 hr | Unknown |

**INDICATIONS & DOSAGE**
*Management of signs and symptoms of psychotic disorders—*
**Adults:** initially, 25 mg b.i.d., with increases in increments of 25 to 50 mg b.i.d. or t.i.d. on days 2 and 3, as tolerated. Target dose range is 300 to 400 mg daily divided into two or three doses by day 4.

Further dosage adjustments, if indicated, should generally occur at intervals of not less than 2 days. Dosages can be increased or decreased by 25 to 50 mg b.i.d. Antipsychotic efficacy is generally in the range of 150 to 750 mg/day. Safety of dosages above 800 mg/day hasn't been evaluated.
**Elderly:** lower dosages, slower adjustment, and careful monitoring in initial dosing period.
*Adjust-a-dose:* For patients with hepatic impairment or hypotension or in debilitated patients, consider lower dosages and slower adjustment.

**ADVERSE REACTIONS**
**CNS:** *dizziness, headache, somnolence,* hypertonia, dysarthria, asthenia.
**CV:** orthostatic hypotension, tachycardia, palpitations, peripheral edema.
**EENT:** ear pain, pharyngitis, rhinitis.
**GI:** dry mouth, dyspepsia, abdominal pain, constipation, anorexia.
**Hematologic:** *leukopenia.*
**Hepatic:** elevated liver enzyme levels.
**Metabolic:** *weight gain,* increased total cholesterol and triglyceride levels; decreased $T_4$ and thyroid-stimulating hormone levels.
**Musculoskeletal:** back pain.
**Respiratory:** increased cough, dyspnea.
**Skin:** rash, diaphoresis.
**Other:** fever, flulike syndrome.

**INTERACTIONS**
**Drug-drug.** *Antihypertensives:* increased effects. Monitor blood pressure.
*Carbamazepine, glucocorticoids, phenobarbital, phenytoin, rifampin:* increased quetiapine clearance. Adjust quetiapine dose as needed.
*CNS depressants:* increased CNS effects. Use cautiously.
*Erythromycin, fluconazole, itraconazole, ketoconazole:* decreased quetiapine clearance. Use cautiously.
*Lorazepam:* reduced clearance of lorazepam. Monitor patient for increased CNS effects.
**Drug-lifestyle.** *Alcohol use:* increased CNS effects. Use cautiously.

**EFFECTS ON DIAGNOSTIC TESTS**
None reported.

---

Reactions may be *common,* uncommon, *life-threatening,* or COMMON AND LIFE-THREATENING.

## CONTRAINDICATIONS

Contraindicated in patients with hypersensitivity to drug or its ingredients.

## NURSING CONSIDERATIONS

• Use with caution in patients with CV or cerebrovascular disease or conditions that predispose to hypotension, in those with a history of seizures or conditions that lower the seizure threshold, and in patients who will be experiencing conditions in which the core body temperature may be elevated.

• *Alert:* Watch for symptoms of neuroleptic malignant syndrome (extrapyramidal effects, hyperthermia, autonomic disturbance), which is rare but frequently fatal. It isn't necessarily related to length of drug use or type of neuroleptic; however, more than 60% of affected patients are men.

• Monitor patient for tardive dyskinesia, which may occur after prolonged use. It may not appear until months or years later, and may disappear spontaneously or persist for life, despite discontinuation of drug.

• Dispense lowest appropriate quantity of drug to reduce risk of overdose.

☑ **Patient teaching**
• Advise patient of risk of orthostatic hypotension. The risk is greatest during the 3- to 5-day period of initial dose adjustment, when reinitiating treatment, or when increasing dosages.

• Tell patient to avoid becoming overheated or dehydrated.

• During initial dose adjustment period or dosage increases, warn patient to avoid activities that require mental alertness until CNS effects of drug are known.

• Remind patient to have an eye examination at beginning of therapy and every 6 months while on drug to monitor for potential cataract formation.

• Tell patient to notify doctor of other drugs (prescription or OTC) he is taking or plans to take.

• Tell woman to notify doctor if she becomes pregnant or intends to become pregnant during drug therapy. Advise her not to breast-feed during therapy.

• Advise patient to avoid alcohol while taking drug.

---

## risperidone
Risperdal

*Pregnancy Risk Category C*

### HOW SUPPLIED
*Tablets:* 1 mg, 2 mg, 3 mg, 4 mg

### ACTION
Blocks dopamine and serotonin receptors; also blocks alpha$_1$, alpha$_2$, and H$_1$ receptors in the CNS.

| Route | Onset | Peak | Duration |
|-------|-------|------|----------|
| P.O. | Unknown | 1 hr | Unknown |

### INDICATIONS & DOSAGE
*Psychosis—*
**Adults:** initially, 1 mg P.O. b.i.d. Increased in increments of 1 mg b.i.d. on days 2 and 3 of treatment to a target dose of 3 mg b.i.d. At least 1 week must pass before dosage is adjusted further. Safety of dosages exceeding 16 mg/day hasn't been evaluated.
**Elderly:** initially, 0.5 mg P.O. b.i.d. Increased in increments of 0.5 mg b.i.d. on days 2 and 3 of treatment to a target dose of 1.5 mg P.O. b.i.d. At least 1 week must pass before dosage is increased further.
*Adjust-a-dose:* For patients with severe renal or hepatic impairment or hypotension or in debilitated patients, initially, 0.5 mg P.O. b.i.d. Increased in increments of 0.5 mg b.i.d. on days 2 and 3 of treatment to a target dosage of 1.5 mg P.O. b.i.d. At least 1 week must pass before dosage is increased further.

### ADVERSE REACTIONS
**CNS:** *somnolence, extrapyramidal symptoms,* headache, *insomnia, agitation, anxiety,* tardive dyskinesia, aggressiveness.
**CV:** tachycardia, chest pain, orthostatic hypotension, *prolonged QT interval.*
**EENT:** *rhinitis,* sinusitis, pharyngitis, abnormal vision.
**GI:** *constipation, nausea, vomiting, dyspepsia.*

---

**Metabolic:** fever, increased serum prolactin levels.
**Musculoskeletal:** arthralgia, back pain.
**Respiratory:** coughing, upper respiratory tract infection.
**Skin:** rash, dry skin, photosensitivity.

## INTERACTIONS
**Drug-drug.** *Carbamazepine:* increased clearance of risperidone, leading to decreased effectiveness. Monitor patient closely.
*Clozapine:* decreased clearance of risperidone, increasing toxicity. Monitor patient closely.
*CNS depressants:* additive CNS depression. Avoid concomitant use.
*Levodopa:* antagonized effects. Avoid concomitant use.
**Drug-lifestyle.** *Alcohol use:* additive CNS depression. Avoid concomitant use.
*Sun exposure:* photosensitivity reactions may occur. Take precautions.

## EFFECTS ON DIAGNOSTIC TESTS
None reported.

## CONTRAINDICATIONS
Contraindicated in patients with hypersensitivity to drug and in breast-feeding women.

## NURSING CONSIDERATIONS
• Use cautiously in patients with prolonged QT interval, CV disease, cerebrovascular disease, dehydration, hypovolemia, history of seizures, or conditions that may affect metabolism or hemodynamic responses; also use cautiously in those exposed to extreme heat
• *Alert:* Obtain baseline blood pressure measurements before starting therapy, and monitor regularly. Watch for orthostatic hypotension, especially during initial dosage adjustment.
• Monitor patient for tardive dyskinesia, which may occur after prolonged use. It may not appear until months or years later, and may disappear spontaneously or persist for life, despite discontinuation of drug.
• *Alert:* Watch for symptoms of neuroleptic malignant syndrome (extrapyramidal effects, hyperthermia, autonomic distur-

bance), which is rare but frequently fatal. It isn't necessarily related to length of drug use or type of neuroleptic; however, more than 60% of patients are men.
• *Alert:* Don't confuse risperidone with reserpine.

### ✓ Patient teaching
• Warn patient to avoid activities that require alertness until CNS effects of drug are known.
• Warn patient to rise slowly, avoid hot showers, and use extra caution during first few days of therapy to avoid fainting.
• Advise patient to use caution in hot weather to prevent heatstroke.
• Tell patient to avoid alcohol.
• Tell patient to use sunblock and to wear protective clothing outdoors.
• Advise woman to notify doctor if she is or plans to become pregnant during therapy.

---

## thioridazine hydrochloride
Aldazine‡, Apo-Thioridazine†, Mellaril*, Mellaril Concentrate, Novo-Ridazine†, PMS-Thioridazine†

*Pregnancy Risk Category C*

### HOW SUPPLIED
*Tablets:* 10 mg, 15 mg, 25 mg, 50 mg, 100 mg, 150 mg, 200 mg
*Oral suspension:* 25 mg/5 ml, 100 mg/5 ml
*Oral concentrate:* 30 mg/ml, 100 mg/ml (3% to 4.2% alcohol)

### ACTION
Unknown. A piperidine phenothiazine that probably blocks postsynaptic dopamine receptors in the brain.

| Route | Onset | Peak | Duration |
|-------|-------|------|----------|
| P.O. | Unknown | Unknown | Unknown |

### INDICATIONS & DOSAGE
*Psychosis—*
**Adults:** initially, 50 to 100 mg P.O. t.i.d., increased gradually to 800 mg daily in divided doses, if needed. Dosage varies.

---

Reactions may be *common*, uncommon, *life-threatening*, or COMMON AND LIFE-THREATENING.

*Short-term treatment of moderate to marked depression with variable degrees of anxiety; treatment of multiple symptoms, such as agitation, anxiety, depressed mood, tension, sleep disturbances, and fears—*
**Adults:** initially, 25 mg P.O. t.i.d. Maximum daily dose is 200 mg.
**Elderly:** initially, 25 mg P.O. t.i.d. Maximum daily dose is 200 mg.
**Children ages 2 to 12:** 0.5 to 3 mg/kg P.O. daily in divided doses.

## ADVERSE REACTIONS
**CNS:** extrapyramidal reactions (low incidence), *tardive dyskinesia, sedation (high incidence),* EEG changes, dizziness.
**CV:** *orthostatic hypotension,* tachycardia, ECG changes.
**EENT:** *ocular changes, blurred vision,* retinitis pigmentosa.
**GI:** *dry mouth, constipation.*
**GU:** *urine retention,* dark urine, menstrual irregularities, gynecomastia, inhibited ejaculation.
**Hematologic:** *transient leukopenia, agranulocytosis,* hyperprolactinemia.
**Hepatic:** elevated test results for liver enzymes, cholestatic jaundice.
**Metabolic:** weight gain, increased appetite, elevated protein-bound iodine test results.
**Skin:** *mild photosensitivity,* allergic reactions.
**After abrupt withdrawal of long-term therapy:** gastritis, nausea, vomiting, dizziness, tremor, feeling of warmth or cold, diaphoresis, tachycardia, headache, insomnia.

## INTERACTIONS
**Drug-drug.** *Antacids:* inhibited absorption of oral phenothiazines. Separate antacid and phenothiazine doses by at least 2 hours.
*Barbiturates, lithium:* may decrease phenothiazine effect. Observe patient.
*Centrally acting antihypertensives:* decreased antihypertensive effect. Monitor blood pressure.
*Other CNS depressants:* increased CNS depression. Use together cautiously.
**Drug-lifestyle.** *Alcohol use:* increased CNS depression. Avoid concomitant use.

*Sun exposure:* photosensitivity reactions may occur. Take precautions.

## EFFECTS ON DIAGNOSTIC TESTS
Drug causes false-positive test results for urinary porphyrins, urobilinogen, amylase, and 5-hydroxyindoleacetic acid because of darkening of urine by metabolites; it also causes false-positive urine pregnancy results in tests using human chorionic gonadotropin.

## CONTRAINDICATIONS
Contraindicated in patients with hypersensitivity to drug and in those experiencing coma, severe hypertensive or hypotensive cardiac disease, or CNS depression.

## NURSING CONSIDERATIONS
• Use cautiously in elderly or debilitated patients and in patients with hepatic disease, CV disease, respiratory disorder, hypocalcemia, seizure disorder, or severe reactions to insulin or electroconvulsive therapy; also use cautiously in those exposed to extreme heat or cold (including antipyretic therapy) or organophosphate insecticides.
• **Alert:** Different liquid formulations have different concentrations. Check dosage carefully.
• Prevent contact dermatitis by keeping drug away from skin and clothes. Wear gloves when preparing liquid forms.
• Dilute liquid concentrate with water or fruit juice just before giving.
• Shake suspension well before using.
• Monitor patient for tardive dyskinesia, which may occur after prolonged use. It may not appear until months or years later, and disappear spontaneously or persist for life, despite discontinuation of drug.
• **Alert:** Watch for symptoms of neuroleptic malignant syndrome (extrapyramidal effects, hyperthermia, autonomic disturbance), which is rare but frequently fatal. It isn't necessarily related to length of drug use or type of neuroleptic; however, more than 60% of patients are men.
• Monitor therapy with weekly bilirubin tests during first month, periodic blood tests (CBC and liver function), and ophthalmic tests (long-term use).

---

*Liquid contains alcohol.  **May contain tartrazine.  †Canada  ‡Australia  §U.K.  ◇OTC

• Don't stop drug abruptly unless required by severe adverse reactions.
• Withhold dose and notify doctor if jaundice, blood dyscrasia (fever, sore throat, infection, cellulitis, weakness), or persistent extrapyramidal reactions develop, especially in children or pregnant women.
• *Alert:* Don't confuse thioridazine with Thorazine, or Mellaril with Elavil.

☑ **Patient teaching**
• Tell patient to shake suspension before use.
• Warn patient to avoid activities that require alertness until CNS effects of drug are known.
• Tell patient to watch for orthostatic hypotension, especially with parenteral administration. Advise patient to change positions slowly.
• Tell patient to avoid alcohol.
• Have patient report signs of urine retention, constipation, or blurred vision.
• Tell patient that drug may discolor the urine.
• Advise patient to relieve dry mouth with sugarless gum or hard candy.
• Instruct patient to use sunblock and to wear protective clothing outdoors.

---

**thiothixene**
Navane

**thiothixene hydrochloride**
Navane*

*Pregnancy Risk Category C*

## HOW SUPPLIED
**thiothixene**
*Capsules:* 1 mg, 2 mg, 5 mg, 10 mg, 20 mg
**thiothixene hydrochloride**
*Oral concentrate:* 5 mg/ml (7% alcohol)
*Injection:* 2 mg/ml, 5 mg/ml

## ACTION
Unknown. A thioxanthene that probably blocks postsynaptic dopamine receptors in the brain.

| Route | Onset | Peak | Duration |
| --- | --- | --- | --- |
| P.O., I.M. | Unknown | Unknown | Unknown |

## INDICATIONS & DOSAGE
*Mild to moderate psychosis—*
**Adults:** initially, 2 mg P.O. t.i.d. Increased gradually to 15 mg daily, p.r.n.
*Severe psychosis—*
**Adults:** initially, 5 mg P.O. b.i.d. Increased gradually to 20 to 30 mg daily, p.r.n. Maximum recommended dose is 60 mg daily. Or, 4 mg I.M. b.i.d. to q.i.d. Maximum dose is 30 mg I.M. daily. Switch to oral form as soon as possible.

## ADVERSE REACTIONS
**CNS:** *extrapyramidal reactions,* drowsiness, restlessness, agitation, insomnia, *tardive dyskinesia,* sedation, pseudoparkinsonism, EEG changes, dizziness.
**CV:** *hypotension,* tachycardia, ECG changes.
**EENT:** ocular changes, *blurred vision,* nasal congestion.
**GI:** *dry mouth, constipation.*
**GU:** *urine retention,* menstrual irregularities, gynecomastia, inhibited ejaculation.
**Hematologic:** *transient leukopenia,* leukocytosis, *agranulocytosis.*
**Hepatic:** elevated test results for liver enzymes, jaundice.
**Metabolic:** weight gain, elevated protein-bound iodine test results.
**Skin:** *mild photosensitivity,* allergic reactions, pain at I.M. injection site, sterile abscess.
**After abrupt withdrawal of long-term therapy:** gastritis, nausea, vomiting, dizziness, tremor, feeling of warmth or cold, diaphoresis, tachycardia, headache, insomnia.

## INTERACTIONS
**Drug-drug.** *CNS depressants:* increased CNS depression. Avoid concomitant use.
**Drug-herb.** *Nutmeg:* may reduce effectiveness or interfere with drug therapy. Avoid concomitant use.
**Drug-lifestyle.** *Alcohol use:* increased CNS depression. Avoid concomitant use.
*Sun exposure:* photosensitivity reactions may occur. Take precautions.

## EFFECTS ON DIAGNOSTIC TESTS
Drug causes false-positive test results for urinary porphyrins, urobilinogen, amylase, and 5-hydroxyindoleacetic acid be-

---

Reactions may be *common,* uncommon, *life-threatening*, or COMMON AND LIFE-THREATENING.

cause of darkening of urine by metabolites; it also causes false-positive urine pregnancy results in tests using human chorionic gonadotropin.

## CONTRAINDICATIONS
Contraindicated in patients with hypersensitivity to drug and in those experiencing circulatory collapse, coma, CNS depression, or blood dyscrasia.

## NURSING CONSIDERATIONS
• Use with extreme caution in patients with history of seizure disorder or in a state of alcohol withdrawal.
• Use cautiously in elderly or debilitated patients and in those with CV disease (may cause sudden drop in blood pressure), hepatic disease, heat exposure, glaucoma, or prostatic hyperplasia.
• Prevent contact dermatitis by keeping drug off skin and clothes. Wear gloves when preparing liquid forms.
• Dilute liquid concentrate with fruit juice, milk, or semisolid food just before administering.
• Slight yellowing of injection or concentrate is common and doesn't affect potency. Discard markedly discolored solutions.
• Give I.M. only in upper outer quadrant of buttocks or midlateral thigh. Massage slowly afterward to prevent sterile abscess. Keep in mind that injection may sting.
• Monitor patient for tardive dyskinesia, which may occur after prolonged use; it may not appear until months or years later, and may disappear spontaneously or persist for life, despite discontinuation of drug.
• *Alert:* Watch for symptoms of neuroleptic malignant syndrome (extrapyramidal effects, hyperthermia, autonomic disturbance), which is rare but frequently fatal. It's necessarily related to length of drug use or type of neuroleptic; however, more than 60% of patients are men.
• Don't withdraw drug abruptly unless necessitated by severe adverse reactions.
• Withhold dose and notify doctor if jaundice, blood dyscrasia (fever, sore throat, infection, cellulitis, weakness), or persistent extrapyramidal reactions develop, especially in pregnant women.
• Monitor therapy with weekly bilirubin tests during first month, periodic blood tests (CBC and liver function), and ophthalmic tests (long-term use).
• Watch for orthostatic hypotension, especially with parenteral administration. Keep patient supine for 1 hour after drug administration and tell him to change positions slowly.
• *Alert:* Don't confuse Navane with Nubain or Norvasc.

✓ **Patient teaching**
• Warn patient to avoid activities that require alertness until CNS effects of drug are known.
• Tell patient to watch for orthostatic hypotension. Advise him to change positions slowly.
• Instruct patient to dilute liquid appropriately.
• Tell patient to avoid alcohol.
• Have him report signs of urine retention, constipation, or blurred vision.
• Instruct patient to use sunblock and to wear protective clothing outdoors.

## trifluoperazine hydrochloride
Apo-Trifluoperazine†, Novo-Flurazine†, PMS Trifluoperazine†, Solazine†, Stelazine, Stelazine Concentrate, Terfluzine†, Terfluzine Concentrate†

*Pregnancy Risk Category NR*

## HOW SUPPLIED
*Tablets (regular and film-coated):* 1 mg, 2 mg, 5 mg, 10 mg
*Oral concentrate:* 10 mg/ml
*Injection:* 2 mg/ml

## ACTION
Unknown. A piperazine phenothiazine that probably blocks postsynaptic dopamine receptors in the brain.

| Route | Onset | Peak | Duration |
|-------|-------|------|----------|
| P.O., I.M. | Unknown | Unknown | Unknown |

## INDICATIONS & DOSAGE

*Anxiety states—*
**Adults:** 1 to 2 mg P.O. b.i.d. Maximum dose is 6 mg/day. Don't use drug for more than 12 weeks for this indication.
*Schizophrenia; other psychotic disorders—*
**Adults:** 2 to 5 mg P.O. b.i.d., gradually increased until therapeutic response. Or, 1 to 2 mg deeply I.M. q 4 to 6 hours, p.r.n. Most patients respond to 15 to 20 mg P.O. daily, although some may need dosages of 40 mg/day or more. More than 6 mg I.M. in 24 hours is rarely needed.
**Children ages 6 to 12 (hospitalized or under close supervision):** 1 mg P.O. daily or b.i.d.; may increase gradually to 15 mg daily, if needed.

## ADVERSE REACTIONS

**CNS:** *extrapyramidal reactions, tardive dyskinesia,* pseudoparkinsonism, dizziness, drowsiness, insomnia, fatigue, headache.
**CV:** *orthostatic hypotension,* tachycardia, ECG changes.
**EENT:** ocular changes, *blurred vision.*
**GI:** *dry mouth, constipation,* nausea.
**GU:** *urine retention,* menstrual irregularities, gynecomastia, inhibited lactation.
**Hematologic:** *transient leukopenia, agranulocytosis.*
**Hepatic:** elevated liver enzyme test results, cholestatic jaundice.
**Metabolic:** weight gain, elevated protein-bound iodine test results.
**Skin:** *photosensitivity,* allergic reactions, pain at I.M. injection site, sterile abscess, rash.
**After abrupt withdrawal of long-term therapy:** gastritis, nausea, vomiting, dizziness, tremor, feeling of warmth or cold, diaphoresis, tachycardia, headache, insomnia, anorexia, muscle rigidity, altered mental status, evidence of autonomic instability.

## INTERACTIONS

**Drug-drug.** *Antacids:* inhibited absorption of oral phenothiazines. Separate antacid and phenothiazine doses by at least 2 hours.
*Barbiturates, lithium:* may decrease phenothiazine effect. Monitor patient.

*Centrally acting antihypertensives:* decreased antihypertensive effect. Monitor blood pressure.
*CNS depressants:* increased CNS depression. Use together cautiously.
*Propranolol:* increased levels of both propranolol and trifluoperazine. Monitor closely.
*Warfarin:* decreased effect of oral anticoagulants. Monitor PT and INR.
**Drug-lifestyle.** *Alcohol use:* increased CNS depression. Avoid concomitant use.
*Sun exposure:* photosensitivity reactions may occur. Take precautions.

## EFFECTS ON DIAGNOSTIC TESTS

Drug causes false-positive test results for urinary porphyrins, urobilinogen, amylase, and 5-hydroxyindoleacetic acid because of darkening of urine by metabolites; it also causes false-positive urine pregnancy results in tests using human chorionic gonadotropin.

## CONTRAINDICATIONS

Contraindicated in patients with hypersensitivity to phenothiazines and in those experiencing coma, CNS depression, bone marrow suppression, or liver damage.

## NURSING CONSIDERATIONS

• Use cautiously in elderly or debilitated patients and in patients with CV disease (may cause drop in blood pressure), seizure disorder, glaucoma, or prostatic hyperplasia; also use cautiously in those exposed to extreme heat.
• Wear gloves when preparing liquid forms.
• Dilute liquid concentrate with 60 ml of tomato or fruit juice, carbonated beverages, coffee, tea, milk, water, or semisolid food just before giving.
• Protect drug from light. Slight yellowing of injection or concentrate is common and doesn't affect potency. Discard markedly discolored solutions.
• Give deeply I.M. only in upper outer quadrant of buttocks. Massage slowly afterward to prevent sterile abscess. Keep in mind that injection may sting.
• Watch for orthostatic hypotension, especially with parenteral administration.

---

Reactions may be *common,* uncommon, *life-threatening,* or COMMON AND LIFE-THREATENING.

Keep patient supine for 1 hour after drug administration, and tell him to change positions slowly.

• Monitor patient for tardive dyskinesia, which may occur after prolonged use. It may not appear until months or years later, and may disappear spontaneously or persist for life, despite discontinuation of drug.

• *Alert:* Watch for symptoms of neuroleptic malignant syndrome (extrapyramidal effects, hyperthermia, autonomic disturbance), which is rare but frequently fatal. It isn't necessarily related to length of drug use or type of neuroleptic; however, more than 60% of patients are men.

• Don't withdraw drug abruptly unless severe reactions occur.

• Withhold dose and notify doctor if jaundice, symptoms of blood dyscrasia (fever, sore throat, infection, cellulitis, weakness), or persistent extrapyramidal reactions (longer than a few hours) develop, especially in children or pregnant women.

• Monitor therapy with weekly bilirubin tests during first month, periodic blood tests (CBC and liver function), and ophthalmic tests (long-term use).

• *Alert:* Don't confuse trifluoperazine with triflupromazine.

**✓ Patient teaching**
• Warn patient to avoid activities that require alertness until CNS effects of drug are known.
• Tell patient to avoid alcohol.
• Instruct patient to properly dilute liquid.
• Tell patient to report signs of urine retention or constipation.
• Tell patient to use sunblock and to wear protective clothing outdoors.
• Advise patient to relieve dry mouth with sugarless gum or hard candy.

**amphetamine sulfate**
**caffeine**
**dextroamphetamine sulfate**
**doxapram hydrochloride**
**methamphetamine hydrochloride**
**methylphenidate hydrochloride**
**modafinil**
**pemoline**
**phentermine hydrochloride**

## COMBINATION PRODUCTS

ADDERALL 5 MG: amphetamine aspartate 1.25 mg, amphetamine sulfate 1.25 mg, dextroamphetamine saccharate 1.25 mg, dextroamphetamine sulfate 1.25 mg, total amphetamine base equivalence 3.13 mg.
ADDERALL 10 MG: amphetamine aspartate 2.5 mg, amphetamine sulfate 2.5 mg, dextroamphetamine saccharate 2.5 mg, dextroamphetamine sulfate 2.5 mg, total amphetamine base equivalence 6.3 mg.
ADDERALL 20 MG: amphetamine aspartate 5 mg, amphetamine sulfate 5 mg, dextroamphetamine saccharate 5 mg, dextroamphetamine sulfate 5 mg, total amphetamine base equivalence 12.6 mg.
ADDERALL 30 MG: amphetamine aspartate 7.5 mg, amphetamine sulfate 7.5 mg, dextroamphetamine saccharate 7.5 mg, dextroamphetamine sulfate 7.5 mg, total amphetamine base equivalence 18.8 mg.

---

## amphetamine sulfate

*Controlled Substance Schedule II*
*Pregnancy Risk Category C*

### HOW SUPPLIED
*Tablets:* 5 mg, 10 mg

### ACTION
Unknown. Probably promotes nerve impulse transmission by releasing stored norepinephrine from nerve terminals in the brain. Main sites of activity appear to be the cerebral cortex and the reticular activating system.

| Route | Onset | Peak | Duration |
|-------|-------|------|----------|
| P.O. | Unknown | Unknown | Unknown |

### INDICATIONS & DOSAGE
*Attention deficit disorder with hyperactivity—*
**Children ages 3 to 5:** 2.5 mg P.O. daily, with dosage increases in 2.5-mg increments weekly, p.r.n.
**Children ages 6 and older:** 5 mg P.O. daily to b.i.d., with dosage increases in 5-mg increments weekly, p.r.n. Give first dose on awakening; additional doses (one or two) given at intervals of 4 to 6 hours. Dosage rarely exceeds 40 mg/day.
*Narcolepsy—*
**Adults and children ages 12 and older:** 10 mg P.O. daily. Dosage increased in 10-mg increments weekly, p.r.n. Daily dosage may be divided, with first dose given on awakening; additional doses given at intervals of 4 to 6 hours.
**Children ages 6 to 12:** 5 mg P.O. daily. Dosage increased in 5-mg increments weekly, p.r.n. Daily dosage may be divided, with first dose given on awakening; additional doses given at intervals of 4 to 6 hours.
*Short-term adjunct in exogenous obesity—*
**Adults:** 5 to 30 mg P.O. daily in divided doses 30 to 60 minutes before meals.

### ADVERSE REACTIONS
**CNS:** *restlessness,* tremor, *hyperactivity, talkativeness, insomnia,* irritability, dizziness, headache, chills, dysphoria, euphoria.
**CV:** *tachycardia, palpitations,* hypertension, **arrhythmias.**
**GI:** dry mouth, metallic taste, diarrhea, constipation, anorexia.
**GU:** impotence.
**Metabolic:** weight loss.
**Skin:** urticaria.
**Other:** altered libido.

---

Reactions may be *common,* uncommon, *life-threatening*, or COMMON AND LIFE-THREATENING.

## INTERACTIONS
**Drug-drug.** *Acetazolamide, antacids, sodium bicarbonate:* increased renal reabsorption. Monitor for enhanced effect.
*Ammonium chloride, ascorbic acid:* decreased serum levels and increased renal excretion of amphetamine. Monitor for decreased amphetamine effect.
*Antihypertensives:* reversal of antihypertensive action. Monitor blood pressure.
*Haloperidol, phenothiazines, tricyclic antidepressants:* altered CNS effect. Avoid concomitant use.
*Insulin, oral antidiabetics:* may decrease antidiabetic requirements. Monitor blood glucose level.
*MAO inhibitors:* may cause severe hypertension, possibly hypertensive crisis. Don't use together or within 14 days of discontinuation of MAO inhibitor therapy.
**Drug-food.** *Caffeine:* may increase amphetamine and related amine effects. Avoid concomitant use.

## EFFECTS ON DIAGNOSTIC TESTS
Amphetamines may elevate plasma corticosteroid levels and may interfere with urinary corticosteroid determinations.

## CONTRAINDICATIONS
Contraindicated in patients with hypersensitivity or idiosyncrasy to sympathomimetic amines and in those with symptomatic CV disease, hyperthyroidism, moderate to severe hypertension, glaucoma, advanced arteriosclerosis, or history of drug abuse; also contraindicated within 14 days of MAO inhibitor therapy and in agitated patients.

## NURSING CONSIDERATIONS
• Use cautiously in elderly, debilitated, or hyperexcitable patients and in those with psychopathic personalities or history of suicidal or homicidal tendencies.
• Drug isn't recommended for first-line treatment of obesity or for treatment of obesity in children under age 12. Use as an anorexigenic is prohibited in some states.
• Drug shouldn't be used to combat fatigue.
• Make sure that obese patient is on a weight-reduction program. Give drug 30 to 60 minutes before meals. Monitor dietary intake and count calories, if needed.
• If tolerance to anorexigenic effect develops, drug should be discontinued. Notify doctor.

### ✅ Patient teaching
• To avoid sleep interference, tell patient to take drug at least 6 hours before bedtime.
• Warn patient to avoid activities that require alertness or good psychomotor coordination until CNS effects of drug are known.
• Tell patient to report signs and symptoms of excessive stimulation.
• Inform patient that fatigue may result as drug effects wear off.
• Advise patient to avoid caffeine while taking drug.
• Warn patient with seizure disorder that drug may decrease seizure threshold. Instruct him to notify doctor if seizure occurs.

---

## caffeine
Caffedrine Caplets◇, Dexitac◇, NoDoz◇, Quick Pep◇, Tirend◇, Vivarin◇

*Pregnancy Risk Category C*

## HOW SUPPLIED
*Tablets:* 100 mg◇, 150 mg◇, 200 mg◇
*Tablets (timed-release):* 200 mg◇
*Capsules (timed-release):* 200 mg◇
*Injection:* caffeine (250 mg/ml) with sodium benzoate (250 mg/ml)

## ACTION
Inhibits phosphodiesterase, the enzyme that degrades cAMP.

| Route | Onset | Peak | Duration |
|---|---|---|---|
| P.O. | Unknown | 50-75 min | Unknown |
| I.M., I.V. | Unknown | Unknown | Unknown |

## INDICATIONS & DOSAGE
*CNS stimulant—*
**Adults:** 100 to 200 mg anhydrous caffeine P.O. q 3 to 4 hours, p.r.n. Or, 500 mg to 1 g I.M. (or slow I.V.). Total daily dose should seldom exceed 2.5 g.

---

## ADVERSE REACTIONS

**CNS:** *insomnia,* restlessness, nervousness, headache, excitement, agitation, muscle tremor, twitching.
**CV:** *tachycardia, palpitations,* extrasystoles.
**EENT:** tinnitus.
**GI:** nausea, vomiting, diarrhea, stomach pain.
**GU:** *diuresis.*
**Other:** irritability after abrupt withdrawal.

## INTERACTIONS

**Drug-drug.** *Beta agonists, cimetidine, fluoroquinolones, oral contraceptives, phenylpropanolamine, theophylline:* excessive CNS stimulation. Avoid concomitant use.
**Drug-food.** *Caffeine-containing beverages:* excessive CNS stimulation. Use cautiously.

## EFFECTS ON DIAGNOSTIC TESTS

Caffeine may increase blood glucose levels and cause false-positive urate levels; it may also cause false-positive test results for pheochromocytoma or neuroblastoma by increasing certain urinary catecholamines.

## CONTRAINDICATIONS

Contraindicated in patients with hypersensitivity to drug.

## NURSING CONSIDERATIONS

• Use cautiously in patients with history of peptic ulcer, symptomatic arrhythmias, or palpitations, and during the first several days to weeks after an acute MI.
• Caffeine doesn't reverse alcohol intoxication or CNS depressant effects of alcohol. Overly vigorous therapy with caffeine may aggravate depression in an already depressed patient.
• *Alert:* A single dose shouldn't exceed 1 g.
• Watch for signs and symptoms of overdose, such as GI pain, mild delirium, insomnia, diuresis, dehydration, and fever. Treat with short-acting barbiturates, gastric emesis, or lavage, as ordered.
• Monitor patient for tolerance or psychological dependence.
• Sudden discontinuation of caffeine may cause headache and irritability.

## ◻ I.V. administration

• May be given I.V. in emergencies, for treatment of respiratory depression associated with overdose of CNS depressants (including opiate analgesics and alcohol) and electric shock.

## ☑ Patient teaching

• Stress importance of not exceeding recommended dosage.
• Instruct patient to stop taking caffeine if increased or abnormal heart rate, dizziness, or palpitations occur.
• Inform patient that caffeine isn't a substitute for sleep.
• Advise patient to minimize use of caffeine-containing beverages while taking drug.
• Tell patient to take drug at least 6 hours before bedtime to avoid sleep interference.
• Warn patient with seizure disorder that drug may decrease seizure threshold. Instruct him to notify doctor if seizure occurs.

---

## dextroamphetamine sulfate
Dexedrine* **, Dexedrine Spansule

*Controlled Substance Schedule II*
*Pregnancy Risk Category C*

## HOW SUPPLIED

*Tablets:* 5 mg, 10 mg
*Capsules (extended-release):* 5 mg, 10 mg, 15 mg

## ACTION

Unknown. Probably promotes nerve impulse transmission by releasing stored norepinephrine from nerve terminals in the brain. Main sites of activity appear to be the cerebral cortex and the reticular activating system. In children with hyperkinesis, dextroamphetamine has a paradoxical calming effect.

| Route | Onset | Peak | Duration |
|-------|-------|------|----------|
| P.O. | Unknown | 2 hr | Unknown |
| P.O. (extended) | Unknown | 8-10 hr | Unknown |

---

Reactions may be *common,* uncommon, *life-threatening,* or **COMMON AND LIFE-THREATENING.**

## INDICATIONS & DOSAGE

*Narcolepsy—*
**Adults:** 5 to 60 mg P.O. daily in divided doses.
**Children ages 6 to 12:** 5 mg P.O. daily. Dosage increased in 5-mg increments weekly, p.r.n.
**Children ages 12 and older:** 10 mg P.O. daily. Dosage increased in 10-mg increments weekly, p.r.n. Give first dose on awakening; additional doses (one or two) given at intervals of 4 to 6 hours.
*Short-term adjunct in exogenous obesity—*
**Adults and children ages 12 and older:** 5 to 30 mg P.O. daily 30 to 60 minutes before meals in divided doses of 5 to 10 mg. Or, one 10- or 15-mg extended-release capsule daily as a single dose in the morning.
*Attention deficit disorder with hyper-activity—*
**Children ages 3 to 5:** 2.5 mg P.O. daily. Dosage increased in 2.5-mg increments weekly, p.r.n.
**Children ages 6 and older:** 5 mg P.O. once daily or b.i.d. Dosage increased in 5-mg increments weekly, p.r.n. Only in rare cases is it necessary to exceed a total dose of 40 mg/day.

## ADVERSE REACTIONS

**CNS:** *restlessness,* tremor, *insomnia,* dizziness, headache, chills, overstimulation, dysphoria, euphoria.
**CV:** *tachycardia, palpitations,* hypertension, **arrhythmias.**
**GI:** dry mouth, unpleasant taste, diarrhea, constipation, anorexia, other GI disturbances.
**GU:** impotence.
**Metabolic:** weight loss.
**Skin:** urticaria.
**Other:** altered libido.

## INTERACTIONS

**Drug-drug.** *Acetazolamide, alkalizing agents, antacids, sodium bicarbonate:* increased renal reabsorption. Monitor for enhanced amphetamine effects.
*Acidifying agents, ammonium chloride, ascorbic acid:* decreased blood levels and increased renal clearance of dextroamphetamine. Monitor for decreased amphetamine effects.

*Adrenergic blockers:* adrenergic blockers inhibited by amphetamines. Avoid concomitant use.
*Chlorpromazine:* inhibits the central stimulant effects of amphetamines. Can be used to treat amphetamine poisoning.
*Haloperidol, phenothiazines, tricyclic antidepressants:* increased CNS effects. Avoid concomitant use.
*Insulin, oral antidiabetics:* may decrease antidiabetic requirements. Monitor blood glucose levels.
*Lithium carbonate:* may inhibit antiobesity and stimulating effects of amphetamines. Monitor patient closely.
*MAO inhibitors:* may cause severe hypertension, possibly hypertensive crisis. Don't use together or within 14 days of discontinuation of MAO inhibitor therapy.
*Meperidine:* amphetamines potentiate analgesic effect. Use together cautiously.
*Methenamine:* increased urinary excretion of amphetamines and reduced efficacy. Monitor effects.
*Norepinephrine:* amphetamines enhance the adrenergic effect of norepinephrine. Monitor patient.
*Phenobarbital, phenytoin:* amphetamines may delay absorption. Monitor patient closely.
**Drug-food.** *Caffeine:* may increase amphetamine and related amine effects. Use cautiously.

## EFFECTS ON DIAGNOSTIC TESTS

Drug may elevate plasma corticosteroid levels and interfere with urinary corticosteroid determinations.

## CONTRAINDICATIONS

Contraindicated in patients with hypersensitivity or idiosyncrasy to sympathomimetic amines and in those with hyperthyroidism, moderate to severe hypertension, symptomatic CV disease, glaucoma, advanced arteriosclerosis, or history of drug abuse; also contraindicated within 14 days of MAO inhibitor therapy.

## NURSING CONSIDERATIONS

• Use cautiously in patients with motor and phonic tics or Tourette syndrome, and agitated patients.

---

*Liquid contains alcohol.   **May contain tartrazine.   †Canada   ‡Australia   §U.K.   ◇OTC

• Drug isn't recommended for first-line treatment of obesity. Use as an anorexigenic is prohibited in some states.
• Drug isn't to be used to prevent fatigue.
• Make sure the obese patient is on a weight-reduction program.
• Drug may cause dependence.
• *Alert:* Overdose may cause seizures.
• If tolerance to anorexigenic effect develops, drug should be discontinued. Notify doctor.
• *Alert:* Don't confuse Dexedrine with dextran or Excedrin.

☑ **Patient teaching**
• Tell patient to take drug 30 to 60 minutes before meals if used for weight reduction and at least 6 hours before bedtime to avoid sleep interference.
• Warn patient to avoid activities that require alertness or good psychomotor coordination until CNS effects of drug are known.
• Tell patient that fatigue may result as drug effects wear off.
• Ask patient to report signs of excessive stimulation.
• Advise patient to use products containing caffeine cautiously.
• Warn patient with seizure disorder that drug may decrease seizure threshold. Instruct him to notify doctor if seizure occurs.

---

**doxapram hydrochloride**
Dopram

*Pregnancy Risk Category B*

**HOW SUPPLIED**
*Injection:* 20 mg/ml (benzyl alcohol 0.9%)

**ACTION**
Not clearly defined. Directly stimulates the central respiratory centers in the medulla and may indirectly act on carotid, aortic, or other peripheral chemoreceptors.

| Route | Onset | Peak | Duration |
|-------|-------|------|----------|
| I.V. | 20-40 sec | 1-2 min | 5-12 min |

**INDICATIONS & DOSAGE**
*Postanesthesia respiratory stimulation—*
**Adults:** 0.5 to 1 mg/kg as a single I.V. injection (not to exceed 1.5 mg/kg) or as multiple injections q 5 minutes, total not to exceed 2 mg/kg. Or, 250 mg in 250 ml of normal saline solution or $D_5W$ infused at initial rate of 5 mg/minute I.V. until satisfactory response is achieved. Maintain at 1 to 3 mg/minute. Recommended total dose for infusion shouldn't exceed 4 mg/kg.
*Drug-induced CNS depression—*
**Adults:** for injection, priming dose of 2 mg/kg I.V., repeated in 5 minutes and again q 1 to 2 hours until patient awakens (and if relapse occurs). Maximum daily dose is 3 g.

For infusion, priming dose of 2 mg/kg I.V., repeated in 5 minutes and again in 1 to 2 hours, if needed. If response occurs, give I.V. infusion (1 mg/ml) at 1 to 3 mg/minute until patient awakens. Don't infuse for longer than 2 hours or administer more than 3 g/day. May resume I.V. infusion after rest period of 30 minutes to 2 hours, if needed.
*Chronic pulmonary disease associated with acute hypercapnia—*
**Adults:** 1 to 2 mg/minute by I.V. infusion (using 2 mg/ml solution). Maximum dose is 3 mg/minute for a maximum duration of 2 hours.

**ADVERSE REACTIONS**
**CNS:** *seizures,* headache, dizziness, apprehension, disorientation, hyperactivity, bilateral Babinski's signs, paresthesia.
**CV:** *chest pain and tightness, variations in heart rate,* hypertension, **arrhythmias,** T-wave depression on ECG, flushing.
**EENT:** sneezing, *laryngospasm.*
**GI:** nausea, vomiting, diarrhea.
**GU:** urine retention, bladder stimulation with incontinence, increased BUN levels, albuminuria.
**Hematologic:** decreased erythrocyte and leukocyte counts, reduced hemoglobin levels and hematocrit.
**Musculoskeletal:** muscle spasms.
**Respiratory:** cough, *bronchospasm, dyspnea,* rebound hypoventilation, hiccups.
**Skin:** pruritus, diaphoresis.

---

Reactions may be *common,* uncommon, *life-threatening,* or COMMON AND LIFE-THREATENING.

## INTERACTIONS
**Drug-drug.** *MAO inhibitors, sympathomimetics:* potentiate adverse CV effects. Use together cautiously.

## EFFECTS ON DIAGNOSTIC TESTS
None reported.

## CONTRAINDICATIONS
Contraindicated in patients with seizure disorders; head injury; CV disorders; frank, uncompensated heart failure; severe hypertension; CVA; respiratory failure or incompetence secondary to neuromuscular disorders, muscle paresis, flail chest, obstructed airway, pulmonary embolism, pneumothorax, restrictive respiratory disease, acute bronchial asthma, or extreme dyspnea; or hypoxia not associated with hypercapnia.

## NURSING CONSIDERATIONS
• Use cautiously in patients with bronchial asthma, severe tachycardia or arrhythmias, cerebral edema or increased CSF pressure, hyperthyroidism, pheochromocytoma, or metabolic disorders.
• Drug is used only in surgical or emergency department situations.
• Separate discontinuation of anesthetics and initiation of doxapram by at least 10 minutes.
• *Alert:* Establish an adequate airway before administering drug. Prevent patient from aspirating vomitus by placing him on his side.
• Monitor blood pressure, heart rate, deep tendon reflexes, and arterial blood gases before giving drug and every 30 minutes afterward.
• Be alert for signs of overdose, such as hypertension, tachycardia, arrhythmias, skeletal muscle hyperactivity, and dyspnea. Discontinue drug and notify doctor if patient shows signs of increased arterial carbon dioxide or oxygen tension, or if mechanical ventilation is needed.
• *Alert:* Don't confuse doxapram with doxorubicin, doxepin, doxacurium, or doxazosin.

## I.V. administration
• Administer slowly; rapid infusion may cause hemolysis. Doxapram is physically incompatible with strongly alkaline drugs, such as thiopental sodium, aminophylline, and sodium bicarbonate. Drug is compatible with $D_5W$ or $D_{10}W$ and normal saline.
• Avoid extravasation, which may lead to thrombophlebitis and local skin irritation.

## ☑ Patient teaching
• Inform patient, if alert, and family of need for drug.
• Answer patient's questions and address his concerns.

---

## methamphetamine hydrochloride
Desoxyn, Desoxyn Gradumet

*Controlled Substance Schedule II*
*Pregnancy Risk Category C*

## HOW SUPPLIED
*Tablets:* 5 mg
*Tablets (extended-release):* 5 mg, 10 mg, 15 mg**

## ACTION
Unknown. Probably promotes nerve impulse transmission by releasing stored norepinephrine from nerve terminals in the brain. Main sites of activity appear to be the cerebral cortex and the reticular activating system. In children with hyperkinesis, methamphetamine has a paradoxical calming effect.

| Route | Onset | Peak | Duration |
|-------|-------|------|----------|
| P.O. | Unknown | Unknown | 24 hr |

## INDICATIONS & DOSAGE
*Attention deficit disorder with hyperactivity—*
**Children ages 6 and older:** 2.5 to 5 mg P.O. once daily or b.i.d. Dosage increased by 5-mg increments weekly, p.r.n. Usual effective dose is 20 to 25 mg daily.
*Short-term adjunct in exogenous obesity—*
**Adults:** 2.5 to 5 mg P.O. b.i.d. or t.i.d. 30 minutes before meals; or 10- to 15-mg long-acting tablet daily before breakfast.

---

*Liquid contains alcohol.  **May contain tartrazine.  †Canada  ‡Australia  §U.K.  ◇OTC

## ADVERSE REACTIONS

**CNS:** *nervousness, insomnia,* irritability, *talkativeness,* dizziness, headache, hyperexcitability, tremor, euphoria.
**CV:** hypertension, *tachycardia, palpitations, arrhythmias.*
**EENT:** blurred vision, mydriasis.
**GI:** dry mouth, metallic taste, diarrhea, constipation, anorexia.
**GU:** impotence.
**Skin:** urticaria.
**Other:** altered libido.

## INTERACTIONS

**Drug-drug.** *Acetazolamide, antacids, sodium bicarbonate:* increased renal reabsorption. Monitor for enhanced effects.
*Ammonium chloride, ascorbic acid:* decreased serum levels and increased renal excretion of methamphetamine. Monitor for decreased methamphetamine effects.
*Haloperidol, phenothiazines, tricyclic antidepressants:* altered CNS effects. Avoid concomitant use.
*Insulin, oral antidiabetic:* may decrease antidiabetic requirements. Monitor blood glucose levels.
*MAO inhibitors:* may cause severe hypertension, possibly hypertensive crisis. Don't use together or within 14 days of discontinuation of MAO inhibitor therapy.
**Drug-herb.** *Melatonin:* enhanced monoaminergic effects of methamphetamine; may exacerbate insomnia. Avoid concomitant use.
**Drug-food.** *Caffeine-containing beverages:* may increase amphetamine and related amine effects. Avoid concomitant use.

## EFFECTS ON DIAGNOSTIC TESTS

Drug may elevate plasma corticosteroid levels and also interfere with urinary corticosteroid determinations.

## CONTRAINDICATIONS

Contraindicated in patients with hypersensitivity or idiosyncrasy to sympathomimetic amines and in those with moderate to severe hypertension, hyperthyroidism, symptomatic CV disease, advanced arteriosclerosis, glaucoma, or history of drug abuse; also contraindicated within 14 days of MAO inhibitor therapy and in agitated patients.

## NURSING CONSIDERATIONS

● Use cautiously in patients who are elderly, debilitated, asthenic, psychopathic, or who have a history of suicidal or homicidal tendencies.
● Drug isn't recommended for first-line treatment of obesity. Use as an anorexigenic is prohibited in some states.
● When used for obesity, make sure patient is on a weight-reduction program.
● Monitor for tolerance or dependence.
● *Alert:* Don't confuse Desoxyn with digitoxin or digoxin.

### ☑ Patient teaching

● Tell patient to take drug at least 6 hours before bedtime to avoid sleep interference.
● Warn patient of high potential for abuse. Advise him that drug shouldn't be used to prevent fatigue.
● If tolerance to anorexigenic effect develops, notify doctor because drug will need to be discontinued.
● Tell patient never to crush extended-release tablets.
● Warn patient to avoid activities that require alertness or good psychomotor coordination until CNS effects of drug are known.
● Tell patient to avoid drinks containing caffeine, which increase the effects of amphetamines and related amines. Ask him to report signs and symptoms of excessive stimulation.
● Warn patient with seizure disorder that drug may decrease seizure threshold. Instruct him to notify doctor if seizure occurs.

---

## methylphenidate hydrochloride
PMS-Methylphenidate†, Ritalin, Ritalin-SR

*Controlled Substance Schedule II*
*Pregnancy Risk Category C*

---

## HOW SUPPLIED

*Tablets:* 5 mg, 10 mg, 20 mg
*Tablets (sustained-release):* 20 mg

---

## ACTION

Unknown. Probably promotes nerve impulse transmission by releasing stored norepinephrine from nerve terminals in the brain. Main site of activity appears to be the cerebral cortex and the reticular activating system. In children with hyperkinesis, methylphenidate has a paradoxical calming effect.

| Route | Onset | Peak | Duration |
|-------|-------|------|----------|
| P.O. | Unknown | 2-5 hr | Unknown |

## INDICATIONS & DOSAGE

*Attention deficit disorder with hyperactivity—*
**Children ages 6 and older:** initial dose, 5 to 10 mg P.O. daily before breakfast and lunch. Dosage increased in 5- to 10-mg increments weekly, p.r.n., up to 60 mg daily.
*Narcolepsy—*
**Adults:** 10 mg P.O. b.i.d. or t.i.d. 30 to 45 minutes before meals. Dosage varies with patient needs.

## ADVERSE REACTIONS

**CNS:** *nervousness, insomnia,* Tourette syndrome, dizziness, headache, akathisia, dyskinesia, *seizures,* drowsiness.
**CV:** *palpitations,* angina, *tachycardia,* changes in blood pressure and pulse rate, *arrhythmias.*
**GI:** nausea, abdominal pain, anorexia.
**Hematologic:** *thrombocytopenia,* thrombocytopenic purpura, *leukopenia,* anemia.
**Metabolic:** weight loss.
**Skin:** rash, urticaria, *exfoliative dermatitis, erythema multiforme.*

## INTERACTIONS

**Drug-drug.** *Centrally acting antihypertensives:* decreased antihypertensive effect. Monitor blood pressure.
*MAO inhibitors:* may cause severe hypertension, possibly hypertensive crisis. Don't use together or within 14 days of discontinuation of MAO inhibitor therapy.
*Tricyclic antidepressants:* increased plasma levels of these drugs. Avoid concomitant use.
**Drug-food.** *Beverages containing caffeine:* may increase amphetamine and related amine effects. Avoid concomitant use.

## EFFECTS ON DIAGNOSTIC TESTS

None reported.

## CONTRAINDICATIONS

Contraindicated in patients with hypersensitivity to drug and in those with glaucoma, motor tics, family history or diagnosis of Tourette syndrome, or history of marked anxiety, tension, or agitation.

## NURSING CONSIDERATIONS

• Use cautiously in patients with history of drug abuse, hypertension, seizures, or EEG abnormalities.
• Drug isn't used to prevent fatigue.
• Drug may precipitate Tourette syndrome in children. Monitor patient, especially at start of therapy.
• Observe for signs of excessive stimulation. Monitor blood pressure.
• Monitor results of periodic CBC, differential, and platelet counts with long-term use.
• Monitor height and weight in children on long-term therapy. Drug may delay growth spurt, but children will attain normal height when drug is stopped.
• Monitor patient for tolerance or psychological dependence.
• **Alert:** Don't confuse Ritalin with Rifadin.

☑ **Patient teaching**
• Tell patient to take drug at least 6 hours before bedtime to prevent insomnia and after meals to reduce appetite-suppressant effects.
• Warn patient against chewing sustained-release tablets.
• Caution patient to avoid activities that require alertness or good psychomotor coordination until CNS effects of drug are known.
• Warn patient with seizure disorder that drug may decrease seizure threshold. Instruct him to notify doctor if seizure occurs.
• Inform patient that he'll need more rest as drug effects wear off.
• Advise patient to avoid caffeine-containing beverages while taking drug.

---

✸ *NEW DRUG*

## modafinil
Provigil

*Controlled Substance Schedule IV*
*Pregnancy Risk Category C*

### HOW SUPPLIED
*Tablets:* 100 mg, 200 mg

### ACTION
Unknown. Drug's wake-promoting actions are similar to those of sympathomimetics, including amphetamines, but drug is structurally distinct from amphetamines and doesn't appear to alter release of either dopamine or norepinephrine to produce CNS stimulation.

| Route | Onset | Peak | Duration |
|-------|-------|------|----------|
| P.O. | Unknown | 2-4 hr | Unknown |

### INDICATIONS & DOSAGE
*Improvement of wakefulness in patients with excessive daytime sleepiness associated with narcolepsy—*
**Adults:** 200 mg P.O. daily, given as a single dose in the morning.
*Adjust-a-dose:* In patients with severe hepatic impairment, 100 mg P.O. daily, given as a single dose in the morning.

### ADVERSE REACTIONS
**CNS:** *headache,* nervousness, dizziness, depression, anxiety, cataplexy, insomnia, paresthesia, dyskinesia, hypertonia, confusion, syncope, amnesia, emotional lability, ataxia, tremor.
**CV:** hypotension, hypertension, vasodilation, **arrhythmias,** chest pain.
**EENT:** *rhinitis,* pharyngitis, epistaxis, amblyopia, abnormal vision, thirst.
**GI:** *nausea,* diarrhea, dry mouth, anorexia, vomiting, mouth ulcer, gingivitis.
**GU:** abnormal urine, urine retention, abnormal ejaculation, albuminuria.
**Hematologic:** eosinophilia.
**Hepatic:** elevated GGT and AST levels.
**Metabolic:** hyperglycemia.
**Musculoskeletal:** joint disorder, neck pain, neck rigidity.

**Respiratory:** lung disorder, dyspnea, asthma.
**Skin:** herpes simplex, dry skin.
**Other:** chills, fever.

### INTERACTIONS
**Drug-drug.** *Carbamazepine, phenobarbital, rifampin, other inducers of CYP3A4:* altered levels of modafinil. Monitor patient closely.
*Cyclosporine, theophylline:* reduced serum levels of these drugs. Use together cautiously.
*Diazepam, phenytoin, propranolol, other drugs metabolized by CYP2C19:* modafinil is a reversible inhibitor of cytochrome P-450 isoenzyme CYP2C19 and thus may lead to increases in serum levels of drugs metabolized by this enzyme. Use together cautiously. Adjust dosage as needed.
*Itraconazole, ketoconazole, other inhibitors of CYP3A4:* altered levels of modafinil. Monitor patient closely.
*Methylphenidate:* 1-hour delay in absorption of modafinil when administered concurrently. Separate administration times.
*Phenytoin, warfarin:* level-dependent inhibition of CYP2C9 activity and increased serum levels of phenytoin and warfarin. Monitor patient closely for signs of toxicity.
*Steroidal contraceptives:* reduced contraceptive effectiveness. Recommend alternative or concomitant method of contraception during modafinil therapy and for 1 month after drug is discontinued.
*Tricyclic antidepressants (such as clomipramine, desipramine):* increased tricyclic antidepressant levels. Reduce dosage of these drugs as needed.

### EFFECTS ON DIAGNOSTIC TESTS
None reported.

### CONTRAINDICATIONS
Contraindicated in patients with known hypersensitivity to drug and in those with a history of left ventricular hypertrophy or ischemic ECG changes, chest pain, arrhythmias, or other signs or symptoms of mitral valve prolapse associated with CNS stimulant use.

---

Reactions may be *common,* uncommon, *life-threatening,* or COMMON AND LIFE-THREATENING.

## NURSING CONSIDERATIONS

• Use with caution in patients with recent history of an MI or unstable angina and in those with history of psychosis. Use cautiously and reduce dosage in patients with severe hepatic impairment, with or without cirrhosis. Also use cautiously in patients concurrently treated with MAO inhibitors.

• Safety and efficacy in patients with severe renal impairment haven't been determined.

• Monitor hypertensive patients closely.

• Although single, daily, 400-mg doses have been well tolerated, the larger dose offers no additional benefit beyond that of the 200-mg dose.

• Even though food has no effect on overall bioavailability, food may delay absorption of drug by 1 hour.

☑ **Patient teaching**

• Advise woman to notify doctor if she becomes pregnant or intends to become pregnant during drug therapy.

• Advise woman to notify doctor if she's breast-feeding.

• Caution patient that concurrent use of steroidal contraceptives (including depot or implantable contraceptives) with modafinil tablets may increase risk of pregnancy. Recommend an alternative or concomitant method of contraception during modafinil therapy and for 1 month after drug is discontinued.

• Instruct patient to confer with doctor before taking prescription or OTC drugs to avoid drug interactions.

• Tell patient to avoid alcohol while taking drug.

• Tell patient to notify doctor if rash, hives, or related allergic reaction develops.

• Warn patient to avoid activities that require alertness or good psychomotor coordination until CNS effects of drug are known.

## pemoline
Cylert, Cylert Chewable

*Controlled Substance Schedule IV*
*Pregnancy Risk Category B*

### HOW SUPPLIED
*Tablets:* 18.75 mg, 37.5 mg, 75 mg
*Tablets (chewable):* 37.5 mg

### ACTION
Unknown. Probably promotes nerve impulse transmission by releasing stored norepinephrine from nerve terminals in the brain. Main sites of activity appear to be the cerebral cortex and the reticular activating system.

| Route | Onset | Peak | Duration |
|-------|-------|------|----------|
| P.O. | Unknown | 2-4 hr | Unknown |

### INDICATIONS & DOSAGE
*Attention deficit disorder with hyperactivity—*
**Children ages 6 and older:** initially, 37.5 mg P.O. in the morning with daily dose raised by 18.75 mg weekly, p.r.n. Usual effective dose is 56.25 to 75 mg daily; maximum dose is 112.5 mg daily.

### ADVERSE REACTIONS
**CNS:** *insomnia,* dyskinetic movements, irritability, fatigue, mild depression, dizziness, headache, drowsiness, hallucinations, **seizures,** *Tourette syndrome,* abnormal oculomotor function.
**GI:** anorexia, abdominal pain, nausea.
**Hematologic:** *aplastic anemia.*
**Hepatic:** *acute hepatic failure, hepatitis,* jaundice, *elevated liver enzyme levels.*
**Skin:** rash.

### INTERACTIONS
**Drug-drug.** *Insulin, oral antidiabetics:* may decrease antidiabetic requirements. Monitor blood glucose levels.

### EFFECTS ON DIAGNOSTIC TESTS
None reported.

## CONTRAINDICATIONS
Contraindicated in patients with hypersensitivity or idiosyncrasy to drug and in those with hepatic dysfunction.

## NURSING CONSIDERATIONS
• Use cautiously in patients with impaired renal function.
• Liver function tests should be performed before starting, and periodically during, therapy; however, they may not predict onset of acute liver failure. Treatment should be initiated only in patients without liver disease and with normal baseline liver function tests.
• Closely monitor patients on long-term therapy for possible blood or hepatic function abnormalities and for growth suppression.
• *Alert:* Discontinue drug if patient experiences significant hepatic dysfunction during its use.
• Drug is structurally dissimilar to amphetamines or methylphenidate; however, it may produce similar adverse reactions. Drug has greater potential for abuse and dependence than previously thought.
• Drug may precipitate Tourette syndrome in children. Monitor patient, especially at start of therapy.
• *Alert:* Don't confuse pemoline with Pelamine.

☑ **Patient teaching**
• Tell patient to take drug at least 6 hours before bedtime to avoid sleep interference.
• Tell patient to avoid activities that require alertness or good psychomotor coordination until CNS effects of drug are known.
• Warn patient with seizure disorder that drug may decrease seizure threshold. Instruct him to notify doctor if seizure occurs.

---

## phentermine hydrochloride
Adipex-P, Duromine‡, Fastin, Obe-Nix, OBY-CAP, Phentercot, Phentride, T-Diet

*Controlled Substance Schedule IV*
*Pregnancy Risk Category NR*

### HOW SUPPLIED
*Tablets:* 8 mg, 30 mg, 37.5 mg
*Capsules:* 15 mg, 18.75 mg, 30 mg, 37.5 mg
*Capsules (resin complex, sustained-release):* 15 mg, 30 mg

### ACTION
Unknown. Drug probably promotes nerve impulse transmission by releasing stored norepinephrine from nerve terminals in the brain. Main sites of activity appear to be the cerebral cortex and the reticular activating system.

| Route | Onset | Peak | Duration |
|-------|-------|------|----------|
| P.O. | Unknown | Unknown | 12-14 hr |

### INDICATIONS & DOSAGE
*Short-term adjunct in exogenous obesity—*
**Adults:** 8 mg P.O. t.i.d. 30 minutes before meals. Or, 15 to 30 mg (resin complex) or 15 to 37.5 mg (phentermine hydrochloride) P.O. daily as a single dose in the morning.

### ADVERSE REACTIONS
**CNS:** overstimulation, headache, euphoria, dysphoria, dizziness, *insomnia.*
**CV:** *palpitations, tachycardia,* increased blood pressure.
**GI:** dry mouth, dysgeusia, constipation, diarrhea, other GI disturbances.
**GU:** impotence.
**Skin:** urticaria.
**Other:** altered libido.

### INTERACTIONS
**Drug-drug.** *Acetazolamide, antacids, sodium bicarbonate:* increased renal reabsorption. Monitor for enhanced effects.
*Ammonium chloride, ascorbic acid:* decreased plasma levels and increased renal excretion of phentermine. Monitor for decreased phentermine effects.
*Haloperidol, phenothiazines, tricyclic antidepressants:* altered CNS effects. Avoid concomitant use.
*Insulin, oral antidiabetics:* may alter antidiabetic requirements. Monitor blood glucose levels.
*MAO inhibitors:* may cause severe hypertension, possibly hypertensive crisis. Don't use together or within 14 days of discontinuation of MAO inhibitor therapy.

---

Reactions may be *common,* uncommon, *life-threatening*, or **COMMON AND LIFE-THREATENING.**

**Drug-food.** *Caffeine:* may increase CNS stimulation. Avoid concomitant use.

**EFFECTS ON DIAGNOSTIC TESTS**
None reported.

**CONTRAINDICATIONS**
Contraindicated in patients with hypersensitivity or idiosyncrasy to sympathomimetic amines and in those with hyperthyroidism, moderate to severe hypertension, advanced arteriosclerosis, symptomatic CV disease, or glaucoma; also contraindicated within 14 days of MAO inhibitor therapy and in agitated patients.

**NURSING CONSIDERATIONS**
• Use cautiously in patients with mild hypertension.
• Use drug with a weight-reduction program.
• Monitor for tolerance or dependence.
• *Alert:* Don't confuse phentermine with phentolamine.

**✓ Patient teaching**
• Tell patient to take drug at least 6 hours before bedtime to avoid sleep interference.
• Advise patient to avoid drinks containing caffeine. Tell him to report signs of excessive stimulation.
• Warn patient that fatigue may result as drug effects wear off and that he'll need more rest.
• Warn patient that drug may lose its effectiveness over time.

# 35

## Antiparkinsonians

**amantadine hydrochloride**
  (See Chapter 17, ANTIVIRALS.)
**benztropine mesylate**
**biperiden hydrochloride**
**biperiden lactate**
**bromocriptine mesylate**
**carbidopa-levodopa**
**entacapone**
**levodopa**
**pergolide mesylate**
**pramipexole dihydrochloride**
**ropinirole hydrochloride**
**selegiline hydrochloride**
**tolcapone**
**trihexyphenidyl hydrochloride**

### COMBINATION PRODUCTS
MADOPAR‡: levodopa 200 mg and benserazide 50 mg.
MADOPAR HBS‡: levodopa 100 mg and
benserazide 25 mg.
MADOPAR Q‡: levodopa 50 mg and
benserazide 12.5 mg.
SINEMET 10-100: carbidopa 10 mg and
levodopa 100 mg.
SINEMET 25-100: carbidopa 25 mg and
levodopa 100 mg.
SINEMET 25-250: carbidopa 25 mg and
levodopa 250 mg.
SINEMET CR: carbidopa 50 mg and levodopa 200 mg, in extended-release
tablets.

---

**benztropine mesylate**
Apo-Benztropine†, Cogentin,
PMS-Benztropine†

*Pregnancy Risk Category NR*

### HOW SUPPLIED
*Tablets:* 0.5 mg, 1 mg, 2 mg
*Injection:* 1 mg/ml in 2-ml ampules

### ACTION
Unknown. May block central cholinergic
receptors, helping to balance cholinergic
activity in the basal ganglia.

| Route | Onset | Peak | Duration |
|-------|-------|------|----------|
| P.O. | 1-2 hr | Unknown | 24 hr |
| I.V., I.M. | 15 min | Unknown | 24 hr |

### INDICATIONS & DOSAGE
*Drug-induced extrapyramidal disorders
(except tardive dyskinesia)—*
**Adults:** 1 to 4 mg P.O. or I.M. once or
twice daily.
*Acute dystonic reaction—*
**Adults:** 1 to 2 mg I.V. or I.M.; then 1 to
2 mg P.O. b.i.d. to prevent recurrence.
*Parkinsonism—*
**Adults:** 0.5 to 6 mg P.O. or I.M. daily.
Initial dose is 0.5 mg to 1 mg, increased
by 0.5 mg q 5 to 6 days. Dosage adjusted
to meet individual requirements. Maxi-
mum daily dose is 6 mg.

### ADVERSE REACTIONS
**CNS:** disorientation, hallucinations, de-
pression, toxic psychosis, confusion,
memory impairment, nervousness.
**CV:** tachycardia.
**EENT:** dilated pupils, blurred vision.
**GI:** *dry mouth, constipation,* nausea,
vomiting, paralytic ileus.
**GU:** urine retention, dysuria.
**Skin:** decreased sweating.

### INTERACTIONS
**Drug-drug.** *Amantadine, phenothiazines,
tricyclic antidepressants:* additive anticholinergic adverse reactions, such as
confusion and hallucinations. Reduce
dosage before administering.
**Drug-herb.** *Jimsonweed:* may adversely
affect CV function. Avoid concomitant
use.

### EFFECTS ON DIAGNOSTIC TESTS
None reported.

### CONTRAINDICATIONS
Contraindicated in patients with hypersensitivity to drug or its components, in
those with angle-closure glaucoma, and in
children under age 3.

---

Reactions may be *common,* uncommon, *life-threatening,* or COMMON AND LIFE-THREATENING.

## NURSING CONSIDERATIONS

• Use cautiously in hot weather, in patients with mental disorders, and in children ages 3 and older. Also use cautiously in patients with prostatic hyperplasia, arrhythmias, and seizure disorders.
• Monitor vital signs carefully. Watch closely for adverse reactions, especially in elderly or debilitated patients. Call doctor promptly if they occur.
• Some adverse reactions may result from atropine-like toxicity and are dose-related.
• Drug produces atropine-like adverse reactions and may aggravate tardive dyskinesia.
• Watch for intermittent constipation and abdominal distention and pain; these symptoms may indicate onset of paralytic ileus.
• *Alert:* Never discontinue drug abruptly. Reduce dosage gradually.
• *Alert:* Don't confuse benztropine with bromocriptine.

### I.V. administration

• I.V. route is seldom used because of small difference in onset when compared with I.M. route.

### Patient teaching

• Warn patient to avoid activities that require alertness until CNS effects of drug are known. If patient is to receive a single daily dose, tell him to take it at bedtime.
• Advise patient to report signs of urinary hesitancy or urine retention.
• Tell patient to relieve dry mouth with cool drinks, ice chips, sugarless gum, or hard candy.
• Advise patient to limit his activities during hot weather because drug-induced anhidrosis may cause hyperthermia.

---

## biperiden hydrochloride
Akineton

## biperiden lactate
Akineton Lactate

*Pregnancy Risk Category C*

## HOW SUPPLIED
**biperiden hydrochloride**
*Tablets:* 2 mg

**biperiden lactate**
*Injection:* 5 mg/ml in 1-ml ampules

## ACTION
Unknown. Blocks central cholinergic receptors, helping to balance cholinergic activity in the basal ganglia.

| Route | Onset | Peak | Duration |
|-------|-------|------|----------|
| P.O. | 1 hr | Unknown | 6-12 hr |
| I.V. | < Few min | Unknown | 1-8 hr |
| I.M. | 10-30 min | Unknown | Unknown |

## INDICATIONS & DOSAGE
*Drug-induced extrapyramidal disorders—*
**Adults:** 2 mg P.O. once daily, b.i.d., or t.i.d., depending on severity. Usual dosage is 2 mg daily, or 2 mg I.M. or I.V. q 30 minutes, not to exceed four doses or 8 mg daily.
*Parkinsonism—*
**Adults:** 2 mg P.O. t.i.d. or q.i.d. Dosage is individualized and adjusted to maximum of 16 mg in 24 hours.

## ADVERSE REACTIONS
**CNS:** disorientation, euphoria, drowsiness, agitation.
**CV:** transient orthostatic hypotension (with parenteral use).
**EENT:** blurred vision.
**GI:** *dry mouth, constipation.*
**GU:** urine retention.

## INTERACTIONS
**Drug-drug.** *Amantadine, phenothiazines, tricyclic antidepressants:* excessive CNS anticholinergic effects. Avoid concomitant use.
*Antacids:* decreased biperiden absorption. Administer antacids at least 1 hour after biperiden.
**Drug-lifestyle.** *Alcohol use:* increased sedative effects. Avoid concomitant use.

## EFFECTS ON DIAGNOSTIC TESTS
None reported.

## CONTRAINDICATIONS
Contraindicated in patients with hypersensitivity to drug and in those with angle-closure glaucoma, bowel obstruction, or megacolon.

---

## NURSING CONSIDERATIONS
• Use cautiously in patients with prostatic hyperplasia, arrhythmias, manifest glaucoma, and seizure disorder.
• To decrease adverse GI effects, give oral doses with or after meals.
• When giving drug parenterally, keep patient in supine position. Parenteral administration may cause transient orthostatic hypotension and coordination disturbances.
• Monitor vital signs carefully. Watch closely for adverse reactions, especially in elderly or debilitated patients. Call doctor promptly if they occur.
• If tolerance develops, notify doctor because dosage will need to be increased.
• In severe parkinsonism, tremors may increase as spasticity is relieved.
• Adverse reactions are dose-related and may resemble atropine toxicity.

**◐ I.V. administration**
• Administer drug very slowly.

**☑ Patient teaching**
• Tell patient to take oral form with or after meals to decrease adverse GI effects.
• Warn patient to avoid activities that require alertness until CNS effects of drug are known.
• Advise patient to report signs of urinary hesitancy or urine retention.
• Instruct patient to relieve dry mouth with cool drinks, ice chips, sugarless gum, or hard candy.
• Advise patient to avoid alcohol while taking drug.

---

## bromocriptine mesylate
Parlodel

*Pregnancy Risk Category B*

### HOW SUPPLIED
*Tablets:* 2.5 mg
*Capsules:* 5 mg

### ACTION
Inhibits secretion of prolactin and acts as a dopamine-receptor agonist by activating postsynaptic dopamine receptors.

| Route | Onset | Peak | Duration |
|---|---|---|---|
| P.O. | 2 hr | 8 hr | 24 hr |

### INDICATIONS & DOSAGE
*Parkinson's disease—*
**Adults:** 1.25 mg P.O. b.i.d. with meals. Dosage increased by 2.5 mg/day q 14 to 28 days, up to 100 mg daily.
*Amenorrhea and galactorrhea associated with hyperprolactinemia; female infertility—*
**Adults:** 1.25 to 2.5 mg P.O. daily, increased by 2.5 mg daily at 3- to 7-day intervals until desired effect is achieved. Therapeutic daily dose is 2.5 to 15 mg. Safety and efficacy of doses exceeding 100 mg daily haven't been established.
*Acromegaly—*
**Adults:** 1.25 to 2.5 mg P.O. with h.s. snack for 3 days. An additional 1.25 to 2.5 mg may be added q 3 to 7 days until patient experiences therapeutic benefit. Maximum daily dose is 100 mg.

### ADVERSE REACTIONS
**CNS:** *dizziness, headache, fatigue,* mania, light-headedness, drowsiness, delusions, nervousness, insomnia, depression, ***seizures.***
**CV:** *hypotension, **stroke, acute MI.***
**EENT:** nasal congestion, blurred vision.
**GI:** *nausea,* vomiting, *abdominal cramps, constipation,* diarrhea, anorexia.
**GU:** urine retention, urinary frequency, transient elevation of BUN levels.
**Hepatic:** transient elevation of liver enzyme levels.
**Metabolic:** transient elevation of CK, alkaline phosphatase, and uric acid levels.
**Skin:** coolness and pallor of fingers and toes.

### INTERACTIONS
**Drug-drug.** *Antihypertensives:* increased hypotensive effects. Adjust dosage of antihypertensive.
*Erythromycin:* increased bromocriptine levels and potential adverse reactions. Use cautiously.
*Estrogens, oral contraceptives, progestins:* interfere with effects of bromocriptine. Concurrent use not recommended.

---

Reactions may be *common,* uncommon, *life-threatening*, or COMMON AND LIFE-THREATENING.

*Haloperidol, loxapine, methyldopa, metoclopramide, MAO inhibitors, phenothiazines, reserpine:* interferes with bromocriptine's effects. Bromocriptine dosage may need to be increased.
*Levodopa:* may have additive effects. Adjust dosage of levodopa if needed.
**Drug-lifestyle.** *Alcohol use:* disulfiram-like reaction. Avoid concomitant use.

**EFFECTS ON DIAGNOSTIC TESTS**
None reported.

**CONTRAINDICATIONS**
Contraindicated in patients with hypersensitivity to ergot derivatives and in those with uncontrolled hypertension, toxemia of pregnancy, severe ischemic heart disease, or peripheral vascular disease.

**NURSING CONSIDERATIONS**
• Use cautiously in patients with impaired renal or hepatic function and history of MI with residual arrhythmias.
• For Parkinson's disease, bromocriptine usually is given in addition to either levodopa or carbidopa-levodopa. The carbidopa-levodopa dose may need to be reduced.
• Drug may be taken with meals to reduce nausea.
• *Alert:* Monitor patient for adverse reactions. Adverse reactions occur in about 68% of patients, particularly at beginning of therapy; however, most reactions are mild to moderate, with nausea the most common. Minimize adverse reactions by gradually adjusting dosages to effective levels, as ordered. Adverse reactions are more common when drug is used for Parkinson's disease.
• Baseline and periodic evaluations of cardiac, hepatic, renal, and hematopoietic function are recommended during prolonged therapy.
• Drug may lead to early postpartum conception. Test for pregnancy every 4 weeks or whenever period is missed after menses resumes.
• *Alert:* Don't confuse bromocriptine with benztropine or brimonidine, or Parlodel with pindolol.

✓ **Patient teaching**
• Instruct patient to take drug with meals.
• Advise patient to use contraceptive methods other than oral contraceptives or subdermal implants during treatment.
• Instruct patient to avoid dizziness and fainting by rising slowly to an upright position and avoiding sudden position changes.
• Inform patient that it may take 8 weeks or longer for menses to resume and galactorrhea to be suppressed.
• Advise patient to avoid alcohol while taking drug.

## carbidopa-levodopa
Sinemet, Sinemet CR

*Pregnancy Risk Category C*

**HOW SUPPLIED**
*Tablets:* carbidopa 10 mg with levodopa 100 mg (Sinemet 10-100), carbidopa 25 mg with levodopa 100 mg (Sinemet 25-100), carbidopa 25 mg with levodopa 250 mg (Sinemet 25-250)
*Tablets (extended-release):* carbidopa 50 mg with levodopa 200 mg (Sinemet CR); carbidopa 25 mg with levodopa 100 mg.

**ACTION**
Levodopa is converted to dopamine in the CNS, increasing dopamine levels in the brain. Carbidopa inhibits the peripheral decarboxylation of levodopa without affecting levodopa's metabolism within the CNS. Therefore, more levodopa is available to be decarboxylated to dopamine in the brain.

| Route | Onset | Peak | Duration |
|-------|-------|------|----------|
| P.O. | Unknown | 40-150 min | Unknown |

**INDICATIONS & DOSAGE**
*Idiopathic Parkinson's disease, post-encephalitic parkinsonism, and symptomatic parkinsonism resulting from carbon monoxide or manganese intoxication—*
**Adults:** 1 tablet of 25 mg carbidopa and 100 mg levodopa P.O. t.i.d.; then an increase of 1 tablet daily or every other day, p.r.n., to maximum daily dose of 8 tablets. 25 mg carbidopa and 250 mg levodopa or

10 mg carbidopa and 100 mg levodopa tablets are substituted, as needed, to obtain maximum response. Optimum daily dose must be determined by careful adjustment for each patient.

Patients given conventional tablets may receive extended-release tablets; dosage is calculated on current levodopa intake. Initially, extended-release tablets given should amount to 10% more levodopa per day increased, as needed and tolerated, to 30% more levodopa per day. Administered in divided doses at intervals of 4 to 8 hours.

## ADVERSE REACTIONS
**CNS:** *choreiform, dystonic, dyskinetic movements; involuntary grimacing, head movements, myoclonic body jerks, ataxia,* tremor, muscle twitching; bradykinetic episodes; psychiatric disturbances, anxiety, disturbing dreams, euphoria, malaise, fatigue; severe depression, **suicidal tendencies,** dementia, delirium, hallucinations (may necessitate reduction or withdrawal of drug), confusion, insomnia, agitation.
**CV:** *orthostatic hypotension,* **cardiac irregularities.**
**EENT:** blepharospasm, blurred vision, diplopia, mydriasis or miosis, oculogyric crises, excessive salivation.
**GI:** dry mouth, bitter taste, *nausea, vomiting, anorexia;* constipation; flatulence; diarrhea; abdominal pain.
**GU:** urinary frequency, urine retention, urinary incontinence, darkened urine, priapism.
**Hematologic:** *hemolytic anemia,* **thrombocytopenia, leukopenia, agranulocytosis.**
**Hepatic:** *hepatotoxicity.*
**Metabolic:** weight loss (may occur at start of therapy).
**Respiratory:** hiccups, hyperventilation.
**Skin:** dark perspiration.
**Other:** phlebitis.

## INTERACTIONS
**Drug-drug.** *Antihypertensives:* additive hypotensive effects. Use together cautiously.
*Iron salts:* may reduce bioavailability of levodopa and carbidopa. Administer iron 1 hour before or 2 hours after Sinemet dose.
*MAO inhibitors:* risk of severe hypertension. Avoid concomitant use.

*Papaverine, phenytoin:* antagonism of antiparkinsonian actions. Don't use together.
*Phenothiazines, other antipsychotics:* may antagonize antiparkinsonian actions. Use together cautiously.
**Drug-herb.** *Octacosanol:* may promote worsening of dyskinesias. Avoid concomitant use.
**Drug-food.** *Foods high in protein:* decreased absorption of levodopa. Don't give levodopa with high-protein foods.

## EFFECTS ON DIAGNOSTIC TESTS
Drug elevates serum and urinary uric acid levels when colorimetric test methods are used; it may produce false-positive test results for urinary glucose when cupric sulfate reagent is used and false-negative results in tests using glucose oxidase. False-positive results may occur for urine ketone tests using sodium nitroprusside reagent. Levodopa interferes with urine screening tests for phenylketonuria, falsely elevates urinary catecholamine levels, and may falsely decrease urinary vanillylmandelic acid levels.

## CONTRAINDICATIONS
Contraindicated in patients with hypersensitivity to drug and in those with angle-closure glaucoma, melanoma, or undiagnosed skin lesions; also contraindicated within 14 days of MAO inhibitor therapy.

## NURSING CONSIDERATIONS
• Use cautiously in patients with severe CV, renal, hepatic, endocrine, or pulmonary disorders; history of peptic ulcer; psychiatric illness; MI with residual arrhythmias; bronchial asthma; emphysema; and well-controlled, chronic openangle glaucoma.
• If patient is being given levodopa, discontinue drug at least 8 hours before starting carbidopa-levodopa.
• Carbidopa-levodopa typically decreases amount of levodopa needed by 75%, reducing incidence of adverse reactions.
• Therapeutic and adverse reactions occur more rapidly with carbidopa-levodopa than with levodopa alone. Observe and monitor vital signs, especially while adjusting dosage. Report significant changes.

---

• *Alert:* Muscle twitching and blepharospasm may be early signs of drug overdose; report immediately.

• Patients receiving long-term therapy should be tested regularly for diabetes and acromegaly and have periodic tests of liver, renal, and hematopoietic function, as ordered.

• An accurate measure for urine glucose can be obtained if the paper strip is only partially immersed in the urine sample. Urine migrates up the strip, as with an ascending chromatographic system. Read only the top of the strip.

✅ **Patient teaching**

• Tell patient to take drug with food to minimize GI upset. However, taking drug with high-protein meals can impair absorption and reduce effectiveness.

• Tell patient not to chew or crush extended-release form.

• Warn patient and caregivers not to increase dosage without doctor's orders.

• Caution patient of possible dizziness and orthostatic hypotension, especially at start of therapy. Tell him to change position slowly and dangle legs before getting out of bed. Elastic stockings may control these adverse reactions in some patients.

• Instruct patient to report adverse reactions and therapeutic effects.

• Inform patient that pyridoxine (vitamin $B_6$) doesn't reverse beneficial effects of carbidopa-levodopa. Multivitamins can be taken without reversal of levodopa's effects.

✳ *NEW DRUG*

## entacapone
Comtan

*Pregnancy Risk Category C*

### HOW SUPPLIED
*Tablets:* 200 mg

### ACTION
A reversible catechol-O-methyltransferase (COMT) inhibitor that's administered with carbidopa-levodopa. Coadministration is thought to result in higher serum

levels of levodopa and optimal control of parkinsonian symptoms.

| Route | Onset | Peak | Duration |
|-------|-------|------|----------|
| P.O.  | 1 hr  | 1 hr | 6 hr     |

### INDICATIONS & DOSAGE
*Adjunct to carbidopa-levodopa for treatment of idiopathic Parkinson's disease in patients who experience signs and symptoms of end-of-dose wearing-off—*
**Adults:** 200 mg P.O. with each dose of carbidopa-levodopa to maximum of eight times daily. Maximum daily dose is 1,600 mg/day. Reductions in daily levodopa dose or extending the interval between doses may be needed to optimize patient's response.

### ADVERSE REACTIONS
**CNS:** *dyskinesia, hyperkinesia,* hypokinesia, dizziness, anxiety, somnolence, agitation, fatigue, asthenia, hallucinations.
**GI:** *nausea, diarrhea,* abdominal pain, constipation, vomiting, dry mouth, dyspepsia, flatulence, gastritis, taste perversion.
**GU:** *urine discoloration.*
**Hematologic:** purpura.
**Musculoskeletal:** back pain.
**Respiratory:** dyspnea.
**Skin:** sweating.
**Other:** bacterial infection.

### INTERACTIONS
**Drug-drug.** *Ampicillin, chloramphenicol, cholestyramine, erythromycin, probenecid:* may block biliary excretion, resulting in higher serum levels of entacapone. Use cautiously.
*CNS depressants:* additive effect. Use cautiously.
*Drugs metabolized by COMT (bitolterol, dobutamine, dopamine, epinephrine, isoetharine, isoproterenol, norepinephrine):* may cause higher serum levels of these drugs, resulting in increased heart rate, changes in blood pressure, or possibly arrhythmias. Use cautiously.
*Nonselective MAO inhibitors (such as phenelzine, tranylcypromine):* may inhibit normal catecholamine metabolism. Avoid concomitant use.
**Drug-lifestyle.** *Alcohol use:* may cause additive CNS effects. Avoid concomitant use.

---

*Liquid contains alcohol.   **May contain tartrazine.   †Canada   ‡Australia   §U.K.   ◊OTC

## EFFECTS ON DIAGNOSTIC TESTS
None reported.

## CONTRAINDICATIONS
Contraindicated in patients with hypersensitivity to drug.

## NURSING CONSIDERATIONS
• Use cautiously in patients with hepatic impairment, biliary obstruction, or orthostatic hypotension.
• Drug should only be used with carbidopa-levodopa; no antiparkinsonian effects will occur when drug is given as monotherapy.
• Carbidopa-levodopa dosage requirements are usually lower when given with entacapone; carbidopa-levodopa dose should be lowered or dosing interval increased to avoid adverse effects.
• Drug may cause or exacerbate preexisting dyskinesia, despite reduction of levodopa dose.
• Hallucinations may occur or worsen when taking this drug.
• Monitor blood pressure closely. Observe for orthostatic hypotension.
• Diarrhea most commonly begins within 4 to 12 weeks of starting therapy, but may begin as early as first week or as late as many months after starting treatment.
• Drug may cause urine discoloration.
• Rarely, rhabdomyolysis has occurred with drug use.
• Rapid withdrawal or abrupt reduction in dose could lead to signs and symptoms of Parkinson's disease; it may also lead to hyperpyrexia and confusion, a symptom complex resembling neuroleptic malignant syndrome. Discontinue drug slowly and monitor patient closely. Adjust other dopaminergic treatments, as needed.
• Drug can be given with immediate or sustained-release carbidopa-levodopa and can be taken with or without food.

☑ **Patient teaching**
• Instruct patient not to crush or break tablet and to take it at same time as carbidopa-levodopa.
• Warn patient to avoid potentially hazardous activities, such as driving or operating heavy machinery, until CNS effects of drug are known.

• Advise patient to avoid alcohol during treatment.
• Instruct patient to use caution when standing after a prolonged period of sitting or lying down because dizziness may occur. This effect is more common during initial therapy.
• Warn patient that hallucinations, increased dyskinesia, nausea, and diarrhea could occur.
• Inform patient that drug may cause urine to turn brownish orange.
• Advise patient to notify doctor if she's pregnant or breast-feeding or if she plans to become pregnant.

## levodopa
Dopar, Larodopa

*Pregnancy Risk Category NR*

## HOW SUPPLIED
*Tablets:* 100 mg, 250 mg, 500 mg
*Capsules:* 100 mg**, 250 mg**, 500 mg**

## ACTION
Unknown. May be decarboxylated to dopamine, countering the depletion of striatal dopamine in extrapyramidal centers; this depletion is thought to produce parkinsonism.

| Route | Onset | Peak | Duration |
|-------|-------|------|----------|
| P.O. | Unknown | 1-3 hr | 5 hr |

## INDICATIONS & DOSAGE
*Idiopathic parkinsonism, postencephalitic parkinsonism, and symptomatic parkinsonism after carbon monoxide or manganese intoxication or in association with cerebral arteriosclerosis*—
**Adults and children over age 12:** initially, 0.5 to 1 g P.O. daily, divided in two or more doses with food; increased by no more than 0.75 g daily q 3 to 7 days until maximum response is achieved. Don't exceed 8 g/day. Dosage adjusted to patient requirements, tolerance, and response. Higher dosage needs close supervision.

## ADVERSE REACTIONS

**CNS:** *aggressive behavior; choreiform, dystonic, and dyskinetic movements; involuntary grimacing, head movements, myoclonic body jerks,* **seizures,** *ataxia, tremor, muscle twitching; bradykinetic episodes; psychiatric disturbances; mood changes, nervousness, anxiety, disturbing dreams, euphoria, malaise, fatigue; severe depression,* **suicidal tendencies,** *dementia, delirium, hallucinations.*

**CV:** *orthostatic hypotension,* cardiac irregularities.

**EENT:** blepharospasm, blurred vision, diplopia, mydriasis or miosis, activation of latent Horner's syndrome, oculogyric crises, excessive salivation.

**GI:** dry mouth, bitter taste, *nausea, vomiting, anorexia,* constipation, flatulence, diarrhea, abdominal pain.

**GU:** urinary frequency, urine retention, transient elevation in BUN level, incontinence, darkened urine, priapism.

**Hematologic:** *hemolytic anemia, leukopenia, agranulocytosis.*

**Hepatic:** transient elevations in liver enzyme levels, *hepatotoxicity.*

**Metabolic:** transient elevations in protein-bound iodine levels, weight loss.

**Respiratory:** hiccups, hyperventilation.

**Skin:** dark perspiration.

**Other:** phlebitis.

## INTERACTIONS

**Drug-drug.** *Antacids:* increased absorption of levodopa. Administer antacids 1 hour after levodopa.

*Inhalation anesthetics, sympathomimetics:* increased risk of arrhythmias. Monitor closely.

*MAO inhibitors, furazolidone, procarbazine:* risk of severe hypertension. Avoid concomitant use.

*Metoclopramide:* accelerated gastric emptying of levodopa. Give metoclopramide 1 hour after levodopa.

*Papaverine, phenothiazines, other antipsychotics, phenytoin, rauwolfia alkaloids:* decreased levodopa effect. Avoid concomitant use, if possible.

*Pyridoxine:* reversal of antiparkinsonian effects. Check vitamin preparations and nutritional supplements for pyridoxine (vitamin $B_6$) content. Don't give together.

**Drug-herb.** *Jimsonweed:* may adversely affect CV function. Avoid concomitant use.

*Kava:* increased parkinsonian symptoms. Avoid concomitant use.

**Drug-food.** *Foods high in protein:* decreased absorption of levodopa. Don't give levodopa with high-protein foods.

**Drug-lifestyle.** *Cocaine use:* increased risk of arrhythmias. Monitor closely.

## EFFECTS ON DIAGNOSTIC TESTS

Coombs' test occasionally becomes positive during extended therapy. Colorimetric test for uric acid has shown false elevations. Copper-reduction method has shown false-positive results for urine glucose; glucose oxidase method has shown false-negative results. Levodopa also may interfere with tests for urine ketones. Levodopa interferes with urine screening tests for phenylketonuria, falsely elevates urinary catecholamine levels, and may falsely decrease urinary vanillylmandelic acid levels.

## CONTRAINDICATIONS

Contraindicated in patients with hypersensitivity to drug and in those with acute angle-closure glaucoma, melanoma, or undiagnosed skin lesions; also contraindicated during and within 14 days of MAO inhibitor therapy.

## NURSING CONSIDERATIONS

• Use cautiously in severe CV, renal, liver, and pulmonary disorders; peptic ulcer; psychiatric illness; MI with residual arrhythmias; bronchial asthma; emphysema; and endocrine disease.

• Patients who must undergo surgery should continue levodopa therapy as long as oral intake is permitted, generally 6 to 24 hours before surgery. Resume therapy as soon as patient is able to take drug orally.

• Carbidopa-levodopa typically decreases amount of levodopa needed by 75%, reducing incidence of adverse reactions.

• Monitor vital signs, especially while adjusting dosage. Report changes.

• *Alert:* Watch for muscle twitching and blepharospasm, which may be early signs of drug overdose; report immediately.

• *Alert:* The appearance of hallucinations may require reduction or withdrawal of drug.

• An accurate measure for urine glucose can be obtained if paper strip is only partially immersed in the urine sample. Urine migrates up the strip, as with an ascending chromatographic system. Read only the top of the strip.

• Patients receiving long-term therapy should be tested regularly for diabetes and acromegaly; periodically monitor renal, liver, and hematopoietic function, as ordered.

☑ **Patient teaching**

• Tell patient to take drug with food to minimize GI upset. However, taking drug with high-protein meals can impair absorption and reduce effectiveness.

• For patient who has difficulty swallowing pills, tell him or caregiver to crush tablets and mix with applesauce or baby food fruits.

• Warn patient or caregiver not to increase dosage unless ordered. Daily dosage shouldn't exceed 8 g.

• Tell patient to protect drug from heat, light, and moisture. If preparation darkens, it has lost potency and should be discarded.

• Warn patient of possible dizziness and orthostatic hypotension, especially at start of therapy. Tell him to change position slowly and dangle legs before rising. Elastic stockings may control these adverse reactions.

• Advise patient and caregivers that multivitamin preparations, fortified cereals, and certain OTC drugs may contain pyridoxine (vitamin $B_6$), which can block the effects of levodopa by enhancing its peripheral metabolism.

---

**pergolide mesylate**
Celance§, Permax

*Pregnancy Risk Category B*

**HOW SUPPLIED**
*Tablets:* 0.05 mg, 0.25 mg, 1 mg

**ACTION**
Dopamine agonist that directly stimulates dopamine receptors in the nigrostriatal system.

| Route | Onset | Peak | Duration |
|-------|-------|------|----------|
| P.O. | Unknown | Unknown | Unknown |

**INDICATIONS & DOSAGE**
*Adjunctive treatment with carbidopa-levodopa in management of symptoms in Parkinson's disease—*
**Adults:** initially, 0.05 mg P.O. daily for first 2 days; then increased dosage of 0.1 to 0.15 mg q third day over 12 days. Subsequent dosage increased by 0.25 mg q third day, if needed, until optimum response is seen. Drug usually is administered in divided doses t.i.d. Gradual reductions in carbidopa-levodopa dosage may be needed during dosage adjustment.

**ADVERSE REACTIONS**
**CNS:** headache, asthenia, *dyskinesia, dizziness, hallucinations, dystonia, confusion, somnolence,* insomnia, anxiety, depression, tremor, abnormal dreams, personality disorder, psychosis, abnormal gait, akathisia, extrapyramidal syndrome, incoordination, akinesia, hypertonia, neuralgia, speech disorder, syncope, twitching.
**CV:** *orthostatic hypotension,* vasodilation, palpitations, hypotension, hypertension, *arrhythmias, MI.*
**EENT:** *rhinitis,* epistaxis, abnormal vision, diplopia, eye disorder.
**GI:** dry mouth, taste perversion, abdominal pain, *nausea, constipation,* diarrhea, dyspepsia, anorexia, vomiting.
**GU:** urinary frequency, urinary tract infection, hematuria.
**Metabolic:** weight gain.
**Musculoskeletal:** chest, neck, and back pain; arthralgia; bursitis; myalgia.
**Respiratory:** dyspnea.
**Skin:** rash, diaphoresis, paresthesia.
**Other:** flulike syndrome; chills; infection; facial, peripheral, or generalized edema.

**INTERACTIONS**
**Drug-drug.** *Butyrophenones, dopamine antagonists, metoclopramide, phenothiazines, thioxanthenes:* may antagonize

---

effects of pergolide. Avoid concomitant use.

**EFFECTS ON DIAGNOSTIC TESTS**
None reported.

**CONTRAINDICATIONS**
Contraindicated in patients with hypersensitivity to drug or ergot alkaloids.

**NURSING CONSIDERATIONS**
• Use cautiously in patients prone to arrhythmias.
• *Alert:* Monitor blood pressure. Symptomatic orthostatic or sustained hypotension may occur, especially at start of therapy.
• Orthostatic or sustained hypotension, although not always attributable to pergolide, occurred in more than 1% of the population.

☑ **Patient teaching**
• Inform patient of potential adverse reactions, especially hallucinations and confusion.
• Warn patient to avoid activities that could result in injury from orthostatic hypotension and syncope.
• Advise patient to take drug with food.

---

**pramipexole dihydrochloride**
Mirapex

*Pregnancy Risk Category C*

**HOW SUPPLIED**
*Tablets:* 0.125 mg, 0.25 mg, 0.5 mg, 1 mg, 1.5 mg

**ACTION**
Unknown. Non-ergot-derivative dopamine receptor agonist that's thought to stimulate dopamine ($D_2$) receptors in striatum.

| Route | Onset | Peak | Duration |
|-------|-------|------|----------|
| P.O. | Rapid | 2 hr | 8-12 hr |

**INDICATIONS & DOSAGE**
*Signs and symptoms of idiopathic Parkinson's disease—*
**Adults:** initially, 0.375 mg P.O. daily in three divided doses; don't increase more

frequently than q 5 to 7 days. Maintenance dose is 1.5 to 4.5 mg/day in three divided doses.
*Adjust-a-dose:* For patients with normal to mild renal impairment (creatinine clearance over 60 ml/minute), initial dose 0.125 mg P.O. t.i.d., up to 1.5 mg t.i.d.; for those with moderate impairment (creatinine clearance between 35 and 59 ml/minute), initial dose 1.25 mg P.O. b.i.d. up to 1.5 mg b.i.d.; and for those with severe impairment (creatinine clearance between 15 and 34 ml/minute), initial dose 0.125 mg P.O. daily, up to 1.5 mg daily.

**ADVERSE REACTIONS**
**CNS:** akathisia, amnesia, *asthenia, confusion,* delusions, *dizziness, dream abnormalities, dyskinesia,* dystonia, *extrapyramidal syndrome,* gait abnormalities, *hallucinations,* hypoesthesia, hypertonia, *insomnia,* myoclonus, paranoid reaction, malaise, *somnolence,* sleep disorders, thought abnormalities.
**CV:** chest pain, peripheral edema, *orthostatic hypotension.*
**EENT:** accommodation abnormalities, diplopia, dry mouth, rhinitis, vision abnormalities.
**GI:** anorexia, *constipation,* dysphagia, *nausea.*
**GU:** decreased libido, impotence, urinary frequency, urinary tract infection, urinary incontinence.
**Metabolic:** weight loss, fever.
**Musculoskeletal:** arthritis, bursitis, myasthenia, twitching.
**Respiratory:** dyspnea, pneumonia.
**Skin:** skin disorders.
**Other:** *accidental injury,* general edema.

**INTERACTIONS**
**Drug-drug.** *Butyrophenones, metoclopramide, phenothiazines, thiothixenes:* may diminish the effectiveness of pramipexole. Monitor closely.
*Cimetidine, diltiazem, quinidine, quinine, ranitidine, triamterene, verapamil:* decreased clearance of pramipexole. Adjust dose as needed.
*Levodopa:* increased adverse effects of levodopa. Adjust levodopa dose as needed.

---

## EFFECTS ON DIAGNOSTIC TESTS
None reported.

## CONTRAINDICATIONS
Contraindicated in patients with hypersensitivity to drug or its components.

## NURSING CONSIDERATIONS
• Dosage may need to be adjusted in patients with renal impairment.
• It's unknown if drug appears in breast milk. Use with caution.
• If drug needs to be discontinued, withdraw over a 1-week period.
• Drug may cause orthostatic hypotension, especially during dosage increases. Monitor patient carefully.
• Adjust dosage gradually. Increase dosage to achieve maximum therapeutic effect, balanced against the main adverse effects of dyskinesia, hallucinations, somnolence, and dry mouth.

☑ **Patient teaching**
• Instruct patient not to rise rapidly after sitting or lying down because of risk of orthostatic hypotension.
• Caution patient not to drive a car or operate complex machinery until CNS response to drug is known.
• Tell patient to use caution before taking drug with other CNS depressants.
• Tell patient that hallucinations may occur, especially if he is elderly.
• Advise patient to take drug with food if nausea develops.
• Tell woman to notify doctor if she is breast-feeding or intends to do so.
• Advise patient that it may take 4 weeks for effects of drug to be noticed because of slow adjustment schedule.

---

**ropinirole hydrochloride**
Requip

*Pregnancy Risk Category C*

## HOW SUPPLIED
*Tablets:* 0.25 mg, 0.5 mg, 1 mg, 2 mg, 5 mg

## ACTION
Unknown. Non-ergot-derivative dopamine receptor agonist that's thought to stimulate dopamine ($D_2$) receptors in striatum.

| Route | Onset | Peak | Duration |
|-------|-------|------|----------|
| P.O. | Unknown | 1-2 hr | 6 hr |

## INDICATIONS & DOSAGE
*Idiopathic Parkinson's disease—*
**Adults:** initially, 0.25 mg t.i.d. Dosages can be adjusted on a weekly basis. After week 4, dosage may be increased by 1.5 mg/day on a weekly basis up to a dose of 9 mg/day; then increased weekly by up to 3 mg/day to maximum of 24 mg/day.
**Elderly:** clearance is reduced in patients over age 65; however, dosages are individually adjusted to clinical response.

## ADVERSE REACTIONS
*Early Parkinson's disease (without levodopa)—*
**CNS:** hallucinations, *dizziness,* aggravated Parkinson's disease, *somnolence,* headache, confusion, hyperkinesia, hypoesthesia, vertigo, amnesia, impaired concentration, *syncope, fatigue,* malaise, asthenia.
**CV:** orthostatic hypotension, orthostatic symptoms, hypertension, edema, chest pain, extrasystoles, ***atrial fibrillation,*** palpitation, tachycardia, flushing.
**EENT:** pharyngitis, dry mouth, abnormal vision, eye abnormality, xerophthalmia, rhinitis, sinusitis.
**GI:** *nausea, vomiting, dyspepsia,* flatulence, abdominal pain, anorexia, constipation.
**GU:** urinary tract infection, impotence.
**Respiratory:** bronchitis, dyspnea.
**Other:** *viral infection,* pain, increased sweating, yawning, peripheral ischemia.
*Advanced Parkinson's disease (with levodopa)—*
**CNS:** *dizziness,* aggravated parkinsonism, *somnolence, headache,* insomnia, *hallucinations,* abnormal dreaming, confusion, tremor, anxiety, nervousness, amnesia, paresis, paresthesia, syncope.
**CV:** hypotension.
**EENT:** diplopia.

---

Reactions may be *common,* uncommon, *life-threatening,* or **COMMON AND LIFE-THREATENING.**

**GI:** *nausea,* abdominal pain, dry mouth, vomiting, constipation, diarrhea, dysphagia, flatulence.
**GU:** urinary tract infection, pyuria, urinary incontinence, increased BUN.
**Hematologic:** anemia.
**Metabolic:** weight decrease, suppressed serum prolactin, increased alkaline phosphatase.
**Musculoskeletal:** arthralgia, arthritis, *dyskinesia,* hypokinesia.
**Respiratory:** upper respiratory infection, dyspnea.
**Skin:** increased sweating.
**Other:** injury, *falls,* viral infection, increased drug level, increased saliva, pain.

## INTERACTIONS
**Drug-drug.** *Ciprofloxacin, inhibitors or substrates of cytochrome P-450:* altered clearance. Adjust ropinirole dose if drugs are started or stopped during treatment with ropinirole.
*CNS depressants:* increased CNS effects. Use cautiously.
*Estrogens:* reduced clearance of ropinirole. Adjust ropinirole dose if estrogens are started or stopped during treatment with ropinirole.
**Drug-lifestyle.** *Alcohol use:* increased sedative effects. Use cautiously.
*Smoking:* may increase clearance of ropinirole. Monitor closely.

## EFFECTS ON DIAGNOSTIC TESTS
None reported.

## CONTRAINDICATIONS
Contraindicated in patients with hypersensitivity to drug.

## NURSING CONSIDERATIONS
• Use cautiously in patients with severe hepatic or renal impairment.
• *Alert:* Monitor patient carefully for orthostatic hypotension, especially during dosage increases.
• Drug can potentiate the dopaminergic adverse effects of levodopa and may cause or exacerbate existing dyskinesia. Dosage of drug may be decreased.
• Other adverse events reported with dopaminergic therapy could occur with ropinirole (but haven't been reported):

withdrawal emergent hyperpyrexia and confusion; fibrotic complications.
• Syncope, with or without bradycardia, has been reported. Monitor patient carefully, especially for 4 weeks after initiation of therapy and with dosage increases.
• Withdraw drug gradually over 7 days.

### ☑ Patient teaching
• Advise patient to take drug with food if nausea is a problem.
• Advise patient that hallucinations can occur, especially if he is elderly.
• Instruct patient not to rise rapidly after sitting or lying down because of risk of orthostatic hypotension, which may occur more frequently during initial therapy or with an increase in dosage.
• Warn patient to use caution when driving or operating machinery until CNS effects are known.
• Advise patient to avoid alcohol.
• Tell woman to notify doctor if pregnancy is suspected or is being planned; also tell her to inform doctor if she's breast-feeding.
• Advise patient not to double a dose if one is missed.

---

## selegiline hydrochloride (L-deprenyl hydrochloride)
Eldepryl

*Pregnancy Risk Category C*

## HOW SUPPLIED
*Capsules:* 5 mg

## ACTION
Unknown. May selectively inhibit MAO type B (found mostly in the brain) and dopamine metabolism. At higher-than-recommended doses, it's a nonselective inhibitor of MAO, including MAO type A (found in the GI tract). May also directly increase dopaminergic activity by decreasing the reuptake of dopamine into nerve cells.

| Route | Onset | Peak | Duration |
|-------|-------|------|----------|
| P.O. | Unknown | 0.5-2 hr | Unknown |

## INDICATIONS & DOSAGE
*Adjunctive treatment with carbidopa-levodopa in management of symptoms in Parkinson's disease—*
**Adults:** 10 mg P.O. daily, taken as 5 mg at breakfast and 5 mg at lunch. After 2 or 3 days, gradual decrease of carbidopa-levodopa dosage may be needed.

## ADVERSE REACTIONS
**CNS:** *dizziness,* increased tremor, chorea, loss of balance, restlessness, increased bradykinesia, facial grimacing, stiff neck, dyskinesia, involuntary movements, twitching, increased apraxia, behavioral changes, fatigue, headache, confusion, hallucinations, vivid dreams, anxiety, insomnia, lethargy, malaise, syncope.
**CV:** orthostatic hypotension, hypertension, hypotension, *arrhythmias,* palpitations, new or increased anginal pain, tachycardia, peripheral edema.
**EENT:** blepharospasm.
**GI:** dry mouth, *nausea,* vomiting, constipation, weight loss, abdominal pain, anorexia or poor appetite, dysphagia, diarrhea, heartburn.
**GU:** slow urination, transient nocturia, prostatic hyperplasia, urinary hesitancy, urinary frequency, urine retention, sexual dysfunction.
**Skin:** rash, hair loss, diaphoresis.

## INTERACTIONS
**Drug-drug.** *Adrenergics:* possible increased pressor response, particularly in patients who have taken an overdose of selegiline. Use together cautiously.
*Meperidine:* may cause stupor, muscle rigidity, severe agitation, and elevated temperature. Avoid concomitant use.
**Drug-herb.** *Cacao tree:* potential vasopressor effects. Avoid concomitant use.
*Ginseng:* adverse reactions including headache, tremors, mania. Avoid concomitant use.
**Drug-food.** *Foods high in tyramine:* possible hypertensive crisis. Monitor blood pressure.

## EFFECTS ON DIAGNOSTIC TESTS
None reported.

## CONTRAINDICATIONS
Contraindicated in patients with hypersensitivity to drug and in those receiving meperidine.

## NURSING CONSIDERATIONS
• *Alert:* Some patients experience increased adverse reactions with levodopa when used with selegiline and require a 10% to 30% reduction of carbidopa-levodopa dosage.
• *Alert:* Don't confuse selegiline with Stelazine, or Eldepryl with enalapril.

### ☑ Patient teaching
• Warn patient to move cautiously at start of therapy because he may experience dizziness.
• Advise patient not to take more than 10 mg daily. A greater amount may increase adverse reactions.

---

## tolcapone
Tasmar

*Pregnancy Risk Category C*

## HOW SUPPLIED
*Tablets:* 100 mg, 200 mg

## ACTION
Unknown. May reversibly inhibit catechol-O-methyltransferase (COMT) when given with carbidopa-levodopa, resulting in an increase in levodopa bioavailability, which causes a more constant dopaminergic stimulation in the brain.

| Route | Onset | Peak | Duration |
|-------|-------|------|----------|
| P.O. | Unknown | 2 hr | Unknown |

## INDICATIONS & DOSAGE
*Adjunct to levodopa and carbidopa for treatment of signs and symptoms of idiopathic Parkinson's disease—*
**Adults:** initially, 100 mg P.O. t.i.d. (with carbidopa-levodopa). Recommended daily dose is 100 mg P.O. t.i.d., although 200 mg P.O. t.i.d. can be given if anticipated clinical benefit is justified. Reduction of levodopa dosage by 20% to 30% may be needed to minimize risk of dyskinesias. Maximum daily dose is 600 mg. Discon-

tinue drug if patient shows no benefit within 3 weeks.

*Adjust-a-dose:* Don't use doses over 100 mg t.i.d. in patients with severe renal dysfunction.

## ADVERSE REACTIONS
**CNS:** *dyskinesia, sleep disorder, dystonia, excessive dreaming, somnolence,* dizziness, *confusion, headache, hallucinations,* hyperkinesia, hypertonia, fatigue, falling, syncope, balance loss, depression, tremor, speech disorder, paresthesia, agitation, irritability, mental deficiency, hyperactivity, hypokinesia.
**CV:** *orthostatic complaints,* chest pain, chest discomfort, palpitation, hypotension.
**EENT:** pharyngitis, tinnitus, sinus congestion.
**GI:** *nausea, anorexia, diarrhea,* flatulence, *vomiting,* constipation, abdominal pain, dyspepsia, dry mouth.
**GU:** urinary tract infection, urine discoloration, hematuria, micturition disorder, urinary incontinence, impotence.
**Hematologic:** bleeding.
**Hepatic:** elevated liver function test results.
**Musculoskeletal:** *muscle cramps,* stiffness, arthritis, neck pain.
**Respiratory:** bronchitis, dyspnea, upper respiratory tract infections.
**Skin:** increased sweating, rash.
**Other:** burning, fever, influenza.

## INTERACTIONS
**Drug-drug.** *Desipramine:* increased incidence of adverse effects. Use cautiously.
*Nonselective MAO inhibitors (phenelzine, tranylcypromine):* possible hypertensive crisis. Avoid concomitant use.

## EFFECTS ON DIAGNOSTIC TESTS
None reported.

## CONTRAINDICATIONS
Contraindicated in patients with hypersensitivity to drug or its components and in those with liver disease, elevated ALT or AST levels, or history of nontraumatic rhabdomyolysis or hyperpyrexia and confusion possibly related to drug; also contraindicated in those who were withdrawn from tolcapone because of evidence of drug-induced hepatocellular injury.

## NURSING CONSIDERATIONS
• Use cautiously in patients with severe renal impairment and in breast-feeding women.
• Because of risk of liver toxicity, stop treatment if patient shows no benefit within 3 weeks.
• Use drug only in patients on carbidopa-levodopa who don't respond to or who aren't appropriate candidates for other adjunctive therapies because of risk of potentially fatal liver failure.
• *Alert:* Make sure patient provides a written, informed consent before using the drug.
• Monitor liver function test results before starting drug, every 2 weeks for first year of therapy, then every 4 weeks for next 6 months, and every 8 weeks thereafter. Stop drug if results are outside the normal limits or if patient appears jaundiced.
• Because of highly protein-bound nature of tolcapone, drug isn't significantly removed during dialysis.
• Monitor for orthostatic hypotension and syncope.
• Administer first dose of day with first daily dose of carbidopa-levodopa.
• Diarrhea is common, sometimes occurring 2 to 12 weeks after therapy begins. Although diarrhea usually resolves with drug discontinuation, patient may need hospitalization in rare cases.

☑ **Patient teaching**
• Advise patient to take drug exactly as prescribed.
• Teach patient signs and symptoms of liver injury (jaundice, fatigue, loss of appetite, persistent nausea, pruritus, dark urine, or right upper quadrant tenderness) and instruct him to report them immediately.
• Warn patient about risk of orthostatic hypotension; tell him to use caution when rising from a seated or recumbent position.
• Advise patient to avoid hazardous activities until CNS effects of drug are known.
• Tell patient that nausea may occur upon initiation of therapy.
• Advise patient about risk of increased dyskinesia or dystonia.

- Inform patient that hallucinations may occur.
- Tell woman to report if pregnancy is being planned or suspected during therapy.
- Tell patient to report adverse effects, including diarrhea, to doctor. Inform patient that diarrhea may occur from 2 to 12 weeks after initiation of therapy.
- Inform patient that drug may be taken without regard to meals.

---

## trihexyphenidyl hydrochloride
Apo-Trihex†, Artane*, Artane Sequels, Trihexane, Trihexy

*Pregnancy Risk Category NR*

### HOW SUPPLIED
*Tablets:* 2 mg, 5 mg
*Capsules (sustained-release):* 5 mg
*Elixir:* 2 mg/5 ml

### ACTION
Unknown. Drug blocks central cholinergic receptors, helping to balance cholinergic activity in the basal ganglia.

| Route | Onset | Peak | Duration |
|-------|-------|------|----------|
| P.O. | 1 hr | Unknown | 6-12 hr |

### INDICATIONS & DOSAGE
*All forms of parkinsonism, drug-induced parkinsonism, adjunctive treatment to levodopa in management of parkinsonism—*
**Adults:** 1 mg P.O. on day 1, 2 mg on day 2; then increased in 2-mg increments q 3 to 5 days until total of 6 to 10 mg is given daily. Usually given t.i.d. with meals, sometimes given q.i.d. (last dose h.s.) or switched to extended-release form b.i.d.

Patients with postencephalitic parkinsonism may need total daily dose of 12 to 15 mg.

### ADVERSE REACTIONS
**CNS:** nervousness, dizziness, headache, hallucinations, drowsiness, weakness.
**CV:** tachycardia.
**EENT:** blurred vision, mydriasis, increased intraocular pressure.
**GI:** *dry mouth,* constipation, *nausea,* vomiting.
**GU:** urinary hesitancy, urine retention.

### INTERACTIONS
**Drug-drug.** *Amantadine:* additive anticholinergic adverse reactions, such as confusion and hallucinations. Reduce dose of trihexyphenidyl before administering.
*Levodopa:* decreased total bioavailability of levodopa. May require lower doses of both drugs.
**Drug-lifestyle.** *Alcohol use:* increased sedative effects. Avoid concomitant use.

### EFFECTS ON DIAGNOSTIC TESTS
None reported.

### CONTRAINDICATIONS
Contraindicated in patients with hypersensitivity to drug.

### NURSING CONSIDERATIONS
- Use cautiously in glaucoma; cardiac, hepatic, or renal disorders; obstructive disease of GI and GU tracts; and prostatic hyperplasia.
- Dosage may need to be gradually increased in patients who develop a tolerance to drug.
- Monitor patient. Adverse reactions are dose-related and transient.
- ***Alert:*** Make sure gonioscopic evaluation is performed and intraocular pressure is monitored, especially in patients over age 40.
- ***Alert:*** Don't confuse Artane with Anturane or Altace.

☑ **Patient teaching**
- Advise patient that drug may cause nausea if given before meals.
- Tell patient to avoid activities that require alertness until CNS effects of drug are known.
- Advise patient to report signs of urinary hesitancy or urine retention.
- Tell patient to relieve dry mouth with cool drinks, ice chips, or sugarless gum or hard candy.
- Advise patient to avoid alcohol while taking drug.
- Advise patient to avoid OTC sleep aids or cold medicines because of possibility of increased anticholinergic effects.

---

Reactions may be *common,* uncommon, *life-threatening,* or COMMON AND LIFE-THREATENING.

bupropion hydrochloride
donepezil hydrochloride
droperidol
fluvoxamine maleate
lithium carbonate
lithium citrate
naratriptan hydrochloride
nicotine polacrilex
nicotine transdermal system
propofol
rizatriptan benzoate
sibutramine hydrochloride
  monohydrate
sumatriptan succinate
tacrine hydrochloride
zolmitriptan

**COMBINATION PRODUCTS**
None.

---

## bupropion hydrochloride
Zyban

*Pregnancy Risk Category B*

### HOW SUPPLIED
*Tablets (sustained-release):* 150 mg

### ACTION
Unknown. Relatively weak inhibitor of the neuronal uptake of norepinephrine, serotonin, and dopamine. It doesn't inhibit MAO.

| Route | Onset | Peak | Duration |
|-------|-------|------|----------|
| P.O. | Unknown | 3 hr | Unknown |

### INDICATIONS & DOSAGE
*Aid to smoking cessation treatment—*
**Adults:** 150 mg P.O. daily for 3 days; increased to maximum of 300 mg P.O. daily in two divided doses at least 8 hours apart.

### ADVERSE REACTIONS
**CNS:** agitation, asthenia, depression, *dizziness,* headache, *insomnia,* irritability, somnolence, tremor, thinking or dream abnormalities, disturbed concentration, anxiety, nervousness.
**CV:** *complete AV block,* hypertension, hypotension, tachycardia, palpitations, hot flashes.
**EENT:** amblyopia, epistaxis, pharyngitis, sinusitis, tinnitus, *rhinitis.*
**GI:** anorexia, dyspepsia, increased appetite, abdominal pain, nausea, constipation, diarrhea, flatulence, vomiting, *dry mouth,* taste perversion, mouth ulcer.
**GU:** urinary frequency.
**Musculoskeletal:** arthralgia, leg cramps and twitching, myalgia.
**Respiratory:** bronchitis, increased cough, dyspnea.
**Musculoskeletal:** neck pain.
**Skin:** dry skin, pruritus, rash, urticaria.
**Other:** allergic reactions, injury, fever.

### INTERACTIONS
**Drug-drug.** *Antipsychotics, antidepressants, systemic corticosteroids, theophylline, treatment regimens (such as abrupt discontinuation of benzodiazepines):* may lower seizure threshold. Use cautiously.
*Carbamazepine, phenobarbital, phenytoin:* may induce metabolism of bupropion and decrease its effect. Monitor closely.
*Cimetidine:* may inhibit metabolism of bupropion and lead to increased levels. Monitor closely.
*Levodopa:* may lead to an increased incidence of adverse reactions when given with bupropion. If used concurrently, give small initial doses of bupropion and increase dosage gradually.
*MAO inhibitors (phenelzine):* increased toxicity. Avoid concurrent use and allow at least 14 days to elapse between discontinuation of MAO inhibitor and initiation of bupropion therapy.
*Other drugs containing bupropion (Wellbutrin, Wellbutrin SR):* contain same active ingredient as Zyban. Avoid concomitant use.
**Drug-lifestyle.** *Alcohol:* may increase risk of seizures. Avoid concomitant use.

**EFFECTS ON DIAGNOSTIC TESTS**
None reported.

**CONTRAINDICATIONS**
Contraindicated in patients with seizure disorders or a current or prior diagnosis of bulimia or anorexia nervosa. Also contraindicated in patients allergic to drug or its components and in those being treated with other drugs containing bupropion (such as Wellbutrin and Wellbutrin SR) or MAO inhibitors. Allow at least 14 days to elapse between discontinuation of MAO inhibitors and initiation of drug therapy.

**NURSING CONSIDERATIONS**
• Use cautiously in patients with recent history of MI or unstable heart disease. Also use cautiously in patients with history of seizures, head trauma, or other predisposition to seizures, and in those being treated with drugs that lower seizure threshold.
• *Alert:* Increased risk of seizures is associated with excessive use of alcohol, abrupt withdrawal from alcohol or other sedatives, and addiction to cocaine, opiates, or stimulants. Seizure risk is also associated with OTC stimulants and anorectics. Diabetic patients being treated with oral antidiabetics or insulin are also at risk for seizures.
• To reduce seizure risk, daily dose of 300 mg shouldn't be exceeded. Divide dose (150 mg twice daily) so that no single dose exceeds 150 mg.
• Therapy should be discontinued if patient hasn't made progress toward abstinence by week 7 of therapy.
• Dose doesn't need tapering before discontinuation of treatment.
• *Alert:* Therapy should begin while patient is still smoking; about 1 week is needed to achieve steady-state plasma drug levels.
• *Alert:* Don't confuse bupropion with buspirone.

☑ **Patient teaching**
• Stress importance of combining behavioral interventions, counseling, and support services with drug therapy.

• Advise patient to take doses at least 8 hours apart. If insomnia occurs, tell him not to take dose at bedtime.
• Tell patient not to chew, divide, or crush tablets.
• Advise patient that it may take 1 week for effects of drug to be evident. Also, tell him to set a target date for cessation of smoking during the second week of therapy.
• Tell patient that treatment usually lasts for 7 to 12 weeks.
• Inform patient that tablets may have a characteristic odor.
• Advise patient to avoid alcohol while taking drug.
• Advise patient to avoid activities that require mental alertness, such as driving or operating machinery, until drug's CNS effects are known.
• Warn patient not to use drug with nicotine patches unless directed to do so by his doctor. Doing so may lead to an increase in blood pressure.
• Inform patient that risk of seizures is increased if he has a seizure or eating disorder, exceeds the recommended dose, or takes other drugs that contain bupropion or lower seizure threshold.
• Advise patient to read accompanying patient information before starting drug.
• Advise patient to notify doctor if she is pregnant or plans to become pregnant while taking drug.

---

## donepezil hydrochloride
Aricept

*Pregnancy Risk Category C*

**HOW SUPPLIED**
*Tablets:* 5 mg, 10 mg

**ACTION**
Inhibits the enzyme acetylcholinesterase in the CNS, increasing the level of acetylcholine. Drug may temporarily improve cognitive function in patients with Alzheimer's disease.

| Route | Onset | Peak | Duration |
|-------|-------|------|----------|
| P.O. | Unknown | 3-4 hr | Unknown |

## INDICATIONS & DOSAGE
*Mild to moderate dementia of the Alzheimer's type—*
**Adults:** initially, 5 mg P.O. daily h.s. After 4 to 6 weeks, dosage may be increased to 10 mg daily.

## ADVERSE REACTIONS
**CNS:** *headache, insomnia,* dizziness, fatigue, depression, abnormal dreams, somnolence, *seizures,* tremor, irritability, paresthesia, aggression, vertigo, ataxia, restlessness, abnormal crying, nervousness, aphasia, syncope, pain.
**CV:** chest pain, hypertension, vasodilation, *atrial fibrillation,* hot flashes, hypotension.
**EENT:** cataract, blurred vision, eye irritation, sore throat.
**GI:** *nausea, diarrhea,* vomiting, anorexia, fecal incontinence, GI bleeding, bloating, epigastric pain.
**GU:** frequent urination.
**Hematologic:** ecchymosis.
**Metabolic:** weight loss, dehydration.
**Musculoskeletal:** muscle cramps, arthritis, toothache, bone fracture.
**Respiratory:** dyspnea, bronchitis.
**Skin:** pruritus, urticaria, diaphoresis.
**Other:** influenza, increased libido.

## INTERACTIONS
**Drug-drug.** *Anticholinergics:* drug may interfere with anticholinergic activity. Monitor patient.
*Anticholinesterases, cholinomimetics:* synergistic effect. Monitor patient closely.
*Bethanechol, succinylcholine:* additive effects. Monitor patient closely.
*Carbamazepine, dexamethasone, phenytoin, phenobarbital, rifampin:* may increase rate of elimination of donepezil. Monitor patient.
**Drug-herb.** *Jaborandi tree:* may have additive effect when used concomitantly. Use cautiously to avoid risk of toxicity.
*Pill-bearing spurge:* additive effects may occur and risk of toxicity may be increased. Use together cautiously.

## EFFECTS ON DIAGNOSTIC TESTS
None reported.

## CONTRAINDICATIONS
Contraindicated in patients with hypersensitivity to drug or piperidine derivatives.

## NURSING CONSIDERATIONS
● Use cautiously in patients with CV disease, asthma or obstructive pulmonary disease, urinary outflow impairment, or history of ulcer disease, and in those presently taking NSAIDs.
● Drug should be used in pregnancy only if benefit justifies risk to fetus. Breast-feeding should be avoided.
● Monitor for symptoms of active or occult GI bleeding.
● *Alert:* Don't confuse Aricept with Ascriptin.

☑**Patient teaching**
● Emphasize that drug doesn't alter underlying degenerative disease but can temporarily stabilize or relieve symptoms. Effect of therapy depends on taking drug at regular intervals.
● Tell caregiver to give drug in the evening, just before bedtime.
● Advise patient and caregiver to immediately report significant adverse effects or changes in overall health status and to inform health care team that patient is taking drug before he receives anesthesia.
● Tell patient to avoid OTC cold or sleep remedies because of the potential for increased anticholinergic effects.

---

## droperidol
Droleptan§, Inapsine

*Pregnancy Risk Category C*

---

## HOW SUPPLIED
*Injection:* 2.5 mg/ml in 1-, 2- and 5-ml ampules, and 2-, 5-, and 10-ml vials

## ACTION
Unknown. Produces marked tranquilization, sedation, and antiemetic effects while allowing for reflex alertness. It also causes mild alpha blockade.

| Route | Onset | Peak | Duration |
|-------|-------|------|----------|
| I.V., I.M. | 3-10 min | 30 min | 2-4 hr |

## INDICATIONS & DOSAGE
*Premedication—*
**Adults and children over age 12:** 2.5 to 10 mg I.M. 30 to 60 minutes preoperatively.
**Children ages 2 to 12:** 1 to 1.5 mg/9 to 11 kg (20 to 24 lb) of body weight I.M.
**Elderly:** reduce dose.
*Adjust-a-dose:* For debilitated patients and those who have received other depressant drugs, use reduced dose.
*For induction as an adjunct to general anesthesia—*
**Adults and children over age 12:** 2.5 mg/9 to 11 kg of body weight I.V. For maintenance, 1.25 to 2.5 mg, usually I.V.
**Children ages 2 to 12:** 1 to 1.5 mg/9 to 11 kg of body weight I.V.
*Use without a general anesthetic in diagnostic procedures—*
**Adults and children over age 12:** 2.5 to 10 mg I.M. 30 to 60 minutes before procedure. Additional doses of 1.25 to 2.5 mg, usually I.V., may be given.
*Adjunct to regional anesthesia when additional sedation is needed—*
**Adults:** 2.5 to 5 mg I.M. or slow I.V.

## ADVERSE REACTIONS
**CNS:** drowsiness, restlessness, hyperactivity, anxiety, extrapyramidal symptoms, dizziness, hallucinations, dysphoria, *neuroleptic malignant syndrome.*
**CV:** hypotension, tachycardia.
**Respiratory:** *laryngospasm, bronchospasm.*
**Other:** chills, shivering.

## INTERACTIONS
**Drug-drug.** *CNS depressants:* additive CNS effects. Adjust dose as needed.
*Fentanyl citrate:* may cause hypertension, respiratory depression. Use together cautiously.

## EFFECTS ON DIAGNOSTIC TESTS
None reported.

## CONTRAINDICATIONS
Contraindicated in patients with hypersensitivity to drug.

## NURSING CONSIDERATIONS
• Use cautiously in patients with hepatic or renal dysfunction and in breast-feeding patients.
• Use with caution in patients with suspected or diagnosed pheochromocytoma because severe hypertension and tachycardia can occur.
• When used for induction of general anesthesia, use with an analgesic.
• If used in procedures such as bronchoscopy, appropriate topical anesthesia is still needed
• *Alert:* Have fluids and other measures to manage hypotension readily available.
• Monitor vital signs routinely.
• *Alert:* Monitor for symptoms of neuroleptic malignant syndrome (fever, altered consciousness, extrapyramidal symptoms, tachycardia).
• *Alert:* Don't confuse droperidol with dronabinol.

🔲 **I.V. administration**
• Administer I.V. doses slowly.
• For high-risk patients, dilute calculated dose in $D_5W$ or lactated Ringers injection and administer as a slow I.V. infusion.

☑ **Patient teaching**
• Warn patient to rise slowly to prevent orthostatic hypotension.
• Advise patient to avoid alcohol for 24 hours after receiving droperidol.

---

fluvoxamine maleate
Faverin§, Luvox

*Pregnancy Risk Category C*

## HOW SUPPLIED
*Tablets:* 50 mg, 100 mg

## ACTION
Unknown. Selectively inhibits the presynaptic neuronal uptake of serotonin, which is thought to improve obsessive-compulsive disorders.

| Route | Onset | Peak | Duration |
|-------|-------|------|----------|
| P.O. | Unknown | 3-8 hr | Unknown |

---

Reactions may be *common,* uncommon, *life-threatening,* or COMMON AND LIFE-THREATENING.

## INDICATIONS & DOSAGE
*Obsessive-compulsive disorder—*
**Adults:** initially, 50 mg P.O. daily h.s., increased in 50-mg increments q 4 to 7 days until maximum benefit achieved. Maximum daily dose is 300 mg. Total daily doses of more than 100 mg should be given in two divided doses.

## ADVERSE REACTIONS
**CNS:** *headache, asthenia, somnolence, insomnia, nervousness,* dizziness, tremor, anxiety, hypertonia, *agitation,* depression, CNS stimulation, taste perversion.
**CV:** palpitations, vasodilation.
**EENT:** amblyopia.
**GI:** *nausea, diarrhea, constipation, dyspepsia,* anorexia, *vomiting,* flatulence, tooth disorder, dysphagia, *dry mouth.*
**GU:** abnormal ejaculation, urinary frequency, impotence, anorgasmia, urine retention.
**Respiratory:** upper respiratory tract infection, dyspnea, yawning.
**Skin:** sweating.
**Other:** flulike syndrome, chills, decreased libido.

## INTERACTIONS
**Drug-drug.** *Benzodiazepines, theophylline, warfarin:* reduced clearance of these drugs by fluvoxamine. Use together cautiously (except for diazepam, which shouldn't be administered with fluvoxamine). Dosage adjustments may be needed.
*Carbamazepine, clozapine, methadone, metipranolol, propranolol, tricyclic antidepressants:* elevated serum levels of these drugs caused by fluvoxamine. Use together cautiously. Monitor patient closely for adverse reactions. Dosage adjustments may be needed.
*Diltiazem:* bradycardia may occur. Monitor heart rate.
*Lithium, tryptophan:* may enhance effects of fluvoxamine. Use together cautiously.
*MAO inhibitors:* may cause severe excitation, hyperpyrexia, myoclonus, delirium, and coma. Avoid concomitant use.
**Drug-lifestyle.** *Smoking:* decreased effectiveness of drug. Encourage patient to stop smoking.

## EFFECTS ON DIAGNOSTIC TESTS
None reported.

## CONTRAINDICATIONS
Contraindicated in patients with hypersensitivity to drug or to other phenylpiperazine antidepressants and within 14 days of MAO inhibitor therapy.

## NURSING CONSIDERATIONS
• Use cautiously in patients with hepatic dysfunction, concomitant conditions that may affect hemodynamic responses or metabolism, or history of mania or seizures.
• *Alert:* Record mood changes. Monitor patient for suicidal tendencies, and allow only a minimum supply of drug.
• *Alert:* Don't confuse Luvox with Lasix.

### ☑ Patient teaching
• Warn patient not to engage in hazardous activity until drug's CNS effects are known.
• Instruct woman who becomes pregnant or intends to become pregnant during therapy to notify doctor.
• Tell patient who develops a rash, hives, or a related allergic reaction to notify doctor.
• Inform patient that several weeks of therapy may be needed to obtain the full antidepressant effect. Once improvement is seen, advise patient not to discontinue drug until directed by doctor.
• Advise patient to check with doctor before taking OTC drugs; drug interactions can occur.

---

## lithium carbonate
Camcolit§, Carbolith†, Duralith†, Eskalith, Eskalith CR, Lithane**, Lithicarb‡, Lithizine†, Lithobid, Lithonate, Lithotabs, Priadel§

## lithium citrate
Cibalith-S*

*Pregnancy Risk Category D*

## HOW SUPPLIED
**lithium carbonate**
*Tablets:* 250 mg‡, 300 mg (300 mg equals 8.12 mEq lithium)

---

*Tablets (controlled-release):* 300 mg, 400 mg‡, 450 mg
*Capsules:* 150 mg, 300 mg, 600 mg
**lithium citrate**
*Syrup (sugarless):* 8 mEq (lithium)/5 ml
*Note:* 5 ml of lithium citrate (liquid) contains 8 mEq lithium, equal to 300 mg lithium carbonate.

## ACTION

Unknown. Probably alters chemical transmitters in the CNS, possibly by interfering with ionic pump mechanisms in brain cells, and may compete with or replace sodium ions.

| Route | Onset | Peak | Duration |
|---|---|---|---|
| P.O. | Unknown | 0.5-3 hr | Unknown |

## INDICATIONS & DOSAGE

*Prevention or control of mania—*
**Adults:** 300 to 600 mg P.O. up to q.i.d. or 900 mg P.O. q 12 hours of controlled-release tablets; increase based on blood levels to achieve optimal dosage. Recommended therapeutic lithium blood levels are 1.5 mEq/L for acute mania, 0.6 to 1.2 mEq/L for maintenance therapy, and 2 mEq/L as maximum level.

## ADVERSE REACTIONS

**CNS:** tremors, drowsiness, headache, confusion, restlessness, dizziness, psychomotor retardation, lethargy, *coma,* blackouts, *epileptiform seizures,* EEG changes, worsened organic mental syndrome, impaired speech, ataxia, muscle weakness, incoordination.
**CV:** reversible ECG changes, *arrhythmias,* hypotension, *bradycardia, peripheral vascular collapse (rare).*
**EENT:** tinnitus, blurred vision.
**GI:** dry mouth, metallic taste, nausea, vomiting, anorexia, diarrhea, *thirst,* abdominal pain, flatulence, indigestion.
**GU:** *polyuria,* glycosuria, decreased creatinine clearance, albuminuria; *renal toxicity (with long-term use).*
**Hematologic:** *leukocytosis with leukocyte count of 14,000 to 18,000/mm³ (reversible);* elevated neutrophil count.
**Metabolic:** transient hyperglycemia, goiter, hypothyroidism (lowered $T_3$, $T_4$, and

protein-bound iodine, but elevated $^{131}I$ uptake), hyponatremia.
**Skin:** pruritus, rash, diminished or absent sensation, drying and thinning of hair, psoriasis, acne, alopecia.
**Other:** ankle and wrist edema.

## INTERACTIONS

**Drug-drug.** *Aminophylline, sodium bicarbonate, urine alkalinizers:* increased lithium excretion. Avoid excessive salt and monitor lithium levels.
*Carbamazepine, fluoxetine, methyldopa, NSAIDs, probenecid:* increased effect of lithium. Monitor for lithium toxicity.
*Diuretics:* increased reabsorption of lithium by kidneys, with possible toxic effect. Use with extreme caution and monitor lithium and electrolyte levels (especially sodium).
*Neuroleptics:* may cause encephalopathy. Watch for signs and symptoms (lethargy, tremor, extrapyramidal symptoms), and stop drug if encephalopathy occurs.
*Neuromuscular blockers:* may cause prolonged paralysis or weakness. Monitor patient closely.
*Thyroid hormones:* may induce hypothyroidism. Monitor thyroid function.
**Drug-herb.** *Parsley:* may promote or produce serotonin syndrome. Avoid concomitant use.
*Plantains:* psyllium seed has been known to inhibit GI absorption. Avoid concomitant use.

## EFFECTS ON DIAGNOSTIC TESTS

Lithium causes false-positive test results on thyroid function tests.

## CONTRAINDICATIONS

Contraindicated if therapy can't be closely monitored.

## NURSING CONSIDERATIONS

• Don't administer drug during pregnancy.
• Use with extreme caution in patients receiving neuroleptics, neuromuscular blockers, and diuretics; in elderly or debilitated patients; and in patients with thyroid disease, seizure disorder, concomitant infection, renal or CV disease, severe debilitation or dehydration, or sodium depletion.

---

Reactions may be *common,* uncommon, *life-threatening,* or COMMON AND LIFE-THREATENING.

• **Alert:** Determination of lithium blood level is crucial to safe use of drug. Don't use drug in patients who can't have regular lithium blood level checks. Monitor lithium blood level 8 to 12 hours after first dose, usually before morning dose, the morning before second dose is given, two or three times weekly for the first month, then weekly to monthly during maintenance therapy.

• When blood levels of lithium are below 1.5 mEq/L, adverse reactions are usually mild.

• Monitor baseline ECG and thyroid and renal studies as well as electrolyte levels, as ordered.

• Check fluid intake and output, especially when surgery is scheduled.

• Weigh patient daily; check for signs of edema or sudden weight gain.

• Adjust fluid and salt ingestion to compensate if excessive loss occurs as a result of protracted diaphoresis or diarrhea. Under normal conditions, patient should have fluid intake of 2,500 to 3,000 ml daily and a balanced diet with adequate salt intake.

• Check urine specific gravity and report level below 1.005, which may indicate diabetes insipidus.

• Drug alters glucose tolerance in diabetics. Monitor blood glucose level closely.

• Perform outpatient follow-up of thyroid and renal functions every 6 to 12 months. Palpate thyroid to check for enlargement.

• **Alert:** Don't confuse Lithobid with Levbid; Lithonate with Lithostat; or Lithotabs with Lithobid or Lithostat.

☑ **Patient teaching**
• Tell patient to take drug with plenty of water and after meals to minimize GI upset.

• Explain that lithium has a narrow therapeutic margin of safety. A blood level that is even slightly high can be dangerous.

• Warn patient and caregivers to watch for evidence of toxicity (diarrhea, vomiting, tremor, drowsiness, muscle weakness, ataxia) and to expect transient nausea, polyuria, thirst, and discomfort during first few days of therapy.

• Instruct patient to withhold one dose and call doctor if toxic symptoms appear, but not to stop drug abruptly.

• Warn ambulatory patient to avoid hazardous activities that require alertness and good psychomotor coordination until CNS effects of drug are known.

• Tell patient not to switch brands of lithium or take other prescription or OTC drugs without doctor's guidance.

• Tell patient to carry medical identification at all times.

## naratriptan hydrochloride
Amerge

*Pregnancy Risk Category C*

### HOW SUPPLIED
*Tablets:* 1 mg, 2.5 mg

### ACTION
May selectively activate serotonin receptors located in intracranial blood vessels, resulting in vasoconstriction and migraine headache relief. Another theory is that activation of receptors on sensory nerve endings in the trigeminal system causes inhibition of proinflammatory neuropeptide release.

| Route | Onset | Peak | Duration |
|-------|-------|------|----------|
| P.O. | Unknown | 2-3 hr | Unknown |

### INDICATIONS & DOSAGE
*Acute migraine attacks with or without aura—*

**Adults:** 1 or 2.5 mg P.O. as a single dose. If headache returns or if only partial response occurs, dose may be repeated after 4 hours, for maximum dose of 5 mg within 24 hours.

*Adjust-a-dose:* For patients with mild to moderate renal or hepatic impairment, a lower initial dose is recommended. Don't exceed maximum dose of 2.5 mg within a 24-hour period.

### ADVERSE REACTIONS
**CNS:** paresthesia, dizziness, drowsiness, malaise, fatigue, vertigo, syncope.
**CV:** palpitation, increased blood pressure, *tachyarrhythmias, abnormal ECG changes (PR, QTc prolongation; ST/T wave abnormalities; PVCs; atrial flutter or fibrillation), coronary vasospasm.*

**EENT:** ear, nose and throat infections; photophobia.
**GI:** nausea, hyposalivation, vomiting.
**Other:** warm or cold sensations; pressure, tightness, heaviness sensations.

## INTERACTIONS

**Drug-drug.** *Ergot-containing or ergot-type drugs (methysergide, dihydroergotamine), other 5-HT$_1$ agonists:* prolonged vasospastic reactions. Don't give within 24 hours of naratriptan.
*Oral contraceptives:* slightly higher levels of naratriptan. Monitor patient.
*Selective serotonin reuptake inhibitors (fluoxetine, fluvoxamine, paroxetine, sertraline):* may cause weakness, hyperreflexia, and incoordination. Monitor patient.
**Drug-lifestyle.** *Smoking:* increased clearance of naratriptan. Discourage concomitant use.

## EFFECTS ON DIAGNOSTIC TESTS
None reported.

## CONTRAINDICATIONS
Contraindicated in patients with hypersensitivity to drug or its components and in those with a history, symptoms, or signs of cardiac ischemia and cerebrovascular or peripheral vascular syndromes or history of uncontrolled hypertension. Also contraindicated in the elderly and in patients with severe renal impairment (creatinine clearance below 15 ml/minute) or severe hepatic impairment (Child-Pugh grade C) and in those who have received ergot-containing, ergot-type, or other 5-HT$_1$ agonists within the past 24 hours.

## NURSING CONSIDERATIONS
● Use cautiously in patients with risk factors for coronary artery disease, such as hypertension, hypercholesterolemia, obesity, diabetes, or strong family history of coronary artery disease. Also use cautiously in women with surgical or physiologic menopause, in men over 40, and in patients who smoke unless a CV evaluation has determined patient to be free from cardiac disease. For patient with cardiac risk factors who has had a satisfactory CV evaluation, monitor closely after first dose.

● Use cautiously in patients with impaired renal or hepatic function.
● Assess cardiac status in patients who develop risk factors for coronary artery disease.
● *Alert:* Drug can cause coronary artery vasospasm and increased risk of cerebrovascular events.
● Drug isn't intended for prophylactic therapy of migraines or for use in managing hemiplegic or basilar migraine.
● Safety and effectiveness of drug haven't been established for cluster headaches or for treating more than four headaches in a 30-day period.
● Use drug after a definite diagnosis of migraine has been established.

### ☑ Patient teaching
● Instruct patient to take drug only as prescribed, and to read the accompanying patient instruction leaflet before using drug.
● Tell patient that drug is intended to relieve, not prevent, migraines.
● Instruct patient to take dose soon after headache starts. If no response occurs with first tablet, tell patient to seek medical approval before taking second tablet. Tell patient that if more relief is needed after first tablet (when a partial response occurs or if headache returns), and doctor has medically approved a second dose, he may take a second tablet but not sooner than 4 hours after first tablet. Inform him not to exceed two tablets within 24 hours.
● Instruct patient not to use drug during pregnancy or if pregnancy is suspected.
● Tell patient to alert doctor if bothersome adverse effects occur.

---

# nicotine polacrilex (nicotine-polacrilin resin complex)
Nicorette ◇ , Nicotinell§

*Pregnancy Risk Category X*

## HOW SUPPLIED
*Chewing gum:* 2 mg/square, 4 mg/square

## ACTION
Provides nicotine, which stimulates nicotinic acetylcholine receptors in the CNS,

---

neuromuscular junction, autonomic ganglia, and adrenal medulla.

| Route | Onset | Peak | Duration |
|-------|-------|------|----------|
| P.O. | Unknown | 15-30 min | Unknown |

## INDICATIONS & DOSAGE
*Relief of nicotine withdrawal symptoms in patients undergoing smoking cessation—*
**Adults:** initially, one 2-mg square; highly dependent patients should start treatment with 4-mg squares. Patient should chew 1 piece of gum slowly and intermittently for 30 minutes whenever the urge to smoke occurs. Most patients need 9 to 12 pieces of gum daily during the first month. For patients using 4-mg squares, maximum dose is 20 pieces daily. For patients using 2-mg squares, maximum dose is 30 pieces daily.

## ADVERSE REACTIONS
**CNS:** dizziness, light-headedness, irritability, insomnia, headache.
**CV:** *atrial fibrillation.*
**EENT:** *throat soreness, jaw muscle ache from chewing.*
**GI:** nausea, vomiting, indigestion, eructation, anorexia, excessive salivation.
**Respiratory:** *hiccups.*

## INTERACTIONS
**Drug-drug.** *Beta blockers, methylxanthines, propoxyphene, propranolol:* decreased metabolism of these drugs, increasing therapeutic effects. Dosage adjustments of these drugs may be needed.
**Drug-lifestyle.** *Smoking:* reduced effectiveness of drug. Warn patient to avoid smoking while taking drug.

## EFFECTS ON DIAGNOSTIC TESTS
None reported.

## CONTRAINDICATIONS
Contraindicated in nonsmokers and in patients with recent MI, life-threatening arrhythmias, severe or worsening angina pectoris, or active temporomandibular joint disease; also contraindicated during pregnancy.

## NURSING CONSIDERATIONS
• Use cautiously in patients with hyperthyroidism, pheochromocytoma, type 1 diabetes mellitus, peptic ulcer disease, history of esophagitis, oral or pharyngeal inflammation, or dental conditions that might be exacerbated by chewing gum.
• Smokers most likely to benefit from nicotine gum are those with high physical nicotine dependence—those who smoke more than 15 cigarettes daily, prefer brands of cigarettes with high nicotine levels, usually inhale the smoke, smoke the first cigarette within 30 minutes of rising, find the first morning cigarette the hardest to give up, smoke most frequently during the morning, find it difficult to refrain from smoking in places where it's forbidden, or smoke even when ill and confined to bed during the day.
• *Alert:* Don't confuse Nicorette with Nordette.

### Patient teaching
• Instruct patient to chew gum slowly and intermittently (chew several times; then place between cheek and gum) for about 30 minutes to promote slow and even buccal absorption of nicotine. Gum must be chewed to release nicotine. Swallowing gum is ineffective. Fast chewing tends to produce more adverse reactions.
• Make sure that patient reads and understands instructions included in the package.
• Emphasize importance of withdrawing gum gradually.
• Tell patient to gradually withdraw gum usage after 3 months. Use of gum for longer than 6 months isn't recommended. For gradual withdrawal, cut gum in halves or quarters and mix with other sugarless gum.

## nicotine transdermal system
Habitrol ◇, Nicoderm, Nicotrol, ProStep

*Pregnancy Risk Category D*

## HOW SUPPLIED
*Transdermal system:* designed to release nicotine at a fixed rate.

Habitrol ◇—21 mg/day, 14 mg/day, 7 mg/day
Nicoderm—21 mg/day, 14 mg/day, 7 mg/day
Nicotrol—15 mg/16 hours, 10 mg/16 hours, 5 mg/16 hours
ProStep—22 mg/day, 11 mg/day

## ACTION
Provides nicotine, which stimulates nicotinic acetylcholine receptors in the CNS, neuromuscular junction, autonomic ganglia, and adrenal medulla.

| Route | Onset | Peak | Duration |
|-------|-------|------|----------|
| Trans-dermal | Unknown | 3-9 hr | Unknown |

## INDICATIONS & DOSAGE
*Relief of nicotine withdrawal symptoms in patients undergoing smoking cessation—*
**Adults:** initially, one transdermal system, delivering the largest available dose of nicotine in its dosage series, applied once daily to nonhairy part of body. For Habitrol, Nicoderm, and ProStep, patch should be kept on for 24 hours, then removed and a new system applied to an alternate skin site. For Nicotrol, the patch should be applied upon awakening and removed h.s. After 4 to 12 weeks (depending on brand used), dose tapered to next lowest available dose of nicotine in its dosage series, followed in 2 to 4 weeks by lowest nicotine dosage system in series being used. Drug is then stopped in 2 to 4 weeks.

## ADVERSE REACTIONS
**CNS:** somnolence, dizziness, *headache, insomnia,* paresthesia, abnormal dreams, nervousness.
**CV:** hypertension.
**EENT:** pharyngitis, sinusitis.
**GI:** abdominal pain, constipation, dyspepsia, nausea, diarrhea, vomiting, dry mouth.
**GU:** dysmenorrhea.
**Musculoskeletal:** back pain, myalgia.
**Respiratory:** increased cough.
**Skin:** *local or systemic erythema, pruritus, burning at application site,* cutaneous hypersensitivity, rash, diaphoresis.

## INTERACTIONS
**Drug-drug.** *Acetaminophen, imipramine, oxazepam, pentazocine, propranolol, theophylline:* may decrease induction of hepatic enzymes that help metabolize certain drugs. Dosage reductions may be needed
*Adrenergic agonists, such as isoproterenol and phenylephrine:* may decrease circulating catecholamines. Dosage increases may be needed.
*Adrenergic antagonists such as labetalol and prazosin:* may decrease circulating catecholamines. Dosage reductions may be needed.
*Insulin:* may increase amount of S.C. insulin absorbed. Dosage reduction of insulin may be needed.
**Drug-herb.** *Blue cohosh:* increased effects of nicotine. Avoid concomitant use.
**Drug-food.** *Caffeine:* may decrease induction of hepatic enzymes that help metabolize certain drugs. Dosage reductions may be needed.

## EFFECTS ON DIAGNOSTIC TESTS
None reported.

## CONTRAINDICATIONS
Contraindicated in patients with hypersensitivity to nicotine or any component of transdermal system. Also contraindicated in nonsmokers and in patients with recent MI, life-threatening arrhythmias, or severe or worsening angina pectoris.

## NURSING CONSIDERATIONS
• Use cautiously in patients with hyperthyroidism, pheochromocytoma, hypertension, type 1 diabetes mellitus, or peptic ulcer disease.
• Health care workers' exposure to nicotine within transdermal systems is probably minimal; however, avoid unnecessary contact with system. Wash hands with water alone because soap may enhance absorption.
• *Alert:* Don't confuse Nicoderm with Nitro-Derm.

### ✓ Patient teaching
• Inform patient that using transdermal system for more than 3 months isn't rec-

---

Reactions may be *common,* uncommon, *life-threatening,* or COMMON AND LIFE-THREATENING.

ommended. Warn patient that long-term nicotine consumption by any route can be dangerous and habit forming.

• *Alert:* Warn patient not to smoke. If he continues to smoke while using system, he may experience serious adverse effects because peak serum nicotine levels will be substantially higher than those achieved by smoking alone.

• Make sure that patient reads and understands information that's dispensed with drug.

• Advise patient to apply patch promptly because nicotine can evaporate from transdermal system once it's removed from its protective packaging. Patch shouldn't be folded or cut before application and shouldn't be stored at temperatures above 86° F (30° C).

• Teach patient proper disposal of transdermal system. After removal, fold patch in half, bringing adhesive sides together. If patch came in a protective pouch, place used patch in same pouch. Careful disposal is needed to prevent accidental poisoning of children or pets.

• Tell patient who experiences persistent or severe local skin reactions or generalized rash to immediately discontinue use of patch and notify doctor.

• Inform patient that those who can't stop cigarette smoking during initial 4 weeks of therapy probably won't benefit from continued use of drug. Such patients may benefit from counseling to identify factors that led to treatment failure. Encourage patient to minimize or eliminate factors contributing to treatment failure and to try again, possibly after some time has passed.

## propofol
Diprivan

*Pregnancy Risk Category B*

### HOW SUPPLIED
*Injection:* 10 mg/ml in 20-ml ampules; 50-ml prefilled syringes; 50-, 100-ml infusion vials

### ACTION
Unknown. Rapidly acting I.V. sedative-hypnotic.

| Route | Onset | Peak | Duration |
|-------|-------|------|----------|
| I.V. | < 40 sec | Unknown | 10-15 min |

### INDICATIONS & DOSAGE
*Induction of general anesthesia—*
**Adults under age 55:** 40 mg I.V. q 10 seconds until induction onset (2 to 2.5 mg/kg). In patients receiving cardiac anesthesia, 20 mg q 10 seconds (0.5 to 1.5 mg/kg) until induction onset. In neurosurgical patients, 20 mg q 10 seconds until induction onset (1 to 2 mg/kg).
**Children ages 3 and older:** in healthy children, 2.5 to 3.5 mg/kg administered over 20 to 30 seconds.
**Elderly:** 20 mg q 10 seconds until induction onset (1 to 1.5 mg/kg).
*Adjust-a-dose:* For debilitated patients or in patients classified as class III or IV by the American Society of Anesthesiologists (ASA), 20 mg q 10 seconds until induction onset (1 to 1.5 mg/kg).
*Maintenance of general anesthesia: infusion—*
**Adults under age 55:** 100 to 200 mcg/kg/minute. In patients receiving cardiac anesthesia, 50 to 150 mcg/kg/minute. In neurosurgical patients, 100 to 200 mcg/kg/minute.
**Children ages 3 and older:** in healthy children, 125 to 300 mcg/kg/minute.
**Elderly:** 50 to 100 mcg/kg/minute.
*Adjust-a-dose:* For debilitated or ASA class III or IV patients, 50 to 100 mcg/kg/minute.
*Maintenance of general anesthesia—*
**Adults under age 55:** intermittent bolus in increments of 20 to 50 mg I.V., p.r.n.
*Initiation of monitored anesthesia care sedation—*
**Adults under age 55:** dosage individualized; 100 to 150 mcg/kg/minute infusion for 3 to 5 minutes, or slow injection of 0.5 mg/kg over 3 to 5 minutes followed immediately by I.V. infusion.
*Maintenance of monitored anesthesia care sedation—*
**Adults under age 55:** 25 to 75 mcg/kg/minute infusion or incremental bolus doses of 10 to 20 mg I.V.

**Elderly:** 80% of healthy adult dose.
*Adjust-a-dose:* For debilitated, neurosurgical, or ASA class III or IV patients, 80% of healthy adult dose.
*Initiation and maintenance of intensive care unit (ICU) sedation in intubated, mechanically ventilated patients—*
**Adults:** dosage individualized; initial infusion usually 5 mcg/kg/minute for 5 minutes. May increase rate at 5- to 10-minute intervals in increments of 5 to 10 mcg/kg/minute until desired level of sedation is achieved. Rates of 5 to 50 mcg/kg/minute or higher may be needed.

**ADVERSE REACTIONS**
**CNS:** movement.
**CV:** *bradycardia,* hypotension, hypertension, decreased cardiac output.
**Metabolic:** hyperlipemia.
**Respiratory:** APNEA, respiratory acidosis.
**Skin:** rash.
**Other:** *burning or stinging at injection site.*

**INTERACTIONS**
**Drug-drug.** *Inhaled anesthetics (such as enflurane, halothane, isoflurane), opioids (fentanyl, meperidine, morphine), sedatives (such as barbiturates, benzodiazepines, chloral hydrate, droperidol):* may increase anesthetic and sedative effects and may also result in a more pronounced decrease in blood pressure and cardiac output. Monitor closely.

**EFFECTS ON DIAGNOSTIC TESTS**
None reported.

**CONTRAINDICATIONS**
Contraindicated in patients with hypersensitivity to drug or its components (including egg lecithin, soybean oil, and glycerol) or when general anesthesia or sedation is contraindicated.

**NURSING CONSIDERATIONS**
• Use cautiously in patients with seizures, disorders of lipid metabolism, and increased intracranial pressure, and in patients who are hemodynamically unstable.
• Drug isn't recommended for obstetric use because it crosses the placenta and may cause neonatal depression.

• Because drug appears in breast milk, use isn't recommended in breast-feeding patients.
• Urine may turn green if drug is used for prolonged sedation in ICU.
• Always use strict aseptic technique during handling. Propofol can support the growth of microorganisms; don't use if contamination is suspected. Discard tubing and unused portions of drug after 12 hours.
• Don't use if there is evidence of separation of phases of emulsion.
• Titrate drug daily to achieve only minimum effective drug level.
• For general anesthesia or MAC sedation, drug should be administered by trained personnel not involved in the surgical or diagnostic procedure. For ICU sedation, drug should be administered by persons skilled in the management of critically ill patients and trained in cardiopulmonary resuscitation and airway management.
• Continuously monitor vital signs.
• Monitor patient at risk for hyperlipidemia for increases in serum triglycerides levels.
• Drug contains 0.1 g of fat (1.1 kcal)/ml. A reduction in concurrently administered lipids is needed.
• Propofol contains ethylenediaminetetraacetic acid, a strong metal chelator. Consider supplemental zinc during prolonged therapy.
• When drug is given in the ICU, assess patient's CNS function daily to determine minimum dose needed.
• Drug should be discontinued slowly to prevent abrupt awakening and increased agitation.

⬛**I.V. administration**
• Strict aseptic technique must be maintained when handling the solution.
• Allow an adequate time interval (3 to 5 minutes) between dosage adjustments to assess effects.
• Protect drug from light. Shake well. Dilute only with $D_5W$. Don't dilute to a concentration below 2 g/ml. Don't infuse through a filter with a pore size smaller than 5 microns. Administer via larger

---

Reactions may be *common,* uncommon, *life-threatening,* or COMMON AND LIFE-THREATENING.

veins of upper extremities to decrease injection site pain.
• Drug shouldn't be mixed with other therapeutic drugs before infusion.
• Don't administer drug in same I.V. line with blood or plasma.

☑ **Patient teaching**
• Advise patient that performance of activities requiring mental alertness, such as operating a motor vehicle or hazardous machinery, may be impaired for some time after drug use.

---

### rizatriptan benzoate
Maxalt, Maxalt-MLT

*Pregnancy Risk Category C*

#### HOW SUPPLIED
*Tablets:* 5 mg, 10 mg
*Tablets (orally disintegrating):* 5 mg, 10 mg

#### ACTION
May act as an agonist at serotonin receptors on the extracerebral intracranial blood vessels, which results in vasoconstriction of the affected vessels, inhibition of neuropeptide release, and reduction of pain transmission in the trigeminal pathways.

| Route | Onset | Peak | Duration |
|-------|-------|------|----------|
| P.O. | Unknown | 1-1.5 hr | Unknown |

#### INDICATIONS & DOSAGE
*Acute migraine headaches with or without aura—*
**Adults:** initially, 5 or 10 mg P.O. If first dose is ineffective, another dose can be given at least 2 hours after first dose. Maximum dose is 30 mg within a 24-hour period. For patients receiving propranolol, 5 mg P.O. up to maximum of three doses (15 mg) in 24 hours.

#### ADVERSE REACTIONS
**CNS:** dizziness, headache, somnolence, paresthesia, asthenia, fatigue, hypesthesia, decreased mental acuity, euphoria, tremor, pain.

**CV:** chest pain, pressure or heaviness, palpitations, flushing.
**EENT:** neck, throat, and jaw pain.
**GI:** dry mouth, nausea, diarrhea, vomiting.
**Respiratory:** dyspnea.
**Other:** warm or cold sensations, hot flashes.

#### INTERACTIONS
**Drug-drug.** *Ergot-containing or ergot-type drugs (dihydroergotamine, methysergide), other 5-HT₁ agonists:* prolonged vasospastic reactions. Don't use within 24 hours of rizatriptan.
*MAO inhibitors (moclobemide), nonselective MAO inhibitors (types A and B): isocarboxazid, phenelzine, tranylcypromine):* increased plasma levels of rizatriptan. Avoid concurrent use and allow at least 14 days to elapse between discontinuation of an MAO inhibitor and initiation of rizatriptan.
*Propranolol:* increased rizatriptan levels. Reduce rizatriptan dose to 5 mg.
*Selective serotonin reuptake inhibitors (fluoxetine, fluvoxamine, paroxetine, sertraline):* weakness, hyperreflexia, incoordination may occur. Monitor patient.

#### EFFECTS ON DIAGNOSTIC TESTS
None reported.

#### CONTRAINDICATIONS
Contraindicated in patients with hypersensitivity to drug or its inactive ingredients and in those with ischemic heart disease (angina pectoris, history of MI, or documented silent ischemia) or symptoms or findings consistent with ischemic heart disease, coronary artery vasospasm (Prinzmetal's variant angina), or other significant underlying CV disease. Also contraindicated in patients with uncontrolled hypertension or within 24 hours of treatment with another 5-HT₁ agonist or ergotamine-containing or ergot-type drug, such as dihydroergotamine or methysergide. Don't use within 2 weeks of discontinuation of MAO inhibitor.

#### NURSING CONSIDERATIONS
• Use cautiously in patients with hepatic or renal impairment.

---

• Use with caution in patients with risk factors for coronary artery disease (hypertension, hypercholesterolemia, smoking, obesity, diabetes, strong family history of coronary artery disease, women with surgical or physiologic menopause, or men over 40), unless a cardiac evaluation provides evidence that patient is free from cardiac disease. Monitor closely after first dose.

• Assess CV status in patients who develop risk factors for coronary artery disease during treatment.

• Drug should be used only after a definite diagnosis of migraine is established.

• Don't use for prophylactic therapy of migraines or in patients with hemiplegic or basilar migraine or cluster headaches.

• Safety of treating, on average, more than four headaches in a 30-day period hasn't been established.

• Safety and effectiveness of drug haven't been evaluated in children under age 18.

• The orally disintegrating tablets contain phenylalanine.

✔ **Patient teaching**
• Inform patient that drug doesn't prevent migraine headache.

• For Maxalt-MLT, tell patient to remove blister pack from pouch, then remove drug from blister pack immediately before use. Tablet shouldn't be popped out of blister pack; pack should be carefully peeled away with dry hands, and tablet placed on tongue and allowed to dissolve. Tablet is then swallowed with saliva. No water is needed or recommended. Tell patient that orally dissolving tablet doesn't provide more rapid headache relief.

• Advise patient that, if headache returns after initial dose, a second dose may be taken with medical approval at least 2 hours after the first dose. Don't take more than 30 mg in a 24-hour period.

• Inform patient that drug may cause somnolence and dizziness and warn him to avoid hazardous activities until effects are known.

• Tell patient that food may delay drug's onset of action.

• Advise patient to notify doctor if pregnancy occurs or is suspected.

• Instruct patient not to breast-feed because effects on the infant are unknown.

## sibutramine hydrochloride monohydrate
Meridia

*Controlled Substance Schedule IV*
*Pregnancy Risk Category C*

### HOW SUPPLIED
*Capsules:* 5 mg, 10 mg, 15 mg

### ACTION
Inhibits reuptake of norepinephrine, serotonin, and dopamine.

| Route | Onset | Peak | Duration |
|-------|-------|------|----------|
| P.O. | Unknown | 3-4 hr | Unknown |

### INDICATIONS & DOSAGE
*Management of obesity—*
**Adults:** 10 mg P.O. administered once daily with or without food. May increase dose to 15 mg P.O. daily after 4 weeks if there is inadequate weight loss. Patients who don't tolerate the 10-mg dose may receive 5 mg P.O. daily. Doses above 15 mg daily aren't recommended.

### ADVERSE REACTIONS
**CNS:** headache, *insomnia*, dizziness, nervousness, anxiety, depression, paresthesia, somnolence, CNS stimulation, emotional lability, asthenia, migraine.
**CV:** tachycardia, vasodilation, hypertension, palpitation, chest pain.
**EENT:** thirst, *rhinitis, pharyngitis*, sinusitis, ear disorder, ear pain.
**GI:** *anorexia, constipation*, increased appetite, nausea, dyspepsia, gastritis, vomiting, *dry mouth,* taste perversion, abdominal pain, rectal disorder.
**GU:** dysmenorrhea, urinary tract infection, vaginal candidiasis, metrorrhagia.
**Hepatic:** elevated liver function tests results.
**Musculoskeletal:** arthralgia, myalgia, tenosynovitis, joint disorder, neck or back pain.
**Respiratory:** cough increase, laryngitis.
**Skin:** rash, sweating, herpes simplex, acne.
**Other:** flulike syndrome, injury, accident, ***allergic reaction,*** generalized edema.

---

Reactions may be *common,* uncommon, ***life-threatening***, or COMMON AND LIFE-THREATENING.

## INTERACTIONS

**Drug-drug.** *CNS depressants:* may enhance CNS depression. Use with caution.
*Dextromethorphan, dihydroergotamine, fentanyl, fluoxetine, fluvoxamine, lithium, MAO inhibitors, meperidine, paroxetine, pentazocine, sertraline, sumatriptan, tryptophan, venlafaxine:* may cause hyperthermia, tachycardia, and loss of consciousness. Avoid concomitant use.
*Ephedrine, phenylpropanolamine, pseudoephedrine:* may increase blood pressure or heart rate. Use with caution.
**Drug-lifestyle.** *Alcohol use:* enhanced CNS depression. Use with caution.

## EFFECTS ON DIAGNOSTIC TESTS
None reported.

## CONTRAINDICATIONS
Contraindicated in patients with hypersensitivity to drug or its active ingredients, in those taking MAO inhibitors or other centrally acting appetite suppressant drugs, and in those with anorexia nervosa. Don't use in patients with severe renal or hepatic dysfunction, history of hypertension, coronary artery disease, heart failure, arrhythmias, or stroke.

## NURSING CONSIDERATIONS
• Use cautiously in patients with history of seizures or angle-closure glaucoma.
• Drug is recommended for obese patients with an initial body mass index of 30 kg/$m^2$ or more or 27 kg/$m^2$ or more in the presence of other risk factors (such as hypertension, diabetes, or dyslipidemia).
• Rule out organic causes of obesity before starting therapy.
• Measure blood pressure and pulse before starting therapy, with dosage changes, and at regular intervals during therapy.
• At least 2 weeks should elapse between stopping an MAO inhibitor and starting drug therapy, and vice versa.

☑ **Patient teaching**
• Advise patient to report rash, hives, or other allergic reactions immediately.
• Instruct patient to inform doctor before taking prescription or OTC drugs.

• Advise patient to have blood pressure and pulse monitored at regular intervals. Stress importance of regular follow-up visits with doctor.
• Advise patient to use drug with reduced-calorie diet.
• Tell patient that weight loss can precipitate gallstone formation. Teach him its signs and symptoms and tell him to report to doctor promptly if they occur.

---

## sumatriptan succinate
Imigran§, Imitrex

*Pregnancy Risk Category C*

### HOW SUPPLIED
*Tablets:* 25 mg, 50 mg, 100 mg (base)†
*Injection:* 6 mg/0.5 ml (12 mg/ml) in 0.5-ml prefilled syringes and vials
*Nasal solution:* 5 mg/0.1 ml; 20 mg/0.1 ml

### ACTION
Unknown. May selectively activate vascular serotonin (5-hydroxytryptamine, 5-HT) receptors. Stimulation of the specific receptor subtype 5-HT$_1$, present on cranial arteries and the dura mater, causes vasoconstriction of cerebral vessels but has minimal effects on systemic vessels, tissue perfusion, and blood pressure.

| Route | Onset | Peak | Duration |
|-------|-------|------|----------|
| P.O. | 0.5 hr | 1.5 hr | Unknown |
| S.C. | 10-20 min | 12 min | Unknown |
| Intranasal | Rapid | 1 to 2 hr | Unknown |

### INDICATIONS & DOSAGE
*Acute migraine attacks (with or without aura)—*
**Adults:** 6 mg S.C. Maximum recommended dose is two 6-mg injections daily, with at least 1 hour between injections. Or, initially 25 to 100 mg P.O. and a second dose of up to 100 mg in 2 hours, if needed. Additional doses may be given q 2 hours, p.r.n., to maximum P.O. dose of 300 mg/day. Intranasal dosage is 5 to 20 mg sprayed into one nostril (if a 10-mg dose is needed, 5 mg is sprayed into each nostril). If needed, dosing may be repeated after 2 hours, to maximum of 40 mg daily.

---

*Liquid contains alcohol.   **May contain tartrazine.   †Canada   ‡Australia   §U.K.   ◊OTC

## ADVERSE REACTIONS

**CNS:** *dizziness, vertigo,* drowsiness, headache, anxiety, malaise, fatigue, *burning sensation, tingling, warm or hot sensation,* feeling of strangeness, tight feeling in head, cold sensation; *heaviness, pressure, or tightness.*
**CV:** pressure or tightness in chest, ***atrial fibrillation, ventricular fibrillation, ventricular tachycardia, MI,*** flushing.
**EENT:** discomfort of throat, nasal cavity or sinus, mouth, jaw, or tongue; altered vision.
**GI:** abdominal discomfort, dysphagia.
**Musculoskeletal:** myalgia, muscle cramps, neck pain.
**Skin:** diaphoresis.
**Other:** *injection site reaction.*

## INTERACTIONS

**Drug-drug.** *Ergot and ergot derivatives:* prolonged vasospastic effects. Don't use these drugs and sumatriptan within the same 24-hour period.
*MAO inhibitors:* increased effects of sumatriptan. Avoid concomitant use or using within 2 weeks of discontinuing MAO inhibitor therapy.
**Drug-herb.** *Horehound:* may enhance serotonergic effects. Avoid concomitant use.

## EFFECTS ON DIAGNOSTIC TESTS
None reported.

## CONTRAINDICATIONS

Contraindicated in patients with hypersensitivity to drug and in those with uncontrolled hypertension or ischemic heart disease (such as angina pectoris, Prinzmetal's angina, history of MI, or documented silent ischemia), or hemiplegic or basilar migraine. Also contraindicated in those taking ergotamine or within 14 days of MAO inhibitor therapy.

## NURSING CONSIDERATIONS

• Use cautiously in patient who is or intends to become pregnant.
• Also use cautiously in patients who may have unrecognized coronary artery disease(such as postmenopausal women, men over 40, or patients with risk factors such as hypertension, hypercholesterol-

emia, obesity, diabetes, smoking, or family history of coronary artery disease).
• *Alert:* When giving drug to patients at risk for unrecognized coronary artery disease, consider administering first dose in doctor's office. Serious adverse cardiac effects can follow S.C. administration of drug, but such events are rare.
• After S.C. injection, most patients experience relief within 1 to 2 hours.
• Redness or pain at injection site should subside within 1 hour after injection.
• *Alert:* Don't confuse sumatriptan with somatropin.

### ☑ Patient teaching
• Inform patient that drug is intended only to treat migraine attacks, not to prevent or reduce their occurrence.
• Tell patient who is pregnant or intends to become pregnant not to use drug. Advise her to discuss with doctor risks and benefits of using drug during pregnancy.
• Tell patient that drug may be given any time during a migraine attack, but should be given as soon as symptoms appear.
• Review information about drug's injectable form, which is available in a spring-loaded injector system that facilitates self-administration. Make sure patient understands how to load the injector, administer the injection, and dispose of used syringes.
• *Alert:* Tell patient to notify doctor immediately of persistent or severe chest pain. Warn him to stop using drug and call doctor if he experiences pain or tightness in the throat, wheezing, heart throbbing, rash, lumps, hives, or swollen eyelids, face, or lips.

---

## tacrine hydrochloride
Cognex

*Pregnancy Risk Category C*

## HOW SUPPLIED
*Capsules:* 10 mg, 20 mg, 30 mg, 40 mg

## ACTION
Reversibly inhibits the enzyme cholinesterase in the CNS, preventing or blocking the breakdown of acetylcholine and there-

by temporarily improving cognitive function in patients with Alzheimer's disease.

| Route | Onset | Peak | Duration |
|-------|-------|------|----------|
| P.O. | Unknown | 0.5-3 hr | Unknown |

## INDICATIONS & DOSAGE
*Mild to moderate dementia of the Alzheimer's type—*
**Adults:** initially, 10 mg P.O. q.i.d. After 6 weeks and if patient tolerates treatment and there are no elevations in transaminase levels, dosage increased to 20 mg q.i.d. After 6 weeks, dosage adjusted upward to 30 mg q.i.d. If still tolerated, dosage increased to 40 mg q.i.d. after another 6 weeks.

## ADVERSE REACTIONS
**CNS:** agitation, ataxia, insomnia, abnormal thinking, somnolence, depression, anxiety, *headache,* fatigue, *dizziness,* confusion.
**CV:** chest pain.
**GI:** *nausea, vomiting, diarrhea,* dyspepsia, loose stools, changes in stool color, anorexia, abdominal pain, flatulence, constipation.
**Hepatic:** elevated liver function test results.
**Metabolic:** weight loss.
**Musculoskeletal:** myalgia.
**Respiratory:** rhinitis, upper respiratory tract infection, cough.
**Skin:** rash, jaundice, facial flushing.

## INTERACTIONS
**Drug-drug.** *Anticholinergics:* may decrease effectiveness of anticholinergics. Monitor patient closely.
*Cholinergics such as bethanechol, anticholinesterases:* additive effects. Monitor for toxicity.
*Succinylcholine:* enhanced neuromuscular blockade and prolonged duration of action. Monitor patient closely.
*Theophylline:* increased serum theophylline levels and prolonged theophylline half-life. Carefully monitor theophylline plasma levels and adjust dosage, as ordered.
**Drug-food.** *Any food:* delayed absorption of drug. Give drug 1 hour before meals.

**Drug-lifestyle.** *Smoking:* decreased plasma levels of drug. Monitor response.

## EFFECTS ON DIAGNOSTIC TESTS
None reported.

## CONTRAINDICATIONS
Contraindicated in patients with hypersensitivity to drug or acridine derivatives. Also contraindicated in patients in whom tacrine-related jaundice has previously developed and which has been confirmed with a total bilirubin level of more than 3 mg/dl.

## NURSING CONSIDERATIONS
• Use cautiously in patients with sick sinus syndrome or bradycardia, in patients at risk for peptic ulceration (including those taking NSAIDs or those with history of peptic ulcer), and in those with history of hepatic disease. Also use cautiously in patients with renal disease, asthma, prostatic hyperplasia, or other urinary outflow impairment.
• Monitor serum ALT levels weekly during first 18 weeks of therapy, as ordered. If ALT is modestly elevated (twice the upper limit of normal range) after first 18 weeks, continue weekly monitoring. If no problems are detected, frequency of serum level determinations is decreased to once every 3 months. On each occasion that dosage is increased, resume weekly monitoring for at least 6 weeks, as ordered.
• If drug is discontinued for 4 weeks or more, full dosage adjustment and monitoring schedule must be restarted.

☑ **Patient teaching**
• Stress that drug doesn't alter the underlying degenerative disease, but can stabilize or alleviate symptoms. Effect of therapy depends on drug administration at regular intervals.
• *Alert:* Remind caregiver that dosage adjustment is an integral part of the safe use of drug. Abrupt discontinuation or a large reduction in daily dosage (80 mg/day or more) may precipitate behavioral disturbances and a decline in cognitive function.
• Tell caregiver to give patient drug between meals whenever possible. If GI upset becomes a problem, drug may be tak-

en with meals, although doing so may reduce plasma levels by 30% to 40%.
• Advise patient and caregiver to immediately report significant adverse reactions or changes in status.

# zolmitriptan
Zomig

*Pregnancy Risk Category C*

## HOW SUPPLIED
*Tablets (immediate-release):* 2.5 mg, 5 mg

## ACTION
Selective serotonin receptor agonist that can abort migraine headaches by causing constriction of cranial blood vessels and inhibition of proinflammatory neuropeptide release.

| Route | Onset | Peak | Duration |
|-------|---------|------|----------|
| P.O. | Unknown | 2 hr | 3 hr |

## INDICATIONS & DOSAGE
*Acute migraine headaches—*
**Adults:** initially, 2.5 mg or lower P.O. increased to 5 mg per dose, p.r.n. If headache returns after initial dose, second dose may be administered after 2 hours. Maximum dose is 10 mg in 24-hour period.
*Adjust-a-dose:* For patients with moderate to severe hepatic impairment, use a lower dose.

## ADVERSE REACTIONS
**CNS:** somnolence, vertigo, hyperesthesia, paresthesia, asthenia, *dizziness,* syncope.
**CV:** pain or heaviness in chest; *arrhythmias;* hypertension; *pain, tightness, or pressure in the neck, throat, or jaw.*
**GI:** dyspepsia, dysphagia, nausea.
**Metabolic:** hyperglycemia.
**Musculoskeletal:** myalgia.
**Other:** warm or cold sensations.

## INTERACTIONS
**Drug-drug.** *Cimetidine:* doubles half-life of zolmitriptan. Monitor patient.
*Ergot-containing drugs:* may cause additive vasospastic reactions. Avoid concomitant use.

*Fluoxetine, fluvoxamine, paroxetine, sertraline:* may cause weakness, hyperreflexia, and incoordination. Use cautiously.
*MAO inhibitors:* increased effects of drug. Avoid concomitant use.

## EFFECTS ON DIAGNOSTIC TESTS
None reported.

## CONTRAINDICATIONS
Contraindicated in patients with hypersensitivity to drug and in those with ischemic heart disease or other significant heart disease (including Wolff-Parkinson-White syndrome), or uncontrolled hypertension. Don't give within 24 hours of ergot-containing drugs or within 2 weeks of discontinuing MAO inhibitor therapy.

## NURSING CONSIDERATIONS
• Use cautiously in patients with liver disease.
• Drug isn't intended for prophylactic therapy of migraines or for use in hemiplegic or basilar migraines.
• Safety of drug hasn't been established for cluster headaches.
• Don't administer to patient who is or may be pregnant or is breast-feeding.

☑ **Patient teaching**
• Tell patient that drug is intended to relieve, not prevent, symptoms of migraine.
• Advise patient to take drug as prescribed, and that he shouldn't take a second dose unless instructed by doctor. Tell patient that, if a second dose is indicated and permitted, to only take it 2 hours after initial dose.
• Advise patient to report pain or tightness in the chest or throat, heart throbbing, rash, skin lumps, or swelling of the face, lips or eyelids immediately.
• Tell patient not to take drug if pregnancy is being planned or is suspected.

---

Reactions may be *common,* uncommon, *life-threatening,* or COMMON AND LIFE-THREATENING.

bethanechol chloride
edrophonium chloride
neostigmine bromide
neostigmine methylsulfate
physostigmine salicylate
pyridostigmine bromide

## COMBINATION PRODUCTS
None.

## bethanechol chloride
Duvoid, Myotonachol,
Myotonine§, Urabeth, Urecholine,
Urocarb‡, Urocarb‡

*Pregnancy Risk Category C*

### HOW SUPPLIED
*Tablets:* 5 mg, 10 mg, 25 mg, 50 mg
*Injection:* 5 mg/ml

### ACTION
Directly stimulates primarily muscarinic cholinergic receptors, mimicking the action of acetylcholine, producing increased tone and peristalsis in the GI tract and increasing contraction of the detrusor muscle of the urinary bladder.

| Route | Onset | Peak | Duration |
|-------|-------|------|----------|
| P.O. | 30-90 min | 1 hr | 6 hr |
| S.C. | 5-15 min | 15-30 min | 2 hr |

### INDICATIONS & DOSAGE
*Acute postoperative and postpartum nonobstructive (functional) urine retention, neurogenic atony of urinary bladder with urine retention—*
**Adults:** 10 to 50 mg P.O. t.i.d. to q.i.d. Or, 2.5 to 5 mg S.C. Never give I.M. or I.V. When used for urine retention, some patients may need 50 to 100 mg P.O. per dose. Use such doses with extreme caution.

Test dose is 2.5 mg S.C., repeated at 15- to 30-minute intervals to total of four doses to determine the minimal effective dose; then minimal effective dose used q

6 to 8 hours. All doses must be adjusted individually.

### ADVERSE REACTIONS
**CNS:** headache, malaise.
**CV:** *bradycardia,* profound hypotension with reflexive tachycardia, flushing.
**EENT:** lacrimation, miosis.
**GI:** *abdominal cramps, diarrhea,* excessive salivation, nausea, belching, borborygmus, elevated amylase, lipase.
**GU:** urinary urgency.
**Hepatic:** elevated liver enzyme levels.
**Respiratory:** *bronchoconstriction,* increased bronchial secretions.
**Skin:** diaphoresis.

### INTERACTIONS
**Drug-drug.** *Anticholinergics, atropine, procainamide, quinidine:* may reverse cholinergic effects. Observe for lack of drug effect.
*Anticholinesterases, cholinergic agonists:* may cause additive effects or increase toxicity. Avoid concomitant use.
*Ganglionic blockers:* may cause critical decrease in blood pressure, usually preceded by severe abdominal pain. Avoid concomitant use.

### EFFECTS ON DIAGNOSTIC TESTS
Drug increases sulfobromophthalein retention time.

### CONTRAINDICATIONS
Contraindicated in patients with hypersensitivity to drug or its components and in those with uncertain strength or integrity of bladder wall, mechanical obstructions of the GI or urinary tract, hyperthyroidism, peptic ulceration, latent or active bronchial asthma, obstructive pulmonary disease, pronounced bradycardia or hypotension, vasomotor instability, cardiac or coronary artery disease, hypertension, seizure disorder, Parkinson's disease, spastic GI disturbances, acute inflammatory lesions of the GI tract, peritonitis, or marked vagotonia. Also contraindicated

for I.M. or I.V. use or when increased muscular activity of the GI or urinary tract is harmful.

## NURSING CONSIDERATIONS
• Use cautiously in pregnant patient.
• Give drug on empty stomach; otherwise, it may cause nausea and vomiting.
• *Alert:* Never give I.M. or I.V.; could cause circulatory collapse, hypotension, severe abdominal cramping, bloody diarrhea, shock, or cardiac arrest.
• Monitor vital signs frequently, especially respirations. Always have atropine injection available and be prepared to give 0.6 mg S.C. or by slow I.V. push, as ordered. Provide respiratory support if needed.
• Watch for toxicity, especially with S.C. administration. Edrophonium isn't effective against muscle relaxation caused by bethanechol.
• Watch closely for adverse reactions that may indicate drug toxicity.
• Oral drug absorption is poor and variable, requiring larger oral doses. Oral and S.C. doses aren't interchangeable.

✅ **Patient teaching**
• Instruct patient to take oral form on an empty stomach and at regular intervals.
• Inform patient that drug is usually effective within 30 to 90 minutes after oral administration and 5 to 15 minutes after S.C. administration.

---

## edrophonium chloride
Enlon, Reversol, Tensilon

*Pregnancy Risk Category C*

## HOW SUPPLIED
*Injection:* 10 mg/ml in 1-ml ampules or in 10-ml or 15-ml vials

## ACTION
Rapidly reversible inhibitor of acetylcholinesterase, thus blocking destruction of acetylcholine released from the parasympathetic and somatic efferent nerves. Acetylcholine accumulates, promoting increased stimulation of the receptors.

| Route | Onset | Peak | Duration |
|-------|-------|------|----------|
| I.V. | < 1 min | Unknown | 5-20 min |
| I.M. | 2-10 min | Unknown | 10-40 min |

## INDICATIONS & DOSAGE
*As curare antagonist (to reverse nondepolarizing neuromuscular blocking action)—*
**Adults:** 10 mg I.V. given over 30 to 45 seconds. Dose may be repeated, p.r.n., to maximum of 40 mg. Larger dosages may potentiate effect of curare.
*Diagnostic aid in myasthenia gravis (Tensilon test)—*
**Adults:** 1 to 2 mg I.V. over 15 to 30 seconds; then 8 mg if no response (increase in muscular strength and no cholinergic reaction) occurs. Or, 10 mg I.M. If cholinergic reaction occurs, 2 mg I.M. 30 minutes later is given to rule out false-negative response.
**Children weighing over 34 kg (75 lb):** 2 mg I.V. If no response within 45 seconds, 1 mg q 45 seconds to maximum of 10 mg.
**Children weighing up to 34 kg:** 1 mg I.V. If no response within 45 seconds, 1 mg q 45 seconds to maximum of 5 mg.

I.M. route may be used in children because of difficulty with I.V. route: for children under 34 kg, 2 mg I.M.; for children over 34 kg, 5 mg I.M. Expect same reactions as with I.V. test, but these appear after 2- to 10-minute delay.
*To differentiate myasthenic crisis from cholinergic crisis—*
**Adults:** 1 mg I.V. If there is no response in 1 minute, dose is repeated once. Increased muscular strength confirms myasthenic crisis; no increase or exaggerated weakness confirms cholinergic crisis.

## ADVERSE REACTIONS
**CNS:** *seizures,* weakness, dysarthria, dysphonia, dizziness, drowsiness, headache, syncope.
**CV:** hypotension, bradycardia, flushing, AV block, *cardiac arrest.*

---

**EENT:** excessive lacrimation, diplopia, miosis, conjunctival hyperemia.
**GI:** nausea, vomiting, *diarrhea, abdominal cramps,* excessive salivation, dysphagia.
**GU:** urinary frequency, incontinence.
**Musculoskeletal:** muscle cramps, muscle fasciculation.
**Respiratory:** *paralysis of respiratory muscles, central respiratory paralysis, bronchospasm, laryngospasm,* increased bronchial secretions, *respiratory depression, respiratory arrest,* dyspnea.
**Skin:** rash, diaphoresis.

**INTERACTIONS**
**Drug-drug.** *Aminoglycosides:* prolonged or enhanced muscle weakness. Monitor closely.
*Cardiac glycosides:* may increase the heart's sensitivity to edrophonium. Use together cautiously.
*Cholinergics:* increased effects. Stop all other cholinergics before giving drug, as ordered.
*Corticosteroids, magnesium, procainamide, quinidine:* may antagonize cholinergic effects. Observe for lack of drug effect.
*Depolarizing muscle relaxants (decamethonium, succinylcholine):* increased neuromuscular blocking effects, prolonged respiratory depression. Monitor closely.
*Local and general anesthetics:* may antagonize cholinergic effects. Observe for lack of drug effect.
**Drug-herb.** *Jaborandi tree, pill-bearing spurge:* may have an additive effect when used concomitantly. Use with caution to avoid risk of toxicity.

**EFFECTS ON DIAGNOSTIC TESTS**
None reported.

**CONTRAINDICATIONS**
Contraindicated in patients with hypersensitivity to anticholinesterases and in those with mechanical obstruction of the intestine or urinary tract.

**NURSING CONSIDERATIONS**
• Use cautiously in patients with bronchial asthma or cardiac arrhythmias.
• *Alert:* Watch closely for adverse reactions; they may indicate toxicity.

• Keep in mind that drug isn't effective against neuromuscular block induced by decamethonium bromide and succinylcholine chloride.
• This cholinergic has the most rapid onset but shortest duration; therefore, it isn't used to treat myasthenia gravis.
• When giving drug to differentiate myasthenic crisis from cholinergic crisis, observe patient's muscle strength closely.

🔲 **I.V. administration**
• For easier parenteral administration, use tuberculin syringe with an I.V. needle.
• *Alert:* Monitor vital signs frequently, especially respirations. Always have atropine injection available and be prepared to give 0.5 to 1 mg S.C. or by slow I.V. push, as ordered. Provide respiratory support as needed.
• If using as a test to distinguish myasthenic crisis from cholinergic crisis, secure controlled ventilation if patient is apneic before administering drug.

☑ **Patient teaching**
• Teach patient to report adverse reactions promptly.
• Tell patient to alert nurse if discomfort occurs at I.V. site.

---

**neostigmine bromide**
Prostigmin

**neostigmine methylsulfate**
Prostigmin

*Pregnancy Risk Category C*

**HOW SUPPLIED**
**neostigmine bromide**
*Tablets:* 15 mg
**neostigmine methylsulfate**
*Injection:* 0.25 mg/ml, 0.5 mg/ml, 1 mg/ml

**ACTION**
Competitive inhibitor of acetylcholinesterase, thus blocking the destruction of acetylcholine released from the parasympathetic and somatic efferent nerves.

Acetylcholine accumulates, promoting increased stimulation of the receptors.

| Route | Onset | Peak | Duration |
|---|---|---|---|
| P.O. | 45-75 min | 1-2 hr | 2-4 hr |
| I.V. | 4-8 min | 1-2 hr | 2-4 hr |
| I.M., S.C. | 20-30 min | 1-2 hr | 2-4 hr |

## INDICATIONS & DOSAGE
*Myasthenia gravis—*
**Adults:** initially, 15 mg P.O. t.i.d.; increase gradually, p.r.n. Range is 15 to 375 mg/day (average dose is 150 mg/day) with intervals individualized. Or, 0.5 to 2.5 mg S.C., I.M.; subsequent parenteral doses should be based on patient's response.
**Children:** 7.5 to 15 mg P.O. t.i.d. or q.i.d. or 0.01 to 0.04 mg/kg/dose I.M. or S.C. q 2 to 3 hours, p.r.n.

Dosage must be highly individualized, depending on response and tolerance of adverse effects. Therapy may be needed day and night.
*Diagnosis of myasthenia gravis—*
**Adults:** 0.022 mg/kg I.M. 30 minutes after 0.011 mg/kg of atropine sulfate I.M.
**Children:** 0.025 to 0.04 mg/kg I.M. after 0.011 mg/kg atropine sulfate S.C.
*Postoperative abdominal distention and bladder atony—*
**Adults:** 0.5 to 1 mg I.M. or S.C. q 3 hours for 5 doses after bladder has emptied (treatment); 0.25 mg I.M. or S.C. q 4 to 6 hours for 2 to 3 days (prevention).
*Antidote for nondepolarizing neuromuscular blockers—*
**Adults:** 0.5 to 2.5 mg I.V. slowly. Repeat, p.r.n., to total of 5 mg. Before antidote dose, give 0.6 to 1.2 mg atropine sulfate I.V. if patient is bradycardic.

## ADVERSE REACTIONS
**CNS:** dizziness, headache, muscle weakness, loss of consciousness, drowsiness, syncope, *seizures.*
**CV:** *bradycardia,* hypotension, tachycardia, AV block, flushing, *cardiac arrest.*
**EENT:** blurred vision, lacrimation, miosis.
**GI:** *nausea, vomiting, diarrhea, abdominal cramps,* excessive salivation, flatulence, increased peristalsis.
**GU:** urinary frequency.

**Musculoskeletal:** *muscle cramps,* muscle fasciculations, arthralgia.
**Respiratory:** *bronchospasm,* dyspnea, *respiratory depression, respiratory arrest,* increased secretions, *laryngospasm, paralysis of respiratory muscles, central respiratory paralysis.*
**Skin:** rash, urticaria, diaphoresis.
**Other:** *hypersensitivity reactions, anaphylaxis.*

## INTERACTIONS
**Drug-drug.** *Aminoglycosides, anticholinergics, atropine, corticosteroids, local and general anesthetics, magnesium sulfate, procainamide, quinidine:* may reverse cholinergic effects. Observe for lack of drug effect. Stop all other cholinergics before giving this drug, as ordered.
*Succinylcholine:* may worsen blockade produced by succinylcholine when used to reverse the effects of nondepolarizing neuromuscular blockers in patients who have undergone surgery. Monitor patient.

## EFFECTS ON DIAGNOSTIC TESTS
None reported.

## CONTRAINDICATIONS
Contraindicated in patients with hypersensitivity to cholinergics or bromides and in those with peritonitis or mechanical obstruction of the intestinal or urinary tract.

## NURSING CONSIDERATIONS
• Use cautiously in patients with bronchial asthma, bradycardia, seizure disorders, recent coronary occlusion, vagotonia, hyperthyroidism, arrhythmias, and peptic ulcer.
• In myasthenia gravis, schedule doses before periods of fatigue. For example, if patient has dysphagia, schedule dose 30 minutes before each meal.
• *Alert:* Monitor vital signs frequently, especially respirations. Have atropine injection available and be prepared to give, as ordered; provide respiratory support as needed.
• Monitor and document patient's response after each dose. Optimum dosage is difficult to judge. Observe closely for

---

Reactions may be *common,* uncommon, *life-threatening,* or COMMON AND LIFE-THREATENING.

improvement in strength, vision, and ptosis 45 to 60 minutes after each dose.

• I.M. neostigmine may be used instead of edrophonium to diagnose myasthenia gravis and may be preferable to edrophonium for lengthy procedures involving testing of limb strength.

• When drug is used to prevent abdominal distention and GI distress, doctor may order insertion of a rectal tube to help passage of gas.

• When drug is given for postoperative abdominal distention and bladder atony, mechanical obstruction should be ruled out before treatment doses are given. If there is no response within 1 hour after first dose, patient should be catheterized.

• Patient sometimes develops resistance to neostigmine.

• If appropriate, obtain doctor's order for hospitalized patient to have bedside supply of tablets. Many patients with long-standing disease insist on self-administration.

**◖ I.V. administration**

• Give at a slow, controlled rate, not exceeding 1 mg/minute in adults.

• If patient's muscle weakness is severe, doctor will determine if severity is caused by drug-induced toxicity or exacerbation of myasthenia gravis. Test dose of edrophonium I.V. will aggravate drug-induced weakness but will temporarily relieve weakness caused by disease.

**☑ Patient teaching**

• Tell patient to take drug with food or milk to reduce adverse GI reactions.

• When using for myasthenia gravis, explain that drug will relieve ptosis, double vision, difficulty in chewing and swallowing, and trunk and limb weakness. Stress importance of taking drug exactly as ordered, including nighttime doses. Explain that drug may have to be taken for life.

• Show patient how to observe and record variations in muscle strength.

• Advise patient to wear medical identification bracelet indicating myasthenia gravis.

## physostigmine salicylate (eserine salicylate)
Antilirium

*Pregnancy Risk Category C*

### HOW SUPPLIED
*Injection:* 1 mg/ml

### ACTION
Reversible inhibitor of acetylcholinesterase, thus blocking the destruction of acetylcholine released from the parasympathetic and somatic efferent nerves. Acetylcholine accumulates, promoting increased stimulation of the receptor.

| Route | Onset | Peak | Duration |
|-------|-------|------|----------|
| I.V. | 3-5 min | 5 min | 0.5-5 hr |
| I.M. | 3-5 min | 20-30 min | 0.5-5 hr |

### INDICATIONS & DOSAGE
*To reverse CNS toxicity associated with clinical or toxic dosages of drugs capable of producing anticholinergic syndrome—*
**Adults:** 0.5 to 2 mg I.M. or I.V. (1 mg/ minute I.V.) repeated q 20 minutes as needed until response or adverse cholinergic effects occur. Additional doses of 1 to 4 mg I.M. or I.V. q 30 to 60 minutes may be given if life-threatening signs recur (coma, seizures, arrhythmias).
**Children:** reserved for life-threatening situations only. 0.02 mg/kg I.M. or slow I.V., repeated q 5 to 10 minutes until response occurs. Maximum dose is 2 mg.

### ADVERSE REACTIONS
**CNS:** *seizures,* muscle weakness, *restlessness, excitability.*
**CV:** *bradycardia,* hypotension.
**EENT:** miosis.
**GI:** nausea, vomiting, epigastric pain, *diarrhea, excessive salivation.*
**GU:** urinary urgency.
**Respiratory:** *bronchospasm,* bronchial constriction, dyspnea, *respiratory paralysis.*
**Skin:** diaphoresis.

### INTERACTIONS
**Drug-drug.** *Anticholinergics, atropine, local and general anesthetics, procain-*

---

*amide, quinidine:* may reverse cholinergic effects. Observe for lack of drug effect.
*Ganglionic blockers:* may decrease blood pressure. Avoid concomitant use.
*Neuromuscular blockers (succinylcholine):* increased neuromuscular blockade, respiratory depression. Use cautiously.
**Drug-herb.** *Jaborandi tree, pill-bearing spurge:* may have an additive effect when used concomitantly. Use with caution to avoid risk of toxicity.

## EFFECTS ON DIAGNOSTIC TESTS
None reported.

## CONTRAINDICATIONS
Contraindicated in patients with mechanical obstruction of the intestine or urogenital tract, asthma, gangrene, diabetes, CV disease, or vagotonia and in those receiving choline esters or depolarizing neuromuscular blockers.

## NURSING CONSIDERATIONS
• Use cautiously in pregnant patients and in patients with epilepsy, parkinsonian syndrome, or bradycardia.
• Use only clear solution. Darkening may indicate loss of potency.
• *Alert:* Watch closely for adverse reactions, particularly CNS disturbances. Raise side rails if patient becomes restless or hallucinates. Adverse reactions may indicate drug toxicity.
• Effectiveness is generally immediate and dramatic but it may be transient and need repeated doses.

### I.V. administration
• Give I.V. at controlled rate; use direct injection at no more than 1 mg/minute in adults or 0.5 mg/minute in children.
• Monitor vital signs frequently, especially respirations. Position patient to ease breathing. Have atropine injection available and be prepared to give 0.5 mg S.C. or by slow I.V. push, as ordered. Provide respiratory support as needed. Best administered in presence of doctor.

### Patient teaching
• Inform patient of need for drug, explain its use and adverse reactions, and answer any questions or concerns.

• Tell patient to report adverse reactions promptly.
• Instruct patient to alert nurse if discomfort occurs at I.V. site.

# pyridostigmine bromide
Mestinon*, Mestinon-SR†, Mestinon Timespans, Regonol

*Pregnancy Risk Category C*

## HOW SUPPLIED
*Tablets:* 60 mg
*Tablets (extended-release):* 180 mg
*Syrup:* 60 mg/5 ml
*Injection:* 5 mg/ml in 2-ml ampules or 5-ml vials

## ACTION
Competitive inhibitor of acetylcholinesterase, thus blocking the destruction of acetylcholine released from the parasympathetic and somatic efferent nerves. Acetylcholine accumulates, promoting increased stimulation of the receptors.

| Route | Onset | Peak | Duration |
|---|---|---|---|
| P.O. | 20-30 min | 1-2 hr | 3-6 hr |
| P.O. (extended) | 30-60 min | 1-2 hr | 6-12 hr |
| I.V. | 2-5 min | Unknown | 2-4 hr |
| I.M. | 15 min | Unknown | 2-4 hr |

## INDICATIONS & DOSAGE
*Antidote for nondepolarizing neuromuscular blockers—*
**Adults:** 10 to 20 mg I.V. preceded by atropine sulfate 0.6 to 1.2 mg I.V.
*Myasthenia gravis—*
**Adults:** 60 to 120 mg P.O. q 3 or 4 hours. Usual dose is 600 mg daily but higher doses may be needed (up to 1,500 mg daily). For I.M. or I.V. use, 1/30 of oral dose is given. Dosage must be adjusted for each patient, based on patient's response and tolerance. Or, 180 to 540 mg extended-release tablets (1 to 3 tablets) P.O. b.i.d., with at least 6 hours between doses.
**Children:** 7 mg/kg or 200 mg/m² daily in five or six divided doses.

---

Reactions may be *common*, uncommon, *life-threatening*, or COMMON AND LIFE-THREATENING.

*Supportive treatment of neonates born to myasthenic mothers—*
**Neonates:** 0.05 to 0.15 mg/kg I.M. q 4 to 6 hours. Dosage decreased daily until drug can be withdrawn.

## ADVERSE REACTIONS
**CNS:** headache (with high doses), weakness, syncope.
**CV:** *bradycardia,* hypotension, *cardiac arrest,* thrombophlebitis.
**EENT:** miosis.
**GI:** abdominal cramps, nausea, vomiting, diarrhea, excessive salivation, increased peristalsis.
**Musculoskeletal:** muscle cramps, muscle fasciculations.
**Respiratory:** *bronchospasm, bronchoconstriction,* increased bronchial secretions.
**Skin:** rash, diaphoresis.

## INTERACTIONS
**Drug-drug.** *Aminoglycosides:* prolonged or enhanced muscle weakness. Use together cautiously.
*Anticholinergics, atropine, corticosteroids, general or local anesthetics, magnesium, procainamide, quinidine:* may antagonize cholinergic effects. Observe for lack of drug effect.
*Ganglionic blockers:* increased risk of hypotension. Monitor closely.

## EFFECTS ON DIAGNOSTIC TESTS
None reported.

## CONTRAINDICATIONS
Contraindicated in patients with hypersensitivity to anticholinesterases or bromides and in those with mechanical obstruction of the intestinal or urinary tract.

## NURSING CONSIDERATIONS
• Use cautiously in patients with bronchial asthma, bradycardia, arrhythmias, epilepsy, recent coronary occlusion, vagotonia, hyperthyroidism, or peptic ulcer. Also use cautiously in pregnant women.
• Stop all other cholinergics before giving this drug, as ordered.
• Don't crush extended-release tablets.

• When using sweet syrup for patients who have difficulty swallowing, give over ice chips if patient can't tolerate flavor.
• Monitor and document patient's response after each dose. Optimum dosage is difficult to judge.
• *Alert:* In the United States, Regonol contains benzyl ethanol preservative, which may cause toxicity in neonates if administered in high doses. The Canadian formulation of this drug doesn't contain benzyl ethanol.
• If appropriate, obtain doctor's order for hospitalized patient to have bedside supply of tablets. Many patients with long-standing disease insist on self-administration.
• *Alert:* Don't confuse Mestinon with Mesantoin or Metatensin.

### I.V. administration
• *Alert:* Administer I.V. injection no faster than 1 mg/minute. With rapid I.V. infusion, bradycardia and seizures may result. Monitor vital signs frequently, especially respirations. Position patient to ease breathing. Have atropine injection available and be prepared to give, as ordered; provide respiratory support as needed.
• If patient's muscle weakness is severe, keep in mind that doctor determines if severity is caused by drug-induced toxicity or exacerbation of myasthenia gravis. Test dose of edrophonium I.V. will aggravate drug-induced weakness, but will temporarily relieve weakness caused by disease.

### ☑ Patient teaching
• When using for myasthenia gravis, stress importance of taking drug exactly as ordered, on time, in evenly spaced doses. If doctor has ordered extended-release tablets, explain that patient must take tablets at same time each day, at least 6 hours apart.
• Advise patient not to crush or chew extended-release tablets.
• Explain that patient may have to take drug for life.
• Advise patient to wear a medical identification bracelet indicating he has myasthenia gravis.

---

**atropine sulfate**
(See Chapter 21, ANTIARRHYTHMICS.)
**dicyclomine hydrochloride**
**glycopyrrolate**
**hyoscyamine**
**hyoscyamine sulfate**
**propantheline bromide**
**scopolamine**
**scopolamine butylbromide**
**scopolamine hydrobromide**

## COMBINATION PRODUCTS
BARBIDONNA No. 2 TABLETS: atropine sulfate 0.025 mg, scopolamine hydrobromide 0.0074 mg, hyoscyamine hydrobromide or sulfate 0.1286 mg, and phenobarbital 32 mg.
BARBIDONNA TABLETS: atropine sulfate 0.025 mg, scopolamine hydrobromide 0.0074 mg, hyoscyamine hydrobromide or sulfate 0.1286 mg, and phenobarbital 16 mg.
DONNATAL ELIXIR*: atropine sulfate 0.0194 mg/5 ml, scopolamine hydrobromide 0.0065 mg/5 ml, ethanol 23%, hyoscyamine hydrobromide or sulfate 0.1037 mg/5 ml, and phenobarbital 16 mg/5 ml.
DONNATAL EXTENTABS: atropine sulfate 0.0582 mg, scopolamine hydrobromide 0.0195 mg, hyoscyamine sulfate 0.3111 mg, and phenobarbital 48.6 mg.
DONNATAL TABLETS AND CAPSULES: atropine sulfate 0.0194 mg, scopolamine hydrobromide 0.0065 mg, hyoscyamine hydrobromide or sulfate 0.1037 mg, and phenobarbital 16.2 mg.

---

**dicyclomine hydrochloride**
Antispas, A-Spas, Bentyl, Bentylol†, Byclomine, Dibent, Di-Spaz, Formulex†, Lominet†, Merbentyl‡, Or-Tyl, Spasmoban†

*Pregnancy Risk Category B*

## HOW SUPPLIED
*Tablets:* 10 mg‡, 20 mg
*Capsules:* 10 mg, 20 mg
*Syrup:* 5 mg/5 ml‡, 10 mg/5 ml
*Injection:* 10 mg/ml

## ACTION
Inhibits action of acetylcholine on post-ganglionic, parasympathetic muscarinic receptors, decreasing GI motility. Also, possesses local anesthetic properties that may be partly responsible for spasmolysis.

| Route | Onset | Peak | Duration |
|-------|-------|------|----------|
| P.O., I.M. | Unknown | 1-1.5 hr | Unknown |

## INDICATIONS & DOSAGE
*Irritable bowel syndrome, other functional GI disorders—*
**Adults:** initially, 20 mg P.O. q.i.d., increased to 40 mg q.i.d., or 20 mg I.M. q.i.d.

## ADVERSE REACTIONS
**CNS:** *headache; dizziness;* insomnia; light-headedness; drowsiness; nervousness, confusion, excitement (in elderly patients).
**CV:** *palpitations,* tachycardia.
**EENT:** blurred vision, increased intraocular pressure, mydriasis, photophobia.
**GI:** nausea, vomiting, *constipation, dry mouth, thirst,* abdominal distention, heartburn, paralytic ileus.
**GU:** *urinary hesitancy, urine retention,* impotence.
**Skin:** urticaria, decreased sweating or possible anhidrosis, other dermal signs and symptoms, local irritation.
**Other:** fever, *allergic reactions.*

## INTERACTIONS
**Drug-drug.** *Amantadine, antihistamines, antiparkinsonians, disopyramide, glutethimide, meperidine, phenothiazines, procainamide, quinidine, tricyclic antidepressants:* additive adverse effects. Avoid concomitant use.
*Antacids:* decreased absorption of oral anticholinergics. Separate administration times by 2 to 3 hours.

---

Reactions may be *common*, uncommon, *life-threatening*, or COMMON AND LIFE-THREATENING.

*Ketoconazole:* anticholinergics may interfere with ketoconazole absorption. Separate administration times by 2 to 3 hours.
*Methotrimeprazine:* anticholinergics may enhance risk of extrapyramidal reactions. Avoid concomitant use.

**EFFECTS ON DIAGNOSTIC TESTS**
None reported.

**CONTRAINDICATIONS**
Contraindicated in patients with hypersensitivity to anticholinergics and in those with obstructive uropathy, obstructive disease of the GI tract, reflux esophagitis, severe ulcerative colitis, toxic megacolon, myasthenia gravis, unstable CV status in acute hemorrhage, tachycardia secondary to cardiac insufficiency or thyrotoxicosis, or glaucoma; also contraindicated in breast-feeding patients and in children under age 6 months.

**NURSING CONSIDERATIONS**
• Use cautiously in patients with autonomic neuropathy, hyperthyroidism, coronary artery disease, arrhythmias, heart failure, hypertension, hiatal hernia, hepatic or renal disease, prostatic hyperplasia, known or suspected GI infection, and ulcerative colitis. Also use cautiously in patients in hot or humid environment. Drug-induced heat stroke can develop.
• Give drug 30 minutes to 1 hour before meals and at bedtime. Bedtime dose can be larger; give at least 2 hours after last meal of day.
• *Alert:* Don't give S.C. or I.V.
• Be prepared to adjust dosage based on patient's needs and response, as ordered. Doses up to 40 mg P.O. q.i.d. have been used in adults, but safety and efficacy for more than 2 weeks haven't been established.
• Dicyclomine is a synthetic tertiary derivative that may have atropine-like adverse reactions.
• Overdose may cause curare-like effects, such as respiratory paralysis.
• Monitor patient's vital signs and urine output carefully.
• *Alert:* The dicyclomine labeling may be misleading. The ampule label reads 10 mg/ml, but doesn't indicate that the ampule contains 2 ml of solution and, therefore, 20 mg of drug.
• *Alert:* Don't confuse dicyclomine with dyclonine or doxycycline, or Bentyl with Aventyl or Benadryl.

☑ **Patient teaching**
• Instruct patient when to take drug and stress importance of taking drug on time and in evenly spaced intervals.
• Advise patient to avoid driving and other hazardous activities if drowsiness, dizziness, or blurred vision occurs; to drink plenty of fluids to help prevent constipation; and to report rash or other skin eruption.

## glycopyrrolate
Robinul, Robinul Forte

*Pregnancy Risk Category B*

**HOW SUPPLIED**
*Tablets:* 1 mg, 2 mg
*Injection:* 0.2 mg/ml

**ACTION**
Inhibits cholinergic (muscarinic) actions of acetylcholine on autonomic effectors innervated by postganglionic cholinergic nerves.

| Route | Onset | Peak | Duration |
|---|---|---|---|
| P.O. | Unknown | Unknown | 8-12 hr |
| I.V. | 1 min | Unknown | 3-7 hr |
| I.M., S.C. | 15-30 min | 30-45 min | 3-7 hr |

**INDICATIONS & DOSAGE**
*Blockade of adverse cholinergic effects caused by anticholinesterases used to reverse neuromuscular blockade—*
**Adults and children:** 0.2 mg I.V. for each 1 mg neostigmine or 5 mg of pyridostigmine. May be given I.V. without dilution or may be added to dextrose injection and given by infusion.
*Preoperatively to diminish secretions and block cardiac vagal reflexes—*
**Adults and children ages 2 and older:** 0.0044 mg/kg of body weight I.M. 30 to 60 minutes before anesthesia.
**Children under age 2:** 0.0088 mg/kg I.M. 30 to 60 minutes before anesthesia.

*Adjunctive therapy in peptic ulcerations
and other GI disorders—*
**Adults:** 1 to 2 mg P.O. t.i.d. or 0.1 to
0.2 mg I.M. or I.V. t.i.d. or q.i.d. Dosage
must be individualized. Maximum daily
oral dose is 8 mg.

## ADVERSE REACTIONS
**CNS:** weakness, nervousness, insomnia,
drowsiness, dizziness, headache, confusion or excitement (in elderly patients).
**CV:** palpitations, tachycardia.
**EENT:** *dilated pupils, blurred vision,*
photophobia, increased intraocular pressure.
**GI:** *constipation, dry mouth,* nausea, loss
of taste, abdominal distention, vomiting,
epigastric distress.
**GU:** urinary hesitancy, urine retention,
impotence.
**Skin:** urticaria, decreased sweating or anhidrosis, other dermal signs and symptoms.
**Other:** *allergic reactions (anaphylaxis),*
fever.

## INTERACTIONS
**Drug-drug.** *Amantadine, antihistamines,
antiparkinsonians, disopyramide, glutethimide, meperidine, phenothiazines, procainamide, quinidine, tricyclic antidepressants:* additive adverse effects.
Avoid concomitant use.
*Antacids:* decreased absorption of oral
anticholinergics. Separate administration
times by 2 to 3 hours.
*Ketoconazole:* anticholinergics may interfere with ketoconazole absorption. Separate administration times by 2 to 3 hours.
*Methotrimeprazine:* anticholinergics may
enhance risk of extrapyramidal reactions.
Avoid concomitant use.

## EFFECTS ON DIAGNOSTIC TESTS
None reported.

## CONTRAINDICATIONS
Contraindicated in patients with hypersensitivity to drug and in those with glaucoma, obstructive uropathy, obstructive
disease of the GI tract, myasthenia gravis,
paralytic ileus, intestinal atony, unstable
CV status in acute hemorrhage, tachycardia secondary to cardiac insufficiency or

thyrotoxicosis, severe ulcerative colitis,
toxic megacolon, or known or suspected
GI infection.

## NURSING CONSIDERATIONS
● Use cautiously in patients with autonomic neuropathy, hyperthyroidism, coronary artery disease, arrhythmias, heart
failure, hypertension, hiatal hernia, hepatic or renal disease, ulcerative colitis and
known or suspected GI infection. Also
use cautiously in patients in hot or humid
environment. Drug-induced heatstroke is
possible.
● Administer oral form 30 minutes to 1
hour before meals.
● *Alert:* Check all dosages carefully; slight
overdose can lead to toxicity.
● Overdose may cause curare-like effects,
such as respiratory paralysis.
● Monitor vital signs carefully. Watch
closely for adverse reactions, especially in
elderly or debilitated patients. Call doctor
promptly if they occur.
● Elderly patients typically receive smaller dosages.

### ◨ I.V. administration
● Administer by direct injection without
dilution. Or, inject into tubing of a free-
flowing I.V. solution.
● Don't mix with I.V. solution containing
sodium bicarbonate or alkaline solutions
with a pH higher than 6. Alkaline drugs,
such as barbiturates, chloramphenicol,
dexamethasone, dimenhydrinate, diazepam, methylprednisolone, and pentazocine, are incompatible with glycopyrrolate.

### ☑ Patient teaching
● Instruct patient to take oral drug 30 to
60 minutes before meals.
● Warn patient to avoid activities that require alertness until drug's CNS effects
are known.
● Advise patient to report signs of urinary
hesitancy or urine retention.

## hyoscyamine
Cystospaz

## hyoscyamine sulfate
Anaspaz, Cystospaz, Cystospaz-M, Gastrosed, Levbid, Levsin*, Levsin Drops*, Levsin/SL, Levsinex Timecaps, Neoquess

*Pregnancy Risk Category C*

### HOW SUPPLIED
**hyoscyamine**
*Tablets:* 0.15 mg
**hyoscyamine sulfate**
*Tablets:* 0.125 mg, 0.13 mg, 0.15 mg
*Capsules (extended-release):* 0.375 mg
*Elixir:* 0.125 mg/5 ml
*Oral solution:* 0.125 mg/ml
*Injection:* 0.5 mg/ml

### ACTION
Competitively blocks the action of acetylcholine at muscarinic receptors, which decreases GI motility and inhibits gastric acid secretion.

| Route | Onset | Peak | Duration |
|---|---|---|---|
| P.O. | 20-30 min | 0.5-1 hr | 4-12 hr |
| P.O. (extended) | 20-30 min | 40-90 min | 12 hr |
| I.V. | 2 min | 15-30 min | 4 hr |
| I.M., S.C. | Unknown | 15-30 min | 4-12 hr |
| S.L. | 5-20 min | 0.5-1 hr | 4 hr |

### INDICATIONS & DOSAGE
*GI tract disorders due to spasm; to diminish secretions and block cardiac vagal reflexes preoperatively; adjunctive therapy for peptic ulcerations, cystitis, renal colic; as a "drying agent" in relief of symptoms of allergic rhinitis—*
**Adults and children ages 12 and older:**
0.125 to 0.25 mg P.O. or S.L. t.i.d. or q.i.d. before meals and h.s.; 0.375 to 0.75 mg extended-release form P.O. q 8 to 12 hours; or 0.25 to 0.5 mg (1 or 2 ml) I.M., I.V., or S.C. b.i.d. to q.i.d. (Oral drug substituted when symptoms are controlled.) Maximum daily dose is 1.5 mg.
**Children under age 12:** dosage individualized according to weight.

### ADVERSE REACTIONS
**CNS:** headache, insomnia, drowsiness, dizziness, *confusion or excitement (in elderly patients),* nervousness, weakness.
**CV:** *palpitations,* tachycardia.
**EENT:** *blurred vision,* mydriasis, increased intraocular pressure, cycloplegia, photophobia.
**GI:** *dry mouth,* dysphagia, *constipation,* heartburn, loss of taste, nausea, vomiting, *paralytic ileus.*
**GU:** *urinary hesitancy, urine retention,* impotence.
**Skin:** urticaria, decreased or lack of sweating, other skin conditions.
**Other:** fever, *allergic reactions.*

### INTERACTIONS
**Drug-drug.** *Amantadine, antihistamines, antiparkinsonians, disopyramide, glutethimide, meperidine, phenothiazines, procainamide, quinidine, tricyclic antidepressants:* additive adverse effects. Avoid concomitant use.
*Antacids:* decreased absorption of oral anticholinergics. Separate administration times by 2 to 3 hours.
*Ketoconazole:* anticholinergics may interfere with ketoconazole absorption. Separate administration times by 2 to 3 hours.
*Methotrimeprazine:* anticholinergics may enhance risk of extrapyramidal reactions. Avoid concomitant use.
**Drug-herb.** *Jimsonweed:* may adversely affect CV function system. Avoid concomitant use.

### EFFECTS ON DIAGNOSTIC TESTS
None reported.

### CONTRAINDICATIONS
Contraindicated in patients with hypersensitivity to anticholinergics and in those with glaucoma, obstructive uropathy, obstructive disease of GI tract, severe ulcerative colitis, myasthenia gravis, paralytic ileus, intestinal atony, unstable CV status in acute hemorrhage, tachycardia secondary to cardiac insufficiency of thyrotoxicosis, or toxic megacolon.

### NURSING CONSIDERATIONS
• Use cautiously in patients with autonomic neuropathy, hyperthyroidism, coronary

artery disease, arrhythmias, heart failure, hypertension, hiatal hernia associated with reflux esophagitis, hepatic or renal disease, known or suspected GI infection, and ulcerative colitis. Also use cautiously in patients in hot or humid environment. Drug-induced heat stroke can develop.

• Give drug 30 minutes to 1 hour before meals and at bedtime. Bedtime dose can be larger; give at least 2 hours after last meal of day.

• *Alert:* Overdose may cause curare-like effects such as respiratory paralysis.

• Monitor patient's vital signs and urine output carefully.

• Injection contains sodium metabisulfite, which may cause allergic reaction in certain individuals.

**I.V. administration**
• I.V. form used when oral or S.L. therapy isn't feasible or when rapid effect is needed.

**✓ Patient teaching**
• Instruct patient to take drug as prescribed.

• Advise patient not to crush or chew extended-release tablets.

• Advise patient to avoid driving and other hazardous activities if drowsiness, dizziness, or blurred vision occurs; to drink plenty of fluids to help prevent constipation; and to report rash or other skin eruption.

---

## propantheline bromide
Pro-Banthine, Propanthel†

*Pregnancy Risk Category C*

### HOW SUPPLIED
*Tablets:* 7.5 mg, 15 mg

### ACTION
Competitively blocks the action of acetylcholine at muscarinic receptors, which decreases GI motility and inhibits gastric acid secretion.

| Route | Onset | Peak | Duration |
|-------|-------|------|----------|
| P.O. | 1.5 hr | 2-6 hr | 6 hr |

### INDICATIONS & DOSAGE
*Adjunctive treatment of peptic ulceration—*
**Adults:** 15 mg P.O. t.i.d. before meals and 30 mg h.s.
**Elderly:** 7.5 mg P.O. t.i.d. before meals.

### ADVERSE REACTIONS
**CNS:** headache, insomnia, drowsiness, dizziness, *confusion or excitement in elderly patients,* nervousness, weakness.
**CV:** *palpitations,* tachycardia.
**EENT:** *blurred vision,* mydriasis, increased intraocular pressure, cycloplegia, drying of salivary secretions.
**GI:** *dry mouth,* constipation, loss of taste, nausea, vomiting, paralytic ileus, bloated feeling.
**GU:** *urinary hesitancy, urine retention,* impotence.
**Skin:** urticaria, decreased sweating or possible anhidrosis, other dermal signs and symptoms.
**Other:** *allergic reactions (anaphylaxis).*

### INTERACTIONS
**Drug-drug.** *Amantadine, antihistamines, antiparkinsonians, disopyramide, glutethimide, meperidine, phenothiazines, procainamide, quinidine, tricyclic antidepressants:* additive adverse effects. Avoid concomitant use.
*Antacids:* decreased absorption of oral anticholinergics. Separate administration times by 2 to 3 hours.
*Digoxin:* increased serum digoxin levels. Monitor closely for digitalis toxicity.
*Ketoconazole:* anticholinergics may interfere with ketoconazole absorption. Separate administration times by 2 to 3 hours.
*Methotrimeprazine:* anticholinergics may enhance risk of extrapyramidal reactions. Avoid concomitant use.

### EFFECTS ON DIAGNOSTIC TESTS
None reported.

### CONTRAINDICATIONS
Contraindicated in patients with hypersensitivity to anticholinergics and in those with angle-closure glaucoma, obstructive uropathy, obstructive disease of GI tract, severe ulcerative colitis, myasthenia gravis, paralytic ileus, intestinal atony, un-

---

stable CV status in acute hemorrhage, tachycardia secondary to cardiac insufficiency or thyrotoxicosis, or toxic megacolon.

## NURSING CONSIDERATIONS
• Use cautiously in patients with autonomic neuropathy, hyperthyroidism, coronary artery disease, arrhythmias, heart failure, hypertension, hiatal hernia associated with reflux esophagitis, hepatic or renal disease, known or suspected GI infection, and ulcerative colitis. Also use cautiously in patients in hot or humid environment. Drug-induced heat stroke can develop.
• Give drug 30 minutes to 1 hour before meals and at bedtime. Bedtime doses can be larger; give at least 2 hours after last meal of day.
• *Alert:* Overdose may cause curare-like effects such as respiratory paralysis.
• Monitor patient's vital signs and urine output carefully.
• Safety and efficacy of drug haven't been established in children.

### ☑ Patient teaching
• Instruct patient when to take drug.
• Advise patient to avoid driving and other hazardous activities if drowsiness, dizziness, or blurred vision occurs; to drink plenty of fluids to help prevent constipation; and to report rash or other skin eruption.

---

**scopolamine (hyoscine)**
Transderm-Scop, Transderm-V

**scopolamine butylbromide
(hyoscine butylbromide)**
Buscopan†

**scopolamine hydrobromide
(hyoscine hydrobromide)**
Scopolamine Hydrobromide Injection

*Pregnancy Risk Category C*

---

## HOW SUPPLIED
**scopolamine**
*Transdermal patch:* 1.5 mg/2.5 cm²
(1 mg/72 hours)

**scopolamine butylbromide**
*Capsules:* 0.25 mg
*Suppositories:* 10 mg†
*Tablets:* 10 mg†
**scopolamine hydrobromide**
*Injection:* 0.3 mg, 0.4 mg, 0.5 mg, 0.6 mg, and 1 mg/ml in 1-ml vials and ampules; 0.86 mg/ml in 0.5-ml ampules

## ACTION
Inhibits muscarinic actions of acetylcholine on autonomic effectors innervated by postganglionic cholinergic neurons. Also, may affect neural pathways originating in the labyrinth (inner ear) to inhibit nausea and vomiting.

| Route | Onset | Peak | Duration |
|-------|-------|------|----------|
| I.V. | 10 min | 50-80 min | 2 hr |
| P.O., I.M. | 1 hr | 1-2 hr | 4-6 hr |
| P.R. | Unknown | Unknown | Unknown |
| S.C. | Unknown | Unknown | Unknown |
| Trans-dermal | 4 hr | Unknown | 72 hr |

## INDICATIONS & DOSAGE
*Spastic states—*
**Adults:** 10 to 20 mg P.O. t.i.d. or q.i.d. or 10 mg P.R. t.i.d. or q.i.d. Dosage adjusted, p.r.n. Or, 10 to 20 mg (butylbromide) S.C., I.M., or I.V. t.i.d. or q.i.d.
*Delirium, preanesthetic sedation, and obstetric amnesia with analgesics—*
**Adults:** 0.3 to 0.65 mg I.M., S.C., or I.V. Dilute solution with sterile water for injection before administering I.V.
**Children:** 0.006 mg/kg I.M., S.C., or I.V.; maximum dose is 0.3 mg. Dilute solution with sterile water for injection before administering I.V.
*Prevention of nausea and vomiting associated with motion sickness—*
**Adults:** one Transderm-Scop or Transderm-V patch (a circular flat unit) programmed to deliver 0.5 mg scopolamine daily over 3 days (72 hours), applied to the skin behind the ear at least 4 hours before antiemetic is needed. Or, 300 to 600 mcg (hydrobromide) S.C., I.M., or I.V.
**Children:** 6 mcg/kg or 200 mcg/m² of body surface area (hydrobromide) S.C., I.M., or I.V.

---

## ADVERSE REACTIONS

**CNS:** disorientation, restlessness, irritability, dizziness, drowsiness, headache, confusion, hallucinations, delirium.
**CV:** palpitations, tachycardia, paradoxical *bradycardia,* flushing.
**EENT:** dilated pupils, blurred vision, photophobia, increased intraocular pressure, difficulty swallowing.
**GI:** *constipation, dry mouth, nausea, vomiting, epigastric distress.*
**GU:** urinary hesitancy, urine retention.
**Respiratory:** bronchial plugging, depressed respirations.
**Skin:** rash, dryness, contact dermatitis (with transdermal patch).
**Other:** fever.

## INTERACTIONS

**Drug-drug.** *Amantadine, antihistamines, antiparkinsonians, disopyramide, glutethimide, meperidine, phenothiazines, procainamide, quinidine, tricyclic antidepressants:* increased incidence of adverse CNS reactions. Avoid concomitant use.
*Antacids:* decreased oral absorption of anticholinergics. Separate administration times by 2 to 3 hours.
*CNS depressants:* increased incidence of CNS depression. Monitor patient closely.
*Digoxin:* increased digoxin levels. Monitor for digitalis toxicity.
*Ketoconazole:* anticholinergics may interfere with ketoconazole absorption. Separate administration times by 2 to 3 hours.
*Methotrimeprazine:* enhanced risk of extrapyramidal reactions. Avoid concomitant use.
**Drug-herb.** *Squaw vine:* tannic acid may decrease metabolic breakdown. Monitor patient.
*Jaborandi tree:* effects of these drugs may be decreased with concomitant administration. Monitor closely.
*Pill-bearing spurge:* choline may decrease effect of scopolamine. Use cautiously.
**Drug-lifestyle.** *Alcohol use:* increased incidence of CNS depression. Monitor patient closely.

## EFFECTS ON DIAGNOSTIC TESTS

None reported.

## CONTRAINDICATIONS

Contraindicated in patients with angle-closure glaucoma, obstructive uropathy, obstructive disease of GI tract, asthma, chronic pulmonary disease, myasthenia gravis, paralytic ileus, intestinal atony, unstable CV status in acute hemorrhage, tachycardia secondary to cardiac insufficiency, or toxic megacolon.

## NURSING CONSIDERATIONS

• Use cautiously in patients with autonomic neuropathy, hyperthyroidism, coronary artery disease, arrhythmias, heart failure, hypertension, hiatal hernia associated with reflux esophagitis, hepatic or renal disease, known or suspected GI infection, or ulcerative colitis and in children under age 6. Also use cautiously in patients in hot or humid environment. Drug-induced heat stroke is possible.
• Raise the bed's side rails as a precaution because some patients become temporarily excited or disoriented or develop amnesia or drowsiness. Reorient patient as needed.
• Tolerance may develop when drug is given over a long time.
• Adverse reactions may be caused by pending atropine-like toxicity and are dose-related. Individual tolerance varies greatly.
• *Alert:* Overdose may cause curare-like effects such as respiratory paralysis.

### 🔷 I.V. administration

• Intermittent and continuous infusions aren't recommended. For direct injection, dilute with sterile water and inject diluted drug at ordered rate through patent I.V. line.
• Protect I.V. solutions from freezing and light, and store at room temperature.

### ☑ Patient teaching

• Advise patient to apply patch the night before a planned trip. Transdermal method releases a controlled therapeutic amount of scopolamine. Transderm-Scop is effective if applied 2 to 3 hours before experiencing motion, but is more effective if applied 12 hours before.
• Instruct patient to wash and dry hands thoroughly before and after applying the

---

*Reactions may be* common, *uncommon,* **life-threatening**, *or* **COMMON AND LIFE-THREATENING**.

transdermal patch (on dry skin behind the ear) and before touching the eye because pupil may dilate. After removing patch, discard it. Wash hands and application site thoroughly.

• Tell patient that, if patch becomes displaced, he should remove it and apply another patch on a fresh skin site behind the ear.

• Alert patient to possible withdrawal signs or symptoms (nausea, vomiting, headache, dizziness) when transdermal system is used for more than 72 hours.

• Advise patient that eyes may be more sensitive to light as a result of wearing patch.

• Warn patient to avoid activities that require alertness until drug's CNS effects are known.

• Instruct patient to ask pharmacist for brochure that comes with the transdermal product.

• Advise patient to report signs of urinary hesitancy or urine retention.

# Adrenergics (sympathomimetics)

**dobutamine hydrochloride**
**dopamine hydrochloride**
**metaraminol bitartrate**
**norepinephrine bitartrate**
**phenylephrine hydrochloride**
**pseudoephedrine hydrochloride**
**pseudoephedrine sulfate**

## COMBINATION PRODUCTS

ENTEX: phenylephrine hydrochloride 5 mg, phenylpropanolamine hydrochloride 45 mg, and guaifenesin 200 mg.
ENTEX LIQUID*: phenylephrine hydrochloride 5 mg/5 ml, phenylpropanolamine hydrochloride 20 mg/5 ml, and guaifenesin 100 mg/5 ml (alcohol 5%).
ENTEX PSE: pseudoephedrine 120 mg and guaifenesin 600 mg.
SEMPREX-D: acrivastine 8 mg and pseudoephedrine hydrochloride 60 mg.

---

**dobutamine hydrochloride**
Dobutrex

*Pregnancy Risk Category B*

## HOW SUPPLIED
*Injection:* 12.5 mg/ml in 20-ml vials (parenteral)

## ACTION
Directly stimulates beta$_1$ receptors of heart to increase myocardial contractility and stroke volume. At therapeutic dosages, drug decreases peripheral vascular resistance (afterload), reduces ventricular filling pressure (preload), and may facilitate AV node conduction. Net result is increased cardiac output.

| Route | Onset | Peak | Duration |
|-------|-------|------|----------|
| I.V. | 1-2 min | 10 min | < 5 min after infusion ends |

## INDICATIONS & DOSAGE
*Increase cardiac output in short-term treatment of cardiac decompensation due to depressed contractility, such as during refractory heart failure; adjunct in cardiac surgery—*
**Adults:** 2.5 to 15 mcg/kg/minute I.V. infusion. Infusion rates up to 40 mcg/kg/minute may be needed (rare).

## ADVERSE REACTIONS
**CNS:** headache.
**CV:** *increased heart rate, hypertension, PVC,* angina, nonspecific chest pain, palpitations, hypotension.
**GI:** nausea, vomiting.
**Respiratory:** shortness of breath, *asthmatic episodes.*
**Other:** phlebitis, *hypersensitivity reactions, anaphylaxis.*

## INTERACTIONS
**Drug-drug.** *Beta blockers:* may antagonize dobutamine effects. Don't use together.
*Bretylium:* may potentiate action of vasopressors on adrenergic receptors. Monitor closely for arrhythmias.
*General anesthetics:* greater incidence of ventricular arrhythmias. Monitor ECG closely.
*Guanethidine, oxytocic drugs:* may increase pressor response, possibly resulting in severe hypertension. Monitor closely.
*Tricyclic antidepressants:* may potentiate pressor response. Use with caution.
**Drug-herb.** *Rue:* increased inotropic potential. Use cautiously.

## EFFECTS ON DIAGNOSTIC TESTS
None reported.

## CONTRAINDICATIONS
Contraindicated in patients with hypersensitivity to drug or its ingredients and in those with idiopathic hypertrophic subaortic stenosis.

## NURSING CONSIDERATIONS
• Use cautiously in patients with history of hypertension. Drug may precipitate an exaggerated pressor response. Also use

cautiously in patients with history of sulfite sensitivity.

• Before initiating therapy with dobutamine, correct hypovolemia with plasma volume expanders, as ordered.

• Administer a cardiac glycoside before dobutamine, as ordered. Because drug increases AV node conduction, patients with atrial fibrillation may develop a rapid ventricular rate.

• Continuously monitor ECG, blood pressure, pulmonary artery wedge pressure, cardiac output, and urine output.

• Monitor serum electrolytes, as ordered. Drug may lower serum potassium levels.

• *Alert:* Don't confuse dobutamine with dopamine.

◖ **I.V. administration**

• Don't mix with sodium bicarbonate injection because drug is incompatible with alkaline solutions.

• Dilute concentrate for injection before administration. Compatible solutions include $D_5W$, half-normal or normal saline for injection and lactated Ringer's injection. The contents of one vial (250 mg) diluted with 1,000 ml of solution yields a concentration of 250 mcg/ml; diluted with 500 ml, a concentration of 500 mcg/ml; diluted with 250 ml, a concentration of 1,000 mcg/ml. Maximum concentration shouldn't exceed 5 mg/ml.

• Oxidation of drug may slightly discolor admixtures containing dobutamine. This doesn't indicate a significant loss of potency provided drug is used within 24 hours of reconstitution.

• Administer through a central venous catheter or large peripheral vein. Titrate infusion according to doctor's orders and patient's condition. Use an infusion pump. Infusions for up to 72 hours produce no more adverse effects than shorter infusions.

• Avoid extravasation; may cause an inflammatory response. Change I.V. sites regularly to avoid phlebitis.

• Don't administer through same I.V. line with other drugs. Drug is incompatible with heparin, hydrocortisone sodium succinate, cefazolin, cefamandole, neutral cephalothin, penicillin, and ethacrynate sodium.

• I.V. solutions remain stable for 24 hours.

✓ **Patient teaching**

• Tell patient to report adverse reactions promptly, especially dyspnea and drug-induced headache.

• Instruct patient to report discomfort at I.V. insertion site.

---

## dopamine hydrochloride
Intropin, Revimine†

*Pregnancy Risk Category C*

### HOW SUPPLIED
*Injection:* 40 mg/ml, 80 mg/ml, 160 mg/ml parenteral concentrate for injection for I.V. infusion; 0.8 mg/ml (200 or 400 mg) in dextrose 5%; 1.6 mg/ml (400 or 800 mg) in dextrose 5%, 3.2 mg/ml (800 mg) in dextrose 5% parenteral injection for I.V. infusion

### ACTION
Dose-related. Drug stimulates dopaminergic and alpha and beta receptors of the sympathetic nervous system. High dose results primarily in alpha stimulation.

| Route | Onset | Peak | Duration |
|-------|-------|------|----------|
| I.V. | 5 min | Unknown | < 10 min after infusion ends |

### INDICATIONS & DOSAGE
*To treat shock and correct hemodynamic imbalances, to improve perfusion to vital organs, to increase cardiac output, to correct hypotension—*
**Adults:** initially, 1 to 5 mcg/kg/minute by I.V. infusion. Dosage titrated to desired hemodynamic or renal response; infusion may be increased by 1 to 4 mcg/kg/minute at 10- to 30-minute intervals.

### ADVERSE REACTIONS
**CNS:** headache.
**CV:** ectopic beats, tachycardia, anginal pain, palpitations, *hypotension*. Less frequently, *bradycardia*, widening of QRS complex, conduction disturbances, vasoconstriction, hypertension.
**GI:** nausea, vomiting.
**GU:** elevated urinary catecholamine levels.

---

**Metabolic:** azotemia, hyperglycemia.
**Respiratory:** dyspnea, *asthmatic episodes.*
**Skin:** necrosis and tissue sloughing with extravasation, piloerection.
**Other:** *anaphylactic reactions.*

## INTERACTIONS
**Drug-drug.** *Alpha blockers, beta blockers:* may antagonize dopamine's effects. Don't use together.
*Ergot alkaloids:* extreme elevations in blood pressure. Don't use together.
*Inhalation anesthetics:* increased risk of arrhythmias or hypertension. Monitor closely.
*MAO inhibitors:* may cause hypertensive crisis. Avoid if possible.
*Oxytocics:* may cause severe, persistent hypertension. Use cautiously.
*Phenytoin:* may cause seizures, severe hypotension, and bradycardia. Monitor carefully.
*Tricyclic antidepressants:* decreased pressor response. Higher doses of dopamine may be needed.

## EFFECTS ON DIAGNOSTIC TESTS
None reported.

## CONTRAINDICATIONS
Contraindicated in patients with uncorrected tachyarrhythmias, pheochromocytoma, or ventricular fibrillation.

## NURSING CONSIDERATIONS
• Use cautiously in patients with occlusive vascular disease, cold injuries, diabetic endarteritis, and arterial embolism; in pregnant patients; in those with a history of sulfite sensitivity, and in those taking MAO inhibitors.
• Remember that drug isn't a substitute for blood or fluid volume deficit. If deficit exists, replace fluid before administering vasopressors, as ordered.
• Discard after 24 hours (dopamine solutions deteriorate after 24 hours) or earlier if solution is discolored.
• During infusion, frequently monitor ECG, blood pressure, cardiac output, central venous pressure, pulmonary artery wedge pressure, pulse rate, urine output, and color and temperature of extremities.

• If disproportionate rise in diastolic pressure (a marked decrease in pulse pressure) is observed in patients receiving dopamine, decrease infusion rate, as ordered, and observe carefully for further evidence of predominant vasoconstrictor activity, unless such an effect is desired.
• Observe patient closely for adverse reactions; doctor may adjust dosage or discontinue drug.
• Check urine output often. If urine flow decreases without hypotension, notify doctor because dosage may need to be reduced.
• *Alert:* After drug is stopped, watch closely for sudden decrease in blood pressure. Taper dosage slowly to evaluate stability of blood pressure, as ordered.
• Acidosis decreases effectiveness of dopamine.
• *Alert:* Don't confuse dopamine with dobutamine.

## I.V. administration
• Use a central line or large vein, such as in the antecubital fossa, to minimize risk of extravasation. Watch infusion site carefully for signs of extravasation; if it occurs, stop infusion immediately and call doctor. Extravasation may require treatment by infiltration of the area with 5 to 10 mg phentolamine in 10 to 15 ml normal saline solution.
• Don't mix with alkaline solutions, oxidizing drugs, or iron salts. Use $D_5W$, normal saline solution, or a combination of $D_5W$ and normal saline solution. Mix just before use.
• Use a continuous infusion pump to regulate flow rate. Patient response depends on dosage and pharmacologic effects. Dosages of 0.5 to 2 mcg/kg/minute predominantly stimulate dopamine receptors and produce vasodilation of the renal vasculature. Dosages of 2 to 10 mcg/kg/minute stimulate beta receptors for a positive inotropic effect. Higher dosages also stimulate alpha receptors, causing vasoconstriction and increased blood pressure. Most patients are satisfactorily maintained on dosages less than 20 mcg/kg/minute.

---

Reactions may be *common,* uncommon, *life-threatening,* or COMMON AND LIFE-THREATENING.

• Don't mix other drugs in I.V. container with dopamine. Don't give alkaline drugs through I.V. line containing dopamine.

☑ **Patient teaching**
• Tell patient to report adverse reactions promptly.
• Instruct patient to alert nurse if discomfort occurs at I.V. insertion site.

## metaraminol bitartrate
Aramine

*Pregnancy Risk Category D*

### HOW SUPPLIED
*Injection:* 10 mg/ml

### ACTION
Stimulates alpha and beta$_1$ receptors within the sympathetic nervous system, causing an increase in both systolic and diastolic blood pressure as a result of vasoconstriction.

| Route | Onset | Peak | Duration |
|-------|-------|------|----------|
| I.V. | 1-2 min | Unknown | 20 min |
| I.M. | 10 min | Unknown | < 90 min |
| S.C. | 5-20 min | Unknown | < 90 min |

### INDICATIONS & DOSAGE
*Prevention of hypotension associated with spinal anesthesia—*
**Adults:** 2 to 10 mg I.M. or S.C.
*Hypotension associated with spinal anesthesia, hemorrhage, drug reaction, surgical complications, or shock associated with brain damage due to trauma or tumor—*
**Adults:** 0.5 to 5 mg by direct I.V. injection; then I.V. infusion titrated to maintain blood pressure.
**Children:** 0.01 mg/kg as single I.V. injection; 1 mg/25 ml of D$_5$W as I.V. infusion. Rate titrated to maintain blood pressure within normal range. Or, 0.1 mg/kg I.M. as single dose, p.r.n. At least 10 minutes should elapse before dosage is increased because maximum effect isn't immediately apparent.

### ADVERSE REACTIONS
**CNS:** apprehension, dizziness, headache, tremor.
**CV:** hypertension; hypotension; palpitations; flushing; ***arrhythmias,*** including sinus or ***ventricular tachycardia, cardiac arrest.***
**GI:** nausea.
**Skin:** diaphoresis; abscess, necrosis, sloughing upon extravasation.

### INTERACTIONS
**Drug-drug.** *Beta blockers:* mutual inhibition of drug effects, with possible hypertension, bradycardia, and heart block. Avoid concomitant use.
*Cardiac glycosides, doxapram, ergot alkaloids, general anesthetics, levodopa, maprotiline, thyroid hormones, tricyclic antidepressants, other sympathomimetics:* increased risk of adverse cardiac effects. Monitor closely.
*Furazolidone, MAO inhibitors, procarbazine:* may cause severe hypertension (hypertensive crisis) and increase action of metaraminol. Avoid this combination.
*Guanadrel, guanethidine:* metaraminol may decrease hypotensive effect of these drugs; guanadrel and guanethidine may enhance pressor effect of metaraminol. Avoid concomitant use.
*Oxytocics:* may cause severe, persistent hypertension. Use cautiously.
**Drug-lifestyle.** *Cocaine use:* increased risk of adverse cardiac effects. Monitor closely.

### EFFECTS ON DIAGNOSTIC TESTS
None reported.

### CONTRAINDICATIONS
Contraindicated in patients with hypersensitivity to drug and in those receiving anesthesia with cyclopropane and halogenated hydrocarbon anesthetics.

### NURSING CONSIDERATIONS
• Use cautiously in patients with heart disease, hypertension, peripheral vascular disease, thyroid disease, diabetes, cirrhosis, history of malaria, or sulfite sensitivity and in patients receiving cardiac glycosides.

• Drug isn't a substitute for blood or fluid volume deficit. If deficit exists, replace fluid before administering vasopressors, as ordered.
• Don't mix metaraminol with other drugs.
• During infusion, check blood pressure every 5 minutes until stabilized; then check every 15 minutes. Frequently monitor ECG, blood pressure, cardiac output, central venous pressure, pulmonary artery wedge pressure, pulse rate, urine output, and color and temperature of extremities. Titrate infusion rate according to findings and doctor's guidelines.
• *Alert:* Blood pressure should be raised to slightly less than the patient's normal level. Avoid excessive blood pressure response. Headache may be a symptom of hypertension. Rapidly induced hypertensive response can cause acute pulmonary edema, arrhythmias, and cardiac arrest.
• Allow at least 10 minutes between doses. Drug effects aren't always immediately apparent.
• Because of prolonged action, a cumulative effect is possible. With an excessive vasopressor response, elevated blood pressure may persist after drug is stopped.
• Observe patient closely for adverse effects; doctor may adjust dosage or discontinue drug.
• Keep emergency drugs on hand to reverse effects of metaraminol: atropine for reflex bradycardia, phentolamine to decrease vasopressor effects, and propranolol for arrhythmias.
• Report persistent decreased urine output. Urine output may decrease initially, then increase as blood pressure returns to normal level.
• Closely monitor patients with diabetes; insulin dosage may need to be adjusted.
• Keep solution in light-resistant container, away from heat. Use within 24 hours.

 **I.V. administration**
• To prepare an I.V. infusion, mix 15 to 100 mg in 500 ml of normal saline solution or $D_5W$. Aramine may be added to less than 500 ml of fluid if a smaller volume is desired. Titrate rate to maintain blood pressure.
• Use a central venous catheter or large vein, such as in the antecubital fossa, to minimize risk of extravasation. Use a continuous infusion pump to regulate infusion flow rate and a piggyback setup so I.V. line remains open if drug is stopped. Watch infusion site carefully for signs of extravasation. If it occurs, stop infusion immediately and notify doctor.
• To treat extravasation, infiltrate site promptly with 10 to 15 ml of normal saline for injection containing 5 to 10 mg phentolamine. Use a fine needle.
• When discontinuing drug, gradually slow infusion rate, as ordered. Continue monitoring vital signs, watching for possible severe drop in blood pressure. Keep equipment nearby to resume drug, if needed. Don't reinstate vasopressor therapy until systolic blood pressure falls below 70 to 80 mm Hg, as ordered.

 **Patient teaching**
• Tell patient to report adverse reactions promptly.
• Instruct patient to alert nurse if discomfort occurs at I.V. site.

## norepinephrine bitartrate (levarterenol bitartrate, noradrenaline acid tartrate)
Levophed

*Pregnancy Risk Category C*

**HOW SUPPLIED**
*Injection:* 1 mg/ml

**ACTION**
Stimulates alpha and beta$_1$ receptors within the sympathetic nervous system, primarily producing vasoconstriction and cardiac stimulation.

| Route | Onset | Peak | Duration |
|-------|-------|------|----------|
| I.V. | Immediate | Immediate | 1-2 min after infusion ends |

**INDICATIONS & DOSAGE**
*To restore blood pressure in acute hypotensive states—*
**Adults:** initially, 8 to 12 mcg/minute I.V. infusion; then titrated to maintain normal

blood pressure. Average maintenance dose is 2 to 4 mcg/minute.
**Children:** 2 mcg/m²/minute I.V. infusion; dosage adjusted based on patient response.
*Severe hypotension during cardiac arrest—*
**Children:** initial I.V. infusion rate is 0.1 mcg/kg/minute. Rate titrated based on patient response.

### ADVERSE REACTIONS
**CNS:** *headache,* anxiety, weakness, dizziness, tremor, restlessness, insomnia.
**CV:** *bradycardia, severe hypertension, arrhythmias.*
**Respiratory:** respiratory difficulties, *asthmatic episodes.*
**Skin:** irritation with extravasation, necrosis and gangrene secondary to extravasation.
**Other:** *anaphylaxis.*

### INTERACTIONS
**Drug-drug.** *Alpha blockers:* may antagonize drug effects. Avoid concomitant use.
*Antihistamines, ergot alkaloids, guanethidine, MAO inhibitors, methyldopa, oxytocics, tricyclic antidepressants:* when given with sympathomimetics, may cause severe hypertension (hypertensive crisis). Don't give together.
*Bretylium, inhalation anesthetics:* increased risk of arrhythmias. Monitor closely.

### EFFECTS ON DIAGNOSTIC TESTS
None reported.

### CONTRAINDICATIONS
Contraindicated in patients with mesenteric or peripheral vascular thrombosis, profound hypoxia, hypercarbia, or hypotension resulting from blood volume deficit and during cyclopropane and halothane anesthesia.

### NURSING CONSIDERATIONS
• Use with extreme caution in patients receiving MAO inhibitors or triptyline- or imipramine-type antidepressants. Use cautiously in patients with sulfite sensitivity.

• Drug isn't substitute for blood or fluid replacement therapy. If volume deficit exists, replace fluid before administering vasopressors.
• *Alert:* Never leave patient unattended during infusion. Also, check blood pressure every 2 minutes until stabilized; then check every 5 minutes. In previously hypertensive patients, blood pressure should be raised no higher than 40 mm Hg below preexisting systolic pressure.
• During infusion, frequently monitor ECG, cardiac output, central venous pressure, pulmonary artery wedge pressure, pulse rate, urine output, and color and temperature of extremities. Titrate infusion rate according to findings and doctor's guidelines.
• Keep emergency drugs on hand to reverse effects of norepinephrine: atropine for reflex bradycardia, phentolamine for increased vasopressor effects, and propranolol for arrhythmias.
• Notify doctor immediately of decreased urine output.
• When discontinuing drug, gradually slow infusion rate, as ordered. Continue monitoring vital signs, watching for possible severe drop in blood pressure.

### I.V. administration
• Avoid mixing with alkaline solutions, oxidizing drugs, or iron salts.
• Use a central venous catheter or a large vein, such as in the antecubital fossa, to minimize risk of extravasation. Administer in dextrose 5% in normal saline for injection; normal saline for injection alone isn't recommended. Use continuous infusion pump to regulate infusion flow rate and a piggyback setup so I.V. line remains open if norepinephrine is stopped.
• Check site frequently for signs of extravasation. If it occurs, stop infusion immediately and call doctor. He may counteract effect by infiltrating area with 5 to 10 mg phentolamine in 10 to 15 ml of normal saline solution. Also check for blanching along course of infused vein; may progress to superficial sloughing.
• Protect drug from light. Discard discolored solutions or solutions that contain a precipitate. Norepinephrine solutions deteriorate after 24 hours.

---

*Liquid contains alcohol.   **May contain tartrazine.   †Canada   ‡Australia   §U.K.   ◇OTC

• If prolonged I.V. therapy is needed, change injection site frequently.

☑ **Patient teaching**
• Tell patient to report adverse reactions promptly.
• Advise patient to alert nurse if discomfort occurs at I.V. insertion site.

## phenylephrine hydrochloride
Neo-Synephrine

*Pregnancy Risk Category C*

### HOW SUPPLIED
*Injection:* 10 mg/ml

### ACTION
Predominantly stimulates alpha receptors in the sympathetic nervous system, causing vasoconstriction.

| Route | Onset | Peak | Duration |
|-------|-------|------|----------|
| I.V. | Immediate | Unknown | 15-20 min |
| I.M. | 10-15 min | Unknown | 0.5-2 hr |
| S.C. | 10-15 min | Unknown | 50-60 min |

### INDICATIONS & DOSAGE
*Hypotensive emergencies during spinal anesthesia—*
**Adults:** initially, 0.2 mg I.V.; subsequent doses shouldn't exceed the preceding dose by more than 0.2 mg. Maximum single dose is 0.5 mg.
*Maintenance of blood pressure during spinal or inhalation anesthesia—*
**Adults:** 2 to 3 mg S.C. or I.M. 3 to 4 minutes before anesthesia.
**Children:** 0.044 mg to 0.088 mg/kg S.C. or I.M.
*Prolongation of spinal anesthesia—*
**Adults:** 2 to 5 mg added to anesthetic solution.
*Vasoconstrictor for regional anesthesia—*
**Adults:** 1 mg phenylephrine added to 20 ml local anesthetic.
*Mild to moderate hypotension—*
**Adults:** 2 to 5 mg S.C. or I.M.; repeated in 1 to 2 hours as needed and tolerated. Initial dose shouldn't exceed 5 mg. Or, 0.1 to 0.5 mg slow I.V., not to be repeated more often than 10 to 15 minutes.

**Children:** 0.1 mg/kg I.M. or S.C.; repeated in 1 to 2 hours as needed and tolerated.
*Severe hypotension and shock (including drug induced)—*
**Adults:** 10 mg in 250 to 500 ml of $D_5W$ or normal saline for injection. I.V. infusion started at 100 to 180 mcg/minute; then decreased to maintenance infusion of 40 to 60 mcg/minute when blood pressure stabilizes.
*Paroxysmal supraventricular tachycardia—*
**Adults:** initially, 0.5 mg rapid I.V.; subsequent doses shouldn't exceed preceding dose by more than 0.1 to 0.2 mg and shouldn't exceed 1 mg.

*Note:* Also used in eyedrops and OTC cold preparations for decongestant effects.

### ADVERSE REACTIONS
**CNS:** *headache,* excitability.
**CV:** **bradycardia, arrhythmias,** hypertension.
**Respiratory:** **asthmatic episodes.**
**Skin:** tissue sloughing with extravasation.
**Other:** possible tachyphylaxis with continued use, **anaphylaxis,** decreased organ perfusion with prolonged use.

### INTERACTIONS
**Drug-drug.** *Alpha blockers, phenothiazines:* decreased vasopressor response. Monitor closely.
*Beta blockers:* blocked cardiostimulatory effects. Monitor closely.
*Bretylium, halogenated hydrocarbon anesthetics, sympathomimetics:* may cause serious arrhythmias. Use with extreme caution.
*Guanethidine, oxytocics, tricyclic antidepressants:* increased pressor response. Observe patient.
*MAO inhibitors:* may cause severe hypertension (hypertensive crisis). Don't use together.

### EFFECTS ON DIAGNOSTIC TESTS
Drug may lower intraocular pressure in normal eyes or in open-angle glaucoma. It also may cause false-normal tonometry readings.

---

Reactions may be *common,* uncommon, *life-threatening,* or **COMMON AND LIFE-THREATENING.**

## CONTRAINDICATIONS

Contraindicated in patients with hypersensitivity to drug and in those with severe hypertension or ventricular tachycardia.

## NURSING CONSIDERATIONS

• Use with extreme caution in patients with heart disease, hyperthyroidism, severe atherosclerosis, bradycardia, partial heart block, myocardial disease, or sulfite sensitivity and in elderly patients.
• Drug causes little or no CNS stimulation.
• Drug is incompatible with butacaine sulfate, alkalis, ferric salts, and oxidizing drugs.

### ☑ I.V. administration

• For direct injection, dilute 10 mg (1 ml) with 9 ml sterile water for injection to provide a solution containing 1 mg/ml. I.V. infusions are usually prepared by adding 10 mg of drug to 500 ml of D₅W or normal saline for injection. The initial infusion rate is usually 100 to 180 mcg/minute; the maintenance infusion rate is usually 40 to 60 mcg/minute.
• Use a central venous catheter or a large vein, as in the antecubital fossa, to minimize risk of extravasation. Use a continuous infusion pump to regulate infusion flow rate.
• To treat extravasation, infiltrate site promptly with 10 to 15 ml of normal saline for injection containing 5 to 10 mg phentolamine, as ordered. Use a fine needle.
• With prolonged I.V. infusions, avoid abrupt withdrawal. During infusion, frequently monitor ECG, blood pressure, cardiac output, central venous pressure, pulmonary artery wedge pressure, pulse rate, urine output, and color and temperature of extremities. Titrate infusion rate according to findings and doctor's guidelines. Use a continuous infusion pump to regulate flow rate and avoid severe increase. Maintain blood pressure slightly below patient's normal level, as ordered. In previously normotensive patients, maintain systolic blood pressure at 80 to 100 mm Hg; in previously hypertensive patients, maintain systolic blood pressure at 30 to 40 mm Hg below usual level.

### ☑ Patient teaching

• Tell patient to report adverse reactions promptly.
• Instruct patient to alert nurse if discomfort occurs at I.V. insertion site.

## pseudoephedrine hydrochloride

Allermed ◇ , Cenafed ◇ , Children's Congestion Relief ◇ , Children's Sudafed Liquid ◇ , Congestion Relief ◇ , Decofed ◇ , Defed-60 ◇ , Dorcol Children's Decongestant Liquid ◇ , Drixoral Non-Drowsy Formula ◇ , Efidac/24 ◇ , Eltor 120† ◇ , Galpseud§, Genaphed ◇ , Halofed ◇ , Halofed Adult Strength ◇ , Maxenal† ◇ , Myfedrine ◇ , Novafed ◇ , Ornex ◇ , Pedia Care Infant's Decongestant ◇ , Pedia Care Infants' Oral Decongestant Drops ◇ , Pseudo ◇ , Pseudo-Gest ◇ , Seudotabs ◇ , Sinufed Timecelles ◇ , Sinustop Pro ◇ , Sudafed ◇ , Sudafed 12 Hour ◇ , Sufedrin ◇

## pseudoephedrine sulfate

Afrin ◇ , Drixoral†, Drixoral Non-Drowsy Formula ◇

*Pregnancy Risk Category C*

## HOW SUPPLIED

**pseudoephedrine hydrochloride**
*Tablets:* 30 mg ◇ , 60 mg ◇
*Tablets (extended-release):* 120 mg ◇ , 240 mg ◇
*Capsules:* 60 mg
*Capsules (extended-release):* 120 mg
*Oral solution:* 7.5 mg/0.8 ml ◇ , 15 mg/5 ml ◇ , 30 mg/5 ml ◇
*Syrup:* 30 mg/5 ml
**pseudoephedrine sulfate**
*Tablets (extended-release):* 120 mg (60 mg immediate-release, 60 mg delayed-release) ◇

---

*Liquid contains alcohol.     **May contain tartrazine.     †Canada     ‡Australia     §U.K.     ◇OTC

## ACTION
Stimulates alpha receptors in the respiratory tract, producing vasoconstriction, causing shrinkage of swollen nasal mucous membranes; reduction of tissue hyperemia, edema, and nasal congestion; and an increase in airway patency.

| Route | Onset | Peak | Duration |
|-------|-------|------|----------|
| P.O. | 0.5 hr | 0.5-1 hr | 4-12 hr |

## INDICATIONS & DOSAGE
*Nasal and eustachian tube decongestion—*
**Adults:** 60 mg P.O. q 4 hours. Maximum dose is 240 mg daily. Or, 120 mg extended-release tablet P.O. q 12 hours or 240 mg extended-release (Efidac/24) once daily.
**Children over age 12:** 60 mg P.O. q 4 to 6 hours. Maximum dose is 240 mg daily. Or, 120 mg extended-release tablet P.O. q 12 hours or 240 mg extended-release (Efidac/24) once daily.
**Children ages 6 to 12:** 30 mg P.O. regular-release form q 4 to 6 hours. Maximum dose is 120 mg daily.
**Children ages 2 to 5:** 15 mg P.O. regular-release form q 4 to 6 hours. Maximum dose is 60 mg daily.
**Children ages 1 to 2:** 7 drops (0.2 ml)/kg P.O. q 4 to q 6 hours, up to four doses daily.
**Children ages 3 to 12 months:** 3 drops/kg P.O. q 4 to 6 hours, up to four doses daily.

## ADVERSE REACTIONS
**CNS:** *anxiety,* transient stimulation, tremor, dizziness, headache, insomnia, *nervousness.*
**CV:** **arrhythmias,** *palpitations,* tachycardia, **CV collapse.**
**GI:** anorexia, nausea, vomiting, dry mouth.
**GU:** difficulty urinating.
**Respiratory:** respiratory difficulties.
**Skin:** pallor.

## INTERACTIONS
**Drug-drug.** *Antihypertensives:* may attenuate hypotensive effect. Monitor blood pressure closely.

*MAO inhibitors:* may cause severe hypertension (hypertensive crisis). Don't use together.
*Methyldopa:* may result in increased pressor response. Monitor closely.

## EFFECTS ON DIAGNOSTIC TESTS
None reported.

## CONTRAINDICATIONS
Contraindicated in patients with severe hypertension or severe coronary artery disease, in those receiving MAO inhibitors, and in breast-feeding women. Extended-release preparations are contraindicated in children under age 12.

## NURSING CONSIDERATIONS
● Use cautiously in patients with hypertension, cardiac disease, diabetes, glaucoma, hyperthyroidism, and prostatic hyperplasia.
● Elderly patients are more sensitive to drug's effects. Extended-release tablets shouldn't be administered to them until safety with short-acting preparations has been established.

☑**Patient teaching**
● Tell patient not to crush or break extended-release forms.
● Warn against using OTC products containing other sympathomimetics.
● Instruct patient not to take drug within 2 hours of bedtime because it can cause insomnia.
● Tell patient to stop drug if he becomes unusually restless, and to notify doctor promptly.

---

Reactions may be *common,* uncommon, **life-threatening,** or COMMON AND LIFE-THREATENING.

**dihydroergotamine mesylate**
**ergotamine tartrate**
**methysergide maleate**
**propranolol hydrochloride**
(See Chapter 22, ANTIANGINALS.)

## COMBINATION PRODUCTS
BELLERGAL-S**, BEL-PHEN-ERGOT-SR,
PHENERBEL-S: ergotamine tartrate 0.6 mg,
levorotatory belladonna alkaloids 0.2 mg,
and phenobarbital 40 mg.
CAFERGOT, ERCAF, WIGRAINE: ergotamine
tartrate 1 mg and caffeine 100 mg.
CAFERGOT SUPPOSITORIES: ergotamine tartrate 2 mg and caffeine 100 mg.
HYDERGINE: dihydroergocornine mesylate
0.167 mg, dihydroergocristine mesylate
0.167 mg, and dihydroergocryptine mesylate 0.167 mg.

---

## dihydroergotamine mesylate
D.H.E. 45, Dihydergot‡,
Dihydroergotamine-Sandoz†,
Migranal

*Pregnancy Risk Category X*

### HOW SUPPLIED
*Injection*: 1 mg/ml
*Intranasal solution*: 0.5 mg/metered spray
(4 mg/ml)

### ACTION
Causes peripheral vasoconstriction primarily by stimulating alpha receptors;
may abort vascular headaches by direct
vasoconstriction of dilated carotid artery
bed with a decline in amplitude of pulsations. Also causes antagonistic effect of
serotonin $5HT_2$ receptors.

| Route | Onset | Peak | Duration |
|---|---|---|---|
| I.V. | 5 min | 15 min | 8 hr |
| I.M. | 15-30 min | 30 min | 3-4 hr |
| Intranasal | Rapid | 0.5-1 hr | Unknown |

### INDICATIONS & DOSAGE
*To prevent or abort vascular or migraine
headache—*
**Adults:** 1 mg I.M. or I.V. repeated q 1 to
2 hours, p.r.n., up to total of 2 mg I.V. or
3 mg I.M. per attack. Maximum weekly
dose is 6 mg.
**Nasal spray:** 1 spray into each nostril
(1 mg total) initially, and then repeat in 15
minutes for a total dose of 2 mg.

### ADVERSE REACTIONS
**CV:** transient tachycardia or ***bradycardia,***
precordial distress and pain, increased ar-
terial pressure.
**GI:** *nausea, vomiting.*
**GU:** uterine contractions.
**Musculoskeletal:** weakness in legs, mus-
cle pain in extremities, numbness and tin-
gling in fingers and toes.
**Skin:** itching.
**Other:** localized edema.

### INTERACTIONS
**Drug-drug.** *Erythromycin, other
macrolides:* may cause symptoms of ergot
toxicity (severe peripheral vasospasm
with possible ischemia, cyanosis and
numbness). Vasodilators (nitroprusside,
nifedipine, or prazosin) may be ordered to
treat such an attack. Monitor closely.
*Propranolol, other beta blockers:* blocked
natural pathway for vasodilation in patients receiving ergot alkaloids; may result in excessive vasoconstriction and
cold extremities. Watch closely if drugs
are used together.

### EFFECTS ON DIAGNOSTIC TESTS
None reported.

### CONTRAINDICATIONS
Contraindicated in patients with hypersensitivity to drug and in those with peripheral and occlusive vascular disease,
coronary artery disease, uncontrolled hypertension, severe hepatic or renal dysfunction, malnutrition, severe pruritus, or

---

*Liquid contains alcohol.   **May contain tartrazine.   †Canada   ‡Australia   §U.K.   ◇OTC

sepsis; also contraindicated in pregnant or breast-feeding patients.

## NURSING CONSIDERATIONS
• Drug is most effective when used at first sign of migraine or soon after onset.
• Avoid prolonged administration; don't exceed recommended dosage, as ordered. Adjust to most effective minimal dosage, as ordered, for best results.
• Intranasal solution isn't intended for prolonged daily use.
• *Alert:* Watch for ergotamine rebound, or an increase in frequency and duration of headache, which may occur when drug is stopped.

### I.V. administration
• Directly inject solution into the vein over 3 minutes. Continuous and intermittent infusion aren't recommended.
• Protect ampules from heat and light. Discard if solution is discolored.

### ☑ Patient teaching
• Instruct patient to lie down and relax in a quiet, low-light environment after administration of drug.
• Tell patient to report feeling of coldness in extremities or of tingling in fingers and toes. Severe vasoconstriction may result in tissue damage. Keep extremities warm and administer vasodilators, as ordered.
• Help patient evaluate underlying causes of stress, which may precipitate attacks.
• Advise patient to notify doctor if she's pregnant or if she plans to become pregnant.

---

## ergotamine tartrate
Ergodryl Mono‡, Ergomar, Ergostat, Gynergen†, Lingraine§, Medihaler Ergotamine

*Pregnancy Risk Category X*

### HOW SUPPLIED
*Capsules:* 1 mg‡
*Tablets:* 1 mg†
*Tablets (S.L.):* 2 mg
*Aerosol inhaler:* 360 mcg/metered spray

## ACTION
Stimulates alpha receptors, causing peripheral vasoconstriction. May abort vascular headaches by direct vasoconstriction of the dilated carotid artery bed with a concomitant decrease in the amplitude of pulsations. Also, inhibits reuptake of norepinephrine, increasing vasoconstrictor activity, and acts as an antagonist of serotonin receptors.

| Route | Onset | Peak | Duration |
|-------|-------|------|----------|
| P.O. | Variable | 0.5-3 hr | Variable |
| S.L., inhalation | Variable | Unknown | Variable |

## INDICATIONS & DOSAGE
*To abort or prevent vascular or migraine headache—*
**Adults:** initially, 2 mg P.O. or S.L., then 1 to 2 mg P.O. q hour or S.L. q 30 minutes, to maximum of 6 mg daily and 10 mg weekly. Or, use aerosol inhaler: 1 spray (360 mcg) initially, repeated q 5 minutes, p.r.n., to maximum of 6 sprays (2.16 mg) per 24 hours or 15 sprays (5.4 mg) per week.
*Daily cluster headaches—*
**Adults:** 1 to 2 mg P.O. h.s. for 10 to 14 days to help terminate a series of attacks.

## ADVERSE REACTIONS
**CV:** transient tachycardia or ***bradycardia,*** precordial distress and pain, increased arterial pressure, angina pectoris, peripheral vasoconstriction.
**GI:** nausea, *vomiting.*
**GU:** uterine contractions.
**Musculoskeletal:** weakness in legs, muscle pain in extremities, numbness and tingling in fingers and toes.
**Skin:** pruritus, localized edema.

## INTERACTIONS
**Drug-drug.** *Erythromycin, other macrolides:* may cause symptoms of ergot toxicity (severe peripheral vasospasm with possible ischemia, cyanosis, and numbness). Monitor closely. Administer vasodilators (nifedipine, nitroprusside, or prazosin), as ordered.
*Propranolol, other beta blockers:* blocked natural pathway for vasodilation in patients receiving ergot alkaloids; may re-

---

sult in excessive vasoconstriction. Watch closely if drugs are used together.

**EFFECTS ON DIAGNOSTIC TESTS**
None reported.

**CONTRAINDICATIONS**
Contraindicated in patients with hypersensitivity to ergot alkaloids and in those with peripheral and occlusive vascular diseases, coronary artery disease, hypertension, hepatic or renal dysfunction, malnutrition, severe pruritus, or sepsis; also contraindicated during pregnancy.

**NURSING CONSIDERATIONS**
• Obtain an accurate dietary history from the patient to determine whether a relationship exists between certain foods and onset of headache.
• Drug is most effective when used during prodromal stage of headache or as soon as possible after onset.
• Avoid prolonged administration; don't exceed recommended dose.
• Provide a quiet, low-light environment to help the patient relax.
• *Alert:* Watch for ergotamine rebound, or an increase in frequency and duration of headache, which may occur if drug is suddenly discontinued.

☑ **Patient teaching**
• Advise patient to dissolve S.L. tablet under tongue, and not to chew or swallow it.
• Tell patient not to eat, drink, or smoke while the tablet is dissolving. S.L. tablet is preferred during early stage of attack because of its rapid absorption.
• Instruct patient to lie down and relax in a quiet, low-light environment after administration of drug.
• Warn patient not to increase dosage without first consulting doctor.
• Advise patient to avoid prolonged exposure to cold weather whenever possible. Cold may increase many of the adverse reactions to drug.
• Instruct patient on long-term therapy to check for and report feeling of coldness in extremities or of tingling in fingers and toes. Severe vasoconstriction may result

in tissue damage. Keep extremities warm and administer vasodilators, as ordered.
• Instruct patient how to use inhaler correctly.
• Help patient evaluate underlying causes of stress, which may precipitate attacks.
• Advise patient to notify doctor if she becomes pregnant or is planning to become pregnant.

---

**methysergide maleate**
Deseril‡, Sansert**

*Pregnancy Risk Category X*

**HOW SUPPLIED**
*Tablets:* 1 mg‡, 2 mg

**ACTION**
Unknown. Specifically blocks serotonin (a neurotransmitter) in the peripheral nervous system. In CNS, drug may act as a serotonin agonist.

| Route | Onset | Peak | Duration |
|-------|-------|------|----------|
| P.O. | 1-2 days | Unknown | 1-2 days after initiation |

**INDICATIONS & DOSAGE**
*Prevention of frequent, severe, uncontrollable, or disabling migraine or other vascular headaches—*
**Adults:** 4 to 8 mg P.O. daily with meals. There must be a drug-free interval of 3 to 4 weeks following each 6-month course of treatment.

**ADVERSE REACTIONS**
**CNS:** insomnia, drowsiness, *euphoria, vertigo,* ataxia, *light-headedness,* hyperesthesia, weakness, hallucinations or feelings of dissociation, rapid speech, lethargy.
**CV:** *fibrotic thickening of cardiac valves and aorta, inferior vena cava, and common iliac branches (retroperitoneal fibrosis);* vasoconstriction, causing chest pain, vascular insufficiency of lower limbs; cold, numb, painful extremities with or without paresthesia and diminished or absent pulses; orthostatic hypotension;

---

flushing; tachycardia; peripheral edema; murmurs; bruits.
**GI:** abdominal pain, nausea, vomiting, diarrhea, constipation, heartburn.
**Hematologic:** *neutropenia,* eosinophilia.
**Metabolic:** weight gain.
**Musculoskeletal:** arthralgia, myalgia.
**Respiratory:** *pulmonary fibrosis (causing dyspnea, tightness and pain in chest, pleural friction rubs, and effusion).*
**Skin:** hair loss, rash.

### INTERACTIONS
**Drug-drug.** *Beta blockers:* may result in peripheral ischemia, cold extremities and possible gangrene. Monitor closely.

### EFFECTS ON DIAGNOSTIC TESTS
None reported.

### CONTRAINDICATIONS
Contraindicated in patients with severe hypertension or arteriosclerosis, peripheral vascular insufficiency, renal or hepatic disease, coronary artery disease, pulmonary disease, serious infections, phlebitis or cellulitis of lower limbs, collagen diseases, fibrotic processes, or valvular heart disease and in debilitated or pregnant patients.

### NURSING CONSIDERATIONS
• Use cautiously in patients with peptic ulcerations or suspected coronary artery disease. ECG and cardiac status evaluation advisable before giving to patients over age 40. Also use cautiously in patients sensitive to aspirin or tartrazine.
• *Alert:* Drug is indicated only for patients who are unresponsive to other drugs and who can be kept under close medical supervision.
• Gradually introduce drug, as ordered, and administer with meals to prevent GI effects.
• Give drug, as ordered, for 3 weeks before evaluating effectiveness. If patient shows no response after 3 weeks, the drug is unlikely to be beneficial.
• Monitor laboratory studies of cardiac and renal function, CBC, and erythrocyte sedimentation rate before and during therapy.

• Drug shouldn't be used to treat migraine or vascular headache or tension (muscle contraction) headaches.
• Drug may be withdrawn gradually every 6 months, then restarted after at least 3 weeks.

### ✓ Patient teaching
• Instruct patient to take drug with meals.
• Instruct patient to keep daily weight record and report unusually rapid weight gain. Teach patient to check for peripheral edema. Explain and suggest low-sodium diet if needed.
• Stress importance of keeping regular medical appointments as scheduled.
• Tell patient not to stop drug abruptly; may cause rebound headaches. Stop gradually over 2 to 3 weeks.
• Instruct patient to promptly notify doctor if the following symptoms occur: cold, numb, or painful hands and feet; leg cramps when walking; and pelvic, chest, or flank pain.
• Advise patient to notify doctor if pregnancy occurs or if she's planning to become pregnant.

baclofen
carisoprodol
chlorzoxazone
cyclobenzaprine hydrochloride
dantrolene sodium
methocarbamol
tizanidine hydrochloride

### COMBINATION PRODUCTS
NORGESIC: orphenadrine citrate 25 mg, aspirin 385 mg, and caffeine 30 mg.
NORGESIC FORTE: orphenadrine citrate 50 mg, aspirin 770 mg, and caffeine 60 mg.
ROBAXISAL: methocarbamol 400 mg and aspirin 325 mg.
SOMA COMPOUND: carisoprodol 200 mg and aspirin 325 mg.
SOMA COMPOUND/CODEINE: carisoprodol 200 mg, aspirin 325 mg, and codeine phosphate 16 mg.

## baclofen
Clofen‡, Lioresal, Lioresal Intrathecal

*Pregnancy Risk Category C*

### HOW SUPPLIED
*Tablets:* 10 mg, 20 mg, 25 mg‡
*Intrathecal injection:* 500 mcg/ml, 2,000 mcg/ml

### ACTION
Hyperpolarizes fibers to reduce impulse transmission. Appears to reduce transmission of impulses from the spinal cord to skeletal muscle, thus decreasing the frequency and amplitude of muscle spasms in patients with spinal cord lesions.

| Route | Onset | Peak | Duration |
|---|---|---|---|
| P.O. | Hrs-wks | 2-3 hr | Unknown |
| Intrathecal | 0.5-1 hr | 4 hr | 4-8 hr |

### INDICATIONS & DOSAGE
*Spasticity in multiple sclerosis; spinal cord injury—*

**Adults:** initially, 5 mg P.O. t.i.d. for 3 days, then 10 mg t.i.d. for 3 days, 15 mg t.i.d. for 3 days, 20 mg t.i.d. for 3 days. Dosage increase based on response, up to maximum of 80 mg daily.
*Management of severe spasticity in patients who don't respond to or can't tolerate oral baclofen therapy—*
**Adults:** *screening phase*—after test dose to check responsiveness, give drug by an implantable infusion pump. Administer test dose of 1 ml of 50-mcg/ml dilution into intrathecal space by barbotage over 1 minute or more. Significantly decreased severity or frequency of muscle spasm or reduced muscle tone should appear within 4 to 8 hours. If response is inadequate, give second test dose of 75 mcg/1.5 ml 24 hours after the first. If response is still inadequate, give final test dose of 100 mcg/2 ml after 24 hours. Patients unresponsive to the 100-mcg dose shouldn't be considered candidates for implantable pump.

*Maintenance therapy*—adjust initial dose based on screening dose that elicited an adequate response. Double this effective dose and administer over 24 hours. However, if screening dose efficacy was maintained for 12 hours or more, don't double the dose. After the first 24 hours, increase dose slowly as needed and tolerated by 10% to 30% daily. During prolonged maintenance therapy, daily dose may be increased by 10% to 40% if needed; if patient experiences adverse effects, dosage may be decreased by 10% to 20%. Maintenance doses have ranged from 12 mcg to 2,000 mcg daily; however, experience with dosages over 1,000 mcg daily is limited. Most patients need 300 to 800 mcg daily.
*Adjust-a-dose:* For patients with impaired renal function, oral and intrathecal dose is decreased.

### ADVERSE REACTIONS
**CNS:** *drowsiness, dizziness,* headache, *weakness, fatigue,* hypotonia, *confusion,*

insomnia, dysarthria, *seizures with in-trathecal use.*
**CV:** hypotension, hypertension.
**EENT:** blurred vision, nasal congestion, slurred speech.
**GI:** *nausea,* constipation, *vomiting.*
**GU:** urinary frequency.
**Hepatic:** increased AST and alkaline phosphatase levels.
**Metabolic:** hyperglycemia, weight gain.
**Respiratory:** dyspnea.
**Skin:** rash, pruritus, excessive perspiration.

### INTERACTIONS
**Drug-drug.** *CNS depressants:* increased CNS depression. Avoid concomitant use.
**Drug-lifestyle.** *Alcohol use:* increased CNS depression. Avoid concomitant use.

### EFFECTS ON DIAGNOSTIC TESTS
None reported.

### CONTRAINDICATIONS
Contraindicated in patients with hypersensitivity to drug.

### NURSING CONSIDERATIONS
• Use cautiously in patients with impaired renal function or seizure disorder or when spasticity is used to maintain motor function.
• Give oral form with meals or with milk to prevent GI distress.
• *Alert:* Don't use oral drug to treat muscle spasm caused by rheumatic disorders, cerebral palsy, Parkinson's disease, or CVA because efficacy hasn't been established. Don't administer intrathecal injection by I.V., I.M., S.C., or epidural route.
• Watch for sensitivity reactions, such as fever, skin eruptions, and respiratory distress.
• Look for increased risk of seizures in patients with seizure disorder.
• The amount of relief determines whether dosage (and drowsiness) can be reduced.
• Don't withdraw drug abruptly after long-term use unless required by severe adverse reactions; may precipitate hallucinations or rebound spasticity.
• Experience with long-term intrathecal use suggests that about 5% of patients

may develop tolerance to drug. In some cases, this may be treated by hospitalizing patient and slowly withdrawing drug over a 2-week period.
• *Alert:* Don't confuse baclofen with Bactroban.

### ✓ Patient teaching
• Instruct patient to take oral form with meals or milk.
• Tell patient to avoid activities that require alertness until drug's CNS effects are known. Drowsiness usually is transient.
• Tell patient to avoid alcohol and OTC antihistamines while taking drug.
• Advise patient to follow doctor's orders regarding rest and physical therapy.

---

## carisoprodol
Carisoma§, Soma, Vanadom

*Pregnancy Risk Category C*

### HOW SUPPLIED
*Tablets:* 350 mg

### ACTION
Unknown. Appears to modify central perception of pain without modifying pain reflexes. Muscle relaxant effects may be related to its sedative properties.

| Route | Onset | Peak | Duration |
|-------|-------|------|----------|
| P.O. | 0.5 hr | 4 hr | 4-6 hr |

### INDICATIONS & DOSAGE
*As an adjunct in acute, painful musculo-skeletal conditions—*
**Adults:** 350 mg P.O. t.i.d. and h.s.

### ADVERSE REACTIONS
**CNS:** *drowsiness, dizziness,* vertigo, ataxia, tremor, agitation, irritability, headache, depressive reactions, insomnia.
**CV:** *orthostatic hypotension,* tachycardia, facial flushing.
**GI:** nausea, vomiting, epigastric distress.
**Hematologic:** eosinophilia.
**Respiratory:** asthmatic episodes, hiccups.
**Skin:** rash, *erythema multiforme,* pruritus.
**Other:** fever, *angioedema, anaphylaxis.*

---

Reactions may be *common,* uncommon, *life-threatening,* or **COMMON AND LIFE-THREATENING.**

## INTERACTIONS
**Drug-drug.** *CNS depressants:* increased CNS depression. Avoid concomitant use.
**Drug-lifestyle.** *Alcohol use:* increased CNS depression. Avoid concomitant use.

## EFFECTS ON DIAGNOSTIC TESTS
None reported.

## CONTRAINDICATIONS
Contraindicated in patients with hypersensitivity to related compounds (such as meprobamate or tybamate) and in those with intermittent porphyria.

## NURSING CONSIDERATIONS
• Use cautiously in patients with impaired hepatic or renal function.
• *Alert:* Watch for idiosyncratic reactions after first to fourth doses (weakness, ataxia, visual and speech difficulties, fever, skin eruptions, and mental changes) and for severe reactions, including bronchospasm, hypotension, and anaphylactic shock. Withhold dose and notify doctor immediately of unusual reactions.
• Record amount of relief to help doctor determine whether dosage can be reduced.
• Don't stop drug abruptly; mild withdrawal effects, such as insomnia, headache, nausea, and abdominal cramps, may result.
• Safety and efficacy in children under age 12 haven't been established.

☑ **Patient teaching**
• Warn patient to avoid activities that require alertness until drug's CNS effects are known. Drowsiness is transient.
• Advise patient to avoid combining drug with alcohol or other CNS depressants.
• Tell patient to ask doctor before using OTC cold or hay fever remedies.
• Instruct patient to follow doctor's orders regarding rest and physical therapy.
• Advise patient to avoid sudden changes in posture if dizziness occurs.
• Tell patient to take drug with food or milk if GI upset occurs.

## chlorzoxazone
Paraflex, Parafon Forte DSC, Remular-S

*Pregnancy Risk Category C*

## HOW SUPPLIED
*Tablets:* 250 mg, 500 mg
*Caplets:* 250 mg, 500 mg

## ACTION
Unknown. Appears to modify central perception of pain without modifying pain reflexes. Inhibits reflex arcs in the spinal cord and subcortical areas of the brain to reduce muscle spasm, relieve pain, and increase mobility.

| Route | Onset | Peak | Duration |
|-------|-------|------|----------|
| P.O. | 1 hr | 1-2 hr | 3-4 hr |

## INDICATIONS & DOSAGE
*As an adjunct in acute, painful musculoskeletal conditions—*
**Adults:** 250 to 750 mg P.O. t.i.d. or q.i.d.

## ADVERSE REACTIONS
**CNS:** *drowsiness, dizziness, light-headedness,* malaise, headache, overstimulation, tremor.
**GI:** anorexia, nausea, vomiting, heartburn, abdominal distress, constipation, diarrhea.
**GU:** urine discoloration (orange or purple-red).
**Hepatic:** hepatic dysfunction.
**Skin:** urticaria, redness, pruritus, petechiae, bruising.
**Other:** angioneurotic edema, ***anaphylaxis.***

## INTERACTIONS
**Drug-drug.** *CNS depressants:* increased CNS depression. Avoid concomitant use.
**Drug-lifestyle.** *Alcohol use:* increased CNS depression. Avoid concomitant use.

## EFFECTS ON DIAGNOSTIC TESTS
None reported.

## CONTRAINDICATIONS
Contraindicated in patients with hypersensitivity to drug and in those with impaired hepatic function.

## NURSING CONSIDERATIONS
• Use cautiously in patients with history of drug allergies.
• The amount of relief determines whether dosage (and drowsiness) can be reduced.
• *Alert:* Monitor patient's liver enzyme levels, as ordered. Watch for early signs of hepatic dysfunction or abnormal liver enzyme levels. If they occur, withhold dose and notify doctor. Serious (including fatal) hepatocellular toxicity has been reported in patients receiving drug.

☑ **Patient teaching**
• Tell patient to take drug with meals or milk.
• Warn patient to avoid activities that require alertness until drug's CNS effects are known.
• Instruct patient to notify doctor immediately if fever, rash, anorexia, nausea, vomiting, fatigue, right upper quadrant pain, dark urine, or jaundice occurs because these may be signs or symptoms of hepatocellular toxicity, which warrants immediate discontinuation of drug.
• Warn patient to avoid alcohol and other CNS depressants; concomitant use with drug may increase risk of hepatocellular toxicity.
• Tell patient that drug may discolor urine orange or purple-red.
• Advise patient to follow doctor's orders regarding physical activity.

## cyclobenzaprine hydrochloride
Flexeril

*Pregnancy Risk Category B*

## HOW SUPPLIED
*Tablets:* 10 mg

## ACTION
Unknown. Relieves skeletal muscle spasm of local origin without interfering with muscle function.

| Route | Onset | Peak | Duration |
|-------|-------|------|----------|
| P.O. | 1 hr | 3-8 hr | 12-24 hr |

## INDICATIONS & DOSAGE
*Short-term treatment of muscle spasm—*
**Adults:** 10 mg P.O. t.i.d. Maximum daily dose is 60 mg; maximum duration of treatment is 2 to 3 weeks.

## ADVERSE REACTIONS
**CNS:** *drowsiness,* headache, insomnia, fatigue, asthenia, nervousness, confusion, paresthesia, *dizziness,* depression, **seizures,** dysarthria, ataxia, syncope.
**CV:** tachycardia, **arrhythmias,** palpitations, hypotension, vasodilation.
**EENT:** blurred vision, visual disturbances.
**GI:** dyspepsia, abnormal taste, constipation, *dry mouth,* nausea.
**GU:** urine retention, urinary frequency.
**Skin:** rash, urticaria, pruritus.
**Other:** with high doses, adverse reactions similar to those of other tricyclic antidepressants.

## INTERACTIONS
**Drug-drug.** *Anticholinergics:* additive anticholinergic effects. Avoid concomitant use.
*CNS depressants:* increased CNS depression. Avoid concomitant use.
*MAO inhibitors:* Hyperpyretic crisis, seizures and death have occurred with concomitant administration of MAO inhibitors and tricyclics; the potential for this interaction with cyclobenzaprine also exists. Don't give within 14 days after discontinuing MAO inhibitors.
**Drug-lifestyle.** *Alcohol use:* increased CNS depression. Avoid concomitant use.

## EFFECTS ON DIAGNOSTIC TESTS
None reported.

## CONTRAINDICATIONS
Contraindicated in patients with hypersensitivity to drug and in those with hyperthyroidism, heart block, arrhythmias, conduction disturbances, or heart failure; also contraindicated in those who have received MAO inhibitors within 14 days or who are in the acute recovery phase of an MI.

## NURSING CONSIDERATIONS
• Use cautiously in patients with history of urine retention, acute angle-closure

glaucoma, and increased intraocular pressure and in elderly or debilitated patients.
• Be alert for nausea, headache, and malaise, which may occur if drug is stopped abruptly after long-term use.
• *Alert:* Watch for symptoms of overdose, including possible cardiac toxicity. Notify doctor immediately.
• Safety and efficacy in children under age 15 haven't been established.
• *Alert:* Don't confuse Flexeril with Floxin or Flaxedil.

☑ **Patient teaching**
• Advise patient to report urinary hesitancy or urine retention. If constipation is a problem, increase fluid intake and suggest a stool softener.
• Warn patient to avoid activities that require alertness until drug's CNS effects are known.
• Warn patient not to combine with alcohol or other CNS depressants, including OTC cold or allergy remedies.

## dantrolene sodium
Dantrium, Dantrium Intravenous

*Pregnancy Risk Category C*

### HOW SUPPLIED
*Capsules:* 25 mg, 50 mg, 100 mg
*Injection:* 20 mg/vial

### ACTION
Acts directly on skeletal muscle to decrease excitation and contraction coupling and reduce muscle strength by interfering with intracellular calcium movement.

| Route | Onset | Peak | Duration |
|-------|-------|------|----------|
| P.O. | Unknown | 5 hr | Unknown |
| I.V. | Unknown | Unknown | 3 hr after infusion ends |

### INDICATIONS & DOSAGE
*Spasticity and sequelae secondary to severe chronic disorders (such as multiple sclerosis, cerebral palsy, spinal cord injury, CVA)—*
**Adults:** 25 mg P.O. daily. Increased gradually in 25-mg increments, up to 100 mg

b.i.d. to q.i.d., to maximum of 400 mg daily. Maintain each dosage level for 4 to 7 days to determine response.
**Children:** initially, 0.5 mg/kg P.O. b.i.d.; increased to t.i.d. then q.i.d. Dosage increased, p.r.n., by 0.5 mg/kg daily up to dose of 3 mg/kg b.i.d. to q.i.d. Maximum dose is 100 mg q.i.d.
*Management of malignant hyperthermia crisis—*
**Adults and children:** 1 mg/kg I.V. push initially; dose repeated, p.r.n., up to cumulative dose of 10 mg/kg.
*Prevention or attenuation of malignant hyperthermia crisis in susceptible patients who need surgery—*
**Adults:** 4 to 8 mg/kg P.O. daily in three to four divided doses for 1 to 2 days before procedure. Final dose administered 3 to 4 hours before procedure.
*Prevention of recurrence of malignant hyperthermia crisis—*
**Adults:** 4 to 8 mg/kg/day P.O. in four divided doses for up to 3 days after hyperthermic crisis.

### ADVERSE REACTIONS
**CNS:** *muscle weakness, drowsiness, dizziness,* light-headedness, *malaise, fatigue,* headache, confusion, nervousness, insomnia, *seizures.*
**CV:** tachycardia, blood pressure changes, phlebitis, thrombophlebitis.
**EENT:** excessive lacrimation, speech disturbance, diplopia, visual disturbances.
**GI:** anorexia, constipation, cramping, dysphagia, metallic taste, severe diarrhea, GI bleeding.
**GU:** urinary frequency, hematuria, incontinence, nocturia, dysuria, crystalluria, difficult erection, urine retention, increased BUN level.
**Hepatic:** increased liver function test results and total serum bilirubin levels, *hepatitis.*
**Musculoskeletal:** myalgia, back pain.
**Respiratory:** pleural effusion with pericarditis, pulmonary edema.
**Skin:** eczematous eruption, pruritus, urticaria, abnormal hair growth, diaphoresis.
**Other:** chills, fever.

## INTERACTIONS
**Drug-drug.** *Clofibrate, warfarin:* may decrease plasma protein binding of dantrolene. Use together cautiously.
*CNS depressants:* increased CNS depression. Avoid concomitant use.
*Estrogens:* may increase risk of hepatotoxicity. Use together cautiously.
*I.V. verapamil:* may result in CV collapse. Stop verapamil before administering I.V. dantrolene.
**Drug-lifestyle.** *Alcohol use:* increased CNS depression. Avoid concomitant use.

## EFFECTS ON DIAGNOSTIC TESTS
None reported.

## CONTRAINDICATIONS
Contraindicated in patients when spasticity is used to maintain motor function or for spasms in rheumatic disorders; in those with upper motor neuron disorders or active hepatic disease; and in breast-feeding patients.

## NURSING CONSIDERATIONS
• Use cautiously in patients with severely impaired cardiac or pulmonary function or preexisting hepatic disease, in women, and in patients over age 35.
• Because of risk of liver damage with long-term use, therapy should be discontinued within 45 days if benefits aren't seen.
• Obtain liver function tests at beginning of therapy.
• Prepare oral suspension for single dose by dissolving capsule contents in juice or other liquid. For multiple doses, use acid vehicle, and refrigerate. Use within several days.
• *Alert:* Watch for hepatitis (fever and jaundice), severe diarrhea, severe weakness, or sensitivity reactions (fever and skin eruptions). Withhold dose and notify doctor.
• The amount of relief in patient determines whether dosage (and drowsiness) can be reduced.
• *Alert:* Don't confuse Dantrium with Daraprim.

## 🔲 I.V. administration
• Give as soon as malignant hyperthermia reaction is recognized, as ordered. Reconstitute drug by adding 60 ml of sterile water for injection and shaking vial until clear. Don't use a diluent that contains a bacteriostatic drug. Protect contents from light, and use within 6 hours. Avoid extravasation.

## ✅ Patient teaching
• Instruct patient to take drug with meals or milk in four divided doses.
• Tell patient to use caution when eating to avoid choking. Some patients may experience difficulty swallowing during therapy.
• Warn patient to avoid driving and other hazardous activities until drug's CNS effects are known.
• Advise patient to avoid combining drug with alcohol and other CNS depressants.
• Advise patient to notify doctor if skin or eyes turn yellow, skin is itchy, or fever develops.
• Tell patient to avoid photosensitivity reactions by using sunblock and wearing protective clothing, to report abdominal discomfort or GI problems immediately, and to follow doctor's orders regarding rest and physical therapy.

---

## methocarbamol
Carbacot, Robaxin, Robaxin-750, Skelex

*Pregnancy Risk Category C*

### HOW SUPPLIED
*Tablets:* 500 mg, 750 mg
*Injection:* 100 mg/ml

### ACTION
Unknown. Probably modifies central perception of pain through sedative effects without modifying pain reflexes.

| Route | Onset | Peak | Duration |
|-------|-------|------|----------|
| P.O. | 0.5 hr | 2 hr | Unknown |
| I.V. | Immediate | Immediate | Unknown |
| I.M. | Unknown | Unknown | Unknown |

---

Reactions may be *common*, uncommon, ***life-threatening***, or **COMMON AND LIFE-THREATENING**.

## INDICATIONS & DOSAGE
*As an adjunct in acute, painful musculoskeletal conditions—*
**Adults:** 1.5 g P.O. q.i.d. for 2 to 3 days, then 1 g P.O. q.i.d.; or not more than 500 mg (5 ml) I.M. into each gluteal region repeated q 8 hours, p.r.n. Or 1 to 3 g daily (10 to 30 ml) I.V. directly into vein at 3 ml/minute, or 10 ml may be added to no more than 250 ml of D₅W or normal saline solution. Maximum I.V. or I.M. dose is 3 g daily for not more than 3 days.
*Supportive therapy in tetanus management—*
**Adults:** 1 to 2 g by direct I.V. or 1 to 3 g as infusion q 6 hours until nasogastric tube can be inserted; then give oral doses through NG tube. Maximum 24 g/day.
**Children:** 15 mg/kg I.V. q 6 hours.

## ADVERSE REACTIONS
**CNS:** *drowsiness, dizziness, lightheadedness,* headache, syncope, mild muscular incoordination with I.M. or I.V. use, *seizures with I.V. use,* vertigo.
**CV:** hypotension, *bradycardia* with I.M. or I.V. use, thrombophlebitis, flushing.
**EENT:** blurred vision, conjunctivitis, nystagmus, diplopia.
**GI:** nausea, GI upset, metallic taste.
**GU:** hematuria with I.V. use, discoloration of urine.
**Skin:** urticaria, pruritus, rash.
**Other:** extravasation with I.V. use, fever, *anaphylactic reactions with I.M. or I.V. use.*

## INTERACTIONS
**Drug-drug.** *CNS depressants:* increased CNS depression. Avoid concomitant use.
**Drug-lifestyle.** *Alcohol use:* increased CNS depression. Avoid concomitant use.

## EFFECTS ON DIAGNOSTIC TESTS
Drug therapy alters laboratory test results for urine 5-hydroxyindoleacetic acid using quantitative method of Udenfriend (false-positive) and urine vanillylmandelic acid (false-positive when Gitlow screening test used; no problem when quantitative method of Sunderman used).

## CONTRAINDICATIONS
Contraindicated in patients with hypersensitivity to drug and in those with impaired renal function (injectable form), or seizure disorder (injectable form).

## NURSING CONSIDERATIONS
• For nasogastric tube administration, prepare liquid by crushing tablets into water or NaCl solution.
• In tetanus management, methocarbamol is used with tetanus antitoxin, penicillin, tracheotomy, and aggressive supportive care. Long course of I.V. methocarbamol therapy is needed.
• Give I.M. deeply, only into upper outer quadrant of buttocks, with maximum of 5 ml in each buttock.
• Don't give S.C.
• Watch for orthostatic hypotension, especially with parenteral administration. Keep the patient in a supine position for 15 minutes afterward, and supervise ambulation. Have patient get up slowly.
• Watch for sensitivity reactions, such as fever and skin eruptions.
• Have epinephrine, antihistamines, and corticosteroids available.
• *Alert:* Don't confuse methocarbamol with mephobarbital.

### 🔾 I.V. administration
• Dilute 10 ml of drug in not more than 250 ml of solution. Use D₅W or normal saline for injection. Infuse slowly; maximum rate is 300 mg (3 ml)/minute.
• Drug irritates veins, may cause phlebitis, aggravate seizures, and cause fainting if injected rapidly. Make sure patient remains in a supine position during infusion. Drug is an irritant; avoid extravasation.

### ✅ Patient teaching
• Instruct patient to take drug with food or milk at evenly spaced intervals, as ordered.
• Tell patient that a metallic taste may develop and urine may turn green, black, or brown.
• Advise patient to follow doctor's orders regarding physical activity.

- Warn patient to avoid activities that require alertness until drug's CNS effects are known.
- Advise patient to avoid combining drug with alcohol or other CNS depressants.

---

## tizanidine hydrochloride
Zanaflex

*Pregnancy Risk Category C*

### HOW SUPPLIED
*Tablets:* 4 mg

### ACTION
Unknown. Acts as an alpha2 agonist. May reduce spasticity by increasing presynaptic inhibition of motor neurons at the level of the spinal cord.

| Route | Onset | Peak | Duration |
|-------|-------|------|----------|
| P.O. | Unknown | 1-2 hr | 3-6 hr |

### INDICATIONS & DOSAGE
*Acute and intermittent management of increased muscle tone associated with spasticity—*
**Adults:** initially, 4 mg P.O. q 6 to 8 hours, p.r.n., to maximum of three doses in 24 hours. Dosage can be increased gradually in 2- to 4-mg increments. Maximum daily dose is 36 mg.
*Adjust-a-dose:* For patients with renal failure, reduce dosage. If higher dosages are needed, individual doses rather than frequency should be increased.

### ADVERSE REACTIONS
**CNS:** *somnolence, sedation, asthenia, dizziness,* speech disorder, dyskinesia, nervousness, hallucinations.
**CV:** *hypotension.*
**EENT:** amblyopia, pharyngitis, rhinitis.
**GI:** *dry mouth,* constipation, vomiting.
**GU:** *urinary tract infection,* urinary frequency.
**Hepatic:** elevated liver function test results, hepatic injury.
**Other:** infection, flulike syndrome.

### INTERACTIONS
**Drug-drug.** *Antihypertensives, other alpha₂ agonists such as clonidine:* may cause hypotension. Monitor patient closely. Don't use with other alpha₂ agonists.
*Baclofen, benzodiazepines, other CNS depressants:* additive CNS depressant effects. Avoid concomitant use.
*Oral contraceptives:* decreased clearance of tizanidine. Dose of tizanidine may be reduced.
**Drug-lifestyle.** *Alcohol use:* increased CNS depression. Avoid concomitant use.

### EFFECTS ON DIAGNOSTIC TESTS
None reported.

### CONTRAINDICATIONS
Contraindicated in patients with known hypersensitivity to drug.

### NURSING CONSIDERATIONS
- Use cautiously in patients who are taking antihypertensives, in those with renal and hepatic impairment, and in the elderly.
- Drug should be used in pregnancy only if the benefit justifies the risk to the fetus. Women taking drug shouldn't breast-feed.
- Safety and effectiveness in children haven't been established.
- Obtain baseline liver function test results, as ordered, before treatment; during treatment at 1, 3, and 6 months; and then periodically thereafter.

### ☑ Patient teaching
- Caution patient that drug may cause drowsiness and to avoid alcohol and activities such as driving and operating machinery that require alertness.
- Inform patient that orthostatic hypotension can be minimized by rising slowly and avoiding sudden position changes.

---

# Neuromuscular blockers

atracurium besylate
cisatracurium besylate
doxacurium chloride
mivacurium chloride
pancuronium bromide
pipecuronium bromide
rapacuronium bromide
rocuronium bromide
succinylcholine chloride
tubocurarine chloride
vecuronium bromide

**COMBINATION PRODUCTS**
None.

---

## atracurium besylate
Tracrium

*Pregnancy Risk Category C*

### HOW SUPPLIED
*Injection:* 10 mg/ml

### ACTION
Nondepolarizing drug that prevents acetylcholine from binding to receptors on motor end plate, thus blocking neuromuscular transmission.

| Route | Onset | Peak | Duration |
|-------|-------|------|----------|
| I.V. | 2 min | 3-5 min | 35-70 min |

### INDICATIONS & DOSAGE
*Adjunct to general anesthesia to facilitate endotracheal intubation and to provide skeletal muscle relaxation during surgery or mechanical ventilation—*
Dosage depends on anesthetic used, individual needs, and response. Dosages given here are representative only.
**Adults and children over age 2:** 0.4 to 0.5 mg/kg by I.V. bolus. Maintenance dose of 0.08 to 0.10 mg/kg within 20 to 45 minutes should be given during prolonged surgery. Maintenance doses may be given q 12 to 25 minutes in patients receiving balanced anesthesia. For pro-

longed procedures, a constant infusion of 5 to 9 mcg/kg/minute may be used.
**Children ages 1 month to 2 years:** initial dose, 0.3 to 0.4 mg/kg. Frequent maintenance doses may be needed.

### ADVERSE REACTIONS
**CV:** *bradycardia,* hypotension, tachycardia.
**Respiratory:** *prolonged, dose-related apnea;* wheezing; increased bronchial secretions; dyspnea; *bronchospasm; laryngospasm.*
**Skin:** *skin flushing,* erythema, pruritus, urticaria, rash.
**Other:** *anaphylaxis.*

### INTERACTIONS
**Drug-drug.** *Aminoglycoside antibiotics (amikacin, gentamicin, kanamycin, neomycin, streptomycin), clindamycin; general anesthetics (enflurane, halothane, isoflurane), polymyxin antibiotics (colistin, polymyxin B sulfate), procainamide, quinidine, thiazide diuretics, trimethaphan, verapamil:* potentiated neuromuscular blockade, leading to increased skeletal muscle relaxation and prolonged effect. Use cautiously during and after surgery.
*Corticosteroids:* prolonged weakness may occur. Monitor closely.
*Edrophonium, neostigmine, pyridostigmine:* inhibition of drug and reversed neuromuscular block. Monitor closely.
*General anesthetics (cyclopropane, enflurane, ether, halothane, methoxyflurane):* potentiated effects of atracurium. Consider dosage reduction of inhaled anesthetics.
*Lithium, magnesium salts, opioid analgesics:* potentiated neuromuscular blockade, leading to increased skeletal muscle relaxation and possible respiratory paralysis. Reduce dose of atracurium.
*Phenytoin, theophylline:* resistance to or reversal of neuromuscular blockade. Monitor closely.
*Succinylcholine:* quickens onset and may increase depth of neuromuscular blockade. Monitor patient.

---

## EFFECTS ON DIAGNOSTIC TESTS
None reported.

## CONTRAINDICATIONS
Contraindicated in patients with hypersensitivity to drug.

## NURSING CONSIDERATIONS
• Use cautiously in those with CV disease; severe electrolyte disorder; bronchogenic carcinoma; hepatic, renal, or pulmonary impairment; neuromuscular disease; or myasthenia gravis and in elderly or debilitated patients.
• Administer analgesics, as ordered, for pain. Remember that patient may have pain but not be able to express it.
• Don't give by I.M. injection.
• Once spontaneous recovery starts, be prepared to reverse atracurium-induced neuromuscular blockade with an anticholinesterase (such as neostigmine or edrophonium), as ordered. Usually given together with an anticholinergic (such as atropine). Complete reversal of neuromuscular blockade is generally achieved within 8 to 10 minutes after administration of an anticholinesterase.
• Monitor respirations and vital signs closely until patient has fully recovered from neuromuscular blockade, as evidenced by tests of muscle strength (hand grip, head lift, and ability to cough).
• A nerve stimulator and train-of-four monitoring are recommended to confirm antagonism of neuromuscular blockade and recovery of muscle strength. Evidence of spontaneous recovery should be seen before attempting reversal with neostigmine.
• Prior administration of succinylcholine doesn't prolong duration of action but quickens onset and may deepen neuromuscular blockade.
• *Alert:* Careful drug calculation is essential. Always verify with a second individual.

## I.V. administration
• Use drug only under direct medical supervision by personnel skilled in the use of neuromuscular blockers and techniques for maintaining a patent airway. Have emergency respiratory support (endotracheal equipment, ventilator, oxygen, atropine, edrophonium, neostigmine, and epinephrine) available.
• Administer sedatives or general anesthetics before neuromuscular blockers, which don't obtund consciousness or alter pain threshold.
• Drug usually is administered by rapid I.V. bolus injection but may be given by intermittent infusion or continuous infusion. At concentrations of 0.2 mg/ml to 0.5 mg/ml, atracurium is compatible for 24 hours in $D_5W$, normal saline for injection, or dextrose 5% in normal saline for injection.
• Don't use lactated Ringer's solution. In lactated Ringer's injection, atracurium is stable for 8 hours at a concentration of 0.5 mg/ml. However, because of increased degradation in this solution, it isn't recommended.
• Don't mix with alkaline solutions such as barbiturates because precipitates may form.

### ✓ Patient teaching
• Explain all events and procedures to patient because he can still hear.

---

## cisatracurium besylate
Nimbex

*Pregnancy Risk Category B*

### HOW SUPPLIED
*Injection:* 2 mg/ml, 10 mg/ml

### ACTION
Nondepolarizing drug that binds to cholinergic receptors on the motor end plate, antagonizing acetylcholine and blocking neuromuscular transmission.

| Route | Onset | Peak | Duration |
|-------|-------|------|----------|
| I.V. | 1-3.3 min | 2-5 min | 25-44 min |

### INDICATIONS & DOSAGE
Dosage requirements vary widely among patients.
*Adjunct to general anesthesia; to facilitate tracheal intubation; to provide skeletal muscle relaxation during surgery—*
**Adults:** initial dose of 0.15 mg/kg I.V., followed by maintenance doses of 0.03 mg/kg I.V. q 40 to 50 minutes, p.r.n.

---

Reactions may be *common,* uncommon, *life-threatening*, or COMMON AND LIFE-THREATENING.

(or initial dose of 0.20 mg/kg I.V., followed by maintenance doses of 0.03 mg/kg I.V. q 50 to 60 minutes, p.r.n.). Or, after initial dose, a maintenance infusion may be given at 3 mcg/kg/minute, reduced to 1 to 2 mcg/kg/minute, p.r.n.

**Children ages 2 to 12:** 0.1 mg/kg I.V. over 5 to 10 seconds. After initial dose, a maintenance infusion may be given at 3 mcg/kg/minute, reduced to 1 to 2 mcg/kg/minute, p.r.n.

*Maintenance of neuromuscular blockade during mechanical ventilation in intensive care unit—*

**Adults:** The principles for infusion in the OR are also applicable to use in the ICU. After initial dose, 3 mcg/kg/minute (range, 0.5 to 10.2 mcg/kg/minute) I.V. infusion.

## ADVERSE REACTIONS

**CV:** bradycardia, hypotension.
**Respiratory:** *bronchospasm; prolonged apnea.*
**Skin:** flushing, rash.

## INTERACTIONS

**Drug-drug.** *Aminoglycosides, bacitracin, clindamycin, colistimethate sodium, colistin, lincomycin, lithium, local anesthetics, magnesium salts, polymyxins, procainamide, quinidine, tetracyclines:* may enhance neuromuscular blocking action of cisatracurium. Use together cautiously.
*Carbamazepine, phenytoin:* may cause slightly shorter duration of neuromuscular block, requiring higher infusion rate. Monitor closely.
*Enflurane or isoflurane administered with nitrous oxide or oxygen:* may prolong duration of action of cisatracurium. Patient may need less frequent maintenance dosing, lower maintenance doses, or reduced infusion rate of cisatracurium.
*Succinylcholine:* shorter time to onset of maximum neuromuscular block. Monitor patient.

## EFFECTS ON DIAGNOSTIC TESTS
None reported.

## CONTRAINDICATIONS
Contraindicated in patients with hypersensitivity to drug, other bis-benzyliso-quinolinium drugs, or benzyl alcohol (found in 10-ml vial).

## NURSING CONSIDERATIONS
• Drug isn't recommended for rapid-sequence endotracheal intubation because of its intermediate onset.
• Use cautiously in pregnant or breast-feeding women.
• Monitor neuromuscular function with nerve stimulator during administration. If stimulation doesn't elicit a response, stop infusion until response returns.
• To avoid inaccurate dosing, perform neuromuscular monitoring on a nonparetic limb in patients with hemiparesis or paraparesis.
• In patients with neuromuscular disease (myasthenia gravis and myasthenic syndrome [Eaton-Lambert syndrome]), prolonged neuromuscular block is possible. Use of a peripheral nerve stimulator and a dose of not more than 0.02 mg/kg is recommended to assess the level of neuromuscular block and to monitor dosage requirements.
• Because patients with burns have been shown to develop resistance to nondepolarizing neuromuscular blockers, they may need increased dosing. Monitor closely.
• Monitor acid-base balance and electrolyte levels, as ordered. Abnormalities may potentiate or antagonize the action of cisatracurium.
• Monitor patient for malignant hyperthermia.
• Administer analgesics, if appropriate. Patient can feel pain but can't indicate its presence.
• **Alert:** Careful drug calculation is essential. Always verify with another health care professional.

## I.V. administration
• Use only under direct medical supervision by personnel skilled in the use of neuromuscular blockers and techniques for maintaining airway patency. Don't use unless facilities and equipment for artificial respiration, mechanical ventilation and oxygen therapy are within reach.
• Drug has no known effect on consciousness, pain threshold, or cerebration. To

avoid patient distress, don't induce neuromuscular block before unconsciousness.
• The 20-ml vial is intended for use in intensive care unit only. Drug isn't compatible with propofol injection or ketorolac injection for Y-site administration. Drug is acidic and may not be compatible with an alkaline solution having a pH greater than 8.5 (such as barbiturate solutions for Y-site administration). Drug shouldn't be diluted in lactated Ringer's injection because of chemical instability.
• Drug is colorless to slightly yellow or green-yellow. Inspect vials for particulate and discoloration before administration. Unclear solutions or those with visible particulate shouldn't be used.

### ☑ Patient teaching
• Explain drug's purpose.
• Assure patient that monitoring will be continuous.
• Explain all procedures and events; drug doesn't interfere with patient's ability to hear.

---

## doxacurium chloride
Nuromax

*Pregnancy Risk Category C*

### HOW SUPPLIED
*Injection:* 1 mg/ml

### ACTION
Nondepolarizing neuromuscular blocker that competes with acetylcholine for receptor sites at the motor end plate; because this action may be antagonized by anticholinesterases, doxacurium is considered a competitive antagonist.

| Route | Onset | Peak | Duration |
|-------|-------|------|----------|
| I.V. | Variable | Variable | Variable |

### INDICATIONS & DOSAGE
*To provide skeletal muscle relaxation during surgery as an adjunct to general anesthesia—*
Dosage is highly individualized. All times of onset and duration are averages; considerable individual variation is normal.

**Adults:** 0.05 mg/kg rapid I.V. produces adequate conditions for endotracheal intubation in 5 minutes in about 90% of patients when used as part of a thiopental-narcotic induction technique. Lower doses may need longer delay before intubation is possible. Neuromuscular blockade at this dose lasts for an average of 100 minutes.
**Children over age 2:** an initial dose of 0.03 mg/kg I.V. given during halothane anesthesia produces effective blockade in 7 minutes with duration of 30 minutes. Under the same conditions, 0.05 mg/kg produces blockade in 4 minutes with duration of 45 minutes.
*Maintenance of neuromuscular blockade during long procedures—*
**Adults:** after initial dose of 0.05 mg/kg I.V., maintenance doses of 0.005 to 0.01 mg/kg will prolong neuromuscular blockade for an average of 30 to 45 minutes.

### ADVERSE REACTIONS
**Musculoskeletal:** prolonged muscle weakness.
**Respiratory:** dyspnea, *respiratory depression, respiratory insufficiency or apnea.*

### INTERACTIONS
**Drug-drug.** *Alkaline solutions:* physically incompatible; precipitate may form. Don't administer through same I.V. line.
*Aminoglycosides (gentamicin, kanamycin, neomycin, and streptomycin), bacitracin, clindamycin, colistimethate sodium, colistin, lincomycin, polymyxin B, tetracyclines:* potentiated neuromuscular blockade leading to increased skeletal muscle relaxation and prolonged effect. Use together cautiously.
*Carbamazepine, phenytoin:* may prolong the time to maximal block or shorten the duration of block with neuromuscular blockers. Monitor patient.
*Inhalation anesthetics:* may enhance or prolong action of nondepolarizing neuromuscular blockers. Monitor patient.
*Lithium, local anesthetics, magnesium salts, procainamide, quinidine:* may enhance neuromuscular blockade. Monitor for excessive weakness.

---

Reactions may be *common,* uncommon, *life-threatening,* or **COMMON AND LIFE-THREATENING.**

**EFFECTS ON DIAGNOSTIC TESTS**
None reported.

**CONTRAINDICATIONS**
Contraindicated in patients with hypersensitivity to drug; also contraindicated in neonates because drug contains benzyl alcohol, which has been associated with fatalities in newborns.

**NURSING CONSIDERATIONS**
• Use cautiously, possibly at reduced dosage, in elderly or debilitated patients; in patients with metastatic cancer, severe electrolyte disturbances, renal or hepatic impairment, or neuromuscular diseases; and in those in whom potentiation or difficulty in reversal of neuromuscular blockade is anticipated. Patients with myasthenia gravis or myasthenic syndrome (Eaton-Lambert syndrome) are particularly sensitive to the effects of nondepolarizing relaxants. Shorter-acting drugs are recommended for use in such patients.
• Because of lack of data supporting drug's safety, it isn't recommended for use in patients requiring prolonged mechanical ventilation in the intensive care unit, before or after administration of nondepolarizing neuromuscular blockers, or during cesarean section.
• Drug isn't metabolized; it's excreted in urine and bile. Patients with renal or hepatic insufficiency may need dosage adjustment.
• Dosage should be adjusted to ideal body weight in obese patients (patients 30% or more above their ideal weight) to avoid prolonged neuromuscular blockade.
• Higher initial doses may be needed in patients with severe burns and in some patients with severe liver disease. Higher doses (0.8 mg/kg) will produce intubating conditions more rapidly (4 minutes), with neuromuscular blockade for 160 minutes or more. Consequently, these higher doses should be reserved for long procedures. Administration during steady-state anesthesia with enflurane, halothane, or isoflurane may allow 33% reduction of dose.
• A nerve stimulator and train-of-four monitoring are recommended to document antagonism of neuromuscular blockade and recovery of muscle strength. Before attempting pharmacologic reversal with neostigmine, some evidence of spontaneous recovery should be present.
• Because drug has minimal vagolytic action, monitor for bradycardia, which may occur during anesthesia.
• Monitor respirations until patient is fully recovered from neuromuscular blockade, as evidenced by tests of muscle strength (hand grip, head lift, and ability to cough).
• Experimental evidence suggests that acid-base and electrolyte balance may influence the actions of nondepolarizing neuromuscular blockers. Alkalosis may counteract paralysis; acidosis may enhance it.
• *Alert:* Careful drug calculation is essential. Always verify with another health care professional.
• *Alert:* Don't confuse doxacurium with doxapram or doxorubicin.

**I.V. administration**
• Use drug only under direct medical supervision by personnel skilled in the use of neuromuscular blockers and techniques for maintaining a patent airway. Don't use unless facilities and equipment for mechanical ventilation, oxygen therapy, and intubation and an antagonist are within reach.
• To avoid patient distress, don't give drug until patient's consciousness is obtunded by general anesthetic. Drug has no effect on consciousness or pain threshold.
• Prepare drug for I.V. use with $D_5W$, normal saline for injection, dextrose 5% in normal saline for injection, lactated Ringer's injection, and dextrose 5% in lactated Ringer's injection.
• Administer product immediately after reconstitution. Diluted solutions are stable for 24 hours at room temperature; however, because reconstitution dilutes the preservative, risk of contamination increases. Discard unused solutions after 8 hours.
• When diluted as directed, remember that drug is compatible with alfentanil, fentanyl, and sufentanil.

☑ **Patient teaching**
- Explain drug's purpose.
- Assure patient that monitoring will be continuous.
- Explain all procedures and events; drug doesn't interfere with patient's ability to hear.

---

## mivacurium chloride
Mivacron

*Pregnancy Risk Category C*

---

### HOW SUPPLIED
*Injection:* 2 mg/ml in 5-ml and 10-ml vials
*Infusion:* 0.5 mg/ml in 50 ml of $D_5W$

### ACTION
Nondepolarizing drug that competes with acetylcholine for receptor sites at the motor end plate, blocking neuromuscular transmission. Because this action may be antagonized by anticholinesterases, mivacurium is considered a competitive antagonist. Drug is a mixture of three stereoisomers, each possessing neuromuscular blocking activity.

| Route | Onset | Peak | Duration |
|-------|-------|------|----------|
| I.V. | 1-2 min | 2-5 min | 20-35 min |

### INDICATIONS & DOSAGE
*Adjunct to general anesthesia; to facilitate endotracheal intubation; to relax skeletal muscles during surgery or mechanical ventilation—*
**Adults:** dosage is highly individualized. Usually, 0.15 mg/kg I.V. push over 5 to 15 seconds provides adequate muscle relaxation within 2½ to 3 minutes for endotracheal intubation. Supplemental doses of 0.1 mg/kg I.V. q 15 minutes are usually sufficient to maintain muscle relaxation.

Or, maintain neuromuscular blockade with a continuous infusion of 4 mcg/kg/ minute begun simultaneously with the initial dose, or 9 to 10 mcg/kg/minute started after spontaneous recovery caused by the initial dose is evident. When used with isoflurane or enflurane anesthesia, dosage usually is reduced up to 40%.

**Children ages 2 to 12:** 0.2 mg/kg I.V. push administered over 5 to 15 seconds. Neuromuscular blockade is usually evident in less than 2 minutes. Maintenance doses are generally needed more frequently in children.

Or, neuromuscular blockade can be maintained with a continuous I.V. infusion titrated to effect. Most children respond to 5 to 31 mcg/kg/minute (average, 14 mcg/kg/minute).

### ADVERSE REACTIONS
**CNS:** dizziness.
**CV:** *flushing,* tachycardia, **bradycardia, arrhythmias,** hypotension, phlebitis.
**Musculoskeletal:** prolonged muscle weakness, muscle spasms.
**Respiratory:** **bronchospasm,** wheezing, ***respiratory insufficiency or apnea.***
**Skin:** rash, urticaria, erythema.

### INTERACTIONS
**Drug-drug.** *Alkaline solutions such as barbiturate solutions:* physically incompatible; precipitate may form. Don't administer through same I.V. line.
*Aminoglycosides (gentamicin, kanamycin, neomycin, streptomycin), bacitracin, clindamycin, colistimethate, colistin, lincomycin, polymyxin B sulfate, tetracyclines:* potentiated neuromuscular blockade, leading to increased skeletal muscle relaxation and prolonged effect. Use together cautiously.
*Carbamazepine, phenytoin:* may prolong time to maximal blockade or shorten duration of blockade with neuromuscular blockers. Monitor patient.
*Inhalation anesthetics (especially enflurane, isoflurane):* may enhance or prolong action of nondepolarizing neuromuscular blockers. Monitor for excessive weakness.
*Lithium, local anesthetics, magnesium salts, procainamide, quinidine:* may enhance neuromuscular blockade. Monitor for excessive weakness.

### EFFECTS ON DIAGNOSTIC TESTS
None reported.

---

## CONTRAINDICATIONS

Contraindicated in patients with hypersensitivity to drug, other bis-benzylisoquinolinium drugs, or benzyl alcohol.

## NURSING CONSIDERATIONS

• Use cautiously in patients with significant CV disease and in those who may be adversely affected by release of histamine (such as asthmatic patients). To avoid hypotension, use lower initial dose of drug or give drug over longer period (60 seconds).

• Use cautiously, possibly at reduced dosage, in debilitated patients; in those with metastatic cancer, severe electrolyte disturbances, or neuromuscular diseases; and in those in whom potentiation or difficulty in reversal of neuromuscular blockade is anticipated. Patients with myasthenia gravis or myasthenic syndrome (Eaton-Lambert syndrome) are particularly sensitive to effects of nondepolarizing relaxants. Test dose of 0.015 to 0.02 mg/kg may be used to assess the patient's sensitivity to drug.

• *Alert:* Use very cautiously, if at all, in patients who are homozygous for the atypical plasma pseudocholinesterase gene. Drug is metabolized to inactive compound by plasma pseudocholinesterase.

• Administer a test dose to assess patient's sensitivity to drug. Patients with severe burns are known to develop resistance to nondepolarizing neuromuscular blockers; however, they also may have reduced plasma pseudocholinesterase activity.

• Dosage should be adjusted to ideal body weight in obese patients (patients 30% or more above their ideal weight) to avoid prolonged neuromuscular blockade.

• Like other neuromuscular blockers, dosage requirements for children are higher on a milligram per kilogram basis than those for adults. Onset and recovery of neuromuscular blockade occur more rapidly in children.

• A nerve stimulator and train-of-four monitoring are recommended to document antagonism of neuromuscular blockade and recovery of muscle strength. Before attempting pharmacologic reversal with neostigmine or edrophonium, some signs of spontaneous recovery should be evident.

• Monitor respirations closely until patient is fully recovered from neuromuscular blockade, as evidenced by tests of muscle strength (hand grip, head lift, and ability to cough).

• Experimental evidence suggests that acid-base and electrolyte balances may influence the actions of nondepolarizing neuromuscular blockers. Alkalosis may counteract the paralysis; acidosis may enhance it.

• Duration of drug effect is increased about 150% in patients with end-stage renal disease and 300% in patients with hepatic dysfunction.

• *Alert:* Careful drug calculation is essential. Always verify with another health care professional.

• *Alert:* Don't confuse Mivacron with Mazicon or Mevacor.

## ⬛ I.V. administration

• Use only under direct medical supervision by personnel skilled in the use of neuromuscular blockers and techniques for maintaining a patent airway. Don't use unless facilities and equipment for artificial respiration, mechanical ventilation, oxygen therapy, and intubation and an antagonist are within reach.

• To avoid patient distress, don't administer until patient's consciousness is obtunded by general anesthetic because drug has no effect on consciousness or pain threshold.

• Prepare drug for I.V. use with $D_5W$, normal saline for injection, dextrose 5% in normal saline for injection, lactated Ringer's injection, and dextrose 5% in lactated Ringer's injection. Diluted solutions are stable for 24 hours at room temperature.

• For drug available as premixed infusion in $D_5W$, remove the protective outer wrap, then check container for minor leaks by squeezing the bag before administering. Don't add other drugs to the container, and don't use the container in series connections.

• When diluted as directed, mivacurium is compatible with alfentanil, fentanyl, sufentanil, droperidol, and midazolam.

☑ **Patient teaching**
- Explain drug's purpose.
- Assure patient that monitoring will be continuous.
- Explain all procedures and events; drug doesn't interfere with patient's ability to hear.

---

## pancuronium bromide
Pavulon

*Pregnancy Risk Category C*

### HOW SUPPLIED
*Injection:* 1 mg/ml, 2 mg/ml

### ACTION
Nondepolarizing drug that prevents acetylcholine from binding to receptors on the motor end plate, thus blocking neuromuscular transmission.

| Route | Onset | Peak | Duration |
|-------|-------|------|----------|
| I.V. | 30-45 sec | 3-4.5 min | 35-65 min |

### INDICATIONS & DOSAGE
*Adjunct to anesthesia to induce skeletal muscle relaxation; to facilitate intubation; to assist with mechanical ventilation—*
Dosage depends on anesthetic used, individual needs, and response. Dosages are representative only.
**Adults and children age 1 month and over:** initially, 0.04 to 0.1 mg/kg I.V.; then 0.01 mg/kg q 30 to 60 minutes.
**Neonates:** individualized.

### ADVERSE REACTIONS
**CV:** tachycardia, increased blood pressure.
**EENT:** excessive salivation.
**Musculoskeletal:** residual muscle weakness.
**Respiratory:** *prolonged respiratory insufficiency or apnea.*
**Skin:** transient rashes.
**Other:** *allergic or idiosyncratic hypersensitivity reactions.*

### INTERACTIONS
**Drug-drug.** *Aminoglycoside antibiotics (including amikacin, gentamicin, kanamycin, neomycin, streptomycin);* *clindamycin; general anesthetics (such as enflurane, halothane, isoflurane); lincomycin; magnesium sulfate, polymyxin antibiotics (colistin, polymyxin B sulfate); quinidine:* potentiated neuromuscular blockade, leading to increased skeletal muscle relaxation and prolonged effect. Use cautiously during surgical and postoperative periods.
*Azathioprine:* may reverse neuromuscular blockade induced by pancuronium. Monitor patient.
*Lithium, opioid analgesics:* potentiated neuromuscular blockade, leading to increased skeletal muscle relaxation and possible respiratory paralysis. Use with extreme caution, and reduce dose of pancuronium.
*Succinylcholine:* increased intensity and duration of neuromuscular blockade. Allow effects of succinylcholine to subside before administering pancuronium.

### EFFECTS ON DIAGNOSTIC TESTS
None reported.

### CONTRAINDICATIONS
Contraindicated in patients with hypersensitivity to bromides or preexisting tachycardia and in those for whom even a minor increase in heart rate is undesirable.

### NURSING CONSIDERATIONS
- Use cautiously in elderly or debilitated patients; in patients with renal, hepatic, or pulmonary impairment; and in those with respiratory depression, myasthenia gravis, myasthenic syndrome (Eaton-Lambert syndrome) of lung cancer or bronchogenic carcinoma, dehydration, thyroid disorders, CV disease, collagen diseases, porphyria, electrolyte disturbances, hyperthermia, and toxemic states. Also use large doses cautiously in patients undergoing cesarean section.
- Drug should be used only by personnel skilled in airway management.
- Allow succinylcholine effects to subside before giving pancuronium.
- Monitor baseline electrolyte determinations (electrolyte imbalance can potentiate neuromuscular effects) and vital signs, especially respirations and heart rate.

---

Reactions may be *common,* uncommon, *life-threatening,* or COMMON AND LIFE-THREATENING.

• Measure fluid intake and output; renal dysfunction may prolong duration of action because 25% of the drug is excreted unchanged in the urine.

• A nerve stimulator and train-of-four monitoring are recommended to confirm antagonism of neuromuscular blockade and recovery of muscle strength. Before attempting pharmacologic reversal with neostigmine, some evidence of spontaneous recovery should be seen.

• Monitor respirations closely until patient has fully recovered from neuromuscular blockade, as evidenced by tests of muscle strength (hand grip, head lift, and ability to cough).

• Once spontaneous recovery starts, pancuronium-induced neuromuscular blockade may be reversed with an anticholinesterase (such as neostigmine or edrophonium), which is usually administered with an anticholinergic (such as atropine).

• Drug doesn't cause histamine release or hypotension but may raise heart rate and blood pressure.

• Give analgesics, as ordered, for pain.

• **Alert:** Careful drug calculation is essential. Always verify with another health care professional.

• **Alert:** Don't confuse pancuronium with pipecuronium or Pavulon with Peptavlon.

**I.V. administration**
• Administer sedatives or general anesthetics before neuromuscular blockers, as ordered. Neuromuscular blockers don't obtund consciousness or alter the pain threshold.

• Have emergency respiratory support equipment (endotracheal equipment, ventilator, oxygen, atropine, edrophonium, epinephrine, and neostigmine) immediately available.

• Don't mix with alkaline solutions, such as barbiturate solutions, because precipitate will form; use only fresh solutions.

• Store in refrigerator. Don't store in plastic containers or syringes, although plastic syringes may be used for administration.

**Patient teaching**
• Explain all events and procedures to patient because he can still hear.

## pipecuronium bromide
Arduan

*Pregnancy Risk Category C*

**HOW SUPPLIED**
*Powder for injection:* 10-mg vial

**ACTION**
Nondepolarizing neuromuscular blocker that competes with acetylcholine for receptor sites at the motor end plate. Because this action may be antagonized by anticholinesterases, pipecuronium is considered a competitive antagonist.

| Route | Onset | Peak | Duration |
|---|---|---|---|
| I.V. | 1-2 min | 5 min | 24 min |

**INDICATIONS & DOSAGE**
*To provide skeletal muscle relaxation during surgery as adjunct to general anesthesia for procedures expected to last 90 minutes or more—*
Dosage is highly individualized. The following doses may serve as a guide for use in nonobese patients with normal renal function.
**Adults and children:** initially, 70 to 85 mcg/kg I.V. provides conditions considered ideal for endotracheal intubation and maintains paralysis for 1 to 2 hours. If succinylcholine is used for endotracheal intubation, initial dose of 50 mcg/kg I.V. provides good relaxation for 45 minutes or more. Maintenance dose of 10 to 15 mcg/kg provides relaxation for about 50 minutes.
**Adjust-a-dose:** For renally impaired patients, dosage adjustment is needed.

**ADVERSE REACTIONS**
**CV:** *hypotension, bradycardia,* hypertension, myocardial ischemia, *CVA,* thrombosis, atrial fibrillation, *ventricular extrasystole.*
**GU:** increased creatinine levels, anuria.
**Musculoskeletal:** prolonged muscle weakness.

**Respiratory:** dyspnea, *respiratory depression, respiratory insufficiency or apnea.*
**Skin:** rash, urticaria.

## INTERACTIONS
**Drug-drug.** *Aminoglycosides (gentamicin, kanamycin, neomycin, streptomycin), bacitracin, colistimethate, colistin, polymyxin B sulfate, tetracyclines:* potentiated neuromuscular blockade, leading to increased skeletal muscle relaxation and prolonged effect. Use together cautiously.
*Inhalation anesthetics, quinidine:* enhances or prolongs action of nondepolarizing neuromuscular blockers. Monitor patient.
*Magnesium salts:* may enhance neuromuscular blockade. Monitor for excessive weakness.

## EFFECTS ON DIAGNOSTIC TESTS
None reported.

## CONTRAINDICATIONS
Contraindicated in patients with hypersensitivity to drug.

## NURSING CONSIDERATIONS
• Use cautiously and with dosage adjustments in patients with renal failure because drug is excreted by the kidneys. No information is available regarding use of drug in patients with hepatic disease.
• Because of lack of data supporting drug's safety, it isn't recommended for use in patients requiring prolonged mechanical ventilation in the intensive care unit, before or after administration of other nondepolarizing neuromuscular blockers, or during cesarean section.
• Patients with myasthenia gravis or myasthenic syndrome (Eaton-Lambert syndrome) are particularly sensitive to the effects of nondepolarizing relaxants. Shorter-acting drugs are recommended.
• Drug isn't recommended for use in neonates and infants under 3 months. Limited evidence suggests that infants and children (ages 1 to 14) under balanced anesthesia or halothane anesthesia may be less sensitive than adults.
• Dosage should be adjusted to ideal body weight in obese patients (30% or more over their ideal weight) to avoid prolonged neuromuscular blockade.
• *Alert:* Because of its prolonged duration of action, pipecuronium is recommended only for procedures that take 90 minutes or longer.
• Monitor respirations closely until patient is fully recovered from neuromuscular blockade, as evidenced by tests of muscle strength (hand grip, head lift, and ability to cough).
• Monitor for bradycardia during anesthesia.
• A nerve stimulator and train-of-four monitoring are recommended to document antagonism of neuromuscular blockade and recovery of muscle strength. Before attempting pharmacologic reversal with neostigmine, some evidence of spontaneous recovery should be present.
• Experimental evidence suggests that acid-base and electrolyte balances may influence the actions of nondepolarizing neuromuscular blockers. Alkalosis may counteract the paralysis, and acidosis may enhance it.
• *Alert:* Careful drug calculation is essential. Always verify with another health care professional.
• *Alert:* Don't confuse pipecuronium with pancuronium.

## I.V. administration
• Use drug under direct medical supervision by personnel skilled in use of neuromuscular blockers and techniques for maintaining a patent airway. Don't use drug unless facilities and equipment for artificial respiration, mechanical ventilation, oxygen therapy, and intubation and an antagonist are within reach.
• Give patient sedatives or general anesthetics before neuromuscular blockers are administered, as ordered. Neuromuscular blockers don't obtund consciousness or alter pain threshold.
• Reconstitute with 10 ml solution before use to yield a solution of 1 mg/ml. Using a large volume of diluent or adding drug to a hanging I.V. solution isn't recommended.
• After reconstitution with sterile water for injection or other compatible I.V. solutions (such as normal saline for injection,

$D_5W$, lactated Ringer's injection, dextrose 5% in normal saline for injection), drug is stable for 24 hours if refrigerated.
• After reconstitution with bacteriostatic water for injection, drug is stable for 5 days at room temperature or in the refrigerator. Bacteriostatic water contains benzyl alcohol and isn't intended for use in neonates.
• After reconstitution with solutions other than bacteriostatic water for injection, discard unused drug.
• Administer pipecuronium after succinylcholine when the latter is used to facilitate intubation.
• Store powder at room temperature or in refrigerator (36° to 86° F [2° to 30° C]).

☑ **Patient teaching**
• Explain drug's purpose.
• Assure patient that monitoring will be continuous.
• Explain all procedures and events; drug doesn't interfere with patient's ability to hear.

✹ NEW DRUG

## rapacuronium bromide
Raplon

*Pregnancy Risk Category C*

### HOW SUPPLIED
*Injection:* 20 mg/ml

### ACTION
Competes with acetylcholine for cholinergic receptors at the motor end plate, thus blocking depolarization. Action can be reversed by neostigmine, an acetylcholinesterase inhibitor.

| Route | Onset | Peak | Duration |
|-------|-------|------|----------|
| I.V. | 60-90 sec | 90 sec | 15 min |

### INDICATIONS & DOSAGE
*Adjunct to general anesthesia to facilitate tracheal intubation and to provide skeletal muscle relaxation during short surgical procedures—*
Dosage is highly individualized. The following dosages should serve as a guide only.

**Adults:** initially, 1.5 mg/kg I.V. provides conditions considered ideal for tracheal intubation within 60 to 90 seconds and maintains paralysis for about 15 minutes. Following intubating dose, up to three maintenance doses of 0.5 mg/kg I.V. may be administered, as needed. Repeat dosing is based on clinical duration of previous dose and shouldn't be administered until recovery of neuromuscular function is evident.
**Adults undergoing cesarean section with thiopental induction:** 2.5 mg/kg I.V. is recommended intubating dose.
**Children ages 13 to 17:** individualize dose considering physical maturity, height, and weight and using the other recommendations as a guide.
**Children ages 1 month to 12 years:** 2 mg/kg I.V. bolus produces acceptable intubating conditions within 60 to 90 seconds; muscle paralysis should last about 15 minutes.

### ADVERSE REACTIONS
**CV:** hypotension, tachycardia, ***bradycardia.***
**GI:** vomiting, nausea.
**Respiratory:** *bronchospasm.*
**Skin:** rash.

### INTERACTIONS
**Drug-drug.** *Anticonvulsants (carbamazepine, phenytoin):* may reduce duration of action of rapacuronium, resulting in higher infusion rates and development of resistance. Monitor patient.
*Certain antibiotics (aminoglycosides, bacitracin, polymyxin, tetracyclines, vancomycin), inhalation anesthetics (desflurane, enflurane, halothane, isoflurane, sevoflurane), lithium, local anesthetics, magnesium salts, procainamide, quinidine:* may enhance neuromuscular blocking action of rapacuronium. Use together cautiously; consider lower doses of rapacuronium.

### EFFECTS ON DIAGNOSTIC TESTS
None reported.

### CONTRAINDICATIONS
Contraindicated in patients with hypersensitivity to drug. Repeat dosing in pedi-

---

atric patients or adults who have been given intubating doses greater than 1.5 mg/kg isn't recommended.

## NURSING CONSIDERATIONS
• Use cautiously in patients with myasthenia gravis, myasthenic syndrome, renal or hepatic dysfunction, acid-base abnormalities, electrolyte disturbances, burns, disuse atrophy, cachexia, and carcinomatosis. Also use cautiously in breast-feeding patients, debilitated patients, and patients with neuromuscular disease.
• Adequate anesthesia or sedating drugs must accompany administration of rapacuronium because drug has no effect on consciousness or pain.
• Use a peripheral nerve stimulator to measure neuromuscular function during administration in order to monitor drug effect, determine need for additional doses, and confirm recovery from neuromuscular block.
• Don't administer additional doses until there is a definite response to nerve stimulation.
• Assess baseline electrolyte levels (electrolyte imbalance can potentiate neuromuscular blocking effects).
• Monitor vital signs, especially respirations and heart rate.
• For morbidly obese patients (body mass index greater than 40 kg/m$^2$), base initial dose on ideal body weight. For all other patients, base dose on actual body weight.
• For patients with end-stage renal disease, watch closely for return of neuromuscular function because condition increases clearance time of drug.
• Profound neuromuscular blockade can be reversed by neostigmine.

### 🔷 I.V. administration
• Use only under direct medical supervision by experienced clinicians skilled in use of neuromuscular blockers and techniques of airway management. Don't administer unless an antagonist and equipment for artificial respiration, oxygen therapy, and intubation are within reach.
• Drug shouldn't be administered by infusion, particularly during long surgical procedures or in ICU setting.

• Reconstitute drug with sterile water for injection or other compatible I.V. solutions, such as normal saline, 5% dextrose in water, 5% dextrose in saline, lactated Ringer's, or bacteriostatic water for injection.
• Use within 24 hours of reconstitution. Prepared solutions may be stored at room temperature or refrigerated (36° to 77° F [2° to 25° C]). Don't use if particulates are present.

### ✅ Patient teaching
• Explain all events and procedures to patient.
• Reassure patient and family that he will be monitored at all times.

---

## rocuronium bromide
Zemuron

*Pregnancy Risk Category B*

### HOW SUPPLIED
*Injection:* 10 mg/ml

### ACTION
Nondepolarizing drug that prevents acetylcholine from binding to receptors on the motor end plate, thus blocking neuromuscular transmission.

| Route | Onset | Peak | Duration |
|-------|-------|------|----------|
| I.V. | 1 min | 2 min | 22-67 min |

### INDICATIONS & DOSAGE
*Adjunct to general anesthesia to facilitate endotracheal intubation and to provide skeletal muscle relaxation during surgery or mechanical ventilation—*
Dosage depends on anesthetic used, individual needs, and response. Dosages are representative and must be adjusted.
**Adults:** initially, 0.6 mg/kg I.V. bolus. In most patients, tracheal intubation may be performed within 2 minutes; muscle paralysis should last about 31 minutes. A maintenance dose of 0.1 mg/kg should provide an additional 12 minutes of muscle relaxation; 0.15 mg/kg will add 17 minutes; or 0.2 mg/kg will add 24 minutes to the duration of effect.

## ADVERSE REACTIONS

**CV:** tachycardia, abnormal ECG, transient hypotension, hypertension.
**GI:** nausea, vomiting.
**Respiratory:** asthma, hiccups, *respiratory insufficiency, apnea.*
**Skin:** rash, edema, pruritus.

## INTERACTIONS

**Drug-drug.** *Aminoglycoside antibiotics (including amikacin, gentamicin, kanamycin, neomycin, streptomycin); anticonvulsants; clindamycin; general anesthetics (such as enflurane, halothane, isoflurane); magnesium salts, opiate analgesics; polymyxin antibiotics (colistin, polymyxin B sulfate); quinidine; succinylcholine; tetracyclines:* potentiated neuromuscular blockade, leading to increased skeletal muscle relaxation and potentiated effect. Use cautiously during surgical and postoperative periods.

## EFFECTS ON DIAGNOSTIC TESTS

None reported.

## CONTRAINDICATIONS

Contraindicated in patients with hypersensitivity to drug or bromides.

## NURSING CONSIDERATIONS

• Use cautiously in patients with altered circulation time caused by CV disease, old age, and edematous states; hepatic disease; severe obesity; bronchogenic carcinoma; electrolyte disturbances; and neuromuscular disease.
• Drug isn't recommended for use during rapid sequence induction for cesarean section.
• Drug should be used only by personnel skilled in airway management.
• Rocuronium provides conditions for intubation within 3 minutes.
• A nerve stimulator and train-of-four monitoring are recommended to confirm antagonism of neuromuscular blockade and recovery of muscle strength. Before attempting pharmacologic reversal with neostigmine, some evidence of spontaneous recovery should be present.
• Prior administration of succinylcholine may enhance neuromuscular blocking effect and duration of action.

• Monitor patients with liver disease because they may need higher doses of drug to achieve adequate muscle relaxation. However, such patients exhibit prolonged effects from drug.
• Monitor respirations closely until patient is fully recovered from neuromuscular blockade, as evidenced by tests of muscle strength (hand grip, head lift, and ability to cough).
• Rocuronium is well tolerated in patients with renal failure.
• Give analgesics, as ordered, for pain.
• *Alert:* Careful drug calculation is essential. Always verify with a second individual.

### I.V. administration

• Administer sedatives or general anesthetics before neuromuscular blockers, as ordered. Neuromuscular blockers don't obtund consciousness or alter the pain threshold.
• Administer by rapid I.V. injection. Or, give by continuous I.V. infusion. Infusion rates are highly individualized. Compatible solutions include $D_5W$, normal saline for injection, dextrose 5% in normal saline for injection, sterile water for injection, and lactated Ringer's injection.
• Keep airway clear. Have emergency respiratory support (endotracheal equipment, ventilator, oxygen, atropine, edrophonium, epinephrine, and neostigmine) available.
• Store vials at room temperature for up to 30 days. Use diluted infusion solutions within 24 hours.

### Patient teaching

• Explain all events and procedures to patient because he can still hear.

---

## succinylcholine chloride (suxamethonium chloride)
Anectine, Anectine Flo-Pack, Quelicin, Scoline‡, Sucostrin

*Pregnancy Risk Category C*

## HOW SUPPLIED

*Injection:* 20 mg/ml, 50 mg/ml, 100 mg/ml; 100-mg vial, 500-mg vial, 1-g vial

---

## ACTION
Binds with a high affinity to cholinergic receptors, prolonging depolarization of the motor end plate and ultimately producing muscle paralysis.

| Route | Onset | Peak | Duration |
|-------|-------|------|----------|
| I.V. | 0.5-1 min | 1-2 min | 4-10 min |
| I.M. | 2-3 min | Unknown | 10-30 min |

## INDICATIONS & DOSAGE
*Adjunct to anesthesia to induce skeletal muscle relaxation for surgery and orthopedic manipulations; to facilitate intubation and assist with mechanical ventilation; to lessen muscle contractions in pharmacologically or electrically induced seizures—*
Dosage depends on anesthetic used, individual needs, and response. Dosages are representative only.
**Adults:** 0.6 mg/kg I.V. given over 10 to 30 seconds. For longer response, administer continuous infusion at rate of 0.5 to 10 mg/minute or 0.04 to 0.07 mg/kg intermittently, p.r.n., to maintain relaxation.
**Children:** 1 to 2 mg/kg I.V. or 3 to 4 mg/kg I.M. Maximum I.M. dose is 150 mg. (Children may be less sensitive to succinylcholine than adults.)

## ADVERSE REACTIONS
**CV:** *bradycardia,* tachycardia, hypertension, hypotension, *arrhythmias,* flushing, *cardiac arrest.*
**EENT:** increased intraocular pressure.
**Metabolic:** myoglobinemia, hyperkalemia.
**Musculoskeletal:** muscle fasciculation, *postoperative muscle pain.*
**Respiratory:** *prolonged respiratory depression, apnea, bronchoconstriction.*
**Other:** *malignant hyperthermia, rhabdomyolysis (with possible myoglobinuric acute renal failure, excessive salivation, hyperkalemia, rash), allergic or idiosyncratic hypersensitivity reactions, anaphylaxis.*

## INTERACTIONS
**Drug-drug.** *Aminoglycoside antibiotics (including amikacin, gentamicin, kanamycin, neomycin, streptomycin); anticholinesterases (such as echothiophate,* edrophonium, neostigmine, physostigmine, pyridostigmine); general anesthetics (such as enflurane, halothane, isoflurane); polymyxin antibiotics (colistin, polymyxin B sulfate): potentiated neuromuscular blockade, leading to increased skeletal muscle relaxation and potentiated effect.* Use cautiously during and after surgery.
*Cardiac glycosides:* may cause arrhythmias. Use together cautiously.
*Cyclophosphamide, lithium, MAO inhibitors:* prolonged apnea. Use with caution.
*Methotrimeprazine, opioid analgesics:* potentiated neuromuscular blockade, leading to increased skeletal muscle relaxation and possible respiratory paralysis. Use with extreme caution.
*Parenteral magnesium sulfate:* potentiated neuromuscular blockade, increased skeletal muscle relaxation, and possible respiratory paralysis. Use with caution, preferably with reduced doses.
**Drug-herb.** *Melatonin:* potentiates blocking properties of succinylcholine. Avoid concomitant use.

## EFFECTS ON DIAGNOSTIC TESTS
None reported.

## CONTRAINDICATIONS
Contraindicated in patients with hypersensitivity to drug and in those with abnormally low plasma pseudocholinesterase, angle-closure glaucoma, personal or family history of malignant hyperthermia, myopathies associated with elevated CK, or penetrating eye injuries.

## NURSING CONSIDERATIONS
• Use cautiously in elderly or debilitated patients; in patients receiving quinidine or cardiac glycoside therapy; in patients with hepatic, renal, or pulmonary impairment; in those with respiratory depression, severe burns or trauma, electrolyte imbalances, hyperkalemia, paraplegia, spinal neuraxis injury, CVA, degenerative or dystrophic neuromuscular disease, myasthenia gravis, myasthenic syndrome (Eaton-Lambert syndrome) of lung cancer or bronchogenic carcinoma, dehydration, thyroid disorders, collagen diseases, por-

---

Reactions may be *common,* uncommon, *life-threatening,* or **COMMON AND LIFE-THREATENING.**

phyria, fractures, muscle spasms, eye surgery, and pheochromocytoma. Also use large doses cautiously in patients undergoing cesarean section.
• Succinylcholine is the drug of choice for short procedures (less than 3 minutes) and for orthopedic manipulations; use caution in fractures or dislocations.
• Succinylcholine should be used only by personnel skilled in airway management.
• When giving drug I.M., inject deeply, preferably high into deltoid muscle.
• Store injectable form in refrigerator. Store powder form at room temperature in tightly closed container. Use immediately after reconstitution. Don't mix with alkaline solutions (thiopental sodium, sodium bicarbonate, or barbiturates).
• Monitor baseline electrolyte determinations and vital signs (check respirations every 5 to 10 minutes during infusion).
• Monitor respirations closely until patient is fully recovered from neuromuscular blockade, as evidenced by tests of muscle strength (hand grip, head lift, and ability to cough).
• *Alert:* Don't use reversing drugs. Unlike nondepolarizing drugs, neostigmine or edrophonium may worsen neuromuscular blockade.
• Repeated or continuous infusions of succinylcholine aren't advisable; they may cause reduced response or prolonged muscle relaxation and apnea.
• Give analgesics, as ordered, for pain.
• Keep airway clear. Have emergency respiratory support equipment (endotracheal equipment, ventilator, oxygen, atropine, and epinephrine) immediately available.
• *Alert:* Careful drug calculation is essential. Always verify with another health care professional.

**I.V. administration**
• Administer sedatives or general anesthetics before neuromuscular blockers, which don't obtund consciousness or alter the pain threshold.
• Give test dose (5 to 10 mg I.V.) after patient has been anesthetized. Normal response (no respiratory depression or transient depression for up to 5 minutes) indicates drug may be given. Don't give if patient develops respiratory paralysis suf-

ficient to permit endotracheal intubation. (Recovery within 30 to 60 minutes.)

☑**Patient teaching**
• Explain all events and procedures to patient because he can still hear.
• Reassure patient that postoperative stiffness is normal and will soon subside.

## tubocurarine chloride
Tubarine†

*Pregnancy Risk Category C*

**HOW SUPPLIED**
*Injection:* 3 mg (20 U)/ml

**ACTION**
Nondepolarizing neuromuscular blocker that prevents acetylcholine from binding to receptors on the motor end plate, thus blocking neuromuscular transmission.

| Route | Onset | Peak | Duration |
|---|---|---|---|
| I.V. | 1 min | 2-5 min | 25-90 min |

**INDICATIONS & DOSAGE**
*Adjunct to anesthesia to induce skeletal muscle relaxation; to facilitate intubation, orthopedic manipulations; as an adjunct during pharmacologically or electrically induced convulsive therapy—*
Dosage depends on anesthetic used, individual needs, and response. Dosages listed are representative and must be adjusted.
**Adults:** 1.1 U/kg or 0.165 mg/kg I.V. slowly over 60 to 90 seconds. Average dose is initially 40 to 60 U. I.V. May give 20 to 30 U in 3 to 5 minutes. For longer procedures, give 20 U, p.r.n.
*To assist with mechanical ventilation—*
**Adults and children:** 0.0165 mg/kg I.V. (average: 1 mg or 7 U); then adjust subsequent doses to patient response.
*To lessen muscle contractions in pharmacologically or electrically induced seizures—*
**Adults and children:** 1.1 U/kg or 0.165 mg/kg over 60 to 90 seconds. As a precaution, initial dose should be 20 U (3 mg) less than calculated dose.

*Diagnosis of myasthenia gravis—*
**Adults:** 4 to 33 mcg/kg as a single I.V. dose.

## ADVERSE REACTIONS
**CV:** hypotension, *arrhythmias, cardiac arrest, bradycardia.*
**EENT:** increased salivation.
**Musculoskeletal:** profound and prolonged muscle relaxation, residual muscle weakness.
**Respiratory:** *respiratory depression or apnea, bronchospasm.*
**Other:** *hypersensitivity reactions,* idiosyncrasy.

## INTERACTIONS
**Drug-drug.** *Aminoglycoside antibiotics (including amikacin, gentamicin, kanamycin, neomycin, streptomycin); clindamycin, general anesthetics (such as enflurane, halothane, isoflurane); lincomycin, magnesium salts, polymyxin antibiotics (colistin, polymyxin B sulfate):* potentiated neuromuscular blockade, leading to increased skeletal muscle relaxation and potentiated effect. Use cautiously during and after surgery.
*Amphotericin B, ethacrynic acid, furosemide, methotrimeprazine, opioid analgesics, propranolol, thiazide diuretics, verapamil:* potentiated neuromuscular blockade, leading to increased skeletal muscle relaxation and possible respiratory paralysis. Use with extreme caution during surgical and postoperative periods.
*Quinidine:* prolonged neuromuscular blockade. Use together with caution. Monitor closely.

## EFFECTS ON DIAGNOSTIC TESTS
Large doses result in production of a factor that interferes with the detection of urinary catecholamines by fluorometric measures in patients with tetanus.

## CONTRAINDICATIONS
Contraindicated in patients with hypersensitivity to drug and in those for whom histamine release is a hazard (asthmatic patients).

## NURSING CONSIDERATIONS
• Use cautiously in elderly or debilitated patients and in those with hepatic or pulmonary impairment, hypothermia, respiratory depression, myasthenia gravis, myasthenic syndrome (Eaton-Lambert syndrome) of lung cancer or bronchogenic carcinoma, in those with sulfite sensitivity, dehydration, thyroid disorders, collagen diseases, porphyria, electrolyte disturbances, fractures, and muscle spasms. Also use large doses cautiously in patients undergoing cesarean section.
• Only personnel skilled in airway management should administer tubocurarine.
• Assess baseline electrolyte determinations (electrolyte imbalance can potentiate neuromuscular blocking effects).
• Check vital signs every 15 minutes. Notify doctor at once of changes.
• Measure fluid intake and output; renal dysfunction prolongs duration of action because much of drug is excreted unchanged in urine.
• A nerve stimulator and train-of-four monitoring are recommended to confirm antagonism of neuromuscular blockade and recovery of muscle strength. Before attempting pharmacologic reversal with neostigmine, some evidence of spontaneous recovery should be present.
• Monitor respirations closely until patient is fully recovered from neuromuscular blockade, as evidenced by tests of muscle strength (hand grip, head lift, and ability to cough).
• Give analgesics, as ordered, for pain.
• Premedication with an antihistamine will decrease the release of histamine-associated hypotension.
• *Alert:* Careful drug calculation is essential. Always verify with another health care professional.

## I.V. administration
• Administer sedatives or general anesthetics before neuromuscular blockers, which don't obtund consciousness or alter the pain threshold.
• Keep airway clear. Have emergency respiratory support (endotracheal equipment, ventilator, oxygen, atropine, edrophonium, epinephrine, and neostigmine) available.

---

*Reactions may be* common, uncommon, **life-threatening**, *or* COMMON AND LIFE-THREATENING.

- Allow succinylcholine effects to subside before giving tubocurarine.
- Give I.V. over 60 to 90 seconds.
- Don't mix with barbiturates or other alkaline solutions because a precipitate will form. Use only fresh solutions and discard if discolored.

☑**Patient teaching**
- Explain all events and procedures to patient because he still can hear.

---

## vecuronium bromide
Norcuron

*Pregnancy Risk Category C*

**HOW SUPPLIED**
*Injection:* 10-mg, 20-mg vials

**ACTION**
Nondepolarizing drug that prevents acetylcholine from binding to receptors on the motor end plate, thus blocking neuromuscular transmission.

| Route | Onset | Peak | Duration |
|-------|-------|------|----------|
| I.V. | 1 min | 3-5 min | 15-25 min |

**INDICATIONS & DOSAGE**
*Adjunct to general anesthesia to facilitate endotracheal intubation and to provide skeletal muscle relaxation during surgery or mechanical ventilation—*
Dosage depends on anesthetic used, individual needs, and response. Dosages are representative and must be adjusted.
**Adults and children over age 9:** initially, 0.08 to 0.1 mg/kg I.V. bolus. Maintenance doses of 0.01 to 0.015 mg/kg within 25 to 40 minutes of initial dose should be administered during prolonged surgical procedures. Maintenance doses may be given q 12 to 15 minutes in patients receiving balanced anesthesia.
**Children ages 1 to 9:** may need a slightly higher initial dose and may need supplementation slightly more often than adults. Or, drug may be given by continuous I.V. infusion of 1 mcg/kg/minute initially, then 0.8 to 1.2 mcg/kg/minute.
**Children ages 7 weeks to 1 year:** doses comparable to those used in adults are ap-

propriate, but less frequent administration of maintenance doses may be needed.

**ADVERSE REACTIONS**
**Musculoskeletal:** skeletal muscle weakness.
**Respiratory:** *prolonged respiratory insufficiency or apnea.*

**INTERACTIONS**
**Drug-drug.** *Aminoglycoside antibiotics (including amikacin, gentamicin, kanamycin, neomycin, streptomycin); bacitracin; clindamycin; general anesthetics (such as enflurane, halothane, isoflurane); magnesium salts, other skeletal muscle relaxants; polymyxin antibiotics (colistin, polymyxin B sulfate); quinidine; succinylcholine, tetracyclines:* potentiated neuromuscular blockade, leading to increased skeletal muscle relaxation and potentiated effect. Use cautiously during and after surgery.
*Opioid analgesics:* potentiated neuromuscular blockade, leading to increased skeletal muscle relaxation and possible respiratory paralysis. Use with extreme caution, and reduce dose of vecuronium.

**EFFECTS ON DIAGNOSTIC TESTS**
None reported.

**CONTRAINDICATIONS**
Contraindicated in patients with hypersensitivity to drug or bromides.

**NURSING CONSIDERATIONS**
- Use cautiously in elderly patients; in patients with altered circulation caused by CV disease and edematous states; and in those with hepatic disease, severe obesity, bronchogenic carcinoma, electrolyte disturbances, and neuromuscular disease.
- Drug should be used only by personnel skilled in airway management.
- A nerve stimulator and train-of-four monitoring are recommended to confirm antagonism of neuromuscular blockade and recovery of muscle strength. Before attempting pharmacologic reversal with neostigmine, some evidence of spontaneous recovery should be seen.
- Monitor respirations closely until patient has fully recovered from neuromus-

---

cular blockade as evidenced by tests of muscle strength (hand grip, head lift, and ability to cough).

• Prior administration of succinylcholine may enhance the neuromuscular blocking effect and duration of action.

• Vecuronium is well tolerated in patients with renal failure.

• Give analgesics, as ordered, for pain.

• *Alert:* Careful drug calculation is essential. Always verify with another health care professional.

## 🔲 I.V. administration

• Administer sedatives or general anesthetics before neuromuscular blockers, which don't obtund consciousness or alter the pain threshold.

• Keep airway clear. Have emergency respiratory support (endotracheal equipment, ventilator, oxygen, atropine, edrophonium, epinephrine, and neostigmine) available.

• Administer by rapid I.V. injection. Or, 10 to 20 mg may be added to 100 ml of a compatible solution and given by I.V. infusion. Compatible solutions include $D_5W$, normal saline for injection, dextrose 5% in normal saline for injection, and lactated Ringer's injection.

• Don't mix with alkaline solutions such as barbiturates.

• Store reconstituted solution in refrigerator. Discard after 24 hours.

## ✅ Patient teaching

• Explain all events and procedures to patient because he can still hear.

**brompheniramine maleate**
**cetirizine hydrochloride**
**chlorpheniramine maleate**
**clemastine fumarate**
**cyproheptadine hydrochloride**
**diphenhydramine hydrochloride**
**fexofenadine hydrochloride**
**loratadine**
**promethazine hydrochloride**
**promethazine theoclate**
**triprolidine hydrochloride**

## COMBINATION PRODUCTS

ALLEREST MAXIMUM STRENGTH
TABLETS ◊ : pseudoephedrine hydrochloride 30 mg and chlorpheniramine maleate 2 mg.
CHLOR-TRIMETON ALLERGY 4-HOUR DECONGESTANT ◊ : chlorpheniramine maleate 4 mg and pseudoephedrine sulfate 60 mg.
CHLOR-TRIMETON 12 HOUR RELIEF
TABLETS ◊ : chlorpheniramine maleate 8 mg and pseudoephedrine sulfate 120 mg.
CLARITIN-D: loratadine 5 mg and pseudoephedrine sulfate 120 mg.
CONTAC 12-HOUR ◊ : phenylpropanolamine 75 mg and chlorpheniramine maleate 8 mg.
CONTAC MAXIMUM STRENGTH 12-HOUR
CAPLETS ◊ : phenylpropanolamine 75 mg and chlorpheniramine maleate 12 mg.
CORICIDIN "D" DECONGESTANT TABLETS ◊ : chlorpheniramine maleate 2 mg, acetaminophen 325 mg, and phenylpropanolamine hydrochloride 12.5 mg.
DECONAMINE: pseudoephedrine hydrochloride 60 mg and chlorpheniramine maleate 4 mg.
DIMETAPP EXTENTABS: brompheniramine maleate 12 mg and phenylpropanolamine hydrochloride 75 mg.
DRIZE: phenylpropanolamine hydrochloride 75 mg and chlorpheniramine maleate 12 mg.
FEDAHIST: pseudoephedrine hydrochloride 60 mg and chlorpheniramine maleate 4 mg.
NALDECON: phenylephrine hydrochloride 10 mg, phenylpropanolamine hydrochloride 40 mg, phenyltoloxamine citrate 15 mg, and chlorpheniramine maleate 5 mg.
NOLAMINE: chlorpheniramine maleate 4 mg, phenindamine tartrate 24 mg, and phenylpropanolamine hydrochloride 50 mg.
NOVAFED A: pseudoephedrine hydrochloride 120 mg and chlorpheniramine maleate 8 mg.
NOVAHISTINE ELIXIR ◊ *: phenylephrine 5 mg, chlorpheniramine maleate 2 mg, and alcohol 5% per 5 ml.
ORNADE SPANSULES: phenylpropanolamine hydrochloride 75 mg and chlorpheniramine maleate 12 mg.
P-V-TUSSIN SYRUP*: chlorpheniramine maleate 2 mg/5 ml, phenindamine tartrate 5 mg/5 ml, phenylephrine hydrochloride 5 mg/5 ml, and pyrilamine maleate 6 mg/5 ml.
SUDAFED PLUS ◊ : pseudoephedrine hydrochloride 60 mg and chlorpheniramine maleate 4 mg.
TAVIST-D ◊ : clemastine fumarate 1.34 mg and phenylpropanolamine 75 mg.
TRIAMINIC-12: phenylpropanolamine hydrochloride 75 mg and chlorpheniramine maleate 12 mg.
TRINALIN REPETABS: azatadine maleate 1 mg and pseudoephedrine sulfate 120 mg.

---

**brompheniramine maleate**
Bromphen* ◊ , Chlorphed ◊ ,
Codimal-LA, Cophene-B, Dehist,
Diamine T.D., Dimetane* ◊ ,
Dimetane Extentabs ◊ ,
Dimotane§, Histaject, Nasahist B,
ND-Stat, Oraminic II

*Pregnancy Risk Category C*

## HOW SUPPLIED
*Tablets:* 4 mg ◊ , 8 mg, 12 mg
*Tablets (extended-release):* 8 mg ◊ ,
12 mg ◊

---

*Liquid contains alcohol.   **May contain tartrazine.   †Canada   ‡Australia   §U.K.   ◊OTC

*Elixir:* 2 mg/5 ml* ◊
*Injection:* 10 mg/ml

## ACTION
Competes with histamine for $H_1$-receptor sites on effector cells. Prevents, but doesn't reverse, histamine-mediated responses.

| Route | Onset | Peak | Duration |
|---|---|---|---|
| P.O. | 15-60 min | 2-5 hr | 3-24 hr |
| I.V., I.M., S.C. | Unknown | Unknown | Unknown |

## INDICATIONS & DOSAGE
*Rhinitis, allergy symptoms—*
**Adults:** 4 to 8 mg P.O. t.i.d. or q.i.d.; or 8 to 12 mg extended-release P.O. b.i.d. or t.i.d. Maximum oral dose is 24 mg daily. Or, 5 to 20 mg q 6 to 12 hours I.M., I.V., or S.C. Maximum parenteral dose is 40 mg daily.
**Children ages 6 to 12:** 2 to 4 mg P.O. t.i.d. or q.i.d.; or 8 to 12 mg extended-release P.O. q 12 hours; or 0.5 mg/kg I.M., I.V., or S.C. daily in divided doses t.i.d. or q.i.d.
**Children under age 6:** 0.5 mg/kg P.O., I.M., I.V., or S.C. daily in divided doses t.i.d. or q.i.d.
*Note:* Children under age 12 should use only as directed by doctor.

## ADVERSE REACTIONS
**CNS:** dizziness, tremors, irritability, insomnia, syncope, *drowsiness, stimulation.*
**CV:** hypotension, palpitations.
**GI:** anorexia, nausea, vomiting, *dry mouth and throat.*
**GU:** urine retention.
**Hematologic:** *thrombocytopenia, agranulocytosis.*
**Skin:** urticaria, rash.
**Other:** local stinging, diaphoresis after parenteral administration.

## INTERACTIONS
**Drug-drug.** *CNS depressants:* increased sedation. Use together cautiously.
*MAO inhibitors:* increased anticholinergic effects. Don't use together.
**Drug-lifestyle.** *Alcohol use:* increased CNS depression. Use cautiously.

## EFFECTS ON DIAGNOSTIC TESTS
Discontinue drug 4 days before performing diagnostic skin tests. Drug can prevent, reduce, or mask positive skin test response.

## CONTRAINDICATIONS
Contraindicated in patients with hypersensitivity to drug's ingredients and in those with acute asthma, severe hypertension, coronary artery disease, angle-closure glaucoma, urine retention, symptomatic prostatic hyperplasia, pyloroduodenal obstruction, or peptic ulcer; also contraindicated within 14 days of MAO inhibitor therapy.

## NURSING CONSIDERATIONS
• Use cautiously in elderly patients and in those with increased intraocular pressure, diabetes, ischemic heart disease, hyperthyroidism, hypertension, bronchial asthma, and prostatic hyperplasia.
• Monitor blood count during long-term therapy, as ordered; observe for signs of blood dyscrasias.

### I.V. administration
• Injectable form containing 10 mg/ml can be given undiluted or diluted with $D_5W$ or normal saline solution very slowly I.V., preferably with the patient in supine position.

### Patient teaching
• Instruct patient to reduce GI distress by taking drug with food or milk.
• Warn patient to avoid alcohol and activities that require alertness until drug's CNS effects are known.
• Advise patient to notify doctor if unusual bleeding or bruising occurs.
• Tell patient that coffee or tea may reduce drowsiness and to use cautiously if palpitations develop. Causes less drowsiness than some other antihistamines.
• Inform patient that sugarless gum, sugarless sour hard candy, or ice chips may relieve dry mouth.
• Tell patient to notify doctor if tolerance develops because a different antihistamine may need to be prescribed.

---

Reactions may be *common,* uncommon, *life-threatening,* or COMMON AND LIFE-THREATENING.

## cetirizine hydrochloride
Zyrtec

*Pregnancy Risk Category B*

### HOW SUPPLIED
*Tablets:* 5 mg, 10 mg
*Oral solution:* 5 mg/5 ml

### ACTION
Drug is a nonsedating antihistamine that selectively inhibits peripheral $H_1$ receptors.

| Route | Onset | Peak | Duration |
|-------|-------|------|----------|
| P.O. | 20-60 min | 0.5-1.5 hr | 24 hr |

### INDICATIONS & DOSAGE
*Seasonal allergic rhititis, perennial allergic rhinitis, chronic urticaria—*
**Adults and children ages 12 and older:** 5 or 10 mg P.O. daily depending on symptom severity.
**Children ages 6 to 11:** 5 or 10 mg (1 or 2 tsp) P.O. once daily depending on symptom severity.
*Adjust-a-dose:* For renally impaired patients with creatinine clearance of 11 to 31 ml/minute, those on dialysis (creatinine clearance less than 7 ml/minute), or those with hepatic impairment, 5 mg P.O. daily.

### ADVERSE REACTIONS
**CNS:** *somnolence,* fatigue, dizziness, headache.
**EENT:** pharyngitis.
**GI:** dry mouth, nausea, vomiting, abdominal distress.

### INTERACTIONS
**Drug-drug.** *CNS depressants:* possible additive effect. Avoid concomitant use.
*Theophylline:* may cause decreased clearance of cetirizine. Monitor patient closely.
**Drug-lifestyle.** *Alcohol use:* possible additive effect. Avoid concomitant use.

### EFFECTS ON DIAGNOSTIC TESTS
Discontinue drug 4 days before performing diagnostic skin tests. Drug can prevent, reduce, or mask positive skin test response.

### CONTRAINDICATIONS
Contraindicated in patients with hypersensitivity to drug or hydroxyzine.

### NURSING CONSIDERATIONS
• Use cautiously in patients with renal impairment or liver impairment.
• Drug isn't recommended for use in breast-feeding women.
• Safety of drug hasn't been established in children under age 6.
• *Alert:* Don't confuse Zyrtec with Zyprexa.

☑ **Patient teaching**
• Warn patient not to drive or perform hazardous activities if he experiences somnolence, a common adverse reaction.
• Advise patient not to use alcohol or other CNS depressants while taking drug.
• Warn patient to avoid driving or other activities that require alertness until drug's CNS effects are known.
• Tell patient that coffee or tea may reduce drowsiness.
• Inform patient that sugarless gum, sugarless sour hard candy, or ice chips may relieve dry mouth.

## chlorpheniramine maleate
Aller-Chlor* ◇ , Chlo-Amine ◇ ,
Chlorate ◇ , Chlor-Niramine ◇ ,
Chlor-100 ◇ , Chlor-Pro,
Chlor-Pro 10, Chlor-Trimeton* ◇ ,
Chlor-Trimeton 12 Hour Relief ◇ ,
Chlor-Tripolon† ◇ , Chlorspan-12,
Chlortab-4, Chlortab-8,
GenAllerate ◇ , Novo-Pheniram† ◇ ,
Pfeiffer's Allergy ◇ , Phenetron*,
Piriton§, Telachlor, Teldrin ◇

*Pregnancy Risk Category B*

### HOW SUPPLIED
*Tablets:* 4 mg ◇ , 8 mg ◇ , 12 mg ◇
*Tablets (chewable):* 2 mg ◇
*Tablets (timed-release):* 8 mg ◇ , 12 mg ◇
*Capsules (timed-release):* 6 mg ◇ ,
8 mg ◇ , 12 mg ◇
*Syrup:* 2 mg/5 ml* ◇
*Injection:* 10 mg/ml, 100 mg/ml

---

## ACTION

Competes with histamine for $H_1$-receptor sites on effector cells. It prevents, but doesn't reverse, histamine-mediated responses.

| Route | Onset | Peak | Duration |
|---|---|---|---|
| P.O. | 15-60 min | 2-6 hr | 24 hr |
| I.V. | 15-60 min | Immediate | 24 hr |
| I.M., S.C. | 15-60 min | Unknown | 24 hr |

## INDICATIONS & DOSAGE

*Rhinitis, allergy symptoms—*
**Adults:** 4 mg P.O. q 4 to 6 hours, not to exceed 24 mg/day; or 8 to 12 mg timed-release P.O. q 8 to 12 hours, not to exceed 24 mg daily. Or, 5 to 20 mg I.M., I.V., or S.C. as a single dose. Maximum recommended parenteral dose is 40 mg per 24 hours.
**Children ages 6 to 12:** 2 mg P.O. q 4 to 6 hours, not to exceed 12 mg daily. Or, may give 8 mg timed-release P.O. h.s.
**Children ages 2 to 6:** 1 mg P.O. q 4 to 6 hours, not to exceed 4 mg daily.
**Children under age 2:** 0.35 mg/kg/day in divided doses q 4 to 6 hours.

## ADVERSE REACTIONS

**CNS:** *stimulation,* sedation, *drowsiness,* excitability (in children).
**CV:** hypotension, palpitations, weak pulse.
**GI:** epigastric distress, *dry mouth.*
**GU:** urine retention.
**Respiratory:** thick bronchial secretions.
**Skin:** rash, urticaria.
**Other:** local stinging, burning sensation (after parenteral administration), pallor.

## INTERACTIONS

**Drug-drug.** *CNS depressants:* increased sedation. Use together cautiously.
*MAO inhibitors:* increased anticholinergic effects. Don't use together.
**Drug-lifestyle.** *Alcohol use:* increased CNS depression. Use cautiously.

## EFFECTS ON DIAGNOSTIC TESTS

Discontinue drug 4 days before performing diagnostic skin tests. Antihistamines can prevent, reduce, or mask positive skin test response.

## CONTRAINDICATIONS

Contraindicated in patients having acute asthmatic attacks and in those with angle-closure glaucoma, symptomatic prostatic hyperplasia, pyloroduodenal obstruction, or bladder neck obstruction; also contraindicated in those taking MAO inhibitors. Antihistamines aren't recommended for breast-feeding women because small amounts of drug appear in breast milk.

## NURSING CONSIDERATIONS

• Use cautiously in elderly patients and in those with increased intraocular pressure, hyperthyroidism, CV or renal disease, hypertension, bronchial asthma, urine retention, prostatic hyperplasia, and stenosing peptic ulcerations.
• Injectable form contains benzyl alcohol. Avoid use in infants.
• If symptoms occur during or after parenteral dose, discontinue drug and notify doctor.

### I.V. administration

• Drug is available in 10-mg/ml ampules for I.V. use. It's compatible with most I.V. solutions. Check with pharmacist before mixing with I.V. solutions to verify specific compatibilities. Give injection over 1 minute.
• *Alert:* Don't give the 100 mg/ml strength I.V.

### Patient teaching

• Warn patient to avoid alcohol and driving or other activities that require alertness until drug's CNS effects are known.
• Tell patient that coffee or tea may reduce drowsiness.
• Inform patient that sugarless gum, sugarless sour hard candy, or ice chips may relieve dry mouth.
• Instruct patient to notify doctor if tolerance develops because a different antihistamine may need to be prescribed.
• Tell parent that drug, including extended-release products, shouldn't be used in children under age 12 unless directed by doctor.

---

Reactions may be *common,* uncommon, *life-threatening,* or COMMON AND LIFE-THREATENING.

## clemastine fumarate
Tavist, Tavist-1 ◇, Antihist-1

*Pregnancy Risk Category B*

### HOW SUPPLIED
*Tablets:* 1.34 mg ◇, 2.68 mg
*Syrup\*:* 0.67 mg/5 ml

### ACTION
Competes with histamine for $H_1$-receptor sites on effector cells. It prevents, but doesn't reverse, histamine-mediated responses.

| Route | Onset | Peak | Duration |
|-------|-------|------|----------|
| P.O. | 15-60 min | 5-7 hr | 12 hr |

### INDICATIONS & DOSAGE
*Rhinitis, allergy symptoms—*
**Adults and children age 12 and over:** 1.34 mg P.O. q 12 hours, or 2.68 mg P.O. once to three times daily, p.r.n. Don't exceed daily dose of 8.04 mg.
**Children ages 6 to 12:** 0.67 to 1.34 mg P.O. b.i.d. Don't exceed daily dose of 4.02 mg.

### ADVERSE REACTIONS
**CNS:** *sedation, drowsiness, seizures,* nervousness, tremor, confusion, restlessness, vertigo, headache, *sleepiness, dizziness, incoordination,* fatigue.
**CV:** hypotension, palpitations, tachycardia.
**GI:** *epigastric distress,* anorexia, diarrhea, nausea, vomiting, constipation, *dry mouth.*
**GU:** urine retention, urinary frequency.
**Hematologic:** hemolytic anemia, ***thrombocytopenia, agranulocytosis.***
**Respiratory:** *thick bronchial secretions.*
**Skin:** rash, urticaria, photosensitivity, diaphoresis.
**Other:** *anaphylactic shock.*

### INTERACTIONS
**Drug-drug.** *CNS depressants:* increased sedation. Use together cautiously.
*MAO inhibitors:* increased anticholinergic effects. Don't use together.
**Drug-lifestyle.** *Alcohol use:* increased CNS depression. Use cautiously.

*Sun exposure:* photosensitivity reactions may occur. Avoid prolonged or unprotected sun exposure.

### EFFECTS ON DIAGNOSTIC TESTS
Discontinue drug 4 days before performing diagnostic skin tests. Antihistamines can prevent, reduce, or mask positive skin test response.

### CONTRAINDICATIONS
Contraindicated in patients with hypersensitivity to drug or other antihistamines of similar chemical structure and in those with acute asthma, angle-closure glaucoma, stenosing peptic ulcer, symptomatic prostatic hyperplasia, bladder neck obstruction, or pyloroduodenal obstruction. Also contraindicated in neonates, premature infants, or breast-feeding women. Avoid use in those taking MAO inhibitors.

### NURSING CONSIDERATIONS
• Use cautiously in elderly patients and in those with increased intraocular pressure, hyperthyroidism, CV disease, hypertension, bronchial asthma, and prostatic hyperplasia.
• Children under age 12 should use only as directed by a doctor.
• Monitor blood counts during long-term therapy, as ordered; observe for signs of blood dyscrasias.

☑ **Patient teaching**
• Warn patient to avoid alcohol and driving or other activities that require alertness until drug's CNS effects are known.
• Tell patient that coffee or tea may reduce drowsiness and to use cautiously if palpitations develop.
• Inform patient that sugarless gum, sugarless sour hard candy, or ice chips may relieve dry mouth.
• Warn patient of possible photosensitivity reactions. Advise use of a sunblock.
• Tell patient to notify doctor if tolerance develops because a different antihistamine may need to be prescribed.

---

\*Liquid contains alcohol.     \*\*May contain tartrazine.     †Canada     ‡Australia     §U.K.     ◇OTC

## cyproheptadine hydrochloride
Periactin

*Pregnancy Risk Category B*

### HOW SUPPLIED
*Tablets:* 4 mg
*Syrup:* 2 mg/5 ml

### ACTION
Competes with histamine for $H_1$-receptor sites on effector cells. It prevents, but doesn't reverse, histamine-mediated responses; also has antiserotonergic activity.

| Route | Onset | Peak | Duration |
|-------|-------|------|----------|
| P.O. | 15-60 min | 6-9 hr | Unknown |

### INDICATIONS & DOSAGE
*Allergy symptoms, pruritus—*
**Adults:** 4 to 20 mg P.O. daily in divided doses. Maximum dose is 0.5 mg/kg daily.
**Children ages 7 to 14:** 4 mg P.O. b.i.d. or t.i.d. Maximum dose is 16 mg/day.
**Children ages 2 to 6:** 2 mg P.O. b.i.d. or t.i.d. Maximum dose is 12 mg daily.
**Children under age 2:** 0.25 mg/kg/day in two or three divided doses.

### ADVERSE REACTIONS
**CNS:** *drowsiness,* dizziness, headache, fatigue, sedation, sleepiness, incoordination, confusion, restlessness, insomnia, nervousness, tremor, *seizures.*
**CV:** hypotension, palpitations, tachycardia.
**GI:** nausea, vomiting, epigastric distress, *dry mouth,* diarrhea, constipation.
**GU:** urine retention, urinary frequency.
**Hematologic:** hemolytic anemia, *leukopenia, agranulocytosis, thrombocytopenia.*
**Metabolic:** weight gain.
**Skin:** rash, urticaria, photosensitivity.
**Other:** *anaphylactic shock.*

### INTERACTIONS
**Drug-drug.** *CNS depressants:* increased sedation. Use together cautiously.
*MAO inhibitors:* increased anticholinergic effects. Don't use together.
**Drug-lifestyle.** *Alcohol use:* increased CNS depression. Use cautiously.

*Sun exposure:* photosensitivity reactions may occur. Avoid prolonged or unprotected sun exposure.

### EFFECTS ON DIAGNOSTIC TESTS
Discontinue drug 4 days before performing diagnostic skin tests. Antihistamines can prevent, reduce, or mask positive skin test response.

### CONTRAINDICATIONS
Contraindicated in patients with hypersensitivity to drug or other drugs of similar chemical structure and in those with acute asthma, angle-closure glaucoma, stenosing peptic ulcer, symptomatic prostatic hyperplasia, bladder-neck obstruction, or pyloroduodenal obstruction. Also contraindicated in those taking MAO inhibitors and in neonates or premature infants, in elderly or debilitated patients, and breast-feeding women.

### NURSING CONSIDERATIONS
• Use cautiously in patients with increased intraocular pressure, hyperthyroidism, CV disease, hypertension, or bronchial asthma.
• Children under age 14 should use only as directed by a doctor.
• *Alert:* Don't confuse cyproheptadine with cyclobenzaprine.

### ☑Patient teaching
• Tell patient that GI distress can be reduced by taking drug with food or milk.
• Warn patient to avoid alcohol and driving or other activities that require alertness until drug's CNS effects are known.
• Tell patient that coffee or tea may reduce drowsiness and to use cautiously if palpitations develop.
• Inform patient that sugarless gum, sugarless sour hard candy, or ice chips may relieve dry mouth.
• Warn patient of possible photosensitivity reactions. Advise use of a sunblock.
• Instruct patient to notify doctor if tolerance develops because a different antihistamine may need to be prescribed.

---

Reactions may be *common,* uncommon, *life-threatening,* or COMMON AND LIFE-THREATENING.

## diphenhydramine hydrochloride

Allerdryl†◇, AllerMax Allergy and Cough Formula, AllerMax Caplets◇, Allermed◇, Banophen◇, Banophen Caplets◇, Beldin◇, Belix◇, Ben-Allergin-50, Bena-D 10, Bena-D 50, Benadryl◇, Benadryl Allergy, Benadryl 25◇, Benadryl Kapseals◇, Benahist 10, Benahist 50, Benoject-10, Benoject-50, Benylin Cough◇, Bydramine Cough◇, Compoz◇, Diphenacen-50, Diphen Cough◇, Diphenadryl◇, Diphenhist◇, Diphenhist Captabs◇, Dormarex 2◇, Genahist◇, Gen-D-phen◇, Hydramine◇, Hydramine Cough◇, Hydramyn◇, Hyrexin-50, Nervine Nighttime Sleep-Aid◇, Nidryl◇, Nordryl◇, Nordryl Cough◇, Nytol Maximum Strength◇, Sleep-eze 3◇, Sominex◇, Tusstat◇, Twilite Caplets◇, Uni-Bent Cough◇, Wehdryl

*Pregnancy Risk Category B*

## HOW SUPPLIED

*Tablets:* 25 mg◇, 50 mg◇
*Capsules:* 25 mg◇, 50 mg◇
*Elixir*:* 12.5 mg/5 ml (14% alcohol)◇
*Liquid:* 6.25 mg/5 ml
*Syrup*:* 12.5 mg/5 ml◇
*Injection:* 10 mg/ml, 50 mg/ml

## ACTION

Competes with histamine for $H_1$-receptor sites on effector cells. Prevents, but doesn't reverse, histamine-mediated responses, particularly histamine's effects on the smooth muscle of the bronchial tubes, GI tract, uterus, and blood vessels. Structurally related to local anesthetics, diphenhydramine provides local anesthesia by preventing initiation and transmission of nerve impulses. Also suppresses cough reflex by a direct effect in the medulla of the brain.

| Route | Onset | Peak | Duration |
|-------|-------|------|----------|
| P.O. | 15 min | 1-4 hr | 6-8 hr |
| I.V. | Immediate | 1-4 hr | 6-8 hr |
| I.M. | Unknown | 1-4 hr | 6-8 hr |

## INDICATIONS & DOSAGE

*Rhinitis, allergy symptoms, motion sickness, Parkinson's disease—*
**Adults and children ages 12 and over:** 25 to 50 mg P.O. t.i.d. or q.i.d.; or 10 to 50 mg deep I.M. or I.V. Maximum I.M. or I.V. dose is 400 mg daily.
**Children under age 12:** 5 mg/kg/day P.O., deep I.M., or I.V. in divided doses q.i.d. Maximum dose is 300 mg daily.
*Sedation—*
**Adults:** 25 to 50 mg P.O., or deep I.M., p.r.n.
*Nighttime sleep aid—*
**Adults:** 25 to 50 mg P.O. h.s.
*Nonproductive cough—*
**Adults:** 25 mg P.O. q 4 to 6 hours (not to exceed 150 mg daily).
**Children ages 6 to 12:** 12.5 mg P.O. q 4 to 6 hours (not to exceed 75 mg daily).
**Children ages 2 to 6:** 6.25 mg P.O. q 4 to 6 hours (not to exceed 25 mg daily).

## ADVERSE REACTIONS

**CNS:** *drowsiness,* confusion, insomnia, headache, vertigo, *sedation, sleepiness, dizziness, incoordination,* fatigue, restlessness, tremor, nervousness, *seizures.*
**CV:** palpitations, hypotension, tachycardia.
**EENT:** diplopia, blurred vision, nasal congestion, tinnitus.
**GI:** *nausea,* vomiting, diarrhea, *dry mouth,* constipation, *epigastric distress,* anorexia.
**GU:** dysuria, urine retention, urinary frequency.
**Hematologic:** hemolytic anemia, ***thrombocytopenia, agranulocytosis.***
**Respiratory:** *thickening of bronchial secretions.*
**Skin:** urticaria, photosensitivity, rash.
**Other:** *anaphylactic shock.*

## INTERACTIONS

**Drug-drug.** *CNS depressants:* increased sedation. Use together cautiously.

---

*Liquid contains alcohol.    **May contain tartrazine.    †Canada    ‡Australia    §U.K.    ◇OTC

*MAO inhibitors:* increased anticholinergic effects. Don't use together.
**Drug-lifestyle.** *Alcohol use:* increased CNS depression. Use cautiously.
*Sun exposure:* photosensitivity reactions may occur. Avoid prolonged or unprotected sun exposure.

### EFFECTS ON DIAGNOSTIC TESTS
Discontinue drug 4 days before performing diagnostic skin tests. Antihistamines can prevent, reduce, or mask positive skin test response.

### CONTRAINDICATIONS
Contraindicated in patients with hypersensitivity to drug and in those with angle-closure glaucoma, stenosing peptic ulcer, symptomatic prostatic hyperplasia, bladder neck obstruction, or pyloroduodenal obstruction; also contraindicated during acute asthmatic attacks and in newborns, premature neonates, or breastfeeding women. Avoid use in patients taking MAO inhibitors.

### NURSING CONSIDERATIONS
• Use with extreme caution in patients with prostatic hyperplasia, asthma or COPD, increased intraocular pressure, hyperthyroidism, CV disease and hypertension.
• Children under age 12 should use only as directed by a doctor.
• Alternate injection sites to prevent irritation. Administer I.M. injection deeply into large muscle.
• *Alert:* Don't confuse diphenhydramine with dimenhydrinate, or Benadryl with Bentyl, Benylin, or benazepril.

### I.V. administration
• Make sure the I.V. site is patent. Drug given perivascularly causes tissue irritation.

### Patient teaching
• Instruct patient to take drug 30 minutes before travel to prevent motion sickness.
• Tell patient to take diphenhydramine with food or milk to reduce GI distress.
• Warn patient to avoid alcohol and driving or other hazardous activities that require alertness until drug's CNS effects are known.

• Tell patient that coffee or tea may reduce drowsiness and to use cautiously if palpitations develop.
• Inform patient that sugarless gum, sugarless sour hard candy, or ice chips may relieve dry mouth.
• Tell patient to notify doctor if tolerance develops because a different antihistamine may need to be prescribed.
• Diphenhydramine is contained in many OTC sleep and cold products. Advise patient to consult doctor before using these products.
• Warn patient of possible photosensitivity reactions. Advise use of a sunblock.

---

## fexofenadine hydrochloride
Allegra, Telfast‡

*Pregnancy Risk Category C*

---

### HOW SUPPLIED
*Capsules:* 60 mg

### ACTION
Nonsedating antihistamine in which the principal effects are mediated through a selective inhibition of peripheral $H_1$ receptors.

| Route | Onset | Peak | Duration |
|-------|-------|------|----------|
| P.O. | Unknown | 3 hr | 14 hr |

### INDICATIONS & DOSAGE
*Seasonal allergic rhinitis—*
**Adults and children ages 12 and over**: 60 mg P.O. b.i.d.
*Adjust-a-dose:* For patients with impaired renal function or on dialysis, 60 mg daily.

### ADVERSE REACTIONS
**CNS:** fatigue, drowsiness.
**GI:** nausea, dyspepsia.
**GU:** dysmenorrhea.
**Other:** viral infection.

### INTERACTIONS
**Drug-lifestyle.** *Alcohol use:* increased CNS depression. Use cautiously.

### EFFECTS ON DIAGNOSTIC TESTS
Drug can prevent, reduce, or mask positive skin test response.

---

Reactions may be *common*, uncommon, *life-threatening*, or COMMON AND LIFE-THREATENING.

## CONTRAINDICATIONS
Contraindicated in patients with hypersensitivity to drug or its components.

## NURSING CONSIDERATIONS
• Use cautiously in patients with impaired renal function.
• Discontinue drug 4 days before performing diagnostic skin tests.
• Safety and effectiveness in children under age 12 haven't been established.
• It isn't known whether drug is excreted in breast milk; caution is recommended when administering drug to breast-feeding women. Advise women taking drug to avoid breast-feeding.

### ☑ Patient teaching
• Caution patient not to perform hazardous activities if drowsiness occurs as a result of drug use.
• Instruct patient not to exceed prescribed dosage and to take drug only when needed.
• Warn patient to avoid alcohol and driving or other activities that require alertness until drug's CNS effects are known.
• Tell patient that coffee or tea may reduce drowsiness.
• Inform patient that sugarless gum, sugarless sour hard candy, or ice chips may relieve dry mouth.

---

## loratadine
Claratyne‡, Clarinase‡, Claritin, Claritin Reditabs, Claritin Syrup

*Pregnancy Risk Category B*

### HOW SUPPLIED
*Tablets:* 10 mg
*Tablets (rapidly disintegrating):* 10 mg
*Syrup:* 1 mg/ml

### ACTION
Blocks effects of histamine at $H_1$-receptor sites. Loratadine is a nonsedating antihistamine; its chemical structure prevents entry into the CNS.

| Route | Onset | Peak | Duration |
|-------|-------|------|----------|
| P.O. | 1-3 hr | 8-10 hr | 24 hr |

## INDICATIONS & DOSAGE
*Symptomatic treatment of seasonal allergic rhinitis, chronic urticaria—*
**Adults and children ages 6 and over:**
10 mg P.O. daily.
*Adjust-a-dose:* For renally impaired patients with glomerular filtration rate below 30 ml/minute and for those with hepatic failure, initial dose is 10 mg every other day.

## ADVERSE REACTIONS
**CNS:** headache, somnolence, fatigue.
**GI:** dry mouth.
**Skin:** photosensitivity reactions.

## INTERACTIONS
**Drug-drug.** *Cimetidine, macrolide antibiotics (clarithromycin, erythromycin, troleandomycin):* increased loratadine plasma levels. Monitor patient closely.
**Drug-herb.** *Licorice:* may prolong the QT interval and be potentially additive. Use together cautiously.
**Drug-lifestyle.** *Alcohol use:* increased CNS depression. Use cautiously.
*Sun exposure:* photosensitivity reactions may occur. Avoid prolonged or unprotected sun exposure.

## EFFECTS ON DIAGNOSTIC TESTS
Drug can prevent, reduce, or mask positive skin test response.

## CONTRAINDICATIONS
Contraindicated in patients with hypersensitivity to drug.

## NURSING CONSIDERATIONS
• Use cautiously in patients with liver impairment and in breast-feeding patients.
• Discontinue drug 4 days before performing diagnostic skin tests;

### ☑ Patient teaching
• Make sure that patient understands that drug should only be taken once daily. If symptoms persist or worsen, tell him to contact the doctor.
• Advise patients taking Claritin Reditabs to place tablet on the tongue, where it disintegrates within a few seconds. It can be swallowed with or without water.

---

*Liquid contains alcohol.   **May contain tartrazine.   †Canada   ‡Australia   §U.K.   ◇OTC

- Warn patient to avoid alcohol and driving or other activities that require alertness until drug's CNS effects are known.
- Warn patient of possible photosensitivity reactions. Advise use of a sunblock.
- Tell patient that dry mouth can be relieved with sugarless gum, sugarless sour hard candy, or ice chips.

---

## promethazine hydrochloride
Anergan 25, Anergan 50, Histantil†, Pentazine, Phencen-50, Phenergan*, Phenergan Fortis*, Phenergan Plain*, Phenoject-50, PMS-Promethazine†, Pro-50, Promethegan, Prorex-25, Prorex-50, Prothazine*, Prothazine Plain, V-Gan-25, V-Gan-50

## promethazine theoclate
Avomine‡

*Pregnancy Risk Category C*

## HOW SUPPLIED
**promethazine hydrochloride**
*Tablets:* 12.5 mg, 25 mg, 50 mg
*Syrup:* 5 mg/5 ml‡*, 6.25 mg/5 ml*, 10 mg/5 ml†*, 25 mg/5 ml*
*Injection:* 25 mg/ml, 50 mg/ml
*Suppositories:* 12.5 mg, 25 mg, 50 mg
**promethazine theoclate**
*Tablets:* 25 mg‡

## ACTION
Phenothiazine derivative that competes with histamine for $H_1$-receptor sites on effector cells. Prevents, but doesn't reverse, histamine-mediated responses. At high doses, also exhibits local anesthetic effects.

| Route | Onset | Peak | Duration |
|---|---|---|---|
| P.O. | 15-60 min | Unknown | < 12 hr |
| I.V. | 3-5 min | Unknown | < 12 hr |
| I.M., P.R. | 20 min | Unknown | < 12 hr |

## INDICATIONS & DOSAGE
*Motion sickness—*
**Adults:** 25 mg P.O. b.i.d.
**Children:** 12.5 to 25 mg P.O. or P.R. b.i.d. Or 0.5 mg/kg 30 minutes to 1 hour before departure.

*Nausea—*
**Adults:** 12.5 to 25 mg P.O., I.M., or P.R. q 4 to 6 hours, p.r.n.
**Children:** 12.5 to 25 mg P.O. or P.R. q 4 to 6 hours, p.r.n. Or 0.25 to 1 mg/kg q 4 to 6 hours, p.r.n. Or 6.25 to 12.5 mg I.M. q 4 to 6 hours, p.r.n.
*Rhinitis, allergy symptoms—*
**Adults:** 12.5 mg P.O. q.i.d.; or 25 mg P.O. h.s.
**Children:** 6.25 to 12.5 mg P.O. t.i.d. or 25 mg P.O. or P.R. h.s. Or, 0.1 mg/kg q 6 hours during the day and 0.5 mg/kg h.s.
*Sedation—*
**Adults:** 25 to 50 mg P.O. or I.M. h.s. or p.r.n.
**Children:** 12.5 to 25 mg P.O., I.M., or P.R. h.s. Or 0.5 to 1 mg/kg q 6 hours, p.r.n.
*Routine preoperative or postoperative sedation, adjunct to analgesics—*
**Adults:** 25 to 50 mg I.M., I.V., or P.O.
**Children:** 12.5 to 25 mg I.M., I.V., or P.O.

## ADVERSE REACTIONS
**CNS:** *sedation,* confusion, sleepiness, dizziness, disorientation, extrapyramidal symptoms, *drowsiness.*
**CV:** hypotension, hypertension.
**EENT:** blurred vision.
**GI:** nausea, vomiting, *dry mouth.*
**GU:** urine retention.
**Hematologic:** *leukopenia, agranulocytosis, thrombocytopenia.*
**Metabolic:** hyperglycemia.
**Skin:** photosensitivity, rash.

## INTERACTIONS
**Drug-drug.** *Anticholinergics, phenothiazines, tricyclic antidepressants:* increased effects. Don't give together.
*CNS depressants:* increased sedation. Use together cautiously.
*Epinephrine:* may block or reverse the effects of epinephrine. Use other pressor drugs instead.
*Levodopa:* may decrease levodopa's antiparkinsonian action. Avoid concomitant use.
*Lithium:* may reduce GI absorption or enhance renal elimination of lithium. Avoid concomitant use.

---

Reactions may be *common,* uncommon, *life-threatening,* or COMMON AND LIFE-THREATENING.

*MAO inhibitors:* increased extrapyramidal effects. Don't use together.

**Drug-lifestyle.** *Alcohol use:* increased sedation. Use together cautiously.

*Sun exposure:* photosensitivity reactions may occur. Avoid prolonged and unprotected sun exposure.

## EFFECTS ON DIAGNOSTIC TESTS
Discontinue drug 4 days before performing diagnostic skin tests. Antihistamines can prevent, reduce, or mask positive skin test response. Drug may cause either false-positive or false-negative pregnancy test results. It may also interfere with blood grouping in the ABO system.

## CONTRAINDICATIONS
Contraindicated in patients with hypersensitivity to drug and in those with intestinal obstruction, prostatic hyperplasia, bladder-neck obstruction, angle-closure glaucoma, seizure disorders, coma, CNS depression, stenosing or peptic ulcerations; also contraindicated in newborns, premature neonates, breast-feeding women; and acutely ill or dehydrated children.

## NURSING CONSIDERATIONS
• Use cautiously in patients with pulmonary, hepatic, CV disease, or asthma.
• Pronounced sedative effect limits use in many ambulatory patients.
• Promethazine is used as an adjunct to analgesics (usually to increase sedation); it has no analgesic activity.
• Reduce GI distress by giving drug with food or milk.
• Inject deep I.M. into large muscle mass. Rotate injection sites.
• *Alert:* Don't administer S.C.
• Drug may be mixed with meperidine in same syringe.
• In patients scheduled for a myelogram, discontinue drug 48 hours before procedure and don't resume drug until 24 hours after procedure, as ordered, because of the risk of seizures.
• *Alert:* Don't confuse promethazine with promazine.

## I.V. administration
• Don't give in a concentration greater than 25 mg/ml or at a rate exceeding 25 mg/minute. Shield I.V. infusion from direct light.

## ☑ Patient teaching
• Tell patient to take oral form with food or milk.
• When treating motion sickness, tell patient to take first dose 30 to 60 minutes before travel. On succeeding days of travel, patient should take dose upon rising and with evening meal.
• Warn patient to avoid alcohol and driving or other activities that require alertness until drug's CNS effects are known.
• Tell patient that coffee or tea may reduce drowsiness.
• Inform patient that sugarless gum, sugarless sour hard candy, or ice chips may relieve dry mouth.
• Warn patient about possible photosensitivity reactions. Advise use of a sunblock.

---

## triprolidine hydrochloride
Actidil ◇, Myidyl

*Pregnancy Risk Category C*

## HOW SUPPLIED
*Tablets:* 2.5 mg ◇
*Syrup\*:* 1.25 mg/5 ml ◇

## ACTION
Competes with histamine for $H_1$-receptor sites on effector cells and prevents, but doesn't reverse, histamine-mediated responses.

| Route | Onset | Peak | Duration |
| --- | --- | --- | --- |
| P.O. | 15-60 min | 2-3 hr | 4-8 hr |

## INDICATIONS & DOSAGE
*Colds and seasonal allergy symptoms, chronic urticaria—*
**Adults and children ages 12 and over:** 2.5 mg P.O. q 4 to 6 hours. Maximum daily dose is 10 mg.
**Children ages 6 to 12:** 1.25 mg P.O. q 4 to 6 hours. Maximum daily dose is 5 mg.
**Children ages 4 to 6:** 0.938 mg P.O. q 4 to 6 hours. Maximum daily dose is 3.744 mg.

---

\*Liquid contains alcohol.   \*\*May contain tartrazine.   †Canada   ‡Australia   §U.K.   ◇OTC

**Children ages 2 to 4:** 0.625 mg P.O. q 4 to 6 hours. Maximum daily dose is 2.5 mg.
**Children ages 4 months to 2 years:** 0.313 mg P.O. q 4 to 6 hours. Maximum daily dose is 1.252 mg.

## ADVERSE REACTIONS
**CNS:** *drowsiness, dizziness,* confusion, restlessness, insomnia, headache, *sedation, sleepiness, incoordination,* fatigue, anxiety, nervousness, tremor, **seizures, stimulation.**
**CV:** hypotension, palpitations, tachycardia.
**EENT:** *dry nose and throat.*
**GI:** anorexia, diarrhea, constipation, nausea, vomiting, *dry mouth,* epigastric distress.
**GU:** urinary frequency, urine retention.
**Hematologic:** hemolytic anemia, ***thrombocytopenia, agranulocytosis.***
**Respiratory:** thickening of bronchial secretions.
**Skin:** urticaria, rash, photosensitivity, diaphoresis.
**Other:** **anaphylactic shock,** chills.

## INTERACTIONS
**Drug-drug.** *CNS depressants:* increased sedation. Use together cautiously.
*MAO inhibitors:* increased anticholinergic effects. Don't use together.
**Drug-lifestyle.** *Alcohol use:* increased CNS depression. Use cautiously.
*Sun exposure:* photosensitivity reactions may occur. Avoid prolonged or unprotected sun exposure.

## EFFECTS ON DIAGNOSTIC TESTS
Discontinue drug 4 days before performing diagnostic skin tests. Antihistamines can prevent, reduce, or mask positive skin test response.

## CONTRAINDICATIONS
Contraindicated in patients with hypersensitivity to drug and in those with acute asthma, angle-closure glaucoma, stenosing peptic ulcer, symptomatic prostatic hyperplasia, bladder neck obstruction, or pyloroduodenal obstruction; also contraindicated in neonates, premature infants, and breast-feeding women. Avoid use in patients taking MAO inhibitors.

## NURSING CONSIDERATIONS
• Use with extreme caution in patients with increased intraocular pressure, hyperthyroidism, CV disease, hypertension, bronchial asthma, and prostatic hyperplasia.
• Children under age 12 should use only as directed by a doctor.

☑ **Patient teaching**
• Tell patient to take drug with food or milk to reduce GI distress.
• Warn patient to avoid alcohol and driving or other activities that require alertness until drug's CNS effects are known.
• Tell patient that coffee or tea may reduce drowsiness.
• Inform patient that sugarless gum, sugarless sour hard candy, or ice chips may relieve dry mouth.
• Warn patient of possible photosensitivity reactions. Advise use of a sunblock.

---

Reactions may be *common,* uncommon, *life-threatening,* or COMMON AND LIFE-THREATENING.

**albuterol**
**albuterol sulfate**
**aminophylline**
**atropine sulfate**
   (See Chapter 21, ANTIARRHYTHMICS.)
**ephedrine sulfate**
**epinephrine**
**epinephrine bitartrate**
**epinephrine hydrochloride**
**ipratropium bromide**
**isoproterenol**
**isoproterenol hydrochloride**
**isoproterenol sulfate**
**levalbuterol hydrochloride**
**metaproterenol sulfate**
**oxtriphylline**
**pirbuterol acetate**
**salmeterol xinafoate**
**terbutaline sulfate**
**theophylline**

## COMBINATION PRODUCTS
**Inhalants**
COMBIVENT: ipratropium bromide 18 mcg and albuterol sulfate 103 mcg per dose.
DUO-MEDIHALER: isoproterenol hydrochloride 0.16 mg and phenylephrine bitartrate 0.24 mg per dose.
**Oral bronchodilators**
ASBRON G INLAY-TABS: theophylline 150 mg and guaifenesin 100 mg.
BRONCHIAL CAPSULES: theophylline 150 mg and guaifenesin 90 mg.
DILOR-G TABLETS: dyphylline 200 mg and guaifenesin 200 mg.
DYFLEX-G TABLETS: dyphylline 200 mg and guaifenesin 200 mg.
DYLINE-GG TABLETS: dyphylline 200 mg and guaifenesin 200 mg.
GLYCERYL-T CAPSULES: theophylline 150 mg and guaifenesin 90 mg.
MARAX*: theophylline 130 mg, ephedrine sulfate 25 mg, and hydroxyzine hydrochloride 10 mg.
MUDRANE GG-2 TABLETS: theophylline 111 mg and guaifenesin 100 mg.
NEOTHYLLINE-GG: dyphylline 200 mg and guaifenesin 200 mg.

QUIBRON CAPSULES: theophylline 150 mg and guaifenesin 90 mg.
QUIBRON-300 CAPSULES: theophylline 300 mg and guaifenesin 180 mg.
SLO-PHYLLIN GG SYRUP: theophylline 150 mg and guaifenesin 90 mg.
SYNOPHYLATE-GG SYRUP*: guaifenesin 33.3 mg/5 ml and theophylline sodium glycinate 100 mg/5 ml.
**Decongestants**
ACTIFED ◊: pseudoephedrine hydrochloride 60 mg and triprolidine hydrochloride 2.5 mg.
DRISTAN COLD MULTI-SYMPTOM FORMULA ◊: phenylephrine hydrochloride 5 mg, chlorpheniramine maleate 2 mg, and acetaminophen 325 mg.
ELIXOPHYLLIN-KI ELIXIR: theophylline 80 mg, potassium iodide 130 mg.
MARAX-DF SYRUP: theophylline 97.5 mg, ephedrine sulfate 18.75 mg, hydroxyzine hydrochloride 7.5 mg.
NALDECON SYRUP: 10 ml contains phenylpropanolamine hydrochloride 40 mg, phenylephrine hydrochloride 10 mg, chlorpheniramine maleate 5 mg, and phenyltoloxamine citrate 15 mg.
SEMPREX-D CAPSULES: acrivastine 8 mg and pseudoephedrine hydrochloride 60 mg.

---

**albuterol (salbutamol)**
Asmol‡, Proventil, Ventolin

**albuterol sulfate (salbutamol sulfate)**
Aerolin Autoinhaler Airomir§, Proventil, Proventil Repetabs, Respolin Autohaler‡, Respolin Inhaler‡, Respolin Respirator Solution‡, Steri-Neb Salamol§, Ventolin, Ventolin Obstetric Injection‡, Ventolin Rotacaps, Volmax

*Pregnancy Risk Category C*

---

## HOW SUPPLIED
**albuterol**
*Aerosol inhaler:* 90 mcg/metered spray, 100 mcg/metered spray‡
**albuterol sulfate**
*Capsules for inhalation:* 200 mcg
*Tablets:* 2 mg, 4 mg
*Tablets (extended-release):* 4 mg, 8 mg
*Syrup:* 2 mg/5 ml
*Solution for inhalation:* 0.083%, 0.5%
*Injection:* 1 mg/ml‡

## ACTION
Relaxes bronchial, uterine, and vascular smooth muscle by stimulating beta$_2$ receptors.

| Route | Onset | Peak | Duration |
|---|---|---|---|
| P.O. | 15-30 min | 2-3 hr | 6-12 hr |
| P.O. (extended) | Unknown | Unknown | 12 hr |
| I.V. | Variable | Unknown | 4-6 hr |
| Inhalation | 5-15 min | 0.5-2 hr | 2-6 hr |

## INDICATIONS & DOSAGE
*To prevent or treat bronchospasm in patients with reversible obstructive airway disease—*
**Adults and children ages 4 and older:** dosage and frequency vary with dosage form.
*Aerosol inhalation*—1 or 2 inhalations q 4 to 6 hours. More frequent administration or more inhalations isn't recommended.
*Capsules for inhalation*—200 mcg inhaled q 4 to 6 hours using a Rotahaler inhalation device. Some patients may need 400 mcg q 4 to 6 hours.
**Adults and children ages 12 and older:**
*Solution for inhalation*—2.5 mg t.i.d. or q.i.d. by nebulizer. To prepare solution, use 0.5 ml of the 0.5% solution diluted with 2.5 ml of normal saline. Or, use 3 ml of the 0.083% solution.
**Children ages 2 to 12:** *Solution for inhalation*—initially, 0.1 to 0.15 mg/kg by nebulizer, with subsequent dosing titrated to response. Don't exceed 2.5 mg t.i.d. or q.i.d. by nebulization.
**Adults and children ages 14 and older:**
*Syrup*—2 to 4 mg (1 to 2 tsp) P.O. t.i.d. or q.i.d. Maximum dose is 8 mg q.i.d.

**Children ages 6 to 14:** *Syrup*—2 mg (1 tsp) P.O. t.i.d. or q.i.d. Maximum dose is 24 mg daily given in divided doses.
**Children ages 2 to 6:** *Syrup*—initially, 0.1 mg/kg P.O. t.i.d. Starting dose shouldn't exceed 2 mg (1 tsp) t.i.d. Maximum dose is 4 mg (2 tsp) t.i.d.
**Adults and children ages 12 and older:**
*Oral tablets*—2 to 4 mg P.O. t.i.d. or q.i.d. Maximum dose is 8 mg q.i.d. *Extended-release tablets*—4 to 8 mg P.O. q 12 hours. Maximum dose is 16 mg b.i.d.
**Children ages 6 to 11:** *Oral tablets*—2 mg P.O. t.i.d. or q.i.d. Maximum dose is 6 mg q.i.d. *Extended-release tablets*—4 mg P.O. q 12 hours. Maximum dose is 12 mg b.i.d.
**Elderly:** 2 mg P.O. t.i.d. or q.i.d. as oral tablets or syrup. Maximum dose is 8 mg t.i.d. or q.i.d.
*Adjust-a-dose:* For those sensitive to beta stimulators: 2 mg P.O. t.i.d. or q.i.d. as oral tablets or syrup. Maximum dose is 8 mg t.i.d. or q.i.d.
*Prevention of exercise-induced bronchospasm—*
**Adults and children ages 4 and older:** 2 aerosol inhalations 15 to 30 minutes before exercise; or 200 mcg (capsule for inhalation) inhaled using a Rotahaler inhalation device 15 minutes before exercise.
*Prevention of premature labor‡—*
**Adults:** initially, 10 mcg/minute by continuous I.V. infusion (via an infusion pump). Dosage should be increased at 10-minute intervals until desired response is achieved.

## ADVERSE REACTIONS
**CNS:** *tremor, nervousness,* dizziness, insomnia, *headache, hyperactivity,* weakness, CNS stimulation, malaise.
**CV:** *tachycardia, palpitations,* hypertension.
**EENT:** dry and irritated nose and throat (with inhaled form), nasal congestion, epistaxis, hoarseness.
**GI:** heartburn, *nausea, vomiting,* anorexia, bad taste in mouth, increased appetite.
**Metabolic:** hypokalemia.
**Musculoskeletal:** muscle cramps.

---

Reactions may be *common,* uncommon, *life-threatening,* or COMMON AND LIFE-THREATENING.

**Respiratory:** *bronchospasm,* cough, wheezing, dyspnea, bronchitis, increased sputum.
**Other:** *hypersensitivity reactions.*

## INTERACTIONS
**Drug-drug.** *CNS stimulants:* increased CNS stimulation. Avoid concomitant use.
*Digoxin:* digoxin serum levels may be decreased. Monitor closely.
*MAO inhibitors, tricyclic antidepressants:* increased adverse CV effects. Monitor patient closely.
*Propranolol, other beta blockers:* mutual antagonism. Monitor patient carefully.

## EFFECTS ON DIAGNOSTIC TESTS
Albuterol may decrease sensitivity of spirometry used for diagnosis of asthma.

## CONTRAINDICATIONS
Contraindicated in patients with hypersensitivity to drug or its ingredients.

## NURSING CONSIDERATIONS
• Use cautiously in patients with CV disorders (including coronary insufficiency and hypertension), hyperthyroidism, or diabetes mellitus and in those who are unusually responsive to adrenergics.
• Use extended-release tablets cautiously in patients with preexisting GI narrowing.
• When switching from regular release to extended-release tablets, a regular release 2-mg tablet every 6 hours is equivalent to an extended release 4-mg tablet every 12 hours.
• Pleasant-tasting syrup may be taken by children as young as age 2; it contains no alcohol or sugar.
• Rarely, erythema mutiforme and Stevens-Johnson syndrome have been associated with the use of syrup in children.
• Aerosol form may be used 15 minutes before exercise to prevent exercise-induced bronchospasm.
• **Alert:** Patient may use tablets and aerosol concomitantly. Monitor closely for toxicity.
• If drug is used to prevent premature labor, monitor maternal heart rate closely. Heart rate shouldn't exceed 140 beats/ minute.

• **Alert:** Don't confuse albuterol with atenolol or Albutein.

### I.V. administration
• Where available, I.V. form may be used to prepare infusion using NaCl for injection, dextrose for injection, or NaCl and dextrose for injection. Don't administer drug without dilution. Don't mix with other drugs. Discard unused diluted solution after 24 hours.
• After uterine contractions have ceased, maintain drip rate for 1 hour; then gradually taper at 50% increments in six hourly intervals. Don't continue infusions for more than 48 hours. If therapy must continue for more than 48 hours, doctor may prescribe 4 to 8 mg P.O. q.i.d.

### Patient teaching
• Warn patient about possibility of paradoxical bronchospasm. If this occurs, discontinue drug immediately.
• Teach patient to perform oral inhalation correctly. Give the following instructions for using metered-dose inhaler:
–Shake the inhaler.
–Clear nasal passages and throat.
–Breathe out, expelling as much air from lungs as possible.
–Place mouthpiece well into mouth as dose from inhaler is released, and inhale deeply.
–Hold breath for several seconds, remove mouthpiece, and exhale slowly.
   Or, inhaler may be held about 1 inch (two finger widths) from open mouth; inhale while dose is released.
• If more than 1 inhalation is ordered, advise patient to wait at least 2 minutes before repeating procedure.
• Tell patient that use with an aerochamber may improve drug delivery to the lungs.
• If patient is also using a steroid inhaler, instruct him to use the bronchodilator first and then wait about 5 minutes before using the steroid. This allows the bronchodilator to open the air passages for maximum effectiveness.
• Tell patient to remove canister and wash inhaler with warm, soapy water at least once a week.

---

*Liquid contains alcohol.    **May contain tartrazine.    †Canada    ‡Australia    §U.K.    ◇ OTC

## aminophylline (theophylline ethylenediamine)
Aminophylline, Pecram§, Phyllocontin, Phyllocontin Continus§, Phyllocontin-350, Truphylline

*Pregnancy Risk Category C*

### HOW SUPPLIED
*Tablets:* 100 mg, 200 mg
*Tablets (extended-release):* 225 mg, 350 mg†
*Oral liquid:* 105 mg/5 ml
*Injection:* 250 mg/10 ml, 500 mg/20 ml, 100 mg/100 ml in half-normal saline, 200 mg/100 ml in half-normal saline
*Rectal suppositories:* 250 mg, 500 mg

### ACTION
Inhibits phosphodiesterase, the enzyme that degrades cAMP, resulting in relaxation of smooth muscle of the bronchial airways and pulmonary blood vessels.

| Route | Onset | Peak | Duration |
|---|---|---|---|
| P.O. (solution) | 15-60 min | 1-7 hr | Variable |
| P.O. (extended) | Variable | Variable | Variable |
| I.V. | 15 min | Immediate | Variable |
| P.R. | Unknown | Unknown | Unknown |

### INDICATIONS & DOSAGE
*Symptomatic relief of bronchospasm—*
**Patients not currently receiving theophylline products who need rapid relief of symptoms:** loading dose is 6 mg/kg (equivalent to 4.7 mg/kg anhydrous theophylline) I.V. (25 mg/minute or less); then maintenance infusion.
**Adults (nonsmokers):** 0.7 mg/kg/hour I.V. for 12 hours; then 0.5 mg/kg/hour.
**Children ages 9 to 16:** 1 mg/kg/hour I.V. for 12 hours; then 0.8 mg/kg/hour.
**Children ages 6 months to 9 years:** 1.2 mg/kg/hour for 12 hours; then 1 mg/kg/hour.
**Elderly:** 0.6 mg/kg/hour I.V. for 12 hours; then 0.3 mg/kg/hour.
*Adjust-a-dose:* For otherwise healthy adult smokers, 1 mg/kg/hour I.V. for 12 hours; then 0.8 mg/kg/hour. For adults

with cor pulmonale, 0.6 mg/kg/hour I.V. for 12 hours; then 0.3 mg/kg/hour. For adults with heart failure or liver disease, 0.5 mg/kg/hour I.V. for 12 hours; then 0.1 to 0.2 mg/kg/hour.
**Patients currently receiving theophylline products:** first determine time, amount, route of administration, and dosage form of patient's last theophylline dose. Aminophylline infusions of 0.63 mg/kg (0.5 mg/kg anhydrous theophylline) will increase plasma levels of theophylline by 1 mcg/ml. Some doctors recommend a dose of 3.1 mg/kg (2.5 mg/kg anhydrous theophylline) if no obvious signs of theophylline toxicity are present.
*Chronic bronchial asthma—*
Dosage is highly individualized.
**Adults and children:** usual initial oral dose is 16 mg/kg or 400 mg (whichever is less) P.O. daily in three or four divided doses q 6 to 8 hours if using rapidly absorbed dosage forms. Dosage may be increased, if tolerated, in increments of 25% q 2 to 3 days. Or, if using extended-release preparations, 12 mg/kg or 400 mg (whichever is less) P.O. daily in two to three divided doses q 8 to 12 hours. Dosage may be increased, if tolerated, by 2 to 3 mg/kg daily q 3 days.

Regardless of dosage form, the following are recommended maximum doses. For adults and children ages 16 and older, 13 mg/kg daily or 900 mg/day, whichever is less; children ages 12 to 16, 18 mg/kg daily; children ages 9 to 12, 20 mg/kg daily; and children ages 1 to 9, 24 mg/kg daily.

When recommended maximum dose is reached, dosage adjustment is based on measurement of peak serum theophylline levels. Target theophylline levels are generally between 10 and 20 mcg/ml.

*Note:* P.R. dosage is same as that recommended for P.O. dosage.

### ADVERSE REACTIONS
**CNS:** *nervousness, restlessness,* headache, *insomnia,* **seizures,** muscle twitching, irritability, *dizziness.*
**CV:** *palpitations, sinus tachycardia,* extrasystoles, flushing, marked hypotension, **arrhythmias.**

---

Reactions may be *common*, uncommon, *life-threatening*, or COMMON AND LIFE-THREATENING.

**GI:** *nausea, vomiting,* diarrhea, epigastric pain, hematemesis.

**Metabolic:** hyperglycemia, increased plasma levels of free fatty acids and urinary catecholamines.

**Respiratory:** tachypnea, *respiratory arrest.*

**Skin:** urticaria.

**Other:** irritation (with rectal suppositories), fever, *hypersensitivity reactions.*

## INTERACTIONS

**Drug-drug.** *Adenosine:* decreased antiarrhythmic effectiveness. Higher doses of adenosine may be needed.

*Alkali-sensitive drugs:* reduced activity. Don't add to I.V. fluids containing aminophylline.

*Barbiturates, nicotine, phenytoin, rifampin:* enhanced metabolism and decreased theophylline blood levels. Monitor for decreased aminophylline effect.

*Beta blockers:* antagonism. *Nadolol and propranolol,* especially, may cause bronchospasm in sensitive patients. Use together cautiously.

*Calcium channel blockers, cimetidine, disulfiram, influenza virus vaccine, interferon, macrolide antibiotics (such as erythromycin), methotrexate, oral contraceptives, quinolone antibiotics (such as ciprofloxacin):* decreased hepatic clearance of theophylline; elevated theophylline levels. Monitor for signs of toxicity.

*Carbamazepine, isoniazid, loop diuretics:* may increase or decrease theophylline levels. Monitor closely.

*Ephedrine, other sympathomimetics:* theophylline may exhibit synergistic toxicity with these drugs, predisposing patients to arrhythmias. Monitor patient closely.

*Lithium:* theophylline may increase excretion of lithium. Monitor patient closely.

**Drug-lifestyle.** *Smoking:* increased elimination of theophylline, increasing dosing requirements. Monitor theophylline response and serum levels.

## EFFECTS ON DIAGNOSTIC TESTS

Aminophylline may alter the assay for uric acid, depending on method used. Theophylline levels are falsely elevated in the presence of furosemide, phenylbuta-zone, probenecid, theobromine, caffeine, tea, chocolate, cola beverages, and acetaminophen, depending on type of assay used.

## CONTRAINDICATIONS

Contraindicated in patients with hypersensitivity to xanthine compounds (caffeine, theobromine) and ethylenediamine and in those with active peptic ulcer disease and seizure disorders (unless adequate anticonvulsant therapy is given). Rectal suppositories are also contraindicated in patients who have an irritation or infection of the rectum or lower colon.

## NURSING CONSIDERATIONS

● Use cautiously in neonates and infants under age 1, young children, and elderly patients; also use cautiously in patients with heart failure or other cardiac or circulatory impairment, COPD, cor pulmonale, renal or hepatic disease, hyperthyroidism, diabetes mellitus, glaucoma, peptic ulcer, severe hypoxemia, and hypertension.

● Relieve GI symptoms by giving oral drug with full glass of water at meals, although food in stomach delays absorption. No evidence exists that antacids reduce adverse GI reactions. Enteric-coated tablets also may delay and impair absorption.

● *Alert:* Before giving loading dose, make sure that patient hasn't had recent theophylline therapy.

● Suppositories are slowly and erratically absorbed. Administer rectal suppository if patients can't take drug orally, as ordered. Schedule after evacuation, if possible; may be retained better if given before meal. Have patients remain recumbent 15 to 20 minutes after insertion.

● Monitor vital signs; measure and record fluid intake and output. Expected clinical effects include improved quality of pulse and respirations.

● Aminophylline is a soluble salt of theophylline. Dosage is adjusted by monitoring response, tolerance, pulmonary function, and serum theophylline levels. Theophylline levels should range from 10 to 20 mcg/ml; toxicity has been reported with levels above 20 mcg/ml.

• *Alert:* Signs of toxicity include tachycardia, anorexia, nausea, vomiting, diarrhea, restlessness, irritability and headache. The presence of any of these signs in patients taking theophylline warrants checking theophylline levels and dosage adjustment as indicated.

• Patients who experience urticaria may still tolerate other theophylline preparations. Urticaria may be caused by the ethylenediamine salt.

• *Alert:* Don't confuse aminophylline with amitriptyline or ampicillin.

### I.V. administration

• I.V. drug administration can cause burning; dilute with compatible I.V. solution, and inject at a rate no faster than 25 mg/minute. Drug is compatible with most I.V. solutions except invert sugar, fructose, and fat emulsions.

### Patient teaching

• Supply instructions for home care administration of form prescribed and dosage schedule. Some patients may need an around-the-clock dosage schedule.

• Warn elderly patient that dizziness, a common adverse reaction at start of therapy, may occur.

• Warn patient to check with the doctor or pharmacist before combining aminophylline with other drugs. Prescription or OTC remedies may contain ephedrine in combination with theophylline salts; excessive CNS stimulation may result.

• Advise patient to avoid switching brand without first checking with doctor.

• Tell patient who is a smoker to notify doctor if he has quit smoking.

---

ephedrine sulfate
Pretz-D ◇

*Pregnancy Risk Category C*

### HOW SUPPLIED
*Capsules:* 25 mg, 50 mg
*Nasal spray:* 0.25% ◇
*Injection:* 25 mg/ml, 30 mg/ml‡,
50 mg/ml

### ACTION
Stimulates alpha and beta receptors and is a direct- and indirect-acting sympathomimetic. Relaxes bronchial smooth muscle by beta$_2$-receptor stimulation.

| Route | Onset | Peak | Duration |
|---|---|---|---|
| P.O. | 15-60 min | Unknown | 3-5 hr |
| I.V. | 5 min | Unknown | 1 hr |
| I.M., S.C. | 10-20 min | Unknown | 0.5-1 hr |

### INDICATIONS & DOSAGE
*To correct hypotension—*
**Adults:** 25 mg one to four times daily P.O.; 25 to 50 mg I.M. or S.C.; or 10 to 25 mg I.V., p.r.n., to maximum of 150 mg/24 hours.
**Children:** 3 mg/kg or 25 to 100 mg/m$^2$ S.C. or I.V. daily, in four to six divided doses.
*Bronchodilation, nasal decongestion—*
**Adults and children over age 12:** 12.5 to 50 mg P.O. q 3 to 4 hours ,p.r.n., not to exceed 150 mg in 24 hours. As a nasal decongestant, 2 to 3 sprays in each nostril not more often that q 4 hours.
**Children ages 6 to 12:** 6.25 to 12.5 mg P.O. q 4 hours, not to exceed 75 mg in 24 hours. As a nasal decongestant, 1 to 2 sprays in each nostril not more often that q 4 hours.
**Children over age 2:** 2 to 3 mg/kg or 100 mg/m$^2$ P.O. daily in four to six divided doses.

### ADVERSE REACTIONS
**CNS:** *insomnia, nervousness,* dizziness, headache, muscle weakness, euphoria, confusion, delirium, tremor, *cerebral hemorrhage.*
**CV:** *palpitations,* tachycardia, hypertension, precordial pain, *arrhythmias.*
**EENT:** dry nose and throat.
**GI:** nausea, vomiting, anorexia.
**GU:** urine retention, painful urination due to visceral sphincter spasm.
**Skin:** diaphoresis.

### INTERACTIONS
**Drug-drug.** *Acetazolamide:* increased serum ephedrine levels. Monitor for toxicity.

---

Reactions may be *common,* uncommon, *life-threatening,* or COMMON AND LIFE-THREATENING.

*Alpha blockers:* unopposed beta-adrenergic effects, resulting in hypotension. Avoid concomitant use.
*Antihypertensives:* decreased effects. Monitor blood pressure.
*Beta blockers:* unopposed alpha-adrenergic effects, resulting in hypertension. Monitor blood pressure.
*Cardiac glycosides, general anesthetics (halogenated hydrocarbons):* increased risk of ventricular arrhythmias. Monitor ECG closely.
*Ergot alkaloids:* decreased vasoconstrictor activity. Monitor patient closely.
*Guanadrel, guanethidine:* decreased pressor effects of ephedrine. Monitor patient closely.
*Levodopa:* enhanced risk of ventricular arrhythmias. Monitor ECG closely.
*MAO inhibitors, tricyclic antidepressants:* when given with sympathomimetics, may cause severe hypertension (hypertensive crisis). Monitor patient and blood pressure closely.
*Methyldopa, reserpine:* may inhibit ephedrine effects. Use cautiously.

**EFFECTS ON DIAGNOSTIC TESTS**
None reported.

**CONTRAINDICATIONS**
Contraindicated in patients with hypersensitivity to ephedrine and other sympathomimetics and in those with porphyria, severe coronary artery disease, arrhythmias, angle-closure glaucoma, psychoneurosis, angina pectoris, substantial organic heart disease, or CV disease; also contraindicated in those receiving MAO inhibitors or general anesthesia with cyclopropane or halothane.

**NURSING CONSIDERATIONS**
• Use with extreme caution in elderly patients and in those with hypertension, hyperthyroidism, nervous or excitable states, diabetes, or prostatic hyperplasia.
• *Alert:* Hypoxia, hypercapnia, and acidosis, which may reduce effectiveness or increase adverse reactions, must be identified and corrected before or during ephedrine therapy.
• Drug isn't a substitute for blood or fluid volume replenishment. Volume deficit

must be corrected before administering vasopressors.
• To prevent insomnia, avoid giving within 2 hours of bedtime.
• Effectiveness decreases after 2 to 3 weeks, as tolerance develops. Doctor may need to increase dosage. Drug isn't addictive.
• Ephedrine should be used in children under age 12 only under the direction of a doctor.
• Rebound congestion and tachyphylaxis may occur with topical decongestant formulations.
• *Alert:* Don't confuse ephedrine with epinephrine.

**I.V. administration**
• Give 10 to 25 mg by I.V. injection slowly; repeat in 5 to 10 minutes if needed. Compatible with most common I.V. solutions.

**Patient teaching**
• Tell patient taking oral form of drug at home to take last dose of day at least 2 hours before bedtime.
• Warn patient not to take OTC drugs or herbs that contain ephedrine without informing doctor.

---

**epinephrine (adrenaline)**
Bronkaid Mist◇, Bronkaid Mistometer†, Primatene Mist◇

**epinephrine bitartrate**
AsthmaHaler Mist◇, Bronitin Mist◇, Bronkaid Mist◇, Primatene Mist*, Primatene Mist Suspension◇

**epinephrine hydrochloride**
Adrenalin Chloride, AsthmaNefrin◇, Epi-Pen, Epi-Pen Jr., microNefrin◇, Nephron◇, Sus-Phrine, Vaponefrin

*Pregnancy Risk Category C*

**HOW SUPPLIED**
*Aerosol inhaler:* 160 mcg◇, 200 mcg◇, 220 mcg◇, 250 mcg/metered spray◇

*Nebulizer inhaler:* 1% (1:100)†◊, 1.25%†◊, 2.25%†◊

*Injection:* 0.01 mg/ml (1:100,000), 0.1 mg/ml (1:10,000), 0.5 mg/ml (1:2,000), 1 mg/ml (1:1,000) parenteral; 5 mg/ml (1:200) parenteral suspension

## ACTION

Stimulates alpha and beta receptors within the sympathetic nervous system. Relaxes bronchial smooth muscle by beta$_2$ receptor stimulation.

| Route | Onset | Peak | Duration |
|---|---|---|---|
| I.V. | Immediate | 5 min | Short |
| I.M. | Variable | Unknown | 1-4 hr |
| S.C. | 5-15 min | 0.5 hr | 1-4 hr |
| Inhalation | 1-5 min | Unknown | 1-3 hr |

## INDICATIONS & DOSAGE

*Bronchospasm, hypersensitivity reactions, anaphylaxis—*

**Adults:** 0.1 to 0.5 ml of 1:1,000 S.C. or I.M. Repeated q 10 to 15 minutes, p.r.n. Or 0.1 to 0.25 ml of 1:1,000 (1 to 2.5 ml of a commercially available 1:10,000 injection or of a 1:10,000 dilution prepared by diluting 1 ml of a commercially available 1:1,000 injection with 10 ml of water for injection or normal saline for injection) I.V. slowly over 5 to 10 minutes.

**Children:** 0.01 ml/kg (10 mcg) of 1:1,000 solution S.C.; repeated q 20 minutes to 4 hours, p.r.n. Maximum single dose shouldn't exceed 0.5 mg. Or, 0.004 to 0.005 ml/kg of 1:200 (Sus-Phrine) S.C.; repeated q 8 to 12 hours, p.r.n. Maximum single dose shouldn't exceed 0.75 mg.

*Hemostasis—*

**Adults:** 1:50,000 to 1:1,000, sprayed or applied topically.

*Acute asthma attacks—*

**Adults and children ages 4 and over:** 160 to 250 mcg (metered aerosol) which is equivalent to 1 inhalation, repeated once if needed after at least 1 minute; subsequent doses shouldn't be administered for at least 3 hours. Or, 1% (1:100) solution of epinephrine or 2.25% solution of racepinephrine administered with a hand-bulb nebulizer as 1 to 3 deep inhalations, repeated q 3 hours, p.r.n.

*To prolong local anesthetic effect—*

**Adults and children:** with local anesthetics, may be used in concentrations of 1:500,000 to 1:50,000. The most commonly used concentration is 1:200,000.

*To restore cardiac rhythm in cardiac arrest—*

**Adults:** usual adult dose is 0.5 to 1 mg I.V. Doses may be repeated q 3 to 5 minutes if needed. Higher dose epinephrine may be used if 1-mg doses fail: 3 to 5 mg (approximately 0.1 mg/kg) doses of epinephrine repeated q 3 to 5 minutes.

**Children:** usual dose is 0.01 mg/kg (0.1 ml/kg of 1:10,000 injection) I.V. Usual initial dose through an endotracheal tube is 0.1 mg/kg (0.1 ml/kg of a 1:1,000 injection) diluted in 1 to 2 ml of 0.45% or normal saline solution. Subsequent I.V. or intratracheal doses range from 0.1 to 0.2 mg/kg (0.1 to 0.2 ml/kg of a 1:1,000 injection). I.V. or intratracheal doses may be repeated q 3 to 5 minutes if needed.

*Note:* 1 mg equals 1 ml of 1:1,000 or 10 ml of 1:10,000.

## ADVERSE REACTIONS

**CNS:** *nervousness, tremor,* vertigo, pain, *headache,* disorientation, agitation, *drowsiness,* fear, pallor, dizziness, weakness, **cerebral hemorrhage, CVA.**

**CV:** *palpitations;* widened pulse pressure; hypertension; tachycardia; ***ventricular fibrillation; shock;*** anginal pain; ECG changes, including a decreased T-wave amplitude.

**GI:** *nausea, vomiting.*

**GU:** increased BUN level.

**Metabolic:** increased blood glucose and serum lactic acid levels.

**Respiratory:** dyspnea.

**Skin:** urticaria, hemorrhage at injection site.

**Other:** tissue necrosis.

## INTERACTIONS

**Drug-drug.** *Alpha blockers:* hypotension due to unopposed beta-adrenergic effects. Avoid concomitant use.

*Antihistamines, thyroid hormones, tricyclic antidepressants:* when given with sympathomimetics, may cause severe adverse cardiac effects. Avoid giving together.

---

Reactions may be *common,* uncommon, *life-threatening,* or COMMON AND LIFE-THREATENING.

*Beta blockers such as propranolol:* may cause vasoconstriction and reflex bradycardia. Monitor patient carefully.
*Cardiac glycosides, general anesthetics (halogenated hydrocarbons):* increased risk of ventricular arrhythmias. Monitor ECG closely.
*Doxapram, mazindol, methylphenidate:* enhanced CNS stimulation or pressor effects. Monitor patient closely.
*Ergot alkaloids:* decreased vasoconstrictor activity. Monitor patient closely.
*Guanadrel, guanethidine:* enhanced pressor effects of epinephrine. Monitor patient closely.
*Levodopa:* enhanced risk of arrhythmias. Monitor ECG closely.
*MAO inhibitors:* increased risk of hypertensive crisis. Monitor blood pressure closely.

## EFFECTS ON DIAGNOSTIC TESTS
Epinephrine therapy interferes with tests for urinary catecholamines.

## CONTRAINDICATIONS
Contraindicated in patients with angle-closure glaucoma, shock (other than anaphylactic shock), organic brain damage, cardiac dilation, arrhythmias, coronary insufficiency, or cerebral arteriosclerosis. Also contraindicated in patients receiving general anesthesia with halogenated hydrocarbons or cyclopropane and in patients in labor (may delay second stage).

Some commercial products contain sulfites and are contraindicated in patients with sulfite allergies except when epinephrine is being used for treatment of serious allergic reactions or other emergency situations.

With local anesthetics, epinephrine is contraindicated for use in fingers, toes, ears, nose, or genitalia.

## NURSING CONSIDERATIONS
• Use with extreme caution in patients with long-standing bronchial asthma and emphysema who have developed degenerative heart disease. Also use cautiously in elderly patients and in those with hyperthyroidism, CV disease, hypertension, psychoneurosis, and diabetes.

• In patients with Parkinson's disease, drug increases rigidity and tremor.
• Epinephrine is drug of choice in emergency treatment of acute anaphylactic reactions.
• Discard epinephrine solutions after 24 hours or if solution is discolored or contains precipitate. Keep solution in light-resistant container, and don't remove before use.
• *Alert:* Avoid I.M. administration of parenteral suspension into buttocks. Gas gangrene may occur because epinephrine reduces oxygen tension of the tissues, encouraging the growth of contaminating organisms.
• Massage site after I.M. injection to counteract possible vasoconstriction. Repeated local injection can cause necrosis resulting from vasoconstriction at injection site.
• Observe patient closely for adverse reactions. Notify doctor if adverse reactions develop; dose adjustment or drug discontinuance may be warranted.
• If a sharp blood pressure increase occurs, rapid-acting vasodilators, such as nitrates or alpha blockers, can be given to counteract the marked pressor effect of large doses of epinephrine.
• Epinephrine is rapidly destroyed by oxidizing agents, such as iodine, chromates, nitrites, oxygen, and salts of easily reducible metals (such as iron).
• *Alert:* Don't confuse epinephrine with ephedrine.

### I.V. administration
• Don't mix with alkaline solutions. Use $D_5W$, normal saline for injection, lactated Ringer's injection, or combinations of dextrose in NaCl. Mix just before use.
• When administering I.V., monitor blood pressure, heart rate, and ECG when therapy is initiated and frequently thereafter.

### Patient teaching
• Teach patient to perform oral inhalation correctly. Give the following instructions for using a metered-dose inhaler:
–Shake canister.
–Clear nasal passages and throat.
–Breathe out, expelling as much air from lungs as possible.

---

–Place mouthpiece well into mouth as dose from inhaler is released, and inhale deeply.

–Hold breath for several seconds, remove mouthpiece, and exhale slowly.

Or, inhaler may be held about 1 inch (two finger widths) from open mouth; inhale while dose is released.

• If more than 1 inhalation is ordered, advise patient to wait at least 2 minutes before repeating procedure.

• Tell patient that use with an aerochamber may improve drug delivery to the lungs.

• If patient is also using a steroid inhaler, instruct him to use the bronchodilator first and then wait about 5 minutes before using the steroid. This allows the bronchodilator to open the air passages for maximum effectiveness.

• Instruct patient to wash inhaler with warm, soapy water at least once weekly. Remove canister before washing.

• If patient has acute hypersensitivity reactions, such as to bee stings, it may be necessary to instruct him to self-inject epinephrine at home.

---

## ipratropium bromide
Atrovent

*Pregnancy Risk Category B*

### HOW SUPPLIED
*Inhaler:* each metered dose supplies 18 mcg
*Solution (for inhalation):* 0.02% (500 mcg/vial)
*Solution (for nebulizer):* 0.025% (250 mcg/ml)‡
*Nasal spray:* 0.03% (each metered dose supplies 21 mcg), 0.06% (each metered dose supplies 42 mcg)

### ACTION
Inhibits vagally mediated reflexes by antagonizing acetylcholine at muscarinic receptors on bronchial smooth muscle.

| Route | Onset | Peak | Duration |
|---|---|---|---|
| Inhalation | 5-15 min | 1-2 hr | 3-6 hr |

### INDICATIONS & DOSAGE
*Bronchospasm associated with COPD—*
**Adults and children over age 12:** 1 to 2 inhalations q.i.d. Additional inhalations may be needed. However, total inhalations shouldn't exceed 12 in 24 hours. Or, use inhalation solution. Give 500 mcg dissolved in normal saline and administer by nebulizer q 6 to 8 hours.
**Children ages 5 to 12:** give 125 to 250 mcg nebulizer solution dissolved in normal saline and administer by nebulizer q 4 to 6 hours.
*Perennial rhinitis—*
**Adults and children ages 6 and older:** usual dosage of 0.03% nasal spray is 2 sprays (42 mcg) per nostril b.i.d. or t.i.d. (total dose 168 to 252 mcg/day).
*Common cold-induced rhinorrhea—*
**Adults and children over age 12:** usual dosage of 0.06% nasal spray is 2 sprays (84 mcg) per nostril t.i.d. or q.i.d.
**Infants and children:** nebulization 25 mcg/kg t.i.d.
✷ *NEW INDICATION: Symptomatic relief of rhinorrhea associated with the common cold—*
**Children ages 5 to 11:** 2 sprays of the 0.06% nasal spray (84 mcg) per nostril three times daily.

### ADVERSE REACTIONS
**CNS:** dizziness, pain, headache, nervousness.
**CV:** palpitations, hypertension, chest pain.
**EENT:** blurred vision, rhinitis, pharyngitis, sinusitis, epistaxis.
**GI:** nausea, GI distress, dry mouth.
**Musculoskeletal:** back pain.
**Respiratory:** *upper respiratory tract infection, bronchitis,* cough, dyspnea, **bronchospasm,** increased sputum.
**Skin:** rash.
**Other:** flulike symptoms, ***hypersensitivity reactions.***

### INTERACTIONS
**Drug-drug.** *Anticholinergics:* increased anticholinergic effects. Avoid concomitant use.
**Drug-herb.** *Jaborandi tree:* effects of ipratropium may be decreased with concurrent administration. Monitor closely.

---

Reactions may be *common,* uncommon, *life-threatening,* or COMMON AND LIFE-THREATENING.

*Pill-bearing spurge:* choline, a chemical component of the herb, may decrease effect of ipratropium. Use together cautiously.

**EFFECTS ON DIAGNOSTIC TESTS**
None reported.

**CONTRAINDICATIONS**
Contraindicated in patients with hypersensitivity to drug, atropine, or its derivatives and in those with history of hypersensitivity to soy lecithin or related food products, such as soybeans and peanuts.

**NURSING CONSIDERATIONS**
• Use cautiously in patients with angle-closure glaucoma, prostatic hyperplasia, and bladder-neck obstruction.
• If using a facemask for a nebulizer, take care to avoid leakage around the mask; temporary blurring of vision or eye pain may occur.
• Safety and efficacy of use beyond 4 days in patients with the common cold haven't been established.
• *Alert:* A patient with a severe peanut allergy could potentially have an anaphylactic reaction after using Atrovent inhalation aerosol (metered-dose inhaler). Take a thorough allergy history from patient before administering any drug.
• *Alert:* Don't confuse Atrovent with Alupent.

☑**Patient teaching**
• Warn patient that drug isn't effective for treating acute episodes of bronchospasm where rapid response is needed.
• Teach patient to perform oral inhalation correctly. Give the following instructions for using a metered-dose inhaler:
–Shake canister.
–Clear nasal passages and throat.
–Breathe out, expelling as much air from lungs as possible.
–Place mouthpiece well into mouth as dose from inhaler is released, and inhale deeply.
–Hold breath for several seconds, remove mouthpiece, and exhale slowly.
• Inform patient that use of aerochamber with metered-dose inhaler may improve drug delivery to lungs.

• Warn patient to avoid accidentally spraying into eyes. Temporary blurring of vision may result.
• If more than 1 inhalation is ordered, tell patient to wait at least 2 minutes before repeating procedure.
• Instruct patient to wash inhaler in warm, soapy water at least once weekly. Remove canister before washing.
• Tell patient who is also using a steroid inhaler to use ipratropium first, then wait about 5 minutes before using the steroid. This allows the bronchodilator to open air passages for maximum effectiveness.
• Inform patient to take missed dose as soon as remembered unless it's almost time for the next dose. In that case, he should skip the missed dose and never double the dose.

---

**isoproterenol (isoprenaline)**
Isuprel, Medihaler-Iso

**isoproterenol hydrochloride**
Isuprel, Isuprel Mistometer

**isoproterenol sulfate**
Medihaler-Iso

*Pregnancy Risk Category C*

**HOW SUPPLIED**
**isoproterenol**
*Nebulizer inhaler:* 0.25%, 0.5%, 1%
**isoproterenol hydrochloride**
*Tablets (S.L.):* 10 mg, 15 mg
*Aerosol inhaler:* 131 mcg/metered spray
*Injection:* 20 mcg/ml, 200 mcg/ml
**isoproterenol sulfate**
*Aerosol inhaler:* 80 mcg/metered spray

**ACTION**
Relaxes bronchial smooth muscle by stimulating $beta_2$ receptors. As a cardiac stimulant, acts on $beta_1$ receptors in the heart.

| Route | Onset | Peak | Duration |
|---|---|---|---|
| I.V. | Immediate | Unknown | < 1 hr |
| S.L. | 15-30 min | Unknown | 1-2 hr |
| Inhalation | 2-5 min | Unknown | 0.5-2 hr |

## INDICATIONS & DOSAGE

*Bronchial asthma, reversible bronchospasm—*

**Adults:** 10 to 20 mg hydrochloride S.L. t.i.d. or q.i.d. Don't exceed daily S.L. dose of 60 mg.

**Children:** 5 to 10 mg hydrochloride S.L. t.i.d. Don't exceed daily S.L. dose of 30 mg.

*Bronchospasm—*

**Adults and children:** acute dyspneic episodes: 1 inhalation of sulfate form initially. Repeated if needed after 2 to 5 minutes. No more than 6 inhalations should be taken during any single hour in a 24-hour period.

Maintenance dose is 1 to 2 inhalations four to six times daily.

*Bronchospasm in COPD—*

Administered via IPPB or for nebulization by compressed air or oxygen.

**Adults:** 2 ml of 0.125% or 2.5 ml of 0.1% solution (prepared by diluting 0.5 ml of 0.5% solution to 2 or 2.5 ml, respectively; or by diluting 0.25 ml of 1% solution to 2 or 2.5 ml, respectively, with water or half-normal or normal saline solution) up to five times daily.

**Children:** 2 ml of a 0.0625% solution or 2.5 ml of 0.05% solution (prepared by diluting 0.25 ml of 0.5% solution to 2 or 2.5 ml, respectively, with water or half-normal or normal saline solution) up to five times daily.

*Heart block, ventricular arrhythmias—*

**Adults:** (hydrochloride) initially, 0.02 to 0.06 mg I.V. Subsequent doses 0.01 to 0.2 mg I.V. or 5 mcg/minute I.V.; or 0.2 mg I.M. initially, then 0.02 to 1 mg, p.r.n.

**Children:** (hydrochloride) I.V. infusion of 2.5 mcg/minute or 0.1 mcg/kg/minute. Dosage is adjusted based on patient's response.

*Shock—*

**Adults and children:** (hydrochloride) 0.5 to 5 mcg/minute by continuous I.V. infusion. Usual concentration is 1 mg (5 ml) in 500 ml D₅W. Rate titrated according to heart rate, CVP, blood pressure, and urine flow.

## ADVERSE REACTIONS

**CNS:** *headache, mild tremor,* weakness, dizziness, *nervousness,* insomnia, **Stokes-Adams seizures.**

**CV:** *palpitations, tachycardia, anginal pain,* **arrhythmias, cardiac arrest,** *rapid rise and fall in blood pressure.*

**EENT:** pharyngitis.

**GI:** *nausea, vomiting, heartburn.*

**Metabolic:** hyperglycemia.

**Respiratory:** *bronchospasm,* bronchitis, sputum increase, pulmonary edema.

**Skin:** diaphoresis.

**Other:** swelling of parotid glands with prolonged use.

## INTERACTIONS

**Drug-drug.** *Epinephrine, other sympathomimetics:* increased risk of arrhythmias. Use together cautiously.

*Halogenated general anesthetics or cyclopropane:* increased risk of arrhythmias. Avoid concomitant use.

*Propranolol, other beta blockers:* blocked bronchodilating effect of isoproterenol. Monitor patient carefully if used together.

## EFFECTS ON DIAGNOSTIC TESTS

Drug may reduce sensitivity of spirometry in the diagnosis of asthma.

## CONTRAINDICATIONS

Contraindicated in patients with tachycardia or AV block caused by digitalis intoxication, preexisting arrhythmias (other than those that may respond to treatment with isoproterenol), angina pectoris, or angle-closure glaucoma; also contraindicated with concurrent use of general anesthetics with halogenated drugs or cyclopropane.

## NURSING CONSIDERATIONS

• Use cautiously in elderly patients and in those with renal or CV disease, coronary insufficiency, diabetes, hyperthyroidism, or history of sensitivity to sympathomimetic amines.

• Drug isn't a substitute for blood or fluid volume deficit. Volume deficit should be corrected before administering vasopressors.

---

Reactions may be *common,* uncommon, *life-threatening,* or COMMON AND LIFE-THREATENING.

• Don't use injection or inhalation solution if it's discolored or contains precipitate.
• *Alert:* If heart rate exceeds 110 beats/minute with I.V. infusion, notify doctor. Doses sufficient to increase the heart rate to more than 130 beats/minute may induce ventricular arrhythmias.
• Don't administer S.L. doses more frequently than every 3 to 4 hours or more than three times daily.
• If drug is administered via inhalation with oxygen, make sure oxygen level won't suppress respiratory drive.
• Follow same instructions for metered powder nebulizer, although deep inhalation isn't needed.
• Drug may aggravate ventilation-perfusion abnormalities; even while ease of breathing is improved, arterial oxygen tension may fall paradoxically.
• Isoproterenol may cause a slight increase in systolic blood pressure and a slight to marked decrease in diastolic blood pressure.
• Monitor patient for adverse reactions.
• *Alert:* Don't confuse Isuprel with Ismelin or Isordil.

**I.V. administration**
• Give by direct injection or I.V. infusion. For infusion, drug may be diluted with most common I.V. solutions. However, don't use with sodium bicarbonate injection; drug decomposes rapidly in alkaline solutions.
• When administering I.V. isoproterenol to treat shock, closely monitor blood pressure, CVP, ECG, arterial blood gas measurements, and urine output. Carefully titrate infusion rate according to these measurements, as ordered. Use a continuous infusion pump to regulate flow rate.

**Patient teaching**
• Teach patient to perform oral inhalation correctly. Give the following instructions for using a metered-dose inhaler:
–Shake canister.
–Clear nasal passages and throat.
–Breathe out, expelling as much air from lungs as possible.

–Place mouthpiece well into mouth as dose from inhaler is released, and inhale deeply.
–Hold breath for several seconds, remove mouthpiece, and exhale slowly.
• Or, inhaler may be held about 1 inch (two finger widths) from open mouth; inhale as dose is released.
• If more than 1 inhalation is ordered, tell patient to wait at least 2 minutes before repeating procedure.
• Use of aerochamber may improve drug delivery to the lungs.
• If patient is also using a steroid inhaler, instruct him to use the bronchodilator first and then wait about 5 minutes before using the steroid. This allows the bronchodilator to open the air passages for maximum effectiveness.
• Instruct patient to wash inhaler with warm, soapy water at least once weekly. Remove canister before washing.
• Warn patient using oral inhalant that drug may turn sputum and saliva pink.
• Teach patient to take S.L. tablet properly. Instruct patient to hold tablet under tongue and not to swallow saliva until tablet dissolves and is absorbed. Instruct him to rinse mouth with water between doses to help prevent oropharyngeal dryness.
• Caution patient that prolonged use of S.L. tablets can cause tooth decay.
• Tell patient not to use drug at bedtime, if possible; it interrupts sleep patterns.
• Inform patient to discontinue drug immediately and notify doctor if drug causes precordial distress or anginal pain or if an increase in chest tightness or dyspnea occurs.
• Warn patient against overuse; tolerance may develop.

**✳ NEW DRUG**

## levalbuterol hydrochloride
## Xopenex

*Pregnancy Risk Category C*

**HOW SUPPLIED**
*Solution for inhalation:* 0.63 mg or 1.25 mg in 3-ml vials

## ACTION
Relaxes smooth muscle of the airways by acting on beta$_2$ receptors. Also, inhibits release of mediators from mast cells in the airway.

| Route | Onset | Peak | Duration |
|-------|-------|------|----------|
| Inhalation | 10-17 min | 1.5 hr | 5-8 hr |

## INDICATIONS & DOSAGE
*To prevent or treat bronchospasm in patients with reversible obstructive airway disease—*
**Adults and adolescents ages 12 and older:** 0.63 mg administered t.i.d. every 6 to 8 hours, by oral inhalation via a nebulizer. Patients with more severe asthma who don't respond adequately to a dosage of 0.63 mg may benefit from a dosage of 1.25 mg t.i.d.

## ADVERSE REACTIONS
**CNS:** dizziness, migraine, nervousness, pain, tremor, anxiety.
**CV:** tachycardia.
**EENT:** *rhinitis*, sinusitis, turbinate edema.
**GI:** dyspepsia.
**Musculoskeletal:** leg cramps.
**Respiratory:** increased cough, *viral infection.*
**Other:** flulike syndrome, accidental injury.

## INTERACTIONS
**Drug-drug.** *Beta blockers:* blocked pulmonary effect of the drug and, possibly, severe bronchospasm. Don't use together, if possible. If concomitant use is needed, a cardioselective beta blocker could be considered, but should be administered with caution.
*Digoxin:* decreased digoxin levels (up to 22%). Monitor serum digoxin levels.
*Loop or thiazide diuretics:* ECG changes and hypokalemia from concurrent administration of these non-potassium-sparing diuretics. Use together cautiously.
*MAO inhibitors, tricyclic antidepressants:* potentiated action of levalbuterol on the vascular system. Administer with extreme caution to patients being treated with monoamine oxidase inhibitors or tricyclic antidepressants, or within 2 weeks of discontinuation of these drugs.
*Other short-acting sympathomimetic aerosol bronchodilators, epinephrine:* increased adrenergic adverse effects. To avoid serious cardiovascular effects, additional adrenergics should be used with caution.

## EFFECTS ON DIAGNOSTIC TESTS
None reported.

## CONTRAINDICATIONS
Contraindicated in patients with hypersensitivity to drug or racemic albuterol.

## NURSING CONSIDERATIONS
• Use cautiously in patients with cardiovascular disorders, especially coronary insufficiency, hypertension, and arrhythmias. Also use cautiously in patients with seizure disorders, hyperthyroidism, or diabetes mellitus and in patients who are unusually responsive to sympathomimetic amines.
• *Alert:* Like other inhaled beta agonists, levalbuterol can produce paradoxical bronchospasm, which may be life-threatening. If this occurs, discontinue levalbuterol immediately and institute alternative therapy, as ordered.
• *Alert:* Like all other beta agonists, levalbuterol can produce significant CV effects in some patients. Although such effects are uncommon at recommended doses, if CV effects occur, the drug may be discontinued, as ordered.
• Drug may worsen preexisting diabetes mellitus and ketoacidosis.
• Serum potassium levels may be transiently decreased, but potassium supplementation is usually unnecessary.
• The compatibility, efficacy, and safety of levalbuterol when mixed with other drugs in a nebulizer haven't been established.

☑ **Patient teaching**
• Warn patient that he may experience paradoxical bronchospasm (worsening breathing). Tell him to discontinue drug and contact doctor immediately if this occurs.

---

Reactions may be *common,* uncommon, *life-threatening,* or **COMMON AND LIFE-THREATENING.**

- Inform patient not to increase the dosage or frequency of dosing without consulting his doctor.
- Inform patient to seek medical attention immediately if levalbuterol becomes less effective for treating signs and symptoms, signs and symptoms become worse, or he is using levalbuterol more frequently than usual.
- Tell patient that the effects of levalbuterol may last up to 8 hours.
- Tell patient that if a dose is missed, the next dose shouldn't be doubled. Doses should be at least 6 hours apart.
- Advise patient to use other inhalations and antasthmatics only as directed while taking levalbuterol.
- Inform patient that common adverse reactions include palpitations, rapid heart rate, headache, dizziness, tremor, and nervousness.
- Inform patient to contact doctor about the use of levalbuterol if she becomes pregnant or is breast-feeding.
- Tell patient to keep unopened vials in foil pouch. Once the foil pouch is opened, the vials should be used within 2 weeks. Inform patient that vials removed from the pouch, if not used immediately, should be protected from light and excessive heat and used within 1 week.
- Teach patient to correctly administer drug by oral inhalation via a nebulizer.
- Inform patient to breathe as calmly, deeply, and evenly as possible until no more mist is formed in the nebulizer reservoir (5 to 15 minutes).

---

## metaproterenol sulfate
Alupent, Arm-A-Med
Metaproterenol, Dey-Lute
Metaproterenol, Metaprel

*Pregnancy Risk Category C*

### HOW SUPPLIED
*Tablets:* 10 mg, 20 mg
*Syrup:* 10 mg/5 ml
*Aerosol inhaler:* 0.65 mg/metered spray
*Nebulizer inhaler:* 0.4%, 0.6%, 5% solution

### ACTION
Relaxes bronchial smooth muscle by stimulating beta$_2$ receptors.

| Route | Onset | Peak | Duration |
|-------|-------|------|----------|
| P.O. | 15 min | 1 hr | 1-4 hr |
| Inhalation | 1 min | 1 hr | 1-2.5 hr |
| Nebulizer | 5-30 min | 1 hr | 1-2.5 hr |

### INDICATIONS & DOSAGE
*Acute episodes of bronchial asthma—*
**Adults and children ages 12 and over:** 2 to 3 inhalations. Don't repeat inhalations more often than q 3 to 4 hours. Don't exceed 12 inhalations daily.
*Bronchial asthma and reversible bronchospasm—*
**Adults:** 20 mg P.O. q 6 to 8 hours.
**Children over age 9 or weighing over 27 kg (60 lb):** 20 mg P.O. q 6 to 8 hours.
**Children ages 6 to 9 or weighing less than 27 kg:** 10 mg P.O. q 6 to 8 hours.
**Children under age 6:** 1.3 to 2.6 mg/kg/day in divided doses of syrup.
Doses below are for IPPB or nebulizer:
**Adults and children ages 12 and over:** 0.2 to 0.3 ml of 5% solution diluted in approximately 2.5 ml of half-normal or normal saline; or 2.5 ml of a commercially available 0.4% or 0.6% solution q 4 hours, p.r.n.
**Children ages 6 to 12:** 0.1 to 0.2 ml of a 5% solution diluted in normal saline to final volume of 3 ml q 4 hours, p.r.n.

### ADVERSE REACTIONS
**CNS:** *nervousness,* weakness, drowsiness, *tremor,* vertigo, headache.
**CV:** *tachycardia,* hypertension, palpitations, *cardiac arrest (with excessive use).*
**EENT:** dry and irritated throat.
**GI:** *vomiting, nausea,* heartburn, dry mouth.
**Respiratory:** paradoxical bronchiolar constriction (with excessive use), cough.
**Skin:** rash, *hypersensitivity reactions.*

### INTERACTIONS
**Drug-drug.** *Epinephrine, other sympathomimetics:* increased risk of arrhythmias. Use together cautiously.
*MAO inhibitors, tricyclic antidepressants:* may potentiate the effect of metapro-

---

\*Liquid contains alcohol.   \*\*May contain tartrazine.   †Canada   ‡Australia   §U.K.   ◇OTC

terenol on the vascular system. Use together cautiously.
*Propranolol, other beta blockers:* blocked bronchodilating effect of metaproterenol. Monitor patient carefully if used together.

## EFFECTS ON DIAGNOSTIC TESTS
Drug may reduce the sensitivity of spirometry in the diagnosis of asthma.

## CONTRAINDICATIONS
Contraindicated in patients with hypersensitivity to drug or its ingredients and in those with tachycardia or arrhythmias associated with tachycardia, peripheral or mesenteric vascular thrombosis, profound hypoxia or hypercapnia; also contraindicated in those receiving anesthesia with cyclopropane or halogenated hydrocarbon general anesthetics.

## NURSING CONSIDERATIONS
• Use cautiously in patients with hypertension, hyperthyroidism, heart disease, diabetes, or cirrhosis and in those who are receiving cardiac glycosides.
• Patients may use tablets and aerosol concomitantly. Monitor closely for toxicity.
• Inhalant solution can be administered by IPPB with drug diluted in normal saline solution or with a hand nebulizer at full strength.
• *Alert:* Don't confuse metaproterenol with metoprolol or metipranolol, or Alupent with Atrovent.

### ✓ Patient teaching
• Teach patient to perform oral inhalation correctly. Give the following instructions for using a metered-dose inhaler:
–Shake canister.
–Clear nasal passages and throat.
–Breathe out, expelling as much air from lungs as possible.
–Place mouthpiece well into mouth as dose from inhaler is released, and inhale deeply.
–Hold breath for several seconds, remove mouthpiece, and exhale slowly. Allow 2 minutes between inhalations.
   Or, inhaler may be held about 1 inch (two finger widths) from open mouth; inhale while dose is released.

• Inform patient that use of aerochamber with metered-dose inhalers may improve drug delivery to lungs.
• Advise patient to store drug in light-resistant container.
• Tell patient who is also using a steroid inhaler to use bronchodilator first, then wait about 5 minutes before using the steroid. This allows bronchodilator to open air passages for maximum effectiveness.
• Tell patient to wash inhaler in warm, soapy water at least once weekly; remove canister before washing.
• Warn patient to discontinue immediately if paradoxical bronchospasm occurs and to notify doctor.
• Warn patient to notify doctor if no response is derived from dosage or to request dosage adjustment.

---

## oxtriphylline
## (choline salt of theophyllinate)
Choledyl SA

*Pregnancy Risk Category C*

### HOW SUPPLIED
*Tablets:* 100 mg, 200 mg
*Tablets (extended-release):* 400 mg, 600 mg
*Syrup:* 50 mg/5 ml
*Elixir\*:* 100 mg/5 ml

### ACTION
Inhibits phosphodiesterase, the enzyme that degrades cAMP, resulting in relaxation of smooth muscle of the bronchial airways and pulmonary blood vessels. Oxtriphylline is equivalent to 64% anhydrous theophylline.

| Route | Onset | Peak | Duration |
|-------|-------|------|----------|
| P.O. | Unknown | 2 hr | Unknown |
| P.O. (extended) | Variable | Variable | Variable |

### INDICATIONS & DOSAGE
*Acute bronchial asthma and reversible bronchospasm associated with chronic bronchitis and emphysema—*
**Adults (nonsmokers):** 4.7 mg/kg P.O. q 8 hours.

---

**Adults (smokers) and children ages 9 to 16:** 4.7 mg/kg q 6 hours.
**Children ages 1 to 9:** 6.2 mg/kg P.O. q 6 hours.

*Note:* If total daily maintenance dose is established at 800 to 1,200 mg, one sustained-action tablet q 12 hours may be substituted.

## ADVERSE REACTIONS

**CNS:** *restlessness, dizziness,* headache, *insomnia,* irritability, **seizures,** muscle twitching.
**CV:** *palpitations, sinus tachycardia,* extrasystoles, flushing, marked hypotension, **arrhythmias.**
**GI:** *nausea, vomiting,* epigastric pain, diarrhea.
**Respiratory:** tachypnea, *respiratory arrest.*

## INTERACTIONS

**Drug-drug.** *Adenosine:* decreased antiarrhythmic effectiveness. Higher doses of adenosine may be needed.
*Allopurinol (high-dose):* increased serum theophylline levels. Monitor for toxicity.
*Barbiturates, nicotine, phenytoin, rifampin:* enhanced metabolism and decreased theophylline blood levels. Monitor for decreased effect.
*Beta blockers (such as nadolol and propranolol):* may cause bronchospasm in sensitive patients. Use together cautiously.
*Calcium channel blockers, cimetidine, influenza virus vaccine, macrolide antibiotics (such as erythromycin), oral contraceptives, quinolone antibiotics (such as ciprofloxacin):* decreased hepatic clearance of theophylline; elevated theophylline levels. Monitor for signs of toxicity.
*Carbamazepine, isoniazid, loop diuretics:* may increase or decrease theophylline levels. Monitor closely.
*Lithium:* increased renal excretion of lithium. Monitor for decreased effect.

## EFFECTS ON DIAGNOSTIC TESTS

Drug may falsely elevate serum uric acid levels measured by colorimetric methods. Theophylline levels may be falsely elevated in patients using furosemide, phenylbutazone, probenecid, some cephalosporins, sulfa drugs, theobromine, caffeine, tea, chocolate, cola beverages, and acetaminophen, depending on assay method used.

## CONTRAINDICATIONS

Contraindicated in patients with hypersensitivity to xanthines (caffeine, theobromine) and in those with preexisting arrhythmias (especially tachyarrhythmias), active peptic ulcer disease, or poorly controlled seizure disorders.

## NURSING CONSIDERATIONS

• Use cautiously in young children, in elderly patients, and in those with peptic ulceration, COPD, heart failure, cor pulmonale, renal or hepatic impairment, glaucoma, severe hypoxemia, hypertension, compromised cardiac or circulatory function, angina, acute MI, sulfite sensitivity, hyperthyroidism, and diabetes.
• **Alert:** Don't combine with products containing ephedrine; excessive CNS stimulation (nervousness, tremor, akathisia) may result.
• Administer drug after meals and at bedtime.
• Oxtriphylline is a soluble salt of theophylline. Dosage is adjusted by monitoring response, tolerance, pulmonary function, and serum theophylline levels. Ensure that theophylline levels range from 10 to 20 mcg/ml; toxicity has been reported with levels above 20 mcg/ml.
• **Alert:** Signs and symptoms of toxicity include tachycardia, anorexia, nausea, vomiting, diarrhea, restlessness, irritability, and headache. The presence of any of these signs in patients taking theophylline warrants checking theophylline levels and adjusting dose as indicated.
• Monitor therapy carefully. Individuals metabolize theophyllines at different rates. Dosage adjustments are needed in elderly patients; in those with heart failure, cor pulmonale, and hepatic disease; and in smokers.
• Store at 59° to 86° F (15° to 30° C). Protect elixir from light and tablets from moisture.

### ☑ Patient teaching

• Tell patient to report GI distress, palpitations, irritability, restlessness, nervous-

---

*Liquid contains alcohol.  **May contain tartrazine.  †Canada  ‡Australia  §U.K.  ◇OTC

ness, or insomnia; may indicate excessive CNS stimulation.

• Inform patient that tablets shouldn't be chewed, crushed, or dissolved. Instruct him when to take drug.

• Inform elderly patients that dizziness, a common adverse reaction at the start of therapy, may occur.

## pirbuterol acetate
Maxair, Maxair Autohaler

*Pregnancy Risk Category C*

### HOW SUPPLIED
*Inhaler:* 0.2 mg/metered dose

### ACTION
Relaxes bronchial smooth muscle by stimulating beta$_2$ receptors.

| Route | Onset | Peak | Duration |
|---|---|---|---|
| Inhalation | 5 min | 0.5-1 hr | 5 hr |

### INDICATIONS & DOSAGE
*Prevention and reversal of bronchospasm; asthma—*
**Adults and children ages 12 and older:** 1 or 2 inhalations (0.2 to 0.4 mg) repeated q 4 to 6 hours. Don't to exceed 12 inhalations daily.

### ADVERSE REACTIONS
**CNS:** tremor, nervousness, dizziness, insomnia, headache, vertigo.
**CV:** tachycardia, palpitations, chest tightness.
**EENT:** dry or irritated throat.
**GI:** nausea, vomiting, diarrhea, dry mouth.
**Respiratory:** cough.

### INTERACTIONS
**Drug-drug.** *Beta blockers, propranolol:* decreased bronchodilating effects. Avoid concomitant use.
*MAO inhibitors, tricyclic antidepressants:* may potentiate action of beta agonist on vascular system. Use together cautiously.

### EFFECTS ON DIAGNOSTIC TESTS
None reported.

### CONTRAINDICATIONS
Contraindicated in patients with hypersensitivity to drug.

### NURSING CONSIDERATIONS
• Use cautiously in patients with CV disorders, hyperthyroidism, diabetes, and seizure disorders or in those who are unusually responsive to sympathomimetic amines.

### ☑ Patient teaching
• Teach patient to perform oral inhalation correctly. Give the following instructions for using a metered-dose inhaler:
–Shake canister.
–Clear nasal passages and throat.
–Breathe out, expelling as much air from lungs as possible.
–Place mouthpiece well into mouth as dose from inhaler is released, and inhale deeply.
–Hold breath for several seconds, remove mouthpiece, and exhale slowly.
• If more than one inhalation is ordered, tell patient to wait at least 2 minutes before repeating procedure.
• Give the following instructions for using an autohaler:
–Remove mouthpiece cover by pulling down lip on back cover. Inspect mouthpiece for foreign objects. Locate "Up" arrows and air vents.
–Hold autohaler upright so that arrows point up while raising lever until it snaps into place.
–Hold autohaler around the middle, and shake gently several times.
–Continue to hold upright and not block air vents at bottom. Exhale normally before use.
–Seal lips around mouthpiece. Inhale deeply through mouthpiece with steady, moderate force. A click will be heard and a soft puff will be felt when inhaling triggers the release of drug. Continue to take a full, deep breath.
–Take autohaler away from mouth when done inhaling. Hold breath for 10 seconds; then exhale slowly.
–Continue to hold autohaler upright while lowering lever. Lower lever after each puff. If additional puffs are ordered, wait

1 minute between each puff and repeat process.

• Tell patient who is also using a steroid inhaler to use bronchodilator first, then wait about 5 minutes before using the steroid. This allows the bronchodilator to open air passages for maximum effectiveness.

• Instruct patient who experiences increased bronchospasm after using drug to call doctor.

• Advise patient to seek medical attention if a previously effective dosage doesn't control symptoms; this may signify worsening of disease.

## salmeterol xinafoate
Serevent, Serevent Diskus

*Pregnancy Risk Category C*

### HOW SUPPLIED
*Inhalation aerosol:* 21 mcg/metered spray
*Inhalation powder:* 50 mcg/blister

### ACTION
Not clearly defined. Selectively activates beta$_2$ receptors, which results in bronchodilation. Also, blocks the release of allergic mediators from mast cells lining the respiratory tract.

| Route | Onset | Peak | Duration |
|-------|-------|------|----------|
| Inhalation | 10-20 min | 3 hr | 12 hr |

### INDICATIONS & DOSAGE
*Long-term maintenance treatment of asthma; prevention of bronchospasm in patients with nocturnal asthma or reversible obstructive airway disease who need regular treatment with short-acting beta agonists—*
For inhalation aerosol—
**Adults and children over age 12:** 2 inhalations q 12 hours, in the morning and evening.
For inhalation powder—
**Adults and children over age 4:** 1 inhalation q 12 hours, in the morning and evening.

*Prevention of exercise-induced bronchospasm—*
For inhalation aerosol—
**Adults and children ages 12 and over:** 2 inhalations at least 30 to 60 minutes before exercise.
For inhalation powder—
**Adults and children ages 4 and older:** 1 inhalation at least 30 minutes before exercise.
*Maintenance treatment of bronchospasm associated with COPD (including emphysema and chronic bronchitis)—*
**Adults:** 2 inhalations (42 mcg; inhalation aerosol) q 12 hours, in the morning and evening.

### ADVERSE REACTIONS
**CNS:** headache, sinus headache, tremor, nervousness, giddiness, dizziness.
**CV:** tachycardia, palpitations, *ventricular arrhythmias.*
**EENT:** *nasopharyngitis,* pharyngitis, nasal cavity or sinus disorder.
**GI:** nausea, vomiting, diarrhea, heartburn.
**Musculoskeletal:** joint and back pain, myalgia.
**Respiratory:** cough, lower respiratory infection, *upper respiratory tract infection, bronchospasm.*
**Other:** *hypersensitivity reactions* (rash, urticaria).

### INTERACTIONS
**Drug-drug.** *Beta agonists, other methylxanthines, theophylline:* possible adverse cardiac effects with excessive use. Monitor closely.
*MAO inhibitors:* risk of severe adverse CV effects. Avoid use within 14 days of MAO therapy.
*Tricyclic antidepressants:* risk of moderate to severe adverse CV effects. Use with extreme caution.

### EFFECTS ON DIAGNOSTIC TESTS
None reported.

### CONTRAINDICATIONS
Contraindicated in patients with hypersensitivity to drug or its ingredients.

---

*Liquid contains alcohol.   **May contain tartrazine.   †Canada   ‡Australia   §U.K.   ◇OTC

## NURSING CONSIDERATIONS

• Use cautiously in patients with coronary insufficiency, arrhythmias, hypertension, other CV disorders, thyrotoxicosis, or seizure disorders and in those who are unusually responsive to sympathomimetics.
• **Alert:** Don't confuse Serevent with Serentil.

### ☑ Patient teaching

• Remind patient to take drug at about 12-hour intervals for optimum effect and to take the drug even when feeling better.
• If patient is taking drug to prevent exercise-induced bronchospasm, tell him he should take it 30 to 60 minutes before exercise.
• **Alert:** Tell patient that, although drug is a beta agonist, it shouldn't be used to treat acute bronchospasm. He must be provided with a short-acting beta agonist such as albuterol to treat such exacerbations.
• Tell patient to contact doctor if the short-acting agonist no longer provides sufficient relief or if more than 4 inhalations are needed daily. This may be a sign that the asthma symptoms are worsening. Tell him not to increase the dosage of salmeterol.
• If patient is taking an inhaled corticosteroid, he should continue to use it on a regular basis. Warn patient not to take other drugs without doctor's consent.
• If taking the inhalation powder (diskus device), instruct patient not to exhale into the device. The device should only be activated and used in a level, horizontal position.
• Tell patient not to use diskus device with a spacer.
• Instruct patient never to wash the mouthpiece or any part of the diskus device; it must be kept dry.

---

## terbutaline sulfate
Brethaire, Brethine, Bricanyl

*Pregnancy Risk Category B*

## HOW SUPPLIED
*Tablets:* 2.5 mg, 5 mg
*Aerosol inhaler:* 200 mcg/metered spray
*Injection:* 1 mg/ml

## ACTION
Relaxes bronchial smooth muscle by stimulating beta$_2$ receptors and relaxes uterine smooth muscle.

| Route | Onset | Peak | Duration |
|---|---|---|---|
| P.O. | 30 min | 2-3 hr | 4-8 hr |
| S.C. | 15 min | 30 min | 1.5-4 hr |
| Inhalation | 5-30 min | 1-2 hr | 3-6 hr |

## INDICATIONS & DOSAGE
*Bronchospasm in patients with reversible obstructive airway disease—*
**Adults and children ages 12 and older:** dosage varies with dosage form.
*Aerosol inhaler*—2 inhalations separated by 60-second interval, repeated q 4 to 6 hours.
*Injection*—0.25 mg S.C. May be repeated in 15 to 30 minutes, p.r.n. Dosage shouldn't exceed 0.5 mg in 4 hours.
*Tablets in adults*—2.5 to 5 mg P.O. q 6 hours t.i.d. during waking hours. Maximum dose is 15 mg/day.
*Tablets in children ages 12 to 15* —2.5 mg P.O. q 6 hours t.i.d. during waking hours. Maximum dose is 7.5 mg/day.
*Note:* Drug isn't recommended for children under age 12.

## ADVERSE REACTIONS
**CNS:** *nervousness, tremor, drowsiness, dizziness, headache,* weakness.
**CV:** *palpitations,* tachycardia, ***arrhythmias,*** flushing.
**EENT:** dry and irritated nose and throat (with inhaled form).
**GI:** *vomiting, nausea,* heartburn.
**Metabolic:** hypokalemia.
**Respiratory:** ***paradoxical bronchospasm with prolonged usage,*** dyspnea.
**Skin:** diaphoresis.

## INTERACTIONS
**Drug-drug.** *Cardiac glycosides, cyclopropane, halogenated inhalation anesthetics, levodopa:* increased risk of arrhythmias. Monitor closely, and avoid concomitant use with levodopa.
*CNS stimulants:* increased CNS stimulation. Avoid concomitant use.
*MAO inhibitors:* when given with sympathomimetics, may cause severe hyperten-

---

sion (hypertensive crisis). Avoid concomitant use.

*Propranolol, other beta blockers:* blocked bronchodilating effects of terbutaline. Avoid concomitant use.

**EFFECTS ON DIAGNOSTIC TESTS**
Terbutaline may reduce the sensitivity of spirometry for the diagnosis of bronchospasm.

**CONTRAINDICATIONS**
Contraindicated in patients with hypersensitivity to drug or sympathomimetic amines.

**NURSING CONSIDERATIONS**
• Use cautiously in patient with CV disorders, hyperthyroidism, diabetes, or seizure disorders.
• Give S.C. injections in lateral deltoid area.
• Protect injection from light. Don't use if discolored.
• Patient may use tablets and aerosol concomitantly. Monitor closely for toxicity.
•*Alert:* Don't confuse terbutaline with tolbutamide or terbinafine.

☑ **Patient teaching**
• Ensure that patient and caregivers understand why drug is needed.
• Teach patient to perform oral inhalation correctly. Give the following instructions for using a metered-dose inhaler:
–Shake canister.
–Clear nasal passages and throat.
–Breathe out, expelling as much air from lungs as possible.
–Place mouthpiece well into mouth as dose from inhaler is released, and inhale deeply.
–Hold breath for several seconds, remove mouthpiece, and exhale slowly.
 Or, inhaler may be held about 1 inch (two finger widths) from open mouth; inhale while drug is released.
• If more than one inhalation is ordered, tell patient to wait at least 2 minutes before repeating procedure.
• Tell patient that use of an aerochamber may improve drug delivery to the lungs.
• Tell patient who is also using a steroid inhaler to use bronchodilator first, then

wait about 5 minutes before using steroid. This allows bronchodilator to open air passages for maximum effectiveness.
• Instruct patient to wash inhaler with warm, soapy water at least once a week; remove canister before washing.
• Warn patient to discontinue drug immediately and notify doctor if paradoxical bronchospasm occurs.
• Warn patient that tolerance may develop with prolonged use.

---

**theophylline**
*Immediate-release liquids:*
Accurbron*, Aerolate, Aquaphyllin, Asmalix*, Bronkodyl*, Elixomin*, Elixophyllin*, Lanophyllin*, Slo-Phyllin, Theoclear-80, Theolair Liquid, Theostat 80*

*Immediate-release tablets and capsules:*
Bronkodyl, Elixophyllin, Nuelin‡, Quibron-T Dividose, Slo-Phyllin

*Timed-release tablets:*
Constant-T, Lasma§, Quibron-T/SR, Respbid, Sustaire, Theochron, Theo-Dur, Theolair-SR, Theo-Sav, Theo-Time, T-Phyl, Uni-Dur, Uniphyl, Uniphyllin Continus§

*Timed-release capsules:*
Aerolate, Elixophyllin SR, Nuelin-SR‡, Slo-bid Gyrocaps, Slo-Phyllin, Theobid Duracaps, Theochron, Theoclear L.A., Theo-Dur Sprinkle, Theospan-SR, Theo-24, Theovent Long-Acting

*Pregnancy Risk Category C*

**HOW SUPPLIED**
*Tablets:* 100 mg, 125 mg, 200 mg, 250 mg, 300 mg
*Tablets (chewable):* 100 mg
*Tablets (extended-release):* 100 mg, 200 mg, 250 mg, 300 mg, 400 mg, 450 mg, 500 mg, 600 mg
*Capsules:* 100 mg, 200 mg
*Capsules (extended-release):* 50 mg, 60 mg, 65 mg, 75 mg, 100 mg, 125 mg,

---

*Liquid contains alcohol.   **May contain tartrazine.   †Canada   ‡Australia   §U.K.   ◇OTC

130 mg, 200 mg, 250 mg, 260 mg, 300 mg
*Elixir:* 27 mg/5 ml*, 50 mg/5 ml*
*Oral solution:* 27 mg/5 ml, 50 mg/5 ml
*Syrup:* 27 mg/5 ml, 50 mg/5 ml
*Dextrose 5% injection:* 200 mg in 50 ml or 100 ml; 400 mg in 100 ml, 250 ml, 500 ml, or 1,000 ml; 800 mg in 500 ml or 1,000 ml

## ACTION
Inhibits phosphodiesterase, the enzyme that degrades cAMP, resulting in relaxation of smooth muscle of the bronchial airways and pulmonary blood vessels.

| Route | Onset | Peak | Duration |
|---|---|---|---|
| P.O. | 15-60 min | 1-2 hr | Unknown |
| P.O. (extended) | 15-60 min | 4-7 hr | Unknown |
| I.V. | 15 min | 15-30 min | Unknown |

## INDICATIONS & DOSAGE
Extended-release preparations shouldn't be used to treat acute bronchospasm.
*Oral theophylline for acute bronchospasm in patients not currently receiving theophylline—*
**Adults (nonsmokers):** 5 mg/kg P.O., followed by 3 mg/kg q 6 hours for two doses. Maintenance dose is 3 mg/kg q 8 hours.
**Children ages 9 to 16:** 5 mg/kg P.O., followed by 3 mg/kg q 4 hours for three doses. Maintenance dose is 3 mg/kg q 6 hours.
**Children ages 6 months to 9 years:** 5 mg/kg P.O., followed by 4 mg/kg q 4 hours for three doses. Maintenance dose is 4 mg/kg q 6 hours.
*Adjust-a-dose:* For otherwise healthy adult smokers, 5 mg/kg P.O., followed by 3 mg/kg q 4 hours for three doses. Maintenance dose is 3 mg/kg q 6 hours.
For older adults and patients with cor pulmonale, 5 mg/kg P.O., followed by 2 mg/kg q 6 hours for two doses. Maintenance dose is 2 mg/kg q 8 hours.
For adults with heart failure or liver disease, 5 mg/kg P.O., followed by 2 mg/kg q 8 hours for two doses. Maintenance dose is 1 to 2 mg/kg q 12 hours.

*Parenteral theophylline for patients not currently receiving theophylline—*
**Loading dose:** 4.7 mg/kg I.V. slowly; then maintenance infusion.
**Adults (nonsmokers):** 0.55 mg/kg/hour I.V. for 12 hours; then 0.39 mg/kg/hour.
**Children ages 9 to 16:** 0.79 mg/kg/hour I.V. for 12 hours; then 0.63 mg/kg/hour.
**Children ages 6 months to 9 years:** 0.95 mg/kg/hour I.V. for 12 hours; then 0.79 mg/kg/hour.
*Adjust-a-dose:* For otherwise healthy adult smokers, 0.79 mg/kg/hour I.V. for 12 hours; then 0.63 mg/kg/hour.
For older adults and patients with cor pulmonale, 0.47 mg/kg/hour I.V. for 12 hours; then 0.24 mg/kg/hour.
For adults with heart failure or liver disease, 0.39 mg/kg/hour I.V. for 12 hours; then 0.08 to 0.16 mg/kg/hour.
*Oral and parenteral theophylline for acute bronchospasm in patients currently receiving theophylline—*
**Adults and children:** each 0.5 mg/kg I.V. or P.O. (loading dose) will increase plasma levels by 1 mcg/ml. Ideally, dose is based on current theophylline level. In emergency situations, some clinicians recommend a 2.5 mg/kg P.O. dose of rapidly absorbed form if no obvious signs of theophylline toxicity are present.
*Chronic bronchospasm—*
**Adults and children:** initially, 16 mg/kg or 400 mg P.O. daily (whichever is less) given in three or four divided doses at 6- to 8-hour intervals. Or, 12 mg/kg or 400 mg P.O. daily (whichever is less) in an extended-release preparation given in two or three divided doses at 8- or 12-hour intervals. Dosage may be increased as tolerated at 2- to 3-day intervals to maximum dose as follows:
**Adults and children ages 16 and older:** 13 mg/kg or 900 mg P.O. daily (whichever is less).
**Children ages 12 to 16:** 18 mg/kg P.O. daily.
**Children ages 9 to 12:** 20 mg/kg P.O. daily.
**Children under age 9:** 24 mg/kg P.O. daily.

---

Reactions may be *common*, uncommon, *life-threatening*, or COMMON AND LIFE-THREATENING.

## ADVERSE REACTIONS
**CNS:** *restlessness, dizziness,* headache, *insomnia,* irritability, **seizures,** muscle twitching.
**CV:** *palpitations, sinus tachycardia,* extrasystoles, flushing, marked hypotension, **arrhythmias.**
**GI:** *nausea, vomiting,* diarrhea, epigastric pain.
**Metabolic:** increased plasma levels of free fatty acids and urinary catecholamines.
**Respiratory:** tachypnea, *respiratory arrest.*

## INTERACTIONS
**Drug-drug.** *Adenosine:* decreased antiarrhythmic effectiveness. Higher doses of adenosine may be needed.
*Allopurinol, calcium channel blockers, cimetidine, disulfiram, influenza virus vaccine, interferon, macrolide antibiotics (such as erythromycin), methotrexate, oral contraceptives, quinolone antibiotics (such as ciprofloxacin):* decreased hepatic clearance of theophylline; elevated theophylline levels. Monitor for signs of toxicity.
*Barbiturates, nicotine, phenytoin, rifampin:* enhanced metabolism and decreased theophylline blood levels. Monitor for decreased effect.
*Beta blockers:* antagonism. Nadolol and propranolol, especially, may cause bronchospasm in sensitive patients. Use together cautiously.
*Carbamazepine, isoniazid, loop diuretics:* may increase or decrease theophylline levels. Monitor closely.
*Ephedrine, other sympathomimetics:* may exhibit synergistic toxicity with these drugs, predisposing patients to arrhythmias. Monitor patient closely.
*Lithium:* may increase lithium excretion. Monitor patient closely.
**Drug-herb.** *Cacao tree:* possible inhibition of theophylline metabolism. Avoid concomitant ingestion of large amounts of cocoa.
*Guarana:* may cause additive CNS and CV effects. Avoid concomitant use of guarana and other sources of caffeine.
**Drug-food.** *Any food:* accelerated release of theophylline from SR products. Tell patient to take Theo-24 on an empty stomach.
*Caffeine:* decreased hepatic clearance of theophylline; elevated theophylline levels. Monitor for signs of toxicity.
**Drug-lifestyle.** *Smoking:* increased elimination of theophylline, increasing dosage requirements. Monitor theophylline response and serum levels.

## EFFECTS ON DIAGNOSTIC TESTS
Depending on assay used, theophylline levels may be falsely elevated in the presence of furosemide, phenylbutazone, probenecid, theobromine, caffeine, tea, chocolate, cola beverages, and acetaminophen.

## CONTRAINDICATIONS
Contraindicated in patients with hypersensitivity to xanthine compounds (caffeine, theobromine) and in those with active peptic ulcer or poorly controlled seizure disorders.

## NURSING CONSIDERATIONS
• Use cautiously in young children, infants under age 1, and neonates; in elderly patients; and in those with COPD, cardiac failure, cor pulmonale, renal or hepatic disease, peptic ulceration, hyperthyroidism, diabetes mellitus, glaucoma, severe hypoxemia, hypertension, compromised cardiac or circulatory function, angina, acute MI, or sulfite sensitivity.
• *Alert:* Don't confuse extended-release forms with regular-release forms.
• Dosage may need to be increased in cigarette smokers and in habitual marijuana smokers because smoking causes the drug to be metabolized faster.
• Give drug around-the-clock, using extended-release product at bedtime, as ordered.
• Monitor vital signs; measure and record fluid intake and output. Expected clinical effects include improved quality of pulse and respirations.
• People metabolize xanthines at different rates; dosage is determined by monitoring response, tolerance, pulmonary function, and serum theophylline levels. Serum theophylline levels should range from 10

---

to 20 mcg/ml; toxicity has been reported with levels above 20 mcg/ml.

• *Alert:* Signs and symptoms of toxicity include tachycardia, anorexia, nausea, vomiting, diarrhea, restlessness, irritability, and headache. The presence of any of these signs in patients taking theophylline warrants checking theophylline levels and adjusting dose as indicated.

• *Alert:* Don't confuse Theolair with Thyrolar.

## I.V. administration
• Use commercially available infusion solution, or mix in $D_5W$. Use infusion pump for continuous infusion.

## Patient teaching
• Supply instructions for home care and dosage schedule.

• Warn patient not to dissolve, crush, or chew extended-release products. Small children unable to swallow these can ingest (without chewing) the contents of capsules sprinkled over soft food.

• Tell patient to relieve GI symptoms by taking oral drug with full glass of water after meals, although food in stomach delays absorption.

• Warn patient to take drug regularly, as directed. Patients tend to want to take extra "breathing pills."

• Inform elderly patient that dizziness, a common adverse reaction at start of therapy, may occur.

• Warn patient to check with doctor or pharmacist about *any* other drugs used. OTC remedies may contain ephedrine in combination with theophylline salts; excessive CNS stimulation may result.

**benzonatate**
**codeine phosphate**
  (See Chapter 28, NARCOTIC AND OPIOID ANALGESICS
**codeine sulfate**
  (See Chapter 28, NARCOTIC AND OPIOID ANALGESICS.)
**dextromethorphan hydrobromide**
**diphenhydramine hydrochloride**
  (See Chapter 43, ANTIHISTAMINES.)
**guaifenesin**
**hydromorphone hydrochloride**
  (See Chapter 28, NARCOTIC AND OPIOID ANALGESICS.)

## COMBINATION PRODUCTS
Preparations are available in the following combinations:
• expectorants with decongestants or antihistamines, or both
• antitussives with decongestants or antihistamines, or both
• expectorants and antitussives
• expectorants and antitussives with decongestants or antihistamines, or both

---

**benzonatate**
Tessalon Perles

*Pregnancy Risk Category C*

## HOW SUPPLIED
*Capsules:* 100 mg

## ACTION
Chemical relative of tetracaine that suppresses the cough reflex by direct action on the cough center in the medulla and through an anesthetic action on stretch receptors of vagal afferent fibers in the respiratory passages, lungs, and pleura.

| Route | Onset | Peak | Duration |
|-------|-------|------|----------|
| P.O. | 15-20 min | Unknown | 3-8 hr |

## INDICATIONS & DOSAGE
*Symptomatic relief of cough—*
**Adults and children over age 10:** 100 mg P.O. t.i.d.; up to 600 mg daily may be needed.
**Children ages 10 and younger:** 8 mg/kg daily in three to six divided doses.

## ADVERSE REACTIONS
**CNS:** dizziness, headache, sedation.
**EENT:** nasal congestion, burning sensation in eyes.
**GI:** nausea, constipation, GI upset.
**Other:** chills, *hypersensitivity reactions.*

## INTERACTIONS
None significant.

## EFFECTS ON DIAGNOSTIC TESTS
None reported.

## CONTRAINDICATIONS
Contraindicated in patients with hypersensitivity to drug or related compounds.

## NURSING CONSIDERATIONS
• Use cautiously in patients hypersensitive to PABA anesthetics (procaine, tetracaine) because cross-sensitivity reactions may occur.
• Don't use benzonatate when cough is a valuable diagnostic sign or is beneficial (as after thoracic surgery).
• Monitor cough type and frequency.
• Use with percussion and chest vibration.

### ☑ Patient teaching
• Warn patient not to chew capsules or dissolve in mouth. Produces either local anesthesia that may result in aspiration or CNS stimulation that may cause restlessness, tremor, and seizures.
• Instruct patient to report adverse reactions.
• Instruct patient to protect drug from light and moisture.
• *Alert:* Make sure patient understands that persistent cough may indicate a serious condition and that he should contact a doctor if cough lasts longer than 1 week, recurs frequently, or is associated with high fever, rash, or severe headache.

# dextromethorphan hydrobromide

Balminil D.M.◇, Benylin DM◇, Broncho-Grippol-DM†, Buckley's Mixture, Children's Hold◇, Delsym, DM Syrup◇, Hold◇, Koffex DM†, Mediquell◇, Neo-DM†, Ornex-DM 15◇, Ornex-DM 30◇, Pertussin Cough Suppressant◇, Pertussin CS◇, Pertussin ES◇, Robidex†, Robitussin Pediatric◇, Sedatuss†, St. Joseph Cough Suppressant for Children◇, Sucrets Cough Control Formula◇, Trocal◇, Vicks Formula 44 Pediatric Formula◇

*More available in combination products, such as* Anti-Tuss DM Expectorant◇, Benylin Expectorant◇, Cheracol D Cough◇, Extra Action Cough◇, Glycotuss-dM◇, Guiamid D.M. Liquid◇, Guiatuss-DM◇, Halotussin-DM◇, Kolephrin GG/DM◇, Mytussin DM◇, Naldecon Senior DX◇, Pertussin CS◇, Rhinosyn-DMX Expectorant◇, Robitussin-DM◇, Scot-Tussin DM Cough Chasers◇, Silexin Cough◇, Tolu-Sed DM◇, Tuss-DM◇, Unproco◇, Vicks Pediatric Formula 44e◇

*Pregnancy Risk Category C*

## HOW SUPPLIED
*Liquid (extended-release):* 30 mg/5 ml◇
*Lozenges:* 5 mg◇, 7.5 mg◇
*Solution:* 3.5 mg/5 ml, 5 mg/5 ml*◇, 7.5 mg/5 ml◇, 10 mg/5 ml*◇, 15 mg/5 ml*◇, 15 mg/15 ml*◇, 12.5 mg/5 ml

## ACTION
Antitussive that suppresses the cough reflex by direct action on the cough center in the medulla.

| Route | Onset | Peak | Duration |
|-------|-------|------|----------|
| P.O. | < 0.5 hr | Unknown | 3-6 hr |

## INDICATIONS & DOSAGE
*Nonproductive cough—*
**Adults and children ages 12 and older:** 10 to 20 mg P.O. q 4 hours, or 30 mg q 6 to 8 hours. Or, 60 mg extended-release liquid b.i.d. Maximum dose is 120 mg daily.
**Children ages 6 to 12:** 5 to 10 mg P.O. q 4 hours, or 15 mg q 6 to 8 hours. Or, 30 mg extended-release liquid b.i.d. Maximum dose is 60 mg daily.
**Children ages 2 to 6:** 2.5 to 5 mg P.O. q 4 hours, or 7.5 mg q 6 to 8 hours. Or, 15 mg extended-release liquid b.i.d. Maximum dose is 30 mg daily.
**Children under age 2:** dosages must be individualized.

## ADVERSE REACTIONS
**CNS:** drowsiness, dizziness.
**GI:** nausea, vomiting, stomach pain.

## INTERACTIONS
**Drug-drug.** *MAO inhibitors:* risk of hypotension, coma, hyperpyrexia, and death. Avoid concomitant use.
*Selegiline:* risk of confusion, coma, hyperpyrexia. Avoid concurrent use.
**Drug-herb.** *Parsley:* may promote or produce serotonin syndrome. Avoid concomitant use.

## EFFECTS ON DIAGNOSTIC TESTS
None reported.

## CONTRAINDICATIONS
Contraindicated in patients currently taking MAO inhibitors or within 2 weeks of discontinuing MAO inhibitors.

## NURSING CONSIDERATIONS
• Use with caution in atopic children, sedated or debilitated patients, and patients confined to the supine position. Also use cautiously in patients with sensitivity to aspirin or tartrazine dyes.
• Don't use dextromethorphan when cough is a valuable diagnostic sign or is beneficial (as after thoracic surgery).
• Dextromethorphan 15 to 30 mg is equivalent to 8 to 15 mg codeine as an antitussive.
• Drug produces no analgesia or addiction and little or no CNS depression.

• Use drug with chest percussion and vibration.
• Monitor cough type and frequency.

### ☑ Patient teaching
• Instruct patient to take exactly as prescribed.
• Tell patient to report adverse reactions.
• *Alert:* Make sure patient understands that persistent cough may indicate a serious condition and that he should contact a doctor if cough lasts longer than 1 week, recurs frequently, or is associated with high fever, rash, or severe headache.

---

## guaifenesin
## (glyceryl guaiacolate)
Anti-Tuss* ◊, Balminil Expectorant†, Breonesin ◊, Fenesin, Gee-Gee ◊, GG-CEN* ◊, Glyate* ◊, Glycotuss ◊, Glytuss ◊, Guiatuss* ◊, Halotussin, Humibid L.A., Humibid Sprinkle, Hytuss ◊, Hytuss-2X ◊, Naldecon Senior EX ◊, Resyl† ◊, Robitussin* ◊, Scot-Tussin Expectorant ◊, Uni-tussin* ◊

*Pregnancy Risk Category C*

### HOW SUPPLIED
*Tablets:* 100 mg ◊, 200 mg ◊
*Tablets (extended-release):* 600 mg
*Capsules:* 200 mg ◊
*Capsules (extended-release):* 300 mg
*Solution:* 100 mg/5 ml* ◊, 200 mg/5 ml ◊

### ACTION
Increases production of respiratory tract fluids to help liquefy and reduce the viscosity of tenacious secretions.

| Route | Onset | Peak | Duration |
| --- | --- | --- | --- |
| P.O. | Unknown | Unknown | Unknown |

### INDICATIONS & DOSAGE
*Expectorant—*
**Adults and children ages 12 and older:** 200 to 400 mg P.O. q 4 hours, or 600 to 1,200 mg extended-release capsules or tablets q 12 hours. Maximum dose is 2,400 mg daily.

**Children ages 6 to 12:** 100 to 200 mg P.O. q 4 hours. Maximum dose is 1,200 mg daily.
**Children ages 2 to 6:** 50 to 100 mg P.O. q 4 hours. Maximum dose is 600 mg daily.

### ADVERSE REACTIONS
**CNS:** dizziness, headache.
**GI:** vomiting, nausea.
**Skin:** rash.

### INTERACTIONS
None significant.

### EFFECTS ON DIAGNOSTIC TESTS
Drug may cause color interference with tests for 5-hydroxyindoleacetic acid and vanillylmandelic acid.

### CONTRAINDICATIONS
Contraindicated in patients with hypersensitivity to drug.

### NURSING CONSIDERATIONS
• Drug is used to liquefy thick, tenacious sputum. There is evidence that guaifenesin is effective as an expectorant but no evidence to support its role as an antitussive.
• Monitor cough type and frequency.
• *Alert:* Don't confuse guaifenesin with guanfacine.

### ☑ Patient teaching
• *Alert:* Make sure patient understands that persistent cough may indicate a serious condition and that he should contact a doctor if cough lasts longer than 1 week, recurs frequently, or is associated with high fever, rash, or severe headache.
• Inform patient that drug shouldn't be used for chronic or persistent cough such as that occurring with smoking, asthma, chronic bronchitis, or emphysema.
• Advise patient to take each dose with one glass of water; increasing fluid intake may prove beneficial.
• Encourage deep-breathing exercises.

---

acetylcysteine
beclomethasone dipropionate
beractant
budesonide
calfactant
cromolyn sodium
dornase alfa
epoprostenol sodium
flunisolide
fluticasone propionate
montelukast sodium
nedocromil sodium
palivizumab
triamcinolone acetonide
zafirlukast
zileuton

**COMBINATION PRODUCTS**
None.

---

## acetylcysteine
Mucomyst, Mucomyst-10,
Mucosil-10, Mucosil-20,
Parvolex†‡

*Pregnancy Risk Category B*

**HOW SUPPLIED**
*Solution:* 10%, 20%
*Injection:* 200 mg/ml‡

**ACTION**
Mucolytic that reduces the viscosity of pulmonary secretions by splitting disulfide linkages between mucoprotein molecular complexes. Also, restores liver stores of glutathione to treat acetaminophen toxicity.

| Route | Onset | Peak | Duration |
|-------|-------|------|----------|
| P.O., I.V., inhalation | Unknown | Unknown | Unknown |

**INDICATIONS & DOSAGE**
*Adjuvant therapy for abnormal viscid or inspissated mucus secretions in patients with pneumonia, bronchitis, bronchiectasis, primary amyloidosis of the lung, tuberculosis, cystic fibrosis, emphysema, atelectasis (adjunct), pulmonary complications of thoracic surgery, and CV surgery—*
**Adults and children:** 1 to 2 ml 10% or 20% solution by direct instillation into trachea as often as q hour; or 1 to 10 ml of 20% solution or 2 to 20 ml of 10% solution by nebulization q 2 to 6 hours, p.r.n.
*Acetaminophen toxicity—*
P.O.—
**Adults and children:** initially, 140 mg/kg P.O., followed by 70 mg/kg P.O. q 4 hours for 17 doses.
I.V.‡—
**Adults:** dilute initial dose (150 mg/kg) in 200 ml of $D_5W$ and infuse over 15 minutes. Dilute second dose of 50 mg/kg in 500 ml of $D_5W$ and give over 4 hours. Dilute final dose of 100 mg/kg in 1,000 ml of $D_5W$ and infuse over 16 hours.

**ADVERSE REACTIONS**
**CV:** tachycardia, hypotension, hypertension, chest tightness.
**EENT:** *rhinorrhea.*
**GI:** *stomatitis, nausea, vomiting.*
**Respiratory:** *bronchospasm* (especially in asthmatic patients).
**Skin:** rash.
**Other:** fever, clamminess, *angioedema.*

**INTERACTIONS**
**Drug-drug.** *Activated charcoal:* limits acetylcysteine's effectiveness. Avoid concomitant use in treating acetaminophen toxicity or lavage before administering acetylcysteine.

**EFFECTS ON DIAGNOSTIC TESTS**
None reported.

**CONTRAINDICATIONS**
Contraindicated in patients with hypersensitivity to drug.

---

Reactions may be *common*, uncommon, *life-threatening*, or COMMON AND LIFE-THREATENING.

## NURSING CONSIDERATIONS

• Use cautiously in elderly or debilitated patients with severe respiratory insufficiency.

• Use plastic, glass, stainless steel, or another nonreactive metal when administering by nebulization. Hand-bulb nebulizers aren't recommended because output is too small and particle size too large.

• Drug is physically or chemically incompatible with tetracyclines, erythromycin lactobionate, amphotericin B, and ampicillin sodium. If administered by aerosol inhalation, these drugs should be nebulized separately. Iodized oil, trypsin, and hydrogen peroxide are physically incompatible with acetylcysteine; don't add to nebulizer.

• Monitor cough type and frequency.

• After opening, store in refrigerator; use within 96 hours.

• *Alert:* Acetylcysteine is administered to treat acetaminophen overdose within 24 hours after ingestion. Start treatment immediately as prescribed; don't wait for results of acetaminophen blood levels.

• When used orally to treat acetaminophen overdose, dilute oral doses with cola, fruit juice, or water before administering. Dilute the 20% solution to a concentration of 5% (add 3 ml of diluent to each ml of acetylcysteine). If patient vomits within 1 hour of receiving loading or maintenance dose, repeat dose.

• *Alert:* Don't confuse acetylcysteine with acetylcholine.

### ⬛ I.V. administration‡

• To prepare I.V. infusion, dilute calculated dose in $D_5W$.

### ☑ Patient teaching

• Warn patient that drug may have a foul taste or smell that some patients find distressing.

• For maximum effect, instruct patient to clear his airway by coughing before aerosol administration.

# beclomethasone dipropionate
Beclodisk†, Becloforte Inhaler‡, Beclovent, Beclovent Rotacaps†, Vanceril

*Pregnancy Risk Category C*

## HOW SUPPLIED
*Oral inhalation aerosol:* 42 mcg/metered spray, 50 mcg/metered spray‡

## ACTION
Unknown. May decrease inflammation by decreasing the number and activity of inflammatory cells, inhibiting bronchoconstrictor mechanisms producing direct smooth-muscle relaxation, and decreasing airway hyperresponsiveness.

| Route | Onset | Peak | Duration |
|-------|-------|------|----------|
| Inhalation | 1-4 wk | Unknown | Unknown |

## INDICATIONS & DOSAGE
*Chronic asthma—*
**Adults and children ages 12 and older:** 2 inhalations t.i.d. or q.i.d.; or 4 inhalations b.i.d. Maximum dose is 20 inhalations daily (840 mcg).
**Children ages 6 to 12:** 1 to 2 inhalations t.i.d. or q.i.d.; or 2 to 4 inhalations b.i.d. Maximum dose is 10 inhalations daily (420 mcg).

## ADVERSE REACTIONS
**EENT:** *hoarseness,* fungal infection of throat, *throat irritation.*
**GI:** dry mouth, *fungal infection of mouth.*
**Respiratory:** *bronchospasm,* wheezing, cough.
**Other:** *angioedema, hypersensitivity reactions,* suppression of hypothalamic-pituitary-adrenal function, *adrenal insufficiency,* facial edema.

## INTERACTIONS
None significant.

## EFFECTS ON DIAGNOSTIC TESTS
None reported.

## CONTRAINDICATIONS
Contraindicated in patients with hypersensitivity to drug or its ingredients (fluo-

rocarbons, oleic acid) and in those with status asthmaticus.

## NURSING CONSIDERATIONS

• Use with extreme caution, if at all, in patients with tuberculosis, fungal or bacterial infections, ocular herpes simplex, or systemic viral infections.
• Don't use drug in patients with asthma controlled by bronchodilators or other noncorticosteroids alone or for those with nonasthmatic bronchial diseases.
• Use with caution in patients receiving systemic corticosteroid therapy.
• A spacer device may help ensure delivery of the proper dose and decrease local (oral) adverse effects.
• Check mucous membranes frequently for signs of fungal infection.
• During times of stress (trauma, surgery, or infection), systemic corticosteroids may be needed to prevent adrenal insufficiency in previously steroid-dependent patients.
• Periodic measurement of growth and development may be needed during high-dose or prolonged therapy in children.
• *Alert:* Taper oral glucocorticoid therapy slowly, as ordered. Acute adrenal insufficiency and death have occurred in asthmatics who changed abruptly from oral corticosteroids to beclomethasone.
• *Alert:* Don't confuse Vanceril with Vansil.

### ✓ Patient teaching

• Inform patient that drug doesn't provide relief for acute asthma attacks.
• Tell patient requiring a bronchodilator to use it several minutes before beclomethasone.
• Instruct patient to carry a medical identification card indicating his need for supplemental systemic glucocorticoids during stress.
• If using a metered-dose inhaler, instruct patient to shake canister well before use.
• Advise patient to allow 1 minute to elapse before taking subsequent puffs of drug and to hold his breath for a few seconds to enhance action of drug.
• Instruct patient to contact his doctor if response to therapy decreases or if symptoms don't improve within 3 weeks; dosage may need to be adjusted. Tell him

not to exceed recommended dosage on his own.
• Tell patient to keep inhaler clean and unobstructed. He should wash it with warm water and dry it thoroughly.
• Advise patient to prevent oral fungal infections by gargling or rinsing mouth with water after each use, but not to swallow the water.
• Tell patient to report symptoms associated with corticosteroid withdrawal, including fatigue, weakness, arthralgia, orthostatic hypotension, and dyspnea.
• Instruct patient to store drug between 59° and 86° F (15° and 30° C). Advise patient to ensure delivery of proper dose by gently warming canister to room temperature before using.

---

## beractant
## (natural lung surfactant)
Survanta

*Pregnancy Risk Category NR*

## HOW SUPPLIED
*Suspension for intratracheal instillation:* 25 mg/ml

## ACTION
Lowers the surface tension on alveolar surfaces during respiration and stabilizes the alveoli against collapse. It's an extract of bovine lung containing neutral lipids, fatty acids, surfactant-associated proteins, and phospholipids, which mimics naturally occurring surfactant; palmitic acid, tripalmitin, and colfosceril palmitate are added to standardize the solution's composition.

| Route | Onset | Peak | Duration |
|-------|-------|------|----------|
| Intra-tracheal | 0.5-2 hr | Unknown | 2-3 days |

## INDICATIONS & DOSAGE
*Prevention of respiratory distress syndrome (RDS), also known as hyaline membrane disease, in premature neonates weighing 1,250 g (2 lb, 12 oz) or less at birth or having symptoms consistent with surfactant deficiency—*
**Neonates:** 4 ml/kg intratracheally. Divide each dose into four quarter-doses and ad-

minister each quarter-dose with infant in a different position to ensure homogenous distribution of drug; between quarter-doses, use a handheld resuscitation bag at a rate of 60 breaths/minute and sufficient oxygen to prevent cyanosis. Give drug as soon as possible, preferably within 15 minutes of birth. Repeat in 6 hours if respiratory distress continues. Give no more than four doses in 48 hours.

*Rescue treatment of RDS in premature infants—*
**Neonates:** 4 ml/kg intratracheally; before administering, increase ventilator rate to 60 breaths/minute with an inspiratory time of 0.5 second and a fraction of inspired oxygen of 1. Divide each dose into four quarter-doses and administer each quarter-dose with infant in a different position to ensure homogenous distribution of drug; between quarter-doses, continue mechanical ventilation for at least 30 seconds or until stable. Give dose as soon as RDS is confirmed by X-ray, preferably within 8 hours of birth. Repeat in 6 hours if respiratory distress continues. Give no more than four doses in 48 hours.

**ADVERSE REACTIONS**
**CV:** *transient bradycardia,* vasoconstriction, hypotension.
**Hematologic:** decreased oxygen saturation, hypocapnia, hypercapnia.
**Respiratory:** endotracheal tube reflux or blockage, *apnea.*
**Skin:** pallor.

**INTERACTIONS**
None significant.

**EFFECTS ON DIAGNOSTIC TESTS**
None reported.

**CONTRAINDICATIONS**
No known contraindications.

**NURSING CONSIDERATIONS**
• Beractant should be administered only by personnel experienced in the care of clinically unstable premature neonates. Such personnel should have knowledge of neonatal intubation and airway management.

• Accurate determination of weight is essential to proper measurement of dosage.
• Continuously monitor neonate before, during, and after beractant administration. The endotracheal tube may be suctioned before giving drug; allow neonate to stabilize before proceeding with administration.
• Refrigerate at 36° to 46° F (2° to 8° C). Warm before administration by allowing drug to stand at room temperature for at least 20 minutes or by holding in hand for at least 8 minutes. Don't use artificial warming methods. Unopened vials that have been warmed to room temperature may be returned to the refrigerator within 8 hours; however, warm and return drug to the refrigerator only once. Vials are for single use only—discard unused drug.
• Beractant doesn't need sonication or reconstitution before use. Inspect contents before giving; ensure that the color is off-white to light brown and the contents are uniform. If settling occurs, swirl vial gently; don't shake. Some foaming is normal.
• Use a large-bore needle (20G or larger) to draw up drug; don't use a filter. Administer drug using a #5 French end-hole catheter. Premeasure and shorten catheter before use. Fill catheter with beractant and discard excess drug so that only total dose to be given remains in the syringe. Insert catheter into neonate's endotracheal tube; make sure catheter tip protrudes just beyond end of tube above neonate's carina. Don't instill drug into a mainstream bronchus.
• Homogeneous distribution of drug is important. For example, give each dose of drug in four quarter-doses, with each quarter-dose being given over 2 to 3 seconds and with the patient positioned differently after each administration. Between administration of quarter-doses, remove the catheter and ventilate the patient. Give the first quarter-dose with the patient's head and body inclined slightly downward, and the head turned to the right; give the second quarter-dose with the head turned to the left. Then, incline the head and body slightly upward with the head turned to the right to give

the third quarter-dose; turn the head to the left for the fourth quarter-dose.
• Immediately after administration, moist breath sounds and crackles can occur. Don't suction the neonate for 1 hour unless other signs of airway obstruction are evident.
• Continuous monitoring of ECG and transcutaneous oxygen saturation are essential; frequent arterial blood pressure monitoring and frequent arterial blood gas sampling are highly desirable.
• Transient bradycardia and oxygen desaturation are common after dosing.
• *Alert:* Beractant can rapidly affect oxygenation and lung compliance. Peak ventilator inspiratory pressures may need to be adjusted if chest expansion improves substantially after drug administration. Notify doctor and adjust immediately as directed because lung overdistention and fatal pulmonary air leakage may result.
• Audiovisual materials that describe dosage and administration procedures are available from the manufacturer.
• *Alert:* Don't confuse Survanta with Sufenta.

☑**Patient teaching**
• Inform parents of need for drug and explain drug action and administration.
• Encourage parents to ask questions and address any concerns raised by them.

---

# budesonide
Pulmicort Turbuhaler

*Pregnancy Risk Category C*

## HOW SUPPLIED
*Dry powder inhaler:* 200 mcg/dose

## ACTION
Anti-inflammatory corticosteroid that exhibits potent glucocorticoid activity and weak mineralocorticoid activity. The exact mechanism of the corticosteroids isn't known, but they have been shown to have a wide range of inhibitory activities against such cell types as mast cells and macrophages and mediators such as leukotrienes involved in allergic and non-allergic inflammation.

| Route | Onset | Peak | Duration |
|-------|-------|------|----------|
| Inhalation | 24 hr | 1-2 wk | Unknown |

## INDICATIONS & DOSAGE
*Prophylactic therapy in maintenance treatment of asthma—*
In all patients, use lowest effective dose after stabilization of asthma has occurred.
**Adults previously on bronchodilators alone:** initially, inhaled dose of 200 to 400 mcg b.i.d. to maximum of 400 mcg b.i.d.
**Adults previously on inhaled corticosteroids:** initially, inhaled dose of 200 to 400 mcg b.i.d. to maximum of 800 mcg b.i.d.
**Adults previously on oral corticosteroids:** initially, inhaled dose of 400 to 800 mcg b.i.d. to maximum of 800 mcg b.i.d.
**Children over age 6 previously on bronchodilators alone or inhaled corticosteroids:** initially, inhaled dose of 200 mcg b.i.d. to maximum of 400 mcg b.i.d.
**Children over age 6 previously on oral corticosteroids:** highest recommended dose is 400 mcg b.i.d.

## ADVERSE REACTIONS
**CNS:** *headache,* asthenia, pain, insomnia, syncope, hypertonia.
**EENT:** *sinusitis, pharyngitis,* rhinitis, voice alteration.
**GI:** oral candidiasis, dyspepsia, gastroenteritis, nausea, dry mouth, taste perversion, vomiting, abdominal pain.
**Metabolic:** weight gain.
**Musculoskeletal:** back pain, fractures, myalgia.
**Respiratory:** *respiratory tract infections,* increased cough, **bronchospasm.**
**Other:** ecchymosis, flulike symptoms, fever, **hypersensitivity reactions.**

## INTERACTIONS
**Drug-drug.** *Ketoconazole:* may inhibit metabolism of budesonide and increase plasma levels. Monitor patient.

---

**EFFECTS ON DIAGNOSTIC TESTS**
None reported.

**CONTRAINDICATIONS**
Contraindicated in patients with hypersensitivity to drug and in the treatment of status asthmaticus or other acute episodes of asthma.

**NURSING CONSIDERATIONS**
• Use cautiously, if at all, in patients with active or quiescent tuberculosis of the respiratory tract; untreated systemic fungal, bacterial, viral, or parasitic infections; or ocular herpes simplex.
• When transferring from systemic steroid to budesonide, use caution and gradually decrease steroid dose to prevent adrenal insufficiency.
• Drug doesn't replace the need for systemic corticosteroid therapy in some situations.
• If bronchospasm occurs after using the budesonide, stop therapy and treat with a bronchodilator.
   *Note:* Improved lung function has been observed within 24 hours of initiating treatment with budesonide, although the maximum benefit may not be achieved for 1 to 2 weeks or longer.
• Watch for *Candida* infections of the mouth or pharynx.
• *Alert:* Corticosteroids may increase risk of developing serious or fatal infections in individuals exposed to viral illnesses, such as chickenpox or measles.
• In rare cases, inhaled steroids have been associated with increased intraocular pressure and cataract development. If local irritation occurs with use, the product should be discontinued.

☑ **Patient teaching**
• Tell patient that the budesonide inhaler isn't a bronchodilator and isn't intended to treat acute episodes of asthma.
• Instruct patient to use the inhaler at regular intervals as follows because effectiveness depends on twice-daily administration on a regular basis:
–Pulmicort Turbuhaler must be in the upright position (mouthpiece on top) during the loading in order to provide the correct dose.

–Turbuhaler must be primed when the unit is used for the very first time. To prime, hold the unit in an upright position and turn the brown grip fully to the right, then fully to the left until it clicks. Repeat.
–To load the first dose, turn grip to the right and fully to the left until it clicks.
–On subsequent doses, load in the upright position, turn the brown grip fully to the right and then the left until it clicks.
–During inhalation, Turbuhaler must be in the upright or horizontal position.
–Don't shake inhaler.
–Place mouthpiece between lips and inhale forcefully and deeply.
–Tell patient that he may not taste the drug but this doesn't mean it isn't effective.
–Tell patient not to exhale through the Turbuhaler.
–Because of the small volume of powder, patient may not taste or sense the drug entering the lungs.
–Rinse the mouth with water without swallowing after each dose to decrease the risk of developing oral candidiasis.
–When there are 20 doses remaining in the Turbuhaler, a red mark appears in the indicator window.
–Don't use with a spacer device.
–Don't chew or bite the mouthpiece.
–Replace mouthpiece cover after use and keep it clean and dry at all times.
• Improvement in asthma control may be seen within 24 hours, although the maximum benefit may not be evident for 1 to 2 weeks. If symptoms worsen during this time, patient should contact doctor.
• Advise patient to avoid exposure to chickenpox or measles and contact doctor if there is exposure.
• Instruct patient to carry medical identification indicating need for supplementary steroids during periods of stress or an asthma attack.
• Tell patient to read and follow the patient information leaflet contained in the package.

## calfactant
Infasurf

*Pregnancy Risk Category NR*

### HOW SUPPLIED
*Intratracheal suspension:* 35 mg phospholipids and 0.65 mg proteins/ml; 6-ml vial

### ACTION
Nonpyrogenic lung surfactant that modifies alveolar surface tension, thereby stabilizing the alveoli.

| Route | Onset | Peak | Duration |
|-------|-------|------|----------|
| Intra-tracheal | 24-48 hr | Unknown | Unknown |

### INDICATIONS & DOSAGE
*Prevention of respiratory distress syndrome (RDS) in premature infants under 29 weeks of gestational age at high risk for RDS; treatment of infants under 72 hours of age in whom RDS develops (confirmed by clinical and radiologic findings) and who need endotracheal intubation—*
**Newborns:** 3 ml/kg body weight at birth intratracheally, administered in two aliquots of 1.5 ml/kg each, q 12 hours for total of three doses.

### ADVERSE REACTIONS
**CV:** BRADYCARDIA.
**Respiratory:** AIRWAY OBSTRUCTION, APNEA, *hypoventilation, cyanosis.*
**Other:** *reflux of drug into endotracheal tube,* dislodgment of endotracheal tube.

### INTERACTIONS
None significant.

### EFFECTS ON DIAGNOSTIC TESTS
None reported.

### CONTRAINDICATIONS
No known contraindications.

### NURSING CONSIDERATIONS
• Drug should be administered under supervision of doctors experienced in the acute care of newborn infants with respiratory failure who need intubation.

• Store drug at 36° to 46° F (2° to 8° C). It isn't necessary to warm drug before use.
• Unopened, unused vials that have warmed to room temperature can be returned to refrigerated storage within 24 hours for future use. Avoid repeated warming to room temperature.
• Suspension settles during storage. Gentle swirling or agitation of the vial is often needed for redispersion. *Don't shake.* Visible flecks in the suspension and foaming at the surface are normal.
• *Alert:* Drug is intended for intratracheal use only; administer to infants for prophylaxis of RDS as soon as possible after birth, preferably within 30 minutes.
• Withdraw dose into a syringe from single-use vial using a 20G or larger needle; avoid excessive foaming.
• Administer through a side-port adapter into the endotracheal tube. Two medical personnel should be present during dosing. Administer dose in two aliquots of 1.5 ml/kg each. After each aliquot is instilled, infant should be positioned on either side. Administration is made while ventilation is continued over 20 to 30 breaths for each aliquot, with small bursts timed only during the inspiratory cycles. Evaluate respiratory status and reposition infant between each aliquot.
• Monitor for reflux of drug into endotracheal tube, cyanosis, bradycardia, or airway obstruction during the dosing procedure. If these occur, stop drug and take appropriate measures to stabilize infant. After infant is stable, resume dosing with appropriate monitoring.
• After giving drug, carefully monitor infant so that oxygen therapy and ventilatory support can be modified in response to improvements in oxygenation and lung compliance.
• Each single-use vial should be entered only once; discard unused material.

### ☑ Patient teaching
• Explain to parents reason for use of drug for the prevention and treatment of RDS.
• Notify parents that although infant may improve rapidly after treatment, he may continue to need intubation and mechanical ventilation.

---

Reactions may be *common,* uncommon, *life-threatening,* or COMMON AND LIFE-THREATENING.

• Notify parents of the potential adverse effects of drug, including bradycardia, reflux into endotracheal tube, airway obstruction, cyanosis, dislodgment of endotracheal tube, and hypoventilation.
• Reassure parents that infant will be carefully monitored.

---

## cromolyn sodium (sodium cromoglycate)
Crolom, Gastrocrom, Intal, Intal Nebulizer Solution, Intal Aerosol Spray, Nasalcrom, Rynacrom†

*Pregnancy Risk Category B*

### HOW SUPPLIED
*Capsules (for oral solution):* 100 mg
*Aerosol:* 800 mcg/metered spray
*Nasal solution:* 5.2 mg/metered spray (40 mg/ml)
*Solution (for nebulization):* 20 mg/2 ml
*Ophthalmic solution:* 4%

### ACTION
Inhibits the degranulation of sensitized mast cells that occurs after a patient's exposure to specific antigens. Also inhibits release of histamine and slow-reacting substance of anaphylaxis.

| Route | Onset | Peak | Duration |
|---|---|---|---|
| P.O., inhalation, intranasal, ophthalmic | Unknown | Unknown | Unknown |

### INDICATIONS & DOSAGE
*Mild to moderate persistent asthma—*
**Adults and children ages 5 and older:** 2 metered sprays using inhaler q.i.d. at regular intervals. Or, 20 mg via nebulization q.i.d. at regular intervals.
*Prevention and treatment of seasonal and perennial allergic rhinitis—*
**Adults and children over age 6:** 1 spray in each nostril t.i.d. or q.i.d. Maximal administration is six times daily.
*Prevention of exercise-induced bronchospasm—*
**Adults and children ages 5 and older:** 2 metered sprays inhaled no more than 1 hour before anticipated exercise.

*Conjunctivitis—*
**Adults and children ages 4 and older:** 1 to 2 drops in each eye four to six times daily at regular intervals.
*Systemic mastocytosis—*
**Adults and children over age 12:** 200 mg P.O. q.i.d. before meals and h.s.
**Children ages 2 to 12:** 100 mg P.O. q.i.d. 30 minutes before meals or h.s.

### ADVERSE REACTIONS
**CNS:** dizziness, headache.
**EENT:** *irritated throat and trachea,* lacrimation, nasal congestion, pharyngeal irritation, *sneezing,* nasal burning and irritation, epistaxis.
**GI:** nausea, esophagitis, abdominal pain, *bad taste in mouth.*
**GU:** dysuria, urinary frequency.
**Musculoskeletal:** joint swelling and pain.
**Respiratory:** *bronchospasm* (after inhalation of dry powder), *cough,* wheezing, eosinophilic pneumonia.
**Skin:** rash, urticaria.
**Other:** swollen parotid gland, *angioedema.*

### INTERACTIONS
None significant.

### EFFECTS ON DIAGNOSTIC TESTS
None reported.

### CONTRAINDICATIONS
Contraindicated in patients with hypersensitivity to drug and in those experiencing acute asthma attacks and status asthmaticus.

### NURSING CONSIDERATIONS
• Administer with caution in children. Use of cromolyn oral inhalation solution isn't recommended in children under age 2; cromolyn powder or aerosol for oral inhalation, not recommended in children under age 5; cromolyn ophthalmic solution, not recommended in children under age 4; and cromolyn nasal solution, not recommended in children under age 6.
• Use inhalation form cautiously in patients with coronary artery disease or a history of arrhythmias.
• Drug (except for ophthalmic solution) should be used only when acute episode of asthma has been controlled, airway is

---

cleared, and the patient can breathe independently.
- *Alert:* Use oral cromolyn sodium in full-term neonates and infants *only* for a severe, incapacitating disease when benefits clearly outweigh risks.
- Dissolve powder in capsules for oral dose in hot water, and further dilute with cold water before ingestion. Don't mix with fruit juice, milk, or food.
- Discontinue drug if eosinophilic pneumonia (indicated by eosinophilia and infiltrates on chest X-ray) develops.
- Watch for recurrence of asthmatic symptoms when dosage is decreased, especially when corticosteroids are also used.

### ☑ Patient teaching
- Instruct patient how to administer form of drug prescribed.
- Instruct patient that full effects of drug may not be noted for 4 weeks.
- Tell patient that esophagitis may be relieved by antacids or a glass of milk.
- Warn patient using nasal solution that stinging or sneezing may occur.

---

## dornase alfa
Pulmozyme

*Pregnancy Risk Category B*

---

### HOW SUPPLIED
*Inhalation solution:* 2.5-mg ampule (1 mg/ml)

### ACTION
Hydrolyzes DNA in sputum of cystic fibrosis patients, causing decreased viscosity and elasticity of pulmonary secretions.

| Route | Onset | Peak | Duration |
|-------|-------|------|----------|
| Inhalation | 3-7 days | 9 days | Unknown |

### INDICATIONS & DOSAGE
*To improve pulmonary function and decrease the frequency of moderate to severe respiratory tract infections in patients with cystic fibrosis—*
**Adults and children ages 5 and older:** 1 ampule (2.5 mg) inhaled once daily. Treatment usually takes 10 to 15 minutes. Use drug only with an approved nebulizer.

### ADVERSE REACTIONS
**CV:** *chest pain.*
**EENT:** *pharyngitis, voice alteration,* laryngitis, conjunctivitis.
**Skin:** *rash,* urticaria.

### INTERACTIONS
None significant.

### EFFECTS ON DIAGNOSTIC TESTS
None reported.

### CONTRAINDICATIONS
Contraindicated in patients with hypersensitivity to drug or products derived from the Chinese hamster ovary cell.

### NURSING CONSIDERATIONS
- Drug is used in conjunction with other standard therapies for cystic fibrosis.
- Some patients (those over age 21 or those with forced vital capacity exceeding 85%) may benefit from twice-daily administration.
- Safety and efficacy in children under age 5 or with forced vital capacity of less than 40% of normal value, or use for more than 12 months haven't been established.
- *Alert:* Administer only with the following nebulizers and compressors: the Hudson T Up-draft II disposable jet nebulizer and the Marquest Acorn II disposable jet nebulizer along with the Pulmo-Aide compressor or the PARI LC Jet+ reusable nebulizer along with the PARI PRONEB compressor.
- Discard cloudy or discolored solution.
- Don't mix with other drugs in the nebulizer. Doing so could lead to a physical or chemical reaction that may inactivate dornase alfa.
- Refrigerate drug in its protective foil pouch to protect it from strong light.
- Once opened, the entire ampule must be used or discarded.

### ☑ Patient teaching
- Instruct patient how to administer drug at home.
- Remind patient to breathe only through his mouth when using the nebulizer. If this is difficult, suggest use of a nose clip.

---

• Tell patient that if he begins coughing during treatment to turn off nebulizer without spilling drug. To resume, he should turn on nebulizer and continue breathing through the mouthpiece until the nebulizer cup is empty or mist is no longer produced.

---

## epoprostenol sodium
Flolan

*Pregnancy Risk Category B*

### HOW SUPPLIED
*Injection:* 0.5 mg (500,000 ng)/17 ml, 1.5 mg (1,500,000 ng)/17 ml

### ACTION
Causes direct vasodilation of pulmonary and systemic arterial vascular beds and inhibits platelet aggregation.

| Route | Onset | Peak | Duration |
|-------|-------|------|----------|
| I.V. | Unknown | Unknown | Unknown |

### INDICATIONS & DOSAGE
*Long-term I.V. treatment of primary pulmonary hypertension in New York Heart Association classes III and IV patients—*
**Adults:** initially, 2 ng/kg/minute as I.V. infusion, increased in increments of 2 ng/kg/minute q 15 minutes or longer until dose-limiting pharmacologic effects are elicited. Maintenance dosing is begun with 4 ng/kg/minute less than the maximum tolerated rate determined during initial dosing. If the maximum rate is less than 5 ng/kg/minute, the maintenance infusion is started at 50% the maximum rate. Subsequent adjustments are made based on persistence, recurrence, or worsening of symptoms; such increases should be made gradually in 1- to 2-ng/kg/minute increments q 15 minutes or longer. Occurrence of adverse events from excessive doses may necessitate a gradual decrease in dosage in 2-ng/kg/minute increments q 15 minutes or longer.

### ADVERSE REACTIONS
*After initial dosing—*
**CNS:** *headache, anxiety, nervousness, agitation,* dizziness, hypoesthesia, paresthesia.
**CV:** *hypotension, chest pain,* **bradycardia,** tachycardia, *flushing.*
**GI:** *nausea, vomiting,* abdominal pain, dyspepsia.
**Musculoskeletal:** musculoskeletal pain, back pain.
**Respiratory:** dyspnea.
**Skin:** sweating.
*During maintenance dosing—*
**CNS:** *headache, anxiety, nervousness, dizziness, hypoesthesia, hyperesthesia, paresthesia, tremor.*
**CV:** *tachycardia.*
**GI:** *nausea, vomiting, diarrhea.*
**Hematologic:** *thrombocytopenia.*
**Musculoskeletal:** *jaw pain, myalgia, nonspecific musculoskeletal pain.*
**Skin:** *flushing.*
**Other:** *flulike symptoms, chills, fever,* **sepsis.**

### INTERACTIONS
**Drug-drug.** *Anticoagulants, antiplatelet drugs:* may increase risk of bleeding. Monitor closely for bleeding.
*Antihypertensives, diuretics, other vasodilators:* additional reductions in blood pressure may occur. Monitor blood pressure closely.

### EFFECTS ON DIAGNOSTIC TESTS
None reported.

### CONTRAINDICATIONS
Contraindicated in patients with hypersensitivity to drug or structurally related compounds. Long-term use is contraindicated in patients with heart failure due to severe left ventricular systolic dysfunction and in patients who develop pulmonary edema during initial dosing.

### NURSING CONSIDERATIONS
• Use cautiously in elderly patients and in pregnant or breast-feeding women.
• Safety and efficacy in children haven't been established.
• Drug should be used only by clinicians experienced in diagnosis and treatment of primary pulmonary hypertension. The appropriate dose must be determined in a setting with adequate personnel and equipment for physiologic monitoring and emergency care.

---

• Reconstituted solutions must be protected from light and refrigerated at 36° to 46° F (2° to 8° C) if not used immediately. Don't freeze reconstituted solutions. Discard frozen solution or solution that has been refrigerated for more than 48 hours.

• To facilitate extended use at ambient temperatures above 77° F (25° C), a cold pouch with frozen gel packs can be used. The pouch must be able to maintain the drug at a temperature of 36° to 46° F for 12 hours. When such a pouch is used, reconstituted solution may be administered up to 24 hours with use of two pouches.

• Administer anticoagulant therapy during maintenance infusion, unless contraindicated. Monitor PT closely.

• To reduce risk of infection, aseptic technique must be used when reconstituting and administering the drug and when performing routine catheter care.

• All orders for epoprostenol are distributed only by Olsten Health Services, Inc. To order the drug or request reimbursement assistance, call 1-800-622-1820.

**⬛ I.V. administration**

• *Alert:* Reconstitute drug only as directed, using sterile diluent for Flolan. Don't reconstitute or mix drug with other parenteral drugs or solutions before or during administration.

• Follow manufacturer guidelines for reconstituting drug. The prescribed concentration should be compatible with the infusion pump's minimum and maximum flow rates and reservoir capacity and with other criteria recommended by manufacturer. When used for maintenance infusion, drug should be prepared in a drug delivery reservoir appropriate for the infusion pump, with a total reservoir volume of at least 100 ml. Drug should be prepared using two vials of sterile diluent for use during 24 hours.

• Maintenance dosing should be given by continuous I.V. infusion via a permanent indwelling central venous catheter using an ambulatory infusion pump. During establishment of dosing range, drug may be administered peripherally.

• After establishment of a maintenance infusion rate, observe patient closely and monitor standing and supine blood pressure and heart rate for several hours to ensure tolerance.

• *Alert:* Avoid abrupt withdrawal of drug or sudden, large reductions in infusion rate. Ensure that a backup infusion pump and I.V. infusion set are available to avoid potential interruptions in drug delivery. A multilumen catheter should be considered if other I.V. therapies are routinely administered.

• Titrate infusion rates only under doctor's direction, except in life-threatening situations.

**☑ Patient teaching**

• Discuss patient's long-term need for drug. Ensure that patient or family member can care for a permanent I.V. catheter and infusion pump.

• Show patient and family how to reconstitute, administer, and store drug; how to use the infusion pump; and how to switch to a new pump in the event of pump failure. Stress importance of maintaining continuous drug therapy.

• Urge patient to report adverse reactions immediately; dosage adjustments may be needed.

• Provide patient with the telephone number of an organization that offers 24-hour support.

## flunisolide
AeroBid, AeroBid-M, Bronalide†

*Pregnancy Risk Category C*

### HOW SUPPLIED
*Oral inhalant:* 250 mcg/metered spray (at least 100 metered inhalations/container)

### ACTION
Unknown. May decrease inflammation through inhibitory activities against such cell types as mast cells and macrophages and mediators such as leukotrienes.

| Route | Onset | Peak | Duration |
|---|---|---|---|
| Inhalation | 1-4 wk | Unknown | Unknown |

## INDICATIONS & DOSAGE
*Chronic asthma—*
**Adults:** 2 inhalations (500 mcg) b.i.d.
Maximum total daily dose is 2,000 mcg
(8 inhalations daily).
**Children ages 6 to 15:** 2 inhalations
(500 mcg) b.i.d. Higher dosages haven't
been studied. Maximum total daily dose
is 1,000 mcg.

## ADVERSE REACTIONS
**CNS:** dizziness, irritability, nervousness.
**CV:** palpitations, chest pain.
**EENT:** throat irritation, hoarseness, nasopharyngeal fungal infections, *sore throat, nasal congestion.*
**GI:** *nausea, vomiting,* dry mouth, *unpleasant taste, diarrhea, upset stomach,* abdominal pain, decreased appetite.
**Respiratory:** *upper respiratory tract infection, cold symptoms.*
**Skin:** rash, pruritus.
**Other:** *flu,* edema, fever.

## INTERACTIONS
None significant.

## EFFECTS ON DIAGNOSTIC TESTS
None reported.

## CONTRAINDICATIONS
Contraindicated in patients with hypersensitivity to drug and in those with status asthmaticus or respiratory tract infections.

## NURSING CONSIDERATIONS
• Drug isn't recommended in patients with asthma controlled by bronchodilators or other noncorticosteroids alone or for those with nonasthmatic bronchial diseases.
• A spacer device may help to ensure proper dosage administration and decrease local (oral) adverse effects.
• Store drug between 59° and 86° F (15° and 30° C).
• *Alert:* Withdraw drug slowly, as ordered, in patients who have received long-term oral corticosteroid therapy.
• After withdrawal of systemic corticosteroids, patient may still need supplementation of systemic steroids if patient show signs and symptoms of adrenal insufficiency when exposed to trauma, surgery, or infections.
• *Alert:* Don't confuse flunisolide with fluocinonide.

☑ **Patient teaching**
• Warn patient that flunisolide doesn't relieve emergency asthma attacks.
• Advise patient to ensure delivery of proper dose by gently warming the canister to room temperature before using. Some patients carry the canister in a pocket to keep it warm.
• Tell patient who also is using a bronchodilator to use it several minutes before he uses flunisolide.
• Instruct patient to allow 1 minute to elapse before repeating inhalations and to hold his breath for a few seconds to enhance drug action.
• Teach patient to keep inhaler clean and unobstructed. He should wash it with warm water and dry it thoroughly after use.
• Teach patient to check mucous membranes frequently for signs of fungal infection.
• Advise patient to prevent oral fungal infections by gargling or rinsing mouth with water after each inhaler use. Caution him not to swallow the water.
• Advise parents of children receiving long-term therapy that the child should have periodic growth measurements and be checked for evidence of hypothalamic-pituitary-adrenal axis suppression.

## fluticasone propionate
Flixotide§, Flovent Inhalation
Aerosol, Flovent Rotadisk

*Pregnancy Risk Category C*

## HOW SUPPLIED
*Oral inhalation aerosol:* 44 mcg,
110 mcg, 220 mcg
*Oral inhalation powder:* 50 mcg,
100 mcg, 250 mcg, 500 mcg§

## ACTION
Synthetic glucocorticoid with potent anti-inflammatory activity. Inflammation is an important component in the pathogenesis

---

of asthma. Glucocorticoids inhibit many cell types and mediator production or secretion involved in the asthmatic response. These anti-inflammatory actions of fluticasone may contribute to its efficacy in asthma.

| Route | Onset | Peak | Duration |
|-------|-------|------|----------|
| Inhalation | 24 hr | 1-2 wk | Several days |

## INDICATIONS & DOSAGE
*Maintenance treatment of asthma as prophylactic therapy and for patients requiring oral corticosteroid treatment for chronic asthma—*
Flovent Inhalation Aerosol—

**Adults and children ages 12 and over:** in those previously taking bronchodilators alone, initially, inhaled dose of 88 mcg b.i.d. to maximum of 440 mcg b.i.d.
**Patients previously taking inhaled corticosteroids:** initially, inhaled dose of 88 to 220 mcg b.i.d. to maximum of 440 mcg b.i.d.
**Patients previously taking oral corticosteroids:** inhaled dose of 880 mcg b.i.d.
Flovent Rotadisk—
**Adults and adolescents:** in patients previously taking bronchodilators alone, initially, inhaled dose of 100 mcg b.i.d. to maximum of 500 mcg b.i.d.
**Patients previously taking inhaled corticosteroids:** initially, inhaled dose of 100 to 250 mcg b.i.d. to maximum of 500 mcg b.i.d.
**Patients previously taking oral corticosteroids:** inhaled dose of 1,000 mcg b.i.d.
**Children ages 4 to 11:** For patients previously on bronchodilators alone or on inhaled corticosteroids, initially, inhaled dose of 50 mcg b.i.d. to maximum of 100 mcg b.i.d.

## ADVERSE REACTIONS
**CNS:** *headache,* dizziness, migraine, nervousness.
**EENT:** *pharyngitis,* acute nasopharyngitis, nasal congestion, sinusitis, dysphonia, rhinitis, otitis media, tonsillitis, nasal discharge, earache, laryngitis, epistaxis, sneezing, hoarseness, conjunctivitis, eye irritation, dental problems.

**GI:** mouth irritation, *oral candidiasis,* diarrhea, abdominal pain, viral gastroenteritis, colitis, abdominal discomfort, nausea, vomiting.
**GU:** dysmenorrhea, candidiasis of vagina, pelvic inflammatory disease, vaginitis, vulvovaginitis, irregular menstrual cycle.
**Metabolic:** cushingoid features, growth retardation in children, weight gain.
**Musculoskeletal:** pain in joint, aches and pains, disorder or symptoms of neck sprain or strain, muscular soreness.
**Respiratory:** *upper respiratory tract infection,* influenza, bronchitis, chest congestion, dyspnea, irritation due to inhalant.
**Skin:** dermatitis, urticaria.
**Other:** fever.

## INTERACTIONS
**Drug-drug.** *Ketoconazole:* increased mean fluticasone levels. Use care when coadministering fluticasone with long-term ketoconazole and other known cytochrome P-450 3A4 inhibitors.

## EFFECTS ON DIAGNOSTIC TESTS
Some patients on high doses of fluticasone may have an abnormal response to the 6-hour cosyntropin stimulation test.

## CONTRAINDICATIONS
Contraindicated in patients with hypersensitivity to ingredients in these preparations. Also contraindicated in primary treatment of patients with status asthmaticus or other acute episodes of asthma in which intensive measures are needed.

## NURSING CONSIDERATIONS
• Use cautiously in breast-feeding patients.
• Because of risk of systemic absorption of inhaled corticosteroids, observe patient carefully for evidence of systemic corticosteroid effects.
• Monitor patient especially postoperatively or during periods of stress for evidence of inadequate adrenal response.
• During withdrawal from oral corticosteroids, some patients may experience symptoms of systemically active corticosteroid withdrawal, such as joint or mus-

---

Reactions may be *common,* uncommon, *life-threatening,* or **COMMON AND LIFE-THREATENING.**

cular pain, lassitude, and depression, despite maintenance or even improvement of respiratory function.
• For patients starting therapy who are currently receiving oral corticosteroid therapy, reduce dose of prednisone to no more than 2.5 mg/day on a weekly basis, beginning after at least 1 week of therapy with fluticasone.
• *Alert:* As with other inhaled asthma drugs, bronchospasm may occur with an immediate increase in wheezing after dosing. If bronchospasm occurs following dosing with fluticasone inhalation aerosol, it should be treated immediately with a fast-acting inhaled bronchodilator.

☑ **Patient teaching**
• Tell patient that drug isn't indicated for the relief of acute bronchospasm.
• For proper use of drug and to attain maximum improvement, tell patient to follow carefully the accompanying patient instructions.
• Advise patient to use drug at regular intervals as directed.
• Instruct patient not to increase dosage but to contact doctor if symptoms don't improve or if condition worsens.
• Instruct patient to contact doctor immediately when episodes of asthma that aren't responsive to bronchodilators occur during course of treatment with fluticasone. During such episodes, patients may need therapy with oral corticosteroids.
• Warn patient to avoid exposure to chickenpox or measles and, if exposed, to consult doctor immediately.
• Tell patient to carry medical identification indicating he may need supplementary corticosteroids during stress or a severe asthma attack.
• During periods of stress or a severe asthma attack, instruct patient who has been withdrawn from systemic corticosteroids to resume oral corticosteroids (in large doses) immediately and to contact doctor for further instruction. Instruct him to rinse his mouth after inhalation.
• Advise patient to avoid spraying inhalation aerosol into eyes.
• Instruct patient to shake canister well before using inhalation aerosol.

• Advise patient to store fluticasone powder in a dry place.

---

## montelukast sodium
Singulair

*Pregnancy Risk Category B*

### HOW SUPPLIED
*Tablets (film-coated):* 10 mg
*Tablets (chewable):* 5 mg

### ACTION
Causes inhibition of airway cysteinyl leukotriene ($CysLT_1$) receptors. Binds with high affinity and selectivity to the $CysLT_1$ receptor and inhibits physiologic action of the cysteinyl leukotriene $LTD_4$. This receptor inhibition reduces early- and late-phase bronchoconstriction due to antigen challenge.

| Route | Onset | Peak | Duration |
|---|---|---|---|
| P.O. (film-coated) | Unknown | 3-4 hr | Unknown |
| P.O. (chewable) | Unknown | 2-2.5 hr | Unknown |

### INDICATIONS & DOSAGE
*For prophylaxis and long-term treatment of asthma—*
**Adults and children ages 15 and older:** 10 mg (film-coated tablet) P.O. once daily in evening.
**Children ages 6 to 14:** 5 mg (chewable tablet) P.O. once daily in evening.

### ADVERSE REACTIONS
**CNS:** *headache,* dizziness, fatigue, asthenia.
**EENT:** nasal congestion, dental pain.
**GI:** dyspepsia, infectious gastroenteritis, abdominal pain.
**GU:** pyuria.
**Hepatic:** increased ALT and AST levels.
**Respiratory:** cough.
**Skin:** rash.
**Other:** fever, trauma, influenza.

### INTERACTIONS
**Drug-drug.** *Phenobarbital, rifampin:* may decrease bioavailability of mon-

---

telukast because of induction of hepatic metabolism. Monitor closely.

## EFFECTS ON DIAGNOSTIC TESTS
None reported.

## CONTRAINDICATIONS
Contraindicated in patients with hypersensitivity to drug or its ingredients.

## NURSING CONSIDERATIONS
• Use cautiously and with appropriate monitoring in patients whose dosages of systemic corticosteroids are reduced.
• Assess patient's underlying condition and monitor for effectiveness.
• Safety and efficacy for patients under age 6 haven't been established.
• *Alert:* Although dose of inhaled corticosteroids may be reduced gradually, don't abruptly substitute drug for inhaled or oral corticosteroids.
• Drug isn't indicated for use in patients with acute asthmatic attacks, status asthmaticus, or as monotherapy for management of exercise-induced bronchospasm. Appropriate rescue drug should be continued for acute exacerbations.

## ☑ Patient teaching
• Advise patient to take drug daily, even if asymptomatic, and to contact doctor if asthma isn't well controlled.
• Warn patient not to reduce or stop taking other prescribed antiasthma drugs without doctor's approval.
• Advise patient to seek medical attention if short-acting inhaled bronchodilators are needed more often than usual during drug therapy.
• Warn patient that drug isn't beneficial in acute asthma attacks or in exercise-induced bronchospasm, and advise him to keep appropriate rescue drugs available.
• Advise patient with known aspirin sensitivity to continue to avoid using aspirin and NSAIDs during drug therapy.
• Advise patient with phenylketonuria that chewable tablet contains phenylalanine.

# nedocromil sodium
Tilade

*Pregnancy Risk Category B*

## HOW SUPPLIED
*Inhalation aerosol:* 1.75 mg/metered spray (from the mouthpiece)

## ACTION
Reduces inflammatory changes in the airway by blocking the release of inflammation mediators (such as leukotrienes, histamine, and prostaglandins) from mast cells, eosinophils, monocytes, neutrophils, macrophages, and other immune cells.

| Route | Onset | Peak | Duration |
|-------|-------|------|----------|
| Inhalation | Unknown | 30 min | 3.5 hr |

## INDICATIONS & DOSAGE
*Maintenance in mild to moderate bronchial asthma—*
**Adults and children ages 12 and older:** 2 inhalations q.i.d. at regular intervals.

## ADVERSE REACTIONS
**CNS:** headache, dysphonia, fatigue.
**CV:** chest pain.
**EENT:** pharyngitis, rhinitis.
**GI:** nausea, vomiting, dyspepsia, abdominal pain, *unpleasant taste,* dry mouth.
**Respiratory:** upper respiratory tract infection, cough, increased sputum, bronchitis, dyspnea, **bronchospasm.**
**Other:** viral infection.

## INTERACTIONS
None significant.

## EFFECTS ON DIAGNOSTIC TESTS
None reported.

## CONTRAINDICATIONS
Contraindicated in patients with hypersensitivity to drug and its components and in those experiencing an acute asthmatic attack or acute bronchospasm.

## NURSING CONSIDERATIONS
• Drug shouldn't be used during acute bronchospasm because drug action has a

slow onset and isn't therapeutic in aborting an acute attack.

### ☑ Patient teaching
• Warn patient that drug has no direct bronchodilating action and can't replace bronchodilators during an acute asthma attack.
• Tell patient that drug is an adjunct to the regular bronchodilator regimen and may reduce the need for corticosteroids or bronchodilators.
• Emphasize that regular use of drug will help him feel better. Most patients report benefits after 1 week of use; some need longer treatment before improvement occurs.
• Teach patient how to use inhaler. Instruct him to shake canister before use and to invert it just before actuation.
• Advise patient that the use of an aerochamber may improve drug delivery to the lungs.
• Advise patient to clean inhaler at least twice weekly and to remove canister before rinsing inhaler in hot running water. Then let inhaler air-dry overnight.

---

## palivizumab
Synagis

*Pregnancy Risk Category C*

---

### HOW SUPPLIED
*Injection:* 100 mg vial

### ACTION
Exhibits neutralizing and fusion-inhibitory activity against respiratory syncytial virus (RSV), which inhibits RSV replication.

| Route | Onset | Peak | Duration |
|-------|-------|------|----------|
| I.M. | Unknown | Unknown | Unknown |

### INDICATIONS & DOSAGE
*Prevention of serious lower respiratory tract disease due to RSV in children at high risk—*
**Children:** 15 mg/kg I.M. monthly throughout RSV season. Administer first dose before beginning of RSV season.

### ADVERSE REACTIONS
**CNS:** nervousness, pain.
**EENT:** *otitis media, rhinitis,* pharyngitis, sinusitis, conjunctivitis, oral candidiasis.
**GI:** diarrhea, vomiting, gastroenteritis.
**Hematologic:** anemia.
**Hepatic:** liver function abnormality (increased ALT and AST levels).
**Respiratory:** *upper respiratory tract infection,* cough, wheeze, bronchiolitis, *apnea,* pneumonia, bronchitis, asthma, croup, dyspnea.
**Skin:** *rash,* fungal dermatitis, eczema, seborrhea.
**Other:** hernia, failure to thrive, injection site reaction, viral infection, flulike syndrome.

### INTERACTIONS
None significant.

### EFFECTS ON DIAGNOSTIC TESTS
None reported.

### CONTRAINDICATIONS
Contraindicated in children with hypersensitivity to drug or its components.

### NURSING CONSIDERATIONS
• Use cautiously in patients with thrombocytopenia or other coagulation disorders.
• Patients should receive monthly doses throughout RSV season, even if RSV infection develops. In the northern hemisphere, RSV season typically lasts from November to April.
• To reconstitute, slowly add 1 ml of sterile water for injection into a 100-mg vial. Gently swirl the vial for 30 seconds to avoid foaming. Don't shake vial. Let reconstituted solution stand at room temperature for 20 minutes. Administer within 6 hours of reconstitution.
• Administer drug in anterolateral aspect of thigh. Don't use gluteal muscle routinely as an injection site because of risk of damage to sciatic nerve. Injection volumes over 1 ml should be given as a divided dose.
• *Alert:* Anaphylactoid reactions after administration of drug haven't been observed, but can occur following the administration of proteins. If anaphylaxis or

---

severe allergic reaction occurs, administer epinephrine (1:1,000) and provide supportive care as needed.

### ✓ Patient teaching
• Explain to parent or caregiver that drug is used to prevent RSV and not to treat it.
• Advise parent that monthly injections are recommended throughout RSV season (November to April in the northern hemisphere).
• Advise parent to report adverse reactions immediately or any unusual bruising, bleeding or weakness.

---

## triamcinolone acetonide
Azmacort

*Pregnancy Risk Category C*

### HOW SUPPLIED
*Inhalation aerosol:* 100 mcg/metered spray

### ACTION
Unknown. May decrease inflammation through inhibitory activities against such cell types as mast cells and macrophages and mediators such as leukotrienes.

| Route | Onset | Peak | Duration |
|-------|-------|------|----------|
| Inhalation | 1-4 wk | Unknown | Unknown |

### INDICATIONS & DOSAGE
*Persistent asthma—*
**Adults:** 2 inhalations t.i.d. to q.i.d. Maximum dose is 16 inhalations daily. In some patients, maintenance can be accomplished when total daily dose is given b.i.d.
**Children ages 6 to 12:** 1 to 2 inhalations t.i.d. to q.i.d. Maximum dose is 12 inhalations daily.

### ADVERSE REACTIONS
**EENT:** dry or irritated nose or throat, hoarseness, *pharyngitis,* oral candidiasis, dry or irritated tongue or mouth.
**Metabolic:** hypothalamic-pituitary-adrenal function suppression, adrenal insufficiency.
**Respiratory:** cough, wheezing.

**Other:** facial edema.

### INTERACTIONS
None significant.

### EFFECTS ON DIAGNOSTIC TESTS
None reported.

### CONTRAINDICATIONS
Contraindicated in patients with hypersensitivity to drug or its ingredients and in those with status asthmaticus.

### NURSING CONSIDERATIONS
• Use with extreme caution, if at all, in patients with tuberculosis of the respiratory tract; untreated fungal, bacterial, or systemic viral infections; or ocular herpes simplex.
• Unlike other available corticosteroids, drug has a spacer built into the drug-delivery device.
• Use cautiously in patients receiving systemic corticosteroids.
• Most adverse reactions to corticosteroids are dose- or duration-dependent.
• Patients who have recently been switched from systemic administration of steroids to oral inhaled steroids may need to resume systemic steroid therapy during periods of stress or severe asthma attacks.
• Taper oral therapy slowly, as ordered.
• Store drug between 59° and 86° F (15° and 30° C).
• It isn't known whether drug appears in breast milk. Because of risk of severe adverse effects, breast-feeding isn't recommended during therapy.
• *Alert:* Don't confuse triamcinolone with Triaminicin or Triaminicol.

### ✓ Patient teaching
• Inform patient that inhaled corticosteroids don't provide relief for emergency asthma attacks.
• Advise patient to warm canister to room temperature before using. Some patients carry canister in a pocket to keep it warm.
• Tell patient requiring a bronchodilator to use it several minutes before triamcinolone. Tell patient to allow 1 minute to elapse before repeat inhalations and to hold breath for a few seconds to enhance drug action.

---

Reactions may be *common*, uncommon, *life-threatening*, or COMMON AND LIFE-THREATENING.

• Teach patient to check mucous membranes frequently for signs of fungal infection.

• Tell patient to prevent oral fungal infections by gargling or rinsing mouth with water after each use of the inhaler, but not to swallow the water.

• Tell patient to keep inhaler clean and unobstructed and to wash it with warm water and dry it thoroughly after use.

• Instruct patient to contact doctor if response to therapy decreases; dosage may need adjustment. Tell him not to exceed recommended dosage on his own.

• Instruct patient to carry a card indicating his need for supplemental systemic glucocorticoids during periods of stress.

---

## zafirlukast
Accolate

*Pregnancy Risk Category B*

### HOW SUPPLIED
*Tablets:* 20 mg

### ACTION
Selectively competes for leukotriene receptor sites, blocking inflammatory action.

| Route | Onset | Peak | Duration |
|-------|-------|------|----------|
| P.O. | Rapid | 3 hr | Unknown |

### INDICATIONS & DOSAGE
*Prophylaxis and maintenance treatment of asthma—*
**Adults and children age 12 and older:** 20 mg P.O. b.i.d. taken 1 hour before or 2 hours after meals.

### ADVERSE REACTIONS
**CNS:** *headache,* asthenia, dizziness, pain.
**GI:** nausea, diarrhea, abdominal pain, vomiting, dyspepsia.
**Hepatic:** elevated liver enzyme levels.
**Musculoskeletal:** myalgia, back pain.
**Other:** infection, accidental injury, fever.

### INTERACTIONS
**Drug-drug.** *Aspirin:* increased plasma levels of zafirlukast. Monitor patient.

*Erythromycin, theophylline:* decreased plasma levels of zafirlukast. Monitor patient.
*Warfarin:* increased PT. Monitor PT and INR levels, and adjust dosage of anticoagulant, as ordered.

### EFFECTS ON DIAGNOSTIC TESTS
None reported.

### CONTRAINDICATIONS
Contraindicated in patients with hypersensitivity to drug.

### NURSING CONSIDERATIONS
• Drug isn't indicated for use in the reversal of bronchospasm in acute asthma attacks.

• Administer with caution in patients with hepatic impairment and in the elderly.

• Use drug in pregnant patients only if clearly needed. Don't use in breastfeeding women.

• *Alert:* Reduction of oral steroid dose has been followed in rare cases by eosinophilia, vasculitic rash, worsening pulmonary symptoms, cardiac complications, or neuropathy, sometimes presenting as Churg-Strauss syndrome.

• Safety and effectiveness in patients under age 12 haven't been established.

### ✓ Patient teaching
• Tell patient that drug is used for long-term treatment of asthma and to keep taking drug even if symptoms disappear.

• Advise patient to continue taking other antiasthma drugs, as ordered.

• Instruct patient not to take drug with food. Drug should be taken 1 hour before or 2 hours after meals.

---

## zileuton
Zyflo

*Pregnancy Risk Category C*

### HOW SUPPLIED
*Tablets:* 600 mg

---

## ACTION
Inhibits enzyme responsible for the formation of leukotrienes, thus reducing inflammatory response.

| Route | Onset | Peak | Duration |
|-------|-------|------|----------|
| P.O. | Rapid | 2 hr | Unknown |

## INDICATIONS & DOSAGE
*Prophylaxis and maintenance treatment of asthma—*
**Adults and children ages 12 and older:** 600 mg P.O. q.i.d.

## ADVERSE REACTIONS
**CNS:** *headache,* asthenia, dizziness, pain, insomnia, nervousness, somnolence, malaise.
**CV:** chest pain.
**EENT:** conjunctivitis.
**GI:** dyspepsia, nausea, abdominal pain, constipation, flatulence, vomiting.
**GU:** urinary tract infection, vaginitis.
**Hematologic:** *leukopenia.*
**Hepatic:** elevated liver enzyme levels.
**Musculoskeletal:** myalgia, arthralgia, hypertonia, neck pain, rigidity.
**Skin:** pruritus.
**Other:** accidental injury, fever, lymphadenopathy.

## INTERACTIONS
**Drug-drug.** *Propranolol, other beta blockers:* increased beta-blocker effect. Monitor patient and reduce dosage of beta blocker as needed.
*Theophylline:* decreased theophylline clearance (on average, serum theophylline levels double). Reduce theophylline dose, as ordered, and monitor serum levels.
*Warfarin:* increased PT. Monitor PT and INR and adjust dosage of anticoagulant, as ordered.

## EFFECTS ON DIAGNOSTIC TESTS
None reported.

## CONTRAINDICATIONS
Contraindicated in patients with hypersensitivity to drug and in those with active liver disease or transaminase elevations at least three times the upper limit of normal.

## NURSING CONSIDERATIONS
• *Alert:* Drug isn't indicated for use in the reversal of bronchospasm in acute asthma attacks.
• Administer with caution in patients with hepatic impairment or history of heavy alcohol use.
• Drug should be used in pregnancy only if the benefit of use outweighs the potential risk to the fetus. Breast-feeding women shouldn't take drug.
• Safety and effectiveness in patients under age 12 haven't been established.
• Obtain baseline and periodic liver enzyme levels, as ordered.

### ☑ Patient teaching
• Tell patient that drug is used for long-term treatment of asthma and to keep taking drug even if symptoms disappear.
• Caution patient that drug isn't a bronchodilator and shouldn't be used to treat an acute asthma attack.
• Advise patient to continue taking other antiasthma drugs, as ordered.
• Instruct patient to notify doctor if his short-acting bronchodilator doesn't relieve symptoms.
• Inform patient that he must undergo periodic testing of liver enzyme levels.
• Tell patient to notify doctor immediately if he develops signs and symptoms of liver dysfunction (right upper quadrant pain, nausea, fatigue, pruritus, jaundice, malaise).
• Tell patient to avoid alcohol and to consult his doctor first before taking OTC or new prescription drugs.
• Instruct patient to report flulike symptoms.

---

Reactions may be *common,* uncommon, ***life-threatening,*** or COMMON AND LIFE-THREATENING.

**aluminum carbonate**
**aluminum hydroxide**
**calcium carbonate**
**magaldrate**
**magnesium hydroxide**
(See Chapter 50, LAXATIVES.)
**magnesium oxide**
**simethicone**
**sodium bicarbonate**
(See Chapter 64, ACIDIFIERS AND ALKALINIZERS.)

## COMBINATION PRODUCTS

ALKA-SELTZER GOLD ◇: sodium bicarbonate 958 mg, citric acid 832 mg, and potassium bicarbonate 312 mg.
ALKA-SELTZER ORIGINAL ◇: aspirin 325 mg, citric acid 1,000 mg and phenylalanine 9 mg.
ALUDROX ◇: aluminum hydroxide 307 mg and magnesium hydroxide 103 mg.
DI-GEL ADVANCED FORMULA ◇: magnesium hydroxide 128 mg, and calcium carbonate 280 mg.
EXTRA STRENGTH ALKA-SELTZER ◇: aspirin 500 mg and citric acid 1,000 mg.
GAVISCON TABLETS ◇: aluminum hydroxide 80 mg and magnesium trisilicate 20 mg.
GELUSIL ◇: aluminum hydroxide 200 mg, magnesium hydroxide 200 mg, and simethicone 25 mg.
MAALOX TABLETS ◇: aluminum hydroxide 200 mg, magnesium hydroxide 200 mg, and simethicone 25 mg.
MAALOX EXTRA STRENGTH TABLETS ◇: aluminum hydroxide 350 mg, magnesium hydroxide 350 mg and simethicone 30 mg.
MAALOX PLUS ◇: aluminum hydroxide 200 mg, magnesium hydroxide 200 mg, and simethicone 25 mg.
MAALOX THERAPEUTIC CONCENTRATE SUSPENSION: aluminum hydroxide 600 mg and magnesium hydroxide 300 mg/5 ml.
MYLANTA LIQUID: aluminum hydroxide 200 mg, magnesium hydroxide 200 mg, and simethicone 20 mg/5 ml.

MYLANTA TABLETS ◇: aluminum hydroxide 200 mg, magnesium hydroxide 200 mg, and simethicone 20 mg.
RIOPAN PLUS CHEWABLE TABLETS ◇: magaldrate 480 mg and simethicone 20 mg.
RIOPAN PLUS DOUBLE STRENGTH CHEWABLE TABLETS: magaldrate 1,080 mg and simethicone 20 mg.
RIOPAN PLUS DOUBLE STRENGTH SUSPENSION: magaldrate 1,080 mg and simethicone 40 mg/5 ml.
RIOPAN PLUS SUSPENSION ◇: magaldrate 540 mg and simethicone 40 mg/5 ml.
TITRALAC PLUS ◇: calcium carbonate 420 mg and simethicone 21 mg.
UNIVOL† ◇: aluminum hydroxide and magnesium carbonate co-dried gel 300 mg and magnesium hydroxide 100 mg.

---

## aluminum carbonate
### Basaljel ◇

*Pregnancy Risk Category NR*

### HOW SUPPLIED
*Tablets or capsules:* equivalent to aluminum hydroxide 500 mg ◇
*Oral suspension:* equivalent to aluminum hydroxide 400 mg/5 ml ◇

### ACTION
Antacid that reduces total acid load in the GI tract, elevates gastric pH to reduce pepsin activity, strengthens the gastric mucosal barrier, and increases esophageal sphincter tone.

| Route | Onset | Peak | Duration |
|-------|-------|------|----------|
| P.O. | 20 min | Unknown | 20-180 min |

### INDICATIONS & DOSAGE
*Antacid—*
**Adults:** 5 to 10 ml of suspension P.O. q 2 hours, p.r.n.; or 1 to 2 tablets or capsules P.O. q 2 hours, p.r.n. Maximum dose is 24 capsules, tablets, or teaspoonfuls per 24 hours.

*To prevent formation of urinary phosphate stones (in conjunction with low-phosphate diet)—*
**Adults:** 15 to 30 ml of suspension in water or juice P.O. 1 hour after meals and h.s.; or 2 to 6 tablets or capsules 1 hour after meals and h.s.

## ADVERSE REACTIONS
**CNS:** encephalopathy.
**GI:** *constipation,* intestinal obstruction.
**Metabolic:** hypophosphatemia, increased serum gastrin levels.
**Musculoskeletal:** osteomalacia.

## INTERACTIONS
**Drug-drug.** *Allopurinol, antibiotics (including quinolones, tetracyclines), corticosteroids, diflunisal, digoxin, ethambutol, H$_2$ antagonists, iron salts, isoniazid, penicillamine, phenothiazines, thyroid hormones, ticlopidine:* decreased pharmacologic effect because of possible impaired absorption. Separate administration times by 1 to 2 hours.
*Enteric-coated drugs:* may be released prematurely in stomach. Separate doses by at least 1 hour.

## EFFECTS ON DIAGNOSTIC TESTS
Aluminum carbonate may interfere with imaging techniques using sodium pertechnetate Tc99m and thus impair evaluation of Meckel's diverticulum. It may also interfere with reticuloendothelial imaging of liver, spleen, or bone marrow using technetium Tc99m sulfur colloid. It may antagonize pentagastrin's effect during gastric acid secretion tests.

## CONTRAINDICATIONS
No known contraindications.

## NURSING CONSIDERATIONS
• Use cautiously in patients with chronic renal disease.
• When administering through nasogastric tube, make sure tube is placed correctly and is patent; after instilling, flush tube with water to ensure passage to stomach and to clear tube.
• *Alert:* Monitor long-term, high-dose use in patients on restricted sodium intake.

Each tablet, capsule, or 5 ml of suspension contains about 3 mg of sodium.
• Record stool amount and consistency. Manage constipation with laxatives or stool softeners, as ordered. Alternate with magnesium-containing antacids (unless patient has renal disease).
• Monitor serum phosphate levels.
• Watch for symptoms of hypophosphatemia (anorexia, malaise, muscle weakness) with prolonged use; can also lead to resorption of calcium and bone demineralization.
• Because drug contains aluminum, keep in mind that it is used in patients with renal failure to help control hyperphosphatemia by binding with phosphate in the GI tract.
• Basaljel liquid contains no sugar.

☑ **Patient teaching**
• Warn patient not to take aluminum carbonate indiscriminately or to switch antacids without doctor's advice.
• Tell patient to shake suspension well and to take with small amount of water or fruit juice to facilitate passage.
• Instruct patient to notify doctor of signs of bleeding, tarry stools, or coffee-ground vomitus.
• Instruct pregnant patient to seek medical advice before taking drug.

---

## aluminum hydroxide
AlternaGEL ◇, Alu-Cap§ ◇,
Aluminum Hydroxide Gel ◇,
Aluminum Hydroxide Gel
Concentrated ◇, Alu-Tab ◇,
Amphojel ◇, Dialume ◇

*Pregnancy Risk Category NR*

## HOW SUPPLIED
*Tablets:* 300 mg ◇, 500 mg ◇, 600 mg ◇
*Capsules:* 400 mg ◇, 500 mg ◇
*Oral suspension:* 320 mg/5 ml ◇,
450 mg/5 ml ◇, 600 mg/5 ml ◇,
675 mg/5 ml ◇

## ACTION
Antacid that reduces total acid load in the GI tract, elevates gastric pH to reduce pepsin activity, strengthens the gastric

---

mucosal barrier, and increases esophageal sphincter tone.

| Route | Onset | Peak | Duration |
|-------|-------|------|----------|
| P.O. | Variable | Unknown | 20-180 min |

## INDICATIONS & DOSAGE
*Antacid—*
**Adults:** 500 to 1,500 mg P.O. (5 to 30 ml of most suspension products) 1 hour after meals and h.s.; Or, 300-mg tablet or 600-mg tablet (chewed before swallowing) taken with milk or water five to six times daily after meals and h.s.

## ADVERSE REACTIONS
**CNS:** encephalopathy.
**GI:** *constipation,* intestinal obstruction.
**Metabolic:** hypophosphatemia, increased serum gastrin levels.
**Musculoskeletal:** osteomalacia.

## INTERACTIONS
**Drug-drug.** *Allopurinol, antibiotics (including quinolones, tetracyclines), corticosteroids, diflunisal, digoxin, ethambutol, $H_2$ antagonists, iron salts, isoniazid, penicillamine, phenothiazines, thyroid hormones, ticlopidine:* decreased pharmacologic effect because of possible impaired absorption. Separate administration times.
*Enteric-coated drugs:* may be released prematurely in stomach. Separate doses by at least 1 hour.

## EFFECTS ON DIAGNOSTIC TESTS
Aluminum hydroxide therapy may interfere with imaging techniques using sodium pertechnetate Tc99m and thus impair evaluation of Meckel's diverticulum. It may also interfere with reticuloendothelial imaging of liver, spleen, or bone marrow using technetium Tc99m sulfur colloid. It may antagonize pentagastrin's effect during gastric acid secretion tests.

## CONTRAINDICATIONS
No known contraindications.

## NURSING CONSIDERATIONS
• Use cautiously in patients with chronic renal disease.

• When administering through nasogastric tube, make sure tube is placed correctly and is patent; after instilling, flush tube with water to ensure passage to stomach and to clear tube.
• *Alert:* Monitor long-term, high-dose use in patient on restricted sodium intake. Each tablet, capsule, or 5 ml of suspension contains 2 to 3 mg of sodium.
• Record amount and consistency of stools. Manage constipation with laxatives or stool softeners, as ordered; alternate with magnesium-containing antacids (if patient doesn't have renal disease).
• Monitor serum phosphate levels.
• Watch for symptoms of hypophosphatemia (anorexia, malaise, and muscle weakness) with prolonged use; can also lead to resorption of calcium and bone demineralization.
• Because drug contains aluminum, keep in mind that it is used in patients with renal failure to help control hyperphosphatemia by binding with phosphate in the GI tract.

### ☑ Patient teaching
• Instruct patient to shake suspension well and to follow with small amount of milk or water to facilitate passage.
• Advise patient not to take aluminum hydroxide indiscriminately or to switch antacids without doctor's advice.
• Instruct patient to notify doctor of signs of bleeding, tarry stools, or coffee-ground vomitus.
• Instruct pregnant patient to seek medical advice before taking drug.

## calcium carbonate
Alka-Mints◇, Amitone◇, Cal-Sup‡, Chooz◇, Dicarbosil◇, Maalox Antacid Caplets◇, Rolaids Calcium Rich◇, Tums◇, Tums E-X◇, Tums Ultra◇

*Pregnancy Risk Category NR*

## HOW SUPPLIED
Calcium carbonate contains 40% calcium; 20 mEq calcium per gram.

---

*Liquid contains alcohol.   **May contain tartrazine.   †Canada   ‡Australia   §U.K.   ◇OTC

*Tablets (chewable):* 350 mg ◇, 420 mg ◇, 500 mg ◇, 750 mg, 850 mg, 1,000 mg, 1,250 mg‡
*Tablets:* 500 mg ◇, 600 mg ◇, 650 mg ◇, 1,000 mg ◇, 1,250 mg ◇
*Chewing gum:* 500 mg/piece
*Oral suspension:* 1,250 mg/5 ml
*Lozenges:* 600 mg ◇

## ACTION
Antacid that reduces total acid load in the GI tract, elevates gastric pH to reduce pepsin activity, strengthens the gastric mucosal barrier, and increases esophageal sphincter tone.

| Route | Onset | Peak | Duration |
|-------|-------|------|----------|
| P.O. | 20 min | Unknown | 20-180 min |

## INDICATIONS & DOSAGE
*Antacid, calcium supplement—*
**Adults:** 350 mg to 1.5 g P.O. or 2 pieces of chewing gum 1 hour after meals and h.s., p.r.n.

## ADVERSE REACTIONS
**CNS:** headache, irritability, weakness.
**GI:** rebound hyperacidity, *nausea.*
**Metabolic:** altered serum phosphate levels.

## INTERACTIONS
**Drug-drug.** *Antibiotics (including quinolones, tetracyclines), hydantoins, iron salts, isoniazid, salicylates:* decreased pharmacologic effect because of possible impaired absorption. Separate administration times.
*Enteric-coated drugs:* may be released prematurely in stomach. Separate doses by at least 1 hour.
**Drug-food.** *Milk, other foods high in vitamin D:* possible milk-alkali syndrome (headache, confusion, distaste for food, nausea, vomiting, hypercalcemia, hypercalciuria). Avoid concomitant use.

## EFFECTS ON DIAGNOSTIC TESTS
None reported.

## CONTRAINDICATIONS
Contraindicated in patients with ventricular fibrillation or hypercalcemia.

## NURSING CONSIDERATIONS
● Use cautiously, if at all, in patients with sarcoidosis or renal or cardiac disease, and in patients receiving cardiac glycosides.
● Record amount and consistency of stools. Manage constipation with laxatives or stool softeners, as ordered.
● Monitor serum calcium levels, especially in patients with mild renal impairment.
● Watch for signs and symptoms of hypercalcemia (nausea, vomiting, headache, confusion, and anorexia).

### ✓ Patient teaching
● Advise patient not to take calcium carbonate indiscriminately or to switch antacids without doctor's advice.
● Tell patient taking chewable tablets to chew thoroughly before swallowing and follow with a glass of water.
● Tell patient using suspension form to shake well and take with a small amount of water to facilitate passage.
● Instruct patient to notify doctor of signs of bleeding, tarry stools, or coffee-ground vomitus.

---

## magaldrate (aluminum-magnesium complex)
Lowsium ◇, Riopan ◇

*Pregnancy Risk Category NR*

## HOW SUPPLIED
*Oral suspension:* 540 mg/5 ml ◇

## ACTION
Antacid that reduces total acid load in the GI tract, elevates gastric pH to reduce pepsin activity, strengthens the gastric mucosal barrier, and increases esophageal sphincter tone.

| Route | Onset | Peak | Duration |
|-------|-------|------|----------|
| P.O. | 20 min | Unknown | 20-180 min |

## INDICATIONS & DOSAGE
*Antacid—*
**Adults:** 540 to 1,080 mg (5 to 10 ml) of suspension P.O. with water between meals and h.s.

---

Reactions may be *common,* uncommon, **life-threatening**, or COMMON AND LIFE-THREATENING.

## ADVERSE REACTIONS
**GI:** mild constipation, diarrhea.
**GU:** increased urine pH levels.
**Metabolic:** hypokalemia, increased serum gastrin levels.

## INTERACTIONS
**Drug-drug.** *Allopurinol, antibiotics (including quinolones, tetracyclines), diflunisal, digoxin, iron salts, isoniazid, penicillamine, phenothiazines, quinidine, salicylates, ticlopidine:* decreased pharmacologic effect because of possible impaired absorption. Separate administration times by 1 to 2 hours.
*Enteric-coated drugs:* may be released prematurely in stomach. Separate doses by at least 1 hour.

## EFFECTS ON DIAGNOSTIC TESTS
Drug may antagonize pentagastrin's effect during gastric acid secretion tests.

## CONTRAINDICATIONS
Contraindicated in patients with severe renal disease.

## NURSING CONSIDERATIONS
• Use cautiously in patients with mild kidney impairment.
• When giving through nasogastric tube, make sure tube is placed properly and is patent. After instilling, flush tube with water to ensure passage to stomach and to clear tube.
• Monitor serum magnesium level in patients with mild kidney impairment. Symptomatic hypermagnesemia usually occurs only in severe renal failure.
• *Alert:* Drug isn't typically used in patients with renal failure to help control hypophosphatemia because it contains magnesium, which may accumulate.
• Drug has a low sodium content and is good for patients on restricted sodium intake.

☑ **Patient teaching**
• Instruct patient to shake suspension well and to follow with water.
• Tell patient taking chewable tablets to chew thoroughly and to follow with a glass of water.

• Advise patient not to take magaldrate indiscriminately or to switch antacids without doctor's advice.
• Instruct patient to notify doctor of signs of bleeding, tarry stools, or coffee-ground vomitus.

---

## magnesium oxide
Mag-Ox 400◇, Maox◇,
Uro-Mag◇

*Pregnancy Risk Category NR*

### HOW SUPPLIED
*Tablets:* 400 mg◇, 420 mg◇, 500 mg
*Capsules:* 140 mg◇

### ACTION
Reduces total acid load in the GI tract, elevates gastric pH, strengthens the gastric mucosal barrier, and increases esophageal sphincter tone.

| Route | Onset | Peak | Duration |
|-------|-------|------|----------|
| P.O. | 20 min | Unknown | 20-180 min |

### INDICATIONS & DOSAGE
*Antacid—*
**Adults:** 140 mg P.O. with water or milk after meals and h.s.
*Laxative—*
**Adults:** 4 g P.O. with water or milk, usually h.s.
*Oral replacement therapy in mild hypomagnesemia—*
**Adults:** 400 to 840 mg P.O. daily. Monitor serum magnesium level.

### ADVERSE REACTIONS
**GI:** *diarrhea,* nausea, abdominal pain.
**Metabolic:** hypermagnesemia.

### INTERACTIONS
**Drug-drug.** *Allopurinol, antibiotics, digoxin, iron salts, penicillamine, phenothiazines:* decreased effect because of possible impaired absorption. Separate administration times by 1 to 2 hours.
*Enteric-coated drugs:* may be released prematurely in stomach. Separate doses by at least 1 hour.

---

*Liquid contains alcohol.   **May contain tartrazine.   †Canada   ‡Australia   §U.K.   ◇OTC

**EFFECTS ON DIAGNOSTIC TESTS**
None reported.

**CONTRAINDICATIONS**
Contraindicated in patients with severe renal disease.

**NURSING CONSIDERATIONS**
• Use cautiously in patients with mild renal impairment.
• When used as laxative, don't give within 1 to 2 hours of other oral drugs.
• *Alert:* Monitor serum magnesium levels. With prolonged use and renal impairment, watch for signs and symptoms of hypermagnesemia (hypotension, nausea, vomiting, depressed reflexes, respiratory depression, and coma).
• If diarrhea occurs, be prepared to suggest alternative preparation.

☑ **Patient teaching**
• Advise patient not to take magnesium oxide indiscriminately or to switch antacids without doctor's advice.
• Instruct patient to report bleeding, tarry stools, or coffee-ground vomitus.

---

**simethicone**
Flatulex◇, Gas Relief◇, Gas-X◇, Gas-X Extra Strength◇, Mylanta Gas◇, Mylanta Gas Maximum Strength◇, Mylicon◇, Ovol†, Ovol-40†, Ovol-80†, Phazyme◇, Phazyme-95◇, Phazyme-125 Maximum Strength◇

*Pregnancy Risk Category NR*

**HOW SUPPLIED**
*Tablets:* 40 mg◇, 55 mg†◇, 60 mg◇, 80 mg◇, 95 mg◇, 125 mg◇
*Capsules:* 125 mg
*Drops:* 40 mg/0.6 ml◇

**ACTION**
By its defoaming action, drug disperses or prevents formation of mucus-surrounded gas pockets in the GI tract.

| Route | Onset | Peak | Duration |
|-------|-------|------|----------|
| P.O. | Immediate | Immediate | Unknown |

**INDICATIONS & DOSAGE**
*Flatulence, functional gastric bloating—*
**Adults and children over age 12:** 40 to 125 mg P.O. after each meal and h.s., up to 500 mg daily. For drops, 40 to 80 mg P.O. after each meal and h.s., up to 500 mg daily.

**ADVERSE REACTIONS**
**GI:** expulsion of excessive liberated gas as belching, rectal flatus.

**INTERACTIONS**
None significant.

**EFFECTS ON DIAGNOSTIC TESTS**
None reported.

**CONTRAINDICATIONS**
Contraindicated in patients with hypersensitivity to drug.

**NURSING CONSIDERATIONS**
• Drug isn't recommended for treating infant colic because of limited information on safety in children.
• Drug doesn't prevent formation of gas.
• *Alert:* Don't confuse simethicone with cimetidine.

☑ **Patient teaching**
• Tell patient to chew tablet before swallowing.
• Advise patient to change positions often and ambulate to aid flatus passage.

---

Reactions may be *common*, uncommon, *life-threatening*, or COMMON AND LIFE-THREATENING.

**pancreatin**
**pancrelipase**
**ursodiol**

## COMBINATION PRODUCTS

DONNAZYME TABLETS: pancreatin 300 mg, pepsin 150 mg, bile salts 150 mg, hyoscyamine sulfate 0.0518 mg, atropine sulfate 0.0097 mg, scopolamine hydrobromide 0.0033 mg, and phenobarbital 8.1 mg.
PANCREASE CAPSULES; lipase 4,000 U, protease 25,000 U, and amylase 20,000 U in enteric-coated microspheres.

---

## pancreatin

Creon, Donnazyme, Hi-Vegi-Lip Tablets ◊ , 4X Pancreatin 600 mg ◊ , 8X Pancreatin 900 mg ◊ , Pancrezyme 4X Tablets ◊

*Pregnancy Risk Category C*

---

## HOW SUPPLIED

**Creon**
*Microspheres (enteric-coated):* 300 mg pancreatin, 8,000 U lipase, 13,000 U protease, 30,000 U amylase
**Donnazyme**
*Tablets:* 500 mg pancreatin, 1,000 U lipase, 12,500 U protease, and 12,500 U amylase
**Hi-Vegi-Lip Tablets**
*Tablets (enteric-coated):* 2,400 mg pancreatin, 4,800 U lipase, 60,000 U protease, and 60,000 U amylase ◊
**4X Pancreatin 600 mg**
*Tablets (enteric-coated):* 2,400 mg pancreatin, 12,000 U lipase, 60,000 U protease, and 60,000 U amylase ◊
**8X Pancreatin 900 mg**
*Tablets (enteric-coated):* 7,200 mg pancreatin, 22,500 U lipase, 180,000 U protease, and 180,000 U amylase ◊
**Pancrezyme 4X Tablets**
*Tablets (enteric-coated):* 2,400 mg pancreatin, 12,000 U lipase, 60,000 U protease, and 60,000 U amylase ◊

## ACTION

Replaces endogenous exocrine pancreatic enzymes and aids digestion of starches, fats, and proteins.

| Route | Onset | Peak | Duration |
|-------|-------|------|----------|
| P.O. | Unknown | Unknown | 1-2 hr |

## INDICATIONS & DOSAGE

*Exocrine pancreatic secretion insufficiency; digestive aid in diseases associated with deficiency of pancreatic enzymes, such as cystic fibrosis—*
**Adults and children:** dosage varies with condition being treated. Usual initial dose is 8,000 to 24,000 U of lipase activity P.O. before or with each meal or snack. Total daily dose may also be given in divided doses at 1- to 2-hour intervals throughout day.

## ADVERSE REACTIONS

**GI:** nausea, diarrhea with high doses.
**Metabolic:** increased serum uric acid levels.
**Skin:** perianal irritation.
**Other:** *allergic reactions.*

## INTERACTIONS

**Drug-drug.** *Antacids:* may negate pancreatin's beneficial effect. Avoid concomitant use.

## EFFECTS ON DIAGNOSTIC TESTS

None reported.

## CONTRAINDICATIONS

Contraindicated in patients with hypersensitivity to drug, pork protein, or enzymes and in those with acute pancreatitis or acute exacerbations of chronic pancreatitis.

## NURSING CONSIDERATIONS

• Use with caution in pregnant or breast-feeding patients.
• Minimal USP standards dictate that each milligram of bovine or porcine pancreatin contains lipase 2 U, protease 25 U, and amylase 25 U.

---

• To avoid indigestion, monitor patient's dietary intake to ensure a proper balance of fat, protein, and starch intake. Dosage varies according to degree of maldigestion and malabsorption, amount of fat in diet, and enzyme activity of individual preparations.

• Fewer bowel movements and improved stool consistency indicate effective therapy.

• Drug isn't effective in GI disorders unrelated to pancreatic enzyme deficiency.

• Enteric coating on some products may reduce available enzyme in upper portion of jejunum.

☑ **Patient teaching**

• Instruct patient to take before or with meals and snacks.

• Tell patient not to crush or chew enteric-coated forms. Capsules containing enteric-coated microspheres may be opened and sprinkled on a small quantity of cooled, soft food. Stress importance of swallowing immediately without chewing and following with glass of water or juice.

• Warn patient not to inhale powder form or powder from capsules; may irritate skin or mucous membranes.

• Tell patient to store in airtight containers at room temperature.

• Instruct patient not to change brands without consulting doctor.

---

### pancrelipase

Cotazym Capsules, Cotazym-S Capsules, Creon 5 Capsules, Creon 10 Minimicrospheres, Creon 20 Minimicrospheres, Ilozyme Tablets, Ku-Zyme HP Capsules, Pancrease Capsules, Pancrease MT4, Pancrease MT10, Pancrease MT16, Pancrease MT20, Pancrelipase Capsules, Protilase Capsules, Ultrase MT12, Ultrase MT18, Ultrase MT20, Viokase Powder, Viokase Tablets, Zymase Capsules

*Pregnancy Risk Category C*

---

**HOW SUPPLIED**
**Cotazym**
*Capsules:* 8,000 U lipase, 30,000 U protease, 30,000 U amylase, and 25 mg calcium carbonate

**Cotazym-S**
*Capsules (enteric-coated spheres):* 5,000 U lipase, 20,000 U protease, and 20,000 U amylase

**Creon 5**
*Capsules (delayed-release):* 5,000 U lipase, 18,750 U protease, and 16,600 U amylase

**Creon 10**
*Capsules (delayed-release):* 10,000 U lipase, 37,500 U protease, and 33,200 U amylase

**Creon 20**
*Capsules (delayed-release):* 20,000 U lipase, 75,000 U protease, and 66,400 U amylase

**Ilozyme**
*Tablets:* 11,000 U lipase, 30,000 U protease, and 30,000 U amylase

**Ku-Zyme HP**
*Capsules:* 8,000 U lipase, 30,000 U protease, and 30,000 U amylase

**Pancrease**
*Capsules (enteric-coated microspheres):* 4,000 U lipase, 25,000 U protease, and 20,000 U amylase

**Pancrease MT4**
*Capsules (enteric-coated microtablets):* 4,500 U lipase, 12,000 U protease, and 12,000 U amylase

**Pancrease MT10**
*Capsules (enteric-coated microtablets):* 10,000 U lipase, 30,000 U protease, and 30,000 U amylase

**Pancrease MT16**
*Capsules (enteric-coated microtablets):* 16,000 U lipase, 48,000 U protease, and 48,000 U amylase

**Pancrease MT20**
*Capsules (enteric-coated microtablets):* 20,000 U lipase, 44,000 U protease, and 56,000 U amylase

**Pancrelipase**
*Capsules (enteric-coated pellets):* 4,000 U lipase, 25,000 U protease, and 20,000 U amylase

**Protilase**
*Capsules (enteric-coated spheres):* 4,000 U lipase, 25,000 U protease, and 20,000 U amylase

**Ultrase MT12**
*Capsules (delayed-release):* 12,000 U lipase, 39,000 U protease, and 39,000 U amylase
**Ultrase MT18**
*Capsules (delayed-release):* 18,000 U lipase, 58,500 U protease, and 58,000 U amylase
**Ultrase MT20**
*Capsules (delayed-release):* 20,000 U lipase, 65,000 U protease, and 65,000 U amylase
**Viokase**
*Powder:* 16,800 U lipase, 70,000 U protease, and 70,000 U amylase per 0.7 g powder
*Tablets:* 8,000 U lipase, 30,000 U protease, and 30,000 U amylase
**Zymase**
*Capsules (enteric-coated spheres):* 12,000 U lipase, 24,000 U protease, and 24,000 U amylase

## ACTION
Replaces endogenous exocrine pancreatic enzymes and aids digestion of starches, fats, and proteins.

| Route | Onset | Peak | Duration |
|-------|-------|------|----------|
| P.O. | Variable | Variable | Variable |

## INDICATIONS & DOSAGE
*Exocrine pancreatic secretion insufficiency; cystic fibrosis in adults and children; steatorrhea and other disorders of fat metabolism secondary to insufficient pancreatic enzymes—*
**Adults and children ages 12 and older:** dosage adjusted to patient's response. Usual initial dose 4,000 to 48,000 U of lipase with each meal.
**Children ages 7 to 12:** 4,000 to 12,000 U (more, if needed) of lipase activity with each meal or snack.
**Children ages 1 to 6:** 4,000 to 8,000 U of lipase with each meal and 4,000 U of lipase with each snack.
**Children ages 6 months to 1 year:** 2,000 U of lipase with each meal.
**Children under age 6 months:** dosage not established.

## ADVERSE REACTIONS
**GI:** *nausea,* cramping, diarrhea (high doses).
**Metabolic:** increased serum uric acid levels.

## INTERACTIONS
**Drug-drug.** *Antacids:* may destroy enteric coating and result in enhanced degradation of pancrelipase. Avoid concomitant use.
*Oral iron:* may decrease serum iron response. Monitor for decreased effectiveness.

## EFFECTS ON DIAGNOSTIC TESTS
None reported.

## CONTRAINDICATIONS
Contraindicated in patients with severe hypersensitivity to pork and in those with acute pancreatitis or acute exacerbations of chronic pancreatic diseases.

## NURSING CONSIDERATIONS
● *Alert:* Use drug only for confirmed exocrine pancreatic insufficiency. It isn't effective in GI disorders unrelated to enzyme deficiency.
● Lipase activity is greater than with other pancreatic enzymes.
● For infants, mix powder with applesauce and give with meals. Avoid contact with or inhalation of powder because it may be very irritating. Older children may take capsules with food.
● Monitor patient's stools. Adequate replacement decreases number of bowel movements and improves stool consistency.
● Minimal USP standards dictate that each milligram of pancrelipase contains 24 U lipase, 100 U protease, and 100 U amylase.
● Dosage varies with degree of maldigestion and malabsorption, amount of fat in diet, and enzyme activity of individual preparations.
● Enteric coating on some products may reduce available enzyme in upper portion of jejunum.

☑**Patient teaching**
● Instruct patient to take before or with meals and snacks.

• Advise patient not to crush or chew enteric-coated forms. Capsules containing enteric-coated microspheres may be opened and sprinkled on a small quantity of cooled, soft food. Stress importance of swallowing immediately without chewing and following with glass of water or juice.
• Warn patient not to inhale powder form or powder from capsules; it may irritate skin or mucous membranes.
• Tell patient to store in airtight containers at room temperature.
• Instruct patient not to change brands without consulting doctor.

---

## ursodiol
Actigall

*Pregnancy Risk Category B*

### HOW SUPPLIED
*Capsules:* 300 mg

### ACTION
Unknown. Drug is a naturally occurring bile acid that probably suppresses hepatic synthesis and secretion of cholesterol as well as intestinal cholesterol absorption. After long-term use, ursodiol can solubilize cholesterol from gallstones.

| Route | Onset | Peak | Duration |
|-------|-------|------|----------|
| P.O. | Unknown | 1-3 hr | Unknown |

### INDICATIONS & DOSAGE
*Dissolution of gallstones less than 20 mm in diameter when surgery precluded—*
**Adults:** 8 to 10 mg/kg P.O. daily in two or three divided doses.
*Prevention of gallstone formation in obese patients with rapid weight loss—*
**Adults:** 300 mg P.O. b.i.d.

### ADVERSE REACTIONS
**CNS:** *headache,* fatigue, anxiety, depression, *dizziness,* sleep disorders.
**EENT:** rhinitis.
**GI:** *nausea, vomiting, dyspepsia,* metallic taste, *abdominal pain,* biliary pain, cholecystitis, *diarrhea, constipation,* stomatitis, flatulence.
**GU:** *urinary tract infection.*

**Musculoskeletal:** arthralgia, myalgia, *back pain.*
**Respiratory:** cough.
**Skin:** pruritus, rash, dry skin, urticaria, hair thinning, diaphoresis.

### INTERACTIONS
**Drug-drug.** *Aluminum-containing antacids, cholestyramine, colestipol:* bind ursodiol and prevent its absorption. Avoid concomitant use.
*Clofibrate, estrogens, oral contraceptives:* increased hepatic cholesterol secretion; may counteract the effects of ursodiol. Avoid concomitant use.

### EFFECTS ON DIAGNOSTIC TESTS
None reported.

### CONTRAINDICATIONS
Contraindicated in patients with hypersensitivity to ursodiol or other bile acids and in those with chronic hepatic disease, unremitting acute cholecystitis, cholangitis, biliary obstruction, gallstone-induced pancreatitis, or biliary fistula.

### NURSING CONSIDERATIONS
• Drug won't dissolve calcified cholesterol stones, radiolucent bile pigment stones, or radiopaque stones.
• *Alert:* Monitor liver function test results, including AST and ALT, at the start of therapy and after 1 month, 3 months, and then every 6 months during therapy, as ordered. Abnormal tests may indicate a worsening of the disease. A theoretical risk exists that a hepatotoxic metabolite of ursodiol may form in some patients.
• Therapy usually is long-term, with ultrasound images of the gallbladder taken every 6 months. If stones don't partially dissolve within 12 months, eventual success is unlikely. Safety of use for longer than 24 months hasn't been established.

### ☑ Patient teaching
• Advise patient about alternative therapies, including "watchful waiting" (no intervention) and cholecystectomy because the relapse rate may be as high as 50% after 5 years.
• Tell patient to report adverse effects.

---

Reactions may be *common,* uncommon, *life-threatening*, or COMMON AND LIFE-THREATENING.

**attapulgite**
**bismuth subsalicylate**
**calcium polycarbophil**
  (See Chapter 50, LAXATIVES.)
**diphenoxylate hydrochloride and
  atropine sulfate**
**loperamide**
**octreotide acetate**
**opium tincture**
**opium tincture, camphorated**

## COMBINATION PRODUCTS
KAODENE NON-NARCOTIC ◊ : 3.9 g kaolin and 194.4 mg pectin in 30-ml bismuth subsalicylate liquid.
KAPECTOLIN: 90 g kaolin and 2 g pectin in 30-ml suspension.
K-C SUSPENSION ◊ : 5.2 g kaolin, 260 mg pectin, 260 mg bismuth subsalicylate in 30-ml suspension.

---

### attapulgite
Diasorb, Donnagel, Fowler's†, Kaopectate Advanced Formula, Kaopectate Maximum Strength, K-Pek, Parepectolin, Rheaban Maximum Strength

*Pregnancy Risk Category NR*

## HOW SUPPLIED
*Tablets:* 300 mg, 600 mg†, 630 mg†, 750 mg
*Oral suspension:* 600 mg/15 ml, 750 mg/5 ml, 750 mg/15 ml†, 900 mg/15 ml†
*Caplets:* 750 mg

## ACTION
Hydrated magnesium aluminum silicate that's thought to adsorb large numbers of bacteria and toxins and reduce water loss.

| Route | Onset | Peak | Duration |
|-------|-------|------|----------|
| P.O. | Unknown | Unknown | Unknown |

## INDICATIONS & DOSAGE
*Acute, nonspecific diarrhea—*
**Adults and children over age 12:** 1.2 to 1.5 g (up to 3 g if using Diasorb) P.O. after each loose bowel movement, not to exceed 9 g in 24 hours.
**Children ages 6 to 12:** 600 mg (suspension) or 750 mg (tablet) P.O. after each loose bowel movement, not to exceed 4.2 g (suspension) or 4.5 g (tablet) in 24 hours.
**Children ages 3 to 6:** 300 mg P.O. after each loose bowel movement, not to exceed 2.1 g in 24 hours.

## ADVERSE REACTIONS
**GI:** constipation.

## INTERACTIONS
**Drug-drug.** *Oral drugs:* potential for impaired absorption of oral drugs. Administer attapulgite not less than 2 hours before or 3 hours after these drugs, and monitor for decreased effectiveness.

## EFFECTS ON DIAGNOSTIC TESTS
None reported.

## CONTRAINDICATIONS
Contraindicated in patients with dysentery or suspected bowel obstruction.

## NURSING CONSIDERATIONS
• Use cautiously in patients with dehydration. Promote adequate fluid intake to compensate for fluid loss from diarrhea.
• Drug shouldn't be used if diarrhea is accompanied by fever or blood or mucus in the stool. If these signs occur during treatment, withhold drug and notify doctor.

☑**Patient teaching**
• Tell patient to take drug after each loose bowel movement until diarrhea is controlled.
• Instruct patient to notify doctor if diarrhea isn't controlled within 48 hours or if fever develops.

---

*Liquid contains alcohol.  **May contain tartrazine.  †Canada  ‡Australia  §U.K.  ◊ OTC

## bismuth subsalicylate
Bismatrol◇, Bismatrol Extra
Strength◇, Pepto-Bismol◇,
Pepto-Bismol Maximum Strength
Liquid◇, Pink Bismuth◇

*Pregnancy Risk Category NR*

### HOW SUPPLIED
*Tablets (chewable):* 262 mg◇
*Oral suspension:* 262 mg/15 ml◇,
524 mg/15 ml◇

### ACTION
Unknown. Has a mild water-binding capacity; and may adsorb toxins and provide
protective coating for mucosa.

| Route | Onset | Peak | Duration |
|-------|-------|------|----------|
| P.O. | 1 hr | Unknown | Unknown |

### INDICATIONS & DOSAGE
*Mild, nonspecific diarrhea—*
**Adults:** 30 ml or 2 tablets P.O. q 30 min-
utes to 1 hour, up to maximum of eight
doses and for no longer than 2 days.
**Children ages 9 to 12:** 15 ml or 1 tablet
P.O.
**Children ages 6 to 9:** 10 ml or ⅔ tablet
P.O.
**Children ages 3 to 6:** 5 ml or ⅓ tablet
P.O.

### ADVERSE REACTIONS
**GI:** temporary darkening of tongue and
stools.
**Other:** salicylism with high doses.

### INTERACTIONS
**Drug-drug.** *Aspirin, other salicylates:*
risk of salicylate toxicity. Monitor closely.
*Oral anticoagulants, oral antidiabetics:*
theoretical risk of increased effects of
these drugs after high doses of bismuth
subsalicylate. Monitor patient closely.
*Tetracycline:* decreased tetracycline absorption. Separate administration times by
at least 2 hours.

### EFFECTS ON DIAGNOSTIC TESTS
Because bismuth is radiopaque, it may interfere with radiologic examination of GI
tract.

### CONTRAINDICATIONS
Contraindicated in patients with hypersensitivity to salicylates.

### NURSING CONSIDERATIONS
• Use cautiously in patients taking aspirin.
Discontinue if tinnitus occurs.
• Salicylate absorption may occur from
bismuth subsalicylate. Use cautiously in
patients with bleeding disorders or salicylate sensitivity and in children.
• Avoid use before GI radiologic procedures because bismuth is radiopaque and
may interfere with X-rays.

### ☑ Patient teaching
• Advise patient that bismuth subsalicylate contains salicylate (each tablet has
102 mg salicylate; the regular-strength
liquid has 130 mg/15 ml, and the extra-
strength liquid has 230 mg/15 ml).
• Instruct patient to chew tablets well before swallowing or to shake liquid before
measuring dose.
• Tell patient to call doctor if diarrhea
persists for more than 2 days or is accompanied by high fever.
• Tell patient to consult with doctor before giving bismuth subsalicylate to children or teenagers during or after recovery
from the flu or chickenpox.
• Inform patient that all forms of Pepto-
Bismol are effective against traveler's diarrhea. Tablets and caplets may be more
convenient to carry.

## diphenoxylate hydrochloride and atropine sulfate
Logen, Lomanate, Lomotil*, Lonox

*Controlled Substance Schedule V*
*Pregnancy Risk Category C*

### HOW SUPPLIED
*Tablets:* 2.5 mg (with atropine sulfate
0.025 mg)
*Liquid:* 2.5 mg/5 ml (with atropine sulfate
0.025 mg/5 ml)*

### ACTION
Unknown. Probably increases smooth
muscle tone in GI tract, inhibits motility

---

Reactions may be *common*, uncommon, ***life-threatening***, or **COMMON AND LIFE-THREATENING**.

and propulsion, and diminishes secretions.

| Route | Onset | Peak | Duration |
|-------|-------|------|----------|
| P.O. | 45-60 min | 3 hr | 3-4 hr |

## INDICATIONS & DOSAGE
*Acute, nonspecific diarrhea—*
**Adults:** initially, 5 mg P.O. q.i.d.; then adjusted, p.r.n.
**Children ages 2 to 12:** 0.3 to 0.4 mg/kg liquid form P.O. daily in four divided doses. For maintenance, initial dose reduced, p.r.n., up to 75%.

## ADVERSE REACTIONS
**CNS:** *sedation, dizziness,* headache, drowsiness, lethargy, restlessness, depression, euphoria, malaise, confusion, numbness in extremities.
**CV:** tachycardia.
**EENT:** mydriasis.
**GI:** *dry mouth,* nausea, vomiting, abdominal discomfort or distention, *paralytic ileus,* anorexia, fluid retention in bowel or megacolon (may mask depletion of extracellular fluid and electrolytes, especially in young children treated for acute gastroenteritis), pancreatitis, swollen gums, possible physical dependence with long-term use.
**GU:** urine retention.
**Respiratory:** *respiratory depression.*
**Skin:** pruritus, rash, dry skin.
**Other:** *angioedema, anaphylaxis.*

## INTERACTIONS
**Drug-drug.** *Barbiturates, CNS depressants, narcotics, tranquilizers:* enhanced CNS depression. Closely monitor patient.
*MAO inhibitors:* possible hypertensive crisis. Avoid concomitant use.
**Drug-lifestyle.** *Alcohol use:* enhanced CNS depression. Closely monitor patient.

## EFFECTS ON DIAGNOSTIC TESTS
None reported.

## CONTRAINDICATIONS
Contraindicated in patients with hypersensitivity to diphenoxylate or atropine, in those with jaundice, and in children under age 2. Also contraindicated in those with acute diarrhea resulting from poison (until toxic material is eliminated from GI tract), from organisms that penetrate intestinal mucosa, or from antibiotic-induced pseudomembranous enterocolitis.

## NURSING CONSIDERATIONS
• Use cautiously in children age 2 and older; in patients with hepatic disease, narcotic dependence, or acute ulcerative colitis; and in pregnant patients. Stop therapy immediately if abdominal distention or other signs of toxic megacolon develop and notify doctor.
• *Alert:* Monitor fluid and electrolyte balance. Correct fluid and electrolyte disturbances before starting drug. Dehydration, especially in young children, may increase risk of delayed toxicity.
• Drug isn't indicated for treating antibiotic-induced diarrhea.
• Drug is unlikely to be effective if no response occurs within 48 hours.
• Risk of physical dependence increases with high dosage and long-term use. Atropine sulfate helps discourage abuse.

## ✅Patient teaching
• Tell patient not to exceed recommended dosage.
• Warn patient not to use drug to treat acute diarrhea for longer than 2 days and to seek medical attention if diarrhea continues.
• Advise patient to avoid hazardous activities, such as driving, until CNS effects of drug are known.

---

## loperamide
Imodium, Imodium A-D ◇,
Kaopectate II Caplets ◇,
Maalox Anti-Diarrheal Caplets ◇,
Pepto Diarrhea Control ◇

*Pregnancy Risk Category B*

## HOW SUPPLIED
*Caplets:* 2 mg ◇
*Capsules:* 2 mg
*Oral liquid:* 1 mg/5 ml ◇

---

## ACTION
Inhibits peristaltic activity, prolonging transit of intestinal contents.

| Route | Onset | Peak | Duration |
|-------|-------|------|----------|
| P.O. | Unknown | 2.5-5 hr | 24 hr |

## INDICATIONS & DOSAGE
*Acute, nonspecific diarrhea—*
**Adults:** initially, 4 mg P.O.; then 2 mg after each unformed stool. Maximum dose is 16 mg daily.
**Children ages 8 to 12:** 10 ml (2 mg) t.i.d. P.O. on first day. (Subsequent doses of 5 ml [1 mg]/10 kg of body weight may be administered after each unformed stool.) Maximum dose is 6 mg daily.
**Children ages 6 to 8:** 10 ml (2 mg) P.O. b.i.d. on first day. If diarrhea persists, contact doctor. Don't exceed 4 mg daily.
**Children ages 2 to 5:** 5 ml P.O. t.i.d. on first day. If diarrhea persists, contact doctor.
*Chronic diarrhea—*
**Adults:** initially, 4 mg P.O.; then 2 mg after each unformed stool until diarrhea subsides. Dosage adjusted to individual response.

## ADVERSE REACTIONS
**CNS:** drowsiness, fatigue, dizziness.
**GI:** dry mouth; abdominal pain, distention, or discomfort; *constipation;* nausea; vomiting.
**Skin:** rash, *hypersensitivity reactions.*

## INTERACTIONS
None significant.

## EFFECTS ON DIAGNOSTIC TESTS
None reported.

## CONTRAINDICATIONS
Contraindicated in patients with hypersensitivity to drug and when constipation must be avoided. Also contraindicated in children under age 2.

## NURSING CONSIDERATIONS
• Use cautiously in patients with hepatic disease.
• Drug produces antidiarrheal action similar to diphenoxylate but without as many adverse CNS effects.

• *Alert:* Monitor children closely for CNS effects; they may be more sensitive than adults to these effects.
• *Alert:* Don't confuse Imodium with Ionamin.

## ✓ Patient teaching
• Advise patient not to exceed recommended dosage.
• Tell patient with acute diarrhea to discontinue drug and seek medical attention if no improvement occurs within 48 hours; in chronic diarrhea, tell him to notify doctor and discontinue drug if no improvement occurs after taking 16 mg daily for at least 10 days.
• Advise patient with acute colitis to stop drug immediately if abdominal distention or other symptoms develop and notify doctor.
• Warn patient to avoid activities that require mental alertness until CNS effects of drug are known.
• Tell patient to report nausea, abdominal pain, or abdominal discomfort.
• Advise patient to relieve dry mouth with ice chips or sugarless gum.

---

# octreotide acetate
## Sandostatin

*Pregnancy Risk Category B*

## HOW SUPPLIED
*Injection ampules:* 0.05 mg, 0.1 mg, 0.5 mg
*Injection-multidose vials:* 0.2 mg/ml, 1 mg/ml

## ACTION
Mimics action of naturally occurring somatostatin.

| Route | Onset | Peak | Duration |
|-------|-------|------|----------|
| S.C. | 0.5 hr | 0.5 hr | < 12 hr |

## INDICATIONS & DOSAGE
*Flushing and diarrhea associated with carcinoid tumors—*
**Adults:** 0.1 to 0.6 mg daily S.C. in two to four divided doses for first 2 weeks of therapy (usual daily dosage is 0.3 mg).

---

Reactions may be *common*, uncommon, *life-threatening*, or COMMON AND LIFE-THREATENING.

Subsequent dosage based on individual response.

*Watery diarrhea associated with vasoactive intestinal polypeptide secreting tumors (VIPomas)—*
**Adults:** 0.2 to 0.3 mg daily S.C. in two to four divided doses for first 2 weeks of therapy. Subsequent dosage based on individual response; typically, don't exceed 0.45 mg daily.

*Acromegaly—*
**Adults:** initially, 50 mcg S.C. t.i.d., then adjusted based on somatomedin C levels q 2 weeks.

**ADVERSE REACTIONS**
**CNS:** dizziness, light-headedness, fatigue, headache.
**CV:** *sinus bradycardia,* edema, conduction abnormalities, *arrhythmias.*
**EENT:** blurred vision.
**GI:** *nausea, diarrhea, abdominal pain or discomfort, loose stools,* vomiting, fat malabsorption, *gallbladder abnormalities*, flatulence, constipation.
**GU:** pollakiuria, urinary tract infection.
**Metabolic:** hyperglycemia, hypoglycemia, hypothyroidism; suppressed secretion of growth hormone and of the gastroenterohepatic peptides gastrin, vasoactive intestinal polypeptide, insulin, glucagon, secretin, motilin, and pancreatic polypeptide.
**Musculoskeletal:** backache, joint pain.
**Skin:** flushing, wheal, erythema or pain at injection site, alopecia.
**Other:** pain or burning at the S.C. injection site, cold symptoms, flulike symptoms.

**INTERACTIONS**
**Drug-drug.** *Cyclosporine:* may decrease plasma levels of cyclosporine. Monitor patient closely.

**EFFECTS ON DIAGNOSTIC TESTS**
None reported.

**CONTRAINDICATIONS**
Contraindicated in patients with hypersensitivity to drug or its components.

**NURSING CONSIDERATIONS**
• Monitor baseline thyroid function tests, as ordered.
• Monitor somatomedin C levels every 2 weeks, as ordered. Dosage adjustments are based on this level.
• Monitor laboratory tests periodically, such as thyroid function tests, blood glucose, urine 5-hydroxyindoleacetic acid, plasma serotonin, and plasma substance P (for carcinoid tumors).
• Monitor patient regularly for gallbladder disease. Octreotide therapy may be associated with development of cholelithiasis because of its effect on gallbladder motility or fat absorption.
• Monitor closely for symptoms of glucose imbalance. Patients with type 1 diabetes mellitus and patients receiving oral antidiabetics or oral diazoxide may need dosage adjustments during therapy. Monitor blood glucose levels.
• Octreotide therapy may alter fluid and electrolyte balance and may need adjustment of other drugs used to control symptoms of the disease, such as beta blockers.
• Half-life may be altered in patients in end-stage renal failure who are receiving dialysis.
• *Alert:* Don't confuse Sandostatin with Sandimmune or Sandoglobulin.

☑ **Patient teaching**
• Instruct patient to report signs of abdominal discomfort immediately.
• Stress importance of need for periodic laboratory testing during octreotide therapy.

**opium tincture***

*Controlled Substance Schedule II*

**opium tincture, camphorated*** **(paregoric)**

*Controlled Substance Schedule III*
*Pregnancy Risk Category NR*

**HOW SUPPLIED**
**opium tincture**
*Oral solution:* equivalent to morphine 10 mg/ml*

## opium tincture, camphorated

*Oral solution:* each 5 ml contains morphine, 2 mg; anise oil, 0.2 ml; benzoic acid, 20 mg; camphor, 20 mg; glycerin, 0.2 ml; and ethanol to make 5 ml*

### ACTION

Increases smooth muscle tone in GI tract, inhibits motility and propulsion, and diminishes secretions.

| Route | Onset | Peak | Duration |
|-------|-------|------|----------|
| P.O. | Unknown | Unknown | Unknown |

### INDICATIONS & DOSAGE

*Acute, nonspecific diarrhea—*
**opium tincture**
**Adults:** 0.6 ml (range 0.3 to 1 ml) P.O. q.i.d. Maximum dose is 6 ml daily.
**opium tincture, camphorated**
**Adults:** 5 to 10 ml P.O. once daily, b.i.d., t.i.d., or q.i.d. until diarrhea subsides.
**Children:** 0.25 to 0.5 ml/kg P.O. once daily, b.i.d., t.i.d., or q.i.d. until diarrhea subsides.

### ADVERSE REACTIONS

**CNS:** dizziness, light-headedness.
**GI:** nausea, vomiting, physical dependence after long-term use.
**Metabolic:** elevated serum amylase and lipase levels.

### INTERACTIONS

None significant.

### EFFECTS ON DIAGNOSTIC TESTS

Opium tincture and camphorated opium tincture may prevent delivery of Tc99m disofenin to small intestine during hepatobiliary imaging tests; delay test until 24 hours after last dose.

### CONTRAINDICATIONS

Contraindicated in patients with acute diarrhea due to poisoning until toxic material is removed from GI tract and in those with diarrhea due to organisms that penetrate intestinal mucosa.

### NURSING CONSIDERATIONS

• Use cautiously in patients with asthma, prostatic hyperplasia, hepatic disease, and history of opioid dependence.

• *Alert:* Opium tincture has 25 times more opium content than camphorated opium tincture. Camphorated opium tincture is more dilute, and teaspoon doses are easier to measure than dropper quantities of opium tincture.

• *Alert:* For overdose, use the narcotic antagonist naloxone, as ordered, to reverse respiratory depression.

• Mix with sufficient water to ensure passage to stomach.

• A milky fluid forms when camphorated opium tincture is added to water.

• Store in tightly capped, light-resistant container.

• *Alert:* Don't confuse opium tincture with camphorated opium tincture.

### ☑ Patient teaching

• Advise patient against long-term use of drug; risk of physical dependence increases with long-term use.

• Instruct patient to measure dose carefully to avoid overdose.

• Tell patient to notify doctor if diarrhea persists.

---

Reactions may be *common,* uncommon, *life-threatening,* or COMMON AND LIFE-THREATENING.

bisacodyl
calcium polycarbophil
cascara sagrada
cascara sagrada aromatic
 fluidextract
cascara sagrada fluidextract
castor oil
docusate calcium
docusate sodium
glycerin
lactulose
magnesium citrate
magnesium hydroxide
magnesium sulfate
methylcellulose
mineral oil
polyethylene glycol and
 electrolyte solution
psyllium
senna
sodium phosphates

## COMBINATION PRODUCTS
DIALOSE PLUS ◊: docusate sodium
100 mg and casanthranol 30 mg.
DOXIDAN ◊: docusate sodium 100 mg and
casanthranol 30 mg.
HALEY'S M-O ◊: mineral oil 3.75 ml and
magnesium hydroxide 900 mg per 15 ml.
PERI-COLACE CAPSULES ◊: docusate sodium 100 mg and casanthranol 30 mg.
PERI-COLACE SYRUP ◊: docusate sodium
60 mg and casanthranol 30 mg/15 ml.
SENOKOT-S ◊: docusate sodium 50 mg
and standardized senna concentrate
187 mg.

---

## bisacodyl
Bisacolax† ◊, Bisalax‡,
Bisco-Lax** ◊, Dulcagen ◊,
Dulcolax ◊, Durolax‡, Fleet
Bisacodyl ◊, Fleet Bisacodyl
Prep ◊, Fleet Laxative ◊, Laxit† ◊

*Pregnancy Risk Category NR*

## HOW SUPPLIED
*Tablets (enteric-coated):* 5 mg ◊

*Enema:* 0.33 mg/ml ◊, 10 mg/5 ml
(microenema)‡
*Powder for rectal solution (bisacodyl tan-
nex):* 1.5 mg bisacodyl and 2.5 g tannic
acid
*Suppositories:* 5 mg ◊, 10 mg ◊

## ACTION
Unknown. Stimulant laxative that increases peristalsis, probably by direct effect on
smooth muscle of the intestine. It is
thought to either irritate the musculature
or stimulate the colonic intramural plexus.
Drug also promotes fluid accumulation in
colon and small intestine.

| Route | Onset | Peak | Duration |
|-------|-------|------|----------|
| P.O. | 6-12 hr | Variable | Variable |
| P.R. | 15-60 min | Variable | Variable |

## INDICATIONS & DOSAGE
*Chronic constipation; preparation for de-
livery, surgery, or rectal or bowel examination—*
**Adults and children ages 12 and over:**
10 to 15 mg P.O. in evening or before
breakfast. Up to 30 mg P.O. as needed and
ordered; or 10 mg P.R. for evacuation before examination or surgery.
**Children ages 6 to 12:** 5 mg P.O. or P.R.
h.s. or before breakfast. Oral dose isn't
recommended if child can't swallow
tablet whole.

## ADVERSE REACTIONS
**CNS:** muscle weakness with excessive
use, dizziness, faintness.
**GI:** *nausea, vomiting, abdominal cramps,*
diarrhea with high doses, *burning sensation in rectum* (with suppositories), laxative dependence with long-term or excessive use, protein-losing enteropathy with
excessive use.
**Metabolic:** alkalosis, hypokalemia, fluid
and electrolyte imbalance.
**Musculoskeletal:** tetany.

---

*Liquid contains alcohol.   **May contain tartrazine.   †Canada   ‡Australia   §U.K.   ◊OTC

## INTERACTIONS
**Drug-drug.** *Antacids:* gastric irritation or dyspepsia from premature dissolution of enteric coating. Don't administer together.
**Drug-food.** *Milk:* gastric irritation or dyspepsia from premature dissolution of enteric coating. Don't administer together.

## EFFECTS ON DIAGNOSTIC TESTS
None reported.

## CONTRAINDICATIONS
Contraindicated in patients with hypersensitivity to drug or its components and in those with rectal bleeding, gastroenteritis, intestinal obstruction, abdominal pain, nausea, vomiting, or other symptoms of appendicitis or acute surgical abdomen.

## NURSING CONSIDERATIONS
• Time administration of drug so as not to interfere with scheduled activities or sleep. Soft, formed stools are usually produced 15 to 60 minutes after rectal administration.
• Before giving for constipation, determine if patient has adequate fluid intake, exercise, and diet.
• Tablets and suppositories are used together to clean the colon before and after surgery and before barium enema.
• Insert suppository as high as possible into the rectum, and try to position suppository against the rectal wall. Avoid embedding within fecal material because this may delay onset of action.

### ☑ Patient teaching
• Advise patient to swallow enteric-coated tablet whole to avoid GI irritation. Don't give within 1 hour of milk or antacid intake.
• Tell patient that drug is for short-term (1 week) treatment only (stimulant laxatives are frequently abused). Discourage excessive use.
• Advise patient to report adverse effects to doctor.
• Teach patient about dietary sources of bulk, including bran and other cereals, fresh fruit, and vegetables.
• Tell patient to take drug with a full glass of water or juice.

# calcium polycarbophil
Equalactin ◇, Fiberall ◇, FiberCon ◇, Fiber-Lax ◇, Mitrolan ◇

*Pregnancy Risk Category NR*

## HOW SUPPLIED
*Tablets:* 500 mg ◇, 625 mg ◇
*Tablets (chewable):* 500 mg ◇, 1,250 mg ◇

## ACTION
Bulk-forming laxative that absorbs water and expands to increase bulk and moisture content of stools. The increased bulk encourages peristalsis and bowel movement. As an antidiarrheal, drug absorbs free fecal water, thereby producing formed stools.

| Route | Onset | Peak | Duration |
|-------|-------|------|----------|
| P.O. | 12-24 hr | 3 days | Variable |

## INDICATIONS & DOSAGE
*Constipation—*
**Adults:** 1 g P.O. q.i.d., p.r.n. Maximum dose is 6 g in 24-hour period.
**Children ages 3 to 6:** use must be directed by doctor; 500 mg P.O. b.i.d., p.r.n. Maximum dose is 1.5 g in 24-hour period.
**Children ages 6 to 12:** 500 mg P.O. one to three times daily, p.r.n. Maximum dose is 3 g in 24-hour period.
*Diarrhea associated with irritable bowel syndrome; acute, nonspecific diarrhea—*
**Adults:** 1 g P.O. q.i.d., p.r.n. Maximum dose is 6 g in 24-hour period.
**Children ages 2 to 6:** use must be directed by doctor; 500 mg P.O. b.i.d., p.r.n. Maximum dose is 1.5 g in 24-hour period.
**Children ages 6 to 12:** 500 mg P.O. t.i.d., p.r.n. Maximum dose is 3 g in 24-hour period.

## ADVERSE REACTIONS
**GI:** abdominal fullness and increased flatus, intestinal obstruction.
**Other:** laxative dependence with long-term or excessive use.

---

Reactions may be *common*, uncommon, *life-threatening*, or COMMON AND LIFE-THREATENING.

## INTERACTIONS
**Drug-drug.** *Tetracyclines:* impaired absorption of tetracyclines. Avoid concomitant use.

## EFFECTS ON DIAGNOSTIC TESTS
None reported.

## CONTRAINDICATIONS
Contraindicated in patients with signs of GI obstruction.

## NURSING CONSIDERATIONS
• Before giving for constipation, determine if patient has adequate fluid intake, exercise, and diet.
• *Alert:* Rectal bleeding or failure to respond to therapy may indicate need for surgery.

☑ **Patient teaching**
• Advise patient to chew Equalactin or Mitrolan tablets thoroughly before swallowing and to drink a full glass of water with each dose. When drug is used as an antidiarrheal, tell patient not to drink a glass of water.
• Teach patient about dietary sources of bulk, including bran and other cereals, fresh fruit, and vegetables.
• For severe diarrhea, advise patient to repeat dose every 30 minutes, but not to exceed maximum daily dose.

---

cascara sagrada ◊

cascara sagrada aromatic fluidextract* ◊

cascara sagrada fluidextract* ◊

*Pregnancy Risk Category C*

## HOW SUPPLIED
*Tablets:* 325 mg ◊
*Aromatic fluidextract:* 1 g/ml* ◊
*Fluidextract:* 1 g/ml* ◊

## ACTION
Unknown. Stimulant laxative that increases peristalsis, probably by direct effect on smooth muscle of the intestine. It's thought to either irritate the musculature or stimulate the colonic intramural plexus. Drug also promotes fluid accumulation in colon and small intestine.

| Route | Onset | Peak | Duration |
|-------|-------|------|----------|
| P.O. | 6-10 hr | Variable | Variable |

## INDICATIONS & DOSAGE
*Acute constipation, preparation for bowel or rectal examination—*
**Adults and children ages 12 and older:** one 325-mg tablet of cascara sagrada P.O. once daily h.s.; 0.5 to 1.5 ml of cascara sagrada fluidextract P.O. once daily, or 2 to 6 ml of aromatic cascara fluidextract P.O. once daily.
**Children ages 2 to 12:** one-half adult dosage.
**Children under age 2:** one-quarter adult dosage.

## ADVERSE REACTIONS
**GI:** *nausea;* vomiting; diarrhea; loss of normal bowel function with excessive use; *abdominal cramps,* especially in severe constipation; malabsorption of nutrients; cathartic colon (syndrome resembling ulcerative colitis radiologically and pathologically) with long-term misuse; discoloration of rectal mucosa after long-term use; protein enteropathy; laxative dependence with long-term or excessive use.
**Metabolic:** hypokalemia, electrolyte imbalance with excessive use.

## INTERACTIONS
None significant.

## EFFECTS ON DIAGNOSTIC TESTS
Drug turns alkaline urine pink to red, red to violet, or red to brown and turns acidic urine yellow to brown in the phenolsulfonphthalein excretion test.

## CONTRAINDICATIONS
Contraindicated in patients with abdominal pain, nausea, vomiting, or other symptoms of appendicitis or acute surgical abdomen; acute surgical delirium; fecal impaction; or intestinal obstruction or perforation.

---

*Liquid contains alcohol.    **May contain tartrazine.    †Canada    ‡Australia    §U.K.    ◊OTC

## NURSING CONSIDERATIONS

• *Alert:* Use cautiously when rectal bleeding is present.
• Before giving for constipation, determine if patient has adequate fluid intake, exercise, and diet.
• Monitor serum electrolyte levels during prolonged use.
• Cascara sagrada aromatic fluidextract is less active and less bitter than the nonaromatic fluidextract.
• Liquid preparations are more reliable than solid dosage forms.

### ☑ Patient teaching

• Warn patient that drug may turn alkaline urine red-pink and acidic urine yellow-brown.
• Teach patient about dietary sources of bulk, including bran and other cereals, fresh fruit, and vegetables.
• Tell patient to take drug with a full glass of water.

---

## castor oil
Emulsoil◇, Fleet Flavored Castor Oil◇, Purge◇

*Pregnancy Risk Category X*

### HOW SUPPLIED
*Capsules:* 0.62 ml
*Oral liquid:* 67% (Fleet◇), 95% (Emulsoil◇, Purge◇)

### ACTION
Unknown. Stimulant laxative that increases peristalsis, probably by direct effect on smooth muscle of the intestine. It's thought to either irritate the musculature or stimulate the colonic intramural plexus. Drug also promotes fluid accumulation in colon and small intestine.

| Route | Onset | Peak | Duration |
|-------|-------|------|----------|
| P.O. | 2-6 hr | Variable | Variable |

### INDICATIONS & DOSAGE
*Preparation for rectal or bowel examination or for surgery—*
**Adults and children ages 12 and older:** 15 to 60 ml P.O.
**Children ages 2 to 12:** 5 to 15 ml P.O.

**Children under age 2:** 2.5 to 7.5 ml P.O. Increased dosage produces no greater effect.

For all patients, administered as a single dose about 16 hours before surgery or procedure.

### ADVERSE REACTIONS
**GI:** *nausea;* vomiting; diarrhea; loss of normal bowel function with excessive use; *abdominal cramps,* especially in severe constipation; malabsorption of nutrients; cathartic colon (syndrome resembling ulcerative colitis radiologically and pathologically) with long-term misuse; protein-losing enteropathy; laxative dependence with long-term or excessive use; possible constipation after catharsis.
**Metabolic:** hypokalemia, other electrolyte imbalances with excessive use.

### INTERACTIONS
None significant.

### EFFECTS ON DIAGNOSTIC TESTS
None reported.

### CONTRAINDICATIONS
Contraindicated in patients with ulcerative bowel lesions; abdominal pain, nausea, vomiting, or other symptoms of appendicitis or acute surgical abdomen; anal or rectal fissures, fecal impaction, or intestinal obstruction or perforation; also contraindicated during menstruation or pregnancy.

### NURSING CONSIDERATIONS
• Use cautiously in patients with rectal bleeding.
• Give castor oil with juice or carbonated beverage to mask oily taste. Have patient stir mixture and drink it promptly. Ice held in the mouth before taking drug will help prevent tasting it.
• Shake emulsion well before measuring dose. Emulsion is better tolerated but is more expensive. Store below 40° F (4.4° C). Don't freeze.
• Give on empty stomach for best results.
• Time drug administration so that it doesn't interfere with scheduled activities or sleep.

---

Reactions may be *common,* uncommon, *life-threatening,* or COMMON AND LIFE-THREATENING.

• Increased intestinal motility lessens absorption of concomitantly administered oral drugs. Separate administration times.
• *Alert:* Failure of patient to respond to drug may indicate acute condition requiring surgery.

☑ **Patient teaching**
• Tell patient not to expect another bowel movement for 1 to 2 days after castor oil has emptied bowel.
• Warn patient about potential adverse reactions.

---

**docusate calcium (dioctyl calcium sulfosuccinate)**
DC Softgels ◇, Pro-Cal-Sof ◇, Sulfalax Calcium ◇, Surfak ◇

**docusate sodium (dioctyl sodium sulfosuccinate)**
Colace ◇, Coloxyl‡, Coloxyl Enema Concentrate‡, Diocto ◇, Dioctyl§, Dioeze ◇, Diosuccin ◇, Disonate ◇, Di-Sosul ◇, DOS ◇, D-S-S ◇, Duosol ◇, Fletcher's Enemette§, Modane Soft ◇, Norgalax Micro-enema§, Pro-Sof ◇, Regulax SS ◇, Regulex† ◇

*Pregnancy Risk Category C*

**HOW SUPPLIED**
**docusate calcium**
*Capsules:* 50 mg ◇, 240 mg ◇
**docusate sodium**
*Tablets:* 100 mg ◇, 50 mg ◇
*Capsules:* 50 mg ◇, 100 mg ◇, 240 mg ◇, 250 mg ◇
*Oral liquid:* 150 mg/15 ml ◇
*Oral solution:* 50 mg/ml ◇, 10 mg/ml ◇
*Syrup:* 20 mg/5 ml, 50 mg/15 ml ◇, 60 mg/15 ml ◇
*Enema concentrate:* 18 g/100 ml (must be diluted)‡

**ACTION**
Stool softener that reduces surface tension of interfacing liquid contents of the bowel. This detergent activity promotes incor-

poration of additional liquid into stools, thus forming a softer mass.

| Route | Onset | Peak | Duration |
|---|---|---|---|
| P.O., P.R. | 24-72 hr | 24-72 hr | 24-72 hr |

**INDICATIONS & DOSAGE**
*Stool softener—*
**Adults and children over age 12:** 50 to 500 mg P.O. daily until bowel movements are normal. Or, give enema (where available). Dilute 1:24 with sterile water before administration, and give 100 to 150 ml (retention enema), 300 to 500 ml (evacuation enema), or 0.5 to 1.5 L (flushing enema) P.R.
**Children ages 6 to 12:** 40 to 120 mg docusate sodium P.O. daily.
**Children ages 3 to 6:** 20 to 60 mg docusate sodium P.O. daily.
**Children under age 3:** 10 to 40 mg docusate sodium P.O. daily.
  Higher dosages used for initial therapy. Dosage adjusted to individual response. Usual dosage in children and adults with minimal needs is 50 to 150 mg (calcium) P.O. daily.

**ADVERSE REACTIONS**
**GI:** bitter taste, mild abdominal cramping, diarrhea, laxative dependence with long-term or excessive use.

**INTERACTIONS**
**Drug-drug.** *Mineral oil:* may increase mineral oil absorption and cause toxicity and lipoid pneumonia. Separate administration times.

**EFFECTS ON DIAGNOSTIC TESTS**
None reported.

**CONTRAINDICATIONS**
Contraindicated in patients with hypersensitivity to drug and in those with intestinal obstruction, undiagnosed abdominal pain, vomiting or other signs of appendicitis, fecal impaction, or acute surgical abdomen.

**NURSING CONSIDERATIONS**
• Give liquid in milk, fruit juice, or infant formula to mask bitter taste.

---

*Liquid contains alcohol.   **May contain tartrazine.   †Canada   ‡Australia   §U.K.   ◇OTC

• Before giving for constipation, determine if patient has adequate fluid intake, exercise, and diet.

• Drug isn't for use in treating existing constipation but prevents constipation from developing.

• Drug is laxative of choice for patients who shouldn't strain during defecation, including patients recovering from MI or rectal surgery, those with rectal or anal disease that makes passage of firm stools difficult, and those with postpartum constipation.

• Store drug at 59° to 86° F (15° to 30° C), and protect liquid from light.

☑ **Patient teaching**
• Teach patient about dietary sources of bulk, including bran and other cereals, fresh fruit, and vegetables.
• Instruct patient to use drug only occasionally and not for more than 1 week without doctor's knowledge.
• Tell patient to discontinue drug if severe cramping occurs and to notify doctor.
• Notify patient that it may take from 1 to 3 days to soften stools.

## glycerin
Fleet Babylax◇, Sani-Supp◇

*Pregnancy Risk Category NR*

### HOW SUPPLIED
*Enema (pediatric):* 4 ml/applicator◇
*Suppositories:* adult, children, and infant sizes◇

### ACTION
Hyperosmolar laxative that draws water from the tissues into the feces, thus stimulating evacuation.

| Route | Onset | Peak | Duration |
|-------|-------|------|----------|
| P.R. | 15-60 min | 15-60 min | 15-60 min |

### INDICATIONS & DOSAGE
*Constipation—*
**Adults and children age 6 and older:** 2 to 3 g as rectal suppository; or 5 to 15 ml as enema.
**Children ages 2 to 6:** 1 to 1.7 g as rectal suppository; or 2 to 5 ml as enema.

### ADVERSE REACTIONS
**GI:** *cramping pain,* rectal discomfort, hyperemia of rectal mucosa.

### INTERACTIONS
None significant.

### EFFECTS ON DIAGNOSTIC TESTS
None reported.

### CONTRAINDICATIONS
Contraindicated in patients with hypersensitivity to drug and in those with intestinal obstruction, undiagnosed abdominal pain, vomiting or other signs of appendicitis, fecal impaction, or acute surgical abdomen.

### NURSING CONSIDERATIONS
• Drug is used mainly to reestablish proper toilet habits in laxative-dependent patients.

☑ **Patient teaching**
• Tell patient that drug must be retained for at least 15 minutes and that it usually acts within 1 hour. Entire suppository need not melt to be effective.
• Warn patient about adverse GI reactions.

## lactulose
Cephulac, Cholac, Chronulac, Constilac, Constulose, Duphalac, Enulose, Evalose, Heptalac, Lactulax†

*Pregnancy Risk Category B*

### HOW SUPPLIED
*Syrup:* 10 g/15 ml

### ACTION
Produces an osmotic effect in colon; resulting distention promotes peristalsis. Also, decreases blood ammonia, probably as a result of bacterial degradation, which decreases the pH of colon contents.

| Route | Onset | Peak | Duration |
|-------|-------|------|----------|
| P.O. | 24-48 hr | Variable | Variable |
| P.R. | Unknown | Unknown | Unknown |

## INDICATIONS & DOSAGE
*Constipation—*
**Adults:** 10 to 20 g (15 to 30 ml) P.O. daily, increased to 60 ml/day if needed.
*To prevent and treat hepatic encephalopathy, including hepatic precoma and coma in patients with severe hepatic disease—*
**Adults:** initially, 20 to 30 g (30 to 45 ml) P.O. t.i.d. or q.i.d., until two or three soft stools are produced daily. Usual dose is 60 to 100 g daily in divided doses. Or, 200 g (300 ml) diluted with 700 ml of water or normal saline solution and given as retention enema P.R. q 4 to 6 hours, p.r.n.

## ADVERSE REACTIONS
**GI:** *abdominal cramps, belching, diarrhea, gaseous distention, flatulence,* nausea, vomiting.

## INTERACTIONS
**Drug-drug.** *Antacids, antibiotics, oral neomycin:* decreased effectiveness of lactulose. Avoid concomitant use.

## EFFECTS ON DIAGNOSTIC TESTS
None reported.

## CONTRAINDICATIONS
Contraindicated in patients on a low-galactose diet.

## NURSING CONSIDERATIONS
• Use cautiously in patients with diabetes mellitus.
• To minimize sweet taste, dilute with water or fruit juice or give with food.
• Prepare enema (not commercially available) by adding 200 g (300 ml) to 700 ml of water or normal saline solution. The diluted solution is administered as retention enema for 30 to 60 minutes. Use a rectal balloon.
• If enema isn't retained for at least 30 minutes, be prepared to repeat dose.
• Monitor serum sodium level for possible hypernatremia, especially when giving in higher doses to treat hepatic encephalopathy.
• Monitor mental status when giving to patients with hepatic encephalopathy.
• Be prepared to replace fluid loss.

• *Alert:* Don't confuse lactulose with lactose.

### ✅ Patient teaching
• Show home care patient how to mix and then administer drug.
• Inform patient about adverse reactions and tell him to notify doctor if reactions become bothersome or if diarrhea occurs.
• Instruct patient not to take other laxatives while on lactulose therapy.

---

## magnesium citrate
### (citrate of magnesia)
Citroma ◊ , Citro-Mag†

## magnesium hydroxide
### (milk of magnesia)
Milk of Magnesia ◊ , Milk of Magnesia Concentrate ◊ , Phillips' Milk of Magnesia ◊

## magnesium sulfate
### (epsom salts) ◊

*Pregnancy Risk Category NR*

---

## HOW SUPPLIED
**magnesium citrate**
*Oral solution:* about 168 mEq magnesium/240 ml ◊
**magnesium hydroxide**
*Oral suspension:* 7% to 8.5% (about 80 mEq magnesium/30 ml) ◊
**magnesium sulfate**
*Granules:* about 40 mEq magnesium/5 g ◊

## ACTION
Saline laxative that produces an osmotic effect in the small intestine by drawing water into the intestinal lumen.

| Route | Onset | Peak | Duration |
|-------|-------|------|----------|
| P.O. | 0.5-3 hr | Variable | Variable |

## INDICATIONS & DOSAGE
*Constipation, to evacuate bowel before surgery—*
**Adults and children ages 12 and older:** 11 to 25 g magnesium citrate P.O. daily as a single dose or divided; 2.4 to 4.8 g (30 to 60 ml) magnesium hydroxide P.O. daily

as a single dose or divided; 10 to 30 g magnesium sulfate P.O. daily as a single dose or divided.

**Children ages 6 to 12:** 5.5 to 12.5 g magnesium citrate P.O. daily as a single dose or divided; 1.2 to 2.4 g (15 to 30 ml) magnesium hydroxide P.O. daily as a single dose or divided; 5 to 10 g magnesium sulfate P.O. daily as a single dose or divided.

**Children ages 2 to 6:** 2.7 to 6.25 g magnesium citrate P.O. daily as a single dose or divided; 0.4 to 1.2 g (5 to 15 ml) magnesium hydroxide P.O. daily as a single dose or divided; 2.5 to 5 g magnesium sulfate P.O. daily as a single dose or divided.
*Antacid—*
**Adults:** 5 to 15 ml milk of magnesia P.O. t.i.d. or q.i.d.

## ADVERSE REACTIONS
**GI:** *abdominal cramping, nausea, diarrhea,* laxative dependence with long-term or excessive use.
**Metabolic:** fluid and electrolyte disturbances with daily use.

## INTERACTIONS
**Drug-drug.** *Oral drugs:* impaired absorption. Separate administration times.

## EFFECTS ON DIAGNOSTIC TESTS
None reported.

## CONTRAINDICATIONS
Contraindicated in patients with abdominal pain, nausea, vomiting, or other symptoms of appendicitis or acute surgical abdomen; myocardial damage; heart block; fecal impaction; rectal fissures; intestinal obstruction or perforation; or renal disease; also contraindicated in pregnant patients about to deliver.

## NURSING CONSIDERATIONS
• Use cautiously in patients with rectal bleeding.
• Time drug administration so that it doesn't interfere with scheduled activities or sleep. Drug produces watery stools in 3 to 6 hours.

• Before giving for constipation, determine if patient has adequate fluid intake, exercise, and diet.
• Chill magnesium citrate before use to make it more palatable.
• Shake suspension well; give with large amount of water when used as laxative. When administering through nasogastric tube, make sure tube is placed properly and is patent. After instilling, flush tube with water to ensure passage to stomach and maintain tube patency.
• *Alert:* Monitor serum electrolyte levels, as ordered, during prolonged use. Magnesium may accumulate in patient with renal insufficiency.
• Drug is for short-term therapy only.
• Magnesium sulfate is more potent than other saline laxatives.

☑ **Patient teaching**
• Instruct patient on drug administration.
• Teach patient about dietary sources of bulk, including bran and other cereals, fresh fruit, and vegetables.
• Warn patient that frequent or prolonged use as a laxative may cause dependence.

---

**methylcellulose**
Citrucel ◇, Citrucel Orange
Flavor ◇, Citrucel Sugar-Free
Orange Flavor ◇

*Pregnancy Risk Category NR*

## HOW SUPPLIED
*Powder:* 2 g/tbs (heaping) ◇

## ACTION
Bulk-forming laxative that absorbs water and expands to increase bulk and moisture content of stools. The increased bulk encourages peristalsis and bowel movement.

| Route | Onset | Peak | Duration |
|-------|-------|------|----------|
| P.O. | 12-24 hr | < 3 days | Variable |

## INDICATIONS & DOSAGE
*Chronic constipation—*
**Adults:** 1 to 3 tbs (heaping) in 8 oz (240 ml) of cold water daily to t.i.d. Usual dose is up to 6 g daily (3 tbs).

**Children ages 6 to 12:** 1 to 1½ level tbs in 4 oz (120 ml) of cold water daily to t.i.d. Usual dose up to 3 g daily (1½ tbs).

## ADVERSE REACTIONS
**GI:** *nausea,* vomiting, diarrhea with excessive use; esophageal, gastric, small intestinal, or colonic strictures when drug is chewed or taken in dry form; *abdominal cramps,* especially in severe constipation; laxative dependence with long-term or excessive use.

## INTERACTIONS
None significant.

## EFFECTS ON DIAGNOSTIC TESTS
None reported.

## CONTRAINDICATIONS
Contraindicated in patients with abdominal pain, nausea, vomiting, or other symptoms of appendicitis or acute surgical abdomen and in those with intestinal obstruction or ulceration, disabling adhesions, or difficulty swallowing.

## NURSING CONSIDERATIONS
• Before giving for constipation, determine if patient has adequate fluid intake, exercise, and diet.
• Drug is especially useful in debilitated patients and in those with postpartum constipation, irritable bowel syndrome, diverticulitis, and colostomies. It's also used to treat laxative abuse and to empty colon before barium enema examinations.
• Drug isn't absorbed systemically and is nontoxic.
• *Alert:* Don't confuse Citrucel with Citracal.

### ✓ Patient teaching
• Tell patient to take drug with at least 8 oz (240 ml) of liquid to mask grittiness.
• Teach patient about dietary sources of bulk, including bran and other cereals, fresh fruit, and vegetables.
• Tell patient to increase fluid intake.

## mineral oil (liquid petrolatum)
Fleet Enema Mineral Oil◊, Kondremul◊, Kondremul Plain◊, Lansoÿl†, Liqui-Doss◊, Milkinol◊, Neo-Cultol◊, Petrogalar Plain◊

*Pregnancy Risk Category C*

## HOW SUPPLIED
*Emulsion:* 2.75 ml/5 ml◊, 4.75 ml/5 ml◊
*Oral liquid:* in pints, quarts, gallons◊
*Enema:* 120 ml◊, 133 ml◊

## ACTION
Lubricant laxative that increases water retention in stools by creating a barrier between colon wall and feces that prevents colonic reabsorption of fecal water.

| Route | Onset | Peak | Duration |
|-------|-------|------|----------|
| P.O. | 6-8 hr | Variable | Variable |
| P.R. | 2-15 min | Unknown | Unknown |

## INDICATIONS & DOSAGE
*Constipation, preparation for bowel studies or surgery—*
**Adults and children ages 12 and older:** 15 to 45 ml P.O. h.s.; or 120 ml P.R. (as enema).
**Children ages 6 to 12:** 5 to 20 ml P.O. h.s.; or 30 to 60 ml P.R. (as enema).
**Children ages 2 to 6:** 30 to 60 ml P.R. (as enema).

## ADVERSE REACTIONS
**GI:** *nausea;* vomiting; diarrhea with excessive use; *abdominal cramps,* especially in severe constipation; hemorrhoids; decreased absorption of nutrients and fat-soluble vitamins, resulting in deficiency; slowed healing after hemorrhoidectomy; laxative dependence with long-term or excessive use.
**Respiratory:** *lipid pneumonia.*
**Skin:** anal pruritus, anal irritation, perianal discomfort.

## INTERACTIONS
**Drug-drug.** *Docusate salts:* may increase mineral oil absorption and cause lipid

pneumonia. Separate administration times.

*Fat-soluble vitamins (A, D, E, K):* possible decreased absorption after prolonged administration. Monitor for vitamin deficiency.

**EFFECTS ON DIAGNOSTIC TESTS**
None reported.

**CONTRAINDICATIONS**
Contraindicated in patients with abdominal pain, nausea, vomiting, or other symptoms of appendicitis or acute surgical abdomen and in those with fecal impaction or intestinal obstruction or perforation.

**NURSING CONSIDERATIONS**
• Use cautiously in young children; in elderly or debilitated patients because of susceptibility to lipid pneumonia through aspiration, absorption, and transport from intestinal mucosa; and in patients with rectal bleeding.
• Before giving for constipation, determine if patient has adequate fluid intake, exercise, and diet.
• Give drug on an empty stomach because it delays passage of food from stomach; drug is more active on an empty stomach.
• Give with fruit juice or carbonated drink to disguise taste.
• Drug may be used when patient needs to ease strain of evacuation.

☑ **Patient teaching**
• Advise patient to take drug only at bedtime on an empty stomach and not to take it for more than 1 week. Tell him to take drug with fruit juice or carbonated drink to disguise taste.
• To avoid soiling clothing, advise patient of possible rectal leakage from excessive dosages.
• Teach patient about dietary sources of bulk, including bran and other cereals, fresh fruit, and vegetables.

## polyethylene glycol and electrolyte solution
Co-Lav, Colovage, CoLyte, Glycoprep‡, Go-Evac, GoLYTELY, NuLYTELY, OCL

*Pregnancy Risk Category C*

**HOW SUPPLIED**
*Powder for oral solution:* polyethylene glycol (PEG) 3350 (6 g), anhydrous sodium sulfate (568 mg), NaCl (146 mg), potassium chloride (74.5 mg)/100 ml (Colovage); PEG 3350 (120 g), sodium sulfate (3.36 g), NaCl (2.92 g), potassium chloride (1.49 g)/2 L (CoLyte); PEG 3350 (60 g), NaCl (1.46 g), potassium chloride (0.745 g), sodium bicarbonate (1.68 g), sodium sulfate (5.68 g)/L (Co-Lav); PEG 3350 (60 g), NaCl (1.46 g), potassium chloride (745 mg), sodium bicarbonate (1.68 g), sodium sulfate (5.68 g)/L (Glycoprep‡); PEG 3350 (236 g), sodium sulfate (22.74 g), sodium bicarbonate (6.74 g), NaCl (5.86 g), potassium chloride (2.97 g)/4.8 L (GoLYTELY); PEG 3350 (59 g), sodium sulfate (5.685 g), sodium bicarbonate (1.685 g), NaCl (1.465 g), potassium chloride (0.743 g)/L (Go-Evac); PEG 3350 (420 g), sodium bicarbonate (5.72 g), NaCl (11.2 g), potassium chloride (1.48 g)/4 L (NuLYTELY); PEG 3350 (6 g), sodium sulfate decahydrate (1.29 g), NaCl (146 mg), potassium chloride (75 mg), polysorbate-80 (30 mg)/100 ml (OCL)

**ACTION**
PEG 3350, a nonabsorbable solution, acts as an osmotic agent. Sodium sulfate greatly reduces sodium absorption. The electrolyte level causes virtually no net absorption or secretion of ions.

| Route | Onset | Peak | Duration |
|-------|-------|------|----------|
| P.O. | 1 hr | Variable | Variable |

**INDICATIONS & DOSAGE**
*Bowel preparation before GI examination—*
**Adults:** 240 ml P.O. q 10 minutes until 4 L are consumed or until watery stool is clear. Typically, administer 4 hours before

examination, allowing 3 hours for drinking and 1 hour for bowel evacuation.

## ADVERSE REACTIONS
**EENT:** rhinorrhea.
**GI:** *nausea, bloating, cramps, vomiting, abdominal fullness.*
**Skin:** urticaria, dermatitis, *allergic reaction,* anal irritation.

## INTERACTIONS
**Drug-drug.** *Oral drugs:* decreased absorption if administered within 1 hour of starting therapy. Administer at least 2 to 3 hours before starting therapy.

## EFFECTS ON DIAGNOSTIC TESTS
Patient preparation for barium enema may be less satisfactory with this solution because it may interfere with the barium coating of the colonic mucosa using the double-contrast technique.

## CONTRAINDICATIONS
Contraindicated in patients with GI obstruction or perforation, gastric retention, toxic colitis, or megacolon.

## NURSING CONSIDERATIONS
• Use tap water to reconstitute powder. Shake vigorously to ensure that all powder is dissolved. Refrigerate reconstituted solution but use within 48 hours.
• *Alert:* Don't add flavoring or additional ingredients to the solution or administer chilled solution. Hypothermia has been reported after ingestion of large amounts of chilled solution.
• Administer solution early in the morning if patient is scheduled for a midmorning examination. Orally administered solution induces diarrhea (onset 30 to 60 minutes) that rapidly cleans the bowel, usually within 4 hours.
• When used as preparation for barium enema, administer solution the evening before the examination to avoid interfering with barium coating of the colonic mucosa.
• If administered to semiconscious patient or to patient with impaired gag reflex, take care to prevent aspiration.
• No major shifts in fluid or electrolyte balance have been reported.

### ✓ Patient teaching
• Tell patient to fast for 3 to 4 hours before taking the solution and thereafter ingest only clear fluids until examination is complete.
• Warn patient about adverse reactions.

---

## psyllium
Effer-Syllium Instant Mix ◇ ,
Fiberall ◇ , Genfiber ◇ , Hydrocil
Instant ◇ , Konsyl ◇ , Konsyl-D ◇ ,
Maalox Daily Fiber Therapy ◇ ,
Metamucil ◇ , Metamucil
Effervescent Sugar Free ◇ ,
Metamucil Sugar-Free ◇ , Modane
Bulk ◇ , Muci-Lax ◇ , Mylanta
Natural Fiber Supplement ◇ ,
Perdiem Fiber ◇ , Prodiem
Plain† ◇ , Reguloid Natural ◇ ,
Restore ◇ , Serutan ◇ , Siblin ◇ ,
Syllact ◇ , Unilax ◇ , V-Lax ◇

*Pregnancy Risk Category NR*

## HOW SUPPLIED
*Chewable pieces:* 1.7 g/piece ◇ ,
3.4 g/piece ◇
*Effervescent powder:* 3.4 g/packet ◇ ,
3.7 g/packet ◇
*Granules:* 2.5 g/tsp ◇ , 4.03 g/tsp ◇
*Powder:* 3.3 g/tsp ◇ , 3.4 g/tsp ◇ ,
3.5 g/tsp ◇ , 4.94 g/tsp ◇
*Wafers:* 3.4 g/wafer ◇

## ACTION
Bulk-forming laxative that absorbs water and expands to increase bulk and moisture content of stool, thus encouraging peristalsis and bowel movement.

| Route | Onset | Peak | Duration |
|-------|-------|------|----------|
| P.O. | 12-24 hr | 3 days | Variable |

## INDICATIONS & DOSAGE
*Constipation, bowel management—*
**Adults:** 1 to 2 tsp (rounded) P.O. in full glass of liquid once daily, b.i.d., or t.i.d., followed by second glass of liquid; or 1 packet dissolved in water once daily, b.i.d., or t.i.d.
**Children over age 6:** 1 tsp (level) P.O. in half a glass of liquid h.s.

---

\*Liquid contains alcohol.     \*\*May contain tartrazine.     †Canada     ‡Australia     §U.K.     ◇OTC

## ADVERSE REACTIONS

**GI:** nausea, vomiting, diarrhea with excessive use; esophageal, gastric, small intestine, and rectal obstruction when drug is taken in dry form; abdominal cramps, especially in severe constipation.

## INTERACTIONS
None significant.

## EFFECTS ON DIAGNOSTIC TESTS
None reported.

## CONTRAINDICATIONS
Contraindicated in patients with hypersensitivity to drug and in those with abdominal pain, nausea, vomiting, or other symptoms of appendicitis; intestinal obstruction or ulceration; disabling adhesions; or difficulty swallowing.

## NURSING CONSIDERATIONS
• Before giving for constipation, determine if patient has adequate fluid intake, exercise, and diet.
• Mix with at least 8 oz (240 ml) of cold, pleasant-tasting liquid such as orange juice to mask grittiness, and stir only a few seconds. Have patient drink mixture immediately so it doesn't congeal. Follow with additional glass of liquid.
• For dosages in children under age 6, consult doctor.
• Drug may reduce appetite if taken before meals.
• Drug isn't absorbed systemically and is nontoxic. It's especially useful in debilitated patients and in those with postpartum constipation, irritable bowel syndrome, or diverticular disease. It's also used to treat chronic laxative abuse and with other laxatives to empty colon before barium enema examinations.

## ✅ Patient teaching
• Teach patient how to properly mix drug. Tell him to take drug with plenty of water. Advise patient that inhaling powder may cause allergic reactions.
• Tell patient that laxative effect usually occurs in 12 to 24 hours but may be delayed 3 days.

• Advise diabetic patient to check label and use a brand of psyllium that doesn't contain sugar.
• Teach patient about dietary sources of bulk, including bran and other cereals, fresh fruit, and vegetables.

---

## senna
Black-Draught ◇, Fletcher's Castoria ◇, Senexon ◇, Senna-Gen ◇, Senokot ◇, Senokotxtra ◇, X-Prep Liquid* ◇

*Pregnancy Risk Category C*

## HOW SUPPLIED
*Tablets:* 187 mg ◇, 217 mg ◇, 600 mg ◇
*Granules:* 326 mg/tsp ◇, 1.65 g/1/2 tsp ◇
*Suppositories:* 652 mg ◇
*Syrup:* 218 mg/5 ml ◇

## ACTION
Unknown. Stimulant laxative that increases peristalsis, probably by direct effect on smooth muscle of the intestine. It's thought to either irritate the musculature or stimulate the colonic intramural plexus. Drug also promotes fluid accumulation in colon and small intestine.

| Route | Onset | Peak | Duration |
|-------|-------|------|----------|
| P.O. | 6-10 hr | Variable | Variable |
| P.R. | 0.5-2 hr | Unknown | Unknown |

## INDICATIONS & DOSAGE
*Acute constipation, preparation for bowel or rectal examination—*
**Adults:** dosage range for Senokot is 1 to 8 tablets P.O.; ½ to 4 tsp of granules added to liquid P.O.; 1 to 2 suppositories P.R. h.s.; or 1 to 4 tsp syrup P.O. h.s. Dosage for Black-Draught is 2 tablets or ¼ to ½ tsp (level) of granules mixed with water.

X-Prep Liquid is used solely as single dose for preradiographic bowel evacuation. Give 20 g powder dissolved in juice or 75 ml liquid P.O. between 2 p.m. and 4 p.m. on day before X-ray procedure. Use in divided doses, if needed, for elderly or debilitated patients.

**Children weighing over 27 kg (60 lb):** one-half adult dose of tablets, granules, or

---

syrup (except Black-Draught tablets and granules—not recommended for children).

**Children ages 1 month to 1 year:** 1.25 to 2.5 ml Senokot syrup P.O. h.s.

## ADVERSE REACTIONS
**GI:** *nausea;* vomiting; diarrhea; loss of normal bowel function with excessive use; *abdominal cramps,* especially in severe constipation; malabsorption of nutrients; cathartic colon (syndrome resembling ulcerative colitis radiologically) with long-term misuse; possible constipation after catharsis; yellow or yellow-green cast to feces; diarrhea in breast-feeding infants of mothers receiving senna; darkened pigmentation of rectal mucosa with long-term use (usually reversible within 4 to 12 months after stopping drug); protein-losing enteropathy; laxative dependence with excessive use.
**GU:** red-pink discoloration in alkaline urine; yellow-brown discoloration in acidic urine.
**Metabolic:** electrolyte imbalance such as hypokalemia.

## INTERACTIONS
None significant.

## EFFECTS ON DIAGNOSTIC TESTS
In phenolsulfonphthalein excretion test, senna may turn urine pink to red, red to violet, or red to brown.

## CONTRAINDICATIONS
Contraindicated in patients with ulcerative bowel lesions; nausea, vomiting, abdominal pain, or other symptoms of appendicitis or acute surgical abdomen; fecal impaction; or intestinal obstruction or perforation.

## NURSING CONSIDERATIONS
• Before giving for constipation, determine if patient has adequate fluid intake, exercise, and diet.
• Limit diet to clear liquids after X-Prep Liquid is taken.
• Avoid exposing product to excessive heat or light.
• Drug is used for short-term therapy.

• Senna is one of the most effective laxatives for counteracting constipation caused by narcotic analgesics.

✅ **Patient teaching**
• Teach patient about dietary sources of bulk, including bran and other cereals, fresh fruit, and vegetables.
• Tell patient to report persistent or severe reactions.

---

## sodium phosphates
Fleet Phospho-Soda ◇

*Pregnancy Risk Category NR*

## HOW SUPPLIED
*Liquid:* 2.4 g/5 ml sodium phosphate and 900 mg sodium biphosphate/5 ml ◇
*Enema:* 160 mg/ml sodium phosphate and 60 mg/ml sodium biphosphate ◇

## ACTION
Saline laxative that produces an osmotic effect in the small intestine by drawing water into the intestinal lumen.

| Route | Onset | Peak | Duration |
|-------|-------|------|----------|
| P.O. | 0.5-3 hr | Variable | Variable |
| P.R. | 5-10 min | With effect | With effect |

## INDICATIONS & DOSAGE
*Constipation—*
**Adults:** 20 to 30 ml solution mixed with 120 ml cold water P.O.; or 60 to 135 ml P.R. (as enema).
**Children:** 5 to 15 ml solution mixed with 120 ml cold water P.O.; or 67.5 ml P.R. (as enema).

## ADVERSE REACTIONS
**GI:** *abdominal cramping,* laxative dependence with long-term or excessive use.
**Metabolic:** fluid and electrolyte disturbances, such as hypernatremia and hyperphosphatemia, with daily use.

## INTERACTIONS
None significant.

## EFFECTS ON DIAGNOSTIC TESTS
None reported.

---

## CONTRAINDICATIONS

Contraindicated in patients with abdominal pain, nausea, vomiting, or other symptoms of appendicitis or acute surgical abdomen; intestinal obstruction or perforation; edema; heart failure; megacolon; or impaired renal function; also contraindicated in patients on sodium-restricted diets.

## NURSING CONSIDERATIONS

• Use cautiously in patients with large hemorrhoids or anal excoriations.
• Before giving for constipation, determine if patient has adequate fluid intake, exercise, and diet.
• *Alert:* Up to 10% of sodium content of drug may be absorbed.
• *Alert:* Severe electrolyte imbalances may occur if recommended dosage is exceeded.

### ☑ Patient teaching

• Teach patient about dietary sources of bulk, including bran and other cereals, fresh fruit, and vegetables.
• Warn patient about adverse reactions and stress importance of using drug only for short-term therapy.

---

Reactions may be *common*, uncommon, *life-threatening*, or COMMON AND LIFE-THREATENING.

**chlorpromazine hydrochloride**
(See Chapter 33, ANTIPSYCHOTICS.)
**dimenhydrinate**
**dolasetron mesylate**
**dronabinol**
**granisetron hydrochloride**
**meclizine hydrochloride**
**metoclopramide hydrochloride**
**ondansetron hydrochloride**
**perphenazine**
(See Chapter 33, ANTIPSYCHOTICS.)
**prochlorperazine**
**prochlorperazine edisylate**
**prochlorperazine maleate**
**promethazine hydrochloride**
(See Chapter 43, ANTIHISTAMINES.)
**scopolamine**
(See Chapter 38, ANTICHOLINERGICS.)
**thiethylperazine maleate**
**trimethobenzamide hydrochloride**

**COMBINATION PRODUCTS**
None.

---

### dimenhydrinate
Andrumin‡, Apo-Dimenhydrinate†,
Calm-X◊, Children's
Dramamine◊, Dimetabs, Dinate,
Dramamine◊*, Dramamine
Chewable◊**, Dramamine
Liquid◊*, Dramanate, Dymenate,
Gravol†, Gravol L/A†, Hydrate,
PMS-Dimenhydrinate†, Triptone
Caplets◊

*Pregnancy Risk Category B*

#### HOW SUPPLIED
*Tablets:* 50 mg◊
*Tablets (chewable):* 50 mg◊
*Elixir:* 15 mg/5 ml†
*Syrup:* 12.5 mg/4 ml*◊, 15.62 mg/5 ml
*Injection:* 50 mg/ml

#### ACTION
Unknown. Antihistamine that may
affect neural pathways originating in
the labyrinth to inhibit nausea and vomiting.

| Route | Onset | Peak | Duration |
|-------|-------|------|----------|
| P.O. | 15-30 min | Unknown | 3-6 hr |
| I.V. | Immediate | Unknown | 3-6 hr |
| I.M. | 20-30 min | Unknown | 3-6 hr |

#### INDICATIONS & DOSAGE
*Prevention and treatment of motion sickness—*
**Adults and children ages 12 and older:**
50 to 100 mg P.O. q 4 to 6 hours; 50 mg
I.M., p.r.n.; or 50 mg I.V. diluted in 10 ml
normal saline for injection, injected over
2 minutes. Maximum dose is 400 mg daily. For prevention, take 30 minutes before
motion exposure.
**Children ages 6 to 12:** 25 to 50 mg P.O. q
6 to 8 hours, not to exceed 150 mg in 24
hours. Or, 1.25 mg/kg or 37.5 mg/m$^2$ I.M.
q.i.d. Maximum dose is 300 mg daily.
**Children ages 2 to 6:** 12.5 to 25 mg P.O.
q 6 to 8 hours, not to exceed 75 mg in 24
hours. Or, 1.25 mg/kg or 37.5 mg/m$^2$ I.M.
q.i.d. Maximum dose is 300 mg daily.

#### ADVERSE REACTIONS
**CNS:** *drowsiness,* headache, dizziness,
confusion, nervousness, vertigo, tingling
and weakness of hands, lassitude, excitation, insomnia, especially in children.
**CV:** palpitations, hypotension, tachycardia.
**EENT:** blurred vision, dry respiratory
passages, diplopia, nasal congestion.
**GI:** dry mouth, nausea, vomiting, diarrhea, epigastric distress, constipation,
anorexia.
**Respiratory:** wheezing, thickened
bronchial secretions.
**Skin:** photosensitivity, urticaria, rash.
**Other:** *anaphylaxis,* tightness of chest.

#### INTERACTIONS
**Drug-drug.** *CNS depressants:* additive
CNS depression. Avoid concomitant use.
**Drug-lifestyle.** *Alcohol use:* additive
CNS depression. Avoid concomitant use.

---

*Liquid contains alcohol.    **May contain tartrazine.    †Canada    ‡Australia    §U.K.    ◊OTC

## EFFECTS ON DIAGNOSTIC TESTS
Drug may alter or confuse test results for xanthines (caffeine, aminophylline) because of its 8-chlorotheophylline content.

## CONTRAINDICATIONS
Contraindicated in patients with hypersensitivity to drug or its components.

## NURSING CONSIDERATIONS
• Use cautiously in patients with seizures, acute angle-closure glaucoma, or enlarged prostate gland, and in patients receiving ototoxic drugs.
• Elderly patients may be more susceptible to CNS adverse effects.
• Undiluted solution irritates veins and may cause sclerosis.
• Because incompatibilities are common, avoid mixing parenteral preparation with other drugs.
• Discontinue drug 4 days before diagnostic skin tests to avoid preventing, reducing, or masking test response.
• *Alert:* Drug may mask symptoms of ototoxicity, brain tumor, or intestinal obstruction.
• *Alert:* Don't confuse dimenhydrinate with diphenhydramine.

### I.V. administration
• Before administration, dilute each ml of drug with 10 ml of sterile water for injection, $D_5W$, or normal saline for injection. Give by direct injection over not less than 2 minutes.
• *Alert:* Most I.V. products contain benzyl alcohol, which has been associated with a fatal gasping syndrome in premature infants and low-birth-weight infants.

### Patient teaching
• Advise patient to avoid activities that require alertness until CNS effects of drug are known.
• Instruct patient to report adverse reactions promptly.

## dolasetron mesylate
Anzemet

*Pregnancy Risk Category B*

## HOW SUPPLIED
*Tablets:* 50 mg, 100 mg
*Injection:* 20 mg/ml as 12.5 mg/0.625 ml ampule or 100 mg/5 ml vials

## ACTION
Selective serotonin 5-$HT_3$ receptor antagonist that blocks the action of serotonin. Blocking the activity of the serotonin receptors prevents serotonin from stimulating the vomiting reflex.

| Route | Onset | Peak | Duration |
|-------|-------|------|----------|
| P.O. | Rapid | 1 hr | 8 hr |
| I.V. | Rapid | 36 min | 7 hr |

## INDICATIONS & DOSAGE
*Prevention of nausea and vomiting associated with cancer chemotherapy—*
**Adults:** 100 mg P.O. given as a single dose 1 hour before chemotherapy; or 1.8 mg/kg (or a fixed dose of 100 mg) as a single I.V. dose given 30 minutes before chemotherapy.
**Children ages 2 to 16:** 1.8 mg/kg P.O. given 1 hour before chemotherapy; or 1.8 mg/kg as a single I.V. dose given 30 minutes before chemotherapy. Injectable formulation can be mixed with apple juice and administered P.O. Maximum dose is 100 mg.
*Prevention of postoperative nausea and vomiting—*
**Adults:** 100 mg P.O. within 2 hours before surgery; or, 12.5 mg as a single I.V. dose about 15 minutes before cessation of anesthesia.
**Children ages 2 to 16:** 1.2 mg/kg P.O. given within 2 hours before surgery, to maximum of 100 mg; or 0.35 mg/kg (up to 12.5 mg) given as a single I.V. dose about 15 minutes before cessation of anesthesia. Injectable formulation can be mixed with apple juice and administered P.O.
*Postoperative nausea and vomiting—*
**Adults:** 12.5 mg as a single I.V. dose as soon as nausea or vomiting occurs.

**Children ages 2 to 16:** 0.35 mg/kg, to maximum dose of 12.5 mg, given as a single I.V. dose as soon as nausea or vomiting occurs.

**ADVERSE REACTIONS**
**CNS:** *headache*, dizziness, drowsiness, fatigue.
**CV:** *arrhythmias,* ECG changes, hypotension, hypertension, tachycardia.
**GI:** *diarrhea*, dyspepsia, abdominal pain, constipation, anorexia.
**GU:** oliguria, urine retention.
**Hepatic:** elevation of liver function tests results.
**Skin:** pruritus, rash.
**Other:** fever, chills, pain at injection site.

**INTERACTIONS**
**Drug-drug.** *Drugs such as antiarrhythmics that prolong ECG intervals:* increased risk of arrhythmia. Monitor patient closely
*Drugs such as cimetidine that inhibit P-450 enzymes:* increased hydrodolasetron levels. Monitor patient for adverse effects.
*Drugs such as rifampin that induce P-450 enzymes:* decreased hydrodolasetron levels. Monitor patient for decreased efficacy of antiemetic.

**EFFECTS ON DIAGNOSTIC TESTS**
None reported.

**CONTRAINDICATIONS**
Contraindicated in patients with hypersensitivity to drug.

**NURSING CONSIDERATIONS**
• *Alert:* Administer with caution in patients who have or may develop prolonged cardiac conduction intervals, such as those with electrolyte abnormalities, history of arrhythmia, and cumulative high-dose anthracycline therapy.
• Drug isn't recommended for use in children under age 2. Use cautiously in breast-feeding women.
• Injection for oral administration is stable in apple or apple-grape juice for 2 hours at room temperature.
• *Alert:* Don't confuse Anzemet with Aldomet.

**I.V. administration**
• Injection can be infused as rapidly as 100 mg/30 seconds or diluted in 50 ml compatible solution and infused over 15 minutes.

**✓ Patient teaching**
• Tell patient about potential adverse effects.
• Instruct patient not to mix injection in juice for oral administration until just before dosing.
• Tell patient to report nausea or vomiting.

---

**dronabinol**
**(delta-9-tetrahydrocannabinol)**
Marinol

*Controlled Substance Schedule III*
*Pregnancy Risk Category B*

**HOW SUPPLIED**
*Capsules:* 2.5 mg, 5 mg, 10 mg

**ACTION**
Unknown. A derivative of marijuana.

| Route | Onset | Peak | Duration |
|-------|-------|------|----------|
| P.O. | Unknown | 2-4 hr | 4-6 hr |

**INDICATIONS & DOSAGE**
*Nausea and vomiting associated with cancer chemotherapy—*
**Adults:** 5 mg/m² P.O. 1 to 3 hours before administration of chemotherapy. Then same dose q 2 to 4 hours after chemotherapy for total of four to six doses daily. If needed, dosage increased in 2.5-mg/m² increments to maximum of 15 mg/m² per dose.
*Anorexia and weight loss in patients with AIDS—*
**Adults:** 2.5 mg P.O. b.i.d. before lunch and dinner. If patient unable to tolerate, decrease dose to 2.5 mg P.O. given as a single dose daily in evening or h.s. May gradually increase dose to maximum of 20 mg/day.

**ADVERSE REACTIONS**
**CNS:** *dizziness, drowsiness, euphoria, ataxia,* depersonalization, hallucinations,

---

somnolence, headache, muddled thinking, asthenia, amnesia, confusion, *paranoia.*
**CV:** tachycardia, orthostatic hypotension, palpitations, vasodilation.
**EENT:** visual disturbances.
**GI:** *dry mouth, nausea, vomiting, abdominal pain,* diarrhea.

## INTERACTIONS
**Drug-drug.** *CNS depressants, psychotomimetic substances, sedatives:* additive CNS depression. Avoid concomitant use.
**Drug-lifestyle.** *Alcohol use:* additive CNS depression. Avoid concomitant use.

## EFFECTS ON DIAGNOSTIC TESTS
None reported.

## CONTRAINDICATIONS
Contraindicated in patients with hypersensitivity to sesame oil or cannabinoids.

## NURSING CONSIDERATIONS
• Use cautiously in elderly, pregnant, or breast-feeding patients and in those with heart disease, psychiatric illness, or history of drug abuse.
• Expect drug to be prescribed only for patients who haven't responded satisfactorily to other antiemetics.
• *Alert:* Dronabinol is the principal active substance in *Cannabis sativa* (marijuana). This substance can produce both physical and psychological dependence and has a high potential for abuse.
• CNS effects are intensified at higher drug dosages.
• Drug's effects may persist for days after treatment ends.
• *Alert:* Don't confuse dronabinol with droperidol.

### ☑ Patient teaching
• Tell patient that drug may induce unusual changes in mood or other adverse behavioral effects.
• Advise patient against activities that require alertness until CNS effects of drug are known.
• Warn caregivers to supervise patient during and immediately after treatment.
• Advise patient to take drug 1 to 3 hours before chemotherapy administration.

# granisetron hydrochloride
Kytril

*Pregnancy Risk Category B*

## HOW SUPPLIED
*Tablets:* 1 mg
*Injection:* 1 mg/ml

## ACTION
Selective antagonist of a specific type of serotonin receptor ($5-HT_3$) located in the CNS in the chemoreceptor trigger zone and in the peripheral nervous system on nerve terminals of the vagus nerve. Drug's blocking action may occur at both sites.

| Route | Onset | Peak | Duration |
|-------|-------|------|----------|
| P.O., I.V. | Unknown | Unknown | Unknown |

## INDICATIONS & DOSAGE
*Prevention of nausea and vomiting associated with emetogenic cancer chemotherapy—*
**Adults and children ages 2 to 16:**
10 mcg/kg I.V. infused over 5 minutes. Begin infusion within 30 minutes before administration of chemotherapy. Or, 1 mg P.O. up to 1 hour before chemotherapy and dose repeated 12 hours later; or 2 mg P.O. daily given up to 1 hour before chemotherapy.
✳ *NEW INDICATION: Prevention of nausea and vomiting associated with radiation, including total body irradiation and fractionated abdominal radiation—*
**Adults:** 2 mg P.O. once daily within 1 hour of radiation.

## ADVERSE REACTIONS
**CNS:** *headache, asthenia,* somnolence, dizziness, anxiety.
**CV:** hypertension.
**GI:** diarrhea, *constipation,* abdominal pain, *nausea,* vomiting, decreased appetite.
**Hematologic:** *leukopenia,* anemia, ***thrombocytopenia.***
**Hepatic:** elevated liver function tests results.
**Skin:** alopecia.
**Other:** fever.

## INTERACTIONS
**Drug-herb.** *Horehound*: may enhance serotoninergic effects. Avoid concomitant use.

## EFFECTS ON DIAGNOSTIC TESTS
None reported.

## CONTRAINDICATIONS
Contraindicated in patients with hypersensitivity to drug.

## NURSING CONSIDERATIONS
• Drug regimen is given only on days when chemotherapy is given. Treatment at other times hasn't been found to be useful.
• *Alert:* Don't mix with other drugs; data regarding compatibility are limited.

### I.V. administration
• Dilute drug with normal saline for injection or $D_5W$ to a volume of 20 to 50 ml. Infuse over 5 minutes, beginning within 30 minutes before chemotherapy, and only on days chemotherapy is given. Diluted solutions are stable for 24 hours at room temperature.

### ✓ Patient teaching
• Stress importance of taking second dose of oral drug 12 hours after first for maximum effectiveness.
• Instruct patient to report adverse reactions immediately.

---

## meclizine hydrochloride
## (meclozine hydrochloride)
Antivert, Antivert/25 ◊, Antivert/50, Bonamine†, Bonine ◊, Dizmiss ◊, Meni-D, Ru-Vert-M, Vergon ◊

*Pregnancy Risk Category B*

## HOW SUPPLIED
*Tablets:* 12.5 mg, 25 mg ◊, 50 mg
*Tablets (chewable):* 25 mg ◊
*Capsules:* 25 mg

## ACTION
Unknown. Antihistamine that may affect neural pathways originating in the labyrinth to inhibit nausea and vomiting.

| Route | Onset | Peak | Duration |
|-------|-------|------|----------|
| P.O. | 1 hr | Unknown | 8-24 hr |

## INDICATIONS & DOSAGE
*Vertigo—*
**Adults:** 25 to 100 mg P.O. daily in divided doses. Dosage varies with response.
*Motion sickness—*
**Adults:** 25 to 50 mg P.O. 1 hour before travel; then daily for duration of trip.

## ADVERSE REACTIONS
**CNS:** *drowsiness,* restlessness, excitation, nervousness, auditory and visual hallucinations.
**CV:** hypotension, palpitations, tachycardia.
**EENT:** blurred vision, diplopia, tinnitus, dry nose and throat.
**GI:** dry mouth, constipation, anorexia, nausea, vomiting, diarrhea.
**GU:** urine retention, urinary frequency.
**Skin:** urticaria, rash.

## INTERACTIONS
**Drug-drug.** *CNS depressants:* increased drowsiness. Use together cautiously.

## EFFECTS ON DIAGNOSTIC TESTS

## CONTRAINDICATIONS
Contraindicated in patients with hypersensitivity to drug.

## NURSING CONSIDERATIONS
• Use cautiously in patients with asthma, glaucoma, or prostatic hyperplasia.
• Drug may mask symptoms of ototoxicity, brain tumor, or intestinal obstruction.
• Discontinue drug 4 days before diagnostic skin tests to avoid interference with test response.

### ✓ Patient teaching
• Advise patient to avoid hazardous activities that require alertness until CNS effects of drug are known.

---

*Liquid contains alcohol.    **May contain tartrazine.    †Canada    ‡Australia    §U.K.    ◊OTC

• Instruct patient to report persistent or serious adverse reactions promptly.

---

# metoclopramide hydrochloride
Apo-Metoclop†, Clopra, Emex†, Maxeran†, Maxolon‡, Octamide PFS, Pramin‡, Reclomide, Reglan

*Pregnancy Risk Category B*

---

## HOW SUPPLIED
*Tablets:* 5 mg, 10 mg
*Syrup:* 5 mg/5 ml
*Injection:* 5 mg/ml

## ACTION
Stimulates motility of upper GI tract and increases lower esophageal sphincter tone and blocks dopamine receptors at the chemoreceptor trigger zone.

| Route | Onset | Peak | Duration |
|-------|-------|------|----------|
| P.O. | 0.5-1 hr | 1-2 hr | 1-2 hr |
| I.V. | 1-3 min | Unknown | 1-2 hr |
| I.M. | 10-15 min | Unknown | 1-2 hr |

## INDICATIONS & DOSAGE
*Prevention or reduction of nausea and vomiting associated with emetogenic cancer chemotherapy—*
**Adults:** 1 to 2 mg/kg I.V. 30 minutes before cancer chemotherapy; then repeated q 2 hours for two doses, then q 3 hours for three doses.
*Prevention or reduction of postoperative nausea and vomiting—*
**Adults:** 10 to 20 mg I.M. near end of surgical procedure, repeated q 4 to 6 hours, p.r.n.
*To facilitate small-bowel intubation, to aid in radiologic examinations—*
**Adults and children over age 14:** 10 mg (2 ml) I.V. as a single dose over 1 to 2 minutes.
**Children under age 6:** 0.1 mg/kg I.V.
**Children ages 6 to 14:** 2.5 to 5 mg I.V. (0.5 to 1 ml).
*Delayed gastric emptying secondary to diabetic gastroparesis—*
**Adults:** 10 mg P.O. for mild symptoms, slow I.V. (1 to 2 minutes) for severe symptoms 30 minutes before meals and

h.s. I.V. dose may be needed for up to 10 days; then P.O. dose may be started and continued for rest of 2 to 8 weeks.
*Gastroesophageal reflux disease—*
**Adults:** 10 to 15 mg P.O. q.i.d., p.r.n., 30 minutes before meals and h.s.
*Adjust-a-dose:* For renally impaired patients with creatinine clearance below 40 ml/minute, decrease initial dosage by half the recommended dose.

## ADVERSE REACTIONS
**CNS:** *restlessness, anxiety, drowsiness, fatigue, lassitude,* depression, akathisia, insomnia, confusion, **suicide ideation, seizures,** hallucinations, headache, dizziness, extrapyramidal symptoms, tardive dyskinesia, *dystonic reactions.*
**CV:** transient hypertension, hypotension.
**GI:** nausea, bowel disorders, diarrhea.
**GU:** urinary frequency, incontinence.
**Hematologic:** *neutropenia, agranulocytosis.*
**Skin:** rash, urticaria.
**Other:** fever, prolactin secretion, loss of libido.

## INTERACTIONS
**Drug-drug.** *Anticholinergics, opioid analgesics:* antagonized GI motility effects of metoclopramide. Use together cautiously.
*CNS depressants:* additive CNS effects. Avoid concomitant use.
*Phenothiazines:* increased risk of extrapyramidal effects. Monitor closely.
**Drug-lifestyle.** *Alcohol use:* additive CNS effects. Avoid concomitant use.

## EFFECTS ON DIAGNOSTIC TESTS
Drug may increase serum aldosterone and prolactin levels.

## CONTRAINDICATIONS
Contraindicated in patients with hypersensitivity to drug and in those with pheochromocytoma or seizure disorders; also contraindicated in those in whom stimulation of GI motility might be dangerous (for example, those with hemorrhage, obstruction, or perforation).

---

Reactions may be *common,* uncommon, *life-threatening,* or COMMON AND LIFE-THREATENING.

## NURSING CONSIDERATIONS
• Use cautiously in patients with history of depression, Parkinson's disease, and hypertension.
• Monitor bowel sounds.
• Drug is compatible with $D_5W$, normal saline for injection, dextrose 5% in half-normal saline, Ringer's injection, and lactated Ringer's injection. Normal saline is the preferred diluent because the drug is most stable in this solution.
• Safety and effectiveness of drug haven't been established for therapy that continues longer than 12 weeks.

### I.V. administration
• Give lower doses (10 mg or less) by direct injection over 1 to 2 minutes. Dilute doses larger than 10 mg in 50 ml of compatible diluent, and infuse over at least 15 minutes. Protection from light is unnecessary if infusion mixture is administered within 24 hours. If infusion mixture is protected from light and refrigerated, it's stable for 48 hours.
• Closely monitor blood pressure.
• *Alert:* Use diphenhydramine 25 mg I.V., as ordered, to counteract extrapyramidal adverse effects associated with high metoclopramide doses.

### ✓ Patient teaching
• Tell patient to avoid activities requiring alertness for 2 hours after doses.
• Instruct patient to report persistent or serious adverse reactions promptly.
• Advise patient to avoid alcohol ingestion.

---

## ondansetron hydrochloride
Zofran

*Pregnancy Risk Category B*

### HOW SUPPLIED
*Tablets:* 4 mg, 8 mg
*Injection:* 2 mg/ml
*Premixed injection:* 32 mg/50 ml

### ACTION
Selective antagonist of a specific type of serotonin receptor ($5-HT_3$) located in the CNS at the chemoreceptor trigger zone and in the peripheral nervous system on nerve terminals of the vagus nerve. Drug's blocking action may occur at both sites.

| Route | Onset | Peak | Duration |
|-------|-------|------|----------|
| P.O., I.V. | Unknown | Unknown | Unknown |

### INDICATIONS & DOSAGE
*Prevention of nausea and vomiting associated with emetogenic chemotherapy—*
**Adults and children ages 12 and older:** 8 mg P.O. 30 minutes before chemotherapy. Then, 8 mg P.O. 8 hours after first dose. Then, 8 mg q 12 hours for 1 to 2 days. Or, administer a single dose of 32 mg by I.V. infusion over 15 minutes beginning 30 minutes before chemotherapy; or three divided doses of 0.15 mg/kg I.V. Give first dose 30 minutes before chemotherapy; administer subsequent doses 4 and 8 hours after first dose. Infuse drug over 15 minutes.
**Children ages 4 to 12:** 4 mg P.O. 30 minutes before chemotherapy. Then, 4 mg P.O. 4 and 8 hours after first dose. Then, 4 mg q 8 hours for 1 to 2 days. Or, three doses of 0.15 mg/kg I.V. Give first dose 30 minutes before chemotherapy; administer subsequent doses 4 and 8 hours after first dose. Infuse drug over 15 minutes.
*Prevention of postoperative nausea and vomiting—*
**Adults:** 4 mg I.V. (undiluted) over 2 to 5 minutes. Or, 16 mg P.O. 1 hour before induction of anesthesia.
*Prevention of nausea and vomiting associated with radiotherapy in patients receiving total body irradiation, single high-dose fraction to abdomen, or daily fractions to abdomen—*
**Adults:** 8 mg P.O. t.i.d.
*Adjust-a-dose:* For patients with severe liver failure, total daily dose shouldn't exceed 8 mg.

### ADVERSE REACTIONS
**CNS:** *headache, malaise, fatigue, dizziness,* sedation.
**CV:** chest pain.
**GI:** *diarrhea, constipation,* abdominal pain, xerostomia.
**GU:** urine retention, gynecologic disorders.

---

**Hepatic:** transient elevations in AST and ALT levels.
**Musculoskeletal:** *pain.*
**Respiratory:** hypoxia.
**Skin:** rash.
**Other:** chills, injection-site reaction, fever.

## INTERACTIONS
**Drug-drug.** *Drugs that alter hepatic drug metabolizing enzymes, such as cimetidine, phenobarbital:* may alter pharmacokinetics of ondansetron. No dosage adjustment appears necessary.
**Drug-herb.** *Horehound:* may enhance serotoninergic effects. Avoid concomitant use.

## EFFECTS ON DIAGNOSTIC TESTS
None reported.

## CONTRAINDICATIONS
Contraindicated in patients with hypersensitivity to drug.

## NURSING CONSIDERATIONS
• Use cautiously in patients with liver failure. Monitor liver function test results. Dose shouldn't exceed 8 mg in this population.
• *Alert:* Don't confuse Zofran with Zosyn or Zantac.

### I.V. administration
• Dilute drug in 50 ml of $D_5W$ injection or normal saline for injection before administration.
• Drug is stable for up to 48 hours after dilution in 5% dextrose in normal saline for injection, 5% dextrose in half-normal saline for injection, and 3% NaCl for injection.
• *Alert:* Administer as I.V. infusion over 15 minutes.

### Patient teaching
• Instruct patient to alert nurse immediately if difficulty in breathing occurs after drug administration.
• Tell patient receiving drug I.V. to report discomfort at insertion site.

## prochlorperazine
Compazine,
PMS Prochlorperazine†,
Prorazin†, Stemetil†

## prochlorperazine edisylate
Compazine, Compazine Syrup

## prochlorperazine maleate
Compazine,
Compazine Spansule,
PMS Prochlorperazine†,
Prorazin†, Stemetil†

*Pregnancy Risk Category C*

## HOW SUPPLIED
**prochlorperazine**
*Tablets:* 5 mg, 10 mg
*Injection:* 5 mg/ml
*Suppositories:* 2.5 mg, 5 mg, 25 mg
**prochlorperazine edisylate**
*Syrup:* 5 mg/5 ml
*Injection:* 5 mg/ml
**prochlorperazine maleate**
*Tablets:* 5 mg, 10 mg, 25 mg
*Capsules (extended-release):* 10 mg, 15 mg, 30 mg

## ACTION
Acts on the chemoreceptor trigger zone to inhibit nausea and vomiting; in larger doses, it partially depresses vomiting center.

| Route | Onset | Peak | Duration |
|---|---|---|---|
| P.O. | 30-40 min | Unknown | 3-12 hr |
| P.O. (extended) | 30-40 min | Unknown | Unknown |
| I.V. | Unknown | Unknown | Unknown |
| I.M. | 10-20 min | Unknown | 3-4 hr |
| P.R. | 1 hr | Unknown | 3-4 hr |

## INDICATIONS & DOSAGE
*Preoperative nausea control—*
**Adults:** 5 to 10 mg I.M. 1 to 2 hours before induction of anesthesia; repeat once in 30 minutes, if needed. Or, 5 to 10 mg I.V. 15 to 30 minutes before induction of anesthesia; repeat once, if needed.
*Severe nausea and vomiting—*
**Adults:** 5 to 10 mg P.O., t.i.d. or q.i.d.; 15 mg sustained-release form P.O. on rising; 10 mg sustained-release form P.O. q

# Nursing2001 Drug Handbook
## Photoguide to tablets and capsules

This photoguide provides full-color photographs of some of the most commonly prescribed tablets and capsules in the United States. Shown in actual size, the drugs are organized alphabetically by trade or generic name for quick reference. Page numbers refer to full drug entries.

**Accupril**
(page 302)

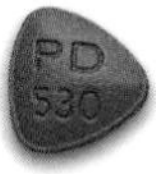

10 mg 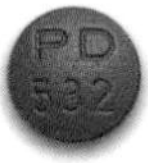        20 mg

**Adalat CC**
(extended-release)
(page 250)

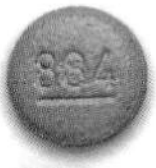

30 mg

**Allegra**
(page 592)

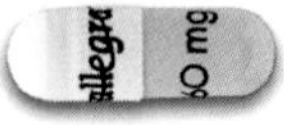

60 mg

**Altace**
(page 304)

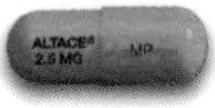

2.5 mg 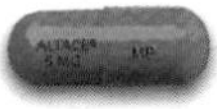        5 mg

**Ambien**
(page 403)

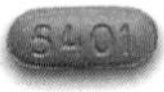

5 mg        10 mg

**amitriptyline hydrochloride**
(page 424)

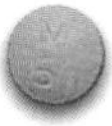

25 mg 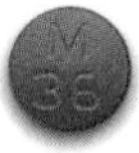        50 mg 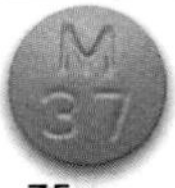        75 mg

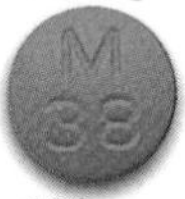

100 mg

**amoxicillin trihydrate**
(page 73)

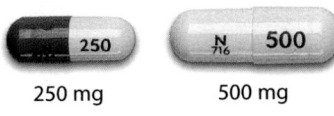

250 mg        500 mg

**Amoxil**
(page 73)

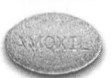

125 mg
(chewable)

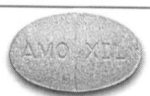

250 mg
(chewable)

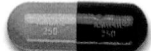

250 mg

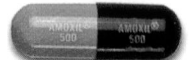

500 mg

**atenolol**
(page 261)

25 mg

**Ativan**
(page 456)

0.5 mg

1 mg

**Augmentin**
(page 72)

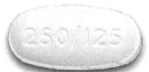

250 mg/125 mg

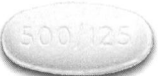

500 mg/125 mg

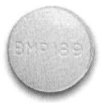

125 mg/31.25 mg
(chewable)

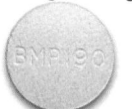

250 mg/62.5 mg
(chewable)

**Axid**
(page 689)

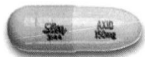

150 mg

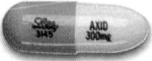

300 mg

**Biaxin**
(page 196)

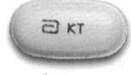

250 mg

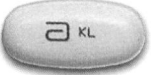

500 mg

**Bumex**
(page 800)

0.5 mg

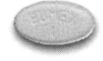

1 mg

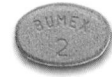

2 mg

**BuSpar**
(page 449)

5 mg

10 mg

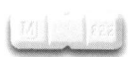

15 mg

| **Calan** (page 256) | 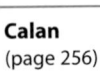 40 mg |  80 mg | 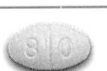 120 mg |
|---|---|---|---|
| **Capoten** (page 266) |  12.5 mg | 25 mg | |
| **Carafate** (page 694) |  1 g | | |
| **Cardizem** (page 245) | 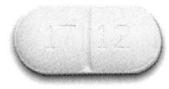 30 mg | 60 mg | 90 mg |
| **Cardizem CD** (extended-release) (page 245) | 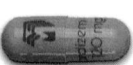 120 mg | 180 mg | 240 mg |
| **Cardura** (page 273) |  1 mg | 2 mg | 4 mg |
| **Ceclor** (page 97) | 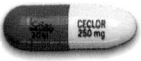 250 mg | 500 mg | |
| **Ceftin** (page 121) | 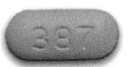 250 mg | 500 mg | |
| **Cefzil** (page 114) | 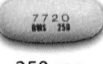 250 mg | | |
| **Celebrex** (page 346) |  100 mg | 200 mg | |
| **cephalexin** (page 123) | 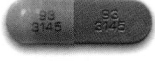 250 mg | 500 mg | |

**cimetidine**
(page 684)

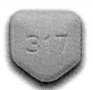

300 mg

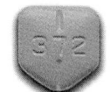

400 mg

**Cipro**
(page 143)

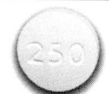

250 mg

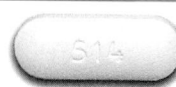

500 mg

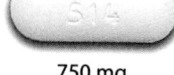

750 mg

**Claritin**
(page 593)

10 mg

**Compazine**
(page 680)

5 mg

10 mg

**Cordarone**
(page 220)

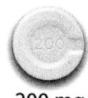

200 mg

**Coreg**
(page 269)

3.125 mg

6.25 mg

12.5 mg

25 mg

**Coumadin**
(page 849)

1 mg

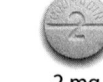

2 mg

2.5 mg

5 mg

7.5 mg

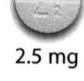

10 mg

**Cozaar**
(page 288)

25 mg

50 mg

**cyclobenzaprine hydrochloride**
(page 562)

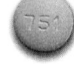

10 mg

**Darvocet-N 100**
(page 368)

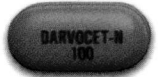

100 mg/650 mg

**Daypro**
(page 362)

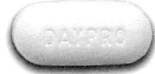

600 mg

**Deltasone**
(page 711)

2.5 mg

5 mg

10 mg

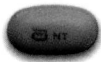

20 mg

**Depakote**
(page 422)

125 mg

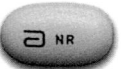

250 mg

500 mg

**Depakote Sprinkle**
(delayed-release)
(page 422)

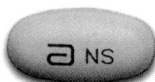

125 mg

**DiaBeta**
(page 758)

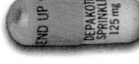

1.25 mg

2.5 mg

5 mg

**Diflucan**
(page 38)

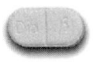

100 mg

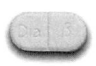

150 mg

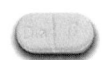

200 mg

**Dilantin Infatabs**
(page 416)

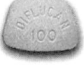

50 mg

**Dilantin Kapseals**
(page 416)

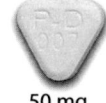

100 mg

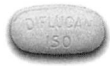

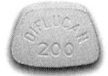

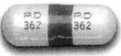

**doxepin hydrochloride**
(page 432)

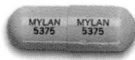

75 mg

**Duricef**
(page 98)

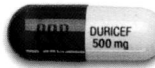

500 mg

**Dyazide**
(page 797)

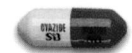

25 mg/37.5 mg

**E.E.S.**
(page 198)

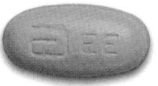

400 mg

**Effexor**
(page 446)

25 mg

37.5 mg

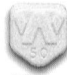

50 mg

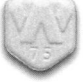

75 mg

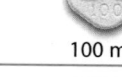

100 mg

**Ery-Tab**
(delayed-release)
(page 198)

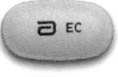

250 mg

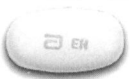

333 mg

**Erythrocin Stearate Filmtab**
(page 198)

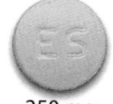

250 mg

**Erythromycin Base Filmtab**
(page 198)

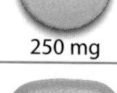

250 mg

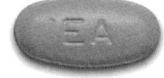

500 mg

**Estrace**
(page 726)

1 mg

2 mg

**Fiorinal with Codeine**
(page 368)

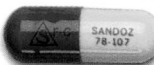

325 mg aspirin, 50 mg butalbital, 40 mg caffeine, 30 mg codeine phosphate

| **Floxin**<br>(page 152) | 200 mg | 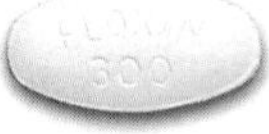 300 mg | 400 mg |
|---|---|---|---|

| **Fosamax**<br>(page 1203) | 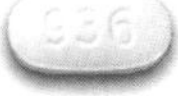 10 mg | 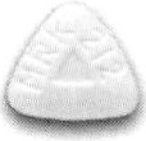 40 mg | |

| **furosemide**<br>(page 804) | 20 mg | | |

| **glipizide**<br>(page 755) | 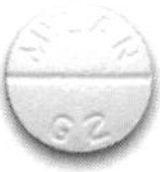 10 mg | | |

| **Glucophage**<br>(page 763) | 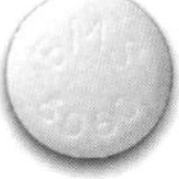 500 mg | 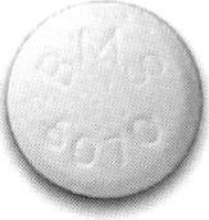 850 mg | |

| **Glucotrol**<br>(page 755) | 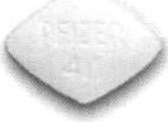 5 mg | 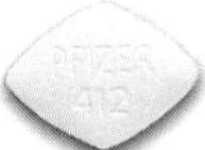 10 mg | |

| **Glucotrol XL**<br>(page 755) | 5 mg | 10 mg | |

| **Glynase**<br>(page 758) | 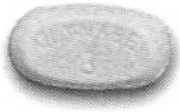 3 mg | 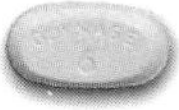 6 mg | |

| **hydrocodone bitartrate and acetaminophen**<br>(page 368) | 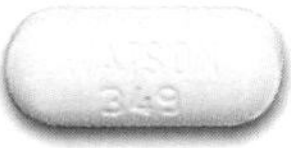 5 mg/500 mg | 7.5 mg/500 mg | 7.5 mg/750 mg |

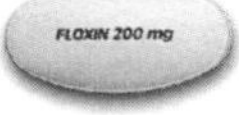

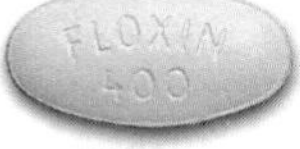

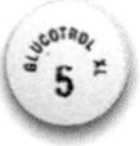

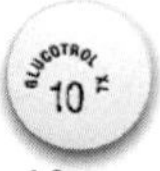

**Hytrin**
(page 306)

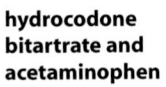 1 mg

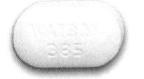 2 mg

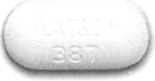 5 mg

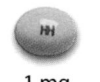 10 mg

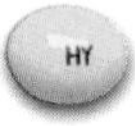

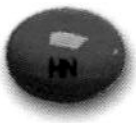

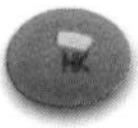

**Inderal**
(page 254)

10 mg  20 mg  40 mg

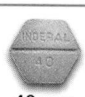

60 mg

**K-Dur**
(page 826)

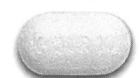 

10 mEq  20 mEq

**Klonopin**
(page 406)

 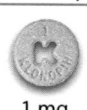 

0.5 mg  1 mg  2 mg

**Lanoxin**
(page 216)

0.125 mg  0.25 mg

**Lasix**
(page 804)

 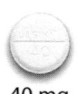

20 mg  40 mg

**Levaquin**
(page 146)

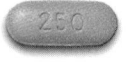 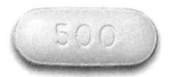

250 mg  500 mg

**Levoxyl**
(page 772)

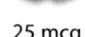  

25 mcg  50 mcg  75 mcg

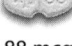  

88 mcg  100 mcg  112 mcg

125 mcg  137 mcg  150 mcg

175 mcg  200 mcg  300 mcg

**Lipitor**
(page 311)

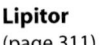 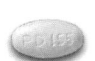 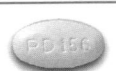

| 10 mg | 20 mg | 40 mg |

**Lodine**
(page 349)

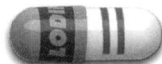 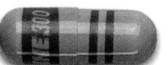 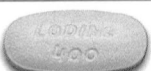

| 200 mg | 300 mg | 400 mg |

**Lopid**
(page 318)

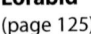

600 mg

**Lorabid**
(page 125)

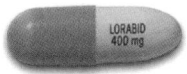

400 mg

**Lorcet 10/650**
(page 369)

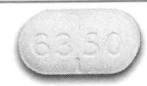

10 mg/650 mg

**Lotensin**
(page 262)

 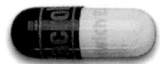 

| 5 mg | 10 mg | 20 mg |

40 mg

**Macrobid**
(page 201)

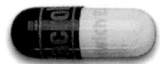

75 mg/25 mg

**methylphenidate
hydrochloride**
(page 492)

  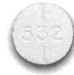

| 5 mg | 10 mg | 20 mg |

20 mg
(sustained-release)

**Mevacor**
(page 319)

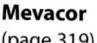 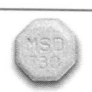 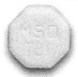 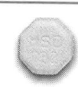

10 mg     20 mg     40 mg

**Micro-K Extencaps**
(controlled-release)
(page 826)

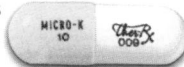

10 mEq (750 mg)

**Micronase**
(page 758)

 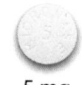

2.5 mg     5 mg

**Monopril**
(page 279)

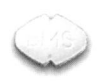 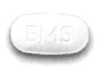 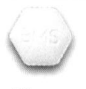

10 mg     20 mg     40 mg

**Motrin**
(page 353)

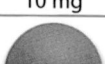 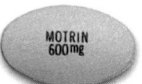 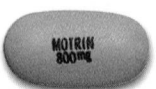

400 mg     600 mg     800 mg

**Naprosyn**
(page 361)

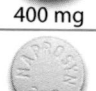 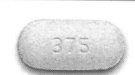 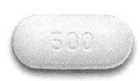

250 mg     375 mg     500 mg

**naproxen**
(page 361)

375 mg     500 mg

**Nitrostat**
(page 251)

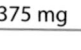  

0.3 mg     0.4 mg     0.6 mg

**Nolvadex**
(page 930)

10 mg

**nortriptyline
hydrochloride**
(page 438)

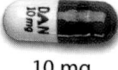 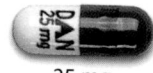 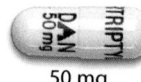

10 mg     25 mg     50 mg

**Norvasc**
(page 242)

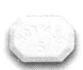

5 mg                    10 mg

**Oruvail**
(page 357)

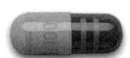   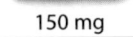   

100 mg                  150 mg                  200 mg

**Pamelor**
(page 438)

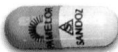   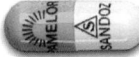   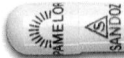

10 mg                   25 mg                   50 mg

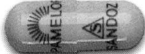

75 mg

**Paxil**
(page 439)

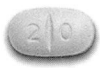   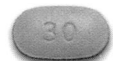

20 mg                   30 mg

**PCE**
(page 198)

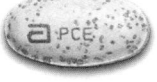   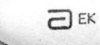

333 mg                  500 mg

**Pepcid**
(page 686)

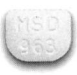   

20 mg                   40 mg

**Percocet 5/325**
(page 368)

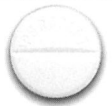

5 mg/325 mg

**potassium
chloride**
(controlled-release)
(page 826)

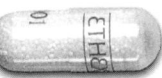

10 mEq

**Pravachol**
(page 320)

      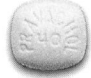

10 mg                   20 mg                   40 mg

**Premarin**
(page 730)

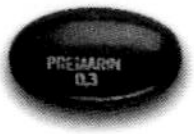

0.3 mg 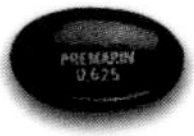     0.625 mg 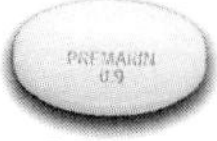     0.9 mg

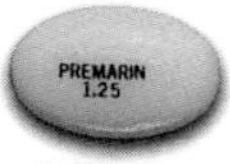

1.25 mg 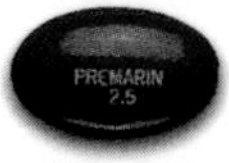     2.5 mg

**Prevacid**
(page 687)

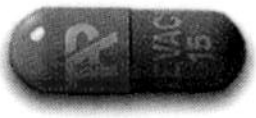

15 mg 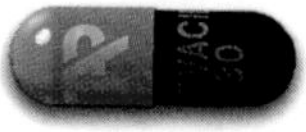     30 mg

**Prilosec**
(page 690)

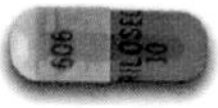

10 mg 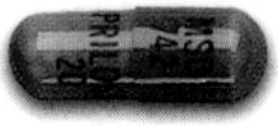     20 mg

**Prinivil**
(page 287)

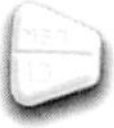

5 mg 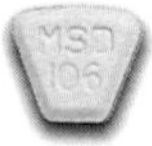     10 mg 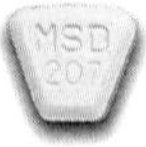     20 mg

**Procardia XL**
(extended-release)
(page 250)

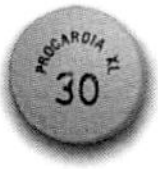

30 mg 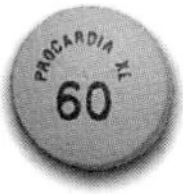     60 mg 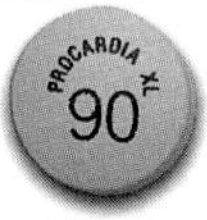     90 mg

**propoxyphene
napsylate with
acetaminophen**
(page 368)

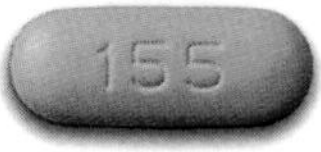

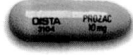

100 mg/650 mg

**Propulsid**
(page 1214)

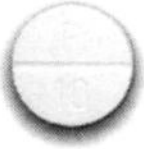

10 mg

**Provera**
(page 741)

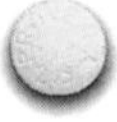

2.5 mg 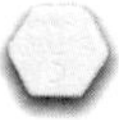     5 mg 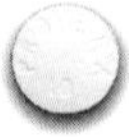     10 mg

**Prozac**
(page 433)

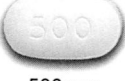 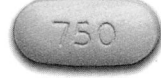

10 mg     20 mg

**Relafen**
(page 360)

500 mg     750 mg

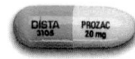
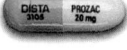
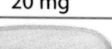

**Risperdal**
(page 479)

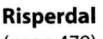

1 mg

2 mg

3 mg

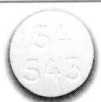

4 mg

**Roxicet**
(page 368)

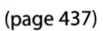

5 mg/325 mg

**Serzone**
(page 437)

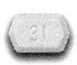

50 mg

100 mg

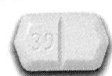

150 mg

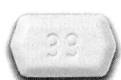

300 mg

**Sinemet**
(page 498)

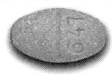

10 mg/100 mg

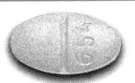

25 mg/250 mg

**Sinemet CR**
(extended-release)
(page 498)

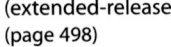

25 mg/100 mg

**Slo-bid Gyrocaps**
(extended-release)
(page 617)

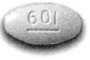

50 mg

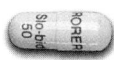

75 mg

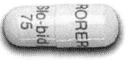

100 mg

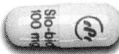

200 mg

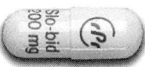

300 mg

**Sumycin**
(page 133)

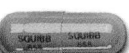

250 mg

**Tagamet**
(page 684)

200 mg

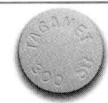

300 mg

**Tenormin**
(page 261)

25 mg  50 mg  100 mg

**Theo-Dur**
(extended-release)
(page 617)

  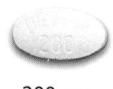  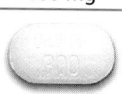

100 mg  200 mg  300 mg

450 mg

**Ticlid**
(page 334)

250 mg

**Toprol XL**
(page 291)

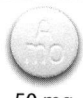  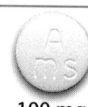  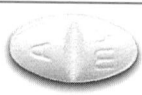

50 mg  100 mg  200 mg

**Toradol**
(page 358)

10 mg

**Trental**
(page 333)

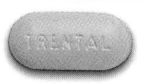

400 mg

**Trimox**
(page 73)

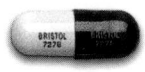  

250 mg  500 mg

**Tylenol with
Codeine No. 3**
(page 369)

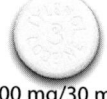

300 mg/30 mg

**Ultram**
(page 391)

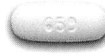

50 mg

**Valium**
(page 452)

  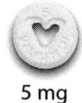  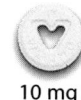

2 mg  5 mg  10 mg

**Vasotec**
(page 274)

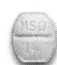  

2.5 mg      5 mg      10 mg

20 mg

**Veetids**
(page 90)

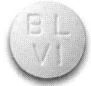 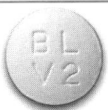

250 mg      500 mg

**verapamil
hydrochloride**
(extended-release)
(page 256)

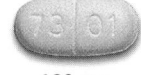

180 mg

**Verelan**
(extended-release)
(page 256)

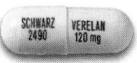 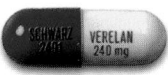

120 mg      240 mg

**Viagra**
(page 1236)

  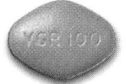

25 mg      50 mg      100 mg

**Vioxx**
(page 365)

 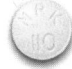

12.5 mg      25 mg

**Xanax**
(page 448)

0.25 mg      0.5 mg      1 mg

**Zantac**
(page 693)

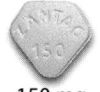 

150 mg      300 mg

**Zantac EFFERdose**
(page 693)

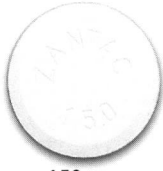

150 mg

**Zestril**
(page 287)

 5 mg

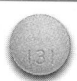 10 mg

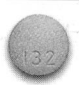 20 mg

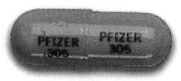 40 mg

**Zithromax**
(page 194)

250 mg

**Zocor**
(page 322)

 5 mg

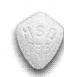 10 mg

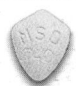 20 mg

**Zoloft**
(page 442)

 50 mg

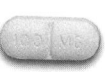 100 mg

**Zovirax**
(page 158)

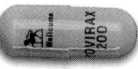 200 mg

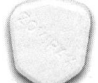 400 mg

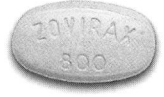 800 mg

**Zyrtec**
(page 587)

 5 mg

 10 mg

12 hours; 25 mg P.R., b.i.d.; or 5 to 10 mg I.M. repeated q 3 to 4 hours, p.r.n. Maximum I.M. dose is 40 mg daily. Or, 2.5 to 10 mg I.V. at a rate not to exceed 5 mg/minute.

**Children weighing 18 to 39 kg (40 to 86 lb):** 2.5 mg P.O. or P.R., t.i.d.; or 5 mg P.O. or P.R., b.i.d. Maximum dose is 15 mg daily. Or, 0.132 mg/kg by deep I.M. injection. Control usually is obtained with one dose.

**Children weighing 14 to 17 kg (31 to 37 lb):** 2.5 mg P.O. or P.R., b.i.d. or t.i.d. Maximum dose is 10 mg daily. Or, 0.132 mg/kg by deep I.M. injection. Control usually is obtained with one dose.

**Children weighing 9 to 13 kg (20 to 29 lb):** 2.5 mg P.O. or P.R. once daily or b.i.d. Maximum dose is 7.5 mg daily. Or, 0.132 mg/kg by deep I.M. injection. Control usually is obtained with one dose.

*To manage symptoms of psychotic disorders—*
**Adults:** 5 to 10 mg P.O., t.i.d. or q.i.d.
**Children ages 2 to 12:** 2.5 mg P.O. or P.R., b.i.d. or t.i.d. Don't exceed 10 mg on day 1. Increase dosage gradually to recommended maximum (if needed). In children ages 2 to 5, maximum daily dose is 25 mg. In children ages 6 to 10, maximum daily dose is 25 mg.

*To manage symptoms of severe psychosis—*
**Adults:** 10 to 20 mg I.M. repeated in 1 to 4 hours, if needed. Rarely, patients may receive 10 to 20 mg q 4 to 6 hours. Institute oral therapy after symptoms are controlled.
**Children ages 2 to 12:** 0.13 mg/kg I.M.

*Nonpsychotic anxiety—*
**Adults:** 5 to 10 mg by deep I.M. injection q 3 to 4 hours, not to exceed 20 mg daily and not to be given for more than 12 weeks; or 5 to 10 mg P.O., t.i.d. or q.i.d. Or, 15 mg extended-release capsule once daily or 10 mg extended-release capsule q 12 hours.

## ADVERSE REACTIONS
**CNS:** *extrapyramidal reactions,* sedation, pseudoparkinsonism, EEG changes, dizziness.
**CV:** *orthostatic hypotension,* tachycardia, ECG changes.
**EENT:** *ocular changes, blurred vision.*

**GI:** *dry mouth, constipation,* increased appetite, weight gain.
**GU:** *urine retention,* dark urine, menstrual irregularities, gynecomastia, inhibited ejaculation.
**Hematologic:** *transient leukopenia,* **agranulocytosis.**
**Hepatic:** cholestatic jaundice, elevated liver enzyme levels.
**Skin:** *mild photosensitivity,* allergic reactions, **exfoliative dermatitis.**
**Other:** hyperprolactinemia.

## INTERACTIONS
**Drug-drug.** *Antacids:* inhibited absorption of oral phenothiazines. Separate antacid and phenothiazine doses by at least 2 hours.
*Anticholinergics, including antidepressants and antiparkinsonians:* increased anticholinergic activity and aggravated parkinsonian symptoms. Use together cautiously.
*Barbiturates:* may decrease phenothiazine effect. Monitor patient for decreased antiemetic effect.

## EFFECTS ON DIAGNOSTIC TESTS
Drug causes false-positive results for urinary porphyrins, urobilinogen, amylase, and 5-hydroxyindoleacetic acid; it also causes false-positive urine pregnancy results in tests using human chorionic gonadotropin.

## CONTRAINDICATIONS
Contraindicated in patients with hypersensitivity to phenothiazines and in those with CNS depression, including coma; also contraindicated during pediatric surgery; when using spinal or epidural anesthetic, adrenergic blockers, or ethanol; and in children under age 2.

## NURSING CONSIDERATIONS
• Use cautiously in patients with impaired CV function, glaucoma, seizure disorders, and Parkinson disease; in those who have been exposed to extreme heat; and in children with acute illness.
• Dilute oral solution with tomato or fruit juice, milk, coffee, carbonated beverage, tea, water, or soup or mix with pudding.

---

*Liquid contains alcohol.    **May contain tartrazine.    †Canada    ‡Australia    §U.K.    ◊OTC

- For I.M. use, inject deeply into upper outer quadrant of gluteal region.
- Don't give S.C. or mix in syringe with another drug.
- To prevent contact dermatitis, avoid getting concentrate or injection solution on hands or clothing.
- Monitor CBC and liver function studies during long-term therapy, as ordered.
- *Alert:* Use drug only when vomiting can't be controlled by other measures or when only a few doses are needed. If more than four doses are needed in 24 hours, notify doctor.
- Store in light-resistant container. Slight yellowing doesn't affect potency; discard extremely discolored solutions.

 **I.V. administration**
- Add 20 mg prochlorperazine/L $D_5W$ and normal saline solution15 to 30 minutes before induction. Infusion rate shouldn't exceed 5 mg/minute. Maximum parenteral dose is 40 mg daily. Infuse slowly, never as a bolus.
- Watch for orthostatic hypotension, especially when giving drug I.V.

 **Patient teaching**
- Teach patient what to use to dilute oral solution.
- Advise patient to wear protective clothing when exposed to sunlight.
- Tell patient to call doctor if more than four doses are needed within 24 hours.

---

### thiethylperazine maleate
Norzine, Torecan**

*Pregnancy Risk Category X*

#### HOW SUPPLIED
*Tablets:* 10 mg
*Injection:* 5 mg/ml

#### ACTION
Unknown. Probably acts on the chemoreceptor trigger zone to inhibit nausea and vomiting.

| Route | Onset | Peak | Duration |
|-------|-------|------|----------|
| P.O., I.M. | 0.5 hr | Unknown | 4 hr |

#### INDICATIONS & DOSAGE
*Nausea and vomiting—*
**Adults:** 10 mg P.O. or I.M., once daily, b.i.d., or t.i.d.

#### ADVERSE REACTIONS
**CNS:** *extrapyramidal reactions* (high incidence), sedation (low incidence), pseudoparkinsonism, EEG changes, dizziness, confusion, especially in elderly patients.
**CV:** *orthostatic hypotension,* tachycardia, ECG changes.
**EENT:** *ocular changes, blurred vision.*
**GI:** *dry mouth, constipation,* increased appetite, weight gain.
**GU:** *urine retention,* dark urine, menstrual irregularities, inhibited ejaculation, gynecomastia.
**Hematologic:** *transient leukopenia, agranulocytosis.*
**Hepatic:** cholestatic jaundice.
**Skin:** *mild photosensitivity,* allergic reactions.
**Other:** hyperprolactinemia.

#### INTERACTIONS
**Drug-drug.** *Antacids:* inhibited absorption of oral phenothiazines. Separate antacid and phenothiazine doses by at least 2 hours.
*Anticholinergics, including antidepressants and antiparkinsonians:* increased anticholinergic activity and increased risk of parkinsonian-like symptoms. Use together cautiously.
*Barbiturates:* may decrease phenothiazine effect. Monitor patient for decreased antiemetic effect.

#### EFFECTS ON DIAGNOSTIC TESTS
Drug may alter immunologic urine pregnancy test results.

#### CONTRAINDICATIONS
Contraindicated in patients with hypersensitivity to phenothiazines and in those with severe CNS depression or hepatic disease; also contraindicated in patients experiencing coma and during pregnancy.

#### NURSING CONSIDERATIONS
- Use cautiously in patients with aspirin or tartrazine hypersensitivity.

---

Reactions may be *common,* uncommon, *life-threatening,* or COMMON AND LIFE-THREATENING.

• **Alert:** Don't give I.V. May cause severe hypotension.
• For nausea and vomiting associated with anesthesia and surgery, give deep I.M. injection shortly before or when terminating anesthesia.
• If drug gets on skin, wash off at once to prevent contact dermatitis.
• Use only when vomiting can't be controlled by other measures or when only a few doses are needed.

### ☑ Patient teaching
• Warn patient about hypotension; suggest that he stay in bed for 1 hour after receiving drug.
• Instruct patient to report decreased urine output, visual changes, and CNS effects immediately.

## trimethobenzamide hydrochloride
Arrestin, Tebamide, Tegamide, T-Gen, Ticon, Tigan, Triban, Trimazide

*Pregnancy Risk Category C*

### HOW SUPPLIED
*Capsules:* 100 mg, 250 mg
*Injection:* 100 mg/ml
*Suppositories:* 100 mg, 200 mg

### ACTION
Unknown. Probably acts on the chemoreceptor trigger zone to inhibit nausea and vomiting.

| Route | Onset | Peak | Duration |
|-------|-------|------|----------|
| P.O. | 10-20 min | Unknown | 3-4 hr |
| I.M. | 15-35 min | Unknown | 2-3 hr |
| P.R. | Unknown | Unknown | Unknown |

### INDICATIONS & DOSAGE
*Nausea and vomiting—*
**Adults:** 250 mg P.O. t.i.d. or q.i.d.; or 200 mg I.M. or P.R. t.i.d. or q.i.d.
**Children weighing under 13 kg (29 lb):** 100 mg P.R. t.i.d. or q.i.d.
**Children weighing 13 to 40 kg (29 to 88 lb):** 100 to 200 mg P.O. or P.R. t.i.d. or q.i.d.

### ADVERSE REACTIONS
**CNS:** *drowsiness,* dizziness with large doses, headache, disorientation, depression, parkinsonian-like symptoms, ***coma, seizures.***
**CV:** hypotension.
**EENT:** blurred vision.
**GI:** diarrhea.
**Hepatic:** jaundice.
**Musculoskeletal:** muscle cramps.
**Other:** *hypersensitivity reactions* (pain, stinging, burning, redness, swelling at I.M. injection site).

### INTERACTIONS
**Drug-drug.** *CNS depressants:* additive CNS depression. Avoid concomitant use.
**Drug-lifestyle.** *Alcohol use:* additive CNS depression. Avoid concomitant use.

### EFFECTS ON DIAGNOSTIC TESTS
None reported.

### CONTRAINDICATIONS
Contraindicated in patients with hypersensitivity to drug. Suppositories contraindicated in patients with hypersensitivity to benzocaine hydrochloride or similar local anesthetic.

### NURSING CONSIDERATIONS
• Use cautiously in children; drug may be associated with Reye's syndrome.
• For I.M. administration, inject deeply into upper outer quadrant of gluteal region to reduce pain and local irritation.
• Drug may mask evidence of overdose of toxic drugs or of intestinal obstruction, brain tumor, or other conditions.
• Withhold drug if skin hypersensitivity reaction occurs.
• **Alert:** Don't confuse Tigan with Ticar.

### ☑ Patient teaching
• Instruct patient to refrigerate suppositories.
• Advise patient of possible drowsiness and dizziness; caution against driving or other activities requiring alertness until CNS effects of drug are known.

**cimetidine**
**cimetidine hydrochloride**
**famotidine**
**lansoprazole**
**misoprostol**
**nizatidine**
**omeprazole**
**rabeprazole sodium**
**ranitidine bismuth citrate**
**ranitidine hydrochloride**
**sucralfate**

## COMBINATION PRODUCTS

ARTHROTEC: 50 mg diclofenac sodium and 200 mcg misoprostol; 75 mg diclofenac sodium and 200 mcg misoprostol

---

## cimetidine
Tagamet, Tagamet HB ◇

## cimetidine hydrochloride
Tagamet HCl

*Pregnancy Risk Category B*

## HOW SUPPLIED
*Tablets:* 100 mg ◇, 200 mg, 300 mg, 400 mg, 800 mg
*Oral liquid:* 300 mg/5 ml
*Injection:* 300 mg/2 ml; 300 mg in 50 ml normal saline solution

## ACTION
Competitively inhibits action of $H_2$ at receptor sites of the parietal cells, decreasing gastric acid secretion.

| Route | Onset | Peak | Duration |
|-------|-------|------|----------|
| P.O. | Unknown | 45-90 min | 4-5 hr |
| I.V. | Unknown | Immediate | Unknown |
| I.M. | Unknown | Unknown | Unknown |

## INDICATIONS & DOSAGE
*Short-term treatment and maintenance of duodenal ulcer—*
**Adults and children ages 16 and older:** 800 mg P.O. h.s. Or, 400 mg P.O. b.i.d. or 300 mg q.i.d. (with meals and h.s.) or 200 mg t.i.d. with a 400-mg h.s. dose. Treatment continued for 4 to 6 weeks unless endoscopy shows healing. For maintenance therapy, 400 mg h.s. For parenteral therapy, 300 mg diluted to 20 ml with normal saline solution or other compatible I.V. solution by I.V. push over at least 5 minutes q 6 hours; or 300 mg diluted in 50 ml $D_5W$ or other compatible I.V. solution by I.V. infusion over 15 to 20 minutes q 6 hours; or 300 mg I.M. q 6 hours (no dilution needed). Parenteral dosage increased by giving 300-mg doses more frequently to maximum daily dose of 2,400 mg, p.r.n.; or, 900 mg/day (37.5 mg/hour) I.V. diluted in 100 to 1,000 ml of compatible solution by continuous I.V. infusion.
*Active benign gastric ulceration—*
**Adults:** 800 mg P.O. h.s., or 300 mg P.O. q.i.d. (with meals and h.s.) for up to 6 weeks.
*Pathologic hypersecretory conditions (such as Zollinger-Ellison syndrome, systemic mastocytosis, and multiple endocrine adenomas)—*
**Adults and children ages 16 and older:** 300 mg P.O. q.i.d. with meals and h.s.; adjusted to patient needs. Maximum oral daily dose is 2,400 mg.
   For parenteral therapy, 300 mg diluted to 20 ml with normal saline solution or other compatible I.V. solution by I.V. push over at least 5 minutes q 6 hours; or 300 mg diluted in 50 ml $D_5W$ or other compatible I.V. solution by I.V. infusion over 15 to 20 minutes q 6 hours. Parenteral dosage increased by giving 300-mg doses more frequently to maximum daily dose of 2,400 mg, p.r.n.
*Gastroesophageal reflux disease—*
**Adults:** 800 mg P.O. b.i.d. or 400 mg q.i.d. before meals and h.s. for up to 12 weeks.
*Prevention of upper GI bleeding in critically ill patients—*
**Adults:** 50 mg/hour by continuous I.V. infusion for up to 7 days; 25 mg/hour to pa-

tients with creatinine clearance below 30 ml/minute.

*Heartburn—*

**Adults:** 200 mg (Tagamet HB only) P.O. with water as symptoms occur, or as directed, up to b.i.d. Maximum daily dose is 400 mg. Drug shouldn't be taken daily for more than 2 weeks.

*Adjust-a-dose:* For patients with creatinine clearance less than 30 ml/minute, decrease dosage to 300 mg P.O. or I.V. q 12 hours.

## ADVERSE REACTIONS

**CNS:** confusion, dizziness, headache, peripheral neuropathy, somnolence, hallucinations.

**GI:** *mild and transient diarrhea.*

**GU:** transient elevations in serum creatinine levels, impotence, mild gynecomastia if used longer than 1 month.

**Hepatic:** increased serum alkaline phosphatase levels.

**Musculoskeletal:** muscle pain, arthralgia.

**Other:** *hypersensitivity reactions.*

## INTERACTIONS

**Drug-drug.** *Antacids:* interference with cimetidine absorption. Separate administration by at least 1 hour if possible.

*Lidocaine, phenytoin, propranolol, some benzodiazepines, theophylline, warfarin:* inhibited hepatic microsomal enzyme metabolism of these drugs. Monitor serum levels.

**Drug-herb.** *Guarana:* may increase caffeine serum levels or prolong serum caffeine half-life. Monitor patient.

*Pennyroyal:* may change rate of formation of toxic metabolites of pennyroyal. Monitor patient.

*Yerba maté:* may decrease clearance of yerba maté methylxanthines and cause toxicity. Use together cautiously.

## EFFECTS ON DIAGNOSTIC TESTS

Drug may antagonize pentagastrin's effect during gastric acid secretion tests; it may cause false-negative results in skin tests using allergen extracts.

FD and C blue dye #2 used in Tagamet tablets may impair interpretation of Hemoccult and Gastroccult tests on gastric content aspirate. Wait at least 15 minutes

after tablet administration before drawing sample and follow test manufacturer's instructions closely.

## CONTRAINDICATIONS

Contraindicated in patients with hypersensitivity to drug.

## NURSING CONSIDERATIONS

• Use cautiously in elderly or debilitated patients because they may be more susceptible to cimetidine-induced confusion.
• Assess for abdominal pain. Note blood in emesis, stool, or gastric aspirate.
• Identify tablet strength when obtaining a drug history.
• Schedule cimetidine dose at end of hemodialysis treatment because hemodialysis reduces blood levels of cimetidine. Adjust dosage, as ordered, for patients with renal failure.
• I.M. injection may be given undiluted.
• Effectiveness for treatment of gastric ulcer isn't as great as for duodenal ulcer.
• Up to 10 g overdose can occur without adverse reactions.

### 🜀 I.V. administration

• Dilute I.V. solutions with normal saline solution, $D_5W$, and $D_{10}W$ (and combinations of these), lactated Ringer's solution, or 5% sodium bicarbonate injection. Don't dilute with sterile water for injection. Cimetidine is also frequently added to total parenteral nutrition solutions with or without fat emulsion.
• *Alert:* Dilute drug before direct injection and give over 5 minutes. Rapid I.V. injection may result in arrhythmias and hypotension. Infuse drug over at least 30 minutes to minimize risk of adverse cardiac effects. If cimetidine is given as continuous I.V. infusion, use infusion pump if giving in a total volume of 250 ml over 24 hours or less.
• *Alert:* Don't confuse cimetidine with simethicone.

### ☑ Patient teaching

• Remind patient taking cimetidine once daily to take it at bedtime. If drug is being taken more than once a day, instruct him to take it with meals.

• Instruct patient taking Tagamet HB not to exceed recommended dosage and not to take daily for longer than 14 days.
• Warn patient receiving drug I.M. that injection may be painful.
• Urge patient to avoid cigarette smoking because it may increase gastric acid secretion and worsen disease.
• Advise patient to report abdominal pain and blood in stools or emesis.

## famotidine
Pepcid, Pepcid AC◇, Pepcidine‡

*Pregnancy Risk Category B*

### HOW SUPPLIED
*Tablets:* 10 mg, 20 mg, 40 mg
*Powder for oral suspension:* 40 mg/5 ml after reconstitution
*Injection:* 10 mg/ml
*Premixed injection:* 20 mg/50 ml in normal saline

### ACTION
Competitively inhibits action of $H_2$ at receptor sites of the parietal cells, decreasing gastric acid secretion.

| Route | Onset | Peak | Duration |
|-------|-------|------|----------|
| P.O. | 1 hr | 1-3 hr | 12 hr |
| I.V. | Unknown | 30 min | 12 hr |

### INDICATIONS & DOSAGE
*Duodenal ulcer (short-term treatment)—*
**Adults:** for acute therapy, 40 mg P.O. once daily h.s. or 20 mg P.O. b.i.d. For maintenance therapy, 20 mg P.O. once daily h.s.
*Benign gastric ulcer (short-term treatment)—*
**Adults:** 40 mg P.O. daily h.s. for 8 weeks.
*Pathologic hypersecretory conditions (such as Zollinger-Ellison syndrome)—*
**Adults:** 20 mg P.O. q 6 hours, up to 160 mg q 6 hours.
*Hospitalized patients with intractable ulcerations or hypersecretory conditions or who can't take oral drug—*
**Adults:** 20 mg I.V. q 12 hours.

*Gastroesophageal reflux disease (GERD)—*
**Adults:** 20 mg P.O. b.i.d. for up to 6 weeks. For esophagitis caused by GERD, 20 to 40 mg b.i.d. for up to 12 weeks.
*Prevention or treatment of heartburn—*
**Adults:** 10 mg (Pepcid AC only) P.O. 1 hour before meals (prevention) or 10 mg (Pepcid AC only) P.O. with water when symptoms occur. Maximum daily dose is 20 mg. Drug shouldn't be taken daily for more than 2 weeks.
*Adjust-a-dose:* For patients with severe renal insufficiency and creatinine clearance below 10 ml/minute, 20 mg I.V. or P.O. h.s., or prolong dosing interval to q 36 to 48 hours.

### ADVERSE REACTIONS
**CNS:** *headache,* dizziness, vertigo, malaise, paresthesia.
**CV:** palpitations, flushing.
**EENT:** tinnitus, orbital edema.
**GI:** diarrhea, constipation, anorexia, taste perversion, dry mouth.
**GU:** increased BUN and creatinine levels.
**Hepatic:** elevated hepatic enzyme levels.
**Musculoskeletal:** bone and muscle pain.
**Skin:** acne, dry skin.
**Other:** transient irritation at I.V. site, fever.

### INTERACTIONS
None significant.

### EFFECTS ON DIAGNOSTIC TESTS
Drug may antagonize pentagastrin during gastric acid secretion tests. In skin tests using allergen extracts, drug may cause false-negative results.

### CONTRAINDICATIONS
Contraindicated in patients with hypersensitivity to drug.

### NURSING CONSIDERATIONS
• Assess for abdominal pain. Note blood in emesis, stool, or gastric aspirate.
• Oral suspension must be reconstituted and shaken before use.
• Store reconstituted suspension below 86° F (30° C). Discard after 30 days.

---

Reactions may be *common,* uncommon, *life-threatening,* or COMMON AND LIFE-THREATENING.

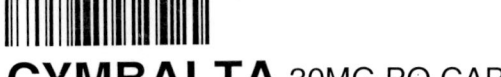

# CYMBALTA 30MG PO CAP

GENERIC NAME: DULOXETINE (doo–LOX–e–teen)

COMMON USES: This medicine is a serotonin and norepinephrine reuptake inhibitor (SNRI) used for treating depression and generalized anxiety disorder. It is used for managing pain caused by fibromyalgia and diabetic peripheral neuropathy (DPNP). It may also be used to treat other conditions as determined by your doctor.

HOW TO USE THIS MEDICINE: Follow the directions for using this medicine provided by your doctor. This medicine comes with a MEDICATION GUIDE approved by the U.S. Food and Drug Administration. Read it carefully each time you refill this medicine. Ask your doctor, nurse, or pharmacist any questions that you may have about this medicine. THIS MEDICINE MAY BE TAKEN on an empty stomach or with food. Taking it with food may help to decrease the chance of nausea or stomach upset. SWALLOW THIS MEDICINE WHOLE. Do not break, crush, or chew before swallowing. Do not open the capsule and sprinkle the contents of the capsule on food or mix with liquids. STORE THIS MEDICINE at 77 degrees F (25 degrees C). Brief storage between 59 and 86 degrees F (15 and 30 degrees C) is permitted. Store away from heat, moisture, and light. Do not store in the bathroom. TAKE THIS MEDICINE on a regular schedule to get the most benefit from it. Taking this medicine at the same time each day will help you to remember. CONTINUE TO TAKE THIS MEDICINE even if you feel well. Do not miss any doses. DO NOT SUDDENLY STOP TAKING THIS MEDICINE without checking with your doctor. Some conditions may become worse when the medicine is suddenly stopped or if the dose of this medicine is decreased. Side effects may occur. They may include mental or mood changes, numbness or tingling of the skin, diarrhea, dizziness, confusion, headache, increased sweating, nausea, nightmare, ringing in the ears, seizures, trouble sleeping, unusual tiredness, or vomiting. You will be closely monitored when you start this medicine and whenever a change in dose is made. If your doctor wants you to stop taking this medicine, your dose may need to be slowly lowered to decrease the risk of side effects. IF YOU MISS A DOSE OF THIS MEDICINE, take it as soon as possible. If it is almost time for your next dose, skip the missed dose and go back to your regular dosing schedule. DO NOT take 2 doses at once.

CAUTIONS: DO NOT USE THIS MEDICINE IF you are allergic to any ingredient in this medicine. LAB TESTS may be performed while you use this medicine. These tests may be used to monitor your condition or check for side effects. KEEP ALL DOCTOR AND LAB APPOINTMENTS. THIS MEDICINE MAY CAUSE DROWSINESS, DIZZINESS, LIGHTHEADEDNESS, FAINTING, OR BLURRED VISION; alcohol, hot weather, exercise, or fever may increase these effects. To prevent them, sit up or stand slowly, especially in the morning. Sit or lie down at the first sign of any of these effects. These effects may be worse if you take it with alcohol or certain medicines. Use this medicine with caution. DO NOT DRIVE OR PERFORM OTHER POSSIBLY UNSAFE TASKS until you know how you react to it. CHECK WITH YOUR DOCTOR before you drink alcohol or use medicines that may cause drowsiness (eg, sleep aids, muscle relaxers) while you are using this medicine; it may add to their effects. Ask your pharmacist if you have questions about which medicines may cause drowsiness. CHILDREN, TEENAGERS, AND YOUNG ADULTS who take this medicine may be at increased risk for suicidal thoughts or actions. Watch all patients who take this medicine closely. Contact the doctor at once if new, worsened, or sudden symptoms such as depressed mood; anxious, restless, or irritable behavior; panic attacks; any unusual change in mood or behavior; or signs of suicidal thoughts or actions occur. SEROTONIN SYNDROME and NEUROLEPTIC MALIGNANT SYNDROME (NMS) are possibly fatal syndromes that can be caused by this medicine. Your risk may be greater if you take this medicine with certain other medicines (eg, MAOIs, SSRIs, "triptans"). Symptoms may include blood pressure changes; agitation; confusion; hallucinations; other mental or mood changes; coma; fever; fast or irregular heartbeat; tremor; excessive sweating; rigid muscles; nausea; vomiting; or diarrhea. Contact your doctor at once if you have any of these symptoms. IF YOUR DOCTOR TELLS YOU TO STOP TAKING THIS MEDICINE, you will need to wait for at least 5 days before beginning to take certain other medicines (eg, MAOIs). Ask your doctor when you should start to take your new medicines after you have stopped taking this medicine. BEFORE YOU BEGIN TAKING ANY NEW MEDICINES, either prescription or over–the–counter, check with your doctor or pharmacist. USE THIS MEDICINE WITH CAUTION IN THE ELDERLY; they may be more sensitive to its effects, especially low blood sodium levels. CAUTION IS ADVISED WHEN USING THIS MEDICINE IN CHILDREN; they may be more sensitive to its effects, especially increased risk of suicidal thoughts or actions. FOR WOMEN: THIS MEDICINE MAY CAUSE HARM TO THE FETUS if it is used during the last 3 months of pregnancy. If you become pregnant, contact your doctor. You will need to discuss the benefits and risks of using this medicine while you are pregnant. THIS MEDICINE IS FOUND in breast milk. DO NOT BREAST–FEED while taking this medicine.

POSSIBLE SIDE EFFECTS: SIDE EFFECTS that may occur while taking this medicine include constipation, decreased sexual desire or ability, diarrhea, dizziness, drowsiness, dry mouth, headache, increased sweating, loss of appetite, nausea, sore throat, tiredness, trouble sleeping, vomiting, or weakness. If they continue or are bothersome, check with your doctor. CONTACT YOUR DOCTOR IMMEDIATELY if you experience bizarre behavior; bloody or black, tarry stools; blurred vision; confusion; dark urine; excessive sweating; fainting; fast or irregular heartbeat; fever or chills; hallucinations; loss of coordination; new or worsening agitation, anxiety, panic attacks, aggressiveness, impulsiveness, irritability, hostility, restlessness, or inability to sit still; pale stools; red, swollen, blistered, or peeling skin; ringing in the ears; seizures; severe or persistent dizziness or headache; severe or persistent nausea, vomiting, or diarrhea; severe or persistent trouble sleeping; severe or persistent tiredness or weakness; stomach pain; suicidal thoughts or attempts; tremor; trouble urinating or change in the amount of urine produced; unusual bruising or bleeding; unusual or severe mental or mood changes; vomit that looks like coffee grounds; worsening of depression; or yellowing of the skin or eyes. AN ALLERGIC REACTION to this medicine is unlikely, but seek immediate medical attention if it occurs. Symptoms of an allergic reaction include rash; hives; itching; difficulty breathing; tightness in the chest; or swelling of the mouth, face, lips, or tongue; unusual hoarseness. This is not a complete list of all side effects that may occur. If you have questions about side effects, contact your healthcare provider. Call your doctor for medical advice about side effects. You may report side effects to FDA at 1–800–FDA–1088.

# DECATUR PHARM

Call your doctor for medical advice about side effects. You may r

The information in this monograph is not intended to cover all possible uses, directions, precautions, drug interactions, or adverse
If you have questions about the medicines you are taking or would like more information, check with your doctor, pharmacist, or nu

BEFORE USING THIS MEDICINE: WARNING: Antidepressants may increase the risk of suicidal thoughts or actions in children, teenagers, and young adults. However, depression and certain other mental problems may also increase the risk of suicide. Talk with the patient's doctor to be sure that the benefits of using this medicine weigh the risks. FAMILY AND CAREGIVERS MUST CLOSELY WATCH PATIENTS who take this medicine. It is tant to keep in close contact with the patient's doctor. Tell the doctor right away if the patient has symptoms e worsened depression, suicidal thoughts, or changes in behavior. Discuss any questions with the patient's doctor. Some medicines or medical conditions may interact with this medicine. INFORM YOUR DOCTOR OR PHARMACIST of all prescription and over-the-counter medicine that you are taking. DO NOT TAKE THIS MEDICINE IF you are taking a quinolone antibiotic (eg, ciprofloxacin), a selective serotonin reuptake inhibitor (SSRI) (eg, fluoxetine, fluvoxamine), an SNRI (eg, venlafaxine), thioridazine, or tryptophan. DO NOT TAKE THIS MEDICINE IF you are taking or have taken a monoamine oxidase inhibitor (MAOI) (eg, phenelzine) within the last 14 days. ADDITIONAL MONITORING OF YOUR DOSE OR CONDITION may be needed if you are taking 5-HT1 receptor agonists (eg, sumatriptan), linezolid, lithium, quinidine, rasagiline, St. John's wort, tramadol, anticoagulants (eg, warfarin), aspirin, nonsteroidal anti-inflammatory drugs (NSAIDs) (eg, ibuprofen), diuretics (eg, furosemide, hydrochlorothiazide), cimetidine, medicines for high blood pressure, certain antiarrhythmics (eg, flecainide, propafenone), phenothiazines (eg, chlorpromazine), or tricyclic antidepressants (eg, amitriptyline). DO NOT START OR STOP any medicine without doctor or pharmacist approval. Inform your doctor of any other medical conditions, including a history of seizures, heart problems (eg, heart failure, irregular heartbeat), recent heart attack, high blood pressure, kidney problems, diabetes, stomach or bowel problems (eg, slowed emptying), increased eye pressure (eg, glaucoma), allergies, pregnancy, or breast-feeding. Tell your doctor if you or a family member has a history of bipolar disorder (manic-depression), other mental or mood problems, suicidal thoughts or attempts, or alcohol or substance abuse. Tell your doctor if you are dehydrated, have trouble urinating, have low blood sodium levels, or drink alcohol. USE OF THIS MEDICINE IS NOT RECOMMENDED if you have uncontrolled narrow-angle glaucoma; liver problems; severe kidney problems; or you are having dialysis. Contact your doctor or pharmacist if you have any questions or concerns about using this medicine.

OVERDOSE: IF OVERDOSE IS SUSPECTED, contact your local poison control center or emergency room immediately. Symptoms of overdose may include agitation; blurred vision; confusion; coma; fast or irregular heartbeat; excessive sweating; fever; hallucinations; seizures; and severe or persistent diarrhea, dizziness, drowsiness, headache, nausea, or vomiting; or severe or persistent tiredness or weakness.

ADDITIONAL INFORMATION: SEVERAL WEEKS MAY PASS before your symptoms improve. Do NOT take more than the recommended dose or use for longer than prescribed without checking with your doctor. DIABETES PATIENTS – This medicine may affect your blood sugar. Check blood sugar levels closely. Ask your doctor before you change the dose of your diabetes medicine. DO NOT SHARE THIS MEDICINE with others for whom it was not prescribed. DO NOT USE THIS MEDICINE for other health conditions. KEEP THIS MEDICINE out of the reach of children and pets. IF USING THIS MEDICINE FOR AN EXTENDED PERIOD OF TIME, be sure to obtain refills before your supply runs out.

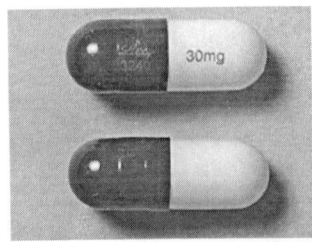

NDC: 00002-3240-30

## ⚫ I.V. administration

• To prepare I.V. injection, dilute 2 ml (20 mg) famotidine with compatible I.V. solution to a total volume of either 5 or 10 ml, and inject over at least 2 minutes. Compatible solutions include sterile water for injection, normal saline for injection, $D_5W$ or $D_{10}W$ injection, 5% sodium bicarbonate injection, and lactated Ringer's injection. Famotidine can also be added to total parenteral nutrition solutions.

• Or, give drug by intermittent I.V. infusion. Dilute 20 mg (2 ml) famotidine in 100 ml compatible solution, and infuse over 15 to 30 minutes. After dilution, solution is stable for 48 hours at room temperature.

• Store I.V. injection in refrigerator at 36° to 46° F (2° to 8° C).

## ☑ Patient teaching

• Instruct patient on proper use of OTC product (Pepcid AC), if appropriate.

• Tell patient to take prescription drug with a snack, if desired.

• Remind patient that prescription drug is most effective if taken at bedtime. Tell patient taking 20 mg b.i.d. to take at least one dose at bedtime

• Advise patient not to take prescription drug for more than 8 weeks, unless ordered by doctor, and to limit use of OTC drug to no more than 2 weeks.

• With doctor's knowledge, allow patient to take antacids concomitantly, especially at beginning of therapy when pain is severe.

• Urge patient to avoid cigarette smoking because it may increase gastric acid secretion and worsen disease.

• Advise patient to report abdominal pain and blood in stools or emesis.

---

**lansoprazole**
Prevacid, Zoton§

*Pregnancy Risk Category B*

## HOW SUPPLIED
*Capsules (delayed-release):* 15 mg, 30 mg

## ACTION
Inhibits activity of proton pump and binds to hydrogen-potassium adenosine triphosphatase, located at secretory surface of the gastric parietal cells, to block secretion of gastric acid.

| Route | Onset | Peak | Duration |
|-------|-------|------|----------|
| P.O. | Unknown | 1.7 hr | Unknown |

## INDICATIONS & DOSAGE
*Short-term treatment of active duodenal ulcer—*
**Adults:** 15 mg P.O. daily before eating for 4 weeks.
*Short-term treatment of active benign gastric ulcer—*
**Adults:** 30 mg P.O. once daily for up to 8 weeks.
*Short-term treatment of erosive esophagitis—*
**Adults:** 30 mg P.O. daily before eating for up to 8 weeks. If healing doesn't occur, 8 more weeks of therapy may be given. Maintenance dose for healing is 15 mg P.O. daily.
*Maintenance of healing of erosive esophagitis—*
**Adults:** 15 mg P.O. once daily.
*Long-term treatment of pathologic hypersecretory conditions, including Zollinger-Ellison syndrome—*
**Adults:** initially, 60 mg P.O. once daily. Dosage increased, p.r.n. Daily doses of more than 120 mg should be given in evenly divided doses.
*Maintenance of healed duodenal ulcers—*
**Adults:** 15 mg P.O. daily.
Helicobacter pylori *eradication to reduce risk of duodenal ulcer recurrence—*
**Adults:** for patients receiving dual therapy, 30 mg P.O. lansoprazole with 1 g P.O. amoxicillin, each given q 8 hours for 14 days. For patients receiving triple therapy, 30 mg P.O. lansoprazole with 1 g P.O. amoxicillin and 500 mg P.O. clarithromycin, all given q 12 hours for 14 days.
*Short-term treatment of symptomatic gastroesophageal reflux disease—*
**Adults:** 15 mg P.O. once daily for up to 8 weeks.

## ADVERSE REACTIONS
**GI:** diarrhea, nausea, abdominal pain.

---

*Liquid contains alcohol.    **May contain tartrazine.    †Canada    ‡Australia    §U.K.    ◊OTC

## INTERACTIONS
**Drug-drug.** *Ampicillin esters, digoxin, iron salts, ketoconazole:* lansoprazole may inhibit absorption. Monitor patient closely.
*Sucralfate:* delayed lansoprazole absorption. Give lansoprazole at least 30 minutes before sucralfate.
*Theophylline:* may cause mild increase in theophylline clearance. Use together cautiously. Dosage adjustment of theophylline may be needed when lansoprazole is started or stopped.
**Drug-herb.** *Male fern:* male fern is inactivated in alkaline environments. Don't give concurrently.

## EFFECTS ON DIAGNOSTIC TESTS
None reported.

## CONTRAINDICATIONS
Contraindicated in patients with hypersensitivity to drug.

## NURSING CONSIDERATIONS
• No dosage adjustment is needed for patients with renal insufficiency or in elderly patients. For patients with severe liver disease, dosage adjustment may be needed.
• A symptomatic response to lansoprazole therapy doesn't preclude presence of gastric malignancy.
• Safety and efficacy of drug haven't been established in children.
• For patients who have an NG tube in place, capsules can be opened and the intact granules mixed in 40 ml of apple juice and administered through the tube into the stomach. After administering the granules, the tube should be flushed with additional apple juice to clear it.
• Because it's unknown if lansoprazole appears in breast milk, a decision to discontinue breast-feeding or drug should be made when drug is prescribed for breast-feeding women.

### ✓ Patient teaching
• For best effect, instruct patient to take drug no more than 30 minutes before eating.
• Tell patient who has trouble swallowing capsules to open and sprinkle contents over applesauce, and to swallow immediately. The contents shouldn't be chewed or crushed.

# misoprostol
Cytotec

*Pregnancy Risk Category X*

## HOW SUPPLIED
*Tablets:* 100 mcg, 200 mcg

## ACTION
A synthetic prostaglandin $E_1$ analogue that replaces gastric prostaglandins depleted by NSAID therapy. Also decreases basal and stimulated gastric acid secretion and may increase gastric mucus and bicarbonate production.

| Route | Onset | Peak | Duration |
|-------|-------|------|----------|
| P.O. | 30 min | 10-15 min | 3 hr |

## INDICATIONS & DOSAGE
*Prevention of NSAID-induced gastric ulcer in elderly or debilitated patients at high risk for complications from gastric ulcer and in patients with history of NSAID-induced ulcer—*
**Adults:** 200 mcg P.O. q.i.d. with food; if not tolerated, may be decreased to 100 mcg P.O. q.i.d. Dosage should be given for duration of NSAID therapy. Last dose should be given h.s.

## ADVERSE REACTIONS
**CNS:** headache.
**GI:** *diarrhea, abdominal pain,* nausea, flatulence, dyspepsia, vomiting, constipation.
**GU:** hypermenorrhea, dysmenorrhea, spotting, cramps, menstrual disorders.

## INTERACTIONS
**Drug-drug.** *Antacids:* reduced plasma levels when administered concomitantly. Not considered significant.
**Drug-food.** *Any food:* Food may decrease rate of absorption. Give on empty stomach if possible.

## EFFECTS ON DIAGNOSTIC TESTS
Drug causes modest decrease in basal pepsin secretion.

---

Reactions may be *common,* uncommon, *life-threatening,* or COMMON AND LIFE-THREATENING.

## CONTRAINDICATIONS
Contraindicated in pregnant or breast-feeding women.

## NURSING CONSIDERATIONS
• Drug shouldn't be routinely given to women of childbearing age unless they are at high risk for developing ulcers or complications from NSAID-induced ulcers.
• **Alert:** Take special precautions to prevent use of drug during pregnancy. Make sure patient understands dangers of drug to fetus and that she receives both oral and written warnings about these dangers. Also ensure that she can comply with effective contraception and that she has a negative serum pregnancy test within 2 weeks of initiating therapy. Patient shouldn't breast-feed during therapy.

☑ **Patient teaching**
• Instruct patient not to share misoprostol. Remind pregnant patient that drug may cause miscarriage, often with potentially life-threatening bleeding.
• Advise woman not to begin therapy until second or third day of next normal menstrual period.
• Advise patient to take drug as prescribed for duration of NSAID therapy.

---

## nizatidine
Axid, Axid AR, Tazac‡

*Pregnancy Risk Category C*

## HOW SUPPLIED
*Tablets:* 75 mg
*Capsules:* 150 mg, 300 mg

## ACTION
Competitively inhibits action of $H_2$ at receptor sites of the parietal cells, decreasing gastric acid secretion.

| Route | Onset | Peak | Duration |
|-------|-------|------|----------|
| P.O. | 0.5 hr | 0.5-3 hr | 12 hr |

## INDICATIONS & DOSAGE
*Active duodenal ulcer—*
**Adults:** 300 mg P.O. daily h.s. Or, 150 mg P.O. b.i.d.

*Maintenance therapy for duodenal ulcer—*
**Adults:** 150 mg P.O. daily h.s.
*Benign gastric ulcer—*
**Adults:** 150 mg P.O. b.i.d. or 300 mg h.s. for 8 weeks.
*Gastroesophageal reflux disease (GERD)—*
**Adults:** 150 mg P.O. b.i.d. for up to 12 weeks.
*Adjust-a-dose:* For renally impaired patients with creatinine clearance of 20 to 50 ml/minute, 150 mg P.O. daily for treatment of active duodenal ulcer, benign gastric ulcer, or GERD; or 150 mg every other day for maintenance therapy. If creatinine clearance is below 20 ml/minute, 150 mg P.O. every other day for treatment, or 150 mg every third day for maintenance.

## ADVERSE REACTIONS
**CNS:** *somnolence.*
**CV:** *arrhythmias.*
**Hematologic:** eosinophilia.
**Hepatic:** elevated liver function tests results, hepatocellular injury.
**Metabolic:** hyperuricemia.
**Skin:** *diaphoresis,* rash, urticaria.
**Other:** fever.

## INTERACTIONS
**Drug-drug.** *Aspirin:* possibly elevated serum salicylate levels (with high doses). Monitor closely.
**Drug-food.** *Tomato-based vegetable juices:* may decrease potency of drug when used concomitantly. Don't use together.

## EFFECTS ON DIAGNOSTIC TESTS
False-positive test results for urobilinogen may occur during drug therapy.

## CONTRAINDICATIONS
Contraindicated in patients with hypersensitivity to $H_2$-receptor antagonists.

## NURSING CONSIDERATIONS
• If needed, open capsules and mix contents with apple juice. However, drug loses some potency when mixed with tomato-based vegetable juices. Ask pharmacist about compatibility.

---

*Liquid contains alcohol.     **May contain tartrazine.     †Canada     ‡Australia     §U.K.     ◊OTC

• Assess patient for abdominal pain. Note presence of blood in emesis, stool, or gastric aspirate.

### ☑ Patient teaching
• Tell patient who has difficulty swallowing capsules that contents may be mixed with apple juice but not with tomato-based vegetable juices.
• Urge patient to avoid cigarette smoking because it may increase gastric acid secretion and worsen disease.
• Advise patient to report abdominal pain and blood in stools or emesis.

## omeprazole
Losect†‡, Prilosec

*Pregnancy Risk Category C*

### HOW SUPPLIED
*Capsules (delayed-release):* 10 mg, 20 mg, 40 mg

### ACTION
Inhibits activity of acid (proton) pump, and binds to hydrogen-potassium adenosine triphosphatase, located at secretory surface of the gastric parietal cells, to block formation of gastric acid.

| Route | Onset | Peak | Duration |
|-------|-------|------|----------|
| P.O. | 1 hr | 2 hr | < 3 days |

### INDICATIONS & DOSAGE
*Symptomatic gastroesophageal reflux disease (GERD) without esophageal lesions—*
**Adults:** 20 mg P.O. daily for 4 to 8 weeks for patients poorly responsive to customary medical treatment usually including an adequate course of $H_2$-receptor antagonists.
*Erosive esophagitis and accompanying symptoms due to GERD—*
**Adults:** 20 mg P.O. daily for 4 to 8 weeks.
*Maintenance of healing erosive esophagitis—*
**Adults:** 20 mg P.O. daily.
*Pathologic hypersecretory conditions (such as Zollinger-Ellison syndrome)—*
**Adults:** initially, 60 mg P.O. daily; dosage adjusted based on patient response. If daily dose exceeds 80 mg, administer in divided doses. Doses up to 120 mg t.i.d. have been given. Continue therapy as long as clinically indicated.
*Duodenal ulcer (short-term treatment)—*
**Adults:** 20 mg P.O. daily for 4 to 8 weeks. Helicobacter pylori *infection and duodenal ulcer disease, to eradicate* H. pylori *with clarithromycin (dual therapy)—*
**Adults:** 40 mg P.O. every morning with clarithromycin 500 mg P.O. t.i.d for days 1 to 14. For patients with an ulcer present at initiation of therapy, an additional 14 days of omeprazole 20 mg P.O. once daily is recommended.
H. pylori *infection and duodenal ulcer disease, to eradicate* H. pylori *with clarithromycin and amoxicillin (triple therapy)—*
**Adults:** 20 mg P.O. with clarithromycin 500 mg P.O. and amoxicillin 1,000 mg P.O., each given b.i.d. for 10 days. For patients with an ulcer present at initiation of therapy, an additional 18 days of omeprazole 20 mg P.O. once daily is recommended.
*Short-term treatment of active benign gastric ulcer—*
**Adults:** 40 mg P.O. once daily for 4 to 8 weeks.

### ADVERSE REACTIONS
**CNS:** headache, dizziness, asthenia.
**GI:** diarrhea, abdominal pain, nausea, vomiting, constipation, flatulence.
**Musculoskeletal:** back pain.
**Respiratory:** cough, upper respiratory tract infection.
**Skin:** rash.

### INTERACTIONS
**Drug-drug.** *Ampicillin esters, iron derivatives, ketoconazole:* may exhibit poor bioavailability in patients taking omeprazole because optimal absorption of these drugs needs a low gastric pH. Avoid concomitant use.
*Diazepam, phenytoin, warfarin:* decreased hepatic clearance, possibly leading to increased serum levels. Monitor closely.
**Drug-herb.** *Male fern:* male fern is inactivated in alkaline environments. Separate administration.

---

Reactions may be *common*, uncommon, *life-threatening*, or COMMON AND LIFE-THREATENING.

*Pennyroyal*: may change rate of formation of toxic metabolites of pennyroyal. Avoid concurrent use.

**EFFECTS ON DIAGNOSTIC TESTS**
Serum gastrin levels rise in most patients during the first 2 weeks of therapy.

**CONTRAINDICATIONS**
Contraindicated in patients with hypersensitivity to drug or its components.

**NURSING CONSIDERATIONS**
• Dosage adjustments aren't needed for patients with renal or hepatic impairment.
• Omeprazole increases its own bioavailability with repeated dosages. Drug is labile in gastric acid; less drug is lost to hydrolysis because drug increases gastric pH.
• *Alert:* Don't confuse Prilosec with Prozac, Prilocaine, or Prinivil.

☑ **Patient teaching**
• Tell patient to swallow capsules whole and not to open, crush, or chew them.
• Instruct patient to take drug 30 minutes before meals.
• Caution patient not to perform hazardous activities if dizziness occurs.

✳ *NEW DRUG*

**rabeprazole sodium**
Aciphex

*Pregnancy Risk Category B*

**HOW SUPPLIED**
*Tablets (delayed-release):* 20 mg

**ACTION**
Blocks activity of acid (proton) pump by inhibiting gastric hydrogen-potassium adenosine triphosphatase at secretory surface of the gastric parietal cell, thereby blocking gastric acid secretion.

| Route | Onset | Peak | Duration |
|-------|-------|------|----------|
| P.O. | < 1 hr | 2-5 hr | > 24 hr |

**INDICATIONS & DOSAGE**
*Healing of erosive or ulcerative gastroesophageal reflux disease (GERD)—*
**Adults:** 20 mg P.O. daily for 4 to 8 weeks. Additional 8-week course may be considered, if needed.
*Maintenance of healing of erosive or ulcerative GERD—*
**Adults:** 20 mg P.O. daily.
*Healing of duodenal ulcers—*
**Adults:** 20 mg P.O. daily after morning meal for up to 4 weeks.
*Pathologic hypersecretory conditions, including Zollinger-Ellison syndrome—*
**Adults:** 60 mg P.O. daily; may be increased, p.r.n., to 100 mg P.O. daily or 60 mg P.O. b.i.d.

**ADVERSE REACTIONS**
**CNS:** headache, dizziness, malaise, asthenia, migraine, syncope, insomnia, anxiety, depression, nervousness, somnolence, neuralgia, vertigo, *seizures,* abnormal dreams, neuropathy, paresthesia, tremor.
**CV:** substernal chest pain, hypertension, *MI*, ECG abnormalities, angina, bundle-branch block, palpitations, *sinus bradycardia,* tachycardia, edema.
**EENT:** epistaxis, cataracts, amblyopia, glaucoma, dry eyes, abnormal vision, tinnitus, otitis media.
**GI:** diarrhea, nausea, abdominal pain, vomiting, dyspepsia, flatulence, constipation, dry mouth, eructation, gastroenteritis, rectal hemorrhage, melena, anorexia, cholelithiasis, mouth ulceration, stomatitis, dysphagia, gingivitis, cholecystitis, increased appetite, abnormal stools, colitis, esophagitis, glossitis, *pancreatitis,* proctitis.
**GU:** cystitis, urinary frequency, dysmenorrhea, dysuria, renal calculi, metrorrhagia, polyuria.
**Hematologic:** anemia.
**Metabolic:** hyperthyroidism, hypothyroidism, weight loss or gain.
**Musculoskeletal:** neck rigidity, myalgia, arthritis, leg cramps, bone pain, arthrosis, bursitis, hypertonia.
**Respiratory:** bronchitis, dyspnea, asthma, laryngitis, hiccups, hyperventilation.
**Skin:** rash, pruritus, sweating, urticaria, alopecia, photosensitivity reaction.

**Other:** infection, fever, allergic reaction, chills, lymphadenopathy, dehydration, decreased libido, ecchymosis, gout.

**INTERACTIONS**
**Drug-drug.** *Cyclosporine:* may inhibit cyclosporine metabolism. Use together cautiously.
*Digoxin, ketoconazole, other gastric pH-dependent drugs:* decreased or increased drug absorption at increased pH values. Monitor patient closely during use with rabeprazole.

**EFFECTS ON DIAGNOSTIC TESTS**
None reported.

**CONTRAINDICATIONS**
Contraindicated in patients with hypersensitivity to drug, other benzimidazoles (lansoprazole, omeprazole), or components in these formulations.

**NURSING CONSIDERATIONS**
• Use cautiously in patients with severe hepatic impairment.
• Consider additional courses of therapy when duodenal ulcers or GERD isn't healed after first course of therapy.
• Symptomatic response to therapy doesn't preclude presence of gastric malignancy.

☑ **Patient teaching**
• Explain importance of taking drug exactly as prescribed for treatment course.
• Advise patient that delayed-release tablets should be swallowed whole and not crushed, chewed, or split.
• Advise patient that drug may be taken without regard to meals.

---

**ranitidine bismuth citrate**
Tritec

*Pregnancy Risk Category C*

**HOW SUPPLIED**
*Tablets:* 400 mg

**ACTION**
Competitively inhibits histamine at the $H_2$ receptor of the gastric parietal cells. Disrupts integrity of bacterial cell walls and prevents adhesion of *Helicobacter pylori* to gastric epithelium.

| Route | Onset | Peak | Duration |
|-------|-------|------|----------|
| P.O. | Unknown | Variable | Variable |

**INDICATIONS & DOSAGE**
*With clarithromycin for treatment of active duodenal ulcer associated with* H. pylori *infection—*
**Adults:** 400 mg P.O. b.i.d for 28 days with clarithromycin 500 mg P.O. t.i.d. for first 14 days.

**ADVERSE REACTIONS**
**CNS:** headache.
**GI:** constipation, darkening of tongue and stool, diarrhea.

**INTERACTIONS**
**Drug-drug.** *Delavirdine, enoxacin, itraconazole, ketoconazole:* decreased absorption with use of ranitidine which increases gastric pH. Avoid concomitant use.
*Glipizide:* possible increased hypoglycemic effect. Monitor glucose levels.
*Warfarin:* concomitant use may increase warfarin's hypoprothrombinemic effects. Monitor PT and INR and adjust dose if needed.

**EFFECTS ON DIAGNOSTIC TESTS**
Drug may cause false-positive results in urine protein tests using Multistix; test with sulfosalicylic acid if needed.

**CONTRAINDICATIONS**
Contraindicated in patients with hypersensitivity to drug or its components.

**NURSING CONSIDERATIONS**
• Don't use drug with clarithromycin in patients with history of acute porphyria.
• Drug isn't recommended for patients with creatinine clearance below 25 ml/minute.
• Drug shouldn't be prescribed alone for treatment of active duodenal ulcers.
• If clarithromycin doesn't eradicate *H. pylori* infection, patient has clarithromycin-resistant *H. pylori* and

---

shouldn't be retreated with a regimen containing clarithromycin.

• Drug may cause a temporary and harmless darkening of tongue or stool. Don't confuse with blood in stool.

• It isn't known if drug appears in breast milk. Use cautiously in breast-feeding women.

☑ **Patient teaching**

• Inform patient that drug may be administered without regard to food.

• Instruct patient to take drug as directed, even after pain has subsided.

• Tell patient that it's important to take clarithromycin with drug for specified length of time.

• Inform patient that a temporary and harmless darkening of tongue or stool may occur.

• *Alert:* Don't confuse ranitidine with ritodrine or rimantadine.

---

**ranitidine hydrochloride**
Apo-Ranitidine†, Zantac*,
Zantac-C†, Zantac 75◇, Zantac
150, Zantac 150 EFFERdose,
Zantac 150 GELdose, Zantac
300, Zantac 300 GELdose

*Pregnancy Risk Category B*

### HOW SUPPLIED
*Tablets:* 75 mg◇, 150 mg, 300 mg
*Tablets (dispersible):* 150 mg‡
*Tablets (effervescent):* 150 mg
*Granules (effervescent):* 150 mg
*Syrup:* 15 mg/ml*
*Injection:* 25 mg/ml
*Infusion:* 0.5 mg/ml in 100-ml containers

### ACTION
Competitively inhibits action of $H_2$ at receptor sites of the parietal cells, decreasing gastric acid secretion.

| Route | Onset | Peak | Duration |
|-------|-------|------|----------|
| P.O. | 1 hr | 1-3 hr | 13 hr |
| I.V. | Unknown | Unknown | Unknown |

### INDICATIONS & DOSAGE
*Duodenal and gastric ulcer (short-term treatment); pathologic hypersecretory conditions, such as Zollinger-Ellison syndrome—*
**Adults:** 150 mg P.O. b.i.d. or 300 mg daily h.s. Or, 50 mg I.V. or I.M. q 6 to 8 hours. Patients with Zollinger-Ellison syndrome may need doses up to 6 g P.O. daily.
*Maintenance therapy for duodenal or gastric ulcer—*
**Adults:** 150 mg P.O. h.s.
*Gastroesophageal reflux disease—*
**Adults:** 150 mg P.O. b.i.d.
*Erosive esophagitis—*
**Adults:** 150 mg P.O. q.i.d. Maintenance dose is 150 mg P.O. b.i.d.
*Heartburn—*
**Adults:** 75 mg (Zantac 75 only) P.O. as symptoms occur, not to exceed 150 mg daily.
*Adjust-a-dose:* For renally impaired patients with creatinine clearance below 50 ml/minute, 150 mg P.O. q 24 hours or 50 mg I.V. q 18 to 24 hours.

### ADVERSE REACTIONS
**CNS:** vertigo, malaise.
**EENT:** blurred vision.
**GU:** increased serum creatinine levels.
**Hematologic:** reversible *leukopenia*, pancytopenia.
**Hepatic:** elevated liver enzymes, jaundice.
**Other:** burning and itching at injection site, *anaphylaxis,* angioneurotic edema.

### INTERACTIONS
**Drug-drug.** *Antacids:* may interfere with ranitidine absorption. Stagger doses if possible.
*Diazepam:* decreased absorption of diazepam. Monitor closely.
*Glipizide:* possible increased hypoglycemic effect. Adjust glipizide dosage as needed.
*Procainamide:* possible decreased renal clearance of procainamide. Monitor patient closely for toxicity.
*Warfarin:* possible interference with warfarin clearance. Monitor closely.

### EFFECTS ON DIAGNOSTIC TESTS
Drug may cause false-positive results in urine protein tests using Multistix.

---

*Liquid contains alcohol.    **May contain tartrazine.    †Canada    ‡Australia    §U.K.    ◇OTC

## CONTRAINDICATIONS
Contraindicated in patients with hypersensitivity to drug.

## NURSING CONSIDERATIONS
• Use cautiously in patients with hepatic dysfunction. Adjust dosage in patients with impaired renal function, as ordered.
• Assess patient for abdominal pain. Note presence of blood in emesis, stool, or gastric aspirate.
• Ranitidine may be added to total parenteral nutrition solutions.
• *Alert:* Don't confuse ranitidine with ritodrine or rimantadine; or Zantac with Xanax.

### 🖐 I.V. administration
• When administering by I.V. push, dilute to a total volume of 20 ml, and inject over a period of 5 minutes. No dilution is needed when administering I.M.
• When giving by intermittent I.V. infusion, dilute 50 mg (2 ml) ranitidine in 100 ml compatible solution, and infuse over 15 to 20 minutes. Compatible solutions include normal saline for injection, $D_5W$ or $D_{10}W$ injection, 5% sodium bicarbonate injection, and lactated Ringer's injection. Or, give by continuous I.V. infusion: 150 mg in 250 ml of compatible solution. Administer at 6.25 mg/hour using an infusion pump.
• When administering premixed I.V. infusion, give by slow I.V. drip (over 15 to 20 minutes). Don't add other drugs to solution. If used with a primary I.V. fluid system, discontinue primary solution during infusion.

### ☑ Patient teaching
• Instruct patient on proper use of OTC preparation, as indicated.
• Remind patient taking prescription drug once daily to take it at bedtime for best results.
• Instruct patient to take without regard to meals because absorption isn't affected by food.
• Tell patient taking EFFERdose to dissolve drug in 6 to 8 oz of water before taking.

• Urge patient to avoid cigarette smoking because it may increase gastric acid secretion and worsen disease.
• Advise patient to report abdominal pain and blood in stool or emesis.

---

## sucralfate
Antepsin§, Carafate

*Pregnancy Risk Category B*

### HOW SUPPLIED
*Tablets:* 1 g
*Suspension:* 1 g/10 ml

### ACTION
Unknown. Probably adheres to and protects the ulcer's surface by forming a barrier.

| Route | Onset | Peak | Duration |
|-------|-------|------|----------|
| P.O. | Unknown | Unknown | 6 hr |

### INDICATIONS & DOSAGE
*Short-term (up to 8 weeks) treatment of duodenal ulcer—*
**Adults:** 1 g P.O. q.i.d. 1 hour before meals and h.s.
*Maintenance therapy for duodenal ulcer—*
**Adults:** 1 g P.O. b.i.d.

### ADVERSE REACTIONS
**CNS:** dizziness, sleepiness, headache, vertigo.
**GI:** *constipation,* nausea, gastric discomfort, diarrhea, bezoar formation, vomiting, flatulence, dry mouth, indigestion.
**Musculoskeletal:** back pain.
**Skin:** rash, pruritus.

### INTERACTIONS
**Drug-drug.** *Antacids:* may decrease binding of drug to gastroduodenal mucosa, impairing effectiveness. Don't administer within 30 minutes of each other.
*Cimetidine, ciprofloxacin, digoxin, ketoconazole, norfloxacin, phenytoin, quinidine, ranitidine, tetracycline, theophylline:* decreased absorption. Separate administration times by at least 2 hours.

---

**EFFECTS ON DIAGNOSTIC TESTS**
None reported.

**CONTRAINDICATIONS**
No known contraindications.

**NURSING CONSIDERATIONS**
• Use cautiously in patients with chronic renal failure.
• Reconstitute drug before instillation through an NG tube. Flush tube with water to ensure passage into stomach.
• Drug is minimally absorbed and has few adverse reactions.
• Monitor for severe, persistent constipation.
• Sucralfate has proved as effective as cimetidine in healing duodenal ulcer.
• Drug contains aluminum but isn't classified as an antacid. Monitor patient with renal insufficiency for aluminum toxicity.

☑ **Patient teaching**
• Tell patient to take sucralfate on an empty stomach (1 hour before each meal and at bedtime).
• Instruct patient to continue prescribed regimen to ensure complete healing. Pain and ulcerative symptoms may subside within first few weeks of therapy.
• Urge patient to avoid cigarette smoking because it may increase gastric acid secretion and worsen disease.

# 53
## Corticosteroids

betamethasone
betamethasone acetate and
  betamethasone sodium
  phosphate
betamethasone sodium
  phosphate
cortisone acetate
dexamethasone
dexamethasone acetate
dexamethasone sodium
  phosphate
fludrocortisone acetate
hydrocortisone
hydrocortisone acetate
hydrocortisone cypionate
hydrocortisone sodium
  phosphate
hydrocortisone sodium
  succinate
methylprednisolone
methylprednisolone acetate
methylprednisolone sodium
  succinate
prednisolone
prednisolone acetate
prednisolone sodium
  phosphate
prednisolone tebutate
prednisone
triamcinolone
triamcinolone acetonide
triamcinolone diacetate

### COMBINATION PRODUCTS
DECADRON PHOSPHATE WITH XYLOCAINE:
dexamethasone phosphate 4 mg and lidocaine hydrochloride 10 mg per ml.
PREDNISOLONE ACETATE AND PREDNISOLONE SODIUM PHOSPHATE: prednisolone acetate 80 mg/ml and prednisolone sodium phosphate 20 mg/ml.

**betamethasone**
Betnelan†, Celestone*

**betamethasone acetate and betamethasone sodium phosphate**
Celestone Chronodose‡,
Celestone Soluspan

**betamethasone sodium phosphate**
Betnesol§, Celestone Phosphate,
Selestoject

*Pregnancy Risk Category C*

### HOW SUPPLIED
**betamethasone**
*Tablets:* 600 mcg, 500 mcg
*Tablets (effervescent):* 500 mcg†
*Syrup:* 600 mcg/5 ml
**betamethasone acetate and betamethasone sodium phosphate**
*Injection (suspension):* betamethasone acetate 3 mg and betamethasone sodium phosphate (equivalent to 3-mg base) per ml
**betamethasone sodium phosphate**
*Injection:* 4 mg (equivalent to 3-mg base)/ml in 5-ml vials

### ACTION
Not completely defined. Decreases inflammation, mainly by stabilizing leukocyte lysosomal membranes; suppresses immune response; stimulates bone marrow; and influences protein, fat, and carbohydrate metabolism.

| Route | Onset | Peak | Duration |
|-------|-------|------|----------|
| P.O. | Rapid | Unknown | 3-25 days |
| I.M. | Unknown | Unknown | 7-14 days |

### INDICATIONS & DOSAGE
Betamethasone sodium phosphate and betamethasone acetate suspension combination product should *not* be used for I.V. administration.

Reactions may be *common*, uncommon, *life-threatening*, or COMMON AND LIFE-THREATENING.

*Conditions with severe inflammation, conditions requiring immunosuppression—*
**Adults:** 0.6 to 7.2 mg P.O. daily; or 0.5 to 9 mg I.M., or into joint or soft tissue daily. Betamethasone sodium phosphate-acetate suspension 1.5 to 12 mg injected into large joints or 1.5 to 6 mg injected into smaller joints. Both injections may be given q 1 to 2 weeks, p.r.n.

**Children:** not recommended for long-term use; especially likely to inhibit growth. 17.5 mcg/kg or 500 mcg/m$^2$ of body surface area; given in three divided doses q 3 days. Or, 5.8 to 8.75 mcg/kg or 166 to 250 mcg/m$^2$ of body surface area once daily.

## ADVERSE REACTIONS

**CNS:** *euphoria, insomnia,* psychotic behavior, pseudotumor cerebri, vertigo, headache, paresthesia, **seizures.**

**CV:** **heart failure,** hypertension, edema, **arrhythmias,** thrombophlebitis, **thromboembolism.**

**EENT:** cataracts, glaucoma.

**GI:** *peptic ulceration,* GI irritation, increased appetite, **pancreatitis**, nausea, vomiting.

**GU:** menstrual irregularities.

**Metabolic:** hypokalemia, hyperglycemia, and carbohydrate intolerance; increased serum cholesterol levels; decreased serum calcium levels.

**Musculoskeletal:** muscle weakness, osteoporosis; growth suppression in children.

**Skin:** hirsutism, delayed wound healing, acne, various skin eruptions.

**Other:** susceptibility to infections; *acute adrenal insufficiency after increased stress or abrupt withdrawal after long-term therapy,* cushingoid state (moonface, buffalo hump, central obesity).

**After abrupt withdrawal:** rebound inflammation, fatigue, weakness, arthralgia, fever, dizziness, lethargy, depression, fainting, orthostatic hypotension, dyspnea, anorexia, hypoglycemia. *After prolonged use, sudden withdrawal may be fatal.*

## INTERACTIONS

**Drug-drug.** *Antidiabetics, including insulin:* decreased response. May need dosage adjustment.

*Aspirin, indomethacin, other NSAIDs:* increased risk of GI distress and bleeding. Give together cautiously.

*Barbiturates, phenytoin, rifampin:* decreased corticosteroid effect. Corticosteroid dosage may need to be increased.

*Cardiac glycosides:* increased risk of arrhythmia resulting from hypokalemia. May need dosage adjustment.

*Oral anticoagulants:* altered dosage requirements. Monitor PT and INR closely.

*Potassium-depleting drugs such as thiazide diuretics:* enhanced potassium-wasting effects of betamethasone. Monitor serum potassium levels.

*Salicylates:* reduced serum salicylate levels with corticosteroids. Monitor for lack of salicylate effectiveness.

*Skin-test antigens:* decreased response. Defer skin testing until therapy is completed.

*Toxoids, vaccines:* decreased antibody response and increased risk of neurologic complications. Avoid concomitant use.

**Drug-lifestyle.** *Alcohol use:* increased risk of gastric irritation and GI ulceration. Advise patient to avoid alcohol use.

## EFFECTS ON DIAGNOSTIC TESTS

Adrenocorticoid therapy suppresses reactions to skin tests, causes false-negative results in the nitroblue tetrazolium tests for systemic bacterial infections, and decreases $^{131}$I uptake and protein-bound iodine levels in thyroid function tests.

## CONTRAINDICATIONS

Contraindicated in patients with hypersensitivity to drug and in those with viral or bacterial infections (except in life-threatening situations) or systemic fungal infections.

## NURSING CONSIDERATIONS

• Use with extreme caution in patient with recent MI or active peptic ulcer (use only in life-threatening situations).

• Use cautiously in patients with renal disease, hypertension, osteoporosis, diabetes mellitus, hypothyroidism, cirrhosis, diverticulitis, nonspecific ulcerative colitis, recent intestinal anastomoses, thromboembolic disorders, seizures, myasthenia gravis, heart failure, tuberculosis, ocular herpes simplex, emotional instability, and psychotic tendencies. Because some formulations contain sulfite preservatives, also use cautiously in patients with hypersensitivity to sulfites.

• Check for sensitivity to other corticosteroid drugs.

• *Alert:* Don't use drug for alternate-day therapy.

• *Alert:* Avoid using wrong salt formulation of drug; salt formulations aren't interchangeable.

• Obtain baseline weight before starting therapy, and weigh patient daily; report sudden weight gain to doctor.

• For better results and less toxicity, give once-daily dose in morning.

• Most adverse reactions to corticosteroids are dose- or duration-dependent.

• To reduce GI irritation, give with milk or food.

• To prevent muscle atrophy, give I.M. injection deeply. Rotate injection sites.

• Always adjust drug to lowest effective dose.

• Monitor blood glucose level and serum potassium levels regularly, as ordered. Diabetic patient may need adjustments in insulin dosage.

• Watch for depression or mood changes, especially in patient receiving long-term therapy.

• A calorie- or sodium-restricted diet with protein supplementation may be needed for patient receiving long-term therapy.

• Elderly patient may be more susceptible to osteoporosis with long-term use.

• Adrenal suppression may last up to 1 year after drug is stopped.

• Gradually reduce drug dosage after long-term therapy, as ordered.

• Observe for signs of infection, especially after corticosteroid withdrawal.

✔ **Patient teaching**

• Tell patient not to stop drug abruptly or without doctor's consent.

• Instruct patient to take drug with food or milk; tell patient using effervescent tablets to dissolve them in water immediately before ingestion.

• Teach patient about drug's effects. Warn patient on long-term therapy about cushingoid signs and symptoms (moon-face, buffalo hump) and to notify doctor of sudden weight gain or swelling.

• Instruct patient to report symptoms associated with corticosteroid withdrawal, including fatigue, weakness, arthralgia, orthostatic hypotension, and dyspnea.

• Tell patient to contact doctor if symptoms worsen or drug is no longer effective. Tell him not to increase dose without doctor's consent.

• Advise elderly patient receiving long-term therapy to consider exercise or physical therapy. Tell him to ask doctor about vitamin D or calcium supplement.

• Advise patient receiving prolonged therapy to have periodic ophthalmic examinations.

• Tell patient to report slow healing of wounds.

• Instruct patient to carry card indicating his need for supplemental glucocorticoids during stress. This card should contain doctor's name, name of drug, and dose being taken.

• Advise patient to avoid exposure to infections (such as chickenpox or measles) and to notify doctor if exposure occurs.

## cortisone acetate
Cortate‡, Cortisyl§, Cortone Acetate

*Pregnancy Risk Category C*

### HOW SUPPLIED
*Tablets:* 5 mg, 10 mg, 25 mg
*Injection (suspension):* 50 mg/ml

### ACTION
Not completely defined. Decreases inflammation, mainly by stabilizing leukocyte lysosomal membranes; suppresses immune response; stimulates bone marrow; and influences protein, fat, and carbohydrate metabolism.

| Route | Onset | Peak | Duration |
|---|---|---|---|
| P.O., I.M. | Variable | Variable | Variable |

## INDICATIONS & DOSAGE
*Adrenal insufficiency, allergy, inflammation—*
**Adults:** 25 to 300 mg P.O. or 20 to 300 mg I.M. daily. Dosages are highly individualized, depending on severity of disease.

## ADVERSE REACTIONS
**CNS:** *euphoria, insomnia,* psychotic behavior, pseudotumor cerebri, vertigo, headache, paresthesia, *seizures.*
**CV:** *heart failure,* hypertension, edema, *arrhythmias,* thrombophlebitis, *thromboembolism.*
**EENT:** cataracts, glaucoma.
**GI:** *peptic ulceration,* GI irritation, increased appetite, *pancreatitis,* nausea, vomiting.
**GU:** menstrual irregularities.
**Metabolic:** possible hypokalemia, hyperglycemia, and carbohydrate intolerance; increased serum cholesterol levels; decreased serum calcium, $T_3$, and $T_4$ levels; increased urine glucose and calcium levels.
**Musculoskeletal:** growth suppression in children, muscle weakness, osteoporosis.
**Skin:** hirsutism, delayed wound healing, acne, various skin eruptions; atrophy at I.M. injection site.
**Other:** susceptibility to infections; *acute adrenal insufficiency after increased stress or abrupt withdrawal after long-term therapy,* cushingoid state (moon-face, buffalo hump, central obesity).
**After abrupt withdrawal:** rebound inflammation, fatigue, weakness, arthralgia, fever, dizziness, lethargy, depression, fainting, orthostatic hypotension, dyspnea, anorexia, hypoglycemia. *After prolonged use, sudden withdrawal may be fatal.*

## INTERACTIONS
**Drug-drug.** *Antidiabetics, including insulin:* decreased response. May need dosage adjustment.
*Aspirin, indomethacin, other NSAIDs:* increased risk of GI distress and bleeding. Give together cautiously.
*Barbiturates, phenytoin, rifampin:* decreased corticosteroid effect. Increase corticosteroid dosage, as ordered.

*Live attenuated virus vaccines, other toxoids and vaccines:* decreased antibody response and increased risk of neurologic complications. Avoid concomitant use.
*Oral anticoagulants:* altered dosage requirements. Monitor PT and INR closely.
*Potassium-depleting drugs such as thiazide diuretics:* enhanced potassium-wasting effects of cortisone. Monitor serum potassium levels.
*Salicylates:* decreased serum salicylate levels with corticosteroids. Watch for lack of salicylate effectiveness.
*Skin-test antigens:* decreased response. Defer skin testing until therapy is completed.
**Drug-lifestyle.** *Alcohol use:* increased risk of gastric irritation and GI ulceration. Advise patient to avoid alcohol use.

## EFFECTS ON DIAGNOSTIC TESTS
Cortisone therapy suppresses reactions to skin tests, causes false-negative results in the nitroblue tetrazolium test for systemic bacterial infections, and decreases $^{131}$I uptake and protein-bound iodine levels in thyroid function tests.

## CONTRAINDICATIONS
Contraindicated in patients with hypersensitivity to drug or its ingredients and in those with systemic fungal infections.

## NURSING CONSIDERATIONS
• Use with extreme caution in patient with recent MI.
• Use cautiously in patients with GI ulcer, renal disease, hypertension, osteoporosis, diabetes mellitus, hypothyroidism, cirrhosis, diverticulitis, nonspecific ulcerative colitis, recent intestinal anastomoses, thromboembolic disorders, seizures, myasthenia gravis, heart failure, tuberculosis, ocular herpes simplex, emotional instability, or psychotic tendencies.
• Check for sensitivity to other corticosteroid drugs.
• Most adverse reactions to corticosteroids are dose- or duration-dependent.
• To reduce GI irritation, give with milk or food. Patient may need medication to prevent GI irritation.
• For better results and less toxicity, give a once-daily dose in morning.

• I.M. route causes slow onset of action and shouldn't be used in acute conditions in which rapid effect is needed. I.M. route may be used on a twice-daily schedule matching diurnal variation. Rotate injection sites to prevent muscle atrophy.

• Mixing or diluting parenteral suspension may alter absorption rate and decrease drug's effectiveness.

• *Alert:* Drug isn't for I.V. use.

• Drug should always be adjusted to lowest effective dose.

• Monitor serum electrolyte and blood glucose levels, as ordered. Diabetic patient may need adjustment in insulin dosage.

• Monitor patient for fluid and electrolyte imbalances. Patient may need low-sodium diet and potassium supplements.

• Elderly patient may be more susceptible to osteoporosis with long-term administration.

• Gradually reduce drug dosage after long-term therapy, as ordered.

• Observe for signs and symptoms of infection, especially after corticosteroid withdrawal.

☑ **Patient teaching**

• Tell patient not to discontinue drug abruptly or without doctor's consent.

• Instruct patient to take drug with milk or food.

• Advise patient receiving long-term therapy to consider exercise or physical therapy. Also tell him to ask doctor about vitamin D or calcium supplement.

• Tell patient to report slow healing of wounds.

• Warn patient on long-term therapy about cushingoid symptoms (moonface, buffalo hump) and to notify doctor of sudden weight gain or swelling.

• Instruct patient to carry card indicating his need for supplemental glucocorticoids during stress. This card should contain doctor's name, name of drug, and dose taken.

• Instruct patient to avoid exposure to infections (such as measles and chickenpox) and to notify doctor if such exposure occurs.

## dexamethasone
Decadron*, Deronil†, Dexasone†, Dexone 0.5, Dexone 0.75, Dexone 1.5, Dexone 4, Hexadrol*, Mymethasone*

## dexamethasone acetate
Cortastat L.A., Dalalone D.P., Dalalone L.A., Decadron-LA, Decaject-L.A., Dexacen LA-8, Dexasone-LA, Dexone LA, Solurex-LA

## dexamethasone sodium phosphate
Cortastat, Dalalone, Decadron Phosphate, Decaject, Dexacen-4, Dexacort Phosphate in Respihaler, Dexasone, Hexadrol Phosphate, Solurex

*Pregnancy Risk Category C*

## HOW SUPPLIED
**dexamethasone**
*Tablets:* 0.25 mg, 0.5 mg, 0.75 mg, 1 mg, 1.5 mg, 2 mg, 4 mg, 6 mg
*Oral solution:* 0.5 mg/5 ml, 1 mg/ml
*Elixir:* 0.5 mg/5 ml*
**dexamethasone acetate**
*Injection:* 8 mg/ml, 16 mg/ml suspension
**dexamethasone sodium phosphate**
*Injection:* 4 mg/ml, 10 mg/ml, 20 mg/ml, 24 mg/ml
*Oral inhalation aerosol:* 84 mcg/spray

## ACTION
Not clearly defined. Decreases inflammation, mainly by stabilizing leukocyte lysosomal membranes; suppresses immune response; stimulates bone marrow; and influences protein, fat, and carbohydrate metabolism.

| Route | Onset | Peak | Duration |
|---|---|---|---|
| P.O. | 1-2 hr | 1-2 hr | 2.5 days |
| P.O. inhalation | Unknown | Unknown | Unknown |
| I.V. | 1 hr | 1 hr | Variable |
| I.M. | 1 hr | 1 hr | 6 days |
| I.M. (acetate) | 1 hr | 8 hr | Unknown |

## INDICATIONS & DOSAGE

*Cerebral edema—*
**Adults:** initially, 10 mg (phosphate) I.V.; then 4 to 6 mg I.M. q 6 hours until symptoms subside (usually 2 to 4 days); then tapered over 5 to 7 days.

*Inflammatory conditions, allergic reactions; neoplasias—*
**Adults:** 0.75 to 9 mg/day P.O. or 0.5 to 9 mg/day (phosphate) I.M.; or 4 to 16 mg (acetate) I.M. into joint or soft tissue q 1 to 3 weeks; or 0.8 to 1.6 mg (acetate) into lesions q 1 to 3 weeks.

*Shock—*
**Adults:** 20 mg (phosphate) as single initial dose; then 3 mg/kg/24 hours via continuous I.V. infusion, or 1 to 6 mg/kg (phosphate) I.V. as single dose; or 40 mg I.V. q 2 to 6 hours, p.r.n.; continued only until patient is stabilized (usually not longer than 48 to 72 hours).

*Dexamethasone suppression test for Cushing's syndrome—*
**Adults:** after determining baseline 24-hour urine levels of 17-hydroxycorticosteroids, 0.5 mg P.O. q 6 hours for 48 hours; or 1 mg as single dose at 11:00 pm. Twenty-four-hour urine collection made again for determination of 17-hydroxycorticosteroid excretion during second 24 hours of dexamethasone administration.

*Adrenocortical insufficiency—*
**Children:** 23.3 mcg/kg daily in three divided doses.

*Bronchial asthma, bronchospasm—*
**Adults:** 3 sprays P.O. t.i.d. or q.i.d.
**Children:** 2 sprays t.i.d. or q.i.d.

## ADVERSE REACTIONS

**CNS:** *euphoria, insomnia,* psychotic behavior, pseudotumor cerebri, vertigo, headache, paresthesia, *seizures.*
**CV:** *heart failure,* hypertension, edema, *arrhythmias,* thrombophlebitis, *thromboembolism.*
**EENT:** cataracts, glaucoma.
**GI:** *peptic ulceration,* GI irritation, increased appetite, *pancreatitis,* nausea, vomiting.
**GU:** menstrual irregularities.
**Metabolic:** hypokalemia, hyperglycemia, and carbohydrate intolerance; increased serum cholesterol levels; decreased serum calcium, $T_3$, and $T_4$ levels; increased urine glucose and calcium levels.

**Musculoskeletal:** growth suppression in children, muscle weakness, osteoporosis.
**Skin:** hirsutism, delayed wound healing, acne, various skin eruptions; atrophy at I.M. injection site.
**Other:** cushingoid state (moonface, buffalo hump, central obesity), susceptibility to infections; *acute adrenal insufficiency after increased stress or abrupt withdrawal after long-term therapy.*
**After abrupt withdrawal:** rebound inflammation, fatigue, weakness, arthralgia, fever, dizziness, lethargy, depression, fainting, orthostatic hypotension, dyspnea, anorexia, hypoglycemia. *After prolonged use, sudden withdrawal may be fatal.*

## INTERACTIONS

**Drug-drug.** *Antidiabetics, including insulin:* decreased response. May need dosage adjustment.
*Aspirin, indomethacin, other NSAIDs:* increased risk of GI distress and bleeding. Give together cautiously.
*Barbiturates, phenytoin, rifampin:* decreased corticosteroid effect. Increase corticosteroid dosage, as ordered.
*Cardiac glycosides:* increased risk of arrhythmia resulting from hypokalemia. May warrant dosage adjustment.
*Oral anticoagulants:* altered dosage requirements. Monitor PT and INR closely.
*Potassium-depleting drugs such as thiazide diuretics:* enhanced potassium-wasting effects of dexamethasone. Monitor serum potassium levels.
*Salicylates:* decreased serum salicylate levels. Monitor for lack of salicylate effectiveness.
*Skin-test antigens:* decreased response. Defer skin testing until therapy is completed.
*Toxoids, vaccines:* decreased antibody response and increased risk of neurologic complications. Avoid concomitant use.
**Drug-lifestyle.** *Alcohol use:* increased risk of gastric irritation and GI ulceration. Advise patient to avoid alcohol use.

## EFFECTS ON DIAGNOSTIC TESTS

Drug suppresses reactions to skin tests, causes false-negative results in the nitroblue tetrazolium test for systemic bacterial infections, and decreases $^{131}$I uptake

---

*Liquid contains alcohol.  **May contain tartrazine.  †Canada  ‡Australia  §U.K.  ◊OTC

and protein-bound iodine levels in thyroid function tests.

## CONTRAINDICATIONS
Contraindicated in patients with hypersensitivity to drug or its ingredients and in those with systemic fungal infections.

## NURSING CONSIDERATIONS
• Use with extreme caution in patient with recent MI.
• Use cautiously in patients with GI ulcer, renal disease, hypertension, osteoporosis, diabetes mellitus, hypothyroidism, cirrhosis, diverticulitis, nonspecific ulcerative colitis, recent intestinal anastomoses, thromboembolic disorders, seizures, myasthenia gravis, heart failure, tuberculosis, ocular herpes simplex, emotional instability, or psychotic tendencies. Because some formulations contain sulfite preservatives, also use cautiously in patients sensitive to sulfites.
• Determine if patient is sensitive to other corticosteroid drugs.
• Most adverse reactions to corticosteroids are dose- or duration-dependent.
• For better results and less toxicity, give once-daily dose in morning.
• Give oral dose with food when possible. Patient may need medication to prevent GI irritation.
• Give I.M. injection deeply into gluteal muscle. Rotate injection sites to prevent muscle atrophy. Avoid S.C. injection because atrophy and sterile abscesses may occur.
• Always adjust to lowest effective dose, as ordered.
• Monitor patient's weight, blood pressure, and serum electrolyte levels.
• Watch for depression or psychotic episodes, especially in high-dose therapy.
• Diabetic patient may need increased insulin; monitor blood glucose levels.
• Drug may mask or exacerbate infections, including latent amebiasis.
• Elderly patient may be more susceptible to osteoporosis with long-term use.
• Inspect patient's skin for petechiae.
• Gradually reduce drug dosage after long-term therapy, as ordered.
• *Alert:* Don't confuse dexamethasone with desoximetasone.

## I.V. administration
• When administering as direct injection, inject undiluted over at least 1 minute. When administering as intermittent or continuous infusion, dilute solution according to manufacturer's instructions and give over prescribed duration. If used for continuous infusion, change solution every 24 hours.

## Patient teaching
• Tell patient not to discontinue drug abruptly or without doctor's consent.
• Instruct patient to take drug with food or milk.
• Teach patient symptoms of early adrenal insufficiency: fatigue, muscular weakness, joint pain, fever, anorexia, nausea, dyspnea, dizziness, and fainting.
• Instruct patient to carry card indicating his need for supplemental systemic glucocorticoids during stress, especially when dosage is decreased. This card should contain doctor's name, name of drug, and dose taken.
• Warn patient on long-term therapy about cushingoid symptoms (moonface, buffalo hump) and to notify doctor of sudden weight gain or swelling.
• Warn patient about easy bruising.
• Advise patient receiving long-term therapy to consider exercise or physical therapy. Give vitamin D or calcium supplement, as ordered.
• Instruct patient receiving long-term therapy to have periodic ophthalmic examinations.
• Advise patient to avoid exposure to infections (such as measles and chickenpox) and to notify doctor if such exposure occurs.

---

## fludrocortisone acetate
Florinef

*Pregnancy Risk Category C*

## HOW SUPPLIED
*Tablets:* 0.1 mg

## ACTION
Increases sodium reabsorption and potassium and hydrogen secretion

---

Reactions may be *common*, uncommon, *life-threatening*, or COMMON AND LIFE-THREATENING.

at the nephrons' distal convoluted tubules.

| Route | Onset | Peak | Duration |
|-------|-------|------|----------|
| P.O. | Variable | 2 hr | 1-2 days |

## INDICATIONS & DOSAGE
*Salt-losing adrenogenital syndrome—*
**Adults:** 0.1 to 0.2 mg P.O. daily.
*Addison's disease (adrenocortical insufficiency)—*
**Adults:** 0.1 mg P.O. daily. Usual dosage range is 0.1 mg three times weekly to 0.2 mg daily. Decrease dosage to 0.05 mg daily if transient hypertension develops as a result of drug therapy.

## ADVERSE REACTIONS
**CV:** hypertension, cardiac hypertrophy, edema, ***heart failure.***
**Metabolic:** *sodium and water retention,* hypokalemia.
**Skin:** bruising, diaphoresis, urticaria, allergic rash.

## INTERACTIONS
**Drug-drug.** *Barbiturates, phenytoin, rifampin:* increased clearance of fludrocortisone acetate. Monitor for possible diminished effect of corticosteroid. Corticosteroid dose may need to be increased.
*Potassium-depleting drugs such as thiazide diuretics:* enhanced potassium-wasting effects of fludrocortisone. Monitor serum potassium levels.
**Drug-food.** *Sodium-containing drugs or foods:* may increase blood pressure. Sodium intake may need adjustment.

## EFFECTS ON DIAGNOSTIC TESTS
Glucose tolerance tests should be performed only if needed because addisonian patients tend to develop severe hypoglycemia within 3 hours of the test.

## CONTRAINDICATIONS
Contraindicated in patients with hypersensitivity to drug and in those with systemic fungal infections.

## NURSING CONSIDERATIONS
• Use cautiously in patients with hypothyroidism, cirrhosis, ocular herpes simplex, emotional instability, psychotic tendencies, diverticulitis, fresh intestinal anastomoses, active or latent peptic ulcer, renal insufficiency, hypertension, osteoporosis, myasthenia gravis, or nonspecific ulcerative colitis.
• Drug is used with cortisone or hydrocortisone in adrenal insufficiency.
• *Alert:* Monitor patient's blood pressure and serum electrolyte levels. If hypertension occurs, notify doctor and expect dosage to be decreased by 50%.
• Weigh patient daily; notify doctor of sudden weight gain.
• Unless contraindicated, give low-sodium diet that's high in potassium and protein. Potassium supplements may be needed.

☑**Patient teaching**
• Tell patient to notify doctor if such symptoms as hypotension, weakness, cramping, and palpitations worsen.
• Warn patient that mild peripheral edema is common.

---

## hydrocortisone
Cortef, Cortenema, Hydrocortone

## hydrocortisone acetate
Cortifoam, Hydrocortone Acetate

## hydrocortisone cypionate
Cortef

## hydrocortisone sodium phosphate
Hydrocortone Phosphate

## hydrocortisone sodium succinate
A-hydroCort, Solu-Cortef

*Pregnancy Risk Category C*

## HOW SUPPLIED
**hydrocortisone**
*Tablets:* 5 mg, 10 mg, 20 mg
*Enema:* 100 mg/60 ml
**hydrocortisone acetate**
*Injection:* 25 mg/ml\*, 50 mg/ml\* suspension
*Enema:* 10% aerosol foam (provides 90 mg/application)

---

**hydrocortisone cypionate**
*Oral suspension:* 2 mg/ml
**hydrocortisone sodium phosphate**
*Injection:* 50 mg/ml solution
**hydrocortisone sodium succinate**
*Injection:* 100-mg vial*, 250-mg vial*,
500-mg vial*, 1,000-mg vial*

## ACTION
Not clearly defined. Decreases inflammation, mainly by stabilizing leukocyte lysosomal membranes; suppresses immune response; stimulates bone marrow; and influences protein, fat, and carbohydrate metabolism.

| Route | Onset | Peak | Duration |
|-------|-------|------|----------|
| P.O., I.V., I.M., P.R. | Variable | Variable | Variable |

## INDICATIONS & DOSAGE
*Severe inflammation, adrenal insufficiency—*
**Adults:** 5 to 30 mg P.O. b.i.d., t.i.d., or q.i.d. (as much as 80 mg q.i.d. may be given in acute situations); or initially, 100 to 500 mg succinate I.M. or I.V., then 50 to 100 mg I.M., as indicated; or 15 to 240 mg phosphate I.M. or I.V. daily in divided doses q 12 hours; or 5 to 75 mg acetate into joints or soft tissue repeated at 2- to 3-week intervals. Dosage varies with size of joint. Local anesthetics frequently are injected with dose.
*Shock—*
**Adults:** initially, 50 mg/kg succinate I.V., repeated in 4 hours. Repeat dosage q 24 hours, p.r.n.; or, 100 to 500 mg to 2 g q 2 to 6 hours, continued until patient is stabilized (usually not longer than 48 to 72 hours).
**Children:** phosphate (I.M.) or succinate (I.M. or I.V.) 0.186 to 0.28 mg/kg or 10 to 12 (base) mg/m² daily in three divided doses.
*Adjunct for ulcerative colitis and proctitis—*
**Adults:** 1 enema (100 mg) P.R. nightly for 21 days. Or, 1 applicator (90-mg foam) P.R. daily or b.i.d. for 14 to 21 days.

## ADVERSE REACTIONS
**CNS:** *euphoria, insomnia,* psychotic behavior, pseudotumor cerebri, vertigo, headache, paresthesia, *seizures.*

**CV:** *heart failure,* hypertension, edema, *arrhythmias,* thrombophlebitis, *thromboembolism.*
**EENT:** cataracts, glaucoma.
**GI:** *peptic ulceration,* GI irritation, increased appetite, *pancreatitis,* nausea, vomiting.
**GU:** menstrual irregularities.
**Metabolic:** hypokalemia, hyperglycemia, and carbohydrate intolerance; increased serum cholesterol levels; decreased serum calcium levels; increased urine calcium levels.
**Musculoskeletal:** growth suppression in children, muscle weakness, osteoporosis.
**Skin:** hirsutism, delayed wound healing, acne, various skin eruptions, easy bruising.
**Other:** cushingoid state (moonface, buffalo hump, central obesity); susceptibility to infections; *acute adrenal insufficiency after increased stress or abrupt withdrawal after long-term therapy.*
**After abrupt withdrawal:** rebound inflammation, fatigue, weakness, arthralgia, fever, dizziness, lethargy, depression, fainting, orthostatic hypotension, dyspnea, anorexia, hypoglycemia. *After prolonged use, sudden withdrawal may be fatal.*

## INTERACTIONS
**Drug-drug.** *Aspirin, indomethacin, other NSAIDs:* increased risk of GI distress and bleeding. Give together cautiously.
*Barbiturates, phenytoin, rifampin:* decreased corticosteroid effect. Increase corticosteroid dosage, as ordered.
*Live attenuated virus vaccines, other toxoids and vaccines:* decreased antibody response and increased risk of neurologic complications. Avoid concomitant use.
*Oral anticoagulants:* altered dosage requirements. Monitor PT and INR closely.
*Potassium-depleting drugs such as thiazide diuretics:* enhanced potassium-wasting effects of hydrocortisone. Monitor serum potassium levels.
*Skin-test antigens:* decreased response. Defer skin testing until after therapy.

## EFFECTS ON DIAGNOSTIC TESTS
Drug suppresses reactions to skin tests, causes false-negative results in the nitro-

---

*Reactions may be* common, *uncommon,* ***life-threatening,*** *or* COMMON AND LIFE-THREATENING.

blue tetrazolium test for systemic bacterial infections, and decreases $^{131}$I uptake and protein-bound iodine levels in thyroid function tests.

## CONTRAINDICATIONS
Contraindicated in patients with hypersensitivity to drug or its ingredients, in those with systemic fungal infections, and in premature infants (succinate).

## NURSING CONSIDERATIONS
• Use with extreme caution in patient with recent MI.
• Use cautiously in patients with GI ulcer, renal disease, hypertension, osteoporosis, diabetes mellitus, hypothyroidism, cirrhosis, diverticulitis, nonspecific ulcerative colitis, recent intestinal anastomoses, thromboembolic disorders, seizures, myasthenia gravis, heart failure, tuberculosis, ocular herpes simplex, emotional instability, and psychotic tendencies.
• Determine if patient is sensitive to other corticosteroid drugs.
• Most adverse reactions to corticosteroids are dose- or duration-dependent.
• For better results and less toxicity, give a once-daily dose in morning.
• Give oral dose with food when possible. Patient may need medication to prevent GI irritation.
• Different salt formulations aren't interchangeable.
• Give I.M. injection deeply into gluteal muscle. Rotate injection sites to prevent muscle atrophy. Avoid S.C. injection because atrophy and sterile abscesses may occur.
• Injectable forms aren't used for alternate-day therapy.
• Enema may produce same systemic effects as other forms of hydrocortisone. If enema therapy must exceed 21 days, discontinue gradually by reducing administration to every other night for 2 to 3 weeks, as ordered.
• High-dose therapy usually isn't continued beyond 48 hours.
• Always adjust to lowest effective dose, as ordered.
• Monitor patient's weight, blood pressure, and serum electrolyte levels.

• Unless contraindicated, give low-sodium diet that's high in potassium and protein. Administer potassium supplements, as ordered.
• Drug may mask or exacerbate infections, including latent amebiasis.
• Stress (fever, trauma, surgery, and emotional problems) may increase adrenal insufficiency. Increase dosage, as ordered.
• Watch for depression or psychotic episodes, especially during high-dose therapy.
• Inspect patient's skin for petechiae.
• Diabetic patient may need increased insulin; monitor blood glucose levels.
• Periodic measurement of growth and development may be needed during high-dose or prolonged therapy in children.
• Elderly patient may be more susceptible to osteoporosis with prolonged use.
• Gradually reduce drug dosage after long-term therapy, as ordered.
• *Alert:* Don't confuse Solu-Cortef with Solu-Medrol (methylprednisolone sodium succinate), or hydrocortisone with hydroxychloroquine.

## I.V. administration
• Don't use acetate or suspension form for I.V. use. When administering as direct injection, inject directly into vein or an I.V. line containing free-flowing compatible solution over 30 seconds to several minutes. When administering as intermittent or continuous infusion, dilute solution according to manufacturer's instructions, and give over prescribed duration. If used for continuous infusion, change solution every 24 hours.
• Hydrocortisone sodium phosphate may be added directly to $D_5W$ or normal saline for I.V. administration.
• Reconstitute hydrocortisone sodium succinate with bacteriostatic water or bacteriostatic NaCl solution before adding to I.V. solutions. When giving by direct I.V. injection, inject over period of 30 seconds to 10 minutes. For infusion, dilute with $D_5W$, normal saline, or dextrose 5% in normal saline to concentration of 1 mg/ml or less.

## Patient teaching
• Tell patient not to discontinue drug abruptly or without doctor's consent.

• Instruct patient to take oral form of drug with milk or food.
• Warn patient on long-term therapy about cushingoid symptoms (moonface, buffalo hump) and to notify doctor of sudden weight gain or swelling.
• Teach patient signs of early adrenal insufficiency: fatigue, muscular weakness, joint pain, fever, anorexia, nausea, dyspnea, dizziness, and fainting.
• Instruct patient to carry a card identifying his need for supplemental systemic glucocorticoids during stress. This card should contain doctor's name, name of drug, and dose taken.
• Warn patient about easy bruising.
• Advise patient receiving long-term therapy to consider exercise or physical therapy. Also tell him to ask doctor about vitamin D or calcium supplement.
• Advise patient receiving long-term therapy to have periodic ophthalmic examinations.
• Advise patient to avoid exposure to infections (such as chickenpox or measles) and to notify doctor if such exposure occurs.

## methylprednisolone
Medrol**, Medrone§

## methylprednisolone acetate
depMedalone 40, depMedalone 80, Depoject-40, Depoject-80, Depo-Medrol, Depo-Medrone§, Depopred-40, Depopred-80, Depo-Predate 40, Depo-Predate 80, Duralone-40, Duralone-80, Medralone-40, Medralone-80, Rep-Pred 40, Rep-Pred 80

## methylprednisolone sodium succinate
A-methaPred, Solu-Medrol

*Pregnancy Risk Category C*

## HOW SUPPLIED
**methylprednisolone**
*Tablets:* 2 mg, 4 mg, 8 mg, 16 mg, 24 mg, 32 mg

**methylprednisolone acetate**
*Injection (suspension):* 20 mg/ml, 40 mg/ml, 80 mg/ml
**methylprednisolone sodium succinate**
*Injection:* 40-mg vial, 125-mg vial, 500-mg vial, 1,000-mg vial, 2,000-mg vial

## ACTION
Not clearly defined. Decreases inflammation, mainly by stabilizing leukocyte lysosomal membranes; suppresses immune response; stimulates bone marrow; and influences protein, fat, and carbohydrate metabolism.

| Route | Onset | Peak | Duration |
|-------|-------|------|----------|
| P.O. | Rapid | 2-3 hr | 30-36 hr |
| I.V. | Rapid | Immediate | 7 days |
| I.M. | 6-48 hr | 4-8 days | 1-4 wk |
| Intra-articular | Rapid | 7 days | 1-5 wk |

## INDICATIONS & DOSAGE
*Severe inflammation or immunosuppression—*
**Adults:** 4 to 48 mg as single dose or in divided doses; 10 to 80 mg acetate I.M. daily, or 10 to 250 mg succinate I.M., 10 to 40 mg (base) repeated as needed or I.V. up to q 4 hours; or 4 to 40 mg acetate into smaller joints or 20 to 80 mg acetate into larger joints. Intralesional administration is usually 20 to 60 mg acetate. Intralesional and intra-articular injections may be repeated q 1 to 5 weeks.
**Children:** 0.03 to 0.2 mg/kg succinate or 1 to 6.25 mg/m$^2$ I.M. once daily or b.i.d.
*Shock—*
**Adults:** 100 to 250 mg succinate I.V. at 2- to 6-hour intervals; or 30 mg/kg I.V. initially, repeated q 4 to 6 hours, p.r.n. Continue therapy for 2 to 3 days or until patient is stable.

## ADVERSE REACTIONS
**CNS:** *euphoria, insomnia,* psychotic behavior, pseudotumor cerebri, vertigo, headache, paresthesia, *seizures.*
**CV:** *heart failure,* hypertension, edema, *arrhythmias,* thrombophlebitis, *thromboembolism, fatal arrest, circulatory collapse after rapid administration of large I.V. doses.*
**EENT:** cataracts, glaucoma.

---

Reactions may be *common*, uncommon, *life-threatening*, or COMMON AND LIFE-THREATENING.

**GI:** *peptic ulceration,* GI irritation, increased appetite, ***pancreatitis,*** nausea, vomiting.
**GU:** menstrual irregularities.
**Metabolic:** hypokalemia, hyperglycemia, and carbohydrate intolerance; increased serum cholesterol levels; decreased serum calcium levels; increased urine calcium levels.
**Musculoskeletal:** growth suppression in children, muscle weakness, osteoporosis.
**Skin:** hirsutism, delayed wound healing, acne, various skin eruptions.
**Other:** cushingoid state (moonface, buffalo hump, central obesity), susceptibility to infections, *acute adrenal insufficiency after increased stress or abrupt withdrawal after long-term therapy.*
**After abrupt withdrawal:** rebound inflammation, fatigue, weakness, arthralgia, fever, dizziness, lethargy, depression, fainting, orthostatic hypotension, dyspnea, anorexia, hypoglycemia. *After prolonged use, sudden withdrawal may be fatal.*

## INTERACTIONS
**Drug-drug.** *Aspirin, indomethacin, other NSAIDs:* increased risk of GI distress and bleeding. Give together cautiously.
*Barbiturates, phenytoin, rifampin:* decreased corticosteroid effect. Increase corticosteroid dosage, as ordered.
*Oral anticoagulants:* altered dosage requirements. Monitor PT and INR closely.
*Potassium-depleting drugs such as thiazide diuretics:* enhanced potassium-wasting effects of methylprednisolone. Monitor serum potassium levels.
*Salicylates:* decreased serum salicylate levels. Monitor for lack of salicylate effectiveness.
*Skin-test antigens:* decreased response. Defer skin testing until after therapy.
*Toxoids, vaccines:* decreased antibody response and increased risk of neurologic complications. Avoid concomitant use.

## EFFECTS ON DIAGNOSTIC TESTS
Methylprednisolone suppresses reactions to skin tests, causes false-negative results in the nitroblue tetrazolium test for systemic bacterial infections, and decreases $^{131}$I uptake and protein-bound iodine levels in thyroid function tests.

## CONTRAINDICATIONS
Contraindicated in patients with hypersensitivity to drug or its ingredients and in those with systemic fungal infections; also contraindicated in premature infants (acetate and succinate).

## NURSING CONSIDERATIONS
● Use cautiously in patients with GI ulceration or renal disease, hypertension, osteoporosis, diabetes mellitus, hypothyroidism, cirrhosis, diverticulitis, nonspecific ulcerative colitis, recent intestinal anastomoses, thromboembolic disorders, seizures, myasthenia gravis, heart failure, tuberculosis, ocular herpes simplex, emotional instability, and psychotic tendencies.
● Determine if patient is sensitive to other corticosteroids.
● Drug may be used for alternate-day therapy.
● Most adverse reactions to corticosteroids are dose- or duration-dependent.
● For better results and less toxicity, give a once-daily dose in the morning.
● Give oral dose with food when possible. Critically ill patients may need concomitant antacid or $H_2$-receptor antagonist therapy.
● Different salt formulations aren't interchangeable.
● *Alert:* Don't give Solu-Medrol intrathecally because severe adverse reactions have been reported.
● Give I.M. injection deeply into gluteal muscle. Avoid S.C. injection because atrophy and sterile abscesses may occur.
● Dermal atrophy may occur with large doses of acetate salt. Use multiple small injections rather than a single large dose and rotate injection sites.
● Don't use acetate when immediate onset of action is needed.
● Discard reconstituted solution after 48 hours.
● Always adjust to lowest effective dose, as ordered.
● Monitor patient's weight, blood pressure, serum electrolyte levels, and sleep patterns. Euphoria may initially interfere

with sleep, but patients generally adjust to therapy after 1 to 3 weeks.
• Drug may mask or exacerbate infections, including latent amebiasis.
• Watch for depression or psychotic episodes, especially in high-dose therapy.
• Diabetic patient may need increased insulin; monitor blood glucose levels.
• Watch for an enhanced response to drug in patients with hypothyroidism or cirrhosis.
• Watch for allergic reaction to tartrazine in patients with sensitivity to aspirin.
• Unless contraindicated, give low-sodium diet that's high in potassium and protein. Administer potassium supplements as needed.
• Elderly patient may be more susceptible to osteoporosis with prolonged use.
• Gradually reduce drug dosage after long-term therapy, as ordered.
• *Alert:* Don't confuse Solu-Medrol with Solu-Cortef (hydrocortisone sodium succinate) or methylprednisolone with medroxyprogesterone.

**◘ I.V. administration**
• Use only methylprednisolone sodium succinate for I.V. use; never use acetate form. Reconstitute according to manufacturer's directions using supplied diluent, or use bacteriostatic water for injection with benzyl alcohol.
• When administering as direct injection, inject diluted drug into vein or free-flowing compatible I.V. solution over at least 1 minute. For treatment of shock, give massive doses over at least 10 minutes to prevent arrhythmias and circulatory collapse. When administering as an intermittent or continuous infusion, dilute solution according to manufacturer's instructions, and give over prescribed duration. If used for continuous infusion, change solution every 24 hours.
• Compatible solutions include $D_5W$, normal saline, and dextrose 5% in normal saline.

**☑ Patient teaching**
• Tell patient not to discontinue drug abruptly or without doctor's consent.
• Instruct patient to take oral form of drug with milk or food.

• Teach patient symptoms of early adrenal insufficiency: fatigue, muscular weakness, joint pain, fever, anorexia, nausea, dyspnea, dizziness, and fainting.
• Instruct patient to carry a card identifying his need for supplemental systemic glucocorticoids during stress. This card should contain doctor's name, name of drug, and dose taken.
• Warn patient on long-term therapy about cushingoid symptoms (moonface, buffalo hump) and to notify doctor of sudden weight gain or swelling.
• Advise patient receiving long-term therapy to consider exercise or physical therapy. Also tell patient to ask doctor about vitamin D or calcium supplement.
• Instruct patient to avoid exposure to infections (such as chickenpox or measles) and to contact doctor if such exposure occurs.

---

## prednisolone
Delta-Cortef, Panafcortelone‡, Precortisyl Forte§, Predenema§, Prelone, Solone‡

## prednisolone acetate
Key-Pred, Predate, Predalone

## prednisolone sodium phosphate
Hydeltrasol, Key-Pred-SP, Pediapred, Predate S, Predicort-RP, Predsol Retention Enema‡, Predsol Suppositories‡

## prednisolone tebutate
Hydeltra-T.B.A., Nor-Pred T.B.A., Predalone T.B.A., Predate TBA, Predcor-TBA

*Pregnancy Risk Category C*

---

**HOW SUPPLIED**
**prednisolone**
*Tablets:* 1 mg‡, 5 mg, 25 mg‡
*Syrup:* 15 mg/5 ml
**prednisolone acetate**
*Injection (suspension):* 25 mg/ml, 50 mg/ml
**prednisolone sodium phosphate**
*Oral solution:* 5 mg/5 ml

---

*Injection:* 20 mg/ml
*Retention enema:* 20 mg/100 ml‡
*Suppositories:* 5 mg‡
**prednisolone tebutate**
*Injection (suspension):* 20 mg/ml

## ACTION
Not clearly defined. Decreases inflammation, mainly by stabilizing leukocyte lysosomal membranes; suppresses immune response; stimulates bone marrow; and influences protein, fat, and carbohydrate metabolism.

| Route | Peak | Onset | Duration |
|-------|------|-------|----------|
| P.O. | Rapid | 1-2 hr | 3-36 hr |
| I.V. | Rapid | 1 hr | Unknown |
| I.M. | Rapid | 1 hr | 4 wk |
| Intra-articular | 1-2 days | Unknown | < 4 wk |
| P.R. | Unknown | Unknown | Unknown |

## INDICATIONS & DOSAGE
*Severe inflammation, immunosuppression—*
**Adults:** 2.5 to 15 mg P.O. b.i.d., t.i.d., or q.i.d.; 2 to 30 mg I.M. (phosphate or acetate) or I.V. (phosphate) q 12 hours; or 2 to 30 mg (phosphate) into joints (depending on joint size), lesions, or soft tissue; or 4 to 40 mg (tebutate) into joints (depending on joint size) and lesions, p.r.n.
*Adrenocortical insufficiency—*
**Children:** 0.14 mg/kg or 4 mg/m² of body surface area daily in three divided doses.
*Proctitis‡—*
**Adults:** 1 suppository b.i.d., preferably in the morning and h.s.
*Ulcerative colitis‡—*
**Adults:** 1 retention enema h.s. nightly for 2 to 4 weeks. Contents of enema should be retained overnight.
*Acute exacerbations of multiple sclerosis—*
**Adults:** 200 mg/day as single or divided dose for 7 days; then 80 mg every other day for 1 month.

## ADVERSE REACTIONS
**CNS:** *euphoria, insomnia,* psychotic behavior, pseudotumor cerebri, vertigo, headache, paresthesia, *seizures.*

**CV:** *heart failure,* hypertension, edema, *arrhythmias,* thrombophlebitis, *thromboembolism.*
**EENT:** cataracts, glaucoma.
**GI:** *peptic ulceration,* GI irritation, increased appetite, *pancreatitis,* nausea, vomiting.
**GU:** menstrual irregularities.
**Metabolic:** hypokalemia, hyperglycemia, and carbohydrate intolerance; increased serum cholesterol levels; decreased serum potassium and calcium levels; increased urine calcium levels.
**Musculoskeletal:** growth suppression in children, muscle weakness, osteoporosis.
**Skin:** hirsutism, delayed wound healing, acne, various skin eruptions.
**Other:** susceptibility to infections, cushingoid state (moonface, buffalo hump, central obesity), *acute adrenal insufficiency after increased stress or abrupt withdrawal after long-term therapy.*
**After abrupt withdrawal:** rebound inflammation, fatigue, weakness, arthralgia, fever, dizziness, lethargy, depression, fainting, orthostatic hypotension, dyspnea, anorexia, hypoglycemia. *After prolonged use, sudden withdrawal may be fatal.*

## INTERACTIONS
**Drug-drug.** *Aspirin, indomethacin, other NSAIDs:* increased risk of GI distress and bleeding. Give together cautiously.
*Barbiturates, phenytoin, rifampin:* decreased corticosteroid effect. Increase corticosteroid dosage, as ordered.
*Oral anticoagulants:* altered dosage requirements. Monitor PT and INR closely.
*Potassium-depleting drugs such as thiazide diuretics:* enhanced potassium-wasting effects of prednisolone. Monitor serum potassium levels.
*Salicylates:* decreased serum salicylate levels. Monitor for lack of salicylate effectiveness.
*Skin-test antigens:* decreased response. Defer skin testing until therapy is completed.
*Toxoids, vaccines:* decreased antibody response and increased risk of neurologic complications. Avoid concomitant use.

---

*Liquid contains alcohol.    **May contain tartrazine.    †Canada    ‡Australia    §U.K.    ◇OTC

## EFFECTS ON DIAGNOSTIC TESTS

Drug suppresses reactions to skin tests, causes false-negative results in the nitro-blue tetrazolium test for systemic bacterial infections, and decreases $^{131}I$ uptake and protein-bound iodine levels in thyroid function tests.

## CONTRAINDICATIONS

Contraindicated in patients with hypersensitivity to drug or its ingredients and in those with systemic fungal infections.

## NURSING CONSIDERATIONS

• Use with extreme caution in patients with recent MI.
• Use cautiously in patients with GI ulcer, renal disease, hypertension, osteoporosis, diabetes mellitus, hypothyroidism, cirrhosis, diverticulitis, nonspecific ulcerative colitis, recent intestinal anastomoses, thromboembolic disorders, seizures, myasthenia gravis, heart failure, tuberculosis, ocular herpes simplex, emotional instability, and psychotic tendencies.
• Determine if patient is sensitive to other corticosteroids.
• Always adjust to lowest effective dose, as ordered.
• Prednisolone salts (sodium phosphate and tebutate) are used parenterally less often than other corticosteroids that have more potent anti-inflammatory action.
• Drug may be used for alternate-day therapy.
• Most adverse reactions to corticosteroids are dose- or duration-dependent.
• Give oral dose with food when possible to reduce GI irritation. Patient may need medication to prevent GI irritation.
• Give I.M. injection deeply into gluteal muscle. Rotate injection sites to prevent muscle atrophy. Avoid S.C. injection because atrophy and sterile abscesses may occur.
• Monitor patient's weight, blood pressure, and serum electrolyte levels.
• Watch for depression or psychotic episodes, especially in high-dose therapy.
• Diabetic patient may need increased insulin; monitor blood glucose levels.
• Unless contraindicated, give low-sodium diet that's high in potassium and protein.

Administer potassium supplements as needed.
• Drug may mask or exacerbate infections, including latent amebiasis.
• Elderly patient may be more susceptible to osteoporosis with long-term use.
• Gradually reduce drug dosage after long-term therapy, as ordered.
• *Alert:* Don't confuse prednisolone with prednisone.

### I.V. administration

• Use only prednisolone sodium phosphate. When administering as direct injection, inject undiluted over at least 1 minute. When administering as intermittent or continuous infusion, dilute solution according to manufacturer's instructions, and give over prescribed duration. $D_5W$ or normal saline is recommended diluent for I.V. infusion.

### Patient teaching

• Tell patient not to discontinue drug abruptly or without doctor's consent.
• Instruct patient to take oral form of drug with food or milk.
• Tell patient symptoms of early adrenal insufficiency: fatigue, muscular weakness, joint pain, fever, anorexia, nausea, dyspnea, dizziness, and fainting.
• Instruct patient to carry a card identifying his need for supplemental systemic glucocorticoids during stress. This card should contain doctor's name, name of drug, and dose taken.
• Warn patient on long-term therapy about cushingoid symptoms (moonface, buffalo hump) and to notify doctor of sudden weight gain or swelling.
• Tell patient to report slow healing.
• Advise patient receiving long-term therapy to consider exercise or physical therapy. Also tell him to ask doctor about vitamin D or calcium supplement.
• Instruct patient to avoid exposure to infections and to notify doctor if exposure occurs.
• Tell patient to avoid immunizations while taking drug.

---

Reactions may be *common*, uncommon, *life-threatening*, or COMMON AND LIFE-THREATENING.

## prednisone
Apo-Prednisone†, Deltasone,
Liquid Pred*, Meticorten, Orasone,
Panafcort‡, Prednicen-M,
Prednisone Intensol*, Sone‡,
Sterapred, Winpred†

*Pregnancy Risk Category C*

### HOW SUPPLIED
*Tablets:* 1 mg, 2.5 mg, 5 mg, 10 mg,
20 mg, 50 mg
*Tablets (film-coated):* 5 mg
*Oral solution:* 5 mg/5 ml*, 5 mg/ml (concentrate)*
*Syrup:* 5 mg/5 ml*

### ACTION
Not clearly defined. Decreases inflammation, mainly by stabilizing leukocyte lysosomal membranes; suppresses immune response; stimulates bone marrow; and influences protein, fat, and carbohydrate metabolism.

| Route | Onset | Peak | Duration |
|-------|-------|------|----------|
| P.O. | Variable | Variable | Variable |

### INDICATIONS & DOSAGE
*Severe inflammation, immunosuppression—*
**Adults:** 5 to 60 mg P.O. daily in single dose or as two to four divided doses. Maintenance dose given once daily or every other day. Dosage must be individualized.
**Children:** 0.14 to 2 mg/kg or 4 to 60 mg/m² daily P.O. in four divided doses.
*Acute exacerbations of multiple sclerosis—*
**Adults:** 200 mg P.O. daily for 7 days; then 80 mg P.O. every other day for 1 month.

### ADVERSE REACTIONS
**CNS:** *euphoria, insomnia,* psychotic behavior, pseudotumor cerebri, vertigo, headache, paresthesia, *seizures.*
**CV:** *heart failure,* hypertension, edema, *arrhythmias,* thrombophlebitis, *thromboembolism.*
**EENT:** cataracts, glaucoma.

**GI:** *peptic ulceration,* GI irritation, increased appetite, *pancreatitis,* nausea, vomiting.
**GU:** menstrual irregularities.
**Metabolic:** hypokalemia, hyperglycemia, and carbohydrate intolerance; increased serum cholesterol levels; decreased serum calcium levels; increased urine calcium levels.
**Musculoskeletal:** growth suppression in children, muscle weakness, osteoporosis.
**Skin:** hirsutism, delayed wound healing, acne, various skin eruptions.
**Other:** cushingoid state (moonface, buffalo hump, central obesity ), susceptibility to infections, *acute adrenal insufficiency after increased stress or abrupt withdrawal after long-term therapy.*
**After abrupt withdrawal:** rebound inflammation, fatigue, weakness, arthralgia, fever, dizziness, lethargy, depression, fainting, orthostatic hypotension, dyspnea, anorexia, hypoglycemia. *After prolonged use, sudden withdrawal may be fatal.*

### INTERACTIONS
**Drug-drug.** *Aspirin, indomethacin, other NSAIDs:* increased risk of GI distress and bleeding. Give together cautiously.
*Barbiturates, phenytoin, rifampin:* decreased corticosteroid effect. Increase corticosteroid dosage, as ordered.
*Oral anticoagulants:* altered dosage requirements. Monitor PT and INR closely.
*Potassium-depleting drugs such as thiazide diuretics:* enhanced potassium-wasting effects of prednisone. Monitor serum potassium levels.
*Salicylates:* decreased serum salicylate levels. Monitor for lack of salicylate effectiveness.
*Skin-test antigens:* decreased response. Defer skin testing until therapy is completed.
*Toxoids, vaccines:* decreased antibody response and increased risk of neurologic complications. Avoid concomitant use.

### EFFECTS ON DIAGNOSTIC TESTS
Drug suppresses reactions to skin tests, causes false-negative results in the nitro-blue tetrazolium test for systemic bacterial infections, and decreases ¹³¹I uptake

---

*Liquid contains alcohol.   **May contain tartrazine.   †Canada   ‡Australia   §U.K.   ◇OTC

and protein-bound iodine levels in thyroid function tests.

## CONTRAINDICATIONS

Contraindicated in patients with hypersensitivity to drug and in those with systemic fungal infections.

## NURSING CONSIDERATIONS

• Use cautiously in patients with GI ulcer, renal disease, hypertension, osteoporosis, diabetes mellitus, hypothyroidism, cirrhosis, diverticulitis, nonspecific ulcerative colitis, recent intestinal anastomoses, thromboembolic disorders, seizures, myasthenia gravis, heart failure, tuberculosis, ocular herpes simplex, emotional instability, and psychotic tendencies.
• Determine if patient is sensitive to other corticosteroids.
• Drug may be used for alternate-day therapy.
• Always adjust to lowest effective dose, as ordered.
• Most adverse reactions to corticosteroids are dose- or duration-dependent.
• For better results and less toxicity, give a once-daily dose in the morning.
• Unless contraindicated, give oral dose with food when possible to reduce GI irritation. Patient may need medication to prevent GI irritation.
• Monitor patient's blood pressure, sleep patterns, and serum potassium levels.
• Weigh patient daily; report sudden weight gain to doctor.
• Watch for depression or psychotic episodes, especially in high-dose therapy.
• Diabetic patient may need increased insulin; monitor blood glucose levels.
• Elderly patient may be more susceptible to osteoporosis with long-term use.
• Drug may mask or exacerbate infections, including latent amebiasis.
• Unless contraindicated, give low-sodium diet that's high in potassium and protein. Administer potassium supplements as needed.
• Gradually reduce drug dosage after long-term therapy, as ordered.
• *Alert:* Don't confuse prednisolone with primidone or prednimustine.

### ☑ Patient teaching

• Tell patient not to discontinue drug abruptly or without doctor's consent.
• Instruct patient to take drug with food or milk.
• Teach patient signs of early adrenal insufficiency: fatigue, muscular weakness, joint pain, fever, anorexia, nausea, dyspnea, dizziness, and fainting.
• Instruct patient to carry a card identifying his need for supplemental systemic glucocorticoids during stress. This card should contain doctor's name, name of drug, and dose taken.
• Warn patient on long-term therapy about cushingoid symptoms (moonface, buffalo hump) and to notify doctor of sudden weight gain or swelling.
• Advise patient receiving long-term therapy to consider exercise or physical therapy. Also tell patient to ask doctor about vitamin D or calcium supplement.
• Tell patient to report slow healing.
• Advise patient receiving long-term therapy to have periodic ophthalmic examinations.
• Instruct patient to avoid exposure to infections and to contact doctor if exposure occurs.

## triamcinolone
Adcortyl Intra-articular/
Intradermal§, Aristocort,
Aristo-Pak, Atolone, Kenacort**

## triamcinolone acetonide
Azmacort, Cenocort A-40,
Cinonide 40, Kenaject-40,
Kenalog-10, Kenalog-40, Tac-3,
Triam-A, Triamonide 40, Tri-Kort,
Trilog

## triamcinolone diacetate
Amcort, Aristocort Forte,
Aristocort Intralesional, Cinalone,
Triam-Forte, Tristoject

*Pregnancy Risk Category C*

## HOW SUPPLIED
**triamcinolone**
*Tablets:* 1 mg, 2 mg, 4 mg, 8 mg

---

Reactions may be *common*, uncommon, *life-threatening*, or COMMON AND LIFE-THREATENING.

**triamcinolone acetonide**
*Injection (suspension):* 3 mg/ml,
10 mg/ml, 40 mg/ml
*Metered spray:* 100 mcg/spray
**triamcinolone diacetate**
*Injectable suspension:* 25 mg/ml, 40
mg/ml

## ACTION
Not clearly defined. Decreases inflammation, mainly by stabilizing leukocyte lysosomal membranes; suppresses immune response; stimulates bone marrow; and influences protein, fat, and carbohydrate metabolism.

| Route | Onset | Peak | Duration |
|---|---|---|---|
| P.O., I.M., intralesion, intra-articular, inhalation | Variable | Variable | Variable |

## INDICATIONS & DOSAGE
*Severe inflammation, immunosuppression—*
**Adults:** 4 to 48 mg P.O. daily in single dose or divided doses; 40 to 80 mg I.M. (acetonide) at 4-week intervals; 1 mg (acetonide) into lesions; 2.5 to 15 mg (acetonide) into joints (depending on joint size) or soft tissue. A local anesthetic frequently is injected with triamcinolone into the joint.
*Adrenocortical insufficiency—*
**Children:** 0.117 mg/kg/day or
3.3 mg/m$^2$/day P.O. as one dose or in divided doses.
*Asthma—*
**Adults:** 2 inhalations t.i.d or q.i.d. Maximum dose is 16 inhalations daily.
**Children ages 6 to 12:** 1 to 2 inhalations t.i.d or q.i.d. Maximum dose is 12 inhalations daily.

## ADVERSE REACTIONS
**CNS:** *euphoria, insomnia,* psychotic behavior, pseudotumor cerebri, vertigo, headache, paresthesia, *seizures.*
**CV:** *heart failure,* hypertension, edema, *arrhythmias,* thrombophlebitis, *thromboembolism.*
**EENT:** cataracts, glaucoma.
**GI:** *peptic ulceration,* GI irritation, increased appetite, *pancreatitis,* nausea, vomiting.

**GU:** menstrual irregularities.
**Metabolic:** hypokalemia, hyperglycemia, and carbohydrate intolerance; increased serum cholesterol levels; decreased serum potassium and calcium levels; increased urine calcium levels.
**Musculoskeletal:** growth suppression (in children), muscle weakness, osteoporosis.
**Skin:** hirsutism, delayed wound healing, acne, various skin eruptions.
**Other:** cushingoid state (moonface, buffalo hump, central obesity), susceptibility to infections, *acute adrenal insufficiency after increased stress or abrupt withdrawal after long-term therapy.*
**After abrupt withdrawal:** rebound inflammation, fatigue, weakness, arthralgia, fever, dizziness, lethargy, depression, fainting, orthostatic hypotension, dyspnea, anorexia, hypoglycemia. *After prolonged use, sudden withdrawal may be fatal.*

## INTERACTIONS
**Drug-drug.** *Aspirin, indomethacin, other NSAIDs:* increased risk of GI distress and bleeding. Give together cautiously.
*Barbiturates, phenytoin, rifampin:* decreased corticosteroid effect. Increase corticosteroid dosage, as ordered.
*Oral anticoagulants:* altered dosage requirements. Monitor PT and INR closely.
*Potassium-depleting drugs such as thiazide diuretics:* enhanced potassium-wasting effects of triamcinolone. Monitor serum potassium levels.
*Salicylates:* decreased serum salicylate levels. Monitor for lack of salicylate effectiveness.
*Skin-test antigens:* decreased response. Defer skin testing until after therapy.
*Toxoids, vaccines:* decreased antibody response and increased risk of neurologic complications. Avoid concomitant use.

## EFFECTS ON DIAGNOSTIC TESTS
Drug suppresses reactions to skin tests, causes false-negative results in the nitro-blue tetrazolium test for systemic bacterial infections, and decreases $^{131}$I uptake and protein-bound iodine levels in thyroid function tests.

---

*Liquid contains alcohol.    **May contain tartrazine.    †Canada    ‡Australia    §U.K.    ◊OTC

## CONTRAINDICATIONS
Contraindicated in patients with hypersensitivity to drug or its ingredients and in those with systemic fungal infections.

## NURSING CONSIDERATIONS
- Use cautiously in patients with GI ulcer, renal disease, hypertension, osteoporosis, diabetes mellitus, hypothyroidism, cirrhosis, diverticulitis, nonspecific ulcerative colitis, recent intestinal anastomoses, thromboembolic disorders, seizures, myasthenia gravis, heart failure, tuberculosis, ocular herpes simplex, emotional instability, and psychotic tendencies.
- Determine if patient is sensitive to other corticosteroids.
- Drug isn't used for alternate-day therapy.
- Always adjust to lowest effective dose, as ordered.
- Most adverse reactions to corticosteroids are dose- or duration-dependent.
- For better results and less toxicity, give a once-daily oral dose in the morning with food.
- Parenteral form isn't for I.V. use. Different salt formulations aren't interchangeable.
- Don't use 40 mg/ml strength for intradermal or intralesion administration.
- Don't use 10 mg/ml strength for I.M. administration.
- Don't use diluents that contain preservatives; flocculation may occur.
- Give I.M. injection deeply into gluteal muscle. Rotate injection sites to prevent muscle atrophy.
- Monitor patient's weight, blood pressure, and serum electrolyte levels.
- Watch for allergic reaction to tartrazine in patients with sensitivity to aspirin.
- Watch for depression or psychotic episodes, especially in high-dose therapy.
- Diabetic patient may need increased insulin; monitor blood glucose levels.
- Drug may mask or exacerbate infections, including latent amebiasis.
- Elderly patient may be more susceptible to osteoporosis with long-term use.
- Unless contraindicated, give low-sodium diet that's high in potassium and protein. Administer potassium supplements as needed.

- Gradually reduce drug dosage after long-term therapy, as ordered. Drug may affect patient's sleep.
- *Alert:* Don't confuse triamcinolone with Triaminicin or Triaminicol.

### ☑ Patient teaching
- Tell patient not to discontinue drug abruptly or without doctor's consent.
- Instruct patient to take drug with food or milk.
- Teach patient symptoms of early adrenal insufficiency: fatigue, muscular weakness, joint pain, fever, anorexia, nausea, dyspnea, dizziness, and fainting.
- Instruct patient to carry a card identifying his need for supplemental systemic glucocorticoids during stress. This card should contain doctor's name, name of drug, and dose taken.
- Warn patient on long-term therapy about cushingoid symptoms (moonface, buffalo hump) and to notify doctor of sudden weight gain and swelling.
- Tell patient to report slow healing.
- Advise patient receiving long-term therapy to consider exercise or physical therapy. Also tell patient to ask doctor about vitamin D or calcium supplement.
- Instruct patient to avoid exposure to infections and to notify doctor if exposure occurs.

---

Reactions may be *common*, uncommon, *life-threatening*, or COMMON AND LIFE-THREATENING.

danazol
fluoxymesterone
methyltestosterone
nandrolone decanoate
nandrolone phenpropionate
testosterone
testosterone cypionate
testosterone enanthate
testosterone propionate
testosterone transdermal
    system

## COMBINATION PRODUCTS

ANDROGYN L.A., DELADUMONE,
VALERTEST NO. 1: testosterone enanthate
90 mg/ml and estradiol valerate 4 mg/ml
in sesame oil.
DEPANDROGYN, DEPO-TESTADIOL, DE-
POTESTOGEN, DUO-CYP, DURATESTRIN,
TEST-ESTRO CYPIONATE (oil): testosterone
cypionate 50 mg and estradiol cypionate
2 mg.
ESTRATEST: esterified estrogens 1.25 mg
and methyltestosterone 2.5 mg.
ESTRATEST H.S.: esterified estrogens
0.625 mg and methyltestosterone
1.25 mg.
HALODRIN: fluoxymesterone 1 mg with
ethinyl estradiol 0.02 mg.
PREMARIN WITH METHYLTESTOSTERONE:
conjugated estrogens 0.625 mg and
methyltestosterone 5 mg; or conjugated
estrogens 1.25 mg and methyltestosterone
10 mg.

---

danazol
Cyclomen†, Danocrine, Danol§

*Pregnancy Risk Category X*

## HOW SUPPLIED
*Capsules:* 50 mg, 100 mg, 200 mg

## ACTION
Binds to receptor sites of gonadal steroids
at target organs. Thus suppresses the
pituitary-ovarian axis and depresses output of follicle-stimulating and luteinizing
hormones.

| Route | Onset | Peak | Duration |
|-------|-------|------|----------|
| P.O. | 1 mo | 6-8 wk | Variable |

## INDICATIONS & DOSAGE
*Mild endometriosis—*
**Women:** initially, 100 to 200 mg P.O.
b.i.d. uninterrupted for 3 to 6 months;
may be continued for 9 months. Subsequent dosage based on patient response.
*Moderate to severe endometriosis—*
**Women:** 400 mg P.O. b.i.d. uninterrupted
for 3 to 6 months; may be continued for 9
months.
*Fibrocystic breast disease—*
**Women:** 100 to 400 mg P.O. daily in two
divided doses uninterrupted for 2 to 6
months.
*Prevention of hereditary angioedema—*
**Adults:** 200 mg P.O. b.i.d. to t.i.d., continued until favorable response is achieved.
Then dosage decreased by 50% at 1- to 3-
month intervals.

## ADVERSE REACTIONS
**CNS:** dizziness, headache, sleep disorders,
fatigue, tremor, irritability, excitation,
lethargy, mental depression, paresthesia.
**CV:** elevated blood pressure.
**EENT:** visual disturbances.
**GI:** gastric irritation, nausea, vomiting,
diarrhea, constipation, change in appetite.
**GU:** hematuria, hypoestrogenic effects
(flushing, diaphoresis, vaginitis [including
itching, dryness, burning], vaginal bleeding, nervousness, emotional lability, menstrual irregularities), testicular atrophy.
**Hepatic:** reversible jaundice, elevated liver enzyme levels, hepatic dysfunction.
**Musculoskeletal:** muscle cramps or
spasms.
**Other:** androgenic effects in women,
chills, *allergic reactions.*

## INTERACTIONS
**Drug-drug.** *Carbamazepine:* may increase
carbamazepine levels. Monitor closely.

---

*Liquid contains alcohol.     **May contain tartrazine.     †Canada     ‡Australia     §U.K.     ◇OTC

*Cyclosporine:* can increase cyclosporine levels and increase chance of nephrotoxicity. Monitor patient closely.
*Warfarin:* may prolong PT in patients stabilized on warfarin. Monitor PT and INR.

**EFFECTS ON DIAGNOSTIC TESTS**
None reported.

**CONTRAINDICATIONS**
Contraindicated in patients with undiagnosed abnormal genital bleeding, porphyria, or impaired renal, cardiac, or hepatic function; also contraindicated in pregnant and breast-feeding women.

**NURSING CONSIDERATIONS**
• Therapy should begin during menstruation.
• Use cautiously in patients with seizure disorders or migraine.
• *Alert:* Don't use in women of childbearing age until pregnancy is ruled out.
• Unless contraindicated, use with diet high in calories and protein.
• Watch closely for signs and symptoms of virilization. Some androgenic effects, such as deepening of voice, may not be reversible upon discontinuation of drug. Other androgenic effects include weight gain, hirsutism, hoarseness, clitoral enlargement, decreased breast size, acne, edema, changes in libido, and oily skin or hair.
• Periodically evaluate hepatic function, as ordered. Semen evaluation is routinely performed every 3 to 4 months, especially in adolescent boys.
• When stopping drug, periodic dosage decreases or gradual withdrawal is best.
• After withdrawal of treatment, ovulation and cyclic menstrual bleeding usually return in 2 to 3 months; fibrocystic disease symptoms return within 1 year for 50% of patients.
• Patient with diabetes may need increased dosages of insulin.
• Watch for symptoms of pseudotumor cerebri: headache, nausea, vomiting, and visual disturbances. Drug may need to be discontinued.

✓ **Patient teaching**
• Advise patient taking drug for fibrocystic breast disease to examine breasts regularly and to notify doctor immediately if breast nodules enlarge.
• Make sure patient understands importance of using an effective nonhormonal contraceptive during therapy.
• Instruct patient to report adverse reactions, especially signs of virilization, promptly.
• Advise woman to wash after intercourse to decrease risk of vaginitis. Instruct her to wear only cotton underwear.

---

**fluoxymesterone**
Android-F, Halotestin**

*Controlled Substance Schedule III*
*Pregnancy Risk Category X*

**HOW SUPPLIED**
*Tablets:* 2 mg, 5 mg, 10 mg

**ACTION**
Stimulates target tissues to develop normally in androgen-deficient men.

| Route | Onset | Peak | Duration |
|-------|-------|------|----------|
| P.O. | Unknown | Unknown | 9 hr |

**INDICATIONS & DOSAGE**
*Hypogonadism due to testicular deficiency—*
**Adults:** 5 to 20 mg P.O. daily.
*Delayed puberty—*
**Adolescent:** highly individualized; usually 2.5 to 10 mg daily for 4 to 6 months.
*Palliation of breast cancer in women—*
**Adults:** 10 to 40 mg P.O. daily in divided doses. All dosages are individualized and reduced to minimum when effect is noted.

**ADVERSE REACTIONS**
**CNS:** headache, anxiety, depression, paresthesia, sleep apnea syndrome.
**CV:** edema.
**GI:** nausea.
**GU:** *hypoestrogenic effects in women;* excessive hormonal effects in men (prepubertal—*premature epiphyseal closure,* acne, priapism, *growth of body and facial hair,* phallic enlargement; postpubertal—testicular atrophy, oligospermia, decreased ejaculatory volume, impotence, gynecomastia, epididymitis).

---

**Hematologic:** polycythemia, suppression of clotting factors.
**Hepatic:** reversible jaundice, *peliosis hepatitis,* elevated liver enzyme levels, *liver cell tumors.*
**Metabolic:** elevated serum lipid levels, hypercalcemia.
**Skin:** *hypersensitivity reactions.*
**Other:** androgenic effects in women.

## INTERACTIONS
**Drug-drug.** *Hepatotoxic drugs:* increased risk of hepatotoxicity. Monitor closely.
*Insulin, oral antidiabetics:* altered dosage requirements. Monitor blood glucose levels in diabetic patients.
*Oral anticoagulants:* increased sensitivity to oral anticoagulants; altered dosage requirements. Monitor INR.

## EFFECTS ON DIAGNOSTIC TESTS
Drug may cause abnormal results of the glucose tolerance test. Thyroid function test results (protein-bound iodine, radioactive iodine uptake, thyroid-binding capacity) may decrease.

## CONTRAINDICATIONS
Contraindicated in patients with hypersensitivity to drug; in males with breast cancer or known or suspected prostate cancer; in those with cardiac, hepatic, or renal decompensation; and in pregnant or breast-feeding women.

## NURSING CONSIDERATIONS
• Use cautiously in prepubertal boys or patients with BPH or aspirin sensitivity.
• *Alert:* Don't use in women of childbearing age until pregnancy is ruled out.
• Monitor INR in patients on oral anticoagulant therapy because dosage may need adjustment.
• Unless contraindicated, use with diet high in calories and protein. Give small, frequent feedings.
• Watch for signs and symptoms of jaundice and periodically evaluate hepatic function, as ordered. Dosage adjustment may reverse condition. If liver function test results are abnormal, notify doctor because therapy should be stopped.

• Edema can be controlled with sodium restriction or diuretics. Monitor weight routinely.
• Monitor men for signs and symptoms of excessive sexual stimulation or priapism.
• Semen evaluation is routinely performed every 3 to 4 months, especially in adolescent boys.
• *Alert:* Hypercalcemia symptoms may be difficult to distinguish from symptoms associated with condition being treated, unless anticipated and thought of as a symptom cluster. Hypercalcemia is particularly likely to occur in immobilized patients or in women with metastatic breast cancer, and may indicate bone metastases.
• *Alert:* Don't use drug for enhancement of athletic performance or physique.
• Watch for signs and symptoms of hypoglycemia in diabetic patients. Check blood glucose levels. Dosage of antidiabetic may need adjustment.
• When used in breast cancer, subjective effects may not occur for about 1 month; objective effects on clinical symptoms may take 3 months.
• Hypoestrogenic effects in women include flushing; diaphoresis; vaginitis, including itching, dryness, and burning; vaginal bleeding; nervousness; emotional lability, and menstrual irregularities.

☑ **Patient teaching**
• If GI upset occurs, tell patient to take drug with food or meals.
• Make sure patient understands importance of using an effective nonhormonal contraceptive during therapy.
• Advise woman to wash after intercourse to decrease risk of vaginitis. Instruct her to wear only cotton underwear.
• Tell woman to report menstrual irregularities and to discontinue therapy pending etiologic determination.
• Explain to patient taking drug for palliation of breast cancer that virilization usually occurs. Give emotional support. Tell patient to immediately report androgenic effects (acne, edema, weight gain, hirsutism, hoarseness, clitoral enlargement, deepening voice, decreased breast size, changes in libido, male-pattern baldness, and oily skin or hair).

• Tell patient that stopping drug will prevent further androgenic changes but probably won't reverse existing effects.
• Warn patient with diabetes to be alert for signs and symptoms of hypoglycemia, and to notify doctor if these occur.
• Tell patient to report sudden weight gain.

## methyltestosterone
Android, Metandren†**, Oreton Methyl, Testred, Virilon

*Controlled Substance Schedule III*
*Pregnancy Risk Category X*

### HOW SUPPLIED
*Tablets:* 10 mg, 25 mg
*Tablets (buccal):* 10 mg
*Capsules:* 10 mg

### ACTION
Stimulates target tissues to develop normally in androgen-deficient men.

| Route | Onset | Peak | Duration |
|-------|-------|------|----------|
| P.O. | Unknown | 2 hr | Unknown |
| Buccal | Unknown | 1 hr | Unknown |

### INDICATIONS & DOSAGE
*Breast cancer in women 1 to 5 years postmenopausal—*
**Women:** 50 to 200 mg P.O. daily; or 25 to 100 mg buccally daily.
*Male hypogonadism—*
**Adults:** 10 to 50 mg P.O. daily; or 5 to 25 mg buccally daily.
*Postpubertal cryptorchidism—*
**Adults:** 30 mg P.O. daily; or 15 mg buccally daily.
*Prevention of postpartum breast engorgement—*
**Women:** 80 mg daily in divided doses for 3 to 5 days.

### ADVERSE REACTIONS
**CNS:** headache, anxiety, depression, paresthesia.
**CV:** edema.
**GI:** irritation of oral mucosa with buccal administration, nausea.
**GU:** *hypoestrogenic effects in women (flushing; diaphoresis; vaginitis, including itching, dryness, and burning; vaginal* bleeding; nervousness; emotional lability; menstrual irregularities); excessive hormonal effects in men (prepubertal—*premature epiphyseal closure, acne,* priapism, *growth of body and facial hair,* phallic enlargement; postpubertal—testicular atrophy, oligospermia, decreased ejaculatory volume, impotence, gynecomastia, epididymitis).
**Hematologic:** suppression of clotting factors, polycythemia.
**Hepatic:** reversible jaundice, cholestatic hepatitis, abnormal liver enzyme levels.
**Metabolic:** increased serum sodium, potassium, calcium, phosphate, and cholesterol levels; hypercalcemia.
**Musculoskeletal:** muscle cramps or spasms.
**Skin:** hypersensitivity reactions.
**Other:** androgenic effects in women.

### INTERACTIONS
**Drug-drug.** *Hepatotoxic drugs:* increased risk of hepatotoxicity. Monitor closely.
*Insulin, oral antidiabetics:* decreased serum glucose may alter dosage requirements. Monitor blood glucose levels in diabetic patients.
*Oral anticoagulants:* increased sensitivity to oral anticoagulants may alter dosage requirements. Monitor PT and INR.

### EFFECTS ON DIAGNOSTIC TESTS
Drug may cause abnormal results of the glucose tolerance test.

### CONTRAINDICATIONS
Contraindicated in pregnant or breastfeeding women and in men with breast cancer or known or suspected prostate cancer.

### NURSING CONSIDERATIONS
• Use cautiously in elderly patients; patients with cardiac, renal, or hepatic disease; or healthy men with delayed puberty.
• Don't use in women of childbearing age until pregnancy is ruled out.
• In children, X-rays of the wrist bones should be taken before therapy begins to establish level of bone maturation. During treatment, bone maturation may proceed more rapidly than linear growth. Periodically review X-ray results to monitor bone maturation.

---

Reactions may be *common,* uncommon, *life-threatening,* or COMMON AND LIFE-THREATENING.

• Drug is typically used only for intermittent therapy. Because of potential hepatotoxicity, watch closely for jaundice.
• Promptly report signs and symptoms of virilization in women.
• Unless contraindicated, use with diet high in calories and protein. Give small, frequent feedings.
• Periodically check hemoglobin level and hematocrit, serum cholesterol and calcium levels, and cardiac and liver function test results, as ordered.
• Check weight regularly. Edema can be controlled with sodium restriction or diuretics.
• *Alert:* Therapeutic response in breast cancer is usually apparent within 3 months. Therapy should be stopped if signs of disease progression appear.
• Report signs of hypercalcemia. In metastatic breast cancer, hypercalcemia may indicate progression of bone metastases.
• Semen evaluation is routinely performed every 3 to 4 months, especially in adolescent boys.
• *Alert:* Drug shouldn't be used for enhancement of athletic performance or physique.
• *Alert:* Testosterone and methyltestosterone aren't interchangeable. Don't confuse methyltestosterone with medroxyprogesterone.

☑ **Patient teaching**
• Make sure patient understands importance of using an effective nonhormonal contraceptive during therapy.
• Buccal tablets are twice as potent as oral tablets. Tell patient to avoid eating, drinking, chewing, or smoking while buccal tablet is in place and not to swallow tablet. Place in upper or lower buccal pouch between cheek and gum; tablet needs 30 to 60 minutes to dissolve.
• Instruct patient to change tablet absorption site with each dose to minimize risk of buccal irritation. Advise patient to rinse mouth after using buccal tablet.
• Tell patient to immediately report signs and symptoms of virilization (acne, edema, weight gain, hirsutism, hoarseness, clitoral enlargement, decreased breast size, deepening voice, changes in libido,

male-pattern baldness, and oily skin or hair).
• Teach patient signs of hypoglycemia and method for checking blood glucose level; drug enhances hypoglycemia. Instruct patient to report hypoglycemia immediately.
• Advise woman to wash after intercourse to decrease risk of vaginitis. Instruct her to wear only cotton underwear.

---

## nandrolone decanoate
Androlone-D, Deca-Durabolin, Hybolin Decanoate, Kabolin, Neo-Durabolic

## nandrolone phenpropionate
Durabolin, Hybolin Improved

*Controlled Substance Schedule III*
*Pregnancy Risk Category X*

---

### HOW SUPPLIED
**nandrolone decanoate**
*Injection (in oil):* 50 mg/ml, 100 mg/ml, 200 mg/ml
**nandrolone phenpropionate**
*Injection (in oil):* 25 mg/ml, 50 mg/ml

### ACTION
An anabolic steroid that promotes tissue-building processes, reverses catabolism, and stimulates erythropoiesis.

| Route | Onset | Peak | Duration |
|---|---|---|---|
| I.M. (decanoate) | Unknown | 3-6 days | Unknown |
| I.M. (phenpropionate) | Unknown | 1-2 days | Unknown |

### INDICATIONS & DOSAGE
*Severe debility or disease states, refractory anemias—*
**Adults:** 50 to 100 mg decanoate I.M. at 1- to 4-week intervals for females; 50 to 200 mg decanoate I.M. at 1- to 4-week intervals for men. Therapy should be intermittent and discontinued if no improvement in 6 months.
**Children ages 2 to 13:** 25 to 50 mg decanoate I.M. q 3 to 4 weeks.
*Control of metastatic breast cancer—*
**Adults:** 25 to 100 mg phenpropionate I.M. weekly.

---

## ADVERSE REACTIONS

**CNS:** excitation, insomnia, habituation, depression.
**CV:** edema.
**GI:** nausea, vomiting, diarrhea.
**GU:** bladder irritability, *hypoestrogenic effects in women (flushing; diaphoresis; vaginitis, including itching, dryness, and burning; vaginal bleeding; nervousness; emotional lability; menstrual irregularities),* excessive hormonal effects in men (prepubertal—*premature epiphyseal closure, acne,* priapism, *growth of body and facial hair;* phallic enlargement; postpubertal—testicular atrophy, oligospermia, decreased ejaculatory volume, impotence, gynecomastia, epididymitis), increased serum-creatinine level.
**Hematologic:** elevated serum lipid levels, suppression of clotting factors.
**Hepatic:** reversible jaundice, *peliosis hepatitis,* elevated liver enzyme levels, *liver cell tumors.*
**Metabolic:** increased serum sodium, potassium, calcium, phosphate, and cholesterol levels.
**Skin:** pain, induration at injection site.
**Other:** androgenic effects in women.

## INTERACTIONS

**Drug-drug.** *Hepatotoxic drugs:* increased risk of hepatotoxicity. Monitor closely.
*Insulin, oral antidiabetics:* altered dosage requirements. Monitor blood glucose levels in diabetic patients.
*Oral anticoagulants:* altered dosage requirements. Monitor PT and INR.

## EFFECTS ON DIAGNOSTIC TESTS

Drug may cause abnormal results of fasting plasma glucose, glucose tolerance, and metyrapone tests.

## CONTRAINDICATIONS

Contraindicated in patients with hypersensitivity to anabolic steroids, in those with nephrosis or experiencing the nephrotic phase of nephritis, in men with breast cancer or known or suspected prostate cancer, in women with breast cancer and hypercalcemia, and in pregnant or breast-feeding women.

## NURSING CONSIDERATIONS

• Use cautiously in patients with diabetes; cardiac, renal, or hepatic disease; epilepsy; or migraine or other conditions that may be aggravated by fluid retention.
• Don't use in women of childbearing age until pregnancy is ruled out.
• In children, X-rays of the wrist bones should be taken before surgery to establish level of bone maturation. During treatment, bone maturation may proceed more rapidly than linear growth; periodically review X-ray results to monitor bone maturation.
• Inject I.M. drug deeply, preferably into upper outer quadrant of gluteal muscle in adults. Rotate injection sites to prevent muscle atrophy.
• Unless contraindicated, use with diet high in calories and protein. Give small, frequent feedings.
• Watch for signs of virilization, which may be irreversible despite prompt discontinuation of therapy. Androgenic effects in women include acne, edema, weight gain, hirsutism, hoarseness, clitoral enlargement, decreased breast size, changes in libido, male-pattern baldness, and oily skin or hair.
• Closely observe boys under age 7 for precocious development of male sexual characteristics.
• Semen evaluation is routinely performed every 3 or 4 months, especially in adolescent boys.
• *Alert:* Periodically evaluate hepatic function, as ordered. Watch for jaundice; dosage adjustment may reverse condition. If liver function test results are abnormal, therapy should be stopped.
• Check weight regularly. Edema generally can be controlled with sodium restrictions or diuretics.
• Watch for signs and symptoms of hypoglycemia in diabetic patients. Check blood glucose levels. Adjust dosage of antidiabetic, as ordered.
• Check quantitative urine and serum calcium levels. Hypercalcemia is most likely to occur in patients with breast cancer.
• When used to promote erythropoiesis in patient with refractory anemias, make sure he has adequate daily iron intake.

---

Reactions may be *common,* uncommon, *life-threatening,* or COMMON AND LIFE-THREATENING.

• Anabolic steroids may alter results of laboratory studies performed during therapy and for 2 to 3 weeks after therapy ends.

### ✓ Patient teaching
• Make sure patient understands importance of using an effective nonhormonal contraceptive during therapy.
• Review signs and symptoms of virilization with woman, and instruct her to notify doctor immediately if they occur.
• Advise woman to wash after intercourse to decrease risk of vaginitis. Instruct her to wear only cotton underwear.
• Warn diabetic patient to be alert for signs and symptoms of hypoglycemia, and tell him to notify doctor if they occur.
• Tell patient to report sudden weight gain to doctor.
• Tell woman to report menstrual irregularities and to discontinue therapy pending etiologic determination.

---

### testosterone
Andro 100, Histerone-50, Histerone 100, Testamone 100, Testaqua, Testoject-50, Testopel Pellets

### testosterone cypionate
Andronate 100, Andronate 200, depAndro 100, depAndro 200, Depotest, Depo-Testadiol, Depo-Testosterone, Duratest-100, Duratest-200, T-Cypionate, T-E Cypionate, Testred Cypionate 200, Virilon IM

### testosterone enanthate
Andro-LA, Delatest, Delatestryl, Everone 200

### testosterone propionate
Malogen†, Testex, Virormone§

*Controlled Substance Schedule III*
*Pregnancy Risk Category X*

### HOW SUPPLIED
**testosterone**
*Injection (aqueous suspension):*
25 mg/ml, 50 mg/ml, 100 mg/ml

*Pellets (S.C. implant):* 75 mg
**testosterone cypionate**
*Injection (in oil):* 100 mg/ml, 200 mg/ml
**testosterone enanthate**
*Injection (in oil):* 100 mg/ml, 200 mg/ml
**testosterone propionate**
*Injection (in oil):* 50 mg/ml, 100 mg/ml

### ACTION
Stimulates target tissues to develop normally in androgen-deficient men. Testosterone may have some antiestrogen properties, making it useful in treating certain estrogen-dependent breast cancers. Its action in postpartum breast engorgement isn't known because testosterone doesn't suppress lactation.

| Route | Onset | Peak | Duration |
|-------|-------|------|----------|
| I.M. | Unknown | 10-100 min | Unknown |

### INDICATIONS & DOSAGE
*Male hypogonadism—*
**Adult men:** 10 to 25 mg (testosterone) I.M. two to three times weekly; or 50 to 400 mg (cypionate or enanthate) I.M. q 2 to 4 weeks.
*Metastatic breast cancer in women 1 to 5 years postmenopausal—*
**Women:** 50 to 100 mg I.M. three times weekly; or 200 to 400 mg (enanthate) I.M. q 2 to 4 weeks.
*Postpartum breast pain and engorgement—*
**Women:** 25 to 50 mg I.M. of testosterone or testosterone propionate daily for 3 to 4 days.

### ADVERSE REACTIONS
**CNS:** headache, anxiety, depression, paresthesia, sleep apnea syndrome.
**CV:** edema.
**GI:** nausea.
**GU:** hypoestrogenic effects in women (flushing; diaphoresis; vaginitis, including itching, drying, and burning; vaginal bleeding; menstrual irregularities), excessive hormonal effects in men (prepubertal—premature epiphyseal closure, *acne,* priapism, *growth of body and facial hair,* phallic enlargement; postpubertal—testicular atrophy, oligospermia, decreased ejaculatory volume, impotence, gynecomastia, epididymitis), elevated creatinine levels.

**Hematologic:** polycythemia, suppression of clotting factors.
**Hepatic:** reversible jaundice, cholestatic hepatitis, abnormal liver enzyme levels.
**Metabolic:** increased serum sodium, potassium, calcium, phosphate, and cholesterol levels.
**Skin:** pain, induration at injection site; local edema; hypersensitivity reactions.
**Other:** androgenic effects in women.

## INTERACTIONS
**Drug-drug.** *Hepatotoxic drugs:* increased risk of hepatotoxicity. Monitor closely.
*Insulin, oral antidiabetics:* decreased serum glucose levels may alter dosage requirements. Monitor blood glucose levels in diabetic patients.
*Oral anticoagulants:* increased sensitivity may alter dosage requirements. Monitor PT and INR.

## EFFECTS ON DIAGNOSTIC TESTS
Testosterone may cause abnormal glucose tolerance test results.

## CONTRAINDICATIONS
Contraindicated in patients with hypersensitivity to drug and in those with hypercalcemia or cardiac, hepatic, or renal decompensation; also contraindicated in men with breast or known or suspected prostate cancer and in pregnant or breast-feeding women.

## NURSING CONSIDERATIONS
• Use cautiously in elderly patients.
• Don't use in women of childbearing age until pregnancy is ruled out.
• Store I.M. preparations at room temperature. If crystals appear, warm and shake bottle to disperse them.
• Inject deep into upper outer quadrant of gluteal muscle. Rotate injection sites. Report soreness at site.
• Unless contraindicated, administer with diet high in calories and protein. Provide small, frequent feedings to help avoid nausea.
• Monitor patient's liver function test results.
• In patients with metastatic breast cancer, hypercalcemia usually indicates progression of bone metastases. Report signs and symptoms of hypercalcemia.
• Report signs and symptoms of virilization in women. Androgenic effects include acne, edema, weight gain, hirsutism, hoarseness, clitoral enlargement, decreased breast size, changes in libido, male-pattern baldness, and oily skin or hair.
• Monitor patient's weight and blood pressure routinely.
• Monitor prepubertal boys by X-ray for rate of bone maturation.
• *Alert:* Therapeutic response in breast cancer is usually apparent within 3 months. Therapy should be stopped if disease progresses.
• Androgens may alter results of laboratory studies during therapy and for 2 to 3 weeks after therapy ends.
• *Alert:* Testosterone and methyltestosterone aren't interchangeable. Don't confuse testosterone with testolactone.

☑ **Patient teaching**
• Make sure patient understands importance of using an effective nonhormonal contraceptive during therapy.
• Review signs and symptoms of virilization with woman and instruct her to notify doctor if they occur.
• Advise woman to wash after intercourse to decrease risk of vaginitis. Instruct her to wear cotton underwear.
• Instruct man to report priapism, reduced ejaculatory volume, and gynecomastia, and to notify doctor if these occur.
• Warn diabetic patient to be alert for signs and symptoms of hypoglycemia, and to notify doctor if they occur.
• Tell patient to report sudden weight gain.
• Warn patient that drug shouldn't be used for enhancement of athletic performance.

## testosterone transdermal system
Androderm, Testoderm

*Controlled Substance Schedule III*
*Pregnancy Risk Category X*

## HOW SUPPLIED
*Transdermal system:* 2.5 mg/day, 4 mg/day, 5 mg/day, 6 mg/day

## ACTION
Releases testosterone, which stimulates target tissues to develop normally in androgen-deficient men.

| Route | Onset | Peak | Duration |
|-------|-------|------|----------|
| Trans-dermal | Unknown | 2-4 hr | 2 hr |

## INDICATIONS & DOSAGE
*Primary or hypogonadotropic hypogonadism in men—*
**Adult men:** *Testoderm*—one 6-mg/day patch applied to scrotal area daily. If scrotal area is too small for 6-mg/day patch, therapy started with 4-mg/day patch. Patch is worn for 22 to 24 hours daily. *Androderm*—two systems applied h.s. for total dose of 5 mg/day. Apply to clean, dry skin on back, abdomen, upper arms, or thigh.

## ADVERSE REACTIONS
**CNS:** headache, depression.
**CV:** *CVA.*
**GI:** GI bleeding.
**GU:** gynecomastia, prostatitis, prostate abnormalities, urinary tract infection, breast tenderness.
**Skin:** acne irritation; *pruritus; blister under system;* allergic contact dermatitis; burning, induration at injection site.

## INTERACTIONS
**Drug-drug.** *Insulin:* altered insulin dosage requirements. Monitor blood glucose levels.
*Oral anticoagulants:* altered anticoagulant dosage requirements. Monitor PT and INR.
*Oxyphenbutazone:* may increase oxyphenbutazone levels. Monitor patient.

## EFFECTS ON DIAGNOSTIC TESTS
None reported.

## CONTRAINDICATIONS
Contraindicated in patients with hypersensitivity to drug, in women, and in men with known or suspected breast or prostate cancer.

## NURSING CONSIDERATIONS
● Use cautiously in elderly men and in patients with preexisting renal, hepatic, or cardiac disease.
● Periodically assess liver function tests, serum lipid profiles, hemoglobin level and hematocrit (with long-term use), and prostatic acid phosphatase and prostate-specific antigen levels, as ordered.
● *Alert:* Don't confuse Testoderm with Estraderm.

### ☑ Patient teaching
● Teach patient how to apply transdermal system. Warn him that adequate serum levels won't be attained if Testoderm patch isn't applied to genital skin. Tell patient using Androderm that patch isn't to be applied to scrotum. Application site should be rotated, with an interval of 7 days between applications to same site. Avoid bony prominences. Don't interchange patch brands.
● Warn diabetic patient that testosterone may decrease serum glucose levels and that he should be alert for signs and symptoms of hypoglycemia.
● Tell man that topical testosterone has caused virilization in women partners, who should report acne or changes in body hair distribution.
● Advise patient to report persistent erections, nausea, vomiting, changes in skin color, ankle edema, or sudden weight gain to doctor.
● Tell patient that Androderm doesn't have to be removed during sexual intercourse or while showering.

---

esterified estrogens
estradiol
estradiol cypionate
estradiol/norethindrone acetate
    transdermal system
estradiol valerate
estrogens, conjugated
estropipate
ethinyl estradiol
ethinyl estradiol and desogestrel
ethinyl estradiol and ethynodiol
    diacetate
ethinyl estradiol and
    levonorgestrel
ethinyl estradiol and
    norethindrone
ethinyl estradiol and
    norethindrone acetate
ethinyl estradiol and norgestimate
ethinyl estradiol and norgestrel
ethinyl estradiol, norethindrone
    acetate, and ferrous fumarate
levonorgestrel
medroxyprogesterone acetate
mestranol and norethindrone
norethindrone
norethindrone acetate
norgestrel
progesterone

### COMBINATION PRODUCTS
ESTRATEST: esterified estrogens 1.25 mg
and methyltestosterone 1.25 mg.
PMB 200: conjugated estrogens 0.45 mg
and meprobamate 200 mg.
PMB 400: conjugated estrogens 0.45 mg
and meprobamate 400 mg.
PREMPHASE: conjugated estrogens
0.625 mg and conjugated estrogens 0.625
mg/medroxyprogesterone acetate 5 mg.
PREMPRO 0.625 mg/2.5 mg: conjugated
estrogens 0.625 mg/medroxyprogesterone
acetate 2.5 mg.
PREMPRO 0.625 mg/5 mg: conjugated estrogens 0.625 mg/medroxyprogesterone
acetate 5 mg.
PREVEN EMERGENCY: ethinyl estradiol (50
mcg) and levonorgestrel (0.25 mg).

## esterified estrogens
Estratab, Menest, Neo-Estrone†

*Pregnancy Risk Category X*

### HOW SUPPLIED
*Tablets:* 0.3 mg, 0.625 mg, 1.25 mg,
2.5 mg
*Tablets (film-coated):* 0.3 mg, 0.625 mg,
1.25 mg, 2.5 mg

### ACTION
Increases synthesis of DNA, RNA, and
protein in responsive tissues. Also reduces
release of follicle-stimulating and
luteinizing hormones from the pituitary
gland.

| Route | Onset | Peak | Duration |
|-------|-------|------|----------|
| P.O. | Unknown | Unknown | Unknown |

### INDICATIONS & DOSAGE
*Inoperable prostate cancer—*
**Men:** 1.25 to 2.5 mg P.O. t.i.d.
*Breast cancer—*
**Men and postmenopausal women:**
10 mg P.O. t.i.d. for 3 or more months.
*Female hypogonadism—*
**Women:** 2.5 to 7.5 mg daily in divided
doses in cycles of 20 days on, 10 days off.
*Castration, primary ovarian failure—*
**Women:** 1.25 mg daily in cycles of 3
weeks on, 1 week off. Adjust for symp-
toms. Can be given continuously.
*Vasomotor menopausal symptoms—*
**Women:** average dosage is 1.25 mg P.O.
daily in cycles of 3 weeks on, 1 week off.
Dose may be increased to 2.5 to 3.75 mg
P.O. daily if needed.
*Atrophic vaginitis, atrophic urethritis—*
**Women:** 0.3 to 1.25 mg or more P.O. dai-
ly in cycles of 3 weeks on, 1 week off.
*Prevention of osteoporosis (Estratab,
Neo-Estrone†)—*
**Women:** initially, 0.3 mg P.O. daily; may
be increased to maximum daily dose of
1.25 mg.

---

Reactions may be *common,* uncommon, *life-threatening,* or COMMON AND LIFE-THREATENING.

## ADVERSE REACTIONS
**CNS:** headache, dizziness, chorea, depression, *seizures.*
**CV:** thrombophlebitis; *thromboembolism;* hypertension; *edema; increased risk of CVA, pulmonary embolism, MI.*
**EENT:** worsening myopia or astigmatism, intolerance of contact lenses.
**GI:** *nausea,* vomiting, abdominal cramps, bloating, anorexia, increased appetite, *pancreatitis.*
**GU:** breakthrough bleeding, altered menstrual flow, dysmenorrhea, amenorrhea, *increased risk of endometrial cancer,* cervical erosion, altered cervical secretions, enlargement of uterine fibromas, vaginal candidiasis (in women); gynecomastia, testicular atrophy, impotence (in men).
**Hematologic:** increased PT and clotting factors VII to X, and norepinephrine-induced platelet aggregation.
**Hepatic:** cholestatic jaundice, *hepatic adenoma.*
**Metabolic:** hypercalcemia, weight changes.
**Skin:** melasma, rash, hirsutism or hair loss, erythema nodosum, dermatitis.
**Other:** increased risk of gallbladder disease; *breast tenderness, enlargement, or secretion*; *possible increased risk of breast cancer.*

## INTERACTIONS
**Drug-drug.** *Carbamazepine, phenobarbital, rifampin:* decreased effectiveness of estrogen therapy. Monitor closely.
*Corticosteroids:* possible enhanced effects. Monitor closely.
*Cyclosporine:* increased risk of toxicity. Use together with caution and frequently monitor cyclosporine levels.
*Dantrolene, other hepatotoxic drugs:* increased risk of hepatotoxicity. Monitor closely.
*Oral anticoagulants:* effect of anticoagulant may be decreased. Dosage adjustments may be needed. Monitor PT and INR, as ordered.
*Tamoxifen:* estrogens may interfere with effectiveness of tamoxifen. Avoid concomitant use.
**Drug-food.** *Caffeine:* may increase serum caffeine levels. Monitor effects.

**Drug-lifestyle.** *Smoking:* increased risk of adverse CV effects. If smoking continues, may need alternative form of therapy.

## EFFECTS ON DIAGNOSTIC TESTS
Glucose tolerance may be impaired. There may be a reduced response to metyrapone test.

## CONTRAINDICATIONS
Contraindicated in patients with hypersensitivity to drug and in those with breast cancer (except metastatic disease), estrogen-dependent neoplasia, active thrombophlebitis or thromboembolic disorders, undiagnosed abnormal genital bleeding, or history of thromboembolic disease; also contraindicated during pregnancy.

## NURSING CONSIDERATIONS
• Use cautiously in patients with history of hypertension, mental depression, cardiac or renal dysfunction, liver impairment, bone diseases, migraine, seizures, or diabetes mellitus.
• When used for vasomotor symptoms in menstruating women, cyclic administration is started on day 5 of bleeding.
• Ensure that patient has thorough physical examination before initiating estrogen therapy. Patients receiving long-term therapy should have annual examinations. Periodically monitor body weight, blood pressure, serum lipid levels, and hepatic function.
• Notify pathologist of patient receiving estrogen therapy when specimens are obtained and sent to laboratory for evaluation.
• Because of risk of thromboembolism, therapy should be discontinued at least 1 month before procedures associated with prolonged immobilization or thromboembolism, such as knee or hip surgery.
• **Alert:** Don't confuse Estratab with Estratest.

### ✓ Patient teaching
• Tell patient that package insert describing estrogen's adverse effects is available; however, also give patient verbal explanation.
• Emphasize importance of regular physical examinations. Postmenopausal women

who use estrogen replacement for over 5 years to treat menopausal symptoms may be at increased risk for endometrial cancer. This risk is reduced by using cyclic rather than continuous therapy and the lowest possible dosages of estrogen. Adding progestins to the regimen decreases risk of endometrial hyperplasia; however, it isn't known if progestins affect risk of endometrial cancer. No increased risk of breast cancer has been reported.

• *Alert:* Warn patient to immediately report abdominal pain; pain, numbness, or stiffness in legs or buttocks; pressure or pain in chest; shortness of breath; severe headaches; visual disturbances, such as blind spots, flashing lights, or blurriness; vaginal bleeding or discharge; breast lumps; swelling of hands or feet; yellow skin or sclera; dark urine; and light-colored stools.

• Tell diabetic patient to report elevated blood glucose level test results so that antidiabetic dosage can be adjusted.

• Explain to patient on cyclic therapy for postmenopausal symptoms that, although she may experience withdrawal bleeding during week off drug, fertility isn't restored. Pregnancy can't occur because patient doesn't ovulate.

• Teach woman to perform routine breast self-examination.

• Advise woman of childbearing age to consult doctor before taking drug, and to advise doctor immediately if pregnancy occurs.

• Teach patient methods to decrease risk of thromboembolism.

---

### estradiol (oestradiol)
Climara, Estrace**, Estrace Vaginal Cream, Estraderm, FemSeven§, Menorest§, Ovestin§, Vivelle, Zumenon§

### estradiol cypionate
depGynogen, Depo-Estradiol, Depogen, Dura-Estrin, E-Cypionate, Estragyn LA 5, Estro-Cyp, Estrofem

### estradiol valerate (oestradiol valerate)
Clinagen LA 40, Delestrogen, Dioval 40, Dioval XX, Duragen-20, Estra-L 40, Estro-Span, Femogex, Gynogen L.A., Menaval, Primogyn Depot‡, Progynova§, Valergen-10, Valergen-20, Valergen-40

*Pregnancy Risk Category X*

### HOW SUPPLIED
**estradiol**
*Tablets (micronized):* 0.5 mg, 1 mg, 2 mg
*Transdermal:* 0.025 mg/24 hours, 0.0375 mg/24 hours, 0.05 mg/24 hours; 0.075 mg/24 hours; 0.1 mg/24 hours; 4 mg/10 cm$^2$ (delivers 0.05 mg/24 hours); 8 mg/10 cm$^2$
*Vaginal cream (in nonliquefying base):* 0.1 mg/g
**estradiol cypionate**
*Injection (in oil):* 1 mg/ml, 5 mg/ml
**estradiol valerate**
*Injection (in oil):* 10 mg/ml, 20 mg/ml, 40 mg/ml

### ACTION
Increases synthesis of DNA, RNA, and protein in responsive tissues. Also reduces release of follicle-stimulating and luteinizing hormones from the pituitary gland.

| Route | Onset | Peak | Duration |
|---|---|---|---|
| P.O., I.M., transdermal, intravaginal | Unknown | Unknown | Unknown |

### INDICATIONS & DOSAGE
*Vasomotor menopausal symptoms, female hypogonadism, female castration, primary ovarian failure—*
**Women:** 0.5 to 2 mg P.O. (estradiol) daily in cycles of 21 days on and 7 days off; or cycles of 5 days on and 2 days off; or one transdermal system (Estraderm) delivering 0.05 mg/24 hours applied twice weekly; or as a system (Vivelle) delivering either 0.05 mg/24 hours or 0.0375 mg/24 hours applied twice weekly; or as a system (Climara) delivering either 0.05 mg/24 hours or 0.1 mg/24 hours and applied

---

once weekly, in cycles of 3 weeks on and 1 week off.

*Note:* Transdermal systems are sometimes used on a continuous basis (not cyclic). Or, 1 to 5 mg (cipionate) I.M. q 3 to 4 weeks; or 10 to 20 mg (valerate) I.M. q 4 weeks, p.r.n.

*Atrophic vaginitis, kraurosis vulvae—*
**Women:** 0.05 mg/24 hours (Estraderm) applied twice weekly in a cyclic regimen; or 0.05 mg/24 hours (Climara) applied weekly in a cyclic regimen; or 2 to 4 g intravaginal applications of cream daily for 1 to 2 weeks. When vaginal mucosa is restored, maintenance dose is 1 g one to three times weekly in a cyclic regimen.
Or, 10 to 20 mg (valerate) I.M. q 4 weeks, p.r.n.

*Palliative treatment of advanced, inoperable breast cancer—*
**Men and postmenopausal women:**
10 mg P.O. (estradiol) t.i.d. for 3 months.
*Palliative treatment of advanced, inoperable prostate cancer—*
**Men:** 30 mg (valerate) I.M. q 1 to 2 weeks, or 1 to 2 mg P.O. (estradiol) t.i.d.
✳ *NEW INDICATION: Prevention of postmenopausal osteoporosis—*
**Adults:** place a 6.5-cm$^2$ (0.025 mg/day) Climara system once weekly on clean, dry skin area of lower abdomen or upper quadrant of buttock; press firmly in place for about 10 seconds, making sure contact is good, especially around edges.

## ADVERSE REACTIONS
**CNS:** headache, dizziness, chorea, depression, *seizures.*
**CV:** thrombophlebitis, *thromboembolism,* hypertension, *edema; increased risk of CVA, pulmonary embolism, MI.*
**EENT:** worsening myopia or astigmatism, intolerance of contact lenses.
**GI:** *nausea,* vomiting, abdominal cramps, bloating, increased appetite, *pancreatitis,* anorexia.
**GU:** breakthrough bleeding, altered menstrual flow, dysmenorrhea, amenorrhea, *increased risk of endometrial cancer,* cervical erosion, altered cervical secretions, enlargement of uterine fibromas, vaginal candidiasis in women; gynecomastia, testicular atrophy, impotence in men.

**Hematologic**: increased PT and clotting factors VII to X, and norepinephrine-induced platelet aggregation.
**Hepatic:** cholestatic jaundice, *hepatic adenoma.*
**Metabolic:** weight changes.
**Skin:** melasma, urticaria, erythema nodosum, dermatitis, hair loss.
**Other:** gallbladder disease; *breast tenderness, enlargement, or secretion; possible increased risk of breast cancer.*

## INTERACTIONS
**Drug-drug.** *Carbamazepine, phenobarbital, rifampin:* decreased effectiveness of estrogen therapy. Monitor closely.
*Corticosteroids:* possible enhanced effects of corticosteroids. Monitor closely.
*Cyclosporine:* increased risk of toxicity. Use together with caution and monitor cyclosporine levels frequently.
*Dantrolene, other hepatotoxic drugs:* increased risk of hepatotoxicity. Monitor closely.
*Oral anticoagulants:* effect of anticoagulant may be decreased. Dosage adjustments may be needed. Monitor PT and INR, as ordered.
*Tamoxifen:* estrogens may interfere with effectiveness of tamoxifen. Avoid concomitant use.
**Drug-food.** *Caffeine:* may increase serum caffeine levels. Monitor effects.
**Drug-lifestyle.** *Smoking:* increased risk of adverse CV effects. If smoking continues, may need alternative therapy.

## EFFECTS ON DIAGNOSTIC TESTS
Glucose tolerance may be impaired. There may be a reduced response to metyrapone test.

## CONTRAINDICATIONS
Contraindicated in patients with thrombophlebitis or thromboembolic disorders, estrogen-dependent neoplasia, breast or reproductive organ cancer (except for palliative treatment), undiagnosed abnormal genital bleeding, or history of thrombophlebitis or thromboembolic disorders associated with previous estrogen use (except for palliative treatment of breast and prostate cancer); also contraindicated during pregnancy.

---

## NURSING CONSIDERATIONS

• Use cautiously in patients with cerebrovascular or coronary artery disease, asthma, bone diseases, migraine, seizures, or cardiac, hepatic, or renal dysfunction; also use cautiously in women with strong family history of breast cancer or who have breast nodules, fibrocystic breasts, or abnormal mammographic findings.

• Ensure that patient has physical examination before initiating therapy. Patients receiving long-term therapy should be examined yearly. Monitor serum lipid levels, blood pressure, body weight, and hepatic function, as ordered.

• Ask patient about allergies, especially to foods or plants. Estradiol is available as an aqueous solution or as a solution in peanut oil; estradiol cypionate, as a solution in cottonseed oil; estradiol valerate, as a solution in castor oil or sesame oil.

• To administer as I.M. injection, make sure drug is well dispersed in solution by rolling vial between palms. Inject deeply into large muscle. Rotate injection sites to prevent muscle atrophy. Never give drug I.V.

• Apply transdermal patch to clean, dry, hairless, intact skin on abdomen or buttocks. Don't apply it to breasts, waistline, or other areas where clothing can loosen patch. When applying, ensure patch is in good contact with skin, especially around edges, and hold in place with the palm for about 10 seconds. Rotate application sites.

• In women also taking oral estrogen, treatment with the Estraderm transdermal patch can begin 1 week after withdrawal of oral therapy or sooner if menopausal symptoms appear before end of the week.

• Because of risk of thromboembolism, therapy should be discontinued at least 1 month before procedures associated with prolonged immobilization or thromboembolism, such as knee or hip surgery.

• Notify pathologist of patient receiving estrogen therapy when specimens are obtained and sent to laboratory for evaluation.

### ☑ Patient teaching

• Tell patient that package insert describing estrogen's adverse effects is available; however, also give patient verbal explanation.

• Emphasize importance of regular physical examinations. Postmenopausal women who use estrogen replacement for over 5 years may be at increased risk for endometrial cancer. Risk is reduced by using cyclic rather than continuous therapy and the lowest possible dosages of estrogen. Adding progestins to regimen decreases risk of endometrial hyperplasia; however, it isn't known if progestins affect risk of endometrial cancer. No increased risk of breast cancer has been reported.

• Tell patient how to use cream. Patient should wash vaginal area with soap and water before applying and take drug at bedtime or lie flat for 30 minutes after instillation to minimize drug loss.

• Tell patient how to use transdermal system. Rotate sites and don't apply to breasts or waistline.

• *Alert:* Warn patient to immediately report abdominal pain; pain, numbness, or stiffness in legs or buttocks; pressure or pain in chest; shortness of breath; severe headaches; visual disturbances; vaginal bleeding or discharge; breast lumps; swelling of hands or feet; yellow skin or sclera; dark urine; and light-colored stools.

• Explain to patient on cyclic therapy for postmenopausal symptoms that, although withdrawal bleeding may occur during week off drug, fertility isn't restored. Pregnancy can't occur because patient doesn't ovulate.

• Tell diabetic patient to report elevated blood glucose level test results so that antidiabetic dosage can be adjusted.

• Teach woman how to perform routine breast self-examination.

• Teach patient methods to decrease risk of thromboembolism.

• Advise woman not to become pregnant during estrogen therapy.

---

Reactions may be *common*, uncommon, *life-threatening*, or COMMON AND LIFE-THREATENING.

## estradiol/norethindrone acetate transdermal system
CombiPatch

*Pregnancy Risk Category X*

### HOW SUPPLIED
*Transdermal:* 9-cm$^2$ system releasing 0.05 mg estradiol and 0.14 mg norethindrone acetate per day; 16-cm$^2$ system releasing 0.05 mg estradiol and 0.25 mg norethindrone acetate per day

### ACTION
A matrix transdermal system in which estradiol and norethindrone are released continuously. Estrogen replacement therapy can reduce frequency of menopausal symptoms and release of follicle-stimulating and luteinizing hormones from the pituitary gland in postmenopausal women.

| Route | Onset | Peak | Duration |
|---|---|---|---|
| Transdermal | 12-24 hr | Unknown | 3-4 days |

### INDICATIONS & DOSAGE
*Moderate to severe vasomotor symptoms associated with menopause, vulvar and vaginal atrophy, and hypoestrogenemia due to hypogonadism, castration, or primary ovarian failure in women with intact uterus—*
**Women:** *Continuous combined regimen—*9-cm$^2$ patch worn continuously on lower abdomen. Old system should be removed and new system applied twice weekly during a 28-day cycle. May increase to 16-cm$^2$ patch.
*Continuous sequential regimen—*patch can be applied as a sequential regimen with an estradiol transdermal system (such as Alora, Esclim, Estraderm, Vivelle). A 0.05-mg estradiol transdermal patch is worn for first 14 days of a 28-day cycle; replace system twice weekly. For rest of 28-day cycle, 9-cm$^2$ patch system should be worn on lower abdomen. May increase to 16-cm$^2$ patch, p.r.n.
    Women not currently receiving continuous estrogen or estrogen/progestin therapy may start therapy at any time.
    Women currently receiving continuous hormone replacement therapy should complete the current cycle of therapy before initiating therapy. Women often experience withdrawal bleeding at completion of cycle; first day of withdrawal bleeding would be an appropriate time to initiate therapy.

### ADVERSE REACTIONS
**CNS:** *asthenia,* depression, insomnia, nervousness, dizziness, *headache.*
**EENT:** tooth disorder, pharyngitis, *rhinitis, sinusitis.*
**GI:** *abdominal pain, diarrhea,* dyspepsia, flatulence, *nausea,* constipation.
**GU:** *dysmenorrhea, leukorrhea, menstrual disorder,* suspicious Papanicolaou smears, *vaginitis,* menorrhagia, vaginal hemorrhage.
**Musculoskeletal:** arthralgia, *back pain.*
**Respiratory:** *respiratory disorder,* bronchitis.
**Skin:** application site reactions, acne.
**Other:** *accidental injury, flulike syndrome, pain, breast pain,* peripheral edema, breast enlargement, infection.

### INTERACTIONS
None significant.

### EFFECTS ON DIAGNOSTIC TESTS
Drug may cause a reduced response to the metyrapone test.

### CONTRAINDICATIONS
Contraindicated in women with hypersensitivity to estrogen, progestin, or any component of the patch; in those who may be pregnant; and in those with known or suspected breast cancer, known or suspected estrogen-dependent neoplasia, undiagnosed abnormal genital bleeding, active thrombophlebitis, thromboembolic disorders, or stroke.

### NURSING CONSIDERATIONS
• Use cautiously in patients with impaired liver function, asthma, epilepsy, migraine, or cardiac or renal dysfunction, and in breast-feeding women.
• Store norethindrone patches in refrigerator before dispensing. Patient may then store patches at room temperature for up to 3 months.

---

*Liquid contains alcohol.    **May contain tartrazine.    †Canada    ‡Australia    §U.K.    ◊OTC

• Advise patient not to store patches where extreme temperatures can occur.
• Reevaluate therapy at 3- to 6-month intervals. Combination estrogen/progestin regimens are indicated for women with intact uterus.
• Progestins taken with estrogen significantly reduce, but don't eliminate, risk of endometrial cancer associated with use of estrogen.
• Blood pressure increases have been associated with estrogen use. Monitor patient's blood pressure regularly.
• Treatment of postmenopausal symptoms is usually initiated during menopausal stage when vasomotor symptoms occur.
• Apply patch system to a smooth (fold-free), clean, dry, nonirritated area of skin on lower abdomen, avoiding the waistline. Application sites should be rotated, with an interval of at least 1 week between applications to same site.
• Don't apply patch on or near breasts.
• Avoid applying to areas that may get prolonged sun exposure.
• Reapply system, if needed, to another area of lower abdomen. If system fails to adhere, replace with a new one.
• INR, activated PTT, and platelet aggregation times may be altered; platelet count and fibrinogen activity may increase. Increased thyroid-binding globulin may lead to increased $T_3$ and $T_4$ levels and decreased $T_3$ resin uptake. A decrease in serum total cholesterol, high-density lipoprotein cholesterol, low-density lipoprotein cholesterol, and triglyceride levels may also occur.
• *Alert:* Don't interchange CombiPatch with other estrogen patches. Verify therapy before application.

☑ **Patient teaching**
• Teach patient how to apply system properly. Only one system should be worn at any time during the dosing intervals.
• Tell patient an oil-based cream or lotion may help remove adhesive from the skin once system has been removed and the area allowed to dry for 15 minutes.
• Advise patient not to use patch if pregnancy occurs or is being planned.
• Instruct patient that, for the continuous combined regimen, irregular bleeding may occur, particularly in the first 6 months, but generally decreases with time, often to an amenorrheic state.
• Tell patient that, for the continuous sequential regimen, monthly withdrawal bleeding often occurs.
• Advise patient to alert doctor and discontinue patch at first sign of thrombotic disorders (thrombophlebitis, cerebrovascular disorders, and pulmonary embolism).
• Instruct patient to discontinue patch and call doctor if partial or complete loss of vision, sudden onset of proptosis (downward displacement of the eyeball), double vision, or migraine occurs.

---

## estrogens, conjugated (estrogenic substances, conjugated; oestrogens, conjugated)
C.E.S.†, Premarin, Premarin Intravenous

*Pregnancy Risk Category X*

### HOW SUPPLIED
*Tablets:* 0.3 mg, 0.625 mg, 0.9 mg, 1.25 mg, 2.5 mg
*Injection:* 25 mg/5 ml
*Vaginal cream:* 0.625 mg/g

### ACTION
Increases synthesis of DNA, RNA, and protein in responsive tissues. Also reduces release of follicle-stimulating and luteinizing hormones from the pituitary gland.

| Route | Onset | Peak | Duration |
|---|---|---|---|
| P.O., I.V., I.M., intravaginal | Unknown | Unknown | Unknown |

### INDICATIONS & DOSAGE
*Abnormal uterine bleeding (hormonal imbalance)—*
**Women:** 25 mg I.V. or I.M., repeated in 6 to 12 hours, p.r.n.
*Palliative treatment of breast cancer (at least 5 years after menopause)—*
**Men and postmenopausal women:** 10 mg P.O. t.i.d. for 3 months or more.

---

Reactions may be *common*, uncommon, *life-threatening*, or COMMON AND LIFE-THREATENING.

*Female castration, primary ovarian failure—*
**Women:** 1.25 mg P.O. daily in cycles of 3 weeks on and 1 week off. Can be given continuously.
*Osteoporosis—*
**Postmenopausal women:** 0.625 mg P.O. daily in cyclic regimen (3 weeks on, 1 week off). Can be given continuously.
*Hypogonadism—*
**Women:** 2.5 to 7.5 mg daily in divided doses for 20 days followed by 10 days off.
*Vasomotor menopausal symptoms—*
**Women:** 0.3 to 1.25 mg P.O. daily in cycles of 3 weeks on and 1 week off. Can be given continuously.
*Atrophic vaginitis, kraurosis vulvae—*
**Women:** 0.5 to 2 g intravaginally once daily on a cyclical basis (3 weeks on and 1 week off).
*Palliative treatment of inoperable prostate cancer—*
**Men:** 1.25 to 2.5 mg P.O. t.i.d.

## ADVERSE REACTIONS
**CNS:** headache, dizziness, chorea, depression, *seizures.*
**CV:** thrombophlebitis; *thromboembolism;* hypertension; *edema; increased risk of CVA, pulmonary embolism, MI.*
**EENT:** worsening myopia or astigmatism, intolerance of contact lenses.
**GI:** *nausea,* vomiting, abdominal cramps, bloating, anorexia, increased appetite, *pancreatitis.*
**GU:** breakthrough bleeding, altered menstrual flow, dysmenorrhea, amenorrhea, *increased risk of endometrial cancer,* cervical erosion, altered cervical secretions, enlargement of uterine fibromas, vaginal candidiasis; gynecomastia, testicular atrophy, impotence.
**Hematologic:** increased PT and clotting factors VII to X, and norepinephrine-induced platelet aggregation.
**Hepatic:** cholestatic jaundice, *hepatic adenoma.*
**Metabolic:** weight changes.
**Skin:** melasma, urticaria, flushing with rapid I.V. administration, hirsutism or hair loss, erythema nodosum, dermatitis.
**Other:** gallbladder disease; *breast tenderness, enlargement, or secretion; possible increased risk of breast cancer.*

## INTERACTIONS
**Drug-drug.** *Carbamazepine, phenobarbital, rifampin:* decreased effectiveness of estrogen therapy. Monitor closely.
*Corticosteroids:* possible enhanced effects of corticosteroids. Monitor closely.
*Cyclosporine:* increased risk of toxicity. Use together with caution and frequently monitor cyclosporine levels.
*Dantrolene, other hepatotoxic drugs:* increased risk of hepatotoxicity. Monitor closely.
*Oral anticoagulants:* effect of anticoagulant may be decreased. Dosage adjustments may be needed. Monitor PT and INR, as ordered.
*Tamoxifen:* estrogens may interfere with effectiveness of tamoxifen. Avoid concomitant use.
**Drug-food.** *Caffeine:* may increase serum caffeine levels. Monitor effects.
**Drug-lifestyle.** *Smoking:* increased risk of adverse CV effects. If smoking continues, may need alternative therapy.

## EFFECTS ON DIAGNOSTIC TESTS
Glucose tolerance may be impaired. Reduced response to metyrapone test

## CONTRAINDICATIONS
Contraindicated in patients with thrombophlebitis or thromboembolic disorders, estrogen-dependent neoplasia, breast or reproductive cancer (except for palliative treatment), or undiagnosed abnormal genital bleeding; also contraindicated during pregnancy.

## NURSING CONSIDERATIONS
• Use cautiously in patients with cerebrovascular or coronary artery disease, asthma, bone disease, migraine, seizures, or cardiac, hepatic, or renal dysfunction; also use cautiously in women with family history (mother, grandmother, sister) of breast or genital tract cancer or who have breast nodules, fibrocystic breasts, or abnormal mammographic findings.
• Ensure that patient has thorough physical examination before initiating estrogen therapy. Patients receiving long-term therapy should have annual examinations. Periodically monitor serum lipid levels,

blood pressure, body weight, and hepatic function, as ordered.

• I.M. or I.V. use is preferred for rapid treatment of dysfunctional uterine bleeding or reduction of surgical bleeding.

• When administering by I.M. injection, inject deeply into large muscle. Rotate injection sites to prevent muscle atrophy.

• Notify pathologist about patient receiving estrogen therapy when specimens are obtained and sent to laboratory for evaluation.

• Because of risk of thromboembolism, therapy should be discontinued at least 1 month before procedures associated with prolonged immobilization or thromboembolism, such as knee or hip surgery.

• *Alert:* Don't confuse Premarin with Primaxin.

### ◖ I.V. administration

• When giving by direct I.V. injection, administer slowly to avoid flushing reaction. I.V. solution isn't compatible with protein hydrolysate, ascorbic acid, or solutions with an acid pH. Use diluent provided to reconstitute drug. Drug is compatible with normal saline, dextrose, or invert sugar solutions.

• Refrigerate before reconstituting. Agitate gently after adding diluent. Use only diluent provided.

### ☑ Patient teaching

• Tell patient that package insert describing estrogen's adverse effects is available; also explain effects.

• Emphasize importance of regular physical examinations. Postmenopausal women who use estrogen replacement for over 5 years to treat menopausal symptoms may be at increased risk for endometrial cancer. This risk is reduced by using cyclic rather than continuous therapy and lowest possible dosages of estrogen. Adding progestins to the regimen decreases risk of endometrial hyperplasia; however, it isn't known if progestins affect risk of endometrial cancer. No increased risk of breast cancer has been reported.

• Teach patient how to use vaginal cream. Patient should wash the vaginal area with soap and water before applying. Tell her to use drug at bedtime or to lie flat for 30 minutes after instillation to minimize drug loss.

• Explain to patient on cyclic therapy for postmenopausal symptoms that, although withdrawal bleeding may occur during week off drug, fertility isn't restored. Pregnancy can't occur because patient doesn't ovulate.

• *Alert:* Warn patient to immediately report abdominal pain; pain, numbness, or stiffness in legs or buttocks; pressure or pain in chest; shortness of breath; severe headaches; visual disturbances, such as blind spots, flashing lights, or blurriness; vaginal bleeding or discharge; breast lumps; swelling of hands or feet; yellow skin or sclera; dark urine; and light-colored stools.

• Tell diabetic patient to report elevated blood glucose level test results so that antidiabetic dosage can be adjusted.

• Teach woman how to perform routine breast self-examination.

• Advise patient not to become pregnant during estrogen therapy.

---

## estropipate
## (piperazine estrone sulfate)
Harmogen§, Ogen, Ortho-Est

*Pregnancy Risk Category X*

### HOW SUPPLIED
*Tablets:* 0.75 mg, 1.5 mg, 3 mg, 6 mg
*Vaginal cream:* 1.5 mg/g

### ACTION
Increases synthesis of DNA, RNA, and proteins in responsive tissues. Also reduces release of follicle-stimulating and luteinizing hormones from the pituitary gland.

| Route | Onset | Peak | Duration |
|---|---|---|---|
| P.O., intravaginal | Unknown | Unknown | Unknown |

### INDICATIONS & DOSAGE
*Vulval and vaginal atrophy—*
**Women:** 0.75 to 6 mg P.O. daily, 3 weeks on and 1 week off; or 2 to 4 g vaginal cream daily. Typically, dosage given on a

---

Reactions may be *common*, uncommon, *life-threatening*, or COMMON AND LIFE-THREATENING.

cyclical, short-term basis. Can be given continuously.

*Primary ovarian failure, female castration, female hypogonadism—*
**Women:** administered on a cyclical basis—1.5 to 9 mg P.O. daily for first 3 weeks; then a rest period of 8 to 10 days. If bleeding doesn't occur by end of rest period, cycle is repeated. Can be given continuously.

*Vasomotor menopausal symptoms—*
**Women:** 0.75 to 6 mg P.O. daily in cyclic method of 3 weeks on and 1 week off. Can be given continuously.

*Prevention of osteoporosis—*
**Women:** 0.625 mg (0.75 mg estropipate) tablet P.O. daily for 25 days of a 31-day cycle.

## ADVERSE REACTIONS
**CNS:** depression, headache, dizziness, migraine, *seizures.*
**CV:** *edema;* thrombophlebitis; *increased risk of CVA, pulmonary embolism, MI; thromboembolism.*
**GI:** nausea, vomiting, abdominal cramps, bloating.
**GU:** increased size of uterine fibromas, *increased risk of endometrial cancer,* vaginal candidiasis, cystitis-like syndrome, dysmenorrhea, amenorrhea, breakthrough bleeding, condition resembling premenstrual syndrome.
**Hematologic:** increased PT and clotting factors VII to X, and norepinephrine-induced platelet aggregation.
**Hepatic:** cholestatic jaundice, *hepatic adenoma.*
**Metabolic:** weight changes.
**Skin:** hemorrhagic eruption, erythema nodosum, *erythema multiforme,* hirsutism, melasma, hair loss.
**Other:** gallbladder disease, breast engorgement or enlargement; *possible increased risk of breast cancer.*

## INTERACTIONS
**Drug-drug.** *Carbamazepine, phenobarbital, rifampin:* decreased effectiveness of estrogen therapy. Monitor closely.
*Corticosteroids:* possible enhanced effects of corticosteroids. Monitor closely.

*Cyclosporine:* increased risk of toxicity. Use together with caution and frequently monitor serum cyclosporine levels.
*Dantrolene, other hepatotoxic drugs:* increased risk of hepatotoxicity. Monitor closely.
*Oral anticoagulants:* effect of anticoagulant may be decreased. Dosage adjustments may be needed. Monitor PT and INR, as ordered.
*Tamoxifen:* estrogens may interfere with effectiveness of tamoxifen. Avoid concomitant use.
**Drug-food.** *Caffeine:* may increase serum caffeine levels. Monitor effects.
**Drug-lifestyle.** *Smoking:* increased risk of adverse CV effects. If smoking continues, may need alternative therapy.

## EFFECTS ON DIAGNOSTIC TESTS
Glucose tolerance may be impaired. There may be a reduced response to metyrapone test.

## CONTRAINDICATIONS
Contraindicated in patients with active thrombophlebitis or thromboembolic disorders; estrogen-dependent neoplasia; breast, reproductive organ, or genital cancer; and in those with undiagnosed genital bleeding; also contraindicated during pregnancy.

## NURSING CONSIDERATIONS
• Use cautiously in patients with cerebrovascular or coronary artery disease; asthma; mental depression; bone disease; migraine; seizures; or cardiac, hepatic, or renal dysfunction; also use cautiously in women with family history (mother, grandmother, sister) of breast or genital tract cancer or who have breast nodules, fibrocystic breasts, or abnormal mammographic findings.
• Ensure that patient has thorough physical examination before initiating estrogen therapy. Patients receiving long-term therapy should have examinations yearly. Periodically monitor serum lipid levels, blood pressure, body weight, and hepatic function, as ordered.
• When used to treat hypogonadism, duration of therapy needed to produce withdrawal bleeding depends on patient's en-

dometrial response to drug. If satisfactory withdrawal bleeding doesn't occur, an oral progestin is added to the regimen, as ordered. Explain to patient that, despite return of withdrawal bleeding, pregnancy can't occur because she doesn't ovulate.
• Be aware of the following estropipate/ estrone equivalents:
0.75 mg estropipate = 0.625 mg estrone
1.5 mg estropipate = 1.25 mg estrone
3 mg estropipate = 2.5 mg estrone
6 mg estropipate = 5 mg estrone
• Because of risk of thromboembolism, therapy should be discontinued at least 1 month before procedures associated with prolonged immobilization or thromboembolism, such as knee or hip surgery.

☑ **Patient teaching**
• Tell patient that package insert describing estrogen's adverse effects is available; also explain effects.
• Tell diabetic patient to report elevated glucose test results to doctor.
• Stress importance of regular physical examinations. Postmenopausal women who use estrogen replacement for over 5 years may have increased risk of endometrial cancer. Using cyclic therapy and lowest possible estrogen dosage reduces risk. Adding progestins to regimen decreases risk of endometrial hyperplasia; however, it isn't known if progestins affect risk of endometrial cancer. No increased risk of breast cancer has been reported.
• *Alert:* Warn patient to immediately report abdominal pain; pain, stiffness, or numbness in legs or buttocks; pressure or pain in chest; shortness of breath; severe headaches; visual disturbances, such as blind spots or flashing lights; vaginal bleeding or discharge; breast lumps; swelling of hands or feet; yellow skin or sclera; dark urine; and light-colored stools.
• Teach woman how to perform routine breast self-examination.
• Advise patient not to become pregnant while on estrogen therapy.

## ethinyl estradiol (ethinyloestradiol)
Estinyl**

*Pregnancy Risk Category X*

### HOW SUPPLIED
*Tablets:* 0.02 mg, 0.05 mg, 0.5 mg

### ACTION
Increases synthesis of DNA, RNA, and protein in responsive tissues. Also reduces release of follicle-stimulating and luteinizing hormones from the pituitary gland.

| Route | Onset | Peak | Duration |
|-------|-------|------|----------|
| P.O. | Unknown | Unknown | Unknown |

### INDICATIONS & DOSAGE
*Palliative treatment of metastatic breast cancer (at least 5 years after menopause)—*
**Women:** 1 mg P.O. t.i.d. for at least 3 months.
*Female hypogonadism—*
**Women:** 0.05 mg P.O. once daily to t.i.d. 2 weeks per month; then 2 weeks of progesterone therapy. Continued for 3 to 6 monthly dosing cycles; then 2 months off. Can be given continuously.
*Vasomotor menopausal symptoms—*
**Women:** 0.02 to 0.05 mg P.O. daily for cycles of 3 weeks on and 1 week off. Can be given continuously.
*Palliative treatment of metastatic inoperable prostate cancer—*
**Men:** 0.15 to 2 mg P.O. daily.

### ADVERSE REACTIONS
**CNS:** headache, dizziness, chorea, depression, *seizures.*
**CV:** thrombophlebitis; *thromboembolism;* hypertension*; edema, increased risk of CVA, pulmonary embolism, MI.*
**EENT:** worsening myopia or astigmatism, intolerance to contact lenses.
**GI:** nausea, vomiting, abdominal cramps, bloating, anorexia, increased appetite.
**GU:** breakthrough bleeding, altered menstrual flow, dysmenorrhea, amenorrhea, cervical erosion, *increased risk of endometrial cancer,* altered cervical secre-

---

Reactions may be *common,* uncommon, *life-threatening,* or COMMON AND LIFE-THREATENING.

tions, enlargement of uterine fibromas, vaginal candidiasis; gynecomastia, testicular atrophy, impotence.
**Hematologic:** increased PT and clotting factors VII to X, and norepinephrine-induced platelet aggregation.
**Hepatic:** cholestatic jaundice, *hepatic adenoma.*
**Metabolic:** weight changes.
**Skin:** melasma, urticaria, acne, seborrhea, oily skin, hirsutism or hair loss, erythema nodosum, dermatitis.
**Other:** gallbladder disease, *breast tenderness, enlargement, or secretion; possible increased risk of breast cancer.*

## INTERACTIONS
**Drug-drug.** *Carbamazepine, phenobarbital, rifampin:* decreased effectiveness of estrogen therapy. Monitor closely.
*Corticosteroids:* possible enhanced effects of corticosteroids. Monitor closely.
*Cyclosporine:* increased risk of toxicity. Use together with caution and frequently monitor cyclosporine levels.
*Dantrolene, other hepatotoxic drugs:* increased risk of hepatotoxicity. Monitor closely.
*Oral anticoagulants:* effect of anticoagulant may be decreased. Dosage adjustments may be needed. Monitor PT and INR, as ordered.
*Tamoxifen:* estrogens may interfere with effectiveness of tamoxifen. Avoid concomitant use.
**Drug-food.** *Caffeine:* may increase serum caffeine levels. Monitor effects.
**Drug-lifestyle.** *Smoking:* increased risk of adverse CV effects. If smoking continues, may need alternative therapy.

## EFFECTS ON DIAGNOSTIC TESTS
Glucose tolerance may be impaired. Reduced response to metyrapone test.

## CONTRAINDICATIONS
Contraindicated in patients with thrombophlebitis, thromboembolic disorders, estrogen-dependent neoplasia, breast or reproductive organ cancer (except for palliative treatment), or undiagnosed abnormal genital bleeding; also contraindicated during pregnancy.

## NURSING CONSIDERATIONS
● Use cautiously in patients with cerebrovascular or coronary artery disease; asthma; mental depression; bone disease; or cardiac, hepatic, or renal dysfunction; and in women with family history (mother, grandmother, sister) of breast or genital tract cancer or who have breast nodules, fibrocystic breasts, or abnormal mammographic findings.
● Ensure that patient has thorough physical examination before initiating estrogen therapy. Patients receiving long-term therapy should have examinations yearly. Periodically monitor serum lipid levels, blood pressure, body weight, and hepatic function, as ordered.
● Because of risk of thromboembolism, therapy should be discontinued at least 1 month before procedures associated with prolonged immobilization or thromboembolism, such as knee or hip surgery.
● Notify pathologist about patient receiving estrogen therapy when specimens are obtained and sent to laboratory for evaluation.

### ✅ Patient teaching
● Tell patient that package insert describing estrogen's adverse effects is available; however, also give patient verbal explanation.
● Emphasize importance of regular physical examinations. Postmenopausal women who use estrogen replacement for over 5 years to treat menopausal symptoms may be at increased risk for endometrial cancer. This risk is reduced by using cyclic rather than continuous therapy and the lowest possible dosages of estrogen. Adding progestins to the regimen decreases risk of endometrial hyperplasia; however, it isn't known if progestins affect risk of endometrial cancer. No increased risk of breast cancer has been reported.
● Explain to patient on cyclic therapy for postmenopausal symptoms that, although withdrawal bleeding may occur during week off drug, fertility isn't restored. Pregnancy can't occur because patient doesn't ovulate.
● *Alert:* Warn patient to immediately report abdominal pain; pain, numbness, or

stiffness in legs or buttocks; pressure or pain in chest; shortness of breath; severe headaches; visual disturbances such as blind spots, flashing lights, or blurriness; vaginal bleeding or discharge; breast lumps; swelling of hands or feet; yellow skin or sclera; dark urine; or light-colored stools.

• Tell diabetic patient to report elevated blood glucose level test results; antidiabetic dosage may be adjusted.

• Teach woman how to perform routine breast self-examination.

• Teach patient methods to decrease risk of thromboembolism.

---

**ethinyl estradiol and desogestrel**
monophasic: Desogen, Marvelon§, Ortho-Cept

**ethinyl estradiol and ethynodiol diacetate**
monophasic: Demulen 1/35, Demulen 1/50

**ethinyl estradiol and levonorgestrel**
monophasic: Alesse-21, Alesse-28, Levlen, Levora-21, Levora-28, Nordette-21, Nordette-28

triphasic: Microgynon-30§, Ovran-30§, Ovranette§, Tri-Levlen, Triphasil

**ethinyl estradiol and norethindrone**
monophasic: Brevicon, Genora 0.5/35, Genora 1/35, ModiCon, N.E.E. 1/35, Nelova 0.5/35E, Nelova 1/35E, Norethin 1/35E, Norinyl 1 + 35, Ortho-Novum 1/35, Ovcon-35, Ovcon-50

biphasic: Jenest, Nelova 10/11, Ortho-Novum 10/11

triphasic: Ortho-Novum 7/7/7, Tri-Norinyl

**ethinyl estradiol and norethindrone acetate**
monophasic: Loestrin 1/20, Loestrin 1.5/30

**ethinyl estradiol and norgestimate**
monophasic: Ortho-Cyclen

triphasic: Ortho Tri-Cyclen

**ethinyl estradiol and norgestrel**
monophasic: Lo/Ovral, Ovral

**ethinyl estradiol, norethindrone acetate, and ferrous fumarate**
monophasic: Loestrin Fe 1/20, Loestrin Fe 1.5/30

**mestranol and norethindrone**
monophasic: Genora 1/50, Nelova 1/50M, Norethin 1/50M, Norinyl 1/50, Ortho-Novum 1/50

*Pregnancy Risk Category X*

---

**HOW SUPPLIED**
*Monophasic oral contraceptives*
**ethinyl estradiol and desogestrel**
*Tablets:* ethinyl estradiol 30 mcg and desogestrel 0.15 mg (Desogen, Ortho-Cept)
**ethinyl estradiol and ethynodiol diacetate**
*Tablets:* ethinyl estradiol 35 mcg and ethynodiol diacetate 1 mg (Demulen 1/35); ethinyl estradiol 50 mcg and ethynodiol diacetate 1 mg (Demulen 1/50)
**ethinyl estradiol and levonorgestrel**
*Tablets:* ethinyl estradiol 30 mcg and levonorgestrel 0.15 mg (Levlen, Levora, Microgynon-30, Ovran-30, Ovranette, Nordette-21, Nordette-28); ethinyl estradiol 20 mg and levonorgestrel 0.1 mg (Alesse-21, Alesse-28)
**ethinyl estradiol and norethindrone**
*Tablets:* ethinyl estradiol 35 mcg and norethindrone 0.4 mg (Ovcon-35); ethinyl estradiol 35 mcg and norethindrone 0.5 mg (Brevicon, Genora 0.5/35, Modi-Con, Nelova 0.5/35E); ethinyl estradiol 35 mcg and norethindrone 1 mg (Genora 1/35, N.E.E. 1/35, Nelova 1/35E,

---

Norethin 1/35E, Norinyl 1/35, Ortho-Novum 1/35); ethinyl estradiol 50 mcg and norethindrone 1 mg (Ovcon-50)
**ethinyl estradiol and norethindrone acetate**
*Tablets:* ethinyl estradiol 20 mcg and norethindrone acetate 1 mg (Loestrin 1/20); ethinyl estradiol 30 mcg and norethindrone acetate 1.5 mg (Loestrin 1.5/30)
**ethinyl estradiol and norgestimate**
*Tablets:* ethinyl estradiol 35 mcg and norgestimate 0.25 mg (Ortho-Cyclen)
**ethinyl estradiol and norgestrel**
*Tablets:* ethinyl estradiol 30 mcg and norgestrel 0.3 mg (Lo/Ovral); ethinyl estradiol 50 mcg and norgestrel 0.5 mg (Ovral)
**ethinyl estradiol, norethindrone acetate, and ferrous fumarate**
*Tablets:* ethinyl estradiol 20 mcg, norethindrone acetate 1 mg, and ferrous fumarate 75 mg (Loestrin Fe 1/20); ethinyl estradiol 30 mcg, norethindrone acetate 1.5 mg, and ferrous fumarate 75 mg (Loestrin Fe 1.5/30)
**mestranol and norethindrone**
*Tablets:* mestranol 50 mcg and norethindrone 1 mg (Genora 1/50, Nelova 1/50M, Norethin 1/50M, Norinyl 1/50, Ortho-Novum 1/50)
*Biphasic oral contraceptives*
**ethinyl estradiol and norethindrone**
*Tablets:* ethinyl estradiol 35 mcg and norethindrone 0.5 mg during phase 1 (10 days); ethinyl estradiol 35 mcg and norethindrone 1 mg during phase 2 (11 days) (Jenest, Nelova 10/11, Ortho-Novum 10/11)
*Triphasic oral contraceptives*
**ethinyl estradiol and levonorgestrel**
*Tablets:* (Tri-Levlen, Triphasil) ethinyl estradiol 30 mcg and levonorgestrel 0.05 mg during phase 1 (6 days); ethinyl estradiol 40 mcg and levonorgestrel 0.075 mg during phase 2 (5 days); ethinyl estradiol 30 mcg and levonorgestrel 0.125 mg during phase 3 (10 days); ethinyl estradiol 30 mcg and levonorgestrel 0.15 mg (Microgynon-30§, Ovran-30§, Ovranette§)
**ethinyl estradiol and norethindrone**
*Tablets:* (Tri-Norinyl) ethinyl estradiol 35 mcg and norethindrone 0.5 mg during

phase 1 (7 days); ethinyl estradiol 35 mcg and norethindrone 1 mg during phase 2 (9 days); ethinyl estradiol 35 mcg and norethindrone 0.5 mg during phase 3 (5 days); (Ortho-Novum 7/7/7) ethinyl estradiol 35 mcg and norethindrone 0.5 mg during phase 1 (7 days); ethinyl estradiol 35 mcg and norethindrone 0.75 mg during phase 2 (7 days); ethinyl estradiol 35 mcg and norethindrone 1 mg during phase 3 (7 days)
**ethinyl estradiol and norgestimate**
*Tablets:* (Ortho Tri-Cyclen) ethinyl estradiol 35 mcg and norgestimate 0.18 mg during phase 1 (7 days); ethinyl estradiol 35 mcg and norgestimate 0.215 mg during phase 2 (7 days); ethinyl estradiol 35 mcg and norgestimate 0.25 mg during phase 3 (7 days)

## ACTION

Oral contraceptives inhibit ovulation through a negative feedback mechanism directed at the hypothalamus. They also may prevent transport of the ovum through the fallopian tubes.

Estrogen suppresses secretion of follicle-stimulating hormone, blocking follicular development and ovulation.

Progestin suppresses secretion of luteinizing hormone so that ovulation can't occur even if the follicle develops. Progestin thickens cervical mucus, which interferes with sperm migration, and causes endometrial changes that prevent implantation of the fertilized ovum.

| Route | Onset | Peak | Duration |
|-------|-------|------|----------|
| P.O. | Unknown | 0.5-4 hr | Unknown |

## INDICATIONS & DOSAGE

*Contraception—*
**Women:** *Monophasic oral contraceptives:* 1 tablet P.O. daily, beginning on day 5 of menstrual cycle (first day of menstrual flow is day 1). With 20- and 21-tablet packages, new dosing cycle begins 7 days after last tablet taken. With 28-tablet packages, dosage is 1 tablet daily without interruption; extra tablets are placebos or contain iron.
*Biphasic oral contraceptives:* 1 color tablet P.O. daily for 10 days; then next color tablet for 11 days. With 21-tablet

---

*Liquid contains alcohol.  **May contain tartrazine.  †Canada  ‡Australia  §U.K.  ◊OTC

packages, new dosing cycle begins 7 days after last tablet taken. With 28-tablet packages, dose is 1 tablet daily without interruption.

*Triphasic oral contraceptives:* 1 tablet P.O. daily in the sequence specified by the brand. With 21-tablet packages, new dosing cycle begins 7 days after last tablet taken. With 28-tablet packages, dose is 1 tablet daily without interruption.

*Acne vulgaris—*

**Women:** 1 tablet P.O. daily, using the 28-day package of Ortho Tri-Cyclen. Dosage schedule for acne should follow the same guidelines for Ortho Tri-Cyclen as when used for contraception.

## ADVERSE REACTIONS

**CNS:** *headache, dizziness,* depression, lethargy, migraine.

**CV:** *thromboembolism,* hypertension, edema, *pulmonary embolism, CVA.*

**EENT:** worsening myopia or astigmatism, intolerance of contact lenses, exophthalmos, diplopia.

**GI:** *nausea,* vomiting, abdominal cramps, bloating, anorexia, changes in appetite, *pancreatitis.*

**GU:** *breakthrough bleeding, spotting,* granulomatous colitis, dysmenorrhea, amenorrhea, cervical erosion or abnormal secretions, enlargement of uterine fibromas, vaginal candidiasis.

**Hematologic:** increased PT and clotting factors VII to X, and norepinephrine-induced platelet aggregation.

**Hepatic:** cholestatic jaundice, *liver tumors.*

**Metabolic:** weight gain.

**Skin:** rash, acne, *erythema multiforme.*

**Other:** gallbladder disease; breast tenderness, enlargement, or secretion.

## INTERACTIONS

**Drug-drug.** *Carbamazepine, phenobarbital, phenytoin, rifampin:* decreased effectiveness of estrogen therapy. Monitor closely.

*Corticosteroids:* possible enhanced effects of corticosteroids. Monitor closely.

*Griseofulvin, penicillins, sulfonamides, tetracyclines:* may decrease effectiveness of oral contraceptives. Avoid concomitant use, if possible.

*Insulin, sulfonylureas:* glucose intolerance may decrease effects of antidiabetics. Monitor effects.

*Oral anticoagulants:* effect of anticoagulant may be decreased. Dosage adjustments may be needed. Monitor PT and INR, as ordered.

*Tamoxifen:* estrogens may interfere with effectiveness of tamoxifen. Avoid concomitant use.

**Drug-food.** *Caffeine:* may increase serum caffeine levels. Monitor effects.

**Drug-lifestyle.** *Smoking:* increased risk of adverse CV effects. If smoking continues, may need alternative therapy.

## EFFECTS ON DIAGNOSTIC TESTS

Glucose tolerance may be impaired.

## CONTRAINDICATIONS

Contraindicated in patients with thromboembolic disorders, cerebrovascular or coronary artery disease, diplopia or ocular lesions arising from ophthalmic vascular disease, classical migraine, MI, known or suspected breast cancer, known or suspected estrogen-dependent neoplasia, benign or malignant liver tumors, active liver disease or history of cholestatic jaundice with pregnancy or previous use of oral contraceptives, and undiagnosed abnormal vaginal bleeding; also contraindicated in known or suspected pregnancy and in breast-feeding women.

## NURSING CONSIDERATIONS

• Use cautiously in patients with cardiac, renal, or hepatic insufficiency; hyperlipidemia; hypertension; migraine; seizure disorders; or asthma.

• Estrogen-containing oral contraceptives should be used with caution in patients who smoke.

• Triphasic oral contraceptives may cause fewer adverse reactions, such as breakthrough bleeding and spotting.

• The Centers for Disease Control and Prevention reports that use of oral contraceptives may decrease risk of ovarian and endometrial cancers. Also, oral contraceptives don't appear to increase woman's risk of breast cancer. However, the FDA reports that oral contraceptives may be

---

Reactions may be *common,* uncommon, *life-threatening,* or COMMON AND LIFE-THREATENING.

linked to an increased risk of cervical cancer.

• Monitor serum lipid levels, blood pressure, body weight, and hepatic function, as ordered.

• *Alert:* Many oral contraceptives share similar names. Be sure to check the strengths of the hormones for verification.

• Many laboratory tests are affected by oral contraceptives.

• Estrogens and progestins may alter glucose tolerance, thus changing dosage requirements for antidiabetics. Monitor blood glucose levels.

• Discontinue oral contraceptive if patient develops granulomatous colitis, and notify doctor.

• Drug should be discontinued at least 1 week before surgery to decrease risk of thromboembolism. Tell patient to use an alternative method of birth control.

### ☑ Patient teaching

• Tell patient to take tablets at same time each day; nighttime dosing may reduce nausea and headaches.

• Advise patient to use an additional method of birth control, such as condoms or a diaphragm with spermicide, for the first week of administration in the initial cycle.

• Tell patient that missing doses in midcycle greatly increases likelihood of pregnancy.

• If one tablet is missed, tell patient to take it as soon as she remembers or to take two tablets the next day and continue regular schedule. If patient misses 2 consecutive days, instruct her to take two tablets daily for 2 days and then resume normal schedule. Also advise her to use an additional method of birth control for 7 days after two missed doses. If three or more doses are missed, tell patient to discard remaining tablets in monthly package and to substitute another contraceptive method. If next menstrual period doesn't begin on schedule, warn patient to rule out pregnancy before starting new dosing cycle. If menstrual period begins, have patient start new dosing cycle 7 days after last tablet was taken.

• Warn patient that headache, nausea, dizziness, breast tenderness, spotting, and breakthrough bleeding are common initially. These effects should diminish after three to six dosing cycles (months).

• Instruct patient to weigh herself at least twice a week and to report any sudden weight gain or edema to doctor.

• Warn patient to avoid exposure to ultraviolet light or prolonged exposure to sunlight.

• *Alert:* Warn patient to immediately report abdominal pain; numbness, stiffness, or pain in legs or buttocks; pressure or pain in chest; shortness of breath; severe headache; visual disturbances such as blind spots, blurriness, or flashing lights; undiagnosed vaginal bleeding or discharge; two consecutive missed menstrual periods; lumps in the breast; swelling of hands or feet; or severe pain in the abdomen (tumor rupture in liver).

• Advise patient of increased risks associated with simultaneous use of cigarettes and oral contraceptives.

• If one menstrual period is missed and tablets have been taken on schedule, tell patient to continue taking them. If two consecutive menstrual periods are missed, tell patient to stop drug and have pregnancy test. Progestins may cause birth defects if taken early in pregnancy.

• Advise patient not to take same drug for longer than 12 months without consulting doctor. Stress importance of Papanicolaou tests and annual gynecologic examinations.

• Advise patient to check with doctor about how soon pregnancy may be attempted after hormonal therapy is stopped. Many doctors recommend that women not become pregnant within 2 months after stopping drug.

• Warn patient of possible delay in achieving pregnancy when drug is discontinued.

• Tell patient that many doctors advise women on long-term therapy (5 years or longer) to stop drug and use other birth control methods. Periodically reassess patient while off hormone therapy.

• Teach woman how to perform routine breast self-examination.

---

• Teach patient methods to decrease risk of thromboembolism.
• Advise patient taking oral contraceptives to use additional form of birth control during concurrent treatment with certain antibiotics.

---

**levonorgestrel**
Norplant System

*Pregnancy Risk Category X*

---

### HOW SUPPLIED
*Implants:* 36 mg per capsule; each kit contains six capsules

### ACTION
Slowly releases synthetic progestin levonorgestrel into bloodstream. How progestins provide contraception isn't fully understood, but they alter the mucus covering the cervix, prevent implantation of the egg and, in some patients, prevent ovulation.

| Route | Onset | Peak | Duration |
|-------|-------|------|----------|
| Subdermal | 24 hr | 24 hr | Unknown |

### INDICATIONS & DOSAGE
*Prevention of pregnancy—*
**Women:** six capsules implanted subdermally in the midportion of upper arm, about 8 cm above elbow crease, during first 7 days of onset of menses. Capsules are placed in fanlike position, 15 degrees apart (total of 75 degrees). Contraceptive efficacy lasts for 5 years.

### ADVERSE REACTIONS
**CNS:** headache, nervousness, dizziness.
**GI:** nausea, *abdominal discomfort,* appetite change.
**GU:** *amenorrhea, many days of bleeding or prolonged bleeding, spotting,* irregular onset of bleeding, frequent onset of bleeding, scanty bleeding, cervicitis, vaginitis, leukorrhea.
**Metabolic:** weight gain.
**Musculoskeletal:** bone and muscle pain.
**Skin:** dermatitis, acne, hirsutism, hypertrichosis, alopecia; infection, transient pain or itching at implant site.

**Other:** adnexal enlargement, mastalgia, *removal difficulty,* breast discharge.

### INTERACTIONS
**Drug-drug.** *Carbamazepine, phenytoin, rifampin:* may reduce contraceptive efficacy of levonorgestrel implants. Monitor closely.
**Drug-food.** *Caffeine:* may increase serum caffeine levels. Monitor effects.
**Drug-lifestyle.** *Smoking:* increased risk of adverse CV effects. If smoking continues, may need alternative therapy.

### EFFECTS ON DIAGNOSTIC TESTS
None reported.

### CONTRAINDICATIONS
Contraindicated in patients with active thrombophlebitis or thromboembolic disorders, undiagnosed abnormal genital bleeding, acute liver disease, malignant or benign liver tumors, known or suspected breast cancer; also contraindicated in known or suspected pregnancy.

### NURSING CONSIDERATIONS
• Use cautiously in patients with history of depression or hyperlipidemia and in diabetic or prediabetic patients.
• Drug can be used 5 days postpartum after lactation has been established.
• Most patients develop variations in menstrual bleeding patterns, including irregular bleeding, prolonged bleeding, spotting, and amenorrhea. In most patients, these irregularities diminish over time (could last up to 1 year).
• Irregular bleeding may mask symptoms of cervical or endometrial cancer.
• Closely monitor patient with condition that may be aggravated by fluid retention because corticosteroid hormones may cause fluid retention.
• Laboratory tests for sex hormone–binding globulin and $T_4$ levels may show decreased values; for $T_3$ uptake, increased values.
• Implants don't contain estrogen. Levonorgestrel is a totally synthetic progestin.
• Expect implants to be removed if patient develops active thrombophlebitis or thromboembolic disease or will be immo-

---

bilized for a significant length of time because of illness or some other factor.
• If jaundice develops, expect implants to be removed because corticosteroid hormone metabolism is impaired in patients with liver failure.
• Although retinal thrombosis after use of oral contraceptives has been reported, no similar incidents have been documented after use of the implant system. However, patients with sudden unexplained vision problems, including users of contact lenses who develop vision changes or changes in lens tolerance, should be immediately evaluated by an ophthalmologist.

☑ **Patient teaching**
• *Alert:* Tell patient to notify doctor immediately if one of the implanted capsules falls out (before the skin heals over the implant). Contraceptive efficacy may be impaired.
• Warn patient that missed menstrual periods aren't an accurate indicator of early pregnancy because drug may induce amenorrhea. Advise patient that 6 weeks or more of amenorrhea (after a pattern of regular menstrual periods) could indicate pregnancy. If pregnancy is confirmed, implants must be removed.
• Instruct patient to report changes in vision.
• Teach woman how to perform breast self-examination.
• Encourage regular (at least annual) physical examinations.
• Teach patient methods to decrease risk of thromboembolism.

---

**medroxyprogesterone acetate**
Amen, Cycrin, Depo-Provera, Provera

*Pregnancy Risk Category X*

**HOW SUPPLIED**
*Tablets:* 2.5 mg, 5 mg, 10 mg
*Injection (suspension):* 150 mg/ml, 400 mg/ml

**ACTION**
Suppresses ovulation, possibly by inhibiting pituitary gonadotropin secretion, thus preventing follicular maturation and causing endometrial thinning.

| Route | Onset | Peak | Duration |
|-------|-------|------|----------|
| P.O., I.M. | Unknown | Unknown | Unknown |

**INDICATIONS & DOSAGE**
*Abnormal uterine bleeding due to hormonal imbalance—*
**Women:** 5 to 10 mg P.O. daily for 5 to 10 days beginning on day 16 of menstrual cycle. If patient also has received estrogen—10 mg P.O. daily for 10 days beginning on day 16 or 21 of cycle.
*Secondary amenorrhea—*
**Women:** 5 to 10 mg P.O. daily for 5 to 10 days. Start at any time during menstrual cycle (usually during latter half of cycle).
*Endometrial or renal cancer—*
**Adults:** 400 to 1,000 mg I.M. weekly. (Dose may be decreased to 400 mg/month when disease has stabilized.)
*Contraception—*
**Women:** 150 mg I.M. once q 3 months.

**ADVERSE REACTIONS**
**CNS:** depression.
**CV:** thrombophlebitis, *pulmonary embolism,* edema, *thromboembolism, CVA.*
**EENT:** exophthalmos, diplopia.
**GI:** *bloating, abdominal pain.*
**GU:** *breakthrough bleeding,* dysmenorrhea, *amenorrhea,* cervical erosion, abnormal secretions.
**Hepatic:** cholestatic jaundice, increased liver function test results.
**Metabolic:** weight changes.
**Skin:** rash, pain, induration, sterile abscesses, acne, pruritus, melasma, alopecia, hirsutism.
**Other:** breast tenderness, enlargement, or secretion.

**INTERACTIONS**
**Drug-drug.** *Aminoglutethimide, carbamazepine, phenobarbital, phenytoin, rifampin:* decreased progestin effects. Monitor for diminished therapeutic response. Tell patient to use a nonhormonal contraceptive during therapy with these drugs.
**Drug-food.** *Caffeine:* may increase serum caffeine levels. Monitor effects.

---

*Liquid contains alcohol.   **May contain tartrazine.   †Canada   ‡Australia   §U.K.   ◇OTC

**Drug-lifestyle.** *Smoking:* increased risk of adverse CV effects. If smoking continues, may need alternative therapy.

## EFFECTS ON DIAGNOSTIC TESTS
Reduced response to metyrapone test.

## CONTRAINDICATIONS
Contraindicated in patients with hypersensitivity to drug and in those with active thromboembolic disorders or past history of thromboembolic disorders, cerebral vascular disease, apoplexy, breast cancer, undiagnosed abnormal vaginal bleeding, missed abortion, or hepatic dysfunction; also contraindicated during pregnancy. Tablets are contraindicated in patients with liver dysfunction or known or suspected malignant disease of genital organs.

## NURSING CONSIDERATIONS
• Use cautiously in patients with diabetes mellitus, seizures, migraine, cardiac or renal disease, asthma, and mental depression.
• Drug shouldn't be used as test for pregnancy; it may cause birth defects and masculinization of female fetus.
• I.M. injection may be painful. Monitor sites for evidence of sterile abscess. Rotate injection sites to prevent muscle atrophy.

### ☑ Patient teaching
• FDA regulations require that, before receiving first dose, patient reads package insert explaining possible adverse effects of progestins. Also, give patient verbal explanation.
• *Alert:* Tell patient to report unusual symptoms immediately and to stop drug and call doctor if visual disturbances or migraine occur.
• Teach woman how to perform routine breast self-examination.
• Advise patient that injection must be administered every 3 months to maintain adequate contraceptive effects.

# norethindrone
Micronor, Nor-QD

# norethindrone acetate
Aygestin

*Pregnancy Risk Category X*

## HOW SUPPLIED
**norethindrone**
*Tablets:* 0.35 mg
**norethindrone acetate**
*Tablets:* 5 mg

## ACTION
Suppresses ovulation, possibly by inhibiting pituitary gonadotropin secretion, and forms thick cervical mucus.

| Route | Onset | Peak | Duration |
|-------|-------|------|----------|
| P.O. | Unknown | Unknown | Unknown |

## INDICATIONS & DOSAGE
*Amenorrhea, abnormal uterine bleeding—*
**Women:** 2.5 to 10 mg norethindrone acetate P.O. daily on days 5 to 25 of menstrual cycle.
*Endometriosis—*
**Women:** 5 mg norethindrone acetate P.O. daily for 14 days; then increased by 2.5 mg daily q 2 weeks, up to 15 mg daily.
*Contraception—*
**Women:** initially, 0.35 mg norethindrone P.O. on first day of menstruation; then 0.35 mg daily.

## ADVERSE REACTIONS
**CNS:** depression.
**CV:** thrombophlebitis, *pulmonary embolism,* edema, *thromboembolism, CVA.*
**EENT:** exophthalmos, diplopia.
**GI:** *bloating, abdominal pain or cramping.*
**GU:** *breakthrough bleeding,* dysmenorrhea, *amenorrhea,* cervical erosion, abnormal secretions.
**Hepatic:** cholestatic jaundice, increased liver function test results.
**Metabolic:** weight changes.
**Skin:** melasma, rash, acne, pruritus.
**Other:** breast tenderness, enlargement, or secretion.

---

Reactions may be *common,* uncommon, *life-threatening,* or COMMON AND LIFE-THREATENING.

## INTERACTIONS
**Drug-drug.** *Barbiturates, carbamazepine, phenytoin, rifampin:* decreased progestin effects. Monitor for diminished therapeutic response.
**Drug-food.** *Caffeine:* may increase serum caffeine levels. Monitor effects.
**Drug-lifestyle.** *Smoking:* increased risk of adverse CV effects. If smoking continues, may need alternative therapy.

## EFFECTS ON DIAGNOSTIC TESTS
Reduced response to metyrapone test.

## CONTRAINDICATIONS
Contraindicated in patients with hypersensitivity to drug and in those with breast cancer, undiagnosed abnormal vaginal bleeding, severe hepatic disease, or missed abortion; also contraindicated in those with thromboembolic disorders, cerebral apoplexy, or history of these conditions; and during pregnancy.

## NURSING CONSIDERATIONS
• Use cautiously in patients with diabetes mellitus, seizures, migraine, cardiac or renal disease, asthma, and mental depression.
• Norethindrone acetate is twice as potent as norethindrone. Norethindrone acetate shouldn't be used for contraception.
• Use as test for pregnancy isn't appropriate; drug may cause birth defects and masculinization of female fetus.
• Preliminary estrogen treatment is usually needed in menstrual disorders.
• Watch patient carefully for signs of edema.
• Monitor blood pressure.

### ☑ Patient teaching
• FDA regulations require that, before receiving first dose, patient reads package insert explaining possible adverse effects of progestin. Also give patient verbal explanation.
• Tell patient that drug needs to be taken at same time every day when used as a contraceptive.
• *Alert:* Tell patient to report unusual symptoms immediately and to stop drug and call doctor if visual disturbances or migraine occurs.

• Teach woman how to perform routine breast self-examination.
• Inform patient what to do if dose is missed.

## norgestrel
Ovrette**

*Pregnancy Risk Category X*

## HOW SUPPLIED
*Tablets:* 0.075 mg

## ACTION
Unknown. Suppresses ovulation, possibly by inhibiting pituitary gonadotropin secretion, and forms thick cervical mucus.

| Route | Onset | Peak | Duration |
|-------|-------|------|----------|
| P.O. | Unknown | Unknown | Unknown |

## INDICATIONS & DOSAGE
*Contraception—*
**Women:** 0.075 mg P.O. daily starting on first day of menstruation.

## ADVERSE REACTIONS
**CNS:** *cerebral thrombosis or hemorrhage,* migraine, depression.
**CV:** thrombophlebitis, *pulmonary embolism, edema, thromboembolism, CVA,* hypertension.
**EENT:** exophthalmos, diplopia.
**GI:** *bloating, abdominal pain or cramping.*
**GU:** *breakthrough bleeding, change in menstrual flow,* dysmenorrhea, spotting, *amenorrhea,* cervical erosion.
**Hepatic:** cholestatic jaundice, benign hepatic adenomas, increased liver function test results.
**Metabolic:** weight changes.
**Skin:** melasma, rash, acne, pruritus.
**Other:** breast tenderness, enlargement, or secretion.

## INTERACTIONS
**Drug-drug.** *Ampicillin, barbiturates, carbamazepine, griseofulvin, phenylbutazone, phenytoin, rifampin, tetracycline:* decreased progestin effects. Monitor for diminished therapeutic response.

**Drug-food.** *Caffeine:* may increase serum caffeine levels. Monitor effects.

**Drug-lifestyle.** *Smoking:* increased risk of adverse CV effects. If smoking continues, may need alternative therapy.

### EFFECTS ON DIAGNOSTIC TESTS
Reduced response to metyrapone test.

### CONTRAINDICATIONS
Contraindicated in patients with hypersensitivity to drug and in those with thromboembolic disorders, cerebral apoplexy, or history of these conditions; breast cancer; undiagnosed abnormal vaginal bleeding; severe hepatic disease; or missed abortion. Also contraindicated during pregnancy.

### NURSING CONSIDERATIONS
• Use cautiously in patients with diabetes mellitus, seizures, migraine, cardiac or renal disease, asthma, and mental depression.
• Norgestrel is a progestin-only oral contraceptive known as the "minipill."

☑ **Patient teaching**
• FDA regulations require that, before receiving first dose, patient reads package insert explaining possible adverse effects of progestins. Also provide verbal explanation.
• Tell patient to take pill every day, at the same time, even if menstruating.
• Risk of pregnancy increases with each tablet missed. Tell patient who misses one tablet to take it as soon as she remembers and then to take the next tablet at the regular time. Advise patient who misses two tablets to take one as soon as she remembers. She must then take the next regular dose at the usual time and use a nonhormonal method of contraception in addition to norgestrel until 14 tablets have been taken. Instruct patient who misses three or more tablets to discontinue drug and use a nonhormonal method of contraception until after menses. If menstrual period doesn't occur within 45 days, pregnancy testing is needed.
• Advise patient using oral contraceptives of the increased risk of serious adverse CV reactions associated with heavy cigarette smoking (15 or more cigarettes per day). These risks are quite marked in women over age 35.
• Instruct woman to immediately report excessive bleeding or bleeding between menstrual cycles, breast pain or tenderness, vaginal discharge, or swelling of hands or feet.
• *Alert:* Tell patient to report unusual symptoms immediately and to stop drug and call doctor if visual disturbances, migraine, or numbness or tingling in limbs occurs.
• Teach woman how to perform routine breast self-examination.

---

## progesterone
Gesterol 50, Gestone§

*Pregnancy Risk Category X*

### HOW SUPPLIED
*Injection (in oil):* 50 mg/ml

### ACTION
Suppresses ovulation, possibly by inhibiting pituitary gonadotropin secretion, and forms thick cervical mucus.

| Route | Onset | Peak | Duration |
|-------|-------|------|----------|
| I.M. | Unknown | Unknown | Unknown |

### INDICATIONS & DOSAGE
*Amenorrhea—*
**Women:** 5 to 10 mg I.M. daily for 6 to 10 days, usually beginning 8 to 10 days before anticipated start of menstruation. Or as a single 100- to 150-mg I.M. dose.
*Dysfunctional uterine bleeding—*
**Women:** 5 to 10 mg I.M. daily for six doses.

### ADVERSE REACTIONS
**CNS:** depression.
**CV:** thrombophlebitis, *thromboembolism, CVA, pulmonary embolism,* edema, hypertension.
**GU:** *breakthrough bleeding,* dysmenorrhea, *amenorrhea,* cervical erosion, abnormal secretions.
**Hepatic:** abnormal liver function test results, cholestatic jaundice.

---

**Skin:** melasma, rash, acne, pruritus, *pain at injection site.*
**Other:** breast tenderness, enlargement, or secretion.

### INTERACTIONS
**Drug-drug.** *Barbiturates, carbamazepine, phenytoin, rifampin:* decreased progestin effects. Monitor for diminished therapeutic response.

### EFFECTS ON DIAGNOSTIC TESTS
Reduced response to metyrapone test may occur.

### CONTRAINDICATIONS
Contraindicated in patients with hypersensitivity to drug and in those with thromboembolic disorders, cerebral apoplexy, or history of these conditions; breast cancer; undiagnosed abnormal vaginal bleeding; severe hepatic disease; or missed abortion. Also contraindicated during pregnancy. Because of possible allergic reaction, drug shouldn't be given to patients allergic to peanuts or sesame.

### NURSING CONSIDERATIONS
• Use cautiously in patients with diabetes mellitus, seizures, migraine, cardiac or renal disease, asthma, or mental depression.
• Preliminary estrogen treatment is usually needed in menstrual disorders.
• Give oil solutions (peanut oil or sesame oil) via deep I.M. injection. Check sites frequently for irritation. Rotate injection sites.

✅ **Patient teaching**
• FDA regulations require that, before receiving first dose, patient reads package insert explaining possible adverse effects of progestins. Also give patient verbal explanation.
• *Alert:* Tell patient to report unusual symptoms immediately and to stop drug and call doctor if visual disturbances or migraine occurs.
• *Alert:* Tell patient to report increased depression immediately; drug may need to be discontinued.
• Teach woman how to perform routine breast self-examination.

---

*Liquid contains alcohol.     **May contain tartrazine.     †Canada     ‡Australia     §U.K.     ◇OTC

**ganirelix acetate**
**gonadorelin acetate**
**histrelin acetate**
**menotropins**

**COMBINATION PRODUCTS**
None.

❋ *NEW DRUG*

### ganirelix acetate
Antagon

*Pregnancy Risk Category X*

**HOW SUPPLIED**
*Injection:* 250 mcg/0.5 ml in prefilled syringes

**ACTION**
Blocks pituitary gonadotropin-releasing hormone (GnRH) receptors and suppresses physiologic, premature surges of luteinizing hormone (LH) and follicle-stimulating hormone (FSH) in the early to midmenstrual cycle during controlled ovarian hyperstimulation (COH). The lack of physiologic LH and FSH surges may contribute to a satisfactory COH trial.

| Route | Onset | Peak | Duration |
|-------|-------|------|----------|
| S.C. | Unknown | 1 hr | Unknown |

**INDICATIONS & DOSAGE**
*Inhibition of premature LH surges in women undergoing medically supervised COH—*
**Adults:** 250 mcg S.C. once daily during early to midfollicular phase of menstrual cycle. Continue daily until enough follicles of sufficient size are confirmed by ultrasound; human chorionic gonadotropin is then administered to induce final maturation of follicles.

**ADVERSE REACTIONS**
**CNS:** headache.
**GI:** abdominal pain, nausea.
**GU:** vaginal bleeding, gynecologic abdominal pain, ovarian hyperstimulation syndrome.
**Skin:** injection site reaction.
**Other:** *fetal death.*

**INTERACTIONS**
None significant.

**EFFECTS ON DIAGNOSTIC TESTS**
None reported.

**CONTRAINDICATIONS**
Contraindicated in patients with hypersensitivity to drug or its components, GnRH, or GnRH analogues; also contraindicated in pregnant women.

**NURSING CONSIDERATIONS**
• Use cautiously in patients who report previous potential hypersensitivity to GnRH; monitor patient closely after first injection.
• Use cautiously in hypersensitive patients because the natural rubber latex packaging of product may cause allergic reactions.
• Only doctors experienced in infertility treatments should prescribe drug.
• *Alert:* Before starting treatment, ensure that patient isn't pregnant.
• Increased WBC count and decreased bilirubin levels and hematocrit have been observed in patients receiving ganirelix injections.

☑ **Patient teaching**
• Tell patient that the correct use of ganirelix injection is extremely important to success of infertility treatments. Patient should be able to adhere to a strict administration schedule.
• Teach patient proper technique for S.C. administration of drug.
• Advise patient to use abdomen or upper thigh for injection and to vary injection site with each dose.

• Advise patient to store drug at room temperature, away from heat and light, and out of children's reach.
• Inform patient to discontinue drug and report suspected or known pregnancy.

## gonadorelin acetate
Lutrepulse

*Pregnancy Risk Category B*

### HOW SUPPLIED
*Injection:* 0.8 mg/10 ml, 3.2 mg/10-ml vials; supplied as kit with I.V. supplies with or without ambulatory infusion pump

### ACTION
Mimics action of gonadotropin-releasing hormone, resulting in synthesis and release of luteinizing hormone (LH) from anterior pituitary gland. LH then acts upon reproductive organs to regulate hormone synthesis.

| Route | Onset | Peak | Duration |
|-------|-------|------|----------|
| I.V. | Unknown | Unknown | 10-40 min |

### INDICATIONS & DOSAGE
*Induction of ovulation in women with primary hypothalamic amenorrhea—*
**Adults:** 5 mcg I.V. q 90 minutes for 21 days. If no response follows three treatment intervals, increase dosage, as ordered.

### ADVERSE REACTIONS
**Hematologic:** hemoconcentration.
**Metabolic:** fluid and electrolyte imbalance.
**Skin:** hematoma, local infection, inflammation, mild phlebitis, urticaria, pruritus.
**Other:** multiple pregnancy, ovarian hyperstimulation including ascites, pleural effusion.

### INTERACTIONS
**Drug-drug.** *Other ovulation stimulators:* additive effects. Avoid concomitant use.

### EFFECTS ON DIAGNOSTIC TESTS
None reported.

### CONTRAINDICATIONS
Contraindicated in patients with hypersensitivity to drug and in those with ovarian cysts or conditions that could be complicated by pregnancy (such as prolactinoma); also contraindicated in patients who are anovulatory from causes other than a hypothalamic disorder and in those with conditions that may be worsened by reproductive hormones, such as estrogen dependent tumors.

### NURSING CONSIDERATIONS
• Patient usually needs pelvic ultrasound on days 7 and 14 after a baseline scan. Some doctors prefer shorter intervals between scans.

### ◖ I.V. administration
• To mimic the naturally occurring hormone, administer gonadorelin in a pulsatile fashion with available ambulatory infusion pump. Set pulse period at 1 minute (infuse drug over 1 minute) and pulse interval at 90 minutes.
• To give 2.5 mcg/pulse, reconstitute drug in 0.8-mg vial with 8 ml of supplied diluent, and set pump to deliver 25 microliters/pulse. To administer 5 mcg/pulse, use same dosage strength and dilution, but set pump to deliver 50 microliters/pulse.
• Some patients may need higher I.V. doses. To give 10 mcg/pulse, reconstitute drug in 3.2-mg vial with 8 ml of supplied diluent, and set pump to deliver 25 microliters/pulse. To give 20 mcg/pulse, use same dosage strength and dilution, but set pump to deliver 50 microliters/pulse.
• Inspect I.V. site at each visit.

### ☑ Patient teaching
• Ensure that patient understands that multiple pregnancy is possible (incidence is about 12%). Monitoring of dosage and ovarian ultrasonography to monitor drug response are needed.
• Instruct patient about proper aseptic technique and care of I.V. site. Cannula and I.V. site should be changed every 48 hours. Printed instructions are available for patient.
• Anaphylaxis has been reported with similar drugs. Teach patient symptoms of hypersensitivity reactions (rash, hives,

wheezing, difficulty breathing, rapid heartbeat), and encourage her to report these at once.

• Tell patient to report signs of infection, hematoma, inflammation, or phlebitis at injection site. She also should report severe abdominal pain, bloating, swelling of hands or feet, nausea, vomiting, diarrhea, substantial weight gain, or shortness of breath.

• Encourage patient to adhere to close monitoring schedule required by therapy. Regular pelvic examinations, midluteal-phase serum progesterone determinations, and multiple ovarian ultrasound scans are needed.

---

## histrelin acetate
Supprelin

*Pregnancy Risk Category X*

### HOW SUPPLIED
*Injection:* 120 mcg/0.6 ml, 300 mcg/0.6 ml, 600 mcg/0.6 ml

### ACTION
An agonist that mimics effects of gonadotropin-releasing hormone (GnRH; also called luteinizing hormone-releasing hormone) but is more potent. Chronic administration desensitizes responsiveness of pituitary gonadotropin, decreasing sex hormone production by testes or ovaries.

| Route | Onset | Peak | Duration |
|-------|-------|------|----------|
| S.C. | Unknown | Unknown | Unknown |

### INDICATIONS & DOSAGE
*Centrally mediated (idiopathic or neurogenic) precocious puberty—*
**Children (girls ages 2 to 8; boys ages 2 to 9½):** 10 mcg/kg S.C. daily.

### ADVERSE REACTIONS
**CNS:** malaise, *mood changes, nervousness, dizziness, depression, headache, libido changes, insomnia, anxiety,* paresthesia, cognitive changes, syncope, somnolence, lethargy, impaired consciousness, tremor, hyperkinesia, *seizures,* hot flashes, conduct disorder, fatigue.

**CV:** *vasodilation,* edema, palpitations, pallor, tachycardia, hypertension.
**EENT:** epistaxis, ear congestion, abnormal pupillary function, otalgia, visual disturbances, hearing loss, polyopia, photophobia, rhinorrhea, sinusitis, nasal infections.
**GI:** *abdominal pain, nausea, vomiting, diarrhea, flatulence, decreased appetite, dyspepsia,* cramps, constipation, thirst, gastritis, GI distress.
**GU:** *menstrual changes, vaginal dryness, leukorrhea, hypermenorrhea, vaginal bleeding, vaginitis, dysmenorrhea,* tenderness of female genitalia, polyuria, incontinence, dysuria, hematuria, nocturia, glycosuria.
**Hematologic:** hyperlipidemia, anemia, purpura.
**Metabolic:** *weight gain.*
**Musculoskeletal:** *arthralgia, muscle stiffness, muscle cramps.*
**Respiratory:** *upper respiratory infection, respiratory congestion, cough,* asthma, breathing disorder, bronchitis, hyperventilation.
**Skin:** *redness, swelling, acne, rash, diaphoresis,* urticaria, pruritus, alopecia.
**Other:** *breast pain or edema,* breast discharge, decreased breast size, *fever, body pains,* chills, acute hypersensitivity reactions, ***anaphylaxis, angioedema.***

### INTERACTIONS
None significant.

### EFFECTS ON DIAGNOSTIC TESTS
None reported.

### CONTRAINDICATIONS
Contraindicated in patients with hypersensitivity to drug or its ingredients and in pregnant or breast-feeding women.

### NURSING CONSIDERATIONS
• Drug is indicated only for patients who will comply with daily schedule. Noncompliance or inadequate dosing may result in inadequate control of pubertal process, possibly allowing recurrence of symptoms, including onset of menses, breast development, or testicular growth; long-term consequences may involve decreased adult height.

---

Reactions may be *common,* uncommon, *life-threatening,* or COMMON AND LIFE-THREATENING.

• A complete physical and endocrinologic evaluation should be performed before initiating drug therapy; several indices should be reexamined at 3 months, then every 6 to 12 months thereafter. Such evaluations should include determinations of height and weight, hand and wrist X-rays for bone-age determination, sex corticosteroid (estradiol or testosterone) levels, and GnRH stimulation test. Monitor these tests periodically to determine effectiveness of therapy.

• Further tests to rule out other causes of precocious puberty include beta human chorionic gonadotropin levels (to detect chorionic gonadotropin–secreting tumor); pelvic, adrenal, or testicular ultrasound (to detect corticosteroid-secreting tumor); and computed tomography scan of the head (to detect previously undiagnosed intracranial tumors). Workup also sets baseline of gonad size for serial monitoring.

• Refrigerate drug (36° to 46° F [2° to 8° C]) and protect from light in its original container. Use vials only once because drug doesn't contain preservatives. Allow drug to reach room temperature before use.

• Give S.C. and rotate injection sites to minimize local reactions.

• Decreases in follicle-stimulating hormone, luteinizing hormone, and sex corticosteroid levels occur within 3 months.

• Reevaluate patient if prepubertal levels of sex corticosteroids or GnRH test responses aren't achieved within 3 months of therapy.

• Safety and efficacy of drug haven't been established in children under age 2.

☑ **Patient teaching**
• Before therapy, make sure patient and caregiver understand importance of adhering to daily schedules. Tell parents to give drug at same time each day to aid compliance and ensure adequate dosing.

• Drug is dispensed as a 30-day kit that contains a patient information leaflet. Ensure that caregiver reads and understands leaflet.

• Inform patient that, because drug is a peptide, it is destroyed in GI tract and so must be given parenterally.

• Explain importance of rotating injection sites daily. Sites should include upper arms, thighs, and abdomen.

• Warn patient of potential risks and adverse effects of therapy. During first month of treatment, girls commonly experience a slight menstrual flow, which probably is related to decreasing estrogen levels brought on by treatment. As estrogen levels drop, menses begins because estrogens support the endometrium.

• Advise patient to seek medical attention immediately if signs of hypersensitivity reactions occur—sudden rash, difficulty breathing or swallowing, or rapid heartbeat. Also tell her to notify doctor if severe or persistent swelling, redness, or irritation occurs at injection site.

---

## menotropins
Humegon, Menogon§, Pergonal, Repronex

*Pregnancy Risk Category X*

---

### HOW SUPPLIED
*Injection:* 75 IU of luteinizing hormone (LH) and 75 IU of follicle-stimulating hormone (FSH) activity per ampule; 150 IU of LH and 150 IU of FSH activity per ampule

### ACTION
When given to women who haven't had primary ovarian failure, drug mimics FSH in inducing follicular growth and LH in aiding follicular maturation. Drug induces spermatogenesis in men.

| Route | Onset | Peak | Duration |
|-------|-------|------|----------|
| I.M. | 9-12 days | Unknown | Unknown |

### INDICATIONS & DOSAGE
*Anovulation—*
**Women:** 75 IU each of FSH and LH I.M. daily for 9 to 12 days; then 5,000 to 10,000 U of human chorionic gonadotropin (HCG) I.M. 1 day after last dose of menotropins. Repeated for one to three menstrual cycles until ovulation occurs.
*Infertility with ovulation—*
**Women:** 75 IU each of FSH and LH I.M. daily for 9 to 12 days; then 10,000 U

HCG I.M. 1 day after last dose of menotropins. Repeated for two menstrual cycles. Then 150 IU each of FSH and LH daily for 9 to 12 days, followed by 10,000 U HCG I.M. 1 day after last dose of menotropins. Repeated for two menstrual cycles.

*Infertility in men—*

**Men:** prior treatment with HCG of 5,000 U three times a week for 4 to 6 months; then 75 IU each of FSH and LH I.M. three times weekly (given with 2,000 U of HCG twice weekly) for at least 4 months. If increased spermatogenesis doesn't occur, increase to 150 IU each of FSH and LH three times weekly (dose of HCG remains unchanged).

## ADVERSE REACTIONS
**CNS:** headache, malaise, dizziness.
**CV:** tachycardia, venous thrombophlebitis, *CVA.*
**GI:** nausea, vomiting, diarrhea, abdominal cramps, bloating.
**GU:** *gynecomastia, ovarian enlargement with pain and abdominal distention,* multiple births, ovarian hyperstimulation syndrome, ovarian cysts, ectopic pregnancy.
**Musculoskeletal:** musculoskeletal aches, joint pains.
**Respiratory:** *atelectasis, acute respiratory distress syndrome, pulmonary embolism, pulmonary infarction, arterial occlusion,* dyspnea, tachypnea.
**Skin:** rash.
**Other:** fever, *hypersensitivity and anaphylactic reactions,* chills.

## INTERACTIONS
None significant.

## EFFECTS ON DIAGNOSTIC TESTS
None reported.

## CONTRAINDICATIONS
Contraindicated in patients with hypersensitivity to drug and in those with primary ovarian failure, uncontrolled thyroid or adrenal dysfunction, pituitary tumor, abnormal uterine bleeding, uterine fibromas, ovarian cysts or enlargement; also contraindicated during pregnancy and in men with normal pituitary function, primary testicular failure, or infertility disorders other than hypogonadotropic hypogonadism.

## NURSING CONSIDERATIONS
• Monitor closely to ensure adequate ovarian stimulation without hyperstimulation.
• Watch for ovarian hyperstimulation syndrome, which may progress rapidly to a serious medical event characterized by dramatic increase in vascular permeability resulting in rapid accumulation of fluid in the peritoneal cavity, thorax, and pericardium. Clinical signs and symptoms include hypovolemia, hemoconcentration, electrolyte imbalance, ascites, hemoperitoneum, pleural effusion, hydrothorax, and thromboembolitic events. Cases are more common and severe if pregnancy occurs.
• Reconstitute with 1 to 2 ml of sterile normal saline for injection. Use immediately.
• Rotate injection sites.

☑ **Patient teaching**
• Tell patient about possibility of multiple births.
• For patient with infertility, encourage daily intercourse from day before HCG is given until ovulation occurs.
• Tell patient that pregnancy usually occurs 4 to 6 weeks after therapy.
• Instruct patient to immediately report severe abdominal pain, bloating, swelling of hands or feet, nausea, vomiting, diarrhea, substantial weight gain, or shortness of breath.

---

Reactions may be *common*, uncommon, *life-threatening*, or COMMON AND LIFE-THREATENING.

acarbose
chlorpropamide
glimepiride
glipizide
glucagon
glyburide
insulins
metformin hydrochloride
miglitol
pioglitazone hydrochloride
repaglinide
rosiglitazone maleate
troglitazone

### COMBINATION PRODUCTS

HUMULIN 50/50 ◊ : isophane insulin suspension (human) 50% and insulin injection (human) 50%, 100 U/ml.
HUMULIN 70/30 ◊ , NOVOLIN 70/30 ◊ : isophane insulin suspension (human) 70% and insulin injection (human) 30%, 100 U/ml.

---

### acarbose
Glucobay§, Prandaset†, Precose

*Pregnancy Risk Category B*

### HOW SUPPLIED
*Tablets:* 50 mg, 100 mg

### ACTION
An alpha-glucosidase inhibitor that delays digestion of carbohydrates, resulting in a smaller rise in blood glucose level.

| Route | Onset | Peak | Duration |
|-------|-------|------|----------|
| P.O. | Unknown | 1 hr | 2-4 hr |

### INDICATIONS & DOSAGE
*Adjunct to diet to lower blood glucose levels in patients with type 2 non-insulin-dependent diabetes mellitus whose hyperglycemia can't be managed by diet alone or by diet and a sulfonylurea—*
**Adults:** individualized. Initially, 25 mg P.O. t.i.d. with first bite of each main meal. Subsequent dosage adjustment

made q 4 to 8 weeks, based on 1-hour postprandial glucose level and tolerance. Maintenance dose is 50 to 100 mg P.O. t.i.d.
*Adjust-a-dose:* For patients weighing below 60 kg (132 lb), don't exceed 50 mg P.O. t.i.d. For patients weighing over 60 kg, don't exceed 100 mg P.O. t.i.d.
❋ *NEW INDICATION: Adjunct to insulin or metformin therapy in patients with type 2 diabetes mellitus whose hyperglycemia can't be managed by diet, exercise, and insulin or metformin alone—*
**Adults:** initially, 25 mg P.O. t.i.d. with first bite of each main meal. Adjust dosage at 4- to 8-week intervals based on 1-hour postprandial glucose levels and tolerance to determine minimum effective dose of each drug. Maintenance dose is 50 to 100 mg P.O. t.i.d. based on patient's weight. Maximum dose for patients weighing 60 kg or less is 50 mg P.O. t.i.d.; for patients weighing over 60 kg, maximum dose is 100 mg P.O. t.i.d.

### ADVERSE REACTIONS
**GI:** *abdominal pain, diarrhea, flatulence.*
**Metabolic:** elevated serum transaminase level, low serum calcium and plasma vitamin $B_6$ levels.

### INTERACTIONS
**Drug-drug.** *Calcium channel blockers, corticosteroids, estrogens, isoniazid, nicotinic acid, oral contraceptives, phenothiazine, phenytoin, sympathomimetics, thiazides and other diuretics, thyroid products:* may cause hyperglycemia during concomitant use, or hypoglycemia when withdrawn. Monitor blood glucose level.
*Digestive enzyme preparations containing carbohydrate-splitting enzymes (such as amylase, pancreatin), intestinal adsorbents (such as activated charcoal):* may reduce effect of acarbose. Don't administer concomitantly.

### EFFECTS ON DIAGNOSTIC TESTS
None reported.

---

*Liquid contains alcohol.    \*\*May contain tartrazine.    †Canada    ‡Australia    §U.K.    ◊OTC

## CONTRAINDICATIONS

Contraindicated in patients with hypersensitivity to drug and in those with diabetic ketoacidosis, cirrhosis, inflammatory bowel disease, colonic ulceration, partial intestinal obstruction, predisposition to intestinal obstruction, chronic intestinal disease associated with marked disorder of digestion or absorption, or conditions that may deteriorate because of increased intestinal gas formation.

## NURSING CONSIDERATIONS

• Drug isn't recommended for use in patients with cirrhosis or serum creatinine levels over 2 mg/dl and in pregnant or breast-feeding women.
• Use cautiously in patients receiving a sulfonylurea or insulin. Drug isn't recommended for renally impaired patients. Acarbose may increase hypoglycemic potential of the sulfonylurea. Monitor patient receiving both drugs closely. If hypoglycemia occurs, treat patient with oral glucose (dextrose). Severe hypoglycemia may need I.V. glucose infusion or glucagon administration. Because dosage adjustments may be needed to prevent further hypoglycemia, report hypoglycemia and treatment required to doctor. Insulin therapy may be needed during increased stress (infection, fever, surgery, or trauma). Monitor patient closely for hyperglycemia.
• Safety and efficacy of drug haven't been established in children.
• Monitor patient's 1-hour postprandial plasma glucose level to determine therapeutic effectiveness of acarbose and to identify appropriate dose. Report hyperglycemia to doctor. Thereafter, glycosylated hemoglobin should be measured every 3 months.
• Monitor serum transaminase level every 3 months in first year of therapy and periodically thereafter in patients receiving doses in excess of 50 mg t.i.d. Report abnormalities; dosage adjustment or drug withdrawal may be needed.

### ☑ Patient teaching

• Tell patient to take drug daily with first bite of each of three main meals.
• Explain that therapy relieves symptoms but doesn't cure the disease.

• Stress importance of adhering to specific diet, weight reduction, exercise, and hygiene programs. Show patient how to monitor blood glucose level and to recognize and treat hyperglycemia.
• Teach patient taking a sulfonylurea how to recognize hypoglycemia, and to treat symptoms with a form of dextrose rather than with a product containing table sugar.
• Urge patient to carry medical identification at all times.
• Instruct patient about nature of disease, importance of following therapeutic regimen, adhering to specific diet, and weight reduction.

---

## chlorpropamide
Apo-Chlorpropamide†, Diabinese, Novo-Propamide†

*Pregnancy Risk Category C*

## HOW SUPPLIED
*Tablets:* 100 mg, 250 mg

## ACTION
Unknown. A sulfonylurea that probably stimulates insulin release from the pancreatic beta cells and reduces glucose output by the liver. An extrapancreatic effect increases peripheral sensitivity to insulin. Also exerts an antidiuretic effect in patients with diabetes insipidus.

| Route | Onset | Peak | Duration |
|-------|-------|------|----------|
| P.O. | 1 hr | 2-4 hr | 24 hr |

## INDICATIONS & DOSAGE
*Adjunct to diet to lower blood glucose level in patients with type 2 non-insulin-dependent diabetes mellitus—*
**Adults:** 250 mg P.O. daily with breakfast. Initial dosage increased after 5 to 7 days because of extended duration of action; then increased q 3 to 5 days by 50 to 125 mg, if needed, to maximum of 750 mg daily. Some patients with mild diabetes respond well to doses of 100 mg or less daily.
**Elderly:** for patients over age 65, initially 100 to 125 mg P.O. daily; then increase as with adult dose.

---

Reactions may be *common*, uncommon, ***life-threatening***, or **COMMON AND LIFE-THREATENING**.

*Adjust-a-dose:* For patients with renal insufficiency, increase dosage as tolerated.
*To change from insulin to oral therapy—*
**Adults:** if insulin dosage is less than 40 U daily, insulin is stopped and oral therapy started as above. If insulin dosage is 40 U or more daily, oral therapy started as above with insulin reduced 50%. Insulin dosage reduced further according to response.

## ADVERSE REACTIONS
**CNS:** paresthesia, fatigue, dizziness, vertigo, malaise, headache.
**EENT:** tinnitus.
**GI:** nausea, heartburn, epigastric distress.
**GU:** tea-colored urine, elevated BUN and creatinine levels.
**Hematologic:** *leukopenia, thrombocytopenia, aplastic anemia, agranulocytosis,* hemolytic anemia.
**Hepatic:** alterations in cholesterol, alkaline phosphatase, and bilirubin levels; elevated AST and LD levels.
**Metabolic:** *prolonged hypoglycemia, dilutional hyponatremia.*
**Skin:** rash, pruritus, erythema, urticaria.
**Other:** *hypersensitivity reactions.*

## INTERACTIONS
**Drug-drug.** *Anabolic steroids, chloramphenicol, clofibrate, guanethidine, MAO inhibitors, salicylates, sulfonamides:* increased hypoglycemic activity. Monitor blood glucose level.
*Beta blockers:* prolonged hypoglycemic effect and masked symptoms of hypoglycemia. Use together cautiously.
*Corticosteroids, glucagon, rifampin, thiazide diuretics:* decreased hypoglycemic response. Monitor blood glucose level.
*Hydantoins:* increased blood levels of hydantoins. Monitor blood levels.
*Oral anticoagulants:* increased hypoglycemic activity or enhanced anticoagulant effect. Monitor blood glucose level and PT.
**Drug-lifestyle.** *Alcohol use:* altered glycemic control, most commonly hypoglycemia. May also cause a disulfiram-like reaction. Discourage concomitant use.

## EFFECTS ON DIAGNOSTIC TESTS
None reported.

## CONTRAINDICATIONS
Contraindicated in patients with hypersensitivity to drug and in those with type 2 diabetes complicated by ketosis, acidosis, diabetic coma, major surgery, severe infections, or severe trauma; also contraindicated for treating type 1 insulin-dependent diabetes or diabetes that can be adequately controlled by diet and in pregnant or breast-feeding women.

## NURSING CONSIDERATIONS
• Use cautiously in patients with porphyria or impaired hepatic or renal function, or in debilitated, malnourished, or elderly patients. Also use cautiously in patients with known allergy to sulfonamides.
• Elderly patients may be more sensitive to adverse effects.
• Drug may accumulate in patients with renal insufficiency. Watch for and report signs of impending renal insufficiency, such as dysuria, anuria, and hematuria.
• *Alert:* Adverse effects of drug, especially hypoglycemia, may be more frequent or severe than with some other sulfonylureas because of drug's long duration of action. If hypoglycemia occurs, monitor patient closely for minimum of 3 to 5 days.
• Patients transferring from another oral antidiabetic don't usually need a transition period.
• Patients may need hospitalization during transition from insulin therapy to an oral antidiabetic. Monitor patient's blood glucose levels at least t.i.d. before meals.
• *Alert:* Don't confuse chlorpropamide with chlorpromazine.

### ☑ Patient teaching
• Instruct patient about nature of disease, importance of following therapeutic regimen, adhering to specific diet, weight reduction, exercise, and personal hygiene programs, and about avoiding infection. Explain how and when to perform self-monitoring of blood glucose level, and teach recognition of and intervention for hypoglycemia and hyperglycemia.
• Make sure patient understands that therapy only relieves symptoms.

---

• Tell patient not to change drug dosage without doctor's consent and to report abnormal blood or urine glucose test results.
• Teach patient to carry candy or other simple sugars to treat mild hypoglycemic episodes. Patient experiencing severe episode may need hospital treatment.
• Advise patient not to take other drugs, including OTC drugs, without first checking with doctor.
• Advise patient to avoid alcohol consumption. Chlorpropamide-alcohol flush is characterized by facial flushing, light-headedness, headache, and occasional breathlessness. Even very small amounts of alcohol can produce this reaction.
• Advise patient to carry medical identification at all times.
• *Alert:* Tell patient to report rash, skin eruptions, and other signs and symptoms of hypersensitivity to doctor immediately.

---

## glimepiride
Amaryl

*Pregnancy Risk Category C*

### HOW SUPPLIED
*Tablets:* 1 mg, 2 mg, 4 mg

### ACTION
Exact mechanism unknown. Lowers blood glucose levels, possibly by stimulating release of insulin from functioning pancreatic beta cells. Drug can also lead to increased sensitivity of peripheral tissues to insulin.

| Route | Onset | Peak | Duration |
|-------|-------|------|----------|
| P.O. | Unknown | 2-3 hr | > 24 hr |

### INDICATIONS & DOSAGE
*Adjunct to diet and exercise to lower blood glucose levels in patients with type 2 non-insulin-dependent diabetes mellitus whose hyperglycemia can't be managed by diet and exercise alone—*
**Adults:** initially, 1 to 2 mg P.O. once daily with first main meal of day; usual maintenance dose is 1 to 4 mg P.O. once daily. After reaching dosage of 2 mg, dosage is increased in increments not exceeding 2 mg q 1 to 2 weeks, based on patient's

blood glucose level response. Maximum dose is 8 mg/day.
*Adjunct to insulin therapy in patients with type 2 diabetes mellitus whose hyperglycemia can't be managed by diet and exercise with oral hypoglycemics—*
**Adults:** 8 mg P.O. once daily with first main meal of day; used with low-dose insulin. Insulin adjusted upward weekly, p.r.n., based on patient's blood glucose level response.
✳ *NEW INDICATION: Adjunct to metformin therapy in patients with type 2 diabetes mellitus whose hyperglycemia can't be managed by diet, exercise, and glimepiride or metformin alone—*
**Adults:** 8 mg P.O. once daily with first main meal of day with metformin if patient doesn't respond adequately to glimepiride monotherapy. Adjust dosages based on patient's blood glucose level to determine minimum effective dose of each drug.
*Adjust-a-dose:* For renally impaired patients, initial dose 1 mg P.O. once daily with first main meal of day; then appropriate dosage adjusted, p.r.n.

### ADVERSE REACTIONS
**CNS:** dizziness, asthenia, headache.
**EENT:** changes in accommodation.
**GI:** nausea.
**GU:** elevated BUN and creatinine levels.
**Hematologic:** *leukopenia,* hemolytic anemia, *agranulocytosis, thrombocytopenia, aplastic anemia, pancytopenia.*
**Hepatic:** cholestatic jaundice, elevated transaminase and alkaline phosphatase levels.
**Metabolic:** hypoglycemia, dilutional hyponatremia.
**Skin:** pruritus, erythema, urticaria, morbilliform or maculopapular eruptions.

### INTERACTIONS
**Drug-drug.** *Beta blockers:* may mask symptoms of hypoglycemia. Monitor blood glucose level.
*Drugs that tend to produce hyperglycemia (such as corticosteroids, estrogens, isoniazid, nicotinic acid, oral contraceptives, other diuretics, phenothiazines, phenytoin, sympathomimetic thiazides, thyroid*

---

Reactions may be *common,* uncommon, *life-threatening,* or COMMON AND LIFE-THREATENING.

*products):* may lead to loss of glucose control. Adjust dosage, as ordered.
*Insulin:* may increase potential for hypoglycemia. Avoid concomitant use.
*NSAIDs, other drugs that are highly protein-bound (such as beta blockers, chloramphenicol, coumarins, MAO inhibitors, probenecid, salicylates, sulfonamides):* may potentiate hypoglycemic action of sulfonylureas such as glimepiride. Monitor blood glucose levels carefully.
**Drug-lifestyle.** *Alcohol use:* altered glycemic control, most commonly hypoglycemia. May also cause disulfiram-like reaction. Discourage concomitant use.

**EFFECTS ON DIAGNOSTIC TESTS**
None reported.

**CONTRAINDICATIONS**
Contraindicated in patients with hypersensitivity to drug and in those with diabetic ketoacidosis, which should be treated with insulin.

**NURSING CONSIDERATIONS**
● Use cautiously in debilitated or malnourished patients and in those with adrenal, pituitary, hepatic, or renal insufficiency; these patients are more susceptible to the hypoglycemic action of glucose-lowering drugs. Use of drug isn't recommended in elderly patients. Also use caution in patients with known allergy to sulfonamides.
● Glimepiride and insulin may be used concurrently in secondary failure patients (those who lose glucose control after initially responding to therapy).
● Monitor fasting blood glucose level periodically to determine therapeutic response. Also monitor glycosylated hemoglobin, usually every 3 to 6 months, to precisely assess long-term glycemic control.
● Oral hypoglycemics have been associated with an increased risk of CV mortality compared with diet alone or with diet and insulin therapy.
● Safety and effectiveness of drug in children haven't been established.
● It isn't known if drug appears in breast milk. Don't administer drug to breast-

feeding women because of potential for hypoglycemia in breast-fed infants.
● When changing patient from other hypoglycemics (sulfonylureas) to glimepiride, a transition period isn't needed.
● **Alert:** Don't confuse glimepiride with glyburide or glipizide.

**☑ Patient teaching**
● Tell patient to take drug with first meal of the day.
● Make sure patient understands that therapy relieves symptoms but doesn't cure the disease. He should also understand potential risks and advantages of taking drug and other treatment methods.
● Stress importance of adhering to diet, weight reduction, exercise, and personal hygiene programs. Explain to patient and family how and when to perform self-monitoring of blood glucose levels, and teach recognition of and intervention for signs and symptoms of hyperglycemia and hypoglycemia.
● Advise patient to carry medical identification at all times.
● Advise woman planning a pregnancy to consult doctor before becoming pregnant. Insulin may be needed during pregnancy and breast-feeding.
● Teach patient to carry candy or other simple sugars to treat mild hypoglycemic episodes. Patient experiencing severe episode may need hospital treatment.
● Inform patient that alcohol lowers blood glucose level, and therefore should be avoided.

---

**glipizide**
Glibenese§, Glucotrol, Glucotrol XL, Minidiab‡

*Pregnancy Risk Category C*

**HOW SUPPLIED**
*Tablets:* 5 mg, 10 mg
*Tablets (extended-release):* 5 mg, 10 mg

**ACTION**
Unknown. A sulfonylurea that probably stimulates insulin release from the pancreatic beta cells and reduces glucose out-

put by the liver. An extrapancreatic effect increases peripheral sensitivity to insulin.

| Route | Onset | Peak | Duration |
|-------|-------|------|----------|
| P.O. | 15-30 min | 1-3 hr | 4 hr |
| P.O. (extended) | 2-3 hr | 6-12 hr | 24 hr |

## INDICATIONS & DOSAGE

*Adjunct to diet to lower blood glucose level in patients with type 2 non-insulin-dependent diabetes mellitus—*
**Adults:** initially, 5 mg P.O. daily 30 minutes before breakfast. Maximum once-daily dose is 15 mg. Doses above 15 mg should be divided; maximum total daily dose is 40 mg for immediate-release tablets. *Extended-release tablets:* initially, 5 mg P.O. daily. Adjust in 5-mg increments q 3 months depending on level of glycemic control. Maximum daily dose is 20 mg.
**Elderly:** for patients over age 65, initial dose is 2.5 mg P.O. daily.
*Adjust-a-dose:* For patients with liver disease, initial dose is 2.5 mg P.O. daily.
*To replace insulin therapy—*
**Adults:** if insulin dosage is more than 20 U daily, patient is started at usual dosage in addition to 50% of insulin. If insulin dosage is less than 20 U, insulin may be discontinued on initiation of glipizide.

## ADVERSE REACTIONS

**CNS:** dizziness, drowsiness, headache.
**GI:** nausea, constipation, diarrhea.
**GU:** elevated BUN and creatinine levels.
**Hematologic:** *leukopenia,* hemolytic anemia, *agranulocytosis, thrombocytopenia, aplastic anemia.*
**Hepatic:** cholestatic jaundice, alterations in cholesterol, alkaline phosphatase, and AST levels.
**Metabolic:** *hypoglycemia.*
**Skin:** rash, pruritus.

## INTERACTIONS

**Drug-drug.** *Anabolic steroids, chloramphenicol, clofibrate, guanethidine, MAO inhibitors, probenecid, salicylates, sulfonamides:* increased hypoglycemic activity. Monitor blood glucose level.
*Beta blockers:* prolonged hypoglycemic effect and masked symptoms of hypoglycemia. Use together cautiously.

*Corticosteroids, glucagon, rifampin, thiazide diuretics:* decreased hypoglycemic response. Monitor blood glucose level.
*Hydantoins:* increased blood levels of hydantoins. Monitor blood glucose levels.
*Oral anticoagulants:* increased hypoglycemic activity or enhanced anticoagulant effect. Monitor blood glucose levels, PT and INR.
**Drug-lifestyle.** *Alcohol use:* altered glycemic control, most commonly hypoglycemia. May also cause disulfiram-like reaction. Discourage concomitant use.

## EFFECTS ON DIAGNOSTIC TESTS
None reported.

## CONTRAINDICATIONS
Contraindicated in patients with hypersensitivity to drug and in those with diabetic ketoacidosis with or without coma; also contraindicated in pregnant or breast-feeding women.

## NURSING CONSIDERATIONS
• Use cautiously in patients with renal and hepatic disease; in debilitated, malnourished, or elderly patients; and in those with known allergy to sulfonamides.
• Give drug about 30 minutes before meals.
• Some patients may attain effective control on a once-daily regimen, whereas others respond better with divided dosing.
• Glipizide is a second-generation sulfonylurea. The frequency of adverse reactions appears to be lower than with first-generation drugs such as chlorpropamide.
• During periods of increased stress, patient may need insulin therapy. Monitor patient closely for hyperglycemia in these situations.
• Patient transferring from insulin therapy to an oral antidiabetic needs blood glucose level monitoring at least t.i.d. before meals. Patient may need hospitalization during transition.
• *Alert:* Don't confuse glimepiride with glyburide or glipizide.

### ☑ Patient teaching
• Instruct patient about disease, importance of following therapeutic regimen, adhering to diet, weight reduction, exer-

---

cise, personal hygiene programs, and avoiding infection. Explain how and when to perform self-monitoring of blood glucose level, and teach recognition of hypoglycemia and hyperglycemia.

• Tell patient to carry candy or other simple sugars to treat mild hypoglycemic episodes. Patient experiencing severe episode may need hospital treatment.

• Instruct patient not to change drug dosage without doctor's consent and to report abnormal blood or urine glucose test results.

• Tell patient not to take other drugs, including OTC drugs, without first checking with doctor.

• Advise patient to carry medical identification at all times.

• Inform patient that alcohol lowers blood glucose level, and therefore should be avoided.

---

## glucagon

*Pregnancy Risk Category B*

---

### HOW SUPPLIED
*Powder for injection:* 1-mg (1 U) vial, 10-mg (10 U) vial

### ACTION
Raises blood glucose level by promoting catalytic depolymerization of hepatic glycogen to glucose.

| Route | Onset | Peak | Duration |
|---|---|---|---|
| I.V. | Immediate | 0.5 hr | Unknown |
| I.M., S.C. | Unknown | Unknown | Unknown |

### INDICATIONS & DOSAGE
*Hypoglycemia—*
**Adults and children over 20 kg (44 lb):** 1 mg S.C., I.M., or I.V.
**Children 20 kg or less:** 0.025 USP U or 25 mcg/kg S.C., I.M., or I.V.; maximum dose 1 mg.
  *Note:* May repeat in 20 minutes, if needed. I.V. glucose must be given if patient fails to respond. When patient responds, supplemental carbohydrate needs to be given immediately.

*Diagnostic aid for radiologic examination—*
**Adults:** 0.25 to 2 mg I.V. or I.M. before radiologic procedure.

### ADVERSE REACTIONS
**CV:** hypotension.
**GI:** nausea, vomiting.
**Metabolic:** decreased potassium levels.
**Respiratory:** *bronchospasm,* respiratory distress.
**Other:** *hypersensitivity reactions.*

### INTERACTIONS
**Drug-drug.** *Phenytoin:* inhibited glucagon-induced insulin release. Use cautiously.

### EFFECTS ON DIAGNOSTIC TESTS
None reported.

### CONTRAINDICATIONS
Contraindicated in patients with hypersensitivity to drug and in those with pheochromocytoma.

### NURSING CONSIDERATIONS
• Use cautiously in those with history of insulinoma or pheochromocytoma.
• Drug should be used in emergency situations only.
• *Alert:* Arouse patient from coma as quickly as possible and give additional carbohydrates orally to prevent secondary hypoglycemic reactions.
• *Alert:* Don't confuse glucagon with Glaucon.

### I.V. administration
• Reconstitute drug in 1-U vial with 1 ml of diluent; reconstitute drug in 10-U vial with 10 ml of diluent. Use only diluent supplied by manufacturer when preparing doses of 2 mg or less. For larger doses, dilute with sterile water for injection.
• For I.V. drip infusion, use dextrose solution, which is compatible with glucagon (drug forms a precipitate in chloride solutions). Inject directly into vein or into I.V. tubing of a free-flowing compatible solution over 2 to 5 minutes. Interrupt primary infusion during glucagon injection if using same I.V. line.

---

• Unstable hypoglycemic diabetic patients may not respond to glucagon; give dextrose I.V. instead, as ordered.

### ☑ Patient teaching
• Instruct patient and caregivers in proper glucagon administration and recognition of hypoglycemia.
• Explain importance of calling doctor at once in emergencies.

---

## glyburide (glibenclamide)
Daonil§, DiaBeta**, Euglucon†, Glynase PresTab, Micronase, Semi-Daonil§

*Pregnancy Risk Category B*

### HOW SUPPLIED
*Tablets:* 1.25 mg, 2.5 mg, 5 mg
*Tablets (micronized):* 1.5 mg, 3 mg, 6 mg

### ACTION
Unknown. A sulfonylurea that probably stimulates insulin release from the pancreatic beta cells and reduces glucose output by the liver. An extrapancreatic effect increases peripheral sensitivity to insulin and causes a mild diuretic effect.

| Route | Onset | Peak | Duration |
|-------|-------|------|----------|
| P.O. | 1-4 hr | 4 hr | 24 hr |

### INDICATIONS & DOSAGE
*Adjunct to diet to lower blood glucose level in patients with type 2 non-insulin-dependent diabetes mellitus—*
**Adults:** initially, 2.5 to 5 regular tablets P.O. once daily with breakfast or first main meal. Usual maintenance dose is 1.25 to 20 mg daily as a single dose or in divided doses. Or, micronized formulation may be used. Initial dose is 1.5 to 3 mg daily. Usual maintenance dose of micronized formulation is 0.75 to 12 mg/day. Patients receiving more than 6 mg/day may have better response with b.i.d. dosing.
*Adjust-a-dose:* For patients who are more sensitive to antidiabetics, initially 1.25 mg daily. Patients with adrenal or pituitary insufficiency should start with 1.25 mg daily. When using micronized tablets, pa-

tients who are more sensitive to antidiabetics should start with 0.75 mg daily.
*To replace insulin therapy—*
**Adults:** if insulin dosage is below 40 U/day, patient may be switched directly to glyburide when insulin is discontinued. If insulin dosage is 40 or more U/day, initially 5-mg regular tablets or 3-mg micronized formulation can be given P.O. once daily in addition to 50% of insulin dosage.

### ADVERSE REACTIONS
**EENT:** changes in accommodation or blurred vision.
**GI:** nausea, epigastric fullness, heartburn.
**GU:** elevated BUN levels.
**Hematologic:** *leukopenia,* hemolytic anemia, *agranulocytosis, thrombocytopenia, aplastic anemia.*
**Hepatic:** cholestatic jaundice, *hepatitis,* abnormal liver function, alterations in cholesterol and alkaline phosphatase levels.
**Metabolic:** *hypoglycemia.*
**Musculoskeletal:** arthralgia, myalgia.
**Skin:** rash, pruritus, other allergic reactions.
**Other:** *angioedema.*

### INTERACTIONS
**Drug-drug.** *Anabolic steroids, chloramphenicol, clofibrate, guanethidine, MAO inhibitors, salicylates, sulfonamides:* increased hypoglycemic activity. Monitor blood glucose level.
*Beta blockers:* prolonged hypoglycemic effect and masked symptoms of hypoglycemia. Use together cautiously.
*Corticosteroids, glucagon, rifampin, thiazide diuretics:* decreased hypoglycemic response. Monitor blood glucose level.
*Hydantoins:* increased blood levels of hydantoins. Monitor blood levels.
*Oral anticoagulants:* increased hypoglycemic activity or enhanced anticoagulant effect. Monitor blood glucose level, PT, and INR.
**Drug-lifestyle.** *Alcohol use:* altered glycemic control, most commonly hypoglycemia. May also cause disulfiram-like reaction. Discourage concomitant use.

### EFFECTS ON DIAGNOSTIC TESTS
None reported.

---

## CONTRAINDICATIONS

Contraindicated in patients with hypersensitivity to drug and in those with diabetic ketoacidosis with or without coma; also contraindicated in pregnant or breast-feeding women.

## NURSING CONSIDERATIONS

• Use cautiously in patients with hepatic or renal impairment; in debilitated, malnourished, or elderly patients; and in patients with known allergy to sulfonamides.

• *Alert:* Micronized glyburide (Glynase PresTab) contains drug in a smaller particle size and isn't bioequivalent to regular glyburide tablets. Patients who have been taking Micronase or DiaBeta need to be readjusted.

• Although most patients may take drug once daily, those taking more than 10 mg daily may achieve better results with b.i.d. dosage.

• Glyburide is a second-generation sulfonylurea. Frequency of adverse effects appears to be lower than with first-generation drugs such as chlorpropamide.

• During periods of increased stress, such as infection, fever, surgery, or trauma, patients may need insulin therapy. Monitor patient closely for hyperglycemia in these situations.

• Patient transferring from insulin to an oral antidiabetic needs blood glucose level monitoring at least t.i.d. before meals. Patient may need hospitalization during transition.

• *Alert:* Don't confuse glimepiride with glyburide or glipizide.

### ☑ Patient teaching

• Instruct patient about nature of disease, importance of following therapeutic regimen, adhering to specific diet, weight reduction, exercise, and personal hygiene programs, and about avoiding infection. Explain how and when to perform self-monitoring of blood glucose levels, and teach recognition of and intervention for hypoglycemia and hyperglycemia.

• Tell patient not to change drug dosage without doctor's consent and to report abnormal blood or urine glucose test results.

• Teach patient to carry candy or other simple sugars to treat mild hypoglycemic episodes. Patient experiencing severe episode may need hospital treatment.

• Advise patient not to take other drugs, including OTC drugs, without first checking with doctor.

• Advise patient to carry medical identification at all times.

• *Alert:* Instruct patient to report episodes of hypoglycemia to doctor immediately; severe hypoglycemia is sometimes fatal in patients receiving as little as 2.5 to 5 mg glyburide daily.

• Inform patient that alcohol may lower blood glucose levels and therefore should be avoided.

---

## insulins

### insulin injection (regular insulin, crystalline zinc insulin)

Actrapid‡, Actrapid PenFill‡, Humulin-R◊, Hypurin Neutral‡, Insulin 2 Neutral‡, Novolin R◊, Novolin R PenFill◊, Pork Regular Iletin II◊, Regular (Concentrated) Iletin II, Regular Iletin I◊, Regular Purified Pork Insulin◊, Velosulin Human BR†

### insulin (lispro)

Humalog

### insulin zinc suspension, prompt (semilente)

Human Monotard§, Hypurin Lente§, Lentard MC§

### isophane insulin suspension (neutral protamine Hagedorn insulin, NPH)

Humulin N◊, Humulin NPH‡, Hypurin Isophane‡, Isotard MC‡, Novolin N◊, Novolin N PenFill◊, NPH insulin◊, NPH Purified Pork◊, Protaphane‡, Protaphane PenFill‡, Purified Pork NPH Iletin II◊

---

## isophane insulin suspension with insulin injection
Humulin 50/50◇, Humulin 70/30◇, Novolin 70/30, Novolin 70/30 PenFill◇

## insulin zinc suspension (lente)
Humulin L◇, Lente Iletin II◇, Lente Insulin◇, Lente MC‡, Lente Purified Pork Insulin◇, Novolin L◇

## protamine zinc suspension (PZI)
Hypurin Bovine Protamine Zinc§

## insulin zinc suspension, extended (ultralente)
Humulin-U◇, Ultralente Insulin◇

*Pregnancy Risk Category NR*

## HOW SUPPLIED
**insulin injection**
*Injection (human):* 100 U/ml (Humulin-R◇, Novolin R◇, Velosulin Human BR‡); 100 U/ml in 1.5-ml cartridge system◇ (Novolin R PenFill◇)
*Injection (from pork):* 100 U/ml◇
*Injection (purified beef):* 100 U/ml (Hypurin Neutral‡, Insulin 2 Neutral‡)
*Injection (purified pork):* 100 U/ml (Actrapid‡, Pork Regular Iletin II◇, Regular Purified Pork Insulin◇); 100 U/ml in 1.5-ml cartridge system‡ (Actrapid PenFill‡); 100 U/ml in 2-ml cartridge system‡; 500 U/ml (Regular [Concentrated] Iletin II)
**insulin lispro injection**
*Injection (human):* 100 U/ml (Humalog)
**insulin zinc suspension, prompt**
*Injection (purified pork):* 100 U/ml◇
**isophane insulin suspension**
*Injection (from beef):* 100 U/ml◇ (NPH Insulin◇)
*Injection (human, recombinant):* 100 U/ml (Humulin N◇, Humulin NPH‡, Novolin N◇); 100 U/ml in 1.5-ml cartridge system (Novolin N PenFill◇, Protaphane PenFill‡)
*Injection (purified beef):* 100 U/ml (Hypurin Isophane‡, Isotard MC‡)

*Injection (purified pork):* 100 U/ml (NPH Purified Pork◇, Purified Pork NPH Iletin II, Protaphane‡)
**isophane insulin suspension 50% with insulin injection 50%**
*Injection (human):* 100 U/ml (Humulin 50/50◇)
**isophane insulin suspension 70% with insulin injection 30%**
*Injection (human):* 100 U/ml (Humulin 70/30◇, Novolin 70/30◇); 100 U/ml in 1.5-ml cartridge system (Novolin 70/30 PenFill◇)
**insulin zinc suspension**
*Injection (from beef):* 100 U/ml (Lente Insulin◇, Lente MC‡)
*Injection (purified beef):* 100 U/ml (Lente MC‡)
*Injection (purified pork):* 100 U/ml (Lente Iletin II, Lente Purified Pork Insulin◇)
*Injection (human):* 100 U/ml◇ (Humulin L◇, Novolin L◇)
**protamine zinc suspension**
*Injection (purified beef):* 100 U/ml (Hypurin Bovine Protamine Zinc §)
**insulin zinc suspension, extended**
*Injection (from beef):* 100 U/ml◇ (Ultralente Insulin◇)
*Injection (human):* 100 U/ml (Humulin-U◇)

## ACTION
Increases glucose transport across muscle and fat cell membranes to reduce blood glucose level. Promotes conversion of glucose to its storage form, glycogen; triggers amino acid uptake and conversion to protein in muscle cells and inhibits protein degradation; stimulates triglyceride formation and inhibits release of free fatty acids from adipose tissue; and stimulates lipoprotein lipase activity, which converts circulating lipoproteins to fatty acids.

| Route | Onset | Peak | Duration |
|---|---|---|---|
| I.V. (rapid) | 10-30 min | 15-30 min | 0.5-1 hr |
| S.C. (rapid) | 0.5-1.5 hr | 2-3 hr | 5-7 hr |
| S.C. (inter-mediate) | 1-2.5 hr | 4-15 hr | 12-24 hr |
| S.C. (long-acting) | 4-8 hr | 10-30 hr | 36 hr |

---

Reactions may be *common*, uncommon, *life-threatening*, or COMMON AND LIFE-THREATENING.

## INDICATIONS & DOSAGE
*Diabetic ketoacidosis (use regular insulin only)—*
**Adults:** 0.33 U/kg as I.V. bolus; then 0.1 U/kg/hour by continuous infusion. Continue infusion until blood glucose level drops to 250 mg/dl; then S.C. insulin is begun with dosage, and dosage interval is adjusted according to patient's blood glucose level.

Or, 50 to 100 U I.V. and 50 to 100 U S.C. immediately; then additional doses q 2 to 6 hours based on blood glucose levels.

To prepare infusion, add 100 U of regular insulin and 1 g of albumin to 100 ml of normal saline solution. Insulin concentration will be 1 U/ml. (The albumin will adhere to plastic, preventing insulin from adhering to plastic.)
**Children:** 0.1 U/kg as I.V. bolus; then 0.1 U/kg hourly by continuous infusion until blood glucose level drops to 250 mg/dl; then S.C. insulin started. Or, 1 to 2 U/kg in two divided doses, one I.V. and the other S.C., followed by 0.5 to 1 U/kg I.V. q 1 to 2 hours based on blood glucose levels.
*Type 1 insulin-dependent diabetes, adjunct to type 2 non-insulin-dependent diabetes inadequately controlled by diet and oral antidiabetics—*
**Adults and children:** therapeutic regimen is prescribed by doctor and adjusted based on patient's blood glucose levels.

## ADVERSE REACTIONS
**Metabolic:** *hypoglycemia,* hyperglycemia (rebound, or Somogyi effect), decreased serum magnesium, potassium, or inorganic phosphate levels.
**Skin:** rash, urticaria, pruritus, swelling, redness, stinging, warmth at injection site.
**Other:** *lipoatrophy, lipohypertrophy, hypersensitivity reactions, anaphylaxis.*

## INTERACTIONS
**Drug-drug.** *Anabolic steroids, beta blockers, clofibrate, fenfluramine, guanethidine, MAO inhibitors, salicylates, tetracycline:* prolonged hypoglycemic effect. Monitor blood glucose level carefully.
*Corticosteroids, dextrothyroxine, epinephrine, thiazide diuretics, thyroid hormone:* diminished insulin response. Monitor for hyperglycemia.

*Diazoxide, phenytoin (high doses):* may inhibit endogenous insulin secretion and cause hypoglycemia in diabetic patients. Carefully adjust insulin dosage when using with these drugs.
*Oral contraceptives:* may decrease glucose tolerance in diabetic patients. Monitor blood glucose levels and adjust insulin dosage carefully.
**Drug-herb.** *Basil, bay, bee pollen, burdock, sage:* may affect glycemic control. Monitor blood glucose level closely.
*Garlic dust, ginseng:* may decrease blood glucose levels. Monitor for effects.
**Drug-lifestyle.** *Alcohol use:* hypoglycemic effect. Discourage concomitant use.
*Marijuana use:* may increase serum glucose levels. Tell patient to avoid use of marijuana.
*Smoking:* may increase blood glucose levels and decrease response to insulin administration. Monitor blood glucose levels.

## EFFECTS ON DIAGNOSTIC TESTS
None reported.

## CONTRAINDICATIONS
Contraindicated in patients with history of systemic allergic reaction to pork.

## NURSING CONSIDERATIONS
• Insulin is drug of choice to treat diabetes during pregnancy. Insulin requirements increase in pregnant diabetic women and then decline immediately postpartum. Monitor patient closely.
• Dosage is always expressed in USP U. Remember to use only the syringes calibrated for the particular concentration of insulin administered. U-500 insulin must be administered with a U-100 syringe because no syringes are made for this strength.
• Some patients may develop insulin resistance and need large insulin doses to control symptoms of diabetes. U-500 insulin is available as Regular (Concentrated) Iletin II for such patients. Although not every pharmacy may stock it, it's available. Be sure to give the hospital pharmacy sufficient notice before requesting refill of in-house prescription.

Never store U-500 insulin in same area with other insulin preparations because of danger of severe overdose if given accidentally to other patients.

• To mix insulin suspension, swirl vial gently or rotate between palms or between palm and thigh. Don't shake vigorously—this causes bubbling and air in syringe.

• Lente, semilente, and ultralente insulins may be mixed in any proportion. Regular insulin may be mixed with NPH or lente insulins in any proportion. When mixing regular insulin with intermediate or long-acting insulin, always draw up regular insulin into syringe first.

• Switching from separate injections to a prepared mixture may alter patient response. When NPH or lente is mixed with regular insulin in the same syringe, give immediately to avoid loss of potency.

• Lispro insulin may be mixed with Humulin N or Humulin U and should be given within 15 minutes before a meal to prevent a hypoglycemic reaction.

• Don't use insulin that changes color or becomes clumped or granular in appearance.

• Check expiration date on vial before using contents.

• Usual administration route is S.C. For proper S.C. administration, remember to pinch a fold of skin with the fingers at least 3 inches (7.6 cm) apart, and insert needle at a 45- to 90-degree angle.

• Press but don't rub site after injection. Rotate injection sites and chart to avoid overuse of one area. Diabetic patients may achieve better control if injection site is rotated within same anatomic region.

• Store insulin in cool area. Refrigeration is desirable but not essential, except with regular insulin (concentrated).

### 🜂 I.V. administration

• Administer only regular insulin I.V. Inject directly into vein at ordered rate through an intermittent infusion device or into a port close to I.V. access site. Intermittent infusion isn't recommended. If given by continuous infusion, infuse drug diluted in normal saline at prescribed rate.

• *Alert:* Regular insulin is used in patients with circulatory collapse, diabetic ketoacidosis, or hyperkalemia. Don't use regular insulin (concentrated), 500 U/ml, I.V. Don't use intermediate or long-acting insulins for coma or other emergency requiring rapid drug action. Also ketosis-prone type 1, severely ill, and newly diagnosed diabetic patients with very high blood glucose levels may need hospitalization and I.V. treatment with regular fast-acting insulin.

### ✓ Patient teaching

• Make sure patient knows that therapy only relieves symptoms.

• Instruct patient about nature of disease, importance of following therapeutic regimen, adhering to specific diet, weight reduction, exercise, and personal hygiene program, and about avoiding infection. Emphasize importance of timing of injections and eating, and that meals must not be omitted.

• Stress that accuracy of measurement is important, especially with concentrated regular insulin. Aids, such as magnifying sleeve or dose magnifier, may improve accuracy. Show patient and caregivers how to measure and administer insulin.

• Advise patient not to alter order of mixing insulins or change model or brand of insulin, syringe, or needle.

• Teach patient that self-monitoring of blood glucose levels and urine ketone tests are essential guides to dosage and success of therapy. It's important for patient to recognize hyperglycemic and hypoglycemic symptoms. Insulin-induced hypoglycemia is hazardous and may cause brain damage if prolonged; most adverse effects are self-limiting and temporary. Instruct patient in insulin peak times and their importance.

• Instruct patient on proper use of equipment for performing self-monitoring of blood glucose levels.

• Advise patient not to smoke within 30 minutes after insulin injection. Cigarette smoking decreases amount of absorption of insulin administered S.C.

• Inform patient that marijuana use may increase insulin requirements.

• Advise patient to wear a medical identification bracelet at all times, to carry ample insulin and syringes on trips, to have carbohydrates (lump of sugar or candy)

---

Reactions may be *common*, uncommon, *life-threatening*, or COMMON AND LIFE-THREATENING.

on hand for emergencies, and to note time zone changes for dosage schedule when traveling.

# metformin hydrochloride
Glucophage

*Pregnancy Risk Category B*

## HOW SUPPLIED
*Tablets:* 500 mg, 850 mg

## ACTION
Decreases hepatic glucose production and intestinal absorption of glucose and improves insulin sensitivity (increases peripheral glucose uptake and utilization).

| Route | Onset | Peak | Duration |
|-------|-------|------|----------|
| P.O. | Unknown | Unknown | Unknown |

## INDICATIONS & DOSAGE
*Adjunct to diet to lower blood glucose level in patients with type 2 non-insulin-dependent diabetes mellitus—*
**Adults:** initially, 500 mg P.O. b.i.d. given with morning and evening meals, or 850 mg P.O. once daily given with morning meal. When 500-mg form used, dosage increased 500 mg weekly to maximum dose of 2,500 mg P.O. daily in divided doses, p.r.n. When 850-mg form used, dosage increased 850 mg every other week to maximum dose of 2,550 mg P.O. daily in divided doses, p.r.n.
**Elderly:** for patients over age 65, dosing should be conservative because of potential decrease in renal function.
*Adjust-a-dose:* For debilitated patients, dosing should be conservative because of potential decrease in renal function.

## ADVERSE REACTIONS
**GI:** diarrhea, nausea, vomiting, abdominal bloating, flatulence, anorexia, unpleasant or metallic taste.
**Hematologic:** megaloblastic anemia.
**Other:** *lactic acidosis.*

## INTERACTIONS
**Drug-drug.** *Calcium channel blockers, corticosteroids, estrogens, isoniazid, nicotinic acid, oral contraceptives, phenoth-* *iazines, phenytoin, sympathomimetics, thiazide and other diuretics, thyroid drugs:* may produce hyperglycemia. Monitor patient's glycemic control. Metformin dosage may need to be increased.
*Cationic drugs (such as amiloride, cimetidine, digoxin, morphine, procainamide, quinidine, quinine, ranitidine, triamterene, trimethoprim, vancomycin):* have potential to compete for common renal tubular transport systems, which may increase metformin plasma levels. Monitor patient's blood glucose level.
*Nifedipine:* increased metformin plasma levels. Monitor patient closely. Metformin dosage may need to be decreased.
*Radiologic contrast dye:* can result in acute renal failure. Withhold metformin for 24 hours before procedure.
**Drug-lifestyle.** *Alcohol use:* potentiated drug's effects. Avoid concurrent use.

## EFFECTS ON DIAGNOSTIC TESTS
None reported.

## CONTRAINDICATIONS
Contraindicated in patients with hypersensitivity to drug and in those with renal disease or metabolic acidosis. Drug should be temporarily withheld in patients undergoing radiologic studies involving parenteral administration of iodinated contrast materials because use of such products may result in acute renal dysfunction. Drug should be promptly discontinued if patient enters a hypoxic state. Avoid use in patients with hepatic disease.

## NURSING CONSIDERATIONS
• Use caution when giving drug to elderly, debilitated, or malnourished patients and to those with adrenal or pituitary insufficiency because of increased risk of hypoglycemia.
• Before therapy begins, and at least annually thereafter, patient's renal function should be assessed. If renal impairment is detected, expect doctor to switch patient to a different antidiabetic. This is particularly important in elderly patients.
• Administer with meals; once-daily dosage should be given with breakfast and twice-daily dosage with breakfast and dinner.

• When transferring patients from standard oral hypoglycemics (except chlorpropamide) to metformin, no transition period generally is needed. When switching patients from chlorpropamide to metformin, care should be exercised during the first 2 weeks of metformin therapy because the prolonged retention of chlorpropamide increases risk of hypoglycemia during this time.

• Monitor patient's blood glucose levels regularly to evaluate effectiveness of therapy. Notify doctor if they become elevated despite therapy.

• If patient hasn't responded to 4 weeks of therapy using the maximum dose, doctor may add an oral sulfonylurea while continuing metformin at the maximum dose. If patient still doesn't respond after several months of concomitant therapy at maximum doses, doctor may discontinue both drugs and institute insulin therapy.

• Monitor patient closely during times of increased stress, such as infection, fever, surgery, or trauma. Insulin therapy may be needed in these situations.

• Risk of drug-induced lactic acidosis is very low. Reported cases have occurred primarily in diabetic patients with significant renal insufficiency; in those with multiple, concomitant medical or surgical problems; and in those with multiple, concomitant drug regimens. Risk increases with degree of renal impairment and patient's age.

• **Alert:** Discontinue drug immediately and notify doctor if patient develops a condition associated with hypoxemia or dehydration because of risk of lactic acidosis.

• Expect drug therapy to be temporarily suspended for surgical procedures (except minor procedures not associated with restricted intake of food and fluids) and for patients undergoing radiologic studies involving use of contrast media containing iodine. Therapy shouldn't be restarted until patient's oral intake has resumed and renal function has been evaluated as normal by doctor.

• Monitor patient's hematologic status for evidence of megaloblastic anemia. Patients with inadequate vitamin $B_{12}$ or calcium intake or absorption appear to be predisposed to developing subnormal vitamin $B_{12}$ levels. These patients should have routine serum vitamin $B_{12}$ level determinations every 2 to 3 years.

### ✅ Patient teaching

• **Alert:** Instruct patient about nature of diabetes, importance of following therapeutic regimen, adhering to specific diet, weight reduction, exercise, personal hygiene programs, and avoiding infection. Explain how and when to perform self-monitoring of blood glucose level; teach signs and symptoms of hypoglycemia and hyperglycemia, and emergency measures.

• Instruct patient to discontinue drug and notify doctor immediately if unexplained hyperventilation, myalgia, malaise, unusual somnolence, or other nonspecific symptoms of early lactic acidosis occur.

• Warn patient not to consume excessive alcohol while taking drug.

• Tell patient not to change drug dosage without doctor's consent. Encourage patient to report abnormal blood glucose level test results.

• Advise patient not to take other drugs, including OTC drugs, without first checking with doctor.

• Instruct patient to carry medical identification at all times.

✳ *NEW DRUG*

## miglitol
Glyset

*Pregnancy Risk Category B*

### HOW SUPPLIED
*Tablets:* 25 mg, 50 mg, 100 mg

### ACTION
Lowers blood glucose level by inhibiting the alpha-glucosidases in the small intestine. These enzymes convert carbohydrates to glucose. Inhibition of the enzymes delays the digestion of carbohydrates after a meal, resulting in a smaller rise in postprandial blood glucose levels.

| Route | Onset | Peak | Duration |
|-------|-------|------|----------|
| P.O. | Unknown | 2-3 hr | Unknown |

---

Reactions may be *common*, uncommon, *life-threatening*, or COMMON AND LIFE-THREATENING.

## INDICATIONS & DOSAGE
*Adjunct to diet to improve glycemic control in patients with type 2 non-insulin-dependent diabetes mellitus whose hyperglycemia can't be managed with diet alone; with a sulfonylurea when diet plus either miglitol or sulfonylurea doesn't result in adequate glycemic control—*
**Adults:** 25 mg P.O. t.i.d. with first bite of each main meal; dose may be increased after 4 to 8 weeks to 50 mg P.O. t.i.d. Dosage may then be further increased after 3 months, based on glycosylated hemoglobin level, to maximum of 100 mg P.O. t.i.d.

## ADVERSE REACTIONS
**GI:** abdominal pain, diarrhea, flatulence.
**Skin:** rash.
**Other:** decreased serum iron levels.

## INTERACTIONS
**Drug-drug.** *Digoxin, propranolol, ranitidine:* may decrease bioavailability of these drugs. Monitor for loss of efficacy of these drugs and adjust dosage.
*Intestinal absorbents (such as charcoal), digestive enzyme preparations (such as amylase, pancreatin):* may reduce effectiveness of miglitol. Avoid concomitant use.

## EFFECTS ON DIAGNOSTIC TESTS
None reported.

## CONTRAINDICATIONS
Contraindicated in patients with hypersensitivity to drug or its components and in those with diabetic ketoacidosis, inflammatory bowel disease, colonic ulceration, partial intestinal obstruction, chronic intestinal diseases associated with marked disorders of digestion or absorption, or conditions that may deteriorate because of increased gas formation in the intestine; also contraindicated in those predisposed to intestinal obstruction. Drug isn't recommended in patients with significant renal dysfunction (serum creatinine over 2 mg/dl).

## NURSING CONSIDERATIONS
• Use cautiously in patients also receiving insulin or oral sulfonylureas because drug may increase hypoglycemic potential of insulin or sulfonylureas. Increased risk of hypoglycemia can occur when drug is used with insulin or sulfonylureas; dosage adjustments of these drugs may be needed. Monitor patient for increased frequency of hypoglycemia.
• Management of type 2 diabetes should include diet control, exercise program, and regular testing of urine and blood glucose levels.
• Monitor blood glucose level regularly, especially during situations of increased stress, such as infection, fever, surgery, or trauma.
• Besides having blood glucose levels checked regularly, monitor glycosylated hemoglobin level every 3 months, as ordered, for evaluating long-term glycemic control.
• Treat mild to moderate hypoglycemia with a form of dextrose, such as glucose tablets or gel. Severe hypoglycemia may need I.V. glucose or glucagon administration.
• Drug should be given with the first bite of each main meal.

☑**Patient teaching**
• Stress importance of adhering to diet, weight reduction, and exercise instructions and to have blood glucose and glycosylated hemoglobin levels tested regularly.
• Inform patient that drug treatment relieves symptoms but doesn't cure diabetes.
• Teach patient how to recognize signs and symptoms of hyperglycemia and hypoglycemia.
• Instruct patient to treat hypoglycemia with glucose tablets and to have a source of glucose readily available to treat symptoms of hypoglycemia when miglitol is taken with a sulfonylurea or insulin.
• Advise patient to seek medical advice promptly during periods of stress, such as fever, trauma, infection, or surgery, because dosage may have to be adjusted.
• Instruct patient to take drug three times daily with first bite of each main meal.
• Show patient how and when to perform self-monitoring of blood glucose levels.

• Advise patient that adverse GI effects are most common during first few weeks of therapy and should improve over time.
• Urge patient to carry medical identification at all times.

✳ *NEW DRUG*

## pioglitazone hydrochloride
Actos

*Pregnancy Risk Category C*

### HOW SUPPLIED
*Tablets:* 15 mg, 30 mg, 45 mg

### ACTION
Lowers blood glucose levels by decreasing insulin resistance. Improves sensitivity of insulin in muscle and adipose tissue.

| Route | Onset | Peak | Duration |
|-------|-------|------|----------|
| P.O. | Unknown | Within 2 hr | Unknown |

### INDICATION & DOSAGE
*Adjunct to diet and exercise to improve glycemic control in patients with type 2 non-insulin-dependent diabetes mellitus; or when diet, exercise, and either a sulfonylurea, metformin, or insulin doesn't result in adequate glycemic control—*
**Adults:** initially, 15 or 30 mg P.O. once daily. For patients who respond inadequately to initial dose, dosage may be increased in increments; maximum dose is 45 mg/day. If used in combination therapy, maximum dose shouldn't exceed 30 mg/day.

### ADVERSE REACTIONS
**CNS:** headache.
**CV:** *edema.*
**EENT:** sinusitis, pharyngitis.
**Hematologic:** anemia.
**Metabolic:** hypoglycemia with combination therapy, aggravated diabetes mellitus, weight gain.
**Musculoskeletal:** myalgia.
**Respiratory:** upper respiratory tract infection.
**Other:** tooth disorder, decreased triglyceride levels, increased high-density lipoprotein cholesterol levels.

### INTERACTIONS
**Drug-drug.** *Ketoconazole:* may inhibit metabolism of pioglitazone. Monitor patient's blood glucose levels more frequently.
*Oral contraceptives:* may reduce plasma levels of oral contraceptives, resulting in less effective contraception. Advise patients taking drug and oral contraceptives to consider additional birth control measures.

### EFFECTS ON DIAGNOSTIC TESTS
None reported.

### CONTRAINDICATIONS
Contraindicated in patients with hypersensitivity to drug or its components and in those with type 1 insulin-dependent diabetes mellitus, clinical evidence of active liver disease, serum ALT level greater than 2½ times the upper limit of normal, or New York Heart Association class III or IV heart failure; also contraindicated in patients who experienced jaundice while taking troglitazone and in the treatment of diabetic ketoacidosis.

### NURSING CONSIDERATIONS
• Use cautiously in patients with edema or heart failure.
• *Alert:* Measure liver enzymes at start of therapy, every 2 months for first year of therapy, and periodically thereafter. Liver function tests also should be done in patients who develop signs and symptoms of liver dysfunction, such as nausea, vomiting, abdominal pain, fatigue, anorexia, or dark urine. Discontinue drug if patient develops jaundice or if results of liver functions tests show elevations in ALT levels greater than three times upper limit of normal.
• Because ovulation may resume in premenopausal, anovulatory women with insulin resistance, recommend use of additional contraceptive measures.
• Drug should be used in pregnancy only if the benefit justifies risk to fetus. Insulin is the preferred antidiabetic for use during pregnancy.
• Monitor patients with heart failure for increased edema.

---

Reactions may be *common*, uncommon, *life-threatening*, or **COMMON AND LIFE-THREATENING**.

- Hemoglobin level and hematocrit may decrease, usually during first 4 to 12 weeks of therapy.
- Patients with normal liver enzyme levels who are switched from troglitazone therapy should undergo a 1-week washout period before starting pioglitazone.
- Management of type 2 diabetes should include diet control. Because caloric restrictions, weight loss, and exercise help improve insulin sensitivity and help make drug therapy effective, these measures are essential for proper diabetes management.
- Watch for hypoglycemia in patients receiving pioglitazone with insulin or a sulfonylurea. Dosage adjustments of these drugs may be needed.
- Monitor blood glucose levels regularly, especially during situations of increased stress, such as infection, fever, surgery, and trauma.
- Blood glucose and glycosylated hemoglobin levels should be checked periodically, as ordered, to evaluate therapeutic response to drug.
- Safety and efficacy of drug in children haven't been evaluated.
- *Alert:* Don't confuse pioglitazone with troglitazone or rosiglitazone.

☑ **Patient teaching**
- Instruct patient to adhere to dietary instructions and to have blood glucose and glycosylated hemoglobin levels tested regularly.
- Inform patient taking pioglitazone with insulin or oral antidiabetics of signs and symptoms of hypoglycemia.
- Advise patient to notify doctor during periods of stress, such as fever, trauma, infection, or surgery, because dosage may have to be changed.
- Notify patient that blood tests for liver function will be performed before start of therapy, every 2 months for first year, and periodically thereafter.
- Tell patient to report unexplained nausea, vomiting, abdominal pain, fatigue, anorexia, or dark urine immediately because these signs and symptoms may indicate potential liver problems.
- Inform patient that drug can be taken with or without meals. If a dose is missed, it shouldn't be doubled the following day.

- Advise anovulatory, premenopausal women with insulin resistance that therapy may cause resumption of ovulation; recommend use of contraceptive measures.

**repaglinide**
Prandin

*Pregnancy Risk Category C*

**HOW SUPPLIED**
*Tablets:* 0.5 mg, 1 mg, 2 mg

**ACTION**
Stimulates release of insulin from the beta cells in the pancreas by closing ATP-dependent potassium channels in the beta cell membrane, which causes opening of the calcium channels. The increased calcium influx induces insulin secretion; the overall effect is to lower the blood glucose level.

| Route | Onset | Peak | Duration |
|-------|-------|------|----------|
| P.O. | Unknown | 1 hr | Unknown |

**INDICATIONS & DOSAGE**
*Adjunct to diet and exercise in lowering blood glucose levels in patient with type 2 non-insulin-dependent diabetes mellitus whose hyperglycemia can't be controlled by diet and exercise alone; with metformin to lower blood glucose levels in patients whose hyperglycemia can't be controlled by exercise, diet, and either repaglinide or metformin —*
**Adults:** for patients not previously treated or whose glycosylated hemoglobin (HbA$_{1c}$) is below 8%, initially 0.5 mg P.O. taken immediately to 30 minutes before each meal; for those previously treated with glucose-lowering drugs and whose HbA$_{1c}$ is 8% or more, initially 1 to 2 mg P.O. taken immediately to 30 minutes before each meal. Recommended dose range is 0.5 to 4 mg with meals divided b.i.d., t.i.d., or q.i.d. Maximum daily dose is 16 mg.

**ADVERSE REACTIONS**
**CNS:** *headache,* paresthesia.
**CV:** angina, chest pain.

**EENT:** rhinitis, sinusitis, tooth disorder.
**GI:** constipation, diarrhea, dyspepsia, nausea, vomiting.
**GU:** urinary tract infection.
**Metabolic:** HYPOGLYCEMIA, hyperglycemia.
**Musculoskeletal:** arthralgia, back pain.
**Respiratory:** bronchitis, *upper respiratory tract infection.*

## INTERACTIONS

**Drug-drug.** *Barbiturates, carbamazepine, rifampin, troglitazone:* may increase metabolism of repaglinide. Monitor glucose level.
*Beta blockers, chloramphenicol, coumarins, MAO inhibitors, NSAIDs, other drugs that are highly protein-bound, probenecid, salicylates, sulfonamides:* may potentiate hypoglycemic action of repaglinide. Monitor glucose level.
*Calcium channel blockers, corticosteroids, estrogens, isoniazid, nicotinic acid, oral contraceptives, phenothiazines, phenytoin, sympathomimetics, thiazides and other diuretics, thyroid products:* may produce hyperglycemia, resulting in a loss of glycemic control. Monitor glucose level.
*Erythromycin, inhibitors of P-450 cytochrome system 3A4, ketoconazole, miconazole:* may inhibit metabolism of repaglinide. Monitor glucose levels.

## EFFECTS ON DIAGNOSTIC TESTS
None reported.

## CONTRAINDICATIONS
Contraindicated in patients with hypersensitivity to drug or its inactive ingredients and in those with type 1 insulin-dependent diabetes mellitus or diabetic ketoacidosis.

## NURSING CONSIDERATIONS
• Use cautiously in patients with hepatic insufficiency in whom reduced metabolism could cause hypoglycemia and elevated blood levels of repaglinide.
• Use cautiously in elderly, debilitated, or malnourished patients and in those with adrenal or pituitary insufficiency because these patients are more susceptible to hypoglycemic effect of glucose-lowering drugs.

• Make increases in drug dosage carefully in patients with impaired renal function or renal failure requiring dialysis.
• Adjust dosage by blood glucose level response. May double dosage up to 4 mg with each meal until satisfactory blood glucose level response is achieved. At least 1 week should elapse between dosage adjustments to assess response to each dose.
• Metformin may be added if repaglinide monotherapy is inadequate.
• Administration of oral antidiabetics has been associated with increased CV mortality compared with diet alone or diet plus insulin treatment. This association may also apply to repaglinide.
• Loss of glycemic control can occur during stress, such as fever, trauma, infection, or surgery. Discontinue drug, as ordered, and administer insulin.
• Hypoglycemia may be difficult to recognize in the elderly and in patients taking beta blockers.
• When switching to another oral hypoglycemic, begin new drug day after last dose of repaglinide.

### ✅ Patient teaching
• Stress importance of diet and exercise with drug therapy.
• Discuss symptoms of hypoglycemia with patient and family.
• Advise patient to monitor blood glucose level periodically to determine minimum effective dose.
• Encourage patient to keep regular appointments and have his $HbA_{1c}$ levels checked every 3 months to determine long-term glucose control.
• Tell patient to administer drug before meals, usually 15 minutes before start of meal; however, time can vary from immediately preceding meal to up to 30 minutes before meal.
• Tell patient that, if a meal is skipped or an extra meal added, he should skip dose or add an extra dose of drug for that meal.
• Instruct patient to monitor blood glucose level carefully and tell him what to do when he's ill, undergoing surgery, or under added stress.

---

Reactions may be *common*, uncommon, *life-threatening*, or COMMON AND LIFE-THREATENING.

✳ *NEW DRUG*

# rosiglitazone maleate
Avandia

*Pregnancy Risk Category C*

## HOW SUPPLIED
*Tablets:* 2 mg, 4 mg, 8 mg

## ACTION
Lowers blood glucose levels by improving insulin sensitivity.

| Route | Onset | Peak | Duration |
|-------|-------|------|----------|
| P.O. | Unknown | 1 hr | Unknown |

## INDICATIONS & DOSAGE
*Adjunct to diet and exercise to improve glycemic control in patients with type 2 non-insulin-dependent diabetes mellitus; with metformin to lower blood glucose levels in patients whose hyperglycemia can't be controlled by diet, exercise, and either rosiglitazone or metformin—*
**Adults:** initially, 4 mg P.O. daily in the morning or in divided doses b.i.d. in the morning and evening. Dosage may be increased to 8 mg P.O. daily or in divided doses b.i.d. if fasting plasma glucose level doesn't improve after 12 weeks of treatment.

## ADVERSE REACTIONS
**CNS:** headache, fatigue.
**CV:** edema.
**EENT:** sinusitis.
**GI:** diarrhea.
**Hematologic:** anemia.
**Metabolic:** hyperglycemia.
**Musculoskeletal:** back pain.
**Respiratory:** upper respiratory tract infection.
**Other:** injury.

## INTERACTIONS
None significant.

## EFFECTS ON DIAGNOSTIC TESTS
None reported.

## CONTRAINDICATIONS
Contraindicated in patients with known hypersensitivity to drug or its components and in those with New York Heart Association class III and I.V. cardiac status unless expected benefits outweigh potential risks. Also contraindicated in patients with active liver disease, increased baseline liver enzyme levels (ALT level over 2½ times upper limit of normal), type 1 diabetes, or diabetic ketoacidosis and in those who experienced jaundice while taking troglitazone. Because metformin is contraindicated in patients with renal impairment, combination therapy with rosiglitazone is also contraindicated in patients with renal impairment. Rosiglitazone can be used as monotherapy in patients with renal impairment.

## NURSING CONSIDERATIONS
• Use cautiously in patients with edema or heart failure.
• Before starting drug therapy, patient should be treated for secondary causes of poor glycemic control, such as infection.
• *Alert:* Liver enzyme levels should be checked before therapy starts. Drug shouldn't be used in patients with increased baseline liver enzyme levels. In patients with normal baseline liver enzyme levels, monitor these levels every 2 months for first 12 months and periodically thereafter. If ALT level is elevated during treatment, recheck levels as soon as possible. Drug should be discontinued if levels remain elevated.
• Because ovulation may resume in premenopausal, anovulatory women with insulin resistance, recommend use of contraceptives.
• Management of type 2 diabetes should include diet control. Because caloric restriction, weight loss, and exercise help improve insulin sensitivity and help make drug therapy effective, these measures are essential to proper diabetes treatment.
• Blood glucose and glycosylated hemoglobin levels should be checked periodically to monitor therapeutic response to drug.
• Monitor patients with heart failure for increased edema.
• Hemoglobin level and hematocrit may decrease during therapy, usually during first 4 to 8 weeks. Increases in total cholesterol, low-density lipoprotein, and

high-density lipoprotein levels and decreases in free fatty acid levels may also occur.

• Patients with normal hepatic enzyme levels who are switched from troglitazone should undergo a 1-week washout before starting rosiglitazone.

• For patients whose blood glucose levels are inadequately controlled with metformin, rosiglitazone should be added to—not substituted for—metformin.

• *Alert:* Don't confuse rosiglitazone with pioglitazone or troglitazone.

☑ **Patient teaching**
• Advise patient that drug can be taken with or without food.

• Notify patient that blood will be tested to check liver function before therapy starts, every 2 months for first 12 months, and then periodically thereafter.

• Tell patient to immediately notify doctor if unexplained signs and symptoms occur, such as nausea, vomiting, abdominal pain, fatigue, anorexia, or dark urine; these may indicate potential liver problems.

• Recommend use of contraceptives to premenopausal, anovulatory women with insulin resistance because ovulation may resume with therapy.

• Advise patient that management of diabetes should include diet control. Because caloric restriction, weight loss, and exercise help improve insulin sensitivity and help make drug therapy effective, these measures are essential to proper diabetes treatment.

---

**troglitazone**
Rezulin

*Pregnancy Risk Category B*

**HOW SUPPLIED**
*Tablets:* 200 mg, 400 mg

**ACTION**
Inhibits hepatic glucose production and enhances effects of circulating insulin.

| Route | Onset | Peak | Duration |
|-------|-------|------|----------|
| P.O. | Rapid | 2-3 hr | Unknown |

**INDICATIONS & DOSAGE**
*Adjunct to diet and insulin therapy in patients with type 2 non-insulin-dependent diabetes mellitus whose hyperglycemia is inadequately controlled with insulin therapy of over 30 U/day given as multiple injections—*
**Adults:** initially, continue with current insulin and begin concomitant therapy with 200 mg P.O. once daily, taken with a meal. May increase dosage after 2 to 4 weeks if needed. Usual daily dose is 400 mg; maximum daily dose is 600 mg. Insulin dose may be decreased by 10% to 25% when fasting glucose levels are below 120 mg/dl in patients receiving both troglitazone and insulin.
*With sulfonylureas in patients with type 2 diabetes mellitus—*
**Adults:** initially, 200 mg P.O. daily; continue current sulfonylurea dose. Increase dosage after 2 to 4 weeks, p.r.n. to maximum dose of 600 mg/day. Sulfonylurea dose may have to be lowered.
*As monotherapy for patients with type 2 diabetes mellitus not controlled with diet alone—*
**Adults:** initially, 400 mg P.O. once daily. Dosage may be increased to 600 mg after 1 month if needed. For patients not responding to 600 mg after 1 month, discontinue drug and consider alternative therapeutic options.
✳ *NEW INDICATION: Adjunct to sulfonylurea and metformin combination therapy in patients with type 2 non-insulin-dependent diabetes mellitus whose hyperglycemia is inadequately controlled—*
**Adults:** 400 mg P.O. once daily, in addition to sulfonylurea and metformin therapy.

**ADVERSE REACTIONS**
**CNS:** *headache,* asthenia, dizziness.
**CV:** peripheral edema.
**EENT:** rhinitis, pharyngitis.
**GI:** nausea, diarrhea.
**GU:** urinary tract infection.
**Hepatic:** *hepatotoxicity,* transient elevations in AST and ALT levels.
**Musculoskeletal:** back pain.
**Other:** *infection, pain,* accidental injury.

---

Reactions may be *common,* uncommon, *life-threatening,* or COMMON AND LIFE-THREATENING.

## INTERACTIONS
**Drug-drug.** *Cholestyramine:* reduced absorption of troglitazone. Avoid concomitant use.

*Oral contraceptives:* may reduce plasma levels of hormones, resulting in loss of contraceptive properties. Additional form of contraception is recommended.

**Drug-food.** *Any food:* increased absorption. Take drug with food.

## EFFECTS ON DIAGNOSTIC TESTS
None reported

## CONTRAINDICATIONS
Contraindicated in patients with hypersensitivity to drug and in those with active liver disease.

## NURSING CONSIDERATIONS
• Use cautiously in heart failure patients with New York Heart Association class III and I.V. status.

• Rare cases of severe idiosyncratic hepatocellular injury have been reported. The injury is usually reversible, but very rare cases of hepatic failure, including death, have been reported. Injury has occurred after both short- and long-term treatment. Drug shouldn't be initiated in patients with ALT levels over 1½ times upper limit of normal.

• *Alert:* Liver enzyme levels should be measured at start of therapy, every month for first 8 months of treatment, every 2 months for rest of year, and periodically thereafter. In addition, liver function tests should be performed on patient receiving drug who develops symptoms of liver dysfunction, such as nausea, vomiting, fatigue, loss of appetite, jaundice, or dark urine. Discontinue drug if patient has jaundice or if results of liver function tests suggest liver injury.

• Drug should be used in pregnancy only if benefit justifies potential risk to fetus. The preferred antidiabetic to be used during pregnancy is insulin. Breast-feeding women shouldn't take troglitazone.

• Safety and effectiveness of drug in children haven't been established.

• Drug doesn't stimulate insulin secretion; it shouldn't be used to treat patients with type 1 diabetes or ketoacidosis.

• When used with insulin, monitor patient for hypoglycemia; dosage of insulin may need to be reduced.

• Before starting drug therapy, investigate and address secondary causes of poor glycemic control, including infection and poor injection technique.

• Monitor glucose levels, especially during times of increased stress, such as infection, fever, surgery, and trauma.

• *Alert:* Don't confuse troglitazone with rosiglitazone or pioglitazone.

## ✓ Patient teaching
• Instruct patient about nature of diabetes, importance of following treatment, avoiding infection, and adhering to specific diet, weight reduction, exercise, and personal hygiene programs. Explain how and when to perform self-monitoring of blood glucose level; teach patient and family members signs and symptoms of hypoglycemia and hyperglycemia and explain what to do if these conditions occur.

• Tell patient that drug should be taken with a meal; if dose is missed, it may be taken with the next meal, but two doses shouldn't be taken the next day.

• Instruct patient to notify doctor immediately if signs and symptoms of liver injury develop, such as fatigue, nausea, vomiting, yellow skin or eyes, or dark urine.

• Inform premenopausal, anovulatory women that drug may cause resumption of ovulation, increasing risk of pregnancy. Recommend use of contraceptives.

• Instruct patient to carry medical identification at all times.

levothyroxine sodium
liothyronine sodium
liotrix
thyroid

**COMBINATION PRODUCTS**
None.

---

## levothyroxine sodium
($T_4$, L-thyroxine sodium)
Eltroxin†, Levo-T, Levothroid,
Levoxine, Levoxyl, Oroxine‡,
Synthroid**

*Pregnancy Risk Category A*

### HOW SUPPLIED
*Tablets:* 25 mcg, 50 mcg, 75 mcg,
88 mcg, 100 mcg, 112 mcg, 125 mcg,
137 mcg, 150 mcg, 175 mcg, 200 mcg,
300 mcg
*Injection:* 200-mcg vial, 500-mcg vial

### ACTION
Not completely defined. Stimulates metabolism of all body tissues by accelerating rate of cellular oxidation.

| Route | Onset | Peak | Duration |
|-------|-------|------|----------|
| P.O. | 24 hr | Unknown | Unknown |
| I.V. | Unknown | Unknown | Unknown |

### INDICATIONS & DOSAGE
*Cretinism—*
**Children up to age 6 months:** 25 to
50 mcg or 5 to 6 mcg/kg P.O. daily.
**Children ages 6 to 12 months:** 50 to
75 mcg or 5 to 6 mcg/kg P.O. daily.
**Children ages 1 to 5:** 75 to 100 mcg or 3
to 5 mcg/kg P.O. daily.
**Children ages 6 to 12:** 100 to 150 mcg or
4 to 5 mcg/kg P.O. daily.
**Children over age 12:** over 150 mcg or 2
to 3 mcg/kg P.O. daily.
*Myxedema coma—*
**Adults:** 200 to 500 mcg I.V.; then 100 to
300 mcg given on second day, followed
by parenteral maintenance dose of 50 to

200 mcg I.V. daily. Switch patient to oral
maintenance as soon as possible.
*Thyroid hormone replacement—*
**Adults:** initially, 25 to 50 mcg P.O. daily,
increased by 25 mcg P.O. q 2 to 4 weeks
until desired response occurs. Maintenance dose is 75 to 200 mcg P.O. daily.
May administer I.V. or I.M. when P.O. ingestion is precluded for long periods.
However, dosage adjustment is needed.
**Children:** in children under age 1, initial
dose is 25 to 50 mcg P.O. daily; in children ages 1 and older, 3 to 5 mcg/kg P.O.
daily. Gradually increased by 25 to
50 mcg q 2 to 4 weeks until desired response occurs.
**Elderly:** for patients over age 65, 12.5 to
50 mcg P.O. daily. Increased by 12.5 or
25 mcg at 3- to 8-week intervals, depending on response.

### ADVERSE REACTIONS
**CNS:** *nervousness, insomnia, tremor,*
headache.
**CV:** *tachycardia, palpitations,* **arrhythmias,** *angina pectoris,* **cardiac arrest.**
**GI:** diarrhea, vomiting.
**GU:** menstrual irregularities.
**Metabolic:** weight loss.
**Skin:** allergic skin reactions, diaphoresis.
**Other:** heat intolerance, fever.

### INTERACTIONS
**Drug-drug.** *Cholestyramine, colestipol:*
impaired levothyroxine absorption. Separate doses by 4 to 5 hours.
*Estrogens:* decreased free levothyroxines.
Monitor for decreased effectiveness of
thyroid hormone.
*Insulin, oral antidiabetics:* altered serum
glucose levels. Monitor blood glucose levels. Dosage adjustments may be needed.
*I.V. phenytoin:* free thyroid released. Monitor for tachycardia.
*Oral anticoagulants:* altered PT. Monitor
PT and INR. Dosage adjustments may be
needed.

---

Reactions may be *common*, uncommon, **_life-threatening_**, or COMMON AND LIFE-THREATENING.

*Sympathomimetics such as epinephrine:* increased risk of coronary insufficiency. Monitor closely.

**EFFECTS ON DIAGNOSTIC TESTS**
Alterations in radioactive iodine ($^{131}$I) thyroid uptake, protein-bound iodine levels, and liothyronine uptake may occur.

**CONTRAINDICATIONS**
Contraindicated in patients with hypersensitivity to drug and in those with acute MI uncomplicated by hypothyroidism, untreated thyrotoxicosis, or uncorrected adrenal insufficiency.

**NURSING CONSIDERATIONS**
• Use with extreme caution in elderly patients and in those with angina pectoris, hypertension, other CV disorders, renal insufficiency, or ischemia.
• Use cautiously in those with diabetes mellitus, insipidus, or myxedema. Patients with diabetes mellitus may need increased doses of antidiabetic when beginning thyroid hormone replacement.
• Rapid replacement in patients with arteriosclerosis may precipitate angina, coronary occlusion, or CVA. Use cautiously in these patients. In patients with coronary artery disease who must receive thyroid hormone, observe carefully for possible coronary insufficiency.
• Thyroid hormone replacement requirements are about 25% lower in patients over age 60 than in young adults.
• Patients with adult hypothyroidism are unusually sensitive to thyroid hormone. Start at lowest dosage and adjust to higher dosages according to patient's symptoms and laboratory data until euthyroid state is reached.
• When changing from levothyroxine to liothyronine, levothyroxine should be stopped and liothyronine begun. Dosage should be increased in small increments after residual effects of levothyroxine have disappeared. When changing from liothyronine to levothyroxine, levothyroxine is started several days before withdrawing liothyronine to avoid relapse. Drugs aren't interchangeable.
• Thyroid hormones alter thyroid function test results.

• Patients taking levothyroxine who need to have $^{131}$I uptake studies performed must discontinue drug 4 weeks before test.
• Patients on anticoagulant therapy may need their dosage modified; also, careful monitoring of coagulation status is needed.
• **Alert:** Don't confuse levothyroxine with liothyronine.

**◖ I.V. administration**
• Prepare I.V. dose immediately before injection. Don't mix with other solutions. Inject into vein over 1 to 2 minutes.
• Monitor blood pressure and heart rate closely. High initial I.V. dosage is usually well tolerated by patients in myxedema coma. Normal serum levels of $T_4$ should occur within 24 hours, followed by a threefold increase in serum $T_3$ in 3 days.

**☑ Patient teaching**
• Make sure patient understands importance of compliance. Tell him to take thyroid hormones at same time each day, preferably before breakfast, to maintain constant hormone levels. Suggest morning dosage to prevent insomnia.
• Make sure patient understands that replacement therapy is for a lifetime.
• Warn patient (especially elderly patient) to notify doctor at once if chest pain, palpitations, sweating, nervousness, shortness of breath, or other signs and symptoms of overdose or aggravated CV disease occur.
• Advise patient who has achieved stable response not to change brands.
• Tell patient to report unusual bleeding and bruising.

---

**liothyronine sodium ($T_3$)**
Cytomel, Tertroxin‡, Triostat

*Pregnancy Risk Category A*

**HOW SUPPLIED**
*Tablets:* 5 mcg, 25 mcg, 50 mcg
*Injection:* 10 mcg/ml

**ACTION**
Not clearly defined. Enhances oxygen consumption by most tissues of the body;

---

increases the basal metabolic rate and the metabolism of carbohydrates, lipids, and proteins.

| Route | Onset | Peak | Duration |
|-------|-------|------|----------|
| P.O. | Unknown | 2-3 days | 3 days |
| I.V. | Unknown | Unknown | Unknown |

## INDICATIONS & DOSAGE
*Congenital hypothyroidism—*
**Children:** 5 mcg P.O. daily with a 5-mcg increase q 3 to 4 days until desired response achieved.
*Myxedema—*
**Adults:** initially, 2.5 to 5 mcg P.O. daily, increased by 5 to 10 mcg q 1 to 2 weeks until daily dose reaches 25 mcg. Then, increased by 12.5 to 25 mcg daily q 1 to 2 weeks. Maintenance dose is 50 to 100 mcg daily.
*Myxedema coma, premyxedema coma—*
**Adults:** initially, 10 to 20 mcg I.V. for patients with known or suspected CV disease; 25 to 50 mcg I.V. for patients not known to have CV disease. Subsequent dosage adjustments made based on patient's condition and response. Switch patient to oral therapy as soon as possible.
*Nontoxic goiter—*
**Adults:** initially, 5 mcg P.O. daily; may increase by 5 to 10 mcg daily q 1 to 2 weeks, until daily dose reaches 25 mcg. Then, increase by 12.5 to 25 mcg daily q 1 to 2 weeks. Usual maintenance dose is 75 mcg daily.
*Thyroid hormone replacement—*
**Adults:** initially, 25 mcg P.O. daily, increased by 12.5 to 25 mcg q 1 to 2 weeks until satisfactory response occurs. Usual maintenance dose is 25 to 50 mcg daily.
**Elderly:** for patients over age 65, 5 mcg daily, increased in 5-mcg daily increments.
*$T_3$ suppression test to differentiate hyperthyroidism from euthyroidism—*
**Adults:** 75 to 100 mcg P.O. daily for 7 days.

## ADVERSE REACTIONS
**CNS:** *nervousness, insomnia, tremor,* headache.
**CV:** *tachycardia,* **arrhythmias,** angina pectoris, **cardiac decompensation and collapse.**
**GI:** diarrhea, vomiting.
**GU:** menstrual irregularities.
**Metabolic:** weight loss.
**Musculoskeletal:** accelerated bone maturation in infants and children.
**Skin:** skin reactions, diaphoresis.
**Other:** heat intolerance.

## INTERACTIONS
**Drug-drug.** *Cholestyramine, colestipol:* impaired liothyronine absorption. Separate doses by 4 to 5 hours.
*Insulin, oral antidiabetics:* initial thyroid replacement therapy may cause increases in insulin or oral hypoglycemic requirements. Monitor blood glucose levels. Dosage adjustments may be needed.
*Oral anticoagulants:* altered PT. Monitor PT and INR. Dosage adjustments may be needed.
*Sympathomimetics such as epinephrine:* increased risk of coronary insufficiency. Monitor closely.

## EFFECTS ON DIAGNOSTIC TESTS
Alterations in radioactive iodine ($^{131}$I) uptake, protein-bound iodine levels, and liothyronine uptake may occur.

## CONTRAINDICATIONS
Contraindicated in patients with hypersensitivity to drug and in those with acute MI uncomplicated by hypothyroidism, untreated thyrotoxicosis, or uncorrected adrenal insufficiency.

## NURSING CONSIDERATIONS
• Use with extreme caution in elderly patients and in those with angina pectoris, hypertension, other CV disorders, renal insufficiency, or ischemia.
• Use cautiously in patients with diabetes mellitus, insipidus, or myxedema.
• Rapid replacement in patients with arteriosclerosis may precipitate angina, coronary occlusion, or CVA. Use cautiously in these patients. In patients with coronary artery disease who must receive thyroid hormones, observe carefully for possible coronary insufficiency.
• **Alert:** Levothyroxine is usually the preferred drug for thyroid hormone replacement therapy. Liothyronine may be used when a rapid onset or a rapidly reversible

drug is desirable, or in patients with impaired peripheral conversion of levothyroxine to liothyronine.
• Regulation of liothyronine dosage is difficult.
• Thyroid hormone replacement requirements are about 25% lower in patients over age 60 than in young adults.
• Monitor pulse and blood pressure.
• When changing from levothyroxine to liothyronine, levothyroxine should be stopped and liothyronine begun at a low dosage. Dosage should be increased in small increments after residual effects of levothyroxine have disappeared. When changing from liothyronine to levothyroxine, levothyroxine is started several days before withdrawing liothyronine to avoid relapse.
• Patients taking liothyronine who need $^{131}$I uptake studies done must discontinue drug 7 to 10 days before test.
• *Alert:* Don't confuse levothyroxine with liothyronine.

### █ I.V. administration
• Administer repeat dosages more than 4 hours but less than 12 hours apart. Don't administer injection I.M. or S.C.

### ✓ Patient teaching
• Make sure patient understands importance of compliance. Tell him to take thyroid hormones at same time each day, preferably before breakfast, to maintain constant hormone levels. Suggest morning dosage to prevent insomnia.
• Make sure patient understands that replacement therapy is for a lifetime.
• Advise patient who has achieved a stable response not to change brands.
• Warn patient (especially elderly patient) to notify doctor at once if chest pain, palpitations, sweating, nervousness, or other signs of overdose or aggravated CV disease occur.
• Tell patient to report unusual bleeding and bruising.

## liotrix
Euthroid**, Thyrolar

*Pregnancy Risk Category A*

### HOW SUPPLIED
*Tablets:* levothyroxine sodium ($T_4$) 30 mcg and liothyronine sodium ($T_3$) 7.5 mcg (Euthroid-½); levothyroxine sodium 60 mcg and liothyronine sodium 15 mcg (Euthroid-1); levothyroxine sodium 120 mcg and liothyronine sodium 30 mcg (Euthroid-2); levothyroxine sodium 180 mcg and liothyronine sodium 45 mcg (Euthroid-3); levothyroxine sodium 12.5 mcg and liothyronine sodium 3.1 mcg (Thyrolar-¼); levothyroxine sodium 25 mcg and liothyronine sodium 6.25 mcg (Thyrolar-½); levothyroxine sodium 50 mcg and liothyronine sodium 12.5 mcg (Thyrolar-1); levothyroxine sodium 100 mcg and liothyronine sodium 25 mcg (Thyrolar-2); levothyroxine sodium 150 mcg and liothyronine sodium 37.5 mcg (Thyrolar-3)

### ACTION
Not clearly defined. Stimulates metabolism of all body tissues by accelerating the rate of cellular oxidation and provides both $T_3$ and $T_4$ to the tissues.

| Route | Onset | Peak | Duration |
|-------|-------|------|----------|
| P.O. | Unknown | Unknown | Unknown |

### INDICATIONS & DOSAGE
*Hypothyroidism—*
Dosages are expressed in thyroid equivalents and must be individualized to approximate the deficit in patient's thyroid secretion.
**Adults:** initially, a single dose of Thyrolar-¼, Thyrolar-½, or Euthroid-½. Dosage is adjusted at 2-week intervals.

### ADVERSE REACTIONS
**CNS:** *nervousness, insomnia, tremor,* headache.
**CV:** *tachycardia,* **arrhythmias,** angina pectoris, **cardiac decompensation and collapse.**
**GI:** diarrhea, vomiting.
**GU:** menstrual irregularities.

**Metabolic:** weight loss.
**Musculoskeletal:** accelerated rate of bone maturation in infants and children.
**Skin:** allergic skin reactions, diaphoresis.
**Other:** heat intolerance, alterations in radioactive iodine ($^{131}$I) uptake, protein-bound iodine levels, and liothyronine uptake.

## INTERACTIONS
**Drug-drug.** *Cholestyramine, colestipol:* impaired liotrix absorption. Separate doses by 4 to 5 hours.
*Insulin, oral antidiabetics:* altered serum glucose levels. Monitor blood glucose levels. Dosage adjustments may be needed.
*I.V. phenytoin:* free thyroid released. Monitor for tachycardia.
*Oral anticoagulants:* altered PT. Monitor PT and INR. Dosage adjustments may be needed.
*Sympathomimetics such as epinephrine:* increased risk of coronary insufficiency. Monitor closely.

## EFFECTS ON DIAGNOSTIC TESTS
None reported.

## CONTRAINDICATIONS
Contraindicated in patients with hypersensitivity to drug and in those with acute MI uncomplicated by hypothyroidism, untreated thyrotoxicosis, or uncorrected adrenal insufficiency.

## NURSING CONSIDERATIONS
• Use with extreme caution in elderly patients and in those with angina pectoris, hypertension, other CV disorders, renal insufficiency, or ischemia.
• Use cautiously in patients with myxedema, diabetes mellitus, or diabetes insipidus.
• Rapid replacement in patients with arteriosclerosis may precipitate angina, coronary occlusion, or CVA. Use cautiously in these patients.
• In patients with coronary artery disease who must receive thyroid hormones, observe carefully for possible coronary insufficiency. Also observe carefully during surgery because arrhythmias can be precipitated.

• Thyroid hormone replacement requirements are about 25% lower in patients over age 60 than in young adults.
• Monitor pulse and blood pressure.
• Patients taking liotrix who need $^{131}$I uptake studies done must discontinue drug 7 to 10 days before test.
• *Alert:* Don't confuse Thyrolar with thyroid.

☑ **Patient teaching**
• Make sure patient understands importance of compliance. He should take thyroid hormones at same time each day, preferably before breakfast, to maintain constant hormone levels. Morning dosage may prevent insomnia.
• Warn patient (especially elderly patient) to notify doctor at once if chest pain, palpitations, sweating, nervousness, or other signs of overdose or aggravated CV disease occur.
• Tell patient not to switch brands; the two commercially prepared liotrix drugs contain different amounts of each ingredient.
• Tell patient to report unusual bleeding and bruising.

## thyroid
Armour Thyroid, S-P-T, Thyrar, Thyroid Strong, Westhroid

*Pregnancy Risk Category A*

## HOW SUPPLIED
*Tablets:* 15 mg, 30 mg, 60 mg, 65 mg, 90 mg, 120 mg, 130 mg, 180 mg, 240 mg, 300 mg
*Tablets (Thyrar; bovine origin):* 30 mg, 60 mg, 120 mg
*Tablets (S-P-T; pork origin):* 15 mg, 30 mg, 60 mg, 120 mg, 200 mg, 250 mg, 300 mg
*Tablets (enteric-coated):* 60 mg, 120 mg
*Strong tablets (50% stronger than thyroid USP, and containing 0.3% iodine):* 32.5 mg, 65 mg, 130 mg, 200 mg
*Capsules (pork origin):* 60 mg, 120 mg, 180 mg, 300 mg

---

Reactions may be *common*, uncommon, *life-threatening*, OR COMMON AND LIFE-THREATENING.

## ACTION
Not clearly defined. Stimulates metabolism of all body tissues by accelerating the rate of cellular oxidation.

| Route | Onset | Peak | Duration |
|-------|-------|------|----------|
| P.O. | Unknown | Unknown | Unknown |

## INDICATIONS & DOSAGE
*Mild hypothyroidism—*
**Adults:** initially, 60 mg P.O. daily, increased by 60 mg q 30 days until desired response occurs. Usual maintenance dose is 60 to 120 mg daily as single dose.
*Severe hypothyroidism—*
**Adults:** initially, 15 mg P.O. daily, increased by 30 mg daily after 2 weeks, and 2 weeks later increased to 60 mg daily. After 2 months, increased to 120 mg daily, p.r.n., for 2 months; then to 120 mg daily, p.r.n.
*Congenital or severe hypothyroidism in children—*
**Children:** same dosage as for adults with severe hypothyroidism.
**Elderly:** for patients over age 65, 7.5 to 15 mg daily. May double dose q 6 to 8 weeks until desired result is obtained.

## ADVERSE REACTIONS
**CNS:** *nervousness, insomnia,* tremor, headache.
**CV:** *tachycardia,* **arrhythmias,** angina pectoris, **cardiac decompensation and collapse.**
**GI:** diarrhea, vomiting.
**GU:** menstrual irregularities.
**Metabolic:** weight loss.
**Musculoskeletal:** accelerated rate of bone maturation in infants and children.
**Skin:** allergic skin reactions, diaphoresis.
**Other:** heat intolerance, alterations in radioactive iodine ($^{131}$I) uptake, protein-bound iodine levels, and liothyronine uptake.

## INTERACTIONS
**Drug-drug.** *Cholestyramine:* impaired thyroid absorption. Separate doses by 4 to 5 hours.
*Insulin, oral antidiabetics:* altered serum glucose levels. Monitor glucose levels, and adjust dosage as needed.

*Oral anticoagulants:* altered PT. Monitor PT and INR. Adjust dosage as needed.
*Sympathomimetics such as epinephrine:* increased risk of coronary insufficiency. Monitor closely.

## EFFECTS ON DIAGNOSTIC TESTS
None reported.

## CONTRAINDICATIONS
Contraindicated in patients with hypersensitivity to drug and in those with acute MI uncomplicated by hypothyroidism, untreated thyrotoxicosis, or uncorrected adrenal insufficiency.

## NURSING CONSIDERATIONS
• Use with extreme caution in elderly patients and in those with angina pectoris, hypertension, other CV disorders, renal insufficiency, or ischemia.
• Use cautiously in patients with myxedema or diabetes mellitus or insipidus.
• In patients with coronary artery disease, check for coronary insufficiency.
• Thyroid hormone replacement requirements are about 25% lower in patients over age 60 than in young adults.
• Monitor pulse and blood pressure.
• In children, sleeping pulse rate and basal morning temperature guide treatment.
• Thyroid hormones alter thyroid function test results.
• Patient must discontinue thyroid 7 to 10 days before undergoing $^{131}$I studies.
• *Alert:* Don't confuse Thyrolar with thyroid.

### ☑ Patient teaching
• Tell patient to take thyroid hormones at same time each day, preferably before breakfast, to maintain constant hormone levels. Advise patient that taking dose in the morning may prevent insomnia.
• Advise patient who has achieved stable response not to change brands.
• Warn patient (especially elderly patient) to notify doctor at once if chest pain, palpitations, or other signs of overdose or aggravated CV disease occur.
• Tell patient to report unusual bleeding and bruising.

---

**methimazole**
**potassium iodide**
**potassium iodide, saturated solution**
**propylthiouracil**
**radioactive iodine (sodium iodide $^{131}$I)**
**strong iodine solution**

**COMBINATION PRODUCTS**
None.

---

**methimazole**
Tapazole

*Pregnancy Risk Category D*

**HOW SUPPLIED**
*Tablets:* 5 mg, 10 mg

**ACTION**
Inhibits oxidation of iodine in thyroid gland, blocking iodine's ability to combine with tyrosine to form $T_4$. Also may prevent coupling of monoiodotyrosine and diiodotyrosine to form $T_4$ and $T_3$.

| Route | Onset | Peak | Duration |
|-------|-------|------|----------|
| P.O. | < 5 days | 0.5-1 hr | Unknown |

**INDICATIONS & DOSAGE**
*Hyperthyroidism—*
**Adults:** if mild, 15 mg P.O. daily; if moderately severe, 30 to 40 mg daily; if severe, 60 mg daily. Dose once daily or in two divided doses. Maintenance dose is 5 to 15 mg daily.
**Children:** 0.4 mg/kg P.O. once or in divided doses daily. Maintenance dose is 0.2 mg/kg once or in divided doses daily.

**ADVERSE REACTIONS**
**CNS:** headache, drowsiness, vertigo, paresthesia, neuritis, neuropathies, CNS stimulation, depression.
**GI:** diarrhea, nausea, vomiting (may be dose-related), salivary gland enlargement, loss of taste, epigastric distress.
**GU:** nephritis.
**Hematologic:** *agranulocytosis, leukopenia, thrombocytopenia, aplastic anemia.*
**Hepatic:** jaundice, hepatic dysfunction, *hepatitis.*
**Musculoskeletal:** arthralgia, myalgia.
**Skin:** rash, urticaria, discoloration, pruritus, erythema nodosum, exfoliative dermatitis, lupus-like syndrome.
**Other:** fever, lymphadenopathy, hypothyroidism.

**INTERACTIONS**
**Drug-drug.** *Aminophylline, oxtriphylline, theophylline:* decreased clearance. May need dosage adjustment.
*Anticoagulants:* may alter dosage requirements. Monitor PT, PTT, and INR.
*Cardiac glycosides:* increase serum levels. May need to decrease digitalis dose.
*Potassium iodide:* may decrease response to drug. May need to increase dosage of methimazole.

**EFFECTS ON DIAGNOSTIC TESTS**
Drug therapy alters selenomethionine ($^{75}$Se) uptake by the pancreas and $^{123}$I or $^{131}$I uptake by the thyroid.

**CONTRAINDICATIONS**
Contraindicated in patients with hypersensitivity to drug and in breast-feeding women.

**NURSING CONSIDERATIONS**
• Use with extreme caution during pregnancy. Pregnant women may need less drug as pregnancy progresses. Monitor thyroid function studies closely. Thyroid may be added to regimen. Drug may be stopped during last few weeks of pregnancy.
• Monitor CBC periodically, as ordered, to detect impending leukopenia, thrombocytopenia, and agranulocytosis. Also monitor hepatic function.
• *Alert:* Doses over 30 mg/day increase risk of agranulocytosis.

---

Reactions may be *common,* uncommon, *life-threatening,* or COMMON AND LIFE-THREATENING.

- *Alert:* Patients over age 40 may have an increased risk of developing drug-induced agranulocytosis.
- Watch for signs and symptoms of hypothyroidism (mental depression; cold intolerance; hard, nonpitting edema); notify doctor because dosage may need to be adjusted as needed.
- *Alert:* Discontinue drug and notify doctor if severe rash or enlarged cervical lymph nodes develop.
- *Alert:* Don't confuse methimazole with mebendazole or methazolamide.

☑ **Patient teaching**
- Tell patient to take drug with meals to reduce adverse GI reactions.
- Warn patient to report fever, sore throat, mouth sores, skin eruptions, anorexia, pruritus, right upper quadrant pain, yellow skin, or sclera.
- Tell patient to ask doctor about using iodized salt and eating shellfish. The iodine in these may make the drug less effective.
- Warn patient against OTC cough medicines; many contain iodine.
- Instruct patient to store drug in light-resistant container.
- Teach patient to watch for signs and symptoms of hypothyroidism (unexplained weight gain, fatigue, cold intolerance) and to notify doctor if they occur.

---

**potassium iodide**
Iosat, Pima, Thyro-Block

**potassium iodide, saturated solution (SSKI)**

**strong iodine solution (Lugol's solution)**

*Pregnancy Risk Category D*

---

**HOW SUPPLIED**
**potassium iodide**
*Tablets:* 130 mg
*Oral solution:* 500 mg/15 ml
*Syrup:* 325 mg/5 ml
**potassium iodide, saturated solution**
*Oral solution:* 1 g/ml

**strong iodine solution**
*Oral solution:* iodine 50 mg/ml and potassium iodide 100 mg/ml

**ACTION**
Inhibits thyroid hormone formation, limits iodide transport into the thyroid gland, and blocks thyroid hormone release.

| Route | Onset | Peak | Duration |
|-------|-------|------|----------|
| P.O. | < 24 hr | 10-15 days | Unknown |

**INDICATIONS & DOSAGE**
*Preparation for thyroidectomy—*
**Adults and children:** strong iodine solution (USP), 0.1 to 0.3 ml P.O. t.i.d.; or potassium iodide, saturated solution (SSKI), 1 to 5 drops in water P.O. t.i.d. after meals for 10 to 14 days before surgery.
*Thyrotoxic crisis—*
**Adults and children:** 500 mg P.O. q 4 hours (about 10 drops of SSKI); or 1 ml of strong iodine solution t.i.d.
*Radiation protectant for thyroid gland—*
**Adults and children ages 1 and older:** 130 mg P.O. daily for 7 to 14 days after radiation exposure.
**Children up to age 1:** 65 mg P.O. daily for 7 to 14 days after exposure.

**ADVERSE REACTIONS**
**EENT:** periorbital edema.
**GI:** diarrhea, inflammation of salivary glands, burning mouth and throat, sore teeth and gums, *metallic taste.*
**Metabolic:** *potassium toxicity.*
**Skin:** acneiform rash.
**Other:** fever; *hypersensitivity reactions.*

**INTERACTIONS**
**Drug-drug.** *ACE inhibitors, potassium-sparing diuretics:* risk of hyperkalemia. Avoid concomitant use.
*Antithyroid drugs:* potassium iodide may potentiate hypothyroid or goitrogenic effects. Monitor closely.
*Lithium carbonate:* hypothyroidism may occur. Use with caution.

**EFFECTS ON DIAGNOSTIC TESTS**
Potassium iodide may alter the results of thyroid function tests.

---

## CONTRAINDICATIONS

Contraindicated in patients with tuberculosis, acute bronchitis, iodide hypersensitivity, or hyperkalemia. Some formulations contain sulfites, which may precipitate allergic reactions in hypersensitive patients.

## NURSING CONSIDERATIONS

• Use cautiously in patients with hypocomplementemic vasculitis, goiter, or autoimmune thyroid disease.
• Drug is usually given with other antithyroid drugs.
• Doctor may avoid prescribing enteric-coated tablets, which have been associated with small-bowel lesions and can lead to serious complications, including perforation, hemorrhage, or obstruction.
• For thyrotoxicosis, initial iodine dose is given at least 1 hour after initial dose of propylthiouracil and methimazole.
• Dilute oral solution in water, milk, or fruit juice, and give after meals to prevent gastric irritation, hydrate patient, and to mask salty taste.
• Give iodides through straw to avoid tooth discoloration.
• *Alert:* Earliest signs of delayed hypersensitivity reactions caused by iodides are irritation and swollen eyelids.
• Store in light-resistant container.

### ✅ Patient teaching

• Show patient how to mask salty taste of oral solution. Tell him to take all forms of drug after meals.
• Warn patient that sudden withdrawal may precipitate thyroid crisis.
• Teach patient signs and symptoms of potassium toxicity, including confusion, irregular heartbeat, numbness, tingling, pain or weakness of hands or feet, tiredness.
• Tell patient to ask doctor about using iodized salt and eating shellfish. These foods contain iodine and may alter drug's effectiveness.

## propylthiouracil (PTU)
Propyl-Thyracil†

*Pregnancy Risk Category D*

### HOW SUPPLIED
*Tablets:* 50 mg, 100 mg

### ACTION
Inhibits oxidation of iodine in thyroid gland, blocking iodine's ability to combine with tyrosine to form $T_4$, and may prevent coupling of monoiodotyrosine and diiodotyrosine to form $T_4$ and $T_3$.

| Route | Onset | Peak | Duration |
|-------|-------|------|----------|
| P.O. | Unknown | 1-1.5 hr | Unknown |

### INDICATIONS & DOSAGE
*Hyperthyroidism—*
**Adults:** 300 to 900 mg P.O. daily in one to four divided doses; up to 1,200 mg daily have been used in severe cases. Maintenance dose is variable but generally ranges from 100 to 150 mg daily.
**Children over age 10:** 150 to 300 mg P.O. daily in divided doses t.i.d. Maintenance dose determined by patient response.
**Children ages 6 to 10:** 50 to 150 mg P.O. daily in divided doses t.i.d or q.i.d. Maintenance dose determined by patient response.
*Thyrotoxic crisis—*
**Adults and children:** 200 mg P.O. q 4 to 6 hours on first day; once full control of symptoms is achieved, dosage is gradually reduced to usual maintenance levels.

### ADVERSE REACTIONS
**CNS:** headache, drowsiness, vertigo, paresthesia, neuritis, neuropathies, CNS stimulation, depression.
**CV:** vasculitis.
**EENT:** visual disturbances.
**GI:** diarrhea, *nausea, vomiting*, epigastric distress, salivary gland enlargement, loss of taste.
**GU:** nephritis.
**Hematologic:** *agranulocytosis, leukopenia, thrombocytopenia, aplastic anemia.*
**Hepatic:** jaundice, *hepatotoxicity.*
**Musculoskeletal:** arthralgia, myalgia.

**Skin:** rash, urticaria, skin discoloration, pruritus, erythema nodosum, exfoliative dermatitis, lupus-like syndrome.
**Other:** fever, lymphadenopathy; dose-related hypothyroidism.

## INTERACTIONS
**Drug-drug.** *Aminophylline, oxtriphylline, theophylline*: decreased clearance. Dosage may need to be altered.
*Anticoagulants:* anticoagulant effects may be increased. Monitor PT and INR.
*Cardiac glycosides:* increased serum levels of glycosides. May need dosage reduction.
*Potassium iodide:* may decrease response to drug. May need to increase dosage of antithyroid drug.

## EFFECTS ON DIAGNOSTIC TESTS
PTU therapy alters selenomethionine ($^{75}$Se) levels and liothyronine uptake.

## CONTRAINDICATIONS
Contraindicated in patients with hypersensitivity to drug and in breast-feeding women.

## NURSING CONSIDERATIONS
• Use cautiously in pregnant women, who may need less drug as pregnancy progresses. Monitor thyroid function studies closely. Thyroid may be added to regimen. Drug may be stopped during last few weeks of pregnancy.
• *Alert:* Patients over age 40 may have an increased risk of developing agranulocytosis.
• Give drug with meals to reduce adverse GI reactions.
• Watch for signs of hypothyroidism (mental depression; cold intolerance; hard, nonpitting edema); adjust dosage, as ordered.
• Monitor CBC periodically to detect impending leukopenia, thrombocytopenia, and agranulocytosis.
• *Alert:* Discontinue drug and notify doctor if severe rash or enlarged cervical lymph nodes develop.
• Store drug in light-resistant container.

### ✅ Patient teaching
• Instruct patient to take drug with meals.

• Warn patient to report fever, sore throat, mouth sores, and skin eruptions.
• Tell patient to ask doctor about using iodized salt and eating shellfish. These foods contain iodine and may alter the effectiveness of drug.
• Warn patient against taking OTC cough medicines; many contain iodine.
• Teach patient to watch for signs and symptoms of hypothyroidism (unexplained weight gain, fatigue, cold intolerance) and to notify doctor if such occur.

# radioactive iodine (sodium iodide $^{131}$I)
Iodotope, Sodium Iodide $^{131}$I
Therapeutic

*Pregnancy Risk Category X*

## HOW SUPPLIED
All radioactivity concentrations are determined at time of calibration.
**iodotope**
*Capsules:* radioactivity range is 1 to 50 millicuries (mCi)/capsule at time of calibration
*Oral solution:* radioactivity concentration is 7.05 mCi/ml at time of calibration; in vials containing about 7, 14, 28, 70, or 106 mCi at time of calibration
**sodium iodide $^{131}$I therapeutic**
*Capsules:* radioactivity range is 0.8 to 100 mCi/capsule at time of calibration
*Oral solution:* radioactivity range is 3.5 to 150 mCi/vial at time of calibration

## ACTION
Limits thyroid hormone secretion by destroying thyroid tissue. Affinity of thyroid tissue for radioactive iodine facilitates uptake of drug by cancerous thyroid tissue that has metastasized to other sites in the body.

| Route | Onset | Peak | Duration |
|-------|-------|------|----------|
| P.O. | Unknown | 1-1.5 hr | Unknown |

## INDICATIONS & DOSAGE
*Hyperthyroidism—*
**Adults:** usual dosage is 4 to 10 mCi P.O. Dosage is based on estimated weight of thyroid gland and thyroid uptake. Treat-

ment repeated after 6 weeks, based on serum $T_4$ level.

*Thyroid cancer—*

**Adults:** initially, 30 to 100 mCi P.O., with subsequent doses of 100 to 200 mCi. Dosage is based on estimated malignant thyroid tissue and metastatic tissue as determined by total body scan. Treatment repeated according to clinical status.

## ADVERSE REACTIONS
**CV:** chest pain, tachycardia.
**EENT:** *fullness in neck,* pain on swallowing, sore throat, cough.
**Hematologic:** anemia, blood dyscrasia, *leukopenia, thrombocytopenia.*
**Skin:** rash, pruritus, urticaria.
**Other:** hypothyroidism; radiation-induced thyroiditis; radiation sickness, *death,* temporary thinning of hair, allergic-type reactions.

## INTERACTIONS
**Drug-drug.** *Lithium carbonate:* hypothyroidism may occur. Use with caution.

The following drugs can interfere with the action of $^{131}I$ and should be withheld for the specified time before administering the $^{131}I$ dose:

*Adrenocorticoids:* 1 week.
*Benzodiazepines:* 1 month.
*Cholecystographic drugs:* 6 to 9 months.
*Contrast media containing iodine:* 1 to 2 months.
*Products containing iodine, including antitussives, expectorants, topical drugs, and vitamins:* 2 weeks.
*Salicylates:* 1 to 2 weeks.

## EFFECTS ON DIAGNOSTIC TESTS
$^{131}I$ therapy alters $^{131}I$ thyroid uptake and protein-bound iodine levels.

## CONTRAINDICATIONS
Contraindicated during pregnancy (except to treat thyroid cancer) and in breast-feeding women.

## NURSING CONSIDERATIONS
• All antithyroid drugs and thyroid preparations must be stopped 1 week before $^{131}I$ dose. If this isn't possible, patient may receive thyroid-stimulating hormone for 3 days before $^{131}I$ dose. When treating

women of childbearing age, give dose during menstruation or within 7 days afterward.
• After therapy for hyperthyroidism, patient shouldn't resume antithyroid drugs but should continue propranolol or other drugs used to treat symptoms of hyperthyroidism until onset of full $^{131}I$ effect (usually 6 weeks).
• Monitor thyroid function via serum $T_4$ levels, as ordered.
• Institute full radiation precautions. Have patient use proper disposal methods when coughing and expectorating. After dose for hyperthyroidism, patient's urine and saliva are slightly radioactive for 24 hours; vomitus is highly radioactive for 6 to 8 hours.
• After dose for thyroid cancer, patient's urine, saliva, and perspiration are radioactive for 3 days. Isolate patient and observe these precautions: Don't allow pregnant personnel to care for patient; provide disposable eating utensils and linens; instruct patient to save urine in lead container for 24 to 48 hours; limit contact with patient to 30 minutes per shift per person on day 1, and increase time, as needed, to 1 hour on day 2 and longer on day 3.

### ✅ Patient teaching
• Tell patient to fast overnight before administration and to drink as much fluid as possible for 48 hours afterward.
• Instruct patient about appropriate radiation exposure precautions to use after drug administration.
• Warn patient who is discharged less than 7 days after $^{131}I$ dose for thyroid cancer to avoid close contact with small children and not to sleep in same room with spouse for 7 days after treatment.
• Teach patient the signs and symptoms of hypothyroidism (unexplained weight gain, fatigue, cold intolerance) and instruct him to notify doctor if these occur.

---

Reactions may be *common,* uncommon, *life-threatening,* or COMMON AND LIFE-THREATENING.

**corticotropin**
**cosyntropin**
**desmopressin acetate**
**leuprolide acetate**
   (See Chapter 72, ANTINEOPLASTICS
   THAT ALTER HORMONE BALANCE.)
**repository corticotropin**
**somatrem**
**somatropin**
**vasopressin**

**COMBINATION PRODUCTS**
None.

---

## corticotropin (ACTH, adrenocorticotropic hormone)
ACTH, Acthar

## repository corticotropin
Acthar Gel (H.P.)†,
H.P. Acthar Gel

*Pregnancy Risk Category C*

### HOW SUPPLIED
*Aqueous injection:* 25-U vial, 40 U/vial
*Repository injection:* 40 U/ml, 80 U/ml

### ACTION
By replacing the body's own tropic hormone, drug stimulates the adrenal cortex to secrete its entire spectrum of hormones.

| Route | Onset | Peak | Duration |
|---|---|---|---|
| I.V., I.M. | Rapid | 1 hr | 2-4 hr |
| I.M. (repository) | Unknown | Unknown | 3 days |
| S.C. | Unknown | Unknown | Unknown |

### INDICATIONS & DOSAGE
*Diagnostic test of adrenocortical function—*
**Adults:** 40 U I.M. (repository) q 12 hours for 1 to 2 days; or 10 to 25 U aqueous form in 500 ml of D₅W I.V. over 8 hours, between blood samplings.

   Individual dosages vary with sensitivity of adrenal glands to stimulation and with specific disease. Infants and younger children need larger doses per kg than older children and adults.
*For therapeutic use—*
**Adults:** 40 U aqueous form S.C. or I.M. in four divided doses; or 40 to 80 U q 24 to 72 hours (repository form).

### ADVERSE REACTIONS
**CNS:** *seizures,* dizziness, vertigo, *increased intracranial pressure with papilledema,* pseudotumor cerebri.
**CV:** hypertension, *heart failure,* necrotizing vasculitis, *shock.*
**EENT:** cataracts, glaucoma.
**GI:** peptic ulceration with perforation and hemorrhage, *pancreatitis,* abdominal distention, ulcerative esophagitis, nausea, vomiting.
**GU:** menstrual irregularities.
**Metabolic:** activation of latent diabetes mellitus, calcium and potassium loss, *sodium and fluid retention,* hypokalemic alkalosis.
**Musculoskeletal:** suppression of growth in children, muscle weakness, steroid myopathy, loss of muscle mass, osteoporosis, vertebral compression fractures.
**Respiratory:** pneumonia, *bronchospasm.*
**Skin:** impaired wound healing, thin fragile skin, petechiae, ecchymoses, facial erythema, diaphoresis, acne, hyperpigmentation, allergic reactions, hirsutism.
**Other:** cushingoid symptoms, abscess and septic infection, *hypersensitivity reactions.*

### INTERACTIONS
**Drug-drug.** *Amphotericin B, potassium-sparing diuretics:* increased risk of hypokalemia. Monitor serum potassium levels.
*Anticonvulsants, barbiturates, rifampin:* increased metabolism of corticotropin and decreased effectiveness. Watch for lack of effect.

---

*Antidiabetics:* may increase requirements of antidiabetics because of intrinsic hyperglycemic activity of corticotropin. Monitor blood glucose levels closely.
*Estrogens:* may potentiate effects of cortisol. Dosage adjustments may be needed.
*NSAIDs, salicylates:* increased risk of GI bleeding. Avoid concomitant use.
*Oral anticoagulants:* altered PT. Monitor PT and INR. Dosage adjustments may be needed.
*Vaccines:* risk of neurologic complications and lack of antibody response. Smallpox vaccine shouldn't be used and other immunizations should be considered with extreme caution.

**EFFECTS ON DIAGNOSTIC TESTS**
High plasma cortisol levels may be reported erroneously in patients receiving spironolactone, cortisone, or hydrocortisone when fluorometric analysis is used. This doesn't occur with the radioimmunoassay or competitive protein-binding method. However, therapy can be maintained with prednisone, dexamethasone, or betamethasone because they aren't detectable by the fluorometric method. Drug may also alter protein-bound iodine levels and radioactive iodine ($^{131}I$) and $T_3$ uptake.

**CONTRAINDICATIONS**
Contraindicated in patients with hypersensitivity to pork and pork products and in those with peptic ulcer, scleroderma, osteoporosis, systemic fungal infections, ocular herpes simplex, peptic ulceration, heart failure, hypertension, Cushing's syndrome, and adrenocortical hyperfunction or primary insufficiency. Also contraindicated after recent surgery.

**NURSING CONSIDERATIONS**
• Use cautiously during pregnancy and in women of childbearing age. Also use cautiously in patients being immunized and in those with latent tuberculosis or tuberculin reactivity, hypothyroidism, cirrhosis, acute gouty arthritis, psychotic tendencies, renal insufficiency, diverticulitis, nonspecific ulcerative colitis, thromboembolic disorders, seizures, uncontrolled hypertension, or myasthenia gravis.

• Corticotropin treatment should be preceded by verification of adrenal responsiveness and testing for hypersensitivity and allergic reactions.
• If administering gel, warm it to room temperature, draw into large needle, and give slowly as deep I.M. injection with 21G or 22G needle.
• Corticotropin may mask signs of chronic disease and decrease host resistance and ability to localize infection.
• Note and record weight changes, fluid exchange, and resting blood pressures until minimal effective dosage is achieved.
• Watch neonates of corticotropin-treated mothers for signs of hypoadrenalism.
• Unusual stress may require additional use of rapidly acting steroids. When possible, gradually reduce corticotropin dosage to smallest effective dose, as ordered, to minimize induced adrenocortical insufficiency. Therapy can be reinstituted if stressful situation (trauma, surgery, severe illness) occurs shortly after stopping drug.
• *Alert:* Don't confuse corticotropin with cosyntropin.

**I.V. administration**
• Use only aqueous form for I.V. administration. Dilute in 500 ml $D_5W$ and infuse over 8 hours.
• Refrigerate reconstituted solution and use within 24 hours.

**Patient teaching**
• Warn patient that injection is painful.
• Stress importance of informing all members of health care team about therapeutic use of drug because unusual stress may require additional use of rapidly acting steroids.
• Instruct patient how to handle troublesome adverse reactions, such as limiting sodium intake to reduce severity of edema and increasing protein intake to combat nitrogen loss.
• Advise patient about need for close follow-up care.
• Instruct patient to avoid individuals with known or suspected varicella infections.

---

## cosyntropin
Cortrosyn

*Pregnancy Risk Category C*

### HOW SUPPLIED
*Injection:* 0.25-mg vial

### ACTION
By replacing the body's own tropic hormone, drug stimulates the adrenal cortex to secrete its entire spectrum of hormones.

| Route | Onset | Peak | Duration |
|-------|-------|------|----------|
| I.V. | Rapid | 45-60 min | Unknown |
| I.M., S.C. | Unknown | 45-60 min | Unknown |

### INDICATIONS & DOSAGE
*Diagnostic test of adrenocortical function—*
**Adults and children ages 2 and older:** 0.25 mg I.M. or I.V over 2 minutes, or 40 mcg/hour over 6 hours (unless label prohibits I.V. administration) between blood samplings.
**Children under age 2:** 0.125 mg I.M. or I.V.

### ADVERSE REACTIONS
**CNS:** *seizures,* dizziness, vertigo, *increased intracranial pressure with papilledema,* pseudotumor cerebri.
**CV:** flushing.
**EENT:** cataracts, glaucoma.
**GI:** peptic ulceration, *pancreatitis,* abdominal distension, ulcerative esophagitis, nausea, vomiting.
**GU:** menstrual irregularities.
**Musculoskeletal:** muscle weakness, steroid myopathy, loss of muscle mass, osteoporosis, vertebral compression, fractures.
**Skin:** pruritus; impaired wound healing; thin, fragile skin; petechiae; ecchymoses; facial erythema; diaphoresis; acne; hyperpigmentation; hirsutism.
**Other:** cushingoid symptoms, *hypersensitivity reactions.*

### INTERACTIONS
**Drug-drug.** *Blood, plasma products:* inactivates cosyntropin. Avoid concomitant administration.

*Cortisone, hydrocortisone:* may interfere with test results of cortisol levels if administered on test day. Avoid concomitant use.
*Spironolactone:* may interfere with fluorometric analysis of cortisol levels. Avoid concomitant use.

### EFFECTS ON DIAGNOSTIC TESTS
None reported.

### CONTRAINDICATIONS
Contraindicated in patients with hypersensitivity to drug.

### NURSING CONSIDERATIONS
● Use cautiously in patients hypersensitive to natural corticotropin.
● Drug is synthetic duplication of the biologically active part of the corticotropin molecule. It's less likely to produce sensitivity than natural corticotropin derived from animal sources.
● Monitor patient for allergic reactions, rash, dyspnea, wheezing, or evidence of anaphylaxis.
● *Alert:* Don't confuse cosyntropin with corticotropin.

### I.V. administration
● Reconstitute with 1 ml supplied diluent. For direct injection, administer over at least 2 minutes. May be further diluted with $D_5W$ or normal saline and infused over 6 hours. Solution is stable for 12 hours at room temperature.

### ✅ Patient teaching
● Explain test procedure to patient.
● Tell patient to report adverse reactions immediately.

## desmopressin acetate
DDAVP, Desmospray§, Minirin‡, Stimate

*Pregnancy Risk Category B*

### HOW SUPPLIED
*Tablets:* 0.1 mg, 0.2 mg
*Nasal solution:* 0.1 mg/ml, 1.5 mg/ml
*Injection:* 4 mcg/ml, 15 mcg/ml

---

*Liquid contains alcohol.  **May contain tartrazine.  †Canada  ‡Australia  §U.K.  ◊OTC

## ACTION
Increases the permeability of the renal tubular epithelium to adenosine monophosphate and water; the epithelium promotes reabsorption of water and produces a concentrated urine. Also increases factor VIII activity by releasing endogenous factor VIII from plasma storage sites.

| Route | Onset | Peak | Duration |
|-------|-------|------|----------|
| P.O. | 1 hr | 1-1.5 hr | 8-12 hr |
| I.V. | 15-30 min | Unknown | 4-12 hr |
| Nasal | 1 hr | 1-5 hr | 8-12 hr |

## INDICATIONS & DOSAGE
*Nonnephrogenic diabetes insipidus, temporary polyuria and polydipsia associated with pituitary trauma—*
**Adults:** 0.1 to 0.4 ml intranasally daily in one to three doses. Morning and evening doses adjusted separately for adequate diurnal rhythm of water turnover. Most adults need 0.2 ml daily in divided doses. Or, injectable form administered in dose of 0.5 to 1 ml I.V. or S.C. daily, usually in two divided doses.
**Children ages 3 months to 12 years:** 0.05 to 0.3 ml intranasally daily in one or two doses.
*Hemophilia A and von Willebrand's disease—*
**Adults and children:** 0.3 mcg/kg diluted in normal saline and infused I.V. over 15 to 30 minutes. Dose repeated, if needed, as indicated by laboratory response and patient's clinical condition. Or, 300 mcg (one spray in each nostril) of solution containing 1.5 mcg/ml. Dose of 150 mcg (one spray into a single nostril of solution containing 1.5 mg/ml) may be adequate for patients weighing under 50 kg (110 lb). Administer 2 hours before surgery.
*Primary nocturnal enuresis—*
**Children ages 6 and older:** initially, 20 mcg (0.2 ml) intranasally h.s. (10 mcg each nostril). Dosage adjusted based on response; maximum recommended dose is 40 mcg daily. Or, initially 0.2 mg P.O. h.s., may be adjusted up to 0.6 mg to achieve desired response. For patients previously on intranasal DDAVP therapy, start tablet night following (24 hours after) last intranasal dose.

## ADVERSE REACTIONS
**CNS:** headache.
**CV:** slight rise in blood pressure (with high doses).
**EENT:** rhinitis, epistaxis, sore throat.
**GI:** nausea, abdominal cramps.
**GU:** vulval pain.
**Respiratory:** cough.
**Other:** flushing; local erythema, swelling, or burning after injection.

## INTERACTIONS
**Drug-drug.** *Carbamazepine, chlorpropamide:* potentiate ADH, may potentiate effects of desmopressin. Avoid concomitant use.
*Clofibrate:* enhanced and prolonged effects of desmopressin. Monitor carefully.
*Demeclocycline, epinephrine, heparin, lithium:* increased risk of adverse effects. Monitor closely.
**Drug-lifestyle.** *Alcohol use:* increased risk of adverse effects. Avoid concomitant use.

## EFFECTS ON DIAGNOSTIC TESTS
None reported.

## CONTRAINDICATIONS
Contraindicated in patients with hypersensitivity to drug and in those with type IIB von Willebrand's disease.

## NURSING CONSIDERATIONS
• Use cautiously in breast-feeding women; it's not known if drug appears in breast milk.
• Use cautiously in patients with coronary artery insufficiency or hypertensive CV disease and in those with conditions associated with fluid and electrolyte imbalances, such as cystic fibrosis, because these patients are prone to hyponatremia.
• Desmopressin injection shouldn't be used to treat hemophilia A with factor VIII levels of up to 5% or severe cases of von Willebrand's disease.
• Intranasal use can cause changes in the nasal mucosa resulting in erratic, unreliable absorption. Report worsening condition to doctor, who may prescribe injectable DDAVP.

---

Reactions may be *common*, uncommon, *life-threatening*, or COMMON AND LIFE-THREATENING.

• Adjust fluid intake to reduce risk of water intoxication and sodium depletion, especially in children or elderly patients.
• *Alert:* Overdose may cause oxytocic or vasopressor activity. Withhold drug and notify doctor. Use furosemide if fluid retention is excessive, as ordered.
• *Alert:* Don't confuse desmopressin with vasopressin.

**◘ I.V. administration**
• For adults and children over 22 lb (10 kg), dilute with 50 ml sterile physiologic saline. For children under 22 lb, 10 ml of diluent is recommended.
• Monitor blood pressure and pulse during infusion.
• Inspect for particulate matter and discoloration before infusing drug.

**☑ Patient teaching**
• Instruct patient to clear nasal passages before administering drug.
• Some patients may have difficulty measuring and inhaling drug into nostrils. Teach patient and caregivers correct method of administration.
• Advise patient to report nasal congestion, allergic rhinitis, or upper respiratory tract infections to doctor; a dosage adjustment may be needed.
• Teach patient using S.C. desmopressin to rotate injection sites to prevent tissue damage.
• Warn patient to drink only enough water to satisfy thirst.
• Inform patient that, when treating hemophilia A and von Willebrand's disease, taking desmopressin may avoid hazards of using blood products.
• Advise patient to wear medical identification indicating use of drug.

---

**somatrem**
Protropin

*Pregnancy Risk Category C*

**HOW SUPPLIED**
*Injectable lyophilized powder:* 5-mg (about 15-IU) vial, 10-mg (about 30-IU) vial

**ACTION**
Purified growth hormone (GH) of recombinant DNA origin that stimulates linear, skeletal muscle, and organ growth.

| Route | Onset | Peak | Duration |
|-------|-------|------|----------|
| I.M., S.C. | Unknown | 3-5 hr | Unknown |

**INDICATIONS & DOSAGE**
*Long-term treatment of children who have growth failure because of lack of adequate endogenous GH secretion—*
**Children (prepuberty):** highly individualized; up to 0.1 mg/kg S.C. (preferred) or I.M. three times weekly. Don't exceed a weekly dose of 0.3 mg/kg.

**ADVERSE REACTIONS**
**Metabolic:** hypothyroidism, hyperglycemia.
**Other:** *antibodies to GH.*

**INTERACTIONS**
**Drug-drug.** *Glucocorticoids:* may inhibit growth-promoting action of somatrem. Adjust glucocorticoid dosage as needed.

**EFFECTS ON DIAGNOSTIC TESTS**
Drug therapy alters glucose tolerance test (reduced with high doses) and total protein and thyroid function tests. ($T_4$-binding capacity and radioactive uptake may be decreased.)

**CONTRAINDICATIONS**
Contraindicated in patients with hypersensitivity to benzyl alcohol and in those with epiphyseal closure or active neoplasia.

**NURSING CONSIDERATIONS**
• Use cautiously in patients with hypothyroidism and in those whose GH deficiency is caused by an intracranial lesion.
• Be sure to check product's expiration date.
• To prepare solution, inject supplied bacteriostatic water for injection into vial containing drug. Then swirl vial with a gentle rotary motion until contents are completely dissolved. Don't shake vial.
• After reconstitution, vial solution should be clear. Don't inject solution if it's cloudy or contains particles.

---

• If prepared for other than neonatal use, store reconstituted drug in refrigerator; use within 14 days.
• **Alert:** Toxicity in neonates has occurred from exposure to benzyl alcohol used in drug as a preservative. If drug is administered to neonates, reconstitute immediately before use with sterile water for injection (without bacteriostat). Use vial once; then discard.
• Regular checkups, including monitoring of height and blood and radiologic studies, are needed.
• Observe patient for signs and symptoms of glucose intolerance and hyperglycemia.
• Monitor for slipped capital femoral epiphysis or progression of scoliosis in patients with rapid growth.
• Monitor periodic thyroid function tests for hypothyroidism, as ordered; condition may need treatment with a thyroid hormone.
• Funduscopic examination of patient for intracranial hypertension should be done at onset of therapy and periodically thereafter.
• **Alert:** Don't confuse somatrem with somatropin.

☑ **Patient teaching**
• Reassure patient and caregivers that somatrem is pure and safe. Drug replaces pituitary-derived human GH, which was removed from the market in 1985 because of its association with a rare but fatal viral infection (Creutzfeldt-Jakob disease).
• Review signs and symptoms of hypothyroidism and hyperglycemia. Instruct patient and parents to report such signs or symptoms promptly.

---

**somatropin**
Genotropin§, Humatrope, Norditropin, Nutropin, Nutropin AQ, Saizen, Serostim, Zomacton§

*Pregnancy Risk Category C*

**HOW SUPPLIED**
*Injection:* 2-mg (about 6-IU [Humatrope]) vial†, 5-mg (about 15-IU [Huma-

trope]) vial, 10-mg (about 30-IU [Nutropin]) vial
*Genotropin injection:* 1.5 mg (about 4 IU/ml), 5.8 mg (about 15 IU/ml)
*Norditropin injection:* 4 mg (about 12 IU/ml), 8 mg (about 24 IU/ml)
*Nutropin injection:* 5 mg (about 15 IU/vial), 10 mg (about 30 IU/vial)
*Nutropin AQ injection:* 10 mg (about 30 IU/vial)
*Serostim injection:* 5 mg (about 15 IU/vial), 6 mg (about 18 IU/ml)
*Saizen injection:* 5 mg (about 15 IU/vial)

**ACTION**
Purified growth hormone (GH) of recombinant DNA origin that stimulates skeletal, linear, muscle, and organ growth.

| Route | Onset | Peak | Duration |
|-------|-------|------|----------|
| I.M., S.C. | Unknown | 3-5 hr | 12-48 hr |

**INDICATIONS & DOSAGE**
*Long-term treatment of growth failure in children with inadequate secretion of endogenous GH—*
**Children:** 0.18 mg/kg body weight S.C. or I.M. weekly, divided equally, and given on 3 alternate days, six times weekly or daily using Humatrope; or 0.30 mg/kg body weight S.C. weekly in daily divided doses using Nutropin; or 0.06 mg/kg I.M. or S.C. three times weekly using Saizen; or 0.024 to 0.034 mg/kg S.C., six to seven times weekly using Norditropin.
*In children, growth failure associated with chronic renal insufficiency up to time of renal transplantation (Nutropin only)—*
**Children:** weekly dosage of up to 0.35 mg/kg S.C. divided into daily doses.
*Long-term treatment of short stature associated with Turner's syndrome—*
**Children:** up to 0.375 mg/kg/week (about 1.125 IU/kg/week) S.C. divided into equal doses given three to seven times weekly.
*Replacement of endogenous GH in adult patients with GH deficiency—*
**Adults:** initially, not more than 0.006 mg/kg S.C. daily. May be increased to maximum of 0.025 mg/kg daily in patients younger than age 35 or 0.0125 mg/kg daily in patients older than age 35.

---

**ADVERSE REACTIONS**
**CNS:** headache, weakness.
**CV:** mild, transient edema.
**Hematologic:** *leukemia.*
**Metabolic:** mild hyperglycemia.
**Musculoskeletal:** localized muscle pain.
**Other:** injection site pain, hypothyroidism, antibodies to GH.

**INTERACTIONS**
**Drug-drug.** *Corticotropin, steroids:* long-term use inhibits growth response to GH. Monitor for lack of effect.

**EFFECTS ON DIAGNOSTIC TESTS**
Laboratory measurements of thyroid hormone may change.

**CONTRAINDICATIONS**
Contraindicated in patients with closed epiphyses or an active underlying intracranial lesion. Humatrope shouldn't be reconstituted with supplied diluent for patients with known sensitivity to either *m*-cresol or glycerin.

**NURSING CONSIDERATIONS**
• Use cautiously in children with hypothyroidism and in those whose GH deficiency is caused by an intracranial lesion. These children should be examined frequently for progression or recurrence of underlying disease.
• To prepare solution, inject supplied diluent into vial containing drug by aiming stream of liquid against glass wall of vial. Then swirl vial with gentle rotary motion until contents are completely dissolved. Don't shake vial.
• After reconstitution, vial solution should be clear. Don't inject solution if it's cloudy or contains particles.
• Patients on dialysis need changes in drug administration schedule as follows:
–Hemodialysis: administer before bedtime or 3 to 4 hours after dialysis.
–Long-term cycling peritoneal dialysis: administer in the morning after completion of dialysis.
–Long-term ambulatory peritoneal dialysis: administer in the evening at the time of the overnight exchange.
• Store reconstituted drug in refrigerator; use within 14 days.

• If sensitivity to diluent should occur, drug may be reconstituted with sterile water for injection. When drug is reconstituted in this manner, use only 1 reconstituted dose per vial; refrigerate solution if it's not used immediately after reconstitution; use reconstituted dose within 24 hours; and discard unused portion.
• Monitor child's height regularly. Regular checkups, including monitoring of blood and radiologic studies, also are needed.
• Monitor patient's blood glucose levels regularly because GH may induce a state of insulin resistance.
• Excessive glucocorticoid therapy will inhibit growth-promoting effect of somatropin. Patients with coexisting corticotropin deficiency should have their glucocorticoid replacement dosage carefully adjusted to avoid an inhibitory effect on growth.
• Monitor for slipped capital femoral epiphysis or progression of scoliosis in patients with rapid growth.
• Monitor periodic thyroid function tests, as ordered, for hypothyroidism; condition may need treatment with a thyroid hormone.
• Funduscopic examination of patient for intracranial hypertension should be done at onset of, and periodically during, therapy.
• *Alert:* Don't confuse somatropin with somatrem or sumatriptan.

☑ **Patient teaching**
• Inform parents that child with endocrine disorders (including GH deficiency) may develop slipped capital epiphyses more frequently. Tell them to notify doctor if they notice their child limping.
• Stress importance of close follow-up care.

---

**vasopressin (ADH)**
Pitressin

*Pregnancy Risk Category C*

**HOW SUPPLIED**
*Injection:* 0.5-ml and 1-ml ampules, 20 U/ml

---

## ACTION
Increases permeability of the renal tubular epithelium to adenosine monophosphate and water; the epithelium promotes reabsorption of water and produces a concentrated urine.

| Route | Onset | Peak | Duration |
|---|---|---|---|
| I.M., S.C., nasal | 2-8 hr | Unknown | Unknown |

## INDICATIONS & DOSAGE
*Nonnephrogenic, nonpsychogenic diabetes insipidus—*
**Adults:** 5 to 10 U I.M. or S.C. b.i.d. to q.i.d., p.r.n.; or intranasally (aqueous solution used as spray or applied to cotton balls) in individualized dosages, based on response.
**Children:** 2.5 to 10 U I.M. or S.C. b.i.d. to q.i.d., p.r.n.; or intranasally (aqueous solution used as spray or applied to cotton balls) in individualized doses.

## ADVERSE REACTIONS
**CNS:** tremor, headache, vertigo.
**CV:** vasoconstriction, ***arrhythmias, cardiac arrest,*** myocardial ischemia, circumoral pallor, decreased cardiac output, angina in patients with vascular disease.
**GI:** abdominal cramps, nausea, vomiting, flatulence.
**Skin:** diaphoresis, cutaneous gangrene.
**Other:** water intoxication, ***hypersensitivity reactions*** including urticaria, ***angioedema, bronchoconstriction, anaphylaxis.***

## INTERACTIONS
**Drug-drug.** *Carbamazepine, chlorpropamide, clofibrate, fludrocortisone, tricyclic antidepressants:* increased antidiuretic response. Use together cautiously.
*Demeclocycline, heparin, lithium, norepinephrine:* reduced antidiuretic activity. Use together cautiously.
**Drug-lifestyle.** *Alcohol use:* reduced antidiuretic activity. Avoid use.

## EFFECTS ON DIAGNOSTIC TESTS
None reported.

## CONTRAINDICATIONS
Contraindicated in patients with chronic nephritis and nitrogen retention.

## NURSING CONSIDERATIONS
• Use cautiously in children, elderly patients, pregnant women, preoperative and postoperative polyuric patients, and in those with seizure disorders, migraine, asthma, CV disease, heart failure, renal disease, goiter with cardiac complications, arteriosclerosis, or fluid overload.
• Synthetic desmopressin is sometimes preferred because of its longer duration of action and less frequent adverse reactions. Desmopressin also is available commercially as a nasal solution.
• Drug may be used for transient polyuria resulting from ADH deficiency related to neurosurgery or head injury.
• Use minimum effective dose to reduce adverse reactions.
• Give with 1 to 2 glasses of water to reduce adverse reactions and to improve therapeutic response.
• Monitor specific gravity of urine and fluid intake and output to aid evaluation of drug effectiveness.
• To prevent possible seizures, coma, and death, observe patient closely for early signs and symptoms of water intoxication, including drowsiness, listlessness, headache, confusion, and weight gain.
• Monitor blood pressure of patient taking vasopressin b.i.d. Watch for excessively elevated blood pressure or lack of response to drug, which may be indicated by hypotension. Also monitor weight daily.
• *Alert:* Don't confuse vasopressin with desmopressin.

### ☑Patient teaching
• Instruct patient to rotate injection sites to prevent tissue damage.
• Tell patient to report adverse reactions promptly.

---

Reactions may be *common*, uncommon, *life-threatening*, or COMMON AND LIFE-THREATENING.

calcifediol
calcitonin (human)
calcitonin (salmon)
calcitriol
dihydrotachysterol
etidronate disodium

## COMBINATION PRODUCTS
None.

---

## calcifediol
Calderol

*Pregnancy Risk Category C*

---

### HOW SUPPLIED
*Capsules:* 20 mcg, 50 mcg

### ACTION
A vitamin D analogue that stimulates calcium absorption from the GI tract and promotes secretion of calcium from bone to blood.

| Route | Onset | Peak | Duration |
|-------|-------|------|----------|
| P.O. | Unknown | 4 hr | 15-20 days |

### INDICATIONS & DOSAGE
*Metabolic bone disease and hypocalcemia associated with chronic renal failure—*
**Adults:** initially, 300 to 350 mcg P.O. weekly. Dosage increased at 4-week intervals, if needed.

### ADVERSE REACTIONS
Vitamin D intoxication associated with hypercalcemia:
**CNS:** headache, somnolence, weakness, irritability.
**CV:** hypertension, *arrhythmias.*
**EENT:** conjunctivitis, rhinorrhea.
**GI:** constipation, nausea, vomiting, polydipsia, *pancreatitis,* metallic taste, dry mouth, anorexia, diarrhea.
**GU:** polyuria, nocturia.
**Metabolic:** weight loss.
**Musculoskeletal:** bone and muscle pain.
**Skin:** pruritus, photosensitivity reactions.

**Other:** hyperthermia, nephrocalcinosis, decreased libido.

### INTERACTIONS
**Drug-drug.** *Cardiac glycosides:* increased risk of arrhythmias. Avoid concomitant use.
*Cholestyramine, colestipol:* decreased absorption of orally administered vitamin D analogues. Avoid concomitant use.
*Corticosteroids:* counteract vitamin D analogue effects. Don't use together.
*Magnesium-containing antacids:* possible hypermagnesemia, especially in patients with chronic renal failure. Avoid concomitant use.
*Other vitamin D analogues:* increased toxicity. Avoid concomitant use.
*Phenytoin:* may increase metabolism of vitamin to inactive metabolites. Avoid concomitant use.
*Products containing calcium, thiazide diuretics:* increased risk of hypercalcemia. Use with caution.

### EFFECTS ON DIAGNOSTIC TESTS
Drug may falsely elevate cholesterol determinations made using the Zlatkis-Zak reaction.

### CONTRAINDICATIONS
Contraindicated in patients with hypercalcemia or vitamin D toxicity.

### NURSING CONSIDERATIONS
• Monitor serum calcium level as ordered; serum calcium level multiplied by serum phosphate level shouldn't exceed 70. During adjustment, serum calcium level should be determined at least weekly.
• If hypercalcemia occurs, discontinue calcifediol and notify doctor. Drug may be resumed after serum calcium level returns to normal.
• **Alert:** Don't confuse calcifediol with calcitonin or calcitriol.

☑ **Patient teaching**
• Teach patient to report signs and symptoms of hypercalcemia.

---

• Instruct patient about importance of getting an adequate daily intake of calcium. Inform patient about foods high in calcium and how much to consume daily to meet RDA.

---

## calcitonin (human)
Cibacalcin

## calcitonin (salmon)
Calcimar, Calsynar§, Miacalcin, Miacalcin Nasal Spray, Osteocalcin, Salmonine

*Pregnancy Risk Category C*

### HOW SUPPLIED
**calcitonin (human)**
*Injection:* 0.5 mg/vial
**calcitonin (salmon)**
*Injection:* 100 IU/ml, 1-ml ampules; 200 IU/ml, 2-ml ampules
*Nasal spray:* 200 IU/activation in 2-ml bottle

### ACTION
Decreases osteoclastic activity by inhibiting osteocytic osteolysis; decreases mineral release and matrix or collagen breakdown in bone.

| Route | Onset | Peak | Duration |
|-------|-------|------|----------|
| I.M., S.C. | 15 min | 4 hr | 8-24 hr |
| Intranasal | Rapid | 0.5 hr | 1 hr |

### INDICATIONS & DOSAGE
*Paget's disease of bone (osteitis deformans)—*
**Adults:** initially, 100 IU of calcitonin (salmon) daily S.C. or I.M.; maintenance dose is 50 to 100 IU daily S.C. or I.M., every other day, or three times weekly. Or, calcitonin (human) 0.5 mg daily, reduced to 0.25 mg daily. Some patients may need up to 0.5 mg b.i.d.
*Hypercalcemia—*
**Adults:** 4 IU/kg of calcitonin (salmon) q 12 hours I.M. If response inadequate after 1 or 2 days, dosage increased to 8 IU/kg I.M. q 12 hours. If response remains unsatisfactory after 2 more days, dosage increased to maximum of 8 IU/kg I.M. q 6 hours.

*Postmenopausal osteoporosis—*
**Adults:** 100 IU of calcitonin (salmon) daily I.M. or S.C. Or, 200 IU (one activation) of calcitonin (salmon) daily intranasally, alternating nostrils daily. Patients should receive adequate vitamin D and calcium supplements (1.5 g calcium carbonate and 400 U of vitamin D daily).

### ADVERSE REACTIONS
**CNS:** headache, weakness, dizziness, paresthesia.
**EENT:** eye pain, nasal congestion.
**GI:** *transient nausea,* unusual taste, diarrhea, anorexia, *vomiting,* epigastric discomfort, abdominal pain.
**GU:** *increased urinary frequency,* nocturia.
**Respiratory:** chest pressure, shortness of breath.
**Skin:** *facial flushing,* rash, pruritus of ear lobes, *inflammation at injection site.*
**Other:** hypersensitivity reactions *(anaphylaxis),* edema of feet, chills, tender palms and soles.

### INTERACTIONS
None significant.

### EFFECTS ON DIAGNOSTIC TESTS
In Paget's disease, maximum reductions of serum alkaline phosphatase and urinary hydroxyproline excretion may take 6 to 24 months of continuous treatment.

### CONTRAINDICATIONS
Contraindicated in patients with hypersensitivity to salmon calcitonin. Human calcitonin has no contraindications.

### NURSING CONSIDERATIONS
• Skin test is usually done before therapy.
• Systemic allergic reactions are possible because hormone is protein. Keep epinephrine nearby.
• Calcitonin (human) is especially indicated in patients who have developed resistance to calcitonin (salmon). Calcitonin (human) is associated with risk of diminishing efficacy caused by antibody formation or hypersensitivity reactions. The two calcitonins aren't interchangeable.
• Administer at bedtime, when possible, to minimize nausea and vomiting.

---

Reactions may be *common,* uncommon, *life-threatening*, or COMMON AND LIFE-THREATENING.

• I.M. route is preferred if volume of dose to be administered exceeds 2 ml.

• Use freshly reconstituted solution within 2 hours.

• Observe patient for signs of hypocalcemic tetany during therapy (muscle twitching, tetanic spasms, and seizures when hypocalcemia is severe).

• Monitor serum calcium level closely. Watch for symptoms of hypercalcemia relapse: bone pain, renal calculi, polyuria, anorexia, nausea, vomiting, thirst, constipation, lethargy, bradycardia, muscle hypotonicity, pathologic fracture, psychosis, and coma.

• Periodic examinations of urine sediment are recommended.

• Monitor periodic serum alkaline phosphatase and 24-hour urine hydroxyproline levels to evaluate drug effect, as ordered.

• In patients with good initial clinical response to calcitonin who suffer relapse, expect to evaluate for antibody response to the hormone protein.

• If symptoms have been relieved after 6 months, treatment may be discontinued until symptoms or radiologic signs recur.

• Store calcitonin (human) at room temperature (77° F [25° C]) and protect from light; refrigerate calcitonin (salmon) at 36° to 46° F (2° to 8° C).

• *Alert:* Don't confuse calcitonin with calcifediol or calcitriol.

☑ **Patient teaching**
• When drug is administered for postmenopausal osteoporosis, remind patient to take adequate calcium and vitamin D supplements.

• Show home care patient and family member how to administer drug. Tell them to administer drug at bedtime if only one dose is needed daily. If nasal spray is prescribed, tell patient to alternate nostrils daily.

• Inform patient that facial flushing and warmth occur in 20% to 30% of all patients within minutes of injection and usually last about 1 hour. Reassure patient that this is a transient effect.

• Tell patient to report signs and symptoms of hypercalcemia promptly. Inform patient that, if calcitonin loses its hypocalcemic activity, other drugs or increased dosages won't help.

• Advise patient to notify doctor immediately if signs of an allergic response occur.

---

## calcitriol (1,25-dihydroxy-cholecalciferol)
Calcijex, Rocaltrol

*Pregnancy Risk Category C*

### HOW SUPPLIED
*Capsules:* 0.25 mcg, 0.5 mcg
*Oral solution:* 1 mcg/ml
*Injection:* 1 mcg/ml, 2 mcg/ml

### ACTION
A vitamin D analogue that stimulates calcium absorption from the GI tract and promotes secretion of calcium from bone to blood.

| Route | Onset | Peak | Duration |
|-------|-------|------|----------|
| P.O. | 2-6 hr | 3-6 hr | 3-5 days |
| I.V. | Immediate | Unknown | 3-5 days |

### INDICATIONS & DOSAGE
*Hypocalcemia in patients undergoing chronic dialysis—*
**Adults:** initially, 0.25 mcg P.O. daily. Dose may be increased by 0.25 mcg daily at 4- to 8-week intervals. Maintenance dose is 0.5 to 3 mcg daily.

Or, 0.5 mcg I.V. three times weekly about every other day. If response is inadequate to initial dose, may increase by 0.25 to 0.5 mcg at 2- to 4-week intervals. Maintenance dose is 0.5 to 3 mcg I.V. three times weekly.
*Hypoparathyroidism, pseudohypoparathyroidism—*
**Adults and children ages 6 and older:** initially, 0.25 mcg P.O. daily. Dosage may be increased at 2- to 4-week intervals. Maintenance dose is 0.25 to 2.7 mcg P.O. daily.
*Hypoparathyroidism—*
**Children ages 1 to 6:** 0.04 to 0.08 mcg/kg P.O. daily.
✳ *NEW INDICATION: Management of secondary hyperparathyroidism and resultant metabolic bone disease in predialysis patients (moderate to severe chronic renal failure with creatinine clearance of 15 to 55 ml/minute)—*

---

*Liquid contains alcohol.   **May contain tartrazine.   †Canada   ‡Australia   §U.K.   ◇OTC

**Adults and children ages 3 and older:** initially, 0.25 mcg P.O. daily. Dosage may be increased to 0.5 mcg/day if needed.
**Children under age 3:** initially, 10 to 15 ng/kg P.O. daily.

## ADVERSE REACTIONS
Vitamin D intoxication associated with hypercalcemia:
**CNS:** headache, somnolence, weakness, irritability.
**CV:** hypertension, *arrhythmias.*
**EENT:** conjunctivitis, photophobia, rhinorrhea.
**GI:** nausea, vomiting, constipation, polydipsia, *pancreatitis,* metallic taste, dry mouth, anorexia.
**GU:** polyuria, nocturia.
**Metabolic:** weight loss.
**Musculoskeletal:** bone and muscle pain.
**Skin:** pruritus.
**Other:** hyperthermia, nephrocalcinosis, decreased libido.

## INTERACTIONS
**Drug-drug.** *Cardiac glycosides:* increased risk of arrhythmias. Avoid concomitant use.
*Cholestyramine, colestipol, excessive use of mineral oil:* decreased absorption of orally administered vitamin D analogues. Avoid concomitant use.
*Corticosteroids:* counteract vitamin D analogue effects. Don't use together.
*Magnesium-containing antacids:* may induce hypermagnesemia, especially in patients with chronic renal failure. Avoid concomitant use.

## EFFECTS ON DIAGNOSTIC TESTS
Drug therapy may falsely elevate cholesterol determinations made using the Zlatkis-Zak reaction.

## CONTRAINDICATIONS
Contraindicated in patients with hypercalcemia or vitamin D toxicity. Withhold all preparations containing vitamin D.

## NURSING CONSIDERATIONS
• Use cautiously in patients receiving cardiac glycosides and in those with sarcoidosis or hyperparathyroidism.
• Monitor serum calcium level; serum calcium level multiplied by the serum

phosphate level shouldn't exceed 70. During adjustment, determine serum calcium level twice weekly. Discontinue and notify doctor if hypercalcemia occurs, but resume after serum calcium level returns to normal. Patient should receive adequate daily intake of calcium. Observe for hypocalcemia, bone pain, and weakness before and during therapy.
• Protect drug from heat and light.
• *Alert:* Don't confuse calcitriol with calcifediol or calcitonin.

### I.V. administration
• For hypocalcemic patients with chronic renal failure who are undergoing hemodialysis, may give drug by rapid I.V. injection through catheter at end of hemodialysis session.

### Patient teaching
• Tell patient to immediately report early symptoms of vitamin D intoxication: weakness, nausea, vomiting, dry mouth, constipation, muscle or bone pain, or metallic taste.
• Instruct patient to adhere to diet and calcium supplementation and to avoid unapproved OTC drugs and magnesium-containing antacids.
• *Alert:* Tell patient that drug mustn't be taken by anyone for whom it wasn't prescribed. It's the most potent form of vitamin D available.

---

### dihydrotachysterol
AT-10‡, DHT Intensol*, Hytakerol

*Pregnancy Risk Category C*

## HOW SUPPLIED
*Tablets:* 0.125 mg, 0.2 mg, 0.4 mg
*Capsules:* 0.125 mg
*Oral solution:* 0.2 mg/5 ml, 0.2 mg/ml* (DHT Intensol*), 0.25 mg/ml (in sesame oil)
   *Note:* 1 mg dihydrotachysterol is equal to 120,000 U ergocalciferol (vitamin $D_2$).

## ACTION
A vitamin D analogue that stimulates calcium absorption from the GI tract and

promotes secretion of calcium from bone to blood.

| Route | Onset | Peak | Duration |
|-------|-------|------|----------|
| P.O. | Several hr | 1-2 wk | 9 wk |

## INDICATIONS & DOSAGE
*Hypocalcemia associated with hypopara-thyroidism and pseudohypoparathy-roidism—*
**Adults:** initially, 0.75 to 2.5 mg P.O. daily for 3 days. Maintenance dose is 0.2 to 1.0 mg daily.
**Children:** initially, 1 to 5 mg P.O. for 4 days. Maintenance dose is 0.5 to 1.5 mg daily.
*Prophylaxis of hypocalcemic tetany following thyroid surgery—*
**Adults:** initially, 0.75 to 2.5 mg P.O. daily for 3 days. Maintenance dose is 0.25 mg weekly to 1 mg daily, p.r.n. (with calcium supplements).

## ADVERSE REACTIONS
Vitamin D intoxication associated with hypercalcemia:
**CNS:** headache, somnolence, irritability.
**CV:** hypertension, *arrhythmias.*
**EENT:** conjunctivitis, photophobia, rhinorrhea.
**GI:** nausea, vomiting, constipation, polydipsia, *pancreatitis,* metallic taste, dry mouth, anorexia, diarrhea.
**GU:** polyuria, nocturia.
**Metabolic:** weight loss, alterations in serum alkaline phosphatase and cholesterol levels and in magnesium, phosphate, and calcium levels.
**Musculoskeletal:** bone and muscle pain.
**Other:** weakness, hyperthermia, decreased libido, nephrocalcinosis.

## INTERACTIONS
**Drug-drug.** *Cardiac glycosides:* increased risk of arrhythmias. Avoid concomitant use.
*Cholestyramine, colestipol, excessive use of mineral oil:* decreased absorption of orally administered vitamin D analogues. Avoid concomitant use.
*Corticosteroids:* counteract vitamin D analogue effects. Don't use together.
*Magnesium-containing antacids:* possible hypermagnesemia, especially in patients with chronic renal failure. Avoid concomitant use.
*Other vitamin D analogues:* increased toxicity. Avoid concomitant use.
*Thiazide diuretics:* may cause hypercalcemia. Use together cautiously.

## EFFECTS ON DIAGNOSTIC TESTS
None reported.

## CONTRAINDICATIONS
Contraindicated in patients with hypercalcemia or vitamin D toxicity.

## NURSING CONSIDERATIONS
• Monitor serum calcium level, as ordered; serum calcium level multiplied by serum phosphate level shouldn't exceed 70. During adjustment, determine serum calcium level twice weekly. Discontinue and notify doctor if hypercalcemia occurs. Drug can be resumed after serum calcium level returns to normal. Adequate daily intake of calcium is 1,000 mg.
• Monitor urine calcium level.
• Store in tightly closed, light-resistant container. Don't refrigerate.

✓ **Patient teaching**
• Tell patient to promptly report early symptoms of hypercalcemia: thirst, headache, vertigo, tinnitus, or anorexia.
• Instruct patient to adhere to diet and calcium supplementation and to avoid OTC drugs and magnesium-containing antacids unless approved by doctor.

---

## etidronate disodium
Didronel

*Pregnancy Risk Category C*

## HOW SUPPLIED
*Tablets:* 200 mg, 400 mg
*Injection:* 50 mg/ml

## ACTION
Decreases osteoclastic activity by inhibiting osteocytic osteolysis; decreases mineral release and matrix or collagen breakdown in bone.

| Route | Onset | Peak | Duration |
|-------|-------|------|----------|
| P.O. | 1 mo (in Paget's) | Unknown | Unknown |
| I.V. | 24 hr | After 3rd infusion | Unknown |

## INDICATIONS & DOSAGE
*Symptomatic Paget's disease of bone (osteitis deformans)—*
**Adults:** 5 to 10 mg/kg P.O. daily (not to exceed 6 months of therapy) or 11 to 20 mg/kg P.O. daily (not to exceed 3 months of therapy) in single dose 2 hours before meals with water or juice. Treatment is initiated only after an etidronate-free period of at least 90 days and when there is specific evidence of active disease process.
*Heterotopic ossification in spinal cord injuries—*
**Adults:** 20 mg/kg P.O. daily for 2 weeks; then 10 mg/kg daily for 10 weeks. Total treatment period is 12 weeks.
*Heterotopic ossification after total hip replacement—*
**Adults:** 20 mg/kg P.O. daily for 1 month before total hip replacement and for 3 months afterward.
*Malignancy-associated hypercalcemia—*
**Adults:** 7.5 mg/kg I.V. daily for 3 consecutive days; a period of at least 7 days should elapse between courses of I.V. therapy. Maintenance dose is 20 mg/kg P.O. daily for 30 days, initiated day after last I.V. dose. May be used for a maximum of 90 days.

## ADVERSE REACTIONS
**CNS:** *seizures.*
**GI:** diarrhea, increased frequency of bowel movements, nausea, constipation, stomatitis (with dose of 20 mg/kg/day), abnormal hepatic function.
**Metabolic:** *elevated serum phosphate levels,* fluid overload.
**Musculoskeletal:** increased or recurrent bone pain, pain at previously asymptomatic sites, increased risk of fracture.
**Respiratory:** dyspnea.
**Other:** fever, *hypersensitivity reactions.*

## INTERACTIONS
**Drug-drug.** *Antacids containing aluminum, calcium, or magnesium; mineral supplements containing aluminum, calcium, iron, or magnesium:* can inhibit absorption. Avoid use within 2 hours of dose.
**Drug-food.** *Foods containing large amounts of calcium, such as milk and dairy products:* can prevent oral absorption. Avoid use within 2 hours of dose.

## EFFECTS ON DIAGNOSTIC TESTS
None reported.

## CONTRAINDICATIONS
Contraindicated in patients with hypersensitivity to drug and in those with clinically overt osteomalacia. I.V. etidronate is contraindicated in patients with serum creatinine levels of 5 mg/dl or more.

## NURSING CONSIDERATIONS
• Use cautiously in patients with impaired renal function.
• Monitor renal function before and during therapy, as ordered.
• Don't give drug with food, milk, or antacids; it may reduce absorption.
• To monitor drug effects, review serum alkaline phosphatase levels and urinary hydroxyproline excretion.
• Elevated serum phosphate level may occur, especially in patients receiving higher doses. Phosphate level usually returns to normal 2 to 4 weeks after drug is discontinued.
• *Alert:* Don't confuse etidronate with etretinate, etidocaine, or etomidate.

### I.V. administration
• Dilute daily dose in at least 250 ml normal saline solution or D₅W, and infuse over at least 2 hours. Diluted solution may be stored at room temperature for up to 48 hours.
• Some patients may receive I.V. drug for up to 7 days. Risk of hypokalemia increases after 3 days.

### ✓ Patient teaching
• Stress importance of a diet high in calcium and vitamin D.
• Tell patient not to eat for 2 hours after daily dose.
• Tell patient that improvement may not occur for up to 3 months and may continue for months after drug is stopped.

---

Reactions may be *common,* uncommon, *life-threatening,* or COMMON AND LIFE-THREATENING.

acetazolamide
acetazolamide sodium
amiloride hydrochloride
bumetanide
chlorthalidone
ethacrynate sodium
ethacrynic acid
furosemide
hydrochlorothiazide
indapamide
mannitol
metolazone
spironolactone
torsemide
triamterene
urea

## COMBINATION PRODUCTS
ALDACTAZIDE 25/25: spironolactone
25 mg and hydrochlorothiazide 25 mg.
ALDACTAZIDE 50/50: spironolactone
50 mg and hydrochlorothiazide 50 mg.
DYAZIDE: triamterene 37.5 mg and hydrochlorothiazide 25 mg.
MAXZIDE: triamterene 75 mg and hydrochlorothiazide 50 mg.
MAXZIDE-25MG: triamterene 37.5 mg
and hydrochlorothiazide 25 mg.
MODURETIC: amiloride hydrochloride
5 mg and hydrochlorothiazide 50 mg.
ZIAC 2.5: bisoprolol fumarate 2.5 mg and
hydrochlorothiazide 6.25 mg.
ZIAC 5: bisoprolol fumarate 5 mg and hydrochlorothiazide 6.25 mg.
ZIAC 10: bisoprolol fumarate 10 mg and
hydrochlorothiazide 6.25 mg.

---

### acetazolamide
Acetazolam†, Apo-Acetazolamide†,
Dazamide, Diamox, Diamox
Sequels

### acetazolamide sodium
Diamox

*Pregnancy Risk Category C*

## HOW SUPPLIED
**acetazolamide**
*Tablets:* 125 mg, 250 mg
*Capsules (extended-release):* 500 mg
**acetazolamide sodium**
*Injection:* 500-mg vial

## ACTION
Blocks action of carbonic anhydrase, promoting renal excretion of sodium, potassium, bicarbonate, water, and decreases
secretion of aqueous humor in the eye,
thereby lowering intraocular pressure. As
an anticonvulsant, may decrease abnormal
paroxysmal or excessive neuronal discharge. In acute mountain sickness, drug
produces a respiratory and metabolic acidosis that may stimulate ventilation, increase cerebral blood flow, promote the
release of oxygen from hemoglobin, and
increase ventilation.

| Route | Onset | Peak | Duration |
|---|---|---|---|
| P.O. | 1-1.5 hr | 2-4 hr | 8-12 hr |
| P.O. (extended) | 2 hr | 3-6 hr | 18-24 hr |
| I.V. | 2 min | 15 min | 1-5 hr |

## INDICATIONS & DOSAGE
*Secondary glaucoma, preoperative treat-
ment of acute angle-closure glaucoma—*
**Adults:** 250 mg P.O. q 4 hours or 250 mg
P.O. b.i.d. for short-term therapy. In acute
cases, 500 mg P.O.; then 125 to 250 mg
P.O. q 4 hours. To rapidly lower intraocular
pressure, initially, 500 mg I.V., which may
be repeated in 2 to 4 hours, if needed, followed by 125 to 250 mg P.O. q 4 hours.
**Children:** 8 to 30 mg/kg P.O. daily in divided doses. For acute angle-closure glaucoma, 5 to 10 mg/kg I.V. q 6 hours.
*Chronic open-angle glaucoma—*
**Adults:** 250 mg to 1 g P.O. daily in divided doses q.i.d., or 500 mg (extended-
release) P.O. b.i.d.
*Prevention or amelioration of acute
mountain sickness—*
**Adults:** 500 mg to 1 g P.O. daily in divided doses q 8 to 12 hours, or 500 mg

(extended-release) P.O. b.i.d. Treatment started 24 to 48 hours before ascent, and continued for 48 hours while at high altitude.

*Adjunctive treatment of myoclonic, refractory, generalized tonic-clonic, absence, or mixed seizures—*
**Adults and children:** 8 to 30 mg/kg P.O. daily in divided doses. For adults, optimum dose range is 375 mg to 1 g daily. Usually given with other anticonvulsants.

## ADVERSE REACTIONS

**CNS:** drowsiness, paresthesia, confusion, depression, *seizures,* weakness.
**EENT:** transient myopia, hearing dysfunction, tinnitus.
**GI:** nausea, vomiting, anorexia, metallic taste, diarrhea, black tarry stools.
**GU:** polyuria, hematuria, crystalluria, glycosuria, renal calculus.
**Hematologic:** *aplastic anemia,* hemolytic anemia, *leukopenia.*
**Metabolic:** hypokalemia, asymptomatic hyperuricemia, hyperchloremic acidosis.
**Skin:** rash.
**Other:** *pain at injection site,* sterile abscesses.

## INTERACTIONS

**Drug-drug.** *Amphetamines, anticholinergics, mecamylamine, procainamide, quinidine:* decreased renal clearance of these drugs, increasing toxicity. Monitor closely.
*Cyclosporine:* increased cyclosporine levels, which may cause nephrotoxicity and neurotoxicity. Monitor closely.
*Diflunisal:* increased risk of adverse effects of acetazolamide; significant decrease in intracranial pressure if used concurrently. Use with caution.
*Lithium:* increased excretion of lithium resulting in decreased effectiveness. Monitor closely.
*Methenamine:* reduced effectiveness of acetazolamide. Avoid concomitant use.
*Primidone:* serum and urine levels of primidone may be decreased. Monitor patient closely.
*Salicylates:* possible accumulation and toxicity of acetazolamide, including CNS depression and metabolic acidosis. Monitor closely.

## EFFECTS ON DIAGNOSTIC TESTS

Because it alkalinizes urine, acetazolamide may cause false-positive proteinuria in Albustix or Albutest. It may also decrease thyroid iodine uptake.

## CONTRAINDICATIONS

Contraindicated in patients with hypersensitivity to drug and in those with hyponatremia or hypokalemia, renal or hepatic disease or dysfunction, renal calculi, adrenal gland failure, or hyperchloremic acidosis; also contraindicated in those receiving long-term treatment for chronic noncongestive angle-closure glaucoma.

## NURSING CONSIDERATIONS

• Use cautiously in patients with respiratory acidosis, emphysema, or chronic pulmonary disease and in those receiving other diuretics.
• Cross-sensitivity between antibacterial sulfonamides and sulfonamide-derivative diuretics such as acetazolamide has been reported.
• If patient is unable to swallow oral forms, pharmacist may make a suspension using crushed acetazolamide tablets in a highly flavored syrup, such as cherry, raspberry, or chocolate. Although concentrations up to 500 mg/5 ml are feasible, concentrations of 250 mg/5 ml are more palatable. Refrigeration improves palatability but doesn't improve stability. Suspensions are stable for 1 week.
• Monitor fluid intake and output, glucose, and electrolytes, especially serum potassium, bicarbonate, and chloride. When drug is used in diuretic therapy, consult doctor and dietitian about providing a high-potassium diet.
• Monitor elderly patients closely because they are especially susceptible to excessive diuresis.
• Weigh patient daily. Rapid or excessive fluid loss causes weight loss and hypotension.
• Diuretic effect decreases when acidosis occurs but can be reestablished by withdrawing drug, as ordered, for several days and then restarting, or by using intermittent administration schedules.

---

Reactions may be *common,* uncommon, *life-threatening,* or COMMON AND LIFE-THREATENING.

• Because bicarbonate ion excretion makes patient's urine alkaline, drug may cause false-positive urine protein tests.
• Drug may increase blood glucose level and cause glycosuria.
• *Alert:* Don't confuse acetazolamide with acetohexamide.

### I.V. administration
• Reconstitute drug in 500-mg vial with at least 5 ml of sterile water for injection. Use within 24 hours of reconstitution.
• Inject 100 to 500 mg/minute into a large vein using a 21G or 23G needle. Intermittent or continuous infusion isn't recommended.

### ✓ Patient teaching
• Tell patient to take oral form with food if GI upset occurs.
• Caution patient not to perform hazardous activities if adverse CNS reactions occur.
• Tell patient to monitor blood glucose level and urine for sugar.

---

## amiloride hydrochloride
Kaluril‡, Midamor

*Pregnancy Risk Category B*

### HOW SUPPLIED
*Tablets:* 5 mg

### ACTION
A potassium-sparing diuretic that inhibits sodium reabsorption and potassium excretion in the distal tubules.

| Route | Onset | Peak | Duration |
|-------|-------|------|----------|
| P.O. | 2 hr | 6-10 hr | 24 hr |

### INDICATIONS & DOSAGE
*Hypertension; hypokalemia; edema associated with heart failure, usually in patients also taking thiazide or other potassium-wasting diuretics—*
**Adults:** 5 mg P.O. daily, increased to 10 mg daily, if needed; then 15 mg. Maximum dose is 20 mg daily.

### ADVERSE REACTIONS
**CNS:** fatigue, *headache,* weakness, dizziness, encephalopathy.
**CV:** orthostatic hypotension.
**GI:** *nausea, anorexia, diarrhea, vomiting,* abdominal pain, constipation, appetite changes.
**GU:** abnormal renal test results, impotence.
**Hematologic:** *aplastic anemia, neutropenia.*
**Hepatic:** abnormal hepatic function test results.
**Metabolic:** hyperkalemia, hyponatremia.
**Musculoskeletal:** muscle cramps.
**Respiratory:** dyspnea.

### INTERACTIONS
**Drug-drug.** *ACE inhibitors, potassium-sparing diuretics, potassium supplements:* possible hyperkalemia. Avoid concomitant use.
*Lithium:* decreased lithium clearance, increasing risk of lithium toxicity. Monitor lithium level.
*NSAIDs:* decreased diuretic effectiveness. Avoid concomitant use.
**Drug-food.** *Foods high in potassium (such as bananas, oranges), potassium-containing salt substitutes:* possible hyperkalemia. Choose diet with caution. Use low-potassium salt substitutes.

### EFFECTS ON DIAGNOSTIC TESTS
Drug causes severe hyperkalemia in diabetic patients after glucose tolerance testing; discontinue drug at least 3 days before testing.

### CONTRAINDICATIONS
Contraindicated in patients with hypersensitivity to drug and in those with elevated serum potassium level (over 5.5 mEq/L), anuria, acute or chronic renal insufficiency, or diabetic nephropathy. Don't administer to patients receiving other potassium-sparing diuretics, such as spironolactone and triamterene.

### NURSING CONSIDERATIONS
• Use cautiously in patients with diabetes mellitus, cardiopulmonary disease, or severe, existing hepatic insufficiency. Also use cautiously in elderly or debilitated patients.
• To prevent nausea, administer drug with meals.

---

• If drug isn't taken with a potassium-wasting drug, monitor potassium level because of increased risk of hyperkalemia. Alert doctor immediately if potassium level exceeds 6.5 mEq/L, and expect drug to be discontinued.

☑ **Patient teaching**
• Advise patient to avoid sudden postural changes and to rise slowly to avoid orthostatic hypotension.
• Caution patient not to perform hazardous activities if adverse CNS reactions occur.
• To prevent serious hyperkalemia, warn patient to avoid excessive ingestion of potassium-rich foods, potassium-containing salt substitutes, and potassium supplements.
• Advise patient to report signs of hyperkalemia: paresthesia, muscular weakness, fatigue, paralysis of extremities.
• Instruct patient to check with doctor or pharmacist before taking new prescription or OTC drugs.

---

## bumetanide
Bumex, Burinex‡§

*Pregnancy Risk Category C*

### HOW SUPPLIED
*Tablets:* 0.5 mg, 1 mg, 2 mg
*Injection:* 0.25 mg/ml

### ACTION
A potent loop diuretic that inhibits sodium and chloride reabsorption at the ascending loop of Henle.

| Route | Onset | Peak | Duration |
|-------|-------|------|----------|
| P.O. | 0.5-1 hr | 1-2 hr | 4-6 hr |
| I.V. | Within min | 15-30 min | 0.5-1 hr |
| I.M. | 40 min | Unknown | 5-6 hr |

### INDICATIONS & DOSAGE
*Edema in heart failure or hepatic or renal disease—*
**Adults:** 0.5 to 2 mg P.O. once daily. If diuretic response isn't adequate, a second or third dose may be given at 4- to 5-hour intervals. Maximum dose is 10 mg/day. May be administered parenterally if P.O. isn't feasible. Usual initial dose is 0.5 to

1 mg given I.V. or I.M. If response isn't adequate, a second or third dose may be given at 2- to 3-hour intervals. Maximum dose is 10 mg/day.

### ADVERSE REACTIONS
**CNS:** *weakness,* dizziness, headache, vertigo.
**CV:** orthostatic hypotension, ECG changes, chest pain, increased cholesterol levels.
**EENT:** transient deafness, tinnitus.
**GI:** nausea, vomiting, upset stomach, dry mouth, diarrhea, pain.
**GU:** *renal failure,* premature ejaculation, difficulty maintaining erection, oliguria.
**Hematologic:** azotemia, *thrombocytopenia.*
**Metabolic:** volume depletion and dehydration, hypokalemia; hypochloremic alkalosis; hypomagnesemia, asymptomatic hyperuricemia; fluid and electrolyte imbalances, including dilutional hyponatremia, hypocalcemia, hyperglycemia, and glucose intolerance.
**Musculoskeletal:** arthritic pain, muscle pain and tenderness.
**Skin:** rash, pruritus, diaphoresis.

### INTERACTIONS
**Drug-drug.** *Aminoglycoside antibiotics:* potentiated ototoxicity. Use together cautiously.
*Antihypertensives:* increased risk of hypotension. Use together cautiously.
*Cardiac glycosides:* increased risk of digitalis toxicity from bumetanide-induced hypokalemia. Monitor potassium and digitalis levels.
*Indomethacin, NSAIDs, probenecid:* inhibited diuretic response. Use together cautiously.
*Lithium:* decreased lithium clearance, increasing risk of lithium toxicity. Monitor lithium level.
*Metolazone:* profound diuresis and potential electrolyte loss. Monitor patient for fluid and electrolyte disorders.
*Other potassium-wasting drugs, (such as amphotericin B, corticosteroids):* increased risk of hypokalemia. Use together cautiously.

---

Reactions may be *common,* uncommon, *life-threatening*, or COMMON AND LIFE-THREATENING.

**EFFECTS ON DIAGNOSTIC TESTS**
None reported.

**CONTRAINDICATIONS**
Contraindicated in patients with hypersensitivity to drug or sulfonamides (possible cross-sensitivity), anuria, or hepatic coma, and in those in states of severe electrolyte depletion.

**NURSING CONSIDERATIONS**
• Use cautiously in patients with hepatic cirrhosis and ascites, in the elderly, and in those with depressed renal function.
• To prevent nocturia, give drug in the morning. If second dose is needed, give in early afternoon.
• Safest and most effective dosage schedule for control of edema is intermittent dosage given on alternate days, or for 3 to 4 days with 1 or 2 days of rest periods.
• Monitor fluid intake and output, weight, and serum electrolyte, BUN, creatinine, and carbon dioxide levels frequently.
• Watch for evidence of hypokalemia, such as muscle weakness and cramps. Instruct patient to report these symptoms.
• Consult doctor and dietitian about a high-potassium diet. Foods rich in potassium include citrus fruits, tomatoes, bananas, dates, and apricots.
• Monitor blood glucose levels in diabetic patients.
• Monitor blood uric acid levels, especially in patients with history of gout.
• Monitor blood pressure and pulse rate during rapid diuresis. Bumetanide can lead to profound water and electrolyte depletion.
• If oliguria or azotemia develops or increases, doctor may stop drug.
• Bumetanide can be safely used in patients allergic to furosemide; 1 mg of bumetanide equals 40 mg of furosemide.
• *Alert:* Don't confuse Bumex with Buprenex.

**I.V. administration**
• Give I.V. doses directly, using a 21G or 23G needle over 1 to 2 minutes. For intermittent infusion, give diluted drug through an intermittent infusion device or piggyback into an I.V. line containing a free-flowing, compatible solution. Infuse at ordered rate. Continuous infusion isn't recommended.

**☑ Patient teaching**
• Tell patient to take drug in morning to prevent nocturia, and if second dose is prescribed to take it in early afternoon. Also instruct patient to take drug with food or milk if adverse GI reactions occur.
• Advise patient to stand up slowly to prevent dizziness, and to limit alcohol intake and strenuous exercise in hot weather to avoid exacerbating orthostatic hypotension.
• Instruct patient to weigh himself daily to monitor fluid status.

---

**chlorthalidone**
Apo-Chlorthalidone†, Hygroton, Novo-Thalidone†, Thalitone, Uridon†

*Pregnancy Risk Category B*

**HOW SUPPLIED**
*Tablets:* 15 mg, 25 mg, 50 mg, 100 mg

**ACTION**
Acts similarly to thiazide diuretics by increasing sodium and water excretion by inhibiting sodium and chloride reabsorption in the nephron's distal segment.

| Route | Onset | Peak | Duration |
|-------|-------|------|----------|
| P.O. | 2-3 hr | 2-6 hr | 2-3 days |

**INDICATIONS & DOSAGE**
*Edema, hypertension—*
**Adults:** initially, 25 to 100 mg P.O. daily, or up to 200 mg P.O. on alternate days.
**Children:** 2 mg/kg or 60 mg/m$^2$ P.O. three times weekly.

**ADVERSE REACTIONS**
**CNS:** dizziness, vertigo, headache, paresthesia, weakness, restlessness.
**CV:** orthostatic hypotension, vasculitis, increased cholesterol and triglyceride levels.
**GI:** anorexia, nausea, *pancreatitis,* vomiting, abdominal pain, diarrhea, constipation.
**GU:** impotence.

**Hematologic:** *aplastic anemia, agranulocytosis, leukopenia, thrombocytopenia.*
**Hepatic:** jaundice.
**Metabolic:** *hypokalemia;* asymptomatic hyperuricemia; hyperglycemia and impairment of glucose tolerance; fluid and electrolyte imbalances, including dilutional hyponatremia and hypochloremia, metabolic alkalosis, hypercalcemia, volume depletion and dehydration.
**Skin:** dermatitis, photosensitivity, rash, purpura, urticaria.
**Other:** *hypersensitivity reactions,* gout.

### INTERACTIONS
**Drug-drug.** *Amphotericin B:* increased risk of hypokalemia. Monitor closely.
*Antidiabetics:* decreased effectiveness; dosage adjustments may be needed. Monitor blood glucose levels.
*Barbiturates, opiates:* increased orthostatic hypotensive effect. Monitor closely.
*Cardiac glycosides:* increased risk of digitalis toxicity from chlorthalidone-induced hypokalemia. Monitor potassium and digitalis levels.
*Cholestyramine, colestipol:* decreased intestinal absorption of thiazides. Separate doses.
*Corticosteroids:* increased risk of hypokalemia. Monitor closely.
*Diazoxide:* increased antihypertensive, hyperglycemic, and hyperuricemic effects. Use together cautiously.
*Lithium:* decreased lithium clearance, increasing risk of lithium toxicity. Monitor lithium level.
*NSAIDs:* increased risk of NSAID-induced renal failure. Monitor closely.
**Drug-lifestyle.** *Alcohol use:* increased orthostatic hypotensive effect. Monitor closely.
*Sun exposure:* photosensitivity reactions may occur. Take precautions.

### EFFECTS ON DIAGNOSTIC TESTS
Drug may interfere with tests for parathyroid functions and should be discontinued before such tests.

### CONTRAINDICATIONS
Contraindicated in patients with hypersensitivity to thiazides or other sulfonamide-derived drugs and in those with anuria.

### NURSING CONSIDERATIONS
• Use cautiously in patients with severe renal disease and impaired hepatic function.
• To prevent nocturia, give drug in the morning.
• Monitor fluid intake and output, weight, blood pressure, and serum electrolyte levels.
• Watch for signs of hypokalemia, such as muscle weakness and cramps. Drug may be used with potassium-sparing diuretic to prevent potassium loss.
• Consult doctor and dietitian about a high-potassium diet. Foods rich in potassium include citrus fruits, tomatoes, bananas, apricots, and dates.
• Monitor serum creatinine and BUN levels regularly. Cumulative effects of drug may occur with impaired renal function.
• Monitor blood uric acid levels, especially in patients with history of gout.
• Monitor blood glucose levels, and check insulin requirements in diabetic patients.
• Monitor elderly patients, who are especially susceptible to excessive diuresis.
• **Alert:** Don't use Hygroton and Thalitone interchangeably; they have different bioavailabilities.
• As ordered, discontinue thiazides and thiazide-like diuretics before parathyroid function tests.
• In patients with hypertension, therapeutic response may be delayed several weeks.
• **Alert:** Don't confuse Uridon tablets (available in Canada only) with the urinary anti-infective Uridon Modified (available in the United States).

☑ **Patient teaching**
• Instruct patient to take in morning to prevent nocturia.
• Tell patient to avoid sudden posture changes and to rise slowly to avoid orthostatic hypotension.
• Advise patient to use a sunblock to prevent photosensitivity reactions.

---

Reactions may be *common*, uncommon, *life-threatening*, or COMMON AND LIFE-THREATENING.

## ethacrynate sodium
Edecrin Sodium

## ethacrynic acid
Edecril‡, Edecrin

*Pregnancy Risk Category B*

### HOW SUPPLIED
**ethacrynate sodium**
*Injection:* 50 mg (with 62.5 mg of mannitol and 0.1 mg of thimerosal)
**ethacrynic acid**
*Tablets:* 25 mg, 50 mg

### ACTION
A potent loop diuretic that inhibits sodium and chloride reabsorption at the proximal and distal tubules and the ascending loop of Henle.

| Route | Onset | Peak | Duration |
|-------|-------|------|----------|
| P.O. | 30 min | 2 hr | 6-8 hr |
| I.V. | 5 min | 15-30 min | 2 hr |

### INDICATIONS & DOSAGE
*Acute pulmonary edema—*
**Adults:** 50 mg or 0.5 to 1 mg/kg I.V. Usually only one dose is needed, although a second dose may be needed.
*Edema—*
**Adults:** 50 to 200 mg P.O. daily. Refractory cases may need up to 200 mg b.i.d.
**Children:** initial dose is 25 mg P.O., increased cautiously in 25-mg increments daily until desired effect is achieved.

### ADVERSE REACTIONS
**CNS:** malaise, confusion, fatigue, vertigo, headache, nervousness.
**CV:** orthostatic hypotension.
**EENT:** transient or permanent deafness with too-rapid I.V. injection, blurred vision, tinnitus, hearing loss.
**GI:** cramping, diarrhea, anorexia, nausea, vomiting, *GI bleeding, pancreatitis.*
**GU:** oliguria, hematuria, nocturia, polyuria, frequent urination.
**Hematologic:** *agranulocytosis, neutropenia, thrombocytopenia,* azotemia.
**Metabolic:** hypokalemia; hypochloremic alkalosis; fluid and electrolyte imbalances, including dilutional hyponatremia,

hypocalcemia, hypomagnesemia; hyperglycemia and impaired glucose tolerance, volume depletion and dehydration.
**Other:** asymptomatic hyperuricemia, rash, fever, chills.

### INTERACTIONS
**Drug-drug.** *Aminoglycoside antibiotics:* potentiated ototoxic adverse reactions of both drugs. Use together cautiously.
*Antihypertensives:* increased risk of hypotension. Use together cautiously.
*Cardiac glycosides:* increased risk of digitalis toxicity from ethacrynate-induced hypokalemia. Monitor potassium and digitalis levels.
*Cisplatin:* increased risk of ototoxicity. Avoid concomitant use.
*Lithium:* decreased lithium clearance, increasing risk of lithium toxicity. Monitor lithium level.
*Metolazone:* profound diuresis and enhanced electrolyte loss. Use together cautiously.
*NSAIDs:* decreased diuretic effectiveness. Use together cautiously.
*Warfarin:* potentiated anticoagulant effect. Use together cautiously.

### EFFECTS ON DIAGNOSTIC TESTS
None reported.

### CONTRAINDICATIONS
Contraindicated in infants, in patients with hypersensitivity to drug, and in those with anuria.

### NURSING CONSIDERATIONS
• Use cautiously in patients with electrolyte abnormalities or hepatic impairment.
• Give oral doses in the morning to prevent nocturia.
• Don't give S.C. or I.M. because of local pain and irritation.
• Monitor fluid intake and output, weight, blood pressure, and serum electrolyte levels.
• Watch for signs of hypokalemia, such as muscle weakness and cramps.
• Consult doctor and dietitian about providing a high-potassium diet. Foods rich in potassium include citrus fruits, tomatoes, bananas, dates, and apricots. Potassi-

---

*Liquid contains alcohol.    **May contain tartrazine.    †Canada    ‡Australia    §U.K.    ◊OTC

um chloride and sodium supplements may be needed.
• Monitor elderly patients, who are especially susceptible to excessive diuresis.
• Monitor blood uric acid levels, especially in patients with history of gout.
• *Alert:* Discontinue drug if patient has severe diarrhea. Patient shouldn't receive drug again after diarrhea has resolved.

### I.V. administration
• Add to vial 50 ml of $D_5W$ or normal saline solution. Give slowly through tubing of running infusion over several minutes. Discard unused solution after 24 hours. Don't use cloudy or opalescent solutions.
• If more than one I.V. dose is needed, use a new injection site to avoid thrombophlebitis.
• Don't mix with whole blood or its derivatives.

### Patient teaching
• Instruct patient to take oral form of drug in morning to prevent nocturia and, if second dose is needed, to take it in early afternoon. Also tell patient to take drug with food or milk if adverse GI reactions occur.
• Advise patient to avoid sudden posture changes and to rise slowly to avoid orthostatic hypotension.
• Caution patient not to perform hazardous activities if drowsiness occurs.
• Advise diabetic patient to closely monitor blood glucose levels.

---

## furosemide (frusemide†‡)
Apo-Furosemide†, Furoside†, Lasix*, Novo-Semide†, Urex‡, Urex-M‡, Uritol†

*Pregnancy Risk Category C*

### HOW SUPPLIED
*Tablets:* 20 mg, 40 mg, 80 mg, 500 mg†‡
*Oral solution:* 10 mg/ml, 40 mg/5 ml
*Injection:* 10 mg/ml

### ACTION
A potent loop diuretic that inhibits sodium and chloride reabsorption at the proxi-

mal and distal tubules and the ascending loop of Henle.

| Route | Onset | Peak | Duration |
|-------|-------|------|----------|
| P.O. | 20-60 min | 1-2 hr | 6-8 hr |
| I.V. | 5 min | 30 min | 2 hr |

### INDICATIONS & DOSAGE
*Acute pulmonary edema—*
**Adults:** 40 mg I.V. injected slowly over 1 to 2 minutes; then 80 mg I.V. in 1 to 1½ hours if needed.
*Edema—*
**Adults:** 20 to 80 mg P.O. daily in the morning, second dose in 6 to 8 hours; carefully adjusted up to 600 mg daily if needed. Or, 20 to 40 mg I.M. or I.V., increased by 20 mg q 2 hours until desired response is achieved. Give I.V. dose slowly over 1 to 2 minutes.
**Infants and children:** 2 mg/kg P.O. daily, increased by 1 to 2 mg/kg in 6 to 8 hours if needed; carefully adjusted up to 6 mg/kg daily if needed.
*Hypertension—*
**Adults:** 40 mg P.O. b.i.d. Dosage adjusted based on response. May be used as adjunct to other antihypertensives if needed.

### ADVERSE REACTIONS
**CNS:** vertigo, headache, dizziness, paresthesia, weakness; restlessness.
**CV:** orthostatic hypotension, increased cholesterol levels.
**EENT:** transient deafness, blurred or yellowed vision.
**GI:** abdominal discomfort and pain, diarrhea, anorexia, nausea, vomiting, constipation, *pancreatitis.*
**GU:** nocturia, polyuria, frequent urination, oliguria.
**Hematologic:** *agranulocytosis, leukopenia, thrombocytopenia,* azotemia, anemia, *aplastic anemia.*
**Hepatic:** hepatic dysfunction.
**Metabolic:** hypokalemia; hypochloremic alkalosis; fluid and electrolyte imbalances, including dilutional hyponatremia, hypocalcemia, hypomagnesemia; hyperglycemia and impaired glucose tolerance.
**Skin:** dermatitis, purpura, photosensitivity, volume depletion and dehydration.
**Musculoskeletal:** muscle spasm.

---

Reactions may be *common,* uncommon, *life-threatening,* or COMMON AND LIFE-THREATENING.

**Other:** asymptomatic hyperuricemia, gout, fever, transient pain at I.M. injection site, thrombophlebitis with I.V. administration.

## INTERACTIONS
**Drug-drug.** *Aminoglycoside antibiotics, cisplatin:* potentiated ototoxicity. Use together cautiously.
*Amphotericin B, corticosteroids, corticotropin, metolazone:* increased risk of hypokalemia. Monitor potassium levels closely.
*Antidiabetics:* decreased hypoglycemic effects. Monitor blood glucose levels.
*Antihypertensives:* increased risk of hypotension. Use together cautiously.
*Cardiac glycosides, neuromuscular blockers:* increased toxicity of these drugs from furosemide-induced hypokalemia. Monitor potassium levels.
*Ethacrynic acid:* may increase risk of ototoxicity. Don't use concomitantly.
*Lithium:* decreased lithium excretion, resulting in lithium toxicity. Monitor lithium level.
*NSAIDs:* inhibited diuretic response. Use together cautiously.
*Salicylates:* may cause salicylate toxicity. Use together cautiously.
*Sucralfate:* may reduce diuretic and antihypertensive effect. Separate administration time by 2 hours.
**Drug-herb.** *Aloe:* possible increased drug effects. Use together cautiously.
**Drug-lifestyle.** *Sun exposure:* photosensitivity reactions may occur. Take precautions.

## EFFECTS ON DIAGNOSTIC TESTS
None reported.

## CONTRAINDICATIONS
Contraindicated in patients with hypersensitivity to drug and in those with anuria.

## NURSING CONSIDERATIONS
● Use cautiously in patients with hepatic cirrhosis and in those allergic to sulfonamides. Furosemide should be used during pregnancy only if potential benefits clearly outweigh possible risks to fetus.

● To prevent nocturia, give P.O. and I.M. preparations in the morning. Give second dose in early afternoon.
● *Alert:* Monitor weight, blood pressure, and pulse rate routinely with long-term use and during rapid diuresis. Furosemide can lead to profound water and electrolyte depletion.
● If oliguria or azotemia develops or increases, drug may need to be discontinued.
● Monitor fluid intake and output and serum electrolyte, BUN, and carbon dioxide levels frequently.
● Watch for signs of hypokalemia, such as muscle weakness and cramps.
● Consult doctor and dietitian about a high-potassium diet. Foods rich in potassium include citrus fruits, tomatoes, bananas, and dates.
● Monitor blood glucose levels in diabetic patients.
● Furosemide may not be well absorbed orally in patient with severe heart failure. Drug may need to be given I.V. even if patient is taking other oral drugs.
● Monitor blood uric acid level, especially in patients with a history of gout.
● Monitor elderly patients, who are especially susceptible to excessive diuresis, because circulatory collapse and thromboembolic complications are possible.
● Store tablets in light-resistant container to prevent discoloration (doesn't affect potency). Don't use discolored (yellow) injectable preparation. Refrigerate oral furosemide solution to ensure drug stability.
● *Alert:* Don't confuse furosemide with torsemide.

### ◐ I.V. administration
● Give by direct injection over 1 to 2 minutes. Or dilute with $D_5W$, normal saline solution, or lactated Ringer's solution, and infuse no faster than 4 mg/minute to avoid ototoxicity. Use prepared infusion solution within 24 hours.

### ✓ Patient teaching
● Advise patient to take drug with food to prevent GI upset, and to take drug in morning to prevent nocturia. If second dose is needed, tell patient to take second

---

dose in early afternoon, 6 to 8 hours after morning dose.
• Inform patient of possible need for potassium or magnesium supplements.
• Instruct patient to stand slowly to prevent dizziness and to limit alcohol intake and strenuous exercise in hot weather to avoid exacerbating orthostatic hypotension.
• Advise patient to immediately report ringing in ears, severe abdominal pain, or sore throat and fever; these symptoms may indicate furosemide toxicity.
• Discourage patient taking furosemide at home from storing different types of drugs in the same container, increasing the risk of drug errors. The most popular strengths of furosemide and digoxin are white tablets about equal in size.
• Tell patient to check with doctor or pharmacist before taking OTC drugs.
• Teach patient to avoid direct sunlight and to use protective clothing and a sunblock because of risk of photosensitivity.

## hydrochlorothiazide
Apo-Hydro†, Dichlotride‡, Diuchlor H†, Esidrix, Ezide, HydroDIURIL, Hydro-Par, HydroSaluric§, Neo-Codema†, Novo-Hydrazide†, Oretic, Urozide†

*Pregnancy Risk Category B*

### HOW SUPPLIED
*Tablets:* 25 mg, 50 mg, 100 mg
*Oral solution:* 50 mg/5 ml, 100 mg/ml

### ACTION
A thiazide diuretic that increases sodium and water excretion by inhibiting sodium and chloride reabsorption in the nephron's distal segment.

| Route | Onset | Peak | Duration |
|-------|-------|------|----------|
| P.O. | 2 hr | 4-6 hr | 6-12 hr |

### INDICATIONS & DOSAGE
*Edema—*
**Adults:** 25 to 100 mg P.O. daily or intermittently; up to 200 mg initially for several days until dry weight is attained.

**Children ages 2 to 12:** 1 to 2 mg/kg once daily or b.i.d., not to exceed 37.5 to 100 mg daily.
**Children ages 6 months to 2 years:** 1 to 2 mg/kg once daily or b.i.d. within range of 12.5 to 37.5 mg daily.
**Infants under age 6 months:** up to 3 mg/kg P.O. daily in two divided doses. Total daily dose may range from 12.5 to 37.5 mg.
*Hypertension—*
**Adults:** 25 to 50 mg P.O. daily as a single dose or divided b.i.d. Daily dose increased or decreased according to blood pressure.

Doses exceeding 50 mg/day aren't needed when combined with other antihypertensives.

### ADVERSE REACTIONS
**CNS:** dizziness, vertigo, headache, paresthesia, weakness, restlessness.
**CV:** orthostatic hypotension, allergic myocarditis, vasculitis.
**GI:** anorexia, nausea, *pancreatitis,* epigastric distress, vomiting, abdominal pain, diarrhea, constipation.
**GU:** polyuria, frequent urination, *renal failure,* interstitial nephritis.
**Hematologic:** *aplastic anemia, agranulocytosis, leukopenia, thrombocytopenia,* hemolytic anemia.
**Hepatic:** jaundice.
**Metabolic:** hypokalemia, hyperglycemia and impaired glucose tolerance; fluid and electrolyte imbalances, including dilutional hyponatremia and hypochloremia, metabolic alkalosis; increased serum glucose, cholesterol, and triglyceride levels; hypercalcemia, volume depletion and dehydration.
**Musculoskeletal:** muscle cramps.
**Respiratory:** respiratory distress, pneumonitis.
**Skin:** dermatitis, photosensitivity, rash, purpura, alopecia.
**Other:** *hypersensitivity reactions,* asymptomatic hyperuricemia, gout, *anaphylactic reactions.*

### INTERACTIONS
**Drug-drug.** *Amphotericin B, corticosteroids:* increased risk of hypokalemia. Monitor closely.

---

Reactions may be *common,* uncommon, *life-threatening,* or COMMON AND LIFE-THREATENING.

*Antidiabetics:* decreased effectiveness of hypoglycemics; dosage adjustments may be needed. Monitor blood glucose levels.

*Antihypertensives:* additive antihypertensive effect. Use together cautiously.

*Barbiturates, opiates:* increased orthostatic hypotensive effect. Monitor closely.

*Cardiac glycosides:* increased risk of digitalis toxicity from hydrochlorothiazide-induced hypokalemia. Monitor potassium and digitalis levels.

*Cholestyramine, colestipol:* decreased intestinal absorption of thiazides. Separate doses.

*Diazoxide:* increased antihypertensive, hyperglycemic, and hyperuricemic effects. Use together cautiously.

*Lithium:* decreased lithium excretion, increasing risk of lithium toxicity. Monitor lithium level.

*NSAIDs:* increased risk of NSAID-induced renal failure. Monitor closely.

**Drug-lifestyle.** *Alcohol use:* increased orthostatic hypotensive effect. Monitor closely.

**EFFECTS ON DIAGNOSTIC TESTS**
Drug may interfere with tests for parathyroid function.

**CONTRAINDICATIONS**
Contraindicated in patients with hypersensitivity to other thiazides or other sulfonamide derivatives and in those with anuria.

**NURSING CONSIDERATIONS**
• Use cautiously in children and in patients with severe renal disease, impaired hepatic function, or progressive hepatic disease.
• To prevent nocturia, give drug in the morning.
• Monitor fluid intake and output, weight, blood pressure, and serum electrolyte levels.
• Watch for signs of hypokalemia, such as muscle weakness and cramps. Drug may be used with potassium-sparing diuretic to prevent potassium loss.
• Consult doctor and dietitian about a high-potassium diet. Foods rich in potassium include citrus fruits, tomatoes, bananas, apricots, and dates.

• Monitor serum creatinine and BUN levels regularly. Cumulative effects of drug may occur with impaired renal function.
• Monitor blood uric acid levels, especially in patients with history of gout.
• Monitor blood glucose levels, especially in diabetic patients.
• Monitor elderly patients, who are especially susceptible to excessive diuresis.
• Discontinue thiazides and thiazide-like diuretics before parathyroid function tests, as ordered.
• In patients with hypertension, therapeutic response may be delayed several weeks.

☑ **Patient teaching**
• Instruct patient to take drug with food to minimize GI upset. Also tell him to take drug in morning to avoid nocturia; if second dose is needed, have him take it in early afternoon.
• Advise patient to avoid sudden posture changes and to rise slowly to avoid orthostatic hypotension.
• Encourage patient to use a sunblock to prevent photosensitivity reactions.
• Tell patient to check with doctor or pharmacist before taking alcohol or OTC drugs.

# indapamide
Lozide†, Lozol, Natrilix‡

*Pregnancy Risk Category B*

**HOW SUPPLIED**
*Tablets:* 1.25 mg, 2.5 mg

**ACTION**
Unknown. A thiazide-like diuretic that probably inhibits sodium reabsorption in the nephron's distal segment. Also has a direct vasodilating effect, possibly resulting from calcium channel-blocking action.

| Route | Onset | Peak | Duration |
|-------|---------|--------|----------|
| P.O. | Unknown | 2-5 hr | 18 hr |

**INDICATIONS & DOSAGE**
*Edema—*
**Adults:** initially, 2.5 mg P.O. daily in the morning. Increased to 5 mg daily after 1 week, if needed.

*Hypertension—*
**Adults:** initially, 1.25 mg P.O. daily in the morning. Increased to 2.5 mg daily after 4 weeks, if needed. Increased to 5 mg daily after 4 more weeks, if needed.

## ADVERSE REACTIONS
**CNS:** headache, nervousness, dizziness, light-headedness, weakness, vertigo, restlessness, drowsiness, fatigue, anxiety, depression, numbness of extremities, irritability, agitation.
**CV:** volume orthostatic hypotension, palpitations, PVC, irregular heartbeat, vasculitis, flushing.
**EENT:** rhinorrhea.
**GI:** anorexia, nausea, epigastric distress, vomiting, abdominal pain, diarrhea, constipation.
**GU:** nocturia, polyuria, frequent urination, impotence, depletion and dehydration.
**Metabolic:** fluid and electrolyte imbalances, including dilutional hyponatremia and hypochloremia, metabolic alkalosis, hypokalemia; weight loss, volume depletion and dehydration.
**Musculoskeletal:** muscle cramps and spasms.
**Skin:** rash, pruritus, urticaria.
**Other:** asymptomatic hyperuricemia; gout; increased serum glucose, cholesterol, and triglyceride levels.

## INTERACTIONS
**Drug-drug.** *Amphotericin B:* increased risk of hypokalemia. Monitor closely.
*Cardiac glycosides:* increased risk of digitalis toxicity from indapamide-induced hypokalemia. Monitor potassium and digitalis levels.
*Corticosteroids:* increased risk of hypokalemia. Monitor closely.
*Diazoxide:* increased antihypertensive, hyperglycemic, and hyperuricemic effects. Use together cautiously.
*Lithium:* decreased lithium clearance that may increase lithium toxicity. Avoid concomitant use.
*NSAIDs:* increased risk of NSAID-induced renal failure. Monitor patient for signs of renal failure.

## EFFECTS ON DIAGNOSTIC TESTS
Drug therapy may interfere with tests for parathyroid function.

## CONTRAINDICATIONS
Contraindicated in patients with hypersensitivity to other sulfonamide-derived drugs and in those with anuria.

## NURSING CONSIDERATIONS
• Use cautiously in patients with severe renal disease, impaired hepatic function, or progressive hepatic disease.
• To prevent nocturia, give drug in the morning.
• Monitor fluid intake and output, weight, blood pressure, and serum electrolyte levels.
• Watch for signs of hypokalemia, such as muscle weakness and cramps. Drug may be used with potassium-sparing diuretic to prevent potassium loss.
• Consult doctor and dietitian about a high-potassium diet. Foods rich in potassium include citrus fruits, tomatoes, bananas, apricots, and dates.
• Monitor serum creatinine and BUN levels regularly. Cumulative effects of drug may occur with impaired renal function.
• Monitor blood uric acid levels, especially in patients with history of gout.
• Monitor blood glucose levels, especially in diabetic patients.
• Monitor elderly patients, who are especially susceptible to excessive diuresis.
• Discontinue thiazides and thiazide-like diuretics before parathyroid function tests, as ordered.
• Therapeutic response may be delayed several weeks in patients with hypertension. Also, if dose needs to be increased to 5 mg, concomitant therapy may be considered.

### ✅ Patient teaching
• Instruct patient to take drug in morning to prevent nocturia and with food if GI upset occurs.
• Advise patient to avoid sudden posture changes and to rise slowly to avoid orthostatic hypotension.

---

Reactions may be *common,* uncommon, *life-threatening,* or COMMON AND LIFE-THREATENING.

# mannitol
Osmitrol

*Pregnancy Risk Category C*

## HOW SUPPLIED
*Injection:* 5%, 10%, 15%, 20%, 25%

## ACTION
An osmotic diuretic that increases the osmotic pressure of glomerular filtrate, inhibiting tubular reabsorption of water and electrolytes. It elevates blood plasma osmolality, resulting in enhanced water flow into extracellular fluid.

| Route | Onset | Peak | Duration |
|-------|-------|------|----------|
| I.V. | 1-3 hr | 0.5-1 hr | 3-8 hr |

## INDICATIONS & DOSAGE
*Test dose for marked oliguria or suspected inadequate renal function—*
**Adults and children over age 12:**
200 mg/kg or 12.5 g as a 15% to 20% I.V. solution over 3 to 5 minutes. Response is adequate if 30 to 50 ml urine/hour is excreted over 2 to 3 hours; if response is inadequate, a second test dose is given. If still no response after second dose, mannitol shouldn't be continued.
*Oliguria—*
**Adults and children over age 12:** 50 to 100 g I.V. as a 15% to 25% solution over 1½ to several hours.
*Prevention of oliguria or acute renal failure—*
**Adults and children over age 12:** 50 to 100 g I.V. of a concentrated solution; then a 5% to 10% solution. Exact concentration determined by fluid requirements.
*Reduction of intraocular or intracranial pressure—*
**Adults and children over age 12:** 1.5 to 2 g/kg as a 15% to 20% I.V. solution over 30 to 60 minutes.
*Diuresis in drug intoxication—*
**Adults and children over age 12:** 5% to 10% solution continuously up to 200 g I.V., while maintaining 100 to 500 ml urine output/hour and a positive fluid balance.
*Irrigating solution during transurethral resection of prostate gland—*
**Adults:** 2.5% to 5% solution, p.r.n.

## ADVERSE REACTIONS
**CNS:** *seizures,* dizziness, headache.
**CV:** edema, thrombophlebitis, hypotension, hypertension, *heart failure,* tachycardia, angina-like chest pain, vascular overload.
**EENT:** blurred vision, rhinitis.
**GI:** thirst, dry mouth, nausea, vomiting, *diarrhea.*
**GU:** urine retention.
**Metabolic:** fluid and electrolyte imbalance, dehydration.
**Other:** local pain, fever, chills, urticaria.

## INTERACTIONS
**Drug-drug.** *Lithium:* increased urinary excretion of lithium. Monitor closely.

## EFFECTS ON DIAGNOSTIC TESTS
Drug also may interfere with tests for inorganic phosphorus or blood ethylene glycol levels.

## CONTRAINDICATIONS
Contraindicated in patients with hypersensitivity to drug and in those with anuria, severe pulmonary congestion, frank pulmonary edema, severe heart failure, severe dehydration, metabolic edema, progressive renal disease or dysfunction, or active intracranial bleeding except during craniotomy.

## NURSING CONSIDERATIONS
• To redissolve crystallized solution (crystallization occurs at low temperatures or in concentrations greater than 15%), warm bottle in hot water bath and shake vigorously. Cool to body temperature before giving. Don't use solution with undissolved crystals.
• For maximum intraocular pressure reduction before surgery, give 1 to 1½ hours preoperatively, as ordered.
• Monitor vital signs, including central venous pressure, and fluid intake and output hourly. Report increasing oliguria. Check weight, renal function, fluid balance, and serum and urine sodium and potassium levels daily.
• Insert urethral catheter in comatose or incontinent patients because therapy is based on strict evaluation of fluid intake and output. In patients with urethral catheters, use

---

*Liquid contains alcohol.   **May contain tartrazine.   †Canada   ‡Australia   §U.K.   ◊OTC

an hourly urometer collection bag to facilitate accurate evaluation of output.
• Drug can be used to measure glomerular filtration rate.
• To relieve thirst, give frequent mouth care or fluids, as permitted.
• When drug is used as an irrigating solution for prostate surgery, concentrations of 3.5% or greater are needed to avoid hemolysis.
• Drug is commonly used in chemotherapy regimens to enhance diuresis of renally toxic drugs.

**▶ I.V. administration**
• Administer as intermittent or continuous infusion at prescribed rate, using an in-line filter and an infusion pump. Direct injection isn't recommended. Check I.V. line patency at infusion site before and during administration.
• Avoid infiltration; if it occurs, observe for inflammation, edema, and necrosis.

**☑ Patient teaching**
• Tell patient that he may feel thirsty or experience mouth dryness, and emphasize importance of drinking only the amount of fluids ordered.
• Instruct patient to report adverse reactions promptly and to alert nurse if discomfort occurs at I.V. site.

---

## metolazone
Metenix-5§, Mykrox, Zaroxolyn**

*Pregnancy Risk Category B*

### HOW SUPPLIED
*Tablets:* 5 mg (Metenix-5§)
*Tablets (extended-release):* 2.5 mg, 5 mg, 10 mg (Zaroxolyn)
*Tablets (prompt-release):* 0.5 mg (Mykrox)

### ACTION
Increases sodium and water excretion by inhibiting sodium reabsorption in the cortical diluting site of the ascending loop of Henle.

| Route | Onset | Peak | Duration |
|-------|-------|------|----------|
| P.O. | 1 hr | 2-8 hr | 12-24 hr |

### INDICATIONS & DOSAGE
*Edema in heart failure or renal disease—*
**Adults:** 5 to 20 mg (extended-release) P.O. daily.
*Hypertension—*
**Adults:** 2.5 to 5 mg (extended-release) P.O. daily. Maintenance dose based on patient's blood pressure. Or, 0.5 mg (prompt-release) P.O. once daily in morning, increased to 1 mg P.O. daily, p.r.n. If response is inadequate, another antihypertensive is added.

### ADVERSE REACTIONS
**CNS:** *dizziness,* headache, fatigue, vertigo, paresthesia, weakness, restlessness, drowsiness, anxiety, depression, nervousness, blurred vision.
**CV:** orthostatic hypotension, palpitations, vasculitis.
**GI:** anorexia, nausea, *pancreatitis,* epigastric distress, vomiting, abdominal pain, diarrhea, constipation, dry mouth.
**GU:** nocturia, polyuria, frequent urination, impotence.
**Hematologic:** *aplastic anemia, agranulocytosis, leukopenia,* purpura.
**Hepatic:** jaundice, *hepatitis.*
**Metabolic:** hyperglycemia and glucose tolerance impairment; fluid and electrolyte imbalances, including hypokalemia, hypomagnesemia, dilutional hyponatremia and hypochloremia, metabolic alkalosis, hypercalcemia; increased serum glucose, cholesterol, and triglyceride levels, volume depletion and dehydration.
**Musculoskeletal:** muscle cramps.
**Skin:** dermatitis, photosensitivity, rash, pruritus, urticaria.

### INTERACTIONS
**Drug-drug.** *Amphotericin B:* increased risk of hypokalemia. Monitor closely.
*Anticoagulants:* may affect hypoprothrombinemic response. Monitor PT and INR.
*Antidiabetics:* may alter blood glucose level requiring dosage adjustment of antidiabetics. Monitor blood glucose levels.
*Barbiturates, opiates:* increased orthostatic hypotensive effect. Monitor closely.
*Cardiac glycosides:* increased risk of digitalis toxicity from metolazone-induced hypokalemia. Monitor potassium and digitalis levels.

---

*Cholestyramine, colestipol:* decreased intestinal absorption of thiazides. Separate doses.
*Corticosteroids:* increased risk of hypokalemia. Monitor closely.
*Diazoxide:* increased antihypertensive, hyperglycemic, and hyperuricemic effects. Use together cautiously.
*Lithium:* decreased lithium clearance, increasing risk of lithium toxicity. Monitor lithium level.
*NSAIDs:* increased risk of NSAID-induced renal failure. Monitor patient for signs of renal failure.
*Other antihypertensives:* may have additive effects. Use together cautiously.
**Drug-lifestyle.** *Alcohol use:* increased orthostatic hypotensive effect. Monitor closely.
*Sun exposure:* photosensitivity reactions may occur. Take precautions.

**EFFECTS ON DIAGNOSTIC TESTS**
Drug also may interfere with tests for parathyroid function.

**CONTRAINDICATIONS**
Contraindicated in patients with hypersensitivity to thiazides or other sulfonamide-derived drugs and in those with anuria, hepatic coma, or precoma.

**NURSING CONSIDERATIONS**
• Use cautiously in patients with impaired renal or hepatic function.
• To prevent nocturia, give drug in the morning.
• Mykrox (prompt-release) tablets are more rapidly and completely absorbed than other brands, mimicking an oral solution. Don't interchange Mykrox with Zaroxolyn (extended-release) tablets.
• Monitor fluid intake and output, weight, blood pressure, and serum electrolyte levels.
• Watch for signs and symptoms of hypokalemia, such as muscle weakness and cramps. Drug may be used with potassium-sparing diuretic to prevent potassium loss.
• Consult doctor and dietitian about a high-potassium diet. Foods rich in potassium include citrus fruits, tomatoes, bananas, dates, and apricots.

• Monitor blood glucose levels, especially in diabetic patients.
• Monitor blood uric acid levels, especially in patients with history of gout.
• Monitor elderly patients, who are especially susceptible to excessive diuresis.
• In patients with hypertension, therapeutic response may be delayed several weeks.
• Metolazone and furosemide may be used together to enhance diuretic effect.
• Unlike thiazide diuretics, metolazone is effective in patients with decreased renal function.
• Drug is used as an adjunct in furosemide-resistant edema.
• As ordered, discontinue thiazides and thiazide-like diuretics before parathyroid function tests.
• *Alert:* Don't confuse Zaroxolyn with Zarontin.

**☑ Patient teaching**
• Tell patient to take drug in morning to prevent nocturia.
• Advise patient to avoid sudden posture changes and to rise slowly to avoid orthostatic hypotension.
• Instruct patient to use a sunblock to prevent photosensitivity reactions.

---

**spironolactone**
Aldactone, Novo-Spiroton†,
Spiractin‡, Spiroctan§

*Pregnancy Risk Category D*

**HOW SUPPLIED**
*Tablets:* 25 mg, 50 mg, 100 mg

**ACTION**
A potassium-sparing diuretic that antagonizes aldosterone in the distal tubules, increasing sodium and water excretion.

| Route | Onset | Peak | Duration |
|-------|-------|------|----------|
| P.O. | 1-2 days | 2-3 days | 2-3 days |

**INDICATIONS & DOSAGE**
*Edema—*
**Adults:** 25 to 200 mg P.O. daily or in two to four divided doses.
**Children:** 3.3 mg/kg P.O. daily or in divided doses.

*Hypertension—*
**Adults:** 50 to 100 mg P.O. daily or in divided doses.
*Diuretic-induced hypokalemia—*
**Adults:** 25 to 100 mg P.O. daily.
*Detection of primary hyperaldosteronism—*
**Adults:** 400 mg P.O. daily for 4 days (short test) or 3 to 4 weeks (long test). If hypokalemia and hypertension are corrected, a presumptive diagnosis of primary hyperaldosteronism is made.
*Management of primary hyperaldosteronism—*
**Adults:** 100 to 400 mg P.O. daily. Use lowest effective dose.

## ADVERSE REACTIONS
**CNS:** headache, drowsiness, lethargy, confusion, ataxia.
**GI:** diarrhea, gastric bleeding, ulceration, cramping, gastritis, vomiting.
**GU:** transient elevation in BUN levels; inability to maintain erection; gynecomastia, breast soreness, and menstrual disturbances.
**Hematologic:** *agranulocytosis.*
**Metabolic:** hyponatremia, *hyperkalemia,* dehydration, mild acidosis.
**Skin:** urticaria, hirsutism, maculopapular eruptions.
**Other:** drug fever, *anaphylaxis.*

## INTERACTIONS
**Drug-drug.** *ACE inhibitors, indomethacin, other potassium-sparing diuretics, potassium supplements:* increased risk of hyperkalemia. Use together cautiously, especially in patients with renal impairment.
*Aspirin:* possible blocked diuretic effect of spironolactone. Watch for diminished spironolactone response.
*Digoxin:* may alter digoxin clearance, increasing risk of digoxin toxicity. Monitor digoxin levels.
**Drug-food.** *Potassium-containing salt substitutes, potassium-rich foods (such as citrus fruits, tomatoes):* increased risk of hyperkalemia. Use low-potassium salt substitutes. Ingest high-potassium foods cautiously.

**Drug-herb.** *Licorice:* may block ulcer healing and aldosterone-like effects of licorice. Avoid concomitant use.

## EFFECTS ON DIAGNOSTIC TESTS
Drug therapy alters fluorometric determinations of plasma and urinary 17-hydroxycorticosteroid levels and may cause false elevations on radioimmunoassay of serum digoxin.

## CONTRAINDICATIONS
Contraindicated in patients with known hypersensitivity to drug and in those with anuria, acute or progressive renal insufficiency, or hyperkalemia.

## NURSING CONSIDERATIONS
• Use cautiously in patients with fluid or electrolyte imbalances, impaired renal function, or hepatic disease.
• Drug or its metabolites may cross the placental barrier. Use with extreme caution in pregnancy.
• To enhance absorption, give drug with meals.
• Protect drug from light.
• Monitor serum electrolyte levels, fluid intake and output, weight, and blood pressure.
• Monitor elderly patients, who are more susceptible to excessive diuresis.
• Inform laboratory that patient is taking spironolactone because drug may interfere with some tests that measure digoxin levels.
• Drug is less potent than thiazide and loop diuretics, and is useful as an adjunct to other diuretic therapy. Diuretic effect is delayed 2 to 3 days when used alone.
• Maximum antihypertensive response may be delayed for up to 2 weeks.
• Watch for hyperchloremic metabolic acidosis, which may occur during therapy, especially in patients with hepatic cirrhosis.
• Breast cancer has been reported in some patients taking spironolactone, although a causal relationship hasn't been established.
• *Alert:* Don't confuse Aldactone with Aldactazide.

---

Reactions may be *common*, uncommon, *life-threatening*, or COMMON AND LIFE-THREATENING.

### ✅ Patient teaching
• Instruct patient to take drug in morning to prevent nocturia. If second dose is needed, tell him to take it in early afternoon and to take it with food.
• *Alert:* Warn patient to avoid excessive ingestion of potassium-rich foods (such as citrus fruits, tomatoes, bananas, dates, and apricots), potassium-containing salt substitutes, and potassium supplements to prevent serious hyperkalemia.
• Caution patient not to perform hazardous activities if adverse CNS reactions occur.
• Advise man about potential breast tenderness or gynecomastia.

---

## torsemide
Demadex, Torem§

*Pregnancy Risk Category B*

### HOW SUPPLIED
*Tablets:* 5 mg, 10 mg, 20 mg, 100 mg
*Injection:* 10 mg/ml

### ACTION
A loop diuretic that enhances excretion of sodium, chloride, and water by acting on the ascending loop of Henle.

| Route | Onset | Peak | Duration |
|-------|-------|------|----------|
| P.O. | 1 hr | 1-2 hr | 6-8 hr |
| I.V. | 10 min | 1 hr | 6-8 hr |

### INDICATIONS & DOSAGE
*Diuresis in patients with heart failure—*
**Adults:** initially, 10 to 20 mg P.O. or I.V. once daily. If response is inadequate, dose is doubled until response is obtained. Maximum dose is 200 mg daily.
*Diuresis in patients with chronic renal failure—*
**Adults:** initially, 20 mg P.O. or I.V. once daily. If response is inadequate, dose is doubled until response is obtained. Maximum dose is 200 mg daily.
*Diuresis in patients with hepatic cirrhosis—*
**Adults:** initially, 5 to 10 mg P.O. or I.V. once daily with an aldosterone antagonist or a potassium-sparing diuretic. If response is inadequate, dose is doubled until response is obtained. Maximum dose is 40 mg daily.
*Hypertension—*
**Adults:** initially, 5 mg P.O. daily. Increased to 10 mg if needed and tolerated. If response is still inadequate, another antihypertensive should be added.

### ADVERSE REACTIONS
**CNS:** asthenia, dizziness, headache, nervousness, insomnia, syncope.
**CV:** ECG abnormalities, chest pain, edema, increased cholesterol level, orthostatic hypotension.
**EENT:** rhinitis, cough, sore throat.
**GI:** *excessive thirst,* diarrhea, constipation, nausea, dyspepsia, **hemorrhage.**
**GU:** increased uric acid, *excessive urination,* impotence, alters renal function test results.
**Metabolic:** *electrolyte imbalances including hypokalemia and hypomagnesemia, dehydration,* hypochloremic alkalosis.
**Musculoskeletal:** arthralgia, myalgia.
**Skin:** rash.

### INTERACTIONS
**Drug-drug.** *Cholestyramine:* decreased absorption of torsemide. Separate administration times by at least 3 hours.
*Digoxin:* decreased torsemide clearance. No dosage adjustments are needed.
*Indomethacin:* decreased diuretic effectiveness in sodium-restricted patients. Avoid concomitant use.
*Lithium, ototoxic drugs (such as aminoglycosides, ethacrynic acid):* possible increased toxicity of these drugs. Avoid concomitant use.
*NSAIDs:* may potentiate nephrotoxicity of NSAIDs. Use together cautiously.
*Probenecid:* decreased diuretic effectiveness. Avoid concomitant use.
*Salicylates:* decreased excretion, possibly leading to salicylate toxicity. Avoid concomitant use.
*Spironolactone:* decreased renal clearance of spironolactone. No dosage adjustments are needed.

### EFFECTS ON DIAGNOSTIC TESTS
None reported.

---

## CONTRAINDICATIONS
Contraindicated in patients with hypersensitivity to drug or other sulfonamide derivatives and in those with anuria.

## NURSING CONSIDERATIONS
• Use cautiously in patients with hepatic disease and associated cirrhosis and ascites; sudden changes in fluid and electrolyte balance may precipitate hepatic coma in these patients.
• To prevent nocturia, give drug in the morning.
• Monitor fluid intake and output, serum electrolyte levels, blood pressure, weight, and pulse rate during rapid diuresis and routinely with long-term use. Drug can cause profound diuresis and water and electrolyte depletion.
• Watch for signs of hypokalemia, such as muscle weakness and cramps.
• Consult doctor and dietitian about providing a high-potassium diet. Foods rich in potassium include citrus fruits, tomatoes, bananas, dates, and apricots.
• Monitor elderly patients, who are especially susceptible to excessive diuresis with potential for circulatory collapse and thromboembolic complications.
• *Alert:* Don't confuse torsemide with furosemide.

### I.V. administration
• Inspect ampules for precipitate or discoloration before use.
• Drug may be given by direct injection over at least 2 minutes. Rapid injection may cause ototoxicity. Don't give more than 200 mg at a time.

### Patient teaching
• Tell patient to take drug in morning to prevent nocturia.
• Advise patient to change positions slowly to prevent dizziness, and to limit alcohol intake and strenuous exercise in hot weather to prevent orthostatic hypotension.
• Advise patient to immediately report ringing in ears because it may indicate toxicity.
• Tell patient to check with doctor or pharmacist before taking OTC drugs.

# triamterene
Dyrenium, Dytac§

*Pregnancy Risk Category B*

## HOW SUPPLIED
*Capsules:* 50 mg, 100 mg

## ACTION
A potassium-sparing diuretic that inhibits sodium reabsorption and potassium and hydrogen excretion by direct action on the distal tubules.

| Route | Onset | Peak | Duration |
|-------|-------|------|----------|
| P.O. | 2-4 hr | 2-4 hr | 7-9 hr |

## INDICATIONS & DOSAGE
*Edema—*
**Adults:** initially, 100 mg P.O. b.i.d. after meals. Total dose shouldn't exceed 300 mg daily.

## ADVERSE REACTIONS
**CNS:** dizziness, weakness, fatigue, headache.
**CV:** hypotension.
**GI:** dry mouth, nausea, vomiting, diarrhea.
**GU:** interstitial nephritis, nephrolithiasis; transient elevation in BUN or creatinine levels.
**Hematologic:** megaloblastic anemia related to low folic acid levels, ***thrombocytopenia, agranulocytosis.***
**Hepatic:** increased liver enzyme abnormalities.
**Metabolic:** acidosis.
**Musculoskeletal:** muscle cramps.
**Skin:** photosensitivity, rash.
**Other:** ***anaphylaxis, hyperkalemia,*** hypokalemia, hyponatremia, hyperglycemia, azotemia, jaundice.

## INTERACTIONS
**Drug-drug.** *ACE inhibitors, potassium supplements:* increased risk of hyperkalemia. Use together as long as serum potassium level is monitored.
*Amantadine:* increased risk of amantadine toxicity. Don't use together.
*Folic acid:* may antagonize folate. Use leucovorin calcium.

---

Reactions may be *common,* uncommon, *life-threatening,* or COMMON AND LIFE-THREATENING.

*Lithium:* decreased lithium clearance, increasing risk of lithium toxicity. Monitor lithium level.

*NSAIDs:* may enhance risk of nephrotoxicity. Use together cautiously.

*Quinidine:* may interfere with some laboratory tests that measure quinidine levels. Inform laboratory that patient is taking triamterene.

**Drug-food.** *Potassium-containing salt substitutes, potassium-rich foods:* increased risk of hyperkalemia. Use cautiously and monitor serum potassium levels.

**Drug-lifestyle.** *Sun exposure:* photosensitivity reactions may occur. Take precautions.

## EFFECTS ON DIAGNOSTIC TESTS
Drug therapy may interfere with enzyme assays that use fluorometry, such as serum quinidine determinations.

## CONTRAINDICATIONS
Contraindicated in patients with hypersensitivity to drug and in those with anuria, severe or progressive renal disease or dysfunction, severe hepatic disease, or hyperkalemia.

## NURSING CONSIDERATIONS
• Use cautiously in patients with impaired hepatic function or diabetes mellitus and in elderly or debilitated patients.
• To minimize nausea, give drug after meals.
• Monitor blood pressure, blood uric acid, CBC, blood glucose level, BUN, and serum electrolyte levels.
• Watch for blood dyscrasia.
• To minimize excessive rebound potassium excretion, withdraw drug gradually, as ordered.
• Drug is less potent than thiazides and loop diuretics and is useful as an adjunct to other diuretic therapy. It's usually used with potassium-wasting diuretics; full effect is delayed 2 to 3 days when used alone.
• *Alert:* Don't confuse triamterene with trimipramine.

### ☑ Patient teaching
• Tell patient to take drug after meals to minimize nausea.

• If a single daily dose is prescribed, instruct patient to take it in the morning to prevent nocturia.
• *Alert:* Warn patient to avoid excessive ingestion of potassium-rich foods (such as citrus fruits, tomatoes, bananas, dates, and apricots), potassium-containing salt substitutes, and potassium supplements to prevent serious hyperkalemia.
• Teach patient to avoid direct sunlight, wear protective clothing, and use sunblock to prevent photosensitivity reactions.
• Tell patient that urine may turn blue.

---

## urea (carbamide)
Ureaphil

*Pregnancy Risk Category C*

### HOW SUPPLIED
*Injection:* 40 g/150 ml

### ACTION
An osmotic diuretic that increases the osmotic pressure of glomerular filtrate, inhibiting tubular reabsorption of water and electrolytes. It also elevates blood plasma osmolality, resulting in enhanced water flow into extracellular fluid.

| Route | Onset | Peak | Duration |
|-------|-------|------|----------|
| I.V. | 30-45 min | 1-2 hr | 3-10 hr |

### INDICATIONS & DOSAGE
*Elevated intracranial or intraocular pressure—*
**Adults:** 1 to 1.5 g/kg as a 30% solution by slow I.V. infusion over 1 to 2½ hours. Rate shouldn't exceed 4 ml/minute. Maximum dose is 120 g daily.
**Children:** 0.1 to 1.5 g/kg by slow I.V. infusion (rate not to exceed 4 ml/minute) or 35 g/m$^2$ in 24 hours. Children under age 2 may receive as little as 0.1 g/kg by slow I.V. infusion.

### ADVERSE REACTIONS
**CNS:** *headache,* syncope, disorientation.
**CV:** hypotension, tachycardia, dizziness, fluid overload, ECG changes.
**GI:** *nausea, vomiting.*

---

**Hematologic:** hemolysis with rapid administration.
**Metabolic:** hyponatremia, hypokalemia; alterations in electrolytes.
**Skin:** irritation or necrotic sloughing with extravasation.

### INTERACTIONS
**Drug-drug.** *Lithium:* increased lithium clearance and decreased lithium effectiveness. Monitor lithium level.

### EFFECTS ON DIAGNOSTIC TESTS
None reported.

### CONTRAINDICATIONS
Contraindicated in patients with severely impaired renal function, marked dehydration, frank hepatic failure, active intracranial bleeding, or sickle-cell disease with CNS involvement.

### NURSING CONSIDERATIONS
• Use cautiously in patients with cardiac disease or hepatic or renal impairment, and in pregnant or breast-feeding women.
• Assess breath sounds for crackles, indicating pulmonary edema.
• Watch for signs and symptoms of hyponatremia (nausea, vomiting, tachycardia) or hypokalemia (muscle weakness, lethargy), which may indicate electrolyte depletion before serum levels are reduced.
• Maintain adequate hydration; monitor blood pressure, fluid intake and output, and serum electrolyte levels.
• Monitor BUN level in patients with renal disease.
• To ensure bladder emptying in comatose patients, use an indwelling urinary catheter and an hourly urometer collection bag for accurate evaluation of diuresis.
• If satisfactory diuresis doesn't occur in 6 to 12 hours, urea should be discontinued and renal function reevaluated.

### ⬛ I.V. administration
• Avoid rapid I.V. infusion because it may cause hemolysis or increased capillary bleeding. Maximum infusion rate is 4 ml/minute.
• *Alert:* Avoid extravasation; it may cause reactions ranging from mild irritation to necrosis.

• To prepare 135 ml of 30% solution, mix contents of 40-g vial of urea with 105 ml of $D_5W$ or $D_{10}W$ or 10% invert sugar in water. Each ml of 30% solution provides 300 mg urea.
• Use freshly reconstituted urea only for I.V. infusion; solution becomes ammonia upon standing. Use within minutes of reconstitution and discard within 24 hours.

### ✅ Patient teaching
• Instruct patient to report adverse reactions promptly.
• Tell patient to alert nurse if discomfort occurs at I.V. insertion site.

---

# 63

## Electrolytes and replacement solutions

calcium acetate
calcium carbonate
calcium chloride
calcium citrate
calcium glubionate
calcium gluceptate
calcium gluconate
calcium lactate
calcium phosphate, dibasic
calcium phosphate, tribasic
dextran, high-molecular-weight
dextran, low-molecular-weight
hetastarch
magnesium chloride
magnesium sulfate
potassium acetate
potassium bicarbonate
potassium chloride
potassium gluconate
**Ringer's injection**
**Ringer's injection, lactated**
**sodium chloride**

**COMBINATION PRODUCTS**
CITRACAL +D: calcium 316.5 mg with 200 U cholecalciferol.
DICAL-D; DIOSTATE D: calcium 116.7 mg (as phosphate tribasic) with cholecalciferol 133 U.
DICAL-D WAFERS: calcium 232 mg (as phosphate tribasic) with cholecalciferol 200 U.
KLORVESS*: potassium and chloride 20 mEq each (from potassium chloride, potassium bicarbonate, and l-lysine monohydrochloride).
K-LYTE/CL: potassium 25 mEq, chloride 25 mEq (from potassium chloride, potassium bicarbonate, and lysine hydrochloride).
KOLYUM: potassium 20 mEq, chloride 3.4 mEq per 15 ml (from potassium gluconate and potassium chloride).
NEUTRA-PHOS: phosphorus 250 mg, sodium 164 mg, potassium 278 mg (from dibasic and monobasic sodium and potassium phosphate).
POSTURE-D: calcium 600 mg (as phosphate tribasic) with cholecalciferol 125 U.
TWIN-K: 15 ml supplies 20 mEq of potassium ions as a combination of potassium gluconate and potassium citrate.

---

**calcium acetate**
PhosLo

**calcium carbonate**
Apo-Cal†◇, Cal Carb-HD◇, Calci-Chew◇, Calciday-667◇, Calci-Mix◇, Calcite 500†◇, Calcium 600◇, Calglycine◇, Cal-Plus◇, Calsan†◇, Caltrate 600◇, Chooz◇, Dicarbosil◇, Gencalc 600◇, Mallamint◇, Nephro-Calci◇, Nu-Cal†◇, Os-Cal†◇, Os-Cal 500◇, Os-Cal Chewable†◇, Oysco◇, Oysco 500 Chewable◇, Oyst-Cal 500◇, Oystercal 500◇, Oyster Shell Calcium-500◇, Rolaids Calcium Rich◇, Super Calcium '1200'◇, Titralac◇, Tums◇, Tums E-X◇

**calcium chloride** ◇
Calciject†

**calcium citrate** ◇
Citracal◇, Citracal Liquitab†◇

**calcium glubionate**
Calcium-Sandoz†, Neo-Calglucon

**calcium gluceptate** ◇

**calcium gluconate**

**calcium lactate** ◇

**calcium phosphate, dibasic** ◇

**calcium phosphate, tribasic**
Posture◇

*Pregnancy Risk Category C*

**HOW SUPPLIED**
**calcium acetate**
Contains 253 mg or 12.7 mEq of elemental calcium/g

*Tablets:* 250 mg ◊, 500 mg ◊, 667 mg,
668 mg ◊, 1,000 mg ◊
*Injection:* 0.5 mEq Ca$^{++}$ per ml
**calcium carbonate**
Contains 400 mg or 20 mEq of elemental
calcium/g
*Tablets:* 650 mg ◊, 1.25 g ◊, 1.5 g ◊
*Tablets (chewable):* 350 mg ◊, 420 mg ◊,
500 mg ◊, 550 mg ◊, 625 mg ◊ †,
750 mg ◊, 835 mg ◊, 850 mg ◊, 1 g ◊,
1.25 g ◊
*Capsules:* 600 mg ◊, 1.25 g ◊
*Oral suspension:* 1 g/5 ml ◊,
1.25 g/5 ml ◊
*Powder packets:* 6.5 g (2,400 mg calcium) per packet ◊
**calcium chloride**
Contains 270 mg or 13.5 mEq of elemental calcium/g
*Injection:* 10% solution in 10-ml ampules, vials, and syringes
**calcium citrate**
Contains 211 mg or 10.6 mEq of elemental calcium/g
*Tablets:* 950 mg ◊, 1.04 g
*Tablets (effervescent):* 2.376 g ◊
**calcium glubionate**
Contains 64 mg or 3.2 mEq elemental
calcium/g
*Syrup:* 1.8 g/5 ml
**calcium gluceptate**
Contains 82 mg or 4.1 mEq elemental
calcium/g
*Injection:* 1.1 g/5 ml in 5-ml ampules or
10-ml vials
**calcium gluconate**
Contains 90 mg or 4.5 mEq of elemental
calcium/g
*Tablets:* 500 mg ◊, 650 mg ◊, 1 g ◊
*Injection:* 10% solution in 10-ml ampules
and vials, 10-ml or 50-ml vials
**calcium lactate**
Contains 130 mg or 6.5 mEq of elemental
calcium/g
*Tablets:* 325 mg, 650 mg
**calcium phosphate, dibasic**
Contains 230 mg or 11.5 mEq of elemental calcium/g
*Tablets:* 500 mg ◊
**calcium phosphate, tribasic**
Contains 400 mg or 20 mEq of elemental
calcium/g
*Tablets:* 300 mg ◊, 600 mg ◊

## ACTION
Replaces calcium and maintains calcium
level.

| Route | Onset | Peak | Duration |
|---|---|---|---|
| P.O. | Unknown | Unknown | Unknown |
| I.V. | Immediate | Immediate | 0.5-2 hr |

## INDICATIONS & DOSAGE
*Hypocalcemic emergency—*
**Adults:** 7 to 14 mEq calcium I.V. May be
given as a 10% calcium gluconate solution,
2% to 10% calcium chloride solution, or a
22% calcium gluceptate solution.
**Children:** 1 to 7 mEq calcium I.V.
**Infants:** up to 1 mEq calcium I.V.
*Hypocalcemic tetany—*
**Adults:** 4.5 to 16 mEq calcium I.V. Repeated until tetany is controlled.
**Children:** 0.5 to 0.7 mEq/kg calcium I.V.
three to four times a day until tetany is
controlled.
**Neonates:** 2.4 mEq/kg I.V. daily in divided doses.
*Adjunctive treatment of cardiac arrest—*
**Adults:** 0.027 to 0.054 mEq/kg calcium
chloride I.V., 4.5 to 6.3 mEq calcium glu-
ceptate I.V., or 2.3 to 3.7 mEq calcium
gluconate I.V.
**Children:** 0.27 mEq/kg calcium chloride
I.V. Repeated in 10 minutes if needed; determine serum calcium levels before administering further doses.
*Adjunctive treatment of magnesium intox-
ication—*
**Adults:** initially, 7 mEq I.V. Subsequent
doses based on patient's response.
*During exchange transfusions—*
**Adults:** 1.35 mEq I.V. with each 100 ml
citrated blood.
**Neonates:** 0.45 mEq I.V. after each
100 ml citrated blood.
*Hyperphosphatemia—*
**Adults:** 1,334 to 2,000 mg P.O. calcium
acetate or 2 to 5.2 g calcium ion t.i.d. with
meals. Most dialysis patients will need
three to four tablets with each meal.
*Dietary supplement—*
**Adults:** 500 mg to 2 g P.O. daily.

## ADVERSE REACTIONS
**CNS:** tingling sensations, sense of op-
pression or heat waves with I.V. use; syncope with rapid I.V. injection.

---

Reactions may be *common,* uncommon, *life-threatening,* or COMMON AND LIFE-THREATENING.

**CV:** mild fall in blood pressure; vasodilation, ***bradycardia, arrhythmias, cardiac arrest with rapid I.V. injection.***
**GI:** irritation, *constipation*; chalky taste; hemorrhage, nausea, vomiting, thirst, abdominal pain.
**GU:** polyuria, renal calculi.
**Metabolic:** hypercalcemia.
**Skin:** local reactions, including burning, necrosis, tissue sloughing, cellulitis, soft-tissue calcification with I.M. use.
**Other:** pain, irritation at S.C. injection site; *vein irritation.*

## INTERACTIONS
**Drug-drug.** *Atenolol, fluoroquinolones, tetracyclines:* decreased bioavailability of these drugs and calcium when oral preparations are taken together. Separate administration times.
*Calcium channel blockers:* decreased calcium effectiveness. Avoid concomitant use.
*Cardiac glycosides:* increased digitalis toxicity. Give calcium cautiously, if at all, to digitalized patients.
*Phenytoin:* concomitant use decreases absorption of both drugs. Avoid concomitant use or monitor levels carefully.
*Sodium polystyrene sulfonate:* risk of metabolic acidosis in patients with renal disease. Avoid concomitant use.
*Thiazide diuretics:* risk of hypercalcemia. Avoid concomitant use.
**Drug-food.** *Foods containing oxalic acid (rhubarb, spinach), phytic acid (bran, whole cereals), phosphorus (dairy products, milk):* may interfere with calcium absorption. Avoid concomitant use.

## EFFECTS ON DIAGNOSTIC TESTS
I.V. calcium may produce transient elevation of plasma 11-hydroxycorticosteroid levels (Glenn-Nelson technique) and false-negative values for serum and urine magnesium as measured by the Titan yellow method.

## CONTRAINDICATIONS
Contraindicated in patients with ventricular fibrillation, hypercalcemia, hypophosphatemia, or renal calculi and in cancer patients with bone metastases.

## NURSING CONSIDERATIONS
● Use all calcium products with extreme caution in patients with sarcoidosis and renal or cardiac disease, and in digitalized patients. Use calcium chloride cautiously in patients with cor pulmonale, respiratory acidosis, or respiratory failure.
● Give I.M. injection in the gluteal region in adults, lateral thigh in infants. Use I.M. route only in emergencies when no I.V. route is available because of irritability of calcium salts to tissue.
● Ensure that doctor specifies form of calcium to be given; crash carts usually contain both calcium gluconate and calcium chloride.
● Monitor blood calcium levels frequently. Hypercalcemia may result after large doses in chronic renal failure. Report abnormalities.

### 🔋 I.V. administration
● Give calcium chloride I.V. only. When adding to parenteral solutions that contain other additives (especially phosphorus or phosphate), watch for precipitate. Use an in-line filter.
● Give calcium gluconate I.V. only.
● *Alert:* Calcium salts aren't interchangeable; verify preparation before use.
● Monitor ECG when giving calcium I.V. Stop if patient complains of discomfort and notify doctor. After I.V. injection, patient should remain recumbent for 15 minutes.
● *Alert:* Severe necrosis and tissue sloughing can occur after extravasation. Calcium gluconate is less irritating to veins and tissues than calcium chloride.
**Direct injection**
● Warm solutions to body temperature before administration.
● Administer slowly through a small needle into a large vein or through an I.V. line containing a free-flowing, compatible solution at a rate not exceeding 1 ml/minute (1.5 mEq/minute) for calcium chloride, 1.5 to 5 ml/minute for calcium gluconate, and 2 ml/minute for calcium gluceptate. Don't use scalp veins in children.
**Intermittent infusion**
● Infuse diluted solution through an I.V. line containing a compatible solution. Maximum rate of 200 mg/minute sug-

gested for calcium gluceptate and calcium gluconate.
• Drug will precipitate if administered I.V. with sodium bicarbonate or other alkaline drugs.

☑ **Patient teaching**
• Tell patient to take oral calcium 1 to 1½ hours after meals if GI upset occurs.
• Warn patient to avoid oxalic acid (in rhubarb and spinach), phytic acid (in bran and whole cereals), and phosphorus (in dairy products) in the meal preceding calcium consumption; these substances may interfere with calcium absorption.

---

**dextran, low-molecular-weight (dextran 40)**
Dextran 40, Gentran 40,
LMD 10%, Rheomacrodex

*Pregnancy Risk Category C*

## HOW SUPPLIED
*Injection:* 10% dextran 40 in $D_5W$ or normal saline solution

## ACTION
Expands plasma volume via colloidal osmotic effect, drawing fluid from interstitial to intravascular space, providing fluid replacement.

| Route | Onset | Peak | Duration |
|-------|-------|------|----------|
| I.V. | Immediate | Immediate | 3 hr |

## INDICATIONS & DOSAGE
*Plasma volume expansion—*
**Adults:** dosage by I.V. infusion depends on amount of fluid loss. Infuse first 10 ml/kg of dextran rapidly with central venous pressure monitoring; then infuse remaining dose slowly. Total dose not to exceed 20 ml/kg body weight daily. If therapy continues longer than 24 hours, don't exceed 10 ml/kg daily, continued for no longer than 5 days.
*Prophylaxis of venous thrombosis—*
**Adults:** 10 ml/kg (500 to 1,000 ml) I.V. on day of procedure; 500 ml on days 2 and 3.

*Hemodiluent in extracorporeal circulation—*
**Adults:** 10 to 20 ml/kg added to the perfusion circuit, not to exceed total dose of 20 ml/kg.

## ADVERSE REACTIONS
**CV:** thrombophlebitis.
**GI:** nausea, vomiting.
**GU:** tubular stasis and blocking, increased urine viscosity.
**Hematologic:** *decreased hemoglobin and hematocrit levels;* increased bleeding time with higher doses.
**Hepatic:** increased AST and ALT levels.
**Skin:** urticaria.
**Other:** *anaphylaxis, hypersensitivity reactions.*

## INTERACTIONS
None significant.

## EFFECTS ON DIAGNOSTIC TESTS
Falsely elevated blood glucose levels may occur in patients receiving dextran 40 or 70 if the test uses high concentrations of acid. Dextran may cause turbidity, which interferes with bilirubin assays that use alcohol, total protein levels using biuret reagent, and blood glucose levels using the orthotoluidine method. Blood typing and cross-matching using enzyme techniques may give unreliable readings if the samples are taken after the dextran infusion.

## CONTRAINDICATIONS
Contraindicated in patients with hypersensitivity to drug and in those with marked hemostatic defects or cardiac decompensation, or renal disease with severe oliguria or anuria.

## NURSING CONSIDERATIONS
• Use cautiously in patients with active hemorrhage, thrombocytopenia, or diabetes mellitus.
• Assess hydration before starting therapy; otherwise, use urine or serum osmolality because urine specific gravity is affected by urine dextran level.
• Watch for circulatory overload and a rise in central venous pressure. Drug pro-

---

vides plasma expansion slightly greater than volume infused.

• Monitor urine flow rate during administration. If oliguria or anuria occurs or isn't relieved, stop dextran and give loop diuretic, as ordered.

• Check hemoglobin levels and hematocrit; if values fall below 30% by volume, notify doctor.

• Drug may interfere with analyses of blood grouping, cross-matching, bilirubin, blood glucose levels, and protein.

• Monitor blood glucose levels before and during infusion; drug metabolizes to glucose.

• *Alert:* Low- and high-molecular-weight dextrans aren't interchangeable. Verify preparation before use.

### ◐ I.V. administration

• Observe patient closely during early phase of infusion when most anaphylactic reactions occur.

• Use $D_5W$ solution instead of normal saline solution for patients with heart failure, as ordered.

• Doctor may order dextran 1 to protect against dextran-induced anaphylaxis. Administer 20 ml of dextran 1 (containing 150 mg/ml) I.V. over 60 seconds, 1 to 2 minutes before I.V. infusion of dextran.

• Store at constant 77° F (25° C). Drug may precipitate in storage but can be heated to dissolve, if needed.

• Discard partially used containers.

### ☑ Patient teaching

• Explain use and administration of dextran to patient and family.

• Tell patient to report adverse effects.

---

### dextran, high-molecular-weight (dextran 70, dextran 75)
Dextran 75, Gendex 75, Gentran 70, Macrodex

*Pregnancy Risk Category C*

## HOW SUPPLIED
*Injection:* 6% dextran 70 in normal saline solution or dextrose 5%; 6% dextran 75 in normal saline solution or dextrose 5%

## ACTION
Expands plasma volume via colloidal osmotic effect, drawing fluid from interstitial to intravascular space, providing fluid replacement.

| Route | Onset | Peak | Duration |
|-------|-------|------|----------|
| I.V. | Immediate | Immediate | Unknown |

## INDICATIONS & DOSAGE
*Plasma expander—*
**Adults:** 30 g (500 ml of 6% solution) I.V. In emergencies, may be given at 1.2 to 2.4 g (20 to 40 ml)/minute. In normovolemic or nearly normovolemic patients, rate of infusion shouldn't exceed 240 mg (4 ml)/minute.

Total dose during first 24 hours not to exceed 1.2 g/kg; actual dose depends on amount of fluid loss and resultant hemoconcentration and must be determined for each patient.

## ADVERSE REACTIONS
**CV:** fluid overload, thrombophlebitis.
**EENT:** nasal congestion.
**GI:** nausea, vomiting.
**GU:** increased specific gravity and viscosity of urine, tubular stasis and blocking, oliguria, anuria.
**Hematologic:** decreased hemoglobin levels and hematocrit; with doses of 15 ml/kg body weight, prolonged bleeding time and significant suppression of platelet function.
**Hepatic:** increased AST and ALT levels.
**Musculoskeletal:** arthralgia.
**Skin:** urticaria.
**Other:** fever, *anaphylaxis, hypersensitivity reactions.*

## INTERACTIONS
**Drug-drug.** *Abciximab, aspirin, heparin, thrombolytics, warfarin:* increased bleeding if given together. Use together with extreme caution.

## EFFECTS ON DIAGNOSTIC TESTS
Falsely elevated blood glucose levels may occur in patients receiving dextran 40 or 70 if the test uses high concentrations of acid. Dextran may cause turbidity, which interferes with bilirubin assays that use alcohol, total protein levels using biuret

---

reagent, and blood glucose levels using the orthotoluidine method. Blood typing and cross-matching using enzyme techniques may give unreliable readings if the samples are taken after the dextran infusion.

## CONTRAINDICATIONS
Contraindicated in patients with hypersensitivity to dextran and in those with marked hemostatic defects or cardiac decompensation, renal disease with severe oliguria or anuria, hypervolemic conditions, or severe bleeding disorders.

## NURSING CONSIDERATIONS
• Use cautiously in patients with active hemorrhage, thrombocytopenia, impaired renal clearance, chronic liver disease, or abdominal conditions and in patients undergoing bowel surgery.
• Assess hydration before starting therapy; otherwise, use urine or serum osmolality because urine specific gravity is affected by urine dextran level.
• *Alert:* Low- and high-molecular-weight dextrans aren't interchangeable. Verify preparation before use.
• Have blood samples drawn before starting infusion.
• Monitor urine flow rate during administration. If oliguria or anuria occurs or isn't relieved by infusion, stop dextran and give loop diuretic.
• Watch for circulatory overload. Drug provides plasma expansion slightly greater than volume infused.
• Monitor hemoglobin levels and hematocrit; if values fall below 30% by volume, notify doctor.
• Drug may interfere with analyses of blood grouping, cross-matching, bilirubin, blood glucose level, and protein.
• Drug may precipitate in storage but can be heated to dissolve, if needed.
• Monitor blood glucose levels before and during infusion; drug metabolizes to glucose.

## I.V. administration
• *Alert:* Observe patient closely during early phase of infusion when most anaphylactic reactions occur.

• Doctor may order dextran 1 to protect against dextran-induced anaphylaxis. Give 20 ml of dextran 1 (containing 150 mg/ml) I.V. over 60 seconds, 1 to 2 minutes before I.V. infusion of dextran 70.
• As ordered, use $D_5W$ solution instead of normal saline solution for patients with heart failure.

## ☑ Patient teaching
• Explain use and administration of dextran to patient and family.
• Tell patient to report adverse effects.

---

# hetastarch
Hespan

*Pregnancy Risk Category C*

## HOW SUPPLIED
*Injection:* 500 ml (6 g/100 ml in normal saline solution)

## ACTION
Expands plasma volume and provides fluid replacement.

| Route | Onset | Peak | Duration |
|-------|-------|------|----------|
| I.V. | Immediate | Immediate | Unknown |

## INDICATIONS & DOSAGE
*Plasma expander—*
**Adults:** 500 to 1,000 ml I.V., depending on amount of blood lost and resultant hemoconcentration. Total daily dose shouldn't exceed 1,500 ml.

## ADVERSE REACTIONS
**CNS:** headache.
**CV:** fluid overload, peripheral edema of lower extremities.
**EENT:** periorbital edema.
**GI:** nausea, vomiting.
**Musculoskeletal:** muscle pain.
**Respiratory:** wheezing.
**Skin:** rash, urticaria.
**Other:** mild fever, chills, *hypersensitivity reactions,* dilution of clotting factors.

## INTERACTIONS
None significant.

---

Reactions may be *common,* uncommon, *life-threatening*, or COMMON AND LIFE-THREATENING.

## EFFECTS ON DIAGNOSTIC TESTS
When added to whole blood, hetastarch increases the erythrocyte sedimentation rate.

## CONTRAINDICATIONS
Contraindicated in patients with known hypersensitivity to drug and in those with severe bleeding disorders, severe heart failure, or renal failure with oliguria and anuria.

## NURSING CONSIDERATIONS
• Use cautiously in patients with liver disease.
• Hetastarch isn't a substitute for blood or plasma.
• To avoid circulatory overload, monitor patients with impaired renal function carefully.
• When used in continuous-flow centrifugation, leukapheresis ratio is usually one part hetastarch to eight parts venous whole blood.
• Discontinue if allergic or sensitivity reactions occur and notify doctor. If needed, administer an antihistamine, as ordered.

### I.V. administration
• Up to 20 ml/kg hourly may be used in hemorrhagic shock. Slower rates of administration are generally used in patients with burns or septic shock.
• Discard partially used bottles.

### Patient teaching
• Explain use and administration of drug to patient and family.
• Tell patient to report adverse reactions promptly.

---

## magnesium chloride
Slow-Mag ◇

## magnesium sulfate

*Pregnancy Risk Category D*

---

## HOW SUPPLIED
**magnesium chloride**
*Tablets (delayed-release):* 64 mg

**magnesium sulfate**
*Injectable solutions:* 10%, 12.5%, 50% in 2-ml, 5-ml, 10-ml, 20-ml, and 30-ml ampules, vials, and prefilled syringes

## ACTION
Replaces magnesium and maintains magnesium level; as an anticonvulsant, reduces muscle contractions by interfering with release of acetylcholine at myoneural junction.

| Route | Onset | Peak | Duration |
|-------|-------|------|----------|
| P.O. | Unknown | 4 hr | 4-6 hr |
| I.V. | Immediate | Unknown | 30 min |
| I.M. | 1 hr | Unknown | 3-4 hr |

## INDICATIONS & DOSAGE
*Mild hypomagnesemia—*
**Adults:** 1 g I.V. by piggyback or I.M. q 6 hours for four doses, depending on serum magnesium level. Or, 3 g P.O. q 6 hours for four doses.
*Severe hypomagnesemia (serum magnesium 0.8 mEq/L or less, with symptoms)—*
**Adults:** 2 to 5 g I.V. in 1 L of solution over 3 hours. Subsequent doses depend on serum magnesium levels.
*Magnesium supplementation—*
**Adults:** 64 mg (one tablet) P.O. t.i.d.
*Magnesium supplementation in total parenteral nutrition (TPN)—*
**Adults:** 4 to 24 mEq I.V. daily added to TPN solution.
**Infants:** 2 to 10 mEq I.V. daily added to TPN solution. Each 2 ml of 50% solution contains 1 g, or 8.12 mEq, magnesium sulfate.

## ADVERSE REACTIONS
**CNS:** toxicity, *weak or absent deep tendon reflexes*, flaccid paralysis, hypothermia, drowsiness, stupor.
**CV:** slow, weak pulse; ***arrhythmias***; *hypotension*; ***circulatory collapse.***
**GI:** diarrhea.
**Metabolic:** hypocalcemia.
**Respiratory:** *respiratory paralysis.*
**Skin:** flushing, diaphoresis.

## INTERACTIONS
**Drug-drug.** *Alendronate, nitrofurantoin, penicillamine, quinolones, sodium polystyrene sulfonate, tetracyclines:* decreased

---

bioavailability with oral magnesium supplements. Separate administration by 2 to 3 hours.
*Cardiac glycosides:* possible serious cardiac conduction changes. Administer with extreme caution.
*CNS depressants:* may have additive effect. Use cautiously.
*Neuromuscular blockers:* possible increased neuromuscular blockage. Use cautiously.

**EFFECTS ON DIAGNOSTIC TESTS**
None reported.

**CONTRAINDICATIONS**
Contraindicated in patients with myocardial damage or heart block and in those in actively progressing labor.

**NURSING CONSIDERATIONS**
• Use parenteral magnesium with extreme caution in patients with impaired renal function.
• Undiluted 50% solutions may be given by deep I.M. injection to adults. Dilute solutions to 20% or less for use in children.
• Keep I.V. calcium available to reverse magnesium intoxication.
• Test knee-jerk and patellar reflexes before each additional dose. If absent, notify doctor and give no more magnesium until reflexes return; otherwise, patient may develop temporary respiratory failure and need cardiopulmonary resuscitation or I.V. administration of calcium.
• Check magnesium level after repeated doses.
• Monitor fluid intake and output. Output should be 100 ml or more during 4-hour period before dose.
• After giving to toxemic patient within 24 hours before delivery, watch neonate for signs and symptoms of magnesium toxicity, including neuromuscular and respiratory depression.

**◖ I.V. administration**
• Inject I.V. bolus dose slowly, using infusion pump for continuous infusion, if available, to avoid respiratory or cardiac arrest. Maximum infusion rate is 150 mg/minute. Rapid drip causes feeling of heat.

• *Alert:* When giving I.V. for severe hypomagnesemia, watch for respiratory depression and signs and symptoms of heart block. Respirations should be over 16 breaths/minute before dose is given.
• Drug is incompatible with alkalis, including carbonates and bicarbonates. Precipitate may form if mixed with solutions containing ethanol, arsenates, barium, calcium, clindamycin, heavy metals, hydrocortisone sodium succinate, phosphates, polymyxin B sulfate, procaine, salicylates, or tartrates.

**☑ Patient teaching**
• Explain use and administration of drug to patient and family.
• Tell patient to report adverse effects.

## potassium acetate

*Pregnancy Risk Category C*

**HOW SUPPLIED**
*Injection:* 2 mEq/ml in 20-ml, 30-ml vials; 4 mEq/ml in 50-ml vials

**ACTION**
Replaces potassium and maintains potassium level.

| Route | Onset | Peak | Duration |
|-------|-------|------|----------|
| I.V. | Immediate | Immediate | Unknown |

**INDICATIONS & DOSAGE**
*Hypokalemia—*
**Adults:** no more than 20 mEq hourly in concentration of 40 mEq/L or less. Total 24-hour dose shouldn't exceed 150 mEq (3 mEq/kg in children). Potassium replacement should be done with ECG monitoring and frequent serum potassium determinations. I.V. route should be used only for life-threatening hypokalemia or when oral replacement isn't feasible.
*Prevention of hypokalemia—*
**Adults:** dosage is individualized to patient's needs, not to exceed 150 mEq/day. Administered as an additive to I.V. infusions. Usual dose is 20 mEq/L infused at a rate not to exceed 20 mEq/hour.

**Children:** individualized dose not to exceed 3 mEq/kg/day. Administered as an additive to I.V. infusions.

## ADVERSE REACTIONS
*Signs and symptoms of hyperkalemia—*
**CNS:** paresthesia of extremities, listlessness, mental confusion, weakness or heaviness of legs, flaccid paralysis.
**CV:** hypotension, *arrhythmias, heart block,* ECG changes, *cardiac arrest.*
**GI:** nausea, vomiting, abdominal pain, diarrhea.
**Metabolic:** hyperkalemia.
**Respiratory:** *respiratory paralysis.*
**Other:** pain, redness at infusion site; fever.

## INTERACTIONS
**Drug-drug.** *ACE inhibitors, potassium-sparing diuretics:* increased risk of hyperkalemia. Use with extreme caution.

## EFFECTS ON DIAGNOSTIC TESTS
None reported.

## CONTRAINDICATIONS
Contraindicated in patients with severe renal impairment with oliguria, anuria, or azotemia; untreated Addison's disease; or acute dehydration, heat cramps, hyperkalemia, hyperkalemic form of familial periodic paralysis, or conditions associated with extensive tissue breakdown.

## NURSING CONSIDERATIONS
• Use cautiously in patients with cardiac disease or renal impairment.
• During therapy, monitor ECG, renal function, fluid intake and output, and serum potassium, serum creatinine, and BUN levels. Never give potassium postoperatively until urine flow is established.
• *Alert:* Potassium preparations aren't interchangeable; verify preparation before use.

## I.V. administration
• Give by I.V. infusion only, never I.V. push or I.M. Watch for pain and redness at infusion site. Large-bore needle reduces local irritation.

• *Alert:* Give slowly as diluted solution; potentially fatal hyperkalemia may result from too-rapid infusion.

## ☑ Patient teaching
• Explain use and administration to patient and family.
• Tell patient to report adverse effects, especially pain at insertion site.

---

## potassium bicarbonate
K+Care ET, Klor-Con/EF, K-Lyte, K-Vescent

*Pregnancy Risk Category C*

## HOW SUPPLIED
*Tablets (effervescent):* 25 mEq

## ACTION
Replaces potassium and maintains potassium level.

| Route | Onset | Peak | Duration |
|-------|-------|------|----------|
| P.O. | Unknown | 4 hr | Unknown |

## INDICATIONS & DOSAGE
*Hypokalemia—*
**Adults:** 25 to 50 mEq dissolved in 4 to 8 oz (120 to 240 ml) of water once daily to q.i.d.

## ADVERSE REACTIONS
**CNS:** paresthesia of extremities, listlessness, mental confusion, weakness or heaviness of legs, flaccid paralysis.
**CV:** *arrhythmias*, ECG changes, hypotension, *heart block, cardiac arrest.*
**GI:** *nausea, vomiting, abdominal pain,* diarrhea.

## INTERACTIONS
**Drug-drug.** *ACE inhibitors, potassium-sparing diuretics:* risk of hyperkalemia. Use with extreme caution.

## EFFECTS ON DIAGNOSTIC TESTS
None reported.

## CONTRAINDICATIONS
Contraindicated in patients with severe renal impairment with oliguria, anuria, or azotemia; untreated Addison's disease; or

acute dehydration, heat cramps, hyperkalemia, hyperkalemic form of familial periodic paralysis, or other conditions associated with extensive tissue breakdown.

## NURSING CONSIDERATIONS
• Use cautiously in patients with cardiac disease or renal impairment.
• Dissolve potassium bicarbonate tablets completely in 4 to 8 oz of cold water.
• Ask patient's flavor preference. Available in lime, fruit punch, citrus, and orange flavors.
• Don't administer potassium supplements postoperatively until urine flow has been established.
• *Alert:* Potassium preparations aren't interchangeable; verify preparation before use. Never switch potassium products without doctor's order. Potassium chloride can't be given instead of potassium bicarbonate.
• Monitor BUN, serum potassium, and creatinine levels and fluid intake and output.

### ☑ Patient teaching
• Tell patient to take drug with meals and sip slowly over 5 to 10 minutes.
• Tell patient to report adverse effects.
• Warn patient not to use salt substitutes concurrently, except with doctor's permission.

## potassium chloride
Cena-K, K + 10, Kaochlor 10%*, Kaochlor S-F 10%*, Kaon-Cl, Kaon-Cl 20%*, Kay-Cee-L§, Kay Ciel*, K + Care, K-Dur, K-Lease, K-Lor, Klor-Con, Klor-Con/25, Klorvess, Klotrix, K-Lyte/Cl, K-Norm, K-Tab, Micro-K Extencaps, Rum-K, Slow-K, Ten-K

*Pregnancy Risk Category C*

## HOW SUPPLIED
*Tablets (controlled-release):* 6.7 mEq (500 mg), 8 mEq (600 mg), 10 mEq (750 mg), 20 mEq (1,500 mg)
*Tablets (film-coated):* 2.5 mEq (200 mg), 8 mEq (600 mg), 10 mEq (750 mg)
*Capsules (controlled-release):* 8 mEq (600 mg), 10 mEq (750 mg)
*Oral liquid:* 10% (20 mEq/15 ml), 15% (30 mEq/15 ml), 20% (40 mEq/15 ml)
*Powder for oral use:* 15-mEq packet, 20-mEq packet, 25-mEq packet, 25-mEq dose
*Injection:* 20-mEq, 40-mEq ampules; additive syringes containing 30-mEq or 40-mEq; 10-mEq, 20-mEq, 30-mEq, 40-mEq, 60-mEq, 100-mEq, 200-mEq, 400-mEq, or 1,000-mEq vials

## ACTION
Replaces potassium and maintains potassium level.

| Route | Onset | Peak | Duration |
|-------|-------|------|----------|
| P.O. | Unknown | Unknown | Unknown |
| I.V. | Immediate | Immediate | Unknown |

## INDICATIONS & DOSAGE
*Hypokalemia—*
**Adults:** 40 to 100 mEq P.O. daily in three or four divided doses for treatment; 10 to 20 mEq for prevention. Further dosage based on serum potassium level.
**Children:** 3 mEq/kg daily. Total daily dose not to exceed 40 mEq/m$^2$.
   Use I.V. route only when oral replacement isn't feasible or when hypokalemia is life-threatening. If serum potassium level is less than 2 mEq/ml, maximum infusion rate is 40 mEq/hour, maximum infusion concentration is 80 mEq/L, and maximum 24-hour dose is 400 mEq. If serum potassium level is greater than 2 mEq/ml, maximum infusion rate is 10 mEq/hour, maximum infusion concentration is 40 mEq/L, and maximum 24-hour dose is 200 mEq. For routine supplementation, usual dose is 10 to 20 mEq hourly in concentrations of 40 mEq/L or less.

## ADVERSE REACTIONS
*Signs and symptoms of hyperkalemia—*
**CNS:** paresthesia of extremities, listlessness, mental confusion, weakness or heaviness of limbs, flaccid paralysis.
**CV:** *arrhythmias, heart block, possible cardiac arrest*, ECG changes, hypotension, *postinfusion phlebitis*.

---

Reactions may be *common,* uncommon, *life-threatening,* or COMMON AND LIFE-THREATENING.

**GI:** nausea, vomiting, abdominal pain, diarrhea.
**Metabolic:** hyperkalemia.
**Respiratory:** *respiratory paralysis.*

### INTERACTIONS
**Drug-drug.** *ACE inhibitors, potassium-sparing diuretics:* risk of hyperkalemia. Use with extreme caution.

### EFFECTS ON DIAGNOSTIC TESTS
None reported.

### CONTRAINDICATIONS
Contraindicated in patients with severe renal impairment with oliguria, anuria, or azotemia; with untreated Addison's disease; or acute dehydration, heat cramps, hyperkalemia, hyperkalemic form of familial periodic paralysis, or other conditions associated with extensive tissue breakdown.

### NURSING CONSIDERATIONS
• Give oral potassium supplements with extreme caution because different forms deliver varying amounts of potassium. Never switch products without doctor's order.
• *Alert:* Potassium preparations aren't interchangeable; verify preparation before use.
• Make sure powders are completely dissolved before administering.
• Enteric-coated tablets aren't recommended because of increased potential for GI bleeding and small-bowel ulcerations.
• Tablets in wax matrix sometimes lodge in esophagus and cause ulceration in cardiac patients who have esophageal compression from enlarged left atrium. Use liquid form in such patients and in those with esophageal stasis or obstruction.
• Drug is often used orally with potassium-wasting diuretics to maintain potassium levels.
• Sugar-free liquid is available (Kaochlor S-F 10%); use if tablet or capsule passage is likely to be delayed, such as in GI obstruction. Have patient sip slowly to minimize GI irritation.
• Don't crush sustained-release potassium products.

• Monitor ECG and serum electrolyte levels during therapy.
• Monitor renal function. Potassium shouldn't be given during immediate postoperative period until urine flow is established.
• Use cautiously in patients with cardiac disease or renal impairment.

### I.V. administration
*Alert:* Give by infusion only, never I.V. push or I.M. Give slowly as dilute solution; potentially fatal hyperkalemia may result from too-rapid infusion. Decrease I.V. rate if burning during infusion occurs.

### Patient teaching
• Instruct patient how to prepare (powders) and administer drug form prescribed. Tell patient to take with or after meals with full glass of water or fruit juice to lessen GI distress.
• Teach patient signs and symptoms of hyperkalemia, and tell patient to notify doctor if they occur.
• Tell patient to alert nurse if discomfort occurs at I.V. insertion site.
• Warn patient not to use salt substitutes concurrently, except with doctor's permission.

---

### potassium gluconate
Glu-K, Kaon, Kaylixir*, K-G Elixir*

*Pregnancy Risk Category C*

### HOW SUPPLIED
*Tablets:* 500 mg (2 mEq $K^+$)
*Elixir:* 4.68 g (20 mEq $K^+$)/15 ml*

### ACTION
Replaces potassium and maintains intracellular and extracellular potassium levels.

| Route | Onset | Peak | Duration |
|-------|-------|------|----------|
| P.O. | Unknown | Unknown | 4 hr |

### INDICATIONS & DOSAGE
*Hypokalemia—*
**Adults:** 40 to 100 mEq P.O. daily in three or four divided doses for treatment; 10 to 20 mEq daily for prevention. Further

---

dosage adjustments are based on serum potassium determinations.

**ADVERSE REACTIONS**
**CNS:** paresthesia of extremities, listlessness, mental confusion, weakness or heaviness of legs, flaccid paralysis.
**CV:** *arrhythmias,* ECG changes.
**GI:** *nausea, vomiting, abdominal pain,* diarrhea.

**INTERACTIONS**
**Drug-drug.** *ACE inhibitors, potassium-sparing diuretics:* risk of hyperkalemia. Use with extreme caution.

**EFFECTS ON DIAGNOSTIC TESTS**
None reported.

**CONTRAINDICATIONS**
Contraindicated in patients with severe renal impairment with oliguria, anuria, or azotemia; untreated Addison's disease; or acute dehydration, heat cramps, hyperkalemia, hyperkalemic form of familial periodic paralysis, or other conditions associated with extensive tissue breakdown.

**NURSING CONSIDERATIONS**
• Give oral potassium supplements with extreme caution because different forms deliver varying amounts of potassium. Never switch products without doctor's order.
• *Alert:* Potassium preparations aren't interchangeable; verify preparation before use.
• Use cautiously in patients with cardiac disease and in those with renal impairment.
• Don't administer potassium supplements postoperatively until urine flow has been established.
• Monitor ECG, fluid intake and output, and BUN, serum potassium, and creatinine levels.

☑ **Patient teaching**
• Advise patient to sip liquid potassium slowly to minimize GI irritation. Also tell him to take drug with or after meals with a full glass of water or fruit juice.

• Warn patient not to use salt substitutes concurrently, except with doctor's permission.

---

## Ringer's injection

*Pregnancy Risk Category NR*

**HOW SUPPLIED**
*Injection:* 250 ml, 500 ml, 1,000 ml

**ACTION**
Replaces fluids and electrolytes.

| Route | Onset | Peak | Duration |
|-------|-------|------|----------|
| I.V. | Immediate | Immediate | Unknown |

**INDICATIONS & DOSAGE**
*Fluid and electrolyte replacement—*
**Adults and children:** dosage highly individualized, but usually 1.5 to 3 L (2% to 6% body weight), infused I.V. over 18 to 24 hours.

**ADVERSE REACTIONS**
**CV:** fluid overload.
**Metabolic:** electrolyte imbalance.

**INTERACTIONS**
None significant.

**EFFECTS ON DIAGNOSTIC TESTS**
None reported.

**CONTRAINDICATIONS**
Contraindicated in patients with renal failure, except as emergency volume expander.

**NURSING CONSIDERATIONS**
• Use cautiously in patients with heart failure, circulatory insufficiency, renal dysfunction, hypoproteinemia, or pulmonary edema.
• Ringer's injection contains sodium, 147 mEq/L; potassium, 4 mEq/L; calcium, 4.5 mEq/L; and chloride, 155.5 mEq/L.
• Electrolyte content is insufficient for treating severe electrolyte deficiencies but does provide electrolytes in levels about equal to those of the blood.

---

● *Alert:* Don't confuse Ringer's injection with Ringer's lactate solution.

### I.V. administration
● Administer at ordered rate via an infusion device.

### ✓ Patient teaching
● Explain use and administration of drug to patient and family.
● Tell patient to report unusual signs or symptoms promptly.

## Ringer's injection, lactated (Ringer's lactate solution)

*Pregnancy Risk Category NR*

### HOW SUPPLIED
*Injection:* 150 ml, 250 ml, 500 ml, 1,000 ml

### ACTION
Replaces fluids and electrolytes.

| Route | Onset | Peak | Duration |
|-------|-------|------|----------|
| I.V. | Immediate | Immediate | Unknown |

### INDICATIONS & DOSAGE
*Fluid and electrolyte replacement—*
**Adults and children:** dosage highly individualized, but usually 1.5 to 3 L (2% to 6% body weight) infused I.V. over 18 to 24 hours.

### ADVERSE REACTIONS
**CV:** fluid overload.
**Metabolic:** electrolyte imbalance.

### INTERACTIONS
None significant.

### EFFECTS ON DIAGNOSTIC TESTS
None reported.

### CONTRAINDICATIONS
Contraindicated in patients with renal failure, except as emergency volume expander.

### NURSING CONSIDERATIONS
● Use cautiously in patients with heart failure, circulatory insufficiency, renal dysfunction, hypoproteinemia, or pulmonary edema.
● Use with caution in patients with hepatic dysfunction because of possible lactic acid accumulation.
● Lactated Ringer's injection contains sodium, 130 mEq/L; potassium, 4 mEq/L; calcium, 3 mEq/L; chloride, 109.7 mEq/L; and lactate, 28 mEq/L.
● Lactated Ringer's injection more closely approximates electrolyte levels in blood plasma.
● *Alert:* Don't confuse Ringer's injection with Ringer's lactate solution.

### I.V. administration
● Administer at ordered rate via an infusion device.

### ✓ Patient teaching
● Explain use and administration of drug to patient and family.
● Tell patient to report unusual signs or symptoms promptly.

## sodium chloride
Slow-Sodium§

*Pregnancy Risk Category C*

### HOW SUPPLIED
*Tablets:* 650 mg
*Tablets (slow-release):* 600 mg, 1 g, 2.25 g
*Injection:* 0.45% NaCl solution 25 ml, 50 ml, 150 ml, 250 ml, 500 ml, 1,000 ml; normal saline solution 2 ml, 3 ml, 5 ml, 10 ml, 20 ml, 25 ml, 30 ml, 50 ml, 100 ml, 150 ml, 250 ml, 500 ml, 1,000 ml; 3% NaCl solution 500 ml; 5% NaCl solution 500 ml; 14.6% NaCl solution 20 ml, 40 ml, 200 ml; 23.4% NaCl solution 30 ml, 50 ml, 100 ml, and 200 ml

### ACTION
Replaces sodium and chloride and maintains levels.

| Route | Onset | Peak | Duration |
|-------|-------|------|----------|
| P.O. | Unknown | Unknown | Unknown |
| I.V. | Immediate | Immediate | Unknown |

---

## INDICATIONS & DOSAGE

*Fluid and electrolyte replacement in hyponatremia due to electrolyte loss or in severe salt depletion—*
**Adults:** dosage is individualized. 3% or 5% solution used only with frequent electrolyte determination and given only slow I.V. With 0.45% solution: 3% to 8% of body weight, according to deficiencies, over 18 to 24 hours; with 0.9% solution: 2% to 6% of body weight, according to deficiencies, over 18 to 24 hours.
*Management of heat cramp due to excessive perspiration—*
**Adults:** 1 g P.O. with each glass of water.

## ADVERSE REACTIONS

**CV:** aggravation of heart failure; thrombophlebitis; edema when given too rapidly or in excess.
**Metabolic:** hypernatremia, aggravation of existing metabolic acidosis with excessive infusion; serious electrolyte disturbances; loss of potassium.
**Respiratory:** *pulmonary edema when given too rapidly or in excess.*
**Other:** local tenderness, abscess, tissue necrosis at injection site.

## INTERACTIONS

None significant.

## EFFECTS ON DIAGNOSTIC TESTS

None reported.

## CONTRAINDICATIONS

Contraindicated in patients with conditions in which sodium and chloride administration is detrimental. NaCl 3% and 5% injections are contraindicated in patients with increased, normal, or only slightly decreased serum electrolyte levels.

## NURSING CONSIDERATIONS

• Use cautiously in patients with heart failure, circulatory insufficiency, renal dysfunction, or hypoproteinemia and in elderly or postoperative patients.
• Monitor serum electrolyte levels.

## I.V. administration

• Don't confuse concentrates (14.6%, 23.4%) available to add to parenteral nutrient solutions with normal saline injection, and never give without diluting. Read labels carefully.
• *Alert:* Infuse 3% and 5% solutions slowly and cautiously to avoid pulmonary edema. Use only for critical situations, and observe patient continually.
• Never use bacteriostatic NaCl injection with newborns.

## Patient teaching

• Explain use and administration of drug to patient and family.
• Tell patient to report adverse reactions promptly.

---

Reactions may be *common,* uncommon, *life-threatening*, or COMMON AND LIFE-THREATENING.

**sodium bicarbonate**
**sodium lactate**
**tromethamine**

### COMBINATION PRODUCTS
None.

---

### sodium bicarbonate ◊
Arm and Hammer Pure Baking
Soda, Bell/ans, Citrocarbonate,
Soda Mint

*Pregnancy Risk Category C*

---

### HOW SUPPLIED
*Tablets* ◊ : 325 mg, 650 mg
*Injection (powder):* 4% (2.4 mEq/5 ml),
4.2% (5 mEq/10 ml), 5% (297.5 mEq/
500 ml), 7.5% (8.92 mEq/10 ml and 44.6
mEq/50 ml), 8.4% (10 mEq/10 ml and 50
mEq/50 ml)

### ACTION
Restores buffering capacity of the body
and neutralizes excess acid.

| Route | Onset | Peak | Duration |
|-------|-------|------|----------|
| P.O. | Unknown | Unknown | Unknown |
| I.V. | Immediate | Immediate | Unknown |

### INDICATIONS & DOSAGE
*Cardiac arrest—*
**Adults and children:** 1 mEq/kg I.V. of
7.5% or 8.4% solution; then 0.5 mEq/kg
I.V. q 10 minutes, depending on arterial
blood gases (ABG). Further dosages
based on results of ABG analysis. If ABG
results are unavailable, use 0.5 mEq/kg
I.V. q 10 minutes until spontaneous circulation returns.
**Infants up to age 2:** not to exceed
8 mEq/kg I.V. of 4.2% solution daily.
*Metabolic acidosis—*
**Adults and children:** dosage depends on
blood carbon dioxide content, pH, and patient's clinical condition. Generally, 2 to 5
mEq/kg I.V. infused over 4- to 8-hour period.

*Systemic or urinary alkalinization—*
**Adults:** initially, 4 g P.O.; then 1 to 2 g q
4 hours.
**Children:** 84 to 840 mg/kg P.O. daily.
*Antacid—*
**Adults:** 300 mg to 2 g P.O. up to q.i.d.
taken with glass of water.

### ADVERSE REACTIONS
**GI:** gastric distention, belching, flatulence.
**Metabolic:** hypokalemia, *metabolic alkalosis*, hypernatremia, hyperosmolarity
with overdose, increased serum lactate
levels.
**Other:** pain, irritation at injection site.

### INTERACTIONS
**Drug-drug.** *Anorexiants, flecainide,
mecamylamine, methenamine, quinidine,
sympathomimetics:* urine alkalinization
causes decreased renal clearance of these
drugs and increased risk of toxicity. Monitor closely.
*Chlorpropamide, lithium, methotrexate,
salicylates, tetracycline:* increased urine
alkalinization causes increased renal
clearance of these drugs and reduced effectiveness. Monitor closely.
*Enteric-coated drugs:* may be released
prematurely in stomach. Avoid concomitant use.
*Ketoconazole:* concurrent use may decrease absorption. Use with caution.

### EFFECTS ON DIAGNOSTIC TESTS
None reported.

### CONTRAINDICATIONS
Contraindicated in patients with metabolic or respiratory alkalosis and in those
with hypocalcemia in which alkalosis
may produce tetany, hypertension,
seizures, or heart failure. Also contraindicated in patients who are losing chlorides
by vomiting or from continuous GI suction and in those receiving diuretics
known to produce hypochloremic alkalosis. Orally administered sodium bicarbonate is contraindicated for treatment of pa-

---

tients with acute ingestion of strong mineral acids.

## NURSING CONSIDERATIONS
• Use with extreme caution in patients with heart failure or other edematous or sodium-retaining conditions or renal insufficiency.
• To avoid risk of alkalosis, obtain blood pH, partial pressure of arterial oxygen, partial pressure of arterial carbon dioxide, and serum electrolyte levels. Keep doctor informed of serum laboratory results.

### 🔋 I.V. administration
• Drug may be added to other I.V. fluids. Sodium bicarbonate inactivates such catecholamines as norepinephrine and dopamine, and forms precipitate with calcium. Don't mix sodium bicarbonate with I.V. solutions of these drugs, and flush I.V. line adequately.
• *Alert:* Sodium bicarbonate isn't routinely recommended for use in cardiac arrest because it may produce a paradoxical acidosis from carbon dioxide production. It shouldn't be routinely administered during the early stages of resuscitation unless preexisting acidosis is clearly present.
• Four percent sodium bicarbonate is usually used for neutralizing certain I.V. drugs such as erythromycin. Consult pharmacist before use.

### ✅ Patient teaching
• Tell patient not to take drug with milk. Drug may cause hypercalcemia, alkalosis, and possibly renal calculi.

---

## sodium lactate

*Pregnancy Risk Category NR*

### HOW SUPPLIED
*Injection:* 1/6 M solution (167 mEq/L)
*Injection:* 5 mEq/ml

### ACTION
Metabolized to sodium bicarbonate, producing buffering effect.

| Route | Onset | Peak | Duration |
|-------|-------|------|----------|
| I.V. | Immediate | 1-2 hr | Unknown |

## INDICATIONS & DOSAGE
*Alkalinize urine—*
**Adults:** 30 ml of 1/6 M solution/kg of body weight I.V., given in divided doses over 24 hours.
*Metabolic acidosis—*
**Adults:** 1/6 M injection (167 mEq lactate/L I.V.); dosage depends on degree of bicarbonate deficit.

## ADVERSE REACTIONS
**CV:** thrombophlebitis at injection site.
**Metabolic:** *metabolic alkalosis,* hypernatremia; hyperosmolarity with overdose.
**Other:** fever, infection.

## INTERACTIONS
None significant.

## EFFECTS ON DIAGNOSTIC TESTS
None reported.

## CONTRAINDICATIONS
Contraindicated in patients with hypernatremia, severe acidosis, lactic acidosis, or conditions in which sodium administration is detrimental, such as heart failure or corticosteroid administration.

## NURSING CONSIDERATIONS
• Use with extreme caution in patients with metabolic or respiratory alkalosis, severe hepatic or renal disease, heart failure, shock, hypoxia, or beriberi.
• Monitor serum electrolyte levels to avoid alkalosis.

### 🔋 I.V. administration
• Add sodium lactate to other I.V. solutions, or give as an isotonic 1/6 M solution. Drug is compatible with most common I.V. solutions.
• Don't mix with sodium bicarbonate; drugs are incompatible.

### ✅ Patient teaching
• Explain use and administration of drug to patient and family.
• Tell patient to report unusual signs and symptoms.

---

Reactions may be *common,* uncommon, *life-threatening,* or COMMON AND LIFE-THREATENING.

## tromethamine
Tham

*Pregnancy Risk Category C*

### HOW SUPPLIED
*Injection:* 18 g/500 ml

### ACTION
Combines with hydrogen ions and associated acid anions; resulting salts are excreted. Also has osmotic diuretic effect.

| Route | Onset | Peak | Duration |
|-------|-------|------|----------|
| I.V. | Immediate | Immediate | Unknown |

### INDICATIONS & DOSAGE
*Metabolic acidosis associated with cardiac bypass surgery or with cardiac arrest—*
**Adults:** dosage depends on bicarbonate deficit. Calculate as follows: each ml of 0.3 M tromethamine solution needed equals weight in kg multiplied by bicarbonate deficit (mEq/L). Additional therapy based on serial determinations of existing bicarbonate deficit. Administer over at least 1 hour; individual doses shouldn't exceed 500 mg/kg.
*Acidosis during bypass surgery:* average dose of 9 ml/kg (2.7 mEq/kg or 0.32 g/kg); total single dose of 500 ml (150 mEq or 18 g) is adequate for most adults; not to exceed 500 mg/kg over a period of less than 1 hour.
*Cardiac arrest:* 3.6 to 10.8 g (111 to 333 ml) injected into large peripheral vein.

### ADVERSE REACTIONS
**Hepatic:** *hemorrhagic hepatic necrosis.*
**Metabolic:** hypoglycemia; *hyperkalemia with decreased urine output.*
**Respiratory:** *respiratory depression.*
**Other:** venospasm; I.V. thrombosis; inflammation, necrosis, sloughing if extravasation occurs; fever.

### INTERACTIONS
None significant.

### EFFECTS ON DIAGNOSTIC TESTS
None reported.

### CONTRAINDICATIONS
Contraindicated in patients with anuria, uremia, or chronic respiratory acidosis; also contraindicated during pregnancy (except in acute, life-threatening situations).

### NURSING CONSIDERATIONS
• Use cautiously in patients with renal disease and poor urine output. Monitor ECG and serum potassium levels.
• Make these determinations before, during, and after therapy: blood pH, carbon dioxide tension, and bicarbonate, glucose, and electrolyte levels.
• Have mechanical ventilation available for patients with associated respiratory acidosis.
• To prevent blood pH from rising above normal, be prepared to adjust dosage carefully, as ordered.

### I.V. administration
• Give slowly through 18G to 20G needle into largest antecubital vein, or by indwelling I.V. catheter.
• If extravasation occurs, infiltrate area with 1% procaine and 150 U hyaluronidase, as ordered.

### Patient teaching
• Explain use of drug to patient and family.
• Tell patient to report adverse reactions.

---

ferrous fumarate
ferrous gluconate
ferrous sulfate
ferrous sulfate, dried
iron dextran
iron sorbitol
polysaccharide-iron complex
sodium ferric gluconate
    complex

## COMBINATION PRODUCTS
FERRO-DOSS, FERROUS DS, FERRO-DSS: ferrous fumarate 150 mg and docusate sodium 100 mg.
FERRO-SEQUELS ◊: ferrous fumarate 150 mg and docusate sodium 100 mg.

---

### ferrous fumarate
Femiron ◊, Feostat ◊, Feostat Drops ◊, Fersamal§, Hemocyte ◊, Ircon ◊, Nephro-Fer ◊, Novofumar†, Palafer†, Palafer Pediatric Drops†, Span-FF ◊

*Pregnancy Risk Category A*

## HOW SUPPLIED
Each 100 mg of ferrous fumarate provides 33 mg of elemental iron
*Tablets ◊:* 63 mg, 200 mg, 324 mg, 325 mg, 350 mg
*Tablets (chewable):* 100 mg ◊
*Oral suspension:* 100 mg/5 ml ◊
*Drops:* 45 mg/0.6 ml ◊

## ACTION
Provides elemental iron, an essential component in the formation of hemoglobin.

| Route | Onset | Peak | Duration |
|-------|-------|------|----------|
| P.O. | 4 days | 7-10 days | 2-4 mo |

## INDICATIONS & DOSAGE
*Iron deficiency—*
**Adults:** 50 to 100 mg P.O. of elemental iron t.i.d.

**Children:** 4 to 6 mg/kg/day P.O. of elemental iron in three divided doses.

## ADVERSE REACTIONS
**GI:** nausea, epigastric pain, vomiting, constipation, diarrhea, black stools, anorexia.
**Other:** temporarily stained teeth from suspension and drops.

## INTERACTIONS
**Drug-drug.** *Antacids, cholestyramine resin, cimetidine, vitamin E:* decreased iron absorption. Separate doses by at least 2 hours.
*Chloramphenicol:* delayed response to iron therapy. Monitor patient.
*Fluoroquinolones, penicillamine, tetracyclines:* decreased GI absorption, possibly resulting in decreased serum levels or efficacy. Separate doses by 2 to 4 hours.
*Levodopa, methyldopa:* decreased absorption and efficacy of levodopa and methyldopa. Monitor for decreased effect of these drugs.
*L-thyroxine:* decreased L-thyroxine absorption. Separate doses by at least 2 hours. Monitor thyroid function.
*Vitamin C:* may increase iron absorption. Give together.
**Drug-food.** *Cereals, cheese, coffee, eggs, milk, tea, whole-grain breads, yogurt:* may impair oral iron absorption. Don't administer together.
**Drug-herb.** *Oregano:* may reduce iron absorption. Separate administration of oregano by at least 2 hours when given with iron supplements or iron-containing foods.

## EFFECTS ON DIAGNOSTIC TESTS
Ferrous fumarate blackens feces and may interfere with tests for occult blood in the stool; the guaiac test and orthotoluidine tests may yield false-positive results, but benzidine test isn't usually affected. Iron overload may decrease uptake of tech-

---

netium 99m and thus interfere with skeletal imaging.

## CONTRAINDICATIONS
Contraindicated in patients with primary hemochromatosis or hemosiderosis, hemolytic anemia unless iron deficiency anemia is also present, peptic ulcer disease, regional enteritis, or ulcerative colitis; also contraindicated in those receiving repeated blood transfusions.

## NURSING CONSIDERATIONS
• Use cautiously on long-term basis.
• GI upset may be related to dose. Between-meal doses are preferable, but can be given with some foods, although absorption may be decreased. Enteric-coated products reduce GI upset but also reduce amount of iron absorbed.
• Check for constipation; record color and amount of stools.
• Oral iron may turn stools black. Although this unabsorbed iron is harmless, it could mask presence of melena.
• Monitor hemoglobin levels and hematocrit and reticulocyte count during therapy, as ordered.
• Combination products such as Ferro-Sequels contain stool softeners, which help prevent constipation, a common adverse reaction.

### ☑ Patient teaching
• Tell patient to take tablets with juice (preferably orange juice) or water, but not with milk or antacids.
• To avoid staining teeth, tell patient to take suspension with straw and place drops at back of throat.
• Caution patient not to crush tablets or to chew extended-release iron preparations.
• Advise patient not to substitute one iron salt for another; the amount of elemental iron may vary.
• Inform parents that as little as three or four tablets can cause serious poisoning in children.

# ferrous gluconate
Fergon* ◊ , Fertinic†,
Novoferrogluc†

*Pregnancy Risk Category A*

## HOW SUPPLIED
Each 100 mg of ferrous gluconate provides 11.6 mg of elemental iron.
*Tablets:* 240 mg ◊ , 325 mg ◊

## ACTION
Provides elemental iron, an essential component in the formation of hemoglobin.

| Route | Onset | Peak | Duration |
| --- | --- | --- | --- |
| P.O. | 4 days | 7-10 days | 2-4 mo |

## INDICATIONS & DOSAGE
*Iron deficiency—*
**Adults:** 100 to 200 mg P.O. of elemental iron t.i.d.
**Children:** 4 to 6 mg/kg/day P.O. of elemental iron in three divided doses.

## ADVERSE REACTIONS
**GI:** *nausea,* epigastric pain, vomiting, *constipation,* diarrhea, *black stools,* anorexia.

## INTERACTIONS
**Drug-drug.** *Antacids, cholestyramine resin, cimetidine, vitamin E:* decreased iron absorption. Separate doses by at least 2 hours.
*Chloramphenicol:* delayed response to iron therapy. Monitor patient.
*Fluoroquinolones, penicillamine, tetracyclines:* decreased GI absorption, possibly resulting in decreased serum levels or efficacy. Separate doses by 2 to 4 hours.
*Levodopa, methyldopa:* decreased absorption and efficacy of levodopa and methyldopa. Monitor for decreased effect of these drugs.
*L-thyroxine:* decreased L-thyroxine absorption. Separate doses by at least 2 hours. Monitor thyroid function.
*Vitamin C:* may increase iron absorption. Give together.
**Drug-food.** *Cereals, cheese, coffee, eggs, milk, tea, whole-grain breads, yogurt:* may impair oral iron absorption. Don't administer together.

---

*Liquid contains alcohol.   **May contain tartrazine.   †Canada   ‡Australia   §U.K.   ◊ OTC

**Drug-herb.** *Oregano:* may reduce iron absorption. Separate administration of oregano by at least 2 hours when given with iron supplements or iron-containing foods.

### EFFECTS ON DIAGNOSTIC TESTS

Ferrous gluconate blackens feces and may interfere with test for occult blood in the stools; the guaiac and orthotoluidine test may yield false-positive results, but benzidine test isn't usually affected. Iron overload may decrease uptake of technetium 99m and thus interfere with skeletal imaging.

### CONTRAINDICATIONS

Contraindicated in patients with peptic ulceration, regional enteritis, ulcerative colitis, hemosiderosis, primary hemochromatosis, or hemolytic anemia (unless an iron deficiency anemia is also present) and in those receiving repeated blood transfusions.

### NURSING CONSIDERATIONS

• Use cautiously on long-term basis.
• GI upset may be related to dose. Between-meal doses are preferable, but can be given with some foods, although absorption may be decreased. Enteric-coated products reduce GI upset but also reduce amount of iron absorbed.
• Check for constipation; record color and amount of stools.
• Oral iron may turn stools black. Although this unabsorbed iron is harmless, it could mask melena.
• Monitor hemoglobin levels and hematocrit and reticulocyte count during therapy.

### ✓ Patient teaching

• To promote absorption, tell patient to take tablets with orange juice.
• Inform parents that as few as three or four tablets can cause serious iron poisoning in children.
• Caution patient not to substitute one iron salt for another because the amounts of elemental iron vary.

## ferrous sulfate
Apo-Ferrous Sulfate†, Feosol*◇, Fer-gen-sol, Fer-In-Sol Drops*◇, Fer-In-Sol Syrup*◇, Fer-Iron Drops◇, Fero-Grad, Mol-Iron*◇

## ferrous sulfate, dried
Fe⁵⁰, Feosol◇, Feospan§, Feratab, Novoferrosulfat†, PMS-Ferrous Sulfate†, Slow FE◇

*Pregnancy Risk Category A*

### HOW SUPPLIED

Ferrous sulfate is 20% elemental iron; dried and powdered, about 32% elemental iron.
*Tablets:* 324 mg, 325 mg◇; 200 mg (dried)
*Tablets (extended-release):* 160 mg (dried)◇, 525 mg
*Caplets (extended-release):* 160 mg (dried)
*Capsules:* 250 mg◇
*Elixir:* 220 mg/5 ml*◇
*Syrup:* 90 mg/5 ml◇
*Drops:* 125 mg/ml

### ACTION

Provides elemental iron, an essential component in the formation of hemoglobin.

| Route | Onset | Peak | Duration |
|-------|-------|------|----------|
| P.O. | 4 days | 7-10 days | 2-4 mo |

### INDICATIONS & DOSAGE

*Iron deficiency—*
**Adults:** 100 to 200 mg P.O. of elemental iron t.i.d.
**Children:** 4 to 6 mg/kg/day P.O. of elemental iron in three divided doses.

### ADVERSE REACTIONS

**GI:** *nausea,* epigastric pain, vomiting, *constipation, black stools,* diarrhea, anorexia.
**Other:** temporarily stained teeth from liquid forms.

---

Reactions may be *common*, uncommon, *life-threatening*, or COMMON AND LIFE-THREATENING.

## INTERACTIONS
**Drug-drug.** *Antacids, cholestyramine resin, cimetidine, vitamin E:* decreased iron absorption. Separate doses if possible.

*Chloramphenicol:* delayed response to iron therapy. Monitor patient.

*Fluoroquinolones, penicillamine, tetracyclines:* decreased GI absorption, possibly resulting in decreased serum levels or efficacy. Separate doses by 2 to 4 hours.

*Levodopa, methyldopa:* decreased absorption and efficacy of levodopa and methyldopa. Monitor for decreased effect of these drugs.

*L-thyroxine:* decreased L-thyroxine absorption. Separate doses by at least 2 hours. Monitor thyroid function.

*Vitamin C:* may increase iron absorption. Give together.

**Drug-food.** *Cereals, cheese, coffee, eggs, milk, tea, whole-grain breads, yogurt:* may impair oral iron absorption. Don't administer together.

**Drug-herb.** *Oregano:* may reduce iron absorption. Separate administration of oregano by at least 2 hours when given with iron supplements or iron-containing foods.

## EFFECTS ON DIAGNOSTIC TESTS
Ferrous sulfate blackens feces and may interfere with tests for occult blood in the stool; the guaiac test and orthotoluidine test may yield false-positive results, but benzidine test isn't usually affected. Iron overload may decrease uptake of technetium 99m and thus interfere with skeletal imaging.

## CONTRAINDICATIONS
Contraindicated in patients with hemosiderosis, primary hemochromatosis, hemolytic anemia (unless iron deficiency anemia is also present), peptic ulceration, ulcerative colitis, or regional enteritis and in those receiving repeated blood transfusions.

## NURSING CONSIDERATIONS
• Use cautiously on long-term basis.
• GI upset may be related to dose. Between-meal doses are preferable, but can be given with some foods, although absorption may be decreased. Enteric-coated products reduce GI upset but also reduce amount of iron absorbed.
• Oral iron may turn stools black. Although this unabsorbed iron is harmless, it could mask melena.
• Monitor hemoglobin levels and hematocrit and reticulocyte count during therapy, as ordered.
• *Alert:* Don't confuse different iron salts; elemental content may vary.

### ✓ Patient teaching
• Tell patient to take with juice.
• Instruct patient not to crush or chew extended-release preparations.
• Inform parents that as little as three to four tablets can cause serious iron poisoning in children.
• Caution patient not to substitute one iron salt for another because amounts of elemental iron vary.
• Advise patient to report constipation and change in stool color or consistency.

---

## iron dextran
DexFerrum, InFeD

## iron sorbitol

*Pregnancy Risk Category C*

---

## HOW SUPPLIED
1 ml iron dextran provides 50 mg elemental iron
*Injection:* 50 mg elemental iron/ml

## ACTION
Provides elemental iron, an essential component in the formation of hemoglobin.

| Route | Onset | Peak | Duration |
|-------|-------|------|----------|
| I.M. | 72 hr | Unknown | 3-4 wk |

## INDICATIONS & DOSAGE
*Iron deficiency anemia—*
**Adults and children:** I.M. or I.V. test dose needed before administration.

*I.M. (by Z-track method):* 0.5-ml test dose injected. If no reactions occur in 1 hour, remainder of dose is given. Daily dose should ordinarily not exceed 0.5 ml (25 mg) for infants under 5 kg (11 lb);

1 ml (50 mg) for children under 10 kg (22 lb); 2 ml (100 mg) for heavier children and adults.

*I.V.:* 0.5-ml test dose injected over 30 seconds. If no reactions occur in 1 hour, remainder of therapeutic I.V. dose is given. Therapeutic dose repeated I.V. daily. Single dose shouldn't exceed 100 mg. Give slowly (1 ml/minute).

## ADVERSE REACTIONS
**CNS:** headache, transitory paresthesia, arthralgia, myalgia, dizziness, malaise.
**CV:** *hypotensive reaction, peripheral vascular flushing.*
**GI:** nausea, anorexia.
**Respiratory:** *bronchospasm,* dyspnea.
**Skin:** rash; urticaria; *soreness, inflammation, brown skin discoloration at I.M. injection site; local phlebitis at I.V. injection site;* sterile abscess; necrosis; atrophy.
**Other:** fibrosis, *anaphylaxis,* delayed sensitivity reactions, fever, chills.

## INTERACTIONS
None significant.

## EFFECTS ON DIAGNOSTIC TESTS
Large doses (over 250 mg iron) may color the serum brown. Iron dextran prevents meaningful measurement of serum iron level and total iron binding capacity for up to 3 weeks; I.M. injection may cause dense areas of activity for 1 to 6 days on bone scans using technetium 99m diphosphonate.

## CONTRAINDICATIONS
Contraindicated in patients with hypersensitivity to drug and in those with acute infectious renal disease or all anemias except iron-deficiency anemia.

## NURSING CONSIDERATIONS
• Don't administer iron dextran with oral iron preparations.
• Use with extreme caution in patients with serious hepatic impairment, rheumatoid arthritis, or other inflammatory diseases because these patients may be at higher risk for certain delays and reactions.
• Use cautiously in patients with history of significant allergies or asthma.

• I.M. or I.V. injections of iron are advisable only for patients in whom oral administration is impossible or ineffective.
• For I.M. route, inject deeply into upper outer quadrant of buttock—never into arm or other exposed area—with a 2- to 3-inch 19G or 20G needle. Use Z-track method to avoid leakage into subcutaneous tissue and staining of skin. After drawing up drug, use a new sterile needle to administer injection.
• Monitor hemoglobin levels and hematocrit and reticulocyte count, as ordered.

## I.V. administration
• Check hospital policy before administering I.V. Don't mix with other parenteral drug or nutritional solutions containing liquid emulsions.
• Upon completion of I.V. dose, flush the vein with 10 ml of normal saline solution. Patient should rest for 15 to 30 minutes after I.V. administration.

## Patient teaching
• Teach patient signs and symptoms of hypersensitivity or iron toxicity and tell him to report them if they occur.
• Inform patient that drug may stain skin.

---

## polysaccharide-iron complex
Hytinic, Niferex, Niferex-150, Nu-Iron, Nu-Iron 150

*Pregnancy Risk Category NR*

## HOW SUPPLIED
*Tablets (film-coated):* 50 mg
*Capsules:* 150 mg
*Solution:* 100 mg/5 ml

## ACTION
Provides elemental iron, an essential component in the formation of hemoglobin.

| Route | Onset | Peak | Duration |
|-------|-------|------|----------|
| P.O. | Few days | 2-10 days | 2 mo |

## INDICATIONS & DOSAGE
*Uncomplicated iron deficiency anemia—*
**Adults:** 100 to 200 mg P.O. of elemental iron t.i.d.

**Children:** 4 to 6 mg/kg/day P.O. of elemental iron in three divided doses.

## ADVERSE REACTIONS
Although nausea, constipation, black stools, and epigastric pain are common adverse reactions associated with iron therapy, few, if any, occur with polysaccharide iron complex.

## INTERACTIONS
**Drug-drug.** *Antacids, cholestyramine resin, cimetidine, vitamin E:* decreased iron absorption. Separate doses by 2 to 4 hours.
*Chloramphenicol:* delayed response to iron therapy. Monitor patient.
*Fluoroquinolones, penicillamine, tetracyclines:* decreased GI absorption, possibly resulting in decreased serum levels or efficacy. Separate doses if possible.
*Levodopa, methyldopa:* decreased absorption and efficacy of levodopa and methyldopa. Monitor for decreased effect of these drugs.
*Vitamin C:* may increase iron absorption. Give together.
**Drug-food.** *Cereals, cheese, coffee, eggs, milk, tea, whole-grain breads, yogurt:* may impair oral iron absorption. Don't administer together.
**Drug-herb.** *Oregano:* may reduce iron absorption. Separate administration of oregano by at least 2 hours when given with iron supplements or iron-containing foods.

## EFFECTS ON DIAGNOSTIC TESTS
Drug may blacken feces and may interfere with test for occult blood in stool; guaiac and orthotoluidine tests may yield false-positive results. Benzidine test isn't usually affected. Iron overload may decrease uptake of technetium 99m and thus interfere with skeletal imaging.

## CONTRAINDICATIONS
Contraindicated in patients with hypersensitivity to drug or its ingredients and in those with hemochromatosis or hemosiderosis.

## NURSING CONSIDERATIONS
• Oral iron may turn stools black. Although this unabsorbed iron is harmless, it may mask melena.
• Monitor hemoglobin levels and hematocrit and reticulocyte count, as ordered.

☑ **Patient teaching**
• Tell patient to take with juice.
• Inform parents that as few as three tablets can cause serious iron poisoning in children.
• Caution patient not to substitute one iron salt for another because the amounts of elemental iron vary.

✳ *NEW DRUG*

# sodium ferric gluconate complex
**Ferrlecit**

*Pregnancy Risk Category B*

## HOW SUPPLIED
*Injection:* 62.5 mg elemental iron (12.5 mg/ml) in 5-ml ampules

## ACTION
Restores total body iron content, which is critical for normal hemoglobin synthesis and oxygen transport.

| Route | Onset | Peak | Duration |
|-------|-------|------|----------|
| I.V. | Unknown | Unknown | Unknown |

## INDICATIONS & DOSAGE
*Iron deficiency anemia in patients undergoing chronic hemodialysis who are receiving supplemental erythropoietin therapy—*
**Adults:** before initiating therapeutic doses, administer test dose of 2 ml sodium ferric gluconate complex (25 mg elemental iron) diluted in 50 ml normal saline and given I.V. over 1 hour. If test dose is tolerated, give therapeutic dose of 10 ml (125 mg elemental iron) diluted in 100 ml normal saline and given I.V. over 1 hour. Most patients need minimum cumulative dose of 1 g elemental iron administered at more than eight sequential dialysis treatments to achieve a favorable hemoglobin or hematocrit response.

**ADVERSE REACTIONS**

**CNS:** asthenia, headache, fatigue, malaise, dizziness, paresthesia, agitation, insomnia, somnolence, syncope.

**CV:** hypotension, hypertension, tachycardia, *bradycardia,* angina, chest pain, *MI,* edema, flushing.

**EENT:** conjunctivitis, abnormal vision, rhinitis.

**GI:** nausea, vomiting, diarrhea, rectal disorder, dyspepsia, eructation, flatulence, melena, abdominal pain.

**GU:** urinary tract infection.

**Hematologic:** abnormal erythrocytes, anemia.

**Metabolic:** hyperkalemia, hypoglycemia, hypokalemia, hypervolemia.

**Musculoskeletal:** myalgia, arthralgia, back pain, arm pain, cramps.

**Respiratory:** dyspnea, coughing, upper respiratory tract infections, pneumonia, pulmonary edema.

**Skin:** pruritus, increased sweating, rash.

**Other:** injection site reaction, pain, fever, infection, rigors, chills, flulike syndrome, sepsis, *carcinoma, hypersensitivity reactions,* lymphadenopathy.

**INTERACTIONS**
None significant.

**EFFECTS ON DIAGNOSTIC TESTS**
None reported.

**CONTRAINDICATIONS**
Contraindicated in patients with hypersensitivity to drug or its components (such as benzyl alcohol) and in those with anemias not associated with iron deficiency. Don't administer to patients with iron overload.

**NURSING CONSIDERATIONS**
• Use cautiously in elderly patients.
• *Alert:* Dosage is expressed in mg of elemental iron.
• Drug shouldn't be administered to patients with iron overload, which generally occurs in hemoglobinopathies and other refractory anemias.
• *Alert:* Potentially life-threatening hypersensitivity reactions (characterized by CV collapse, cardiac arrest, bronchospasm, oral or pharyngeal edema, dyspnea, an-

gioedema, urticaria, or pruritus sometimes associated with pain and muscle spasm of chest or back) may occur during infusion. Have adequate supportive measures readily available. Monitor patient closely during infusion.

• Monitor hemoglobin levels and hematocrit and serum ferritin and iron saturation levels, as ordered.

• Some adverse reactions in hemodialysis patients may be related to dialysis itself or to chronic renal failure.

• Check with patient about other potential sources of iron, such as OTC iron preparations and iron-containing multiple vitamins with minerals.

**◖ I.V. administration**
• Dilute test dose of sodium ferric gluconate complex in 50 ml normal saline and administer over 1 hour. Dilute therapeutic doses of drug in 100 ml normal saline and give over 1 hour.
• Don't mix sodium ferric gluconate complex with other drugs, or add to parenteral nutrition solutions for I.V. infusion. Use immediately after dilution in normal saline.
• Profound hypotension with flushing, light-headedness, malaise, fatigue, weakness, or severe chest, back, flank, or groin pain has been reported following rapid I.V. administration of iron. These reactions aren't associated with hypersensitivity reactions and may be due to too rapid administration of drug. Don't exceed recommended rate of administration (2.1 mg/minute). Monitor patient closely during infusion.

**✔ Patient teaching**
• Advise patient to notify doctor immediately if abdominal pain, diarrhea, vomiting, drowsiness, or hyperventilation occurs. These symptoms may indicate iron poisoning.

**ardeparin sodium**
**dalteparin sodium**
**danaparoid sodium**
**enoxaparin sodium**
**heparin calcium**
**heparin sodium**
**warfarin sodium**

**COMBINATION PRODUCTS**
None.

---

**ardeparin sodium**
Normiflo Injection

*Pregnancy Risk Category C*

**HOW SUPPLIED**
*Injection:* 5,000 antifactor Xa U/0.5 ml,
10,000 antifactor Xa U/0.5 ml

**ACTION**
A low-molecular-weight heparin that
binds to antithrombin III and accelerates
its activity, resulting in an inactivation of
factor Xa and thrombin, thereby preventing the formation of clots.

| Route | Onset | Peak | Duration |
|-------|-------|------|----------|
| S.C. | Unknown | 3 hr | Unknown |

**INDICATIONS & DOSAGE**
*Prevention of deep venous thrombosis*
*that may lead to pulmonary embolism fol-*
*lowing knee replacement surgery—*
**Adults:** 50 anti-Xa U/kg S.C. q 12 hours
for 14 days or until patient is ambulatory,
whichever is shorter. Give initial dose in
evening of day of surgery or following
morning.

**ADVERSE REACTIONS**
**CNS:** dizziness, headache, insomnia.
**CV:** chest pain, peripheral edema, *CVA.*
**GI:** nausea, vomiting.
**Hematologic:** anemia, ecchymosis, *hem-*
*orrhage, thrombocytopenia.*
**Musculoskeletal:** arthralgia.
**Respiratory:** dyspnea.

**Skin:** injection site hematoma, pruritus,
rash, local reaction, urticaria.
**Other:** fever, pain.

**INTERACTIONS**
**Drug-drug.** *Anticoagulants, antiplatelet*
*drugs, including aspirin, NSAIDs:* concomitant use may increase risk of bleeding. Avoid use together. Monitor patient,
PT, PTT, and INR.

**EFFECTS ON DIAGNOSTIC TESTS**
None reported.

**CONTRAINDICATIONS**
Contraindicated in patients with known
hypersensitivity to drug or pork products
and in those with active major bleeding
or thrombocytopenia associated with
antiplatelet antibodies in presence of
drug.

**NURSING CONSIDERATIONS**
• Use with extreme caution in patients
with history of heparin-induced thrombocytopenia and known hypersensitivity to
parabens or sulfites.
• Use cautiously in patients at increased
risk for hemorrhage, such as those with
bacterial endocarditis, congenital or acquired bleeding disorders, active ulcerative disease, angiodysplastic GI disease,
hemorrhagic stroke, or severe uncontrolled hypertension; in those receiving
concomitant antiplatelet drugs; and shortly after brain, spinal, or ophthalmic
surgery. Monitor vital signs.
• Use cautiously in patients with severe
renal failure.
• It's unknown if drug appears in breast
milk. Use cautiously when administering
to breast-feeding women.
• *Alert:* Bleeding is main sign of drug
overdose. To stop most bleeding, discontinue drug, apply pressure to the site, and
replace hemostatic blood elements, if
needed. Protamine sulfate can also be administered. Dose of protamine should be
equal to dose of drug administered (1 mg

of protamine neutralizes 100 anti-Xa U of ardeparin). If bleeding persists after 2 hours, blood should be drawn and residual anti-Xa levels determined. Administer additional protamine if clinically important bleeding persists or anti-Xa levels remain high.

• Base ardeparin dose on actual body weight.

• *Alert:* Ardeparin can't be used interchangeably (unit for unit) with heparin sodium or other low-molecular-weight heparins.

• Routinely monitor CBC, platelet counts, urinalysis, and occult blood in stools. Routine monitoring of coagulation parameters isn't needed.

• Don't mix with other injections or infusions.

• Administer drug with deep S.C. injection. Injection sites include the abdomen (avoiding the navel), outer aspect of upper arm, and anterior thigh with patient sitting or lying down. Extrude air and excess drug before administration. Introduce full length of needle into skinfold held between the thumb and forefinger. Hold skinfold during injection. Don't rub injection site.

• Rotate injection site.

• Don't give drug I.M. to avoid possible hematoma at injection site.

• Monitor patient closely for bleeding if drug is given during or immediately following spinal or epidural puncture.

### ✅ Patient teaching
• Instruct patient to report abnormal bruising, bleeding, or dark stools.
• Instruct patient to observe for hematoma at injection site.
• Tell patient to avoid use of OTC products such as aspirin or NSAIDs.

---

## dalteparin sodium
Fragmin

*Pregnancy Risk Category B*

### HOW SUPPLIED
*Syringe:* 2,500 antifactor Xa IU/0.2 ml, 5,000 antifactor Xa IU/0.2 ml

### ACTION
A low-molecular-weight heparin derivative that enhances inhibition of factor Xa and thrombin by antithrombin.

| Route | Onset | Peak | Duration |
|-------|---------|------|----------|
| S.C. | Unknown | 4 hr | Unknown |

### INDICATIONS & DOSAGE
*Prophylaxis against deep vein thrombosis (DVT) in patients undergoing abdominal surgery who are at risk for thromboembolic complications—*
**Adults:** 2,500 IU S.C. daily, starting 1 to 2 hours before surgery and repeated once daily for 5 to 10 days postoperatively.
✳ *NEW INDICATION: DVT prophylaxis in patients undergoing hip replacement surgery—*
**Adults:** 2,500 IU S.C. within 2 hours before surgery and second dose 2,500 IU S.C. in the evening of surgery (at least 6 hours after first dose). If surgery is performed in the evening, omit second dose on day of surgery. Starting on first postoperative day, administer 5,000 IU S.C. once daily for 5 to 10 days. Or, 5,000 IU S.C. on the evening before surgery; then 5,000 IU S.C. once daily starting in the evening of surgery for 5 to 10 days postoperatively.
✳ *NEW INDICATION: Unstable angina and non-Q-wave MI—*
**Adults:** 120 IU/kg S.C. q 12 hours with oral aspirin unless contraindicated. Maximum dose 10,000 IU. Usual duration of treatment is 5 to 8 days.

### ADVERSE REACTIONS
**Hematologic:** *thrombocytopenia,* **hemorrhage,** ecchymoses, bleeding complications.
**Hepatic:** falsely elevated AST and ALT levels.
**Skin:** pruritus; rash; pain; *hematoma at injection site.*
**Other:** fever.

### INTERACTIONS
**Drug-drug.** *Antiplatelet drugs, oral anticoagulants:* may increase risk of bleeding. Use together cautiously.

---

Reactions may be *common,* uncommon, **life-threatening**, or COMMON AND LIFE-THREATENING.

**EFFECTS ON DIAGNOSTIC TESTS**
None reported.

**CONTRAINDICATIONS**
Contraindicated in patients with hypersensitivity to drug, heparin, or pork products and in those with active major bleeding or thrombocytopenia associated with positive in vitro tests for antiplatelet antibody in presence of drug.

**NURSING CONSIDERATIONS**
• Use with extreme caution in patients with history of heparin-induced thrombocytopenia and in patients at increased risk for hemorrhage, such as those with severe uncontrolled hypertension, bacterial endocarditis, congenital or acquired bleeding disorders, active ulceration or angiodysplastic GI disease, or hemorrhagic stroke; also use with extreme caution shortly after brain, spinal, or ophthalmic surgery. Monitor vital signs.
• Patients receiving dalteparin who need neuraxial anesthesia or spinal puncture may be at increased risk for developing an epidural or spinal hematoma, which can result in long-term or permanent paralysis. Monitor patient's neurologic status and function frequently.
• Use with caution in patients with bleeding diathesis, thrombocytopenia, platelet defects, severe hepatic or renal insufficiency, hypertensive or diabetic retinopathy, or recent GI bleeding.
• DVT is a risk factor in patients who are candidates for therapy, including those over age 40, those who are obese or are undergoing surgery under general anesthesia lasting over 30 minutes, or have additional risk factors (such as malignancy or history of DVT or pulmonary embolism).
• Have patient assume a sitting or supine position when administering drug. Give S.C. injection deeply. Injection sites include a U-shaped area around the navel, upper outer side of thigh, and upper outer quadrant of buttock. Rotate sites daily. When area around the navel or thigh is used, use thumb and forefinger to lift up a fold of skin while giving injection. The entire length of needle should be inserted at a 45- to 90-degree angle.
• Never administer drug I.M.
• Don't mix with other injections or infusions unless specific compatibility data support such mixing.
• *Alert:* Drug isn't interchangeable (unit for unit) with unfractionated heparin or other low-molecular-weight heparin.
• Periodic, routine CBC and fecal occult blood tests are recommended during therapy. Patients don't need regular monitoring of PT or activated PTT.
• Monitor patient closely for thrombocytopenia.
• Drug should be discontinued if a thromboembolic event occurs despite dalteparin prophylaxis.

✓ **Patient teaching**
• Instruct patient and family to watch for and report signs of bleeding (bruising and blood in stools).
• Tell patient to avoid OTC drugs containing aspirin or other salicylates.

---

**danaparoid sodium**
Orgaran

*Pregnancy Risk Category B*

---

**HOW SUPPLIED**
*Ampule:* 750 anti-Xa U/0.6 ml
*Syringe:* 750 anti-Xa U/0.6 ml

**ACTION**
Prevents fibrin formation by inhibiting generation of thrombin by factor Xa and factor IIa.

| Route | Onset | Peak | Duration |
|-------|-------|------|----------|
| S.C. | Unknown | 2-5 hr | Unknown |

**INDICATIONS & DOSAGE**
*Prophylaxis against postoperative deep vein thrombosis (DVT) in patients undergoing elective hip replacement surgery—*
**Adults:** 750 anti-Xa U S.C. b.i.d. starting 1 to 4 hours preoperatively, and then not sooner than 2 hours after surgery. Treatment continued for 7 to 10 days postoper-

---

atively or until risk of DVT has diminished.

**ADVERSE REACTIONS**
**CNS:** insomnia, headache, asthenia, dizziness.
**CV:** peripheral edema, *hemorrhage.*
**GI:** *nausea, constipation,* vomiting.
**GU:** urinary tract infection, urine retention.
**Hematologic:** anemia.
**Musculoskeletal:** joint disorder.
**Skin:** rash, pruritus.
**Other:** *fever, injection site pain,* infection.

**INTERACTIONS**
**Drug-drug.** *Oral anticoagulants, platelet inhibitors:* may increase risk of bleeding. Use together cautiously. Monitor PT and INR.

**EFFECTS ON DIAGNOSTIC TESTS**
Drug may cause unreliable PT and Thrombotest results within 5 hours after administration.

**CONTRAINDICATIONS**
Contraindicated in patients with hypersensitivity to drug or pork products and in those with severe hemorrhagic diathesis (such as hemophilia or idiopathic thrombocytopenic purpura), active major bleeding, or thrombocytopenia associated with positive in vitro tests for antiplatelet antibody in presence of drug.

**NURSING CONSIDERATIONS**
• Use with extreme caution in patients at increased risk for hemorrhage, such as those with severe uncontrolled hypertension, acute bacterial endocarditis, congenital or acquired bleeding disorders, active ulcerative and angiodysplastic GI disease, nonhemorrhagic stroke, or postoperative indwelling epidural catheter; also use with extreme caution shortly after brain, spinal, or ophthalmic surgery. Monitor vital signs.
• Drug contains sodium sulfite, which can cause allergic reactions in some people, especially asthmatics.

• Use with caution in patients with impaired renal function.
• Drug should be used in pregnancy only if clearly needed. Use cautiously in breast-feeding women.
• Safety and effectiveness of drug in children haven't been established.
• Danaparoid should never be given I.M. To administer drug, have patient lie down. Give S.C. injection deeply, using a 25G to 26G needle. Injection sites should be alternated between the left and right anterolateral and posterolateral abdominal wall. Gently pull up a skinfold with thumb and forefinger and insert entire length of needle into tissue. Don't rub afterward.
• *Alert:* Drug isn't interchangeable (unit for unit) with heparin or low-molecular-weight heparin.
• Periodic, routine CBC (including platelet count) and fecal occult blood tests are recommended during therapy. Patients don't need regular monitoring of PT and PTT.
• Drug has little effect on PT, PTT, fibrinolytic activity, or bleeding time.
• *Alert:* Monitor patient's hematocrit and blood pressure closely; a decrease in either may signal hemorrhage.
• If serious bleeding occurs, drug should be stopped and blood products transfused, as ordered.
• Store ampules at room temperature; syringes should be refrigerated at 36° to 46° F (2° to 8° C). Protect drug from light.

☑ **Patient teaching**
• Instruct patient and family to watch for and report signs of bleeding.
• Tell patient to avoid OTC drugs containing aspirin or other salicylates.

---

**enoxaparin sodium**
Lovenox

*Pregnancy Risk Category B*

**HOW SUPPLIED**
*Injection:* 30 mg/0.3 ml, 40 mg/0.4 ml, 60 mg/0.6 ml, 80 mg/0.8 ml, 100 mg/1 ml

---

## ACTION
A low-molecular-weight heparin derivative that accelerates formation of antithrombin III–thrombin complex and deactivates thrombin, preventing conversion of fibrinogen to fibrin. Has a higher antifactor Xa to antifactor IIa activity ratio.

| Route | Onset | Peak | Duration |
|-------|-------|------|----------|
| S.C. | Unknown | 3-5 hr | 24 hr |

## INDICATIONS & DOSAGE
*Prevention of pulmonary embolism and deep vein thrombosis (DVT) after hip or knee replacement surgery—*
**Adults:** 30 mg S.C. q 12 hours for 7 to 10 days. Initial dose given between 12 and 24 hours postoperatively provided hemostasis has been established. Treatment should continue during postoperative period until risk of DVT has diminished. Hip replacement patients may receive 40 mg S.C. given 12 hours preoperatively. After initial phase of therapy, hip replacement patients should continue with 40 mg S.C. daily for 3 weeks.
*Prevention of pulmonary embolism and DVT after abdominal surgery—*
**Adults:** 40 mg S.C. daily with initial dose 2 hours before surgery. Subsequent dose, provided hemostasis has been established, is given 24 hours after initial preoperative dose and continued once daily for 7 to 10 days. Treatment should continue during postoperative period until risk of DVT has diminished.
*Prevention of ischemic complications of unstable angina and non-Q-wave MI with oral aspirin therapy—*
**Adults:** 1 mg/kg S.C. q 12 hours until clinical stabilization (minimum 2 days) with aspirin 100 to 325 mg P.O. once daily.
✳ *NEW INDICATION: Inpatient treatment of acute DVT with and without pulmonary embolism when administered with warfarin sodium—*
**Adults:** 1 mg/kg S.C. q 12 hours; or, 1.5 mg/kg S.C. once daily (at same time daily) for 5 to 7 days until therapeutic oral anticoagulant effect (INR 2 to 3) has been achieved. Warfarin sodium therapy is usually initiated within 72 hours of enoxaparin injection.

✳ *NEW INDICATION: Outpatient treatment of acute DVT without pulmonary embolism when administered with warfarin sodium—*
**Adults:** 1 mg/kg S.C. q 12 hours for 5 to 7 days until therapeutic oral anticoagulant effect (INR 2 to 3) has been achieved. Warfarin sodium therapy is usually initiated within 72 hours of enoxaparin injection.

## ADVERSE REACTIONS
**CNS:** confusion, *neurologic injury when used with spinal or epidural puncture.*
**CV:** edema, peripheral edema, *CV toxicity (chest pain, dizziness, irregular heartbeat).*
**GI:** nausea.
**Hematologic:** hypochromic anemia, *thrombocytopenia, hemorrhage,* ecchymoses; bleeding complications.
**Hepatic:** increased AST and ALT levels.
**Skin:** irritation, pain, hematoma, erythema at injection site; *rash, hives.*
**Other:** fever, pain, *angioedema.*

## INTERACTIONS
**Drug-drug.** *Anticoagulants, antiplatelet drugs, NSAIDs:* increased risk of bleeding. May also lead to spinal or epidural hematomas in patients with spinal punctures or epidural or spinal anesthesia. Don't use together.
*Plicamycin, valproic acid:* may cause hypoprothrombinemia and inhibit platelet aggregation. Monitor closely.

## EFFECTS ON DIAGNOSTIC TESTS
None reported.

## CONTRAINDICATIONS
Contraindicated in patients with hypersensitivity to drug, heparin, or pork products and in those with active major bleeding, thrombocytopenia, or antiplatelet antibodies in presence of drug.

## NURSING CONSIDERATIONS
• Use with extreme caution in patients with history of heparin-induced thrombocytopenia, aneurysms, cerebrovascular hemorrhage, spinal or epidural punctures (as with anesthesia), uncontrolled hypertension, or threatened abortion.

• The vascular access sheath for instrumentation should remain in place for 6 to 8 hours following a dose and the next dose given no sooner than 6 to 8 hours after sheath removal. Monitor vital signs.

• Use cautiously in elderly patients and in those with conditions that place them at increased risk for hemorrhage, such as bacterial endocarditis; congenital or acquired bleeding disorders; ulcer disease; angiodysplastic GI disease; hemorrhagic stroke; or recent spinal, eye, or brain surgery. Also use cautiously in patients with regional or lumbar block anesthesia, blood dyscrasias, recent childbirth, pericarditis or pericardial effusion, renal insufficiency, or severe CNS trauma.

• *Alert:* Patients receiving low-molecular-weight heparins or heparinoids, who have epidural or spinal anesthesia or spinal puncture, are at risk for developing epidural or spinal hematoma that can result in long-term paralysis. Risk increases with use of epidural catheters, drugs affecting hemostasis, or traumatic or repeated epidural or spinal punctures. Monitor these patients frequently for signs of neurologic impairment. Urgent treatment is needed.

• Draw blood to establish baseline coagulation parameters before therapy.

• Never administer drug I.M.

• Don't massage after S.C. injection. Watch for signs of bleeding at site. Rotate sites and keep record.

• Avoid excessive I.M. injections of other drugs to prevent or minimize hematomas. If possible, don't give I.M. injections at all.

• Monitor platelet counts regularly. Patients with normal coagulation won't need close monitoring of PT or PTT.

• Regularly inspect patient for bleeding gums, bruises on arms or legs, petechiae, nosebleeds, melena, tarry stools, hematuria, hematemesis.

• To treat severe overdose, give protamine sulfate (a heparin antagonist) by slow I.V. infusion at concentration of 1% to equal dose of drug injected, as ordered.

• *Alert:* Heparin and enoxaparin aren't interchangeable.

☑ **Patient teaching**
• Instruct patient and family to watch for signs of bleeding and to notify doctor immediately if any occur.
• Tell patient to avoid OTC drugs containing aspirin or other salicylates.

---

**heparin calcium**
Calcilean†, Uniparin-Ca‡

**heparin sodium**
Hepalean†, Heparin Leo†, Heparin Lock Flush Solution (with Tubex), Heparin Sodium Injection, Hep-Lock, Monoparin§, Multiparin§, Pump-Hep§, Unihep§, Uniparin‡

*Pregnancy Risk Category C*

---

**HOW SUPPLIED**
Products are derived from beef lung or pork intestinal mucosa.
**heparin calcium**
*Ampule:* 12,500 U/0.5 ml; 20,000 U/0.8 ml
*Syringe:* 5,000 U/0.2 ml
**heparin sodium**
*Carpuject:* 5,000 U/ml
*Disposable syringes:* 1,000 U/ml, 2,500 U/ml, 5,000 U/ml, 7,500 U/ml, 10,000 U/ml, 15,000 U/ml, 20,000 U/ml, 40,000 U/ml
*Premixed I.V. solutions:* 1,000 U in 500 ml of normal saline solution; 2,000 U in 1,000 ml of normal saline solution; 12,500 U in 250 ml of 0.45% NaCl solution; 25,000 U in 250 ml of 0.45% NaCl solution; 25,000 U in 500 ml of 0.45% NaCl solution; 10,000 U in 100 ml of $D_5W$; 12,500 U in 250 ml of $D_5W$; 25,000 U in 250 ml $D_5W$; 25,000 U in 500 ml $D_5W$; 20,000 U in 500 ml of $D_5W$
*Unit-dose vials:* 1,000 U/ml, 5,000 U/ml, 10,000 U/ml, 20,000 U/ml, 40,000 U/ml
*Vials:* 1,000 U/ml, 2,000 U/ml, 2,500 U/ml, 5,000 U/ml, 7,500 U/ml, 10,000 U/ml, 20,000 U/ml, 40,000 U/ml
**heparin sodium flush**
*Disposable syringes:* 10 U/ml, 100 U/ml
*Vials:* 10 U/ml, 100 U/ml

---

## ACTION
Accelerates formation of antithrombin III–thrombin complex and deactivates thrombin, preventing conversion of fibrinogen to fibrin.

| Route | Onset | Peak | Duration |
|-------|-------|------|----------|
| I.V. | Immediate | Unknown | Variable |
| S.C. | 20-60 min | 2-4 hr | Variable |

## INDICATIONS & DOSAGE
Dosage is highly individualized, depending upon disease state, age, and renal and hepatic status.

*Full-dose continuous I.V. infusion therapy for deep vein thrombosis (DVT), MI, pulmonary embolism—*
**Adults:** initially, 5,000 U by I.V. bolus; then 750 to 1,500 U/hour by I.V. infusion with pump. Hourly rate titrated 8 hours after bolus dose and based on PTT results.
**Children:** initially, 50 U/kg I.V.; then 25 U/kg/hour or 20,000 U/m$^2$ daily by I.V. infusion pump. Dosage titrated based on PTT.

*Full-dose S.C. therapy for DVT, MI, pulmonary embolism—*
**Adults:** initially, 5,000 U I.V. bolus and 10,000 to 20,000 U in a concentrated solution S.C.; then 8,000 to 10,000 U S.C. q 8 hours or 15,000 to 20,000 U in a concentrated solution q 12 hours.

*Full-dose intermittent I.V. therapy for DVT, MI, pulmonary embolism—*
**Adults:** initially, 10,000 U by I.V. bolus; then titrated according to PTT, and 5,000 to 10,000 U I.V. q 4 to 6 hours.
**Children:** initially, 100 U/kg by I.V. bolus; then 50 to 100 U/kg q 4 hours.

*Fixed low-dose therapy for venous thrombosis, pulmonary embolism, atrial fibrillation with embolism, postoperative DVT, and prevention of embolism—*
**Adults:** 5,000 U S.C. q 12 hours. In surgical patients, first dose given 2 hours before procedure; then 5,000 U S.C. q 8 to 12 hours for 5 to 7 days or until patient can walk.

*Consumptive coagulopathy (such as disseminated intravascular coagulation)—*
**Adults:** 50 to 100 U/kg by I.V. bolus or continuous I.V. infusion q 4 hours.

**Children:** 25 to 50 U/kg by I.V. bolus or continuous I.V. infusion q 4 hours. If no improvement within 4 to 8 hours, discontinue heparin.
*Open-heart surgery—*
**Adults:** (total body perfusion) 150 to 300 U/kg continuous I.V infusion.
*Patency maintenance of I.V. indwelling catheters—*
**Adults:** 10 to 100 U I.V. flush. Use sufficient volume to fill device. Not intended for therapeutic use.

## ADVERSE REACTIONS
**EENT:** rhinitis.
**Hematologic:** *hemorrhage, overly prolonged clotting time, thrombocytopenia.*
**Hepatic:** falsely elevated AST and serum ALT levels.
**Skin:** irritation, mild pain, hematoma, ulceration, cutaneous or S.C. necrosis, pruritus, urticaria.
**Other:** *"white clot" syndrome; hypersensitivity reactions,* including chills, fever, *anaphylactoid reactions*, false elevated in some tests for serum thyroxine levels.

## INTERACTIONS
**Drug-drug.** *Oral anticoagulants:* increased additive anticoagulation. Monitor PT, INR, and PTT.
*Salicylates, other antiplatelet drugs:* increased anticoagulant effect. Don't use together.
*Thrombolytics:* increased risk of hemorrhage. Monitor closely.
**Drug-herb.** *Motherwort, red clover:* risk of increased bleeding. Avoid concomitant use.

## EFFECTS ON DIAGNOSTIC TESTS
None reported.

## CONTRAINDICATIONS
Contraindicated in patients with hypersensitivity to drug. Conditionally contraindicated in patients with active bleeding, blood dyscrasia, or bleeding tendencies, such as hemophilia, thrombocytopenia, or hepatic disease with hypoprothrombinemia; suspected intracranial hemorrhage; suppurative thrombophlebitis; inaccessible ulcerative lesions (especially of GI tract) and open ulcerative

wounds; extensive denudation of skin; ascorbic acid deficiency and other conditions that cause increased capillary permeability. Also conditionally contraindicated during or after brain, eye, or spinal cord surgery; during spinal tap or spinal anesthesia; during continuous tube drainage of stomach or small intestine; in subacute bacterial endocarditis; shock; advanced renal disease; threatened abortion; or severe hypertension.

Although heparin use is clearly hazardous in these conditions, its risks and benefits must be evaluated.

## NURSING CONSIDERATIONS
• Use cautiously during menses and in patients with mild hepatic or renal disease, alcoholism, occupations with high risk of physical injury, or history of allergies, asthma, or GI ulcerations; also use cautiously immediately postpartum.
• Draw blood to establish baseline coagulation parameters before therapy.
• When patient needs anticoagulation during pregnancy, most doctors use heparin.
• Drug requirements are higher in early phases of thrombogenic diseases and febrile states; lower when patient's condition stabilizes.
• Elderly patients should usually start at lower doses.
• Check order and vial carefully; heparin comes in various concentrations.
• Give low-dose injections sequentially between iliac crests in lower abdomen deep into S.C. fat. Inject drug S.C. slowly into fat pad. Leave needle in place for 10 seconds after injection; then withdraw needle. Don't massage after S.C. injection, and watch for signs of bleeding at injection site. Alternate sites every 12 hours—right for morning, left for evening.
• For S.C. injections, PTT should be drawn 4 to 6 hours after dose administered.
• Avoid excessive I.M. injections of other drugs to prevent or minimize hematomas. If possible, don't give I.M. injections at all.
• *Alert:* Heparin and enoxaparin aren't interchangeable.

• Measure PTT carefully and regularly. Anticoagulation is present when PTT values are one and one-half to two times the control values.
• Monitor platelet count regularly. Thrombocytopenia caused by heparin may be associated with a type of arterial thrombosis known as "white clot" syndrome.
• Regularly inspect patient for bleeding gums, bruises on arms or legs, petechiae, nosebleeds, melena, tarry stools, hematuria, and hematemesis.
• Monitor vital signs.
• *Alert:* To treat severe heparin calcium or sodium overdose, use protamine sulfate, a heparin antagonist, as ordered. Dosage is based on the dose of heparin, its route of administration, and the time elapsed since it was given. Generally, 1 to 1.5 mg of protamine/100 U of heparin is given if only a few minutes have elapsed; 0.5 to 0.75 mg protamine/100 U heparin if 30 to 60 minutes have elapsed, 0.25 to 0.375 mg protamine/100 U heparin if 2 hours or more have elapsed. Don't give more than 50 mg protamine in a 10-minute period.
• Abrupt withdrawal may cause increased coagulability; heparin therapy is usually followed by oral anticoagulants for prophylaxis.

## I.V. administration
• Administer I.V. using infusion pump to provide maximum safety because of longterm effect and irregular absorption when given S.C. Check constant I.V. infusions regularly, even when pumps are in good working order, to prevent overdose or underdose. Place notice above patient's bed to inform I.V. team or laboratory personnel to apply pressure dressings after taking blood.
• During intermittent I.V. therapy, always draw blood 30 minutes before next scheduled dose to avoid falsely elevated PTT. Blood for PTT may be drawn any time after 8 hours of initiation of continuous I.V. heparin therapy. Blood for PTT should never be drawn from the I.V. tubing of the heparin infusion or from the infused vein. Falsely elevated PTT will result. Always draw blood from the opposite arm.
• Don't skip a dose or "catch up" with an I.V. containing heparin. If I.V. runs out,

restart it as soon as possible, and reschedule bolus dose immediately.
• Concentrated heparin solutions (over 100 U/ml) can irritate blood vessels.
• Never piggyback other drugs into an infusion line while heparin infusion is running. Never mix another drug and heparin in same syringe when giving a bolus.

✓ **Patient teaching**
• Instruct patient and family to watch for signs of bleeding and notify doctor immediately if any occur.
• Tell patient to avoid OTC drugs containing aspirin, other salicylates, or drugs that may interact with heparin.

## warfarin sodium
Coumadin, Warfilone†

*Pregnancy Risk Category X*

### HOW SUPPLIED
*Tablets:* 1 mg, 2 mg, 2.5 mg, 3 mg, 4 mg, 5 mg, 6 mg, 7.5 mg, 10 mg
*Injection:* 2 mg/ml (powder)

### ACTION
Inhibits vitamin K–dependent activation of clotting factors II, VII, IX, and X, formed in the liver.

| Route | Onset | Peak | Duration |
|-------|-------|------|----------|
| P.O. | 0.5-3 days | Unknown | 2-5 days |
| I.V. | Unknown | Unknown | Unknown |

### INDICATIONS & DOSAGE
*Pulmonary embolism associated with deep vein thrombosis, MI, rheumatic heart disease with heart valve damage, prosthetic heart valves, chronic atrial fibrillation—*
**Adults:** 2 to 5 mg P.O. daily for 2 to 4 days; then dosage based on daily PT and INR. Usual maintenance dose is 2 to 10 mg P.O. daily; I.V. dosage would be same as that used P.O.

### ADVERSE REACTIONS
**GI:** anorexia, nausea, vomiting, cramps, *diarrhea,* mouth ulcerations, sore mouth, melena.

**GU:** hematuria, excessive menstrual bleeding.
**Hematologic:** *hemorrhage;* prolonged PT, INR, and PTT.
**Hepatic:** *hepatitis,* elevated liver function test results, jaundice.
**Skin:** dermatitis, urticaria, necrosis, gangrene, alopecia, *rash.*
**Other:** *fever,* headache; enhanced uric acid excretion.

### INTERACTIONS
**Drug-drug.** *Acetaminophen:* may increase bleeding with long-term therapy (more than 2 weeks) with high doses (more than 2 g/day) of acetaminophen. Monitor very carefully.
*Allopurinol, amiodarone, anabolic steroids, cephalosporins, chloramphenicol, cimetidine, ciprofloxacin, clofibrate, danazol, diazoxide, diflunisal, disulfiram, erythromycin, ethacrynic acid, fenoprofen calcium, fluconazole, fluoroquinolones, glucagon, heparin, ibuprofen, influenza virus vaccine, isoniazid, itraconazole, ketoprofen, lovastatin, meclofenamate, methimazole, methylthiouracil, metronidazole, miconazole, nalidixic acid, neomycin (oral), norfloxacin, ofloxacin, omeprazole, pentoxifylline, propafenone, propoxyphene, propylthiouracil, quinidine, simvastatin, streptokinase, sulfinpyrazone, sulfonamides, sulindac, tamoxifen, tetracyclines, thiazides, thyroid drugs, tricyclic antidepressants, urokinase, vitamin E:* increased PT and INR. Monitor patient carefully for bleeding. Consider anticoagulant dosage reduction.
*Anticonvulsants:* increased serum levels of phenytoin and phenobarbital. Monitor closely.
*Barbiturates, carbamazepine, corticosteroids, corticotropin, dicloxacillin, ethchlorvynol, griseofulvin, haloperidol, meprobamate, mercaptopurine, methaqualone, nafcillin, oral contraceptives containing estrogen, rifampin, spironolactone, sucralfate, trazodone:* decreased PT and INR with reduced anticoagulant effect. Monitor patient carefully.
*Chloral hydrate, glutethimide, propylthiouracil, sulfinpyrazone:* increased or decreased PT. Avoid use, if possible, and monitor patient carefully.

*Cholestyramine:* decreased response when administered too closely together. Administer 6 hours after oral anticoagulants.

*NSAIDs, salicylates:* increased PT and INR; ulcerogenic effects. Don't use together.

*Sulfonylureas (oral antidiabetics):* increased hypoglycemic response. Monitor blood glucose levels.

**Drug-food.** *Foods or enteral products containing vitamin K:* may impair anticoagulation. Patient should maintain consistent daily intake of leafy green vegetables.

**Drug-herb.** *Angelica:* significantly prolonged PT when *Angelica sinensis* is given with warfarin. Avoid concomitant use.

*Motherwort, red clover:* risk of increased bleeding. Avoid concomitant use.

**Drug-lifestyle.** *Alcohol use:* enhanced anticoagulant effects may occur. Tell patient to avoid large amounts of alcohol.

## EFFECTS ON DIAGNOSTIC TESTS

Warfarin can cause false-negative serum theophylline levels.

## CONTRAINDICATIONS

Contraindicated in patients with hypersensitivity to drug and in those with bleeding from the GI, GU, or respiratory tracts; aneurysm; cerebrovascular hemorrhage; severe or malignant hypertension; severe renal or hepatic disease; subacute bacterial endocarditis, pericarditis, or pericardial effusion; or blood dyscrasias or hemorrhagic tendencies. Also contraindicated during pregnancy, threatened abortion, eclampsia, or preeclampsia and after recent surgery involving large open areas, eye, brain, or spinal cord; recent prostatectomy; major regional lumbar block anesthesia, spinal puncture, or diagnostic or therapeutic invasive procedures.

Don't use in patients with a history of warfarin-induced necrosis; in unsupervised patients with senility, alcoholism, or psychosis; or in situations in which there are inadequate laboratory facilities for coagulation testing.

## NURSING CONSIDERATIONS

• Use cautiously in patients with diverticulitis, colitis, mild or moderate hypertension, or mild or moderate hepatic or renal disease; with drainage tubes in any orifice; with regional or lumbar block anesthesia; or in conditions that increase risk of hemorrhage; also use cautiously in breast-feeding women.

• Draw blood to establish baseline coagulation parameters before therapy.

• PT and INR determinations are essential for proper control. Doctors typically try to maintain PT at one and one-half times to twice normal. There is a high risk of bleeding when PT exceeds two and one-half times the control values.

• Give warfarin at same time daily. INR range for chronic atrial fibrillation is 2 to 3.

• I.M. administration isn't recommended.

• Regularly inspect patient for bleeding gums, bruises on arms or legs, petechiae, nosebleeds, melena, tarry stools, hematuria, and hematemesis.

• Observe breast-fed infants of women on drug for unexpected bleeding.

• *Alert:* Withhold drug and call doctor at once if fever or rash (signs of severe adverse reactions) occurs.

• Half-life of warfarin's anticoagulant effect is 36 to 44 hours. Effect can be neutralized by vitamin K injections.

• Drug is best oral anticoagulant for patient taking antacids or phenytoin.

• Elderly patients and patients with renal or hepatic failure are especially sensitive to warfarin effect.

## I.V. administration

• I.V. form may be ordered in rare instances when oral therapy can't be given. Reconstitute powder with 2.7 ml sterile water, or as instructed in manufacturer guidelines. Give I.V. as a slow bolus injection over 1 to 2 minutes into a peripheral vein.

• Because onset of action is delayed, heparin sodium is often given during first few days of treatment. When heparin is being given simultaneously, blood for PT and INR shouldn't be drawn within 5 hours of intermittent I.V. heparin administration. However, blood for PT and INR may be drawn at any time during continuous heparin infusion.

---

### ✓ Patient teaching
- Stress importance of complying with prescribed dosage and follow-up appointments. Tell patient to carry a card that identifies him as a potential bleeder.
- Tell patient and family to watch for signs of bleeding and to call doctor at once if they occur.
- Warn patient to avoid OTC products containing aspirin, other salicylates, or drugs that may interact with warfarin.
- Instruct woman to notify doctor if menses is heavier than usual; may need dosage adjustment.
- Tell patient to use electric razor when shaving to avoid scratching skin, and to use a soft toothbrush.
- Warn patient to read food labels. Food and enteral feedings that contain vitamin K may impair anticoagulation.
- Tell patient to eat a daily, consistent amount of leafy green vegetables, which contain vitamin K. Eating different amounts daily may alter anticoagulant effects.

**albumin 5%**
**albumin 25%**
**antihemophilic factor**
**anti-inhibitor coagulant complex**
**antithrombin III, human**
**factor IX (human)**
**factor IX complex**
**plasma protein fractions**

### COMBINATION PRODUCTS
None.

---

**albumin 5%**
Albuminar-5, Albutein 5%,
Buminate 5%, Plasbumin-5

**albumin 25%**
Albuminar-25, Albutein 25%,
Buminate 25%, Plasbumin-25

*Pregnancy Risk Category C*

### HOW SUPPLIED
**albumin 5%**
*Injection:* 50-ml, 250-ml, 500-ml,
1,000-ml vials
**albumin 25%**
*Injection:* 20-ml, 50-ml, 100-ml vials

### ACTION
Albumin 5% supplies colloid to the blood
and expands plasma volume. Albumin
25% provides intravascular oncotic pressure in a 5:1 ratio, causing a fluid shift
from interstitial spaces to the circulation
and slightly increasing plasma protein
level.

| Route | Onset | Peak | Duration |
|-------|-------|------|----------|
| I.V. | < 15 min | < 15 min | Several hr |

### INDICATIONS & DOSAGE
*Hypovolemic shock—*
**Adults:** initially, 500 to 750 ml 5% solution by I.V. infusion, repeated q 30 min-
utes, p.r.n. Or, 100 to 200 ml I.V. of 25%
solution, repeated after 10 to 30 minutes,
if needed. Dosage varies with patient's
condition and response.
**Children:** 12 to 20 ml 5% solution/kg by
I.V. infusion, repeated in 15 to 30 minutes
if response is inadequate. Or, 2.5 to 5 ml
I.V. of 25% solution/kg, repeated after 10
to 30 minutes, if needed.
*Hypoproteinemia—*
**Adults:** 200 to 300 ml of 25% albumin.
Dosage varies with patient's condition and
response.
*Hyperbilirubinemia—*
**Infants:** 1 g albumin (4 ml 25%)/kg during or 1 to 2 hours before exchange trans-
fusion.

### ADVERSE REACTIONS
**CNS:** headache.
**CV:** *vascular overload after rapid infu-
sion,* hypotension, tachycardia.
**GI:** increased salivation, nausea, vomit-
ing.
**Musculoskeletal:** back pain.
**Respiratory:** altered respiration, dysp-
nea, *pulmonary edema.*
**Skin:** urticaria, rash.
**Other:** chills, fever, increased plasma al-
bumin levels.

### INTERACTIONS
None significant.

### EFFECTS ON DIAGNOSTIC TESTS
Preparations of albumin derived from placental tissue may increase serum alkaline
phosphatase level.

### CONTRAINDICATIONS
Contraindicated in patients with hypersensitivity to drug and in those with severe anemia or cardiac failure.

### NURSING CONSIDERATIONS
• Use with extreme caution in patients
with hypertension, low cardiac reserve,
hypervolemia, pulmonary edema, or hypoalbuminemia with peripheral edema.
• Watch for hemorrhage or shock after
surgery or injury. Rapid rise in blood

---

pressure may cause bleeding from sites that aren't apparent at lower pressures.
• Monitor vital signs carefully.
• Watch for signs of vascular overload (heart failure or pulmonary edema).
• Monitor fluid intake and output; hemoglobin, serum protein, and electrolyte levels; and hematocrit during therapy.
• Follow storage instructions on bottle. Freezing may cause bottle to break.

### I.V. administration
• Make sure patient is properly hydrated before infusion.
• To minimize waste, take care when preparing and administering drug. This product is expensive, and random supply shortages frequently occur.
• Avoid rapid I.V. infusion. Specific rate is individualized based on patient's age, condition, and diagnosis. Albumin 5% is infused undiluted; albumin 25% may be infused undiluted or diluted with normal saline solution or $D_5W$ injection. Use solution promptly. Discard unused solution. Don't use cloudy solutions or those containing sediment. Solution should be a clear amber color.
• *Alert:* Don't give more than 250 g in 48 hours.

### Patient teaching
• Explain use and administration of albumin to patient and family.
• Tell patient to report adverse reactions promptly.

---

## antihemophilic factor (AHF)
Alphanate, Helixate, Hemofil M, Humate-P, Koate-HP, Kogenate, Monoclate-P, Recombinate

*Pregnancy Risk Category C*

### HOW SUPPLIED
*Injection:* vials, with diluent. Units specified on label

### ACTION
Directly replaces deficient clotting factor.

| Route | Onset | Peak | Duration |
|-------|-------|------|----------|
| I.V. | Immediate | 1-2 hr | Unknown |

### INDICATIONS & DOSAGE
*Spontaneous hemorrhage in patients with hemophilia A (factor VIII deficiency)—*
**Adults and children:** calculate dosage using this formula:

$$\text{AHF required (IU)} = \text{body weight (kg)} \times \text{desired factor VIII increase (\% of normal)} \times 0.5$$

To prevent spontaneous hemorrhage, the desired level of factor VIII is 5% of normal; for mild hemorrhage, 30% of normal; for moderate hemorrhage and minor surgery, 30% to 50% of normal; for severe hemorrhage, 80% to 100% of normal.
*Bleeding in patients with hemophilia A (factor VIII deficiency)—*
**Adults and children:** for minor hemorrhage into muscle and joints, 8 to 10 IU/kg I.V. (or calculated dose to raise plasma factor VIII levels to 20% to 40% of normal) q 8 to 12 hours for 1 to 3 days, as needed. For overt bleeding, initial dose of 15 to 25 IU/kg I.V.; then 8 to 15 IU/kg q 8 to 12 hours for 3 to 4 days. To treat massive bleeding or hemorrhage involving major organs, initial dose of 40 to 50 IU/kg I.V.; then 20 to 25 IU/kg I.V. q 8 to 12 hours.
*Prevention of bleeding in hemophilic patients requiring surgery—*
**Adults:** 25 to 30 IU/kg I.V. 1 hour before surgery; then 50% of initial dose 5 hours later. Dosage titrated to achieve a level of AHF 80% to 100% of normal during surgery and maintained at 30% to 60% of normal for at least 10 to 14 days postoperatively.

### ADVERSE REACTIONS
**CV:** tightness in chest, *thrombosis.*
**GI:** nausea.
**Hematologic:** *hemolytic anemia, thrombocytopenia.*
**Respiratory:** wheezing.
**Skin:** *urticaria,* stinging at injection site.
**Other:** *chills, fever, hypersensitivity reactions, anaphylaxis, risk of hepatitis B and HIV.*

### INTERACTIONS
None significant.

---

*Liquid contains alcohol.   **May contain tartrazine.   †Canada   ‡Australia   §U.K.   ◊OTC

**EFFECTS ON DIAGNOSTIC TESTS**
None reported.

**CONTRAINDICATIONS**
Monoclonal prepared AHF is contraindicated in patients with hypersensitivity to drug or murine (mouse) protein.

**NURSING CONSIDERATIONS**
• Use cautiously in neonates, infants, and patients with hepatic disease because of their susceptibility to hepatitis, which may be transmitted in antihemophilic factor.
• Monitor coagulation studies before therapy.
• Monitor patients with blood types A, B, and AB for possible hemolysis.
• Change in urine color to an orange or red hue can signify a hemolytic reaction.
• Administer hepatitis B vaccine before administering antihemophilic factor, as ordered.
• Don't give drug S.C. or I.M.
• Monitor vital signs regularly.
• Monitor coagulation studies frequently during therapy.
• Monitor patient for allergic reactions.
• Some patients develop inhibitors to factor VIII, resulting in decreased response to drug.
• Risk of hepatitis must be weighed against risk of patient not receiving drug.
• Because of manufacturing process, risk of HIV transmission is extremely low.

**◖ I.V. administration**
• Refrigerate concentrate until ready to use. Warm concentrate and diluent bottles to room temperature before reconstituting. To mix drug, gently roll vial between hands.
• Use reconstituted solution within 3 hours. Store away from heat and don't refrigerate. Refrigeration after reconstitution may cause active ingredient to precipitate. Don't shake or mix with other I.V. solutions. Solution should be filtered before administration.
• Take baseline pulse rate before I.V. administration. Use plastic syringe; drug may interact with glass syringe and bind to its surface. If pulse rate increases significantly, flow rate should be reduced or administration stopped.

**☑ Patient teaching**
• Explain use and administration of AHF to patient and family.
• Advise patient to report adverse reactions promptly.
• Advise patient to wear medical identification tag.
• Tell patient to notify doctor if drug seems less effective; a change may signify the development of antibodies.

## anti-inhibitor coagulant complex
Autoplex T, Feiba VH Immuno

*Pregnancy Risk Category C*

**HOW SUPPLIED**
*Injection:* number of units of factor VIII correctional activity indicated on label of vial

**ACTION**
Unknown. Efficacy may be related in part to presence of activated factors, which leads to more complete factor X activation with tissue factor, phospholipid, and ionic calcium and allows the coagulation process to proceed beyond those stages in which factor VIII is needed.

| Route | Onset | Peak | Duration |
|-------|-------|------|----------|
| I.V. | 10-30 min | Unknown | Unknown |

**INDICATIONS & DOSAGE**
*Prevention and control of hemorrhagic episodes in patients with hemophilia A who have developed inhibitor antibodies to antihemophilic factor; management of bleeding in patients with acquired hemophilia who have spontaneously acquired inhibitors to factor VIII—*
**Adults and children:** highly individualized and varies among manufacturers. For Autoplex T, 25 to 100 U/kg I.V., depending on severity of hemorrhage. If no hemostatic improvement occurs within 6 hours after initial administration, dosage repeated. For Feiba VH Immuno, 50 to 100 U/kg I.V. q 6 or 12 hours until clear signs of improvement. Maximum daily dose is 200 U/kg.

Reactions may be *common,* uncommon, *life-threatening*, or COMMON AND LIFE-THREATENING.

**ADVERSE REACTIONS**
**CNS:** headache, lethargy.
**CV:** changes in blood pressure, flushing, *acute MI, thromboembolic events.*
**GI:** nausea, vomiting.
**Hematologic:** *DIC.*
**Skin:** rash, urticaria.
**Other:** fever, chills, *hypersensitivity reactions, anaphylaxis, risk of hepatitis B and HIV.*

**INTERACTIONS**
**Drug-drug.** *Antifibrinolytic drugs:* may alter effects of anti-inhibitor coagulant complex. Don't use together.

**EFFECTS ON DIAGNOSTIC TESTS**
None reported.

**CONTRAINDICATIONS**
Contraindicated in patients with DIC or a normal coagulation mechanism and in those showing signs of fibrinolysis.

**NURSING CONSIDERATIONS**
• Use with caution in patients with liver disease.
• Administer hepatitis B vaccine before giving drug, as ordered.
• Keep epinephrine available to treat anaphylaxis.
• Feiba VH Immuno shouldn't be used with newborns, but Autoplex T can be used with caution.
• Monitor patient closely for hypersensitivity reactions.
• Monitor vital signs regularly, and report significant changes to doctor.
• Reassure patient that, because of manufacturing process, risk of HIV transmission is extremely low.

**I.V. administration**
• Warm drug and diluent to room temperature before reconstitution. Reconstitute according to manufacturer's directions. Use filter needle provided by manufacturer to withdraw reconstituted solution from vial into syringe; filter needle should then be replaced with a sterile injection needle for administration. Administer as soon as possible. If drug is given as an I.V. infusion, administration set must contain a filter. Autoplex T infusions should be com-

pleted within 1 hour after reconstitution; Feiba VH Immuno infusions, within 3 hours.
• Individualize rate of administration based on patient's response. Autoplex T infusions may begin at rate of 2 ml/minute; if well tolerated, infusion rate may be increased gradually to 10 ml/minute. Feiba VH Immuno infusion rate shouldn't exceed 2 U/kg/minute.
• *Alert:* If flushing, lethargy, headache, transient chest discomfort, or changes in blood pressure or pulse rate develop because of a rapid rate of infusion, stop drug and notify doctor. These symptoms usually disappear with cessation of infusion. The infusion may then be resumed at a slower rate, as ordered.

**☑ Patient teaching**
• Explain use and administration of anti-inhibitor coagulant complex to patient and family.
• Tell patient to report adverse reactions promptly.

---

**antithrombin III, human (AT-III, heparin cofactor I)**
ATnativ, Thrombate III

*Pregnancy Risk Category C*

**HOW SUPPLIED**
*Injection:* 500 IU

**ACTION**
Replaces deficient AT-III in patients with hereditary AT-III deficiency, normalizing coagulation inhibition and inhibiting thromboembolism formation. Also deactivates plasmin (to lesser extent than clotting factor).

| Route | Onset | Peak | Duration |
|-------|-------|------|----------|
| I.V. | Immediate | Unknown | 4 days |

**INDICATIONS & DOSAGE**
*Thromboembolism associated with hereditary AT-III deficiency—*
**Adults and children:** initial dose is individualized to quantity needed to increase AT-III activity to 120% of normal activity as determined 30 minutes after adminis-

tration. Usual dose is 50 to 100 IU/minute I.V., not to exceed 100 IU/minute. Dose is calculated based on anticipated 1% increase in plasma AT-III activity produced by 1 IU/kg of body weight using the formula:

$$\text{Dose required (IU)} = \frac{(\text{desired activity [\%]} - \text{baseline activity [\%]}) \times \text{weight (kg)}}{1.4}$$

Maintenance dose is individualized to quantity needed to increase AT-III activity to 80% of normal activity and is administered at 24-hour intervals.

To calculate subsequent dosages, multiply desired AT-III activity (as percentage of normal) minus baseline AT-III activity (as percentage of normal) by body weight (in kg). Divide by actual increase in AT-III activity (as percentage) produced by 1 IU/kg as determined 30 minutes after initial dose is given.

Treatment is usually continued for 2 to 8 days but may be prolonged in pregnancy or when used with surgery or immobilization.

### ADVERSE REACTIONS
**CNS:** dizziness.
**CV:** vasodilation, lowered blood pressure.
**GI:** nausea, foul taste.
**GU:** diuresis.
**Other:** chills.

### INTERACTIONS
**Drug-drug.** *Heparin:* increased anticoagulant effect of both drugs. Heparin dosage reduction may be needed.

### EFFECTS ON DIAGNOSTIC TESTS
Plasma levels of AT-III may be measured with clotting assays or amidolytic assays using synthetic chromogenic substrates. Immunoassays may not detect all congenital AT-III deficiencies.

### CONTRAINDICATIONS
No known contraindications.

### NURSING CONSIDERATIONS
• Use with extreme caution in children and neonates because safety and efficacy haven't been established.

• Use cautiously. Prepared from pooled plasma from human donors, drug carries minimal risk of transmission of viruses, including hepatitis and HIV.
• *Alert:* Because of risk of neonatal thromboembolism (sometimes fatal) in children of parents with hereditary AT-III deficiency, anticipate obtaining AT-III levels immediately after birth.
• Bring solution to room temperature before administration. Use solution within 3 hours of preparation.
• Obtain AT-III activity levels b.i.d. until dosage requirement has stabilized, then daily immediately before dose. Functional assays are preferred because quantitative immunologic test results may be normal despite decreased AT-III activity.
• Watch for dyspnea and increased blood pressure, which may occur if administration rate is too rapid.
• 1 IU is equivalent to quantity of endogenous AT-III present in 1 ml of normal human plasma.
• Heparin binds to AT-III lysine-binding sites, increasing heparin efficacy.
• Drug isn't recommended for long-term prophylaxis of thrombotic episodes.
• Store drug at 36° to 46° F (2° to 8° C).

### I.V. administration
• Reconstitute using 10 ml of sterile water (provided), normal saline solution, or $D_5W$. Don't shake vial. Dilute further in same diluent solution if desired.

### Patient teaching
• Explain use and administration of AT-III to patient and parents.
• Instruct patient to report adverse reactions promptly.

## factor IX (human)
AlphaNine SD, Mononine

## factor IX complex
Konyne 80, Profilnine SD, Proplex T

*Pregnancy Risk Category C*

### HOW SUPPLIED
*Injection:* vials, with diluent. Units specified on label

---

## ACTION
Directly replaces deficient clotting factor.

| Route | Onset | Peak | Duration |
|-------|-------|------|----------|
| I.V. | Immediate | 10-30 min | Unknown |

## INDICATIONS & DOSAGE
*Factor IX deficiency (hemophilia B or Christmas disease), anticoagulant over-dosage—*
**Adults and children:** to calculate approximate units of factor IX needed, use the following equation:
Human product: 1 U/kg × body weight in kilograms × percentage of desired increase of factor IX level; Recombinant product: 1.2 U/kg × body weight in kilograms × percentage of desired increase of factor IX level; Proplex T: 0.5 U/kg × body weight in kilograms × percentage of desired increase of factor IX level. Infusion rates vary with product and patient comfort. Dosage is highly individualized, depending on degree of deficiency, level of factor IX desired, patient weight, and severity of bleeding.

## ADVERSE REACTIONS
**CNS:** headache.
**CV:** *thromboembolic reactions, MI, DIC, pulmonary embolism,* changes in blood pressure, *flushing.*
**GI:** nausea, vomiting.
**Skin:** urticaria.
**Other:** *transient fever, chills, tingling.*

## INTERACTIONS
**Drug-drug.** *Aminocaproic acid:* increased risk of thrombosis. Avoid concomitant use.

## EFFECTS ON DIAGNOSTIC TESTS
None reported.

## CONTRAINDICATIONS
Contraindicated in patients with hepatic disease in whom intravascular coagulation or fibrinolysis is suspected. Mononine is contraindicated in patients with hypersensitivity to murine (mouse) protein.

## NURSING CONSIDERATIONS
• Use cautiously in neonates and infants because of susceptibility to hepatitis, which may be transmitted with factor IX complex.
• Administer hepatitis B vaccine before giving factor IX complex, as ordered.
• Observe patient for allergic reactions, and monitor vital signs regularly.
• Risk of hepatitis must be weighed against risk of not receiving drug.
• Risk of HIV transmission is extremely low because of manufacturing process.

### 🖐 I.V. administration
• Avoid rapid infusion. If tingling sensation, fever, chills, or headache develops, decrease flow rate and notify doctor.
• Reconstitute with 20 ml of sterile water for injection for each vial of lyophilized drug. Keep refrigerated until ready to use; warm to room temperature before reconstituting. Use within 3 hours. Unstable in solution. Don't shake, refrigerate, or mix with other I.V. solutions. Store away from heat.

### ✓ Patient teaching
• Explain use and administration of factor IX to patient and family.
• Tell patient to report adverse reactions promptly and to discontinue drug if they occur.
• Advise patient to report chest tightness, wheezing, or hypotension.

## plasma protein fractions
Plasmanate, Plasma-Plex, Plasmatein, Protenate

*Pregnancy Risk Category C*

## HOW SUPPLIED
*Injection:* 5% solution in 50-ml, 250-ml, 500-ml vials

## ACTION
Supplies colloid to the blood and expands plasma volume.

| Route | Onset | Peak | Duration |
|-------|-------|------|----------|
| I.V. | Immediate | Immediate | Unknown |

---

*Liquid contains alcohol.     **May contain tartrazine.     †Canada     ‡Australia     §U.K.     ◇OTC

## INDICATIONS & DOSAGE
*Shock—*
**Adults:** varies with patient's condition and response, but usual dose is 250 to 500 ml I.V. (12.5 to 25 g protein), usually no faster than 10 ml/minute.
**Children:** 6.6 to 33 ml/kg (0.33 to 1.65 g/kg of protein) I.V., 5 to 10 ml/minute.
*Hypoproteinemia—*
**Adults:** 1,000 to 1,500 ml I.V. daily. Maximum infusion rate is 8 ml/minute.

## ADVERSE REACTIONS
**CNS:** headache.
**CV:** hypotension, *vascular overload,* tachycardia, flushing.
**GI:** nausea, vomiting, hypersalivation.
**Musculoskeletal:** back pain.
**Respiratory:** dyspnea, *pulmonary edema.*
**Skin:** rash.
**Other:** chills, fever.

## INTERACTIONS
None significant.

## EFFECTS ON DIAGNOSTIC TESTS
None reported.

## CONTRAINDICATIONS
Contraindicated in patients with severe anemia or heart failure and in those undergoing cardiac bypass.

## NURSING CONSIDERATIONS
• Use cautiously in patients with hepatic or renal failure, low cardiac reserve, or restricted sodium intake.
• Hypotension risk is greater when infusion rates exceed 10 ml/minute.
• Monitor blood pressure. Be prepared to slow or stop infusion if hypotension suddenly occurs. Vital signs should return to normal gradually; monitor hourly.
• Watch for signs of vascular overload (heart failure or pulmonary edema).
• Watch for hemorrhage or shock after surgery or injury. A rapid rise in blood pressure may cause bleeding from sites that isn't apparent at lower pressures.
• Report decreased urine output.
• Drug contains 130 to 160 mEq sodium/L.

### I.V. administration
• Check expiration date before using. Don't use solutions that are cloudy, contain sediment, or have been frozen. Discard solutions in containers that have been open for more than 4 hours because solution contains no preservatives.
• Don't infuse solutions containing amino acids or alcohol through same I.V. line; proteins may precipitate.
• If patient is dehydrated, give additional fluids either P.O. or I.V., as ordered.
• Don't give more than 250 g or 5,000 ml in 48 hours.

### Patient teaching
• Explain use and administration of drug to patient and family.
• Tell patient to report adverse reactions promptly.

---

Reactions may be *common*, uncommon, *life-threatening*, or COMMON AND LIFE-THREATENING.

alteplase
anistreplase
reteplase, recombinant
streptokinase
urokinase

## COMBINATION PRODUCTS
None.

---

### alteplase (tissue plasminogen activator, recombinant; t-PA)
Actilyse‡, Activase

*Pregnancy Risk Category C*

---

## HOW SUPPLIED
*Injection:* 20-mg (11.6 million–IU), 50-mg (29 million–IU), 100 mg (58 million–IU) vials

## ACTION
Binds to fibrin in a thrombus, and locally converts plasminogen to plasmin, which initiates local fibrinolysis.

| Route | Onset | Peak | Duration |
|-------|-------|------|----------|
| I.V. | Immediate | 45 min | 4 hr |

## INDICATIONS & DOSAGE
*Lysis of thrombi obstructing coronary arteries in acute MI—*
**Adults:** 100 mg I.V. infusion over 3 hours as follows: 60 mg in first hour, of which 6 to 10 mg is given as a bolus over first 1 to 2 minutes. Then 20 mg/hour infusion for 2 hours. Smaller adults (under 65 kg [143 lb]) should receive 1.25 mg/kg in a similar fashion (60% in first hour, 10% as a bolus; then 20% of total dose per hour for 2 hours).
*Management of acute massive pulmonary embolism—*
**Adults:** 100 mg I.V. infusion over 2 hours. Heparin begun at end of infusion when PTT or thrombin time returns to twice normal or less. Don't exceed 100-mg dose. Higher doses may increase risk of intracranial bleeding.

*Acute ischemic stroke—*
**Adults:** 0.9 mg/kg I.V. infusion over 1 hour with 10% of total dose administered as an initial I.V. bolus over 1 minute. Maximum total dose is 90 mg.
   *Note:* Administer within 3 hours after symptoms occur and only when intracranial bleeding has been ruled out.

## ADVERSE REACTIONS
**CNS:** *cerebral hemorrhage,* fever.
**CV:** hypotension, *arrhythmias,* edema.
**GI:** nausea, vomiting.
**Hematologic:** *severe, spontaneous bleeding.*
**Other:** bleeding at puncture sites, *cholesterol embolization, hypersensitivity reactions, anaphylaxis.*

## INTERACTIONS
**Drug-drug.** *Aspirin, coumadin anticoagulants, dipyridamole, heparin:* increased risk of bleeding. Monitor patient carefully.

## EFFECTS ON DIAGNOSTIC TESTS
Altered results may be expected in coagulation and fibrinolytic tests. Use of aprotinin (150 to 200 U/ml) in blood sample may attenuate this interference.

## CONTRAINDICATIONS
Contraindicated in patients with active internal bleeding; intracranial neoplasm; arteriovenous malformation; aneurysm; severe uncontrolled hypertension; or history or current evidence of intracranial hemorrhage, suspicion of subarachnoid hemorrhage, or seizure at onset of stroke when used for acute ischemic stroke. Also contraindicated in patients with history of CVA, intraspinal or intracranial trauma or surgery within 2 months, or known bleeding diathesis.

## NURSING CONSIDERATIONS
• Use cautiously in patients with major surgery within 10 days (when bleeding is difficult to control because of its location); organ biopsy; trauma (including

---

cardiopulmonary resuscitation); GI or GU bleeding; cerebrovascular disease; systolic pressure of 180 mm Hg or higher or diastolic pressure of 110 mm Hg or higher; mitral stenosis, atrial fibrillation or other conditions that may lead to left heart thrombus; acute pericarditis or subacute bacterial endocarditis; hemostatic defects due to hepatic or renal impairment; septic thrombophlebitis; or diabetic hemorrhagic retinopathy. Also use cautiously in patients receiving anticoagulants, in patients ages 75 and older, and during pregnancy and first 10 days postpartum

• Drug may be given to menstruating women.

• Recanalization of occluded coronary arteries and improvement of heart function need initiation of treatment with alteplase as soon as possible after onset of symptoms.

• Anticoagulant and antiplatelet therapy is frequently initiated during or after treatment to decrease risk of rethrombosis.

• Monitor vital signs and neurologic status carefully. Keep patient on strict bed rest.

• Have antiarrhythmics readily available, and carefully monitor ECG. Coronary thrombolysis is associated with arrhythmias induced by reperfusion of ischemic myocardium. Such arrhythmias don't differ from those commonly associated with MI.

• Avoid invasive procedures during thrombolytic therapy. Carefully monitor patient for signs of internal bleeding, and frequently check all puncture sites. Bleeding is the most common adverse effect and may occur internally and at external puncture sites.

• If uncontrollable bleeding occurs, stop infusion (and concomitant heparin) and notify doctor.

**◖ I.V. administration**

• Administer alteplase I.V. only, using a controlled infusion device.

• Reconstitute drug with sterile water for injection (without preservatives) only. (Check manufacturer's labeling for specific information.) Don't use vial if vacuum isn't present in 50-mg vials; 100-mg vials don't have a vacuum. Reconstitute with

large-bore (18G) needle, directing stream of sterile water at lyophilized cake. Don't shake. Slight foaming is common (allow foaming to settle before use), and solution should be clear or pale yellow.

• Drug may be given as reconstituted (1 mg/ml) or diluted with an equal volume of normal saline solution or $D_5W$ to make a 0.5 mg/ml solution. Adding other drugs to the infusion isn't recommended.

• Reconstitute solution immediately before use, and administer within 8 hours.

**☑ Patient teaching**

• Explain use and administration of drug to patient and family.

• Tell patient to report adverse reactions promptly.

## anistreplase (anisoylated plasminogen-streptokinase activator complex; APSAC)
Eminase

*Pregnancy Risk Category C*

**HOW SUPPLIED**
*Injection:* 30 U-vial

**ACTION**
Anistreplase, derived from Lys-plasminogen and streptokinase, is formulated into a fibrinolytic enzyme plus activator complex with the activator temporarily blocked by an anisoyl group. Is activated in vivo by a nonenzymatic process that removes the anisoyl group. Active drug converts plasminogen to plasmin, resulting in thrombolysis.

| Route | Onset | Peak | Duration |
|-------|-------|------|----------|
| I.V. | Immediate | 45 min | 6 hr-2 days |

**INDICATIONS & DOSAGE**
*Lysis of coronary artery thrombi following acute MI—*
**Adults:** 30 U I.V. over 2 to 5 minutes by direct injection.

**ADVERSE REACTIONS**
**CNS:** *intracranial hemorrhage.*
**CV:** ARRHYTHMIAS, *conduction disorders, hypotension,* flushing.

---

**EENT:** hemoptysis, gum or mouth hemorrhage.
**GI:** *hemorrhage.*
**GU:** hematuria.
**Hematologic:** *bleeding tendency,* eosinophilia.
**Musculoskeletal:** arthralgia.
**Skin:** hematoma, urticaria, pruritus, delayed purpuric rash.
**Other:** bleeding at puncture sites.

## INTERACTIONS
**Drug-drug.** *Drugs that alter platelet function (including aspirin, dipyridamole), heparin, oral anticoagulants:* may increase risk of bleeding. Use together cautiously.

## EFFECTS ON DIAGNOSTIC TESTS
Drug prolongs activated PTT, PT, and thrombin time; it remains active in vivo and can cause degeneration of fibrinogen in blood samples drawn for analysis. Decreases in alpha$_2$-antiplasmin, factor V, factor VIII, fibrinogen, and plasminogen activities have been reported as well as moderate reductions in hemoglobin level and hematocrit. Levels of fibrinogen- and fibrin-degeneration products are increased.

## CONTRAINDICATIONS
Contraindicated in patients with history of severe allergic reaction to anistreplase or streptokinase; active internal bleeding, CVA, recent (within past 2 months) intraspinal or intracranial surgery or trauma, aneurysm, arteriovenous malformation, intracranial neoplasm, uncontrolled hypertension, or known bleeding diathesis.

## NURSING CONSIDERATIONS
• Use cautiously in patients with recent (within 10 days) major surgery (when bleeding is difficult to control because of its location); trauma (including cardiopulmonary resuscitation); GI or GU bleeding; cerebrovascular disease; hypertension (systolic pressure of 180 mm Hg or higher or diastolic pressure of 110 mm Hg or higher); mitral stenosis, atrial fibrillation, or other conditions that may lead to left heart thrombus; acute pericarditis or subacute bacterial endocarditis; hemostatic defects due to hepatic or renal impairment; septic thrombophlebitis; diabetic hemorrhagic retinopathy; also contraindicated during pregnancy and first 10 days postpartum; in patients receiving anticoagulants; and in those ages 75 and older.
• Drug may be given to menstruating women.
• Carefully monitor ECG during treatment. Be prepared to treat bradycardia or ventricular irritability. Thrombolytic therapy is associated with reperfusion arrhythmias that may signify successful thrombolysis. These arrhythmias are similar to those seen in the course of an acute MI and may include sinus bradycardia, accelerated idioventricular rhythm, ventricular tachycardia, or premature ventricular depolarizations.
• Carefully monitor patient; avoid I.M. injections and nonessential handling or moving of patient. Bleeding is the most common adverse reaction and may occur internally and at external puncture sites.
• Anticoagulant or antiplatelet therapy may be used with drug treatment to decrease risk of rethrombosis.
• Anistreplase is derived from human plasma. No cases of hepatitis or HIV infection have been reported to date. The manufacturing process is designed to purify the plasma used in preparation of drug.
• *Alert:* Drug efficacy may be limited if antistreptokinase antibodies are present. Antibody levels may be elevated if more than 5 days have elapsed since previous treatment with anistreplase or streptokinase, or if patient has had a recent streptococcal infection.
• In vitro coagulation tests will be affected by presence of anistreplase. This can be attenuated if blood samples are collected in presence of aprotinin (150 to 200 U/ml).
• *Alert:* Don't confuse anistreplase with alteplase.

### ◖ I.V. administration
• Unlike other thrombolytics that must be infused, administer drug by direct injection into an I.V. line over 2 to 5 minutes.
• Reconstitute drug by slowly adding 5 ml of sterile water for injection. Direct

stream against side of vial, not at drug itself. Gently roll vial to mix dry powder and water. To avoid excessive foaming, don't shake vial. Reconstituted solution should be colorless to pale yellow. Inspect for precipitate. If drug isn't administered within 30 minutes of reconstituting, discard vial.

• Don't mix with other drugs; don't dilute solution after reconstitution.

☑ **Patient teaching**
• Explain use and administration of drug to patient and family.
• Tell patient to report adverse reactions promptly.

---

**reteplase, recombinant**
Rapilysin§, Retavase

*Pregnancy Risk Category C*

## HOW SUPPLIED
*Injection:* 10.8 U (18.8 mg)/vial. Supplied in a kit with components for reconstitution for two single-use vials.

## ACTION
Enhances cleavage of plasminogen to generate plasmin, which leads to fibrinolysis.

| Route | Onset | Peak | Duration |
|-------|-------|------|----------|
| I.V. | Unknown | Unknown | Unknown |

## INDICATIONS & DOSAGE
*Management of acute MI—*
**Adults:** double-bolus injection of 10 + 10 U. Give each bolus I.V. over 2 minutes. If complications, such as serious bleeding or an anaphylactoid reaction, don't occur after first bolus, give second bolus 30 minutes after start of first bolus.

## ADVERSE REACTIONS
**CNS:** *intracranial hemorrhage.*
**CV:** *arrhythmias, cholesterol embolization, hemorrhage.*
**GI:** *hemorrhage.*
**GU:** hematuria.
**Hematologic:** *bleeding tendency,* anemia.
**Other:** bleeding at puncture sites.

## INTERACTIONS
**Drug-drug.** *Heparin, oral anticoagulants, platelet inhibitors (abciximab, aspirin, dipyridamole):* may increase risk of bleeding. Use together cautiously.

## EFFECTS ON DIAGNOSTIC TESTS
Reteplase may alter coagulation studies; drug remains active in vitro and can lead to degradation of fibrinogen in sample. Collect blood samples in the presence of PPACK (chloromethylketone) at 2-micromolar concentrations.

## CONTRAINDICATIONS
Contraindicated in patients with active internal bleeding, known bleeding diathesis, history of CVA, recent intracranial or intraspinal surgery or trauma, severe uncontrolled hypertension, intracranial neoplasm, arteriovenous malformation, or aneurysm.

## NURSING CONSIDERATIONS
• Use cautiously in patients with recent (within 10 days) major surgery, obstetric delivery, organ biopsy, GI or GU bleeding, or trauma; previous puncture of noncompressible vessels; cerebrovascular disease; hypertension (systolic pressure of 180 mm Hg or more or diastolic pressure of 110 mm Hg or more); conditions that may lead to left heart thrombus, including mitral stenosis; acute pericarditis or subacute bacterial endocarditis; hemostatic defects; diabetic hemorrhagic retinopathy; septic thrombophlebitis; other conditions in which bleeding would be difficult to manage; also use cautiously in patients ages 75 and older and in breast-feeding women.
• Drug may be given to menstruating women.
• Carefully monitor ECG during treatment. Coronary thrombolysis may result in arrhythmias associated with reperfusion. Be prepared to treat bradycardia or ventricular irritability.
• Carefully monitor patient for bleeding. Avoid I.M. injections, invasive procedures, and nonessential handling of patient. Bleeding is the most common adverse reaction and may occur internally or at external puncture sites. Should local

---

Reactions may be *common,* uncommon, *life-threatening,* or COMMON AND LIFE-THREATENING.

measures not control serious bleeding, discontinue concomitant anticoagulation therapy and notify doctor. Withhold second bolus of reteplase.

• Drug should be used in pregnancy only if benefit justifies potential risk to fetus.

• Safety and efficacy of drug in children haven't been established.

• Potency is expressed in terms of units specific for reteplase and not comparable to other thrombolytic drugs.

• Avoid use of noncompressible pressure sites during therapy. If an arterial puncture is needed, use an upper extremity vessel that can be compressed manually. Apply pressure for at least 30 minutes; then apply a pressure dressing. Check site frequently.

### ⬭ I.V. administration

• Drug is administered I.V. as a double-bolus injection. If bleeding or anaphylactoid reactions occur after first bolus, notify doctor; second bolus may be withheld.

• Reconstitute drug according to manufacturer's instructions using items provided in kit. Reconstitute with sterile water for injection, USP (without preservatives). Reconstituted solution should be colorless; resulting concentration will be 1 U/ml. If foaming occurs, allow vial to stand for several minutes. Inspect for precipitation. Use within 4 hours of reconstitution; discard unused portions.

• Don't administer with other I.V. drugs through same I.V. line. Note that heparin and reteplase are incompatible in solution.

### ☑ Patient teaching

• Explain use and administration of drug to patient and family.

• Tell patient to report adverse reactions immediately.

---

## streptokinase
Kabikinase, Streptase

*Pregnancy Risk Category C*

### HOW SUPPLIED
*Injection:* 250,000 IU, 750,000 IU, 1,500,000 IU in vials for reconstitution

## ACTION
Activates plasminogen in two steps: Plasminogen and streptokinase form a complex that exposes the plasminogen-activating site; plasminogen is then converted to plasmin by cleavage of the peptide bond, which leads to fibrinolysis.

| Route | Onset | Peak | Duration |
|-------|-------|------|----------|
| I.V. | Immediate | 20 min-2 hr | 4 hr |

## INDICATIONS & DOSAGE
*Arteriovenous cannula occlusion—*
**Adults:** 250,000 IU in 2 ml I.V. solution by I.V. pump infusion into each occluded limb of the cannula over 25 to 35 minutes. Clamp off cannula for 2 hours. Then aspirate contents of cannula; flush with saline solution, and reconnect.
*Venous thrombosis, pulmonary embolism, arterial thrombosis and embolism—*
**Adults:** loading dose is 250,000 IU by I.V. infusion over 30 minutes. Sustaining dose is 100,000 IU/hour I.V. infusion for 72 hours for deep vein thrombosis and 100,000 IU/hour over 24 to 72 hours by I.V. infusion pump for pulmonary embolism and arterial thrombosis or embolism.
*Lysis of coronary artery thrombi following acute MI—*
**Adults:** loading dose is 20,000 IU bolus via coronary catheter; then infusion of a maintenance dose of 2,000 IU/minute over 60 minutes. Or, may be administered as an I.V. infusion. Usual adult dose is 1.5 million IU infused I.V. over 60 minutes.

## ADVERSE REACTIONS
**CNS:** polyradiculoneuropathy, headache.
**CV:** *reperfusion arrhythmias, hypotension,* vasculitis, flushing.
**EENT:** periorbital edema.
**GI:** nausea.
**Hematologic:** *bleeding;* increased thrombin time, activated PTT, and PT; moderately decreased hematocrit.
**Musculoskeletal:** pain.
**Respiratory:** minor breathing difficulty, *bronchospasm, pulmonary edema.*
**Skin:** urticaria, pruritus.
**Other:** phlebitis at injection site, *hypersensitivity reactions, anaphylaxis, delayed hypersensitivity reactions, angioedema, fever.*

---

*Liquid contains alcohol.    **May contain tartrazine.    †Canada    ‡Australia    §U.K.    ◊OTC

## INTERACTIONS

**Drug-drug.** *Anticoagulants:* increased risk of bleeding. Monitor patient closely.

*Antifibrinolytic drugs:* streptokinase activity is inhibited and reversed by antifibrinolytic drugs such as aminocaproic acid. Avoid concurrent use.

*Aspirin, dipyridamole, drugs affecting platelet activity, indomethacin, phenylbutazone:* increased risk of bleeding. Monitor patient closely.

## EFFECTS ON DIAGNOSTIC TESTS

None reported.

## CONTRAINDICATIONS

Contraindicated in patients with ulcerative wounds; active internal bleeding; recent CVA; recent trauma with possible internal injuries; visceral or intracranial malignant neoplasms; ulcerative colitis; diverticulitis; severe hypertension; acute or chronic hepatic or renal insufficiency; uncontrolled hypocoagulation; chronic pulmonary disease with cavitation; subacute bacterial endocarditis or rheumatic valvular disease; recent cerebral embolism, thrombosis, or hemorrhage; or previous severe allergic reaction to streptokinase.

Also contraindicated within 10 days after intra-arterial diagnostic procedure or any surgery, including liver or kidney biopsy, lumbar puncture, thoracentesis, paracentesis, or extensive or multiple cutdowns.

I.M. injections and other invasive procedures are contraindicated during streptokinase therapy.

## NURSING CONSIDERATIONS

• Use cautiously when treating arterial embolism that originates from left side of heart because of danger of cerebral infarction.

• Drug may be given to menstruating women.

• Only doctors with wide experience in thrombotic disease management should use streptokinase. Drug should be administered only where clinical and laboratory monitoring can be performed.

• Before using streptokinase to clear an occluded arteriovenous cannula, try flushing with heparinized saline solution, as ordered.

• Keep aminocaproic acid available to treat bleeding, and corticosteroids to treat allergic reactions.

• Before initiating therapy, draw blood for coagulation studies, hematocrit, platelet count, and type and crossmatching. Rate of I.V. infusion depends on thrombin time and streptokinase resistance.

• To check for hypersensitivity reactions, give 100 IU intradermally, as ordered; a wheal and flare response within 20 minutes means patient is probably allergic. Monitor vital signs frequently.

• If patient has had either a recent streptococcal infection or recent treatment with streptokinase, a higher loading dose may be needed.

• Combined therapy with low-dose aspirin (162.5 mg) or dipyridamole has improved acute and long-term results.

• Monitor patient for excessive bleeding every 15 minutes for first hour, every 30 minutes for second through eighth hours, then every 4 hours. If bleeding is evident, stop therapy and notify doctor. Pretreatment with heparin or drugs that affect platelets causes high risk of bleeding, but may improve long-term results. Monitor closely.

• Monitor pulse, color, and sensation of extremities every hour.

• Maintain involved extremity in straight alignment to prevent bleeding from infusion site.

• Avoid unnecessary handling of patient; pad side rails. Bruising is more likely during therapy.

• Keep a laboratory flow sheet on patient's chart to monitor PTT, PT, thrombin time, and hemoglobin level and hematocrit. Monitor vital signs and neurologic status.

• Avoid I.M. injection. Keep venipuncture sites to a minimum; use pressure dressing on puncture sites for at least 15 minutes.

• *Alert:* Watch for signs of hypersensitivity and notify doctor immediately if any occur. Antihistamines or corticosteroids may be used to treat mild allergic reactions. If a severe reaction occurs, stop infusion immediately and notify doctor.

---

Reactions may be *common,* uncommon, *life-threatening,* or COMMON AND LIFE-THREATENING.

• Thrombolytic therapy in patients with acute MI may decrease infarct size, improve ventricular function, and decrease risk of heart failure. For optimal effect, streptokinase must be administered within 6 hours of onset of symptoms.

### I.V. administration

• Reconstitute drug in each vial with 5 ml of normal saline solution for injection or $D_5W$ solution. Further dilute to 45 ml (if needed, total volume may be increased to 500 ml in a glass or 50 ml in a plastic container). Don't shake; roll gently to mix. Some flocculation may be present after reconstituting; discard if large amounts are present. Filter solution with 0.8-micron or larger filter. Use within 8 hours. Store powder at room temperature and refrigerate after reconstitution.
• Don't mix with other drugs or give other drugs through the same I.V. line.
• Heparin by continuous infusion is usually started within 1 to 4 hours after stopping streptokinase. Use infusion pump to administer heparin.

### ☑ Patient teaching

• Explain use and administration of drug to patient and family.
• Tell patient to report adverse reactions promptly.

---

## urokinase
Abbokinase, Abbokinase Open-Cath, Ukidan‡

*Pregnancy Risk Category B*

## HOW SUPPLIED
*Injection:* 5,000 U (IU) per unit-dose vial; 9,000 U (IU) per unit-dose vial; 250,000-IU vial

## ACTION
Activates plasminogen to plasmin by directly cleaving peptide bonds at two different sites, causing fibrinolysis.

| Route | Onset | Peak | Duration |
|-------|-------|------|----------|
| I.V. | Immediate | 20 min-4 hr | 4 hr |

## INDICATIONS & DOSAGE
*Lysis of acute massive pulmonary embolism and lysis of pulmonary embolism accompanied by unstable hemodynamics—*
**Adults:** for I.V. infusion *only* by constant infusion pump. Priming dose: 4,400 IU/kg of urokinase—normal saline or $D_5W$ solution admixture, given over 10 minutes. Then 4,400 IU/kg/hour for 12 hours. Therapy followed by continuous I.V. infusion of heparin, then oral anticoagulants.
*Coronary artery thrombosis—*
**Adults:** after bolus dose of heparin ranging from 2,500 to 10,000 U, 6,000 IU/minute of urokinase is infused into occluded artery for up to 2 hours. Average total dose is 500,000 IU. Urokinase therapy should be initiated within 6 hours of onset of symptoms.
*Venous catheter occlusion—*
**Adults:** solution containing 5,000 IU/ml is instilled into occluded line and, after 5 minutes, is aspirated. Aspiration attempts repeated q 5 minutes for 30 minutes. If not patent after 30 minutes, line is capped and urokinase left to work for 30 to 60 minutes before aspirating again. May require second instillation. Flush with 10 ml normal saline after patency restored.

## ADVERSE REACTIONS
**CV:** *reperfusion arrhythmias,* hypotension.
**Hematologic:** *bleeding.*
**Respiratory:** *bronchospasm,* minor breathing difficulties.
**Other:** phlebitis at injection site, fever, chills, nausea, vomiting, *hypersensitivity reactions.*

## INTERACTIONS
**Drug-drug.** *Anticoagulants:* increased risk of bleeding. Monitor patient closely. *Aspirin, dipyridamole, indomethacin, phenylbutazone, other drugs affecting platelet activity:* increased risk of bleeding. Monitor patient.

## EFFECTS ON DIAGNOSTIC TESTS
Drug increases thrombin time, PT, and activated PTT; it sometimes moderately decreases hematocrit.

---

## CONTRAINDICATIONS

Contraindicated in patients with active internal bleeding, history of CVA, aneurysm, arteriovenous malformation, known bleeding diathesis, recent trauma with possible internal injuries, visceral or intracranial malignancy, ulcerative colitis, diverticulitis, severe hypertension, hemostatic defects including those secondary to severe hepatic or renal insufficiency, uncontrolled hypocoagulation, chronic pulmonary disease with cavitation, subacute bacterial endocarditis or rheumatic valvular disease, and recent cerebral embolism, thrombosis, or hemorrhage.

Also contraindicated within 10 days after intra-arterial diagnostic procedure or surgery (liver or kidney biopsy, lumbar puncture, thoracentesis, paracentesis, or extensive or multiple cutdowns) or within 2 months after intracranial or intraspinal surgery. Don't use during pregnancy or first 10 days postpartum.

I.M. injections and other invasive procedures are contraindicated during urokinase therapy.

## NURSING CONSIDERATIONS

• Have typed and crossmatched RBCs, whole blood, plasma expanders (other than dextran), and aminocaproic acid available to treat bleeding; and corticosteroids, epinephrine, and antihistamines to treat allergic reactions.
• Drug may be given to menstruating women.
• Only doctors with extensive experience in thrombotic disease management should use urokinase in institutions where clinical and laboratory monitoring can be performed.
• Monitor patient for excessive bleeding every 15 minutes for first hour; every 30 minutes for second through eighth hours; then once every 4 hours. Pretreatment with drugs affecting platelets places patient at high risk of bleeding.
• Monitor pulse, color, and sensation of extremities every hour.
• Although risk of hypersensitivity reactions is low, monitor patient.
• Keep a laboratory flow sheet on patient's chart to monitor PTT, PT, thrombin time, and hemoglobin level and hematocrit.
• Monitor vital signs and neurologic status. Don't take blood pressure in lower extremities because this could dislodge a clot.
• Keep venipuncture sites to a minimum; use pressure dressing on puncture sites for at least 15 minutes.
• Maintain involved extremity in straight alignment to prevent bleeding from infusion site.
• Avoid unnecessary handling of patient; pad side rails; bruising is more likely during therapy.

### 🔆 I.V. administration

• Reconstitute according to manufacturer's directions. Gently roll vial; don't shake. Don't use bacteriostatic water for injection to reconstitute; it contains preservatives. Dilute further with normal saline solution or $D_5W$ solution before infusion. Urokinase solutions may be filtered through a 0.45-micron or smaller cellulose-membrane filter before administration. Discard unused solution.
• Don't mix with other drugs. Administer through separate I.V. line.
• Heparin by continuous infusion is usually started within 3 to 4 hours after urokinase has been stopped to prevent recurrent thrombosis.

### ✅ Patient teaching

• Explain use and administration of drug to patient and family.
• Instruct patient to report adverse reactions promptly.

**busulfan**
**carboplatin**
**carmustine**
**chlorambucil**
**cisplatin**
**cyclophosphamide**
**ifosfamide**
**lomustine**
**mechlorethamine hydrochloride**
**melphalan**
**melphalan hydrochloride**
**streptozocin**
**temozolomide**
**thiotepa**

**COMBINATION PRODUCTS**
None.

---

**busulfan**
Myleran

*Pregnancy Risk Category D*

**HOW SUPPLIED**
*Tablets:* 2 mg

**ACTION**
Unknown. Thought to cross-link strands of cellular DNA and interfere with RNA transcription, causing an imbalance of growth that leads to cell death. Cell cycle–nonspecific.

| Route | Onset | Peak | Duration |
|-------|-------|------|----------|
| P.O. | 1-2 wk | Unknown | Unknown |

**INDICATIONS & DOSAGE**
*Chronic myelocytic (granulocytic) leukemia—*
**Adults:** 4 to 8 mg P.O. daily, until WBC count falls to 15,000/mm³; drug stopped until WBC count rises to 50,000/mm³, and then resumed as before; or 4 to 8 mg P.O. daily until WBC count falls to 10,000 to 20,000/mm³; then daily dosage reduced, p.r.n., to maintain WBC count at this level. Dosage highly variable; range is 2 mg/week to 4 mg/day.

**Children:** 0.06 to 0.12 mg/kg/day or 1.8 to 4.6 mg/m²/day P.O.; dosage adjusted to maintain WBC count at 20,000/mm³, but never below 10,000/mm³.

**ADVERSE REACTIONS**
**CNS:** unusual tiredness or weakness, fatigue.
**EENT:** cataracts.
**GI:** cheilosis, dry mouth, anorexia.
**GU:** gynecomastia.
**Hematologic:** *leukopenia, thrombocytopenia, anemia, severe pancytopenia.*
**Hepatic:** jaundice.
**Respiratory:** *irreversible pulmonary fibrosis.*
**Skin:** alopecia, *transient hyperpigmentation,* rash, urticaria, anhidrosis.
**Other:** Addison-like wasting syndrome, profound hyperuricemia.

**INTERACTIONS**
**Drug-drug.** *Anticoagulants, aspirin:* increased risk of bleeding. Avoid concomitant use.
*Cyclophosphamide:* may increase risk of cardiac tamponade in patients with thalassemia. Monitor patient.
*Myelosuppressives:* concomitant use can cause additive myelosuppression. Monitor patient.
*Thioguanine:* may cause hepatotoxicity, esophageal varices, or portal hypertension. Use together cautiously.

**EFFECTS ON DIAGNOSTIC TESTS**
Drug-induced cellular dysplasia may interfere with interpretation of cytologic studies. Busulfan therapy may increase blood and urine levels of uric acid as a result of increased purine catabolism that accompanies cell destruction.

**CONTRAINDICATIONS**
Contraindicated in patients with chronic myelogenous leukemia that has shown prior resistance to drug. Not useful with chronic lymphocytic or acute leukemia or

---

\*Liquid contains alcohol.     \*\*May contain tartrazine.     †Canada     ‡Australia     §U.K.     ◇OTC

in the blastic crisis of chronic myelogenous leukemia.

## NURSING CONSIDERATIONS
• Use cautiously in patients recently given other myelosuppressives or radiation treatment and in those with depressed neutrophil or platelet count. Because high-dose therapy has been associated with seizures, use such therapy cautiously in patients with history of head trauma or seizures and in those receiving other drugs that lower the seizure threshold.
• Follow institutional policy regarding preparation and handling of drug. Label as a hazardous drug.
• Therapeutic effects are often accompanied by toxicity.
• To prevent bleeding, avoid all I.M. injections when platelet count is below 100,000/mm$^3$.
• Monitor patient response (increased appetite and sense of well-being, decreased total WBC count, reduced size of spleen), which usually begins within 1 to 2 weeks.
• Monitor serum uric acid level. To prevent hyperuricemia with resulting uric acid nephropathy, allopurinol may be ordered in addition to keeping patient adequately hydrated.
• Anticipate possible blood transfusion during treatment because of cumulative anemia. Patients may receive injections of RBC colony-stimulating factors to promote RBC production and decrease the need for blood transfusions.
• **Alert:** Pulmonary fibrosis may occur as late as 8 months to 10 years after treatment with busulfan. (Average duration of therapy is 4 years.)

### ☑ Patient teaching
• Advise patient to watch for signs of infection (fever, sore throat, fatigue) and bleeding (easy bruising, nosebleeds, bleeding gums, melena). Tell patient to take temperature daily.
• Instruct patient to report signs and symptoms of toxicity so dosage adjustments can be made. Persistent cough and progressive dyspnea with alveolar exudate, suggestive of pneumonia, may be result of drug toxicity.

• Instruct patient to avoid OTC products containing aspirin.
• Inform patient that drug may cause darkening of skin.
• Advise woman of childbearing age to avoid becoming pregnant during therapy. Recommend that she consult doctor before becoming pregnant.
• Warn breast-feeding woman to discontinue breast-feeding because of risk of infant toxicity.
• Instruct patient to take drug on an empty stomach to decrease nausea and vomiting.
• Because of risk of impotence and male sterility, advise man of childbearing potential about sperm banking before therapy begins.

## carboplatin
Paraplatin, Paraplatin-AQ†

*Pregnancy Risk Category D*

### HOW SUPPLIED
*Injection:* 50-mg, 150-mg, 450-mg vials

### ACTION
Unknown. An alkylating drug that probably produces cross-linking of DNA strands. Cell cycle–nonspecific.

| Route | Onset | Peak | Duration |
|-------|-------|------|----------|
| I.V. | Unknown | Unknown | Unknown |

### INDICATIONS & DOSAGE
*Palliative treatment of ovarian cancer—*
**Adults:** 360 mg/m$^2$ I.V. on day 1 q 4 weeks or 300 mg/m$^2$ when used with other chemotherapy drugs; doses shouldn't be repeated until platelet count exceeds 100,000/mm$^3$ and neutrophil count exceeds 2,000/mm$^3$. Subsequent doses are based on blood counts.
*Adjust-a-dose:* For renally impaired patients with creatinine clearance of 41 to 59 ml/minute, initial dose is 250 mg/m$^2$; if between 16 and 40 ml/minute, initial dose is 200 mg/m$^2$. Drug isn't recommended for patients with creatinine clearance of 15 ml/minute or less.

---

Reactions may be *common*, uncommon, *life-threatening*, or COMMON AND LIFE-THREATENING.

## ADVERSE REACTIONS

**CNS:** *asthenia,* dizziness, confusion, peripheral neuropathy, ototoxicity, central neurotoxicity, paresthesia.
**CV:** *cardiac failure, embolism, CVA.*
**EENT:** visual disturbances.
**GI:** constipation, diarrhea, *nausea, vomiting,* mucositis, change in taste, stomatitis.
**GU:** *increased BUN and creatinine levels.*
**Hematologic:** THROMBOCYTOPENIA, *leukopenia, neutropenia,* anemia, BONE MARROW SUPPRESSION.
**Hepatic:** *increased AST and alkaline phosphatase levels.*
**Metabolic:** *decreased serum electrolyte levels.*
**Skin:** alopecia.
**Other:** *hypersensitivity reactions, pain, anaphylaxis.*

## INTERACTIONS

**Drug-drug.** *Aspirin:* increased risk of bleeding. Avoid concomitant use.
*Bone marrow suppressants, including radiation therapy:* increased hematologic toxicity. Monitor closely.
*Myelosuppressives:* concomitant use can cause additive myelosuppression. Monitor patient.
*Nephrotoxic drugs, especially aminoglycosides:* enhanced nephrotoxicity of carboplatin. Use cautiously.

## EFFECTS ON DIAGNOSTIC TESTS

None reported.

## CONTRAINDICATIONS

Contraindicated in patients with history of hypersensitivity to cisplatin, platinum-containing compounds, or mannitol, and in those with severe bone marrow suppression or bleeding.

## NURSING CONSIDERATIONS

• Determine serum electrolyte, creatinine, and BUN levels; CBC; and creatinine clearance before first infusion and before each course of treatment.
• Bone marrow suppression may be more severe in patients with creatinine clearance below 60 ml/minute; dosage adjustments are recommended for such patients.
• Follow institutional policy to reduce risks because preparation and administra-

tion of parenteral form of drug is associated with mutagenic, teratogenic, and carcinogenic risks for personnel.
• Carefully check ordered dose against laboratory test results. Only one increase in dosage is recommended. Subsequent doses shouldn't exceed 125% of starting dose.
• Therapeutic effects are often accompanied by toxicity.
• To prevent bleeding, avoid all I.M. injections when platelet count is below 100,000/mm³.
• Monitor vital signs during infusion.
• Monitor CBC and platelet count frequently during therapy and, when indicated, until recovery. WBC and platelet count nadirs usually occur by day 21. Levels usually return to baseline by day 28. Dose shouldn't be repeated unless platelet count exceeds 100,000/mm³. Administer WBC colony-stimulating factors, as ordered, to promote cell line growth.
• Administer antiemetic therapy, as ordered. Carboplatin can produce severe vomiting.
• Anticipate possible blood transfusions during treatment because of cumulative anemia. Patient may receive injections of RBC colony-stimulating factors to promote cell production.
• Hydration or diuresis before or after treatment isn't needed.
• Patients over age 65 are at greater risk for neurotoxicity.
• *Alert:* Don't confuse carboplatin with cisplatin.

### ◖ I.V. administration

• *Alert:* Have epinephrine, corticosteroids, and antihistamines available when administering carboplatin because anaphylactoid reactions may occur within minutes of administration.
• Reconstitute with $D_5W$, normal saline solution, or sterile water for injection to make a concentration of 10 mg/ml. Add 5 ml of diluent to 50-mg vial, 15 ml of diluent to 150-mg vial, or 45 ml of diluent to 450-mg vial. Reconstituted drug can then be further diluted for infusion with normal saline solution or $D_5W$. A concentration as low as 0.5 mg/ml can be

prepared. Give drug by continuous or intermittent infusion over at least 15 minutes.

• Don't use needles or I.V. administration sets containing aluminum to administer carboplatin; precipitation and loss of drug's potency may occur.

• Store unopened vials at room temperature. Once reconstituted and diluted as directed, drug is stable at room temperature for 8 hours. Because drug doesn't contain antibacterial preservatives, discard unused drug after 8 hours.

### ✓ Patient teaching

• Advise patient of most common adverse reactions: nausea, vomiting, bone marrow suppression, anemia, and thrombocytopenia.

• Advise patient to watch for signs of infection (fever, sore throat, fatigue) and bleeding (easy bruising, nosebleeds, bleeding gums, melena). Tell patient to take temperature daily.

• Instruct patient to avoid OTC products containing aspirin.

• Because of risk of infant toxicity, advise breast-feeding woman taking drug to discontinue breast-feeding.

• Because of risk of impotence, sterility, and amenorrhea, counsel both men and women of childbearing age before initiating therapy. Also recommend that women consult doctor before becoming pregnant.

---

## carmustine (BCNU)
BiCNU, Gliadel

*Pregnancy Risk Category D*

### HOW SUPPLIED
*Injection:* 100-mg vial (lyophilized), with a 3-ml vial of absolute alcohol supplied as a diluent
*Wafer:* 7.7 mg, for intracavitary use

### ACTION
Inhibits enzymatic reactions involved with DNA synthesis, cross-links strands of cellular DNA, and interferes with RNA transcription, causing an imbalance of growth that leads to cell death. Cell cycle–nonspecific.

| Route | Onset | Peak | Duration |
|---|---|---|---|
| I.V., intra-cavitary | Unknown | Unknown | Unknown |

### INDICATIONS & DOSAGE
*Brain tumors, Hodgkin's disease, malignant lymphoma, multiple myeloma—*
**Adults:** 75 to 100 mg/m² I.V. by slow infusion daily for 2 days; repeated q 6 weeks if platelet count is above 100,000/mm³ and WBC count is above 4,000/mm³.

*Adjust-a-dose:* Dosage is reduced by 50% when WBC count is 3,000 to 3,999/mm³. Dosage is reduced by 75% when WBC count is 2,000 to 2,999/mm³ and platelet count is 25,000 to 75,000/mm³. Dosage is held when WBC count is below 2,000/mm³ and platelet count is below 25,000/mm³.

*Adjunct to surgery to prolong survival in patients with recurrent glioblastoma multiforme for whom surgical resection is indicated—*
**Adults:** recommendation *(for wafer)*—8 wafers placed in the resection cavity if size and shape of cavity allows. If 8 wafers can't be accommodated, use maximum number of wafers allowed.

Or, 150 to 200 mg/m² I.V. by slow infusion as single dose, repeated q 6 to 8 weeks.

### ADVERSE REACTIONS
**CNS:** ataxia, drowsiness.
**EENT:** ocular toxicities.
**GI:** *nausea beginning in 2 to 6 hours (can be severe),* vomiting, stomatitis.
**GU:** *nephrotoxicity,* azotemia, *renal failure.*
**Hematologic:** *cumulative bone marrow suppression, leukopenia, thrombocytopenia, acute leukemia or bone marrow dysplasia,* anemia.
**Hepatic:** increased serum alkaline phosphatase, AST, and bilirubin levels; *hepatotoxicity.*
**Respiratory:** *pulmonary fibrosis.*
**Skin:** *intense pain at infusion site from venous spasm,* facial flushing, hyperpigmentation.

---

Reactions may be *common,* uncommon, *life-threatening,* or COMMON AND LIFE-THREATENING.

## INTERACTIONS
**Drug-drug.** *Anticoagulants, aspirin:* increased risk of bleeding. Avoid concomitant use.
*Cimetidine:* may increase carmustine's bone marrow toxicity. Avoid combination, if possible.
*Myelosuppressives:* concomitant use can cause additive myelosuppression. Monitor patient.

## EFFECTS ON DIAGNOSTIC TESTS
None reported.

## CONTRAINDICATIONS
Contraindicated in patients with hypersensitivity to drug.

## NURSING CONSIDERATIONS
• Pulmonary toxicity appears to be dose-related and may occur 9 days to 15 years after treatment. Obtain pulmonary function tests, as ordered, before and during therapy.
• To reduce nausea, give antiemetic before administering drug, as ordered.
• Avoid contact with skin because carmustine will cause a brown stain. If drug comes into contact with skin, wash off thoroughly.
• Perform liver, renal function, and pulmonary function tests periodically, as ordered.
• Monitor CBC, as ordered.
• Monitor serum uric acid level, as ordered. To prevent hyperuricemia with resulting uric acid nephropathy, allopurinol may be used with adequate hydration.
• Therapeutic effects are often accompanied by toxicity.
• Acute leukemia or bone marrow dysplasia may occur after long-term use.
• To prevent bleeding, avoid all I.M. injections when platelet count is below 100,000/mm$^3$.
• Anticipate possible blood transfusions during treatment because of cumulative anemia. Patient may receive injections of RBC colony-stimulating factors to promote cell production.
• Unopened foil pouches of wafer may be kept at ambient room temperature for a maximum of 6 hours.

• Wafers broken in half may be used; however, discard wafers broken in more than two pieces.

## ◖ I.V. administration
• Follow institutional policy to reduce risks because preparation and administration of parenteral form of this drug are associated with carcinogenic, mutagenic, and teratogenic risks for personnel. Manufacturer recommends wearing gloves when handling either form.
• To reconstitute, dissolve 100 mg of carmustine in 3 ml of absolute alcohol provided by manufacturer. Dilute solution with 27 ml of sterile water for injection. Resultant solution contains 3.3 mg of carmustine/ml in 10% alcohol. Dilute in normal saline solution or $D_5W$ for I.V. infusion. Give at least 250 ml over 1 to 2 hours. To reduce pain on infusion, dilute further or slow infusion rate.
• Discard drug if powder liquefies or appears oily (decomposition has occurred).
• Administer only in glass containers. Solution is unstable in plastic I.V. bags.
• Don't mix with other drugs during administration.
• Store reconstituted solution in refrigerator for 24 hours or at room temperature for 8 hours. May decompose at temperatures above 80° F (27° C).

## ☑ Patient teaching
• Advise patient about common adverse reactions to drug.
• Tell patient to watch for signs and symptoms of infection (fever, sore throat, fatigue) and bleeding (easy bruising, nosebleeds, bleeding gums, melena). Tell him to take temperature daily.
• Instruct patient to avoid OTC products containing aspirin.
• Advise breast-feeding woman to discontinue breast-feeding during therapy because of possible infant toxicity.
• Caution woman of childbearing age to avoid becoming pregnant during therapy. Recommend that she consult doctor before becoming pregnant.

---

*Liquid contains alcohol.     **May contain tartrazine.     †Canada     ‡Australia     §U.K.     ◇OTC

# chlorambucil
Leukeran

*Pregnancy Risk Category D*

## HOW SUPPLIED
*Tablets:* 2 mg

## ACTION
Cross-links strands of cellular DNA and interferes with RNA transcription, causing an imbalance of growth that leads to cell death. Cell cycle–nonspecific.

| Route | Onset | Peak | Duration |
|-------|-------|------|----------|
| P.O. | 3-4 wk | 1 hr | Unknown |

## INDICATIONS & DOSAGE
*Chronic lymphocytic leukemia; malignant lymphomas, including lymphosarcoma, giant follicular lymphoma, and Hodgkin's disease—*
**Adults:** 0.1 to 0.2 mg/kg P.O. daily for 3 to 6 weeks; then adjusted for maintenance (usually 4 to 10 mg daily).

## ADVERSE REACTIONS
**CNS:** *seizures,* peripheral neuropathy, tremor, muscle twitching, confusion, agitation, ataxia, flaccid paresis.
**GI:** *nausea, vomiting,* stomatitis, diarrhea.
**GU:** *azoospermia, infertility,* sterile cystitis.
**Hematologic:** *neutropenia* (delayed up to 3 weeks, lasting up to 10 days after last dose); *bone marrow suppression, thrombocytopenia,* anemia, *myelosuppression.*
**Hepatic:** increased serum alkaline phosphatase and AST levels, *hepatotoxicity.*
**Respiratory:** interstitial pneumonitis, *pulmonary fibrosis* (rare).
**Skin:** rash, including erythema multiforme, epidermal necrolysis, and *Stevens-Johnson syndrome.*
**Other:** allergic febrile reaction, increased blood and urine uric acid levels, *hypersensitivity reactions.*

## INTERACTIONS
**Drug-drug.** *Anticoagulants, aspirin:* increased risk of bleeding. Avoid concomitant use.

*Myelosuppressives:* concomitant use can cause additive myelosuppression. Monitor patient.

## EFFECTS ON DIAGNOSTIC TESTS
None reported.

## CONTRAINDICATIONS
Contraindicated in patients with hypersensitivity or resistance to previous therapy. Patients hypersensitive to other alkylating drugs may also be hypersensitive to chlorambucil.

## NURSING CONSIDERATIONS
• Use cautiously in patients with history of head trauma or seizures and in patients receiving other drugs that lower the seizure threshold. Also use cautiously within 4 weeks of a full course of radiation or chemotherapy.
• Monitor CBC, as ordered.
• Monitor serum uric acid level, as ordered. To prevent hyperuricemia with resulting uric acid nephropathy, allopurinol may be used with adequate hydration.
• If WBC count falls below 2,000/mm$^3$ or granulocyte count falls below 1,000/mm$^3$, follow institutional policy for infection control in immunocompromised patients. Patients may receive injections of WBC colony-stimulating factors to decrease risk of infection. Severe neutropenia is reversible up to cumulative dosage of 6.5 mg/kg in a single course.
• Therapeutic effects are frequently accompanied by toxicity.
• To prevent bleeding, avoid all I.M. injections when platelet count is below 100,000/mm$^3$.
• Anticipate possible blood transfusions during treatment because of cumulative anemia. Patient may receive injections of RBC colony-stimulating factors to promote RBC production and decrease need for blood transfusions.

✓ **Patient teaching**
• Advise patient to watch for signs of infection (fever, sore throat, fatigue) and bleeding (easy bruising, nosebleeds, bleeding gums, melena). Tell patient to take temperature daily.

---

Reactions may be *common,* uncommon, *life-threatening,* or COMMON AND LIFE-THREATENING.

• Instruct patient to avoid OTC products containing aspirin.
• Tell breast-feeding woman to discontinue breast-feeding during therapy because of possible infant toxicity.
• Advise woman of childbearing age to avoid becoming pregnant during therapy and to notify doctor immediately if pregnancy is suspected.

---

## cisplatin (CDDP, cis-platinum†)
Platinol AQ

*Pregnancy Risk Category D*

### HOW SUPPLIED
*Injection:* 0.5 mg/ml†, 1 mg/ml

### ACTION
Unknown. Probably cross-links strands of cellular DNA and interferes with RNA transcription, causing an imbalance of growth that leads to cell death. Cell cycle–nonspecific.

| Route | Onset | Peak | Duration |
|-------|-------|------|----------|
| I.V. | Unknown | Unknown | Several days |

### INDICATIONS & DOSAGE
*Adjunctive therapy in metastatic testicular cancer—*
**Adults:** 20 mg/m² I.V. daily for 5 days. Repeated q 3 weeks for three cycles or longer.
*Adjunctive therapy in metastatic ovarian cancer—*
**Adults:** 100 mg/m² I.V.; repeated q 4 weeks. Or, 50 to 100 mg/m² I.V. once q 3 to 4 weeks with cyclophosphamide.
*Advanced bladder cancer—*
**Adults:** 50 to 70 mg/m² I.V. q 3 to 4 weeks. Patients who have received other antineoplastic drugs or radiation therapy should receive 50 mg/m² q 4 weeks.

### ADVERSE REACTIONS
**CNS:** *peripheral neuritis,* **seizures.**
**EENT:** *tinnitus, hearing loss, ototoxicity,* vestibular toxicity, optic neuritis, papilledema, cerebral blindness, blurred vision.
**GI:** loss of taste, *nausea, vomiting beginning 1 to 4 hours after dose and lasting 24 hours.*
**GU:** MORE PROLONGED AND SEVERE RENAL TOXICITY WITH REPEATED COURSES OF THERAPY.
**Hematologic:** MYELOSUPPRESSION; *leukopenia, thrombocytopenia,* anemia.
**Metabolic:** *hypomagnesemia,* hypokalemia, hypocalcemia, hyponatremia, hypophosphatemia, hyperuricemia.
**Other:** *anaphylactoid reaction.*

### INTERACTIONS
**Drug-drug.** *Aminoglycoside antibiotics:* additive nephrotoxicity. Carefully monitor renal function studies.
*Aspirin:* increased risk of bleeding. Avoid concurrent use.
*Bumetanide, ethacrynic acid, furosemide:* additive ototoxicity. Avoid concomitant use.
*Myelosuppressives:* concomitant use can cause additive myelosuppression. Monitor patient.
*Phenytoin:* decreased serum phenytoin levels. Monitor serum levels.

### EFFECTS ON DIAGNOSTIC TESTS
None reported.

### CONTRAINDICATIONS
Contraindicated in patients with hypersensitivity to drug or other platinum-containing compounds and in those with severe renal disease, hearing impairment, or myelosuppression.

### NURSING CONSIDERATIONS
• Use cautiously in patients previously treated with radiation or cytotoxic drugs and in those with preexisting peripheral neuropathies; also use cautiously with other ototoxic and nephrotoxic drugs.
• Monitor CBC, electrolyte levels (especially potassium and magnesium), platelet count, and renal function studies before initial and subsequent doses, as ordered.
• To detect hearing loss, perform audiometry before initial and subsequent doses, as ordered.
• Prehydration and mannitol diuresis may significantly reduce renal toxicity and ototoxicity.

---

- Therapeutic effects are frequently accompanied by toxicity.
- Check current protocol. Some doctors use I.V. sodium thiosulfate to minimize toxicity.
- Administer antiemetics, as ordered. Nausea and vomiting may be severe and protracted; however, incidence and severity have been significantly reduced with the use of ondansetron and granisetron. Monitor intake and output. Continue I.V. hydration until patient can tolerate adequate oral intake.
- Some doctors combine metoclopramide with dexamethasone and antihistamines, or ondansetron or granisetron with dexamethasone.
- Delayed-onset vomiting (3 to 5 days after treatment) has been reported; patients may need prolonged antiemetic treatment.
- Renal toxicity is cumulative; renal function must return to normal before next dose can be given.
- Dose shouldn't be repeated unless platelet count is over 100,000/mm$^3$, WBC count is over 4,000/mm$^3$, creatinine level is under 1.5 mg/dl, or BUN level is under 25 mg/dl.
- To prevent bleeding, avoid all I.M. injections when platelet count is below 100,000/mm$^3$.
- Anticipate blood transfusions during treatment because of cumulative anemia.
- *Alert:* Immediately administer epinephrine, corticosteroids, or antihistamines for anaphylactoid reactions, as ordered.
- Safety of drug in children hasn't been established.
- *Alert:* Don't confuse cisplatin with carboplatin; they aren't interchangeable.

### I.V. administration
- As ordered, administer mannitol or furosemide boluses or infusions before and with cisplatin infusion to maintain diuresis of 100 to 400 ml/hour during and for 24 hours after therapy.
- Hydrate patient with normal saline solution before giving drug, as ordered. Maintain urine output of at least 100 ml/hour for 4 consecutive hours before therapy and for 24 hours after therapy.
- Follow institutional policy to reduce risks because preparation and administration of parenteral form of drug are associated with carcinogenic, mutagenic, and teratogenic risks for personnel.
- Reconstitute powder using sterile water for injection. Add 10 ml to 10-mg vial or 50 ml to 50-mg vial to make a solution containing 1 mg/ml. If needed, further dilute with dextrose 5% in 0.3% NaCl injection or dextrose 5% in half-normal saline injection. Solutions are stable for 20 hours at room temperature. Don't refrigerate.
- Infusions are most stable in chloride-containing solutions (such as normal or half-normal saline and 0.22% NaCl).
- The manufacturer recommends administering drug as an I.V. infusion in 2 L of dextrose 5% in half-normal saline or dextrose 5% in 0.22% NaCl solution with 37.5 g of mannitol over 6 to 8 hours.
- Don't use needles or I.V. administration sets that contain aluminum because it will displace the platinum, causing loss of potency and formation of a black precipitate.
- To prevent hypokalemia, potassium chloride (10 to 20 mEq/L) is frequently added to I.V. fluids before and after cisplatin therapy.

### Patient teaching
- Advise patient to watch for signs and symptoms of infection (fever, sore throat, fatigue) and bleeding (easy bruising, nosebleeds, bleeding gums, melena). Tell patient to take temperature daily.
- Tell patient to immediately report tinnitus or numbness in hands or feet.
- Instruct patient to avoid OTC products containing aspirin.
- Advise breast-feeding woman taking drug to discontinue breast-feeding because of risk of infant toxicity.
- Advise woman of childbearing age to avoid becoming pregnant during therapy. Recommend that she consult doctor before becoming pregnant.

---

Reactions may be *common*, uncommon, *life-threatening*, or COMMON AND LIFE-THREATENING.

## cyclophosphamide
Cycloblastin‡, Cytoxan**, Cytoxan
Lyophilized, Endoxan-Asta‡,
Neosar, Procytox†

*Pregnancy Risk Category D*

### HOW SUPPLIED
*Tablets:* 25 mg, 50 mg
*Injection:* 100-mg, 200-mg, 500-mg, 1-g,
2-g vials

### ACTION
Cross-links strands of cellular DNA and
interferes with RNA transcription, causing an imbalance of growth that leads to
cell death. Cell cycle–nonspecific.

| Route | Onset | Peak | Duration |
|-------|-------|------|----------|
| P.O., I.V. | Unknown | Unknown | Unknown |

### INDICATIONS & DOSAGE
*Breast and ovarian cancers, Hodgkin's
disease, chronic lymphocytic leukemia,
chronic myelocytic leukemia, acute lymphoblastic leukemia, acute myelocytic
and monocytic leukemia, neuroblastoma,
retinoblastoma, malignant lymphoma,
multiple myeloma, mycosis fungoides,
sarcoma—*
**Adults:** initially for induction, 40 to
50 mg/kg I.V. in divided doses over 2 to 5
days. Or, 10 to 15 mg/kg I.V. q 7 to 10
days, 3 to 5 mg/kg I.V. twice weekly, or 1
to 5 mg/kg P.O. daily, based on patient
tolerance.
**Children:** initially for induction, 2 to 8
mg/kg or 60 to 250 mg/m² P.O. or I.V. daily. Maintenance dose is 2 to 5 mg/kg P.O.
or 50 to 150 mg/m² P.O. twice weekly.
   Subsequent doses adjusted according
to evidence of antitumor activity or
leukopenia.
*"Minimal change" nephrotic syndrome in
children—*
**Children:** 2 to 3 mg/kg P.O. daily for 60
to 90 days.

### ADVERSE REACTIONS
**CV:** *cardiotoxicity with very high doses
and with doxorubicin,* flushing.
**GI:** anorexia, *nausea and vomiting beginning within 6 hours,* abdominal pain,
stomatitis, mucositis.
**GU:** HEMORRHAGIC CYSTITIS, impaired
fertility.
**Hematologic:** *leukopenia (nadir between
days 8 and 15, recovery in 17 to 28 days),
thrombocytopenia,* anemia.
**Hepatic:** *hepatotoxicity.*
**Respiratory:** *pulmonary fibrosis with
high doses.*
**Skin:** *reversible alopecia,* rash, pigmentation, nail changes, itching.
**Other:** *secondary malignant disease,
anaphylaxis, hypersensitivity reactions,*
increased serum uric acid levels, decreased serum pseudocholinesterase levels.

### INTERACTIONS
**Drug-drug.** *Allopurinol:* increased
myelosuppression. Monitor toxicity.
*Aspirin:* increased risk of bleeding. Avoid
concurrent use.
*Barbiturates:* increased pharmacologic effect and enhanced cyclophosphamide toxicity due to induction of hepatic enzymes.
Monitor patient closely.
*Cardiotoxic drugs:* additive adverse cardiac effects. Monitor for toxicity.
*Chloramphenicol, corticosteroids:* reduced activity of cyclophosphamide. Use
cautiously.
*Digoxin:* may decrease serum digoxin
levels. Monitor levels closely.
*Myelosuppressives:* concomitant use can
cause additive myelosuppression. Monitor
patient.
*Succinylcholine:* prolonged neuromuscular blockade. Don't use together.

### EFFECTS ON DIAGNOSTIC TESTS
Drug may suppress positive reaction to
*Candida,* mumps, *Trichophyton,* and tuberculin TB skin test. A false-positive result for the Papanicolaou test may occur.

### CONTRAINDICATIONS
Contraindicated in patients with hypersensitivity to drug and in those with severe bone marrow suppression.

## NURSING CONSIDERATIONS

• Use cautiously in patients with leukopenia, thrombocytopenia, malignant cell infiltration of bone marrow, or hepatic or renal disease and in those who have recently undergone radiation therapy or chemotherapy.
• Don't give drug at bedtime; infrequent urination during the night may increase possibility of cystitis. If cystitis occurs, discontinue drug and notify doctor. Cystitis can occur months after therapy ceases. Mesna may be given to lower incidence and severity of bladder toxicity.
• Use caution to ensure correct dose to decrease risk of cardiac toxicity.
• Monitor CBC and renal and liver function tests, as ordered.
• Monitor serum uric acid level, as ordered. To prevent hyperuricemia with resulting uric acid nephropathy, allopurinol may be used with adequate hydration.
• *Alert:* Monitor for cyclophosphamide toxicity if patient's corticosteroid therapy is discontinued.
• To prevent bleeding, avoid all I.M. injections when platelet count is below 100,000/mm³.
• Anticipate possible blood transfusions because of cumulative anemia. Patients may receive injections of RBC colony-stimulating factors to promote RBC production and decrease need for blood transfusions.
• Therapeutic effects are frequently accompanied by toxicity.

### I.V. administration

• Follow institutional policy to reduce risks. Preparation and administration of parenteral form of this drug are associated with carcinogenic, mutagenic, and teratogenic risks for personnel.
• Reconstitute powder using sterile water for injection or bacteriostatic water for injection containing only parabens. For the nonlyophilized product, add 5 ml to 100-mg vial, 10 ml to 200-mg vial, 25 ml to 500-mg vial, 50 ml to 1-g vial, or 100 ml to 2-g vial to produce a solution containing 20 mg/ml. Shake to dissolve; this may take up to 6 minutes, and it may be difficult to completely dissolve drug. Lyophilized preparation is much easier to reconstitute; check package insert for quantity of diluent needed to reconstitute drug.
• After reconstitution, administer, as ordered, by direct I.V. injection or infusion. For I.V. infusion, further dilute with D₅W, dextrose 5% in normal saline injection, dextrose 5% in Ringer's injection, lactated Ringer's injection, sodium lactate injection, or half-normal saline injection.
• Check reconstituted solution for small particles. Filter solution if needed.
• Reconstituted solution is stable for 6 days refrigerated or 24 hours at room temperature. However, use stored solutions cautiously because drug contains no preservatives.

### ✓ Patient teaching

• Warn patient that alopecia is likely to occur but that it's reversible.
• Advise patient to watch for signs and symptoms of infection (fever, sore throat, fatigue) and bleeding (easy bruising, nosebleeds, bleeding gums, melena). Tell patient to take temperature daily.
• Instruct patient to avoid OTC products containing aspirin.
• To minimize risk of hemorrhagic cystitis, encourage patient to void every 1 to 2 hours while awake and to drink at least 3 L of fluid daily. If patient is taking oral form of drug, instruct him to avoid taking it at bedtime because infrequent urination increases risk of cystitis.
• Advise both men and women to practice contraception during therapy and for 4 months afterward; drug is potentially teratogenic.
• Advise breast-feeding woman taking drug to discontinue breast-feeding because of risk of infant toxicity.
• Drug can cause irreversible sterility in both men and women. Counsel patients of childbearing potential before initiating therapy. Also recommend that women consult doctor before becoming pregnant.

# ifosfamide
Ifex, Mitoxana§

*Pregnancy Risk Category D*

## HOW SUPPLIED
*Injection:* 1 g, 2 g†, 3 g

## ACTION
Cross-links strands of cellular DNA and interferes with RNA transcription, causing an imbalance of growth that leads to cell death. Cell cycle–nonspecific.

| Route | Onset | Peak | Duration |
|-------|-------|------|----------|
| I.V. | Unknown | Unknown | Unknown |

## INDICATIONS & DOSAGE
*Testicular cancer—*
**Adults:** 1.2 g/m$^2$/day I.V. for 5 consecutive days. Treatment is repeated q 3 weeks or after patient recovers from hematologic toxicity.

## ADVERSE REACTIONS
**CNS:** *somnolence, confusion, **coma, seizures,** ataxia, hallucinations,* depressive psychosis, dizziness, disorientation, cranial nerve dysfunction.
**GI:** *nausea, vomiting.*
**GU:** *hemorrhagic cystitis, hematuria, **nephrotoxicity.***
**Hematologic:** *leukopenia, thrombocytopenia, **myelosuppression.***
**Hepatic:** elevated liver enzyme levels, liver dysfunction.
**Metabolic:** *metabolic acidosis.*
**Skin:** *alopecia.*
**Other:** infection, phlebitis.

## INTERACTIONS
**Drug-drug.** *Allopurinol:* may produce excessive ifosfamide effect by prolonging half-life. Monitor for enhanced toxicity.
*Anticoagulants, aspirin:* increased risk of bleeding. Avoid concomitant use.
*Barbiturates, chloral hydrate, phenytoin:* may increase ifosfamide toxicity by inducing hepatic enzymes that hasten formation of toxic metabolites. Monitor patient closely.
*Corticosteroids:* may inhibit hepatic enzymes, reducing ifosfamide's effect. Monitor for enhanced ifosfamide toxicity if concurrent corticosteroid dosage is suddenly reduced or discontinued.
*Cyclophosphamides:* may increase risk of cardiac tamponade in patients with thalassemia. Monitor concomitant use.
*Myelosuppressives:* enhanced hematologic toxicity. Dosage adjustment may be needed.

## EFFECTS ON DIAGNOSTIC TESTS
None reported.

## CONTRAINDICATIONS
Contraindicated in patients with hypersensitivity to drug and in those with severe bone marrow suppression.

## NURSING CONSIDERATIONS
● Use cautiously in patients with renal impairment or compromised bone marrow reserve as indicated by leukopenia, granulocytopenia, extensive bone marrow metastases, previous radiation therapy, or previous therapy with cytotoxic drugs.
● Administer antiemetics, as ordered, before giving ifosfamide to help decrease nausea.
● Don't give drug at bedtime; infrequent voiding during the night may increase possibility of cystitis. If cystitis develops, discontinue drug and notify doctor.
● Bladder irrigation with normal saline solution may decrease possibility of cystitis.
● Monitor CBC and renal and liver function tests, as ordered.
● To prevent bleeding, avoid all I.M. injections when platelet count is below 100,000/mm$^3$.
● Anticipate possible blood transfusions because of cumulative anemia. Patients may receive injections of RBC colony-stimulating factors to promote RBC production and decrease need for blood transfusions.
● Assess patient for mental status changes; dosage may have to be decreased
● *Alert:* Don't confuse ifosfamide with cyclophosphamide.

## ⬛ I.V. administration

• Follow institutional policy to reduce risks. Preparation and administration of parenteral form of drug are associated with carcinogenic, mutagenic, and teratogenic risks for personnel.

• Reconstitute each gram of drug with 20 ml of diluent to yield a solution of 50 mg/ml. Use sterile water for injection or bacteriostatic water for injection. Solutions may then be further diluted with sterile water, dextrose 2.5% or 5% in water, half-normal or normal saline for injection, 5% dextrose and normal saline for injection, or lactated Ringer's injection.

• Infuse each dose over at least 30 minutes.

• As ordered, administer ifosfamide with a protective drug such as mesna to prevent hemorrhagic cystitis. Obtain urinalysis before each dose. If microscopic hematuria is present, mesna must be given with or before ifosfamide to prevent cystitis. (Dosage adjustments of mesna given concomitantly may be needed.) Adequate fluid intake (2 L/day, either P.O. or I.V.) is essential before, and 72 hours after, therapy.

• Ifosfamide and mesna are physically compatible and may be mixed in the same I.V. solution.

• Reconstituted solution is stable for 1 week at room temperature or 6 weeks if refrigerated. However, use solution within 6 hours if drug was reconstituted with sterile water without a preservative (such as benzyl alcohol or parabens).

## ☑ Patient teaching

• Remind patient to void frequently to minimize contact of drug and its metabolites with the bladder mucosa.

• Advise patient to watch for signs and symptoms of infection (fever, sore throat, fatigue) and bleeding (easy bruising, nosebleeds, bleeding gums, melena). Tell patient to take temperature daily.

• Instruct patient to avoid OTC products containing aspirin.

• Advise breast-feeding woman to discontinue breast-feeding during therapy because of possible infant toxicity.

• Caution woman of childbearing age to avoid becoming pregnant during therapy. Recommend that she consult doctor before becoming pregnant.

---

# lomustine (CCNU)
CeeNu

*Pregnancy Risk Category D*

## HOW SUPPLIED
*Capsules:* 10 mg, 40 mg, 100 mg, dose pack (two 10-mg, two 40-mg, two 100-mg capsules)

## ACTION
Cross-links strands of cellular DNA and interferes with RNA transcription, causing an imbalance of growth that leads to cell death. Cell cycle–nonspecific.

| Route | Onset | Peak | Duration |
|-------|-------|------|----------|
| P.O. | Unknown | Unknown | Unknown |

## INDICATIONS & DOSAGE
*Brain tumor, Hodgkin's disease—*
**Adults and children:** 100 to 130 mg/m$^2$ P.O. as single dose q 6 weeks. Repeat doses shouldn't be given until WBC count exceeds 4,000/mm$^3$ and platelet count is over 100,000/mm$^3$.
*Adjust-a-dose:* Dosage reduced according to degree of bone marrow suppression or when used with other myelosuppressive drugs. Dosage should be reduced by 25% for WBC count 3,000 to 3,999/mm$^3$; by 50% for WBC count 2,000 to 2,999/mm$^3$; dosage should be withheld for WBC count below 2,000/mm$^3$.

## ADVERSE REACTIONS
**CNS:** disorientation, lethargy, ataxia.
**GI:** *nausea, vomiting,* stomatitis.
**GU:** *nephrotoxicity,* progressive azotemia, *renal failure.*
**Hematologic:** anemia, *leukopenia (delayed up to 6 weeks, lasting 1 to 2 weeks); thrombocytopenia (delayed up to 4 weeks, lasting 1 to 2 weeks); bone marrow suppression (delayed up to 4 to 6 weeks).*
**Hepatic:** *hepatotoxicity.*
**Skin:** alopecia.

---

Reactions may be *common,* uncommon, **life-threatening,** or COMMON AND **LIFE-THREATENING.**

**Other:** *secondary malignant disease, pulmonary fibrosis.*

## INTERACTIONS
**Drug-drug.** *Anticoagulants, aspirin:* increased risk of bleeding. Avoid concomitant use.
*Myelosuppressives:* concomitant use can cause additive myelosuppression. Monitor patient

## EFFECTS ON DIAGNOSTIC TESTS
None reported.

## CONTRAINDICATIONS
Contraindicated in patients with hypersensitivity to drug.

## NURSING CONSIDERATIONS
• Use cautiously in patients with decreased platelet, WBC, or RBC counts and in those receiving other myelosuppressives.
• To avoid nausea, give antiemetic before administering, as ordered.
• Give 2 to 4 hours after meals; drug will be more completely absorbed if taken when stomach is empty.
• Monitor CBC weekly, as ordered. Usually not administered more often than every 6 weeks; bone marrow toxicity is cumulative and delayed, usually occurring 4 to 6 weeks after drug administration.
• Periodically monitor liver function tests, as ordered.
• To prevent bleeding, avoid all I.M. injections when platelet count is below 100,000/mm³.
• Anticipate possible blood transfusions because of cumulative anemia. Patients may receive RBC colony-stimulating factors to promote RBC production and decrease need for blood transfusions.
• Therapeutic effects are often accompanied by toxicity.
• Store capsules at room temperature. Avoid exposure to moisture and protect from temperatures above 104° F (40° C).

### ✓ Patient teaching
• Advise patient to watch for signs and symptoms of infection (fever, sore throat, fatigue) and bleeding (easy bruising, nosebleeds, bleeding gums, melena). Tell patient to take temperature daily.
• Instruct patient to avoid OTC products containing aspirin.
• Advise breast-feeding woman to discontinue breast-feeding during therapy because of possible infant toxicity.
• Caution woman of childbearing age to avoid becoming pregnant during therapy. Recommend that she consult doctor before becoming pregnant.

---

## mechlorethamine hydrochloride (nitrogen mustard)
Mustargen

*Pregnancy Risk Category D*

### HOW SUPPLIED
*Injection:* 10-mg vials

### ACTION
Cross-links strands of cellular DNA and interferes with RNA transcription, causing an imbalance of growth that leads to cell death. Cell cycle–nonspecific.

| Route | Onset | Peak | Duration |
|-------|-------|------|----------|
| I.V., intra-cavitary | Few seconds-few minutes | Unknown | Unknown |

### INDICATIONS & DOSAGE
*Polycythemia vera, chronic lymphocytic leukemia, chronic myelocytic leukemia, malignant effusions (pericardial, peritoneal, pleural), mycosis fungoides, Hodgkin's disease, lymphosarcoma, bronchogenic cancer—*
**Adults:** 0.4 mg/kg I.V. as single dose or in divided doses of 0.1 to 0.2 mg/kg/day. Given through running I.V. infusion. Subsequent courses of therapy given when patient has recovered hematologically from previous course (usually 3 to 6 weeks).
*Malignant effusions—*
**Adults:** 0.4 mg/kg intracavitarily, although 0.2 mg/kg has been used intrapericardially.

### ADVERSE REACTIONS
**CNS:** weakness, vertigo, neurotoxicity.

---

**CV:** *thrombophlebitis.*
**EENT:** tinnitus; deafness with high doses.
**GI:** *nausea, vomiting, anorexia (beginning within minutes, lasting 8 to 24 hours);* diarrhea, metallic taste.
**GU:** menstrual irregularities, impaired spermatogenesis.
**Hematologic:** *thrombocytopenia,* lymphocytopenia, *agranulocytosis (nadir of myelosuppression occurring between days 4 and 10 and lasting 10 to 21 days);* mild anemia beginning in 2 to 3 weeks.
**Hepatic:** jaundice.
**Skin:** *alopecia,* rash, sloughing; severe skin irritation with extravasation or contact.
**Other:** precipitation of herpes zoster, *anaphylaxis, secondary malignant disease,* hyperuricemia, amyloidosis.

**INTERACTIONS**
**Drug-drug.** *Anticoagulants, aspirin:* increased risk of bleeding. Avoid concomitant use.
*Myelosuppressives:* concomitant use can cause additive myelosuppression. Monitor patient.

**EFFECTS ON DIAGNOSTIC TESTS**
None reported.

**CONTRAINDICATIONS**
Contraindicated in patients with hypersensitivity to drug and in those with known infectious diseases.

**NURSING CONSIDERATIONS**
• Use cautiously in patients with severe anemia, depressed neutrophil or platelet count, and in those who have recently undergone radiation therapy or chemotherapy. Monitor CBC.
• When given intracavitarily for sclerosing effect, dilute using up to 100 ml of normal saline for injection. Turn patient from side to side every 5 to 10 minutes for 1 hour to distribute drug.
• Monitor serum uric acid level, as ordered. To prevent hyperuricemia with resulting uric acid nephropathy, mechlorethamine may be used with adequate hydration.

• Therapeutic effects are frequently accompanied by toxicity.
• Neurotoxicity increases with dosage and patient age.
• To prevent bleeding, avoid all I.M. injections when platelet count is below 100,000/mm$^3$.
• Anticipate possible blood transfusions because of cumulative anemia. Patients may receive RBC colony-stimulating factors to promote RBC cell production and decrease need for blood transfusions.

**I.V. administration**
• Follow institutional policy to reduce risks. Preparation and administration of parenteral form of drug are associated with carcinogenic, mutagenic, and teratogenic risks for personnel.
• Reconstitute drug using 10 ml of sterile water for injection or normal saline injection. Resulting solution contains 1 mg/ml of mechlorethamine. Give by direct injection into a vein or into tubing of a free-flowing I.V. solution.
• Prepare immediately before infusion. Solution is very unstable. Visually inspect before using; use within 15 minutes, and discard unused solution.
• Dispose of equipment used in preparation and administration of mechlorethamine properly and according to institutional policy. Neutralize unused solution with an equal volume of 5% sodium bicarbonate and 5% sodium thiosulfate for 45 minutes.
• *Alert:* Make sure that I.V. solution doesn't infiltrate. Mechlorethamine is a potent vesicant. If drug extravasates, apply cold compresses for 6 to 12 hours, and infiltrate area with isotonic sodium thiosulfate, as ordered.

**Patient teaching**
• Advise patient to watch for signs and symptoms of infection (fever, sore throat, fatigue) and bleeding (easy bruising, nosebleeds, bleeding gums, melena). Tell patient to take temperature daily.
• Instruct patient to avoid OTC products containing aspirin.
• Caution breast-feeding woman taking drug to discontinue breast-feeding because of risk of infant toxicity.

---

Reactions may be *common,* uncommon, *life-threatening,* or COMMON AND LIFE-THREATENING.

• Advise woman of childbearing age to avoid becoming pregnant during therapy. Suggest that she consult doctor before becoming pregnant.

---

## melphalan
### (L-phenylalanine mustard)
Alkeran

## melphalan hydrochloride
Alkeran

*Pregnancy Risk Category D*

### HOW SUPPLIED
*Tablets (scored):* 2 mg
*Injection:* 50 mg

### ACTION
Cross-links strands of cellular DNA and interferes with RNA transcription, causing an imbalance of growth that leads to cell death. Cell cycle–nonspecific.

| Route | Onset | Peak | Duration |
|-------|-------|------|----------|
| P.O., I.V. | Unknown | Unknown | Unknown |

### INDICATIONS & DOSAGE
*Multiple myeloma—*
**Adults:** initially, 6 mg P.O. daily for 2 to 3 weeks; then drug is stopped for up to 4 weeks or until WBC and platelet counts stop dropping and begin to rise again; maintenance dose is 2 mg daily. Or, 0.15 mg/kg P.O. daily for 7 days, or 0.25 mg/kg for 4 days; repeated q 4 to 6 weeks.

Or, administered I.V. to patients who can't tolerate oral therapy, 16 mg/m² given by infusion over 15 to 20 minutes at 2-week intervals for four doses. After patient has recovered from toxicity, drug given at 4-week intervals.
*Adjust-a-dose:* For patients with renal insufficiency, dosage is reduced up to 50%.
*Nonresectable advanced ovarian cancer—*
**Adults:** 0.2 mg/kg P.O. daily for 5 days. Repeated q 4 to 6 weeks, depending on bone marrow recovery.

### ADVERSE REACTIONS
**CV:** hypotension, tachycardia, edema.
**GI:** nausea, vomiting, diarrhea, oral ulceration, stomatitis.
**Hematologic:** *thrombocytopenia, leukopenia, bone marrow suppression,* hemolytic anemia.
**Hepatic:** *hepatotoxicity.*
**Respiratory:** *pneumonitis, pulmonary fibrosis,* dyspnea, *bronchospasm.*
**Skin:** pruritus, alopecia, urticaria; ulceration at injection site.
**Other:** *anaphylaxis, hypersensitivity reactions,* hyperuricemia.

### INTERACTIONS
**Drug-drug.** *Anticoagulants, aspirin:* increased risk of bleeding. Avoid concomitant use.
*Antigout drugs:* decreased effectiveness. Dosage adjustments may be needed.
*Bone marrow suppressants:* additive toxicity. Monitor closely.
*Cyclosporine:* severe renal failure may occur. Monitor closely.
*Myelosuppressives:* concomitant use can cause additive myelosuppression. Monitor patient.
*Vaccines:* decreased effectiveness of killed virus vaccines and increased risk of toxicity from live virus vaccines. Postpone routine immunization for at least 3 months after last dose of melphalan.
**Drug-food.** *Any food:* decreased oral drug absorption. Give oral drug on empty stomach.

### EFFECTS ON DIAGNOSTIC TESTS
None reported.

### CONTRAINDICATIONS
Contraindicated in patients with hypersensitivity to drug and in those whose disease is known to be resistant to drug. Patients hypersensitive to chlorambucil may have cross-sensitivity to melphalan.

### NURSING CONSIDERATIONS
• Drug isn't recommended in patients with severe leukopenia, thrombocytopenia, or anemia or in those with chronic lymphocytic leukemia. Use cautiously in patients receiving concurrent radiation and chemotherapy.
• Dosage may need to be reduced in patients with renal impairment.

---

*Liquid contains alcohol.    **May contain tartrazine.    †Canada    ‡Australia    §U.K.    ◇OTC

• Melphalan is drug of choice with prednisone in patients with multiple myeloma.
• Give oral form on empty stomach. Food decreases drug absorption.
• Monitor serum uric acid level and CBC, as ordered.
• To prevent bleeding, avoid all I.M. injections when platelet count is below 100,000/mm$^3$.
• Anticipate possible blood transfusions because of cumulative anemia. Patients may receive RBC colony-stimulating factors to promote RBC production and decrease need for blood transfusions
• *Alert:* Don't confuse melphalan with Mephyton.

⚡ **I.V. administration**
• Follow institutional policy to reduce risks. Preparation and administration of parenteral form of drug are associated with carcinogenic, mutagenic, and teratogenic risks for personnel.
• Because drug isn't stable in solution, reconstitute immediately before administering with the 10 ml of sterile diluent supplied by manufacturer. Shake vigorously until solution is clear. The resultant solution will contain 5 mg/ml of melphalan. Immediately dilute required dose in normal saline for injection. Final concentration shouldn't exceed 0.45 mg/ml. Give infusion over 15 to 20 minutes.
• Promptly dilute and administer; reconstituted product begins to degrade within 30 minutes. After final dilution, nearly 1% of drug degrades every 10 minutes. Don't refrigerate reconstituted product because a precipitate will form. Administration of drug must be completed within 60 minutes of reconstitution.

✅ **Patient teaching**
• Advise patient to watch for signs and symptoms of infection (fever, sore throat, fatigue) and bleeding (easy bruising, nosebleeds, bleeding gums, melena). Tell patient to take temperature daily.
• Instruct patient to avoid OTC products containing aspirin.
• Caution breast-feeding woman taking drug to discontinue breast-feeding because of risk of infant toxicity.

• Advise woman of childbearing age to avoid becoming pregnant during therapy. Suggest that she consult doctor before becoming pregnant.

## streptozocin
Zanosar

*Pregnancy Risk Category C*

**HOW SUPPLIED**
*Injection:* 1-g vials

**ACTION**
Unknown. Probably cross-links strands of cellular DNA and interferes with RNA transcription, causing an imbalance of growth that leads to cell death. Cell cycle–nonspecific.

| Route | Onset | Peak | Duration |
|-------|-------|------|----------|
| I.V. | Unknown | Unknown | Unknown |

**INDICATIONS & DOSAGE**
*Metastatic islet cell carcinoma of pancreas—*
**Adults:** 500 mg/m$^2$ I.V. for 5 consecutive days q 6 weeks until maximum benefit or toxicity is observed. Or, 1,000 mg/m$^2$ at weekly intervals for first 2 weeks. Not to exceed single dose of 1,500 mg/m$^2$.

**ADVERSE REACTIONS**
**CNS:** confusion, lethargy, depression.
**GI:** *nausea, vomiting,* diarrhea.
**GU:** *renal toxicity (azotemia, glycosuria, and renal tubular acidosis),* mild proteinuria.
**Hematologic:** anemia, *leukopenia, thrombocytopenia.*
**Hepatic:** elevated liver enzyme levels, jaundice, *liver dysfunction.*
**Metabolic:** hyperglycemia, hypoglycemia, diabetes mellitus.

**INTERACTIONS**
**Drug-drug.** *Doxorubicin:* prolonged elimination half-life of doxorubicin. Dosage of doxorubicin should be reduced.
*Other potentially nephrotoxic drugs such as aminoglycosides:* increased risk of renal toxicity. Use cautiously.

---

Reactions may be *common*, uncommon, *life-threatening*, or COMMON AND LIFE-THREATENING.

*Phenytoin:* may decrease effectiveness of streptozocin in patients with pancreatic cancer. Monitor carefully.

*Myelosuppressives:* concomitant use can cause additive myelosuppression. Monitor patient.

## EFFECTS ON DIAGNOSTIC TESTS
None reported.

## CONTRAINDICATIONS
No known contraindications.

## NURSING CONSIDERATIONS
• Use cautiously in patients with renal disease.
• Obtain renal function tests before therapy, as ordered.
• Monitor renal function tests after each course of therapy, as ordered. Renal toxicity resulting from streptozocin therapy is dose-related and cumulative. Urinalysis; BUN, creatinine, and serum electrolyte levels; and creatinine clearance should be obtained at least weekly during drug therapy. Weekly monitoring should continue for 4 weeks after each course.
• Test urine for protein and glucose levels each nursing shift. Notify doctor if mild proteinuria, one of the first signs of renal toxicity, occurs. Dosage may be reduced.
• Monitor CBC and liver function studies at least weekly, as ordered.
• Make sure patients are being treated with an antiemetic. Nausea and vomiting frequently occur.
• Therapeutic effects are frequently accompanied by toxicity.
• *Alert:* Don't confuse streptozocin with streptomycin.

### ⬛ I.V. administration
• Follow institutional policy to reduce risks. Preparation and administration of parenteral form of drug are associated with carcinogenic, mutagenic, and teratogenic risks for personnel.
• Reconstitute streptozocin powder with 9.5 ml of $D_5W$ or normal saline for injection. This will produce a pale gold solution. May be further diluted with $D_5W$ or normal saline for injection. Infuse over at least 15 minutes to minimize risk of phlebitis.

• Refrigerate unopened vials.
• *Alert:* If extravasation occurs, stop infusion at once and notify doctor.
• Use within 12 hours of reconstitution; product contains no preservatives and isn't intended as a multiple-dose vial.

### ✅ Patient teaching
• Advise patient to watch for signs and symptoms of infection (fever, sore throat, fatigue) and bleeding (easy bruising, nosebleeds, bleeding gums, melena). Tell patient to take temperature daily.
• Caution breast-feeding woman taking drug to discontinue breast-feeding because of risk of infant toxicity.

✳ *NEW DRUG*

## temozolomide
Temodar

*Pregnancy Risk Category D*

## HOW SUPPLIED
*Capsules:* 5 mg, 20 mg, 100 mg, 250 mg

## ACTION
Active metabolite of temozolomide is thought to promote alkylation of DNA in rapidly dividing tissues, interfering with DNA replication.

| Route | Onset | Peak | Duration |
|-------|-------|------|----------|
| P.O. | Unknown | 1 hr | Unknown |

## INDICATIONS & DOSAGE
*Refractory anaplastic astrocytoma that has relapsed following chemotherapy regimen containing a nitrosourea and procarbazine—*
**Adults:** initial cycle: 150 mg/m² P.O. once daily for first 5 days of 28-day treatment cycle. Subsequent cycles: 100 to 200 mg/m² P.O. once daily for first 5 days of subsequent 28-day treatment cycles. Timing and dosage of subsequent cycles must be adjusted according to absolute neutrophil count (ANC) and platelet count measured on cycle day 22 (expected nadir) and cycle day 29 (initiation of next cycle).

Dosage adjustments are based on lowest of ANC and platelet results. For ANC below 1,000/mm³ or platelet count below 50,000/mm³, hold therapy until ANC is over 1,500/mm³ and platelet count is over 100,000/mm³. Reduce dose by 50 mg/m² for subsequent cycle. Minimum dose is 100 mg/m².

For ANC of 1,000 to 1,500/mm³ or platelet count of 50,000 to 100,000/mm³, hold therapy until ANC exceeds 1,500/mm³ and platelet count exceeds 100,000/mm³. Maintain prior dose for subsequent cycle.

For ANC over 1,500/mm³ and platelet count over 100,000/mm³, increase dose to, or maintain at, 200 mg/m² for first 5 days of subsequent cycle.

## ADVERSE REACTIONS
**CNS:** amnesia, anxiety, asthenia, ataxia, confusion, SEIZURES, coordination abnormality, depression, dizziness, dysphasia, fatigue, gait abnormality, headache, hemiparesis, insomnia, local seizures, paresis, paresthesia, somnolence.
**CV:** peripheral edema.
**EENT:** abnormal vision, diplopia, pharyngitis, sinusitis.
**GI:** abdominal pain, anorexia, constipation, diarrhea, nausea, vomiting.
**GU:** increased urinary frequency, urinary incontinence, urinary tract infection.
**Hematologic:** anemia, LEUKOPENIA, NEUTROPENIA, THROMBOCYTOPENIA.
**Metabolic:** weight increase.
**Musculoskeletal:** back pain, myalgia.
**Respiratory:** coughing, upper respiratory tract infection.
**Skin:** pruritus, rash.
**Other:** hyperadrenocorticism, breast pain in women, fever, viral infection.

## INTERACTIONS
**Drug-drug.** *Valproic acid:* decreases oral clearance of temozolomide by about 5%. Use cautiously.
**Drug-food.** *Any food:* reduces rate and extent of drug absorption; however, there are no dietary restrictions with drug administration. Give drug on empty stomach to reduce nausea and vomiting.

## EFFECTS ON DIAGNOSTIC TESTS
None reported.

## CONTRAINDICATIONS
Contraindicated in patients with hypersensitivity to drug or its components and in those allergic to dacarbazine, which is structurally similar to temozolomide.

## NURSING CONSIDERATIONS
• Use with caution in elderly patients and in those with severe hepatic or renal impairment.
• A CBC should be drawn on days 22 and 29 of each treatment cycle. If ANC falls below 1,500/mm³ or platelet count falls below 100,000/mm³, a weekly CBC should be obtained until counts have recovered.
• Women and elderly patients are at higher risk for developing myelosuppression.
• Nausea and vomiting, which may be self-limiting, are most common side effects. Administration on an empty stomach or at bedtime may lessen these effects. Usual antiemetics effectively control nausea and vomiting associated with drug use.
• Avoid skin contact with, or inhalation of, capsule contents if capsule is accidentally opened or damaged. Follow procedures for safe handling and disposal of antineoplastics.
• Store capsules at room temperature (59° to 86° F [15° to 30° C]).

## ☑ Patient teaching
• Emphasize importance of taking dose exactly as prescribed, usually on an empty stomach or at bedtime.
• Stress importance of continuing drug despite nausea and vomiting.
• Tell patient to call immediately if vomiting occurs shortly after a dose is taken.
• Tell patient to promptly report sore throat, fever, unusual bruising or bleeding, rash, or seizures.
• Advise patient to avoid exposure to people with infections.
• Advise sexually active patient to use effective birth control measures during treatment because drug may cause birth defects.
• Tell patient to swallow capsules whole and to not break open the capsules.

---

Reactions may be *common*, uncommon, *life-threatening*, or COMMON AND LIFE-THREATENING.

## thiotepa (TESPA, triethylenethiophosphoramide, TSPA)
Thioplex

*Pregnancy Risk Category D*

### HOW SUPPLIED
*Injection:* 15-mg vials

### ACTION
Cross-links strands of cellular DNA and interferes with RNA transcription, causing an imbalance of growth that leads to cell death. Cell cycle–nonspecific.

| Route | Onset | Peak | Duration |
|---|---|---|---|
| I.V., intra-cavitary | Unknown | Unknown | Unknown |

### INDICATIONS & DOSAGE
*Breast and ovarian cancers, lymphoma, Hodgkin's disease—*
**Adults and children over age 12:** 0.3 to 0.4 mg/kg I.V. q 1 to 4 weeks or 0.2 mg/kg for 4 to 5 days at intervals of 2 to 4 weeks.
*Bladder tumor—*
**Adults and children over age 12:** 30 to 60 mg in 30 to 60 ml of saline instilled in bladder for 2 hours once weekly for 4 weeks.
*Neoplastic effusions—*
**Adults and children over age 12:** 0.6 to 0.8 mg/kg intracavitarily q 1 to 4 weeks.

### ADVERSE REACTIONS
**CNS:** headache, dizziness, fatigue, weakness.
**EENT:** blurred vision, laryngeal edema, conjunctivitis.
**GI:** *nausea, vomiting,* abdominal pain, anorexia, stomatitis.
**GU:** amenorrhea, decreased spermatogenesis, dysuria, urine retention, hemorrhagic cystitis.
**Hematologic:** *leukopenia beginning within 5 to 10 days, thrombocytopenia, neutropenia,* anemia.
**Respiratory:** asthma.
**Skin:** hives, rash, dermatitis, alopecia; pain at injection site.

**Other:** fever, *hypersensitivity, anaphylactic shock*; increased blood and urine levels of uric acid, decreased plasma pseudocholinesterase levels.

### INTERACTIONS
**Drug-drug.** *Anticoagulants, aspirin:* increased risk of bleeding. Avoid concomitant use.
*Myelosuppressives:* concomitant use can cause additive myelosuppression. Monitor patient.
*Neuromuscular blockers:* may prolong muscular paralysis. Monitor closely.
*Other alkylating drugs, irradiation therapy:* may intensify toxicity rather than enhance therapeutic response. Avoid concurrent use.
*Succinylcholine:* increased apnea with concomitant use. Avoid concurrent use.

### EFFECTS ON DIAGNOSTIC TESTS
None reported.

### CONTRAINDICATIONS
Contraindicated in patients with hypersensitivity to drug and in those with severe bone marrow, hepatic, or renal dysfunction.

### NURSING CONSIDERATIONS
• Use in pregnant women isn't recommended except in situations in which benefits outweigh risk of teratogenicity.
• Use cautiously in patients with mild bone marrow suppression and renal or hepatic dysfunction.
• For bladder instillation: dehydrate patient 8 to 10 hours before therapy. Instill drug into bladder by catheter; ask patient to retain solution for 2 hours. Volume may be reduced to 30 ml if discomfort is too great with 60 ml. Reposition patient every 15 minutes for maximum area contact.
• Monitor CBC weekly for at least 3 weeks after last dose, as ordered.
• Discontinue drug and notify doctor if patient's WBC count drops below 3,000/mm$^3$ or if platelet count falls below 150,000/mm$^3$. If WBC count falls below 2,000/mm$^3$ or granulocyte count falls below 1,000/mm$^3$, follow institutional policy for infection control in immunocompromised patients.

*Liquid contains alcohol.  **May contain tartrazine.  †Canada  ‡Australia  §U.K.  ◇OTC

• Monitor serum uric acid levels, as ordered. To prevent hyperuricemia with resulting uric acid nephropathy, allopurinol may be used with adequate hydration.
• Therapeutic effects are frequently accompanied by toxicity.
• To prevent bleeding, avoid all I.M. injections when platelet count is below 100,000/mm³.
• Anticipate blood transfusions because of cumulative anemia. Patient may need injections of RBC colony-stimulating factors to promote RBC production and decrease need for blood transfusions.
• Refrigerate and protect dry powder from direct sunlight to avoid possible drug breakdown.

### I.V. administration
• Follow institutional policy to minimize risks. Preparation and administration of parenteral form of drug are linked with mutagenic, teratogenic, and carcinogenic risks to personnel.
• Reconstitute with 1.5 ml of sterile water for injection. Don't reconstitute with other solutions. Further dilute with normal saline for injection, D₅W, dextrose 5% in normal saline for injection, Ringer's injection, or lactated Ringer's injection. Use solutions within 8 hours.
• If pain occurs at insertion site, dilute drug further or use a local anesthetic, as ordered, to reduce pain. Make sure drug doesn't infiltrate.
• Discard if solution appears grossly opaque or has a precipitate. Solutions should be clear to slightly opaque. To eliminate haze, filter solutions through a 0.22-micron filter before use.

### Patient teaching
• Advise patient to watch for signs and symptoms of infection (fever, sore throat, fatigue) and bleeding (easy bruising, nosebleeds, bleeding gums, melena). Tell patient to take temperature daily. Tell patient to report even mild infections.
• Instruct patient to avoid OTC products containing aspirin.
• Advise breast-feeding woman to stop breast-feeding during therapy because of possible infant toxicity.

• Caution woman of childbearing age to avoid becoming pregnant during therapy. Suggest that she consult doctor before becoming pregnant.

---

Reactions may be *common*, uncommon, *life-threatening*, or COMMON AND LIFE-THREATENING.

capecitabine
cladribine
cytarabine
floxuridine
fludarabine phosphate
fluorouracil
hydroxyurea
mercaptopurine
methotrexate
methotrexate sodium
thioguanine

**COMBINATION PRODUCTS**
None.

---

## capecitabine
Xeloda

*Pregnancy Risk Category D*

---

### HOW SUPPLIED
*Tablets:* 150 mg, 500 mg

### ACTION
Converted to active drug 5-fluorouracil (5-FU), which is metabolized by both normal and tumor cells to metabolites that cause cellular injury via two different mechanisms: interference with DNA synthesis to inhibit cell division and interference with RNA processing and protein synthesis.

| Route | Onset | Peak | Duration |
|-------|-------|------|----------|
| P.O. | Unknown | 1.5-2 hr | Unknown |

### INDICATIONS & DOSAGE
*Patients with metastatic breast cancer resistant to both paclitaxel and an anthracycline-containing chemotherapy regimen or resistant to paclitaxel and for whom further anthracycline therapy isn't indicated—*
**Adults:** 2,500 mg/m² P.O. daily in two divided doses (about 12 hours apart) at end of a meal for 2 weeks, followed by a 1-week rest period given as 3-week cycles.

*Adjust-a-dose:* National Cancer Institute of Canada (NCIC) Common Toxicity Criteria: NCIC grade 2: First appearance, interrupt treatment until resolved to grade 0 to 1; then restart at 100% of starting dose for next cycle. Second appearance, interrupt treatment until resolved to grade 0 to 1 and use 75% of starting dose for next cycle. Third appearance, interrupt treatment until resolved to grade 0 to 1 and use 50% of starting dose for next cycle. Fourth appearance, discontinue treatment permanently.

NCIC grade 3: First appearance, interrupt treatment until resolved to grade 0 to 1 and use 75% of starting dose for next cycle. Second appearance, interrupt treatment until resolved to grade 0 to 1 and use 50% of starting dose for next cycle. Third appearance, discontinue treatment permanently.

NCIC grade 4: First appearance, discontinue treatment permanently or interrupt treatment until resolved to grade 0 to 1 and use 50% of starting dose for next cycle.

*Note:* Toxicity criteria relate to degrees of severity of diarrhea, nausea, vomiting, stomatitis, and hand-and-foot syndrome. Refer to drug package insert for specific toxicity definitions.

### ADVERSE REACTIONS
**CNS:** dizziness, *fatigue,* headache, insomnia, *paresthesia.*
**CV:** edema.
**EENT:** eye irritation.
**GI:** *diarrhea, nausea, vomiting, stomatitis, abdominal pain, constipation, anorexia,* intestinal obstruction, *dyspepsia.*
**Hematologic:** NEUTROPENIA, THROMBOCYTOPENIA, anemia, lymphopenia.
**Hepatic:** *hyperbilirubinemia.*
**Musculoskeletal:** myalgia, pain in limb.
**Skin:** *hand-and-foot syndrome, dermatitis,* nail disorder.
**Other:** *pyrexia,* dehydration.

---

*Liquid contains alcohol.   **May contain tartrazine.   †Canada   ‡Australia   §U.K.   ◇OTC

## INTERACTIONS
**Drug-drug.** *Leucovorin*: increased levels of 5-FU with enhanced toxicity. Monitor patient carefully.

## EFFECTS ON DIAGNOSTIC TESTS
None reported.

## CONTRAINDICATIONS
Contraindicated in patients with hypersensitivity to 5-FU.

## NURSING CONSIDERATIONS
• Use cautiously in patients with history of coronary artery disease, mild to moderate hepatic dysfunction due to liver metastases, hyperbilirubinemia, renal insufficiency, and in elderly patients. Safety and efficacy of drug in patients ages 18 or younger haven't been established.
• Patients over age 80 may experience greater incidence of GI adverse effects.
• Monitor for and notify doctor if severe diarrhea occurs. Give fluid and electrolyte replacement, as ordered, if patient becomes dehydrated. Drug may need to be immediately interrupted until diarrhea resolves or decreases in intensity.
• Monitor for hand-and-foot syndrome (numbness, paresthesia, tingling, painless or painful swelling, erythema, desquamation, blistering and severe pain of hands or feet), hyperbilirubinemia, and severe nausea. Drug therapy will need to be immediately adjusted.
• Hyperbilirubinemia may require stopping drug.
• *Alert:* Monitor patient carefully for toxicity. Toxicity may be managed by symptomatic treatment, dose interruptions, and dosage adjustments.

☑ **Patient teaching**
• Inform patient and caregiver of expected adverse effects of drug, especially nausea, vomiting, diarrhea, and hand-and-foot syndrome (pain, swelling or redness of hands or feet). Tell them that patient-specific dose adaptations during therapy are expected and needed.
• *Alert:* Instruct patient to stop taking drug and contact doctor immediately if following occur: diarrhea (over four bowel movements daily or diarrhea at night), vomiting (two to five episodes in 24 hours), nausea, appetite loss or decrease in amount of food taken each day, stomatitis (pain, redness, swelling or sores in mouth), hand-and-foot syndrome, fever of 100.5° F (38° C) or more, or other evidence of infection.
• Tell patient that most adverse effects improve within 2 to 3 days after stopping drug. If improvement doesn't occur, tell him to contact doctor.
• Tell patient how to take drug. Drug is usually taken for 14 days followed by 7-day rest period (no drug) given as a 21-day cycle. Doctor determines number of treatment cycles.
• Instruct patient to take drug with water within 30 minutes after end of a meal (breakfast and dinner).
• If a combination of tablets is prescribed, teach patient importance of correctly identifying the tablets to avoid possible misdosing.
• For missed doses, instruct patient not to take the missed dose and not to double the next one. Instead, he should continue with regular dosing schedule and check with doctor.
• Instruct patient to inform doctor if he's taking folic acid.
• Advise woman of childbearing age to avoid becoming pregnant during therapy.
• Advise breast-feeding woman to discontinue breast-feeding during therapy.

---

## cladribine (CdA, 2-chlorodeoxyadenosine)
Leustat§, Leustatin

*Pregnancy Risk Category D*

## HOW SUPPLIED
*Injection:* 1 mg/ml, 10-mg vial, preservative-free

## ACTION
Unknown. A purine nucleoside analogue that enters tumor cells and is phosphorylated by deoxycytidine kinase and subsequently converted into an active triphosphate deoxynucleotide. This metabolite probably impairs synthesis of new DNA,

inhibits repair of existing DNA, and disrupts cellular metabolism.

| Route | Onset | Peak | Duration |
|-------|-------|------|----------|
| I.V. | 4 mo | Unknown | > 8 mo |

## INDICATIONS & DOSAGE
*Active hairy cell leukemia—*
**Adults:** 0.09 mg/kg daily by continuous I.V. infusion for 7 days.

## ADVERSE REACTIONS
**CNS:** *malaise, headache, fatigue,* dizziness, insomnia, asthenia.
**CV:** tachycardia, edema.
**EENT:** epistaxis.
**GI:** *nausea, decreased appetite, vomiting, diarrhea,* constipation, abdominal pain.
**Hematologic:** NEUTROPENIA, *anemia,* **thrombocytopenia.**
**Musculoskeletal:** *trunk pain, myalgia, arthralgia.*
**Respiratory:** *abnormal breath or chest sounds, cough,* shortness of breath.
**Skin:** *rash, pruritus, erythema, purpura,* petechiae, *diaphoresis.*
**Other:** *fever,* INFECTION, *chills,* hyperuricemia; *local reaction at injection site.*

## INTERACTIONS
None significant.

## EFFECTS ON DIAGNOSTIC TESTS
None reported.

## CONTRAINDICATIONS
Contraindicated in patients with hypersensitivity to drug.

## NURSING CONSIDERATIONS
• Use cautiously in patients with renal or hepatic impairment.
• Because of risk of hyperuricemia from tumor lysis, administer allopurinol, as ordered, during therapy.
• Monitor hematologic function closely, as ordered, especially during first 4 to 8 weeks of therapy. Cladribine is a toxic drug, and some toxicity is expected during treatment. Severe bone marrow suppression, including neutropenia, anemia, and thrombocytopenia, has commonly been observed in patients treated with drug; many patients also have preexisting

hematologic impairment from their disease.
• Fever is common during first month of therapy. Most patients received parenteral antibiotics.
• To prevent bleeding, avoid all I.M. injections when platelet count is below 100,000/mm³.
• If WBC count falls below 2,000/mm³ or granulocyte count falls below 1,000/mm³, follow institutional policy for infection control in immunocompromised patients.
• Anticipate blood transfusions because of cumulative anemia. Patient may receive injections of RBC colony-stimulating factors to promote RBC production and decrease need for blood transfusions.

### ⬤ I.V. administration
• For a 24-hour infusion, add calculated dose to 500-ml infusion bag of normal saline for injection. Once diluted, administer promptly or store in refrigerator for no more than 8 hours. Don't use solutions that contain dextrose because studies have shown increased degradation of drug. Repeat preparation daily for 7 consecutive days.
• *Alert:* Because drug product doesn't contain bacteriostatic drugs, use strict aseptic technique to prepare daily admixture.
• Or, prepare a 7-day infusion solution, using bacteriostatic NaCl for injection, which contains 0.9% benzyl alcohol. Studies have shown acceptable physical and chemical stability using Pharmacia Deltec medication cassettes. First, pass calculated amount of drug through a disposable 0.22-micron hydrophilic syringe filter into a sterile infusion reservoir. Then, add sufficient bacteriostatic NaCl injection to bring total volume to 100 ml. Clamp off the line; then disconnect and discard filter. If needed, aseptically aspirate air bubbles from the reservoir using a new filter or a sterile vent filter assembly.
• Because calculated dose dilutes benzyl alcohol preservative, 7-day infusion solutions prepared for patients over 187 lb may have reduced preservative effectiveness.
• Refrigerate unopened vials at 36° to 46° F (2° to 8° C) and protect from light. Although freezing doesn't adversely af-

fect drug, a precipitate may form; this will disappear if drug is allowed to warm to room temperature gradually and vial is vigorously shaken. Don't heat or microwave; don't refreeze.

### ☑ Patient teaching
• Instruct patient to watch for signs and symptoms of infection and bleeding (easy bruising, nosebleeds, bleeding gums, melena). Tell patient to take temperature daily.
• Caution woman of childbearing age to avoid becoming pregnant during therapy because of risk of fetal malformations.
• Advise breast-feeding woman to discontinue breast-feeding during therapy because of possible infant toxicity.

---

## cytarabine
## (ara-C, cytosine arabinoside)
Cytosar†, Cytosar-U

*Pregnancy Risk Category D*

### HOW SUPPLIED
*Injection:* 100-mg, 500-mg, 1-g, 2-g vials

### ACTION
Inhibits DNA synthesis.

| Route | Onset | Peak | Duration |
|---|---|---|---|
| I.V., intra-thecal | Unknown | Unknown | Unknown |
| S.C. | Unknown | 20-60 min | Unknown |

### INDICATIONS & DOSAGE
*Acute nonlymphocytic leukemia, acute lymphocytic leukemia, blast phase of chronic myelocytic leukemia—*
**Adults and children:** 100 mg/m² daily by continuous I.V. infusion or 100 mg/m² I.V. q 12 hours. Given for 7 days and repeated q 2 weeks. For maintenance, 1 mg/kg S.C. once or twice weekly.
*Meningeal leukemia—*
**Adults and children:** highly variable from 5 to 75 mg/m² intrathecally. Frequency also varies from once daily for 4 days to once q 4 days. The most frequently used dose is 30 mg/m² q 4 days until CSF fluid is normal; then one additional dose.

### ADVERSE REACTIONS
**CNS:** neurotoxicity, malaise, dizziness, headache.
**CV:** *thrombophlebitis*, edema.
**EENT:** conjunctivitis.
**GI:** *nausea, vomiting, diarrhea, anorexia, anal ulceration,* abdominal pain; oral ulcers in 5 to 10 days; projectile vomiting, bowel necrosis with high doses given rapid I.V.
**GU:** urine retention, renal dysfunction.
**Hematologic:** *leukopenia (initial WBC count nadir 7 to 9 days after drug is stopped and a second, more severe, nadir 15 to 24 days after drug is stopped);* anemia; reticulocytopenia; *thrombocytopenia (platelet count nadir occurring on days 12 to 15);* megaloblastosis.
**Hepatic:** *hepatotoxicity,* jaundice.
**Musculoskeletal:** myalgia, bone pain.
**Skin:** *rash,* pruritus, alopecia, freckling.
**Other:** flulike syndrome, hyperuricemia, infection, *fever, anaphylaxis.*

### INTERACTIONS
**Drug-drug.** *Digoxin:* may decrease digoxin absorption. Monitor closely. Digoxin oral liquid and liquid-filled capsules may not be affected.
*Flucytosine:* decreased flucytosine activity. Avoid concomitant use.
*Gentamicin:* decreased activity against *Klebsiella pneumoniae.* Avoid concomitant use.

### EFFECTS ON DIAGNOSTIC TESTS
None reported.

### CONTRAINDICATIONS
Contraindicated in patients with hypersensitivity to drug.

### NURSING CONSIDERATIONS
• Use cautiously in patients with hepatic or renal compromise, gout, or myelosuppression.
• For intrathecal administration, use preservative-free normal saline. Add 5 ml to 100-mg vial or 10 ml to 500-mg vial. Use immediately after reconstitution. Discard unused drug.
• Monitor fluid intake and output carefully. Maintain high fluid intake and give allopurinol, if ordered, to avoid urate nephrop-

---

athy in leukemia-induction therapy. Monitor serum uric acid level, as ordered.
• Monitor hepatic and renal function studies and CBC, as ordered.
• Therapy may be modified or stopped if granulocyte count is below 1,000/mm³ or if platelet count is below 50,000/mm³.
• Corticosteroid eyedrops are prescribed to prevent drug-induced keratitis.
• Provide diligent mouth care to help prevent stomatitis.
• *Alert:* Assess patient receiving high doses for neurotoxicity, which may first appear as nystagmus, but can progress to ataxia and cerebellar dysfunction.
• To prevent bleeding, avoid all I.M. injections when platelet count is below 100,000/mm³.
• Anticipate blood transfusions because of cumulative anemia. Patient may receive RBC colony-stimulating factors to promote RBC production and decrease need for blood transfusions.
• Therapeutic effects are frequently accompanied by toxicity.

**I.V. administration**
• To reduce nausea, give antiemetic before administering, as ordered. Nausea and vomiting are more frequent when large doses are administered rapidly by I.V. push. These reactions are less frequent when given by infusion.
• Follow institutional policy to reduce risks. Preparation and administration of parenteral form are associated with carcinogenic, mutagenic, and teratogenic risks for personnel.
• Reconstitute drug using the provided diluent, which is bacteriostatic water for injection containing benzyl alcohol. Avoid this diluent when preparing drug for neonates or for intrathecal use. Reconstitute drug in 100-mg vial with 5 ml of diluent or 500-mg vial with 10 ml of diluent. Reconstituted solution is stable for 48 hours. Discard cloudy reconstituted solution.
• For I.V. infusion, further dilute using normal saline for injection or D₅W.

**Patient teaching**
• Instruct patient to watch for signs and symptoms of infection (fever, sore throat,

fatigue) and bleeding (easy bruising, nosebleeds, bleeding gums, melena). Tell patient to take temperature daily.
• Advise breast-feeding woman to discontinue breast-feeding during therapy because of possible infant toxicity.
• Caution woman of childbearing age to avoid becoming pregnant during therapy. Recommend that she consult doctor before becoming pregnant. Drug may harm fetus.

**floxuridine (fluorodeoxyuridine)**
FUDR

*Pregnancy Risk Category D*

**HOW SUPPLIED**
*Powder for injection:* 500 mg for reconstitution (5-ml, 10-ml vials)
*Preservative-free injection:* 100 mg/ml (5-ml vials)

**ACTION**
Inhibits DNA synthesis.

| Route | Onset | Peak | Duration |
|---|---|---|---|
| Intra-arterial | Unknown | Unknown | Unknown |

**INDICATIONS & DOSAGE**
*GI adenocarcinoma metastatic to the liver—*
Adults: 0.1 to 0.6 mg/kg daily by intra-arterial infusion for 14 to 21 days or until toxicity occurs; or 0.4 to 0.6 mg/kg daily into hepatic artery.

**ADVERSE REACTIONS**
CNS: malaise, weakness, headache, lethargy, disorientation, confusion, euphoria.
CV: thrombophlebitis, *myocardial ischemia,* angina.
EENT: blurred vision, nystagmus, photophobia, epistaxis.
GI: *anorexia, stomatitis, nausea, vomiting, diarrhea, bleeding, abdominal pain, enteritis,* GI ulceration, intrahepatic and extrahepatic biliary sclerosis, acalculous cholecystitis, hepatotoxicity.

**Hematologic:** *leukopenia, anemia, thrombocytopenia, agranulocytosis.*
**Skin:** *erythema,* dermatitis, pruritus, rash, alopecia, photosensitivity.
**Other:** *anaphylaxis,* fever.

**INTERACTIONS**
**Drug-lifestyle.** *Sun exposure:* may increase skin reaction. Take precautions.

**EFFECTS ON DIAGNOSTIC TESTS**
None reported.

**CONTRAINDICATIONS**
Contraindicated in patients with poor nutritional state, bone marrow suppression, or serious infection.

**NURSING CONSIDERATIONS**
• Use cautiously following high-dose pelvic radiation therapy or use of alkylating drugs and in patients with impaired hepatic or renal function.
• Check line for bleeding, blockage, displacement, or leakage.
• Monitor fluid intake and output, CBC, and renal and hepatic function, as ordered.
• Use of antacid eases but won't prevent GI distress. An $H_2$ antihistamine is recommended to prevent peptic ulcer disease during drug therapy.
• Provide diligent mouth care to help prevent stomatitis.
• Severe skin and adverse GI reactions require stopping drug.
• Discontinue drug and notify doctor if patient's WBC count drops below 3,500/mm³ or if platelet count falls below 100,000/mm³. If WBC count falls below 2,000/mm³ or granulocyte count falls below 1,000/mm³, follow institutional policy for infection control in immunocompromised patients.
• To prevent bleeding, avoid all I.M. injections when platelet count is below 100,000/mm³.
• Anticipate blood transfusions because of cumulative anemia. Patients may receive injections of RBC colony-stimulating factors to promote RBC production and decrease need for blood transfusions.

• **Alert:** Don't confuse floxuridine with fludarabine or flucytosine.

**⚠ I.V. administration**
• Follow institutional policy to reduce risks. Preparation and administration of parenteral form of drug are associated with carcinogenic, mutagenic, and teratogenic risks for personnel.
• Reconstitute with sterile water for injection. To prepare infusion, dilute in $D_5W$ or normal saline solution.
• Refrigerated solution is stable for no more than 2 weeks.
• Use an infusion pump with intra-arterial infusions.

**✓ Patient teaching**
• Inform patient that therapeutic effect may be delayed 1 to 6 weeks.
• Inform patient receiving drug at home to monitor placement of needle into catheter site and to call his infusion provider immediately if needle becomes dislodged.
• Advise patient to watch for signs and symptoms of infection (fever, sore throat, fatigue) and bleeding (easy bruising, nosebleeds, bleeding gums, melena). Tell patient to take temperature daily.
• Tell patient that exposure to sun may initiate or intensify skin reaction.
• Advise breast-feeding woman to discontinue breast-feeding during therapy because of possible infant toxicity.
• Caution woman of childbearing age to avoid becoming pregnant during therapy. Recommend that she consult doctor before becoming pregnant.

---

## fludarabine phosphate
Fludara

*Pregnancy Risk Category D*

**HOW SUPPLIED**
*Powder for injection:* 50 mg

**ACTION**
Unknown. An antineoplastic antimetabolite that may have multifaceted actions. After conversion to its active metabolite, fludarabine interferes with DNA synthesis

by inhibiting DNA polymerase alpha, ribonucleotide reductase, and DNA primase.

| Route | Onset | Peak | Duration |
|-------|-------|------|----------|
| I.V. | 7-21 wk | Unknown | Unknown |

## INDICATIONS & DOSAGE
*B-cell chronic lymphocytic leukemia in patients who have either not responded or responded inadequately to at least one standard alkylating drug regimen—*
**Adults:** 25 mg/m$^2$ I.V. over 30 minutes for 5 consecutive days. Cycle repeated q 28 days.

## ADVERSE REACTIONS
**CNS:** *fatigue, malaise, weakness, paresthesia,* peripheral neuropathy, headache, sleep disorder, depression, cerebellar syndrome, transient ischemic attack, agitation, *confusion, coma, death.*
**CV:** *edema,* angina, phlebitis, ***arrhythmias, heart failure, MI,*** supraventricular tachycardia, deep venous thrombosis, ***aneurysm, hemorrhage, CVA.***
**EENT:** *visual disturbances,* hearing loss, delayed blindness, sinusitis, pharyngitis, epistaxis.
**GI:** *nausea, vomiting, diarrhea,* constipation, *anorexia,* stomatitis, *GI bleeding,* esophagitis, mucositis.
**GU:** dysuria, *urinary infection* or hesitancy, proteinuria, hematuria, ***renal failure.***
**Hematologic:** ***hemolytic anemia,*** MYELOSUPPRESSION.
**Hepatic:** *liver failure,* cholelithiasis.
**Metabolic:** hypocalcemia, hyperkalemia, hyperglycemia, dehydration, hyperuricemia, hyperphosphatemia.
**Musculoskeletal:** *myalgia.*
**Respiratory:** *cough, pneumonia, dyspnea, upper respiratory tract infection,* allergic pneumonitis, hemoptysis, hypoxia, bronchitis.
**Skin:** *rash,* pruritus, alopecia, seborrhea, diaphoresis.
**Other:** *fever, chills, pain,* tumor lysis syndrome, INFECTION, ***anaphylaxis.***

## INTERACTIONS
**Drug-drug.** *Other myelosuppressives:* increased toxicity. Avoid concomitant use.

*Pentostatin:* increases risk of pulmonary toxicity, which can be fatal. Avoid concomitant administration.

## EFFECTS ON DIAGNOSTIC TESTS
None reported.

## CONTRAINDICATIONS
Contraindicated in patients with hypersensitivity to drug or its components.

## NURSING CONSIDERATIONS
• Use cautiously in patients with renal insufficiency.
• *Alert:* Monitor patient closely and expect modified dosage based on toxicity. Most toxic effects are dose-dependent. Advanced age, renal insufficiency, and bone marrow impairment may predispose patients to increased or excessive toxicity.
• Careful hematologic monitoring is needed, especially of neutrophil and platelet counts. Bone marrow suppression can be severe.
• To prevent bleeding, avoid all I.M. injections when platelet count is below 100,000/mm$^3$.
• Anticipate blood transfusions because of cumulative anemia. Patients may receive RBC colony-stimulating factors to promote RBC production and decrease need for blood transfusions.
• Optimal duration of therapy isn't yet determined. Current recommendations suggest three additional cycles after achieving maximal response before discontinuing therapy.
• Take preventive measures before starting drug treatment. Hyperuricemia, hypocalcemia, hyperkalemia, and renal failure may result from rapid lysis of tumor cells.
• Store drug in refrigerator at 36° to 46° F (2° to 8° C).
• *Alert:* Don't confuse fludarabine with floxuridine or flucytosine.

### ⬙ I.V. administration
• Follow institutional policy to reduce risks. Preparation and administration of parenteral form of drug are associated with mutagenic, teratogenic, and carcinogenic risks for personnel.

• To prepare solution, add 2 ml of sterile water for injection to the solid cake of fludarabine. Dissolution should occur within 15 seconds; each milliliter will contain 25 mg of drug. Dilute further in 100 or 125 ml of $D_5W$ or normal saline for injection. Use within 8 hours of reconstitution.

☑ **Patient teaching**
• Instruct patient to watch for signs and symptoms of infection (fever, sore throat, fatigue) and bleeding (easy bruising, nosebleeds, bleeding gums, melena). Tell patient to take temperature daily.
• Advise woman of childbearing age to avoid becoming pregnant during therapy. Recommend that she consult doctor before becoming pregnant.
• Caution breast-feeding woman to discontinue breast-feeding during therapy because of possible infant toxicity.

# fluorouracil
## (5-fluorouracil, 5-FU)
Adrucil, Efudex, Fluoroplex

*Pregnancy Risk Category D (injection); X (topical form)*

## HOW SUPPLIED
*Injection:* 50 mg/ml
*Cream:* 1%, 5%
*Topical solution:* 1%, 2%, 5%

## ACTION
Thought to inhibit DNA and RNA synthesis.

| Route | Onset | Peak | Duration |
|-------|-------|------|----------|
| I.V., topical | Unknown | Unknown | Unknown |

## INDICATIONS & DOSAGE
*Colon, rectal, breast, stomach, and pancreatic cancers—*
**Adults:** initially, 12 mg/kg I.V. daily for 4 days; if no toxicity, 6 mg/kg given on days 6, 8, 10, and 12; then a single weekly maintenance dose of 10 to 15 mg/kg I.V. begun after toxicity (if any) from initial course has subsided. (Dosages recommended based on actual body weight unless patient is obese or retaining fluid.)

Maximum single recommended dose is 800 mg/day.
*Palliative treatment of advanced colorectal cancer—*
**Adults:** 425 mg/m² I.V. daily for 5 consecutive days. Given with 20 mg/m² of leucovorin I.V. Repeated at 4-week intervals for two additional courses; then repeated at intervals of 4 to 5 weeks if tolerated.
*Multiple actinic (solar) keratoses, superficial basal cell carcinoma—*
**Adults:** apply cream or topical solution once daily or b.i.d. Usual duration of treatment is 2 to 6 weeks.

## ADVERSE REACTIONS
**CNS:** acute cerebellar syndrome, confusion, disorientation, euphoria, ataxia, headache, nystagmus, *weakness, malaise.*
**CV:** *myocardial ischemia,* angina, thrombophlebitis.
**EENT:** epistaxis, photophobia, lacrimation, lacrimal duct stenosis, visual changes.
**GI:** *stomatitis, GI ulcer, nausea, vomiting, diarrhea, anorexia,* GI bleeding.
**Hematologic:** *leukopenia, thrombocytopenia, agranulocytosis,* anemia; *WBC count nadir 9 to 14 days after first dose; platelet count nadir in 7 to 14 days.*
**GU:** increased 5-hydroxyindoleacetic acid in urine.
**Hepatic:** may increase alkaline phosphatase, serum transaminases, bilirubin, and LD levels.
**Skin:** *dermatitis; erythema; scaling; pruritus;* nail changes; pigmented palmar creases; erythematous, contact dermatitis, desquamative rash of hands and feet ("hand-and-foot syndrome" with long-term use); photosensitivity, *reversible alopecia.*
**Other:** *pain, burning,* soreness, suppuration, swelling with topical use, *anaphylaxis;* decreased plasma albumin.

## INTERACTIONS
**Drug-drug.** *Leucovorin calcium, previous treatment with alkylating drugs:* increased toxicity of fluorouracil. Use with extreme caution.
**Drug-lifestyle.** *Sun exposure:* photosensitivity reactions may occur. Take precautions.

---

Reactions may be *common,* uncommon, *life-threatening,* or **COMMON AND LIFE-THREATENING.**

## EFFECTS ON DIAGNOSTIC TESTS
None reported.

## CONTRAINDICATIONS
Contraindicated in patients with hypersensitivity to drug and in those with bone marrow suppression (WBC counts of 5,000/mm³ or less or platelet counts of 100,000/mm³ or less) or potentially serious infections; also contraindicated in those who are in a poor nutritional state and in those who have had major surgery within previous month.

## NURSING CONSIDERATIONS
• Use cautiously after high-dose pelvic radiation therapy or use of alkylating drugs, and in patients with impaired hepatic or renal function or widespread neoplastic infiltration of bone marrow.
• Apply topical form with caution near eyes, nose, and mouth.
• Avoid occlusive dressings with topical form because they increase risk of inflammatory reactions in adjacent normal skin.
• Apply topical form with a nonmetal applicator or suitable gloves. Wash hands immediately after handling topical form.
• Expect to use 1% topical concentration on the face. Higher concentrations are used for thicker-skinned areas or resistant lesions.
• Expect to use 5% topical strength for superficial basal cell carcinoma confirmed by biopsy.
• Ingestion and systemic absorption of topical form may cause leukopenia, thrombocytopenia, stomatitis, diarrhea, or GI ulceration, bleeding, and hemorrhage. Application to large ulcerated areas may cause systemic toxicity.
• Watch for stomatitis or diarrhea (signs of toxicity). May use topical oral anesthetic to soothe lesions, as ordered. Discontinue drug and notify doctor if diarrhea occurs.
• Encourage diligent oral hygiene to prevent superinfection of denuded mucosa.
• Monitor WBC and platelet counts daily, as ordered. Watch for ecchymoses, petechiae, easy bruising, and anemia.
• Monitor fluid intake and output, CBC, and renal and hepatic function tests, as ordered.

• Dermatologic adverse effects are reversible when drug is stopped.
• To prevent bleeding, avoid all I.M. injections when platelet count is below 100,000/mm³.
• Anticipate blood transfusions because of cumulative anemia. Patient may receive injections of RBC colony-stimulating factors to promote RBC production and decrease need for blood transfusions.
• *Alert:* Fluorouracil toxicity may be delayed for 1 to 3 weeks.
• Drug is sometimes ordered as 5-fluorouracil or 5-FU. The numeral 5 is part of drug name and shouldn't be confused with dosage units.
• *Alert:* Don't confuse fluorouracil with floxuridine, fludarabine, or flucytosine.

### I.V. administration
• Follow institutional policy to reduce risks. Preparation and administration of parenteral form of drug are associated with carcinogenic, mutagenic, and teratogenic risks for personnel.
• Give antiemetic, as ordered, before administering drug to reduce nausea.
• Drug may be administered by direct injection without dilution. For I.V. infusion, drug may be diluted with $D_5W$, sterile water for injection or normal saline for injection. Discard unused portion of vial after 1 hour.
• Don't use cloudy solution. If crystals form, redissolve by warming.
• Use plastic I.V. containers for administering continuous infusions. Solution is more stable in plastic I.V. bags than in glass bottles.
• Don't refrigerate fluorouracil. Protect drug from sunlight.

### Patient teaching
• Warn patient that alopecia may occur, but that it's reversible.
• Caution patient to avoid prolonged exposure to sunlight or ultraviolet light when topical form is used.
• Tell patient to use highly protective sunblock to avoid inflammatory erythematous dermatitis. Long-term use of drug is associated with erythematous, desquamative rash of the hands and feet. May be

treated with pyridoxine (50 to 150 mg P.O. daily) for 5 to 7 days.
• Warn patient that topically treated area may be unsightly during therapy and for several weeks afterward. Complete healing may take 1 or 2 months.
• Caution woman of childbearing age to avoid becoming pregnant during therapy. Recommend that she consult doctor before becoming pregnant.
• Advise breast-feeding woman to discontinue breast-feeding during therapy because of possible infant toxicity.

---

### hydroxyurea
Droxia, Hydrea**

*Pregnancy Risk Category D*

### HOW SUPPLIED
*Capsules:* 200 mg, 300 mg, 400 mg, 500 mg

### ACTION
Unknown. Thought to inhibit DNA synthesis.

| Route | Onset | Peak | Duration |
|-------|-------|------|----------|
| P.O. | Unknown | 2 hr | 24 hr |

### INDICATIONS & DOSAGE
*Melanoma; resistant chronic myelocytic leukemia; recurrent, metastatic, or inoperable ovarian cancer; head and neck cancers—*
**Adults:** 80 mg/kg P.O. as single dose q 3 days; or 20 to 30 mg/kg P.O. as single daily dose.
*To reduce frequency of painful crises and need for blood transfusions in adult patients with sickle cell anemia with recurrent moderate to severe painful crises—*
**Adults:** 15 mg/kg P.O. once daily. If blood counts are in acceptable range, dose may be increased by 5 mg/kg/day q 12 weeks until maximum tolerated dose or 35 mg/kg/day has been reached. If blood counts are considered toxic, withhold drug until hematologic recovery occurs. Resume treatment after reducing dose by 2.5 mg/kg/day. Every 12 weeks, drug may then be adjusted up or down in 2.5-mg/

kg/day increments until patient is at stable, nontoxic dose for 24 weeks.

### ADVERSE REACTIONS
**CNS:** hallucinations, headache, dizziness, disorientation, *seizures,* malaise.
**GI:** *anorexia, nausea, vomiting, diarrhea,* stomatitis, constipation.
**GU:** increased BUN and serum creatinine levels.
**Hematologic:** *leukopenia, thrombocytopenia, anemia, megaloblastosis; bone marrow suppression (dose-limiting and dose-related with rapid recovery).*
**Skin:** rash, itching.
**Other:** fever, chills, increased serum uric acid levels.

### INTERACTIONS
**Drug-drug.** *Cytotoxic drugs, radiation therapy:* enhanced toxicity of hydroxyurea. Use together cautiously.

### EFFECTS ON DIAGNOSTIC TESTS
None reported.

### CONTRAINDICATIONS
Contraindicated in patients with hypersensitivity to drug and in those with marked bone marrow depression (leukopenia [less than 2,500/mm³ WBCs], thrombocytopenia [less than 100,000/ mm³ platelets], or severe anemia).

### NURSING CONSIDERATIONS
• Use cautiously in patients with renal dysfunction.
• Routinely measure BUN, uric acid, and serum creatinine levels; blood counts must be monitored every 2 weeks.
• Acceptable blood counts during dosage adjustment: neutrophils, 2,500 cells/mm³ or more; platelets, 95,000/mm³ or more; hemoglobin, over 5.3 g/dl; and reticulocytes (if Hg is below 9 g/dl), over 95,000/ mm³. Toxic levels are considered when neutrophil count is below 2,000 cells/ mm³, platelets are below 80,000/mm³, hemoglobin is under 4.5 g/dl, and reticulocytes (if Hg is below 9 g/dl) are below 80,000/mm³.
• Monitor fluid intake and output; keep patient hydrated.

---

- To prevent bleeding, avoid all I.M. injections when platelet count is below 100,000/mm$^3$.
- Anticipate blood transfusions because of cumulative anemia. Patient may receive injections of RBC colony-stimulating factors to promote RBC production and decrease need for blood transfusions.
- Dosage modification may be needed after chemotherapy or radiation therapy.
- Auditory and visual hallucinations and hematologic toxicity increase when renal function decreases.
- Drug crosses blood-brain barrier.
- Concomitant radiation therapy may increase incidence or severity of GI distress or stomatitis.

☑ **Patient teaching**
- Tell patient who can't swallow capsules that he may empty contents into water and take immediately. Patient should rinse mouth with water after taking drug this way. Inform patient that some inert material may not dissolve.
- Advise patient to watch for signs and symptoms of infection (fever, sore throat, fatigue) and bleeding (easy bruising, nosebleeds, bleeding gums, melena). He should also take his temperature daily.
- Caution woman of childbearing age to avoid becoming pregnant during therapy. Recommend that she consult doctor before becoming pregnant.

---

**mercaptopurine**
**(6-mercaptopurine, 6-MP)**
Purinethol

*Pregnancy Risk Category D*

**HOW SUPPLIED**
*Tablets (scored):* 50 mg

**ACTION**
Inhibits RNA and DNA synthesis.

| Route | Onset | Peak | Duration |
|-------|-------|------|----------|
| P.O. | Unknown | Unknown | Unknown |

**INDICATIONS & DOSAGE**
*Acute myeloblastic leukemia, chronic myelocytic leukemia—*
**Adults:** 80 to 100 mg/m$^2$ (rounded to nearest 25 mg) P.O. daily as single dose, up to 5 mg/kg/day.
**Children:** 75 mg/m$^2$ (rounded to nearest 25 mg) P.O. daily.
*Acute lymphoblastic leukemia—*
**Children:** 75 mg/m$^2$ (rounded to nearest 25 mg) P.O. daily.
   *Note:* After remission is attained, usual maintenance dose for adults and children is 1.5 to 2.5 mg/kg/day.

**ADVERSE REACTIONS**
**GI:** nausea, vomiting, anorexia, painful oral ulcers, diarrhea, *pancreatitis,* GI ulceration.
**Hematologic:** *leukopenia, thrombocytopenia,* anemia.
**Hepatic:** *jaundice, hepatotoxicity.*
**Skin:** rash, hyperpigmentation.
**Other:** hyperuricemia.

**INTERACTIONS**
**Drug-drug.** *Allopurinol:* slowed inactivation of mercaptopurine. Decrease mercaptopurine to 25% or 33% of normal dose.
*Co-trimoxazole:* enhanced bone marrow suppression; monitor carefully.
*Hepatotoxic drugs:* may enhance hepatotoxicity of mercaptopurine. Monitor for hepatotoxicity.
*Nondepolarizing neuromuscular blockers:* antagonized muscle relaxant effect. Notify anesthesiologist that patient is receiving mercaptopurine.
*Warfarin:* antagonized or potentiated anticoagulant effect. Monitor PT and INR.

**EFFECTS ON DIAGNOSTIC TESTS**
Drug therapy may cause falsely elevated serum glucose and uric acid levels when sequential multiple analyzer is used.

**CONTRAINDICATIONS**
Contraindicated in patients whose disease has shown resistance to drug.

**NURSING CONSIDERATIONS**
- Dosage modifications may be needed after chemotherapy or radiation therapy in patients with depressed neutrophil or

---

*Liquid contains alcohol.   **May contain tartrazine.   †Canada   ‡Australia   §U.K.   ◇OTC

platelet counts and in those with impaired hepatic or renal function.

• Drug is sometimes ordered as 6-mercaptopurine or 6-MP. The numeral 6 is part of drug name and doesn't signify number of dosage units.

• Monitor blood counts and serum transaminase, alkaline phosphatase, and bilirubin levels weekly during induction and monthly during maintenance, as ordered.

• Leukopenia, thrombocytopenia, or anemia may persist for several days after drug is stopped.

• Observe for signs of bleeding and infection.

• Monitor fluid intake and output. Encourage adequate fluid intake (3 L daily).

• **Alert:** Watch for jaundice, clay-colored stools, and frothy, dark urine. Hepatic dysfunction is reversible when drug is stopped. If hepatic tenderness occurs, drug should be stopped and doctor notified.

• Monitor serum uric acid level, as ordered. If allopurinol is ordered, use cautiously.

• To prevent bleeding, avoid all I.M. injections when platelet count is below 100,000/mm$^3$.

• Anticipate blood transfusions because of cumulative anemia. Patient may receive injections of RBC colony-stimulating factors to promote RBC production and decrease need for blood transfusions.

• GI adverse reactions are less common in children than in adults.

☑ **Patient teaching**
• Instruct patient to watch for signs and symptoms of infection (fever, sore throat, fatigue) and bleeding (easy bruising, nosebleeds, bleeding gums, melena). Tell patient to take temperature daily.

• Caution woman of childbearing age to avoid becoming pregnant during therapy. Recommend that she consult doctor before becoming pregnant.

• Advise breast-feeding woman to discontinue breast-feeding during therapy because of possible infant toxicity.

# methotrexate
# (amethopterin, MTX)

## methotrexate sodium
Folex, Folex PFS, Rheumatrex

*Pregnancy Risk Category X*

## HOW SUPPLIED
*Tablets (scored):* 2.5 mg
*Injection:* 20-mg, 25-mg, 50-mg, 100-mg, 250-mg vials, lyophilized powder, preservative free; 25-mg/ml vials, preservative-free solution; 2.5-mg/ml, 25-mg/ml vials, lyophilized powder, preserved

## ACTION
Prevents reduction of folic acid to tetrahydrofolate by binding to dihydrofolate reductase.

| Route | Onset | Peak | Duration |
|-------|-------|------|----------|
| P.O. | Unknown | 1-2 hr | Unknown |
| I.V. | Unknown | Immediate | Unknown |
| I.M. | Unknown | 0.5-1 hr | Unknown |
| Intrathecal | Unknown | Unknown | Unknown |

## INDICATIONS & DOSAGE
*Trophoblastic tumors (choriocarcinoma, hydatidiform mole)—*
**Adults:** 15 to 30 mg P.O. or I.M. daily for 5 days. Repeated after 1 or more weeks, based on response or toxicity. Number of courses is three to five, not to exceed five.
*Acute lymphocytic leukemia—*
**Adults and children:** 3.3 mg/m$^2$/day P.O., I.M., or I.V. for 4 to 6 weeks or until remission occurs; then 20 to 30 mg/m$^2$ P.O. or I.M. weekly in two divided doses or 2.5 mg/kg I.V. q 14 days.
*Meningeal leukemia—*
**Adults and children:** 12 mg/m$^2$ or less (maximum 15 mg) intrathecally q 2 to 5 days until CSF is normal; then one additional dose.
*Burkitt's lymphoma (stage I, II, or III)—*
**Adults:** 10 to 25 mg P.O. daily for 4 to 8 days with 1-week rest intervals.
*Lymphosarcoma (stage III)—*
**Adults:** 0.625 to 2.5 mg/kg daily P.O., I.M., or I.V.

*Osteosarcoma—*
**Adults:** initially, 12 g/m² I.V. as 4-hour infusion. Subsequent doses 12 to 15 g/m² I.V. as 4-hour infusion given at post-operative weeks 4, 5, 6, 7, 11, 12, 15, 16, 29, 30, 44, and 45. Given with leucovorin, 15 mg P.O., I.M., or I.V. q 6 hours for 10 doses, beginning 24 hours after start of methotrexate infusion.
*Mycosis fungoides—*
**Adults:** 2.5 to 10 mg P.O. daily; or 50 mg I.M. weekly; or 25 mg I.M. twice weekly.
*Psoriasis—*
**Adults:** 10 to 25 mg P.O., I.M., or I.V. as single weekly dose; or 2.5 mg P.O. every 12 hours for three doses. Dosage shouldn't exceed 30 mg/week.
*Rheumatoid arthritis—*
**Adults:** initially, 7.5 mg P.O. weekly, either in single dose or divided as 2.5 mg P.O. q 12 hours for three doses once weekly. Dosage may be gradually increased to maximum of 20 mg weekly.

## ADVERSE REACTIONS
**CNS:** *arachnoiditis within hours of intrathecal use,* subacute neurotoxicity possibly beginning few weeks later, *leukoencephalopathy,* demyelination, malaise, fatigue, dizziness, headache, aphasia, hemiparesis, drowsiness, *seizures.*
**EENT:** pharyngitis, blurred vision.
**GI:** gingivitis, *stomatitis, diarrhea,* abdominal distress, anorexia, GI ulceration and bleeding, enteritis, *nausea, vomiting.*
**GU:** nephropathy, *tubular necrosis, renal failure,* hematuria, menstrual dysfunction, defective spermatogenesis, infertility, abortion, cystitis.
**Hematologic:** *WBC and platelet count nadirs occurring on day 7; anemia, leukopenia, thrombocytopenia.*
**Hepatic:** *acute toxicity, chronic toxicity,* including cirrhosis, and *hepatic fibrosis.*
**Musculoskeletal:** arthralgia, myalgia; osteoporosis in children on long-term therapy.
**Respiratory:** *pulmonary fibrosis; pulmonary interstitial infiltrates;* pneumonitis; dry, nonproductive cough.
**Skin:** *urticaria,* pruritus, hyperpigmentation, erythematous rashes, ecchymoses, rash, photosensitivity, alopecia, acne, pso-

riatic lesions aggravated by exposure to sun.
**Other:** fever, chills, reduced resistance to infection, septicemia, hyperuricemia, diabetes, *sudden death.*

## INTERACTIONS
**Drug-drug.** *Acyclovir:* concurrent use with intrathecal MTX may cause neurologic abnormalities. Monitor closely.
*Digoxin:* may decrease serum digoxin levels. Monitor closely.
*Folic acid derivatives:* antagonized methotrexate effect. Avoid concomitant use, except for leucovorin rescue with high-dose methotrexate therapy.
*Hepatotoxic drugs:* may increase risk of hepatotoxicity. Monitor closely.
*NSAIDs, phenylbutazone, probenecid, salicylates, sulfonamides:* increased methotrexate toxicity. Avoid use together.
*Oral antibiotics:* may decrease absorption of methotrexate. Monitor closely.
*Phenytoin:* may decrease serum phenytoin levels. Monitor closely.
*Theophylline:* may increase level of theophylline. Monitor closely.
*Vaccines:* immunizations may be ineffective; risk of disseminated infection with live virus vaccines. Defer immunization, if possible.
**Drug-food.** *Any food:* may delay absorption and reduce peak level of methotrexate. Avoid concomitant use.
**Drug-lifestyle.** *Alcohol use:* may increase hepatotoxicity. Discourage concomitant use.
*Sun exposure:* photosensitivity reactions may occur. Take precautions.

## EFFECTS ON DIAGNOSTIC TESTS
Drug may alter results of laboratory assay for folate, thus interfering with detection of folic acid deficiency.

## CONTRAINDICATIONS
Contraindicated in patients with hypersensitivity to drug and in those with psoriasis or rheumatoid arthritis who also have alcoholism, alcoholic liver, chronic liver disease, immunodeficiency syndromes, or preexisting blood dyscrasias; also contraindicated in pregnant or breast-feeding women.

---

## NURSING CONSIDERATIONS
• Use cautiously and at modified dosage in patients with impaired hepatic or renal function, bone marrow suppression, aplasia, leukopenia, thrombocytopenia, or anemia. Also use cautiously in patients with infection, peptic ulceration, or ulcerative colitis and in very young, elderly, or debilitated patients.
• Monitor pulmonary function tests periodically, as ordered, and fluid intake and output daily. Encourage fluid intake of 2 to 3 L daily.
• Monitor serum uric acid level, as ordered.
• *Alert:* Alkalinize urine, as ordered, by giving sodium bicarbonate tablets to prevent precipitation of drug, especially with high doses. Maintain urine pH at more than 6.5. Reduce dosage, as ordered, if BUN level is 20 to 30 mg/dl or creatinine level is 1.2 to 2 mg/dl. Stop drug and notify doctor if BUN level exceeds 30 mg/dl or creatinine level is over 2 mg/dl.
• Use preservative-free formulation for intrathecal administration.
• Watch for increases in AST, ALT, and alkaline phosphatase levels, which may signal hepatic dysfunction.
• Watch for signs and symptoms of bleeding (especially GI) and infection.
• To prevent bleeding, avoid all I.M. injections when platelet count is below 100,000/mm$^3$.
• Anticipate blood transfusions because of cumulative anemia. Patient may receive injections of RBC colony-stimulating factors to promote RBC production and decrease need for blood transfusions.
• Rash, redness, or ulcerations in mouth or adverse pulmonary reactions may signal serious complications.
• Leucovorin rescue is needed with high-dose (over 100 mg) protocols and is started 24 hours after beginning methotrexate therapy.
• Monitor methotrexate levels and adjust leucovorin dose, as ordered.

## 🔲 I.V. administration
• Follow institutional policy to reduce risks. Preparation and administration of parenteral form of drug are associated with carcinogenic, mutagenic, and teratogenic risks for personnel.
• Dilution of drug depends on product, and infusion guidelines vary, depending on dose.
• Reconstitute solutions without preservatives immediately before use, and discard unused drug.

## ☑ Patient teaching
• Advise patient to watch for signs and symptoms of infection (fever, sore throat, fatigue) and bleeding (easy bruising, nosebleeds, bleeding gums, melena). Tell patient to take temperature daily.
• Teach and encourage diligent mouth care to reduce risk of superinfection in the mouth.
• Tell patient to use highly protective sunblock when exposed to sunlight.
• Warn patient to avoid conception during and immediately after therapy because of possible abortion or congenital anomalies.
• Advise breast-feeding woman to discontinue breast-feeding during therapy because of possible infant toxicity.

# thioguanine
## (6-TG, 6-thioguanine)
Lanvis†

*Pregnancy Risk Category D*

## HOW SUPPLIED
*Tablets (scored):* 40 mg

## ACTION
Inhibits DNA and (to a lesser degree) RNA synthesis.

| Route | Onset | Peak | Duration |
|-------|-------|------|----------|
| P.O. | Unknown | Unknown | Unknown |

## INDICATIONS & DOSAGE
*Acute nonlymphocytic leukemia, chronic myelogenous leukemia—*
**Adults and children:** initially, 2 mg/kg P.O. daily (usually calculated to nearest 20 mg). If after 4 weeks at 2 mg/kg there is no clinical improvement, dose may be cautiously increased to 3 mg/kg/day if not contraindicated.

---

Reactions may be *common,* uncommon, *life-threatening,* or COMMON AND LIFE-THREATENING.

## ADVERSE REACTIONS
**GI:** nausea, vomiting, stomatitis, diarrhea, anorexia.
**Hematologic:** *leukopenia, anemia, thrombocytopenia occurring slowly over 2 to 4 weeks.*
**Hepatic:** *hepatotoxicity,* jaundice, hepatic fibrosis, *toxic hepatitis.*
**Other:** hyperuricemia.

## INTERACTIONS
**Drug-drug.** *Myelosuppressives:* increased risk of toxicity, especially myelosuppression, bleeding, and hepatotoxicity. Use together cautiously.

## EFFECTS ON DIAGNOSTIC TESTS
None reported.

## CONTRAINDICATIONS
Contraindicated in patients whose disease has shown resistance to drug. There is usually complete cross-resistance between mercaptopurine and thioguanine.

## NURSING CONSIDERATIONS
• Use cautiously and with dosage modification in patients with renal or hepatic dysfunction.
• Monitor CBC daily during induction and then weekly during maintenance therapy, as ordered. Leukocyte or platelet count depression is a contraindication to increasing dosage.
• Monitor serum uric acid level, as ordered. Hyperuricemia can be minimized by increased urine alkalization and administration of allopurinol.
• Watch for jaundice; it may be reversible if drug is stopped promptly.
• To prevent bleeding, avoid all I.M. injections when platelet count is below 100,000/mm$^3$.
• Anticipate blood transfusions because of cumulative anemia. Patient may receive injections of RBC colony-stimulating factors to promote RBC production and decrease need for blood transfusions.
• Drug is sometimes ordered as 6-thioguanine. The numeral 6 is part of drug name and doesn't signify dosage units.

### ☑ Patient teaching
• Instruct patient to watch for signs and symptoms of infection (fever, sore throat, fatigue) and bleeding (easy bruising, nosebleeds, bleeding gums, melena). Tell patient to take temperature daily.
• Caution woman of childbearing age to avoid becoming pregnant during therapy. Recommend that she consult doctor before becoming pregnant.
• Advise breast-feeding woman to discontinue breast-feeding during therapy because of possible infant toxicity.

bleomycin sulfate
dactinomycin
daunorubicin citrate liposomal
daunorubicin hydrochloride
doxorubicin hydrochloride
doxorubicin hydrochloride
  liposomal
epirubicin hydrochloride
idarubicin hydrochloride
mitomycin
pentostatin
plicamycin
valrubicin

**COMBINATION PRODUCTS**
None.

---

## bleomycin sulfate
Blenoxane

*Pregnancy Risk Category D*

### HOW SUPPLIED
*Injection:* 15-U vials, 30-U vials

### ACTION
Unknown. Thought to inhibit DNA synthesis and cause scission of single- and double-stranded DNA.

| Route | Onset | Peak | Duration |
|-------|-------|------|----------|
| I.V., S.C. | Unknown | Unknown | Unknown |
| I.M. | Unknown | 30-60 min | Unknown |

### INDICATIONS & DOSAGE
Dosage and indications may vary. Check treatment protocol with doctor.
*Squamous cell carcinoma (head and neck, skin, penis, cervix, and vulva), lymphosarcoma, reticulum cell carcinoma, testicular carcinoma—*
**Adults:** 10 to 20 U/m² I.V., I.M., or S.C. once or two times weekly to total of 300 to 400 U.
*Hodgkin's disease—*
**Adults:** 10 to 20 U/m² I.V., I.M., or S.C. one or two times weekly. After 50% response, maintenance dose is 1 U I.M. or I.V. daily or 5 U I.M. or I.V. weekly.
*Treatment of malignant pleural effusion, prevention of recurrent pleural effusions—*
**Adults:** 60 U administered as single-dose bolus intrapleural injection.

### ADVERSE REACTIONS
**GI:** *stomatitis, anorexia, nausea, vomiting,* diarrhea.
**Metabolic:** weight loss.
**Respiratory:** PNEUMONITIS, *pulmonary fibrosis.*
**Skin:** *erythema, hyperpigmentation, acne, rash, striae, skin tenderness, pruritus, reversible alopecia,* hyperkeratosis, nail changes.
**Other:** *chills,* fever, *anaphylactoid reactions;* increased blood and urine levels of uric acid.

### INTERACTIONS
**Drug-drug.** *Anesthesia:* may increase oxygen requirements. Monitor closely.
*Cardiac glycosides:* decreased serum digoxin levels. Monitor closely.
*Phenytoin:* decreased serum phenytoin levels. Monitor closely.

### EFFECTS ON DIAGNOSTIC TESTS
None reported.

### CONTRAINDICATIONS
Contraindicated in patients with hypersensitivity to drug.

### NURSING CONSIDERATIONS
• Use cautiously in patients with renal or pulmonary impairment.
• Obtain pulmonary function tests, as ordered. Drug should be stopped if tests show a marked decline.
• For I.M. use, dilute drug in 1 to 5 ml of sterile water for injection, bacteriostatic water for injection, or normal saline for injection.
• For intrapleural use, dissolve drug in 50 to 100 ml normal saline injection and ad-

minister through a thoracotomy tube after drainage of excess pleural fluid and confirmation of complete lung expansion.

• Monitor injection site for irritation.

• *Alert:* Adverse pulmonary reactions are more common in patients over age 70. Pulmonary fibrosis is fatal in 1% of patients, especially when cumulative dosage exceeds 400 U. Also, pulmonary toxic adverse effects may be increased in patients receiving radiation therapy.

• Monitor chest X-ray, as ordered, and listen to lungs regularly.

• If patient's condition requires sclerosis, drug may be instilled when chest tube drainage is 100 to 300 ml/24 hours before therapy; ideally, drainage should be under 100 ml. Following instillation, thoracotomy tube is clamped and patient is moved alternately from the supine to left and right lateral positions for the next 4 hours. The clamp is then removed and suction reestablished. Amount of time chest tube is left in place after sclerosis depends on patient's condition.

• Watch for fever, which may be treated with antipyretics. Fever usually occurs within 3 to 6 hours of administration.

• Watch for hypersensitivity reactions, which may be delayed for several hours, especially in patients with lymphoma. (Test dose of 1 to 2 U should be given before first two doses in these patients. If no reaction occurs, regular dosage is followed.)

• Don't use adhesive dressings on skin.

**◖ I.V. administration**

• Follow institutional policy to reduce risks. Preparation and administration of parenteral form of drug are associated with carcinogenic, mutagenic, and teratogenic risks for personnel.

• Reconstitute drug with 5 ml or more of normal saline for injection. For I.V. infusion, dilute with 50 to 100 ml normal saline for injection. Administer over 10 minutes.

• Refrigerate unopened vials containing dry powder. Refrigerated, reconstituted solution is stable for 4 weeks; at room temperature, for 2 weeks. Bleomycin may adsorb to plastic I.V. bags. For prolonged stability, use glass containers.

**☑ Patient teaching**

• Warn patient that alopecia may occur, but that it's usually reversible.

• Tell patient to report adverse reactions promptly and to take infection-control and bleeding precautions.

• Instruct patient that, if he's to receive anesthesia, he must inform anesthesiologist of previous treatment with bleomycin. Pulmonary toxicity of drug may be enhanced by high inspired oxygen levels during surgery.

## dactinomycin (actinomycin D)
Cosmegen

*Pregnancy Risk Category C*

## HOW SUPPLIED
*Injection:* 500 mcg-vial

## ACTION
May interfere with DNA-dependent RNA synthesis by intercalation.

| Route | Onset | Peak | Duration |
|-------|---------|---------|----------|
| I.V. | Unknown | Unknown | Unknown |

## INDICATIONS & DOSAGE
Dosage and indications vary. Check treatment protocol with doctor.
*Sarcoma, trophoblastic tumors in women, testicular cancer—*
**Adults:** 500 mcg (0.5 mg) I.V. daily for 5 days. Maximum dose is 15 mcg/kg or 400 to 600 mcg/m²/day for 5 days. After bone marrow recovery, and at least 3 weeks, course may be repeated.
*Wilms' tumor, rhabdomyosarcoma, Ewing's sarcoma—*
**Children:** 10 to 15 mcg/kg or 400 to 500 mcg/m²/day I.V. for 5 days. Maximum dose is 500 mcg/day. Or, 2.5 mg/m² I.V. in equally divided daily doses over 7 days. After bone marrow recovery, course may be repeated. Not recommended for infants under age 6 months.

## ADVERSE REACTIONS
**CNS:** malaise, fatigue, lethargy.
**GI:** *anorexia, nausea, vomiting,* abdominal pain, diarrhea, *stomatitis,* ulceration, proctitis.

**Hematologic:** *anemia, leukopenia, thrombocytopenia, pancytopenia, aplastic anemia, agranulocytosis.*
**Hepatic:** *hepatotoxicity.*
**Metabolic:** hypocalcemia.
**Musculoskeletal:** myalgia.
**Skin:** *erythema;* desquamation; reversible alopecia; *hyperpigmentation of skin, especially in previously irradiated areas, acne-like eruptions,* "radiation recall effect."
**Other:** phlebitis and severe damage to soft tissue at injection site, fever, ***anaphylactoid reaction, death,*** increased blood and urine levels of uric acid.

## INTERACTIONS
**Drug-drug.** *Bone marrow suppressants:* additive toxicity. Monitor closely.
*Vitamin K derivatives:* decreased effectiveness. Monitor closely.

## EFFECTS ON DIAGNOSTIC TESTS
Drug may interfere with determination of antibiotic drug levels (peak and trough).

## CONTRAINDICATIONS
Contraindicated in patients with chickenpox or herpes zoster.

## NURSING CONSIDERATIONS
• If skin contact occurs, irrigate with water for at least 15 minutes.
• *Alert:* Dosage must be reduced in patients who have recently been treated with, or who will receive concomitant treatment with, radiation therapy or other chemotherapy drugs.
• In the event of a spill, use a solution of trisodium phosphate 5% to inactivate drug.
• Monitor CBC and platelet counts and renal and hepatic functions, as ordered.
• If WBC count falls below 2,000/mm$^3$ or granulocyte count falls below 1,000/mm$^3$, follow institutional policy for infection control in immunocompromised patients.
• Watch for stomatitis, diarrhea, leukopenia, or thrombocytopenia.
• To reduce nausea, give antiemetic before drug, as ordered.

## I.V. administration
• Follow institutional policy to reduce risks. Preparation and administration of parenteral form of drug are associated with carcinogenic, mutagenic, and teratogenic risks for personnel.
• Use only sterile water (without preservatives) as diluent for reconstitution. Add 1.1 ml to vial to yield gold-colored solution containing 0.5 mg/ml. Give by direct injection into a vein or through tubing of a free-flowing I.V. solution of normal saline for injection or D$_5$W. An in-line cellulose ester membrane filter shouldn't be used during dactinomycin administration.
• For I.V. infusion, dilute with up to 50 ml of D$_5$W or normal saline for injection; infuse over 15 minutes.
• Administer through a running I.V. line with good blood return. Drug is a vesicant; if extravasation occurs, severe tissue necrosis may result. If infiltration occurs, apply cold compresses to area and notify doctor.
• Discard unused solutions.

## Patient teaching
• Advise patient to watch for signs and symptoms of infection (fever, sore throat, fatigue) and bleeding (easy bruising, nosebleeds, bleeding gums, melena), and to take temperature daily.
• Tell patient that alopecia may occur, but that it's usually reversible.
• Inform patient who received a course of radiation therapy that he may experience "radiation recall effect," which is a reactivation of adverse effects, such as erythema at the site of irradiation, followed by hyperpigmentation, edema, desquamation, vesiculation, and necrosis.

---

## daunorubicin citrate liposomal
DaunoXome

*Pregnancy Risk Category D*

## HOW SUPPLIED
*Injection:* 2 mg/ml (equivalent to 50 mg daunorubicin base)

---

Reactions may be *common*, uncommon, ***life-threatening***, or COMMON AND LIFE-THREATENING.

## ACTION

Maximizes selectivity of daunorubicin for solid tumors in situ. After penetrating tumor, drug is released over time to exert its antineoplastic activity by inhibiting DNA synthesis and DNA-dependent RNA synthesis through intercalation.

| Route | Onset | Peak | Duration |
|-------|-------|------|----------|
| I.V. | Unknown | Unknown | Unknown |

## INDICATIONS & DOSAGE

*First-line cytotoxic therapy for advanced HIV-associated Kaposi's sarcoma—*
**Adults:** 40 mg/m$^2$ I.V. over 60 minutes once q 2 weeks. Treatment should be continued until there is evidence of progressive disease or until other complications of HIV preclude continuation of therapy.
*Adjust-a-dose:* For patients with impaired hepatic and renal function, reduce dosage as follows: If serum bilirubin level is 1.2 to 3 mg/dl, give three-fourths normal dose; if serum bilirubin or creatinine level exceeds 3 mg/dl, give one-half normal dose.

## ADVERSE REACTIONS

**CNS:** *headache, neuropathy,* depression, dizziness, syncope, insomnia, amnesia, anxiety, ataxia, confusion, *seizures,* hallucination, tremor, hypertonia, meningitis, *fatigue,* malaise, emotional lability, abnormal gait, hyperkinesia, somnolence, abnormal thinking.
**CV:** *dose-related cardiomyopathy,* chest pain, hypertension, palpitation, *arrhythmias, pericardial effusion, pericardial tamponade, cardiac arrest,* angina pectoris, *pulmonary hypertension,* flushing, edema, tachycardia, *MI.*
**EENT:** *rhinitis,* stomatitis, sinusitis, abnormal vision, conjunctivitis, tinnitus, eye pain, deafness, taste disturbances, earache, gingival bleeding, tooth caries, dry mouth.
**GI:** *nausea, diarrhea, abdominal pain, vomiting, anorexia,* constipation, thirst, *GI hemorrhage,* gastritis, dysphagia, stomatitis, increased appetite, melena, hemorrhoids, tenesmus.
**GU:** dysuria, nocturia, polyuria.
**Hematologic:** NEUTROPENIA.
**Hepatic:** hepatomegaly.

**Metabolic:** dehydration.
**Musculoskeletal:** *rigors, back pain,* arthralgia, myalgia.
**Respiratory:** *cough, dyspnea,* hemoptysis, hiccups, pulmonary infiltration, increased sputum.
**Skin:** alopecia, pruritus, *increased sweating,* dry skin, seborrhea, folliculitis.
**Other:** *fever,* splenomegaly, lymphadenopathy, *opportunistic infections, allergic reactions,* influenza-like symptoms, injection site inflammation.

## INTERACTIONS
None significant.

## EFFECTS ON DIAGNOSTIC TESTS
None reported.

## CONTRAINDICATIONS
Contraindicated in patients who have experienced severe hypersensitivity reaction to drug or its components.

## NURSING CONSIDERATIONS
● Use cautiously in patients with myelosuppression, preexisting cardiac disease, previous radiotherapy encompassing the heart, previous anthracycline use (doxorubicin is 300 mg/m$^2$ or above), or hepatic or renal dysfunction.
● Administer only under supervision of doctor specializing in cancer chemotherapy.
● Monitor cardiac function regularly. Assess patient before administering each dose because of risk of cardiac toxicity and heart failure. Determine left ventricular ejection fraction at total cumulative doses of 320 mg/m$^2$ and every 160 mg/m$^2$ thereafter.
● Careful hematologic monitoring is needed because severe myelosuppression may occur. Repeat blood counts and evaluate before giving each dose. Withhold treatment if absolute granulocyte count is below 750 cells/mm$^3$.
● Monitor patient closely for signs and symptoms of opportunistic infections, especially because patients with HIV infection are immunocompromised.

---

## ⬛ I.V. administration

• Dilute drug with $D_5W$ before use. Withdraw calculated volume of drug from vial and transfer into an equivalent amount of $D_5W$. Recommended concentration after dilution should be 1 mg/ml.
• Don't mix daunorubicin citrate liposomal with bacteriostatic or other drugs, or saline or other solutions.
• After dilution, immediately administer I.V. over 60 minutes. If unable to use immediately, refrigerate at 2° to 8° C (36° to 46° F) for maximum of 6 hours.
• Don't use in-line filters for I.V. infusion.
• *Alert:* A triad of back pain, flushing, and chest tightness may occur within first 5 minutes of infusion. These symptoms subside after stopping infusion and generally don't recur when infusion is given at a slower rate.
• Because local tissue necrosis is possible, monitor I.V. site closely to avoid extravasation.
• Follow procedures for proper handling and disposal of antineoplastics.

## ☑ Patient teaching

• Inform patient that alopecia may occur, but that it's usually reversible.
• Instruct patient to call doctor if sore throat, fever, or other signs or symptoms of infection occur. Tell patient to avoid exposure to people with infections.
• Advise woman to report if pregnancy is suspected or confirmed during therapy.
• Tell patient to report back pain, flushing, and chest tightness during infusion.

---

## daunorubicin hydrochloride
Cerubidine

*Pregnancy Risk Category D*

## HOW SUPPLIED
*Injection:* 20 mg-vial

## ACTION
May interfere with DNA-dependent RNA synthesis by intercalation.

| Route | Onset | Peak | Duration |
|-------|-------|------|----------|
| I.V. | Unknown | Unknown | Unknown |

## INDICATIONS & DOSAGE
Dosage and indications vary. Check treatment protocol with doctor.
*Remission induction in acute nonlymphocytic (myelogenous, monocytic, erythroid) leukemia—*
**Adults:** in combination, 30 to 45 mg/m²/day I.V. on days 1, 2, and 3 of first course and on days 1 and 2 of subsequent courses with cytarabine infusions.
*Remission induction in acute lymphocytic leukemia—*
**Adults:** in combination, 45 mg/m²/day I.V. on days 1, 2, and 3 of first course.
**Children ages 2 and older:** 25 mg/m² I.V. on day 1 q week, for up to 6 weeks, if needed.
**Children under age 2 or body surface area under 0.5 m²:** dose based on body weight (1 mg/kg), not surface area.

## ADVERSE REACTIONS
**CV:** IRREVERSIBLE CARDIOMYOPATHY, ECG changes.
**GI:** *nausea, vomiting,* diarrhea.
**GU:** red urine.
**Hematologic:** *bone marrow suppression, with lowest blood counts 10 to 14 days after administration.*
**Hepatic:** *hepatotoxicity.*
**Skin:** rash, *reversible alopecia,* darkening or redness of previously irradiated areas.
**Other:** *severe cellulitis, tissue sloughing* with drug extravasation; ***anaphylactoid reaction,*** fever, chills, hyperuricemia.

## INTERACTIONS
**Drug-drug.** *Doxorubicin:* additive cardiotoxicity. Monitor closely.
*Hepatotoxic drugs:* increased risk of additive hepatotoxicity. Monitor closely.

## EFFECTS ON DIAGNOSTIC TESTS
None reported.

## CONTRAINDICATIONS
No known contraindications.

## NURSING CONSIDERATIONS
• Use cautiously in patients with myelosuppression or impaired cardiac, renal, or hepatic function.

---

Reactions may be *common,* uncommon, *life-threatening,* or COMMON AND LIFE-THREATENING.

• Take preventive measures (including adequate hydration) before starting treatment. Hyperuricemia may result from rapid lysis of leukemic cells. Allopurinol may be ordered.
• Cardiac function studies, including ECG, should be performed before treatment and then periodically throughout therapy.
• Never give drug I.M. or S.C.
• Cumulative adult dosage is limited to 400 to 550 mg/m² (450 mg/m² when patient is also receiving or has received cyclophosphamide or radiation therapy to cardiac area).
• Therapeutic effects are frequently accompanied by toxicity.
• Monitor CBC and hepatic function tests, as ordered; monitor ECG every month during therapy.
• Monitor pulse rate closely. Notify doctor if light resting pulse rate (a sign of cardiac adverse reactions) occurs.
• *Alert:* Stop drug immediately and notify doctor if signs of heart failure or cardiomyopathy develop.
• Watch for nausea and vomiting, which may last 24 to 48 hours.
• Anticipate the need for blood transfusions to combat anemia. Patient may receive injections of RBC colony-stimulating factors to promote RBC production and decrease need for blood transfusions.
• *Alert:* Reddish color of drug is similar to that of doxorubicin; don't confuse the two.
• Optimally, use within 8 hours of preparation. Reconstituted solution is stable for 24 hours at room temperature or 48 hours if refrigerated.

**I.V. administration**
• Follow institutional policy to reduce risks. Preparation and administration of parenteral form of drug are associated with carcinogenic, mutagenic, and teratogenic risks for personnel.
• Reconstitute drug using 4 ml of sterile water for injection to produce a 5 mg/ml solution.
• Withdraw desired dose into syringe containing 10 to 15 ml of normal saline for injection. Inject into tubing of a free-flowing I.V. solution of D₅W or normal

saline for injection over 2 to 3 minutes. Or, dilute in 50 ml of normal saline for injection and infuse over 10 to 15 minutes, or dilute in 100 ml and infuse over 30 to 45 minutes.
• If extravasation occurs, discontinue I.V. infusion immediately, apply ice to area for 24 to 48 hours, and notify doctor. Because drug is a vesicant, extravasation could cause severe tissue necrosis.
• Dexamethasone and heparin may form a precipitate. Don't mix together.

**Patient teaching**
• Advise patient to watch for signs and symptoms of infection (fever, sore throat, fatigue) and bleeding (easy bruising, nosebleeds, bleeding gums, melena) and to take temperature daily.
• Inform patient that red urine for 1 to 2 days is normal and doesn't indicate the presence of blood in urine.
• Advise patient that alopecia may occur, but that it's usually reversible.
• Caution woman of childbearing age to avoid becoming pregnant during therapy. Recommend that she consult doctor before becoming pregnant.

---

**doxorubicin hydrochloride**
Adriamycin‡, Adriamycin PFS, Adriamycin RDF, Rubex

*Pregnancy Risk Category D*

**HOW SUPPLIED**
*Injection (preservative-free):* 2 mg/ml
*Powder for injection:* 10-mg, 20-mg, 50-mg, 100-mg, 150-mg vials

**ACTION**
May interfere with DNA-dependent RNA synthesis by intercalation.

| Route | Onset | Peak | Duration |
|---|---|---|---|
| I.V. | Unknown | Unknown | Unknown |

**INDICATIONS & DOSAGE**
Dosage and indications vary. Check treatment protocol with doctor.
*Bladder, breast, lung, ovarian, stomach, and thyroid cancers; Hodgkin's disease; acute lymphoblastic and myeloblastic*

*leukemia; Wilms' tumor; neuroblastoma; lymphoma; sarcoma—*

**Adults:** 60 to 75 mg/m² I.V. as single dose q 3 weeks; or 30 mg/m² I.V. in single daily dose, days 1 to 3 of 4-week cycle. Or, 20 mg/m² I.V. once weekly. Maximum cumulative dose is 550 mg/m².

**Elderly:** may need reduced dosage.

*Adjust-a-dose:* For patients with myelosuppression or impaired cardiac or liver function, dosage may be reduced. Be prepared to decrease dosage if serum bilirubin level rises: give 50% of dose when bilirubin level is 1.2 to 3 mg/100 ml; 25% when it's over 3 mg/100 ml.

## ADVERSE REACTIONS

**CV:** cardiac depression, seen in such ECG changes as sinus tachycardia, T-wave flattening, ST-segment depression, voltage reduction; ***arrhythmias; acute left ventricular failure; irreversible cardiomyopathy.***

**EENT:** conjunctivitis.

**GI:** *nausea, vomiting,* diarrhea, *stomatitis,* esophagitis, anorexia.

**GU:** transient red urine.

**Hematologic:** *leukopenia during days 10 to 15 with recovery by day 21, thrombocytopenia,* MYELOSUPPRESSION.

**Skin:** urticaria, facial flushing, *complete alopecia within 3 to 4 weeks,* hyperpigmentation of nail beds and dermal creases, "radiation recall effect."

**Other:** *severe cellulitis, tissue sloughing with drug extravasation;* hyperuricemia; fever; chills; ***anaphylaxis.***

## INTERACTIONS

**Drug-drug.** *Aminophylline, cephalothin, dexamethasone, fluorouracil, heparin, hydrocortisone:* may form a precipitate. Don't mix together.

*Calcium channel blockers:* may potentiate cardiotoxic effects. Monitor closely.

*Digoxin:* may decrease serum digoxin levels. Monitor closely.

*Phenytoin:* decreased serum levels of phenytoin. Check levels.

*Streptozocin:* increased and prolonged blood levels. Dosage may have to be titrated.

**Drug-herb.** *Green tea:* may enhance the antitumor activity of doxorubicin. Monitor patient.

## EFFECTS ON DIAGNOSTIC TESTS
None reported.

## CONTRAINDICATIONS
Contraindicated in patients with marked myelosuppression induced by previous treatment with other antitumor drugs or by radiotherapy and in patients who have received lifetime cumulative dose of 550 mg/m² of doxorubicin or daunorubicin.

## NURSING CONSIDERATIONS

• Cardiac function studies, including ECG, should be performed before treatment and then periodically throughout therapy. Dexrazoxane may be administered with doxorubicin if the accumulated dose of doxorubicin has reached 300 mg/m².

• Take preventive measures, including adequate hydration, before starting treatment. Hyperuricemia may result from rapid lysis of leukemic cells. Allopurinol may be ordered.

• Premedicate with antiemetic, as ordered, to reduce nausea.

• If skin or mucosal contact occurs, immediately wash with soap and water.

• If a leak or spill occurs, inactivate drug with 5% sodium hypochlorite solution (household bleach).

• Never give drug I.M. or S.C.

• Dosage modification may be needed in patients with myelosuppression or impaired cardiac or hepatic function, and in elderly patients.

• Monitor CBC and hepatic function tests, as ordered; monitor ECG monthly during therapy. If WBC count falls below 2,000/mm³ or granulocyte count falls below 1,000/mm³, follow institutional policy for infection control in immunocompromised patients.

• Be prepared to stop drug or slow rate of infusion and notify doctor if tachycardia develops.

• *Alert:* If signs of heart failure develop, stop drug and notify doctor. Heart failure can often be prevented by limiting cumu-

---

lative dose to 550 mg/m² (400 mg/m² when patient is also receiving or has received cyclophosphamide or radiation therapy to cardiac area).
• *Alert:* Reddish color of drug is similar to that of daunorubicin; don't confuse the two drugs.
• *Alert:* Esophagitis is very common in patients who have also received radiation therapy.

### ⬛ I.V. administration
• Follow institutional policy to reduce risks. Preparation and administration of parenteral form of drug are associated with carcinogenic, mutagenic, and teratogenic risks for personnel.
• Reconstitute using preservative-free normal saline for injection. Add 5 ml to 10-mg vial, 10 ml to 20-mg vial, or 25 ml to 50-mg vial. Shake vial and allow drug to dissolve; final concentration will be 2 mg/ml. Give by direct injection into the tubing of a free-flowing I.V. solution containing $D_5W$ or normal saline for injection. Administration rate shouldn't be less than 3 minutes. Drug is a severe vesicant; if extravasation occurs, tissue necrosis may result.
• Don't place I.V. line over joints or in extremities with poor venous or lymphatic drainage. If extravasation occurs, discontinue I.V. infusion immediately, apply ice to area for 24 to 48 hours, and notify doctor. Monitor area closely because extravasation may be progressive. Early consultation with a plastic surgeon may be advisable.
• If vein streaking occurs, slow administration rate. However, if welts occur, stop administration and notify doctor.
• Refrigerated, reconstituted solution is stable for 48 hours; at room temperature, it's stable for 24 hours.

### ✅ Patient teaching
• Advise patient to watch for signs and symptoms of infection (fever, sore throat, fatigue) and bleeding (easy bruising, nosebleeds, bleeding gums, melena) and to take temperature daily.
• Advise patient that orange to red urine for 1 to 2 days is normal and doesn't indicate presence of blood.

• Inform patient that alopecia may occur, but that it's usually reversible. Hair may regrow 2 to 5 months after drug is stopped.

---

## doxorubicin hydrochloride liposomal
Doxil

*Pregnancy Risk Category D*

---

### HOW SUPPLIED
*Injection:* 2 mg/ml

### ACTION
Consists of doxorubicin hydrochloride encapsulated in liposomes. Action possibly related to drug's ability to bind DNA and inhibit nucleic acid synthesis.

| Route | Onset | Peak | Duration |
|-------|-------|------|----------|
| I.V. | Unknown | Unknown | Unknown |

### INDICATIONS & DOSAGE
*Metastatic carcinoma of ovary in patients with disease that's refractory to both paclitaxel- and platinum-based chemotherapy regimen—*
**Adults:** 50 mg/m² (doxorubicin hydrochloride equivalent) I.V. at initial infusion rate of 1 mg/minute once every 4 weeks for minimum of 4 courses. Continue as long as condition doesn't progress and patient shows no evidence of cardiotoxicity and continues to tolerate treatment. If no infusion-related adverse reactions are observed, increase infusion rate to complete administration over 1 hour.
*AIDS-related Kaposi's sarcoma in patients with disease that has progressed on previous combination chemotherapy and in patients intolerant to such therapy—*
**Adults:** 20 mg/m² (doxorubicin hydrochloride equivalent) I.V. over 30 minutes once every 3 weeks. Continue as long as patient responds satisfactorily and tolerates treatment.
*Adjust-a-dose:* For patients with impaired hepatic function, reduce dosage as follows: If serum bilirubin level is 1.2 to 3 mg/dl, give one-half normal dose; if

serum bilirubin level is more than 3 mg/dl, give one-quarter normal dose.

**ADVERSE REACTIONS**
**CNS:** *asthenia,* paresthesia, headache, somnolence, dizziness, depression, insomnia, anxiety, malaise, emotional lability, fatigue.
**CV:** chest pain, hypotension, tachycardia, peripheral edema, cardiomyopathy, *heart failure, arrhythmias,* pericardial effusion.
**EENT:** *mucous membrane disorder,* mouth ulceration, pharyngitis, rhinitis, conjunctivitis, retinitis, optic neuritis.
**GI:** *nausea, vomiting, constipation, anorexia, diarrhea,* abdominal pain, dyspepsia, oral candidiasis, enlarged abdomen, esophagitis, dysphagia, *stomatitis,* taste perversion, glossitis.
**GU:** albuminuria.
**Hematologic:** LEUKOPENIA, NEUTROPENIA, THROMBOCYTOPENIA, *anemia,* increased PT.
**Hepatic:** hyperbilirubinemia.
**Metabolic:** dehydration, weight loss, hypocalcemia, hyperglycemia.
**Musculoskeletal:** myalgia, back pain.
**Respiratory:** dyspnea, increased cough, pneumonia.
**Skin:** *rash, alopecia,* dry skin, pruritus, skin discoloration, skin disorder, exfoliative dermatitis, herpes zoster, sweating, *palmar-plantar erythrodysesthesia,* alopecia.
**Other:** fever, allergic reaction, chills, infection, infusion-related reactions.

**INTERACTIONS**
None reported. However doxorubicin hydrochloride liposomal may interact with drugs known to affect the conventional formulation of doxorubicin hydrochloride.

**EFFECTS ON DIAGNOSTIC TESTS**
None reported.

**CONTRAINDICATIONS**
Contraindicated in patients with hypersensitivity to conventional formulation of doxorubicin hydrochloride or any component in the liposomal formulation and in those with marked myelosuppression. Also contraindicated in patients who have

received a lifetime cumulative dose of 550 mg/m², or 400 mg/m² in patients who have received radiotherapy to the mediastinal area or therapy with other cardiotoxic drugs such as cyclophosphamide.

**NURSING CONSIDERATIONS**
● Don't give I.M. or S.C.
● Use cautiously in patients who have received other anthracyclines. Previous or concomitant therapy with related compounds such as daunorubicin should be considered when calculating total dose of drug to be administered. Heart failure and cardiomyopathy may occur after discontinuation of therapy.
● Administer drug to patient with history of cardiovascular disease only when benefit outweighs risk to patient.
● *Alert:* Monitor patient for signs and symptoms of palmar-plantar erythrodysesthesia, hematologic toxicity, or stomatitis. These adverse reactions may be managed with dosage delays and adjustments, as ordered.
● Evaluate patient's hepatic function before therapy and adjust dosage accordingly.
● Drug exhibits unique pharmacokinetic properties compared to conventional doxorubicin hydrochloride and shouldn't be substituted on a milligram per milligram basis.
● Drug may potentiate toxicity of other antineoplastic therapies.
● Closely monitor cardiac function by endomyocardial biopsy, echocardiography, or gated radionuclide scans. If results indicate possible cardiac injury, the benefit of continued therapy must be weighed against the risk of myocardial injury.
● Monitor CBC, including platelets, before each dose and frequently throughout therapy. Leukopenia is usually transient. Persistent severe myelosuppression may result in superinfection or hemorrhage. Patient may need G-CSF (or GM-CSF) to support blood counts.

🔲 **I.V. administration**
● Follow procedures for proper handling and disposal of antineoplastics.
● Dilute appropriate dose (to maximum of 90 mg) in 250 ml D₅W using aseptic tech-

Reactions may be *common,* uncommon, *life-threatening,* or COMMON AND LIFE-THREATENING.

nique. Refrigerate diluted solution at 36°
to 46° F °(2° to 8°C) and administer within 24 hours.
• Carefully check label on I.V. bag before
administering. Accidental substitution of
doxorubicin hydrochloride liposomal for
conventional doxorubicin hydrochloride
has resulted in severe adverse reactions.
• *Alert:* Don't use with in-line filters.
• Infuse over 30 to 60 minutes depending
on dose. Monitor patient carefully during
infusion. Acute infusion-associated reactions (flushing, shortness of breath, facial
swelling, headache, chills, back pain,
tightness in chest or throat, and hypotension) may occur. Reactions resolve over
several hours to a day once infusion is
stopped, and may resolve when infusion
rate is slowed.
• If signs or symptoms of extravasation
occur, stop infusion immediately and
restart in another vein. Application of ice
over site of extravasation for approximately 30 minutes may help alleviate local reaction.

### ✓ Patient teaching
• Tell patient to notify doctor if he experiences signs and symptoms of hand-foot
syndrome (such as tingling or burning,
redness, flaking, bothersome swelling,
small blisters, or small sores on palms of
hands or soles of feet).
• Advise patient to report signs and symptoms of stomatitis (such as painful redness, swelling, or sores in mouth).
• Warn patient to avoid exposure to people with infections. Tell patient to report
temperature of 100.5° F (38° C) or higher.
• Tell patient to report nausea, vomiting,
tiredness, weakness, rash, or mild hair
loss.
• Advise woman of childbearing age to
avoid pregnancy during therapy.

✳ *NEW DRUG*

## epirubicin hydrochloride
Ellence

*Pregnancy Risk Category D*

### HOW SUPPLIED
*Injection:* 2 mg/ml

### ACTION
Exact mechanism unknown. Thought to
form a complex with DNA by intercalation between nucleotide base pairs; thereby inhibiting DNA, RNA, and protein
synthesis; DNA cleavage occurs, resulting
in cytocidal activity. Drug may also interfere with replication and transcription of
DNA and generate cytotoxic free radicals.

| Route | Onset | Peak | Duration |
|-------|-------|------|----------|
| I.V. | Unknown | Unknown | Unknown |

### INDICATIONS & DOSAGE
*Adjuvant therapy in patients with evi-
dence of axillary node tumor involvement
following resection of primary breast cancer—*
**Adults:** 100 to 120 mg/m$^2$ I.V. infusion
over 3 to 5 minutes via a free-flowing I.V.
solution on day 1 of each cycle or divided
equally in two doses on days 1 and 8 of
each cycle; cycle repeated q 3 to 4 weeks
for 6 cycles; used with regimens containing cyclophosphamide and fluorouracil.

Dosage modification after first cycle is
based on toxicity. For patients with
platelet count below 50,000/mm$^3$, absolute neutrophil count (ANC) below
250/mm$^3$, neutropenic fever, or grade 3 or
4 nonhematologic toxicity, reduce day 1
dose in subsequent cycles to 75% of day 1
dose given in current cycle. Delay day 1
therapy in subsequent cycles until platelet
count is at least 100,000/mm$^3$, ANC is at
least 1,500/mm$^3$, and nonhematologic
toxicities recover to grade 1.

For patients receiving divided doses
(days 1 and 8), day 8 dose should be 75%
of day 1 dose if platelet count is 75,000 to
100,000/mm$^3$ and ANC is 1,000 to
1,499/mm$^3$. If day 8 platelet count is below 75,000/mm$^3$, ANC below 1,000/mm$^3$,
or grade 3 or 4 nonhematologic toxicity
has occurred, omit day 8 dose.
*Adjust-a-dose:* For patients with bone
marrow dysfunction (heavily pretreated
patients, patients with bone marrow depression, or those with neoplastic bone
marrow infiltration), start at lower doses
of 75 to 90 mg/m$^2$. For patients with hepatic dysfunction, if bilirubin is 1.2 to 3
mg/dl or AST is two to four times upper
limit of normal, give one-half recom-

---

*Liquid contains alcohol.   **May contain tartrazine.   †Canada   ‡Australia   §U.K.   ◊OTC

mended starting dose. If bilirubin level is above 3 mg/dl or AST is over four times upper limit of normal, give one-quarter recommended starting dose. For patients with severe renal dysfunction (serum creatinine level over 5 mg/dl), consider lower doses.

## ADVERSE REACTIONS
**CNS:** *lethargy.*
**CV:** *cardiomyopathy, heart failure.*
**EENT:** *conjunctivitis, keratitis.*
**GI:** *nausea, vomiting, diarrhea,* anorexia, *mucositis.*
**GU:** *amenorrhea.*
**Hematologic:** LEUKOPENIA, NEUTROPENIA, *febrile neutropenia, anemia,* THROMBOCYTOPENIA.
**Skin:** *alopecia,* rash, itch, skin changes.
**Other:** *infection,* fever, hot flashes, local toxicity.

## INTERACTIONS
**Drug-drug.** *Calcium channel blockers, other cardioactive compounds:* may increase risk of heart failure. Monitor cardiac function closely.
*Cimetidine:* increased epirubicin levels by 50%. Avoid concomitant use.
*Cytotoxic drugs:* additive toxicities (especially hematologic and GI) may occur. Monitor patient closely.
*Radiation therapy:* effects may be enhanced. Monitor patient carefully.

## EFFECTS ON DIAGNOSTIC TESTS
None reported.

## CONTRAINDICATIONS
Contraindicated in patients with hypersensitivity to drug, other anthracyclines, or anthracenediones, and in those with baseline neutrophil counts below 1,500 cells/mm³, severe myocardial insufficiency, recent MI, or severe hepatic dysfunction; also contraindicated in patients who have previous treatment with anthracyclines to total cumulative doses.

## NURSING CONSIDERATIONS
• Use cautiously in patients with active or dormant cardiac disease, previous or concomitant radiotherapy to mediastinal and pericardial area, or previous therapy with

other anthracyclines or anthracenediones; also use cautiously in patients receiving other cardiotoxic drugs concomitantly.
• Patients receiving 120 mg/m² of epirubicin should also receive prophylactic antibiotic therapy with co-trimoxazole or a fluoroquinolone.
• Antiemetics before epirubicin may be needed to reduce nausea and vomiting.
• Obtain the following measurements before therapy begins: total bilirubin, AST, and creatinine levels; CBC including ANC; and left ventricular ejection fraction (LVEF).
• Monitor LVEF regularly during therapy. Discontinue drug at first sign of impaired cardiac function. Early signs of cardiac toxicity include sinus tachycardia, ECG abnormalities, tachyarrhythmias, bradycardia, AV block, and bundle-branch block.
• Delayed cardiac toxicity may occur 2 to 3 months after treatment ends; indications include reduced LVEF and signs and symptoms of heart failure (tachycardia, dyspnea, pulmonary edema, dependent edema, hepatomegaly, ascites, pleural effusion and gallop rhythm). Delayed cardiac toxicity depends on cumulative dose of epirubicin. Don't exceed cumulative dose of 900 mg/m².
• Obtain total and differential WBC, RBC, and platelet counts before and during each cycle of therapy.
• WBC nadir is usually reached 10 to 14 days after drug administration, and returns to normal by day 21.
• Monitor serum uric acid, potassium, calcium phosphate, and creatinine levels immediately after initial chemotherapy administration in patients susceptible to tumor lysis syndrome. Hydration, urine alkalinization, and prophylaxis with allopurinol may prevent hyperuricemia and minimize potential complications of tumor lysis syndrome.
• Anthracycline-induced leukemia may occur.
• Administration of drug after previous radiation therapy may induce an inflammatory cell reaction at irradiation site.
• Administer drug under supervision of doctor experienced in cancer chemotherapy. Pregnant nurses shouldn't handle drug.

---

Reactions may be *common,* uncommon, *life-threatening*, or COMMON AND LIFE-THREATENING.

• Wear protective clothing (goggles, gown, disposable gloves) when handling drug.

### ⬦ I.V. administration
• **Alert:** Drug is a vesicant. Never give I.M. or S.C. Always administer through free-flowing I.V. solution of normal saline or $D_5W$ over 3 to 5 minutes.
• Facial flushing and local erythematous streaking along vein may indicate excessively rapid administration.
• Avoid veins over joints or in extremities with compromised venous or lymphatic drainage.
• Immediately stop infusion if burning or stinging occurs and restart in another vein.
• Don't mix drug with heparin or fluorouracil because precipitation may result.
• Don't mix in same syringe with other drugs.
• Discard unused solution left in vial 24 hours after vial has been penetrated.

### ☑ Patient teaching
• Advise patient to report nausea, vomiting, stomatitis, dehydration, fever, evidence of infection, or symptoms of heart failure (tachycardia, dyspnea, edema).
• Inform patient of risk of cardiac damage and treatment-related leukemia with use of drug.
• Advise men to use effective contraception during treatment.
• Advise women that irreversible amenorrhea or premature menopause may occur.
• Tell patient that hair regrowth usually occurs within 2 to 3 months after therapy is discontinued.

---

## idarubicin hydrochloride
Idamycin, Zavedos§

*Pregnancy Risk Category D*

### HOW SUPPLIED
*Powder for injection:* 5 mg, 10 mg, 20 mg

### ACTION
Unknown. Probably inhibits nucleic acid synthesis by intercalation and interacts with the enzyme topoisomerase II. It is highly lipophilic, which results in an increased rate of cellular uptake.

| Route | Onset | Peak | Duration |
|-------|-------|------|----------|
| I.V. | Unknown | Few min | Unknown |

### INDICATIONS & DOSAGE
Dosage and indications vary. Check treatment protocol with doctor.
*Acute myeloid leukemia, including FAB (French-American-British) classifications M1 through M7, with other approved antileukemic drugs—*
**Adults:** 12 mg/m²/day for 3 days by slow I.V. injection (over 10 to 15 minutes) with 100 mg/m²/day of cytarabine for 7 days by continuous I.V. infusion. Or as a 25 mg/m² bolus (cytarabine); then 200 mg/m²/day (cytarabine) for 5 days by continuous infusion. A second course may be administered, if needed.
**Adjust-a-dose:** If patient experiences severe mucositis, delay administration until recovery is complete and reduce dosage by 25%. Reduce dosage in patients with hepatic or renal impairment. Don't give idarubicin if bilirubin level exceeds 5 mg/dl.

### ADVERSE REACTIONS
**CNS:** *headache, changed mental status,* peripheral neuropathy, *seizures.*
**CV:** *heart failure,* atrial fibrillation, chest pain, *MI,* asymptomatic decline in left ventricular ejection fraction, *myocardial insufficiency, arrhythmias,* HEMORRHAGE, *myocardial toxicity.*
**GI:** *nausea, vomiting, cramps, diarrhea, mucositis.*
**GU:** decreased renal function, red urine.
**Hematologic:** *myelosuppression.*
**Hepatic:** changes in hepatic function.
**Skin:** *alopecia, rash, urticaria, bullous erythrodermatous rash on palms and soles,* hives at injection site, erythema at previously irradiated sites, tissue necrosis at injection site if extravasation occurs.
**Other:** INFECTION, *fever,* hyperuricemia, *hypersensitivity reactions.*

### INTERACTIONS
**Drug-drug.** *Alkaline solutions, heparin:* incompatibility. Don't mix idarubicin

---

with other drugs unless specific compatibility data are available.

**EFFECTS ON DIAGNOSTIC TESTS**
None reported.

**CONTRAINDICATIONS**
No known contraindications.

**NURSING CONSIDERATIONS**
• Use with extreme caution in patients with bone marrow suppression induced by previous drug therapy or radiotherapy, impaired hepatic or renal function, previous treatment with anthracyclines or cardiotoxic drugs, or a preexisting cardiac condition.
• Cardiotoxicity is the dose-limiting toxicity of drug.
• Take preventive measures, including adequate hydration, before starting treatment. Hyperuricemia may result from rapid lysis of leukemic cells. Allopurinol may be ordered.
• Assess patient for systemic infection and ensure that it's controlled before therapy begins.
• Give antiemetics, as ordered, to prevent or treat nausea and vomiting.
• Drug must never be given I.M. or S.C.
• Monitor hepatic and renal function tests and CBC frequently, as ordered.
• To prevent bleeding, avoid all I.M. injections when platelet count is below 100,000/mm³.
• Anticipate need for blood transfusions to combat anemia. Patient may receive injections of RBC colony-stimulating factors to promote RBC production and decrease need for blood transfusions.
• Notify doctor if signs or symptoms of heart failure occur.
• *Alert:* Don't confuse idarubicin with daunorubicin.

**◑ I.V. administration**
• Follow institutional policy to reduce risks. Preparation and administration of parenteral form of drug are associated with carcinogenic, mutagenic, and teratogenic risks for personnel.
• Reconstitute to final concentration of 1 mg/ml using normal saline for injection without preservatives. Add 5 ml to 5-mg

vial, 10 ml to 10-mg vial, or 20 ml to 20-mg vial. Don't use bacteriostatic NaCl. Vial is under negative pressure.
• Administer over 10 to 15 minutes into a free-flowing I.V. infusion of normal saline or $D_5W$ solution running into a large vein.
• Drug is a vesicant; tissue necrosis may result. If extravasation occurs, discontinue infusion immediately and notify doctor. Treat with intermittent ice packs—for one-half hour immediately, and then for one-half hour q.i.d. for 4 days.
• Reconstituted solutions are stable for 72 hours at room temperature (59° to 86° F [15° to 30° C]); 7 days if refrigerated. Label unused solutions with chemotherapy hazard label.

**☑ Patient teaching**
• Instruct patient to recognize signs and symptoms of extravasation and to notify doctor or nurse if these occur.
• Warn patient to watch for signs and symptoms of infection (fever, sore throat, fatigue) and bleeding (easy bruising, nosebleeds, bleeding gums, melena).
• Advise patient that red urine for several days is normal and doesn't indicate presence of blood.
• Caution woman of childbearing age to avoid becoming pregnant during therapy. Recommend that she consult doctor before becoming pregnant.

## mitomycin (mitomycin-C)
Mutamycin

*Pregnancy Risk Category NR*

**HOW SUPPLIED**
*Injection:* 5-mg, 20-mg, 40-mg vials

**ACTION**
Similar to an alkylating drug, cross-linking strands of DNA and causing an imbalance of cell growth, leading to cell death.

| Route | Onset | Peak | Duration |
|-------|-------|------|----------|
| I.V. | Unknown | Unknown | Unknown |

## INDICATIONS & DOSAGE

Dosage and indications vary. Check treatment protocol with doctor.

*Disseminated adenocarcinoma of stomach or pancreas—*

**Adults:** 10 to 20 mg/m$^2$ as an I.V. single dose. Cycle repeated after 6 to 8 weeks when WBC and platelet counts have returned to normal.

## ADVERSE REACTIONS

**CNS:** headache, neurologic abnormalities, confusion, drowsiness, fatigue.
**EENT:** blurred vision.
**GI:** *nausea, vomiting, anorexia, diarrhea.*
**GU:** *renal toxicity.*
**Hematologic:** THROMBOCYTOPENIA, LEUKOPENIA THAT MAY BE DELAYED UP TO 8 WEEKS AND MAY BE CUMULATIVE WITH SUCCESSIVE DOSES; *microangiopathic hemolytic anemia characterized by thrombocytopenia, renal failure, and hypertension.*
**Respiratory:** *interstitial pneumonitis,* pulmonary edema, dyspnea, nonproductive cough, adult respiratory distress syndrome.
**Skin:** pruritus, *pain at injection site, reversible alopecia,* purple bands on nails, rash, sloughing with extravasation.
**Other:** induration, desquamation, *septicemia;* cellulitis, ulceration, *fever,* pain.

## INTERACTIONS

**Drug-drug.** *Vinca alkaloids:* may cause acute respiratory distress when administered concomitantly. Monitor closely.

## EFFECTS ON DIAGNOSTIC TESTS

None reported.

## CONTRAINDICATIONS

Contraindicated in patients with hypersensitivity to drug and in those with thrombocytopenia, coagulation disorders, or an increase in bleeding tendency due to other causes.

## NURSING CONSIDERATIONS

• Never give drug I.M. or S.C.
• Continue CBC and blood studies, as ordered, at least 8 weeks after therapy is stopped. Leukopenia and thrombocytopenia are cumulative. If WBC count falls below 2,000/mm$^3$ or granulocyte count falls below 1,000/mm$^3$, follow institutional policy for infection control in immunocompromised patients.
• To prevent bleeding, avoid all I.M. injections when platelet count is below 100,000/mm$^3$.
• Anticipate need for blood transfusions to combat anemia. Patients may receive injections of RBC colony-stimulating factors to promote RBC production and decrease need for blood transfusions.
• Monitor patient for dyspnea with nonproductive cough; chest X-ray may show infiltrates.
• Monitor renal function tests, as ordered.
• *Alert:* Don't confuse mitomycin with mithramycin.

## I.V. administration

• Follow institutional policy to reduce risks. Preparation and administration of parenteral form of drug are associated with mutagenic, teratogenic, and carcinogenic risks to personnel.
• Using sterile water for injection, reconstitute drug in 5-mg vials with 10 ml, 20-mg vials with 40 ml, and 40-mg vials with 80 ml. When reconstituted with sterile water, the solution is stable for 14 days under refrigeration and 7 days at room temperature.
• For infusion, dilute with normal saline for injection, D$_5$W, or sodium lactate for injection. After dilution, drug is stable for 3 hours in D$_5$W, 12 hours in normal saline for injection, and 24 hours in sodium lactate for injection at room temperature.
• Avoid extravasation. Stop infusion immediately and notify doctor if extravasation occurs because of potential for severe ulceration and necrosis.

## Patient teaching

• Warn patient to watch for signs and symptoms of infection (fever, sore throat, fatigue) and bleeding (easy bruising, nosebleeds, bleeding gums, melena). Tell patient to take temperature daily.
• Inform patient that alopecia may occur, but that it's usually reversible.

# pentostatin
# (2'-deoxycoformycin)
Nipent

*Pregnancy Risk Category D*

## HOW SUPPLIED
*Powder for injection:* 10 mg-vial

## ACTION
Inhibits the enzyme adenosine deaminase (ADA), causing an increase in intracellular levels of deoxyadenosine triphosphate, which leads to cell damage and death. Because the greatest activity of ADA is in cells of the lymphoid system (especially malignant T cells), pentostatin is useful in treating leukemias.

| Route | Onset | Peak | Duration |
|-------|-------|------|----------|
| I.V. | Unknown | Unknown | Unknown |

## INDICATIONS & DOSAGE
*Alpha interferon–refractory hairy cell leukemia—*
**Adults:** 4 mg/m$^2$ I.V. every other week.

## ADVERSE REACTIONS
**CNS:** *headache, neurologic symptoms, malaise, anxiety, confusion, depression, dizziness, insomnia, nervousness, paresthesia, somnolence, abnormal thinking, fatigue, asthenia.*
**CV:** **arrhythmias,** abnormal ECG, *MI,* angina, **heart failure,** thrombophlebitis, peripheral edema, **hemorrhage.**
**EENT:** abnormal vision, conjunctivitis, ear pain, eye pain, *epistaxis, pharyngitis, rhinitis,* sinusitis.
**GI:** *abdominal pain, nausea, vomiting, anorexia, diarrhea,* constipation, flatulence, *stomatitis.*
**GU:** hematuria, dysuria, increased BUN and creatinine levels.
**Hematologic:** *myelosuppression,* LEUKOPENIA, *anemia,* THROMBOCYTOPENIA, lymphadenopathy.
**Hepatic:** *elevated liver enzyme levels.*
**Metabolic:** weight loss.
**Musculoskeletal:** chest pain, back pain, *myalgia,* arthralgia.

**Respiratory:** *cough, bronchitis, dyspnea,* **pulmonary edema,** pneumonia, *upper respiratory infection.*
**Skin:** *ecchymosis, petechiae, rash,* eczema, dry skin, herpes simplex or zoster, maculopapular rash, vesiculobullous rash, *pruritus, seborrhea, discoloration, diaphoresis.*
**Other:** *fever,* INFECTION, *pain,* HYPERSENSITIVITY REACTIONS, *chills, sepsis,* **death, neoplasm,** flulike syndrome, increased uric acid levels.

## INTERACTIONS
**Drug-drug.** *Cytarabine, vidarabine:* increased incidence or severity of adverse effects associated with either drug. Avoid concomitant use.
*Fludarabine:* risk of severe or fatal pulmonary toxicity. Don't use together.

## EFFECTS ON DIAGNOSTIC TESTS
None reported.

## CONTRAINDICATIONS
Contraindicated in patients with hypersensitivity to drug.

## NURSING CONSIDERATIONS
● Use cautiously and only under supervision of doctor qualified in and experienced with chemotherapeutic drugs. Adverse reactions after pentostatin therapy are common.
● Avoid use in patients with renal damage (creatinine clearance of 60 ml/minute or less).
● Treat all spills and waste products with 5% sodium hypochlorite (household bleach).
● Optimal duration of therapy is unknown. Current recommendations suggest two additional courses of therapy after a complete response. If a partial response isn't evident after 6 months of therapy, drug is discontinued. If partial response occurs, drug is continued for another 6 months.
● *Alert:* Withhold or discontinue drug and notify doctor if there is evidence of CNS toxicity, severe rash, or active infection. Drug may be resumed when the infection clears.

---

Reactions may be *common,* uncommon, **life-threatening**, or COMMON AND LIFE-THREATENING.

• Temporarily withhold drug and notify doctor if absolute neutrophil count falls below 200/mm$^3$ and pretreatment level was over 500/mm$^3$. No recommendations exist regarding dosage adjustments in patients with anemia, neutropenia, or thrombocytopenia.

• If WBC count falls below 2,000/mm$^3$ or granulocyte count falls below 1,000/mm$^3$, follow institutional policy for infection control in immunocompromised patients.

• Anticipate possible blood transfusion during treatment because of cumulative anemia. Patient may receive injections of RBC colony-stimulating factors to promote RBC production and decrease need for blood transfusions.

• Drug should be used only in patients with hairy cell leukemia refractory to alpha interferon. This is defined as disease that progresses after minimum of 3 months of treatment with alpha interferon or disease that doesn't exhibit response after 6 months of therapy.

• Monitor renal function.

• *Alert:* Don't confuse pentostatin with pentosan.

**◖ I.V. administration**

• Make sure patient is adequately hydrated before therapy. Administer 500 to 1,000 ml of D$_5$W in half-normal saline solution, as ordered, for hydration. Ensure at least 2 L of urine output daily during therapy.

• Follow institutional policy to reduce risks. Preparation and administration of parenteral form of drug are associated with mutagenic, teratogenic, and carcinogenic risks to personnel.

• Add 5 ml of sterile water for injection to vial containing pentostatin powder for injection. Mix thoroughly to make a solution of 2 mg/ml. Drug may be administered by I.V. bolus injection or diluted further in 25 or 50 ml of D$_5$W or normal saline for injection and infused over 20 to 30 minutes.

• Use reconstituted solution within 8 hours; it contains no preservatives.

• Give an additional 500 ml of D$_5$W, as ordered, for hydration after drug is administered.

**☑ Patient teaching**

• Advise patient to watch for signs and symptoms of infection (fever, sore throat, fatigue) and bleeding (easy bruising, nosebleeds, bleeding gums, melena), and to take temperature daily.

• Caution woman of childbearing age to avoid becoming pregnant during therapy. Recommend that she consult doctor before becoming pregnant.

## plicamycin (mithramycin)
Mithracin

*Pregnancy Risk Category X*

### HOW SUPPLIED
*Injection:* 2.5-mg vials (contains mannitol 100 mg)

### ACTION
Unknown. Thought to form a complex with DNA, thus inhibiting RNA synthesis. Drug also inhibits osteocytic activity, blocking calcium and phosphorus resorption from bone.

| Route | Onset | Peak | Duration |
|-------|-------|------|----------|
| I.V. | 1-2 days | 3 days | 7-10 days |

### INDICATIONS & DOSAGE
Dosage and indications vary. Check treatment protocol with doctor.

*Hypercalcemia and hypercalciuria associated with advanced malignant disease—*
**Adults:** 15 to 25 mcg/kg/day I.V. over 4 to 6 hours for 3 to 4 days. Dosage repeated at weekly intervals until desired response is obtained.

*Testicular cancer—*
**Adults:** 25 to 30 mcg/kg/day I.V. for 8 to 10 days or until toxicity occurs. Don't use more than 10 daily doses, or 30 mcg/kg individual daily doses.

### ADVERSE REACTIONS
**CNS:** drowsiness, weakness, lethargy, depression, headache, malaise.
**GI:** *nausea, vomiting,* anorexia, diarrhea, stomatitis.
**GU:** increased BUN and serum creatinine levels.

**Hematologic:** *leukopenia, thrombocytopenia; bleeding syndrome.*
**Hepatic:** *elevated liver enzyme levels, hepatotoxicity.*
**Metabolic:** *decreased serum calcium,* potassium, and phosphorus levels.
**Skin:** facial flushing, rash; pain, redness, swelling at injection site, cellulitis with extravasation, phlebitis.
**Other:** *death,* fever.

**INTERACTIONS**
None significant.

**EFFECTS ON DIAGNOSTIC TESTS**
None reported.

**CONTRAINDICATIONS**
Contraindicated in patients with thrombocytopenia, bone marrow suppression, or coagulation and bleeding disorders, and in women who are or may become pregnant.

**NURSING CONSIDERATIONS**
• Use with extreme caution in patients with significant renal or hepatic impairment.
• Obtain baseline platelet count and PT before therapy, as ordered.
• To reduce nausea, give antiemetic before administering, as ordered.
• Use ideal body weight to calculate dose if patient has edema or fluid retention.
• Avoid contact with skin or mucous membranes.
• Monitor platelet count and PT during therapy, as ordered. Discontinue drug and notify doctor if patient's WBC falls below 4,000/mm³, if platelet count falls below 150,000/mm³, or if PT is prolonged more than 4 seconds longer than control.
• *Alert:* Facial flushing is an early indicator of bleeding. The first evidence of a bleeding syndrome may range from epistaxis (nosebleed) to generalized hemorrhage.
• To prevent bleeding, avoid all I.M. injections when platelet count is below 100,000/mm³.
• Anticipate need for blood transfusions to combat anemia. Patient may receive injections of RBC colony-stimulating factors to promote RBC production and decrease need for blood transfusions.

• Monitor LD, AST, ALT, alkaline phosphatase, BUN, creatinine, potassium, calcium, and phosphorus levels, as ordered.
• Monitor patient for tetany, carpopedal spasm, Chvostek's sign, and muscle cramps; check serum calcium level. Precipitous drop in calcium level is possible.
• Patients receiving drug for treatment of testicular cancer may need calcium supplementation.

**⬛ I.V. administration**
• Follow institutional policy to reduce risks. Preparation and administration of parenteral form of drug are associated with carcinogenic, mutagenic, and teratogenic risks for personnel.
• To prepare solution, add 4.9 ml of sterile water for injection to vial and shake to dissolve. Then dilute for I.V infusion in 1,000 ml of D₅W or normal saline. Administer by infusion over 4 to 6 hours. Discard unused drug.
• Slow infusion reduces nausea that develops with I.V. push.
• Avoid extravasation. Plicamycin is a vesicant and tissue necrosis may result. If I.V. solution infiltrates, stop infusion immediately, notify doctor, and use ice packs. Restart I.V. line.
• Store lyophilized powder in refrigerator and protect from light.

**✅ Patient teaching**
• Advise patient to watch for signs and symptoms of infection (fever, sore throat, fatigue) and bleeding (easy bruising, nosebleeds, bleeding gums, melena), and to take temperature daily.
• Caution woman of childbearing age to avoid becoming pregnant during therapy. Recommend that she consult doctor before becoming pregnant.

**✳ NEW DRUG**

## valrubicin
Valstar

*Pregnancy Risk Category C*

**HOW SUPPLIED**
*Solution for intravesical instillation:* 200 mg/5 ml

---

Reactions may be *common,* uncommon, *life-threatening,* or COMMON AND LIFE-THREATENING.

## ACTION

An anthracycline that exerts its cytotoxic activity by penetrating into cells, where it inhibits the incorporation of nucleosides into nucleic acids, causes extensive chromosomal damage, and stops the cell cycle. Also interferes with the normal DNA breaking-resealing, thereby inhibiting DNA synthesis.

| Route | Onset | Peak | Duration |
|-------|-------|------|----------|
| Intra-vesically | Unknown | Unknown | Unknown |

## INDICATIONS & DOSAGE

*Intravesical therapy of bacillus Calmette-Guérin–refractory carcinoma in situ of urinary bladder in patients for whom immediate cystectomy would be associated with unacceptable morbidity or mortality—*
**Adults:** 800 mg intravesically once weekly for 6 weeks.

## ADVERSE REACTIONS

**CNS:** asthenia, headache, malaise, dizziness.
**CV:** vasodilation, chest pain, peripheral edema.
**GI:** diarrhea, flatulence, nausea, vomiting, abdominal pain.
**GU:** urine retention, *urinary tract infection,* urinary frequency, dysuria, urinary urgency, bladder spasm, hematuria, *bladder pain, urinary incontinence,* pelvic pain, urethral pain, nocturia, *cystitis,* local burning symptoms.
**Hematologic:** anemia.
**Metabolic:** hyperglycemia.
**Musculoskeletal:** myalgia, back pain.
**Respiratory:** pneumonia.
**Skin:** rash.
**Other:** fever.

## INTERACTIONS

None significant.

## EFFECTS ON DIAGNOSTIC TESTS

None reported.

## CONTRAINDICATIONS

Contraindicated in patients with hypersensitivity to drug, other anthracyclines, or Cremophor EL (polyoxyethyleneglycol triricinoleate) and in those with concurrent urinary tract infections, small bladder capacity (unable to tolerate a 75-ml instillation), or perforated bladder; also contraindicated in those in whom the integrity of the bladder mucosa has been compromised.

## NURSING CONSIDERATIONS

• Use cautiously in patients with severe irritable bladder symptoms. Bladder spasm and spontaneous discharge of intravesical instillate may occur. Don't clamp the urinary catheter; if absolutely necessary, perform under medical supervision.
• For patients undergoing transurethral resection of the bladder, evaluate status of bladder before intravesical instillation of drug to avoid dangerous systemic exposure. If bladder perforation occurs, delay administration until bladder integrity has been restored.
• If there isn't a complete response of carcinoma in situ (CIS) to drug treatment after 3 months or if CIS recurs, cystectomy must be reconsidered because delaying cystectomy could lead to development of metastatic bladder cancer.
• Myelosuppression is possible if drug is inadvertently administered systemically or if significant systemic exposure occurs after intravesical administration, such as in patients with bladder rupture or perforation. If drug is administered when bladder rupture or perforation is suspected, monitor CBC weekly for 3 weeks. Myelosuppression begins during first week, with nadir by second week, and recovery by third week.
• Monitor patient closely for disease recurrence or progression by cystoscopy, biopsy, and urine cytology every 3 months.
• Drug should be administered intravesically only under supervision of doctors experienced in use of intravesical antineoplastics. Don't give drug I.V. or I.M.
• Use caution when handling and preparing solution. Use gloves during dose preparation and administration. Prepare and store solution in glass, polypropylene, or polyolefin containers and tubing. Use polyethylene-lined administration sets.

---

Don't use with products containing polyvinyl chloride.
• To prepare, warm four vials containing drug slowly to room temperature. Withdraw total of 20 ml from the four vials (200 mg valrubicin in each 5-ml vial), and dilute with 55 ml of normal saline, providing 75 ml of diluted valrubicin solution.
• Use aseptic technique during administration to avoid introducing contaminants into urinary tract or traumatizing urinary mucosa.
• To administer drug, first drain bladder by inserting a urethral catheter into patient's bladder under aseptic conditions. Then, instill solution slowly via gravity flow over period of several minutes. Withdraw catheter. Patient should retain drug for 2 hours before voiding. (Some patients are unable to retain drug for 2 hours.)
• Use procedures for proper handling and disposal of antineoplastics.
• Store unopened vials under refrigeration at 36° to 46° F (2° to 8° C). Diluted valrubicin is stable for 12 hours at temperatures up to 77° F (25° C).

### ✓ Patient teaching
• Inform patient that drug has been shown to induce complete response in only about one in five patients with refractory CIS. If there isn't a complete response of CIS to treatment after 3 months or if CIS recurs, tell patient to discuss with doctor risks of cystectomy versus risks of metastatic bladder cancer.
• Advise patient to retain drug for 2 hours before voiding, if possible, and to void at end of 2 hours.
• Instruct patient to maintain adequate hydration following treatment.
• Inform patient about irritable bladder symptoms, such as bladder spasm, urinary urgency, frequency or pain, that may occur during instillation and retention of drug and for a limited period following voiding. For first 24 hours following administration, red-tinged urine is common. Tell patient to immediately report prolonged irritable bladder symptoms or prolonged passage of red-colored urine.

• Advise woman of childbearing age and their partners to avoid pregnancy during treatment. Recommend use of effective contraception during therapy.

---

# 72

## Antineoplastics that alter hormone balance

**anastrozole**
**bicalutamide**
**estramustine phosphate sodium**
**exemestane**
**flutamide**
**goserelin acetate**
**letrozole**
**leuprolide acetate**
**megestrol acetate**
**nilutamide**
**tamoxifen citrate**
**testolactone**
**toremifene citrate**

**COMBINATION PRODUCTS**
None.

### anastrozole
Arimidex

*Pregnancy Risk Category D*

**HOW SUPPLIED**
*Tablets*: 1 mg

**ACTION**
A selective nonsteroidal aromatase inhibitor that significantly lowers serum estradiol levels, thereby inhibiting stimulation of breast cancer cell growth in postmenopausal women.

| Route | Onset | Peak | Duration |
|---|---|---|---|
| P.O. | < 24 hr | Unknown | < 6 days |

**INDICATIONS & DOSAGE**
*Advanced breast cancer in postmenopausal women with disease progression after tamoxifen therapy—*
**Adults:** 1 mg P.O. daily.

**ADVERSE REACTIONS**
**CNS:** *headache, asthenia,* dizziness, depression, paresthesia.
**CV:** chest pain, edema, thromboembolic disease, peripheral edema.
**EENT:** pharyngitis.
**GI:** *nausea,* vomiting, diarrhea, constipation, abdominal pain, anorexia, dry mouth, weight gain.
**GU:** vaginal hemorrhage, vaginal dryness, pelvic pain.
**Musculoskeletal:** bone pain, *back pain.*
**Respiratory:** dyspnea, increased cough.
**Skin:** *alopecia,* rash, sweating.
**Other:** *pain, hot flashes.*

**INTERACTIONS**
None significant.

**EFFECTS ON DIAGNOSTIC TESTS**
None reported.

**CONTRAINDICATIONS**
No known contraindications.

**NURSING CONSIDERATIONS**
- Use cautiously in breast-feeding women.
- Pregnancy must be ruled out before treatment.
- Administer drug under supervision of a qualified doctor experienced in use of anticancer drugs.

☑ **Patient teaching**
- Instruct patient to report adverse reactions.
- Stress need for follow-up care.
- Counsel woman of childbearing age about potential risks to pregnancy during therapy.

### bicalutamide
Casodex

*Pregnancy Risk Category X*

**HOW SUPPLIED**
*Tablets:* 50 mg

## ACTION

A nonsteroidal antiandrogen that binds to cytosol androgen receptors in target tissue.

| Route | Onset | Peak | Duration |
|-------|-------|------|----------|
| P.O. | Unknown | Unknown | Unknown |

## INDICATIONS & DOSAGE

*Adjunct therapy with a luteinizing hormone–releasing hormone (LH–RH) analogue for treatment of advanced prostate cancer—*
**Adults:** 50 mg P.O. once daily in morning or evening, at same time each day.

## ADVERSE REACTIONS

**CNS:** anxiety, *asthenia,* depression, headache, dizziness, paresthesia, insomnia.
**CV:** hypertension, chest pain, peripheral edema.
**GI:** *constipation, nausea, diarrhea,* abdominal pain, flatulence, vomiting, weight loss.
**GU:** nocturia, hematuria, urinary tract infection, impotence, urinary incontinence, *gynecomastia, breast pain, pelvic pain.*
**Hematologic:** hypochromic anemia, iron deficiency anemia.
**Hepatic:** elevated liver enzyme levels.
**Metabolic:** hyperglycemia.
**Musculoskeletal:** bone pain, *back pain.*
**Respiratory:** dyspnea.
**Skin:** rash, sweating, dry skin, pruritus.
**Other:** *general pain, infection,* flulike syndrome, *hot flashes.*

## INTERACTIONS

**Drug-drug.** *Coumadin anticoagulants:* displacement of these drugs from their protein-binding sites. Monitor PT closely; anticoagulant dosage may need adjustment.

## EFFECTS ON DIAGNOSTIC TESTS

Drug may elevate bilirubin, BUN, and creatinine levels and decrease hemoglobin level and WBC count.

## CONTRAINDICATIONS

Contraindicated in patients with hypersensitivity to drug or its components and during pregnancy.

## NURSING CONSIDERATIONS

• Use cautiously in patients with moderate to severe hepatic impairment (drug is extensively metabolized by the liver).
• Drug is used with an LH–RH analogue. Treatment should begin at same time for both drugs.
• Give drug at same time each day.
• Regularly monitor serum prostate-specific antigen (PSA) levels, as ordered. PSA levels help in assessing response to therapy. Report elevated levels to doctor, who should evaluate patient to determine disease progression.
• Monitor liver function studies, as ordered. When patient develops jaundice or exhibits laboratory evidence of liver injury in the absence of liver metastases, drug should be discontinued. Abnormalities are usually reversible on discontinuation.

☑ **Patient teaching**
• Tell patient to take drug at same time each day, without regard to meals.
• Urge patient not to stop drug therapy without consulting doctor.

---

**estramustine phosphate sodium**
Emcyt, Estracyt‡ , Estracyt§

*Pregnancy Risk Category NR*

## HOW SUPPLIED

*Capsules:* 140 mg

## ACTION

Unknown. A combination of estrogen and an alkylating drug, it probably acts by its ability to bind selectively to a protein present in the prostate gland.

| Route | Onset | Peak | Duration |
|-------|-------|------|----------|
| P.O. | Unknown | Unknown | Unknown |

## INDICATIONS & DOSAGE

*Palliative treatment of metastatic or progressive prostate cancer—*
**Adults:** 10 to 16 mg/kg/day P.O. in three or four divided doses. Usual dose is 14 mg/kg daily. Therapy continued for up to 3 months and, if successful, maintained as long as patient responds.

## ADVERSE REACTIONS

**CNS:** lethargy, insomnia, headache, anxiety.

**CV:** *MI, edema,* chest pain, thrombophlebitis, *heart failure, stroke.*

**GI:** *nausea, vomiting,* diarrhea, anorexia, flatulence, GI bleeding, thirst.

**GU:** *painful gynecomastia,* decreased libido.

**Hematologic:** *leukopenia, thrombocytopenia.*

**Hepatic:** increased AST, ALT, LD, and triglyceride levels.

**Musculoskeletal:** leg cramps.

**Respiratory:** *pulmonary embolism,* dyspnea.

**Skin:** rash, pruritus, dry skin, thinning of hair, flushing.

**Other:** *breast tenderness,* sodium and fluid retention, increased ceruloplasmin, cortisol, phospholipids and prolactin PT levels, decreased serum folate, pregnanediol, pyridoxine, and phosphate levels.

## INTERACTIONS

**Drug-drug.** *Calcium-containing drugs such as antacids:* impaired absorption of estramustine. Don't administer at same time.

**Drug-food.** *Calcium-rich foods, such as dairy products and milk:* impaired absorption of estramustine. Don't administer concurrently.

## EFFECTS ON DIAGNOSTIC TESTS

May increase norepinephrine-induced platelet aggregation and may reduce response to the metyrapone test. Glucose tolerance may be decreased.

## CONTRAINDICATIONS

Contraindicated in patients with hypersensitivity to estradiol or nitrogen mustard and in those with active thrombophlebitis or thromboembolic disorders, except when actual tumor mass is cause of thromboembolic phenomenon.

## NURSING CONSIDERATIONS

• Use cautiously in patients with history of thrombophlebitis or thromboembolic disorders or cerebrovascular or coronary artery disease. Monitor weight regularly in these patients. Drug may exaggerate preexisting peripheral edema or heart failure.

• Also use cautiously in patients with impaired liver function. Monitor liver function periodically throughout therapy.

• Each 140-mg capsule contains 12.5 mg of sodium.

• Drug may increase blood pressure and decrease blood glucose level. Monitor periodically throughout therapy.

• Drug is a combination of estrogen estradiol and a nitrogen mustard, and has been shown to be effective in patients refractory to estrogen therapy alone.

• Patient may continue therapy as long as response is favorable. Some patients have taken drug for over 3 years.

• Store capsules in refrigerator.

### ☑ Patient teaching

• Tell patient to take drug on an empty stomach (1 hour before or 2 hours after meals) and to avoid taking with milk or dairy products.

• Because of risk of mutagenic effects, advise patient and partner to use contraception if woman is of childbearing age.

---

✳ *NEW DRUG*

## exemestane
Aromasin

*Pregnancy Risk Category D*

## HOW SUPPLIED

*Tablets:* 25 mg

## INDICATION AND DOSAGE

*Advanced breast cancer in post-menopausal women whose disease has progressed following treatment with ta-moxifen—*

**Adults:** 25 mg P.O. once daily after food.

## ACTION

A highly protein-bound, irreversible, steroidal aromatase inactivator that leads to reduced levels of circulating estrogens, thereby decreasing cell growth in estrogen-dependent breast cancer.

| Route | Onset | Peak | Duration |
|-------|-------|------|----------|
| P.O. | Unknown | 1.2 hr | 24 hr |

## ADVERSE REACTIONS
**CNS:** *depression, insomnia, anxiety, fatigue, pain,* dizziness, headache, paresthesia, generalized weakness, asthenia, confusion, hypoesthesia.
**CV:** hypertension, edema, chest pain.
**EENT:** sinusitis, rhinitis, pharyngitis.
**GI:** *nausea,* vomiting, abdominal pain, anorexia, constipation, diarrhea, increased appetite, dyspepsia.
**GU:** urinary tract infection.
**Musculoskeletal:** pathological fractures, arthritis, back pain, skeletal pain.
**Respiratory:** *dyspnea,* bronchitis, coughing, upper respiratory tract infection.
**Skin:** rash, increased sweating, alopecia, itching.
**Other:** fever, infection, flulike syndrome, lymphedema, *hot flashes.*

## INTERACTIONS
**Drug-drug.** *Drugs that induce CYP 3A4:* may decrease exemestane plasma levels. Monitor closely.

## EFFECTS ON DIAGNOSTIC TESTS
None reported.

## CONTRAINDICATIONS
Contraindicated in patients with hypersensitivity to drug or its components.

## NURSING CONSIDERATIONS
• Use drug only in postmenopausal women.
• *Alert:* Don't coadminister with estrogen-containing drugs because this may interfere with intended action.
• Treatment should continue until tumor progression is apparent.

### ☑ Patient teaching
• Inform patient to take drug after a meal.
• Tell patient that she may need to take drug for a long time.
• Advise patient to report adverse effects to doctor.

## flutamide
Drogenil§, Euflex†, Eulexin

*Pregnancy Risk Category D*

## HOW SUPPLIED
*Capsules:* 125 mg, 250 mg†

## ACTION
Inhibits androgen uptake or prevents binding of androgens in nucleus of cells within target tissues.

| Route | Onset | Peak | Duration |
|-------|-------|------|----------|
| P.O. | Unknown | 2 hr | Unknown |

## INDICATIONS & DOSAGE
*Metastatic prostate cancer (stages $B_2$, C, $D_2$) with luteinizing hormone–releasing hormone analogues such as leuprolide acetate—*
**Adults:** 250 mg P.O. q 8 hours.

## ADVERSE REACTIONS
**CNS:** drowsiness, confusion, depression, anxiety, nervousness, paresthesia.
**CV:** peripheral edema, hypertension.
**GI:** *diarrhea, nausea, vomiting,* anorexia.
**GU:** *impotence, loss of libido,* gynecomastia.
**Hematologic:** anemia, *leukopenia, thrombocytopenia,* hemolytic anemia.
**Hepatic:** elevated liver enzyme levels, *hepatitis,* encephalopathy.
**Skin:** rash, photosensitivity.
**Other:** *hot flashes.*

## INTERACTIONS
**Drug-drug.** *Warfarin:* may increase PT. Monitor PT and INR.
**Drug-lifestyle.** *Sun exposure:* may cause sensitivity reactions. Warn patient to take appropriate precautions.

## EFFECTS ON DIAGNOSTIC TESTS
Elevation of plasma testosterone and estradiol levels has been reported. Serum ALT, AST, bilirubin, and creatinine levels may be increased.

## CONTRAINDICATIONS
Contraindicated in patients with hypersensitivity to drug.

---

Reactions may be *common,* uncommon, *life-threatening,* or COMMON AND LIFE-THREATENING.

## NURSING CONSIDERATIONS
• Monitor liver function tests and CBC periodically, as ordered.
• Flutamide must be taken continuously with drug used for medical castration (such as leuprolide) to allow full benefit of therapy. Leuprolide suppresses testosterone production while flutamide inhibits testosterone action at cellular level; together, they can impair growth of androgen-responsive tumors.

### ☑ Patient teaching
• Advise patient not to discontinue drug therapy without consulting doctor.
• Instruct patient to report adverse reactions promptly.

---

## goserelin acetate
Zoladex

*Pregnancy Risk Category X (endometriosis and endometrial thinning); D (breast cancer)*

## HOW SUPPLIED
*Implants:* 3.6 mg, 10.8 mg

## ACTION
A luteinizing hormone–releasing hormone (LH–RH) analogue that acts on the pituitary gland to decrease the release of follicle-stimulating hormone and luteinizing hormone, resulting in dramatically lowered serum levels of sex hormones.

| Route | Onset | Peak | Duration |
|-------|-------|------|----------|
| S.C. | 2-4 wk | 12-15 days | Throughout therapy |

## INDICATIONS & DOSAGE
*Endometriosis, palliative treatment of advanced prostate cancer—*
**Adults:** 3.6 mg S.C. q 28 days into upper abdominal wall. For endometriosis, maximum duration of therapy is 6 months. For prostate cancer, 10.8 mg S.C. into upper abdominal wall q 12 weeks.
*Palliative treatment of advanced breast cancer in pre- and perimenopausal women—*
**Adults:** 3.6 mg S.C. q 28 days into upper abdominal wall.

*For endometrial thinning before endometrial ablation—*
**Adults:** 3.6 mg S.C. into upper abdominal wall. One or two depots are recommended (each given 4 weeks apart).

## ADVERSE REACTIONS
**CNS:** lethargy, pain, dizziness, *insomnia,* anxiety, *depression, headache,* chills, *emotional lability asthenia.*
**CV:** edema, *heart failure, arrhythmias, peripheral edema, CVA,* hypertension, *MI,* peripheral vascular disorder, chest pain.
**GI:** nausea, vomiting, diarrhea, constipation, ulcer, anorexia, abdominal pain.
**GU:** *impotence, sexual dysfunction, lower urinary tract symptoms,* renal insufficiency, urinary obstruction, *vaginitis,* urinary tract infection, amenorrhea.
**Hematologic:** anemia.
**Metabolic:** hypercalcemia, hyperglycemia, weight increase.
**Musculoskeletal:** back pain.
**Respiratory:** COPD, upper respiratory tract infection.
**Skin:** rash, *diaphoresis, acne, seborrhea,* hirsutism.
**Other:** *hot flashes,* gout, breast swelling and tenderness, *changes in breast size,* breast pain, *changes in libido, infection.*

## INTERACTIONS
None significant.

## EFFECTS ON DIAGNOSTIC TESTS
Serum testosterone levels increase during first week of therapy and then decrease. Serum acid phosphatase level may increase initially and will decrease by week 4. Serum lipid levels may be increased.

## CONTRAINDICATIONS
Contraindicated in patients with hypersensitivity to LH–RH, LH–RH agonist analogues, or goserelin acetate. Also contraindicated in pregnant or breast-feeding women and in patients with obstructive uropathy or vertebral metastases. The 10.8-mg implant is contraindicated in women because data are insufficient to support reliable suppression of serum estradiol.

---

## NURSING CONSIDERATIONS

• Because use of drug is associated with loss of bone mineral density in women, use cautiously in patients with risk factors for osteoporosis, such as family history of osteoporosis, chronic alcohol or tobacco abuse, or use of drugs, such as corticosteroids or anticonvulsants, that affect bone density.
• Before administering to women, rule out pregnancy.
• Never administer by I.V. injection.
• Administer drug into upper abdominal wall using aseptic technique. After cleaning area with an alcohol swab (and injecting a local anesthetic), stretch patient's skin with one hand while grasping barrel of syringe with the other. Insert needle into the subcutaneous fat; then change direction of needle so that it parallels the abdominal wall. Push needle in until hub touches patient's skin; withdraw about 1 cm (this creates a gap for drug to be injected) before depressing plunger completely.
• To avoid need for a new syringe and injection site, don't aspirate after inserting needle. If needle penetrates a blood vessel, blood will be seen in the syringe chamber. Withdraw needle, and inject elsewhere with a new syringe.
• **Alert:** Implant comes in a preloaded syringe. If package is damaged, don't use the syringe. Make sure that drug is visible in the translucent chamber of the syringe.
• When used for prostate cancer, LH–RH analogues such as goserelin may initially cause a worsening of prostatic cancer symptoms because drug initially increases testosterone serum levels. Some patients may experience increased bone pain. Rarely, disease exacerbation (either spinal cord compression or ureteral obstruction) has occurred.
• When used for endometrial thinning, surgery should be performed at 4 weeks if one depot is administered. When two depots are given, surgery should be performed within 2 to 4 weeks after administration of second depot.

### ☑ Patient teaching
• Advise patient to report every 28 days for a new implant. A delay of a couple of days is permissible.

• Tell patient that pain may worsen for first 30 days of treatment.
• Tell woman to use a nonhormonal form of contraception during treatment. Caution patient about significant risks to fetus should pregnancy occur.
• Tell woman to call doctor if menstruation persists or if breakthrough bleeding occurs. Menstruation should stop during treatment.
• Inform woman that a delayed return of menses may occur after therapy ends. Persistent amenorrhea is rare.

---

## letrozole
Femara

*Pregnancy Risk Category D*

### HOW SUPPLIED
*Tablets:* 2.5 mg

### ACTION
A nonsteroidal competitive inhibitor of the aromatase enzyme system, resulting in the inhibition of the conversion of androgens to estrogens. Decreased estrogens lead to decreased tumor mass or delayed progression of tumor growth in some women.

| Route | Onset | Peak | Duration |
|-------|-------|------|----------|
| P.O. | Unknown | 2 days | Unknown |

### INDICATIONS & DOSAGE
*Metastatic breast cancer in postmenopausal women with disease progression following antiestrogen therapy—*
**Adults:** 2.5 mg P.O. as single daily dose.

### ADVERSE REACTIONS
**CNS:** headache, somnolence, dizziness, fatigue, mood changes.
**CV:** hypertension, *thromboembolism,* chest pain, edema.
**GI:** *nausea,* vomiting, constipation, diarrhea, abdominal pain, anorexia.
**Metabolic:** weight gain.
**Musculoskeletal:** *bone pain, extremities pain, back pain,* arthralgia.
**Respiratory:** dyspnea, coughing.
**Skin:** rash, pruritus.

---

**Other:** hypercholesterolemia, viral infections, hot flashes.

**INTERACTIONS**
None significant.

**EFFECTS ON DIAGNOSTIC TESTS**
None reported.

**CONTRAINDICATIONS**
Contraindicated in patients with known hypersensitivity to drug or its components.

**NURSING CONSIDERATIONS**
• Dosage adjustment isn't needed in renally impaired patients with creatinine clearance of 10 ml/minute or more.
• Use cautiously in patients with severe liver impairment; dosage adjustment isn't needed for mild to moderate liver dysfunction.
• Food doesn't affect drug absorption.

☑ **Patient teaching**
• Instruct patient to take drug exactly as prescribed.
• Tell patient that drug can be taken with or without food.
• Inform patient about potential adverse reactions.

---

**leuprolide acetate**
Lucrin‡, Lupron, Lupron Depot, Lupron Depot-Ped, Lupron Depot-3 Month, Lupron Depot-4 Month, Lupron for Pediatric Use

*Pregnancy Risk Category X*

**HOW SUPPLIED**
*Injection:* 1 mg/0.2 ml (5 mg/ml) in 2.8-ml multiple-dose vials
*Depot injection:* 3.75 mg, 7.5 mg, 11.25 mg, 15 mg, 22.5 mg, 30 mg

**ACTION**
Initially stimulates but then inhibits release of follicle-stimulating hormone and luteinizing hormone, resulting in testosterone suppression.

| Route | Onset | Peak | Duration |
|-------|-------|------|----------|
| I.M., S.C. | < 2-4 wk | 1-2 mo | 60-90 days |

**INDICATIONS & DOSAGE**
*Advanced prostate cancer—*
**Adults:** 1 mg S.C. daily. Or, 7.5 mg I.M. (depot injection) monthly, or 22.5 mg I.M. q 3 months (depot injection), or 30 mg I.M. q 4 months (depot injection).
*Endometriosis—*
**Adults:** 3.75 mg I.M (depot injection only) as single injection once monthly for up to 6 months, or 11.25 mg I.M. q 3 months for up to 6 months.
*Central precocious puberty—*
**Children:** initially, 0.3 mg/kg (minimum 7.5 mg) I.M. (depot injection only) as single injection q 4 weeks. Dosage may be increased in increments of 3.75 mg q 4 weeks, if needed. Therapy should be discontinued before female child reaches age 11 and before male child reaches age 12.

**ADVERSE REACTIONS**
**CNS:** *dizziness, depression, headache, pain,* insomnia, paresthesia, *asthenia.*
**CV:** *arrhythmias,* angina, *MI, peripheral edema, ECG changes,* hypotension, hypertension, murmur.
**GI:** *nausea, vomiting,* anorexia, constipation.
**GU:** *impotence, vaginitis,* urinary frequency, hematuria, urinary tract infection, gynecomastia, amenorrhea.
**Hematologic:** anemia.
**Hepatic:** elevated liver enzyme levels.
**Metabolic:** *weight gain or loss.*
**Musculoskeletal:** transient bone pain during first week of treatment, joint disorder, myalgia, neuromuscular disorder.
**Respiratory:** dyspnea, sinus congestion, pulmonary fibrosis.
**Skin:** reactions at injection site, dermatitis.
**Other:** *hot flashes,* androgen-like effects.

**INTERACTIONS**
None significant.

**EFFECTS ON DIAGNOSTIC TESTS**
Serum acid phosphatase and testosterone levels initially increase; then decrease with continued therapy.

**CONTRAINDICATIONS**
Contraindicated in patients with hypersensitivity to drug or other gonadotropin-releasing hormone analogues, in women

---

with undiagnosed vaginal bleeding, and in pregnant or breast-feeding women. The 30-mg depot injection is contraindicated in women.

## NURSING CONSIDERATIONS
• Use cautiously in patients hypersensitive to benzyl alcohol.
• Never administer by I.V. injection.
• Depot injections should be administered under medical supervision. Use supplied diluent to reconstitute drug (extra diluent is provided and remainder should be discarded). Draw 1 ml into a syringe with a 22G needle. (When preparing Lupron Depot-3 Month 22.5 mg, use a 23G or larger needle.) Withdraw 1.5 ml from ampule for the 3-month formulation. Inject into vial; then shake well. Suspension will appear milky. Although suspension is stable for 24 hours after reconstitution, it contains no bacteriostatic agent. Use immediately.
• When using prefilled dual-chamber syringes: Prepare for injection by screwing white plunger into end stopper until stopper begins to turn. Remove and discard tab around base of needle. Hold syringe upright and release diluent by slowly pushing plunger until first stopper is at blue line in middle of barrel. Gently shake syringe to form a uniform milky suspension. If particles adhere to stopper, tap syringe against your finger. Remove needle guard and advance plunger to expel air from syringe. Inject entire contents I.M. as you would for a normal injection.
• A fractional dose of drug formulated to give q 3 months isn't equivalent to same dose of once-a-month formulation.
• After the start of treatment for central precocious puberty, patient response should be monitored q 1 to 2 months with a gonadotropin-releasing hormone stimulation test and sex corticosteroid level determinations. Measurement of bone age for advancement should be done q 6 to 12 months.
• During first few weeks of therapy, drug may cause an increase in signs and symptoms being treated.

### ✓ Patient teaching
• Before starting child on treatment for central precocious puberty, ensure that parents understand importance of continuous therapy.
• Carefully instruct patient who will self-administer S.C. injection about proper administration techniques and advise her to use only the syringes provided by manufacturer.
• Advise patient that, if another syringe must be substituted, a low-dose insulin syringe (U-100, 0.5 ml) may be an appropriate choice but that needle gauge should be no smaller than 22G (except when using Lupron Depot-3 Month 22.5 mg).
• Instruct patient to store drug at room temperature, protected from heat and light.
• Inform patient with history of undesirable effects from other endocrine therapies that leuprolide is easier to tolerate.
• Reassure patient that adverse effects disappear after about 1 week. Worsening of prostate cancer symptoms or central precocious puberty symptoms may occur initially.
• Advise woman of childbearing age to use a nonhormonal form of contraception during treatment.

---

**megestrol acetate**
Megace, Megostat‡

*Pregnancy Risk Category D*

## HOW SUPPLIED
*Tablets:* 20 mg, 40 mg
*Oral suspension:* 40 mg/ml

## ACTION
A progestin that changes the tumor's hormonal environment and alters the neoplastic process. Mechanism for appetite stimulation is unknown.

| Route | Onset | Peak | Duration |
|-------|-------|------|----------|
| P.O. | Unknown | Unknown | Unknown |

## INDICATIONS & DOSAGE
*Breast cancer—*
**Adults:** 40 mg P.O. q.i.d.
*Endometrial cancer—*
**Adults:** 40 to 320 mg P.O. daily in divided doses.

---

*Anorexia, cachexia, or unexplained significant weight loss in patients with AIDS—*
**Adults:** 800 mg P.O. (oral suspension) daily.

**ADVERSE REACTIONS**
**CV:** thrombophlebitis, *heart failure,* hypertension.
**GI:** nausea, vomiting, diarrhea, flatulence, constipation, dry mouth, increased appetite.
**GU:** breakthrough menstrual bleeding, impotence, vaginal bleeding or discharge, urinary tract infection, gynecomastia.
**Metabolic:** hyperglycemia, weight gain.
**Musculoskeletal:** carpal tunnel syndrome.
**Respiratory:** *pulmonary embolism,* dyspnea.
**Skin:** alopecia, rash.
**Other:** tumor flare.

**INTERACTIONS**
None significant.

**EFFECTS ON DIAGNOSTIC TESTS**
Pregnanediol excretion may decrease; serum alkaline phosphatase and amino acid levels may increase. Glucose tolerance has been shown to decrease in a small percentage of patients.

**CONTRAINDICATIONS**
Contraindicated in patients with hypersensitivity to drug; also contraindicated as a diagnostic test for pregnancy.

**NURSING CONSIDERATIONS**
• Use cautiously in patients with history of thrombophlebitis.
• Blood glucose levels may increase in diabetic patients.
• Drug is relatively nontoxic, with a low risk of adverse effects.
• In patients with cancer, 2 months is an adequate trial period.

✓ **Patient teaching**
• Inform patient that therapeutic response isn't immediate.
• Advise breast-feeding woman to discontinue breast-feeding during therapy because of possible infant toxicity.

• Advise woman of childbearing age to use an effective form of contraception while receiving drug.

---

**nilutamide**
Anandron†, Nilandron

*Pregnancy Risk Category C*

**HOW SUPPLIED**
*Tablets:* 50 mg, 100 mg†

**ACTION**
A nonsteroidal antiandrogen that interacts with the androgen receptor and prevents normal androgenic response.

| Route | Onset | Peak | Duration |
|-------|-------|------|----------|
| P.O. | Unknown | Unknown | Unknown |

**INDICATIONS & DOSAGE**
*Adjunct therapy with surgical castration for treatment of metastatic prostate cancer—*
**Adults:** 300 mg P.O. daily for 30 days; then 150 mg P.O. daily thereafter.

**ADVERSE REACTIONS**
**CNS:** dizziness.
**CV:** hypertension.
**EENT:** *impaired adaptation to darkness,* photophobia, abnormal vision.
**GI:** nausea, constipation, diarrhea.
**GU:** urinary tract infection, impotence.
**Hepatic:** elevated liver enzyme levels.
**Respiratory:** dyspnea, interstitial pneumonitis.
**Other:** *hot flashes.*

**INTERACTIONS**
**Drug-drug.** *Phenytoin, theophylline, vitamin K antagonists:* possible delayed elimination and toxicity. Doses should be modified accordingly.
**Drug-lifestyle.** *Alcohol use:* may cause alcohol intolerance as evidenced by facial flushing, malaise, and hypotension. Avoid concomitant use.

**EFFECTS ON DIAGNOSTIC TESTS**
None reported.

## CONTRAINDICATIONS
Contraindicated in patients with hypersensitivity to drug and in those with severe hepatic or respiratory disease.

## NURSING CONSIDERATIONS
• Drug is used with surgical castration and should begin on same day or on day after surgery for maximum benefit.
• Safety and efficacy of drug in children haven't been determined.
• Obtain baseline liver enzyme levels and at 3-month intervals, as ordered. Drug should be discontinued if transaminase levels exceed three times upper limit of normal.
• A baseline chest X-ray should be obtained before therapy begins. Monitor patient (especially if Asian) for signs and symptoms of interstitial pneumonitis, and notify doctor if they occur. Obtain chest X-ray, as ordered.

☑ **Patient teaching**
• Explain purpose of drug, how it's given, and importance of not stopping treatment without consulting doctor.
• Tell patient to immediately report dyspnea or aggravation of preexisting dyspnea.
• Inform patient of risk of developing hepatitis and to report nausea, vomiting, abdominal pain, or jaundice to doctor. Tell patient to avoid alcohol during therapy.
• Warn patient that visual disturbances, such as a delay in adaptation to darkness, may affect driving at night or through tunnels.

---

## tamoxifen citrate
Nolvadex, Nolvadex-D†‡, Novo-
Tamoxifen†, Tamofen†, Tamone†

*Pregnancy Risk Category D*

## HOW SUPPLIED
*Tablets:* 10 mg, 20 mg
*Tablets (enteric-coated)†:* 10 mg, 20 mg

## ACTION
Exact neoplastic action unknown. Acts as an estrogen antagonist.

| Route | Onset | Peak | Duration |
|-------|-------|------|----------|
| P.O. | 1-several mo | Unknown | Several wk |

## INDICATIONS & DOSAGE
*Advanced breast cancer in women and men—*
**Adults:** 10 to 20 mg P.O. b.i.d.
*Adjunct treatment of breast cancer in women—*
**Adults:** 10 mg P.O. b.i.d. for 5 years.
*Reduction of breast cancer incidence in high-risk women—*
**Adults:** 20 mg P.O. daily for 5 years.

## ADVERSE REACTIONS
**CNS:** confusion, weakness, sleepiness, headache.
**CV:** *fluid retention.*
**EENT:** corneal changes, cataracts, retinopathy.
**GI:** *nausea, vomiting, diarrhea.*
**GU:** *vaginal discharge,* vaginal bleeding, *irregular menses, increased BUN level, amenorrhea.*
**Hematologic: leukopenia, thrombocytopenia.**
**Hepatic:** changes in liver enzyme levels, fatty liver, cholestasis, **hepatic necrosis.**
**Metabolic:** *hypercalcemia, weight gain or loss.*
**Musculoskeletal:** brief exacerbation of pain from osseous metastases.
**Skin:** *skin changes,* rash.
**Other:** temporary bone or tumor pain, *hot flashes.*

## INTERACTIONS
**Drug-drug.** *Antacids:* may affect absorption of enteric-coated tablet. Don't use within 2 hours.
*Bromocriptine:* may elevate tamoxifen levels. Monitor closely.
*Coumadin-type anticoagulants:* may cause significant increase in anticoagulant effect. Monitor patient, PT, and INR closely.

## EFFECTS ON DIAGNOSTIC TESTS
Variations on karyopyknotic index in vaginal smears and various degrees of estrogen effect on Papanicolaou smears have been infrequently seen in postmenopausal patients.

## CONTRAINDICATIONS
Contraindicated in patients with hypersensitivity to drug. Therapy to reduce risk of breast cancer in high-risk women who

---

need concomitant coumarin-type anti-coagulant therapy or in women with history of deep vein thrombosis or pulmonary embolism is also contraindicated.

**NURSING CONSIDERATIONS**
• Use cautiously in patients with existing leukopenia or thrombocytopenia. Monitor CBC closely, as ordered.
• Monitor serum lipid levels, as ordered, during long-term therapy in patients with preexisting hyperlipidemia.
• Monitor serum calcium levels, as ordered. During initiation of therapy, drug may compound hypercalcemia related to bone metastases.
• Drug acts as an antiestrogen. Best results have been reported in patients with positive estrogen receptors.
• Adverse reactions are usually minor and well tolerated.

☑ **Patient teaching**
• Tell patient taking enteric-coated tablets (Nolvadex-D) to swallow tablets whole without crushing or chewing. Tell her not to take antacids within 2 hours of dose.
• Reassure patient that acute exacerbation of bone pain during therapy usually indicates drug will produce good response. Recommend analgesics to relieve pain.
• Strongly encourage woman who is taking or has taken tamoxifen to have regular gynecologic examinations because of increased risk of uterine cancer associated with its use.
• Encourage woman to have annual mammograms and breast examinations.
• Advise patient to use barrier form of contraception because short-term therapy induces ovulation in premenopausal patients.
• Instruct patient to report vaginal bleeding.
• Caution woman of childbearing age to avoid becoming pregnant during therapy and first 2 months after stopping drug. Recommend that she consult doctor before becoming pregnant.
• Advise patient that breast cancer risk assessment tools are available and to discuss her concerns with doctor.

**testolactone**
Teslac

*Controlled Substance Schedule III*
*Pregnancy Risk Category C*

**HOW SUPPLIED**
*Tablets:* 50 mg

**ACTION**
Exact antineoplastic action unknown. Appears to inhibit aromatase activity and decrease estrone synthesis.

| Route | Onset | Peak | Duration |
|---|---|---|---|
| P.O. | 6-12 wk | Unknown | Unknown |

**INDICATIONS & DOSAGE**
*Advanced postmenopausal breast cancer, advanced premenopausal breast cancer in women whose ovarian function has been terminated—*
**Women:** 250 mg P.O. q.i.d.

**ADVERSE REACTIONS**
**CNS:** paresthesia, peripheral neuropathy.
**CV:** increased blood pressure, edema.
**GI:** nausea, vomiting, diarrhea, anorexia, glossitis.
**Skin:** alopecia, erythema, nail changes.

**INTERACTIONS**
**Drug-drug.** *Oral anticoagulants:* increased pharmacologic effects. Monitor patient, PT, and INR carefully.

**EFFECTS ON DIAGNOSTIC TESTS**
Drug therapy may increase levels of serum calcium, urinary creatinine, and urinary 17-ketosteroids. Estradiol levels measured by radioimmunoassay may be decreased.

**CONTRAINDICATIONS**
Contraindicated in patients with hypersensitivity to drug and in men with breast cancer.

**NURSING CONSIDERATIONS**
• Monitor fluid and electrolyte levels, especially calcium level.
• Force fluids to aid calcium excretion and encourage exercise to prevent hyper-

calcemia. Immobilized patients are prone to hypercalcemia.

• Higher-than-recommended doses may increase risk of remission in patients with visceral metastases.

### ✓ Patient teaching
• Inform patient that therapeutic response isn't immediate; 3 months is an adequate trial for drug.
• Tell patient to notify doctor if numbness or tingling occurs in fingers, toes, or face.

---

## toremifene citrate
Fareston

*Pregnancy Risk Category D*

### HOW SUPPLIED
*Tablets:* 60 mg

### ACTION
A nonsteroidal triphenylethylene that exerts its antitumor effect by competing with estrogen for binding sites in the tumor. This blocks the growth-stimulating effects of endogenous estrogen in the tumor, causing an antiestrogenic effect.

| Route | Onset | Peak | Duration |
|-------|-------|------|----------|
| P.O. | Unknown | 3 hr | Unknown |

### INDICATIONS & DOSAGE
*Metastatic breast cancer in postmenopausal women with estrogen-receptor positive or unknown tumors—*
**Adults:** 60 mg P.O. as single daily dose. Treatment is usually continued until disease progression is observed.

### ADVERSE REACTIONS
**CNS:** dizziness, fatigue, depression.
**CV:** edema, *thromboembolism, heart failure, MI, pulmonary embolism.*
**EENT:** visual disturbances, glaucoma, dry eyes, *cataracts.*
**GI:** *nausea*, vomiting.
**GU:** *vaginal discharge*, vaginal bleeding.
**Hepatic:** elevated liver function test results.
**Metabolic:** hypercalcemia.
**Skin:** *sweating.*
**Other:** *hot flashes.*

### INTERACTIONS
**Drug-drug.** *Calcium-elevating drugs such as hydrochlorothiazide:* increased risk of hypercalcemia. Monitor calcium levels closely.
*Coumadin-like anticoagulants such as warfarin:* prolonged PT and INR. Monitor PT and INR closely.
*Cytochrome P-450 3A4 enzyme inducers, such as carbamazepine, phenobarbital, phenytoin:* increased rate of toremifene metabolism. Monitor patient closely.
*Cytochrome P-450 3A4-6 enzyme inhibitors, such as erythromycin, ketoconazole:* decreased toremifene metabolism. Clinical relevance is uncertain.

### EFFECTS ON DIAGNOSTIC TESTS
None reported.

### CONTRAINDICATIONS
Contraindicated in patients with hypersensitivity to drug.

### NURSING CONSIDERATIONS
• Obtain periodic CBC, calcium levels, and liver function tests.
• Monitor calcium levels closely for first weeks of treatment in patients with bone metastases because of increased risk of hypercalcemia.

### ✓ Patient teaching
• Instruct patient to take drug exactly as prescribed.
• Warn patient not to discontinue therapy without consulting doctor.
• Inform patient about vaginal bleeding and other adverse effects; tell her to notify doctor if bleeding occurs.
• Warn patient that disease flare-up may occur during first weeks of therapy. Reassure her that this doesn't indicate treatment failure.
• Advise patient to report leg or chest pain, severe headache, visual changes, or dyspnea.

---

Reactions may be *common*, uncommon, *life-threatening*, or COMMON AND LIFE-THREATENING.

asparaginase
bacillus Calmette-Guérin (BCG),
  live intravesical
dacarbazine
docetaxel
etoposide
etoposide phosphate
gemcitabine hydrochloride
irinotecan hydrochloride
mitotane
mitoxantrone hydrochloride
paclitaxel
pegaspargase
porfimer sodium
procarbazine hydrochloride
rituximab
teniposide
topotecan hydrochloride
trastuzumab
tretinoin
vinblastine sulfate
vincristine sulfate
vinorelbine tartrate

**COMBINATION PRODUCTS**
None.

---

## asparaginase
Elspar, Kidrolase†

*Pregnancy Risk Category C*

**HOW SUPPLIED**
*Injection:* 10,000-IU vial

**ACTION**
Destroys the amino acid asparagine, which is needed for protein synthesis in acute lymphocytic leukemia, leading to death of the leukemic cell.

| Route | Onset | Peak | Duration |
|-------|-------|------|----------|
| I.V. | Immediate | Immediate | 23-33 days |
| I.M. | Unknown | 14-24 hr | 23-33 days |

**INDICATIONS & DOSAGE**
*Acute lymphocytic leukemia (with other drugs)—*
**Adults and children:** 1,000 IU/kg I.V. daily for 10 days, injected over 30 minutes; or 6,000 IU/m² I.M. at intervals specified in protocol.
*Sole induction drug for acute lymphocytic leukemia—*
**Adults and children:** 200 IU/kg I.V. daily for 28 days.

**ADVERSE REACTIONS**
**CNS:** confusion, drowsiness, depression, hallucinations, fatigue, agitation, headache, lethargy, somnolence.
**GI:** *vomiting, anorexia, nausea,* cramps, stomatitis, HEMORRHAGIC PANCREATITIS.
**GU:** *azotemia, renal failure,* glycosuria, polyuria, uric acid nephropathy, elevated BUN levels.
**Hematologic:** *anemia, hypofibrinogenemia,* depression of other clotting factors, *leukopenia.*
**Hepatic:** elevated AST and ALT levels, *hepatotoxicity.*
**Metabolic:** weight loss, *hyperglycemia,* hyperuricemia, hyperammonemia, hypocalcemia, altered thyroid function tests.
**Skin:** *rash, urticaria.*
**Other:** ANAPHYLAXIS, chills, fever, *hypersensitivity reactions.*

**INTERACTIONS**
**Drug-drug.** *Methotrexate:* decreased methotrexate effectiveness. Avoid concomitant use.
*Prednisone, vincristine:* increased toxicity. Monitor patient closely.

**EFFECTS ON DIAGNOSTIC TESTS**
None reported.

**CONTRAINDICATIONS**
Contraindicated in patients with previous hypersensitivity unless desensitized and in those with pancreatitis or history of pancreatitis.

---

## NURSING CONSIDERATIONS
• Use cautiously in patients with preexisting hepatic dysfunction. Drug should be given in hospital setting with close supervision.
• Monitor blood and urine glucose levels before and during therapy. Watch for signs and symptoms of hyperglycemia.
• Allopurinol should be started before therapy begins to help prevent uric acid nephropathy.
• *Alert:* Risk of hypersensitivity increases with repeated doses. An intradermal skin test should be performed before initial dose and when drug is given after an interval of 1 week or more between doses. Give 2 IU asparaginase as I.D. injection, as ordered. Observe site for at least 1 hour for erythema or a wheal, which indicates a positive response. Patient with negative skin test may still develop allergic reaction to drug. Desensitization may be needed before giving first treatment dose and on retreatment of patient. One IU of drug may be ordered I.V. Dose is then doubled every 10 minutes provided no re-action has occurred, until total amount given equals patient's total dose for that day.
• Drug shouldn't be used alone to induce remission unless combination therapy is inappropriate. Drug isn't recommended for maintenance therapy.
• For I.M. injection, reconstitute with 2 ml NaCl to the 10,000-IU vial. Refrigerate and use within 8 hours.
• Don't give more than 2 ml at one injection site.
• Don't use cloudy solutions.
• If drug contacts skin or mucous membranes, wash with a generous amount of water for at least 15 minutes.
• Keep epinephrine, diphenhydramine, and I.V. corticosteroids available for treating anaphylaxis.
• Monitor CBC and bone marrow function tests, as ordered.
• Obtain serum amylase level determinations, as ordered, to check pancreatic status. If levels are elevated, asparaginase should be discontinued.
• Help prevent occurrence of tumor lysis (which can result in uric acid nephropathy) by increasing fluid intake.

• Drug may affect clotting factors, leading to thrombosis or, more commonly, severe bleeding. Monitor patient and bleeding studies closely.
• Because of vomiting, administer parenteral fluids, as ordered, for 24 hours or until oral fluids are tolerated.
• Some patients may develop hypersensitivity to asparaginase, derived from cultures of *Escherichia coli. Erwinia asparaginase,* derived from cultures of *E. carotovora,* has been used in these patients without cross-sensitivity.
• Drug toxicity is more likely in adults than children.
• There are several protocols for use of this drug.

### ◖ I.V. administration
• Follow institutional policy to reduce risks. Preparation and administration of parenteral form of drug are associated with carcinogenic, mutagenic, and teratogenic risks for personnel.
• Reconstitute drug with 5 ml of either sterile water for injection or NaCl for injection.
• Don't vigorously shake vial because foaming may occur.
• Give I.V. injection over 30 minutes through a running infusion of normal saline solution or $D_5W$ solution.
• Refrigerate unopened dry powder. Reconstituted solution is stable for 8 hours if refrigerated. Use only clear solutions.

### ✔ Patient teaching
• Tell patient to watch for signs of infection (fever, sore throat, fatigue) and bleeding (easy bruising, nosebleeds, bleeding gums, melena), and to take temperature daily.
• Stress importance of maintaining adequate fluid intake to help prevent hyperuricemia. If adverse GI reactions prevent patient from drinking fluids, tell patient to notify doctor.

---

Reactions may be *common,* uncommon, *life-threatening,* or COMMON AND LIFE-THREATENING.

# bacillus Calmette-Guérin (BCG), live intravesical
TheraCys, TICE BCG

*Pregnancy Risk Category C*

## HOW SUPPLIED
**TheraCys**
*Suspension (freeze-dried) for bladder instillation:* 81 mg/vial
**TICE BCG**
*Suspension (freeze-dried) for bladder instillation:* about 50 mg/ampule

## ACTION
Unknown. Instillation of the live bacterial suspension causes a local inflammatory response. Local infiltration of histiocytes and leukocytes is followed by a decrease in superficial tumors within the bladder.

| Route | Onset | Peak | Duration |
|-------|-------|------|----------|
| Intravesical | Unknown | Unknown | Unknown |

## INDICATIONS & DOSAGE
*In situ carcinoma of the urinary bladder (primary and relapsed)—*
**Adults:** one reconstituted and diluted vial, 81 mg, administered intravesically once weekly for 6 weeks (induction); then additional treatments at 3, 6, 12, 18, and 24 months (TheraCys). Or, one bladder instillation (one ampule suspended in 50 ml of sterile, preservative-free NaCl solution) once weekly for 6 weeks; then once monthly for 6 to 12 months (TICE BCG).

## ADVERSE REACTIONS
**CNS:** *malaise.*
**CV:** *hypotension.*
**GI:** *nausea, vomiting, anorexia,* diarrhea.
**GU:** *dysuria, urinary frequency, hematuria, cystitis, urinary urgency,* nocturia, urinary incontinence, *urinary tract infection,* cramps, pain, decreased bladder capacity, renal toxicity, genital pain.
**Hematologic:** *anemia, **leukopenia.***
**Hepatic:** elevated liver enzyme levels.
**Musculoskeletal:** myalgia, arthralgia.
**Other:** ***hypersensitivity reaction,*** fever, chills.

## INTERACTIONS
**Drug-drug.** *Antibiotics:* may attenuate response to BCG intravesical. Avoid concomitant use.
*Bone marrow suppressants, immunosuppressants, radiation therapy:* may impair response to BCG intravesical by decreasing the immune response; may also increase the risk of osteomyelitis or disseminated BCG infection. Avoid concomitant use.

## EFFECTS ON DIAGNOSTIC TESTS
Tuberculin sensitivity may be rendered positive by BCG intravesical treatment.

## CONTRAINDICATIONS
Contraindicated in immunocompromised patients, in those receiving immunosuppressive therapy, in asymptomatic carriers with a positive HIV serology, and in those with urinary tract infection, gross hematuria, or fever of unknown origin.

## NURSING CONSIDERATIONS
• Determine patient's reactivity to tuberculin before therapy. Tuberculin sensitivity may be rendered positive by BCG intravesical treatment.
• Drug shouldn't be handled by caregiver with known immunologic deficiency.
• BCG intravesical shouldn't be administered within 7 to 14 days of transurethral resection or biopsy. Fatal disseminated BCG infection has occurred after traumatic catheterization.
• Drug may cause pyuria.
• To administer TheraCys, reconstitute only with 3 ml of provided diluent per vial just before use. Don't remove rubber stopper to prepare solution. Use immediately. Add contents of three reconstituted vials to 50 ml of sterile, preservative-free NaCl solution (final volume, 53 ml). Instill a urethral catheter into bladder under aseptic conditions, drain bladder, and infuse 53 ml of prepared solution by gravity feed. Remove catheter and properly dispose of unused drug.
• To administer TICE BCG, use thermosetting plastic or sterile glass containers and syringes. Draw 1 ml of sterile, preservative-free NaCl solution into a 3-ml syringe. Add to one ampule of drug;

gently expel back into ampule three times to ensure thorough mixing. Use immediately. Dispense cloudy suspension into top end of a catheter-tipped syringe that contains 49 ml of NaCl solution. Gently rotate syringe. Properly dispose of unused drug.

• Don't use reconstituted product with clumping that can't be dispersed with gentle shaking.

• Protect drug from exposure to direct or indirect sunlight.

• Handle drug and material used for instillation as infectious material because it contains live, attenuated mycobacteria. Dispose of associated equipment (syringes, catheters, and containers) as biohazardous waste.

• Use strict aseptic technique to administer drug to minimize trauma to GU tract and to prevent introduction of other contaminants.

• If there is evidence of traumatic catheterization, don't administer drug; notify doctor. Subsequent treatment may resume after 1 week as if no interruption occurred.

• Carefully monitor patient's urinary status because drug causes an inflammatory response in the bladder.

• Closely monitor patient for evidence of systemic BCG infection. BCG infections are rarely detected by positive cultures. Withhold therapy if systemic infection is suspected (short-term high temperature over 103° F [39° C] or persistent temperature over 101° F [38° C] for more than 2 days or with severe malaise). Contact an infectious disease specialist for initiation of fast-acting antituberculosis therapy, as ordered.

• If fever is caused by infection, drug should be withheld until patient recovers.

• Drug isn't used as an immunizing agent to prevent cancer or tuberculosis.

• Drug has the potential to cause hypersensitivity. Manage symptomatically.

• Patients with a small bladder capacity may experience increased local irritation with usual dose of BCG intravesical.

• Be prepared to treat bladder irritation symptomatically with phenazopyridine, acetaminophen, and propantheline, as ordered. Systemic hypersensitivity can be

treated with diphenhydramine. To minimize risk of systemic infection, some clinicians give isoniazid for 3 days starting on first day of treatment.

• *Alert:* Don't confuse BCG intravesical with BCG vaccine.

### ✓ Patient teaching

• Tell patient to retain drug in bladder for 2 hours after instillation (if possible). For first hour, have patient lie 15 minutes prone, 15 minutes supine, and 15 minutes on each side; patient may spend second hour in sitting position.

• Advise patient to sit when voiding.

• Instruct patient to disinfect urine for 6 hours after instillation of drug. Tell him to pour undiluted household bleach (5% sodium hypochlorite solution) in equal volume to voided urine into the toilet and wait 15 minutes before flushing.

• Tell patient to notify doctor if symptoms worsen or if the following symptoms develop: blood in the urine, fever and chills, frequent urge to urinate, painful urination, nausea, vomiting, joint pain, or rash.

• *Alert:* Warn patient that a cough that develops after therapy could indicate a life-threatening BCG infection. Tell him to report it immediately.

• Caution woman of childbearing age not to become pregnant or breast-feed during therapy.

---

## dacarbazine (DTIC)
DTIC†, DTIC-Dome

*Pregnancy Risk Category C*

---

**HOW SUPPLIED**
*Injection:* 100-mg, 200-mg vials

**ACTION**
Unknown. Probably cross-links strands of cellular DNA and interferes with RNA transcription, causing an imbalance of growth that leads to cell death. Cell cycle–nonspecific.

| Route | Onset | Peak | Duration |
|-------|-------|------|----------|
| I.V. | Unknown | Unknown | Unknown |

---

Reactions may be *common*, uncommon, *life-threatening*, or COMMON AND LIFE-THREATENING.

## INDICATIONS & DOSAGE
*Metastatic malignant melanoma—*
**Adults:** 2 to 4.5 mg/kg I.V. daily for 10 days; repeated q 4 weeks, as tolerated. Or 250 mg/m$^2$ I.V. daily for 5 days; repeated at 3-week intervals.
*Hodgkin's disease—*
**Adults:** 150 mg/m$^2$ I.V. daily (with other drugs) for 5 days; repeated q 4 weeks. Or 375 mg/m$^2$ on first day of combination regimen; repeated q 15 days.

## ADVERSE REACTIONS
**CNS:** facial paresthesia.
**GI:** *severe nausea and vomiting, anorexia,* stomatitis.
**GU:** transient increases in serum BUN levels.
**Hematologic:** *leukopenia, thrombocytopenia.*
**Hepatic:** transient increase in liver enzyme levels.
**Skin:** phototoxicity, alopecia, rash, facial flushing.
**Other:** tissue damage; *flulike syndrome, anaphylaxis;* severe pain (with infiltration or if solution is too concentrated).

## INTERACTIONS
**Drug-lifestyle.** *Sun exposure:* photosensitivity reactions may occur especially during first 2 days of therapy. Take precautions.

## EFFECTS ON DIAGNOSTIC TESTS
None reported.

## CONTRAINDICATIONS
Contraindicated in patients with hypersensitivity to drug.

## NURSING CONSIDERATIONS
• Use cautiously in patients with impaired bone marrow function.
• To prevent bleeding, avoid all I.M. injections when platelet count is below 100,000/mm$^3$.
• Anticipate need for blood transfusions to combat anemia. Patient may receive injections of RBC colony-stimulating factors to promote RBC production and decrease need for blood transfusions.
• Therapeutic effects are often accompanied by toxicity. Monitor CBC and platelet count.

• For Hodgkin's disease, drug is usually given with bleomycin, vinblastine, and doxorubicin.

### I.V. administration
• Administer antiemetics, as ordered, before giving dacarbazine. Nausea and vomiting may sometimes subside after several doses.
• Follow institutional policy to reduce risks. Preparation and administration of parenteral form of drug are associated with carcinogenic, mutagenic, and teratogenic risks for personnel.
• Reconstitute drug using sterile water for injection. Add 9.9 ml to 100-mg vial or 19.7 ml to 200-mg vial; resulting solution will be colorless to clear yellow. For infusion, further dilute by using up to 250 ml of normal saline solution or D$_5$W; infuse over 30 minutes.
• Drug may be diluted further or given at a slower infusion rate to decrease pain at insertion site.
• Avoid extravasation during infusion. If I.V. solution infiltrates, discontinue immediately, apply ice to area for 24 to 48 hours, and notify doctor.
• Reconstituted solutions are stable for 8 hours at room temperature and normal lighting conditions, or up to 3 days if refrigerated. Diluted solutions are stable for 8 hours at normal room temperature and light, or up to 24 hours if refrigerated. If solutions turn pink, discard drug because decomposition has occurred.
• Discard refrigerated solution after 24 hours and room temperature solution after 8 hours.

### Patient teaching
• Tell patient to watch for signs and symptoms of infection (fever, sore throat, fatigue) and bleeding (easy bruising, nosebleeds, bleeding gums, melena), and to take temperature daily.
• Instruct patient to avoid OTC products containing aspirin.
• Advise patient to avoid sunlight and sunlamps for first 2 days after treatment.
• Reassure patient that flulike syndrome (fever, malaise; myalgia, beginning 7 days after treatment ends and possibly lasting 7

to 21 days) may be treated with mild antipyretics such as acetaminophen.
• Counsel woman to avoid pregnancy and breast-feeding during therapy.

## docetaxel
Taxotere

*Pregnancy Risk Category D*

### HOW SUPPLIED
*Injection:* 20 mg, 80 mg, in single-dose vials

### ACTION
Disrupts microtubular network in cells essential for mitotic and interphase cellular functions.

| Route | Onset | Peak | Duration |
|-------|-------|------|----------|
| I.V. | Rapid | Unknown | Unknown |

### INDICATIONS & DOSAGE
*Locally advanced or metastatic breast cancer after failure of previous chemotherapy—*
**Adults:** 60 to 100 mg/m² I.V. over 1 hour q 3 weeks.

### ADVERSE REACTIONS
**CNS:** *asthenia,* paresthesia.
**CV:** *fluid retention,* hypotension, flushing, chest tightness.
**GI:** *stomatitis, nausea, vomiting, diarrhea.*
**Hematologic:** *anemia,* NEUTROPENIA, FEBRILE NEUTROPENIA, MYELOSUPPRESSION, LEUKOPENIA, THROMBOCYTOPENIA.
**Hepatic:** *increased liver function test results.*
**Musculoskeletal:** *myalgia,* arthralgia, back pain.
**Respiratory:** dyspnea.
**Skin:** *alopecia,* skin eruptions, desquamation, nail pigmentation alterations, nail pain, rash; reaction at injection site.
**Other:** *hypersensitivity reactions,* infection, drug fever, chills.

### INTERACTIONS
**Drug-drug.** *Compounds that induce, inhibit, or are metabolized by cytochrome P-450 3A4, such as cyclosporine, erythromycin, ketoconazole, troleandomycin:* metabolism of docetaxel may be modified by concomitant administration. Use cautiously when administering these drugs with docetaxel.

### EFFECTS ON DIAGNOSTIC TESTS
None reported.

### CONTRAINDICATIONS
Contraindicated in patients with history of severe hypersensitivity to drug or to other formulations containing polysorbate 80 and in those with neutrophil counts below 1,500 cells/mm³.

### NURSING CONSIDERATIONS
• Don't administer drug in patients with bilirubin levels exceeding upper limit of normal. Also, avoid use of drug in patients with ALT or AST levels above 1.5 times upper limit of normal and alkaline phosphatase levels over 2.5 times upper limit of normal.
• Premedicate all patients with oral corticosteroids such as dexamethasone 16 mg P.O. (8 mg b.i.d.) daily for 3 days starting 1 day before docetaxel administration, to reduce incidence and severity of fluid retention and hypersensitivity reactions.
• Bone marrow toxicity is the most frequent and dose-limiting toxicity. Frequent blood count monitoring is needed during therapy.
• Monitor patient closely for hypersensitivity reactions, especially during first and second infusions.
• Safety and efficacy of drug in children haven't been established.
• Contact of undiluted docetaxel concentrate with polyvinyl chloride equipment or devices isn't recommended.
• *Alert:* Don't confuse dacarbazine with Dicarbosil or procarbazine.

### 🖤 I.V. administration
• Wear gloves during drug preparation and administration. If solution contacts skin, wash immediately and thoroughly with soap and water. If drug contacts mucous membranes, flush thoroughly with water. Mark all waste materials with CHEMOTHERAPY HAZARD labels.
• Prepare and store infusion solutions in bottles (glass or polypropylene) or

---

Reactions may be *common,* uncommon, *life-threatening,* or COMMON AND LIFE-THREATENING.

plastic bags, and administer through polyethylene-lined administration sets. Administer drug as 1-hour infusion; store unopened vials in refrigerator.
• Before administration, dilute drug using diluent supplied. Allow drug and diluent to stand at room temperature for 5 minutes before mixing. After adding all the diluent to drug vial, gently rotate vial for about 15 seconds. Allow solution to stand for a few minutes to enable foam to dissipate. All foam need not fully dissipate before proceeding to the next step.
• Prepare drug infusion solution by withdrawing the needed amount of premixed solution from the vial and injecting it into 250 ml normal saline or $D_5W$ to produce a final concentration of 0.3 to 0.9 mg/ml. Doses exceeding 240 mg need a larger volume of infusion solution so as not to exceed concentration of 0.9 mg/ml of docetaxel. Mix infusion thoroughly by manual rotation.
• Discard solution if it isn't clear or appears to have precipitates.

☑ **Patient teaching**
• Caution woman of childbearing age to avoid pregnancy or breast-feeding during therapy.
• Warn patient that alopecia occurs in almost 80% of patients.
• Tell patient to promptly report sore throat, fever, or unusual bruising or bleeding as well as signs and symptoms of fluid retention, such as swelling or dyspnea.

---

**etoposide (VP-16, VP-16-213)**
VePesid

**etoposide phosphate**
Etopophos

*Pregnancy Risk Category D*

**HOW SUPPLIED**
**etoposide**
*Capsules:* 50 mg
*Injection:* 20 mg/ml in 5-ml vials
**etoposide phosphate**
*Injection:* 119.3-mg vials equivalent to 100 mg etoposide

**ACTION**
Unknown. Thought to damage DNA and inhibit DNA synthesis. Appears to be cell cycle–specific.

| Route | Onset | Peak | Duration |
|-------|-------|------|----------|
| P.O., I.V. | Unknown | Unknown | Unknown |

**INDICATIONS & DOSAGE**
*Testicular cancer—*
**Adults:** 50 to 100 mg/m² I.V. on 5 consecutive days q 3 to 4 weeks; or 100 mg/m² on days 1, 3, and 5 q 3 to 4 weeks.
*Small-cell carcinoma of the lung—*
**Adults:** 35 mg/m²/day I.V. for 4 days; or 50 mg/m²/day I.V. for 5 days. P.O. dose is two times I.V. dose, rounded to nearest 50 mg.

**ADVERSE REACTIONS**
**CNS:** peripheral neuropathy.
**CV:** hypotension.
**GI:** *nausea and vomiting, anorexia, diarrhea,* abdominal pain, stomatitis.
**Hematologic:** *anemia, myelosuppression,* LEUKOPENIA, THROMBOCYTOPENIA, NEUTROPENIA.
**Skin:** *reversible alopecia,* rash.

**INTERACTIONS**
**Drug-drug.** *Warfarin:* may further prolong PT. Monitor closely.

**EFFECTS ON DIAGNOSTIC TESTS**
None reported.

**CONTRAINDICATIONS**
Contraindicated in patients with hypersensitivity to drug.

**NURSING CONSIDERATIONS**
• Use cautiously in patients who have had cytotoxic or radiation therapy.
• Obtain baseline blood pressure before starting therapy.
• Anticipate need for antiemetics.
• Have diphenhydramine, hydrocortisone, epinephrine, and emergency equipment available to establish an airway in case anaphylaxis occurs.
• Store capsules in refrigerator.
• Monitor CBC, as ordered. Observe for signs and symptoms of bone marrow suppression.

---

• Observe oral cavity for signs of ulceration.
• To prevent bleeding, avoid all I.M. injections when platelet count is below 100,000/mm³.
• Anticipate need for blood transfusions to combat anemia. Patient may receive injections of RBC colony-stimulating factors to promote RBC production and decrease need for blood transfusions.
• Etoposide has caused complete remissions in small-cell lung cancer and testicular cancer.
• Dose of etoposide phosphate is expressed as etoposide equivalents; 119.3 mg of etoposide phosphate is equivalent to 100 mg of etoposide.

### ◖ I.V. administration
• Dilute etoposide for infusion in either D₅W or normal saline solution to concentration of 0.2 or 0.4 mg/ml. Higher concentrations may crystallize. Etoposide phosphate may be given without further dilution or may be diluted to concentrations as low as 0.1 mg/ml in either D₅W or normal saline.
• Etoposide diluted to 0.2 mg/ml is stable for 96 hours at room temperature in plastic or glass unprotected from light; solutions diluted to 0.4 mg/ml are stable for 48 hours under same conditions. Diluted solutions of etoposide phosphate are stable at room temperature or under refrigeration for 24 hours.
• Give etoposide by slow I.V. infusion (over at least 30 minutes) to prevent severe hypotension. Etoposide phosphate may be given over 5 to 210 minutes.
• *Alert:* Monitor blood pressure every 15 minutes during infusion. Hypotension can occur with too rapid an infusion. If systolic pressure falls below 90 mm Hg, stop infusion and notify doctor.
• Follow institutional policy to reduce risks. Preparation and administration of parenteral form of drug are associated with carcinogenic, mutagenic, and teratogenic risks for personnel.
• *Alert:* Don't confuse VePesid with Versed.

### ☑ Patient teaching
• Tell patient to watch for signs and symptoms of infection (fever, sore throat, fatigue) and bleeding (easy bruising, nosebleeds, bleeding gums, melena), and to take temperature daily.
• Inform patient of need for frequent blood pressure readings during I.V. administration.
• Caution woman of childbearing age to avoid pregnancy or breast-feeding during therapy.

## gemcitabine hydrochloride
Gemzar

*Pregnancy Risk Category D*

### HOW SUPPLIED
*Powder for injection:* 200-mg, 1-g vials

### ACTION
Cytotoxic and cell cycle–specific; inhibits DNA synthesis and blocks progression of cells through G1/S-phase boundary.

| Route | Onset | Peak | Duration |
|-------|-------|------|----------|
| I.V. | Unknown | Unknown | Unknown |

### INDICATIONS & DOSAGE
*Locally advanced or metastatic adenocarcinoma of pancreas and patients treated previously with fluorouracil—*
**Adults:** 1,000 mg/m² I.V. over 30 minutes once weekly for up to 7 weeks, unless toxicity occurs. Monitor CBC (including differential) and platelet count before giving each dose. If bone marrow suppression is detected, therapy is adjusted. Give full dose if absolute granulocyte count (AGC) is 1,000/mm³ or more and platelet count is 100,000/mm³ or more. If AGC is 500 to 999/mm³ or platelet count is 50,000 to 99,999/mm³, 75% of dose should be given. Withhold dose if AGC is below 500/mm³ or platelet count is below 50,000/mm³. Treatment course of 7 weeks is followed by 1 week rest. Subsequent dosage cycles consist of 1 infusion weekly for 3 of 4 consecutive weeks. Dosage adjustments for subsequent cycles are based on AGC and platelet count nadirs and degree of nonhematologic toxicity.

---

*With cisplatin as first-line treatment of in-operable, locally advanced, or metastatic non-small-cell lung cancer—*
**Adults:** Four-week schedule: 1,000 mg/$m^2$ I.V. over 30 minutes on days 1, 8, and 15 of each 28-day cycle. Cisplatin 100 mg/$m^2$ on day 1 after gemcitabine infusion.

Three-week schedule: 1,250 mg/$m^2$ I.V. over 30 minutes on days 1 and 8 of each 21-day cycle. Cisplatin 100 mg/$m^2$ on day 1 after gemcitabine infusion.

## ADVERSE REACTIONS
**CNS:** *somnolence, paresthesia.*
**CV:** *edema, peripheral edema.*
**GI:** *stomatitis, nausea, vomiting, consti-pation, diarrhea.*
**GU:** *proteinuria, hematuria,* elevated BUN and creatinine levels.
**Hematologic:** *anemia, **leukopenia, neu-tropenia, thrombocytopenia.***
**Hepatic:** *elevated liver enzyme levels.*
**Respiratory:** *dyspnea, **bronchospasm.***
**Skin:** *alopecia, rash.*
**Other:** *pain, fever, flulike syndrome, in-fection;* pain at injection site.

## INTERACTIONS
None significant.

## EFFECTS ON DIAGNOSTIC TESTS
None reported.

## CONTRAINDICATIONS
Contraindicated in patients with hyper-sensitivity to drug.

## NURSING CONSIDERATIONS
• Use cautiously in patients with renal or hepatic impairment.
• Drug isn't recommended for use in pregnant or breast-feeding women.
• Monitor patient closely. Expect dosage modification according to toxicity and de-gree of myelosuppression. Age, gender, and presence of renal impairment may predispose patient to toxicity.
• Careful hematologic monitoring, espe-cially of neutrophil and platelet counts, is needed.
• Obtain baseline and periodic renal and hepatic laboratory tests, as ordered.

• Safety and effectiveness of drug in chil-dren haven't been determined.

### ■ I.V. administration
• Follow institutional policy to reduce risks. Preparation and administration of parenteral form of drug are associated with mutagenic, teratogenic, and carcino-genic risks for personnel.
• To prepare solution, add 5 ml of normal saline injection without preservatives to 200-mg vial or 25 ml of diluent to a 1-g vial. Shake to dissolve. Resulting concen-tration is 40 mg/ml; reconstitution at greater concentrations isn't recommend-ed. Resulting concentration may be fur-ther diluted with normal saline injection to a concentration as low as 0.1 mg/ml, if needed. Solution should be clear to light straw-colored, and be free of particulates. It's stable for 24 hours at room tempera-ture. Don't refrigerate reconstituted drug because crystallization may occur.
• Prolonging infusion time beyond 60 minutes or administering drug more fre-quently than once weekly may increase toxicity.

### ✓ Patient teaching
• Advise patient to watch for signs and symptoms of infection (fever, sore throat, fatigue) and bleeding (easy bruising, nosebleeds, bleeding gums, melena). Tell patient to take temperature daily.
• Caution woman of childbearing age to avoid pregnancy or breast-feeding during therapy.

## irinotecan hydrochloride
Campto§, Camptosar

*Pregnancy Risk Category D*

## HOW SUPPLIED
*Injection:* 100-mg/5-ml vial

## ACTION
A derivative of camptothecin. Camp-tothecins interact specifically with the en-zyme topoisomerase I, which relieves tor-sional strain in DNA by inducing re-versible single-strand breaks. Irinotecan and its active metabolite bind to the topo-

isomerase I-DNA complex and prevent relegation of these single-strand breaks.

| Route | Onset | Peak | Duration |
|-------|-------|------|----------|
| I.V. | Unknown | 1 hr | Unknown |

## INDICATIONS & DOSAGE
*Metastatic carcinoma of the colon or rectum that has recurred or progressed following fluorouracil (5-FU) therapy—*
**Adults:** initially, 125 mg/m$^2$ I.V. infusion over 90 minutes. Recommended treatment is 125 mg/m$^2$ I.V. once weekly for 4 weeks; then 2-week rest period. Thereafter, additional courses of treatment may be repeated q 6 weeks (4 weeks on therapy; then 2 weeks off therapy). Subsequent doses may be adjusted to low of 50 mg/m$^2$ or to maximum of 150 mg/m$^2$ in 25- to 50-mg/m$^2$ increments based on patient's tolerance. Treatment with additional courses may continue indefinitely in patients who respond favorably and in those whose disease remains stable, provided intolerable toxicity doesn't occur.

## ADVERSE REACTIONS
**CNS:** *insomnia, dizziness, asthenia, headache,* akathisia.
**CV:** *vasodilation, edema.*
**GI: *diarrhea,** nausea, vomiting, anorexia, stomatitis, constipation, flatulence, dyspepsia, abdominal cramping and pain, abdominal enlargement.*
**Hematologic: *leukopenia,** anemia, **neutropenia.***
**Hepatic:** *increased alkaline phosphatase and AST levels.*
**Metabolic:** *weight loss, dehydration.*
**Musculoskeletal:** *back pain.*
**Respiratory:** *dyspnea, increased coughing, rhinitis.*
**Skin:** *alopecia, sweating, rash.*
**Other:** *fever, pain, chills, minor infection.*

## INTERACTIONS
**Drug-drug.** *Dexamethasone:* increased risk of irinotecan-induced lymphocytopenia. Monitor closely.
*Diuretics:* increased risk of dehydration and electrolyte imbalance. Consider discontinuing diuretic during active periods of nausea and vomiting.

*Laxative use:* increased risk of diarrhea. Avoid concomitant use.
*Other antineoplastics:* may cause additive adverse effects, such as myelosuppression and diarrhea. Monitor patient closely.
*Pelvic or abdominal irradiation:* increased risk of severe myelosuppression. Avoid use of drug with irradiation.
*Prochlorperazine:* increased risk of akathisia. Monitor patient.

## EFFECTS ON DIAGNOSTIC TESTS
None reported.

## CONTRAINDICATIONS
Contraindicated in patients with hypersensitivity to drug.

## NURSING CONSIDERATIONS
• Use cautiously in elderly patients.
• Drug is packaged in a plastic blister to protect against inadvertent breakage and leakage. Inspect vial for damage and visible signs of leakage before removing blister.
• Store vial at temperature of 59° to 86° F (15° to 30° C). Protect from light.
• Diuretic may be withheld during therapy and periods of active vomiting or diarrhea to decrease risk of dehydration.
• Drug can induce severe diarrhea. Diarrhea occurring within 24 hours of administration may be preceded by diaphoresis and abdominal cramping and may be relieved by 0.25 to 1 mg atropine I.V., unless contraindicated. Diarrhea occurring more than 24 hours after drug administration may be prolonged, leading to dehydration and electrolyte imbalances, and can be life-threatening. Diarrhea occurring after 24 hours should be treated with loperamide, as ordered. Monitor patient's fluid status and serum electrolyte levels.
• Temporarily discontinue therapy if neutropenic fever occurs or if absolute neutrophil count drops below 500/mm$^3$. Dosage should be reduced, as ordered, especially if WBC count is below 2,000/mm$^3$, neutrophil count is below 1,000/mm$^3$, hemoglobin level is below 8 g/dl, or platelet count is below 100,000/mm$^3$.
• Routine administration of a colony-stimulating factor isn't needed but may be

---

helpful in patients with significant neutropenia.
• Monitor WBC count with differential, hemoglobin level, and platelet count before each dose of irinotecan.
• Safety and effectiveness of drug in children haven't been established.

### I.V. administration
• Premedicate patient with antiemetic drugs on day of treatment starting at least 30 minutes before giving irinotecan.
• Wear gloves while handling and preparing infusion solutions. If drug contacts skin, wash thoroughly with soap and water. If drug contacts mucous membranes, flush thoroughly with water.
• Irinotecan must be diluted in $D_5W$ injection (preferred) or normal saline injection before infusion. Final concentration range is 0.12 to 1.1 mg/ml.
• Irinotecan solution is stable for up to 24 hours at temperature of 77° F (25° C) and in ambient fluorescent lighting. Solutions diluted in $D_5W$, stored at refrigerated temperatures of 36° to 46° F (2° to 8° C), and protected from light are stable for 48 hours. However, because of possible microbial contamination during dilution, use admixture within 24 hours if refrigerated or 6 hours if kept at room temperature. Refrigerating admixtures using normal saline isn't recommended because of low and sporadic risk of visible particulate. Don't freeze admixture because drug may precipitate.
• Don't add other drugs to irinotecan infusion.
• Avoid extravasation of drug. If extravasation occurs, flush site with sterile water and apply ice. Notify doctor.

### ✓ Patient teaching
• Inform patient about risk of diarrhea and how to treat it; tell him to avoid laxatives.
• Tell patient to notify doctor if vomiting, fever, signs and symptoms of infection, or symptoms of dehydration (fainting, light-headedness, or dizziness) occur following drug administration.
• Warn patient that alopecia may occur.

• Caution woman of childbearing age to avoid pregnancy or breast-feeding during therapy.

---

## mitotane (o,p'-DDD)
Lysodren

*Pregnancy Risk Category C*

### HOW SUPPLIED
*Tablets (scored):* 500 mg

### ACTION
Unknown. May suppress function of adrenocortical tissue and hinder extra-adrenal metabolism of cortisol.

| Route | Onset | Peak | Duration |
|-------|-------|------|----------|
| P.O. | Unknown | 3-5 hr | Unknown |

### INDICATIONS & DOSAGE
*Inoperable adrenocortical cancer—*
**Adults:** initially, 2 to 6 g P.O. daily in divided doses t.i.d. or q.i.d.; increased to 9 to 10 g P.O. daily in divided doses t.i.d. or q.i.d. Adjust dosage until maximum tolerated dose is achieved (varies from 2 to 16 g/day but is usually 9 to 10 g/day).

### ADVERSE REACTIONS
**CNS:** *depression, somnolence, lethargy, vertigo.*
**CV:** hypertension, orthostatic hypotension, flushing.
**EENT:** visual disturbances, diplopia, lens opacity, toxic retinopathy.
**GI:** *severe nausea, vomiting, diarrhea, anorexia.*
**GU:** hemorrhagic cystitis.
**Musculoskeletal:** myalgia.
**Skin:** dermatitis, *maculopapular rash,* muscle twitching.
**Other:** adrenal insufficiency, fever; increased urinary 17-hydroxycorticosteroid, plasma cortisol, protein-bound iodine, and serum uric acid levels.

### INTERACTIONS
**Drug-drug.** *Corticosteroids:* increased metabolism of corticosteroids requiring higher corticosteroid doses. Monitor carefully.

---

*Warfarin:* increased metabolism, which may require higher warfarin doses. Monitor PT and INR closely.

**EFFECTS ON DIAGNOSTIC TESTS**
None reported.

**CONTRAINDICATIONS**
Contraindicated in patients with hypersensitivity to drug and in those in shock or who have suffered trauma.

**NURSING CONSIDERATIONS**
• Use cautiously in patients with hepatic disease.
• To reduce nausea, give antiemetic before mitotane, as ordered.
• Monitor effectiveness according to reduction in pain, weakness, and anorexia.
• Assess and record behavioral and neurologic signs daily. Prolonged therapy has been associated with significant neurologic impairment.
• Corticosteroids are generally needed, and their use may avoid acute adrenocortical insufficiency. Glucocorticoid dosage should be increased during periods of physiologic stress, such as infection or trauma.
• Because drug distributes mostly to body fat, obese patients may need higher dosage and may have longer-lasting adverse reactions.
• An adequate therapeutic trial is at least 3 months, but treatment can continue if clinical benefits are observed.

☑ **Patient teaching**
• Warn ambulatory patient to avoid activities that require alertness and good motor coordination until CNS effects of drug are known.
• Instruct patient to notify doctor if severe adverse GI or skin reactions occur because dosage adjustment may be needed.
• Counsel woman of childbearing age to avoid pregnancy or breast-feeding during therapy.

## mitoxantrone hydrochloride
Novantrone

*Pregnancy Risk Category D*

**HOW SUPPLIED**
*Injection:* 2 mg/ml in 10-ml, 12.5-ml, 15-ml vials

**ACTION**
Exact mechanism unknown. Probably cell cycle–nonspecific. Reacts with DNA, producing cytotoxic effect.

| Route | Onset | Peak | Duration |
|-------|-------|------|----------|
| I.V. | Unknown | Unknown | Unknown |

**INDICATIONS & DOSAGE**
*Combination initial therapy for acute nonlymphocytic leukemia—*
**Adults:** induction begins with 12 mg/m$^2$ I.V. daily on days 1 to 3, with 100 mg/m$^2$ daily of cytarabine on days 1 to 7. A second induction may be given if response isn't adequate. Maintenance therapy: 12 mg/m$^2$ on days 1 and 2, with cytarabine on days 1 to 5.
*Combination initial therapy for pain related to advanced hormone-refractory prostate cancer—*
**Adults:** 12 to 14 mg/m$^2$ I.V. infusion over 15 to 30 minutes q 21 days as an adjunct to corticosteroid therapy.

**ADVERSE REACTIONS**
**CNS:** *seizures,* headache.
**CV:** *heart failure, arrhythmias,* tachycardia.
**EENT:** conjunctivitis.
**GI:** *bleeding, abdominal pain, diarrhea, nausea, mucositis, vomiting, stomatitis.*
**GU:** *renal failure.*
**Hematologic:** *myelosuppression, sepsis.*
**Hepatic:** jaundice, increased AST, ALT, and bilirubin levels.
**Metabolic:** hyperuricemia.
**Respiratory:** *dyspnea, cough.*
**Skin:** *alopecia,* petechiae, ecchymoses, local irritation or phlebitis.
**Other:** *fungal infections, fever.*

**INTERACTIONS**
None significant.

---

Reactions may be *common,* uncommon, *life-threatening,* or COMMON AND LIFE-THREATENING.

## EFFECTS ON DIAGNOSTIC TESTS
None reported.

## CONTRAINDICATIONS
Contraindicated in patients with hypersensitivity to drug.

## NURSING CONSIDERATIONS
• Use cautiously in patients with previous exposure to anthracyclines or other cardiotoxic drugs, previous radiation therapy to mediastinal area, and preexisting heart disease.
• Patients with significant myelosuppression shouldn't receive drug unless benefits outweigh risks.
• Be prepared to administer allopurinol, as ordered. Uric acid nephropathy can be avoided by hydrating patient before and during therapy.
• Closely monitor hematologic and laboratory chemistry parameters.
• To prevent bleeding, avoid all I.M. injections if platelet count falls below 100,000/mm$^3$.
• Anticipate need for blood transfusion to combat anemia. Patients may receive injections of RBC colony-stimulating factors to promote RBC production and decrease need for blood transfusions.
• Monitor left ventricular ejection fraction.
• Be prepared to treat infections with antibiotics, as ordered. Patients may receive injections of WBC colony-stimulating factors to promote cell growth and decrease risk of infection.
• If severe nonhematologic toxicity occurs during first course, delay second course until patient recovers.

## ◨ I.V. administration
• Follow institutional policy to minimize risks. Preparation and administration of parenteral form are associated with mutagenic, teratogenic, and carcinogenic risks to personnel.
• Dilute dose (available as an aqueous solution of 2 mg/ml in volumes of 10, 12.5, and 15 ml) in at least 50 ml of normal saline injection or D$_5$W injection. Administer by direct injection into free-flowing I.V. line of normal saline or D$_5$W injec-

tion over at least 3 minutes, usually 15 to 30 minutes. Don't mix with other drugs.
• If extravasation occurs, discontinue infusion immediately and notify doctor.
• Once vial is penetrated, undiluted solution may be stored at room temperature for 7 days, or 14 days in refrigerator. Don't freeze.
• Drug is physically incompatible with heparin. Don't mix together.

### ☑ Patient teaching
• Inform patient that urine may appear blue-green within 24 hours after administration and some bluish discoloration of the sclera may occur. These effects aren't harmful and may persist during therapy.
• Advise patient to watch for signs and symptoms of bleeding and infection.
• Caution woman of childbearing age to avoid pregnancy during therapy. Recommend that she consult doctor before becoming pregnant.

---

## paclitaxel
Taxol

*Pregnancy Risk Category D*

## HOW SUPPLIED
*Injection:* 30 mg/5 ml, 100 mg/16.7 ml

## ACTION
Prevents depolymerization of cellular microtubules, thus inhibiting normal reorganization of microtubule network needed for mitosis and other vital cellular functions.

| Route | Onset | Peak | Duration |
|-------|-------|------|----------|
| I.V. | Unknown | Unknown | Unknown |

## INDICATIONS & DOSAGE
*Metastatic ovarian cancer after failure of first-line or subsequent chemotherapy—*
**Adults:** 135 mg/m$^2$ or 175 mg/m$^2$ I.V. over 3 hours q 3 weeks.
*Breast cancer after failure of combination chemotherapy for metastatic disease or relapse within 6 months of adjuvant chemotherapy—*
**Adults:** 175 mg/m$^2$ I.V. over 3 hours q 3 weeks.

*Second-line therapy in patients with AIDS-related Kaposi's sarcoma—*
**Adults:** 135 mg/m$^2$ I.V. over 3 hours q 3 weeks, or 100 mg/m$^2$ I.V. over 3 hours q 2 weeks.
*Adjust-a-dose:* For patients experiencing severe neutropenia (neutrophil count below 500 cells/mm$^3$ for 1 week or more) or severe peripheral neuropathy, reduce subsequent courses of drug by 20%.

## ADVERSE REACTIONS
**CNS:** *peripheral neuropathy.*
**CV:** *bradycardia, hypotension, abnormal ECG.*
**GI:** *nausea, vomiting, diarrhea, mucositis.*
**Hematologic:** NEUTROPENIA, LEUKOPENIA, THROMBOCYTOPENIA, *anemia, bleeding, phlebitis.*
**Hepatic:** *elevated liver enzyme levels.*
**Metabolic:** increased triglyceride levels.
**Musculoskeletal:** *myalgia, arthralgia.*
**Skin:** *alopecia.*
**Other:** *hypersensitivity reactions, **anaphylaxis,** cellulitis at injection site, infections.*

## INTERACTIONS
**Drug-drug.** *Cisplatin:* possible additive myelosuppressive effects. When given together, paclitaxel should be given before cisplatin.
*Doxorubicin:* Plasma levels of doxorubicin and its active metabolite, doxorubicinol, may be increased when coadministered. Use together cautiously.
*Drugs that inhibit cytochrome P-450, such as cyclosporine, dexamethasone, diazepam, etoposide, ketoconazole, quinidine, retinoic acid, teniposide, testosterone, verapamil, vincristine:* may increase paclitaxel levels. Check for toxicity.
*Ketoconazole:* inhibited paclitaxel metabolism. Use together cautiously.

## EFFECTS ON DIAGNOSTIC TESTS
None reported.

## CONTRAINDICATIONS
Contraindicated in patients with hypersensitivity to drug or polyoxyethylated castor oil (a vehicle used in drug solution) and in those with baseline neutrophil counts below 1,500/mm$^3$ or AIDS-related Kaposi's sarcoma with baseline neutrophil counts below 1,000/mm$^3$.

## NURSING CONSIDERATIONS
• Use cautiously in patients with hepatic impairment.
• Some patients experience peripheral neuropathies, which may be cumulative and dose-related. Patients with severe symptoms may need dosage reduction.
• To reduce incidence or severity of hypersensitivity, anticipate pretreating patient with corticosteroids, such as dexamethasone, and antihistamines, as ordered. Both H$_1$-receptor antagonists, such as diphenhydramine, and H$_2$-receptor antagonists, such as cimetidine or ranitidine, may be used. Severe hypersensitivity reactions have occurred in as many as 2% of patients.
• Frequently monitor blood counts during therapy. Bone marrow toxicity is most common and dose-limiting toxicity. Packed RBC or platelet transfusions may be needed in severe cases. Institute bleeding precautions as appropriate.
• Patient may receive injections of RBC colony-stimulating factors to promote RBC production and decrease need for blood transfusions.
• Avoid all I.M. injections when platelet count is below 100,000/mm$^3$.
• If patient develops significant cardiac conduction abnormalities, initiate appropriate therapy and continuous cardiac monitoring during therapy and subsequent infusions.
• Initiate or repeat doses in patient with Kaposi's sarcoma only if neutrophil count exceeds 1,000 cells/mm$^3$; patient may also need reduction in dexamethasone premedication dose and start of a hematopoietic growth factor.
• *Alert:* Don't confuse paclitaxel with paroxetine or Paxil; or Taxol with Paxil.

### ◨ I.V. administration
• Follow institutional protocol for safe handling, preparation, and administration of chemotherapeutic drugs. Preparation and administration of parenteral form of drug are associated with carcinogenic, mutagenic, and teratogenic risks for personnel. Mark all waste materials with CHEMOTHERAPY HAZARD labels.

---

Reactions may be *common*, uncommon, *life-threatening*, or COMMON AND LIFE-THREATENING.

• Dilute concentrate before infusion. Compatible solutions include normal saline injection, $D_5W$, 5% dextrose in normal saline injection, and 5% dextrose in Ringer's lactate injection. Dilute to a final concentration of 0.3 to 1.2 mg/ml. Diluted solutions are stable for 24 hours at room temperature.

• Prepare and store infusion solutions in glass containers. Undiluted concentrate shouldn't contact polyvinyl chloride I.V. bags or tubing. Prepared solution may appear hazy. Store diluted solution in glass or polypropylene bottles, or use polypropylene or polyolefin bags. Administer through polyethylene-lined administration sets, and use an in-line 0.22-micron filter.

• Take care to avoid extravasation.

• Continuously monitor patient for 30 minutes after initiating infusion. Continue close monitoring throughout infusion.

☑ **Patient teaching**

• Tell patient to watch for signs and symptoms of infection (fever, sore throat, fatigue) and bleeding (easy bruising, nosebleeds, bleeding gums, melena), and to take temperature daily.

• Teach patient symptoms of peripheral neuropathy, such as a tingling or burning sensation or numbness in the extremities, and advise her to report these symptoms immediately.

• Warn patient that alopecia is common (up to 82% of patients).

• Caution woman of childbearing age to avoid becoming pregnant during therapy. Recommend that she consult doctor before becoming pregnant.

---

**pegaspargase**
**(PEG-L-asparaginase)**
Oncaspar

*Pregnancy Risk Category C*

**HOW SUPPLIED**
*Injection:* 750 IU/ml

**ACTION**
A modified version of the enzyme L-asparaginase that exerts its cytotoxic activity by inactivating the amino acid as-paragine. Asparagine is needed by tumor cells to synthesize proteins. Because the tumor cells can't synthesize their own asparagine, protein synthesis and, eventually, synthesis of DNA and RNA are inhibited.

| Route | Onset | Peak | Duration |
|-------|-------|------|----------|
| I.V., I.M. | Unknown | Unknown | Unknown |

**INDICATIONS & DOSAGE**
*Acute lymphoblastic leukemia (ALL) in patients who need L-asparaginase but have developed hypersensitivity to the native forms of L-asparaginase—*
**Adults and children with body surface area (BSA) of at least 0.6 m²:** 2,500 IU/m² I.M. or I.V. q 14 days.
**Children with BSA below 0.6 m²:** 82.5 IU/kg I.M. or I.V. q 14 days.

**ADVERSE REACTIONS**
**CNS:** *seizures,* headache, paresthesia, *status epilepticus,* somnolence, *coma,* mental status changes, dizziness, emotional lability, mood changes, parkinsonism, confusion, disorientation, fatigue, malaise.
**CV:** hypotension, tachycardia, chest pain, subacute bacterial endocarditis, hypertension.
**EENT:** epistaxis.
**GI:** nausea, vomiting, abdominal pain, anorexia, diarrhea, constipation, indigestion, flatulence, mucositis, mouth tenderness, *pancreatitis,* increased serum amylase and lipase levels, severe colitis.
**GU:** increased BUN and creatinine levels, increased urinary frequency, hematuria, severe hemorrhagic cystitis, renal dysfunction, *renal failure.*
**Hematologic:** *thrombosis;* prolonged PT, INR, and PTT; decreased antithrombin III; *disseminated intravascular coagulation;* decreased fibrinogen; hemolytic anemia; *leukopenia; pancytopenia; agranulocytosis; thrombocytopenia;* increased thromboplastin; easy bruising; ecchymoses; *hemorrhage.*
**Hepatic:** jaundice, bilirubinemia, increased ALT and AST levels, ascites, hypoalbuminemia, fatty changes in liver, *liver failure.*
**Metabolic:** hyperuricemia, hyponatremia, uric acid nephropathy, hypoproteinemia,

proteinuria, weight loss, metabolic acidosis, increased blood ammonia level, hyperglycemia, hypoglycemia.
**Musculoskeletal:** arthralgia, myalgia, musculoskeletal pain, joint stiffness, cramps, pain in extremities.
**Respiratory:** cough, *severe bronchospasm,* upper respiratory tract infection.
**Skin:** urticaria, itching, alopecia, fever blister, purpura, hand whiteness, fungal changes, nail whiteness and ridging, erythema simplex, petechial rash, injection pain or reaction, localized edema, rash, erythema.
**Other:** *hypersensitivity reactions,* including *anaphylaxis,* edema, pain, fever, chills, dyspnea, or bronchospasm; peripheral edema; night sweats; infection; *sepsis, septic shock.*

## INTERACTIONS
**Drug-drug.** *Aspirin, dipyridamole, heparin, NSAIDs, warfarin:* imbalances in coagulation factors may occur, predisposing patient to bleeding or thrombosis. Use together cautiously.
*Methotrexate:* during period of drug's inhibition of protein synthesis and cell replication, pegaspargase may interfere with action of such drugs as methotrexate, which need cell replication for their lethal effects. Check for decreased effectiveness.
*Protein-bound drugs:* depletion of serum proteins by pegaspargase may increase toxicity of other drugs that bind to proteins. Check for toxicity. Pegaspargase also may interfere with enzymatic detoxification of other drugs, particularly in the liver. Administer concomitantly with caution.

## EFFECTS ON DIAGNOSTIC TESTS
None reported.

## CONTRAINDICATIONS
Contraindicated in patients with pancreatitis or history of pancreatitis; in those who have had significant hemorrhagic events associated with previous treatment with L-asparaginase; and in those with history of serious allergic reactions to drug, such as generalized urticaria, bronchospasm, laryngeal edema, hypotension, or other unacceptable adverse reactions.

## NURSING CONSIDERATIONS
• Use cautiously in patients with liver dysfunction; use only when clearly indicated in pregnant women.
• Use drug as sole induction drug only when combined regimen using other chemotherapeutic drugs is inappropriate because of toxicity or other specific patient-related factors, or in patients refractory to other therapy.
• I.M. route is preferred because it has the lowest risk of hepatotoxicity, coagulopathy, and GI and renal disorders.
• When administering I.M., limit volume administered at a single injection site to 2 ml. If volume to be administered exceeds 2 ml, use multiple injection sites.
• *Alert:* Monitor patient closely for hypersensitivity reactions such as life-threatening anaphylaxis, which may occur during therapy, especially in those with known hypersensitivity to other forms of L-asparaginase. As a routine precaution, keep patient under observation for 1 hour and have resuscitation equipment and other drugs needed to treat anaphylaxis (such as epinephrine, oxygen, and I.V. corticosteroids readily available. Moderate to life-threatening hypersensitivity reactions require discontinuation of L-asparaginase.
• To assess effects of therapy, monitor patient's peripheral blood count and bone marrow, as ordered. A fall in circulating lymphoblasts is often noted after initiating therapy, sometimes accompanied by a marked rise in serum uric acid levels.
• Take preventive measures (including adequate hydration) before starting treatment. Hyperuricemia may result from rapid lysis of leukemic cells. Allopurinol may be ordered.
• Obtain frequent serum amylase determinations, as ordered, to detect pancreatitis. Monitor patient's blood glucose level during therapy to detect hyperglycemia.
• Monitor patient for liver dysfunction when drug is used with hepatotoxic chemotherapeutic drugs.
• Drug may affect several plasma proteins; therefore, monitoring of fibrinogen, PT, INR, and PTT may be indicated. Question doctor if not ordered.

---

Reactions may be *common,* uncommon, *life-threatening,* or COMMON AND LIFE-THREATENING.

## ◀ I.V. administration
• Don't administer if drug has been frozen. Although there may not be a change in drug's appearance, pegaspargase's activity is destroyed after freezing. Obtain new dose from pharmacist.
• Avoid excessive agitation; don't shake. Keep refrigerated at 36° to 46° F (2° to 8° C). Don't use if cloudy or if precipitate is present. Don't use if stored at room temperature for more than 48 hours. Don't freeze. Discard unused portions. Use only one dose per vial; don't reenter vial.
• Drug may be a contact irritant, and solution must be handled and administered with care. Gloves are recommended. Inhalation of vapors and contact with skin or mucous membranes, especially those of the eyes, must be avoided. If contact occurs, wash with generous amounts of water for at least 15 minutes.
• When administering I.V., give over a period of 1 to 2 hours in 100 ml of normal saline or $D_5W$ injection through an infusion that is already running.

## ✔ Patient teaching
• Inform patient of risk of hypersensitivity reactions and importance of alerting nurse immediately if they occur.
• Instruct patient not to take other drugs, including OTC preparations, until approved by doctor because risk of bleeding is higher when pegaspargase is given with drugs such as aspirin. Pegaspargase may also increase toxicity of other drugs.
• Instruct patient to report signs and symptoms of infection (fever, chills, and malaise); drug may have immunosuppressant effect.
• Caution woman of childbearing age to avoid pregnancy and breast-feeding during therapy.

---

## porfimer sodium
Photofrin

*Pregnancy Risk Category C*

## HOW SUPPLIED
*Injection:* 75 mg/vial

## ACTION
Photosensitizing drug that damages cancer cells through propagation of radical reactions. Tumor death occurs through ischemic necrosis secondary to vascular occlusion that appears to be partly mediated by release of thromboxane $A_2$. Cytotoxic and antitumor actions of porfimer depend on light and oxygen.

| Route | Onset | Peak | Duration |
|-------|-------|------|----------|
| I.V. | Unknown | Unknown | Unknown |

## INDICATIONS & DOSAGE
*Palliative treatment for patients with completely obstructing esophageal cancer or for those with partially obstructing esophageal cancer who can't be satisfactorily treated with Nd:YAG laser therapy—*
**Adults:** 2 mg/kg I.V. for 3 to 5 minutes (first stage of therapy); then illumination with laser light 40 to 50 hours later (second stage). A second laser-light application may be given 96 to 120 hours after injection. Total of three courses (each course consisting of both stages) may be given, separated by at least 30 days.
*Microinvasive endobronchial non-small-cell lung cancer in patients for whom surgery and radiotherapy aren't indicated—*
**Adults:** 2 mg/kg I.V. for 3 to 5 minutes (first stage of therapy); then illumination with laser light 40 to 50 hours later (second stage). A second laser-light application may be given 96 to 120 hours after injection. Total of three courses (each course consisting of both stages) may be given, separated by at least 30 days.

## ADVERSE REACTIONS
**CNS:** anxiety, confusion, *insomnia,* asthenia.
**CV:** hypotension, hypertension, ***heart failure,*** atrial fibrillation, tachycardia, edema.
**EENT:** *pharyngitis,* diplopia, discomfort, photophobia.
**GI:** *constipation, abdominal pain, nausea, vomiting,* diarrhea, dyspepsia, dysphagia, eructation, esophageal edema, esophageal tumor bleeding, esophageal stricture, esophagitis, hematemesis, melena, anorexia.

---

**GU:** urinary tract infection, candidiasis.
**Hematologic:** *anemia.*
**Metabolic:** dehydration, weight loss.
**Respiratory:** coughing, *dyspnea, pleural effusion, pneumonia,* respiratory insufficiency, tracheoesophageal fistula.
**Skin:** *photosensitivity.*
**Other:** *back or chest pain,* substantial or general pain, fever, surgical complication.

## INTERACTIONS
**Drug-drug.** *Other photosensitizing drugs (griseofulvin, phenothiazines, sulfonamides, sulfonylurea hypoglycemics, tetracyclines, thiazide diuretics):* may increase photosensitivity reaction. Use together cautiously.
**Drug-lifestyle.** *Sun exposure:* photosensitivity reactions may occur. Take precautions.

## EFFECTS ON DIAGNOSTIC TESTS
None reported.

## CONTRAINDICATIONS
Contraindicated in patients with hypersensitivity to porphyrins and in those with porphyria, tracheoesophageal or bronchoesophageal fistula, or tumor eroding into major blood vessel.

## NURSING CONSIDERATIONS
• Breast-feeding isn't recommended during therapy because it isn't known if drug appears in breast milk.
• Safety and efficacy of drug in children haven't been established.
• Before each course of treatment, patient should be evaluated for a tracheoesophageal or bronchoesophageal fistula.
• Don't allow drug to contact eyes or skin during preparation or administration. Protect an exposed person from bright light.
• Patient may receive 630-nm wavelength laser-light therapy 40 to 50 hours after porfimer injection for drug to be effective. A second laser-light treatment (but not a second injection) may be given as early as 96 hours or as late as 120 hours after injection. Before a second treatment, residual tumor should be debrided; vigorous debridement may cause tumor bleeding. Monitor patient closely.

• Inflammation of treatment area may cause substernal chest pain. Notify doctor if this occurs; pain may be sufficiently intense to warrant short-term use of opiate analgesics.
• Monitor CBC regularly to detect anemia. Drug and laser therapy may cause tumor bleeding.

### ⬛ I.V. administration
• Reconstitute each vial of porfimer with 31.8 ml of $D_5W$ solution or normal saline solution for injection, resulting in final concentration of 2.5 mg/ml. Shake until dissolved. Don't mix porfimer with other drugs in same solution. Reconstituted drug is opaque. Inspect carefully for particulate and discoloration before use. Protect reconstituted drug from bright light, and use immediately.
• Administer drug as a single slow I.V. injection over 3 to 5 minutes.
• Take precautions to prevent extravasation at injection site. If it occurs, protect area from light.

### ✓ Patient teaching
• Instruct patient to avoid direct sunlight and bright indoor light for 30 days after injection, but tell him to expose skin to ambient indoor light. After 30 days, he should expose a small area of skin (not face) to sunlight for 10 minutes. If he doesn't develop a photosensitivity reaction (erythema, edema, blistering) within 24 hours, he can gradually resume outdoor activities while exercising caution. If photosensitivity occurs, he should avoid sunlight and bright indoor light for 2 weeks before retesting.
• Urge patient traveling to an area with stronger sun to retest his photosensitivity level.
• Warn patient that ultraviolet sunscreens don't protect against photosensitivity.
• Advise patient to wear dark sunglasses with an average white light transmittance of less than 4% when outdoors.
• Caution woman of childbearing age to use an effective contraceptive method, avoid pregnancy, and to notify doctor of suspected pregnancy.

---

## procarbazine hydrochloride
Matulane, Natulan†

*Pregnancy Risk Category D*

### HOW SUPPLIED
*Capsules:* 50 mg

### ACTION
Unknown. Thought to inhibit DNA, RNA, and protein synthesis.

| Route | Onset | Peak | Duration |
|-------|-------|------|----------|
| P.O. | Unknown | Unknown | Unknown |

### INDICATIONS & DOSAGE
Dosage and indications vary. Check treatment protocol with doctor.

*Adjunct treatment of Hodgkin's disease (stages III and IV), other cancers using MOPP (nitrogen mustard, vincristine, procarbazine, prednisone) regimen—*
**Adults:** 2 to 4 mg/kg P.O. daily in single dose or divided doses for first week. Then, 4 to 6 mg/kg/day until WBC count falls below 4,000/mm$^3$, platelet count falls below 100,000/mm$^3$, or maximum response is obtained. Maintenance dose is 1 to 2 mg/kg/day after bone marrow recovery. For MOPP regimen, 100 mg/m$^2$/day P.O. for 14 days.
**Children:** 50 mg/m$^2$ P.O. daily for first week; then 100 mg/m$^2$ until response or toxicity occurs. Maintenance dose is 50 mg/m$^2$ P.O. daily after bone marrow recovery.

### ADVERSE REACTIONS
**CNS:** nervousness, depression, headache, dizziness, *coma,* insomnia, nightmares, paresthesia, neuropathy, *hallucinations,* confusion, syncope.
**CV:** hypotension, tachycardia, flushing.
**EENT:** retinal hemorrhage, nystagmus, photophobia.
**GI:** *nausea, vomiting,* abdominal pain, hematemesis, melena, anorexia, stomatitis, dry mouth, dysphagia, diarrhea, constipation.
**GU:** hematuria, urinary frequency, nocturia, gynecomastia.

**Hematologic:** *bleeding tendency, thrombocytopenia, leukopenia, anemia,* hemolytic anemia, *pancytopenia,* eosinophilia.
**Hepatic:** *hepatotoxicity.*
**Respiratory:** *pleural effusion,* cough, pneumonitis.
**Skin:** reversible alopecia, dermatitis, pruritus, rash, hyperpigmentation, herpes.
**Other:** allergic reaction.

### INTERACTIONS
**Drug-drug.** *CNS depressants:* additive depressant effects. Avoid concomitant use.
*Digoxin:* may decrease serum digoxin levels. Monitor closely.
*Drugs high in tyramine, local anesthetics, sympathomimetics, tricyclic antidepressants:* possible tremor, palpitations, increased blood pressure. Monitor closely.
**Drug-food.** *Caffeine:* concurrent use may result in arrhythmias, severe hypertension. Discourage caffeine intake.
*Foods high in tyramine (cheese, Chianti wine):* possible tremor, palpitations, increased blood pressure. Monitor closely.
**Drug-lifestyle.** *Alcohol use:* mild disulfiram-like reaction manifested by flushing, headache, nausea, and hypotension. Warn patient to avoid alcoholic beverages.

### EFFECTS ON DIAGNOSTIC TESTS
None reported.

### CONTRAINDICATIONS
Contraindicated in patients with hypersensitivity to drug and in those with inadequate bone marrow reserve as shown by bone marrow aspiration.

### NURSING CONSIDERATIONS
• Use cautiously in patients with impaired hepatic or renal function.
• Monitor CBC and platelet counts.
• To prevent bleeding, avoid all I.M. injections when platelet count is below 100,000/mm$^3$.
• Anticipate need for blood transfusions to combat anemia. Patients may receive injections of RBC colony-stimulating factors to promote RBC production and decrease need for blood transfusions.
• Be prepared to discontinue drug if patient becomes confused or if paresthesia or other neuropathies develop. Notify doctor.

### ✓ Patient teaching

• To decrease nausea and vomiting, advise patient to take drug at bedtime and in divided doses.

• Tell patient to watch for signs of infection (fever, sore throat, fatigue) and bleeding (easy bruising, nosebleeds, bleeding gums, melena), and to take temperature daily.

• Warn patient to avoid alcohol during therapy. Urge him to stop drug and check with doctor immediately if he experiences a disulfiram-like reaction (chest pains, rapid or irregular heartbeat, severe headache, stiff neck).

• Instruct patient to avoid foods high in tyramine, such as wine, cheese, and bananas, and OTC preparations containing sympathomimetics.

• Warn patient to avoid hazardous activities that require alertness and good motor coordination until CNS effects of drug are known.

• Caution woman of childbearing age to avoid becoming pregnant during therapy and to consult doctor before becoming pregnant.

## rituximab
Rituxan

*Pregnancy Risk Category C*

### HOW SUPPLIED
*Injection:* 10 mg/ml; 10-ml, 50-ml single-use, sterile vials

### ACTION
A murine and human monoclonal antibody directed against CD20 antigen found on the surface of normal and malignant B lymphocytes. Binding to this antigen mediates the lysis of the B cells.

| Route | Onset | Peak | Duration |
|-------|----------|----------|----------|
| I.V. | Variable | Variable | 6-12 mo |

### INDICATIONS & DOSAGE
*B-cell malignant lymphoma with relapsed or refractory, low-grade or follicular, CD20 positive disease—*
**Adults:** 375 mg/m$^2$ given as I.V. infusion once weekly for four doses (days 1, 8, 15,

22). Initial infusion should be started at 50 mg/hour. If hypersensitivity or infusion-related events don't occur, increase rate 50 mg/hour q 30 minutes, to maximum of 400 mg/hour. Subsequent infusions can be administered at initial rate of 100 mg/hour and increased by increments of 100 mg/hour at 30-minute intervals, to maximum of 400 mg/hour as tolerated.

### ADVERSE REACTIONS
**CNS:** dizziness, *asthenia, headache,* fatigue, paresthesia, malaise, agitation, insomnia, hypesthesia, hypertonia, nervousness.
**CV:** *hypotension, arrhythmias,* hypertension, peripheral edema, chest pain, tachycardia, orthostatic hypotension, *bradycardia,* flushing.
**EENT:** sore throat, rhinitis, sinusitis, lacrimation disorder, conjunctivitis.
**GI:** *nausea,* vomiting, abdominal pain or enlargement, diarrhea, dyspepsia, anorexia, increased LD, taste perversion.
**Hematologic:** LEUKOPENIA, *thrombocytopenia, neutropenia,* anemia.
**Metabolic:** hyperglycemia, hypercalcemia.
**Musculoskeletal:** myalgia, back pain.
**Respiratory:** *bronchospasm,* dyspnea, cough increase, bronchitis.
**Skin:** *pruritus, rash,* urticaria.
**Other:** ANGIOEDEMA, *fever, chills, rigor,* pain, pain at injection site, tumor pain.

### INTERACTIONS
None significant.

### EFFECTS ON DIAGNOSTIC TESTS
None reported.

### CONTRAINDICATIONS
Contraindicated in patients with type I hypersensitivity or anaphylactic reactions to murine proteins or components of rituximab.

### NURSING CONSIDERATIONS
• Monitor patient closely for signs and symptoms of a hypersensitivity reaction. Have drugs, such as epinephrine, antihistamine, and corticosteroids, available to immediately treat such a reaction. Consid-

---

Reactions may be *common,* uncommon, *life-threatening,* or COMMON AND LIFE-THREATENING.

er premedicating with acetaminophen and diphenhydramine before each infusion.

• Obtain CBC at regular intervals and more frequently in patients who develop cytopenias.

• Protect vials from direct sunlight.

### 🔲 I.V. administration

• *Alert:* Drug must be given as I.V. infusion; don't give as I.V. push or bolus.

• Dilute to a final concentration of 1 to 4 mg/ml in bag of $D_5W$ or normal saline. Gently invert bag to mix solution. Discard unused portion left in vial.

• Monitor patient's blood pressure closely during infusion. If hypotension, bronchospasm, or angioedema occurs, discontinue infusion and restart at a 50% rate reduction when symptoms resolve.

• Discontinue infusion if serious or life-threatening arrhythmias occur. Patients who develop clinically significant arrhythmias should undergo cardiac monitoring during and after subsequent infusions of rituximab.

### ✅ Patient teaching

• Tell patient to report symptoms of hypersensitivity reaction, such as itching, rash, chills, or rigors, during and after infusion.

• Tell patient to watch for signs and symptoms of infection (fever, sore throat, fatigue) and bleeding (easy bruising, nosebleeds, bleeding gums, melena), and to take temperature daily.

## teniposide (VM-26)
Vumon

*Pregnancy Risk Category D*

### HOW SUPPLIED
*Injection:* 10 mg/ml

### ACTION
A phase-specific cytotoxic drug that acts in the late S or early $G_2$ phase of the cell cycle, thus preventing cells from entering mitosis.

| Route | Onset | Peak | Duration |
|-------|-------|------|----------|
| I.V. | Unknown | Unknown | Unknown |

### INDICATIONS & DOSAGE
*Refractory childhood acute lymphoblastic leukemia—*

**Children:** optimum dosage hasn't been established. Dosages ranging from 165 to 250 mg/m² I.V. once or twice weekly for 4 to 6 weeks have been used. Usually given with other drugs.

*Adjust-a-dose:* Patients with both Down syndrome and leukemia are at higher risk for myelosuppression. Administer first course of treatment at half the dosage.

### ADVERSE REACTIONS
**CV:** hypotension.
**GI:** *nausea, vomiting, mucositis, diarrhea.*
**Hematologic:** MYELOSUPPRESSION, LEUKOPENIA, NEUTROPENIA, THROMBOCYTOPENIA, *anemia*.
**Skin:** rash.
**Other:** *infection,* bleeding, ***hypersensitivity reactions;** phlebitis, extravasation at injection site;* increased blood and urine levels of uric acid.

### INTERACTIONS
**Drug-drug.** *Methotrexate:* may increase clearance and intracellular levels of methotrexate. Avoid concurrent use.
*Sodium salicylate, sulfamethizole, tolbutamide:* may displace teniposide from protein-binding sites and increase toxicity. Don't administer together.

### EFFECTS ON DIAGNOSTIC TESTS
None reported.

### CONTRAINDICATIONS
Contraindicated in patients with hypersensitivity to drug or to polyoxyethylated castor oil, an injection vehicle.

### NURSING CONSIDERATIONS
• Drug may be prescribed despite patient's history of hypersensitivity because therapeutic benefits outweigh risks. Treat such patients with antihistamines and corticosteroids before infusion begins and observe continuously for first hour of infusion and at frequent intervals thereafter.
• Obtain baseline blood counts and renal and hepatic function tests, as ordered.

---

*Liquid contains alcohol.  **May contain tartrazine.  †Canada  ‡Australia  §U.K.  ◇OTC

• Monitor blood pressure before and during therapy. Hypotension can occur from rapid infusion.
• Have on hand diphenhydramine, hydrocortisone, epinephrine, and emergency equipment to establish an airway in case of anaphylaxis. Signs of hypersensitivity reaction include chills, fever, urticaria, tachycardia, bronchospasm, dyspnea, hypotension, flushing.
• Monitor blood counts and renal and hepatic function tests, as ordered.

### ☑I.V. administration
• Dilute drug in either $D_5W$ or normal saline injection to a final concentration of 0.1, 0.2, 0.4, or 1 mg/ml. Don't agitate vigorously; precipitation may occur. Discard cloudy solutions. Prepare and store drug in glass containers. Infuse over 30 to 60 minutes to prevent hypotension.
• Don't mix with other drugs or solutions. Heparin solution can cause precipitation. Flush administration apparatus and catheters with $D_5W$ or normal saline before and after infusion of drug.
• Ensure careful placement of I.V. catheter. Extravasation can result in local tissue necrosis or sloughing.
• Occlusion of catheters, including those centrally placed, can occur, particularly during 24-hour infusions at 0.1 to 0.2 mg/ml. Monitor carefully.
• Don't administer through a membrane-type in-line filter because diluent may dissolve it.
• Monitor blood pressure every 30 minutes during infusion. If systolic blood pressure falls below 90 mm Hg, stop infusion and notify doctor.
• In normal saline or $D_5W$, concentrations of 0.1 to 0.4 mg/ml are chemically stable for at least 24 hours at room or refrigerated temperature in glass containers.
• Follow institutional policy to reduce risks. Preparation and administration of parenteral form of drug are associated with carcinogenic, mutagenic, and teratogenic risks for personnel.
• Use nonDEHP (di[2-ethylhexyl] phthalate) containers and tubing for administration.

### ☑Patient teaching
• Tell patient to report signs and symptoms of infection (fever, sore throat, fatigue) and bleeding (easy bruising, nosebleeds, bleeding gums, melena), and to take temperature daily.
• Caution woman of childbearing age to avoid becoming pregnant during therapy and to consult doctor before becoming pregnant.

## topotecan hydrochloride
Hycamtin

*Pregnancy Risk Category D*

### HOW SUPPLIED
*Injection:* 4-mg single-dose vial

### ACTION
Relieves torsional strain in DNA by inducing reversible single-strand breaks. Binds to the topoisomerase I-DNA complex and prevents relegation of these single-strand breaks. Cytotoxicity of topotecan is thought to be due to double-strand DNA damage produced during DNA synthesis when replication enzymes interact with the ternary complex formed by topotecan, topoisomerase I, and DNA.

| Route | Onset | Peak | Duration |
|-------|-------|------|----------|
| I.V. | Unknown | Unknown | Unknown |

### INDICATIONS & DOSAGE
*Metastatic carcinoma of the ovary after failure of initial or subsequent chemotherapy—*
**Adults:** 1.5 mg/m² I.V. infusion given over 30 minutes daily for 5 consecutive days, starting on day 1 of a 21-day cycle. Minimum of four cycles should be given.
✱*NEW INDICATION: Small-cell lung cancer sensitive disease after failure of first-line chemotherapy—*
**Adults:** 1.5 mg/m² I.V. infusion given over 30 minutes daily for 5 consecutive days, starting on day 1 of 21-day cycle. Minimum of four cycles should be given.
*Adjust-a-dose:* For patients with creatinine clearance of 20 to 39 ml/minute, dosage decreased to 0.75 mg/m². If severe neutropenia occurs, dosage decreased by

0.25 mg/m² for subsequent courses. Or, if severe neutropenia occurs, granulocyte colony–stimulating factor may be administered following subsequent course (before resorting to dosage reduction) starting from day 6 of course (24 hours after completion of topotecan administration).

**ADVERSE REACTIONS**
**CNS:** *fatigue, asthenia, headache.*
**GI:** *nausea, vomiting, diarrhea, constipation, abdominal pain, stomatitis, anorexia.*
**Hematologic:** NEUTROPENIA, LEUKOPENIA, THROMBOCYTOPENIA, *anemia.*
**Hepatic:** transient elevations of AST, ALT, and bilirubin levels.
**Respiratory:** *dyspnea, coughing.*
**Skin:** *alopecia.*
**Other:** *sepsis, fever.*

**INTERACTIONS**
**Drug-drug.** *Cisplatin:* increased severity of myelosuppression, if given together. Use both drugs with extreme caution.
*Granulocyte colony–stimulating factor:* prolonged duration of neutropenia. If granulocyte colony–stimulating factor is to be used, don't start it until day 6 of the course, 24 hours after completion of topotecan treatment.

**EFFECTS ON DIAGNOSTIC TESTS**
None reported.

**CONTRAINDICATIONS**
Contraindicated in patients with hypersensitivity to drug or its components and in those with severe bone marrow depression. Also contraindicated in pregnant or breast-feeding women.

**NURSING CONSIDERATIONS**
• *Alert:* Before first course of therapy is administered, patient must have baseline neutrophil count over 1,500 cells/mm³ and platelet count over 100,000 cells/mm³.
• Drug should be prepared under vertical laminar flow hood; wear gloves and protective clothing. If drug solution contacts skin, wash immediately and thoroughly with soap and water. If mucous membranes are affected, flush areas thoroughly with water.

• Bone marrow suppression (primarily neutropenia) indicates toxic levels of topotecan. The nadir occurs at about 11 days. Neutropenia isn't cumulative over time.
• Duration of thrombocytopenia is about 5 days, with nadir at 15 days. The nadir for anemia is 15 days. Blood or platelet transfusions may be needed.
• Frequent monitoring of peripheral blood cell counts is needed. Don't treat patient with subsequent courses of topotecan until neutrophil count recovers to more than 1,000 cells/mm³, platelet count recovers to more than 100,000 cells/mm³, and hemoglobin level recovers to more than 9 mg/dl (with transfusion, if needed).
• Patient may receive injections of WBC colony-stimulating factors to promote cell growth and decrease risk for infection.
• Safety and effectiveness of drug in children haven't been established.

**◨ I.V. administration**
• Reconstitute each 4-mg vial with 4 ml sterile water for injection. Dilute appropriate volume of reconstituted solution in either normal saline solution or D₅W before administration.
• Because lyophilized dosage form contains no antibacterial preservative, use reconstituted product immediately.
• Protect unopened vials from light. Reconstituted drug stored at 68° to 77° F (20° to 25° C) and exposed to ambient lighting is stable for 24 hours.
• Inadvertent drug extravasation has been associated with mild local reactions, such as erythema and bruising.

**☑ Patient teaching**
• Instruct patient to promptly report sore throat, fever, chills, or unusual bleeding or bruising.
• Caution woman of childbearing age to avoid pregnancy or breast-feeding during therapy.
• Teach patient and family about drug's adverse reactions and need for frequent monitoring of blood counts.

---

## trastuzumab
Herceptin

*Pregnancy Risk Category B*

### HOW SUPPLIED
*Injection:* lyophilized sterile powder containing 440 mg per vial

### ACTION
A recombinant DNA-derived monoclonal antibody that selectively binds to human epidermal growth factor receptor 2 protein (HER2), inhibiting proliferation of human tumor cells that overexpress HER2.

| Route | Onset | Peak | Duration |
|-------|-------|------|----------|
| I.V. | Unknown | Unknown | Unknown |

### INDICATIONS & DOSAGE
*Single-drug treatment of metastatic breast cancer in patients whose tumors overexpress the HER2 protein and who have received one or more chemotherapy regimens for their metastatic disease, or with paclitaxel for metastatic breast cancer in patients whose tumors overexpress the HER2 protein and who haven't received chemotherapy for their metastatic disease—*
**Adults:** initial loading dose is 4 mg/kg I.V. over 90 minutes. Maintenance dose is 2 mg/kg I.V. weekly as 30-minute I.V. infusion if initial loading dose is well tolerated.

### ADVERSE REACTIONS
**CNS:** depression, *dizziness, insomnia,* neuropathy, paresthesia, peripheral neuritis, *asthenia, headache.*
**CV: *heart failure,** peripheral edema,* tachycardia, edema.
**EENT:** *rhinitis, pharyngitis,* sinusitis.
**GI:** *anorexia, abdominal pain, diarrhea, nausea, vomiting.*
**GU:** urinary tract infection.
**Hematologic: *leukopenia,*** anemia.
**Musculoskeletal:** arthralgia, *back pain,* bone pain.
**Respiratory:** *dyspnea, increased cough.*
**Skin:** acne, herpes simplex, *rash.*

**Other:** allergic reaction, *chills, fever, flu-like syndrome, infection, pain.*

### INTERACTIONS
None significant.

### EFFECTS ON DIAGNOSTIC TESTS
None reported.

### CONTRAINDICATIONS
No known contraindications.

### NURSING CONSIDERATIONS
• Use cautiously in elderly patients, in patients with hypersensitivity to drug or its components, and in those with preexisting cardiac dysfunction.
• Safety and effectiveness of drug in children haven't been established.
• Before beginning therapy, patient should undergo thorough baseline cardiac assessment, including history and physical examination and appropriate evaluation methods to identify those at risk for developing cardiotoxicity.
• Assess patient for signs and symptoms of cardiac dysfunction, especially if patient is receiving drug with anthracyclines and cyclophosphamide.
• Check for dyspnea, increased cough, paroxysmal nocturnal dyspnea, peripheral edema, or S3 gallop. Treatment may be stopped in patients who develop a significant decrease in left ventricular function.
• Monitor patient receiving both drug and chemotherapy closely for cardiac dysfunction or failure, anemia, leukopenia, diarrhea, and infection.
• Drug should be used only in patients with metastatic breast cancer whose tumors have HER2 protein overexpression.
• Check for first-infusion symptom complex, commonly consisting of chills or fever. Treat with acetaminophen, diphenhydramine, and meperidine (with or without reducing rate of infusion), as ordered. Other signs or symptoms may include nausea, vomiting, pain, rigors, headache, dizziness, dyspnea, hypotension, rash, and asthenia. These symptoms occur infrequently with subsequent infusions.

---

Reactions may be *common,* uncommon, ***life-threatening,*** or COMMON AND LIFE-THREATENING.

## 🔲 I.V. administration

• Don't administer as an I.V. push or bolus.

• Reconstitute drug in each vial with 20 ml of bacteriostatic water for injection, 1.1% benzyl alcohol preserved, as supplied, to yield a multidose solution containing 21 mg/ml. Immediately upon reconstitution, label vial for drug expiration 28 days from date of reconstitution.

• *Alert:* If patient has known hypersensitivity to benzyl alcohol, reconstitute drug with sterile water for injection, use immediately, and discard unused portion. Avoid use of other reconstitution diluents.

• Determine dose (mg) of drug needed, based on loading dose of 4 mg/kg or maintenance dose of 2 mg/kg. Calculate volume of 21 mg/ml solution and withdraw this amount from vial and add it to an infusion bag containing 250 ml of normal saline. Don't use $D_5W$ solution. Gently invert bag to mix solution.

• Infuse initial loading dose over 90 minutes. If well tolerated, infuse maintenance doses over 30 minutes.

• Don't mix or dilute drug with other drugs.

• Vials of drug are stable at 36° to 46° F (2° to 8° C) before reconstitution. Discard reconstituted solution after 28 days. Don't freeze drug that has been reconstituted. Solution of drug diluted in normal saline for injection should be stored at 36° to 46° F (2° to 8° C) before use, and is stable for up to 24 hours.

## ☑ Patient teaching

• Tell patient about risk of first dose infusion-associated adverse reactions.

• Instruct patient to notify doctor immediately if signs or symptoms of cardiac dysfunction occur, such as shortness of breath, increased cough, or peripheral edema.

• Instruct patient to report adverse effects to doctor.

• Advise breast-feeding woman to discontinue breast-feeding during drug therapy and for 6 months after last dose of drug.

## tretinoin
Vesanoid

*Pregnancy Risk Category D*

**HOW SUPPLIED**
*Capsules:* 10 mg

**ACTION**
Unknown.

| Route | Onset | Peak | Duration |
|-------|-------|------|----------|
| P.O. | Unknown | 1-2 hr | Unknown |

**INDICATIONS & DOSAGE**
*Induction of remission in patients with acute promyelocytic leukemia (APL), French-American-British (FAB) classification $M^3$ (including $M^3$ variant), when anthracycline chemotherapy is contraindicated or unsuccessful—*
**Adults and children ages 1 and older:** 45 mg/m²/day P.O. in two even doses. Therapy should be discontinued 30 days after complete remission is documented or after 90 days of treatment, whichever occurs first.

**ADVERSE REACTIONS**
**CNS:** dizziness, *paresthesia, anxiety, insomnia, depression, confusion, cerebral hemorrhage,* intracranial hypertension, agitation, hallucination, abnormal gait, agnosia, aphasia, asterixis, cerebellar edema, cerebellar disorders, *seizures, coma,* CNS depression, dysarthria, encephalopathy, facial paralysis, hemiplegia, hyporeflexia, hypotaxia, no light reflex, neurologic reaction, spinal cord disorder, tremor, leg weakness, unconsciousness, dementia, forgetfulness, somnolence, slow speech, *fatigue, malaise, weakness, pain.*
**CV:** *chest discomfort,* ARRHYTHMIAS, *hypotension, hypertension, phlebitis, edema, heart failure, MI, pericardial effusions,* impaired myocardial contractility, progressive hypoxemia, enlarged heart, heart murmur, ischemia, myocarditis, pericarditis, secondary cardiomyopathy, *CVA, flushing.*
**EENT:** *earache, ear fullness,* hearing loss, *visual disturbances,* changed visual acuity, visual field defects, *ocular disorders.*

**GI:** *GI hemorrhage, nausea, vomiting, anorexia, abdominal pain, GI disorders, diarrhea, constipation, dyspepsia, abdominal distention,* hepatosplenomegaly, ulcer.
**GU:** *renal insufficiency,* dysuria, **acute renal failure,** urinary frequency, renal tubular necrosis, enlarged prostate.
**Hematologic:** *leukocytosis,* HEMORRHAGE, DISSEMINATED INTRAVASCULAR COAGULATION.
**Hepatic:** **hepatitis,** unspecified liver disorder, *hypercholesterolemia, hypertriglyceridemia, elevated liver function test results.*
**Metabolic:** fluid imbalance, acidosis, *weight gain or loss.*
**Musculoskeletal:** *myalgia, bone pain,* bone inflammation.
**Respiratory:** *pneumonia, upper respiratory tract disorders, dyspnea, respiratory insufficiency, pleural effusion, rales, expiratory wheezing,* lower respiratory tract disorders, pulmonary infiltrates, bronchial asthma, pulmonary edema, laryngeal edema, unspecified pulmonary disease, pulmonary hypertension.
**Skin:** *rash, skin and mucous membrane dryness, pruritus, alopecia, increased sweating, skin changes.*
**Other:** **retinoic acid–APL syndrome, septicemia, multiorgan failure,** *fever, infections, shivering, peripheral edema, injection site reactions, mucositis,* flank pain, cellulitis, facial edema, pallor, lymph disorder, hypothermia, ascites.

## INTERACTIONS
**Drug-drug.** *Ketoconazole:* may enhance tretinoin activity when taken together. Use cautiously.
**Drug-food.** *Any food:* may enhance absorption of tretinoin. Give with food.

## EFFECTS ON DIAGNOSTIC TESTS
None reported.

## CONTRAINDICATIONS
Contraindicated in patients with hypersensitivity to retinoids and in those with sensitivity to parabens, which is used as a preservative in gelatin capsule.

## NURSING CONSIDERATIONS
• Drug isn't recommended for use in pregnant or breast-feeding women.
• Because patient with APL is at high risk and can have severe reactions, give drug under supervision of doctor with experience managing such patients and in a facility able to monitor drug tolerance and protect and maintain patient compromised by toxicity.
• Some patients receiving drug have experienced retinoic acid–APL syndrome, characterized by fever, dyspnea, weight gain, radiographic pulmonary infiltrates, and pleural or pericardial effusions. Notify doctor immediately if these occur because the syndrome has occasionally been accompanied by impaired myocardial contractility and episodic hypotension with or without leukocytosis. Some patients have died from progressive hypoxemia and multiorgan failure. The syndrome generally occurs during first month of therapy. Prompt treatment with high-dose corticosteroids appears to reduce morbidity and mortality.
• Monitor CBC and platelet counts regularly. Patients with high WBC counts at diagnosis are at increased risk for further, rapid elevations. Rapidly evolving leukocytosis is associated with higher risk of life-threatening complications.
• Administer drug for induction of remission only. Patients should receive standard consolidation or maintenance regimen after induction therapy.
• Monitor patient (especially child) for pseudotumor cerebri. Early signs and symptoms include papilledema, headache, nausea, vomiting, and visual disturbances. Notify doctor immediately if these occur.
• Monitor cholesterol and triglyceride levels and liver function studies and report abnormalities to doctor.
• Maintain infection control and bleeding precautions, and provide prompt treatment, as ordered.
• Ensure that pregnancy testing and contraception counseling are repeated monthly throughout therapy and for 1 month after completion of therapy.
• **Alert:** Don't confuse tretinoin with trientine.

---

Reactions may be *common,* uncommon, *life-threatening,* or COMMON AND LIFE-THREATENING.

## ☑ Patient teaching
• Explain infection control and bleeding precautions. Tell patient to notify doctor of signs and symptoms of infection (fever, sore throat, fatigue) or bleeding (easy bruising, nosebleeds, bleeding gums, melena), and to take temperature daily.
• Inform woman that pregnancy test is needed 1 week before therapy begins and that therapy will be delayed, if possible, until a negative result is obtained.
• Instruct woman to use contraception during therapy and for 1 month after completion of therapy, despite history of infertility or menopause, unless a hysterectomy has been performed. Recommend use of two methods of contraception simultaneously, unless abstinence is the chosen method, and to notify doctor if pregnancy is suspected.

## vinblastine sulfate (VLB)
Velban, Velbe†‡

*Pregnancy Risk Category D*

## HOW SUPPLIED
*Injection:* 10-mg vials (lyophilized powder), 1 mg/ml in 10-ml vials

## ACTION
Arrests mitosis in metaphase, blocking cell division.

| Route | Onset | Peak | Duration |
|-------|-------|------|----------|
| I.V. | Unknown | Unknown | Unknown |

## INDICATIONS & DOSAGE
*Breast or testicular cancer, Hodgkin's disease and malignant lymphoma, choriocarcinoma, lymphosarcoma, mycosis fungoides, Kaposi's sarcoma, histiocytosis—*
**Adults:** 3.7 mg/m$^2$ I.V. weekly. May increase to maximum dose of 18.5 mg/m$^2$ I.V. weekly based on response. Don't repeat dose if WBC count is below 4,000/mm$^3$. Increase dosage at weekly intervals in increments of 1.8 mg/m$^2$ until desired therapeutic response is obtained, leukocyte count decreases to 3,000/mm$^3$, or maximum weekly dose of 18.5 mg/m$^2$ is reached.

**Children:** initial dose, 2.5 mg/m$^2$ I.V. weekly. Dosage increased by 1.25 mg/m$^2$ weekly until WBC count is below 3,000/mm$^3$ or tumor response is seen. Maximum dose is 12.5 mg/m$^2$ I.V. weekly.
*Adjust-a-dose:* For patients with direct serum bilirubin over 3 mg/dl, reduce dose by 50%. For patients with recent exposure to radiation therapy or chemotherapy, single doses usually don't exceed 5.5 mg/m$^2$.

## ADVERSE REACTIONS
**CNS:** depression, *paresthesia, peripheral neuropathy and neuritis, numbness, loss of deep tendon reflexes, muscle pain and weakness,* headache.
**CV:** hypertension, *MI, CVA.*
**EENT:** pharyngitis.
**GI:** *nausea, vomiting,* bleeding of ulcer, *constipation, ileus, anorexia,* diarrhea, abdominal pain, *stomatitis.*
**Hematologic:** anemia, *leukopenia,* **thrombocytopenia.**
**Metabolic:** *weight loss.*
**Respiratory:** **acute bronchospasm,** shortness of breath.
**Skin:** reversible alopecia, vesiculation.
**Other:** *irritation, phlebitis,* cellulitis, necrosis with extravasation, hyperuricemia.

## INTERACTIONS
**Drug-drug.** *Erythromycin, other drugs that inhibit cytochrome P-450 pathway:* may increase toxicity of vinblastine. Monitor closely.
*Mitomycin:* increased risk of bronchospasm and shortness of breath. Monitor patient's respiratory status.
*Phenytoin:* decreased plasma phenytoin levels. Monitor closely.

## EFFECTS ON DIAGNOSTIC TESTS
None reported.

## CONTRAINDICATIONS
Contraindicated in patients with severe leukopenia or bacterial infection.

## NURSING CONSIDERATIONS
• Use cautiously in patients with hepatic dysfunction.

---

*Liquid contains alcohol.    **May contain tartrazine.    †Canada    ‡Australia    §U.K.    ◊OTC

• To reduce nausea, give antiemetic before drug, as ordered.

• Don't administer drug into a limb with compromised circulation.

• *Alert:* After administering drug, check for development of life-threatening acute bronchospasm. If this occurs, notify doctor immediately. Reaction is most likely to occur in patients who are also receiving mitomycin.

• Monitor patient for stomatitis. Be prepared to stop drug if stomatitis occurs and notify doctor.

• Assess bowel activity. Give laxatives as needed and ordered. Stool softeners may be used prophylactically.

• Dosage shouldn't be repeated more frequently than every 7 days or severe leukopenia will occur. Nadir occurs days 4 to 10 and lasts another 7 to 14 days.

• Assess patient for numbness and tingling in hands and feet. Assess gait for early evidence of footdrop.

• Drug is less neurotoxic than vincristine.

• Anticipate a decrease in dosage by 50% if bilirubin levels exceed 3 mg/100 ml.

• Discontinue drugs known to cause urine retention for first few days after vinblastine therapy, particularly in elderly patients.

• *Alert:* Don't confuse vinblastine with vincristine, vindesine, or vinorelbine.

**I.V. administration**

• Follow institutional policy to reduce risks. Preparation and administration of parenteral form of drug are associated with carcinogenic, mutagenic, and teratogenic risks for personnel.

• *Alert:* Drug is fatal if given intrathecally; it's for I.V. use only.

• Inject drug directly into vein or tubing of running I.V. line over 1 minute. Drug is a vesicant; if extravasation occurs, stop infusion immediately and notify doctor. The manufacturer recommends that moderate heat be applied to area of leakage. Local injection of hyaluronidase may help disperse drug, as ordered. Moderate heat may be applied on and off every 2 hours for 24 hours, with local injection of hydrocortisone or normal saline.

• Reconstitute drug in 10-mg vial with 10 ml of NaCl injection. This yields 1 mg/ml. Refrigerate reconstituted solution. Protect solution from light and discard after 28 days.

**☑Patient teaching**

• Tell patient to report signs and symptoms of infection (fever, sore throat, fatigue) and bleeding (easy bruising, nosebleeds, bleeding gums, melena), and to take temperature daily.

• Warn patient that alopecia may occur, but explain that it's usually reversible.

• Caution woman of childbearing age to avoid pregnancy during therapy.

• Tell patient that pain in jaw and organ containing tumor may occur.

---

## vincristine sulfate (VCR)
Oncovin, Vincasar PFS

*Pregnancy Risk Category D*

### HOW SUPPLIED
*Injection:* 1 mg/ml in 1-ml, 2-ml, 5-ml multidose vials; 1 mg/ml in 1-ml, 2-ml, 5-ml preservative-free vials

### ACTION
Arrests mitosis in metaphase, blocking cell division.

| Route | Onset | Peak | Duration |
|-------|-------|------|----------|
| I.V. | Unknown | Unknown | Unknown |

### INDICATIONS & DOSAGE
*Acute lymphoblastic and other leukemias, Hodgkin's disease, malignant lymphoma, neuroblastoma, rhabdomyosarcoma, Wilms' tumor—*
**Adults:** 0.4 to 1.4 mg/m$^2$ I.V. weekly. Maximum weekly dose is 2 mg.
**Children weighing more than 10 kg (22 lb):** 1.5 to 2 mg/m$^2$ I.V. weekly.
**Children 10 kg and less or with body surface area below 1 m$^2$:** initially, 0.05 mg/kg I.V. weekly.

### ADVERSE REACTIONS
**CNS:** *peripheral neuropathy,* sensory loss, *loss of deep tendon reflexes, paresthesia, wristdrop and footdrop,* **seizures, coma,** headache, ataxia, cranial nerve

---

palsies, *jaw pain, muscle weakness and cramps.*

**CV:** hypotension, hypertension.

**EENT:** visual disturbances, blindness, diplopia, optic and extraocular neuropathy, ptosis, hoarseness, vocal cord paralysis, photophobia.

**GI:** diarrhea, *constipation, cramps,* ileus that mimics surgical abdomen, paralytic ileus, *nausea, vomiting,* anorexia, dysphagia, *intestinal necrosis, stomatitis.*

**GU:** urine retention, SIADH, dysuria, polyuria.

**Hematologic:** anemia, *leukopenia, thrombocytopenia.*

**Metabolic:** weight loss, hyponatremia.

**Respiratory:** *acute bronchospasm,* dyspnea.

**Skin:** rash, reversible alopecia.

**Other:** fever, severe local reaction following extravasation, *phlebitis,* cellulitis at injection site.

### INTERACTIONS

**Drug-drug.** *Asparaginase:* decreased hepatic clearance of vincristine. Concurrent use may also result in additive neurotoxicity. Check for toxicity.

*Digoxin:* decreased digoxin effects. Monitor serum digoxin level.

*Mitomycin:* possible increased frequency of bronchospasm and acute pulmonary reactions. Monitor patient's respiratory status.

*Ototoxic drugs:* can potentiate loss of hearing. Use concomitantly with extreme caution.

*Phenytoin:* may reduce phenytoin levels. Monitor closely.

### EFFECTS ON DIAGNOSTIC TESTS
None reported.

### CONTRAINDICATIONS

Contraindicated in patients with hypersensitivity to drug and in those with demyelinating form of Charcot-Marie-Tooth syndrome. Don't give to patients who are receiving radiation therapy through ports that include the liver.

### NURSING CONSIDERATIONS

• Use cautiously in patients with hepatic dysfunction, neuromuscular disease, or infection.

• A 50% dosage reduction is recommended if direct serum bilirubin level exceeds 3 mg/dl.

• Don't administer 5-mg vials to one patient as a single dose. The 5-mg vials are for multiple-dose use only.

•*Alert:* After administering drug, check for development of life-threatening acute bronchospasm. If this occurs, notify doctor immediately. This reaction is most likely to occur in those also receiving mitomycin.

• Check for hyperuricemia, especially in patients with leukemia or lymphoma. Maintain hydration and administer allopurinol, as ordered, to prevent uric acid nephropathy. Check for toxicity.

• Monitor fluid intake and output. Fluid restriction may be needed if SIADH develops.

• Because of risk of neurotoxicity, drug shouldn't be given more than once weekly. Children are more resistant to neurotoxicity than adults. Neurotoxicity is dose-related and usually reversible. Some neurotoxicities may be permanent.

• Check for depression of Achilles tendon reflex, numbness, tingling, footdrop or wristdrop, difficulty in walking, ataxia, and slapping gait. Also check ability to walk on heels. Support patient when walking.

• Monitor bowel function. Give stool softener or laxative, as ordered, or water before giving dose. Constipation may be an early sign of neurotoxicity.

• All vials (1-mg, 2-mg, 5-mg) contain 1 mg/ml solution and should be refrigerated.

• Discontinue drugs known to cause urine retention, particularly in elderly patients, for first few days after vincristine therapy.

•*Alert:* Drug is fatal if given intrathecally; it's for I.V. use only.

•*Alert:* Don't confuse vincristine with vinblastine or vindesine.

 **I.V. administration**

• Follow institutional policy to reduce risks. Preparation and administration of

parenteral form of drug are associated with carcinogenic, mutagenic, and teratogenic risks for personnel.
• Inject directly into vein or tubing of running I.V. line slowly over 1 minute. Vincristine is a vesicant; if drug extravasates, stop infusion immediately and notify doctor. Apply heat on and off every 2 hours for 24 hours. Administer 150 U hyaluronidase, as ordered, to area of infiltrate.

☑**Patient teaching**
• Tell patient to report signs and symptoms of infection (fever, sore throat, fatigue) and bleeding (easy bruising, nosebleeds, bleeding gums, melena), and to take temperature daily.
• Warn patient that alopecia may occur, but explain that it's usually reversible.
• Caution woman of childbearing age to avoid becoming pregnant during therapy and to consult doctor before becoming pregnant.

---

**vinorelbine tartrate**
Navelbine

*Pregnancy Risk Category D*

**HOW SUPPLIED**
*Injection:* 10 mg/ml, 50 mg/5 ml

**ACTION**
A semisynthetic vinca alkaloid that exerts its antineoplastic effect by disrupting microtubule assembly, which in turn disrupts spindle formation and prevents mitosis.

| Route | Onset | Peak | Duration |
|-------|---------|---------|----------|
| I.V. | Unknown | Unknown | Unknown |

**INDICATIONS & DOSAGE**
*Alone or as adjunct therapy with cisplatin for first-line treatment of ambulatory patients with nonresectable advanced non-small-cell lung cancer (NSCLC); alone or with cisplatin in stage IV of NSCLC; with cisplatin in stage III of NSCLC—*
**Adults:** 30 mg/m² I.V. weekly. In combination treatment, same dosage with 120 mg/m² of cisplatin given on days 1 and 29, then q 6 weeks.

**ADVERSE REACTIONS**
**CNS:** *peripheral neuropathy, asthenia, fatigue.*
**CV:** chest pain.
**GI:** *nausea, vomiting, anorexia, diarrhea, constipation, stomatitis.*
**Hematologic:** *bone marrow suppression, agranulocytosis,* LEUKOPENIA, *thrombocytopenia, anemia, granulocytopenia.*
**Hepatic:** *abnormal liver function test results, bilirubinemia.*
**Musculoskeletal:** myalgia, arthralgia, jaw pain, loss of deep tendon reflexes.
**Respiratory:** dyspnea.
**Skin:** *alopecia,* rash.
**Other:** *injection pain or reaction.*

**INTERACTIONS**
**Drug-drug.** *Cisplatin:* increased risk of bone marrow suppression when used with cisplatin. Monitor hematologic status closely.
*Mitomycin:* may cause pulmonary reactions. Monitor respiratory status closely.

**EFFECTS ON DIAGNOSTIC TESTS**
None reported.

**CONTRAINDICATIONS**
Contraindicated in patients with pretreatment granulocyte counts below 1,000 cells/mm³.

**NURSING CONSIDERATIONS**
• Use with extreme caution in patients whose bone marrow may have been compromised by previous exposure to radiation therapy or chemotherapy or whose bone marrow is still recovering from chemotherapy.
• Use cautiously in patients with hepatic impairment. Monitor liver enzyme levels.
• Check patient's granulocyte count before administration; count should be 1,000 cells/mm³ or more for drug to be administered. Withhold drug and notify doctor if count is lower.
• **Alert:** Drug is fatal if given intrathecally; it's for I.V. use only.
• Dosage adjustments are made according to hematologic toxicity or hepatic insufficiency, whichever results in the lower dosage. Expect dosage reduction of 50% if granulocyte count falls below 1,500

---

Reactions may be *common,* uncommon, *life-threatening,* or COMMON AND LIFE-THREATENING.

cells/mm³ but is greater than 1,000 cells/mm³. If three consecutive doses are skipped because of agranulocytosis, don't resume vinorelbine therapy.
• Patient may receive injections of WBC colony-stimulating factors to promote cell growth and decrease risk of infection.
• Drug may be a contact irritant, and the solution must be handled and administered with care. Gloves are recommended. Inhalation of vapors and contact with skin or mucous membranes, especially those of the eyes, must be avoided. In case of contact, wash with generous amounts of water for at least 15 minutes.
•*Alert:* Monitor deep tendon reflexes; loss may represent cumulative toxicity.
• Monitor patient closely for hypersensitivity reactions.
• As a guide to the effects of therapy, monitor patient's peripheral blood count and bone marrow, as ordered.

### I.V. administration
• Dilute drug before use to concentration of 1.5 to 3 mg/ml with $D_5W$ or normal saline solution in a syringe. Or, dilute to concentration of 0.5 to 2 mg/ml in an I.V. bag. Administer drug I.V. over 6 to 10 minutes into side port of a free-flowing I.V. line that is closest to I.V. bag; then flush with at least 75 to 125 ml of $D_5W$ or normal saline solution.
• Drug may be used up to 24 hours when stored at room temperature.
• Avoid extravasation when administering vinorelbine because drug can cause considerable irritation, localized tissue necrosis, and thrombophlebitis. If extravasation occurs, stop drug immediately and inject remaining dose portion into a different vein.

### Patient teaching
• Instruct patient not to take other drugs, including OTC preparations, until approved by doctor.
• Tell patient to report signs and symptoms of infection (fever, sore throat, fatigue) and bleeding (easy bruising, nosebleeds, bleeding gums, melena), and to take temperature daily.
• Caution woman of childbearing age to avoid becoming pregnant during therapy.

---

**azathioprine**
**basiliximab**
**cyclosporine**
**daclizumab**
**lymphocyte immune globulin**
**muromonab-CD3**
**mycophenolate mofetil**
**mycophenolate mofetil**
  **hydrochloride**
**sirolimus**
**tacrolimus**

**COMBINATION PRODUCTS**
None.

---

**azathioprine**
Imuran, Thioprine‡

*Pregnancy Risk Category D*

**HOW SUPPLIED**
*Tablets:* 50 mg
*Powder for injection:* 100 mg

**ACTION**
Unknown, but thought to cause variable alterations in antibody production.

| Route | Onset | Peak | Duration |
|-------|-------|------|----------|
| P.O., I.V. | Unknown | Unknown | Unknown |

**INDICATIONS & DOSAGE**
*Immunosuppression in kidney transplantation—*
**Adults:** initially, 3 to 5 mg/kg P.O. or I.V. daily, usually beginning on day of transplantation. Maintained at 1 to 3 mg/kg daily (dosage based on patient response and tolerance).
*Adjust-a-dose:* For patients with oliguria in the posttransplant period and for those with impaired renal function, drug is given in lower doses.
*Severe, refractory rheumatoid arthritis—*
**Adults:** initially, 1 mg/kg P.O. as single dose or divided into two doses. If patient response isn't satisfactory after 6 to 8 weeks, dosage may be increased by

0.5 mg/kg daily (up to maximum of 2.5 mg/kg daily) at 4-week intervals.

**ADVERSE REACTIONS**
**GI:** *nausea, vomiting, **pancreatitis,*** steatorrhea, diarrhea, abdominal pain.
**Hematologic:** LEUKOPENIA, *myelosuppression,* anemia, *pancytopenia,* THROMBOCYTOPENIA, *immunosuppression.*
**Hepatic:** *hepatotoxicity,* jaundice, elevated liver enzyme levels.
**Musculoskeletal:** arthralgia, myalgia.
**Skin:** rash, alopecia.
**Other:** *infections,* fever, *increased risk of neoplasia,* decreased serum uric acid levels.

**INTERACTIONS**
**Drug-drug.** *ACE inhibitors:* combination may cause severe leukopenia. Monitor patient closely.
*Allopurinol:* impaired inactivation of azathioprine. Decrease azathioprine dose to one-third to one-quarter normal dose.
*Cyclosporine:* plasma levels of cyclosporine may be increased. Monitor closely.
*Methotrexate:* may increase plasma levels of methotrexate metabolite. Monitor closely.
*Nondepolarizing neuromuscular blockers:* azathioprine may reverse the neuromuscular blockade. Monitor patient closely.
*Other myelopoiesis drugs:* exaggerated leukopenia, especially in renal transplant patients. Monitor patient closely.
*Warfarin:* azathioprine may decrease action of warfarin. Monitor patient closely.

**EFFECTS ON DIAGNOSTIC TESTS**
None reported.

**CONTRAINDICATIONS**
Contraindicated in patients with hypersensitivity to drug or its components.

**NURSING CONSIDERATIONS**
• Use cautiously in patients with hepatic or renal dysfunction.

---

Reactions may be *common,* uncommon, ***life-threatening,*** or COMMON AND LIFE-THREATENING.

• Administer drug after meals to minimize adverse GI effects.

• To prevent bleeding, avoid all I.M. injections when platelet count is below 100,000/mm³.

• Monitor hemoglobin level and WBC and platelet counts weekly for 1 month; then twice monthly. Notify doctor if counts drop suddenly or become dangerously low. Drug may need to be temporarily withheld.

• Watch for early signs of hepatotoxicity, such as clay-colored stools, dark urine, pruritus, and yellow skin and sclera; and for increased alkaline phosphatase, bilirubin, AST, and ALT levels.

• Therapeutic response usually occurs within 8 weeks.

• Benefits must be weighed against risk when giving to patient with systemic viral infection, such as chickenpox or herpes zoster.

• Patients with rheumatoid arthritis previously treated with alkylating drugs, such as cyclophosphamide, chlorambucil, or melphalan, may have a prohibitive risk of neoplasia if treated with azathioprine.

• Drug shouldn't be used for treating rheumatoid arthritis in pregnant women.

• *Alert:* Don't confuse azathioprine with azidothymidine, Azulfidine, or azatadine; or Imuran with Inderal.

🔳 **I.V. administration**

• Reconstitute drug in 100-mg vial with 10 ml of sterile water for injection. Visually inspect for particles before use. Drug may be administered by direct I.V. injection or further diluted in normal saline for injection or D₅W and infused over 30 to 60 minutes. Use only in patients who are unable to tolerate oral drugs.

✅ **Patient teaching**

• Warn patient to report even mild infections (colds, fever, sore throat, and malaise) because drug is a potent immunosuppressant.

• Instruct patient to avoid conception during therapy and for 4 months after stopping therapy.

• Warn patient that some thinning of hair is possible.

• Tell patient taking drug for refractory rheumatoid arthritis that it may take up to 12 weeks to be effective.

• Advise patient to report unusual bleeding or bruising to doctor.

• Tell patient that drug may be taken with food to decrease nausea.

• Advise patient to use soft toothbrush and perform oral care cautiously.

---

## basiliximab
Simulect

*Pregnancy Risk Category B*

---

**HOW SUPPLIED**
*Injection:* 20-mg vials

**ACTION**
Binds specifically to and blocks the interleukin (IL)-2 receptor alpha chain on the surface of activated T lymphocytes, inhibiting IL-2–mediated activation of lymphocytes, a critical pathway in the cellular immune response involved in allograft rejection.

| Route | Onset | Peak | Duration |
|-------|-------|------|----------|
| I.V. | Unknown | Immediate | Unknown |

**INDICATIONS & DOSAGE**
*Prophylaxis of acute organ rejection in patients receiving renal transplantation when used as part of an immunosuppressive regimen that includes cyclosporine and corticosteroids—*
**Adults:** 20 mg I.V. given within 2 hours before transplant surgery and 20 mg I.V. given 4 days after transplantation.
**Children ages 2 to 15:** 12 mg/m² (to maximum of 20 mg) I.V. given within 2 hours before transplant surgery and 12 mg/m² (to maximum of 20 mg) I.V. given 4 days after transplantation.

**ADVERSE REACTIONS**
**CNS:** agitation, anxiety, *asthenia,* depression, *dizziness, headache,* hypoesthesia, *insomnia,* neuropathy, paresthesia, *tremor,* fatigue.
**CV:** angina pectoris, ***arrhythmias,*** atrial fibrillation, ***cardiac failure,*** chest pain, abnormal heart sounds, aggravated hyper-

---

tension, *hypertension,* hypotension, tachycardia.

**EENT:** abnormal vision, cataract, conjunctivitis, *rhinitis,* sinusitis.

**GI:** *abdominal pain, candidiasis, constipation, diarrhea, dyspepsia,* esophagitis, enlarged abdomen, flatulence, gastroenteritis, GI disorder, **GI hemorrhage,** gum hyperplasia, melena, *nausea,* ulcerative stomatitis, *vomiting.*

**GU:** abnormal renal function, albuminuria, bladder disorder, *dysuria,* frequent micturition, genital edema, hematuria, *increased nonprotein nitrogen,* oliguria, renal tubular necrosis, surgery, ureteral disorder, *urinary tract infection,* urinary retention, impotence.

**Hematologic:** *anemia,* hematoma, **hemorrhage,** polycythemia, purpura, **thrombocytopenia,** thrombosis.

**Metabolic:** *acidosis,* dehydration, diabetes mellitus, fluid overload, hypercalcemia, *hypercholesterolemia, hyperglycemia, hyperkalemia,* hyperlipemia, *hyperuricemia, hypocalcemia, hypokalemia,* hypomagnesemia, *hypophosphatemia,* hypoproteinemia, *weight increase.*

**Musculoskeletal:** arthralgia, arthropathy, *back pain,* bone fracture, cramps, hernia, *leg pain,* myalgia.

**Respiratory:** abnormal chest sounds, bronchitis, **bronchospasm,** *cough, dyspnea, pharyngitis,* pneumonia, pulmonary disorder, **pulmonary edema,** upper respiratory tract infection.

**Skin:** acne, cyst, herpes simplex, herpes zoster, hypertrichosis, pruritus, rash, skin disorder or ulceration.

**Other:** accidental trauma, *viral infection, leg or peripheral edema,* general edema, infection, **sepsis,** *fever, surgical wound complications.*

## INTERACTIONS
None significant.

## EFFECTS ON DIAGNOSTIC TESTS
None reported.

## CONTRAINDICATIONS
Contraindicated in patients with hypersensitivity to drug or its components.

## NURSING CONSIDERATIONS
• Use cautiously and only under supervision of doctor qualified and experienced in immunosuppressive therapy and management of organ transplantation.
• Use cautiously in elderly patients.
• Anaphylactoid reactions may result following administration of proteins. Be sure that drugs for treating severe hypersensitivity reactions are available for immediate use.
• Check for electrolyte imbalances and acidosis during drug therapy.
• Monitor patient's intake and output, vital signs, hemoglobin level, and hematocrit during therapy.
• Be alert for signs and symptoms of opportunistic infections during drug therapy.

### I.V. administration
• Reconstitute with 5 ml sterile water for injection. Shake vial gently to dissolve powder. Dilute reconstituted solution to volume of 50 ml with normal saline or dextrose 5% for infusion. When mixing solution, gently invert bag to avoid foaming. Don't shake.
• Infuse over 20 to 30 minutes via a central or peripheral vein. Don't add or infuse other drugs simultaneously through same I.V. line.
• Use reconstituted solution immediately; may be refrigerated at 36° to 46° F (2° to 8° C) for up to 24 hours or kept at room temperature for 4 hours.

### Patient teaching
• Inform patient of potential benefits and risks associated with immunosuppressive therapy, including decreased risk of graft loss or acute rejection. Advise patient that immunosuppressive therapy increases risks of developing lymphoproliferative disorders and opportunistic infections. Tell him to report signs and symptoms of infection promptly.
• Inform woman of childbearing age to use effective contraception before beginning therapy and for 2 months after completion of therapy.
• Instruct patient to report adverse effects immediately.
• Explain that drug is used with cyclosporine and corticosteroids.

## cyclosporine (cyclosporin A)
Neoral, Sandimmun‡,
Sandimmune

*Pregnancy Risk Category C*

### HOW SUPPLIED
*Oral solution:* 100 mg/ml
*Capsules:* 25 mg, 50 mg, 100 mg
*Capsules for microemulsion:* 25 mg,
50 mg
*Injection:* 50 mg/ml

### ACTION
Unknown. Thought to inhibit proliferation
and function of T lymphocytes and inhibit
production and release of lymphokines.

| Route | Onset | Peak | Duration |
|-------|-------|------|----------|
| P.O. | Unknown | 3.5 hr | Unknown |
| I.V. | Unknown | Unknown | Unknown |

### INDICATIONS & DOSAGE
*Prophylaxis of organ rejection in kidney,
liver, or heart transplantation—*
**Adults and children:** 15 mg/kg P.O. 4 to
12 hours before transplantation and continued daily postoperatively for 1 to 2
weeks. Then dose reduced by 5% each
week to maintenance level of 5 to 10 mg/
kg/day. Or, 5 to 6 mg/kg I.V. concentrate 4
to 12 hours before transplantation given
as a continuous infusion. Postoperatively,
dose repeated daily until patient can tolerate P.O. forms.
**Elderly:** dosage adjustment may be
needed.
*Severe, active rheumatoid arthritis that
hasn't adequately responded to methotrexate (Neoral only)—*
**Adults:** 2.5 mg/kg/day P.O., taken b.i.d.
as divided dose.
*Adjust-a-dose:* For patients with such adverse effects as hypertension, elevations
in serum creatinine level (30% above pretreatment level), or abnormal CBC and
liver function test results, decrease dosage
by 25% to 50%.

### ADVERSE REACTIONS
**CNS:** *tremor, headache,* confusion, pares-
thesia.
**CV:** *hypertension.*

**EENT:** *gum hyperplasia,* oral thrush,
sinusitis.
**GI:** *nausea, vomiting,* diarrhea, abdomi-
nal discomfort.
**GU:** NEPHROTOXICITY, gynecomastia.
**Hematologic:** anemia, *leukopenia,
thrombocytopenia.*
**Hepatic:** *hepatotoxicity.*
**Metabolic:** hyperglycemia.
**Skin:** *hirsutism,* acne, flushing.
**Other:** increased low-density lipoprotein
levels, *infections, anaphylaxis.*

### INTERACTIONS
**Drug-drug.** *Acyclovir, aminoglycosides,
amphotericin B, co-trimoxazole, melphalan, NSAIDs, ranitidine, vancomycin:* increased risk of nephrotoxicity. Avoid concomitant use.
*Azathioprine, corticosteroids, cyclophos-
phamide, verapamil:* increased immunosuppression. Monitor closely.
*Carbamazepine, isoniazid, phenobarbital,
phenytoin, rifabutin, rifampin:* possible
decreased immunosuppressant effect secondary to low cyclosporine levels. Cyclosporine dosage may need to be increased.
*Cimetidine, danazol, diltiazem, ery-
thromycin, fluconazole, imipenem-
cilastatin, ketoconazole, methylprednisolone, metoclopramide, nicardipine,
prednisolone:* may increase blood levels of
cyclosporine. Check for increased toxicity.
*Digoxin:* cyclosporine may elevate digoxin levels. Monitor patient for toxicity.
*Potassium-sparing diuretics:* cyclosporine
may induce hyperkalemia. Monitor patient closely.
*Vaccines:* decreased immune response.
Postpone routine immunization.
**Drug-food.** *Grapefruit juice:* slowed metabolism of drug. Avoid concomitant use.
*High-fat meals:* Neoral absorption may be
decreased by a high-fat meal. Give on
empty stomach.

### EFFECTS ON DIAGNOSTIC TESTS
None reported.

### CONTRAINDICATIONS
Contraindicated in patients with hypersensitivity to drug or polyoxyethylated
castor oil (found in injectable form). Patients who have rheumatoid arthritis and

hypertension, malignancies, or impaired renal function shouldn't receive Neoral.

## NURSING CONSIDERATIONS
• Measure oral solution doses carefully in an oral syringe. To increase palatability, conventional oral solution may be mixed with milk, chocolate milk, or orange juice. Oral cyclosporine solution for emulsion may be mixed with orange or apple juice (avoid grapefruit juice). Solution for emulsion is less palatable when mixed with milk. Use a glass container to mix and have patient drink at once. Don't rinse dosing syringe with water. If syringe needs cleaning, it must be completely dry before reuse.
• Monitor elderly patient for renal impairment and hypotension.
• Dosage is typically given once or twice daily.
• Neoral has greater bioavailability than Sandimmune. Less Neoral may be needed to yield same blood level derived from Sandimmune. Switch patients between these two brands using blood level monitoring, as ordered.
• Always give cyclosporine with adrenal corticosteroids, as ordered.
• Monitor cyclosporine blood levels at regular intervals. Absorption of cyclosporine oral solution can be erratic.
• Monitor BUN and serum creatinine levels. Nephrotoxicity may develop 2 to 3 months after transplant surgery, possibly requiring dosage reduction. Notify doctor of signs or symptoms of nephrotoxicity.
• Doctor must differentiate between transplanted kidney rejection and cyclosporine-induced nephrotoxicity.
• *Alert:* Don't confuse cyclosporine with Cyklokapron, cyclophosphamide, or cycloserine; or Sandimmune with Sandoglobulin or Sandostatin.

## I.V. administration
• Administer cyclosporine I.V. concentrate at one-third oral dose and dilute before use. Dilute each milliliter of concentrate in 20 to 100 ml of $D_5W$ or normal saline for injection. Dilute immediately before use; infuse over 2 to 6 hours. I.V. administration is usually reserved for pa-

tients who can't tolerate oral drugs. Protect I.V. solution from light.

## ✅ Patient teaching
• Encourage patient to take drug at same time each day, and teach him how to measure dosage and mask taste of oral solution, if prescribed. Tell him not to take cyclosporine with grapefruit juice.
• Instruct patient to fill glass with water after dose and drink to assure all drug is consumed.
• Advise patient to take drug with meals if nausea occurs.
• Advise patient to take Neoral on an empty stomach.
• Stress that drug shouldn't be stopped without doctor's approval.
• Advise patient to use mechanical contraceptive measures, such as a diaphragm or condom, during therapy. Tell woman not to use oral contraceptives.

---

## daclizumab
## Zenapax

*Pregnancy Risk Category C*

## HOW SUPPLIED
*Injection:* 25 mg/5 ml

## ACTION
An interleukin (IL)-2 receptor antagonist that inhibits IL-2 binding to prevent IL-2–mediated activation of lymphocytes, a critical pathway in the cellular immune response against allografts. Once in circulation, drug impairs response of immune system to antigenic challenges.

| Route | Onset | Peak | Duration |
|-------|-------|------|----------|
| I.V. | Unknown | Unknown | Unknown |

## INDICATIONS & DOSAGE
*Prophylaxis of acute organ rejection in patients receiving renal transplants with an immunosuppressive regimen that includes cyclosporine and corticosteroids—*
**Adults:** 1 mg/kg I.V. Standard course of therapy is five doses. Administer first dose no more than 24 hours before transplantation; remaining four doses are given at 14-day intervals.

## ADVERSE REACTIONS

**CNS:** tremor, headache, dizziness, insomnia, generalized weakness, prickly sensation, fever, pain, fatigue, depression, anxiety.

**CV:** tachycardia, hypertension, hypotension, aggravated hypertension, edema, fluid overload, chest pain.

**EENT:** blurred vision, pharyngitis, rhinitis.

**GI:** constipation, nausea, diarrhea, vomiting, abdominal pain, dyspepsia, pyrosis, abdominal distention, epigastric pain, flatulence, gastritis, hemorrhoids.

**GU:** *oliguria,* dysuria, *renal tubular necrosis,* renal damage, urinary retention, hydronephrosis, urinary tract bleeding, urinary tract disorder, renal insufficiency.

**Hematologic:** lymphocele; platelet, bleeding, and clotting disorders.

**Metabolic:** diabetes mellitus, dehydration.

**Musculoskeletal:** musculoskeletal or back pain, arthralgia, myalgia, leg cramps.

**Respiratory:** dyspnea, coughing, atelectasis, congestion, *hypoxia,* rales, abnormal breath sounds, pleural effusion, pulmonary edema.

**Skin:** acne, impaired wound healing without infection, pruritus, hirsutism, rash, night sweats, increased sweating.

**Other:** shivering, extremity edema.

## INTERACTIONS
None significant.

## EFFECTS ON DIAGNOSTIC TESTS
None reported.

## CONTRAINDICATIONS
Contraindicated in patients with hypersensitivity to drug or its components.

## NURSING CONSIDERATIONS
• Use cautiously and only under supervision of doctor experienced in immunosuppressive therapy and management of organ transplantation.
• Protect undiluted solution from direct light.
• Drug is used as part of an immunosuppressive regimen that includes corticosteroids and cyclosporine. Check for lipoproliferative disorders and opportunistic infections.

• Anaphylactoid reactions have been reported following administration of proteins. Have drugs used in treatment of anaphylactic reactions immediately available.

### ⬛I.V. administration
• Don't use drug as direct I.V. injection. Dilute in 50 ml of sterile normal saline solution before administration. To avoid foaming, don't shake. Inspect for particulates or discoloration before use. If there are particulates or discoloration, don't use.
• Administer over 15 minutes via a central or peripheral line. Don't add or infuse other drugs simultaneously through same I.V. line.
• Drug may be refrigerated at 36° to 46° F (2° to 8° C) for 24 hours, and is stable at room temperature for 4 hours. Discard solution if not used within 24 hours.

### ☑Patient teaching
• Tell patient to consult doctor before taking other drugs during therapy.
• Advise patient to practice infection prevention precautions.
• Inform patient that neither he nor any household member should receive vaccinations unless medically approved.
• Tell patient to report immediately wounds that fail to heal, unusual bruising or bleeding, or fever.
• Advise patient to drink plenty of fluids during drug therapy, and to report painful urination, blood in the urine, or decrease in urine amount.
• Instruct woman of childbearing age to use effective contraception before beginning therapy and to continue until 4 months after completing therapy.

---

## lymphocyte immune globulin (anti-thymocyte globulin [equine], ATG, LIG)
Atgam

*Pregnancy Risk Category C*

## HOW SUPPLIED
*Injection:* 50 mg of equine IgG/ml in 5-ml ampules

---

## ACTION

Unknown. Inhibits cell-mediated immune responses either by altering T-cell function or eliminating antigen-reactive T cells.

| Route | Onset | Peak | Duration |
|-------|-------|------|----------|
| I.V. | Immediate | 5 days | Unknown |

## INDICATIONS & DOSAGE

*Prevention of acute renal allograft rejection—*

**Adults:** 15 mg/kg/day I.V. daily for 14 days; then alternate-day dosing for 14 days. First dose should be given within 24 hours of transplantation.

**Children:** 5 to 25 mg/kg/day I.V. daily for 14 days; then alternate-day dosing for 14 days. First dose should be given within 24 hours of transplantation.

*Treatment of acute renal allograft rejection—*

**Adults and children:** 10 to 15 mg/kg I.V. daily for 14 days. Additional alternate-day therapy to total of 21 doses can be given. Therapy should be initiated when rejection is diagnosed.

*Aplastic anemia—*

**Adults:** 10 to 20 mg/kg I.V. daily for 8 to 14 days. Additional alternate-day therapy to total of 21 doses can be given.

## ADVERSE REACTIONS

**CNS:** malaise, *seizures,* headache.
**CV:** *hypotension, chest pain,* thrombophlebitis, tachycardia, edema, iliac vein obstruction, renal artery stenosis.
**EENT:** *laryngospasm.*
**GI:** *nausea, vomiting, diarrhea,* hiccups, epigastric pain, abdominal distention, stomatitis.
**Hematologic:** LEUKOPENIA, THROMBOCYTOPENIA, hemolysis, *aplastic anemia.*
**Hepatic:** elevated liver enzyme levels.
**Metabolic:** hyperglycemia.
**Musculoskeletal:** *arthralgia, myalgia.*
**Respiratory:** dyspnea, *pulmonary edema.*
**Skin:** *rash, pruritus, urticaria.*
**Other:** febrile reactions, *hypersensitivity reactions,* serum sickness, *anaphylaxis,* infections, night sweats, lymphadenopathy, chills.

## INTERACTIONS

None significant.

## EFFECTS ON DIAGNOSTIC TESTS

Elevations of hepatic serum enzymes have been reported.

## CONTRAINDICATIONS

Contraindicated in patients with hypersensitivity to drug.

## NURSING CONSIDERATIONS

• Use cautiously in patients receiving additional immunosuppressive therapy (such as corticosteroids or azathioprine) because of increased potential for infection.
• An intradermal skin test is recommended at least 1 hour before first dose. Marked local swelling or erythema larger than 10 mm indicates increased potential for severe systemic reaction such as anaphylaxis. Severe reactions to skin test, such as hypotension, tachycardia, dyspnea, generalized rash, or anaphylaxis, usually preclude further use of drug.
• Don't dilute ATG concentrate with dextrose solutions or solutions with a low salt concentration because a precipitate may form. The proteins in ATG can be denatured by air. ATG is unstable in acidic solutions.
• Monitor patient for hypotension, respiratory distress, and chest, flank, or back pain, which may indicate anaphylaxis or hemolysis.
• Keep airway adjuncts and anaphylaxis drugs at bedside during drug administration.
• Watch for signs and symptoms of infection, such as fever, sore throat, malaise.

### I.V. administration

• Dilute concentrated drug for injection before administration. Dilute required dose in 250 to 1,000 ml of half-normal or normal saline solution. Final concentration of drug shouldn't exceed 1 mg/ml. When adding ATG to infusion solution, make sure container is inverted so that drug doesn't contact air inside container. Gently rotate or swirl container to mix contents; don't shake because this may cause excessive foaming or denature the drug protein. Infuse with an in-line filter

---

Reactions may be *common,* uncommon, *life-threatening,* or COMMON AND LIFE-THREATENING.

with a pore size of 0.2 to 1 micron over no less than 4 hours (most institutions infuse over 4 to 8 hours) into a vascular shunt, arterial venous fistula, or high-flow central vein.
• Don't use solutions that are older than 12 hours, including actual infusion time.
• Refrigerate at 35° to 47° F (2° to 8° C). ATG concentrate is heat-sensitive. Don't freeze. Allow diluted ATG to reach room temperature before infusion.

### ☑Patient teaching
• Instruct patient to report adverse drug reactions promptly, especially signs and symptoms of infection (fever, sore throat, fatigue).
• Tell patient to alert nurse immediately if discomfort occurs at I.V. insertion site because drug can cause a chemical phlebitis.
• Advise woman of childbearing age to avoid pregnancy during therapy.

## muromonab-CD3
Orthoclone OKT3

*Pregnancy Risk Category C*

### HOW SUPPLIED
*Injection:* 1 mg/1 ml in 5-ml ampules

### ACTION
A murine monoclonal antibody that reacts in the T-lymphocyte membrane with a molecule (CD3) needed for antigen recognition. Depletes the blood of $CD3^+$ T cells, which leads to restoration of allograft function and reversal of rejection.

| Route | Onset | Peak | Duration |
|-------|-------|------|----------|
| I.V. | Immediate | Unknown | 1 wk |

### INDICATIONS & DOSAGE
*Acute allograft rejection in renal transplant patients; in corticosteroid-resistant hepatic or cardiac allograft rejection—*
**Adults:** 5 mg I.V. bolus once daily for 10 to 14 days.

### ADVERSE REACTIONS
**CNS:** *tremor, headache,* **seizures, encephalopathy, cerebral edema.**

**CV:** *chest pain, tachycardia,* hypertension, **cardiac arrest,** hypotension, **shock, heart failure.**
**EENT:** *blindness, blurred vision, tinnitus, otitis media, conjunctivitis.*
**GI:** *nausea, vomiting, diarrhea.*
**GU:** oliguria, anuria, increased serum creatinine level.
**Respiratory:** **severe pulmonary edema,** *dyspnea, wheezing,* **adult respiratory distress syndrome.**
**Other:** *fever, chills, tremors,* INFECTION, **anaphylaxis, cytokine release syndrome, aseptic meningitis, risk of neoplasia.**

### INTERACTIONS
**Drug-drug.** *Immunosuppressants:* increased risk of infection. Monitor closely.
*Indomethacin:* increased muromonab-CD3 levels with encephalopathy and other CNS effects. Monitor patient closely.
*Live virus vaccines:* may potentiate replication and increase effects of virus vaccine. Monitor patient.

### EFFECTS ON DIAGNOSTIC TESTS
Drug may increase BUN and serum creatinine levels and cause abnormal urine cytologic study results.

### CONTRAINDICATIONS
Contraindicated in patients with hypersensitivity to drug or other products of murine (mouse) origin and in those who have history of seizures or are predisposed to seizures. Also contraindicated in those who have antimurine antibody titers of 1:1,000 or more or fluid overload, as evidenced by chest X-ray or weight gain greater than 3% within the week before treatment. Don't use in pregnant and breast-feeding women.

### NURSING CONSIDERATIONS
• Obtain chest X-ray within 24 hours before starting drug treatment, as ordered.
• Assess patient for signs and symptoms of fluid overload before treatment.
• Treatment should begin in facility equipped and staffed for cardiopulmonary resuscitation and where patient can be monitored closely.
• Most adverse reactions develop within 30 minutes to 6 hours after first dose.

• Administer an antipyretic, as ordered, before giving drug to help lower risk of expected pyrexia and chills. Treat temperature exceeding 100° F (38° C) with antipyretics before drug administration and evaluate risk of infection.

• Administer corticosteroids, as ordered, before first injection to help decrease risk of adverse reactions. Methylprednisolone sodium succinate (1 mg/kg) before injection, followed by hydrocortisone sodium succinate (100 mg) 30 minutes after injection, have been recommended to alleviate severity of first-dose reaction.

• Patients develop antibodies to muromonab-CD3 that can lead to loss of effectiveness and more severe adverse reactions if a second course of therapy is attempted. Therefore, some doctors believe that drug should be used for only a single course of treatment.

## I.V. administration

• Draw solution into syringe through low protein-binding 0.2- or 0.22-micron filter. Discard filter and attach needle for I.V. bolus injection. Give bolus in less than 1 minute.

## ✓ Patient teaching

• Inform patient of expected adverse reactions.

• Reassure patient that reactions will be less severe as treatment progresses.

• Advise woman to avoid pregnancy during therapy.

---

## mycophenolate mofetil
CellCept

## mycophenolate mofetil hydrochloride
CellCept Intravenous

*Pregnancy Risk Category C*

## HOW SUPPLIED
**mycophenolate mofetil**
*Capsules:* 250 mg
*Tablets:* 500 mg
**mycophenolate mofetil hydrochloride**
*Injection:* 500 mg/vial

## ACTION
Inhibits proliferative response of T and B lymphocytes, suppresses antibody formation by B lymphocytes, and may inhibit recruitment of leukocytes into sites of inflammation and graft rejection.

| Route | Onset | Peak | Duration |
|-------|-------|------|----------|
| P.O. | Unknown | 0.5-1.25 hr | 7.5-18 hr |
| I.V. | Unknown | Unknown | 10-17 hr |

## INDICATIONS & DOSAGE
*Prophylaxis of organ rejection in patients receiving allogenic renal transplants—*
**Adults:** 1 g P.O. or I.V. b.i.d. with corticosteroids and cyclosporine.
*Adjust-a-dose:* For patients with severe chronic renal impairment outside of immediate posttransplant period, avoid doses above 1 g b.i.d. If neutropenia develops, interrupt or reduce dosing.
*Prophylaxis of organ rejection in patients receiving allogenic cardiac transplant—*
**Adults:** 1.5 g P.O. or I.V. b.i.d. with cyclosporine and corticosteroids.

## ADVERSE REACTIONS
**CNS:** *tremor,* insomnia, dizziness, *headache, asthenia.*
**CV:** *chest pain, hypertension, edema.*
**GI:** *diarrhea, constipation, nausea, dyspepsia, vomiting, oral candidiasis, abdominal pain,* **hemorrhage.**
**GU:** *urinary tract infection, hematuria,* kidney tubular necrosis.
**Hematologic:** anemia, LEUKOPENIA, THROMBOCYTOPENIA, hypochromic anemia, leukocytosis.
**Metabolic:** *hypercholesterolemia, hypophosphatemia, hypokalemia, hyperkalemia, hyperglycemia.*
**Musculoskeletal:** *back pain.*
**Respiratory:** *dyspnea, cough, infection, pharyngitis, bronchitis, pneumonia.*
**Skin:** *acne,* rash.
**Other:** *pain, fever, infection,* **sepsis,** *peripheral edema.*

## INTERACTIONS
**Drug-drug.** *Acyclovir, ganciclovir, other drugs known to undergo renal tubular secretion:* increased risk of toxicity for both drugs. Monitor patient closely.

---

Reactions may be *common,* uncommon, *life-threatening*, or COMMON AND LIFE-THREATENING.

*Antacids with magnesium and aluminum hydroxides:* decreased absorption of mycophenolate. Separate administration.

*Azathioprine:* hasn't been clinically studied. Monitor patient closely when used concomitantly.

*Cholestyramine:* may interfere with enterohepatic recirculation, reducing mycophenolate bioavailability. Avoid concurrent use.

*Phenytoin, theophylline:* levels of these drugs may be increased. Monitor closely.

*Probenecid, salicylates:* may increase mycophenolate levels. Monitor closely.

**EFFECTS ON DIAGNOSTIC TESTS**
None reported.

**CONTRAINDICATIONS**
Contraindicated in patients with hypersensitivity to drug, its ingredients, or mycophenolic acid and in patients sensitive to polysorbate 80.

**NURSING CONSIDERATIONS**
• Drug isn't recommended for use in pregnant (unless benefits outweigh risks to fetus) or breast-feeding women.
• Use cautiously in patients with GI disorders.
• Safety and effectiveness of drug in children haven't been established.
• Start drug therapy within 24 hours following transplantation. I.V. form is recommended for patients unable to take capsules or tablets.
• I.V. form can be administered for up to 14 days; switch patient to capsules or tablets as soon as oral drugs can be tolerated.
• Avoid doses above 1 g b.i.d. after immediate posttransplant period in patients with severe chronic renal impairment.
• Because of potential teratogenic effects, don't open or crush capsule. Avoid inhaling powder in capsule or having it contact skin or mucous membranes. If such contact occurs, wash thoroughly with soap and water, and rinse eyes with water.

**I.V. administration**
• CellCept Intravenous must be reconstituted and diluted to a concentration of 6 mg/ml using 14 ml of 5% dextrose injection.
• Never administer drug by rapid or bolus I.V. injection. Give infusion over at least 2 hours.
• Use within 4 hours of reconstitution and dilution.
• Drug is incompatible with other I.V. solutions.

**Patient teaching**
• Warn patient not to open or crush capsules but to swallow them whole on an empty stomach.
• Stress importance of not interrupting or stopping therapy without first consulting doctor.
• Inform woman that pregnancy test is needed 1 week before therapy begins.
• Instruct woman of childbearing age to use contraception during therapy and for 6 weeks after discontinuation, even with a history of infertility, unless a hysterectomy has been performed. Recommend use of two methods of contraception, unless abstinence is the chosen method, and to notify doctor immediately of suspected pregnancy.
• Warn patient that there is an increased risk of lymphoma and other malignancies.

**✴ NEW DRUG**

**sirolimus**
Rapamune

*Pregnancy Risk Category C*

**HOW SUPPLIED**
*Oral solution:* 1 mg/ml

**ACTION**
An immunosuppressant that inhibits T-lymphocyte activation and proliferation that occurs in response to antigenic and cytokine stimulation. Also inhibits antibody formation.

| Route | Onset | Peak | Duration |
|-------|-------|------|----------|
| P.O. | Unknown | 1-3 hr | Unknown |

## INDICATIONS & DOSAGE

*Prophylaxis of organ rejection in patients receiving renal transplants with cyclosporine and corticosteroids—*

**Adults and adolescents:** initially, 6 mg P.O. as one-time dose as soon as possible after transplantation; then maintenance dose of 2 mg P.O. once daily.

*Adjust-a-dose:* For patients ages 13 and older weighing below 40 kg (88 lb), initial dose is 3 mg/m$^2$ P.O. as one-time dose after transplantation; then 1 mg/m$^2$ P.O. once daily. For patients with mild to moderate hepatic impairment, reduce maintenance dose by about one-third. It isn't necessary to reduce loading dose.

## ADVERSE REACTIONS

**CNS:** *headache, insomnia, tremor, anxiety, depression, asthenia,* malaise, syncope, confusion, dizziness, emotional lability, hypertonia, hypesthesia, hypotonia, neuropathy, paresthesia, somnolence.

**CV:** *hypertension,* **heart failure, atrial fibrillation,** tachycardia, hypotension, *chest pain, edema,* **hemorrhage,** palpitations, peripheral vascular disorder, thrombophlebitis, thrombosis, vasodilatation.

**EENT:** facial edema, *pharyngitis,* epistaxis, rhinitis, sinusitis, abnormal vision, cataract, conjunctivitis, deafness, ear pain, otitis media, tinnitus.

**GI:** *diarrhea, nausea, vomiting, constipation, abdominal pain, dyspepsia,* enlarged abdomen, ascites, peritonitis, anorexia, dysphagia, eructation, esophagitis, flatulence, gastritis, gastroenteritis, gingivitis, gum hyperplasia, ileus, mouth ulceration, oral candidiasis, stomatitis.

**GU:** *dysuria, hematuria, albuminuria,* **kidney tubular necrosis,** *increased creatinine, urinary tract infection,* pelvic pain, glycosuria, increased BUN level, bladder pain, hydronephrosis, impotence, kidney pain, nocturia, oliguria, pyuria, scrotal edema, testis disorder, **toxic nephropathy,** urinary frequency, urinary incontinence, urinary retention.

**Hematologic:** *anemia,* **THROMBOCYTOPENIA, leukopenia,** thrombotic thrombocytopenia purpura, ecchymosis, leukocytosis, polycythemia.

**Hepatic:** elevated liver enzyme levels.

**Metabolic:** *hypercholesteremia, hyperlipidemia, hypokalemia, weight gain, hypophosphatemia, hyperkalemia,* hypervolemia, Cushing's syndrome, diabetes mellitus, acidosis, dehydration, hypercalcemia, hyperglycemia, hyperphosphatemia, hypocalcemia, hypoglycemia, hypomagnesemia, hyponatremia, weight loss.

**Musculoskeletal:** *back pain, arthralgia,* myalgia, arthrosis, bone necrosis, leg cramps, osteoporosis, tetany.

**Respiratory:** *dyspnea, cough, atelectasis, upper respiratory infection,* asthma, bronchitis, hypoxia, lung edema, pleural effusion, pneumonia.

**Skin:** *rash, acne,* hirsutism, fungal dermatitis, pruritus, skin hypertrophy, skin ulcer, sweating.

**Other:** *fever, pain, peripheral edema,* abscess, cellulitis, chills, flulike syndrome, hernia, infection, **sepsis,** lymphadenopathy, abnormal healing.

## INTERACTIONS

**Drug-drug.** *Aminoglycosides, amphotericin, other nephrotoxic drugs:* increased risk of nephrotoxicity. Use with caution.

*Bromocriptine, cimetidine, cisapride, clarithromycin, clotrimazole, danazol, erythromycin, fluconazole, indinavir, itraconazole, metoclopramide, nicardipine, ritonavir, verapamil, other drugs that inhibit CYP3A4:* may increase blood levels of sirolimus. Monitor closely.

*Carbamazepine, phenobarbital, phenytoin, rifabutin, rifapentine, other drugs that induce CYP3A4:* may decrease blood levels of sirolimus. Monitor closely.

*Cyclosporine (oral solution and capsules):* increased sirolimus levels. Administer sirolimus 4 hours after cyclosporine. After long-term administration, sirolimus may reduce cyclosporine clearance, requiring reduction in cyclosporine dosage.

*Diltiazem:* increased sirolimus levels. Monitor sirolimus levels, as needed.

*Ketoconazole:* increased rate and extent of sirolimus absorption. Avoid concomitant use.

*Live virus vaccines (BCG; measles, mumps, rubella; oral polio; yellow fever; varicella; TY21a typhoid):* reduced effec-

---

Reactions may be *common,* uncommon, **life-threatening,** or **COMMON AND LIFE-THREATENING.**

tiveness of vaccines. Avoid concomitant use.

*Rifampin:* decreased sirolimus levels. Alternative therapy to rifampin may be prescribed.

**Drug-food.** *Grapefruit juice:* decreased metabolism of sirolimus. Avoid concomitant use.

## EFFECTS ON DIAGNOSTIC TESTS

None reported.

## CONTRAINDICATIONS

Contraindicated in patients with hypersensitivity to active drug, its derivatives, or components of product.

## NURSING CONSIDERATIONS

• Use with caution in patients with hyperlipidemia and impaired liver or renal function.

• Drug should be prescribed only by doctors experienced in immunosuppressive therapy and management of renal transplant patients.

• Drug should be used in regimen with cyclosporine and corticosteroids; it should be taken 4 hours after cyclosporine dose.

• Following transplantation, antimicrobial prophylaxis for *Pneumocystis carinii* and cytomegalovirus should be administered for 1 year and 3 months, respectively.

• *Alert:* Patients on drug are more susceptible to infection and possible development of lymphoma.

• Monitor renal function tests, as ordered, because use with cyclosporine may cause serum creatinine levels to increase. Adjustment of immunosuppressive regimen may be needed.

• Monitor cholesterol and triglyceride levels during drug administration, as ordered. Treatment with lipid-lowering drugs during therapy isn't uncommon. If hyperlipidemia is detected, additional interventions, such as diet and exercise, should be initiated.

• Check for development of rhabdomyolysis.

• Monitor drug levels in patients ages 13 and older weighing under 88 lb; in patients with hepatic impairment; during concurrent administration of drugs that induce or inhibit CYP3A4; or if cyclosporine dosing is markedly reduced or discontinued.

• Drug should be taken consistently with or without food.

• Dilute drug before use. After dilution, use immediately and discard syringe.

• When diluting drug, empty correct amount into glass or plastic (not Styrofoam) container holding at least ¼ cup (60 ml) of water or orange juice only. Don't use grapefruit juice or other liquids. Stir vigorously and have patient drink immediately. Refill container with at least ½ cup (120 ml) of water or orange juice, stir again, and have patient drink all contents.

• A slight haze may develop during refrigeration. This doesn't affect quality of drug. If haze develops, bring to room temperature and shake until haze disappears.

• Store away from light and refrigerate at 36° to 46° F (2° to 8° C). After opening bottle, use contents within 1 month. If needed, store bottles and pouches at room temperature (up to 77° F [25° C]) for several days. Drug may be kept in oral dosing syringe for 24 hours at room temperature.

### ✓Patient teaching

• Inform patient how to properly store, dilute, and administer drug.

• Advise woman of childbearing age of potential risks during pregnancy and to use effective contraception before and during therapy. Contraception should be continued for 12 weeks after stopping drug.

• Tell patient to take drug consistently with or without food to minimize absorption variability.

• Tell patient to take drug 4 hours after taking cyclosporine to avoid drug interactions.

• Advise patient to wash with soap and water if drug solution touches skin or mucous membranes.

# tacrolimus (FK506)
Prograf

*Pregnancy Risk Category C*

## HOW SUPPLIED
*Capsules:* 1 mg, 5 mg
*Injection:* 5 mg/ml

## ACTION
Exact mechanism unknown. Inhibits T-lymphocyte activation, which results in immunosuppression.

| Route | Onset | Peak | Duration |
|-------|-------|------|----------|
| P.O., I.V. | Unknown | 1.5-3.5 hr | Unknown |

## INDICATIONS & DOSAGE
*Prophylaxis of organ rejection in allogenic liver or kidney transplants—*
**Adults:** 0.03 to 0.05 mg/kg/day I.V. as continuous infusion administered no sooner than 6 hours after transplantation. Substitute P.O. therapy as soon as possible, with first oral dose given 8 to 12 hours after discontinuing I.V. infusion. Or, administer P.O. dose within 24 hours of transplantation after renal function has recovered. Recommended initial P.O. dose for allogenic liver transplants is 0.1 to 0.15 mg/kg/day P.O. in two divided doses q 12 hours. Recommended initial P.O. dose for allogenic kidney transplants is 0.2 mg/kg/day P.O. in two divided doses q 12 hours. Dosages should be adjusted based on clinical response.
**Children:** initially, 0.03 to 0.05 mg/kg/day I.V.; then 0.15 to 0.2 mg/kg/day P.O. on schedule similar to adults adjusted, p.r.n.
*Adjust-a-dose:* For patients with renal or hepatic impairment, use lowest recommended doses for I.V. and P.O.

## ADVERSE REACTIONS
**CNS:** *headache, tremor, insomnia, paresthesia, delirium,* **coma,** *asthenia.*
**CV:** *hypertension, peripheral edema.*
**GI:** *diarrhea, nausea, constipation, abnormal liver function tests, anorexia, vomiting, abdominal pain.*
**GU:** *abnormal renal function, increased creatinine or BUN levels, urinary tract infection, oliguria.*
**Hematologic:** *anemia, leukocytosis,* THROMBOCYTOPENIA.
**Metabolic:** *hyperkalemia, hypokalemia, hyperglycemia, hypomagnesemia.*
**Musculoskeletal:** *back pain.*
**Respiratory:** *pleural effusion, atelectasis, dyspnea.*
**Skin:** *pruritus, rash, alopecia, photosensitivity, alopecia.*
**Other:** *pain, fever, ascites,* **anaphylaxis.**

## INTERACTIONS
**Drug-drug.** *Bromocriptine, cimetidine, clarithromycin, clotrimazole, cyclosporine, danazol, diltiazem, erythromycin, fluconazole, itraconazole, ketoconazole, methylprednisolone, metoclopramide, nicardipine, verapamil:* may increase tacrolimus levels. Watch for adverse effects.
*Carbamazepine, phenobarbital, phenytoin, rifabutin, rifampin:* may decrease tacrolimus levels. Monitor effectiveness of tacrolimus.
*Cyclosporine:* increased risk of excess nephrotoxicity. Don't administer together.
*Immunosuppressants (except adrenal corticosteroids):* may oversuppress immune system. Monitor patient closely, especially during times of stress.
*Inducers of cytochrome P-450 enzyme system:* may increase tacrolimus metabolism and decrease blood levels. Dosage adjustment may be needed.
*Inhibitors of cytochrome P-450 enzyme system (phenobarbital, phenytoin, rifampin):* may decrease tacrolimus metabolism and increase blood levels. Dosage adjustment may be needed.
*Nephrotoxic drugs (such as aminoglycosides, amphotericin B, cisplatin, cyclosporine):* may cause additive or synergistic effects. Monitor closely.
*Viral vaccines:* may interfere with immune response to live virus vaccines. Defer routine immunizations.
**Drug-food.** *Any food:* inhibited drug absorption. Take drug on empty stomach.
*Grapefruit juice:* increased drug blood levels. Avoid concomitant use.

---

Reactions may be *common,* uncommon, *life-threatening,* or COMMON AND LIFE-THREATENING.

**EFFECTS ON DIAGNOSTIC TESTS**
None reported.

**CONTRAINDICATIONS**
Contraindicated in patients with hypersensitivity to drug. I.V. form is contraindicated in patients with hypersensitivity to castor oil derivatives.

**NURSING CONSIDERATIONS**
• *Alert:* Because of risk of anaphylaxis, use injection only in patients who can't take oral form.
• Keep epinephrine 1:1,000 and oxygen available to treat anaphylaxis.
• Children with normal renal and hepatic function may need higher dosages than adults.
• Patients with hepatic or renal dysfunction should receive lowest dosage possible.
• Expect to administer adrenal corticosteroids with drug.
• Monitor patient for signs of neurotoxicity and nephrotoxicity, especially in patients receiving a high dose or with renal or hepatic dysfunction.
• Monitor patient for signs and symptoms of hyperkalemia, such as muscle weakness or cramping, palpitations, and obtain serum potassium levels regularly, as ordered. Potassium-sparing diuretics should be avoided during drug therapy.
• Monitor patient's blood glucose level regularly, as ordered. Also monitor patient for signs and symptoms of hyperglycemia, such as dizziness, confusion, and frequent urination. Treatment of hyperglycemia may be needed. Insulin-dependent type 1 posttransplant diabetes may occur; in some cases, it's reversible.
• Patient receiving drug is at increased risk for infections, lymphomas, and other malignant diseases.

**I.V. administration**
• Dilute drug with normal saline for injection or $D_5W$ injection to concentration between 0.004 and 0.02 mg/ml before use. Store diluted infusion solution for no more than 24 hours in glass or polyethylene containers. Don't store drug in a polyvinyl chloride container because of decreased stability and potential for extraction of phthalates.
• Monitor patient continuously during first 30 minutes of I.V. administration and frequently thereafter for signs and symptoms of anaphylaxis.

☑**Patient teaching**
• Instruct patient to check with doctor before taking other drugs during therapy.
• Tell patient to report adverse reactions promptly.

BCG vaccine
cholera vaccine
diphtheria and tetanus toxoids, adsorbed
diphtheria and tetanus toxoids and acellular pertussis vaccine adsorbed
diphtheria and tetanus toxoids and whole-cell pertussis vaccine
*Haemophilus* b conjugate vaccines
hepatitis A vaccine, inactivated
hepatitis B vaccine, recombinant
influenza virus vaccine, 1999-2000 trivalent types A & B (purified surface antigen)
influenza virus vaccine, 1999-2000 trivalent types A & B (subvirion or purified subvirion)
influenza virus vaccine, 1999-2000 trivalent types A & B (whole virion)
Japanese encephalitis virus vaccine, inactivated
Lyme disease vaccine (recombinant OspA)
measles, mumps, and rubella virus vaccine, live
measles and rubella virus vaccine, live attenuated
measles virus vaccine, live attenuated
meningococcal polysaccharide vaccine
mumps virus vaccine, live
plague vaccine
pneumococcal vaccine, polyvalent
poliovirus vaccine, inactivated
poliovirus vaccine, live, oral, trivalent
rabies vaccine, adsorbed
rabies vaccine, human diploid cell
rubella and mumps virus vaccine, live
rubella virus vaccine, live attenuated
tetanus toxoid, adsorbed
tetanus toxoid, fluid
typhoid vaccine, oral
typhoid vaccine, parenteral
typhoid Vi polysaccharide vaccine
varicella virus vaccine
yellow fever vaccine

## COMBINATION PRODUCTS

ACTHIB/DTP: 10 mcg *Haemophilus* b polyribosylribitol phosphate (PRP) conjugated to 24 mcg tetanus toxoid, 6.7 Lf (limit flocculation) units diphtheria toxoid, 5 Lf units tetanus toxoid, and 4 units whole-cell pertussis vaccine per 0.5 ml.
COMVAX: 7.5 mcg *Haemophilus* b PRP, 125 mcg *Neisseria meningitidis* OMPC, and 5 mcg hepatitis B surface antigen per 0.5 ml.
TETRAMUNE: 10 mcg purified *Haemophilus* b saccharide and about 25 mcg $CRM_{197}$ protein, 12.5 Lf units inactivated diphtheria, 5 Lf units inactivated tetanus, and 4 protective units pertussis per 0.5 ml.

---

## BCG vaccine
TICE BCG

*Pregnancy Risk Category C*

### HOW SUPPLIED
*Percutaneous vaccine:* 1 to $8 \times 10^8$ colony-forming units (CFU)/vial (TICE strain)

### ACTION
A live, attenuated bacterial vaccine prepared from *Mycobacterium bovis* that promotes active immunity to tuberculosis (TB).

| Route | Onset | Peak | Duration |
|-------|-------|------|----------|
| Percutaneous | Unknown | Unknown | Unknown |

### INDICATIONS & DOSAGE
*TB exposure—*
**Adults and children ages 1 month and older:** 0.2 to 0.3 ml (percutaneous vaccine) applied to cleaned skin followed by application of multiple-puncture disk.

---

Reactions may be *common*, uncommon, *life-threatening*, or COMMON AND LIFE-THREATENING.

**Infants under age 1 month:** dosage reduced by 50% by using 2 ml of sterile water without preservatives when reconstituting.

**ADVERSE REACTIONS**
**Musculoskeletal:** osteomyelitis.
**Other:** lymphadenopathy, allergic reaction, *anaphylaxis.*

**INTERACTIONS**
**Drug-drug.** *Immunosuppressants:* may reduce response to BCG vaccine. Avoid if possible.
*Isoniazid, rifampin, streptomycin:* inhibited multiplication of BCG. Avoid use together.

**EFFECTS ON DIAGNOSTIC TESTS**
Tuberculin sensitivity may be rendered positive by BCG intravesical treatment. Determine patient's reactivity to tuberculin before initiating therapy.

**CONTRAINDICATIONS**
Contraindicated in patients with hypersensitivity to vaccine. Also contraindicated in patients with hypogammaglobulinemia, in presence of a positive tuberculin reaction (when meant for use as immunoprophylactic after exposure to TB) in immunosuppressed patients, in those with fresh smallpox vaccinations, in those who have suffered burns, and in patients receiving corticosteroid therapy. Avoid use in pregnant women.

**NURSING CONSIDERATIONS**
• Don't inject vaccine I.V., S.C., or I.D.
• Use cautiously in patients with chronic skin disease. Inject in healthy skin only.
• Obtain history of allergies and reaction to immunization.
• Keep epinephrine 1:1,000 available to treat anaphylaxis.
• Don't shake vial after reconstitution. Use within 2 hours.
• Don't administer to febrile patients unless cause is determined.
• Expected lesions in 7 to 14 days. Papules reach maximum diameter of 3 mm, then fade.
• Allow at least 6 to 8 weeks between BCG and live virus vaccines; administer

killed virus vaccines 7 days before or 10 days after BCG, as ordered.
• Vaccine is of no value as immunoprophylactic in patients with positive tuberculin test.
• Destroy live vaccine by autoclaving or treating with formaldehyde solution before disposal.

☑**Patient teaching**
• Advise patient to have tuberculin skin test 2 to 3 months after BCG vaccination.
• Tell patient to report unusual signs and symptoms after vaccination.
• Inform patient to keep site dry for 24 hours and not to expose area to others because live vaccine may infect them.

---

cholera vaccine

*Pregnancy Risk Category C*

**HOW SUPPLIED**
*Injection:* suspension of killed *Vibrio cholerae* (each ml contains 8 U of Inaba and Ogawa serotypes) in 1.5-ml and 20-ml vials

**ACTION**
Promotes active immunity to cholera.

| Route | Onset | Peak | Duration |
|-------|-------|------|----------|
| I.M., S.C., I.D. | After second dose | Unknown | 3-6 mo |

**INDICATIONS & DOSAGE**
*Primary immunization for persons traveling to areas where cholera is endemic or epidemic—*
**Adults and children over age 10:** two doses of 0.5 ml I.M. or S.C., 1 week to 1 month apart, before traveling in cholera area. Booster is 0.5 ml q 6 months, p.r.n.
**Adults and children ages 5 and older:** two doses of 0.2 ml I.D., 1 week to 1 month apart, and q 6 months, p.r.n.
**Children ages 5 to 10:** 0.3 ml I.M. or S.C. Boosters of same dose should be given q 6 months, p.r.n.
**Children ages 6 months to 4 years:** 0.2 ml I.M. or S.C. Boosters of same dose should be given q 6 months, p.r.n.

## ADVERSE REACTIONS
**CNS:** headache, malaise.
**Skin:** *erythema, swelling, pain, induration at injection site.*
**Other:** fever, *anaphylaxis.*

## INTERACTIONS
**Drug-drug.** *Plague, typhoid, other vaccines with systemic adverse reactions:* enhanced toxicity. Don't use together.
*Yellow fever vaccine:* simultaneous administration may interfere with immune response to both vaccines. Administer 3 weeks apart.

## EFFECTS ON DIAGNOSTIC TESTS
None reported.

## CONTRAINDICATIONS
Contraindicated in those with acute illness or history of severe systemic reaction or allergic response to vaccine.

## NURSING CONSIDERATIONS
● Obtain history of allergies and reaction to immunization.
● Keep epinephrine 1:1,000 available to treat anaphylaxis.
● Shake vial vigorously before withdrawing each dose.
● Don't administer vaccine I.M. to patients with thrombocytopenia or other coagulation disorders that contraindicate I.M. injection.
● Administer vaccine I.M. in deltoid muscle in adults and children over age 3.
● I.M. and S.C. routes give higher levels of protection in children under age 5.
● Vaccine is about 50% effective in reducing clinical illness incidence for 3 to 6 months.

### ☑ Patient teaching
● Advise patient that pain, induration, and swelling at injection site are common for 24 to 48 hours.
● Tell traveler to avoid food and water that may be contaminated.
● Advise patient that malaise, headache, and mild to moderate fever may persist for 1 to 2 days.

## diphtheria and tetanus toxoids, adsorbed

*Pregnancy Risk Category C*

## HOW SUPPLIED
Available in pediatric (DT) and adult (Td) strengths
*Injection (for pediatric use):* diphtheria toxoid 6.6 Lf (limit flocculation) units and tetanus toxoid 5 Lf units per 0.5 ml; diphtheria toxoid 7.5 Lf units and tetanus toxoid 7.5 Lf units per 0.5 ml; diphtheria toxoid 10 Lf units and tetanus toxoid 5 Lf units per 0.5 ml; diphtheria toxoid 12.5 Lf units and tetanus toxoid 5 Lf units per 0.5 ml
*Injection (for adult use):* diphtheria toxoid 2 Lf units and tetanus toxoid 2 Lf units per 0.5 ml; diphtheria toxoid 2 Lf units and tetanus toxoid 5 Lf units per 0.5 ml

## ACTION
Promotes immunity to diphtheria and tetanus by inducing production of antitoxins.

| Route | Onset | Peak | Duration |
|-------|-------|------|----------|
| I.M. | Unknown | Unknown | 10 yr |

## INDICATIONS & DOSAGE
*Primary immunization—*
**Adults and children ages 7 and older:** adult strength; 0.5 ml I.M. 4 to 8 weeks apart for two doses and third dose 6 to 12 months after second dose. Booster is 0.5 ml I.M. q 10 years.
**Children ages 1 to 6:** pediatric strength; 0.5 ml I.M. at least 4 weeks apart for two doses. Give booster dose 6 to 12 months after second injection. If final immunizing dose is given after seventh birthday, use adult strength.
**Infants ages 6 weeks to 1 year:** pediatric strength; 0.5 ml I.M. at least 4 weeks apart for three doses. Give booster dose 6 to 12 months after third injection.

## ADVERSE REACTIONS
**CNS:** headache, malaise.
**CV:** tachycardia, hypotension, flushing.
**Skin:** *pain, stinging, edema, erythema, induration at injection site;* urticaria; pruritus.
**Other:** *anaphylaxis,* chills, fever.

---

Reactions may be *common*, uncommon, *life-threatening*, or COMMON AND LIFE-THREATENING.

## INTERACTIONS
None significant.

## EFFECTS ON DIAGNOSTIC TESTS
None reported.

## CONTRAINDICATIONS
Contraindicated in patients with hypersensitivity to vaccine or its components, which include a mercury derivative, thimerosal. Also contraindicated in immunosuppressed patients and in those receiving radiation or corticosteroid therapy. Defer vaccination in patients with respiratory illness and during polio outbreaks; also defer use in those with acute illness except during emergency. When polio is a risk, use single antigen. Use only when diphtheria, tetanus, and pertussis combination is contraindicated in children under age 6 because of pertussis component. Don't use DT in patients over age 7.

## NURSING CONSIDERATIONS
• Obtain history of allergies and reaction to immunization.
• Before injection, verify strength (pediatric or adult) of toxoid used.
• Keep epinephrine 1:1,000 available to treat anaphylaxis.
• Give in site not recently used for vaccines or toxoids.
• Vaccine isn't used to treat an acute diphtheria infection.
• Document manufacturer, lot number, date of injection, and name, address, and title of person administering injection on patient record or log.
• Interruption of recommended dosing schedule doesn't interfere with final immunity achieved.

☑**Patient teaching**
• Advise patient that local reactions, such as pain and pruritus, are common at injection site and that a nodule may be present for a few weeks.
• Review primary immunization schedule with patient or parents, and stress importance of compliance with subsequent injections.

# diphtheria and tetanus toxoids and whole-cell pertussis vaccine (DPT, DTP)
DTwP, Tri-Immunol

# diphtheria and tetanus toxoids and acellular pertussis vaccine adsorbed
Acel-Imune, DTaP, Tripedia

*Pregnancy Risk Category C*

## HOW SUPPLIED
**whole-cell vaccine**
*Injection:* 6.5 Lf (limit flocculation) units inactivated diphtheria, 5 Lf units inactivated tetanus, and 4 protective units pertussis per 0.5 ml, in 2.5-, 5-, and 7.5-ml vials; 10 Lf units inactivated diphtheria, 5.5 Lf units inactivated tetanus, and 4 protective units pertussis per 0.5 ml in 5-ml vials (DTwP); 12.5 Lf units inactivated diphtheria, 5 Lf units inactivated tetanus, and 4 protective units pertussis per 0.5 ml, in 7.5-ml vials (Tri-Immunol)
**acellular vaccine**
*Injection:* 5 Lf units inactivated diphtheria, 5 Lf units inactivated tetanus, and 300 hemagglutinating units of acellular pertussis vaccine per 0.5 ml; 66.7 Lf units inactivated diphtheria, 5 Lf units inactivated tetanus, and 46.8 pertussis antigens per 0.5 ml

## ACTION
Promotes active immunity to diphtheria, tetanus, and pertussis (DTP) by inducing production of antitoxins and antibodies.

| Route | Onset | Peak | Duration |
|-------|-------|------|----------|
| I.M. | 2 wk after last dose | Unknown | 4-6 yr |

## INDICATIONS & DOSAGE
*Primary immunization—*
**Children ages 2 months to 7 years:**
0.5 ml I.M. 4 to 8 weeks apart for three doses and fourth dose after 6 to 12 months. Booster is 0.5 ml I.M. when starting school unless fourth dose in series was administered after child's fourth birthday; then, booster isn't needed at time of school entrance.

## ADVERSE REACTIONS
**CNS:** *seizures, encephalopathy,* peripheral neuropathy, *drowsiness.*
**GI:** *vomiting, anorexia.*
**Skin:** *soreness at injection site, redness,* nodule remaining several weeks at injection site, urticaria.
**Other:** *anaphylaxis, shock,* thrombocytopenic purpura, *fever, hypersensitivity reactions.*

## INTERACTIONS
**Drug-drug.** *Immunosuppressants:* may reduce response to DTP vaccine. Avoid if possible.

## EFFECTS ON DIAGNOSTIC TESTS
None reported.

## CONTRAINDICATIONS
Contraindicated in patients with hypersensitivity to vaccine or its components. Also contraindicated in patients who developed an immediate anaphylactic reaction or encephalopathy within 7 days of DTP dose, in immunosuppressed patients, in those on corticosteroid therapy, and in those with an evolving neurologic condition. Defer vaccination in patients with acute febrile illness of unknown cause. Children with preexisting neurologic disorders shouldn't receive pertussis vaccine. Also, children who exhibit neurologic signs after DTP injection shouldn't receive pertussis component in any succeeding injections; diphtheria and tetanus toxoids (called DT) should be given instead.

## NURSING CONSIDERATIONS
• Vaccine isn't advised for adults or children over age 7.
• Products containing acellular pertussis vaccine may be used for dose in DTP immunization.
• Obtain history of allergies and reaction to immunization.
• Keep epinephrine 1:1,000 available to treat anaphylaxis.
• Shake before using. Refrigerate vaccine.
• Administer only by deep I.M. injection, preferably in thigh or deltoid muscle. Don't give S.C.
• DTP injection may be given at same time as trivalent oral polio vaccine.

• Acellular vaccine may be associated with a lower risk of local pain and fever.

### ✓ Patient teaching
• Make sure parents understand risks and benefits of vaccine before it's administered.
• Tell parents to report systemic reactions promptly; remind them that local reactions are common. Acetaminophen in age-appropriate dosing will decrease occurrence of postvaccination fever in children prone to febrile seizure activity.

---

## *Haemophilus* b conjugate vaccines

### *Haemophilus* b conjugate vaccine, diphtheria CRM$_{197}$ protein conjugate (HbOC)
HibTITER

### *Haemophilus* b conjugate vaccine, diphtheria toxoid conjugate (PRP-D)
ProHIBIT

### *Haemophilus* b conjugate vaccine, meningococcal protein conjugate (PRP-OMP)
PedvaxHIB

*Pregnancy Risk Category C*

---

## HOW SUPPLIED
***Haemophilus* b conjugate vaccine, diphtheria CRM$_{197}$ protein conjugate**
*Injection:* 10 mcg of purified *Haemophilus* b saccharide and about 25 mcg CRM$_{197}$ protein per 0.5 ml
***Haemophilus* b conjugate vaccine, diphtheria toxoid conjugate**
*Injection:* 25 mcg of *Haemophilus influenzae* type B (HIB) capsular polysaccharide and 18 mcg of diphtheria toxoid protein per 0.5 ml
***Haemophilus* b conjugate vaccine, meningococcal protein conjugate**
*Powder for injection:* 15 mcg of *Haemophilus* b PRP, 250 mcg *Neisseria meningitidis* OMPC per dose

---

*Injection:* 7.5 mcg of *Haemophilus* b PRP and 125 mcg *N. meningitidis* OMPC per 0.5 ml

## ACTION
Promotes active immunity to HIB; is a polymer of ribose, ribitol, and phosphate (PRP); and is linked by covalent bonds to highly antigenic substances, enabling the vaccine to promote an immune response in infants.

| Route | Onset | Peak | Duration |
|-------|-------|------|----------|
| I.M. | 2 wk after last dose | Unknown | Several yr |

## INDICATIONS & DOSAGE
*Immunization against HIB infection—*
*Conjugate vaccine, diphtheria CRM₁₉₇*
*protein conjugate*
**Infants:** 0.5 ml I.M. at age 2 months. Repeated at 4 months and 6 months. Booster dose given at age 15 months.
**Previously unvaccinated infants ages 2 to 6 months:** 0.5 ml I.M. Repeated in 2 months and again in 4 months for total of three doses. Booster dose given at age 15 months.
**Previously unvaccinated infants ages 7 to 11 months:** 0.5 ml I.M. Repeated in 2 months, for a total of two doses. Booster dose given at age 15 months (but no sooner than 2 months after last vaccination).
**Previously unvaccinated infants ages 12 to 14 months:** 0.5 ml I.M. Booster dose given at age 15 months (but no sooner than 2 months after first vaccination).
**Previously unvaccinated children ages 15 months to 71 months:** 0.5 ml I.M. Booster dose isn't needed.
*Conjugate vaccine, diphtheria toxoid conjugate*
**Previously unvaccinated children ages 15 to 71 months:** 0.5 ml I.M. Booster dose isn't needed. Not recommended for use in children under age 15 months.
*Conjugate vaccine, meningococcal protein conjugate*
**Infants:** 0.5 ml I.M. at age 2 months. Repeated at 4 months. Booster dose given at age 12 months.
**Previously unvaccinated infants ages 2 to 6 months:** 0.5 ml I.M. Repeated in 2

months. Booster dose given at age 12 months.
**Previously unvaccinated infants ages 7 to 11 months:** 0.5 ml I.M. Repeated in 2 months. Booster dose given at age 15 months (but no sooner than 2 months after last vaccination).
**Previously unvaccinated infants ages 12 to 14 months:** 0.5 ml I.M. Booster dose given at age 15 months (but no sooner than 2 months after first vaccination).
**Previously unvaccinated children ages 15 to 71 months:** 0.5 ml I.M. Booster dose isn't needed.
    Premature infants follow same schedule as full-term infants.

## ADVERSE REACTIONS
**GI:** diarrhea, vomiting.
**Skin:** *erythema, pain at injection site.*
**Other:** *anaphylaxis,* fever, crying.

## INTERACTIONS
**Drug-drug.** *Immunosuppressants:* may suppress antibody response to HIB vaccine. Defer immunization.

## EFFECTS ON DIAGNOSTIC TESTS
Drug may interfere with interpretation of antigen detection tests used to diagnose systemic HIB disease.

## CONTRAINDICATIONS
Contraindicated in patients with hypersensitivity to vaccine or its components and in those with acute illness.

## NURSING CONSIDERATIONS
• Keep epinephrine 1:1,000 available to treat anaphylaxis.
• Don't administer vaccine I.D. or I.V.; must administer I.M.
• Administer vaccine into anterolateral aspect of upper thigh in small children. Injections may be made into deltoid muscle of larger children if sufficient muscle mass is present.
• Vaccine isn't routinely administered to adults or children over age 5 unless they're at high risk for infection (including patients with chronic conditions, such as functional asplenia, splenectomy, Hodgkin's disease, or sickle cell anemia).

• *Alert:* Don't administer to febrile children.
• Immunization against HIB infection is recommended for children with HIV infections. Follow usual immunization schedule.
• Vaccine and DTP may be given simultaneously. A combination product is commercially available.
• Diphtheria toxoid conjugate vaccine (ProHIBIT) isn't recommended in children under age 15 months.
• HIB is an important cause of meningitis in infants and preschool children.

### ☑ Patient teaching
• Warn patient or parents that pain may occur at injection site.
• Tell patient or parents to notify doctor if adverse reactions persist or become severe.

## hepatitis A vaccine, inactivated
Havrix, Vaqta

*Pregnancy Risk Category C*

### HOW SUPPLIED
**Havrix**
*Injection:* 360 ELISA units (EL.U.)/0.5 ml; 720 EL.U./0.5 ml; 1,440 EL.U./ml
**Vaqta**
*Injection:* 25 U/0.5 ml, 50 U/ml

### ACTION
Promotes active immunity to hepatitis A virus.

| Route | Onset | Peak | Duration |
|-------|-------|------|----------|
| I.M. | 1-15 days | Unknown | 6 mo |

### INDICATIONS & DOSAGE
*Active immunization against hepatitis A virus—*
**Adults:** 1,440 EL.U. (Havrix) or 50 U (Vaqta) I.M. as single dose. For booster dose, 1,440 EL.U. (Havrix) or 50 U (Vaqta) I.M. given 6 to 12 months after initial dose. A booster dose is recommended if prolonged immunity is desired.
**Children ages 2 to 18:** 720 EL.U. (Havrix) or 25 U (Vaqta) I.M. as single dose; then booster dose of 720 EL.U.

(Havrix) or 25 U (Vaqta) I.M. given 6 to 12 months after initial dose, or 360 EL.U. I.M. given 1 month apart and 360 EL.U. I.M. 6 to 12 months after primary course. Booster recommended for prolonged immunity.
*Prevention of hepatitis A in patients with chronic liver disease or clotting factor disorders, and in food handlers—*
**Adults:** 1,440 EL.U. (Havrix) I.M. as single dose. For booster dose, 1,440 EL.U. (Havrix) I.M. given 6 to 12 months after initial dose. Booster dose is recommended if prolonged immunity is desired.
**Children ages 2 to 18:** 720 EL.U. (Havrix) I.M. as single dose; then booster dose of 720 EL.U. (Havrix) I.M. given 6 to 12 months after initial dose; or two doses of 360 EL.U. I.M. given 1 month apart and 360 EL.U. I.M. 6 to 12 months after primary course. Booster dose is recommended if prolonged immunity is desired.

### ADVERSE REACTIONS
**CNS:** hypertonia, insomnia, vertigo, *headache, fatigue, malaise,* **seizures,** encephalopathy, dizziness.
**EENT:** pharyngitis, photophobia.
**GI:** *anorexia, nausea,* abdominal pain, diarrhea, dysgeusia, vomiting.
**GU:** menstruation disorders.
**Musculoskeletal:** arthralgia, myalgia.
**Respiratory:** other upper respiratory tract infections.
**Skin:** pruritus, rash, urticaria, *induration, redness, swelling,* hematoma, *injection site soreness,* jaundice.
**Other:** *fever,* lymphadenopathy, ***anaphylaxis,*** elevated CK level.

### INTERACTIONS
**Drug-drug.** *Anticoagulants:* increased risk of bleeding. Administer I.M. injections with caution.

### EFFECTS ON DIAGNOSTIC TESTS
None reported.

### CONTRAINDICATIONS
Contraindicated in patients with hypersensitivity to vaccine's components.

---

Reactions may be *common,* uncommon, *life-threatening,* or COMMON AND LIFE-THREATENING.

## NURSING CONSIDERATIONS

• Use with caution in patients with thrombocytopenia or bleeding disorders and in those who are taking an anticoagulant because bleeding may occur following an I.M. injection.

• As with other vaccines, administration of hepatitis A vaccine should be delayed, if possible, in patient with febrile illness.

• Keep epinephrine 1:1,000 available to treat anaphylaxis.

• If vaccine is administered to immunosuppressed persons or persons receiving immunosuppressants, expected immune response may not be obtained.

• Persons who should receive vaccine include people traveling to or living in areas of high endemicity for hepatitis A (Africa, Asia [except Japan], the Mediterranean basin, Eastern Europe, the Middle East, Central and South America, Mexico, and parts of the Caribbean), military personnel, native peoples of Alaska and the Americas, persons engaging in high-risk sexual activity, and users of illegal injectable drugs. Certain institutional workers, employees of child day-care centers, laboratory workers who handle live hepatitis A virus, and handlers of primate animals also may benefit.

• For I.M. use, shake vial or syringe well before withdrawal. After it has been agitated thoroughly, vaccine is an opaque white suspension. Discard if it appears otherwise. No dilution or reconstitution is needed.

• Administer as I.M. injection into the deltoid region in adults. It shouldn't be administered in the gluteal region; such injections may result in suboptimal response. Never inject I.V., S.C., or I.D.

### ☑ Patient teaching

• Inform patient that vaccine won't prevent hepatitis caused by other drugs or pathogens known to infect the liver.

• Warn patient about local adverse reactions. Tell him to report persistent or severe reactions promptly.

• Alert travelers to dangers of eating raw or undercooked shellfish or consuming food or drink in countries with poor hygienic conditions.

## hepatitis B vaccine, recombinant
Engerix-B, Recombivax HB

*Pregnancy Risk Category C*

### HOW SUPPLIED
*Injection:* 5 mcg HBsAg/0.5 ml (Recombivax HB, pediatric/adolescent formulation with or without preservative); 10 mcg HBsAg/0.5 ml (Engerix-B, adolescent/pediatric formulation); 10 mcg HBsAg/ml (Recombivax HB, adult formulation); 20 mcg HBsAg/ml (Engerix-B, adult formulation); 40 mcg HBsAg/ml (Recombivax HB dialysis formulation)

### ACTION
Promotes active immunity to hepatitis B.

| Route | Onset | Peak | Duration |
|-------|-------|------|----------|
| I.M. | 2 wk after last dose | Unknown | Yrs |

### INDICATIONS & DOSAGE
*Immunization against infection from all known subtypes of hepatitis B virus (HBV), primary preexposure prophylaxis against HBV, postexposure prophylaxis (when given with hepatitis B immune globulin)—Engerix-B*

**Adults ages 20 and older:** initially, 20 mcg I.M.; then second dose of 20 mcg I.M. after 30 days. A third dose of 20 mcg I.M. is given 6 months after the initial dose.

*Adjust-a-dose:* For adults undergoing dialysis or receiving immunosuppressants, initially, 40 mcg I.M. (divided into two 20-mcg doses and administered at different sites). Then second dose of 40 mcg I.M. in 30 days, a third dose after 2 months, and final dose of 40 mcg I.M. 6 months after initial dose.

*Note:* Certain populations (neonates born to infected mothers, persons recently exposed to virus, and travelers to high-risk areas) may receive the four-dose regimen, as above, because immunity can be induced more quickly with this regimen.

**Adolescents ages 11 to 19:** initially, 10 mcg (adolescent/pediatric formulation) I.M.; then second dose of 10 mcg I.M. 30

days later. A third dose of 10 mcg I.M. is given 6 months after initial dose. Or, 20 mcg (adult formulation) is given I.M.; then second dose of 20 mcg I.M. after 30 days. A third dose of 20 mcg I.M. is given 6 months after initial dose.

**Neonates and children up to age 10:** initially, 10 mcg I.M.; then second dose of 10 mcg I.M. after 30 days. A third dose of 10 mcg I.M. is given 6 months after initial dose.

*Recombivax HB*

**Adults ages 20 and older:** initially, 10 mcg I.M.; then second dose of 10 mcg I.M. after 30 days. A third dose of 10 mcg is given I.M. 6 months after initial dose.

*Adjust-a-dose:* For adults undergoing dialysis, initially, 40 mcg I.M. (use dialysis formulation, which contains 40 mcg/ml); then second dose of 40 mcg I.M. in 30 days, and final dose of 40 mcg I.M. 6 months after initial dose. A booster or revaccination may be indicated if anti-HBs level is below 10 mIU/ml 1 to 2 months after third dose.

**Children ages 11 to 19:** initially, 5 mcg I.M.; then second dose of 5 mcg I.M. after 30 days. A third dose of 5 mcg is given I.M. 6 months after initial dose.

**Children ages 1 to 10:** initially, 2.5 mcg I.M.; then second dose of 2.5 mcg I.M. after 30 days. A third dose of 2.5 mcg I.M. is given 6 months after initial dose.

**Infants born of HBsAg-negative mothers:** initially, 2.5 mcg I.M.; then second dose of 0.5 mcg after 30 days. A third dose of 0.5 mcg is given I.M. 6 months after initial dose.

**Infants born of HBsAg-positive mothers:** initially, 5 mcg I.M.; then second dose of 5 mcg I.M. after 30 days. A third dose of 5 mcg is given I.M. 6 months after initial dose.

*Chronic hepatitis C infection— Engerix-B*

**Adults:** initially, 20 mcg is given I.M.; then second dose of 20 mcg I.M. after 30 days. A third dose of 20 mcg I.M. is given 6 months after initial dose.

## ADVERSE REACTIONS
**CNS:** headache, dizziness, insomnia, paresthesia, neuropathy, transient malaise.
**EENT:** pharyngitis.

**GI:** anorexia, diarrhea, nausea, vomiting.
**Musculoskeletal:** myalgia, arthralgia, neck stiffness.
**Skin:** local inflammation, *soreness at injection site,* pruritus.
**Other:** *anaphylaxis,* slight fever, flulike syndrome.

## INTERACTIONS
**Drug-drug.** *Immunosuppressants:* inadequate circulating antibody levels. May need larger than usual doses of hepatitis B vaccine (recombinant).

## EFFECTS ON DIAGNOSTIC TESTS
None reported.

## CONTRAINDICATIONS
Contraindicated in patients with hypersensitivity to yeast or components of vaccine; recombinant vaccines are derived from yeast cultures.

## NURSING CONSIDERATIONS
• Use cautiously in patients with serious, active infections or compromised cardiac or pulmonary status and in those for whom a febrile or systemic reaction could pose a risk.
• The American Academy of Pediatrics recommends hepatitis B vaccination for all neonates and encourages immunization for adolescents when resources allow.
• The Recombivax HB vaccine pediatric/adolescent formulation without preservatives may be used for persons for whom a thimerosal-free vaccine is recommended (such as infants up to age 6 months who may receive other vaccines containing thimerosal).
• Although anaphylaxis hasn't been reported, always keep epinephrine available when giving vaccine to counteract possible reaction.
• Thoroughly agitate vial just before administration to restore suspension.
• Inspect product for particulates or discoloration before administration. Product should be a slightly opaque white suspension. Discard if it appears otherwise.
• Administer vaccine in deltoid muscle for adults and adolescents; for infants and young children, administer in anterolateral aspect of thigh. Never administer I.V.

---

Reactions may be *common,* uncommon, *life-threatening,* or **COMMON AND LIFE-THREATENING.**

• Administer S.C. in patients at risk for hemorrhage, such as hemophiliacs. Otherwise, don't use this route; it may lead to an increased incidence or severity of local reactions.
• Certain health care personnel (especially those working with dialysis patients, with selected patients and patient contacts, in blood banks, in emergency medicine, or among populations in which infection is endemic [Indo-Chinese, native peoples of Alaska, and Haitian refugees]), certain military personnel, morticians and embalmers, sexually active homosexual men, prostitutes, prisoners, and users of illegal injectable drugs are at increased risk for infection and should be considered for vaccine.
• Recombinant hepatitis B vaccine isn't made with human plasma products.

☑ **Patient teaching**
• Warn patient or parents about local adverse reactions such as swelling or redness at injection site. Tell patient to report persistent or severe reactions promptly.
• Review immunization schedule with patient or parents; stress importance of completing series.

---

**influenza virus vaccine, 1999-2000 trivalent types A & B (purified surface antigen)**
Fluvirin

**influenza virus vaccine, 1999-2000 trivalent types A & B (subvirion or purified subvirion)**
Fluogen, Flu-Shield, Fluzone

**influenza virus vaccine, 1999-2000 trivalent types A & B (whole virion)**
Fluzone

*Pregnancy Risk Category C*

**HOW SUPPLIED**
*Injection:* 0.5-ml prefilled syringe; 5 ml vial

**ACTION**
Promotes immunity to influenza by inducing production of antibodies.

| Route | Onset | Peak | Duration |
|-------|-------|------|----------|
| I.M. | 2-4 wk | Unknown | Unknown |

**INDICATIONS & DOSAGE**
*Influenza prophylaxis—*
**Adults and children ages 13 and older:** 0.5 ml (whole virus or split virus) I.M. Only one dose is needed.
**Children ages 9 to 12:** 0.5 ml (split virus only) I.M. Only one dose is needed.
**Children ages 3 to 8:** 0.5 ml (split virus only) I.M. Repeated in 4 weeks unless child has been previously vaccinated.
**Children ages 6 to 35 months:** 0.25 ml (split virus only) I.M. Repeated in 4 weeks unless child has been previously vaccinated.

**ADVERSE REACTIONS**
**CNS:** headache, malaise.
**Musculoskeletal:** myalgia.
**Skin:** erythema, induration; *soreness at injection site.*
**Other:** *anaphylaxis,* fever.

**INTERACTIONS**
**Drug-drug.** *Immunosuppressants:* may reduce immune response to vaccine. Monitor patient closely.
*Theophylline, warfarin:* clearance may be impaired, causing increased levels. Monitor patient closely.

**EFFECTS ON DIAGNOSTIC TESTS**
None reported.

**CONTRAINDICATIONS**
Contraindicated in patients with hypersensitivity to eggs or components of vaccine, including thimerosal. Defer vaccination in patients with acute respiratory or other active infection and in those with active neurologic disorders.

**NURSING CONSIDERATIONS**
• Use cautiously in patients with history of sulfite allergy.
• Fever and malaise reactions occur most often in children and in others not ex-

---

*Liquid contains alcohol.   **May contain tartrazine.   †Canada   ‡Australia   §U.K.   ◊OTC

posed to influenza viruses. Severe reactions in adults are rare.

• Obtain history of allergies, especially to eggs, and reaction to immunization.

• Keep epinephrine 1:1,000 available to treat anaphylaxis.

• Thoroughly agitate vial just before administration to restore suspension.

• Give injections for adults and older children in deltoid muscle; for infants and children under age 3, give in anterolateral aspect of thigh.

• Ideally, administer vaccinations from October to mid-November because outbreaks of influenza generally don't occur until December. Don't give vaccine too early in season because antibody titers may begin to decline before flu season.

• Children ages 12 and under should be given their second dose before December, if possible.

• Give vaccines to both children and adults throughout flu season, even as late as April.

• The American Academy of Pediatrics states that influenza vaccine can be administered simultaneously (but at a different site and with a different syringe) with other routine vaccinations in children.

• *Alert:* Don't give influenza vaccine with, or within 3 days after administration of, whole cell pertussis vaccine or combined diphtheria/tetanus toxoid/whole cell pertussis vaccine, adsorbed.

• Vaccine is considered safe in pregnant women. Vaccination shouldn't be postponed, regardless of stage of pregnancy, in patients who have high-risk conditions and who will be in first trimester of pregnancy when flu season begins.

• Immunodeficient patients may receive two doses 1 month apart; however, there is little evidence that booster doses improve immunogenic response to vaccine. Chemoprophylaxis with amantadine may be helpful.

• Vaccine is strongly recommended for anyone over age 6 months; for patients with chronic disease, metabolic disorders, or medical conditions that put them at risk for complications from influenza; for health care workers, especially doctors, nurses, employees of nursing homes, volunteer workers, and other personnel in both hospital and outpatient settings; and for household members who may contact persons at high risk for medical complications of influenza. Also recommended for anyone who wishes to reduce chance of infection.

• Allergic reactions, which usually occur immediately, are extremely rare and paralysis associated with Guillain-Barré syndrome is rare and has been associated only with the 1976 vaccine.

• Vaccine prepared for a previous influenza season shouldn't be used to provide protection for current season.

• Although there is little information regarding influenza in persons with HIV, it's recommended that these patients receive vaccine. Patients with advanced disease may have a low response; there is no evidence that booster dose will improve immune response.

✅ **Patient teaching**

• Advise patient about risks of vaccination compared with risk of influenza and its complications.

• Ensure that patient understands that annual vaccination with current vaccine is needed because immunity to influenza decreases in year after injection.

• Ensure that patient understands that vaccine can't cause influenza. Fever, malaise, and myalgia may begin 6 to 12 hours after vaccination and last 1 to 2 days. Such systemic reactions aren't common.

• Advise appropriate acetaminophen dose for fever and ice compresses to injection site to minimize discomfort.

## Japanese encephalitis virus vaccine, inactivated
JE-VAX

*Pregnancy Risk Category C*

**HOW SUPPLIED**
*Injection:* 1-ml, 10-ml vials

**ACTION**
Provides active immunity against Japanese encephalitis (JE), a mosquito-borne

---

Reactions may be *common*, uncommon, **life-threatening**, or COMMON AND LIFE-THREATENING.

arboviral flavivirus infection that's the main cause of viral encephalitis in Asia.

| Route | Onset | Peak | Duration |
|-------|-------|------|----------|
| S.C. | Unknown | Unknown | 2 yr |

## INDICATIONS & DOSAGE

*Active immunization against JE—*
Primary immunization schedule:
**Adults and children ages 3 and older:**
1 ml S.C. on days 0, 7, and 30.
**Children ages 1 to 3:** 0.5 ml S.C. on days 0, 7, and 30.
Booster doses:
**Adults and children ages 3 and older:**
1 ml S.C., 2 years after last dose.
**Children ages 1 to 3:** 0.5 ml S.C., 2 years after last dose.

## ADVERSE REACTIONS

**CNS:** *headache, dizziness, malaise.*
**GI:** *nausea, vomiting, abdominal pain.*
**Musculoskeletal:** *myalgia.*
**Respiratory:** *respiratory distress.*
**Skin:** rash, *local tenderness and swelling at injection site,* generalized urticaria.
**Other:** *anaphylaxis, fever, chills, angioedema of the face, oropharynx, extremities, or lips.*

## INTERACTIONS

None significant.

## EFFECTS ON DIAGNOSTIC TESTS

None reported.

## CONTRAINDICATIONS

Contraindicated in patients with hypersensitivity to drug or thimerosal, a preservative, and in those who exhibited severe adverse reactions, such as generalized urticaria or angioedema, to previous dose of vaccine. Because vaccine is derived from mouse brain, its use is contraindicated in patients with hypersensitivity to substances of murine or neural origin.

## NURSING CONSIDERATIONS

• Use cautiously in pregnant or breast-feeding women, elderly patients, and in those with history of urticaria after vaccines, drugs, or insect stings. Advanced age may be a risk factor for developing symptomatic illness after JE infection. JE acquired during pregnancy can cause intrauterine infection and fetal death.

• Use vaccine to provide protection against JE in persons planning to travel 1 month or longer or who reside in areas where virus is endemic. It isn't indicated for all persons traveling to or residing in Asia. For most travelers to Asia, the risk of acquiring JE is extremely low. Contact the Centers for Disease Control and Prevention at (877) FYI-TRIP for current travel advisories.

• Keep epinephrine 1:1,000 and other resuscitation equipment and drugs available to treat anaphylaxis and other adverse reactions.

• To prepare vaccine for injection, use supplied diluent (sterile water for injection). Add 1.3 ml of diluent to single-dose vial and 11 ml of diluent to 10-dose vial. Shake vial thoroughly to ensure dissolution of vaccine. After reconstitution, refrigerate vaccine (36° to 46° F [2° to 8° C]) for up to 8 hours; then discard.

• Follow recommended three-dose schedule for best results. When time constraints prohibit use of schedule, an abbreviated schedule with injections on days 0, 7, and 14 may be used.

• When it isn't possible to follow usual dose schedule, a two-dose regimen with injections on days 0 and 7 may be used. Antibodies will be induced in about 80% of patients with this schedule. A two-dose regimen shouldn't be used unless circumstances are unusual.

• Monitor patient closely for 30 minutes after injection.

• Reactions to first dose have occurred a median of 12 hours after injection (88% occurred within 3 days). The delay between second dose and adverse effects was usually longer, with median of 3 days, and some effects were not seen for 2 weeks. Some patients exhibited adverse reactions to second or third dose, even when first or second dose was well tolerated.

### ✓ Patient teaching

• Warn patient about possibility of delayed generalized urticaria or delayed angioedema of the extremities, face, oropharynx or (especially) the lips. Gen-

eralized urticaria or angioedema may occur within minutes of vaccination. Most reactions occur within 48 hours. However, reactions that may be related to vaccine have occurred as late as 17 days after injection.
• Because of risk of delayed reactions, advise patient to remain in areas where medical care is available for 10 days after injection. Caution against international travel during this time. Advise patient to seek medical assistance as soon as a reaction appears.
• Encourage patient and parents to report adverse effects after vaccination. Health care providers should report these adverse effects to U.S. Department of Health and Human Services Vaccine Adverse Event Reporting System (VAERS). Contact VAERS at (800) 822-7967 for information about the system and reporting forms.
• Teach patient about precautions that may limit exposure to mosquito bites, such as using insect repellents, wearing protective clothing, and avoiding outdoor activities, especially in the evening.

✳ *NEW DRUG*

## Lyme disease vaccine (recombinant OspA)
LYMErix

*Pregnancy Risk Category C*

### HOW SUPPLIED
*Injection:* 30 mcg/0.5 ml single-dose vials and prefilled syringes

### ACTION
Stimulates formation of anti-OspA antibodies, which have demonstrated bactericidal activity against *Borrelia burgdorferi*, the bacterial spirochete that causes Lyme disease.

| Route | Onset | Peak | Duration |
|-------|-------|------|----------|
| I.M. | Unknown | Unknown | Unknown |

### INDICATIONS & DOSAGE
*Active immunization against Lyme disease—*
**Adults and adolescents ages 15 to 70:** 30 mcg I.M. in deltoid region; repeat dose at 1 and 12 months after first dose. Administration of second and third doses should take place several weeks before onset of *B. burgdorferi* transmission season (varies according to geographic area).

### ADVERSE REACTIONS
**CNS:** *headache, fatigue,* dizziness, depression, hypoesthesia, paresthesia.
**EENT:** pharyngitis, rhinitis, sinusitis.
**GI:** diarrhea, nausea.
**Musculoskeletal:** *arthralgia,* back pain, aches, myalgia, arthritis, arthrosis, stiffness, tendinitis.
**Respiratory:** bronchitis, coughing, pharyngitis, rhinitis, sinusitis, upper respiratory tract infection.
**Skin:** *rash,* injection site reaction, contact dermatitis, *injection site pain, redness, soreness, swelling.*
**Other:** chills or rigors, fever, viral infection, flulike syndrome.

### INTERACTIONS
**Drug-drug.** *Immunosuppressants:* expected immune response may not occur. Consider deferring vaccination for 3 months after therapy ends.

### EFFECTS ON DIAGNOSTIC TESTS
Immunization with Lyme disease vaccine may cause a false-positive enzyme-linked immunosorbent assay (ELISA) result for *B. burgdorferi* in the absence of infection. Therefore, it's important to perform Western blot testing if ELISA test is positive or equivocal in vaccinated persons being evaluated for suspected Lyme disease.

### CONTRAINDICATIONS
Contraindicated in patients with hypersensitivity to vaccine or its components. Don't administer vaccine to patients outside indicated age range or to those with treatment-resistant Lyme arthritis (antibiotic refractory) or moderate to severe febrile illness.

### NURSING CONSIDERATIONS
• Use cautiously in patients who may be allergic to the natural rubber packaging for the prefilled syringe. Note that packaging for vial doesn't contain rubber.

---

Reactions may be *common,* uncommon, ***life-threatening,*** or COMMON AND LIFE-THREATENING.

• Use with caution in breast-feeding women because it's unknown whether vaccine appears in breast milk.
• Vaccine is a preventive measure, not a treatment for Lyme disease.
• Before immunization, review patient's history for possible vaccine sensitivity, allergies, previous vaccination-related adverse reactions, and occurrence of adverse event–related signs and symptoms. Epinephrine injection and other drugs appropriate for controlling immediate allergic reactions must be readily available.
• Immunization against Lyme disease is appropriate in persons who live or work in, travel to, or pursue recreational activities in *B. burgdorferi*–infected grassy or wooded areas.
• Patients with a history of Lyme disease may benefit from vaccination because previous infection with *B. burgdorferi* may not provide protective immunity.
• As with other vaccines, Lyme disease vaccine may not protect everyone.
• Refrigerate vaccine between 36° and 46° F (2° and 8° C). Don't freeze; discard if product has been frozen.
• Shake well before use. Inspect visually for particulates or discoloration before administering. With thorough agitation, Lyme disease vaccine is a turbid, white suspension. Discard if it appears otherwise.
• Use vaccine as supplied, without diluting or reconstituting it. The full, recommended dose of the vaccine should be used. Discard vaccine remaining in single-dose vial.
• Lyme disease vaccine should be administered I.M. in deltoid region. Don't administer I.V., I.D., or S.C.
• As with other I.M. injections, vaccine shouldn't be given to persons taking anticoagulants or who have clotting disorders, unless potential benefit clearly outweighs risk.
• No information is available on immune response to Lyme disease vaccine when administered with other vaccines. When vaccine must be given with other vaccines, each should be given with a different syringe and at a different injection site.

• Register pregnant women who receive Lyme disease vaccine by calling Smith-Kline Beecham Pharmaceuticals at 1-800-366-8900, ext. 5231.

☑ **Patient teaching**
• Inform patient that vaccine prevents, not treats, Lyme disease.
• As with other vaccines, inform patient that Lyme disease vaccine may not protect everyone.
• Inform patient of benefits and risks of immunization with vaccine and of importance of completing all three vaccinations several weeks before start of *B. burgdorferi* season in his geographic area.
• Tell patient to report adverse effects.
• Advise patient to take standard preventive measures, such as wearing long-sleeved shirts and long pants, tucking pants into socks, treating clothing with tick repellent, and checking for and removing ticks when in endemic areas.
• Show patient the appropriate way to remove ticks, such as using fine-pointed tweezers and not squeezing the tick before withdrawal.
• Advise patient to notify doctor of immunization with vaccine because it may interfere with laboratory diagnosis of Lyme disease.

## measles, mumps, and rubella virus vaccine, live
### M-M-R II

*Pregnancy Risk Category C*

### HOW SUPPLIED
*Injection:* single-dose vial containing not less than 1,000 $TCID_{50}$ (tissue culture infective doses) of attenuated measles virus derived from Enders' attenuated Edmonston strain (grown in chick embryo culture), 20,000 $TCID_{50}$ of the Jeryl Lynn (B level) mumps strain (grown in chick embryo culture), and 1,000 $TCID_{50}$ of the Wistar RA 27/3 strain of rubella virus (propagated in human diploid cell culture) per 0.5-ml dose. Multidose vial available to institutions or government agencies

---

## ACTION
Promotes immunity to measles, mumps, and rubella virus by inducing production of antibodies.

| Route | Onset | Peak | Duration |
|-------|-------|------|----------|
| S.C. | Unknown | Unknown | < 11 yr |

## INDICATIONS & DOSAGE
*Routine immunization—*
**Adults:** one vial S.C. Patients born after 1957 should receive two doses at least 1 month apart.
**Children:** one vial S.C. A two-dose schedule is recommended, with first dose given at 15 months (12 months in high-risk areas) and second dose given either at ages 4 to 6 or 11 or 12.

## ADVERSE REACTIONS
**GI:** diarrhea.
**Musculoskeletal:** arthritis, arthralgia.
**Skin:** rash, erythema at injection site, urticaria.
**Other:** fever, regional lymphadenopathy, *anaphylaxis.*

## INTERACTIONS
**Drug-drug.** *Immune serum globulin, plasma, whole blood:* antibodies in serum may interfere with immune response. Don't use vaccine within 3 to 11 months of these products, depending on dose of antibody or blood given.
*Immunosuppressants:* may decrease immune response to vaccine. Monitor closely.

## EFFECTS ON DIAGNOSTIC TESTS
Vaccine may temporarily decrease response to tuberculin skin testing.

## CONTRAINDICATIONS
Contraindicated in immunosuppressed patients; in those with cancer, blood dyscrasia, gamma globulin disorders, fever, active untreated tuberculosis, or anaphylactic or anaphylactoid reactions to neomycin or eggs; in those receiving corticosteroid or radiation therapy; and in pregnant women.

## NURSING CONSIDERATIONS
• Obtain history of allergies, especially anaphylactic reactions to antibiotics, or reaction to immunization.

• Keep epinephrine 1:1,000 available to treat anaphylaxis.
• If skin test is needed, administer it either before or simultaneously with vaccine.
• Inject into outer aspect of upper arm with a 25G 5/8-inch needle. Don't give I.V.
• Use only diluent supplied. Discard 8 hours after reconstituting.
• Refrigerate vaccine; protect from light. Solution may be used if red, pink, or yellow, but must be clear.
• Risk of adverse effects is low (0.5% to 4%).
• Treat fever with antipyretics such as acetaminophen.
• Presence of maternal antibodies may prevent response in children under age 12 months.
• The Immunization Practices Advisory Committee recommends that colleges, other post–high school educational institutions, and medical institutions employing health care providers obtain documentation of receipt of two doses of vaccine after age 1 (or other evidence of immunity, such as infection, documented by doctor). Combined measles, mumps, and rubella vaccine is preferred.
• *Alert:* The Centers for Disease Control and Prevention recommends that, during a measles outbreak in a health care facility, susceptible personnel exposed to measles virus (whether or not they received measles vaccine or immunoglobulin) avoid patient contact for days 5 through 21 after such exposure. If personnel become ill, they should avoid patient contact for at least 7 days after developing rash.

### ✓ Patient teaching
• Warn patient or parents about adverse reactions associated with vaccine.
• Review immunization schedule with parents, and stress importance of receiving second injection at the appropriate time to maintain immunization.
• Tell woman of childbearing age to use measures to prevent pregnancy until 3 months after immunization.
• Febrile seizures have rarely occurred in children postvaccination. Tell parents to treat and promptly report fever, especially in patient with family history of seizures.

# measles and rubella virus vaccine, live attenuated
M-R-Vax II

*Pregnancy Risk Category C*

## HOW SUPPLIED
*Injection:* single-dose vial containing not less than 1,000 $TCID_{50}$ (tissue culture infective doses) per 0.5 ml of attenuated measles virus derived from Enders' attenuated Edmonston strain (grown in chick embryo culture); 1,000 $TCID_{50}$ of the Wistar RA 27/3 strain of rubella virus

## ACTION
Promotes immunity to measles and rubella virus by inducing production of antibodies.

| Route | Onset | Peak | Duration |
|-------|-------|------|----------|
| S.C. | Unknown | Unknown | < 11 yr |

## INDICATIONS & DOSAGE
*Immunization—*
**Adults and children ages 15 months and older:** 0.5 ml (1,000 U) S.C.

## ADVERSE REACTIONS
**Musculoskeletal:** arthralgia.
**Skin:** rash; *burning, stinging at injection site.*
**Other:** fever, lymphadenopathy, ***anaphylaxis.***

## INTERACTIONS
**Drug-drug.** *Immune serum globulin, plasma, whole blood:* antibodies in serum may interfere with immune response. Don't use vaccine within 3 months of transfusion.
*Immunosuppressants:* may reduce immune response to vaccine. Monitor closely.

## EFFECTS ON DIAGNOSTIC TESTS
Vaccine may temporarily decrease response to tuberculin skin testing.

## CONTRAINDICATIONS
Contraindicated in immunosuppressed patients; in those with cancer, blood dyscrasia, gamma globulin disorders, fever, active untreated tuberculosis, or anaphylactic or anaphylactoid reactions to eggs or neomycin; in those receiving corticosteroid or radiation therapy; and in pregnant women.

## NURSING CONSIDERATIONS
• Obtain history of allergies, especially anaphylactic reactions to antibiotics.
• Keep epinephrine 1:1,000 available to treat anaphylaxis.
• If skin test is needed, administer it either before or simultaneously with vaccine.
• Use only diluent supplied. Discard 8 hours after reconstituting.
• Inject into outer upper arm. Don't inject I.V.
• Store in refrigerator and protect from light. Reconstituted solution should be clear yellow.
• *Alert:* Vaccine shouldn't be given within 1 month of other live virus vaccines, except oral poliovirus vaccine. Immunization should be deferred in patients with acute illness.
• Allow at least 3 weeks between BCG and rubella vaccines.

### ✅ Patient teaching
• Warn patient or parents about adverse reactions associated with vaccine.
• Caution woman of childbearing age to avoid pregnancy until 3 months post-immunization.
• Advise use of antipyretics to control fever.

# measles virus vaccine, live attenuated
Attenuvax

*Pregnancy Risk Category C*

## HOW SUPPLIED
*Injection:* single-dose vial containing not less than 1,000 $TCID_{50}$ (tissue culture infective doses) of measles virus derived from the more attenuated line of Enders' attenuated Edmonston strain (grown in chick embryo culture). Available in 10- and 50-dose vials

---

## ACTION

Promotes immunity to measles virus by inducing production of antibodies.

| Route | Onset | Peak | Duration |
|-------|-------|------|----------|
| S.C. | Few days | Unknown | ≥ 13 yr |

## INDICATIONS & DOSAGE

*Immunization—*

**Adults and children ages 15 months and older:** 0.5 ml (1,000 U) S.C. A two-dose schedule is recommended, with first dose given at 15 months (12 months in high-risk areas) and second dose given at ages 4 to 6 or 11 or 12.

*Measles outbreak control—*

**Adults:** school personnel born in or after 1957 should be revaccinated if they lack evidence of measles immunity. If outbreak is in a medical facility, all workers born in or after 1957 should be revaccinated if they lack evidence of immunity.

**Children:** if cases occur in children under age 1, children should be vaccinated as young as age 6 months. All students and siblings should be revaccinated if they lack documentation of measles immunity.

## ADVERSE REACTIONS

**CNS:** *febrile seizures in susceptible children.*

**GI:** anorexia.

**Hematologic:** *leukopenia, thrombocytopenia.*

**Skin:** rash, erythema, swelling, tenderness at injection site.

**Other:** fever, lymphadenopathy, *anaphylaxis.*

## INTERACTIONS

**Drug-drug.** *Immune serum globulin, plasma, whole blood:* antibodies in serum may interfere with immune response. Don't use vaccine for at least 3 months after administration of these products.

## EFFECTS ON DIAGNOSTIC TESTS

Vaccine may temporarily decrease response to tuberculin skin test.

## CONTRAINDICATIONS

Contraindicated in immunosuppressed patients; in those with cancer, blood dyscrasia, gamma globulin disorders, fever, active untreated tuberculosis, or anaphylactic or anaphylactoid reactions to neomycin or eggs; in those receiving corticosteroid or radiation therapy; and in pregnant women.

## NURSING CONSIDERATIONS

• Obtain history of allergies, especially anaphylactic reactions to antibiotics, or reaction to immunization. Immunization should be deferred in patients with acute illness or after administration of blood or plasma.

• Keep epinephrine 1:1,000 available to treat anaphylaxis.

• If skin test is needed, administer it either before or simultaneously with vaccine.

• Use only diluent supplied. Discard 8 hours after reconstituting.

• Don't give vaccine I.V.

• Vaccine may be given with oral poliovirus vaccine.

• The Immunization Practices Advisory Committee recommends that colleges, other post–high school educational institutions, and medical institutions employing health care providers obtain documentation of receipt of two doses of vaccine after age 1 (or other evidence of immunity, such as infection, documented by doctor). Combined measles, mumps, and rubella vaccine is preferred.

• Don't give vaccine within 3 months of receiving blood or plasma transfusion or human immune serum globulin.

• *Alert:* The Centers for Disease Control and Prevention recommends that during a measles outbreak in a health care facility, susceptible personnel exposed to the measles virus (whether or not they received measles vaccine or immune globulin) avoid patient contact for days 5 through 21 after such exposure. If personnel become ill, they should avoid patient contact for at least 7 days after developing rash.

• If attenuated measles vaccine is administered immediately after exposure to the disease, some protection may be provided. This level of protection is significantly increased if vaccine is administered even a few days before exposure.

---

Reactions may be *common*, uncommon, *life-threatening*, or COMMON AND LIFE-THREATENING.

### ☑ Patient teaching
• Warn patient or parents about adverse reactions associated with vaccine.
• Review immunization schedule with patient or parents and stress importance of receiving second injection at appropriate time.
• Stress importance of avoiding pregnancy for 3 months after vaccination. Provide contraception information, if needed.

## meningococcal polysaccharide vaccine
Menomune-A/C/Y/W-135

*Pregnancy Risk Category C*

### HOW SUPPLIED
*Injection:* 1-dose, 10-dose, and 50-dose vials with vial of diluent

### ACTION
Promotes active immunity to meningitis.

| Route | Onset | Peak | Duration |
|-------|-------|------|----------|
| S.C. | Unknown | Unknown | 3 yr |

### INDICATIONS & DOSAGE
*Meningococcal meningitis prophylaxis—*
**Adults and children ages 2 and older:**
0.5 ml S.C.

### ADVERSE REACTIONS
**CNS:** headache, malaise.
**Musculoskeletal:** muscle cramps.
**Skin:** *pain, tenderness, erythema, induration at injection site.*
**Other:** chills, fever, ***anaphylaxis,*** mild lymphadenopathy.

### INTERACTIONS
**Drug-drug.** *Immunosuppressants:* may reduce immune response to vaccine. Monitor closely.

### EFFECTS ON DIAGNOSTIC TESTS
None reported.

### CONTRAINDICATIONS
Contraindicated in patients with hypersensitivity to thimerosal or other vaccine components; also contraindicated in pregnant women. Defer vaccination in patients with acute illness. Vaccine isn't contraindicated in immunocompromised patients.

### NURSING CONSIDERATIONS
• Obtain history of allergies and reaction to immunization.
• Keep epinephrine 1:1,000 available to treat anaphylaxis.
• Don't give I.V, I.M., or I.D.
• Vaccine may be given with other immunizations.
• Routine vaccination isn't recommended. Vaccine should be reserved for persons at risk, such as those who live in or are traveling to epidemic or highly endemic areas, household or institutional contacts of meningococcal disease as an adjunct to appropriate antibiotic chemoprophylaxis, medical and laboratory personnel at risk for exposure to meningococcal disease, patients with terminal complement component deficiency, and those with anatomic or functional asplenia.
• Reconstitute vaccine only with supplied diluent.
• Some doctors will revaccinate children if they are at high risk and if they previously received vaccine before age 4.
• Don't give vaccine within 3 months of receiving blood or plasma transfusion or human immune serum globulin administration.

### ☑ Patient teaching
• Warn patient or parents about adverse reactions associated with vaccine.
• Stress importance of avoiding pregnancy for 3 months after vaccination. Provide contraception information, if needed.
• Advise correct acetaminophen dose to control fever.

## mumps virus vaccine, live
Mumpsvax

*Pregnancy Risk Category C*

### HOW SUPPLIED
*Injection:* single-dose vial containing not less than 20,000 $TCID_{50}$ (tissue culture infective doses) of attenuated mumps virus derived from Jeryl Lynn mumps strain

---

(grown in chick embryo culture) per 0.5 ml and vial of diluent; single-dose vial containing not less than 5,000 $TCID_{50}$ of the U.S. Reference Mumps Virus in each 0.5 ml†.

## ACTION
Promotes active immunity to mumps.

| Route | Onset | Peak | Duration |
|-------|-------|------|----------|
| S.C. | Unknown | Unknown | > 15 yr |

## INDICATIONS & DOSAGE
*Immunization—*
**Adults and children ages 1 and older:**
0.5 ml (20,000 U) S.C.

    Although not recommended in children under age 12 months, children vaccinated when under 12 months should be revaccinated.

## ADVERSE REACTIONS
**CNS:** malaise.
**GI:** diarrhea.
**Skin:** rash, injection site reaction.
**Other:** *anaphylaxis, slight fever,* mild allergic reactions, mild lymphadenopathy.

## INTERACTIONS
**Drug-drug.** *Immune serum globulin, plasma, whole blood:* antibodies in serum may interfere with immune response. Don't use vaccine for at least 3 months after administration of these products.

## EFFECTS ON DIAGNOSTIC TESTS
Vaccine may temporarily decrease response to tuberculin skin test.

## CONTRAINDICATIONS
Contraindicated in immunosuppressed patients; in those with cancer, blood dyscrasia, gamma globulin disorders, fever, untreated active tuberculosis, or anaphylactic or anaphylactoid reactions to neomycin or eggs; in those receiving corticosteroid or radiation therapy; and in pregnant women.

## NURSING CONSIDERATIONS
• Obtain history of allergies, especially anaphylactic reactions to antibiotics, and reaction to immunization. Defer use in patients with acute or febrile illness and for at least 3 months after transfusions or treatment with immune serum globulin.
• Keep epinephrine 1:1,000 available to treat anaphylaxis.
• If skin test is needed, administer it either before or simultaneously with vaccine.
• Use only diluent supplied. Discard 8 hours after reconstituting.
• Use a 25G ⅝-inch needle to inject.
• Don't give vaccine I.V.
• Refrigerate and protect from light. Reconstituted solution is clear yellow; don't use if discolored.
• Don't give vaccine less than 1 month before or after immunization with other live virus vaccines; however, trivalent live, oral poliovirus vaccine may be administered simultaneously.
• Administer to asymptomatic HIV-infected children.
• Vaccine isn't recommended for infants under age 12 months because retained maternal mumps antibodies may interfere with immune response.
• Don't use for delayed hypersensitivity (allergy) skin testing. Use mumps skin-test antigen, a killed viral product.

☑ **Patient teaching**
• Warn patient or parents about adverse reactions associated with vaccine.
• Stress importance of avoiding pregnancy for 3 months after vaccination. Provide contraception information, if needed.
• Tell patient to treat fever with antipyretics.

---

## plague vaccine

*Pregnancy Risk Category C*

## HOW SUPPLIED
*Injection:* 1.8 to 2.2 billion killed plague bacilli (*Yersinia pestis*)/ml in 20-ml vials

## ACTION
Promotes active immunity to plague caused by *Y. pestis.*

| Route | Onset | Peak | Duration |
|-------|-------|------|----------|
| I.M. | Unknown | Unknown | 6-12 mo |

## INDICATIONS & DOSAGE
*Primary immunization and booster—*
**Adults:** 1 ml I.M.; then 0.2 ml in 4 to 12 weeks, followed by 0.2 ml 5 to 6 months after second dose. Booster is 0.1 to 0.2 ml q 6 months while in plague area. After 3 boosters, use 1- to 2-year booster cycle.
**Children:** Centers for Disease Control and Prevention doesn't recommend vaccination because data are insufficient in persons below age 18.

## ADVERSE REACTIONS
**CNS:** headache, malaise.
**GI:** nausea, vomiting.
**Musculoskeletal:** arthralgia, myalgia.
**Other:** *slight fever, lymphadenopathy, anaphylaxis,* leukocytosis, swelling, *induration, erythema, tenderness at injection site.*

## INTERACTIONS
**Drug-drug.** *Anticoagulants:* increased risk of bleeding. Administer with caution. *Cholera, typhoid vaccine:* increased risk of adverse effects. Don't give at same time.

## EFFECTS ON DIAGNOSTIC TESTS
None reported.

## CONTRAINDICATIONS
Contraindicated in immunosuppressed patients; in those with hypersensitivity to beef, soy, casein, phenol, sulfite, or formaldehyde; and in pregnant women. Patients who have had severe local or systemic reactions to plague vaccine shouldn't be revaccinated. Also contraindicated in patients with severe thrombocytopenia or other coagulation disorders that would contraindicate I.M. injections.

## NURSING CONSIDERATIONS
• Obtain history of allergies and reaction to immunization. Immunization should be deferred in patients with respiratory infection.
• Keep epinephrine 1:1,000 available to treat anaphylaxis.
• Inject into the deltoid area, the preferred site.

• Vaccination is recommended for all laboratory and field personnel working with *Y. pestis.*

### ☑ Patient teaching
• Warn patient about adverse reactions associated with vaccine.
• Caution woman of childbearing age to notify doctor of suspected pregnancy before administration.
• Tell patient to treat fever with appropriate acetaminophen dose.

# pneumococcal vaccine, polyvalent
Pneumovax 23, Pnu-Imune 23

*Pregnancy Risk Category C*

## HOW SUPPLIED
*Injection:* 25 mcg each of 23 polysaccharide isolates/0.5 ml

## ACTION
Promotes active immunity to infections caused by *Streptococcus pneumoniae.*

| Route | Onset | Peak | Duration |
|-------|-------|------|----------|
| I.M., S.C. | 2-3 wk | Unknown | 5 yr |

## INDICATIONS & DOSAGE
*Pneumococcal immunization—*
**Adults and children ages 2 and older:** 0.5 ml I.M. or S.C.

## ADVERSE REACTIONS
**Musculoskeletal:** myalgia, arthralgia.
**Skin:** injection site rash; *injection site soreness,* severe local reaction associated with revaccination within 3 years.
**Other:** *anaphylaxis,* slight fever.

## INTERACTIONS
**Drug-drug.** *Immunosuppressants:* may reduce immune response to vaccine. Monitor closely.

## EFFECTS ON DIAGNOSTIC TESTS
None reported.

---

## CONTRAINDICATIONS

Contraindicated in patients with hypersensitivity to drug or its components (phenol) and in those with Hodgkin's disease who have received extensive chemotherapy or nodal irradiation. Defer use in patients with acute respiratory distress syndrome.

## NURSING CONSIDERATIONS

• Vaccine isn't recommended for children under age 2.
• Check immunization history to avoid revaccination within 3 years.
• Obtain history of allergies and reaction to immunization. Eggs and egg protein aren't used during the manufacture of vaccine; contains phenol as a preservative.
• Keep epinephrine 1:1,000 available to treat anaphylaxis.
• Inject in deltoid or midlateral thigh. Don't inject I.V or I.D.
• When splenectomy is being considered, vaccine should be given at least 2 weeks before procedure to ensure adequate antibody response. Vaccine may be less effective in splenectomized patients.
• Vaccine protects against 23 pneumococcal types, accounting for 90% of pneumococcal disease.
• Vaccine may be administered to children ages 2 and older to prevent pneumococcal otitis media, although the Centers for Disease Control and Prevention doesn't recommend otitis media as an indicator for vaccine.
• Vaccine is recommended for all adults over age 65.
• Administration with influenza virus vaccine is safe and effective.

### ☑ Patient teaching

• Warn patient about adverse reactions associated with vaccine.
• Tell patient to treat fever with mild antipyretics and local site reaction with cold compresses.
• Warn patient with idiopathic thrombocytopenic purpura that there is possibility of relapse 2 to 14 days after vaccination.

## poliovirus vaccine, live, oral, trivalent (TOPV)
Orimune

## poliovirus vaccine, inactivated (IPV)
IPOL

*Pregnancy Risk Category C*

## HOW SUPPLIED

*Oral vaccine:* mixture of three live viruses (types 1, 2, and 3), grown in monkey kidney tissue culture; in 0.5-ml single-dose Dispettes
*Inactivated virus vaccine injection:* mixture of three types of poliovirus (types 1, 2, and 3) grown in tissue culture. IPOL uses monkey kidney cultures; Poliovax uses human diploid cell cultures. IPV comes in 0.5-ml prefilled syringes

## ACTION

Promotes immunity to poliomyelitis by inducing humoral antibodies and antibodies in the lymphatic tissue.

| Route | Onset | Peak | Duration |
|-------|-------|------|----------|
| P.O. | 7-10 days | 21 days | Yrs |
| S.C. | Unknown | Unknown | Yrs |

## INDICATIONS & DOSAGE

*Poliovirus immunization (IPV)—*
**Adults:** 0.5 ml S.C.; then second dose in 4 to 8 weeks. A third dose is given in 6 to 12 months.
**Children:** 0.5 ml S.C. at 2 and 4 months. A third dose is given at 15 to 18 months. A reinforcing dose of 0.5 ml S.C. should be given before entry into school at ages 4 to 6.

## ADVERSE REACTIONS

**CNS:** sleepiness.
**GI:** decreased appetite.
**Skin:** injection site erythema, induration, *pain.*
**Other:** *poliomyelitis—TOPV only,* fever, crying, **hypersensitivity reaction.**

## INTERACTIONS

**Drug-drug.** *Immune serum globulin, plasma, whole blood:* antibodies in serum

may interfere with immune response. Don't use vaccine within 3 months of transfusion.
*Immunosuppressants:* may reduce immune response to vaccine. Monitor closely.

**EFFECTS ON DIAGNOSTIC TESTS**
Vaccine may temporarily decrease response to tuberculin skin test.

**CONTRAINDICATIONS**
Oral vaccine is contraindicated in immunosuppressed patients; in those with cancer or immunoglobulin abnormalities; in those receiving radiation, antimetabolite, alkylating drug, or corticosteroid therapy; and in those who have a household contact who fits one of these preceding categories. These patients should receive IPV. Injectable vaccine is contraindicated in patients with hypersensitivity to neomycin, streptomycin, or polymyxin B.

**NURSING CONSIDERATIONS**
• TOPV is no longer recommended for routine immunization schedule. Special circumstances when oral vaccine would be appropriate include: imminent travel to a polio-endemic area, "catch-up" immunization, or when a parent objects to number of injections a child needs to receive.
• Don't use TOPV in siblings of child with known immunodeficiency syndrome; IPV is preferred.
• Obtain history of allergies and reaction to immunization.
• If skin test is needed, administer it either before or simultaneously with vaccine
• Keep TOPV frozen until used. Once thawed, if unopened, may refrigerate up to 30 days; if opened, up to 7 days. Thaw before administration.
• Color change of TOPV from pink to yellow has no effect on efficacy of vaccine. Yellow color is caused by storage at low temperatures.
• *Alert:* Parenteral form should be administered to immunodeficient patients or those with altered immune status because they may be at risk for developing the disease if live virus vaccine is administered.
• Keep epinephrine 1:1,000 available to treat anaphylaxis.

• Oral vaccine should be deferred in patients with vomiting or diarrhea. Both forms of vaccine should be deferred in patients with acute illness.
• Don't administer to neonates under age 6 weeks.
• Highest risk of poliovirus infection occurs after first dose of oral vaccine.
• Adults at high risk for exposure who have completed a primary course may receive another dose.
• Vaccine isn't effective in modifying or preventing existing or incubating poliomyelitis.
• Document manufacturer, lot number, date given, and name, address, and title of person administering on patient record or log.

☑ **Patient teaching**
• Instruct patient or parents about risks and benefits of vaccine before administration.
• Warn patient or parents about adverse reactions associated with vaccine.

---

**rabies vaccine, adsorbed**

*Pregnancy Risk Category C*

**HOW SUPPLIED**
*Injection:* single dose 1-ml vial

**ACTION**
Promotes active immunity to rabies.

| Route | Onset | Peak | Duration |
|-------|-------|------|----------|
| I.M. | Unknown | 2 wk after 3 doses | Unknown |

**INDICATIONS & DOSAGE**
*Preexposure prophylaxis rabies immunization for persons in high-risk groups—*
**Adults and children:** 1 ml I.M. at 0, 7, and 21 or 28 days for total of three injections. Patients at increased risk for rabies should be checked q 6 months and given booster vaccination, 1 ml I.M, p.r.n., to maintain adequate serum titer (about q 2 to 5 years based on antibody titers).
*Postexposure rabies prophylaxis—*
**Adults and children not previously vaccinated against rabies:** 20 IU/kg doses

of human rabies immune globulin (HRIG) I.M. and five 1-ml injections of rabies vaccine, adsorbed I.M. given on days 0, 3, 7, 14, and 28.
**Adults and children previously vaccinated against rabies:** two 1-ml injections of rabies vaccine, adsorbed I.M. given on days 0 and 3. HRIG shouldn't be given.

## ADVERSE REACTIONS
**CNS:** *headache, dizziness, fatigue.*
**GI:** *abdominal pain, nausea.*
**Musculoskeletal:** *myalgia,* aching of injected muscle.
**Skin:** *transient pain, erythema, swelling, itching,* mild inflammatory reaction at injection site.
**Other:** *slight fever,* reaction resembling serum sickness, ***anaphylaxis.***

## INTERACTIONS
**Drug-drug.** *Antimalarials, corticosteroids, immunosuppressants:* decreased response to rabies vaccine. Avoid concomitant use.

## EFFECTS ON DIAGNOSTIC TESTS
None reported.

## CONTRAINDICATIONS
Contraindicated in patients who have experienced life-threatening allergic reactions to previous injections of vaccine or to components of vaccine, including thimerosal.

## NURSING CONSIDERATIONS
• Use cautiously in patients with hypersensitivity to monkey-derived proteins, in those with history of non-life-threatening allergic reactions to previous injections of vaccine, and in children.
• Keep epinephrine 1:1,000 available to treat anaphylaxis.
• Administer as I.M. injection into deltoid region in adults and older children. For younger children, the midanterolateral aspect of the thigh also is acceptable. Don't use I.D. route. Take care not to inject vaccine near a peripheral nerve or into adipose or subcutaneous tissue.
• Vaccine is normally a light pink color because of presence of phenol red in suspension.

• **Alert:** If patient experiences serious adverse reaction to vaccine, report reaction promptly to manufacturer: Michigan Department of Public Health, 517-335-8050 during working hours or 517-335-9030 at other times.
• **Alert:** Don't confuse vaccine with rabies immune globulin. Both drugs may be given in some situations.

## ✅ Patient teaching
• Inform patient about adverse reactions associated with vaccine and importance of reporting serious adverse reactions to doctor.
• Caution patient not to perform hazardous activities if dizziness occurs.
• Advise proper antipyretic dose for fever.
• Teach proper wound care and signs and symptoms of infection.

# rabies vaccine, human diploid cell (HDCV)
Imovax Rabies, Imovax Rabies I.D.

*Pregnancy Risk Category C*

## HOW SUPPLIED
*I.M. injection:* 2.5 IU rabies antigen/ml, in single-dose vial with diluent
*I.D. injection:* 0.25 IU rabies antigen/dose

## ACTION
Promotes active immunity to rabies.

| Route | Onset | Peak | Duration |
|-------|-------|------|----------|
| I.M., I.D. | 1 wk | 1-2 mo | > 2 yr |

## INDICATIONS & DOSAGE
*Postexposure antirabies immunization—*
**Adults and children:** five 1-ml doses of HDCV I.M. (for example, in deltoid region). First dose given as soon as possible after exposure; an additional dose given on each of days 3, 7, 14, and 28 after first dose. If no antibody response after this primary series occurs, booster dose is recommended.
*Preexposure prophylaxis immunization for persons in high-risk groups—*
**Adults and children:** three 1-ml injections administered I.M. First dose given

on day 0 (first day of therapy), second dose on day 7, and third dose on either day 21 or 28. Or, 0.1 ml I.D. on same dosage schedule.

**ADVERSE REACTIONS**
**CNS:** *headache,* dizziness, *fatigue.*
**GI:** *nausea,* abdominal pain, diarrhea.
**Musculoskeletal:** muscle aches.
**Skin:** *injection site pain, erythema, swelling, itching.*
**Other:** *fever,* **anaphylaxis,** serum sickness.

**INTERACTIONS**
**Drug-drug.** *Antimalarials, corticosteroids, immunosuppressants:* decreased response to rabies vaccine. Avoid concomitant use.

**EFFECTS ON DIAGNOSTIC TESTS**
None reported.

**CONTRAINDICATIONS**
No contraindications reported for persons after exposure. An acute febrile illness contraindicates use of vaccine for persons previously exposed.

**NURSING CONSIDERATIONS**
• Use cautiously in patients with history of hypersensitivity.
• Keep epinephrine 1:1,000 available to treat anaphylaxis.
• Use vaccine immediately after reconstitution.
• *Alert:* Don't use I.D. route for postexposure rabies vaccination.
• Alternative regimen of 0.1-ml doses is only for preexposure prophylaxis. For postexposure prophylaxis, only use 1-ml doses.
• Be prepared to stop corticosteroid therapy during immunizing period unless therapy is essential for treatment of other conditions.
• Some patients who receive booster doses experience serum sickness–like hypersensitivity reactions. These reactions usually respond to antihistamines.
• All serious reactions should be reported to the State Department of Health.

• *Alert:* Don't confuse vaccine with rabies immune globulin. Both drugs may be given in some situations.

☑ **Patient teaching**
• Inform patient about adverse reactions associated with vaccine. Tell patient to report persistent or severe reactions to doctor.
• Stress importance of receiving booster, if appropriate for patient.
• Tell patient to treat mild reaction with anti-inflammatory or antipyretic at appropriate doses.

# rubella and mumps virus vaccine, live
Biavax II

*Pregnancy Risk Category C*

**HOW SUPPLIED**
*Injection:* single-dose vial containing not less than 1,000 $TCID_{50}$ (tissue culture infective doses) of Wistar RA 27/3 rubella virus (propagated in human diploid cell culture) and not less than 20,000 $TCID_{50}$ of Jeryl Lynn mumps strain (grown in chick embryo cell culture)

**ACTION**
Promotes immunity to rubella and mumps by inducing antibody production.

| Route | Onset | Peak | Duration |
|-------|-------|------|----------|
| S.C. | Unknown | Unknown | 10.5 yr |

**INDICATIONS & DOSAGE**
*Rubella and mumps immunization—*
**Adults and children ages 1 and older:** 0.5 ml S.C.

**ADVERSE REACTIONS**
**GI:** diarrhea.
**Musculoskeletal:** arthritis, arthralgia.
**Skin:** rash, pain, erythema, induration at injection site; thrombocytopenic purpura; urticaria.
**Other:** polyneuritis, fever, **anaphylaxis,** lymphadenopathy.

---

## INTERACTIONS
**Drug-drug.** *Immune serum globulin, plasma, whole blood:* antibodies in serum may interfere with immune response. Don't give vaccine for at least 3 months after use of these products.
*Immunosuppressants:* may reduce immune response to vaccine. Monitor closely.

## EFFECTS ON DIAGNOSTIC TESTS
Vaccine may temporarily decrease response to tuberculin skin test.

## CONTRAINDICATIONS
Contraindicated in immunosuppressed patients; in those with cancer, blood dyscrasia, gamma globulin disorders, fever, active untreated tuberculosis, or history of anaphylaxis or anaphylactoid reactions to neomycin or eggs; in those receiving corticosteroid (except those receiving corticosteroids as replacement therapy) or radiation therapy; and in pregnant women.

## NURSING CONSIDERATIONS
• Obtain history of allergies, especially anaphylactic reaction to antibiotics, and reaction to immunization.
• Keep epinephrine 1:1,000 available to treat anaphylaxis.
• If skin test is needed, administer it either before or simultaneously with vaccine.
• Vaccination should be deferred in patients with acute illness and after administration of immune serum globulin, blood, or plasma.
• Use only diluent supplied. Discard 8 hours after reconstituting.
• Inject into outer upper arm. Don't inject I.V.
• Allow an interval of at least 3 weeks between BCG and rubella vaccines.
• Document drug manufacturer, lot number, date, and name, address, and title of person administering dose on patient record or log.
• Patients born before 1956 are believed to have naturally acquired immunity.

### ☑ Patient teaching
• Inform patient about adverse reactions associated with vaccine.

• Stress importance of avoiding pregnancy for 3 months after vaccination. Provide contraception information, if needed.
• Inform woman over age 12 of risk of self-limited arthralgia or arthritis occurring 2 to 4 weeks postvaccination.

## rubella virus vaccine, live attenuated (RA 27/3)
Meruvax II

*Pregnancy Risk Category C*

## HOW SUPPLIED
*Injection:* single-dose vial containing not less than 1,000 $TCID_{50}$ (tissue culture infective doses) of Wistar RA 27/3 strain of rubella virus (propagated in human diploid cell culture)

## ACTION
Promotes immunity to rubella by inducing production of antibodies.

| Route | Onset | Peak | Duration |
|-------|-------|------|----------|
| S.C. | 2-6 wk | Unknown | > 10 yr |

## INDICATIONS & DOSAGE
*Rubella immunization—*
**Adults and children ages 1 and older:** 0.5 ml (1,000 U) S.C.

## ADVERSE REACTIONS
**CNS:** headache, malaise.
**EENT:** sore throat.
**Musculoskeletal:** arthralgia, arthritis.
**Skin:** rash, pain, erythema, induration at injection site; thrombocytopenic purpura; urticaria.
**Other:** polyneuritis, fever, *anaphylaxis,* lymphadenopathy.

## INTERACTIONS
**Drug-drug.** *Immune serum globulin, plasma, whole blood:* antibodies in serum may interfere with immune response. Don't use vaccine for at least 3 months after use of these products.
*Immunosuppressants, interferon:* may reduce immune response to vaccine. Monitor closely.

---

## EFFECTS ON DIAGNOSTIC TESTS
Vaccine may temporarily decrease response to tuberculin skin test.

## CONTRAINDICATIONS
Contraindicated in immunosuppressed patients; in those with cancer, blood dyscrasia, gamma globulin disorders, fever, active untreated tuberculosis, or history of hypersensitivity to neomycin; in patients receiving corticosteroids (except those receiving corticosteroids as replacement therapy) or radiation therapy; and in pregnant women. Don't vaccinate patients who have AIDS or symptomatic HIV.

## NURSING CONSIDERATIONS
• Obtain history of allergies and reaction to immunization.
• Keep epinephrine 1:1,000 available to treat anaphylaxis.
• If skin test is needed, administer it either before or simultaneously with vaccine.
• Immunization should be deferred in patients with acute illness and after administration of human immune serum globulin, blood, or plasma.
• Use only diluent supplied. Discard 8 hours after reconstituting. Protect from light.
• Inject into outer upper arm. Don't inject vaccine I.V.
• Document drug manufacturer, lot number, date, and name, address, and title of person administering dose on patient record or log.
• Allow at least 3 weeks between BCG and rubella vaccines.

☑ **Patient teaching**
• Inform patient about adverse reactions associated with vaccine.
• Stress importance of avoiding pregnancy for 3 months after vaccination. Provide contraception information, if needed.
• Tell patient to use correct dose of antipyretic for treating fever.

# tetanus toxoid, adsorbed

# tetanus toxoid, fluid

*Pregnancy Risk Category C*

## HOW SUPPLIED
**tetanus toxoid, adsorbed**
*Injection:* 5 to 10 Lf (limit flocculation) units inactivated tetanus/0.5-ml dose, in 0.5-ml syringes and 5-ml vials
**tetanus toxoid, fluid**
*Injection:* 4 to 5 Lf units inactivated tetanus/0.5-ml dose, in 0.5-ml syringes and 7.5-ml vials

## ACTION
Promotes immunity to tetanus by inducing antitoxin production.

| Route | Onset | Peak | Duration |
|-------|-------|------|----------|
| I.M., S.C. | After 2 doses | Unknown | > 10 yr |

## INDICATIONS & DOSAGE
*Primary immunization—*
**Adults and children ages 6 and older:** 0.5 ml (adsorbed) I.M. 4 to 8 weeks apart for two doses; then third dose given 6 to 12 months after second. Or, 0.5 ml (fluid) I.M. or S.C. 4 to 8 weeks apart for three doses; then fourth dose of 0.5 ml 6 to 12 months after third dose.
**Children ages 6 weeks to 6 years:** 0.5 ml (adsorbed) I.M. at ages 2, 4, and 6 months. A fourth dose is given at 15 to 18 months. A fifth dose is given at ages 4 to 6, just before entry into school, if indicated.
*Booster doses—*
**Adults:** 0.5 ml I.M. at 10-year intervals.

## ADVERSE REACTIONS
**CNS:** headache, *seizures,* malaise, encephalopathy.
**CV:** tachycardia, hypotension, flushing.
**Musculoskeletal:** aches, pains.
**Skin:** erythema, induration, nodule at injection site; urticaria; pruritus.
**Other:** slight fever, chills, *anaphylaxis.*

---

*Liquid contains alcohol.    **May contain tartrazine.    †Canada    ‡Australia    §U.K.    ◇OTC

## INTERACTIONS
**Drug-drug.** *Chloramphenicol:* may interfere with response to tetanus toxoid. Watch for effect.
*Cimetidine:* increased levels of tetanus toxoid. Monitor closely.
*Immunosuppressants, tetanus immune globulin:* may reduce immune response to vaccine. Monitor closely.

## EFFECTS ON DIAGNOSTIC TESTS
None reported.

## CONTRAINDICATIONS
Contraindicated in immunosuppressed patients and in those with immunoglobulin abnormalities or severe hypersensitivity or neurologic reactions to toxoid or its ingredients. Also contraindicated in patients with thrombocytopenia or other coagulation disorders that would contraindicate I.M. injection unless potential benefits outweigh risks. Defer vaccination in patients with acute illness and during polio outbreaks, except in emergencies.

## NURSING CONSIDERATIONS
• Use cautiously (adsorbed form) in infants or children with cerebral damage, neurologic disorders, or history of febrile seizures.
• Obtain history of allergies and reaction to immunization.
• Determine date of last tetanus immunization.
• Keep epinephrine 1:1,000 available to treat anaphylaxis.
• Adsorbed form produces longer duration of immunity. Fluid form provides quicker booster effect in patients actively immunized previously.
• Document manufacturer, lot number, date, and name, address, and title of person administering dose on patient record or log.
• *Alert:* Don't confuse drug with tetanus immune globulin, human. Both drugs may be given in some situations.

### ☑ Patient teaching
• Advise patient to avoid using hot or cold compresses at injection site; this may increase severity of local reaction.

• Instruct patient to report persistent or severe adverse reactions.
• Advise patient of proper antipyretic dose for fever reaction.
• Advise patient that nodule at injection site may be present for few weeks.

---

## typhoid vaccine, parenteral

## typhoid vaccine, oral
Vivotif Berna Vaccine

*Pregnancy Risk Category C*

## HOW SUPPLIED
*Injection:* suspension of killed Ty-2 strain of *Salmonella typhi;* 8 U/ml in 5- and 10-ml vials
*Capsules (enteric-coated):* 2 to $6 \times 10^9$ colony-forming U of viable *S. typhi* Ty21a and 5 to $50 \times 10^9$ bacterial cells of nonviable Ty21a2 (four doses of vaccine in a single package)

## ACTION
Provides active immunity to typhoid fever.

| Route | Onset | Peak | Duration |
|-------|-------|------|----------|
| P.O., S.C., I.D. | After last dose | Unknown | 3-5 yr |

## INDICATIONS & DOSAGE
*Primary immunization—*
**Adults:** one capsule P.O. on alternate days 1 hour before meals for four doses. Protocol repeated as booster q 5 years.
**Adults and children over age 10:** 0.5 ml S.C.; repeated in 4 weeks. Protocol repeated as booster q 3 years with either 0.5 ml S.C. or 0.1 ml I.D.
**Children ages 6 months to 10 years:** 0.25 ml S.C.; repeated in 4 weeks. Protocol repeated as booster q 3 years with either 0.25 ml S.C. or 0.1 ml I.D.

## ADVERSE REACTIONS
**CNS:** headache, malaise.
**GI:** nausea, abdominal cramps, vomiting.
**Musculoskeletal:** myalgia.
**Skin:** rash; urticaria; swelling, pain, inflammation at injection site; induration.
**Other:** *fever, anaphylaxis.*

---

Reactions may be *common*, uncommon, *life-threatening*, or COMMON AND LIFE-THREATENING.

## INTERACTIONS
**Drug-drug.** *Immunosuppressants, phenytoin, sulfonamides:* may impair antibody response. Don't use together.
*Other vaccines:* may increase adverse effects. Monitor closely.

## EFFECTS ON DIAGNOSTIC TESTS
None reported.

## CONTRAINDICATIONS
Contraindicated in patients with hypersensitivity to vaccine or its components and in immunosuppressed patients. Defer vaccination in patients with acute illness. Use parenteral, inactivated vaccine in HIV-positive patients.

## NURSING CONSIDERATIONS
• Obtain history of allergies and reaction to immunization. Keep epinephrine 1:1,000 available to treat anaphylaxis.
• Treat fever with antipyretics.
• Shake thoroughly before withdrawing from vial.
• Refrigerate vaccine at 36° to 46° F (2° to 8° C).

### ☑ Patient teaching
• When administering oral vaccine, ensure that patient understands importance of taking all four doses and following alternate-day regimen.
• Tell patient to take oral vaccine with cold or lukewarm water and not to chew or crush enteric-coated capsules. Capsules should be swallowed immediately.
• Tell patient to take oral vaccine 1 hour before meals.
• Inform patient about adverse reactions associated with vaccine; reactions usually appear within 24 hours and last 1 to 2 days.

## typhoid Vi polysaccharide vaccine
Typhim Vi

*Pregnancy Risk Category C*

## HOW SUPPLIED
*Injection:* 0.5-ml syringe, 20-dose vial, 50-dose vial

## ACTION
Promotes active immunity to typhoid fever.

| Route | Onset | Peak | Duration |
|-------|-------|------|----------|
| I.M. | 2 wk | Unknown | 2 yr |

## INDICATIONS & DOSAGE
*Active immunization against typhoid fever—*
**Adults and children ages 2 and older:** 0.5 ml I.M. as single dose. Reimmunization q 2 years with 0.5 ml I.M. as single dose, if needed.

## ADVERSE REACTIONS
**CNS:** *headache,* malaise.
**GI:** nausea, vomiting, abdominal cramps.
**Musculoskeletal:** myalgia.
**Skin:** *pain, tenderness, induration, erythema at injection site;* rash; urticaria.
**Other:** *anaphylaxis,* fever.

## INTERACTIONS
*Anticoagulants:* enhanced effect of anticoagulants. Check for bleeding.

## EFFECTS ON DIAGNOSTIC TESTS
None reported.

## CONTRAINDICATIONS
Contraindicated in patients with hypersensitivity to vaccine's components. Don't use vaccine to treat patients with typhoid fever; don't administer to those who are chronic typhoid carriers.

## NURSING CONSIDERATIONS
• Use cautiously in patients with thrombocytopenia or bleeding disorder and in those taking an anticoagulant; bleeding may occur following an I.M. injection in these patients.
• As with other vaccines, administration should be delayed, if possible, in patients with febrile illness.
• Although anaphylaxis is rare, keep epinephrine available to treat an anaphylactoid reaction.
• Administer as an I.M. injection into deltoid region in adults and into deltoid or vastus lateralis in children. Don't administer in gluteal region or areas where there

may be a nerve trunk. Never inject vaccine I.V.

• Record drug manufacturer, lot number, date, and name, address, and title of person administering dose on patient record or log.

☑ **Patient teaching**
• Advise patient to take all precautions needed to avoid contact with or ingestion of contaminated food and water.
• Inform patient that immunization should be given at least 2 weeks before expected exposure. Although an optimal reimmunization schedule hasn't been established, recommended reimmunization consists of single dose for U.S. travelers every 2 years if exposure to typhoid fever is possible.
• Inform patient about adverse reactions associated with vaccine.

---

## varicella virus vaccine
Varivax

*Pregnancy Risk Category C*

### HOW SUPPLIED
*Injection:* single-dose vial containing 1350 plague-forming units (PFU) of Oka/Merck varicella virus (live)

### ACTION
Prevents chickenpox by inducing production of antibodies to varicella-zoster virus.

| Route | Onset | Peak | Duration |
|-------|-------|------|----------|
| S.C. | 4-6 wk | Unknown | > 2 yr |

### INDICATIONS & DOSAGE
*Prevention of varicella-zoster (chickenpox) infections—*
**Adults and children ages 13 and older:** 0.5 ml S.C.; then second 0.5-ml dose 4 to 8 weeks later.
**Children ages 1 to 12:** 0.5 ml S.C.

### ADVERSE REACTIONS
**Skin:** swelling, redness, pain, rash, varicella-like rash at injection site.
**Other:** *anaphylaxis, fever,* herpes zoster, stiffness.

### INTERACTIONS
**Drug-drug.** *Blood products, immune globulin:* may inactivate vaccine. Defer vaccination for at least 5 months following blood or plasma transfusions or administration of immune globulin or varicella-zoster immune globulin.
*Immunosuppressants:* risk of severe reactions to live virus vaccines. Postpone routine vaccination.
*Salicylates:* Reye's syndrome has been reported after natural varicella infection. Avoid use of salicylates for 6 weeks after varicella immunization.

### EFFECTS ON DIAGNOSTIC TESTS
None reported.

### CONTRAINDICATIONS
Contraindicated in patients with hypersensitivity to drug or history of anaphylactoid reaction to neomycin; in those with blood dyscrasia, leukemia, lymphomas, neoplasms affecting bone marrow or lymphatic system, primary and acquired immunosuppressive states, active untreated tuberculosis, or any febrile respiratory illness or other active febrile infection; and in pregnant women.

### NURSING CONSIDERATIONS
• Vaccine must be stored frozen. Diluent should be stored separately at room temperature or refrigerated.
• To reconstitute vaccine, first withdraw 0.7 ml of diluent into syringe to be used for reconstitution. Inject all diluent in syringe into vial of lyophilized vaccine, and gently agitate to mix thoroughly. Administer immediately after reconstitution. Discard if not used within 30 minutes.
• Have epinephrine available to treat anaphylaxis.
• Vaccine has been safely and effectively used with measles, mumps, and rubella vaccine.
• Document manufacturer, lot number, date, and name, address, and title of person administering dose on patient record or log.
• **Alert:** Vaccine contains live, attenuated virus. Vaccinated individuals who develop rash may be able to transmit virus.

---

Reactions may be *common*, uncommon, *life-threatening*, or COMMON AND LIFE-THREATENING.

### ✓ Patient teaching

• Inform patient or parents of adverse reactions associated with vaccine.

• Caution woman of childbearing age to notify doctor of suspected pregnancy before administration.

• Instruct patient to avoid salicylates for 6 weeks after vaccination to prevent Reye's syndrome.

• Tell patient to avoid pregnancy for 3 months after vaccination.

• Inform patient to avoid postinjection close contact with susceptible high-risk individuals (such as pregnant women or immunocompromised persons).

## yellow fever vaccine
YF-Vax

*Pregnancy Risk Category C*

### HOW SUPPLIED
*Injection:* live, attenuated 17D yellow fever virus in 1-, 5-, and 20-dose vials, with diluent; supplied only to centers authorized to issue yellow fever vaccination certificates

### ACTION
Provides active immunity to yellow fever.

| Route | Onset | Peak | Duration |
|-------|-------|------|----------|
| S.C. | 7-10 days | 28 days | > 10 yr |

### INDICATIONS & DOSAGE
*Primary vaccination—*
**Adults and children ages 9 months and older:** 0.5 ml deep S.C.; booster is 0.5 ml S.C. q 10 years.
**Children ages 6 to 9 months:** same dose as above if they are to be exposed to mosquito bites.

### ADVERSE REACTIONS
**CNS:** headache, *malaise.*
**Musculoskeletal:** myalgia.
**Skin:** mild swelling, pain at injection site.
**Other:** *anaphylaxis, fever.*

### INTERACTIONS
**Drug-drug.** *Cholera vaccine:* concurrent administration may interfere with immune response to both yellow fever and cholera vaccines. Administer 3 weeks apart.
*Immunosuppressants:* may increase viral replication and development of infection with yellow fever virus. Defer immunization until immunosuppressant is stopped.

### EFFECTS ON DIAGNOSTIC TESTS
None reported.

### CONTRAINDICATIONS
Contraindicated in immunosuppressed patients; in those with cancer, gamma globulin deficiency, or hypersensitivity to eggs; and in those receiving corticosteroid or radiation therapy. Also contraindicated in pregnant women and in infants under age 6 months, except in high-risk areas.

### NURSING CONSIDERATIONS
• Obtain history of allergies, especially to eggs, and reaction to immunization.

• Keep epinephrine 1:1,000 available to treat anaphylaxis.

• In patients who have received blood or plasma transfusions, 8 weeks should pass before administering vaccine.

• Reconstitute with NaCl injection that contains no preservatives (they inactivate the yellow fever viruses).

• Keep vaccine frozen. Don't use unless shipping case contains some dry ice on arrival. Avoid vigorous shaking; carefully swirl mixture until suspension is uniform. Use within 1 hour after reconstituting. Discard remainder.

• Yellow fever vaccine shouldn't be given within 1 month of other live virus vaccines; may be given with hepatitis B vaccine.

### ✓ Patient teaching

• Inform patient about adverse reactions associated with vaccine.

• Caution woman of childbearing age to notify doctor of suspected pregnancy before administration.

• Advise patient to avoid bites by using sprays, repellents, protective clothing, and screens.

---

*Liquid contains alcohol.   **May contain tartrazine.   †Canada   ‡Australia   §U.K.   ◇OTC

black widow spider antivenin
Crotalidae antivenom, polyvalent
diphtheria antitoxin, equine
*Micrurus fulvius* antivenin

## COMBINATION PRODUCTS
None.

## black widow spider antivenin
Antivenin *(Latrodectus mactans)*

*Pregnancy Risk Category C*

## HOW SUPPLIED
*Injection:* combination package—one vial of antivenin (6,000-U vial), one 2.5-ml vial of diluent (sterile water for injection), and one 1-ml vial of normal equine serum (1:10 dilution) for sensitivity testing

## ACTION
Unknown.

| Route | Onset | Peak | Duration |
|-------|-------|------|----------|
| I.V. | Immediate | Unknown | Unknown |
| I.M. | Unknown | 2-3 days | Unknown |

## INDICATIONS & DOSAGE
*Black widow spider bite—*
**Adults and children:** 2.5 ml I.M. in anterolateral thigh. Second dose may be needed. In severe cases, antivenin may be given I.V.

Test for sensitivity before giving drug, as ordered; use 0.02 ml of 1:10 antivenin in normal saline. Evaluate result in 10 minutes.

For desensitization, use 1:10 and 1:100 dilutions of antivenin in normal saline for injection and administer, as ordered.

## ADVERSE REACTIONS
**CNS:** *neurotoxicity.*
**Other:** *hypersensitivity reactions, anaphylaxis, serum sickness.*

## INTERACTIONS
**Drug-drug.** *Antihistamines:* may interfere with sensitivity tests. Avoid concomitant use.

## EFFECTS ON DIAGNOSTIC TESTS
None reported.

## CONTRAINDICATIONS
Contraindicated in patients with hypersensitivity to drug or its components (horse serum) when desensitization isn't feasible.

## NURSING CONSIDERATIONS
• Immobilize patient; splint the bitten limb to prevent spread of venom.
• Obtain history of allergies, especially to horses, and reaction to immunization. Have epinephrine 1:1,000 available to treat anaphylaxis.
• For best results, antivenin should be given as soon as possible.
• A skin or conjunctival test should be performed before administration.
• *Alert:* Give I.M. injection in anterolateral thigh so that a tourniquet may be applied if a systemic reaction occurs.
• Watch patient for 2 to 3 days. Venom is neurotoxic and may cause respiratory paralysis and seizures.
• Symptoms usually subside in 1 to 3 hours.
• Refrigerate at 36° to 46° F (2° to 8° C).
• Discard if injection is frozen.

## I.V. administration
• Reconstitute antivenom with 2.5 ml of diluent. Further dilute reconstituted solution in 10 to 50 ml normal saline injection and infuse over 15 minutes.
• I.V. is preferred route in severe cases or in patients in shock or under age 12.

## Patient teaching
• Explain to patient and family how drug will be administered.
• Instruct patient to report adverse reactions promptly.

---

Reactions may be *common*, uncommon, *life-threatening*, or COMMON AND LIFE-THREATENING.

• Tell patient that serum sickness can occur 8 to 12 days after administration.

---

## Crotalidae antivenom, polyvalent

*Pregnancy Risk Category C*

### HOW SUPPLIED
*Injection:* combination package—one vial of lyophilized serum, one vial of diluent (10 ml of bacteriostatic water for injection), and one 1-ml vial of normal horse serum (diluted 1:10) for sensitivity testing

### ACTION
Neutralizes and binds venom of crotalids (pit vipers), including rattlesnakes, water moccasins, and copperheads.

| Route | Onset | Peak | Duration |
|-------|-------|------|----------|
| I.V. | Immediate | Unknown | Unknown |

### INDICATIONS & DOSAGE
*Crotalid (rattlesnake) bites—*
**Adults and children:** initially, 20 to 150 ml I.V., depending on severity of bite and patient response. Minimal envenomation: 20 to 40 ml I.V.; moderate envenomation: 50 to 90 ml I.V.; severe envenomation: 100 to 150 ml I.V. If there is a large amount of venom, more than 150 ml may be given I.V. directly into superficial vein. Subsequent doses are based on patient's response; may need another 10 to 50 ml if swelling progresses, if systemic symptoms increase, or if new signs and symptoms appear.

Test for sensitivity before giving drug. Give 0.02 to 0.03 ml of 1:10 dilution in normal saline solution I.D. Read results after 5 to 10 minutes. Watch carefully for delayed allergic reaction or relapse.

If sensitivity test is positive, desensitize, as ordered; prepare 1:10 and 1:100 dilutions of antivenom in normal saline for injection.

Children, who have less resistance and less body fluid to dilute venom, may need twice adult dose.

### ADVERSE REACTIONS
**Musculoskeletal:** arthralgia.

**Skin:** erythema, urticaria.
**Other:** pain, *hypersensitivity reactions, anaphylaxis, serum sickness,* lymphadenopathy, fever.

### INTERACTIONS
**Drug-drug.** *Antihistamines:* enhanced toxicity of crotaline venoms. Don't use together.

### EFFECTS ON DIAGNOSTIC TESTS
None reported.

### CONTRAINDICATIONS
Contraindicated in patients with hypersensitivity to drug or its components.

### NURSING CONSIDERATIONS
• Use drug cautiously. About 60% of patients treated with antivenom develop hypersensitivity.
• Immobilize patient immediately. Splint bitten extremity.
• Obtain history of allergies, especially to horses, and reaction to immunization. Have epinephrine 1:1,000 ready in case of hypersensitivity reaction.
• *Alert:* Type and crossmatch blood as soon as possible; hemolysis from venom prevents accurate crossmatching.
• For best results, administer antivenom as soon as possible.
• Give corticosteroids, as prescribed. If a large number of vials is administered, serum sickness may result 5 to 24 days postinfusion.
• Antivenom may be stored without refrigeration for 60 days, but it shouldn't be exposed to temperatures over 98.6° F (37° C).

### ⬗ I.V. administration
• Reconstitute drug by adding 10 ml of supplied diluent. Further dilute to make a 1:1 to 1:10 solution using normal saline or 5% dextrose injection. To avoid foaming, don't shake while mixing. Infuse an initial 5 to 10 ml of diluted antivenin over 3 to 5 minutes and observe patient carefully. If no symptoms of immediate systemic reaction occur, infusion may be continued.

---

☑ **Patient teaching**
• Explain to patient and family that test dose will be given first to check for sensitivity to drug.
• Instruct patient to report adverse reactions promptly.

## diphtheria antitoxin, equine

*Pregnancy Risk Category C*

### HOW SUPPLIED
*Injection:* not less than 500 U/ml in 10,000-U and 20,000-U vials

### ACTION
Binds with circulating toxin and prevents disease progression.

| Route | Onset | Peak | Duration |
|-------|-------|------|----------|
| I.V. | Immediate | Unknown | Unknown |
| I.M. | Unknown | 2 days | Unknown |

### INDICATIONS & DOSAGE
*Diphtheria prevention—*
**Adults and children:** 5,000 to 10,000 U I.M.
*Diphtheria treatment—*
**Adults and children:** 20,000 to 120,000 U I.M. or slow I.V. Additional doses may be given in 24 hours. I.M. route may be used in mild cases.

### ADVERSE REACTIONS
**Skin:** erythema, urticaria.
**Other:** pain, *hypersensitivity reactions, anaphylaxis,* serum sickness (urticaria, pruritus, fever, malaise, arthralgia) may occur in 7 to 12 days.

### INTERACTIONS
None significant.

### EFFECTS ON DIAGNOSTIC TESTS
None reported.

### CONTRAINDICATIONS
Contraindicated in patients with hypersensitivity to drug or its components.

### NURSING CONSIDERATIONS
• Obtain history of allergies, especially to horses, and reaction to immunization.

Have epinephrine 1:1,000 ready in case of anaphylaxis. Antitoxin should be used with extreme caution in patients with history of allergic disorders.
• Test for sensitivity before giving drug, as ordered.
• *Alert:* If patient has symptoms of diphtheria (sore throat, fever, tonsillar membrane), therapy should be started immediately, without waiting for culture reports.
• For storage, refrigerate antitoxin at 36° to 50° F (2° to 10° C). Before administering, warm to 90° to 95° F (32° to 35° C), never higher.
• Begin appropriate antimicrobial therapy.

◔ **I.V. administration**
• Dilute appropriate dose in $D_5W$ or normal saline solution to achieve a 1:20 dilution.
• Administer solution by direct infusion at no more than 1 ml/minute.

☑ **Patient teaching**
• Explain to patient and family that test dose will be given first to check for sensitivity to drug.
• Tell patient to report adverse reactions promptly.

## *Micrurus fulvius* antivenin

*Pregnancy Risk Category C*

### HOW SUPPLIED
*Injection:* combination package with 10 ml of diluent

### ACTION
Neutralizes and binds coral snake venom.

| Route | Onset | Peak | Duration |
|-------|-------|------|----------|
| I.V. | Immediate | Unknown | Unknown |

### INDICATIONS & DOSAGE
*Eastern and Texas coral snake bite—*
**Adults and children:** 30 to 50 ml (3 to 5 vials) slow I.V. through running I.V. of normal saline solution. Give 1 to 2 ml over 3 to 5 minutes; monitor closely for allergic reaction. If no signs of allergic reaction develop, injection is continued; 100 ml or more may be needed.

---

Reactions may be *common,* uncommon, *life-threatening,* or COMMON AND LIFE-THREATENING.

Test for sensitivity before giving drug, as ordered. If sensitivity test is positive, prepare to desensitize, as ordered; prepare 1:10 and 1:100 dilutions of antivenin in NaCl for injection.

**ADVERSE REACTIONS**
**Musculoskeletal:** arthralgia.
**Skin:** erythema, urticaria.
**Other:** pain, *hypersensitivity reactions, anaphylaxis,* fever, lymphadenopathy.

**INTERACTIONS**
None significant.

**EFFECTS ON DIAGNOSTIC TESTS**
None reported.

**CONTRAINDICATIONS**
Contraindicated in patients with hypersensitivity to drug or its components.

**NURSING CONSIDERATIONS**
• *Alert:* Drug isn't effective for Sonoran or Arizona coral snake bites.
• Immobilize patient and splint bitten limb to prevent spread of venom.
• Obtain accurate patient history of allergies, especially to horses, and reaction to immunization. Make sure epinephrine 1:1,000 is available to treat anaphylaxis.
• Antivenin should be given as soon as possible (before onset of neurotoxic signs); asymptomatic patients should be treated because systemic symptoms usually develop later.
• Watch patient carefully for 24 hours. Venom is neurotoxic and may cause respiratory paralysis.
• Antivenin can be stored at room temperature for 10 days.

**⬛ I.V. administration**
• Reconstitute antivenin powder with diluent. Further dilute in normal saline to achieve a 1:1 to 1:10 dilution. Gently swirl solution to avoid foaming.
• Infuse initial 1 to 2 ml over 3 to 5 minutes while closely monitoring patient. If no immediate systemic response occurs, continue infusion at maximum safe rate for I.V. fluid administration.

**✅ Patient teaching**
• Explain to patient and family that test dose will be given first to check for sensitivity to drug.
• Tell patient to report adverse reactions promptly.

**cytomegalovirus immune globulin, intravenous**
**hepatitis B immune globulin, human**
**immune globulin intramuscular**
**immune globulin intravenous**
**rabies immune globulin, human**
**respiratory syncytial virus immune globulin intravenous, human**
**Rh₀(D) immune globulin, human**

$Rh_o(D)$ immune globulin, human

**Rh₀(D) immune globulin intravenous, human**

$Rh_o(D)$ immune globulin intravenous, human

**tetanus immune globulin, human**
**varicella-zoster immune globulin**

**COMBINATION PRODUCTS**
None.

---

## cytomegalovirus immune globulin (human), intravenous (CMV-IGIV)
CytoGam

*Pregnancy Risk Category C*

**HOW SUPPLIED**
*Injection:* 2.5 g/50 ml†; 1 g/20 ml

**ACTION**
Provides passive immunity by supplying a relatively high level of immunoglobulin (IgG) antibodies against CMV. Increasing these antibody levels in CMV-exposed patients may attenuate or reduce risk of serious CMV disease.

| Route | Onset | Peak | Duration |
|-------|-------|------|----------|
| I.V. | Unknown | Unknown | Unknown |

**INDICATIONS & DOSAGE**
*To attenuate primary CMV disease in seronegative kidney transplant recipients who receive a kidney from a CMV seropositive donor—*
**Adults:** administered I.V. based on time after transplantation:
within 72 hours: 150 mg/kg
2 weeks after: 100 mg/kg
4 weeks after: 100 mg/kg
6 weeks after: 100 mg/kg
8 weeks after: 100 mg/kg
12 weeks after: 50 mg/kg
16 weeks after: 50 mg/kg.
Initial dose given at 15 mg/kg/hour. Increased to 30 mg/kg/hour after 30 minutes if no untoward reactions occur, then to 60 mg/kg/hour after another 30 minutes if no reactions occur. Volume shouldn't exceed 75 ml/hour. Subsequent doses may be given at 15 mg/kg/hour for 15 minutes, increasing q 15 minutes in a stepwise fashion to 60 mg/kg/hour.
✳ *NEW INDICATION: Prophylaxis of CMV disease associated with lung, liver, pancreas, and heart transplants—*
**Adults:** used with ganciclovir in organ transplants from CMV seropositive donors into seronegative recipients. Maximum total dose per infusion is 150 mg/kg I.V. administered as follows based on time after transplantation:
within 72 hours: 150 mg/kg
2 weeks after: 150 mg/kg
4 weeks after: 150 mg/kg
6 weeks after: 150 mg/kg
8 weeks after: 150 mg/kg
12 weeks after: 100 mg/kg
16 weeks after: 100 mg/kg.
Administer initial dose at 15 mg/kg/hour. If no adverse reactions occur after 30 minutes, increase rate to 30 mg/kg/hour. If no adverse reactions occur after a subsequent 30 minutes, infusion may be increased to 60 mg/kg/hour (volume shouldn't exceed 75 ml/hour). Subsequent doses may be given at 15 mg/kg/hour for 15 minutes, increasing every 15 minutes in a stepwise fashion to maximum rate of 60 mg/kg/hour (volume shouldn't exceed 75 ml/hour). Monitor patient closely during and after each rate change.

**ADVERSE REACTIONS**
**CV:** hypotension, *flushing.*
**GI:** *nausea, vomiting.*
**Musculoskeletal:** muscle cramps, *back pain.*

---

Reactions may be *common,* uncommon, *life-threatening,* or COMMON AND LIFE-THREATENING.

**Respiratory:** *wheezing.*
**Other:** *anaphylaxis,* aseptic meningitis syndrome, *chills,* fever.

## INTERACTIONS
**Drug-drug.** *Live virus vaccines:* may interfere with immune response to live virus vaccines. Defer vaccination for at least 3 months.

## EFFECTS ON DIAGNOSTIC TESTS
None reported.

## CONTRAINDICATIONS
Contraindicated in patients with sensitivity to other human Ig preparations or with selective IgA deficiency.

## NURSING CONSIDERATIONS
• Monitor patient's vital signs closely pre-infusion, midinfusion, postinfusion, and before and after increases in infusion rate.
• *Alert:* If anaphylaxis or drop in blood pressure occurs, discontinue infusion, notify doctor, and be prepared to administer cardiopulmonary resuscitation and such drugs as diphenhydramine and epinephrine.
• Refrigerate drug at 36° to 46° F (2° to 8° C).

⚠ **I.V. administration**
• Prepare for administration as follows: Remove tab portion of vial cap and clean rubber stopper with 70% alcohol or equivalent. To avoid foaming, don't shake vial. Inspect vial for clarity and particles.
• If possible, administer through a separate I.V. line, using a constant infusion pump. Filters aren't needed. If unable to administer through separate line, piggyback into preexisting line of NaCl injection or one of the following dextrose solutions with or without NaCl: $D_{2.5}W$, $D_5W$, $D_{10}W$, or $D_{20}W$. Don't dilute more than 1:2 with any of the above solutions.
• Begin infusion within 6 hours of entering vial; finish within 12 hours.

✅ **Patient teaching**
• Review drug therapy regimen with patient, and stress importance of compliance in follow-up visits.
• Instruct patient to report adverse reactions promptly.

# hepatitis B immune globulin, human
H-BIG, HyperHep

*Pregnancy Risk Category C*

## HOW SUPPLIED
*Injection:* 1-ml, 4-ml, 5-ml vials; 0.5-ml neonatal single-dose syringe

## ACTION
Provides passive immunity to hepatitis B.

| Route | Onset | Peak | Duration |
|-------|-------|------|----------|
| I.M. | 1-6 days | 3-11 days | 2 mo |

## INDICATIONS & DOSAGE
*Hepatitis B exposure in high-risk patients—*
**Adults and children:** 0.06 ml/kg I.M. within 7 days after exposure. Dose repeated 28 days after exposure if patient refuses hepatitis B vaccine.
**Neonates born to patients who test positive for hepatitis B surface antigen (HBsAg):** 0.5 ml I.M. within 12 hours of birth.

## ADVERSE REACTIONS
**Skin:** urticaria; *pain, tenderness at injection site.*
**Other:** *anaphylaxis, angioedema.*

## INTERACTIONS
**Drug-drug.** *Live virus vaccines:* may interfere with response to live virus vaccines. Defer routine immunization for 3 months.

## EFFECTS ON DIAGNOSTIC TESTS
None reported.

## CONTRAINDICATIONS
Contraindicated in patients with history of anaphylactic reactions to immune serum. Administer to patients with coagulation disorders or thrombocytopenia only if benefit outweighs risk.

## NURSING CONSIDERATIONS
• Obtain history of allergies and reaction to immunizations. Make sure epinephrine 1:1,000 is available.

---

*Liquid contains alcohol.    **May contain tartrazine.    †Canada    ‡Australia    §U.K.    ◇OTC

• Inject into anterolateral aspect of thigh or deltoid muscle areas in older children and adults; inject into anterolateral aspect of thigh in neonates and children under age 3.

• Inspect for discoloration or particulates. Drug is clear, slightly amber, and moderately viscous.

• For postexposure prophylaxis (for example, needle stick, direct contact), drug is usually given with hepatitis B vaccine.

• **Alert:** This immune globulin provides passive immunity; don't confuse with hepatitis B vaccine. Both drugs may be given at same time. Don't mix in the same syringe.

• **Alert:** Don't confuse HyperHep with Hyperstat or Hyper-Tet.

☑ **Patient teaching**
• Inform patient that pain and tenderness may occur at injection site.
• Tell patient to report signs of hypersensitivity immediately.

---

**immune globulin intramuscular (gamma globulin, IG, IGIM)**

**immune globulin intravenous (IGIV)**
Gamimune N, Gammagard S/D, Gammar-P I.V., Iveegam, Polygam S/D, Sandoglobulin, Venoglobulin-I, Venoglobulin-S

*Pregnancy Risk Category C*

---

**HOW SUPPLIED**
**immune globulin intramuscular**
*Injection:* 2-ml, 10-ml vials
**immune globulin intravenous**
*Injection:* 5% and 10% in 10-ml, 50-ml, 100-ml, 250-ml vials (Gamimune N) 5% in 2.5-g, 5-g, 10-g vials; 5%, 10% in 5-g, 10-g, 20-g vials (Venoglobulin-S)
*Powder for injection:* 50 mg protein/ml in 2.5-g, 5-g, 10-g vials (Gammagard S/D); 2.5-g, 1-g, 5-g vials (Gammar-P I.V.); 500-mg, 1-g, 2.5-g, 5-g vials (Iveegam); 2.5-g, 5-g, 10-g vials (Polygam S/D); 1-g, 3-g, 6-g, 12-g vials (Sandoglobulin); 500-mg, 2.5-g, 5-g, 10-g vials (Venoglobulin-I)

**ACTION**
Provides passive immunity by increasing antibody titer. The primary component is immunoglobulin (Ig) G. The mechanism for treating idiopathic thrombocytopenic purpura is unknown.

| Route | Onset | Peak | Duration |
|-------|-------|------|----------|
| I.V. | Immediate | Immediate | Unknown |
| I.M. | Unknown | 2-5 hr | Unknown |

**INDICATIONS & DOSAGE**
*Primary humoral immunodeficiency (IGIV)—*
**Adults and children:** *Gamimune N*—100 to 200 mg/kg I.V. monthly, at rate of 0.01 to 0.02 ml/kg/minute for 30 minutes. If no problems, rate can be slowly increased to maximum rate of 0.08 ml/kg/minute.

*Gammagard S/D*—200 to 400 mg/kg I.V.; then monthly doses of 100 mg/kg. Initiate infusion at 0.5 ml/kg/hour and increase to maximum of 4 ml/kg/hour. Dose related to patient response.

*Gammar-P I.V.*—200 to 400 mg/kg infused I.V. at 0.01 ml/kg/minute and increased to 0.02 ml/kg/minute after 15 to 30 minutes if no problems, given q 3 to 4 weeks. Maximum infusion rate is 0.06 ml/kg/minute.

*Iveegam*—200 mg/kg I.V. monthly. May increase dose to maximum of 800 mg/kg or give more frequently to produce desired effect. Infusion rate is 1 to 2 ml/minute for 5% solution.

*Polygam S/D*—initially, 200 to 400 mg/kg I.V. at 0.5 ml/kg/hour, increasing to maximum of 4 ml/kg/hour. Subsequent dose is 100 mg/kg I.V. monthly.

*Sandoglobulin*—200 mg/kg I.V. monthly. Start initially with 0.5 to 1 ml/minute of 3% solution; gradually increase dose to 2.5 ml/minute after 15 to 30 minutes.

*Venoglobulin-I*—initially, 200 mg/kg I.V. monthly at 0.01 to 0.02 ml/kg/minute for 30 minutes; then increase to 0.04 ml/kg/minute or more if no adverse reaction. Dose may be increased to 300 to 400 mg/kg and given more often than once monthly if needed and tolerated.

*Venoglobulin-S*—200 mg/kg I.V. monthly. Dose may be increased to 300 to 400 mg/kg and given more often than

---

Reactions may be *common*, uncommon, **life-threatening**, or **COMMON AND LIFE-THREATENING**.

once monthly if adequate IgG levels haven't occurred. Begin infusion at 0.01 to 0.02 ml/kg/minute for 30 minutes; then increase 5% solutions to 0.04 ml/kg/minute and 10% solutions to 0.05 ml/kg/minute, if tolerated.

*Idiopathic thrombocytopenic purpura (IGIV)—*

**Adults and children:** *Gamimune N—* 400 mg/kg 5% solution I.V. for 5 days; or 1,000 mg/kg 10% solution I.V. for 1 to 2 days with maintenance dose of 10% solution at 400 to 1,000 mg/kg I.V. single infusion to maintain 30,000/mm$^3$ platelet count.

*Sandoglobulin*—0.4 g/kg I.V. for 2 to 5 consecutive days.

*Bone marrow transplant (IGIV)—*

**Adults over age 20:** *Gamimune N—* 500 mg/kg 5% or 10% solution I.V. on days 7 and 2 pretransplantation; then weekly until 90 days posttransplantation.

*B-cell chronic lymphocytic leukemia (IGIV)—*

**Adults:** 400 mg/kg Gammagard S/D or Polygam S/D I.V. q 3 to 4 weeks.

*Hepatitis A exposure (IGIM)—*

**Adults and children:** 0.02 ml/kg I.M. as soon as possible after exposure. Up to 0.1 ml/kg may be administered if prolonged or intense exposure.

*Measles exposure (IGIM)—*

**Adults and children:** 0.25 ml/kg I.M. within 6 days postexposure.

*Postexposure prophylaxis of measles (IGIM)—*

**Children:** 0.5 ml/kg I.M. within 6 days postexposure (maximum 15 ml).

*Chickenpox exposure (IGIM)—*

**Adults and children:** 0.6 to 1.2 ml/kg I.M. as soon as exposed.

*Rubella exposure in first trimester pregnancy (IGIM)—*

**Women:** 0.55 ml/kg I.M. as soon as possible postexposure (within 72 hours).

*Pediatric HIV infection (IGIV)—*

**Children:** 400 mg/kg Gamimune N I.V. q 28 days, at 0.01 to 0.02 ml/kg/minute for 30 minutes; increase to maximum of 0.08 ml/kg/minute.

## ADVERSE REACTIONS

**CNS:** headache, faintness, malaise.
**GI:** nausea, vomiting.

**Musculoskeletal:** hip pain, chest pain, chest tightness.
**Respiratory:** dyspnea.
**Skin:** urticaria; pain, erythema, muscle stiffness at injection site.
**Other:** fever, *anaphylaxis,* chills.

## INTERACTIONS

**Drug-drug.** *Live virus vaccines:* length of time to wait before administering live virus vaccinations varies with dose of immune globulin given. Refer to recommendations by American Academy of Pediatrics.

## EFFECTS ON DIAGNOSTIC TESTS

None reported.

## CONTRAINDICATIONS

Contraindicated in patients with hypersensitivity to drug or its components.

## NURSING CONSIDERATIONS

• Obtain history of allergies and reaction to immunizations. Make sure epinephrine 1:1,000 is available to treat anaphylaxis.
• When giving I.M., use gluteal region. Divide doses over 10 ml and inject into several muscle sites to reduce pain and discomfort.
• Administer drug soon after reconstitution.
• Immune globulin shouldn't be given for prophylaxis against hepatitis A if 6 weeks or more have elapsed since exposure or onset of clinical illness.
• *Alert:* Don't confuse Sandoglobulin with Sandostatin or Sandimmune.

**⚠ I.V. administration**
• When administering Polygam S/D, Gammagard S/D, or Iveegam, use a 15-micron in-line filter.
• Most adverse reactions are related to a rapid infusion rate. If adverse reactions occur, decrease infusion rate or discontinue infusion until reactions subside. Resume infusion at a rate that's tolerated by patient.
• Gamimune N 5% and 10% are incompatible with NaCl solutions. They may be diluted with D$_5$W, if needed.
• Reconstitute Gammagard S/D and Polygam S/D according to package directions with sterile water for injection dilu-

ent and transfer device provided to prepare a solution containing 50 mg of protein per ml for 5% immune globulin solution or 100 mg of protein per ml for 10% immune globulin solution. Warm powder and sterile water for injection to room temperature before reconstitution. Administer no more than 2 hours after reconstitution. Infuse with administration set provided or with an adequate filter.

• Reconstitute Gammar-P I.V. with sterile water for injection diluent provided. Warm powder and diluent to room temperature before reconstitution. After adding diluent, keep vial in upright position and undisturbed for 5 minutes. Gently swirl vial after 5 minutes. Don't shake. Dissolution may take up to 20 minutes.

• Reconstitute Iveegam with sterile water for injection diluent provided. Agitate or rotate vial gently. Don't shake.

• Reconstitute Sandoglobulin with normal saline diluent provided. Or, reconstitute with sterile water for injection or 5% dextrose injection. Consider patient's fluid, electrolyte, and caloric requirements when choosing diluent.

• When preparing Sandoglobulin, don't shake vial. Swirl gently to dissolve drug. Dissolution may take up to 20 minutes. Solution should be clear and at room temperature before use. If large doses are to be given, several reconstituted vials of same concentration and diluent may be pooled into an empty sterile glass or plastic I.V. infusion container using aseptic technique. Filtering isn't needed. If filtering, use a filter with pore size of 15 microns or larger to prevent slowing of infusion. Antibacterial filters may be used. If drug is reconstituted outside of sterile laminar airflow conditions, use promptly. Drug reconstituted in a sterile laminar flow hood and stored under refrigeration is stable for up to 24 hours.

• Don't mix with other drugs or I.V. fluids.

### ☑ Patient teaching
• Explain to patient and family how drug will be administered.

• Tell patient that local reactions may occur at injection site. Instruct him to notify doctor promptly if adverse reactions persist or become severe.

• Inform patient of possible need to have therapy more than once monthly to maintain appropriate IgG levels.

## rabies immune globulin, human
Hyperab, Imogam Rabies

*Pregnancy Risk Category C*

### HOW SUPPLIED
*Injection:* 150 IU/ml in 2-ml, 10-ml vials

### ACTION
Provides passive immunity to rabies.

| Route | Onset | Peak | Duration |
|-------|-------|------|----------|
| I.M. | 24 hr | Unknown | Unknown |

### INDICATIONS & DOSAGE
*Rabies exposure—*
**Adults and children:** 20 IU/kg I.M. at time of first dose of rabies vaccine. Half of dose is used to infiltrate wound area; remainder is given I.M. in a different site.

### ADVERSE REACTIONS
**GU:** *nephrotic syndrome.*
**Skin:** *rash;* pain, redness, induration at injection site.
**Other:** slight fever, *anaphylaxis, angioedema.*

### INTERACTIONS
**Drug-drug.** *Live virus vaccines (measles, mumps, polio, or rubella):* interferes with response to vaccine. Delay immunization if possible.

### EFFECTS ON DIAGNOSTIC TESTS
None reported.

### CONTRAINDICATIONS
No known contraindications.

### NURSING CONSIDERATIONS
• Use with caution in patients with hypersensitivity to thimerosal or history of systemic allergic reactions to human immunoglobulin preparations; also use cautiously in those with IgA deficiency.

• Obtain history of animal bites, allergies, and reaction to immunizations. Have epi-

---

Reactions may be *common,* uncommon, *life-threatening*, or **COMMON AND LIFE-THREATENING**.

nephrine 1:1,000 available to treat anaphylaxis.
• Ask patient when last tetanus immunization was received; many doctors order booster at this time.
• Use only with rabies vaccine and immediate local treatment of wound. Don't give rabies vaccine and rabies immune globulin in same syringe or at same site. Administer as soon as possible after exposure or through day 7. After day 8, antibody response to culture vaccine has occurred.
• Don't administer live virus vaccines within 3 months of rabies immune globulin.
• Don't administer more than 5 ml I.M. at one injection site; divide I.M. doses over 5 ml; administer at different sites.
• Administer large volumes (5 ml) in adults only. Use upper outer quadrant of gluteal area.
• *Alert:* This immune serum provides passive immunity. Don't confuse with rabies vaccine, a suspension of killed microorganisms that confers active immunity. The two drugs are often used together prophylactically after exposure to rabid animals.
• Clean wound thoroughly with soap and water; this is the best prophylaxis against rabies.

✅ **Patient teaching**
• Inform patient that local reactions may occur at injection site. Instruct him to notify doctor promptly if reactions persist or become severe.
• Tell patient that a tetanus shot also may be needed.
• Instruct patient in wound care.

## respiratory syncytial virus immune globulin intravenous, human (RSV-IGIV)
RespiGam

*Pregnancy Risk Category C*

### HOW SUPPLIED
*Injection:* 50 mg ±10 mg/ml in 20-ml, 50-ml single-use vial

### ACTION
Provides passive immunity to RSV.

| Route | Onset | Peak | Duration |
|-------|-------|------|----------|
| I.V. | Unknown | Unknown | ≥ 1 mo |

### INDICATIONS & DOSAGE
*Prevention of serious lower respiratory tract infections due to RSV in children with bronchopulmonary dysplasia (BPD) or history of premature birth (35 weeks' gestation or less)—*
**Premature infants and children under age 2:** single infusion monthly. Give 1.5 ml/kg/hour I.V. for 15 minutes; then, if clinical condition allows higher rate, increase to 3 ml/kg/hour for 15 minutes and then to maximum of 6 ml/kg/hour until infusion ends. Maximum recommended total dose per monthly infusion is 750 mg/kg.

### ADVERSE REACTIONS
**CNS:** dizziness, anxiety.
**CV:** fluid overload, tachycardia, hypertension, palpitations, chest tightness.
**GI:** vomiting, diarrhea, gastroenteritis, abdominal cramps.
**Musculoskeletal:** myalgia, arthralgia.
**Respiratory:** respiratory distress, wheezing, crackles, hypoxia, tachypnea, dyspnea.
**Skin:** rash, flushing, pruritus; inflammation at injection site.
**Other:** fever, overdose effect, *hypersensitivity reactions including anaphylaxis, angioneurotic edema.*

### INTERACTIONS
**Drug-drug.** *Live virus vaccines (such as mumps, rubella, and especially measles):* may interfere with response. If such vaccines are given during or within 10 months after RSV-IGIV, reimmunization is recommended, if appropriate.

### EFFECTS ON DIAGNOSTIC TESTS
None reported.

### CONTRAINDICATIONS
Contraindicated in patients with history of severe hypersensitivity to drug or other human immunoglobulin and selective immunoglobulin (Ig) A deficiency.

---

## NURSING CONSIDERATIONS

• Children with fluid overload shouldn't receive drug.

• First dose should be given before RSV season (November to April) begins; subsequent doses should be given monthly throughout RSV season to maintain protection. Children with RSV should continue to receive monthly doses for duration of RSV season.

• Watch closely for signs of fluid overload. Children with BPD may be more prone to this condition. Report increases in heart rate, respiratory rate, retractions, or crackles. Have a loop diuretic, such as furosemide or bumetanide, available.

### I.V. administration

• Drug doesn't contain a preservative. Enter single-use vial only once; don't shake; avoid foaming. Begin infusion within 6 hours and end within 12 hours after vial is entered. Don't use if solution is turbid. Administer through I.V. line using a constant infusion pump. Predilution of drug before infusion isn't recommended. Although filters aren't needed for infusion, an in-line filter with pore size larger than 15 microns may be used. Give drug separately from other drugs.

• Adhere to infusion rate guidelines; most adverse reactions may be related to rate used. In especially ill children with BPD, slower rates may be indicated.

• Assess cardiopulmonary status and vital signs before beginning infusion, before each rate increase, and every 30 minutes thereafter until 30 minutes after completion of infusion.

• *Alert:* If patient develops hypotension, anaphylaxis, or severe allergic reaction, stop infusion and administer epinephrine (1:1,000), as ordered. Patients with selective IgA deficiency can develop antibodies to IgA and have anaphylactic or allergic reactions to subsequent administration of blood products containing IgA, including RSV-IGIV.

### ✓ Patient teaching

• Explain to parents importance of their child receiving drug monthly throughout RSV season, even if child is already infected.

• Teach parents how drug is administered and which adverse reactions are associated with administration. Instruct parents to report all adverse reactions promptly.

---

# Rh₀(D) immune globulin, human

Gamulin Rh, HypRho-D, HypRho-D Mini-Dose, MICRhoGAM, Mini-Gamulin Rh, RhoGAM

# Rh₀(D) immune globulin intravenous, human

WinRho SD

*Pregnancy Risk Category C*

## HOW SUPPLIED

**Rh₀(D) immune globulin, human**
*Injection:* 300 mcg of Rh₀(D) immune globulin/vial (standard dose); 50 mcg of Rh₀(D) immune globulin/vial (microdose)
**Rh₀(D) immune globulin I.V., human**
*Injection:* 120 mcg, 300 mcg

## ACTION

Suppresses the active antibody response and formation of anti-Rh₀(D) antibodies in Rh₀(D)-negative, Dᵘ-negative persons exposed to Rh-positive blood. Rh₀(D) immune globulin I.V. may form complexes with RBCs blocking platelet destruction in adults who are Rh₀(D) antigen-positive. However, mechanism of action isn't completely known.

| Route | Onset | Peak | Duration |
|---|---|---|---|
| I.V., I.M. | Unknown | Unknown | Unknown |

## INDICATIONS & DOSAGE

*Rh₀ (D) immune globulin, human Rh exposure—*

**Adults (after abortion, miscarriage, ectopic pregnancy; or postpartum):** transfusion unit or blood bank determines fetal packed RBC volume entering patient's blood; then one vial I.M. is given if fetal packed RBC volume is less than 15 ml. More than one vial I.M. may be needed if severe fetomaternal hemorrhage occurs; must be given within 72 hours after delivery or miscarriage.

---

Reactions may be *common,* uncommon, *life-threatening,* or COMMON AND LIFE-THREATENING.

*After abortion or miscarriage to prevent Rh antibody formation—*
**Adults:** consult transfusion unit or blood bank. One microdose vial I.M. will suppress immune reaction to 2.5 ml $Rh_0(D)$-positive RBCs. Ideally, should be given within 3 hours, but may be given up to 72 hours after abortion or miscarriage.

*$Rh_0(D)$ immune globulin I.V., human Rh exposure—*
**Adults (after abortion, amniocentesis [after 34 weeks' gestation], or other manipulations late in pregnancy [after 34 weeks' gestation] associated with increased risk of Rh isoimmunization):** 120 mcg I.M. or I.V.; must be given within 72 hours after delivery, miscarriage, or manipulation.

*Pregnancy—*
**Adults:** 300 mcg (WinRho SD) I.M. or I.V. at 28 weeks' gestation. If administered early in pregnancy, additional doses should be given at 12-week intervals to maintain adequate levels of passively acquired anti-Rh antibodies. Then, within 72 hours of delivery, 120 mcg should be given I.M. or I.V. If 72 hours have elapsed, drug should be given as soon as possible, up to 28 days.

*Transfusion accidents—*
**Adults:** 600 mcg I.V. q 8 hours or 1,200 mcg I.M. q 12 hours until total dose administered. Total dose depends on volume of packed RBCs or whole blood infused. Consult blood bank or transfusion unit at once; must be given within 72 hours.

*Immune thrombocytopenic purpura (ITP) in adults who are $Rh_0(D)$ antigen-positive—*
**Adults:** initially, 50 mcg/kg I.V. If hemoglobin is less than 10 g/dl, reduce initial dose to 25 to 40 mcg/kg. Initial dose may be administered as single dose or divided into two doses and administered on separate days. Then, 25 to 60 mcg/kg I.V. may be administered, p.r.n., to elevate platelet counts with specific dosage that's determined individually.

**ADVERSE REACTIONS**
**Skin:** discomfort at injection site.
**Other:** *anaphylaxis,* slight fever.

**INTERACTIONS**
**Drug-drug.** *Live virus vaccines:* may interfere with response. Delay immunization for 3 months, if possible.

**EFFECTS ON DIAGNOSTIC TESTS**
None reported.

**CONTRAINDICATIONS**
Contraindicated in $Rh_0(D)$-positive or $D^u$-positive patients and in those previously immunized to $Rh_0(D)$ blood factor. Also contraindicated in patients with anaphylactic or severe systemic reaction to human globulin.

**NURSING CONSIDERATIONS**
• Use extreme caution when administering drug to patients with immunoglobulin A (IgA) deficiency. Because of risk of patient developing IgA antibodies and having an anaphylactic reaction, doctor must weigh potential benefits of treatment against potential for hypersensitivity reactions.
• Obtain history of allergies and reaction to immunization. Be sure epinephrine 1:1,000 is available to treat anaphylaxis.
• *Alert:* Immediately after delivery, send a sample of neonate's cord blood to laboratory for typing and crossmatching. Confirm if mother is $Rh_0(D)$-negative and $D^u$-negative. Administer drug to mother, as ordered, only if infant is $Rh_0(D)$-positive or $D^u$-positive. Administration must occur within 72 hours of delivery.
• This immune serum provides passive immunity to patient exposed to $Rh_0(D)$-positive fetal blood during pregnancy and prevents formation of maternal antibodies (active immunity), which would endanger future $Rh_0(D)$-positive pregnancies.
• Defer vaccination with live virus vaccines for 3 months after administration of $Rh_0(D)$ immune globulin.
• Minidose preparations are recommended for every patient undergoing abortion or miscarriage up to 12 weeks' gestation unless she is $Rh_0(D)$-positive or $D^u$-positive or has Rh antibodies, or unless the father or fetus is Rh-negative.

⬭ **I.V. administration**
• Reconstitute only with normal saline solution.
• Reconstitute drug in vials containing 600 or 1,500 U with 2.5 ml of normal saline and vials containing 5,000 U with 8.5 ml of normal saline.
• Slowly inject diluent onto the outside wall of vial and gently swirl vial until lyophilized pellet is dissolved. Don't shake vial.
• Give injection over 3 to 5 minutes.
• Don't administer with other products.

☑ **Patient teaching**
• Explain how drug protects future Rh$_o$(D)-positive fetuses if used because of pregnancy, or explain to patient drug use in condition indicated.
• Warn patient about adverse reactions associated with drug.
• Assure patient receiving this drug that there is no risk of HIV transmission.

---

# tetanus immune globulin, human
Hyper-Tet

*Pregnancy Risk Category C*

## HOW SUPPLIED
*Injection:* 250-U vial or syringe

## ACTION
Provides passive immunity to tetanus.

| Route | Onset | Peak | Duration |
|-------|-------|------|----------|
| I.M. | Unknown | 2-3 days | 4 wk |

## INDICATIONS & DOSAGE
*Tetanus exposure—*
**Adults and children:** 250 U I.M.
*Tetanus treatment—*
**Adults and children:** single doses of 3,000 to 6,000 U I.M. have been used. Optimal dosage schedules haven't been established.

## ADVERSE REACTIONS
**Skin:** pain, stiffness; erythema at injection site.

**Other:** slight fever, *hypersensitivity reactions, anaphylaxis, angioedema,* nephrotic syndrome.

## INTERACTIONS
**Drug-drug.** *Live virus vaccines:* may interfere with response. Defer administration of live virus vaccines for 3 months after administration of tetanus immune globulin.

## EFFECTS ON DIAGNOSTIC TESTS
None reported.

## CONTRAINDICATIONS
Contraindicated in patients with thrombocytopenia or other coagulation disorders that would contraindicate I.M. injection unless potential benefits outweigh risks.

## NURSING CONSIDERATIONS
• Use cautiously in patients with history of previous systemic allergic reactions following administration of human immunoglobulin preparations and in those allergic to thimerosal.
• Obtain history of injury, tetanus immunizations, last tetanus toxoid injection, allergies, and reaction to immunizations. Have epinephrine 1:1,000 available to treat hypersensitivity reaction.
• Don't administer I.V. or I.D. Don't administer in gluteal area.
• Tetanus immune globulin is used only if wound is more than 24 hours old or patient has had fewer than two tetanus toxoid injections.
• Thoroughly clean wound and remove all foreign matter.
• *Alert:* Don't confuse drug with tetanus toxoid. Tetanus immune globulin isn't a substitute for tetanus toxoid, which should be given at same time to produce active immunization. Don't give at same site as toxoid.
• Antibodies remain at effective levels for about 4 weeks, which is several times the duration of equine antitetanus antibodies, therefore protecting patients for incubation period of most tetanus cases.
• Don't administer live virus vaccines for 3 months after administering tetanus immune globulin.

---

Reactions may be *common*, uncommon, *life-threatening*, or COMMON AND LIFE-THREATENING.

• *Alert:* Don't confuse Hyper-Tet with HyperHep or Hyperstat.

☑ **Patient teaching**
• Warn patient about local adverse reactions associated with drug.
• Instruct patient to report serious adverse reactions promptly.
• Advise patient to complete full series of tetanus immunizations.
• Discuss use of acetaminophen for fever reduction and cool compresses at injection site for comfort.

---

## varicella-zoster immune globulin (VZIG)

*Pregnancy Risk Category C*

### HOW SUPPLIED
*Injection:* 10% to 18% solution of the globulin fraction of human plasma containing 125 U of varicella-zoster virus antibody (volume is about 2.5 ml or less)

### ACTION
Provides passive immunity to varicella-zoster virus in immunodeficient patients.

| Route | Onset | Peak | Duration |
|-------|-------|------|----------|
| I.M. | Unknown | Unknown | 1 mo |

### INDICATIONS & DOSAGE
*Passive immunization of susceptible immunodeficient patients after exposure to varicella (chickenpox or herpes zoster)—*
**Adults and children weighing over 40 kg (88 lb):** 625 U I.M.
**Children 30.1 to 40 kg (66 to 88 lb):** 500 U I.M.
**Children 20.1 to 30 kg (44 to 66 lb):** 375 U I.M.
**Children 10.1 to 20 kg (22 to 44 lb):** 250 U I.M.
**Children up to 10 kg (22 lb):** 125 U I.M.

### ADVERSE REACTIONS
**CNS:** headache, malaise.
**GI:** GI distress.
**Respiratory:** respiratory distress.
**Skin:** discomfort at injection site, rash.
**Other:** *anaphylaxis.*

### INTERACTIONS
**Drug-drug.** *Live virus vaccines:* may interfere with response. Defer vaccination for 3 months after administration of VZIG.

### EFFECTS ON DIAGNOSTIC TESTS
None reported.

### CONTRAINDICATIONS
Contraindicated in patients with thrombocytopenia or history of severe reaction to human immune serum globulin or thimerosal; also contraindicated during pregnancy.

### NURSING CONSIDERATIONS
• Obtain accurate patient history of allergies and reaction to immunization. Make sure epinephrine 1:1,000 is available to treat anaphylaxis.
• For maximum benefit, administer as soon as possible after presumed exposure. Drug may be of benefit when given as late as 96 hours after exposure.
• Administer only by deep I.M. injection into a large muscle mass such as gluteal muscle. Never administer I.V.
• Don't give in divided doses.
• Although usually restricted to children under age 15, VZIG may be administered to adolescents and adults, if needed.
• VZIG isn't recommended for non-immunosuppressed patients.
• *Alert:* VZIG provides passive immunity; don't confuse with varicella vaccine. Don't use these two drugs together.
• Drug isn't commercially distributed and is available only from 20 regional United States distribution centers. These centers will distribute to Canada and overseas. Contact the Massachusetts Public Health Biologic Laboratories or The Centers for Disease Control and Prevention at (800) 232-2522 for more information.

☑ **Patient teaching**
• Warn patient about local adverse reactions associated with drug.
• Instruct patient to report serious adverse reactions to doctor promptly.
• Discuss use of acetaminophen for fever reduction and cool compresses at injection site for comfort.

---

**aldesleukin**
**epoetin alfa**
**filgrastim**
**glatiramer acetate for injection**
**interferon alfacon-1**
**interferon alfa-2a, recombinant**
**interferon alfa-2b, recombinant**
**interferon beta-1a**
**interferon beta-1b, recombinant**
**interferon gamma-1b**
**levamisole hydrochloride**
**oprelvekin**
**sargramostim**

**COMBINATION PRODUCTS**
None.

---

**aldesleukin (IL-2, interleukin-2)**
Proleukin

*Pregnancy Risk Category C*

### HOW SUPPLIED
*Powder for injection:* 22 million IU/vial

### ACTION
Unknown. Stimulation of an immunologic host reaction to the tumor may be involved.

| Route | Onset | Peak | Duration |
|-------|-------|------|----------|
| I.V. | 4 wk | Unknown | ≤ 12 mo |

### INDICATIONS & DOSAGE
*Metastatic renal cell carcinoma—*
**Adults:** 600,000 IU/kg (0.037 mg/kg) I.V. over 15 minutes q 8 hours for 5 days (total of 14 doses). After 9-day rest, sequence is repeated for another 14 doses. Repeat courses may be given after rest period of at least 7 weeks.
*Metastatic melanoma—*
**Adults:** 600,000 IU/kg (0.037 mg/kg) I.V. over 15 minutes q 8 hours for total of 14 doses. After 9-day rest, sequence is repeated for another 14 doses. Repeat courses may be given after rest period of at least 7 weeks.

*Adjust-a-dose:* If toxicity occurs, withhold drug rather than administer a reduced dose. Therapy is continued after evaluation of patient.

### ADVERSE REACTIONS
**CNS:** *headache, mental status changes, dizziness, sensory dysfunction,* special senses disorders, syncope, motor dysfunction, **coma,** fatigue, *malaise; weakness.*
**CV:** *hypotension, sinus tachycardia,* **arrhythmias, bradycardia,** *PVC, premature atrial contractions,* myocardial ischemia, **MI, heart failure, cardiac arrest,** myocarditis, endocarditis, **CVA,** pericardial effusion, *phlebitis,* thrombosis, **capillary leak syndrome,** *edema.*
**EENT:** conjunctivitis.
**GI:** *nausea, vomiting, diarrhea, stomatitis, anorexia, bleeding,* dyspepsia, constipation.
**GU:** *oliguria, anuria, proteinuria,* hematuria, dysuria, urine retention, urinary frequency, *elevated BUN and serum creatinine levels.*
**Hematologic:** *anemia,* THROMBOCYTOPENIA, LEUKOPENIA, *coagulation disorders,* leukocytosis, eosinophilia.
**Hepatic:** *jaundice;* ascites; hepatomegaly; *elevated bilirubin, serum transaminase, alkaline phosphatase levels.*
**Metabolic:** *hypomagnesemia; acidosis; hypocalcemia; hypophosphatemia; hypokalemia; hyperuricemia; hypoalbuminemia;* hypoproteinemia; *hyponatremia; hyperkalemia, weight gain;* weight loss.
**Musculoskeletal:** arthralgia; myalgia.
**Respiratory:** *pulmonary congestion, dyspnea, pulmonary edema, hemoptysis,* **respiratory failure, pleural effusion, apnea, pneumothorax,** tachypnea, wheezing.
**Skin:** *pruritus, erythema, rash, dryness, exfoliative dermatitis, purpura, alopecia, petechiae,* persistent, nonprogressive vitiligo (in melanoma patients).
**Other:** *fever; chills; abdominal, chest,* or *back pain; infections at catheter tip; uri-*

---

Reactions may be *common,* uncommon, *life-threatening,* or COMMON AND LIFE-THREATENING.

*nary tract infections; injection site infections;* SEPSIS.

## INTERACTIONS
**Drug-drug.** *Antihypertensives:* increased risk of hypotension. Monitor closely.
*Cardiotoxic, hepatotoxic, myelotoxic, or nephrotoxic drugs:* enhanced toxicity. Avoid concomitant use.
*Corticosteroids:* decreased antitumor effectiveness of aldesleukin. Avoid concomitant use.
*Psychotropic drugs:* unpredictable interaction. Aldesleukin can alter CNS function. Use together cautiously.

## EFFECTS ON DIAGNOSTIC TESTS
None reported.

## CONTRAINDICATIONS
Contraindicated in patients with hypersensitivity to drug or its components and in those with abnormal cardiac (thallium) stress test or pulmonary function tests or organ allografts. Retreatment is contraindicated in patients who experience the following adverse effects: pericardial tamponade; disturbances in cardiac rhythm that were uncontrolled or unresponsive to intervention; sustained ventricular tachycardia (five beats or more); chest pain accompanied by ECG changes, indicating MI or angina pectoris; renal dysfunction requiring dialysis for 72 hours or more; coma or toxic psychosis lasting 48 hours or more; seizures that were repetitive or difficult to control; ischemia or perforation of the bowel; GI bleeding requiring surgery.

## NURSING CONSIDERATIONS
• Don't use drug unless patient has had definitive tests documenting normal cardiac and pulmonary function. Use with extreme caution in patients with history of seizure disorders and in those with normal test results if they have history of cardiac or pulmonary disease.
• Use cautiously and with close monitoring because severe adverse reactions usually accompany therapy at the recommended dosage.

• Use cautiously in patients who need large volumes of fluid (such as patients with hypercalcemia).
• Drug should be administered only in hospital under direction of doctor experienced in use of chemotherapeutic drugs. An intensive care facility and intensive care or cardiopulmonary specialist must be available.
• Monitor hematologic tests, including CBC, differential, and platelet counts; serum electrolyte levels; and renal and liver function tests, and obtain chest X-ray before therapy, as ordered. Repeat daily during therapy.
• Treat patients with bacterial infections before therapy, as ordered.
• Be prepared to titrate dosage of other drugs, as ordered, to compensate for renal and hepatic impairment occurring during treatment. Dosage is modified by withholding a dose or interrupting therapy rather than by reducing dose, as ordered.
• Withhold dose and notify doctor if patient develops moderate to severe lethargy or somnolence; continued administration can result in coma.
• Administer packed RBCs or platelets, as ordered. Severe anemia or thrombocytopenia may occur.
• *Alert:* Drug has been associated with capillary leak syndrome (CLS), a condition caused by loss of vascular tone, in which plasma proteins and fluids escape into the extravascular space. Mean arterial blood pressure begins to drop within 2 to 12 hours of treatment; edema and effusions may be severe, and death can result from hypoperfusion of major organs. Other conditions that accompany CLS include arrhythmias, MI, angina, mental status changes, renal insufficiency, respiratory distress or failure, and GI bleeding or infarction.
• Therapy is associated with impaired neutrophil function, which can lead to disseminated infection. Prophylactic antibiotic therapy with oxacillin, nafcillin, ciprofloxacin, or vancomycin has been used; check protocol and administer antibiotics, as ordered. Watch for infection.
• Patient should be neurologically stable with a negative computed tomography scan for CNS metastases. Drug may exac-

erbate symptoms in patients with unrecognized or undiagnosed CNS metastases.
• Drug may exacerbate preexisting autoimmune disease.

### I.V. administration
• To avoid altering the pharmacologic properties of drug, reconstitute and dilute carefully, and follow manufacturer's recommendations. Don't mix with other drugs or albumin.
• Reconstitute drug in vial containing 22 million IU (1.3 mg) with 1.2 ml of sterile water for injection. *Don't* use bacteriostatic water or normal saline for injection; these diluents increase aggregation of drug. Direct stream at sides of vial and gently swirl to reconstitute. Don't shake. Reconstituted solution will have concentration of 18 million IU (1.1 mg)/ml. It should be particle-free and colorless to slightly yellow.
• Add ordered dose of reconstituted drug to 50 ml of D₅W and infuse over 15 minutes. Don't use an in-line filter. Plastic infusion bags are preferred because they provide consistent drug delivery.
• Refrigerate powder for injection or reconstituted solutions. Return drug to room temperature before administering to patient. After reconstitution and dilution, administer within 48 hours.

### ✅ Patient teaching
• Explain administration schedule to patient and caregivers, and stress importance of compliance.
• Instruct patient to report adverse reactions promptly.

## epoetin alfa (erythropoietin)
Epogen, Eprex§, Procrit

*Pregnancy Risk Category C*

### HOW SUPPLIED
*Injection:* 2,000 U/ml, 3,000 U/ml, 4,000 U/ml, 10,000 U/ml; multidose vials of 10,000 U/ml, 20,000 U/ml

### ACTION
Mimics effects of erythropoietin, a naturally occurring hormone produced by the kidneys. Is one of the factors controlling rate of RBC production. Acts on the erythroid tissues in the bone marrow, stimulating mitotic activity of erythroid progenitor cells and early precursor cells. Functions as a growth factor and as a differentiating factor, enhancing rate of RBC production.

| Route | Onset | Peak | Duration |
|-------|-------|------|----------|
| I.V. | 1-6 wk | Immediate | Unknown |
| S.C. | 1-6 wk | 5-24 hr | Unknown |

### INDICATIONS & DOSAGE
*Anemia due to reduced production of endogenous erythropoietin due to end-stage renal disease—*
**Adults:** dosage is individualized. Starting dose is 50 to 100 U/kg I.V. three times weekly. (Nondialysis patients with chronic renal failure or patients receiving continuous peritoneal dialysis may receive drug by S.C. injection or I.V.) Maintenance dose is highly individualized.
*Adjust-a-dose:* Dosage is reduced when target hematocrit is reached or if hematocrit rises more than 4 points in a 2-week period. Dosage is increased if hematocrit doesn't increase by 5 to 6 points after 8 weeks of therapy.
*Adjunctive treatment of HIV-infected patients with anemia secondary to zidovudine therapy—*
**Adults:** 100 U/kg I.V. or S.C. three times weekly for 8 weeks or until target hemoglobin level is reached. If response isn't satisfactory after 8 weeks, dosage may be increased by 50 to 100 U/kg I.V. or S.C. three times weekly. After 4 to 8 weeks, dosage may be further increased in increments of 50 to 100 U/kg three times weekly, up to maximum of 300 U/kg I.V. or S.C. three times weekly.
*Anemia secondary to cancer chemotherapy—*
**Adults:** 150 U/kg S.C. three times weekly for 8 weeks or until target hemoglobin level is reached. If response isn't satisfactory after 8 weeks, dosage may be increased up to 300 U/kg S.C. three times weekly.
*Adjust-a-dose:* If hematocrit exceeds 40%, drug should be withheld until hematocrit falls to 36%.

---

Reactions may be *common*, uncommon, *life-threatening*, or **COMMON AND LIFE-THREATENING**.

*Reduction of need for allogenic blood transfusion in anemic patients scheduled to undergo elective, noncardiac, nonvascular surgery—*
**Adults:** 300 U/kg/day S.C. daily for 10 days before surgery, on day of surgery, and for 4 days after surgery. Or, 600 U/kg S.C. in once-weekly doses (21, 14, and 7 days before surgery), plus one-quarter dose on day of surgery.

**ADVERSE REACTIONS**
**CNS:** *headache,* **seizures,** *paresthesia, fatigue,* dizziness, *asthenia.*
**CV:** *hypertension, edema.*
**GI:** *nausea, vomiting, diarrhea.*
**GU:** increased BUN and creatinine levels.
**Metabolic:** hyperuricemia, hyperkalemia, hyperphosphatemia.
**Musculoskeletal:** *arthralgia.*
**Respiratory:** *cough, shortness of breath.*
**Skin:** *rash, injection site reactions,* urticaria.
**Other:** increased clotting of arteriovenous grafts, *pyrexia.*

**INTERACTIONS**
None significant.

**EFFECTS ON DIAGNOSTIC TESTS**
None reported.

**CONTRAINDICATIONS**
Contraindicated in patients with hypersensitivity to mammalian cell–derived products or albumin (human) and in those with uncontrolled hypertension.

**NURSING CONSIDERATIONS**
• Use with caution in breast-feeding women.
• Monitor blood pressure before therapy. Up to 80% of patients with chronic renal failure have hypertension. Blood pressure may rise, especially when hematocrit is increasing in the early part of therapy.
• If hematocrit is increasing and approaching 36%, reduce dosage to maintain target hematocrit range. If hematocrit stays after reducing dosage, hold dose temporarily until hematocrit decreases.
• When used in HIV-infected patients, be prepared to individualize dosage based on response, as ordered. Dosage recommen-

dations are for patients with endogenous erythropoietin levels of 500 U/L or less and cumulative zidovudine doses of 4.2 g/week or less.
• Patient treated with epoetin alfa may need additional heparin to prevent clotting during dialysis treatments.
• Monitor blood count, as ordered. Hematocrit may rise and cause excessive clotting. Renal function, uric acid, and potassium levels may rise.
• Institute diet restrictions or drug therapy to control blood pressure. Reduce dosage in patients who exhibit rapid rise in hematocrit (more than 4 points in a 2-week period), as ordered, to prevent hypertension.
• Patient's response to epoetin alfa depends on amount of endogenous erythropoietin in the plasma. Patients with levels of 500 U/L or more usually have transfusion-dependent anemia and probably won't respond to drug. Those with levels below 500 U/L usually respond well.
• Patient should receive adequate iron supplementation beginning no later than when epoetin alfa treatment starts and continuing throughout therapy. Patient may also need vitamin $B_{12}$ and folic acid.
• **Alert:** Don't confuse Epogen with Neupogen.

**I.V. administration**
• Give by direct injection without dilution. Solution contains no preservatives. Discard unused portion. Don't mix with other drugs. Don't shake.
• Drug may be given via the venous return line of dialysis tubing following dialysis to eliminate need for additional I.V. access.

**Patient teaching**
• Inform patient that pain or discomfort in limbs (long bones) and pelvis, and coldness and sweating aren't uncommon after injection (usually occurring within 2 hours). Symptoms may last for 12 hours and then disappear.
• Advise patient that blood specimens will be drawn weekly for blood counts and that dosage adjustments may be made based on results.
• Advise patient to avoid driving or operating heavy machinery during initiation of

therapy. There may be a relationship between excessively rapid hematocrit rise and seizures.
• Tell patient to monitor blood pressure at home and to adhere to dietary restrictions.
• Instruct patient to check that syringes used to administer drug are in tenths of ml.

---

## filgrastim (G-CSF; granulocyte-colony stimulating factor)
Neupogen

*Pregnancy Risk Category C*

### HOW SUPPLIED
*Injection:* 300 mcg/ml

### ACTION
A glycoprotein that stimulates proliferation and differentiation of hematopoietic cells. Is specific for neutrophils.

| Route | Onset | Peak | Duration |
|-------|-------|------|----------|
| I.V. | 5-60 min | 24 hr | 1-7 days |
| S.C. | 5-60 min | 2-8 hr | 1-7 days |

### INDICATIONS & DOSAGE
*To decrease risk of infection in patients with nonmyeloid malignant disease receiving myelosuppressive antineoplastics—*
**Adults and children:** 5 mcg/kg/day I.V. or S.C. as single dose given no sooner than 24 hours after cytotoxic chemotherapy. Doses may be increased in increments of 5 mcg/kg for each chemotherapy cycle depending on duration and severity of the nadir of absolute neutrophil count (ANC).
*To decrease risk of infection in patients with nonmyeloid malignant disease receiving myelosuppressive antineoplastics followed by bone marrow transplantation—*
**Adults and children:** 10 mcg/kg/day I.V. infusion of 4 or 24 hours or as continuous 24-hour S.C. infusion at least 24 hours after cytotoxic chemotherapy and bone marrow infusion. Subsequent dosages adjusted based on neutrophil response.
*Adjust-a-dose:* For patients with ANC over 1,000/mm³ for 3 consecutive days, reduce dose to 5 mcg/kg/day; if ANC remains over 1,000/mm³ for 3 more consecutive days, discontinue drug. If ANC de-

creases to below 1,000/mm³, resume therapy at 5 mcg/kg/day.
*Congenital neutropenia—*
**Adults:** 6 mcg/kg S.C. b.i.d. Dosage adjusted based on patient response.
*Adjust-a-dose:* For patients with a persistently elevated ANC (exceeding 10,000/mm³), reduce dose.
*Idiopathic or cyclic neutropenia—*
**Adults:** 5 mcg/kg S.C. daily. Dosage adjusted based on patient response.
*Peripheral blood progenitor cell (PBPC) collection and therapy in cancer patients—*
**Adults:** 10 mcg/kg/day S.C. Give 4 days before leukapheresis and continue until last leukapheresis.
*Adjust-a-dose:* For patients with WBC count over 100,000/mm³, dosage adjustment may be needed.

### ADVERSE REACTIONS
**CNS:** headache, weakness, *fatigue.*
**CV:** *MI, arrhythmias,* chest pain, hypotension.
**GI:** *nausea, vomiting, diarrhea, mucositis,* stomatitis, constipation.
**GU:** increased serum creatinine.
**Hematologic:** *thrombocytopenia,* leukocytosis.
**Hepatic:** increased alkaline phosphatase levels.
**Musculoskeletal:** *skeletal pain.*
**Respiratory:** dyspnea, cough.
**Skin:** *alopecia,* rash, cutaneous vasculitis.
**Other:** *fever, hypersensitivity reactions,* elevated uric acid and LD levels.

### INTERACTIONS
**Drug-drug.** *Chemotherapeutic drugs:* rapidly dividing myeloid cells are potentially sensitive to cytotoxic drugs. Don't use within 24 hours before or after a dose of one of these drugs. Use with caution in patients taking lithium.

### EFFECTS ON DIAGNOSTIC TESTS
None reported.

### CONTRAINDICATIONS
Contraindicated in patients with hypersensitivity to drug or its components or to proteins derived from *Escherichia coli.*

---

Reactions may be *common,* uncommon, *life-threatening*, or COMMON AND LIFE-THREATENING.

## NURSING CONSIDERATIONS
• Use with caution in breast-feeding women.
• Obtain baseline CBC and platelet count before therapy, as ordered.
• Once a dose is withdrawn, don't reenter vial. Discard unused portion. Vials are for single-dose use and contain no preservatives.
• Obtain CBC and platelet count two to three times weekly during therapy, as ordered. Patients who receive drug may potentially receive high doses of chemotherapy, which may increase risk of toxicities.
• A transiently increased neutrophil count is common 1 or 2 days after initiation of therapy. Give daily for up to 2 weeks or until ANC has returned to 10,000/mm³ after the expected chemotherapy-induced neutrophil nadir, as ordered.
• **Alert:** Don't confuse Neupogen with Epogen.

### ⬛ I.V. administration
• Dilute in 50 to 100 ml of D₅W and give by intermittent infusion over 15 to 60 minutes or continuous infusion over 24 hours. If final concentration of drug is 5 to 15 mcg/ml, add albumin at a concentration of 2 mg/ml (0.2%) to minimize binding of drug to plastic containers or tubing. Don't dilute with normal saline solution. Dilution to final concentration of less than 5 mcg/ml isn't recommended.

### ✅ Patient teaching
• If patient is to self-administer drug, teach him how to administer it and how to dispose of used needles, syringes, drug containers, and unused medicine.
• Instruct patient to report persistent or serious adverse reactions promptly.

---

## glatiramer acetate for injection (formerly copolymer 1)
Copaxone

*Pregnancy Risk Category B*

## HOW SUPPLIED
*Injection:* 20 mg lyophilized glatiramer acetate and 40 mg mannitol, USP, in a single-use 2-ml vial; 1-ml vial of sterile water for injection is included for reconstitution

## ACTION
Unknown. Thought to act by modifying immune processes responsible for the pathogenesis of multiple sclerosis.

| Route | Onset | Peak | Duration |
|-------|-------|------|----------|
| S.C. | Unknown | Unknown | Unknown |

## INDICATIONS & DOSAGE
*To reduce frequency of relapse in patients with relapsing-remitting multiple sclerosis—*
**Adults:** 20 mg S.C. daily.

## ADVERSE REACTIONS
**CNS:** abnormal dreams, agitation, *anxiety, asthenia,* confusion, emotional lability, foot drop, *hypertonia,* migraine, nervousness, nystagmus, speech disorder, stupor, tremor, vertigo, syncope.
**CV:** *chest pain,* hypertension, *palpitations, vasodilation,* tachycardia.
**EENT:** ear pain, eye disorder, *rhinitis.*
**GI:** anorexia, bowel urgency, *diarrhea,* gastroenteritis, GI disorder, *nausea,* oral moniliasis, salivary gland enlargement, tooth caries, ulcerative stomatitis, vomiting.
**GU:** amenorrhea, dysmenorrhea, hematuria, impotence, menorrhagia, suspicious Papanicolaou smear, *urinary urgency,* vaginal candidiasis, vaginal hemorrhage.
**Hematologic:** ecchymosis, *lymphadenopathy.*
**Metabolic:** weight gain.
**Musculoskeletal:** *arthralgia, back pain,* neck pain.
**Respiratory:** bronchitis, *dyspnea,* hyperventilation, laryngismus.
**Skin:** eczema; erythema; herpes simplex and zoster; *pruritus, rash, injection site reaction* or hemorrhage; skin atrophy; skin nodule; *diaphoresis;* urticaria; warts.
**Other:** bacterial infection, chills, cyst, peripheral and facial edema, fever, *flulike syndrome, infection,* pain.

## INTERACTIONS
None significant.

**EFFECTS ON DIAGNOSTIC TESTS**
None reported.

**CONTRAINDICATIONS**
Contraindicated in patients with hypersensitivity to drug or mannitol.

**NURSING CONSIDERATIONS**
• Administer drug by S.C. injection only.
• Store drug in refrigerator (36° to 46° F [2° to 8° C]); diluent can be kept at room temperature.
• Swirl lyophilized material and diluent gently and allow to stand at room temperature until completely dissolved, about 5 minutes.
• Use immediately after reconstitution because drug doesn't contain preservatives; discard unused drug. Use diluent provided for reconstitution.
• Immediate postinjection reactions have occurred in 10% of patients with multiple sclerosis; symptoms include flushing, chest pain, palpitations, anxiety, dyspnea, constriction of the throat, and urticaria. These reactions were transient and self-limiting, and didn't need specific treatment. Onset of postinjection reaction may occur several months after initiation of treatment and patients may have more than one episode.
• About 26% of patients have experienced at least one episode of transient chest pain, which usually begins at least 1 month after initiation of treatment; it isn't accompanied by other symptoms and doesn't appear to be clinically important.
• Because drug can modify immune response, it could interfere with normal immune function. Although evidence is lacking, there has been no evaluation of this risk.
• Drug is antigenic and may lead to induction of unwanted host responses. Systemic study of these effects hasn't been done.
• It isn't known if drug appears in breast milk.
• **Alert:** Don't confuse Copaxone with Compazine.

☑ **Patient teaching**
• Instruct patient how to reconstitute and self-inject drug. Supervise first injection.

• Explain need for aseptic self-injection techniques and warn patient against reuse of needles and syringes. Periodically review proper disposal of needles, syringes, drug containers, and unused drug.
• Tell patient to notify doctor if pregnancy is being planned, is suspected, or occurs.
• Tell woman to notify doctor if she is breast-feeding.
• Advise patient not to change drug or dosing schedule or to stop drug without medical approval.
• Tell patient to notify doctor immediately if dizziness, urticaria, diaphoresis, chest pain, difficulty breathing, or severe pain occurs following drug injection.

# interferon alfacon-1
Infergen

*Pregnancy Risk Category C*

**HOW SUPPLIED**
*Injection:* 9-mcg/0.3 ml, 15-mcg/0.5 ml vials

**ACTION**
Type-I interferons induce genetic-mediated biological responses that include antiviral, antiproliferative, and immunomodulatory effects and regulation of cytokine expression.

| Route | Onset | Peak | Duration |
|-------|-------|------|----------|
| S.C. | Unknown | 24-36 hr | Unknown |

**INDICATIONS & DOSAGE**
*Chronic hepatitis C viral infection—*
**Adults:** 9 mcg S.C. three times weekly for 24 weeks; for nonresponders or those patients who relapse, 15 mcg S.C. three times weekly for 6 months.
*Adjust-a-dose:* For patients intolerant to higher doses, dose may be reduced to 7.5 mcg. Don't give doses below 7.5 mcg because decreased efficacy may result.

**ADVERSE REACTIONS**
**CNS:** *headache, insomnia, dizziness, paresthesia, amnesia, nervousness, depression, anxiety, emotional lability,* confusion, agitation, **suicidal ideation,** *malaise.*

---

**CV:** hypertension, tachycardia, palpitations.
**EENT:** *retinal hemorrhages,* loss of visual acuity or visual field, conjunctivitis, tinnitus, ear pain, taste perversion, *pharyngitis, sinusitis, rhinitis,* epistaxis.
**GI:** *abdominal pain, nausea, diarrhea, anorexia, dyspepsia, vomiting,* constipation, flatulence, toothache, hemorrhoids, decreased saliva.
**GU:** decreased libido, dysmenorrhea, vaginitis.
**Hematologic:** *granulocytopenia, leukopenia, thrombocytopenia,* ecchymosis, lymphadenopathy, lymphocytosis, increased PT.
**Metabolic:** hypothyroidism.
**Respiratory:** *infection, cough, congestion,* dyspnea, bronchitis.
**Skin:** *alopecia, pruritus, rash,* dry skin; pain, erythema at injection site.
**Other:** *hypersensitivity reactions, body pain, flulike symptoms,* increased serum triglycerides.

## INTERACTIONS
**Drug-drug.** *Drugs metabolized by cytochrome P-450:* may alter drug levels. Monitor changes in levels of these drugs.
*Myelosuppressives:* no studies have been conducted; however, use cautiously with interferon alfacon-1. Monitor CBC and therapeutic or toxic levels of concomitant drugs.

## EFFECTS ON DIAGNOSTIC TESTS
None reported.

## CONTRAINDICATIONS
Contraindicated in patients with hypersensitivity to alpha interferons, to *Escherichia coli*–derived products, or to any component of product. Also contraindicated in patients with history of severe psychiatric disorders, autoimmune hepatitis, or decompensated hepatic disease.

## NURSING CONSIDERATIONS
• Use with caution in patients with history of cardiac disease and other autoimmune or endocrine disorders, in those with abnormally low peripheral blood cell counts, or those receiving drugs known to cause myelosuppression.

• Depression and suicidal behavior have been associated with drug.
• The following laboratory tests should be performed before therapy, 2 weeks after initiation, and periodically during therapy: CBC with platelets, serum creatinine, serum albumin, serum bilirubin, thyroid-stimulating hormone, and $T_4$.
• At least 48 hours should elapse between doses.
• Store drug in refrigerator at 36° to 46° F (2° to 8° C); don't freeze. Injection may be allowed to reach room temperature just before use. Avoid vigorous shaking. Discard unused portion.
• *Alert:* If hypersensitivity reaction occurs, stop drug immediately and treat, as ordered.

### ☑ Patient teaching
• If drug is to be used at home, instruct patient on appropriate use, dosage, and administration. A patient information leaflet is available from the manufacturer and should be given to the patient. Also instruct patient on proper disposal procedures for needles, syringes, drug containers, and unused drug.
• Instruct patient not to reuse needles or syringes or reenter vial once initially used.
• Tell patient to discard all syringes and needles in a puncture-resistant container.
• Caution patient to inspect vial for discoloration and particulates before use; don't use if either are observed.
• Tell patient that nonnarcotic analgesics and administration at bedtime may be used to prevent or lessen flulike symptoms (headache, fever, malaise, myalgia) associated with therapy.
• Instruct patient to immediately report symptoms of depression.

---

## interferon alfa-2a, recombinant (rIFN-A)
Roferon-A

*Pregnancy Risk Category C*

### HOW SUPPLIED
*Injection:* 3, 6, 9, 36 million IU/single-use vial; 9, 18 million IU/multidose vial

---

*Sterile powder for injection:* 18 million IU/vial with diluent

## ACTION
Unknown. Appears to involve direct antiproliferative action against tumor or viral cells to inhibit replication and modulation of host immune response by enhancing phagocytic activity of macrophages and augmenting specific cytotoxicity of lymphocytes for target cells.

| Route | Onset | Peak | Duration |
|-------|-------|------|----------|
| I.M. | Unknown | 2-12 hr | Unknown |
| S.C. | Unknown | 3-12 hr | Unknown |

## INDICATIONS & DOSAGE
*Hairy cell leukemia—*
**Adults:** for induction, 3 million IU S.C. or I.M. daily for 16 to 24 weeks. For maintenance, 3 million IU S.C. or I.M. three times weekly.
*AIDS-related Kaposi's sarcoma—*
**Adults:** for induction, 36 million IU S.C. or I.M. daily for 10 to 12 weeks. For maintenance, 36 million IU S.C. or I.M. three times weekly.
*Philadelphia chromosome–positive chronic myelogenous leukemia—*
**Adults:** initially, 3 million IU daily for 3 days; then 6 million IU for 3 days; then 9 million IU for duration of treatment.

## ADVERSE REACTIONS
**CNS:** *dizziness, confusion,* paresthesia, numbness, lethargy, *depression, decreased mental status,* forgetfulness, **coma,** nervousness, insomnia, sedation, apathy, anxiety, irritability, fatigue, vertigo, gait disturbances, incoordination, syncope.
**CV:** hypotension, chest pain, ***arrhythmias,*** palpitations, **heart failure,** hypertension, edema, ***MI.***
**EENT:** *dryness or inflammation of the oropharynx,* rhinorrhea, sinusitis, conjunctivitis, earache, eye irritation.
**GI:** *anorexia, nausea, diarrhea, vomiting,* abdominal fullness, *abdominal pain,* flatulence, constipation, hypermotility, gastric distress, excessive salivation, *change in taste.*
**GU:** transient impotence.

**Hematologic:** *leukopenia, mild thrombocytopenia,* increased PT, INR and PTT.
**Hepatic:** *hepatitis,* increased ALT, AST, LD, and alkaline phosphatase levels.
**Metabolic:** *weight loss,* hypercalcemia, hyperphosphatemia, increased fasting blood glucose level.
**Respiratory:** *cough, dyspnea.*
**Skin:** *rash,* dryness, pruritus, *partial alopecia,* urticaria, flushing, diaphoresis; *inflammation at injection site.*
**Other:** *flulike syndrome,* cyanosis, night sweats, hot flashes.

## INTERACTIONS
**Drug-drug.** *Aminophylline, theophylline:* may reduce theophylline clearance. Monitor serum levels.
*Aspirin:* increased risk of GI bleeding. Avoid use together.
*CNS depressants:* enhanced CNS effects. Avoid concomitant use.
*Live virus vaccine:* increased risk of adverse reactions and decreased antibody response. Don't use together.
**Drug-lifestyle.** *Alcohol use:* increased risk of GI bleeding. Avoid use during drug therapy.

## EFFECTS ON DIAGNOSTIC TESTS
None reported.

## CONTRAINDICATIONS
Contraindicated in patients with hypersensitivity to drug, murine (mouse) immunoglobulin, or other drug components.

## NURSING CONSIDERATIONS
• Use cautiously in patients with severe hepatic or renal function impairment, seizure disorders, compromised CNS function, cardiac disease, or myelosuppression.
• Depression and suicidal behavior have been associated with treatment.
• Obtain allergy history. Drug contains phenol as a preservative and serum albumin as a stabilizer.
• Use S.C. administration route in patients whose platelet count is below 50,000/mm$^3$.
• Administer drug at bedtime to minimize daytime drowsiness.

---

Reactions may be *common,* uncommon, *life-threatening,* or COMMON AND LIFE-THREATENING.

• Make sure patient is well hydrated, especially during initial stages of treatment.
• At beginning of therapy, assess patient for flulike symptoms, which tend to diminish with continued therapy. Premedicate patient with acetaminophen to minimize symptoms.
• Watch for CNS adverse reactions, such as decreased mental status and dizziness, during therapy.
• For patients who develop thrombocytopenia, exercise extreme care in performing invasive procedures; inspect injection site and skin frequently for signs of bruising; limit frequency of I.M. injections; test urine, emesis fluid, stool, and secretions for occult blood.
• *Alert:* Different brands of interferon may not be equivalent and may need different dosages.
• Severe adverse reactions may need dosage reduction to one-half or discontinuation of drug until reactions subside.
• *Alert:* Neurotoxicity and cardiotoxicity are more common in elderly patients, especially those with underlying CNS or cardiac impairment.
• Use with blood dyscrasia–causing drugs, bone marrow suppressant, or radiation therapy may increase bone marrow suppressant effects. Dosage reduction may be needed.
• Keep drug refrigerated. Don't freeze.

✓**Patient teaching**
• Advise patient that laboratory tests will be performed before and periodically during therapy. Tests include CBC with differential, platelet count, blood chemistry and electrolyte studies, liver function tests and, if patient has preexisting cardiac disorder or advanced stages of cancer, ECG.
• Instruct patient in proper oral hygiene during treatment because the bone marrow suppressant effects of interferon may lead to microbial infection, delayed healing, and gingival bleeding. Drug may also decrease salivary flow.
• Emphasize need to follow doctor's instructions about taking and recording temperature and how and when to take acetaminophen.
• Advise patient to check with doctor for instructions after missing dose.

• Tell patient that drug may cause temporary partial hair loss; hair should return when drug is withdrawn.
• If patient will be self-administering drug, teach him how to prepare and administer it and how to dispose of used needles, syringes, containers, and unused drug.
• Instruct patient not to take aspirin or alcohol because concurrent use increases risk of GI bleeding.
• Instruct patient not to change brands of interferon without medical consultation.
• Advise patients against performing tasks that require mental alertness.
• Advise patients to immediately report signs of depression.

## interferon alfa-2b, recombinant (IFN-alpha 2)
Intron-A

*Pregnancy Risk Category C*

### HOW SUPPLIED
*Powder for injection:* 3, 5, 10, 18, 25, 50 million IU/vial with diluent
*Injection:* 3, 5 million IU/0.5-ml vial; 1, 10 million IU/1-ml vial; 18 million IU/3.8-ml vial; 25 million IU/3.2-ml vial

### ACTION
Unknown. Appears to involve direct antiproliferative action against tumor or viral cells to inhibit replication and modulation of host immune response by enhancing phagocytic activity of macrophages and augmenting specific cytotoxicity of lymphocytes for target cells.

| Route | Onset | Peak | Duration |
|---|---|---|---|
| I.V. | Unknown | 15-60 min | 4 hr |
| I.M., S.C. | Unknown | 3-12 hr | 16 hr |

### INDICATIONS & DOSAGE
*Hairy cell leukemia—*
**Adults:** 2 million IU/m$^2$ I.M. or S.C., three times weekly for 6 months or more.
*Condylomata acuminata (genital or venereal warts)—*
**Adults:** 1 million IU for each lesion intralesionally three times weekly for 3 weeks.

*AIDS-related Kaposi's sarcoma—*
**Adults:** 30 million IU/m$^2$ S.C. or I.M. three times weekly.
*Chronic hepatitis B—*
**Adults:** 30 to 35 million IU weekly I.M. or S.C., administered as 5 million IU daily or 10 million IU three times weekly for 16 weeks.
**Children ages 1 and older:** 3 million IU/m$^2$ S.C. three times weekly for first week; then increase to 6 million IU/m$^2$ S.C. three times weekly (maximum is 10 million IU three times weekly) for total of 16 to 24 weeks.
*Chronic hepatitis C—*
**Adults:** 3 million IU I.M. or S.C. three times weekly.
*Adjunct to surgical treatment in patients with malignant melanoma who are asymptomatic after surgery but at high risk for systemic recurrence for up to 8 weeks after surgery—*
**Adults:** initially, 20 million IU/m$^2$ by I.V. infusion 5 consecutive days weekly for 4 weeks; then maintenance dose of 10 million IU/m$^2$ S.C. three times weekly for 48 weeks.

## ADVERSE REACTIONS

**CNS:** *dizziness, confusion, paresthesia,* lethargy, *depression, difficulty in thinking or concentrating, insomnia,* anxiety, *fatigue, hypoesthesia, amnesia,* nervousness, *somnolence,* weakness, *malaise, asthenia.*
**CV:** hypotension, *chest pain,* flushing.
**EENT:** visual disturbances, hearing disorders, pharyngitis, *nasal congestion, sinusitis,* rhinitis, stye.
**GI:** *anorexia, nausea, diarrhea, vomiting,* abdominal pain, *dyspepsia,* constipation, loose stools, eructation, *dry mouth,* dysgeusia, stomatitis, gingivitis.
**GU:** transient impotence, gynecomastia.
**Hematologic:** *leukopenia,* anemia, *thrombocytopenia,* increased PT, INR and PTT.
**Hepatic:** increased ALT, AST, LD, and alkaline phosphatase levels.
**Metabolic:** hypercalcemia, hyperphosphatemia, increased fasting blood glucose level.
**Musculoskeletal:** *arthralgia, back pain.*
**Respiratory:** *dyspnea, coughing.*

**Skin:** *rash, dryness, pruritus, alopecia,* candidiasis, dermatitis, *increased diaphoresis.*
**Other:** *flulike syndrome, rigors.*

## INTERACTIONS

**Drug-drug.** *Aminophylline, theophylline:* may reduce theophylline clearance. Monitor serum levels.
*CNS depressants:* enhanced CNS effects. Avoid concomitant use.
*Live virus vaccines:* risk of enhanced adverse reactions to vaccine or decreased antibody response. Postpone immunization.
*Zidovudine:* synergistic adverse effects (higher risk of neutropenia) may occur. Carefully monitor WBC count.

## EFFECTS ON DIAGNOSTIC TESTS
None reported.

## CONTRAINDICATIONS
Contraindicated in patients with hypersensitivity to drug or its components.

## NURSING CONSIDERATIONS
• Use cautiously in patients with history of CV disease, pulmonary disease, diabetes mellitus, coagulation disorders, and severe myelosuppression.
• Use S.C. administration route in patients whose platelet count is below 50,000/mm$^3$.
• Depression and suicidal behavior have been associated with drug use; patients with preexisting psychotic disorder, especially depression, shouldn't continue drug treatment.
• Administer drug at bedtime to minimize daytime drowsiness.
• When administering interferon for condylomata acuminata, use only 10 million-IU vial because dilution of other strengths needed for intralesional use results in a hypertonic solution. Don't reconstitute drug in 10 million-IU vial with more than 1 ml of diluent. Use tuberculin or similar syringe and 25G to 30G needle. Don't inject too deeply beneath lesion or too superficially. As many as five lesions can be treated at one time. To ease discomfort, administer in evening with acetaminophen.

---

Reactions may be *common,* uncommon, *life-threatening,* or COMMON AND LIFE-THREATENING.

• Make sure patient is well hydrated, especially during initial treatment.

• At beginning of treatment, monitor patient for flulike symptoms, which tend to diminish with continued therapy. Premedicate patient with acetaminophen to minimize these symptoms.

• Periodically check for adverse CNS reactions, such as decreased mental status and dizziness, during therapy.

• For patients who develop thrombocytopenia, exercise extreme care in performing invasive procedures; inspect injection site and skin frequently for signs of bruising; limit frequency of I.M. injections; test urine, emesis fluid, stool, and secretions for occult blood.

• Severe adverse reactions may need dosage reduction to one-half or discontinuation of drug until reactions subside.

• *Alert:* Neurotoxicity and cardiotoxicity are more common in elderly patients, especially those with underlying CNS or cardiac impairment.

• Use with blood dyscrasia–causing drugs, bone marrow suppressants, or radiation therapy may increase bone marrow suppressant effects. Dosage reduction may be needed.

• In treatment of condylomata acuminata, keep in mind that maximum response usually occurs 4 to 8 weeks after initiation of therapy. If results aren't satisfactory after 12 to 16 weeks, a second course may be instituted. Patients with 6 to 10 condylomata may receive a second course of treatment; patients with more than 10 condylomata may receive additional courses.

**I.V. administration**

• Infusion solution should be prepared immediately before use. Based on desired dose, reconstitute appropriate vial strength of drug with diluent provided. Withdraw dose and inject into a 100-ml bag of normal saline. Final concentration of drug shouldn't be less than 10 million IU/100 ml. Infuse over 20 minutes.

**✓ Patient teaching**

• Advise patient to avoid contact with persons with viral illness; patient is at increased risk for infection during therapy.

• Advise patient that laboratory tests will be performed before and periodically during therapy. Tests include CBC with differential, platelet count, blood chemistry and electrolyte studies, liver function tests and, if patient has preexisting cardiac disorder or advanced stages of cancer, ECG.

• Instruct patient in proper oral hygiene during treatment because bone marrow suppressant effects of interferon may lead to microbial infection, delayed healing, and gingival bleeding. Drug may also decrease salivary flow.

• Advise patient to check with doctor for instructions after missing a dose.

• Emphasize need to follow doctor's instructions about taking and recording temperature and how and when to take acetaminophen.

• If patient is to self-administer drug, teach him how to prepare injection and how to use disposable syringe. Give him information on drug stability.

• Tell patient that drug may cause temporary partial hair loss; hair should return after drug is withdrawn.

• Advise patient to notify doctor if signs of depression occur.

## interferon beta-1a
Avonex

*Pregnancy Risk Category C*

### HOW SUPPLIED
*Lyophilized powder for injection:* 33 mcg (6.6 million IU)

### ACTION
Exact mechanism unknown. Its biological response-modifying properties are mediated through its interactions with specific cell receptors found on the surface of human cells. Binding of these receptors induces the expression of a number of interferon-induced gene products believed to mediate the biological actions of interferon beta-1a.

| Route | Onset | Peak | Duration |
|-------|-------|------|----------|
| I.M. | Unknown | 3-15 hr | Unknown |

## INDICATIONS & DOSAGE
*Relapsing forms of multiple sclerosis to slow accumulation of physical disability and decrease frequency of clinical exacerbation—*
**Adults ages 18 and older:** 30 mcg I.M. once weekly.

## ADVERSE REACTIONS
**CNS:** *headache, sleep difficulty, dizziness,* syncope, ***suicidal tendency, seizures,*** speech disorder, ataxia, *asthenia,* malaise.
**CV:** chest pain, vasodilation.
**EENT:** otitis media, decreased hearing, *sinusitis.*
**GI:** *nausea, diarrhea, dyspepsia,* anorexia, abdominal pain.
**GU:** ovarian cyst, vaginitis.
**Hematologic:** anemia, elevated eosinophil levels, decreased hematocrit.
**Hepatic:** elevated AST levels.
**Musculoskeletal:** *muscle ache,* muscle spasm, arthralgia.
**Respiratory:** *upper respiratory tract infection,* dyspnea.
**Skin:** ecchymosis at injection site, injection site reaction, urticaria, alopecia, nevus, herpes zoster, herpes simplex.
**Other:** *flulike syndrome, pain, fever, chills, infection,* ***hypersensitivity reactions.***

## INTERACTIONS
**Drug-lifestyle.** *Sun exposure:* photosensitivity reactions may occur. Take precautions.

## EFFECTS ON DIAGNOSTIC TESTS
None reported.

## CONTRAINDICATIONS
Contraindicated in patients with history of hypersensitivity to natural or recombinant interferon beta, human albumin, or other components of drug.

## NURSING CONSIDERATIONS
• Use cautiously in patients with depression, seizure disorders, or severe cardiac conditions.
• Safety and efficacy of drug in chronic progressive multiple sclerosis or in children under age 18 haven't been established.
• Monitor patient closely for depression and suicidal ideation. It isn't known if these symptoms are related to the underlying neurologic basis of multiple sclerosis or to interferon beta-1a.
• Monitor WBC count, platelet count, and blood chemistries, including liver function tests.
• To reconstitute drug, inject 1.1 ml of supplied diluent (sterile water for injection) into vial and gently swirl to dissolve drug. Don't shake.
• Drug should be used as soon as possible but may be used within 6 hours after being reconstituted if stored at 36° to 46° F (2° to 8° C).
• It isn't known if drug appears in breast milk. Because of potential for serious adverse reactions in breast-fed infants, a decision whether to discontinue breast-feeding or drug must be made.

### ✅ Patient teaching
• Teach patient and family member how to reconstitute drug and administer I.M.
• Caution patient not to change dosage or schedule of administration. If a dose is missed, tell him to take it as soon as he remembers. The regular schedule may then be resumed. Two injections shouldn't be administered within 2 days of each other.
• Show patient how to store drug.
• Inform patient that flulike symptoms, such as fever, fatigue, myalgia, headache, chills, and arthralgia, aren't uncommon following initiation of therapy. Acetaminophen 650 mg P.O. may be taken immediately before injection and for an additional 24 hours after each injection, as ordered, to lessen severity of these symptoms.
• Advise patient to report depression, suicidal ideation, or other adverse reactions.
• Instruct patient to keep syringes and needles away from children. Also instruct him not to reuse needles or syringes and to discard them in a syringe-disposal unit.
• Caution woman of childbearing age not to become pregnant during therapy because of potential of drug to cause spontaneous abortion. If pregnancy occurs, in-

struct patient to notify doctor immediately and to discontinue drug, as ordered.
• Advise patient to use sunscreen and avoid sun exposure while taking drug because photosensitization may occur.

---

## interferon beta-1b, recombinant
Betaferon§, Betaseron

*Pregnancy Risk Category C*

### HOW SUPPLIED
*Powder for injection:* 9.6 million IU (0.3 mg)

### ACTION
A naturally occurring antiviral and immunoregulatory drug derived from human fibroblasts. Attaches to membrane receptors and causes cellular changes, including increased protein synthesis.

| Route | Onset | Peak | Duration |
|-------|-------|------|----------|
| S.C. | Unknown | 1-8 hr | Unknown |

### INDICATIONS & DOSAGE
*To reduce frequency of exacerbations in patients with relapsing-remitting multiple sclerosis—*
**Adults:** 8 million IU (0.25 mg) S.C. every other day.

### ADVERSE REACTIONS
**CNS:** depression, anxiety, emotional lability, depersonalization, ***suicidal tendencies,*** confusion, somnolence, *hypertonia, asthenia, migraine,* **seizures,** *headache, dizziness.*
**CV:** palpitations, hypertension, tachycardia, peripheral vascular disorder, ***hemorrhage.***
**EENT:** laryngitis, *sinusitis, conjunctivitis,* abnormal vision.
**GI:** *diarrhea, constipation, abdominal pain, vomiting.*
**GU:** *menstrual bleeding or spotting, early or delayed menses, fewer days of menstrual flow, menorrhagia.*
**Hematologic:** *decreased WBC and absolute neutrophil counts.*
**Hepatic:** *elevated ALT and bilirubin levels.*

**Respiratory:** dyspnea.
**Skin:** *inflammation, pain, necrosis at injection site, diaphoresis,* alopecia.
**Other:** *flulike syndrome,* breast pain, *pelvic pain, lymphadenopathy, pain,* generalized edema, *myasthenia.*

### INTERACTIONS
None significant.

### EFFECTS ON DIAGNOSTIC TESTS
None reported.

### CONTRAINDICATIONS
Contraindicated in patients with hypersensitivity to interferon beta, human albumin, or components of drug.

### NURSING CONSIDERATIONS
• Use cautiously in women of childbearing age. Inconclusive evidence exists about drug's teratogenic effects, but it may be an abortifacient.
• To reconstitute, inject 1.2 ml of supplied diluent (half normal saline injection) into vial and gently swirl to dissolve drug. Don't shake. Reconstituted solution will contain 8 million IU (0.25 mg)/ml. Discard vial that contains particulates or discolored solution.
• Inject immediately after preparation.
• Rotate injection sites to minimize local reactions and observe site for necrosis.
• Monitor patient for signs of depression.

### ☑ Patient teaching
• Warn woman of childbearing age about dangers to fetus. If pregnancy occurs during therapy, tell her to notify doctor and stop taking drug.
• Teach patient how to self-administer S.C. injections, including solution preparation, use of aseptic technique, rotation of injection sites, and equipment disposal. Periodically reevaluate patient's technique.
• Advise patient to take drug at bedtime to minimize mild flulike symptoms that commonly occur.
• Advise patient to report thoughts of suicidal ideation or depression.
• Tell patient to immediately report signs of necrosis at injection site.

---

*Liquid contains alcohol.   **May contain tartrazine.   †Canada   ‡Australia   §U.K.   ◇OTC

## interferon gamma-1b
Actimmune

*Pregnancy Risk Category C*

### HOW SUPPLIED
*Injection:* 100 mcg (3 million U)/0.5-ml vial

### ACTION
Acts as an interleukin-type lymphokine. Has potent phagocyte-activating properties and enhances the oxidative metabolism of tissue macrophages.

| Route | Onset | Peak | Duration |
|-------|-------|------|----------|
| S.C. | Unknown | 7 hr | Unknown |

### INDICATIONS & DOSAGE
*Chronic granulomatous disease—*
**Adults with body surface area (BSA) over 0.5 m²:** 50 mcg/m² (1.5 million U/m²) S.C. three times weekly, preferably h.s., and in deltoid or anterior thigh muscle.
**Adults with a BSA 0.5 m² or below:** 1.5 mcg/kg S.C. three times weekly.

### ADVERSE REACTIONS
**CNS:** *fatigue,* decreased mental status, gait disturbance, dizziness.
**GI:** *nausea, vomiting, diarrhea,* abdominal pain.
**GU:** proteinuria.
**Hematologic:** *neutropenia, thrombocytopenia.*
**Hepatic:** elevated liver enzyme levels.
**Metabolic:** weight loss.
**Musculoskeletal:** back pain.
**Skin:** *erythema, tenderness at injection site; rash.*
**Other:** *flulike syndrome.*

### INTERACTIONS
**Drug-drug.** *Myelosuppressives:* possible additive myelosuppression. Monitor closely.
*Zidovudine:* increased plasma levels of zidovudine. Dosage adjustments are needed when used concurrently.

### EFFECTS ON DIAGNOSTIC TESTS
None reported.

### CONTRAINDICATIONS
Contraindicated in patients with hypersensitivity to drug or to genetically engineered products derived from *Escherichia coli.*

### NURSING CONSIDERATIONS
• Use cautiously in patients with cardiac disease, including arrhythmias, ischemia, or heart failure. The flulike syndrome commonly seen with high doses of drug can exacerbate these conditions.
• Use cautiously in patients with compromised CNS function or seizure disorders. CNS adverse reactions that may occur at high doses of drug can exacerbate these conditions.
• Use myelosuppressives together with caution.
• Premedicate patient with acetaminophen to minimize symptoms at start of therapy. Flulike symptoms tend to diminish with continued therapy.
• Before beginning therapy and at 3-month intervals, monitor CBC, platelets, renal and hepatic function tests, and urinalysis.
• Discard unused drug. Each vial is for single-dose use only and doesn't contain a preservative.

### ☑ Patient teaching
• If patient is to self-administer drug, teach him how to administer it and how to dispose of used needles, syringes, containers, and unused drug.
• Instruct patient how to manage flulike symptoms (fever, fatigue, myalgia, headache, chills, arthralgia) that commonly occur.
• Advise use of acetaminophen.

## levamisole hydrochloride
Ergamisol

*Pregnancy Risk Category C*

### HOW SUPPLIED
*Tablets:* 50 mg (base)

### ACTION
Unknown. Appears to restore depressed immune function and may potentiate the

actions of monocytes and macrophages and enhance T-cell responses. Also inhibits alkaline phosphatase and cholinergic activity.

| Route | Onset | Peak | Duration |
|-------|-------|------|----------|
| P.O. | Unknown | 1.5-2 hr | Unknown |

## INDICATIONS & DOSAGE
*Adjuvant treatment of Dukes' stage C colon cancer (with fluorouracil) after surgical resection—*
**Adults:** 50 mg P.O. q 8 hours for 3 days, beginning no sooner than 7 days and no later than 30 days after surgery, provided patient is out of the hospital, ambulatory, and maintaining normal oral nutrition; has well-healed wounds; and has recovered from postoperative complications. Fluorouracil (450 mg/m$^2$/day I.V.) is given for 5 days with a 3-day course of levamisole starting 21 to 34 days after surgery.

Maintenance dose is 50 mg P.O. q 8 hours for 3 days q 2 weeks for 1 year. Given with fluorouracil maintenance therapy (450 mg/m$^2$/day by rapid I.V. push once weekly, beginning 28 days after initial 5-day course) for 1 year.
*Adjust-a-dose:* Dosage modifications are based on hematologic parameters. If WBC count is 2,500 to 3,500/mm$^3$, don't administer fluorouracil, as ordered, until WBC count is above 3,500/mm$^3$. When fluorouracil is restarted, reduce dosage by 20%, as ordered. If WBC count stays below 2,500/mm$^3$ for over 10 days after fluorouracil is withdrawn, discontinue levamisole, as ordered. If platelet count is below 100,000/mm$^3$, therapy with both fluorouracil and levamisole should be discontinued.

## ADVERSE REACTIONS
**CNS:** *dizziness, headache, paresthesia, somnolence, depression, nervousness, insomnia, anxiety, fatigue.*
**CV:** chest pain, edema.
**EENT:** blurred vision, conjunctivitis, *stomatitis, dysgeusia, altered sense of smell.*
**GI:** *nausea, diarrhea, vomiting,* anorexia, abdominal pain, constipation, flatulence, dyspepsia.
**GU:** hyperbilirubinemia.

**Hematologic:** *agranulocytosis, leukopenia, thrombocytopenia,* anemia.
**Musculoskeletal:** arthralgia, myalgia.
**Skin:** dermatitis, exfoliative dermatitis, pruritus, urticaria, *alopecia.*
**Other:** rigors, *infection, fever.*

## INTERACTIONS
**Drug-drug.** *Phenytoin:* plasma levels may be elevated when administered with levamisole and fluorouracil. Monitor phenytoin plasma levels.
*Warfarin:* may prolong coagulation times if taken together. Warfarin dose may need to be adjusted.
**Drug-lifestyle.** *Alcohol use:* may precipitate a disulfiram-like reaction. Avoid concomitant use.

## EFFECTS ON DIAGNOSTIC TESTS
None reported.

## CONTRAINDICATIONS
Contraindicated in patients with hypersensitivity to drug or its components.

## NURSING CONSIDERATIONS
● *Alert:* Use cautiously and with close hematologic monitoring because agranulocytosis, which is sometimes fatal, may occur. Neutropenia is usually reversible when therapy is discontinued.
● Obtain baseline CBC with differential, platelet count, and electrolyte levels, and liver function studies, as ordered, immediately before starting therapy.
● If levamisole therapy begins 7 to 20 days after surgery, fluorouracil should be started with second course of levamisole therapy. It should begin no sooner than 21 days and no later than 34 days after surgery. If levamisole is deferred until 21 to 30 days after surgery, fluorouracil therapy should begin with first course of levamisole.
● Recommended doses shouldn't be exceeded. Higher doses are associated with greater risk of agranulocytosis.
● Obtain CBC with differential and platelet count at weekly intervals, as ordered, before treatment with fluorouracil. Obtain electrolyte levels and liver function studies every 3 months for 1 year, as ordered.

---

*Liquid contains alcohol.    **May contain tartrazine.    †Canada    ‡Australia    §U.K.    ◇OTC

## ☑Patient teaching
• Tell patient to promptly report development of stomatitis or diarrhea. If either of these reactions occur during initial course of fluorouracil therapy, drug is discontinued and then weekly fluorouracil therapy is begun 28 days after start of initial course. If stomatitis or diarrhea develops during weekly doses of fluorouracil, fluorouracil therapy is deferred until these symptoms subside. Then fluorouracil therapy is started at dosages reduced by 20%.
• Advise patient to immediately report flulike symptoms, such as fever, malaise, headache, chills, arthralgia, and fatigue.
• Advise breast-feeding woman to discontinue nursing during drug therapy.

## oprelvekin
Neumega

*Pregnancy Risk Category C*

## HOW SUPPLIED
*Injection:* 5 mg single-dose vial with diluent

## ACTION
A thrombopoietic growth factor that directly stimulates proliferation of hematopoietic stem cells and megakaryocyte progenitor cells. Also induces megakaryocyte maturation, resulting in increased platelet production.

| Route | Onset | Peak | Duration |
|-------|-------|------|----------|
| S.C. | Unknown | 3-5 hr | Unknown |

## INDICATIONS & DOSAGE
*Prevention of severe thrombocytopenia and reduction of need for platelet transfusions following myelosuppressive chemotherapy with nonmyeloid malignancies—*
**Adults:** 50 mcg/kg as single daily S.C. injection.

## ADVERSE REACTIONS
**CNS:** *asthenia, headache, insomnia, dizziness,* paresthesia, *syncope.*
**CV:** *tachycardia, palpitations,* ATRIAL FLUTTER OR FIBRILLATION, *edema.*

**EENT:** blurred vision, *conjunctival injection,* eye hemorrhage, pharyngitis.
**GI:** *oral candidiasis, nausea, vomiting, diarrhea.*
**Hematologic:** anemia.
**Metabolic:** dehydration, hypocalcemia.
**Respiratory:** dyspnea, cough, pleural effusions.
**Skin:** *rash,* skin discoloration, exfoliative dermatitis.

## INTERACTIONS
**Drug-drug.** *Diuretics, ifosfamide:* severe hypokalemia resulting in death has occurred in patients concomitantly receiving these drugs and oprelvekin. Use with caution.

## EFFECTS ON DIAGNOSTIC TESTS
None reported.

## CONTRAINDICATIONS
Contraindicated in patients with hypersensitivity to drug or its components.

## NURSING CONSIDERATIONS
• Administer S.C. in the abdomen, thigh, hip, or upper arm.
• Dosing should begin 6 to 24 hours following completion of chemotherapy and end at least 2 days before starting next planned cycle of chemotherapy.
• Each single-dose vial should be reconstituted with 1 ml of supplied diluent. Avoid excessive or vigorous agitation. Discard unused portions.
• Use reconstituted drug within 3 hours.
• Store drug and diluent in refrigerator until ready to use.
• Use drug cautiously in patients with heart failure because of fluid retention.
• Closely monitor fluid and electrolyte status in patients receiving chronic diuretic therapy.
• Obtain a CBC before chemotherapy and at regular intervals during drug therapy.
• Fluid retention can be severe; monitor closely.

## ☑Patient teaching
• Instruct patient about appropriate preparation and administration of drug if he is to self-administer at home.

- Warn patient about potential adverse reactions. Tell him to report if any occur.
- Tell patient to keep drug refrigerated and not to reconstitute until before use.
- Advise patient to call doctor immediately if swelling, rapid heart beat, or difficulty breathing occurs.
- Tell patient to report evidence of increased bleeding or bruising.

# sargramostim (GM-CSF; granulocyte macrophage-colony stimulating factor)
Leukine

*Pregnancy Risk Category C*

## HOW SUPPLIED
*Powder for injection:* 250 mcg, 500 mcg; liquid: 500 mcg/ml

## ACTION
A glycoprotein containing 127 amino acids manufactured by recombinant DNA technology in a yeast expression system. It differs from the natural human granulocyte-macrophage colony-stimulating factor by substitution of leucine for arginine at position 23. The carbohydrate moiety may also be different. Drug induces cellular responses by binding to specific receptors on cell surfaces of target cells.

| Route | Onset | Peak | Duration |
|-------|-------|------|----------|
| I.V., S.C. | 15 min | 2-4 hr | Unknown |

## INDICATIONS & DOSAGE
*Acceleration of hematopoietic reconstitution after autologous bone marrow transplantation in patients with malignant lymphoma or acute lymphoblastic leukemia or during autologous bone marrow transplantation in patients with Hodgkin's disease—*
**Adults:** 250 mcg/m² daily for 21 consecutive days given as 2-hour I.V. infusion beginning 2 to 4 hours after bone marrow transplantation.
*Bone marrow transplantation failure or engraftment delay—*
**Adults:** 250 mcg/m²/day for 14 days as 2-hour I.V. infusion. Dose may be repeated after 7 days of no therapy. If engraft-

ment still hasn't occurred, a third course of 500 mcg/m²/day I.V. for 14 days may be attempted after another therapy-free 7 days.
*Adjust-a-dose:* Stimulation of marrow precursors may result in rapid rise of WBC count. If blast cells appear or increase to 10% or more of WBC count or if progression of the underlying disease occurs, discontinue therapy. If absolute neutrophil count is above 20,000/mm³ or if platelet count is above 50,000/mm³, temporarily discontinue drug or reduce dose by 50%.

## ADVERSE REACTIONS
**CNS:** *malaise, CNS disorders, asthenia.*
**CV:** *blood dyscrasias, edema,* **supraventricular arrhythmias,** pericardial effusion.
**GI:** *nausea, vomiting, diarrhea, anorexia, hemorrhage, GI disorders, stomatitis.*
**GU:** *urinary tract disorder,* abnormal kidney function.
**Hepatic:** *liver damage.*
**Respiratory:** *dyspnea, lung disorders,* pleural effusion.
**Skin:** *alopecia, rash.*
**Other:** *fever, mucous membrane disorder, peripheral edema,* SEPSIS.

## INTERACTIONS
**Drug-drug.** *Corticosteroids, lithium:* may potentiate myeloproliferative effects of sargramostim. Use cautiously together.

## EFFECTS ON DIAGNOSTIC TESTS
None reported.

## CONTRAINDICATIONS
Contraindicated in patients with hypersensitivity to drug or its components or to yeast-derived products and in those with excessive leukemic myeloid blasts in bone marrow or peripheral blood.

## NURSING CONSIDERATIONS
- Use cautiously in patients with preexisting cardiac disease, hypoxia, preexisting fluid retention, pulmonary infiltrates, heart failure, or impaired renal or hepatic function because these conditions may be exacerbated.
- Anticipate reducing dose by 50% or temporarily discontinuing drug if severe

adverse reactions occur; notify doctor. Therapy may be resumed when reactions abate. Transient rash and local reactions at injection site may occur; no serious allergic or anaphylactic reactions have been reported.

• Don't administer within 24 hours of last dose of chemotherapy or within 12 hours of last dose of radiotherapy because rapidly dividing progenitor cells may be sensitive to these cytotoxic therapies and drug would be ineffective.

• Monitor CBC with differential, including examination for presence of blast cells, biweekly, as ordered.

• Drug is effective in accelerating myeloid recovery in patients receiving bone marrow that is either unpurged or purged by anti–B cell monoclonal antibodies compared with patients who receive bone marrow that is chemically purged.

• Drug may have a limited response in transplant patients who have received extensive radiotherapy or in patients who have received multiple myelotoxic drugs.

• Drug can act as a growth factor for any tumor type, particularly myeloid malignant disease.

### I.V. administration

• Reconstitute with 1 ml of sterile water for injection. Direct stream of sterile water against side of vial and gently swirl contents to minimize foaming. Avoid excessive or vigorous agitation or shaking. Dilute in normal saline solution. If final concentration is below 10 mcg/ml, add human albumin at final concentration of 0.1% to NaCl solution before adding sargramostim to prevent adsorption to components of the delivery system. For a final concentration of 0.1% human albumin, add 1 mg human albumin/1 ml NaCl (dilute 1 ml of 5% human albumin in 50 ml of NaCl). Administer as soon as possible after mixing and no later than 6 hours after reconstituting.

• Don't add other drugs to infusion solution because no data exist regarding solution compatibility and stability.

• Don't use in-line filter for I.V. administration.

### ✓ Patient teaching

• Review administration schedule with patient and caregivers, and address their concerns.

• Instruct patient to report adverse reactions promptly.

**bacitracin**
**chloramphenicol**
**ciprofloxacin hydrochloride**
**erythromycin**
**gentamicin sulfate**
**ofloxacin 0.3%**
**polymyxin B sulfate**
**sulfacetamide sodium 10%**
**sulfacetamide sodium 15%**
**sulfacetamide sodium 30%**
**tobramycin**
**vidarabine**

## COMBINATION PRODUCTS

AK-POLY-BAC: polymyxin B sulfate 10,000 U and bacitracin zinc 500 U.

BLEPHAMIDE STERILE OPHTHALMIC OINTMENT: sulfacetamide sodium 10% and prednisolone acetate 0.2%.

CETAPRED OINTMENT: sulfacetamide sodium 10% and prednisolone acetate 0.25%.

CORTISPORIN OPHTHALMIC OINTMENT: polymyxin B sulfate 10,000 U, bacitracin zinc 400 U, neomycin sulfate 0.35%, and hydrocortisone 1%.

CORTISPORIN OPHTHALMIC SUSPENSION: polymyxin B sulfate 10,000 U, neomycin sulfate 0.35%, and hydrocortisone 1%.

ISOPTO CETAPRED: sulfacetamide sodium 10% and prednisolone acetate 0.25%.

MAXITROL OINTMENT/OPHTHALMIC SUSPENSION: dexamethasone 0.1%, neomycin sulfate 0.35%, and polymyxin B sulfate 10,000 U.

METIMYD OPHTHALMIC OINTMENT/SUSPENSION: sulfacetamide sodium 10% and prednisolone acetate 0.5%.

NEOSPORIN OPHTHALMIC OINTMENT: polymyxin B sulfate 10,000 U, neomycin sulfate 3.5 mg, and bacitracin zinc 400 U/g.

NEOSPORIN OPHTHALMIC SOLUTION: polymyxin B sulfate 10,000 U, neomycin sulfate 1.75 mg, and gramicidin 0.025 mg.

POLYSPORIN OPHTHALMIC OINTMENT: polymyxin B sulfate 10,000 U and bacitracin zinc 500 U.

POLYTRIM OPHTHALMIC: trimethoprim sulfate 1 mg and polymyxin B sulfate 10,000 U/ml.

PRED-G S.O.P.: prednisolone acetate 0.6%, gentamicin sulfate equivalent to gentamicin base 0.3%.

TOBRADEX: dexamethasone 0.1%, tobramycin 0.3%.

VASOCIDIN OPHTHALMIC OINTMENT: sulfacetamide sodium 10% and prednisolone acetate 0.5%.

VASOCIDIN OPHTHALMIC SOLUTION: sulfacetamide sodium 10% and prednisolone phosphate 0.25%.

VASOSULF: sulfacetamide sodium 15% and phenylephrine hydrochloride 0.125%.

---

## bacitracin
### AK-Tracin

*Pregnancy Risk Category C*

### HOW SUPPLIED
*Ophthalmic ointment:* 500 U/g

### ACTION
Inhibits bacterial cell-wall synthesis; may be bactericidal or bacteriostatic, depending on concentration and infection.

| Route | Onset | Peak | Duration |
|---|---|---|---|
| Ophthalmic | Unknown | Unknown | Unknown |

### INDICATIONS & DOSAGE
*Surface bacterial infections involving conjunctiva and cornea—*
**Adults and children:** small amount of ointment applied into conjunctival sac one or more times daily or p.r.n. until favorable response is observed.

### ADVERSE REACTIONS
**GU:** increased serum creatinine and BUN levels.
**EENT:** slowed corneal wound healing, temporary visual haze.
**Other:** overgrowth of nonsusceptible organisms.

---

*Liquid contains alcohol.    **May contain tartrazine.    †Canada    ‡Australia    §U.K.    ◇OTC

## INTERACTIONS
**Drug-drug.** *Heavy metals such as silver nitrate:* inactivation of bacitracin. Don't use together.

## EFFECTS ON DIAGNOSTIC TESTS
Urinary sediment tests may show increased protein and cast excretion.

## CONTRAINDICATIONS
Contraindicated in patients with hypersensitivity to drug and in those with atopy.

## NURSING CONSIDERATIONS
• Ophthalmic ointment may be stored at room temperature.
• Clean eye area of excessive exudate before application.
• Watch for signs and symptoms of superinfection.
• **Alert:** Don't confuse bacitracin with Bactrim or Bactroban.

### ☑ Patient teaching
• Teach patient how to apply drug; tell him only small amount of ointment is needed and that it may cause blurred vision. Advise him to wash hands before and after administering and not to touch tip of tube to eye or surrounding tissue.
• Instruct patient to stop drug and notify doctor of signs and symptoms of sensitivity (itching lids, swelling, constant burning, or failure to heal).
• Tell patient not to share drug, washcloths, or towels with family members and to notify doctor if anyone develops same symptoms.
• Stress importance of compliance with recommended therapy.

---

## chloramphenicol
AK-Chlor, Chloromycetin
Ophthalmic, Chloroptic, Chloroptic
S.O.P., Chlorsig‡, Pentamycetin†,
Sno Phenicol§, Sopamycetin†

*Pregnancy Risk Category C*

## HOW SUPPLIED
*Ophthalmic ointment:* 1%
*Ophthalmic solution:* 0.5%

*Powder for ophthalmic solution:*
25 mg/vial

## ACTION
Inhibits protein synthesis; may be bacteriostatic or bactericidal, depending on concentration.

| Route | Onset | Peak | Duration |
|-------|-------|------|----------|
| Ophthalmic | Unknown | Unknown | Unknown |

## INDICATIONS & DOSAGE
*Surface bacterial infection involving conjunctiva or cornea—*
**Adults and children:** 1 or 2 drops of solution in eye q 3 to 6 hours or more frequently, if needed. Or, small amount of ointment applied to lower conjunctival sac q 3 to 6 hours or more frequently, if needed. Continued for at least 48 hours after eye appears normal.

## ADVERSE REACTIONS
**EENT:** optic atrophy in children, stinging or burning of eye after instillation, blurred vision (with ointment).
**GU:** hemoglobinuria.
**Hematologic:** *bone marrow hypoplasia with prolonged use, aplastic anemia.*
**Metabolic:** lactic acidosis.
**Skin:** dermatitis.
**Other:** overgrowth of nonsusceptible organisms; *hypersensitivity reactions,* including itching and burning eye, *angioedema.*

## INTERACTIONS
None significant.

## EFFECTS ON DIAGNOSTIC TESTS
False elevation of urinary PABA levels occurs if drug is administered during a bentiromide test for pancreatic function. Drug therapy causes false-positive results on tests for urine glucose level using cupric sulfate (Clinitest).

## CONTRAINDICATIONS
Contraindicated in patients with hypersensitivity to drug.

## NURSING CONSIDERATIONS
• If chloramphenicol drops are to be given hourly and then tapered, follow order

---

Reactions may be *common,* uncommon, *life-threatening,* or **COMMON AND LIFE-THREATENING.**

closely to ensure adequate anterior chamber levels.

• Reconstitute powder for ophthalmic solution with supplied diluent. Use 5 ml of diluent to make 0.5% solution, 10 ml of diluent to make 0.25% solution, or 15 ml to make 0.16% solution.

• Store drug in tightly closed, light-resistant container.

• If patient has more than a superficial infection, anticipate using systemic therapy as well.

☑ **Patient teaching**

• Teach patient how to instill drops or apply ointment. Advise him to wash hands before and after administering ointment or solution, and warn him not to touch tip of applicator to eye or surrounding tissue.

• Tell patient to clean eye area of excessive exudate before application.

• Instruct patient to apply light finger pressure on lacrimal sac for 1 minute after drops are instilled.

• Tell patient that vision may be blurred for a few minutes after application of ointment.

• Tell patient not to share drug, washcloths, or towels with family members and to notify doctor if anyone develops same symptoms.

• Instruct patient to stop drug and notify doctor of sensitivity (itching lids, swelling, or constant burning).

• Tell patient to notify doctor if improvement doesn't occur within 3 days.

• Stress importance of compliance with recommended therapy.

• Instruct patient to watch for signs and symptoms of superinfection, such as redness, drainage, soreness, or failure to heal.

---

## ciprofloxacin hydrochloride
Ciloxan

*Pregnancy Risk Category C*

### HOW SUPPLIED
*Ophthalmic solution:* 0.3% (base) in 2.5- and 5-ml containers

### ACTION
Inhibits bacterial DNA gyrase, an enzyme needed for bacterial replication. May be bacteriostatic or bactericidal, depending on concentration.

| Route | Onset | Peak | Duration |
|-------|-------|------|----------|
| Ophthalmic | Unknown | Unknown | Unknown |

### INDICATIONS & DOSAGE
*Corneal ulcers due to* Pseudomonas aeruginosa, Staphylococcus aureus, Staphylococcus epidermidis, Streptococcus pneumoniae, *and possibly* Serratia marcescens *and* Streptococcus viridians—
**Adults and children over age 12:** 2 drops in affected eye q 15 minutes for first 6 hours; then 2 drops q 30 minutes for remainder of first day. On day 2, 2 drops hourly. On days 3 to 14, 2 drops q 4 hours.
*Bacterial conjunctivitis due to* Haemophilus influenzae, S. aureus *and* S. epidermidis *and possibly* S. pneumoniae—
**Adults and children over age 12:** 1 or 2 drops into conjunctival sac of affected eye q 2 hours while awake for first 2 days. Then, 1 or 2 drops q 4 hours while awake for next 5 days.

### ADVERSE REACTIONS
**EENT:** *local burning or discomfort, white crystalline precipitate in superficial portion of corneal defect in patients with corneal ulcers, margin crusting, crystals or scales, foreign body sensation, itching, conjunctival hyperemia,* bad or bitter taste in mouth, corneal staining, allergic reactions, keratopathy, lid edema, tearing, photophobia, decreased vision.
**GI:** nausea.

### INTERACTIONS
None significant.

### EFFECTS ON DIAGNOSTIC TESTS
None reported.

### CONTRAINDICATIONS
Contraindicated in patients with history of hypersensitivity to ciprofloxacin or other fluoroquinolone antibiotics.

---

## NURSING CONSIDERATIONS
• It's unknown if drug appears in breast milk after application to eye; however, systemically administered ciprofloxacin has appeared in human milk. Use with caution in breast-feeding women.
• **Alert:** Discontinue drug at first sign of hypersensitivity reaction, such as rash, and notify doctor. Serious hypersensitivity reactions, including anaphylaxis, may occur in patients receiving systemic fluoroquinolone therapy.
• A topical overdose may be flushed from eyes with warm tap water.
• If corneal epithelium is still compromised after 14 days of treatment, continue therapy, as ordered.
• Institute appropriate therapy if superinfection occurs. Prolonged use may result in overgrowth of nonsusceptible organisms, including fungi.
• **Alert:** Don't confuse Ciloxan with Cytoxan or cinoxacin.

### ☑ Patient teaching
• Tell patient to clean eye area of excessive exudate before instilling.
• Teach patient how to instill drops. Advise him to wash hands before and after administering solution and not to touch tip of dropper to eye or surrounding tissues.
• Instruct patient to apply light finger pressure on lacrimal sac for 1 minute after drops are instilled.
• Tell patient not to share drug, washcloths, or towels with family members and to notify doctor if anyone develops same symptoms.
• Stress importance of compliance with recommended therapy.

---

### erythromycin
Ilotycin Ophthalmic Ointment

*Pregnancy Risk Category B*

## HOW SUPPLIED
*Ophthalmic ointment:* 0.5%

## ACTION
Inhibits protein synthesis; usually bacteriostatic, but may be bactericidal in high concentrations or against highly susceptible organisms.

| Route | Onset | Peak | Duration |
|-------|-------|------|----------|
| Ophthalmic | Unknown | Unknown | Unknown |

## INDICATIONS & DOSAGE
*Acute and chronic conjunctivitis, other eye infections—*
**Adults and children:** a ribbon of ointment about 1 cm long applied directly to infected eye up to six times daily, depending on severity of infection.
*Chlamydial ophthalmic infections (trachoma)—*
**Adults and children:** small amount applied to each eye b.i.d. for 2 months or b.i.d. on first 5 days of each month for 6 months.
*Prophylaxis of ophthalmia neonatorum due to* Neisseria gonorrhoeae *or* Chlamydia trachomatis—
**Neonates:** a ribbon of ointment about 1 cm long applied in lower conjunctival sac of each eye shortly after birth.

## ADVERSE REACTIONS
**EENT:** slowed corneal wound healing, blurred vision.
**Skin:** urticaria, dermatitis.
**Other:** overgrowth of nonsusceptible organisms with long-term use, hypersensitivity reactions, including itching and burning eyes.

## INTERACTIONS
None significant.

## EFFECTS ON DIAGNOSTIC TESTS
Drug may interfere with fluorometric determinations of urinary catecholamines.

## CONTRAINDICATIONS
Contraindicated in patients with hypersensitivity to drug.

## NURSING CONSIDERATIONS
• For prophylaxis of ophthalmia neonatorum, apply ointment no later than 1 hour after birth. Drug is used in neonates born by either vaginal delivery or cesarean section. Gently massage eyelids for 1 minute to spread ointment.

---

Reactions may be *common,* uncommon, *life-threatening,* or COMMON AND LIFE-THREATENING.

• Drug should be used only when sensitivity studies show it's effective against infecting organisms; it shouldn't be used in infections of unknown etiology.

• Use cautiously in breast-feeding women.

• Store drug at room temperature in tightly closed, light-resistant container.

### ☑ Patient teaching

• Tell patient to clean eye area of excessive exudate before application.

• Teach patient how to apply drug. Advise him to wash hands before and after administering ointment, and warn him not to touch tip of applicator to eye or surrounding tissue.

• Tell patient that vision may be blurred for a few minutes after application of ointment.

• Advise patient to watch for and report signs and symptoms of sensitivity (itching lids, redness, swelling, or constant burning).

• Tell patient not to share drug, washcloths, or towels with family members and to notify doctor if anyone develops same symptoms.

• Stress importance of compliance with recommended therapy.

---

## gentamicin sulfate
Cidomycin§, Garamycin
Ophthalmic, Genoptic, Gentacidin,
Gentak, Genticin§

*Pregnancy Risk Category C*

### HOW SUPPLIED
*Ophthalmic ointment:* 0.3% (base)
*Ophthalmic solution:* 0.3% (base)

### ACTION
Unknown. Thought to inhibit protein synthesis and is usually bactericidal.

| Route | Onset | Peak | Duration |
|-------|-------|------|----------|
| Ophthalmic | Unknown | Unknown | Unknown |

### INDICATIONS & DOSAGE
*External ocular infections (conjunctivitis, keratoconjunctivitis, corneal ulcers, blepharitis, blepharoconjunctivitis, meibomianitis, and dacryocystitis) due to suscepti-*

*ble organisms, especially* Pseudomonas aeruginosa, Proteus, Klebsiella pneumoniae, Escherichia coli, *and other gram-negative organisms—*
**Adults and children:** 1 to 2 drops in eye q 4 hours. In severe infections, up to 2 drops q hour. Or, ointment applied to lower conjunctival sac b.i.d. or t.i.d.

### ADVERSE REACTIONS
**EENT:** burning, stinging, or blurred vision with ointment, transient irritation from solution, conjunctival hyperemia.
**GU:** *nephrotoxicity (elevated BUN, nonprotein nitrogen, or serum creatinine levels and increased urinary excretion of casts).*
**Other:** hypersensitivity reactions; overgrowth of nonsusceptible organisms with long-term use.

   Systemic absorption from excessive use may cause systemic toxicities.

### INTERACTIONS
None significant.

### EFFECTS ON DIAGNOSTIC TESTS
None reported.

### CONTRAINDICATIONS
Contraindicated in patients with hypersensitivity to drug.

### NURSING CONSIDERATIONS
• Use cautiously in patients with history of sensitivity to aminoglycosides because cross-sensitivity may occur.

• Have culture taken before giving drug. Therapy may begin before culture results are known.

• If ophthalmic gentamicin is given concomitantly with systemic gentamicin, monitor serum gentamicin levels.

• Solution isn't for injection into conjunctiva or anterior chamber of eye.

• Store drug away from heat.

### ☑ Patient teaching
• Tell patient to clean eye area of excessive exudate before administering drug.

• Teach patient how to instill drops or apply ointment. Advise him to wash hands before and after administering ointment

---

or solution and not to touch tip of dropper or tube to eye or surrounding tissues.

• Instruct patient to apply light finger pressure on lacrimal sac for 1 minute after drops are instilled.

• Instruct patient to stop drug and notify doctor if signs and symptoms of sensitivity (itching lids, swelling, or constant burning) occur.

• Advise patient not to share drug, washcloths, or towels with family members and to notify doctor if anyone develops same symptoms.

• Tell patient that vision may be blurred for few minutes after application of ointment.

• *Alert:* Stress importance of following recommended therapy. *Pseudomonas* infections can cause complete vision loss within 24 hours if infection isn't controlled.

---

## ofloxacin 0.3%
Exocin§, Ocuflox

*Pregnancy Risk Category C*

### HOW SUPPLIED
*Ophthalmic solution:* 0.3% in 1-ml and 5-ml solution

### ACTION
Bactericidal. Inhibits bacterial DNA gyrase, an enzyme needed for bacterial replication.

| Route | Onset | Peak | Duration |
|-------|-------|------|----------|
| Ophthalmic | Unknown | Unknown | Unknown |

### INDICATIONS & DOSAGE
*Conjunctivitis due to* Staphylococcus aureus, S. epidermidis, Streptococcus pneumoniae, Enterobacter cloacae, Haemophilus influenzae, Proteus mirabilis, Pseudomonas aeruginosa, *and* Propionibacterium acnes—
**Adults and children over age 1:** 1 to 2 drops in conjunctival sac q 2 to 4 hours daily, while awake, for first 2 days; then q.i.d. for up to 5 additional days.
*Bacterial corneal ulcer due to* S. aureus, S. epidermidis, S. pneumoniae, E. cloacae, H. influenzae, P. mirabilis, P. aeruginosa, Serratia marcescens, *and* P. acnes—

**Adults and children over age 1:** 1 to 2 drops q 30 minutes while awake and 1 to 2 drops 4 to 6 hours after retiring on days 1 and 2. Days 3 to 7, 1 to 2 drops hourly while awake. Days 7 to 9, 1 to 2 drops q.i.d.

### ADVERSE REACTIONS
**EENT:** *transient ocular burning or discomfort,* stinging, redness, itching, photophobia, lacrimation, eye dryness.
**Metabolic:** hyperglycemia.

### INTERACTIONS
None significant.

### EFFECTS ON DIAGNOSTIC TESTS
None reported.

### CONTRAINDICATIONS
Contraindicated in patients with history of hypersensitivity to ofloxacin, other fluoroquinolones, or other components of drug; also contraindicated in breast-feeding women.

### NURSING CONSIDERATIONS
• *Alert:* Don't inject drug into conjunctiva or introduce directly into anterior chamber of eye.

• Discontinue drug if improvement doesn't occur within 7 days. Prolonged use may result in overgrowth of nonsusceptible organisms, including fungi.

• *Alert:* Don't confuse Ocuflox with Ocufen.

### ✅ Patient teaching
• If an allergic reaction occurs, tell patient to discontinue drug and call doctor. Serious acute hypersensitivity reactions may need emergency treatment.

• Teach patient how to instill drops. Advise him to wash hands before and after instilling solution, and warn him not to touch tip of dropper to eye or surrounding tissue.

• Advise patient to apply light finger pressure on lacrimal sac for 1 minute after drug instillation.

• Tell patient not to share drug, washcloths, or towels with family members and to notify doctor if anyone develops same symptoms.

• Stress importance of compliance with recommended therapy.

---

Reactions may be *common,* uncommon, *life-threatening*, or COMMON AND LIFE-THREATENING.

• Warn patient not to use leftover drug for new eye infection.
• Remind patient to discard drug when no longer needed.

---

## polymyxin B sulfate
Polyfax§

*Pregnancy Risk Category C*

### HOW SUPPLIED
*Ophthalmic sterile powder for solution:* 500,000-U vials to be reconstituted to 20 to 50 ml

### ACTION
Bactericidal. Alters osmotic barrier of bacteria cell membrane.

| Route | Onset | Peak | Duration |
|-------|-------|------|----------|
| Ophthalmic | Unknown | Unknown | Unknown |

### INDICATIONS & DOSAGE
*Alone or with other drugs to treat superficial eye infections involving conjunctiva and cornea resulting from infection with* Pseudomonas *or other gram-negative organisms—*
**Adults and children:** 1 to 3 drops of 0.1% to 0.25% (10,000 to 25,000 U/ml) hourly. Interval increased based on patient response; or up to 10,000 U injected subconjunctivally daily.

### ADVERSE REACTIONS
**EENT:** eye irritation, conjunctivitis.
**GU:** increased BUN and serum creatinine levels.
**Other:** overgrowth of nonsusceptible organisms; hypersensitivity reactions, including local burning, itching.

### INTERACTIONS
None significant.

### EFFECTS ON DIAGNOSTIC TESTS
None reported.

### CONTRAINDICATIONS
Contraindicated in patients with hypersensitivity to drug. Drug shouldn't be injected into eye or anterior chamber of eye.

### NURSING CONSIDERATIONS
• Reconstitute carefully to ensure correct drug concentration in solution.
• Drug is often used with neomycin sulfate.
• Drug is one of the most effective antibiotics against gram-negative organisms, especially *Pseudomonas.*
• In severe, life-threatening *Pseudomonas* infections, polymyxin B may be used as an ocular irrigant.

### ☑ Patient teaching
• Tell patient to clean eye area of excessive exudate before application.
• Teach patient how to instill drops. Advise him to wash hands before and after administering solution, and warn him not to touch tip of dropper to eye or surrounding tissue.
• Instruct patient to apply light finger pressure on lacrimal sac for 1 minute after drops are instilled.
• Advise patient to watch for and report signs and symptoms of sensitivity (itching lids, swelling, or constant burning).
• Tell patient not to share drug, washcloths, or towels with family members and to notify doctor if anyone develops same symptoms.
• Stress importance of compliance with recommended therapy.

---

## sulfacetamide sodium 10%
AK-Sulf, Bleph-10, Cetamide Ophthalmic, OcuSulf-10, Sodium Sulamyd 10% Ophthalmic, Sulf-10 Ophthalmic

## sulfacetamide sodium 15%
Isopto Cetamide Ophthalmic

## sulfacetamide sodium 30%
Sodium Sulamyd 30% Ophthalmic

*Pregnancy Risk Category C*

### HOW SUPPLIED
*Ophthalmic ointment:* 10%
*Ophthalmic solution:* 10%, 15%, 30%

### ACTION
Bacteriostatic, although may be bactericidal in high concentrations. Prevents up-

---

take of PABA, a metabolite of bacterial folic acid synthesis.

| Route | Onset | Peak | Duration |
|-------|-------|------|----------|
| Ophthalmic | Unknown | Unknown | Unknown |

## INDICATIONS & DOSAGE

*Inclusion conjunctivitis, corneal ulcers, chlamydial infection—*

**Adults and children:** 1 to 2 drops of 10% solution into lower conjunctival sac q 2 to 3 hours during day, less often at night; or 1 to 2 drops of 15% solution instilled into lower conjunctival sac q 1 to 2 hours initially. Interval increased as condition responds; or 1 drop of 30% solution instilled into lower conjunctival sac q 2 hours. 1.25 to 2.5 cm of 10% ointment applied into conjunctival sac q.i.d. and h.s. Ointment may be used at night along with drops during the day.

*Trachoma—*

**Adults and children:** 2 drops of 30% solution into lower conjunctival sac q 2 hours with systemic sulfonamide or tetracycline.

## ADVERSE REACTIONS

**EENT:** slowed corneal wound healing with ointment, pain on instillation of eyedrops, headache or brow pain, photophobia, periorbital edema.

**Skin:** *Stevens-Johnson syndrome.*

**Other:** hypersensitivity reactions, including itching, burning; overgrowth of nonsusceptible organisms.

## INTERACTIONS

**Drug-drug.** *Gentamicin (ophthalmic):* in vitro antagonism. Avoid concomitant use. *Local anesthetics (procaine, tetracaine), PABA derivatives:* decreased sulfacetamide sodium action. Wait ½ to 1 hour after instilling anesthetic or PABA derivative before instilling sulfacetamide. *Silver preparations:* precipitate formation. Avoid using together.

**Drug-lifestyle.** *Sun exposure:* photophobia may occur. Take precautions.

## EFFECTS ON DIAGNOSTIC TESTS

None reported.

## CONTRAINDICATIONS

Contraindicated in patients with hypersensitivity to sulfonamides. Drug isn't recommended for children under age 2 months.

## NURSING CONSIDERATIONS

• Drug is often used with oral tetracycline in treating trachoma and inclusion conjunctivitis.
• Store drug in tightly closed, light-resistant container away from heat.

### ✅ Patient teaching

• Tell patient to clean eye area of excessive exudate before administering drug.
• Teach patient how to instill drops or apply ointment. Advise him to wash hands before and after administering ointment or solution and not to touch tip of dropper to eye or surrounding tissues.
• Instruct patient to apply light finger pressure on lacrimal sac for 1 minute after drops are instilled.
• Warn patient that eyedrops burn slightly.
• Advise patient to watch for and report signs and symptoms of sensitivity (itching lids, swelling, or constant burning).
• Tell patient to wait at least 5 minutes before administering other eyedrops.
• Warn patient that solution may stain clothing.
• Tell patient to minimize photophobia by wearing sunglasses and avoiding prolonged exposure to sunlight.
• Advise patient not to use discolored solution.
• Tell patient not to share drug, washcloths, or towels with family members and to notify doctor if anyone develops same symptoms.
• Stress importance of compliance with recommended therapy.

---

## tobramycin
AKTob, Tobrex

*Pregnancy Risk Category B*

## HOW SUPPLIED

*Ophthalmic ointment:* 0.3%
*Ophthalmic solution:* 0.3%

---

## ACTION

Unknown. Thought to inhibit protein synthesis; usually bactericidal.

| Route | Onset | Peak | Duration |
|---|---|---|---|
| Ophthalmic | Unknown | Unknown | Unknown |

## INDICATIONS & DOSAGE

*External ocular infections due to susceptible bacteria—*

**Adults and children:** in mild to moderate infections, 1 or 2 drops instilled into affected eye q 4 hours, or thin strip (1 cm long) of ointment applied q 8 to 12 hours. In severe infections, 2 drops instilled into infected eye q 30 to 60 minutes until condition improves; then frequency reduced. Or, thin strip (1 cm long) of ointment applied q 3 to 4 hours until improvement; then frequency reduced.

## ADVERSE REACTIONS

**EENT:** burning or stinging on instillation, lid itching or swelling, conjunctival erythema, blurred vision with ointment.
**GU:** elevated BUN, nonprotein nitrogen, or serum creatinine levels; increased urinary excretion of casts.
**Other:** *hypersensitivity reactions,* overgrowth of nonsusceptible organisms.

## INTERACTIONS

None significant.

## EFFECTS ON DIAGNOSTIC TESTS

None reported.

## CONTRAINDICATIONS

Contraindicated in patients with hypersensitivity to drug or other aminoglycosides.

## NURSING CONSIDERATIONS

• When two different ophthalmic solutions are used, allow at least 5 minutes before instillation.
• *Alert:* Tobramycin ophthalmic solution isn't for injection.
• If topical ocular tobramycin is administered with systemic tobramycin, carefully monitor serum levels.
• Prolonged use may result in overgrowth of nonsusceptible organisms, including fungi.

• *Alert:* Don't confuse tobramycin with Trobicin, or Tobrex with Tobradex.

### ☑ Patient teaching

• Tell patient to clean eye area of excessive exudate before administering drug.
• Teach patient how to instill drops or apply ointment. Advise him to wash hands before and after administering and to avoid touching tip of dropper to eye or surrounding tissue.
• Instruct patient to apply light finger pressure on lacrimal sac for 1 minute after drops are instilled.
• Advise patient to watch for itching lids, swelling, or constant burning. Tell him to discontinue drug and notify doctor if these signs and symptoms develop.
• Tell patient not to share drug, washcloths, or towels with family members and to notify doctor if anyone develops same symptoms.
• Stress importance of compliance with recommended therapy.

## vidarabine
Vira-A

*Pregnancy Risk Category C*

## HOW SUPPLIED

*Ophthalmic ointment:* 3% in 3.5-g tube (equivalent to 2.8% vidarabine)

## ACTION

Unknown. Thought to interfere with DNA synthesis.

| Route | Onset | Peak | Duration |
|---|---|---|---|
| Ophthalmic | Unknown | Unknown | Unknown |

## INDICATIONS & DOSAGE

*Acute keratoconjunctivitis, superficial keratitis, and recurrent epithelial keratitis due to herpes simplex I and II—*

**Adults and children:** 1 cm of ointment into lower conjunctival sac five times daily at 3-hour intervals. If there are no signs of improvement after 7 days, or if complete reepithelialization hasn't occurred in 21 days, consider other forms of therapy. Some cases may need longer treatment if severe. After reepithelialization has occurred, treat for an additional 5 to 7 days at reduced dosage (such as b.i.d.) to prevent recurrence.

**ADVERSE REACTIONS**
**EENT:** temporary burning, itching, mild irritation, pain, lacrimation, foreign body sensation, conjunctival injection, punctal occlusion, sensitivity, superficial punctate keratitis, photophobia.
**Other:** *hypersensitivity reactions.*

**INTERACTIONS**
None significant.

**EFFECTS ON DIAGNOSTIC TESTS**
None reported.

**CONTRAINDICATIONS**
Contraindicated in patients with hypersensitivity to drug.

**NURSING CONSIDERATIONS**
• Use corticosteroids cautiously and monitor closely. Drug therapy should be continued for several days after corticosteroid therapy.
• Drug isn't effective against RNA virus, adenoviral ocular infections, or bacterial, fungal, or chlamydial infections.
• Store drug in tightly closed, light-resistant container.
•*Alert:* Don't confuse vidarabine with cytarabine.

✓ **Patient teaching**
• Tell patient to clean eye area of excessive exudate before application.
• Teach patient how to apply. Advise him to wash hands before and after administering ointment and to avoid touching tip of tube to eye or surrounding tissue.
• Instruct patient to apply light finger pressure on lacrimal sac for 1 minute after drops are instilled.
• Explain that ointment may produce a temporary visual haze.
• Advise patient to watch for signs of sensitivity, such as itching lids, swelling, or constant burning. Tell patient who develops such signs and symptoms to stop drug and notify doctor immediately.

• Tell patient to minimize photophobia by wearing sunglasses and avoiding prolonged exposure to sunlight.
• Tell patient not to share drug, washcloths, or towels with family members and to notify doctor if anyone develops same symptoms.
• Stress importance of compliance with recommended therapy.

---

Reactions may be *common*, uncommon, *life-threatening*, or COMMON AND LIFE-THREATENING.

**dexamethasone**
**dexamethasone sodium phosphate**
**diclofenac sodium 0.1%**
**fluorometholone**
**flurbiprofen sodium**
**ketorolac tromethamine**
**prednisolone acetate (suspension)**
**prednisolone sodium phosphate (solution)**

### COMBINATION PRODUCTS
Corticosteroids for ophthalmic use are commonly used with antibiotics and sulfonamides. See Chapter 79, Ophthalmic anti-infectives.

---

**dexamethasone**
Maxidex Ophthalmic Suspension

**dexamethasone sodium phosphate**
AK-Dex, Decadron Phosphate Ophthalmic, Maxidex Ophthalmic

*Pregnancy Risk Category C*

### HOW SUPPLIED
**dexamethasone**
*Ophthalmic suspension:* 0.1%
**dexamethasone sodium phosphate**
*Ophthalmic ointment:* 0.05%
*Ophthalmic solution:* 0.1%

### ACTION
Unknown. Thought to decrease infiltration of WBCs at inflammation site.

| Route | Onset | Peak | Duration |
|-------|-------|------|----------|
| Ophthalmic | Unknown | Unknown | Unknown |

### INDICATIONS & DOSAGE
*Uveitis; iridocyclitis; inflammatory conditions of eyelids, conjunctiva, cornea, anterior segment of globe; corneal injury from chemical or thermal burns, or penetration of foreign bodies; allergic conjunctivitis; suppression of graft rejection after keratoplasty—*
**Adults and children:** 1 to 2 drops of suspension or solution or 1.25 to 2.5 cm of ointment into conjunctival sac. In severe disease, drops may be used hourly, tapering to discontinuation as condition improves. In mild conditions, drops may be used up to four to six times daily or ointment applied t.i.d. or q.i.d. As condition improves, dosage tapered to b.i.d.; then once daily. Treatment may extend from a few days to several weeks.

### ADVERSE REACTIONS
**EENT:** increased intraocular pressure; thinning of cornea; interference with corneal wound healing; increased susceptibility to viral or fungal corneal infection; corneal ulceration; glaucoma exacerbation, cataracts, defects in visual acuity and visual field, optic nerve damage with excessive or long-term use; mild blurred vision; burning, stinging, or redness of eyes; watery eyes; discharge; discomfort; ocular pain; foreign body sensation.
**Other:** systemic effects, adrenal suppression with excessive or long-term use.

### INTERACTIONS
None significant.

### EFFECTS ON DIAGNOSTIC TESTS
None reported.

### CONTRAINDICATIONS
Contraindicated in patients with hypersensitivity to any component of drug; in those with ocular tuberculosis or acute superficial herpes simplex (dendritic keratitis), vaccinia, varicella, or other fungal or viral diseases of cornea and conjunctiva; in patients with acute, purulent, untreated infections of eye; and after uncomplicated removal of superficial corneal foreign

---

*Liquid contains alcohol.   **May contain tartrazine.   †Canada   ‡Australia   §U.K.   ◇OTC

body. Safe use in pregnant and breast-feeding women hasn't been established.

## NURSING CONSIDERATIONS
• Use cautiously in patients with corneal abrasions that may be infected (especially with herpes).
• Use cautiously in patients with glaucoma (any form) because intraocular pressure may increase. Dosage of glaucoma drugs may need to be increased to compensate.
• Drug isn't for long-term use.
• Watch for corneal ulceration; may require stopping drug.
• Corneal viral and fungal infections may be exacerbated by corticosteroid application.
• *Alert:* Don't confuse dexamethasone with desoximetasone, or Maxidex with Maxzide.

### ✅ Patient teaching
• Tell patient to shake suspension well before use.
• Teach patient how to instill drops or apply ointment. Advise him to wash hands before and after administering ointment or solution, and warn him not to touch tip of dropper to eye or surrounding tissue.
• Tell patient to apply light finger pressure on lacrimal sac for 1 minute after instillation.
• Advise patient that he may use eye pad with ointment.
• Warn patient not to use leftover drug for new eye inflammation; doing so may cause serious problems.
• *Alert:* Warn patient to call doctor immediately and to stop drug if visual acuity changes or visual field diminishes.
• Tell patient not to share drug, washcloths, or towels with family members and to notify doctor if anyone develops same symptoms.
• Stress importance of compliance with recommended therapy.

## diclofenac sodium 0.1%
Voltaren Ophthalmic, Voltarol Ophtha§

*Pregnancy Risk Category B*

### HOW SUPPLIED
*Ophthalmic solution:* 0.1%

### ACTION
Unknown. Thought to inhibit the enzyme cyclooxygenase, which is essential in biosynthesis of prostaglandins. Prostaglandins may be mediators of certain kinds of intraocular inflammation.

| Route | Onset | Peak | Duration |
|-------|-------|------|----------|
| Ophthalmic | Unknown | Unknown | Unknown |

### INDICATIONS & DOSAGE
*Postoperative inflammation following removal of cataract—*
**Adults:** 1 drop in conjunctival sac q.i.d., beginning 24 hours after surgery and continuing throughout first 2 weeks of postoperative period.
*Photophobia in incisional refractive surgery—*
**Adults:** 1 to 2 drops to operative eye 1 hour before surgery. Within 15 minutes after surgery, instill 1 to 2 drops into operative eye. Then 1 drop q.i.d. beginning 4 to 6 hours after surgery up to 3 days, p.r.n.

### ADVERSE REACTIONS
**EENT:** *transient stinging and burning, increased intraocular pressure, keratitis,* anterior chamber reaction, ocular allergy increased bleeding of ocular tissues, including hyphemas with ocular surgery.
**GI:** nausea, vomiting.
**Other:** viral infection.

### INTERACTIONS
None significant.

### EFFECTS ON DIAGNOSTIC TESTS
None reported.

---

Reactions may be *common*, uncommon, *life-threatening*, or COMMON AND LIFE-THREATENING.

## CONTRAINDICATIONS

Contraindicated in patients with hypersensitivity to any component of drug and in those wearing soft contact lenses. Because of known effects of prostaglandin-inhibiting drugs on fetal CV system (closure of ductus arteriosus), avoid use of drug during late pregnancy.

## NURSING CONSIDERATIONS

• Use cautiously in patients with hypersensitivity to acetylsalicylic acid, phenylacetic acid derivatives, and other NSAIDs; potential for cross-sensitivity exists. Also use cautiously in surgical patients with known bleeding tendencies and in those receiving drugs that may prolong bleeding time.
• Drug may slow or delay healing.
• Most cases of increased intraocular pressure have occurred postoperatively and before drug administration.
• *Alert:* Don't confuse diclofenac with Diflucan or Duphalac, or Voltaren with Vontrol or Verelan.

### ☑ Patient teaching

• Teach patient how to instill drops. Advise him to wash hands before and after instilling solution, and warn him not to touch tip of dropper to eye or surrounding tissue.
• Advise patient to apply light finger pressure on lacrimal sac for 1 minute after drug instillation.
• Stress importance of compliance with recommended therapy.
• Warn patient not to use leftover drug for new eye inflammation.
• Remind patient to discard drug when no longer needed.

---

## fluorometholone
Flarex, Fluor-Op, FML Forte, FML Liquifilm Ophthalmic, FML S.O.P.

*Pregnancy Risk Category C*

## HOW SUPPLIED
*Ophthalmic ointment:* 0.1%
*Ophthalmic suspension:* 0.1%, 0.25%

## ACTION
Unknown. Thought to decrease infiltration of WBCs at inflammation site.

| Route | Onset | Peak | Duration |
|-------|-------|------|----------|
| Ophthalmic | Unknown | Unknown | Unknown |

## INDICATIONS & DOSAGE
*Inflammatory and allergic conditions of cornea, conjunctiva, sclera, anterior uvea—*

**Adults and children:** 1 to 2 drops in conjunctival sac b.i.d. to q.i.d. May be given q 2 hours during first 1 to 2 days, if needed. Or, 1.25-cm ribbon of ointment applied to conjunctival sac q 4 hours, decreased to once daily to t.i.d. as inflammation subsides.

## ADVERSE REACTIONS
**EENT:** increased intraocular pressure, thinning of cornea, interference with corneal wound healing, corneal ulceration, increased susceptibility to viral or fungal corneal infections; glaucoma exacerbation, discharge, discomfort, ocular pain, foreign body sensation, cataracts, decreased visual acuity, diminished visual field, optic nerve damage with excessive or long-term use.
**Other:** systemic effects, adrenal suppression with excessive or long-term use.

## INTERACTIONS
None significant.

## EFFECTS ON DIAGNOSTIC TESTS
None reported.

## CONTRAINDICATIONS
Contraindicated in patients with vaccinia, varicella, acute superficial herpes simplex (dendritic keratitis), or other fungal or viral eye diseases; ocular tuberculosis; or acute, purulent, untreated eye infections.

## NURSING CONSIDERATIONS
• Use cautiously in patients with corneal abrasions that may be contaminated (especially with herpes).
• Safety and efficacy of drug in children under age 2 haven't been established.
• Duration of treatment may range from a few days to several weeks; however, long-

---

term use should be avoided. Monitor intraocular pressure.
• Drug is less likely to cause increased intraocular pressure with extended use than other ophthalmic anti-inflammatory drugs (except medrysone).
• Consult doctor if no improvement after 2 days. Don't discontinue treatment prematurely.
• In chronic conditions, withdraw treatment by gradually decreasing frequency of applications.
• Shake well before use.
• Store drug in tightly covered, light-resistant container.

### ✓ Patient teaching
• Teach patient how to instill drops or apply ointment. Advise him to wash hands before and after administering ointment or solution, and warn him not to touch tip of dropper to eye or surrounding tissue.
• Advise patient to apply light finger pressure on lacrimal sac for 1 minute after instillation.
• Advise patient to call doctor immediately and to stop drug if visual acuity decreases or visual field diminishes.
• Tell patient not to share drug, washcloths, or towels with family members and to notify doctor if anyone develops same symptoms.
• Warn patient not to use leftover drug for new eye inflammation; it may cause serious problems.

---

## flurbiprofen sodium
Ocufen

*Pregnancy Risk Category C*

### HOW SUPPLIED
*Ophthalmic solution:* 0.03%

### ACTION
Unknown. An NSAID thought to inhibit the cyclooxygenase enzyme essential in biosynthesis of prostaglandins.

| Route | Onset | Peak | Duration |
|-------|-------|------|----------|
| Ophthalmic | Unknown | Unknown | Unknown |

### INDICATIONS & DOSAGE
*Inhibition of intraoperative miosis—*
**Adults:** 1 drop instilled into affected eye about q 30 minutes, beginning 2 hours before surgery; total of 4 drops is given.

### ADVERSE REACTIONS
**EENT:** transient burning and stinging on instillation, ocular irritation.

### INTERACTIONS
**Drug-drug.** *Acetylcholine, carbachol:* may be rendered ineffective. Avoid concomitant use.
*Anticoagulants:* increased risk of bleeding if significant systemic absorption occurs. Monitor closely.

### EFFECTS ON DIAGNOSTIC TESTS
None reported.

### CONTRAINDICATIONS
Contraindicated in patients with hypersensitivity to drug. Safe use in pregnant and breast-feeding women hasn't been established.

### NURSING CONSIDERATIONS
• Use cautiously in patients who may be allergic to aspirin and other NSAIDs.
• Use cautiously in patients with bleeding tendencies and in those receiving drugs that may prolong clotting times.
• Wound healing may be delayed with drug use.
• *Alert:* Don't confuse Ocufen with Ocuflox.

### ✓ Patient teaching
• Advise patient to alert doctor immediately if visual acuity decreases or visual field diminishes.
• Urge patient to take drug as prescribed.
• Advise patient to report excessive bleeding or bruising.

---

## ketorolac tromethamine
Acular

*Pregnancy Risk Category C*

### HOW SUPPLIED
*Ophthalmic solution:* 0.5%

---

## ACTION
Unknown. An NSAID thought to inhibit the action of cyclooxygenase, an enzyme responsible for prostaglandin synthesis. Prostaglandins mediate the inflammatory response and also cause miosis.

| Route | Onset | Peak | Duration |
|---|---|---|---|
| Ophthalmic | Unknown | Unknown | Unknown |

## INDICATIONS & DOSAGE
*Relief from ocular itching due to seasonal allergic conjunctivitis—*
**Adults:** 1 drop into conjunctival sac in each eye q.i.d.
*Postoperative inflammation in patients who have undergone cataract extraction—*
**Adults:** 1 drop to operative eye or eyes q.i.d. beginning 24 hours after cataract surgery and continuing through first 2 weeks of postoperative period.

## ADVERSE REACTIONS
**EENT:** *transient stinging and burning on instillation,* superficial keratitis, superficial ocular infections, ocular irritation.
**Other:** *hypersensitivity reactions.*

## INTERACTIONS
None significant.

## EFFECTS ON DIAGNOSTIC TESTS
None reported.

## CONTRAINDICATIONS
Contraindicated in patients with hypersensitivity to components of drug and in those wearing soft contact lenses.

## NURSING CONSIDERATIONS
• Use cautiously in patients with bleeding disorders or hypersensitivity to other NSAIDs or aspirin.
• Use with caution in breast-feeding women.
• Store drug away from heat in a dark, tightly closed container and protect from freezing.
• *Alert:* Don't confuse Acular with Acthar.

## ✅ Patient teaching
• Teach patient how to instill drops. Advise him to wash hands before and after instilling solution, and warn him not to touch tip of dropper to eye or surrounding tissue.
• Advise patient to apply light finger pressure on lacrimal sac for 1 minute after instillation.
• Stress importance of compliance with recommended therapy.
• Tell patient not to administer drug while wearing contact lenses.
• Advise patient to report excessive bleeding or bruising to doctor.
• Remind patient to discard drug when it's no longer needed.

## prednisolone acetate (suspension)
Econopred Ophthalmic, Econopred Plus Ophthalmic, Pred Forte, Pred Mild Ophthalmic

## prednisolone sodium phosphate (solution)
AK-Pred, Inflamase Forte, Inflamase Mild, Predsol Eye Drops‡

*Pregnancy Risk Category C*

## HOW SUPPLIED
**prednisolone acetate**
*Ophthalmic suspension:* 0.12%, 0.125%, 1%
**prednisolone sodium phosphate**
*Ophthalmic solution:* 0.125%, 1%

## ACTION
Unknown. Thought to decrease infiltration of WBCs at inflammation site.

| Route | Onset | Peak | Duration |
|---|---|---|---|
| Ophthalmic | Unknown | Unknown | Unknown |

## INDICATIONS & DOSAGE
*Inflammation of palpebral and bulbar conjunctiva, cornea, and anterior segment of globe—*
**Adults and children:** 1 to 2 drops instilled into eye. In severe conditions, may be used hourly, tapering to discontinuation as inflammation subsides. In mild conditions, may be used b.i.d. to q.i.d.

## ADVERSE REACTIONS
**EENT:** increased intraocular pressure; thinning of cornea, interference with corneal wound healing, increased susceptibility to viral or fungal corneal infection, corneal ulceration; discharge, discomfort, foreign body sensation, glaucoma exacerbation, cataracts, visual acuity and visual field defects, optic nerve damage with excessive or long-term use.
**Other:** systemic effects, adrenal suppression with excessive or long-term use.

## INTERACTIONS
None significant.

## EFFECTS ON DIAGNOSTIC TESTS
None reported.

## CONTRAINDICATIONS
Contraindicated in patients with acute, untreated, purulent ocular infections; acute superficial herpes simplex (dendritic keratitis); vaccinia, varicella, or other viral or fungal eye diseases; or ocular tuberculosis.

## NURSING CONSIDERATIONS
• Use cautiously in patients with corneal abrasions that may be contaminated (especially with herpes).
• Shake suspension and check dosage before administering to ensure using correct strength. Store in tightly covered container.
• *Alert:* Don't confuse prednisolone with prednisone.

## ✔ Patient teaching
• Teach patient how to instill drops. Advise him to wash hands before and after instillation, and warn him not to touch tip of dropper to eye or surrounding area.
• Advise patient to apply light finger pressure on lacrimal sac for 1 minute after instillation.
• Tell patient on long-term therapy to have frequent tonometric examinations.
• Tell patient not to share drug, washcloths, or towels with family members and to notify doctor if anyone develops same symptoms.
• Stress importance of compliance with recommended therapy.

• Tell patient to notify doctor if improvement doesn't occur within several days or if pain, itching, or swelling of eye occurs.
• Warn patient not to use leftover drug for new eye inflammation because serious problems may occur.

---

Reactions may be *common,* uncommon, *life-threatening,* or COMMON AND LIFE-THREATENING.

**acetylcholine chloride
carbachol (intraocular)
carbachol (topical)
echothiophate iodide
pilocarpine
pilocarpine hydrochloride
pilocarpine nitrate**

## COMBINATION PRODUCTS
E-PILO: epinephrine bitartrate 1% and pilocarpine hydrochloride 1%, 2%, 3%, 4%, or 6%.

## acetylcholine chloride
Miochol-E

*Pregnancy Risk Category NR*

## HOW SUPPLIED
*Ophthalmic injection:* 1%

## ACTION
A cholinergic that causes contraction of the sphincter muscles of the iris, resulting in miosis, and that produces ciliary spasm, deepening of the anterior chamber, and vasodilation of conjunctival vessels of the outflow tract.

| Route | Onset | Peak | Duration |
|-------|-------|------|----------|
| Ophthalmic | Secs | Unknown | 10 min |

## INDICATIONS & DOSAGE
*Anterior segment surgery—*
**Adults and children:** before or after securing sutures, doctor gently instills 0.5 to 2 ml into anterior chamber.

## ADVERSE REACTIONS
**CV:** bradycardia, hypotension, flushing.
**EENT:** corneal edema, clouding, decompensation.
**Respiratory:** breathing difficulties.
**Skin:** diaphoresis.

## INTERACTIONS
None significant.

## EFFECTS ON DIAGNOSTIC TESTS
None reported.

## CONTRAINDICATIONS
Contraindicated in patients with hypersensitivity to drug or its components.

## NURSING CONSIDERATIONS
● Reconstitute immediately before using, shaking vial gently until clear solution is obtained.
● Discard unused solution.
● Don't gas-sterilize vial. Ethylene oxide may produce formic acid. Watch for hypotension and bradycardia if this occurs.
● *Alert:* Don't confuse acetylcholine with acetylcysteine.

## ☑ Patient teaching
● Inform patient about need for drug during surgical procedure, and answer questions and address concerns.
● Instruct patient to immediately report breathing difficulties.

## carbachol (intraocular)
Miostat

## carbachol (topical)
Carboptic, Isopto Carbachol

*Pregnancy Risk Category C*

## HOW SUPPLIED
*Intraocular injection:* 0.01%
*Topical ophthalmic solution:* 0.75%, 1.5%, 2.25%, 3%

## ACTION
A cholinergic that causes contraction of the sphincter muscles of the iris, resulting in miosis, and that produces ciliary spasm, deepening of the anterior cham-

ber, and vasodilation of conjunctival vessels of the outflow tract.

| Route | Onset | Peak | Duration |
|-------|-------|------|----------|
| Ophthalmic | 10-20 min | 4 hr | 8 hr |
| Intraocular | Unknown | 2-5 min | 24 hr |

## INDICATIONS & DOSAGE
*To produce pupillary miosis in ocular surgery—*
**Adults:** before or after securing sutures, doctor gently instills 0.5 ml (intraocular form) into anterior chamber.
*Open-angle glaucoma—*
**Adults:** 1 to 2 drops (topical form) instilled up to t.i.d.

## ADVERSE REACTIONS
**CNS:** headache, syncope.
**CV:** *arrhythmias,* hypotension, flushing.
**EENT:** spasm of eye accommodation, conjunctival vasodilation, eye and brow pain, transient stinging and burning, corneal clouding, bullous keratopathy, salivation.
**GI:** abdominal cramps, diarrhea.
**GU:** urinary urgency.
**Respiratory:** asthma.
**Skin:** diaphoresis.

## INTERACTIONS
**Drug-drug.** *Pilocarpine:* additive effect. Use together cautiously.

## EFFECTS ON DIAGNOSTIC TESTS
None reported.

## CONTRAINDICATIONS
Contraindicated in patients with hypersensitivity to drug and in conditions in which cholinergic effects such as constriction are undesirable (for example, acute iritis, some forms of secondary glaucoma, pupillary block glaucoma, or acute inflammatory disease of the anterior chamber).

## NURSING CONSIDERATIONS
• Use cautiously in patients with acute heart failure, bronchial asthma, peptic ulcer, hyperthyroidism, GI spasm, Parkinson's disease, and urinary tract obstruction.

• In case of toxicity, give atropine parenterally, as ordered.
• Drug is used in open-angle glaucoma, especially when patients are resistant or allergic to pilocarpine hydrochloride or nitrate.
• *Alert:* Patients with dark eyes (hazel or brown irises) may need stronger solutions or more frequent instillation because eye pigment may absorb drug.
• If tolerance to drug develops, doctor may switch to another miotic for a short time.

### ☑ Patient teaching
• Teach patient how to instill drug. Advise him to wash hands before and after instillation and to apply light finger pressure on lacrimal sac for 1 minute after drops are instilled. Warn him not to exceed recommended dosage.
• Warn patient to avoid hazardous activities, such as operating machinery or driving, until temporary blurring subsides. Reassure patient that blurred vision usually diminishes with prolonged use.
• Tell glaucoma patient that long-term use may be needed. Stress compliance. Tell him to remain under medical supervision for periodic tonometric readings.
• Warn patient to use caution during night driving and while performing other hazardous activities in poor light.

## echothiophate iodide (ecothiopate iodide)
Phospholine Iodide

*Pregnancy Risk Category C*

## HOW SUPPLIED
*Ophthalmic powder for solution:* for reconstitution to make 0.03%, 0.06%, 0.125%, and 0.25% solutions

## ACTION
An anticholinesterase that inhibits the enzymatic destruction of acetylcholine by inactivating cholinesterase, leaving acetylcholine free to act on the effector cells of the iridic sphincter and ciliary

muscles, causing pupillary constriction and spasm of accommodation.

| Route | Onset | Peak | Duration |
|-------|-------|------|----------|
| Ophthalmic | 10 min-8 hr | 0.5-24 hr | Days-4 wk |

## INDICATIONS & DOSAGE
*Primary open-angle glaucoma, conditions obstructing aqueous outflow—*
**Adults and children:** 1 drop of 0.03% to 0.125% solution instilled into conjunctival sac daily. Maximum dose is 1 drop b.i.d. Lowest possible dose used for continuous control of intraocular pressure.
*Diagnosis of convergent strabismus—*
**Adults:** 1 drop of 0.125% solution instilled into each eye daily h.s. for 2 to 3 weeks.
*Treatment of convergent strabismus—*
**Adults:** initially, 1 drop of 0.125% solution instilled into each eye daily h.s. for 2 to 3 weeks. Dosage decreased to 1 drop of 0.125% solution every other day or 1 drop of 0.06% solution daily. The 0.03% solution may be effective for some patients.

## ADVERSE REACTIONS
**CNS:** fatigue, muscle weakness, paresthesia, headache.
**CV:** bradycardia, hypotension, flushing.
**EENT:** ciliary spasm or spasm of eye accommodation, ciliary or circumcorneal injection, nonreversible cataract formation (time- and dose-related), reversible iris cysts, pupillary block, blurred or dimmed vision, eye or brow pain, twitching of eyelids, hyperemia, photophobia, lens opacities, lacrimation, retinal detachment.
**GI:** diarrhea, nausea, vomiting, abdominal pain, intestinal cramps, salivation.
**GU:** frequent urination.
**Respiratory:** *bronchoconstriction.*
**Skin:** diaphoresis.

## INTERACTIONS
**Drug-drug.** *Anticholinergics, cyclopentolate, ophthalmic belladonna alkaloids such as atropine:* antagonized miotic effects. Avoid concomitant use.
*Local anesthetics, ophthalmic tetracaine:* increased rate of systemic toxicity and prolonged ocular anesthesia. Monitor closely.

*Ophthalmic adrenocorticoids:* increased intraocular pressure and decreased antiglaucoma effectiveness. Avoid concomitant use.
*Other cholinesterase inhibitors:* possible additive effect causing systemic effects. Monitor patient closely.
*Succinylcholine:* respiratory and CV collapse. Don't use together.
*Systemic anticholinesterases for myasthenia gravis, pilocarpine:* effects may be additive. Watch for signs of toxicity.
**Drug-lifestyle.** *Cocaine use:* increased risk of cocaine toxicity. Avoid concomitant use.
*Organophosphate insecticides, such as malathion, parathion:* possible additive effect causing systemic effects. Tell at-risk patient to protect himself from exposure.

## EFFECTS ON DIAGNOSTIC TESTS
Drug therapy decreases plasma cholinesterase activity.

## CONTRAINDICATIONS
Contraindicated in patients with hypersensitivity to drug or iodine and in those with uveal inflammation, acute angle-closure glaucoma before iridectomy, or other forms of glaucoma (except for primary open-angle glaucoma).

## NURSING CONSIDERATIONS
• Use with extreme caution, if at all, in patients with seizure disorders, vasomotor instability, parkinsonism, bronchial asthma, spastic GI conditions, urinary tract obstruction, peptic ulcer, severe bradycardia or hypotension, vascular hypertension, MI, or history or risk of retinal detachment.
• Use with caution in patients with corneal abrasion.
• Reconstitute powder, using only diluent provided to avoid contamination. Discard refrigerated, reconstituted solution after 6 months; discard solution stored at room temperature after 1 month.
• Stop drug, as ordered, at least 2 weeks preoperatively if succinylcholine is to be used in surgery.
• Toxicity is cumulative; toxic systemic symptoms may not appear for weeks or

months after start of therapy. Atropine sulfate S.C., I.M., or I.V. is antidote of choice.

### ✅ Patient teaching
• Teach patient how to instill drug. Advise him to wash hands before and after instillation, to avoid touching applicator tip to any surface, and to apply light finger pressure on lacrimal sac for 1 minute after instillation.
• Tell patient to instill drug at bedtime because it causes transient blurred vision. Warn him that transient brow pain or dimmed or blurred vision is common at first but usually disappears within 5 to 10 days.
• Warn patient to notify doctor if salivation, diarrhea, profuse diaphoresis, urinary incontinence, or muscle weakness occurs.
• Tell patient to remain under constant medical supervision and not to exceed recommended dosage.
• Advise patient to avoid driving if visual blurring occurs, particularly at night.
• Advise patient to carry medical identification card at all times during therapy. Drug is potent, long-acting, and irreversible.

---

## pilocarpine
Ocusert Pilo Ocular System

## pilocarpine hydrochloride
Adsorbocarpine, Akarpine, Isopto Carpine, Miocarpine†, Pilocar, Pilogel§, Pilopine HS, Pilopt‡, Pilostat, Sno Pilo§

## pilocarpine nitrate
Pilagan Liquifilm

*Pregnancy Risk Category C*

### HOW SUPPLIED
**pilocarpine**
*Extended-release insert:* 20 mcg/hour, 40 mcg/hour for 7 days
**pilocarpine hydrochloride**
*Ophthalmic solution:* 0.25%, 0.5%, 1%, 2%, 3%, 4%, 5%, 6%, 8%, 10%
*Ophthalmic gel:* 4%

**pilocarpine nitrate**
*Ophthalmic solution:* 1%, 2%, 4%

### ACTION
A cholinergic that causes contraction of iris sphincter muscles, resulting in miosis, and that produces ciliary spasm, deepening of the anterior chamber, and vasodilation of conjunctival vessels of the outflow tract.

| Route | Onset | Peak | Duration |
|-------|-------|------|----------|
| Ophthalmic | 10-30 min | 30-85 min | 4-8 hr |

### INDICATIONS & DOSAGE
*Primary open-angle glaucoma—*
**Adults and children:** 1 to 2 drops instilled up to q.i.d. or 1-cm ribbon of 4% gel applied h.s. Or, one Ocusert Pilo system (20 or 40 mcg/hour) applied q 7 days.
*Emergency treatment of acute angle-closure glaucoma—*
**Adults and children:** 1 drop of 2% solution instilled q 5 to 10 minutes for three to six doses; then 1 drop q 1 to 3 hours until pressure is controlled.
*Mydriasis due to mydriatic or cycloplegic drugs—*
**Adults and children:** 1 drop of 1% solution.

### ADVERSE REACTIONS
**CV:** hypertension, tachycardia, hypotension.
**EENT:** periorbital or supraorbital headache, *myopia,* ciliary spasm, *blurred vision,* conjunctival irritation, transient stinging and burning, keratitis, lens opacity, retinal detachment, lacrimation, changes in visual field, *brow pain.*
**GI:** nausea, vomiting, diarrhea, salivation.
**Respiratory:** *bronchoconstriction, pulmonary edema.*
**Skin:** diaphoresis.
**Other:** *hypersensitivity reactions.*

### INTERACTIONS
**Drug-drug.** *Carbachol, echothiophate:* additive effect. Don't use together.
*Cyclopentolate, ophthalmic belladonna alkaloids, such as atropine, scopolamine:* decreased pilocarpine antiglaucoma effec-

---

tiveness and blocked mydriatic effects of these drugs. Avoid concomitant use.
*Phenylephrine:* decreased dilation by phenylephrine. Don't use together.

**EFFECTS ON DIAGNOSTIC TESTS**
None reported.

**CONTRAINDICATIONS**
Contraindicated in patients with hypersensitivity to drug and in conditions in which cholinergic effects such as constriction are undesirable (for example, acute iritis, some forms of secondary glaucoma, pupillary block glaucoma, acute inflammatory disease of the anterior chamber).

**NURSING CONSIDERATIONS**
• Use cautiously in patients with acute cardiac failure, bronchial asthma, peptic ulcer, hyperthyroidism, GI spasm, urinary tract obstruction, and Parkinson's disease.
• Monitor vital signs.
• *Alert:* Patients with dark eyes (hazel or brown irises) may need stronger solutions or more frequent instillation because eye pigment may absorb drug.

☑ **Patient teaching**
• Instruct patient to apply gel at bedtime because it will blur vision. Warn him to avoid hazardous activities, such as operating machinery or driving, until temporary blurring subsides.
• Teach patient how to instill drug. Advise him to wash hands before and after instillation and to apply light finger pressure on lacrimal sac for 1 minute after drops are instilled. Warn patient not to touch applicator tip to eye or surrounding tissue.
• If Ocusert Pilo system falls out of eye during sleep, tell patient to wash hands, rinse insert in cool tap water, and reposition in eye. Also tell him not to use a deformed insert.
• Warn patient that transient brow pain and myopia are common at first but usually disappear within 10 to 14 days.
• Advise patient to carry medical identification card at all times during therapy.

**atropine sulfate**
**cyclopentolate hydrochloride**
**epinephrine hydrochloride**
**epinephryl borate**
**homatropine hydrobromide**
**phenylephrine hydrochloride**
**scopolamine hydrobromide**
**tropicamide**

### COMBINATION PRODUCTS
CYCLOMYDRIL OPHTHALMIC: cyclopentolate hydrochloride 0.2% and phenylephrine hydrochloride 1%.
MUROCOLL-2: scopolamine hydrobromide 0.3% and phenylephrine hydrochloride 10%.
PAREMYD: tropicamide 0.25% and hydroxyamphetamine hydrobromide 1%.
ZINCFRIN ◊ : phenylephrine hydrochloride 0.12% and zinc sulfate 0.25%.

---

### atropine sulfate
Atropine-1, Atropisol, Atropt‡,
Isopto Atropine

*Pregnancy Risk Category C*

### HOW SUPPLIED
*Ophthalmic ointment:* 1%
*Ophthalmic solution:* 0.5%, 1%, 2%

### ACTION
A potent mydriatic and cycloplegic whose anticholinergic action leaves the pupil under unopposed adrenergic influence, causing it to dilate.

| Route | Onset | Peak | Duration |
|-------|-------|------|----------|
| Ophthalmic | Unknown | 0.5-3 hr | 7-10 days |

### INDICATIONS & DOSAGE
*Acute iritis, uveitis—*
**Adults:** 1 to 2 drops instilled up to q.i.d. or small strip of ointment applied to conjunctival sac up to t.i.d.
**Children:** 1 to 2 drops of 0.5% solution up to t.i.d. or small strip of ointment applied to conjunctival sac up to t.i.d.

*Cycloplegic refraction—*
**Adults:** 1 to 2 drops of 1% solution 1 hour before refraction.
**Children:** 1 to 2 drops of 0.5% solution in each eye b.i.d. for 1 to 3 days before eye examination and 1 hour before refraction.

### ADVERSE REACTIONS
**CNS:** confusion, somnolence, headache.
**CV:** tachycardia.
**EENT:** ocular congestion with long-term use, conjunctivitis, contact dermatitis of eye, ocular edema, *blurred vision,* eye dryness, photophobia, increased intraocular pressure (IOP), transient stinging and burning, irritation, hyperemia.
**GI:** dry mouth; abdominal distention in infants.
**Skin:** dryness.

### INTERACTIONS
**Drug-lifestyle.** *Sun exposure:* photophobia may occur. Take precautions.

### EFFECTS ON DIAGNOSTIC TESTS
None reported.

### CONTRAINDICATIONS
Contraindicated in patients with hypersensitivity to drug or belladonna alkaloids and in those with glaucoma or adhesions between the iris and lens. Atropine shouldn't be used in infants ages 3 months or younger because of possible association between cycloplegia produced and development of amblyopia.

### NURSING CONSIDERATIONS
• Use cautiously in elderly patients and in others in whom increased IOP may be encountered. Excessive use in children or in certain susceptible patients, including those with spastic paralysis, brain damage, or Down syndrome, may produce systemic symptoms of atropine poisoning.
• *Alert:* Treat drops and ointment as poison (not for internal use); signs of poisoning are disorientation and confusion. An-

tidote of choice is physostigmine salicylate I.V. or I.M.
• Watch for signs and symptoms of glaucoma, including increased IOP, ocular pain, headache, and progressive blurring of vision; notify doctor if they occur.
• *Alert:* Don't confuse Atropisol with Aplisol.

### ✅ Patient teaching
• Teach patient how to instill atropine. Advise him to wash hands before and after instillation and to apply light finger pressure on lacrimal sac for 1 minute after instillation. Warn patient not to touch tip of dropper or tube to eye or surrounding tissue.
• Warn patient to avoid hazardous activities, such as operating machinery or driving, until temporary blurring subsides.
• Advise patient to ease photophobia by wearing dark glasses.

---

## cyclopentolate hydrochloride
AK-Pentolate, Cyclogyl,
Mydrilate§, Pentolair

*Pregnancy Risk Category C*

### HOW SUPPLIED
*Ophthalmic solution:* 0.5%, 1%, 2%

### ACTION
A potent mydriatic and cycloplegic whose anticholinergic action leaves the pupil under unopposed adrenergic influence, causing it to dilate.

| Route | Onset | Peak | Duration |
|-------|-------|------|----------|
| Ophthalmic | Rapid | 0.5-1.25 hr | 6-24 hr |

### INDICATIONS & DOSAGE
*Diagnostic procedures requiring mydriasis and cycloplegia—*
**Adults:** 1 or 2 drops of 0.5%, 1%, or 2% solution into each eye; then 1 or 2 drops in 5 to 10 minutes, if needed.
**Children:** 1 drop of 0.5%, 1%, or 2% solution into each eye; then 1 drop of 0.5% or 1% solution in 5 to 10 minutes, if needed.

### ADVERSE REACTIONS
**CNS:** irritability, confusion, somnolence, hallucinations, ataxia, *seizures;* behavioral disturbances in children.
**CV:** tachycardia.
**EENT:** eye burning on instillation, blurred vision, eye dryness, *photophobia,* ocular congestion, contact dermatitis in eye, conjunctivitis, increased intraocular pressure (IOP), transient stinging and burning, irritation, hyperemia.
**GU:** urine retention.
**Skin:** dryness.

### INTERACTIONS
**Drug-drug.** *Carbachol, pilocarpine:* may counteract mydriatic effect. Avoid concomitant use.
*Long-acting cholinergic antiglaucoma drugs:* miotic actions may be inhibited. Avoid concomitant use.
**Drug-lifestyle.** *Sun exposure:* photophobia may occur. Take precautions.

### EFFECTS ON DIAGNOSTIC TESTS
None reported.

### CONTRAINDICATIONS
Contraindicated in patients with hypersensitivity to drug or belladonna alkaloids and in those with glaucoma or adhesions between the iris and lens.

### NURSING CONSIDERATIONS
• Use with extreme caution in infants and young children.
• The combination product containing 1% phenylephrine hydrochloride shouldn't be used in infants under age 1 because of risk of precipitating severe hypertension.
• Use cautiously in elderly patients and in those in whom increased IOP may be encountered.
• Drug is superior to homatropine hydrobromide, and has a shorter duration of action. Physostigmine is antidote of choice.

### ✅ Patient teaching
• Teach patient how to instill drug. Advise him to wash hands before and after instillation and to apply light finger pressure on lacrimal sac for 1 minute after instillation. Warn him not to touch tip of dropper

---

to eye or surrounding tissue and that drug will burn when instilled.
• Warn patient to avoid hazardous activities, such as operating machinery or driving, until temporary blurring subsides.
• Advise patient to ease photophobia by wearing dark glasses.

---

## epinephrine hydrochloride
Epifrin, Eppy§, Glaucon

## epinephryl borate
Epinal

*Pregnancy Risk Category C*

### HOW SUPPLIED
**epinephrine hydrochloride**
*Ophthalmic solution:* 0.1%, 0.5%, 1%, 2%
**epinephryl borate**
*Ophthalmic solution:* 0.5%, 1%

### ACTION
An adrenergic that dilates the pupil by contracting the dilator muscle.

| Route | Onset | Peak | Duration |
|-------|-------|------|----------|
| Ophthalmic | 1 hr | 4-8 hr | 24 hr |

### INDICATIONS & DOSAGE
*Open-angle glaucoma—*
**Adults:** 1 or 2 drops of 1% or 2% solution once daily or b.i.d. Dosage adjusted based on tonometric readings.

### ADVERSE REACTIONS
**CNS:** brow ache, headache, lightheadedness.
**CV:** palpitations, tachycardia, *arrhythmias,* hypertension.
**EENT:** corneal or conjunctival pigmentation, corneal edema with long-term use; follicular hypertrophy; chemosis; conjunctivitis; iritis; hyperemic conjunctiva; maculopapular rash; eye stinging, burning, tearing on instillation; eye pain; allergic lid reaction; ocular irritation.
**GU:** increased BUN levels.
**Metabolic:** hyperglycemia.

### INTERACTIONS
**Drug-drug.** *Antihistamines (dexchlorpheniramine, diphenhydramine), tricyclic antidepressants:* potentiated cardiac effects of epinephrine. Monitor closely.
*Beta blockers, osmotic drugs, systemic carbonic anhydrase inhibitors, topical miotics:* additive lowering of intraocular pressure. Use together cautiously.
*Cardiac glycosides:* increased risk of arrhythmias. Monitor closely.
*Cyclopropane, halogenated hydrocarbons:* arrhythmias, tachycardia. Use together cautiously, if at all.
*Local or systemic sympathomimetics:* additive toxic effects. Avoid concomitant use.
*MAO inhibitors:* exaggerated adrenergic effects. Adjust dosage of epinephrine carefully.

### EFFECTS ON DIAGNOSTIC TESTS
Drug therapy interferes with tests for urinary catecholamines.

### CONTRAINDICATIONS
Contraindicated in patients with hypersensitivity to drug or sulfites and in those with hypertensive CV disease or coronary artery disease. Also contraindicated in patients with angle-closure glaucoma or when nature of glaucoma hasn't been established.

### NURSING CONSIDERATIONS
• Use cautiously in elderly patients and in those with diabetes mellitus, hypertension, Parkinson's disease, hyperthyroidism, aphakia (eye without lens), cardiac disease, cerebral arteriosclerosis, or bronchial asthma.
• Drug can be injected into anterior chamber to produce rapid mydriasis during cataract removal or can be used to control local bleeding during surgery.
• *Alert:* Don't substitute one salt if another one is ordered; epinephrine salts aren't interchangeable.
• Monitor blood pressure and other vital signs.
• *Alert:* Don't confuse epinephrine with ephedrine, or Glaucon with glucagon.

### ☑ Patient teaching
• Teach patient how to instill drug. Advise him to wash hands before and after instillation and to apply light finger pressure

---

on lacrimal sac for 1 minute after drops are instilled. Warn him not to touch tip of dropper to eye or surrounding tissue.
• Instruct patients to report immediately any decrease in visual acuity.
• Advise patient not to use drug while wearing soft contact lenses because discoloration of lenses may occur.
• Tell patient not to use darkened solution.

---

## homatropine hydrobromide
Isopto Homatropine, Minims Homatropine†

*Pregnancy Risk Category C*

### HOW SUPPLIED
*Ophthalmic solution:* 2%, 5%

### ACTION
An anticholinergic that leaves the pupil under unopposed adrenergic influence, causing it to dilate.

| Route | Onset | Peak | Duration |
|---|---|---|---|
| Ophthalmic | Rapid | 40-60 min | 1-3 days |

### INDICATIONS & DOSAGE
*Cycloplegic refraction—*
**Adults and children:** 1 to 2 drops into each eye; if needed, repeated in 5 to 10 minutes for two or three doses.
*Uveitis—*
**Adults and children:** 1 to 2 drops into each eye q 3 to 4 hours.
*Note:* Use only 2% solution with children.

### ADVERSE REACTIONS
**CNS:** confusion, headache, somnolence.
**CV:** tachycardia.
**EENT:** eye irritation, *blurred vision, photophobia,* increased intraocular pressure (IOP), transient stinging and burning, conjunctivitis, vascular congestion, edema.
**GI:** dry mouth.
**Skin:** dryness, rash.

### INTERACTIONS
**Drug-lifestyle.** *Sun exposure:* photophobia may occur. Take precautions.

### EFFECTS ON DIAGNOSTIC TESTS
None reported.

### CONTRAINDICATIONS
Contraindicated in patients with hypersensitivity to drug or other belladonna alkaloids such as atropine and in those with glaucoma or adhesions between the iris and lens.

### NURSING CONSIDERATIONS
• Use cautiously in elderly patients, in those in whom increased IOP may be encountered, and in those with cardiac disease or hypertension.
• In patients with heavily pigmented irises, larger doses may be needed.
• Monitor vital signs.
• *Alert:* Homatropine is similar to atropine but weaker, with a shorter duration of action. Drug may produce symptoms of atropine poisoning, such as severe dryness of mouth or tachycardia.

### ✓ Patient teaching
• Teach patient how to instill drug. Advise him to wash hands before and after instillation and to apply light finger pressure on lacrimal sac for 1 minute after drops are instilled.
• Warn patient not to touch tip of dropper to eye or surrounding tissue.
• Caution patient to avoid hazardous activities, such as operating machinery or driving, until temporary blurring subsides.
• Instruct patient to ease photophobia by wearing dark glasses.
• Advise patient to carry medical identification card during therapy.

---

## phenylephrine hydrochloride
AK-Dilate, AK-Nefrin Ophthalmic◇, Isopto Frin◇, Mydfrin, Phenoptic, Prefrin Liquifilm◇, Relief◇

*Pregnancy Risk Category C*

### HOW SUPPLIED
*Ophthalmic solution:* 0.12%◇, 2.5%, 10%

---

## ACTION
An adrenergic that dilates the pupil by contracting the dilator muscle.

| Route | Onset | Peak | Duration |
|-------|-------|------|----------|
| Ophthalmic | Rapid | 10-90 min | 3-7 hr |

## INDICATIONS & DOSAGE
*Mydriasis without cycloplegia—*
**Adults and children:** 1 drop of 2.5% or 10% solution instilled before examination. May be repeated in 1 hour, if needed.
*Mydriasis and vasoconstriction—*
**Adults and adolescents:** 1 drop of 2.5% or 10% solution.
**Children:** 1 drop of 2.5% solution.
*Chronic mydriasis—*
**Adults and adolescents:** 1 drop of 2.5% or 10% solution b.i.d. or t.i.d.
**Children:** 1 drop of 2.5% solution instilled b.i.d. or t.i.d.
*Posterior synechia (adhesion of iris)—*
**Adults and children:** instill 1 drop of 2.5% or 10% solution. Don't use 10% concentration in infants.

## ADVERSE REACTIONS
**CNS:** brow ache, headache.
**CV:** *hypertension with 10% solution,* tachycardia, palpitations, *PVCs, MI.*
**EENT:** transient eye burning or stinging on instillation, blurred vision, increased intraocular pressure, keratitis, lacrimation, reactive hyperemia of eye, allergic conjunctivitis, rebound miosis.
**Skin:** pallor, dermatitis, diaphoresis.
**Other:** trembling.

## INTERACTIONS
**Drug-drug.** *Beta blockers, MAO inhibitors:* may cause arrhythmias because of increased pressor effect. Use together cautiously.
*Guanethidine:* increased mydriatic and pressor effects of phenylephrine. Use together cautiously.
*Levodopa (systemic):* reduced mydriatic effect of phenylephrine. Use together cautiously.
*Topical atropine, cyclopentolate, homatropine, scopolamine:* may increase dilation of pupil. Use together cautiously.

*Tricyclic antidepressants:* potentiated cardiac effects of epinephrine. Use together cautiously.
**Drug-lifestyle.** *Sun exposure:* photophobia may occur. Take precautions.

## EFFECTS ON DIAGNOSTIC TESTS
Drug may lower intraocular pressure in normal eyes or in open-angle glaucoma; it may also cause false-normal tonometry readings.

## CONTRAINDICATIONS
Contraindicated in patients with hypersensitivity to drug; also contraindicated in those with angle-closure glaucoma and in patients who wear soft contact lenses.

## NURSING CONSIDERATIONS
• Use cautiously in patients with marked hypertension, cardiac disorders, advanced arteriosclerotic changes, type 1 diabetes, or hyperthyroidism; in children of low body weight; and in elderly patients.
• Systemic adverse reactions are least likely with 2.5% solution and most likely with 10% solution.
• *Alert:* Don't confuse Mydfrin with Midrin.

☑ **Patient teaching**
• Teach patient how to instill drug. Advise him to wash hands before and after instillation and to apply light finger pressure on lacrimal sac for 1 minute after drops are instilled. Warn him not to touch tip of dropper to eye or surrounding tissue.
• Warn patient not to exceed recommended dosage because systemic effects can result. Monitor blood pressure and pulse rate.
• Tell patient not to use brown solutions or solutions that contain precipitate.
• Warn patient to avoid hazardous activities, such as operating machinery or driving, until temporary blurring subsides.
• Advise patient to contact doctor if condition persists more than 12 hours after discontinuation of drug.
• Advise patient to ease photophobia by wearing dark glasses.

## scopolamine hydrobromide
Isopto Hyoscine

*Pregnancy Risk Category NR*

### HOW SUPPLIED
*Ophthalmic solution:* 0.25%

### ACTION
An anticholinergic that leaves the pupil under unopposed adrenergic influence, causing it to dilate.

| Route | Onset | Peak | Duration |
|-------|-------|------|----------|
| Ophthalmic | Rapid | 15-45 min | < 1 wk |

### INDICATIONS & DOSAGE
*Cycloplegic refraction—*
**Adults:** 1 to 2 drops of 0.25% solution instilled 1 hour before refraction.
**Children:** 1 drop of 0.25% solution instilled b.i.d. for 2 days before refraction.
*Iritis, uveitis—*
**Adults:** 1 to 2 drops of 0.25% solution instilled once daily to q.i.d.
**Children:** 1 drop of 0.25% solution instilled once daily to q.i.d.

### ADVERSE REACTIONS
**CNS:** confusion, delirium, somnolence, acute psychotic reactions, headache, hallucinations.
**CV:** tachycardia.
**EENT:** ocular congestion with prolonged use, conjunctivitis, *blurred vision,* eye dryness, increased intraocular pressure, *photophobia,* transient stinging and burning, edema.
**GI:** dry mouth.
**Skin:** dryness, contact dermatitis.

### INTERACTIONS
**Drug-lifestyle.** *Sun exposure:* photophobia may occur. Take precautions.

### EFFECTS ON DIAGNOSTIC TESTS
None reported.

### CONTRAINDICATIONS
Contraindicated in patients with hypersensitivity to drug and in those with shallow anterior chamber, angle-closure glaucoma, or adhesions between the iris and lens; also contraindicated in children with previous severe systemic reaction to atropine.

### NURSING CONSIDERATIONS
• Use with extreme caution (if at all) in infants and small children.
• Use cautiously in patients with cardiac disease and in elderly patients.
• Observe patients closely for adverse CNS effects (such as disorientation and delirium).
• Drug may be used in patients sensitive to atropine because it's faster acting and has a shorter duration of action and fewer adverse reactions.

### ☑ Patient teaching
• Teach patient how to instill drug. Advise him to wash hands before and after instillation and to apply light finger pressure on lacrimal sac for 1 minute after drops are instilled. Warn him to avoid touching tip of dropper to eye or surrounding tissue.
• Warn patient to avoid hazardous activities, such as operating machinery or driving, until temporary blurring subsides.
• Advise patient to ease photophobia by wearing dark glasses.
• Instruct patient to carry medical alert card at all times during therapy.

---

## tropicamide
Mydriacyl, Opticyl, Tropicacyl

*Pregnancy Risk Category NR*

### HOW SUPPLIED
*Ophthalmic solution:* 0.5%, 1%

### ACTION
The shortest-acting cycloplegic available, whose anticholinergic action leaves the pupil under unopposed adrenergic influence, causing it to dilate.

| Route | Onset | Peak | Duration |
|-------|-------|------|----------|
| Ophthalmic | Rapid | 20-40 min | 7 hr |

### INDICATIONS & DOSAGE
*Cycloplegic refraction—*
**Adults:** 1 drop of 1% solution; repeated in 5 minutes. If needed, additional drop in 20 to 30 minutes.

---

**Children:** 1 drop of 0.5% or 1% solution; repeated in 5 minutes, if needed.
*Fundus examinations—*
**Adults and children:** 1 to 2 drops of 0.5% solution instilled in each eye 15 to 20 minutes before examination; may be repeated q 30 minutes, p.r.n. Compress lacrimal sac with finger pressure for 1 to 2 minutes after instillation to avoid excessive systemic absorption.

**ADVERSE REACTIONS**
**CNS:** confusion, somnolence, hallucinations; behavioral disturbances in children.
**CV:** tachycardia.
**EENT:** *transient eye stinging on instillation,* increased intraocular pressure, hyperemia, irritation, conjunctivitis, edema, *blurred vision, photophobia; dry throat.*
**GI:** dry mouth.
**Skin:** dryness.

**INTERACTIONS**
**Drug-lifestyle.** *Sun exposure:* photophobia may occur. Take precautions.

**EFFECTS ON DIAGNOSTIC TESTS**
None reported.

**CONTRAINDICATIONS**
Contraindicated in patients with hypersensitivity to drug and in those with shallow anterior chamber or angle-closure glaucoma.

**NURSING CONSIDERATIONS**
• Use cautiously in elderly patients.
• Wash hands before and after instilling drug and apply light finger pressure on lacrimal sac for 1 minute after instillation. Don't touch tip of dropper to eye or surrounding tissue.
• Drug's mydriatic effect is greater than its cycloplegic effect.

☑ **Patient teaching**
• Warn patient that drug causes transient stinging.
• Warn patient to avoid hazardous activities until blurring subsides.
• Advise patient to ease photophobia by wearing dark glasses.

---

Reactions may be *common,* uncommon, *life-threatening,* or COMMON AND LIFE-THREATENING.

**naphazoline hydrochloride**
**oxymetazoline hydrochloride**
**tetrahydrozoline hydrochloride**

### COMBINATION PRODUCTS
VASOCON-A OPHTHALMIC SOLUTION: naphazoline hydrochloride 0.05% and antazoline phosphate 0.5%.

---

### naphazoline hydrochloride
AK-Con, Albalon Liquifilm, Allerest◇, Clear Eyes◇, Comfort Eye Drops◇, Degest 2◇, Nafazair, Naphcon◇, Naphcon Forte, Optazine‡, Vasocon Regular

*Pregnancy Risk Category C*

---

### HOW SUPPLIED
*Ophthalmic solution:* 0.012%◇, 0.02%◇, 0.03%◇, 0.1%

### ACTION
Unknown. Thought to cause vasoconstriction by local adrenergic action on the blood vessels of the conjunctiva.

| Route | Onset | Peak | Duration |
|-------|-------|------|----------|
| Ophthalmic | 10 min | Unknown | 2-6 hr |

### INDICATIONS & DOSAGE
*Ocular congestion, irritation, itching—*
**Adults:** 1 drop of 0.1% solution instilled q 3 to 4 hours or 1 drop of 0.012% to 0.03% solution up to q.i.d.

### ADVERSE REACTIONS
**CNS:** headache, dizziness, nervousness, weakness.
**EENT:** transient eye stinging, pupillary dilation, eye irritation, photophobia, blurred vision, increased intraocular pressure, keratitis, lacrimation.
**GI:** nausea.
**Skin:** diaphoresis.

### INTERACTIONS
**Drug-drug.** *MAO inhibitors, maprotiline, tricyclic antidepressants:* hypertensive crisis if naphazoline is systemically absorbed. Use together cautiously.

### EFFECTS ON DIAGNOSTIC TESTS
None reported.

### CONTRAINDICATIONS
Contraindicated in patients with hypersensitivity to drug's ingredients and in those with acute angle-closure glaucoma. Use of 0.1% solution is contraindicated in infants and small children.

### NURSING CONSIDERATIONS
• Use cautiously in patients with hyperthyroidism, cardiac disease, hypertension, or diabetes mellitus.
• Drug is most widely used ocular decongestant.
• Store drug in tightly closed container.

### ☑ Patient teaching
• Teach patient how to instill drug. Advise him to wash hands before and after instillation and to apply light finger pressure on lacrimal sac for 1 minute after drops are instilled. Warn him not to touch tip of dropper to eye or surrounding tissue.
• Warn patient not to exceed recommended dosage. Rebound congestion and conjunctivitis may occur with frequent or prolonged use.
• Tell patient to notify doctor if photophobia, blurred vision, pain, or lid edema develops.
• Instruct patient not to use OTC preparations longer than 72 hours without consulting doctor.

---

*Liquid contains alcohol.    **May contain tartrazine.    †Canada    ‡Australia    §U.K.    ◇OTC

## oxymetazoline hydrochloride
OcuClear ◊ , Visine L.R. ◊

*Pregnancy Risk Category C*

### HOW SUPPLIED
*Ophthalmic solution:* 0.025%

### ACTION
A direct-acting sympathomimetic amine that acts on alpha-adrenergic receptors in the arterioles of the conjunctiva to produce vasoconstriction, resulting in decreased conjunctival congestion.

| Route | Onset | Peak | Duration |
|-------|-------|------|----------|
| Ophthalmic | 5 min | Unknown | 6 hr |

### INDICATIONS & DOSAGE
*Relief of eye redness due to minor eye irritations—*
**Adults and children ages 6 and older:** 1 to 2 drops instilled into conjunctival sac b.i.d. to q.i.d. (spaced at least 6 hours apart).

### ADVERSE REACTIONS
**CNS:** headache, light-headedness, nervousness, insomnia.
**CV:** palpitations, tachycardia, irregular heartbeat.
**EENT:** *transient stinging on initial instillation;* blurred vision, keratitis, lacrimation, increase in intraocular pressure; reactive hyperemia with excessive doses or prolonged use.
**Other:** trembling.

### INTERACTIONS
**Drug-drug.** *MAO inhibitors, maprotiline, tricyclic antidepressants:* if significant systemic absorption of oxymetazoline occurs, concurrent use may potentiate pressor effect of oxymetazoline. Avoid use together.

### EFFECTS ON DIAGNOSTIC TESTS
None reported.

### CONTRAINDICATIONS
Contraindicated in patients with hypersensitivity to drug or its components and in those with angle-closure glaucoma.

### NURSING CONSIDERATIONS
• Use cautiously in patients with hyperthyroidism, cardiac disease, hypertension, and eye disease, infection, or injury.
• Don't use if solution has become cloudy or changes color.
• *Alert:* Don't confuse Visine with Visken.

### ✅ Patient teaching
• Teach patient how to instill drops. Advise him to wash hands before and after instillation, and warn him not to touch tip of dropper to eye or surrounding tissue.
• Instruct patient to apply light finger pressure on lacrimal sac for 1 minute after drug instillation.
• Advise patient to stop drug and consult doctor if eye pain occurs, if vision changes, or if redness or irritation continues, worsens, or lasts for more than 72 hours.

## tetrahydrozoline hydrochloride
Collyrium Fresh Eye Drops ◊ , Eyesine ◊ , Murine Plus ◊ , Optigene 3 ◊ , Tetrasine ◊ , Visine Moisturizing ◊ , Visine Extra ◊

*Pregnancy Risk Category C*

### HOW SUPPLIED
*Ophthalmic solution:* 0.05% ◊

### ACTION
Unknown. Thought to cause vasoconstriction by local adrenergic action on the blood vessels of the conjunctiva.

| Route | Onset | Peak | Duration |
|-------|-------|------|----------|
| Ophthalmic | Few min | Unknown | 1-4 hr |

### INDICATIONS & DOSAGE
*Conjunctival congestion, irritation, and allergic conditions—*
**Adults and children over age 2:** 1 to 2 drops of 0.05% solution instilled up to q.i.d. or as directed by doctor.

### ADVERSE REACTIONS
**CNS:** headache, drowsiness, insomnia, dizziness, tremor.
**CV:** *arrhythmias.*

---

Reactions may be *common*, uncommon, *life-threatening*, or COMMON AND LIFE-THREATENING.

**EENT:** transient eye stinging, pupillary dilation, increased intraocular pressure, keratitis, lacrimation, eye irritation.

**INTERACTIONS**
**Drug-drug.** *Guanethidine, MAO inhibitors, tricyclic antidepressants:* hypertensive crisis if tetrahydrozoline is systemically absorbed. Don't use together.

**EFFECTS ON DIAGNOSTIC TESTS**
None reported.

**CONTRAINDICATIONS**
Contraindicated in patients with hypersensitivity to drug or its components and in those with angle-closure glaucoma or other serious eye diseases.

**NURSING CONSIDERATIONS**
• Use cautiously in patients with hyperthyroidism, heart disease, hypertension, or diabetes mellitus.
• Rebound congestion may occur with frequent or prolonged use.
• *Alert:* Don't confuse Visine with Visken.

☑ **Patient teaching**
• Teach patient how to instill drug. Advise him to wash hands before and after instillation and to apply light finger pressure on lacrimal sac for 1 minute after drops are instilled. Warn him not to touch tip of dropper to eye or surrounding tissue.
• Warn patient not to exceed recommended dosage.
• Tell patient to stop drug and notify doctor if redness or irritation persists or increases or if no relief occurs within 2 days.
• Warn patient not to share ophthalmic drugs.

**apraclonidine hydrochloride**
**betaxolol hydrochloride**
**brimonidine tartrate**
**carteolol hydrochloride**
**dipivefrin hydrochloride**
**dorzolamide hydrochloride**
**emedastine difumarate**
**fluorescein sodium**
**ketotifen fumarate**
**latanoprost**
**levobunolol hydrochloride**
**metipranolol hydrochloride**
**sodium chloride, hypertonic**
**timolol maleate**

## COMBINATION PRODUCTS
FLUORACAINE: fluorescein sodium 0.25% and proparacaine hydrochloride 0.5%.
FLURESS AND FLU-OXINATE: fluorescein sodium 0.25% and benoxinate hydrochloride 0.4%.

---

## apraclonidine hydrochloride
Iopidine

*Pregnancy Risk Category C*

### HOW SUPPLIED
*Ophthalmic solution:* 0.5%, 1%

### ACTION
Unknown. An alpha agonist that reduces intraocular pressure (IOP), possibly by decreasing production of aqueous humor.

| Route | Onset | Peak | Duration |
|-------|-------|------|----------|
| Ophthalmic | 1 hr | 3-5 hr | 12 hr |

### INDICATIONS & DOSAGE
*Prevention or control of IOP elevation before and after ocular laser surgery—*
**Adults:** 1 drop of 1% solution instilled 1 hour before initiation of laser surgery on anterior segment; then 1 drop immediately after surgery.

*Short-term adjunct therapy in patients who need additional IOP reduction—*
**Adults:** 1 or 2 drops of 0.5% solution instilled into affected eyes t.i.d.

### ADVERSE REACTIONS
**CNS:** insomnia, irritability, dream disturbances, headache, irritability, paresthesia.
**CV:** bradycardia, vasovagal attack, palpitations, hypotension, orthostatic hypotension.
**EENT:** upper eyelid elevation, conjunctival blanching and microhemorrhage, mydriasis, eye burning or discomfort, foreign body sensation in eye, eye dryness and *itching, hyperemia,* conjunctivitis, blurred vision, nasal burning or dryness, increased pharyngeal secretions.
**GI:** abdominal pain, discomfort, diarrhea, vomiting, taste disturbances, dry mouth.
**Skin:** pruritus not associated with rash, sweaty palms.
**Other:** body heat sensation, decreased libido, extremity pain or numbness, allergic response.

### INTERACTIONS
**Drug-drug.** *Beta blockers, topical pilocarpine:* additive effects in lowering IOP. Use together cautiously.

### EFFECTS ON DIAGNOSTIC TESTS
None reported.

### CONTRAINDICATIONS
Contraindicated in patients with hypersensitivity to apraclonidine or clonidine and in those undergoing concurrent MAO inhibitor therapy.

### NURSING CONSIDERATIONS
• Use cautiously in patients with severe cardiac disease including hypertension or history of vasovagal attack.
• Closely monitor patients who tend to develop exaggerated decreases in IOP after drug therapy.
• Observe patients closely for vasovagal attack during laser surgery.

---

Reactions may be *common,* uncommon, *life-threatening*, or COMMON AND LIFE-THREATENING.

• Closely monitor patients with severe systemic disease, including hypertension, even though drug's systemic effects (altered heart rate and blood pressure) are uncommon after usual dose.

### ✓ Patient teaching
• Teach patient how to instill 0.5% solution. Advise him to wash hands before and after instillation and to apply light finger pressure on lacrimal sac for 1 minute after instilling drug.
• Warn patient not to touch tip of dropper to eye or surrounding tissue.
• Tell patient to separate intervals between each ophthalmic product instillation by at least 5 minutes to avoid washing away previous dose.
• Encourage patient to comply with t.i.d. regimen.

## betaxolol hydrochloride
Betoptic, Betoptic S

*Pregnancy Risk Category C*

### HOW SUPPLIED
*Ophthalmic solution:* 0.5%
*Ophthalmic suspension:* 0.25%

### ACTION
Unknown. A cardioselective beta blocker that reduces aqueous formation and possibly increases outflow of aqueous humor.

| Route | Onset | Peak | Duration |
|-------|-------|------|----------|
| Ophthalmic | 0.5-1 hr | 2 hr | > 12 hr |

### INDICATIONS & DOSAGE
*Chronic open-angle glaucoma, ocular hypertension—*
**Adults:** 1 or 2 drops of 0.5% solution or 0.25% suspension instilled b.i.d.

### ADVERSE REACTIONS
**CNS:** insomnia, *CVA,* depressive neurosis.
**CV:** *arrhythmias, heart block, heart failure,* palpitations.
**EENT:** *eye stinging on instillation causing brief discomfort,* photophobia, erythema, itching, keratitis, occasional tearing.
**Respiratory:** asthma, *bronchospasm.*

### INTERACTIONS
**Drug-drug.** *Calcium channel blockers:* AV conduction disturbances, ventricular failure, and hypotension if significant systemic absorption occurs. Monitor closely.
*Cardiac glycosides:* risk of excessive bradycardia. Patient may need ECG monitoring if significant systemic absorption occurs.
*Dipivefrin, ophthalmic epinephrine:* may produce mydriasis. Use together cautiously.
*Inhalation hydrocarbon anesthetics:* prolonged severe hypotension if significant systemic absorption occurs. Tell anesthesiologist that patient is receiving ophthalmic betaxolol.
*Insulin, oral antidiabetics:* risk of hypoglycemia or hyperglycemia if significant systemic absorption occurs. May need to adjust dosage of antidiabetics.
*Phenothiazines:* additive hypotensive effects; increased risk of adverse effects if significant systemic absorption occurs. Monitor closely.
*Reserpine:* excessive beta blockade. Monitor closely.
*Systemic beta blockers:* additive effects. Monitor closely.
**Drug-lifestyle.** *Cocaine use:* may inhibit betaxolol's effects. Avoid concomitant use.
*Sun exposure:* photophobia may occur. Take precautions.

### EFFECTS ON DIAGNOSTIC TESTS
None reported.

### CONTRAINDICATIONS
Contraindicated in patients with hypersensitivity to drug and in those with sinus bradycardia, greater-than-first-degree AV block, cardiogenic shock, or overt heart failure.

### NURSING CONSIDERATIONS
• Use cautiously in patients with restricted pulmonary function, diabetes mellitus, hyperthyroidism, or history of heart failure.
• Some patients may need a few weeks' treatment to stabilize intraocular pressure (IOP)–lowering response. Determine IOP after 4 weeks of treatment.

---

*Liquid contains alcohol. **May contain tartrazine. †Canada ‡Australia §U.K. ◇OTC

### ✓ Patient teaching

• Teach patient how to instill drug. Advise him to wash hands before and after instillation and to apply light finger pressure on lacrimal sac for 1 minute after instilling drug. Warn him not to touch tip of dropper to eye or surrounding tissue. He should shake suspension well before instilling.

• Encourage patient to comply with b.i.d. regimen.

• Tell patient to remove contact lenses before drug administration.

• Advise patient to ease photophobia by wearing dark glasses.

---

## brimonidine tartrate
### Alphagan

*Pregnancy Risk Category B*

---

### HOW SUPPLIED
*Ophthalmic solution:* 0.2%; 5 ml, 10 ml

### ACTION
A selective alpha$_2$-adrenergic agonist that reduces aqueous humor production and increases uveoscleral outflow.

| Route | Onset | Peak | Duration |
|-------|-------|------|----------|
| Ophthalmic | Unknown | 1-4 hr | Unknown |

### INDICATIONS & DOSAGE
*Intraocular pressure (IOP) reduction in open-angle glaucoma or ocular hypertension—*
**Adults:** 1 drop in affected eye t.i.d., about 8 hours apart.

### ADVERSE REACTIONS
**CNS:** anxiety, asthenia, depression, dizziness, *drowsiness, fatigue, headache,* insomnia, syncope.
**CV:** hypertension, palpitations.
**EENT:** abnormal vision or taste; blepharitis; *blurring, burning, stinging;* runny or stuffy nose, sneezing; conjunctival blanching, edema, hemorrhage, discharge, *conjunctival follicles;* corneal staining or erosion; eyelid erythema or eyelid edema; *foreign body sensation;* lid crusting; nasal dryness; *ocular hyperemia, allergic reac-*tions, *pruritus,* ache or pain, *dryness,* tearing, irritation; photophobia.
**GI:** nausea, vomiting, *oral dryness.*
**Musculoskeletal:** muscular pain.

### INTERACTIONS
**Drug-drug.** *Antihypertensives, beta blockers, cardiac glycosides:* may further decrease blood pressure or pulse. Use cautiously.
*CNS depressants:* may have additive effects. Use cautiously.
*Tricyclic antidepressants:* may interfere with brimonidine's IOP-lowering effects. Use cautiously.
**Drug-lifestyle.** *Alcohol use:* may have additive CNS depressant effect. Use cautiously.

### EFFECTS ON DIAGNOSTIC TESTS
None reported.

### CONTRAINDICATIONS
Contraindicated in patients with hypersensitivity to drug or benzalkonium chloride and in those receiving MAO inhibitor therapy.

### NURSING CONSIDERATIONS
• Use cautiously in patients with CV disease, cerebral or coronary insufficiency, hepatic or renal impairment, depression, Raynaud's phenomenon, orthostatic hypotension, or thromboangiitis obliterans.
• Monitor IOP because loss of effects after first month of therapy may occur.
• It's unknown if drug appears in breast milk. Use with caution.

### ✓ Patient teaching
• Tell patient to wait at least 15 minutes after instilling drug before wearing soft contact lenses.
• Caution patient to avoid hazardous activities because of potential for decreased mental alertness, fatigue, or drowsiness.

---

# carteolol hydrochloride
Ocupress, Teoptic§

*Pregnancy Risk Category C*

## HOW SUPPLIED
*Ophthalmic solution:* 1%

## ACTION
Exact mechanism unknown. A nonselective beta blocker that reduces intraocular pressure (IOP).

| Route | Onset | Peak | Duration |
|-------|-------|------|----------|
| Ophthalmic | Unknown | Unknown | Unknown |

## INDICATIONS & DOSAGE
*Chronic open-angle glaucoma, intraocular hypertension—*
**Adults:** 1 drop into conjunctival sac of affected eye b.i.d.

## ADVERSE REACTIONS
**CNS:** headache, dizziness, insomnia, asthenia.
**CV:** *bradycardia,* hypotension, *arrhythmias,* palpitations.
**EENT:** *transient eye irritation, burning, tearing, conjunctival hyperemia, ocular edema,* blurred and cloudy vision, photophobia, decreased night vision, ptosis, blepharoconjunctivitis, abnormal corneal staining, corneal sensitivity, sinusitis, taste perversion.
**Respiratory:** dyspnea.

## INTERACTIONS
**Drug-drug.** *Catecholamine-depleting drugs such as reserpine, oral beta blockers:* may cause additive effects and development of hypotension or bradycardia. Monitor patient closely.
**Drug-lifestyle.** *Sun exposure:* photophobia may occur. Take precautions.

## EFFECTS ON DIAGNOSTIC TESTS
None reported.

## CONTRAINDICATIONS
Contraindicated in patients with hypersensitivity to drug or its components and in those with bronchial asthma, severe COPD, sinus bradycardia, second- or third-degree AV block, overt cardiac failure, or cardiogenic shock.

## NURSING CONSIDERATIONS
• Use with caution in patients with hypersensitivity to other beta blockers; in those with nonallergic bronchospastic disease, diabetes mellitus, hyperthyroidism, or decreased pulmonary function; and in breast-feeding women.
• Monitor vital signs.
• *Alert:* Discontinue drug at first sign of cardiac failure, and notify doctor.
• When used to reduce elevated IOP in angle-closure glaucoma, drug should be given with a miotic and never alone.

### ☑ Patient teaching
• Tell patient that, if more than one topical ophthalmic drug is being used, drugs should be administered at least 10 minutes apart.
• Teach patient how to instill drops. Advise him to wash hands before and after instillation, and warn him not to touch tip of dropper to eye or surrounding tissue.
• Advise patient to apply light finger pressure on lacrimal sac for 1 minute after drug instillation to minimize systemic absorption.
• Instruct patient to keep bottle tightly closed when not in use and to protect it from light.
• Tell patient that drug is a beta blocker and, although it's administered topically, it has the potential to be absorbed systemically.
• Inform patient that adverse reactions that can result from beta blockers can occur with topical administration. Tell him to discontinue drug and notify doctor immediately if signs or symptoms of serious adverse reactions or hypersensitivity occur.
• Advise patient to monitor heart rate and blood pressure closely and to report slow heart rate to doctor.
• Stress importance of compliance with recommended therapy.
• Advise patient to ease photophobia by wearing dark glasses.

## dipivefrin hydrochloride
Propine

*Pregnancy Risk Category B*

### HOW SUPPLIED
*Ophthalmic solution:* 0.1%

### ACTION
A prodrug of epinephrine that is converted to epinephrine in the eye. The liberated epinephrine appears to decrease aqueous production and increase aqueous outflow.

| Route | Onset | Peak | Duration |
|-------|-------|------|----------|
| Ophthalmic | 0.5 hr | 1 hr | > 12 hr |

### INDICATIONS & DOSAGE
*Intraocular pressure (IOP) reduction in chronic open-angle glaucoma—*
**Adults:** for initial glaucoma therapy, 1 drop of 0.1% solution q 12 hours. Dosage adjustments based on patient response as determined by tonometric readings.

### ADVERSE REACTIONS
**CV:** tachycardia, hypertension, *arrhythmias.*
**EENT:** eye burning or stinging, conjunctival injection, conjunctivitis, mydriasis, allergic reaction, photophobia, *macular edema.*

### INTERACTIONS
**Drug-drug.** *Cardiac glycosides, inhalation hydrocarbon anesthetics, tricyclic antidepressants:* increased risk of adverse cardiac effects if significant systemic absorption occurs. Monitor closely.
*Ophthalmic beta blockers, osmotic drugs, systemically administered carbonic anhydrase inhibitors:* additive lowering of IOP. Use together cautiously. Watch for potential adverse effects.
*Systemic sympathomimetics:* possible additive effects if significant systemic absorption occurs. Monitor closely.

### EFFECTS ON DIAGNOSTIC TESTS
None reported.

### CONTRAINDICATIONS
Contraindicated in patients with hypersensitivity to drug and in those with angle-closure glaucoma.

### NURSING CONSIDERATIONS
• Use cautiously in patients with asthma, aphakia, CV disease, or history of hypersensitivity to epinephrine.
• Monitor patient for hypertension.
• Drug is commonly used with other antiglaucoma drugs.
• Drug may have fewer adverse reactions than conventional epinephrine therapy.

### ☑ Patient teaching
• Teach patient how to instill dipivefrin. Advise him to wash hands before and after instillation and to avoid touching tip of dropper to eye or surrounding tissue.
• Instruct patient to promptly report persistent or serious adverse reactions.

## dorzolamide hydrochloride
Trusopt

*Pregnancy Risk Category C*

### HOW SUPPLIED
*Ophthalmic solution:* 2%

### ACTION
Inhibits carbonic anhydrase in the ciliary processes of the eye, which decreases aqueous humor secretion, presumably by slowing the formation of bicarbonate ions, thereby reducing sodium and fluid transport, resulting in a reduction in intraocular pressure (IOP).

| Route | Onset | Peak | Duration |
|-------|-------|------|----------|
| Ophthalmic | Unknown | Unknown | Unknown |

### INDICATIONS & DOSAGE
*Increased IOP in patients with ocular hypertension or open-angle glaucoma—*
**Adults:** 1 drop into conjunctival sac of affected eye t.i.d.

### ADVERSE REACTIONS
**CNS:** headache, asthenia, fatigue.
**EENT:** *ocular burning, stinging, discomfort; superficial punctate keratitis; ocular*

---

*allergic reaction; blurred vision; lacrimation; dryness; photophobia; bitter taste;* iridocyclitis.
**GI:** nausea.
**GU:** urolithiasis.
**Skin:** rash.

### INTERACTIONS
**Drug-drug.** *Oral carbonic anhydrase inhibitors:* may cause additive effects. Don't administer concomitantly.

### EFFECTS ON DIAGNOSTIC TESTS
None reported.

### CONTRAINDICATIONS
Contraindicated in patients with hypersensitivity to drug or its components.

### NURSING CONSIDERATIONS
• Use with caution in patients with hepatic or renal impairment.
• If more than one topical ophthalmic drug is being used, drugs should be administered at least 10 minutes apart.

### ✓ Patient teaching
• Teach patient how to instill drops. Advise him to wash hands before and after instillation, and warn him not to touch tip of dropper to eye or surrounding tissue.
• Tell patient that drug is a sulfonamide and, although it's administered topically, it can be absorbed systemically. Advise patient to apply light finger pressure on lacrimal sac for 1 minute after drug instillation to minimize systemic absorption.
• Tell patient that adverse reactions that can result from sulfonamides may occur with topical administration. Tell him to discontinue drug and notify doctor immediately if signs or symptoms of serious adverse reactions or hypersensitivity occur.
• Advise patient to discontinue drug and notify doctor if ocular reactions, particularly conjunctivitis and eyelid reactions, occur.
• Tell patient not to wear soft contact lenses during therapy.
• Stress importance of compliance with recommended therapy.

## emedastine difumarate
Emadine

*Pregnancy Risk Category B*

### HOW SUPPLIED
*Ophthalmic solution:* 0.05%

### ACTION
A selective $H_1$ receptor antagonist that inhibits histamine-stimulated vascular permeability in the conjunctiva.

| Route | Onset | Peak | Duration |
|---|---|---|---|
| Topical, ophthalmic | Unknown | Unknown | Unknown |

### INDICATIONS & DOSAGE
*Temporary relief from signs and symptoms of allergic conjunctivitis—*
**Adults and children ages 3 and older:** 1 drop instilled into affected eyes up to q.i.d.

### ADVERSE REACTIONS
**CNS:** *headache,* abnormal dreams, asthenia.
**EENT:** blurred vision, burning or stinging, corneal infiltrates, corneal staining, discomfort, dry eye, foreign body sensation, hyperemia, keratitis, tearing, bad taste, sinusitis, rhinitis.
**Skin:** pruritus.

### INTERACTIONS
None significant.

### EFFECTS ON DIAGNOSTIC TESTS
None reported.

### CONTRAINDICATIONS
Contraindicated in patients with hypersensitivity to drug or its components.

### NURSING CONSIDERATIONS
• Drug is for topical use only; not for injection or oral use.
• Avoid touching eyelids or surrounding areas with dropper tip of bottle.
• Keep bottle tightly closed when not in use.
• Don't use if solution is discolored.
• Safety and effectiveness of drug in children under age 3 haven't been established.

### ✅ Patient teaching

• Teach patient how to instill drops. Wash hands before and after instillation. To prevent contaminating dropper tip and solution, tell patient to use care not to touch eyelids or surrounding areas with dropper tip of bottle.

• Tell patient not to wear contact lens if eye is red.

• Instruct patient not to use drug for contact lens–related irritation.

• Tell patient that solution contains a preservative (benzalkonium chloride) that may be absorbed by soft contact lenses. If patient wears soft contact lenses and his eyes aren't red, instruct him to wait at least 10 minutes after instilling drug before inserting contact lenses.

---

## fluorescein sodium
AK-Fluor, Fluorescite, Fluor-I-Strip, Fluor-I-Strip-A.T., Ful-Glo◇, Funduscein-10, Funduscein-25, Ophthifluor

*Pregnancy Risk Category C*

### HOW SUPPLIED
*Ophthalmic solution:* 2%
*Ophthalmic strips:* 0.6 mg, 1 mg, 9 mg
*Parenteral injection:* 10%, 25%

### ACTION
A water-soluble dye that produces an intense green fluorescence in alkaline solution (pH over 5) or a bright yellow fluorescence when viewed under cobalt blue illumination.

| Route | Onset | Peak | Duration |
|-------|-------|------|----------|
| I.V., ophthalmic | Immediate | Unknown | Unknown |

### INDICATIONS & DOSAGE
*As diagnostic in corneal abrasions and foreign bodies, fitting hard contact lenses, lacrimal patency, fundus photography, applanation tonometry—*
**Adults and children:** 1 or 2 drops of 2% solution followed by irrigation. Or strip moistened with sterile water; then conjunctiva or fornix touched with moistened tip, and eye flushed with irrigating solution. Patient should blink several times after application.
*Retinal angiography—*
**Adults:** 5 ml of 10% solution (500 mg) or 3 ml of 25% solution (750 mg) I.V. rapidly injected into antecubital vein.
**Children:** 7.5 mg/kg I.V. injected rapidly into antecubital vein.

### ADVERSE REACTIONS
*Topical use:*
**EENT:** eye stinging or burning, yellow tears.
*I.V. use:*
**CNS:** headache, dizziness, syncope, *seizures.*
**CV:** hypotension, *shock, cardiac arrest, thrombophlebitis.*
**GI:** nausea, vomiting, GI distress.
**GU:** bright yellow urine.
**Respiratory:** transient dyspnea, *bronchospasm.*
**Skin:** temporary yellow skin discoloration, pruritus.
**Other:** *anaphylaxis,* extravasation at injection site, fever, *angioedema, hypersensitivity reactions, including urticaria.*

### INTERACTIONS
None significant.

### EFFECTS ON DIAGNOSTIC TESTS
Bright yellow discoloration of urine may interfere with routine urinalysis.

### CONTRAINDICATIONS
Contraindicated in patients with hypersensitivity to drug.

### NURSING CONSIDERATIONS
• Use cautiously in patients with history of allergy or bronchial asthma.

• Always use aseptic technique; area is easily contaminated by *Pseudomonas aeruginosa.*

• Use topical anesthetic, as ordered, before instillation to relieve burning and irritation.

• Never instill dye while patient is wearing soft contact lenses; fluorescein will ruin them.

• Defects appear green under normal light or bright yellow under cobalt blue illumination. Foreign bodies are surrounded by

---

Reactions may be *common,* uncommon, *life-threatening,* or COMMON AND LIFE-THREATENING.

green ring. Similar lesions of conjunctiva are delineated in orange-yellow.

⚡ **I.V. administration**
• Take care to avoid extravasation.
• Inject contents of ampule or prefilled syringe rapidly into antecubital vein.
• Keep an antihistamine, epinephrine, and oxygen available when giving parenterally. Avoid extravasation during injection.

☑ **Patient teaching**
• Tell patient to promptly report persistent or serious adverse reactions.

✳ *NEW DRUG*

## ketotifen fumarate
Zaditor

*Pregnancy Risk Category C*

### HOW SUPPLIED
*Ophthalmic solution:* 0.025%

### ACTION
Stabilizes mast cells to inhibit release of mediators involved in hypersensitivity reactions and blocks action of histamine at the $H_1$ receptor, temporarily preventing itching of the eye.

| Route | Onset | Peak | Duration |
|-------|-------|------|----------|
| Ophthalmic | Within min | Unknown | Unknown |

### INDICATIONS & DOSAGE
*Temporary prevention of itching of the eye due to allergic conjunctivitis—*
**Adults and children ages 4 and older:** instill 1 drop in affected eyes q 8 to 12 hours.

### ADVERSE REACTIONS
**CNS:** headache.
**EENT:** *conjunctival injection, rhinitis,* ocular allergic reactions, burning or stinging of eyes, conjunctivitis, eye discharge, dry eyes, eye pain, eyelid disorder, itching of eyes, keratitis, lacrimation disorder, mydriasis, photophobia, ocular rash, pharyngitis.
**Other:** flulike syndrome.

### INTERACTIONS
None significant.

### EFFECTS ON DIAGNOSTIC TESTS
None reported.

### CONTRAINDICATIONS
Contraindicated in patients with hypersensitivity to components of drug.

### NURSING CONSIDERATIONS
• Drug is for ophthalmic use only; not for injection or oral use.
• Drug isn't indicated for irritation related to contact lenses.
• Preservative in drug may be absorbed by soft contact lenses. Contact lenses shouldn't be inserted until 10 minutes after drug is instilled.
• To prevent contaminating dropper tip and solution, don't touch eyelids or surrounding areas with dropper tip of bottle.

☑ **Patient teaching**
• Teach patient the proper technique for administering drops.
• Advise patient not to wear contact lens if eye is red. Warn patient not to use drug to treat contact lens–related irritation.
• Instruct patients who wear soft contact lenses and whose eyes aren't red to wait at least 10 minutes after instilling drug before inserting contact lenses.
• Advise patient to report adverse reactions to drops.
• Advise patient to keep bottle tightly closed when not in use.

## latanoprost
Xalatan

*Pregnancy Risk Category C*

### HOW SUPPLIED
*Ophthalmic solution:* 0.005%
(50 mcg/ml)

### ACTION
Exact mechanism unknown. Believed to increase outflow of aqueous humor, thereby lowering intraocular pressure (IOP).

| Route | Onset | Peak | Duration |
|-------|-------|------|----------|
| Ophthalmic | 2-4 hr | 8-12 hr | Unknown |

## INDICATIONS & DOSAGE
*Increased IOP in patients with ocular hypertension or open-angle glaucoma who are intolerant of other IOP-lowering drugs or insufficiently responsive to other IOP-lowering drugs—*
**Adults:** 1 drop in conjunctival sac of affected eye once daily in the evening.

## ADVERSE REACTIONS
**CV:** angina pectoris, chest pain.
**EENT:** *blurred vision, burning, stinging,* conjunctival hyperemia, foreign body sensation, itching, increased brown pigmentation of the iris, dry eye, punctate epithelial keratopathy, lid crusting or edema, lid discomfort, excessive tearing, eye pain, photophobia.
**Musculoskeletal:** muscle, joint, or back pain.
**Respiratory:** upper respiratory tract infection.
**Skin:** rash, allergic skin reaction.
**Other:** cold or flu.

## INTERACTIONS
**Drug-drug.** *Eyedrops containing thimerosal:* precipitation occurs when mixed with latanoprost. If used concomitantly, administer at least 5 minutes apart.

## EFFECTS ON DIAGNOSTIC TESTS
None reported.

## CONTRAINDICATIONS
Contraindicated in patients with hypersensitivity to drug, benzalkonium chloride, or other components of drug.

## NURSING CONSIDERATIONS
• Use cautiously when administering to patients with impaired renal or hepatic function.
• Drug shouldn't be administered while patient is wearing contact lenses.
• More frequent administration than that recommended may decrease IOP-lowering effects of drug.
• Drug may gradually change eye color, increasing amount of brown pigment in iris. This change in iris color occurs slowly and may not be noticeable for months or years. Increased pigmentation may be permanent.

• To avoid ocular infections, don't allow tip of dispenser to contact eye or surrounding structures. Serious damage to eye and subsequent loss of vision may result from using contaminated solutions.
• Safety and efficacy of drug in children haven't been established.
• It isn't known if drug appears in breast milk; use caution when administering drug to breast-feeding women.

### ✔ Patient teaching
• Inform patient of potential for change in iris color. Patients receiving treatment in only one eye should be told about risk of increased brown pigmentation in treated eye.
• Teach patient how to instill drops. Advise him to wash his hands before and after instillation, and warn him not to touch dropper or its tip to eye or surrounding tissue.
• Advise patient to apply light finger pressure on lacrimal sac for 1 minute after instillation to minimize systemic absorption.
• Instruct patient to report ocular reactions, especially conjunctivitis and lid reactions.
• Tell patient who wears contact lenses to remove them before administering solution and not to reinsert the lenses until 15 minutes have elapsed.
• Advise patient that, if more than one topical ophthalmic drug is being used, drugs should be administered at least 5 minutes apart.
• If patient develops another ocular condition (such as trauma or infection) or needs ocular surgery, advise him to contact doctor about continued use of multidose container.
• Stress importance of compliance with recommended therapy.

## levobunolol hydrochloride
AKBeta, Betagan

*Pregnancy Risk Category C*

## HOW SUPPLIED
*Ophthalmic solution:* 0.25%, 0.5%

---

Reactions may be *common*, uncommon, *life-threatening*, or COMMON AND LIFE-THREATENING.

## ACTION

Unknown. A nonselective beta blocker thought to reduce aqueous formation and possibly increase outflow of aqueous humor.

| Route | Onset | Peak | Duration |
|-------|-------|------|----------|
| Ophthalmic | 1 hr | 2-6 hr | 24 hr |

## INDICATIONS & DOSAGE

*Chronic open-angle glaucoma, ocular hypertension—*
**Adults:** 1 to 2 drops once daily (0.5%) or b.i.d. (0.25%).

## ADVERSE REACTIONS

**CNS:** headache, depression, insomnia, *syncope.*
**CV:** slight reduction in resting heart rate, *hypotension, bradycardia, **heart failure.***
**EENT:** *transient eye stinging and burning,* tearing, erythema, itching, keratitis, corneal punctate staining, photophobia; decreased corneal sensitivity.
**GI:** nausea.
**Respiratory:** *asthmatic attacks in patients with history of asthma.*
**Skin:** urticaria.

## INTERACTIONS

**Drug-drug.** *Dipivefrin, epinephrine, systemically administered carbonic anhydrase inhibitors, topical miotics:* additive lowered intraocular pressure. Use together cautiously.
*Metoprolol, propranolol, other oral beta blockers:* increased ocular and systemic effects. Use together cautiously.
*Reserpine, other catecholamine-depleting drugs:* enhanced hypotensive and bradycardiac effects. Monitor closely.
**Drug-lifestyle.** *Sun exposure:* photophobia may occur. Take precautions.

## EFFECTS ON DIAGNOSTIC TESTS

None reported.

## CONTRAINDICATIONS

Contraindicated in patients with hypersensitivity to drug and in those with bronchial asthma, sinus bradycardia, second- or third-degree AV block, cardiac failure, cardiogenic shock, or history of bronchial asthma or severe COPD.

## NURSING CONSIDERATIONS

• Use cautiously in patients with chronic bronchitis and emphysema, diabetes mellitus, hyperthyroidism, and myasthenia gravis.
• Avoid letting dropper touch patient's eye or surrounding tissue.
• Safe use in pregnant or breast-feeding women hasn't been established.
• *Alert:* Don't confuse Betagan with Betapen.

### ☑ Patient teaching

• Teach patient how to instill drug. Advise him to wash hands before and after instillation and to apply light finger pressure on lacrimal sac for 1 minute after drops are instilled.
• Warn patient not to touch dropper to eye or surrounding tissue.
• Advise elderly patient to report signs and symptoms of dyspnea, chest pain, or heart irregularities to doctor. Drug may be absorbed systemically and produce signs and symptoms of beta blockade.
• Advise patient to carry medical alert card at all times during therapy.

---

## metipranolol hydrochloride
OptiPranolol

*Pregnancy Risk Category C*

## HOW SUPPLIED

*Ophthalmic solution:* 0.3% in 5-ml, 10-ml, or 15-ml dropper bottles

## ACTION

Unknown. A noncardioselective beta blocker that appears to reduce aqueous production and reduce elevated and normal intraocular pressure (IOP), with or without glaucoma, with little or no effect on pupil size or accommodation. IOP above 24 mm Hg is usually reduced about 20% to 26%.

| Route | Onset | Peak | Duration |
|-------|-------|------|----------|
| Ophthalmic | 0.5 hr | 2 hr | 12-24 hr |

## INDICATIONS & DOSAGE

*IOP reduction in ocular conditions, including ocular hypertension and chronic open-angle glaucoma—*

**Adults:** 1 drop into affected eye b.i.d. If IOP isn't at satisfactory level, concomitant therapy to lower it may be instituted.

## ADVERSE REACTIONS

**CNS:** headache, anxiety, dizziness, depression, somnolence, nervousness, asthenia, brow ache.
**CV:** hypertension, *MI,* atrial fibrillation, angina, palpitation, *bradycardia.*
**EENT:** transient local eye discomfort, tearing, conjunctivitis, eyelid dermatitis, blurred vision, blepharitis, abnormal vision, photophobia, eye edema, rhinitis, epistaxis.
**GI:** nausea.
**Musculoskeletal:** myalgia.
**Respiratory:** dyspnea, bronchitis, cough.
**Skin:** rash.
**Other:** *hypersensitivity reactions.*

## INTERACTIONS

**Drug-drug.** *Calcium channel blockers, cardiac glycosides, quinidine:* increased risk of adverse cardiac effects if significant amount of drug is systemically absorbed. Use together cautiously.
*Fentanyl, general anesthetics:* excessive hypotension. Monitor closely.
*Metoprolol tartrate, propranolol, other oral beta blockers:* increased ocular and systemic effects. Use together cautiously.
*Reserpine, other catecholamine-depleting drugs:* enhanced hypotensive and bradycardia-induced effects. Avoid concurrent use.

## EFFECTS ON DIAGNOSTIC TESTS

None reported.

## CONTRAINDICATIONS

Contraindicated in patients with hypersensitivity to drug or its components and in those with bronchial asthma, sinus bradycardia, second- or third-degree AV block, cardiac failure, cardiogenic shock, or history of bronchial asthma or severe COPD.

## NURSING CONSIDERATIONS

● Use cautiously in patients with nonallergic bronchospasm, chronic bronchitis, emphysema, diabetes mellitus (especially in those subject to spontaneous hypoglycemia), hyperthyroidism, or cerebrovascular insufficiency.
● Anticipate using pilocarpine, other miotics, or systemic carbonic anhydrase inhibitors concomitantly if IOP isn't adequately controlled.
● Check expiration date on bottle before use. Don't use if drops have changed color.
● A slight increase in outflow facility has been demonstrated with metipranolol. Like other noncardioselective beta blockers, metipranolol doesn't have significant local anesthetic (membrane-stabilizing) actions or intrinsic sympathomimetic activity.
● *Alert:* Don't confuse metipranolol with metaproterenol.

☑ **Patient teaching**
● Teach patient how to instill drug. Instruct him to first wash hands thoroughly and then tilt head back or lie down and gaze upward. Tell patient to gently grasp lower eyelid below eyelashes and pull eyelid away from eye to form a pouch. Then have him place dropper directly over eye, avoiding contact with eye or any surface; look up just before applying drop; and look down for several seconds after instillation and slowly release eyelid.
● Tell patient to close eyes gently for 1 to 2 minutes and to apply gentle pressure to inside corner of eye at bridge of nose to retard draining of solution from intended area. Warn him not to rub eye or rinse dropper.
● Advise patient to report signs and symptoms of dyspnea, bradycardia, or chest pain to his doctor.

---

**sodium chloride, hypertonic**
Adsorbonac, Ak-NaCl◇, Muro-128◇, Muroptic-5◇

*Pregnancy Risk Category NR*

## HOW SUPPLIED

*Ophthalmic ointment:* 5%
*Ophthalmic solution:* 2%, 5%

---

Reactions may be *common,* uncommon, *life-threatening,* or COMMON AND LIFE-THREATENING.

## ACTION
An osmotic drug that removes excess fluid from cornea.

| Route | Onset | Peak | Duration |
|-------|-------|------|----------|
| Ophthalmic | Unknown | Unknown | Unknown |

## INDICATIONS & DOSAGE
*Temporary relief of corneal edema—*
**Adults and children:** 1 to 2 drops q 3 to 4 hours, or ¼-inch (6 mm) of ointment applied q 3 to 4 hours.

## ADVERSE REACTIONS
**EENT:** slight eye stinging.
**Other:** *hypersensitivity reactions.*

## INTERACTIONS
None significant.

## EFFECTS ON DIAGNOSTIC TESTS
None reported.

## CONTRAINDICATIONS
Contraindicated in patients with hypersensitivity to drug or its components.

## NURSING CONSIDERATIONS
• Ophthalmic solution is for topical use only; never inject.
• Check expiration date before use.

## ☑ Patient teaching
• Teach patient how to instill drug. Advise him to wash hands before and after instillation and to apply light finger pressure on lacrimal sac for 1 minute after drops are instilled. Warn patient not to touch dropper to eye or surrounding tissue.
• Tell patient to prevent caking on dropper bottle tip by putting a few drops of sterile irrigation solution inside bottle cap.
• Warn patient that ointment may cause blurred vision.
• If patient experiences severe headache, pain, rapid change in vision, acute redness of eyes, sudden appearance of floating spots, pain on exposure to light, or double vision, tell him to discontinue drug and notify doctor.
• Advise patient to store drug in tightly closed container.

# timolol maleate
Betimol, Timoptic, Timoptic-XE

*Pregnancy Risk Category C*

## HOW SUPPLIED
*Ophthalmic gel:* 0.25%, 0.5%
*Ophthalmic solution:* 0.25%, 0.5%

## ACTION
Unknown. A beta blocker thought to reduce aqueous formation and possibly increase aqueous outflow.

| Route | Onset | Peak | Duration |
|-------|-------|------|----------|
| Ophthalmic | 0.5 hr | 1-2 hr | 12-24 hr |

## INDICATIONS & DOSAGE
*Elevated intraocular pressure (IOP) in ocular hypertension or open-angle glaucoma—*
**Adults:** initially, 1 drop of 0.25% solution in each affected eye b.i.d.; maintenance dose is 1 drop daily. If no response, 1 drop of 0.5% solution in each affected eye b.i.d. If IOP is controlled, dosage reduced to 1 drop daily. Or, 1 drop of gel in each affected eye once daily.

## ADVERSE REACTIONS
**CNS:** depression, fatigue, dizziness, lethargy, hallucinations, confusion, *syncope.*
**CV:** slight reduction in resting heart rate, *arrhythmia, CVA, cardiac arrest, heart block,* palpitations, *hypotension, bradycardia, heart failure.*
**EENT:** minor eye irritation, conjunctivitis, blepharitis, keratitis, visual disturbances, diplopia, ptosis; decreased corneal sensitivity with long-term use.
**GU:** slightly increased BUN levels.
**Hematologic:** anemia.
**Metabolic:** hyperkalemia, hyperglycemia.
**Respiratory:** *asthmatic attacks in patients with history of asthma.*
**Other:** increased uric acid levels.

## INTERACTIONS
**Drug-drug.** *Calcium channel blockers, cardiac glycosides, quinidine:* increased risk of adverse cardiac effects if signifi-

cant amounts of timolol are systemically absorbed. Use together cautiously.
*Fentanyl, general anesthetics:* excessive hypotension. Monitor closely.
*Metoprolol tartrate, propranolol, other oral beta blockers:* increased ocular and systemic effects. Use together cautiously.
*Reserpine, other catecholamine-depleting drugs:* enhanced hypotensive and brady-cardia-induced effects. Avoid concurrent use.

**EFFECTS ON DIAGNOSTIC TESTS**
None reported.

**CONTRAINDICATIONS**
Contraindicated in patients with hyper-sensitivity to drug and in those with bronchial asthma, sinus bradycardia, sec-ond- or third-degree AV block, cardiac failure, cardiogenic shock, or history of bronchial asthma or severe COPD.

**NURSING CONSIDERATIONS**
• Use cautiously in patients with nonaller-gic bronchospasm, chronic bronchitis, emphysema, diabetes mellitus, hyperthy-roidism, or cerebrovascular insufficiency.
• Administer other ophthalmic drugs at least 10 minutes before administering gel form of drug.
• Monitor diabetic patients carefully. Sys-temic beta-blocking effects can mask some signs of hypoglycemia.
• Some patients may need a few weeks' treatment to stabilize pressure-lowering response. Determine IOP after 4 weeks of treatment.
• Drug can be used safely in patients with glaucoma who wear conventional hard contact lenses.
• *Alert:* Don't confuse timolol with atenolol, or Timoptic with Viroptic.

☑ **Patient teaching**
• Teach patient how to instill drug. Advise him to wash hands before and after instil-lation and to apply light finger pressure on lacrimal sac for 1 minute after drops are instilled. Warn patient not to touch dropper to eye or surrounding tissue.
• Instruct patient using gel to invert con-tainer and shake once before each use. Also tell him to administer other oph-thalmic drugs at least 10 minutes before administering gel.
• Advise patient to monitor pulse rate and report slow rate to doctor. Drug may be absorbed systemically and produce signs and symptoms of beta blockade.
• Tell patient to report difficulty breathing or chest pain to doctor.

**boric acid**
**carbamide peroxide**
**chloramphenicol**
**triethanolamine polypeptide**
   **oleate-condensate**

**COMBINATION PRODUCTS**
None.

---

## boric acid
Auro-Dri◇, Dri/Ear◇ Ear-Dry◇

*Pregnancy Risk Category NR*

---

**HOW SUPPLIED**
*Otic solution:* 2.75% boric acid in isopropyl alcohol

**ACTION**
A weak bacteriostatic that inhibits or destroys bacteria in the ear canal. Is also fungistatic.

| Route | Onset | Peak | Duration |
|-------|-------|------|----------|
| Otic | Unknown | Unknown | Unknown |

**INDICATIONS & DOSAGE**
*External ear canal infection—*
**Adults and children:** 3 to 8 drops into ear canal; plug with cotton. Repeated t.i.d. or q.i.d.

**ADVERSE REACTIONS**
**EENT:** ear irritation or itching.
**Skin:** urticaria.
**Other:** overgrowth of nonsusceptible organisms.

**INTERACTIONS**
None significant.

**EFFECTS ON DIAGNOSTIC TESTS**
None reported.

**CONTRAINDICATIONS**
Contraindicated in patients with a perforated eardrum or excoriated membranes.

**NURSING CONSIDERATIONS**
• Watch for signs and symptoms of superinfection.

✅ **Patient teaching**
• Show patient or caregiver how to administer drug.
• To prevent reinfection, warn patient to avoid touching ear with dropper.
• Tell patient using cotton plug to always moisten with drug.

---

## carbamide peroxide
Auro Ear Drops◇, Debrox◇,
Murine Ear◇

*Pregnancy Risk Category NR*

---

**HOW SUPPLIED**
*Otic solution:* 6.5% carbamide in glycerin or glycerin and propylene glycol

**ACTION**
A ceruminolytic that emulsifies and disperses accumulated cerumen.

| Route | Onset | Peak | Duration |
|-------|-------|------|----------|
| Otic | Unknown | Unknown | 15-30 min |

**INDICATIONS & DOSAGE**
*Impacted cerumen—*
**Adults and children:** 5 to 10 drops into ear canal b.i.d. for up to 4 days. Allow solution to remain in ear canal for 15 minutes or longer; remove with warm water.

**ADVERSE REACTIONS**
None reported.

**INTERACTIONS**
None significant.

**EFFECTS ON DIAGNOSTIC TESTS**
None reported.

**CONTRAINDICATIONS**
Contraindicated in patients with perforated eardrum.

---

*Liquid contains alcohol.    **May contain tartrazine.    †Canada    ‡Australia    §U.K.    ◇OTC

## NURSING CONSIDERATIONS
• Use in children under age 12 only under doctor's direction.

### ✅ Patient teaching
• Show patient or caregiver how to administer drug.
• To prevent reinfection, warn patient to avoid touching ear with dropper.
• Instruct patient to flush ear gently with warm water, using a rubber bulb syringe.
• Advise patient to call doctor if redness, pain, or swelling persists.

---

## chloramphenicol
Chloromycetin Otic

*Pregnancy Risk Category NR*

---

### HOW SUPPLIED
*Otic solution:* 0.5%

### ACTION
Inhibits or destroys bacteria in ear canal.

| Route | Onset | Peak | Duration |
|-------|-------|------|----------|
| Otic | Unknown | Unknown | Unknown |

### INDICATIONS & DOSAGE
*External ear canal infection—*
**Adults and children:** 2 to 3 drops into ear canal t.i.d.

### ADVERSE REACTIONS
**EENT:** ear itching or burning.
**GU:** hemoglobinuria.
**Hematologic:** *bone marrow depression*, bone marrow hypoplasia, *aplastic anemia.*
**Metabolic:** lactic acidosis.
**Skin:** pruritus, urticaria.
**Other:** overgrowth of nonsusceptible organisms, burning.

### INTERACTIONS
None significant.

### EFFECTS ON DIAGNOSTIC TESTS
None reported.

### CONTRAINDICATIONS
Contraindicated in patients with hypersensitivity to drug or its components and in those with perforated eardrum.

### NURSING CONSIDERATIONS
• Obtain history of drug use and reactions.
• Watch for signs and symptoms of superinfection. Avoid prolonged use.
• Reculture persistent drainage.
• Watch for signs and symptoms of sore throat (early sign of toxicity).
• *Alert:* Don't confuse Chloromycetin with chlorambucil.

### ✅ Patient teaching
• Show patient or caregiver how to administer drug.
• To avoid reinfection, warn patient to avoid touching ear with dropper.

---

## triethanolamine polypeptide oleate-condensate
Cerumenex

*Pregnancy Risk Category NR*

---

### HOW SUPPLIED
*Otic solution:* 10% in 6-ml, 12-ml bottles with droppers

### ACTION
A ceruminolytic that emulsifies and disperses accumulated cerumen.

| Route | Onset | Peak | Duration |
|-------|-------|------|----------|
| Otic | Unknown | Unknown | 15-30 min |

### INDICATIONS & DOSAGE
*Impacted cerumen—*
**Adults and children:** fill ear canal with solution and insert cotton plug. After 15 to 30 minutes, flush with warm water.

### ADVERSE REACTIONS
**EENT:** ear erythema or itching.
**Skin:** severe eczema.

### INTERACTIONS
None significant.

---

Reactions may be *common*, uncommon, *life-threatening*, or COMMON AND LIFE-THREATENING.

**EFFECTS ON DIAGNOSTIC TESTS**
None reported.

**CONTRAINDICATIONS**
Contraindicated in patients with perforated eardrum, otitis media, or otitis externa.

**NURSING CONSIDERATIONS**
• *Alert:* If hypersensitivity is suspected, anticipate patch test: Place 1 drop of drug on inner forearm; cover with bandage. Read results in 24 hours. If reaction occurs, drug shouldn't be used.

☑ **Patient teaching**
• Teach patient to moisten cotton plug with drug before insertion, leave cotton in place for a maximum of 30 minutes, and flush ear gently with warm water, using a rubber bulb syringe.
• Tell patient not to use drops more often than prescribed.
• Warn patient that drug is for use only in the ears.
• Advise patient to discontinue drug and to contact doctor immediately if adverse reactions occur.
• Tell patient to keep container tightly closed and away from moisture.

beclomethasone dipropionate
budesonide
ephedrine sulfate
epinephrine hydrochloride
flunisolide
fluticasone propionate
naphazoline hydrochloride
oxymetazoline hydrochloride
phenylephrine hydrochloride
tetrahydrozoline hydrochloride
triamcinolone acetonide
xylometazoline hydrochloride

### COMBINATION PRODUCTS
4-WAY FAST ACTING SPRAY ◊: phenyl-ephrine hydrochloride 0.5%, naphazoline hydrochloride 0.05%, and pyrilamine maleate 0.2%.

---

### beclomethasone dipropionate
Beconase, Beconase AQ, Vancenase, Vancenase AQ

*Pregnancy Risk Category C*

### HOW SUPPLIED
*Nasal aerosol:* 42 mcg/metered spray, 50 mcg/metered spray‡
*Nasal spray:* 42 mcg/metered spray, 50 mcg/metered spray‡, 84 mcg/metered spray

### ACTION
A corticosteroid that decreases nasal inflammation, mainly by stabilizing leukocyte lysosomal membranes.

| Route | Onset | Peak | Duration |
|-------|-------|------|----------|
| Nasal | 5-7 days | 3 wk | Unknown |

### INDICATIONS & DOSAGE
*Relief of symptoms of seasonal or perennial rhinitis, prevention of recurrence of nasal polyps after surgical removal—*
**Adults and children over age 12:** usual dosage is 1 or 2 sprays in each nostril, b.i.d., t.i.d., or q.i.d.

**Children ages 6 to 12:** 1 spray into each nostril t.i.d.

### ADVERSE REACTIONS
**CNS:** headache.
**EENT:** *mild transient nasal burning and stinging,* nasal congestion, sneezing, burning, stinging, dryness, epistaxis, nasopharyngeal fungal infections.

### INTERACTIONS
None significant.

### EFFECTS ON DIAGNOSTIC TESTS
None reported.

### CONTRAINDICATIONS
Contraindicated in patients with hypersensitivity to drug and in those with untreated localized infection involving the nasal mucosa.

### NURSING CONSIDERATIONS
• Use cautiously, if at all, in patients with active or quiescent respiratory tract tuberculous infections or untreated fungal, bacterial, or systemic viral or ocular herpes simplex infections. Also use cautiously in patients who have recently had nasal septal ulcers, nasal surgery, or trauma.
• Observe patient for fungal infections.
• Drug isn't effective for acute exacerbations of rhinitis. Decongestants or antihistamines may be needed.
• *Alert:* Don't confuse Vancenase with Vanceril.

☑ **Patient teaching**
• To instill, instruct patient to shake container before use, to blow nose to clear nasal passages, and to tilt head slightly forward and insert nozzle into nostril, pointing away from septum. Tell him to hold other nostril closed and then to inspire gently and spray. Next, have him shake container and repeat in other nostril.
• Advise patient to pump nasal spray three or four times before first use, and

---

Reactions may be *common,* uncommon, *life-threatening*, or COMMON AND LIFE-THREATENING.

once or twice before first use each day. The cap and nosepiece of the activator should be cleaned in warm water every day, then allowed to air-dry.

• Advise patient to use drug regularly, as prescribed, because its effectiveness depends on regular use.

• Explain that drug's therapeutic effects, unlike those of decongestants, aren't immediate. Most patients achieve benefit within a few days, but some may need 2 to 3 weeks.

• Warn patient not to exceed recommended dosage because of risk of hypothalamic-pituitary-adrenal axis suppression.

• Tell patient to notify doctor if symptoms don't improve within 3 weeks or if nasal irritation persists.

• Teach patient good nasal and oral hygiene.

## budesonide
Rhinocort

*Pregnancy Risk Category C*

### HOW SUPPLIED
*Nasal spray:* 32 mcg/metered spray (7-g canister)

### ACTION
Unknown. A corticosteroid that probably decreases nasal inflammation, mainly by inhibiting the activities of specific cells and the mediators involved in the allergic response.

| Route | Onset | Peak | Duration |
|-------|-------|------|----------|
| Nasal | Unknown | Unknown | Unknown |

### INDICATIONS & DOSAGE
*Symptoms of seasonal or perennial allergic rhinitis—*
**Adults and children ages 6 and older:** 2 sprays in each nostril in the morning and evening or 4 sprays in each nostril in the morning. Maintenance dose should be the fewest number of sprays needed to control symptoms.

### ADVERSE REACTIONS
**CNS:** nervousness.
**EENT:** *nasal irritation, epistaxis, pharyngitis,* reduced sense of smell, nasal pain, hoarseness.
**GI:** bad taste, dry mouth, dyspepsia, nausea.
**Musculoskeletal:** myalgia.
**Respiratory:** *cough,* candidiasis, wheezing, dyspnea.
**Skin:** facial edema, rash, pruritus, contact dermatitis.
**Other:** *hypersensitivity reactions.*

### INTERACTIONS
None significant.

### EFFECTS ON DIAGNOSTIC TESTS
None reported.

### CONTRAINDICATIONS
Contraindicated in patients hypersensitive to drug or its components and in those who have had recent septal ulcers, nasal surgery, or nasal trauma until total healing has occurred.

### NURSING CONSIDERATIONS
• Use cautiously in patients with tuberculous infections; untreated fungal, bacterial, or systemic viral infections; or ocular herpes simplex.

• Systemic effects of corticosteroid therapy may occur if recommended daily dose is increased.

☑ **Patient teaching**
• Tell patient to avoid exposure to chickenpox or measles.

• To instill drug, instruct patient to shake container before use, blow nose to clear nasal passages, and tilt head slightly forward and insert nozzle into nostril, pointing away from septum. Tell him to hold other nostril closed; then inspire gently and spray. Next, have him shake container and repeat in other nostril.

• Advise patient not to break, incinerate, or store canister in extreme heat; contents are under pressure.

• Advise patient to store canister with valve upwards.

• Warn patient not to exceed prescribed dosage or use for long periods of time because of risk of hypothalamic-pituitary-adrenal axis suppression.

• Tell patient to contact doctor if symptoms don't improve in 3 weeks or if condition worsens.
• Teach patient good nasal and oral hygiene.
• Tell patient to use drug within 6 months of opening the protective aluminum pouch.
• Instruct patient that product should be used by one person only to prevent spread of infection.

---

## ephedrine sulfate
Pretz-D◊ , Vicks Vatronol◊

*Pregnancy Risk Category NR*

### HOW SUPPLIED
*Nasal jelly:* 1%
*Nasal solution:* 0.5%◊
*Nasal spray:* 0.25%◊

### ACTION
Causes local vasoconstriction of dilated arterioles, reducing blood flow and nasal congestion.

| Route | Onset | Peak | Duration |
|-------|-------|------|----------|
| Nasal | Unknown | Unknown | Unknown |

### INDICATIONS & DOSAGE
*Nasal congestion—*
**Adults and children:** 2 to 3 drops of 0.5% solution into each nostril. Use no more frequently than q 4 hours.

### ADVERSE REACTIONS
**CNS:** nervousness, excitation.
**CV:** *tachycardia.*
**EENT:** rebound nasal congestion, mucosal irritation.

### INTERACTIONS
**Drug-drug.** *MAO inhibitors:* hypertensive crisis if ephedrine is absorbed. Don't use together.

### EFFECTS ON DIAGNOSTIC TESTS
None reported.

### CONTRAINDICATIONS
Contraindicated in patients with hypersensitivity to drug or other sympatho-
mimetics and in those with angle-closure glaucoma, psychoneurosis, angina pectoris, substantial organic heart disease, or CV disease.

### NURSING CONSIDERATIONS
• Use cautiously in patients with hyperthyroidism, hypertension, diabetes mellitus, or prostatic hyperplasia.
• *Alert:* Don't confuse ephedrine with epinephrine.

### ☑ Patient teaching
• Teach patient how to instill nose drops or use nasal spray.
• Instruct patient that product should be used by only one person to prevent spread of infection.
• Tell patient not to exceed recommended dosage and to use only when needed.

---

## epinephrine hydrochloride
Adrenalin Chloride

*Pregnancy Risk Category NR*

### HOW SUPPLIED
*Nasal solution:* 0.1%

### ACTION
Causes local vasoconstriction of dilated arterioles, reducing blood flow and nasal congestion.

| Route | Onset | Peak | Duration |
|-------|-------|------|----------|
| Nasal | 1 min | Unknown | Unknown |

### INDICATIONS & DOSAGE
*Nasal congestion, local superficial bleeding—*
**Adults and children ages 6 and older:** instill 1 or 2 drops of solution.

### ADVERSE REACTIONS
**CNS:** nervousness, excitation.
**CV:** *tachycardia.*
**EENT:** rebound nasal congestion; slight stinging on application.
**GU:** increased BUN levels.
**Metabolic:** hyperglycemia, lactic acidosis.

---

Reactions may be *common,* uncommon, *life-threatening,* or COMMON AND LIFE-THREATENING.

## INTERACTIONS
None significant.

## EFFECTS ON DIAGNOSTIC TESTS
Drug therapy may interfere with tests for urinary catecholamines.

## CONTRAINDICATIONS
Contraindicated in patients with hypersensitivity to drug.

## NURSING CONSIDERATIONS
• Use cautiously in patients with hyperthyroidism, coronary artery disease, hypertension, or diabetes mellitus.
• Monitor heart rate.
• *Alert:* Don't confuse epinephrine with ephedrine.

## ☑ Patient teaching
• Teach patient how to instill nose drops.
• Instruct patient that product should be used by only one person to prevent spread of infection.
• Tell patient not to exceed recommended dosage and to use only when needed.

---

## flunisolide
Nasalide, Nasarel, Rhinalart,
Syntaris§

*Pregnancy Risk Category C*

## HOW SUPPLIED
*Nasal inhalant:* 25 mcg/metered spray, 200 doses/bottle‡
*Nasal solution:* 0.25 mg/ml in pump spray bottle (25 mcg/spray)

## ACTION
Exact mechanism unknown. Decreases nasal inflammation, mainly by stabilizing leukocyte lysosomal membranes.

| Route | Onset | Peak | Duration |
|-------|-------|------|----------|
| Nasal | Unknown | Unknown | Unknown |

## INDICATIONS & DOSAGE
*Symptoms of seasonal or perennial rhinitis—*

**Adults:** starting dose is 2 sprays (50 mcg) in each nostril b.i.d. Total daily dose is 200 mcg. If needed, dosage may be in-

creased to 2 sprays in each nostril t.i.d. Maximum total daily dose is 8 sprays in each nostril (400 mcg daily).
**Children ages 6 to 14:** starting dose is 1 spray (25 mcg) in each nostril t.i.d. or 2 sprays (50 mcg) in each nostril b.i.d. Total daily dose is 150 to 200 mcg. Maximum total daily dose is 4 sprays in each nostril (200 mcg daily).

## ADVERSE REACTIONS
**CNS:** headache.
**EENT:** *mild, transient nasal burning and stinging;* nasal congestion; nasopharyngeal fungal infection; burning; stinging; dryness; sneezing; epistaxis; watery eyes.
**GI:** nausea, vomiting.

## INTERACTIONS
None significant.

## EFFECTS ON DIAGNOSTIC TESTS
None reported.

## CONTRAINDICATIONS
Contraindicated in patients with hypersensitivity to drug and in those with untreated localized infection involving nasal mucosa.

## NURSING CONSIDERATIONS
• Use cautiously, if at all, in patients with active or quiescent respiratory tract tuberculous infections or untreated fungal, bacterial, or systemic viral or ocular herpes simplex infections. Also use cautiously in patients who have recently had nasal septal ulcers, nasal surgery, or nasal trauma.
• Drug isn't effective for acute exacerbations of rhinitis. Decongestants or antihistamines may be needed.
• *Alert:* Don't confuse flunisolide with fluocinonide or Flumadine.

## ☑ Patient teaching
• Tell patient to avoid exposure to chickenpox or measles.
• To instill drug, instruct patient to shake container before use, blow nose to clear nasal passages, and tilt head slightly forward and insert nozzle into nostril, pointing away from septum. Tell him to hold other nostril closed; then inspire gently and spray. Have him repeat procedure in

other nostril. Tell him to clean nosepiece with warm water if it becomes clogged.
• Explain that drug's therapeutic effects aren't immediate. Most patients achieve benefit within few days, but some may need 2 to 3 weeks.
• Advise patient to use drug regularly, as prescribed.
• Warn patient not to exceed recommended dosage to avoid hypothalamic-pituitary-adrenal axis suppression.
• Tell patient to stop drug and notify doctor if symptoms don't diminish in 3 weeks or if nasal irritation persists.

---

## fluticasone propionate
Flixonase§, Flonase

*Pregnancy Risk Category C*

### HOW SUPPLIED
*Nasal spray:* 50 mcg/metered spray (9-g, 16-g bottles)

### ACTION
Exact mechanism unknown. Decreases nasal inflammation.

| Route | Onset | Peak | Duration |
|-------|-------|------|----------|
| Nasal | Unknown | Unknown | Unknown |

### INDICATIONS & DOSAGE
*Seasonal and perennial allergic rhinitis—*
**Adults:** initially, 2 sprays (100 mcg) in each nostril once daily. Or, 1 spray in each nostril b.i.d. After few days, dose may be reduced to 1 spray in each nostril daily. Maximum daily dose is 2 sprays in each nostril.
**Children ages 4 and older:** initially, 1 spray (50 mcg) in each nostril once daily. If patient doesn't respond or symptoms are severe, increase to 2 sprays in each nostril daily. Depending on patient's response, may decrease dose to 1 spray in each nostril daily. Maximum daily dose is 2 sprays in each nostril.

### ADVERSE REACTIONS
**CNS:** headache.
**EENT:** epistaxis, nasal burning, blood in nasal mucus, pharyngitis, nasal irritation.

### INTERACTIONS
None significant.

### EFFECTS ON DIAGNOSTIC TESTS
None reported.

### CONTRAINDICATIONS
Contraindicated in patients with hypersensitivity to drug or its components. Don't use drug in patients with recent nasal septal ulcers, nasal surgery, or nasal trauma until healing has occurred.

### NURSING CONSIDERATIONS
• Use cautiously, if at all, in patients with active or quiescent tuberculous infections; glaucoma; untreated fungal, bacterial, or systemic viral infections; or ocular herpes simplex. Also use cautiously in patients already receiving systemic corticosteroids and in breast-feeding women.
• Although occurrence is rare, watch for signs of immediate hypersensitivity reactions or contact dermatitis after intranasal administration.

### ☑ Patient teaching
• Urge patient to read instruction sheet before using drug for first time.
• To instill drug, tell patient to shake container gently before use, blow nose to clear nasal passages, and tilt head slightly forward and insert nozzle into nostril, pointing away from septum. Tell him to hold other nostril closed; then inspire gently and spray. Next, have patient shake container and repeat procedure in other nostril.
• Stress importance of adhering to a schedule for instillation because drug effectiveness depends on regular use. Caution patient not to exceed recommended dose; doing so may lead to hyperadrenocorticism, hypothalamic-pituitary-adrenal axis suppression, or suppression of growth in children or teenagers.
• Tell patient to notify doctor if symptoms don't improve or condition worsens.
• Warn patient to avoid exposure to chickenpox and measles and, if exposed, to obtain medical advice.
• Instruct patient to watch for and report signs and symptoms of nasal infection.

---

Reactions may be *common*, uncommon, *life-threatening*, or COMMON AND LIFE-THREATENING.

## naphazoline hydrochloride
Privine ◇

*Pregnancy Risk Category NR*

### HOW SUPPLIED
*Nose drops:* 0.05% solution
*Nasal spray:* 0.05% solution

### ACTION
Causes local vasoconstriction of dilated arterioles, reducing blood flow and nasal congestion.

| Route | Onset | Peak | Duration |
|-------|-------|------|----------|
| Nasal | 10 min | Unknown | 2-6 hr |

### INDICATIONS & DOSAGE
*Nasal congestion—*
**Adults and children ages 12 and older:**
1 or 2 drops in each nostril at least 6 hours apart. Or, 1 or 2 sprays in each nostril at least 6 hours apart.
    Don't give to children under age 12 unless directed by doctor.

### ADVERSE REACTIONS
**CNS:** marked sedation.
**EENT:** rebound nasal congestion, sneezing, stinging, dryness of mucosa.
**Other:** systemic effects in children.

### INTERACTIONS
None significant.

### EFFECTS ON DIAGNOSTIC TESTS
None reported.

### CONTRAINDICATIONS
Contraindicated in patients with hypersensitivity to drug.

### NURSING CONSIDERATIONS
• Use cautiously in patients with hyperthyroidism, heart disease, hypertension, or diabetes mellitus and in those who have difficulty urinating because of enlargement of prostate gland.

### ✓ Patient teaching
• Teach patient how to use drug. For nose drops, instruct patient to tilt head back as far as possible, instill drops, then lean head forward while inhaling; then repeat procedure for other nostril. For nasal spray, instruct him to hold spray container and head upright. Tell patient not to shake container.
• Tell patient that product should be used by only one person to prevent spread of infection.
• Warn patient not to exceed recommended dosage.
• Instruct patient to call doctor if nasal congestion persists after 5 days.

## oxymetazoline hydrochloride
Afrin ◇, Afrin Children's Strength Nose Drops ◇, Allerest 12 Hour Nasal Spray ◇, Chlorphed-LA ◇, Dristan Long Lasting ◇, Drixine Nasal‡, Duramist Plus ◇, Duration ◇, 4-Way Long Lasting Spray, Genasal Spray ◇, Neo-Synephrine 12 Hour Nasal Spray ◇, Nostrilla ◇, NTZ Long Acting Decongestant Nasal Spray ◇, Sinarest 12 Hour Nasal ◇, Sinex Long-Acting ◇, Twice-A-Day Nasal ◇

*Pregnancy Risk Category NR*

### HOW SUPPLIED
*Nasal solution:* 0.025% ◇, 0.05% ◇

### ACTION
Unknown. Thought to cause local vasoconstriction of dilated arterioles, reducing blood flow and nasal congestion.

| Route | Onset | Peak | Duration |
|-------|-------|------|----------|
| Nasal | 5-10 min | 6 hr | < 12 hr |

### INDICATIONS & DOSAGE
*Nasal congestion—*
**Adults and children ages 6 and older:** 2 to 3 drops or sprays of 0.05% solution in each nostril b.i.d.
**Children ages 2 to 5:** 2 to 3 drops of 0.025% solution in each nostril b.i.d. Use no longer than 3 to 5 days.

### ADVERSE REACTIONS
**CNS:** headache, drowsiness, dizziness, insomnia, possible sedation.

---

*Liquid contains alcohol.    **May contain tartrazine.    †Canada    ‡Australia    §U.K.    ◇OTC

**CV:** palpitations, *CV collapse,* hypertension.

**EENT:** rebound nasal congestion or irritation, dryness of nose and throat, increased nasal discharge, stinging, sneezing.

**Other:** systemic effects in children.

## INTERACTIONS
None significant.

## EFFECTS ON DIAGNOSTIC TESTS
None reported.

## CONTRAINDICATIONS
Contraindicated in patients with hypersensitivity to drug.

## NURSING CONSIDERATIONS
• Use cautiously in patients with hyperthyroidism, cardiac disease, hypertension, or diabetes mellitus.

☑ **Patient teaching**
• Teach patient how to apply drug. Tell him to hold head upright to minimize swallowing of drug and to sniff spray briskly.
• Tell patient that drug should be used by only one person to prevent spread of infection.
• Tell patient not to exceed recommended dosage and to use only when needed.
• *Alert:* Warn patient that excessive use may cause bradycardia, hypotension, dizziness, and weakness.

---

## phenylephrine hydrochloride
Alconefrin Nasal Drops 12 ◇,
Alconefrin Nasal Drops 25 ◇,
Alconefrin Nasal Drops 50 ◇,
Doktors ◇, Duration ◇,
Neo-Synephrine ◇, Nostril ◇,
Rhinall ◇, Rhinall-10 Children's
Flavored Nose Drops ◇, Sinex ◇

*Pregnancy Risk Category NR*

## HOW SUPPLIED
*Nasal solution:* 0.125%, 0.16%, 0.25%, 0.5%, 1%

## ACTION
Causes local vasoconstriction of dilated arterioles, reducing blood flow and nasal congestion.

| Route | Onset | Peak | Duration |
|-------|-------|------|----------|
| Nasal | Rapid | Unknown | 0.5-4 hr |

## INDICATIONS & DOSAGE
*Nasal congestion—*
**Adults and children ages 12 and older:** 2 to 3 drops or 1 to 2 sprays in each nostril q 4 hours, p.r.n. Don't use for more than 3 to 5 days.
**Children ages 6 to 12:** 2 to 3 drops or 1 to 2 sprays of 0.25% solution in each nostril q 4 hours, p.r.n.
**Children under age 6:** 2 to 3 drops of 0.125% solution q 4 hours, p.r.n.

## ADVERSE REACTIONS
**CNS:** headache, tremor, dizziness, nervousness.
**CV:** *palpitations, tachycardia, PVCs,* hypertension, pallor.
**EENT:** transient burning or stinging, dryness of nasal mucosa; rebound nasal congestion.
**GI:** nausea.

## INTERACTIONS
None significant.

## EFFECTS ON DIAGNOSTIC TESTS
Drug may lower intraocular pressure in normal eyes or in open-angle glaucoma. It may also cause false-normal tonometry readings.

## CONTRAINDICATIONS
Contraindicated in patients with hypersensitivity to drug.

## NURSING CONSIDERATIONS
• Use cautiously in patients with hyperthyroidism, marked hypertension, type 1 diabetes mellitus, cardiac disease, or advanced arteriosclerotic changes; in children of low body weight; and in elderly patients.

☑ **Patient teaching**
• Teach patient how to apply drug. Tell him to hold head upright to minimize

swallowing of drug, then to sniff spray
briskly.
• Inform patient that drug should be used
by only one person to prevent spread of
infection.
• Tell patient not to exceed recommended
dosage and to use only when needed.
• Advise patient to contact doctor if
symptoms persist beyond 3 days.

## tetrahydrozoline hydrochloride
Tyzine, Tyzine Pediatric

*Pregnancy Risk Category C*

### HOW SUPPLIED
*Nasal solution:* 0.05%, 0.1%

### ACTION
Unknown. Thought to cause local vasoconstriction of dilated arterioles, reducing
blood flow and nasal congestion.

| Route | Onset | Peak | Duration |
|-------|-------|------|----------|
| Nasal | Few min | Unknown | 4-8 hr |

### INDICATIONS & DOSAGE
*Nasal congestion—*
**Adults and children over age 6:** 2 to 4
drops of 0.1% solution or spray into each
nostril q 4 to 6 hours, p.r.n.
**Children ages 2 to 6:** 2 to 3 drops of
0.05% solution into each nostril q 4 to 6
hours, p.r.n.

### ADVERSE REACTIONS
**EENT:** transient burning, stinging; sneezing; rebound nasal congestion.

### INTERACTIONS
None significant.

### EFFECTS ON DIAGNOSTIC TESTS
None reported.

### CONTRAINDICATIONS
Contraindicated in patients with hypersensitivity to drug, in those with angle-
closure glaucoma or other serious eye diseases, and in children under age 2. The

0.1% solution is contraindicated in children under age 6.

### NURSING CONSIDERATIONS
• Use cautiously in patients with hyperthyroidism, hypertension, and diabetes
mellitus.

### ☑ Patient teaching
• Teach patient how to apply drug. Tell
him to hold head upright to minimize
swallowing of drug, then to sniff spray
briskly.
• Instruct patient that product should be
used by only one person to prevent spread
of infection.
• Tell patient not to exceed recommended
dosage and to use only as needed for 3 to
5 days.

## triamcinolone acetonide
Nasacort, Nasacort AQ

*Pregnancy Risk Category C*

### HOW SUPPLIED
*Nasal aerosol:* 55 mcg/metered spray
*Nasal spray pump:* 55 mcg/spray

### ACTION
Unknown. A glucocorticoid with anti-
inflammatory properties.

| Route | Onset | Peak | Duration |
|-------|-------|------|----------|
| Nasal | 12 hr | 3-4 days | Unknown |

### INDICATIONS & DOSAGE
*Relief of symptoms of seasonal or peren-
nial allergic rhinitis—*
**Adults and children ages 12 and older:**
initially, 2 sprays (110 mcg) in each nostril once daily. Increased, p.r.n., up to
440 mcg daily either as once-daily dose or
in divided doses up to q.i.d. After desired
effect is obtained, dosage decreased, if
possible, to 1 spray (55 mcg) in each nostril daily.
**Children ages 6 to 11:** initially, 2 sprays
in each nostril (220 mcg), once daily.
Once maximal effect has been obtained,
reduce to effective dose.

## ADVERSE REACTIONS

**CNS:** *headache.*
**EENT:** *nasal irritation,* dry mucous membranes, nasal and sinus congestion, irritation, burning, stinging, throat discomfort, sneezing, epistaxis.

## INTERACTIONS

None significant.

## EFFECTS ON DIAGNOSTIC TESTS

None reported.

## CONTRAINDICATIONS

Contraindicated in patients with hypersensitivity to drug or its components.

## NURSING CONSIDERATIONS

• Use with extreme caution, if at all, in patients with active or quiescent tuberculosis infection of respiratory tract and in patients with untreated fungal, bacterial, or systemic viral infection or ocular herpes simplex.
• Use cautiously in patients already receiving systemic corticosteroids because of increased likelihood of hypothalamic-pituitary-adrenal axis suppression compared with therapeutic dosage of either one alone; in those with recent nasal septal ulcers, nasal surgery, or trauma because of inhibitory effect on wound healing; and in breast-feeding women.
• *Alert:* When excessive doses are used, signs and symptoms of hyperadrenocorticism and adrenal axis suppression may occur; drug should be discontinued slowly.
• *Alert:* Don't confuse triamcinolone with Triaminicin or Triaminicol.

### ☑ Patient teaching

• Urge patient to read patient-instruction sheet contained in each package before using drug for first time.
• To instill, instruct patient to shake container before use, blow nose to clear nasal passages, and tilt head slightly forward and insert nozzle into nostril, pointing away from septum. Tell him to hold other nostril closed; then inspire gently and spray. Next, have patient shake container and repeat procedure in other nostril.
• Tell patient to discard canister after 100 actuations.

• Stress importance of using drug on a regular schedule because its effectiveness depends on regular use. However, caution patient not to exceed dosage prescribed because serious adverse reactions can occur.
• Tell patient to notify doctor if symptoms don't diminish within 2 to 3 weeks or if condition worsens.
• Warn patient to avoid exposure to chickenpox or measles and, if exposed, to obtain medical advice.
• Instruct patient to watch for and report signs and symptoms of nasal infection. Drug may need to be discontinued and appropriate local therapy given.
• Advise patient not to break or incinerate canister or store it in extreme heat; contents are under pressure and may explode.

---

## xylometazoline hydrochloride
Otrivin ◇, Otrivin Pediatric

*Pregnancy Risk Category NR*

### HOW SUPPLIED

*Nasal solution:* 0.05%, 0.1%

### ACTION

Unknown. Thought to cause local vasoconstriction of dilated arterioles, reducing blood flow and nasal congestion.

| Route | Onset | Peak | Duration |
|-------|-------|------|----------|
| Nasal | 5-10 min | Unknown | 5-6 hr |

### INDICATIONS & DOSAGE

*Nasal congestion—*
**Adults and children ages 12 and older:** 2 to 3 drops or sprays of 0.1% solution in each nostril q 8 to 10 hours, not to exceed three times in 24 hours.
**Infants and children ages 6 months to 12 years:** 2 to 3 drops of 0.05% solution in each nostril q 8 to 10 hours, not to exceed three times in 24 hours.
**Infants under age 6 months:** 1 drop of 0.05% solution in each nostril q 6 hours, p.r.n.

### ADVERSE REACTIONS

**EENT:** transient burning, stinging; dryness or ulceration of nasal mucosa; sneez-

---

Reactions may be *common*, uncommon, **life-threatening**, or COMMON AND LIFE-THREATENING.

ing; rebound nasal congestion or irritation.

**INTERACTIONS**
None significant.

**EFFECTS ON DIAGNOSTIC TESTS**
None reported.

**CONTRAINDICATIONS**
Contraindicated in patients with hypersensitivity to drug and in those with angle-closure glaucoma.

**NURSING CONSIDERATIONS**
• Use cautiously in patients with hyperthyroidism, cardiac disease, hypertension, diabetes mellitus, or advanced arteriosclerosis.
• Don't use 0.1% solution in children under age 6.

**☑ Patient teaching**
• Teach patient how to apply drug. Have patient hold head upright to minimize swallowing of drug, then sniff spray briskly.
• Tell patient that drug should be used by only one person.
• Inform patient not to exceed recommended dosage and to use only as needed for 3 to 5 days.

acyclovir
amphotericin B
azelaic acid cream
bacitracin
butoconazole nitrate
clindamycin phosphate
clotrimazole
econazole nitrate
erythromycin
gentamicin sulfate
ketoconazole
mafenide acetate
metronidazole (topical)
miconazole nitrate
mupirocin
naftifine hydrochloride
neomycin sulfate
nitrofurazone
nystatin
silver sulfadiazine
terbinafine hydrochloride
terconazole
tetracycline hydrochloride
tioconazole
tolnaftate

### COMBINATION PRODUCTS
BENZAMYCIN: erythromycin 3% and benzoyl peroxide 5%.
LANABIOTIC ◇ : polymyxin B sulfate 10,000 U, neomycin sulfate 3.5 mg, bacitracin 500 U, and lidocaine 40 mg/g.
LOTRISONE: clotrimazole 1% and betamethasone dipropionate 0.05%.
MYCITRACIN ◇ : polymyxin B sulfate 5,000 U, bacitracin 500 U, and neomycin sulfate 3.5 mg/g.
MYCOLOG II: triamcinolone acetonide 0.1% and nystatin 100,000 U/g.
NEO-CORTEF: hydrocortisone acetate 1% and neomycin sulfate 0.5%.
NEODECADRON: sodium phosphate 0.1% and neomycin sulfate 0.5%.
NEOSPORIN CREAM ◇ : polymyxin B sulfate 10,000 U and neomycin sulfate 3.5 mg/g.
NEOSPORIN OINTMENT ◇ : polymyxin B sulfate 5,000 U, bacitracin zinc 400 U, and neomycin sulfate 3.5 mg/g.

POLYSPORIN OPHTHALMIC OINTMENT ◇ : polymyxin B sulfate 10,000 U and bacitracin zinc 500 U/g.
VIOFORM-HYDROCORTISONE MILD CREAM: iodochlorhydroxyquin 3% and hydrocortisone 0.5%.

---

## acyclovir
Acyclo-V‡, Zovirax

*Pregnancy Risk Category C*

---

### HOW SUPPLIED
*Ointment:* 5%

### ACTION
Inhibits herpes simplex and varicella-zoster viral DNA synthesis by inhibiting viral DNA polymerase action.

| Route | Onset | Peak | Duration |
|-------|-------|------|----------|
| Topical | Unknown | Unknown | Unknown |

### INDICATIONS & DOSAGE
*Initial herpes genitalis; limited, non-life-threatening mucocutaneous herpes simplex virus infections in immunocompromised patients—*
**Adults:** cover all lesions q 3 hours six times daily for 7 days. Although dose varies depending on total lesion area, use about ½-inch (1.3-cm) ribbon of ointment on each 4-inch (10-cm) square of surface area.

### ADVERSE REACTIONS
**Skin:** *transient burning and stinging, rash*, pruritus, vulvitis; edema, pain at application site.

### INTERACTIONS
None significant.

### EFFECTS ON DIAGNOSTIC TESTS
None reported.

---

Reactions may be *common*, uncommon, *__life-threatening__*, or COMMON AND LIFE-THREATENING.

## CONTRAINDICATIONS

Contraindicated in patients with hypersensitivity or chemical intolerance to drug.

## NURSING CONSIDERATIONS

• Start therapy as early as possible after onset of symptoms, as ordered.
• Apply drug with a finger cot or rubber glove to prevent autoinoculation of other body sites and transmission of infection to other persons.
• All lesions must be thoroughly covered.
• Drug is for cutaneous use only; don't apply to eye.
• Drug isn't a cure, but it will help with symptoms.

### ✅ Patient teaching

• Teach patient that virus transmission can occur during treatment.
• Tell patient that there may be some discomfort with application.
• Stress importance of compliance for successful therapy.
• Teach patient that therapy should begin as soon as signs and symptoms appear.
• Tell patient to notify doctor if adverse reactions occur.
• Instruct patient to store drug in a dry place at 59° to 77° F (15° to 25° C).

---

## amphotericin B
Fungizone

*Pregnancy Risk Category B*

---

## HOW SUPPLIED

*Cream:* 3%
*Lotion:* 3%
*Ointment:* 3%

## ACTION

Usually fungistatic; binds to sterols in the fungal cell membrane, resulting in increased membrane permeability and subsequent cell leakage.

| Route | Onset | Peak | Duration |
|-------|-------|------|----------|
| Topical | Unknown | Unknown | Unknown |

## INDICATIONS & DOSAGE

*Cutaneous or mucocutaneous candidal infections—*
**Adults and children:** apply liberally, rubbing in gently b.i.d. to q.i.d. for 1 to 3 weeks. Interdigital lesions and paronychias are treated for 2 to 4 weeks, and onychomycoses for several months because relapses are common.

## ADVERSE REACTIONS

**Skin:** possible dryness, contact sensitivity, erythema, burning, pruritus.

## INTERACTIONS

None significant.

## EFFECTS ON DIAGNOSTIC TESTS

None reported.

## CONTRAINDICATIONS

Contraindicated in patients with hypersensitivity to drug or its components.

## NURSING CONSIDERATIONS

• Clean area before applying drug.
• Report local irritation. Cream may dry skin; ointment may irritate if applied to moist, hairy areas.
• Avoid using occlusive dressings.
• Cream or lotion is preferred for such areas as groin folds, armpits, and neck creases.
• Stop drug if irritation or hypersensitivity occurs, and notify doctor.

### ✅ Patient teaching

• Tell patient to use drug for full treatment period, even if condition has improved.
• Inform patient that skin may become discolored if amphotericin B isn't rubbed in thoroughly; nail lesions may become stained.
• Caution patient against application to eyes.
• Tell patient that fabric discoloration caused by cream or lotion can be removed by washing; discoloration by ointment can be removed with cleaning fluid.
• Instruct patient not to apply occlusive dressing.

---

## azelaic acid cream
Azelex, Skinoren§

*Pregnancy Risk Category B*

**HOW SUPPLIED**
*Cream:* 20%

**ACTION**
Unknown. May inhibit microbial cellular protein synthesis.

| Route | Onset | Peak | Duration |
|-------|-------|------|----------|
| Topical | Unknown | Unknown | Unknown |

**INDICATIONS & DOSAGE**
*Mild to moderate inflammatory acne vulgaris—*
**Adults:** apply thin film and gently but thoroughly massage into affected areas b.i.d., in morning and evening.

**ADVERSE REACTIONS**
**Skin:** pruritus, burning, stinging, tingling.

**INTERACTIONS**
None significant.

**EFFECTS ON DIAGNOSTIC TESTS**
None reported.

**CONTRAINDICATIONS**
Contraindicated in patients with hypersensitivity to drug or its components.

**NURSING CONSIDERATIONS**
• Use cautiously in pregnant and breast-feeding women.
• Monitor patient for early signs of hypopigmentation, especially patient with dark complexion.
• If sensitivity or severe irritation occurs, notify doctor, who may discontinue drug and order appropriate treatment.
• Avoid use of occlusive dressings.

☑ **Patient teaching**
• Instruct patient to wash and pat dry affected areas before applying drug and to wash hands well after application. Warn him not to apply occlusive dressings or wrappings to affected areas.

• Warn patient that skin irritation may occur, usually at start of therapy, when drug is applied to broken or inflamed skin. Tell him to notify doctor if irritation persists.
• Advise patient to keep drug away from mouth, eyes, and other mucous membranes. If contact occurs, tell him to rinse thoroughly with water and to notify doctor if irritation persists.
• Advise patient to report abnormal changes in skin color.
• Urge patient to use drug for full treatment period. In most patients with inflammatory lesions, improvement occurs in 1 to 2 months.
• Instruct patient to store drug at 59° to 86° F (15° to 30° C) and protect it from freezing.

## bacitracin
Baciguent◇

*Pregnancy Risk Category C*

**HOW SUPPLIED**
*Ointment:* 500 U/g

**ACTION**
Bactericidal or bacteriostatic, depending on organism and concentration of drug; inhibits bacterial cell-wall synthesis. Effective against gram-positive organisms.

| Route | Onset | Peak | Duration |
|-------|-------|------|----------|
| Topical | Unknown | Unknown | Unknown |

**INDICATIONS & DOSAGE**
*Topical infections, abrasions, cuts, minor burns or wounds—*
**Adults and children:** apply thin film one to three times daily, based on severity of condition. Drug shouldn't be used for over 1 week.

**ADVERSE REACTIONS**
**Skin:** stinging, rash, other allergic reactions, allergic contact dermatitis; pruritus, burning, swelling of lips or face.
**Other:** *anaphylaxis.*

**INTERACTIONS**
None significant.

## EFFECTS ON DIAGNOSTIC TESTS
None reported.

## CONTRAINDICATIONS
Contraindicated in patients with hypersensitivity to drug and in those with atopy.

## NURSING CONSIDERATIONS
• Use cautiously in patients with neuromuscular disease or myasthenia gravis.
• Clean skin before applying drug, especially if skin is crusted or suppurative.
• Anticipate alternative treatment for burns that cover over 20% of body surface, especially if patient suffers from impaired renal function.
• Prolonged use may result in overgrowth of nonsusceptible organisms, particularly *Candida* species.
• Patients allergic to neomycin may also be sensitive to bacitracin.
• Before applying drug, obtain culture and sensitivity tests, as ordered.
• *Alert:* Don't confuse bacitracin with Bactroban.

☑ **Patient teaching**
• Tell patient to stop using drug and notify doctor if improvement doesn't occur or if condition worsens.
• Instruct patient to report persistent or severe adverse reactions.
• Tell patient to not use drug for more than 1 week, except on doctor's advice.

---

**butoconazole nitrate**
Femstat

*Pregnancy Risk Category C*

## HOW SUPPLIED
*Vaginal cream:* 2% with applicators supplied

## ACTION
Unknown. Thought to control or destroy fungus by disrupting cell membrane permeability, thereby causing osmotic instability.

| Route | Onset | Peak | Duration |
|-------|-------|------|----------|
| Intravaginal | Unknown | Unknown | Unknown |

## INDICATIONS & DOSAGE
*Vulvovaginal mycotic infections caused by* Candida *species—*
**Adults:** for nonpregnant patient, 1 applicator intravaginally h.s. for 3 days. If needed, treat for another 3 days. For pregnant women during second or third trimester, 1 applicator intravaginally h.s. for 6 days.

## ADVERSE REACTIONS
**GU:** vulvovaginal burning and itching, soreness, discharge, swelling.
**Skin:** finger itching.

## INTERACTIONS
None significant.

## EFFECTS ON DIAGNOSTIC TESTS
None reported.

## CONTRAINDICATIONS
Contraindicated in patients with hypersensitivity to drug.

## NURSING CONSIDERATIONS
• Use cautiously in breast-feeding women.
• Confirm diagnosis by smears or cultures, as ordered.
• Use of drug in pregnant women is restricted to second and third trimesters and only when potential benefits outweigh possible risks to fetus.
• Drug may be used with oral contraceptive and antibiotic therapy.

☑ **Patient teaching**
• Teach patient how to apply drug, and tell her not to use tampons during treatment.
• Advise patient to keep affected area cool and dry, wear loose-fitting cotton clothing, avoid feminine hygiene sprays, wash area daily with unscented soap and dry thoroughly with clean towel, and prevent reinfection by wiping perineum from front to back.
• Instruct patient to clean applicator with soap and water after each use.
• Advise patient to use drug for prescribed length of time, even during menses.
• Tell woman that drug should be placed high in the vagina except during pregnancy.
• Advise patient to refrain from sexual intercourse until treatment is complete.

---

Man should consult doctor if penile itching, redness, or discomfort occurs.

• Alert patient that drug base may weaken latex products (such as condom or diaphragm); their use within 3 days of drug administration isn't recommended as method of birth control.

• Tell patient not to store drug in temperatures above 104° F (40° C). Avoid freezing.

## clindamycin phosphate
Cleocin, Cleocin T

*Pregnancy Risk Category B*

### HOW SUPPLIED
*Gel:* 1%
*Lotion:* 1%
*Pledget:* 1%
*Topical solution:* 1%
*Vaginal cream:* 2%

### ACTION
Bacteriostatic or bactericidal, based on drug level and susceptibility of organism; suppresses growth of susceptible organisms in sebaceous glands by blocking protein synthesis.

| Route | Onset | Peak | Duration |
|-------|-------|------|----------|
| Topical, intravaginal | Unknown | Unknown | Unknown |

### INDICATIONS & DOSAGE
*Inflammatory acne vulgaris—*
**Adults and adolescents:** apply to skin b.i.d., morning and evening.
*Bacterial vaginosis—*
**Adults:** 1 applicator intravaginally h.s. for 7 consecutive days.

### ADVERSE REACTIONS
**GI:** GI upset, diarrhea, bloody diarrhea, abdominal pain, colitis including pseudomembranous colitis.
**GU:** *cervicitis, vaginitis, Candida albicans* overgrowth, *vulvar irritation.*
**Hepatic:** abnormal liver function test results.
**Skin:** *dryness,* rash, *redness,* pruritus, swelling, irritation, contact dermatitis, burning.

### INTERACTIONS
**Drug-drug.** *Erythromycin:* may antagonize clindamycin's effect. Separate administration times.
*Isotretinoin:* potential cumulative dryness, resulting in excessive skin irritation. Use cautiously.
*Neuromuscular blockers:* may enhance action of neuromuscular blocker. Use cautiously together.
**Drug-lifestyle.** *Abrasive or medicated soaps or cleansers, acne products or other preparations containing peeling drugs (benzoyl peroxide, resorcinol, salicylic acid, sulfur, tretinoin), alcohol-containing products (aftershave, cosmetics, perfumed toiletries, shaving creams or lotions), astringent soaps or cosmetics, medicated cosmetics or cover-ups:* potential cumulative dryness, resulting in excessive skin irritation. Use cautiously.

### EFFECTS ON DIAGNOSTIC TESTS
None reported.

### CONTRAINDICATIONS
Contraindicated in patients with hypersensitivity to drug and in those with history of ulcerative colitis, regional enteritis, or antibiotic-associated colitis.

### NURSING CONSIDERATIONS
• For treating acne, drug may be used with tretinoin or benzoyl peroxide as well as systemic antibiotics.
• Drug can cause excessive dryness.
• Monitor elderly patients for systemic effects.

### ✓ Patient teaching
• Tell patient to wash area with warm water and soap, to rinse and pat dry, and to wait 30 minutes after washing or shaving to apply.
• Warn patient to avoid too-frequent washing of area. Tell patient to cover entire affected area but to avoid contact with eyes, nose, mouth, and other areas bearing mucous membranes.
• Tell patient to use only as prescribed.
• Instruct patient to dab, not roll, applicator-tipped bottle. If tip becomes dry, patient should invert bottle and depress tip several times to moisten.

- Warn patient not to smoke while applying topical solution.
- For intravaginal application, make sure patient knows how to use applicators that come with drug.
- Advise patient to avoid sexual intercourse during intravaginal treatment.
- Instruct patient to notify doctor immediately if abdominal pain or diarrhea occurs. Inform him that antidiarrheal drug may worsen condition and should only be used as directed by doctor.
- Tell patient to remove pledgets from foil before use.

---

## clotrimazole
Canesten†, Femizol-7◇, Gyne-Lotrimin◇, Lotrimin, Mycelex, Mycelex-7◇, Mycelex-G, Mycelex OTC◇

*Pregnancy Risk Category B (C for troches)*

### HOW SUPPLIED
*Troches:* 10 mg
*Topical cream:* 1%
*Topical lotion:* 1%
*Topical solution:* 1%
*Vaginal cream:* 1%◇
*Vaginal tablets:* 100 mg◇, 200 mg, 500 mg
*Combination pack:* vaginal tablets 100 mg and vulvar cream 1%◇

### ACTION
Fungistatic but may be fungicidal, depending on level. Alters fungal cell-wall permeability and produces osmotic instability.

| Route | Onset | Peak | Duration |
|-------|-------|------|----------|
| P.O. | Unknown | Unknown | 3 hr |
| Topical, intravaginal | Unknown | Unknown | Unknown |

### INDICATIONS & DOSAGE
*Superficial fungal infections (tinea corporis, tinea cruris, tinea pedis, tinea versicolor; candidiasis)—*
**Adults and children:** apply thinly and massage into affected and surrounding area, morning and evening, for 2 to 4

weeks. If improvement doesn't occur after 4 weeks, patient should be reevaluated.
*Vulvovaginal candidiasis—*
**Adults:** one 100-mg vaginal tablet inserted daily h.s. for 7 consecutive days; or one 500-mg vaginal tablet daily h.s. for 1 day; or 1 applicator of vaginal cream daily h.s. for 7 days.
*Oropharyngeal candidiasis—*
**Adults and children ages 3 and older:** dissolve troche over 15 to 30 minutes in mouth five times daily for 14 consecutive days.
*Prevention of oropharyngeal candidiasis in patients immunocompromised by such conditions as chemotherapy, radiotherapy, or corticosteroid therapy in the treatment of leukemia, solid tumors, or renal transplantation—*
**Adults and children:** dissolve troche over 15 to 30 minutes in mouth t.i.d. for duration of chemotherapy or until corticosteroid is reduced to maintenance levels.

### ADVERSE REACTIONS
**GI:** lower abdominal cramps; nausea, vomiting with lozenges.
**GU:** *mild vaginal burning or irritation*, cramping, urinary frequency.
**Hepatic:** elevated liver function test results.
**Skin:** blistering, *erythema*, edema, pruritus, burning, stinging, peeling, urticaria, skin fissures, general irritation.

### INTERACTIONS
None significant.

### EFFECTS ON DIAGNOSTIC TESTS
None reported.

### CONTRAINDICATIONS
Contraindicated in patients with hypersensitivity to drug. Also contraindicated for ophthalmic use.

### NURSING CONSIDERATIONS
- Clean area before applying drug.
- Watch for and report irritation or sensitivity; discontinue if irritation occurs, and notify doctor.
- Improvement usually occurs within 1 week; if no improvement is seen by 4 weeks, diagnosis should be reviewed.

---

*Liquid contains alcohol.   **May contain tartrazine.   †Canada   ‡Australia   §U.K.   ◇OTC

• If compliance is a problem, mild to moderate vaginal candidiasis may be treated with a single 500-mg tablet.
• *Alert:* Don't confuse clotrimazole with co-trimoxazole.

✓ **Patient teaching**
• Reassure patient that hypopigmentation from tinea versicolor will resolve gradually.
• Warn patient not to use occlusive wrappings or dressings.
• Warn patient to avoid drug contact with eyes.
• Caution patient that frequent or persistent yeast infections may be symptomatic of a more serious medical problem such as AIDS.
• Tell patient to refrain from sexual intercourse during intravaginal treatment.
• Warn patient that topical preparation may stain clothing.
• Tell patient with tinea pedis to change shoes and cotton socks daily.
• Emphasize need to continue treatment for full course and to notify doctor if no improvement occurs after 4 weeks.

---

## econazole nitrate
Ecostatin†, Prevaryl§, Spectazole

*Pregnancy Risk Category C*

---

**HOW SUPPLIED**
*Cream:* 1%

**ACTION**
Fungistatic but may be fungicidal, depending on level. Alters fungal cell-wall permeability and produces osmotic instability.

| Route | Onset | Peak | Duration |
|-------|-------|------|----------|
| Topical | Unknown | Unknown | Unknown |

**INDICATIONS & DOSAGE**
*Tinea corporis, tinea cruris, tinea pedis, tinea versicolor; cutaneous candidiasis—*
**Adults and children:** rub into affected areas once daily for at least 2 weeks.
*Cutaneous candidiasis—*
**Adults and children:** rub into affected areas b.i.d.

**ADVERSE REACTIONS**
**Skin:** burning, pruritus, stinging, erythema.

**INTERACTIONS**
None significant.

**EFFECTS ON DIAGNOSTIC TESTS**
None reported.

**CONTRAINDICATIONS**
Contraindicated in patients with hypersensitivity to drug or its components.

**NURSING CONSIDERATIONS**
• Clean affected area before applying.
• Don't use occlusive dressings.

✓ **Patient teaching**
• Tell patient to use drug for entire treatment period, even if symptoms improve. Instruct him to notify doctor if no improvement occurs after 2 weeks (tinea corporis, tinea cruris, and tinea versicolor) or 4 weeks (tinea pedis).
• Reassure patient that hypopigmentation from tinea versicolor will resolve gradually.
• Tell patient to stop drug and call doctor if condition persists or worsens or if irritation occurs.
• Warn patient that drug may stain clothing.
• Tell patient with tinea pedis to change shoes and cotton socks daily.

---

## erythromycin
Akne-mycin, A/T/S, Del-Mycin, Emgel, Erycette, EryDerm, Erygel, Erymax, Erysol†, Erythra-Derm, ETS†, Sans-Acne†, Staticin, T-Stat†

*Pregnancy Risk Category C*

---

**HOW SUPPLIED**
*Ointment:* 2%
*Topical gel:* 2%
*Topical solution:* 1.5%*, 2%*
*Pledgets:* 2%

**ACTION**
Usually bacteriostatic but may be bactericidal in high concentrations or against

---

Reactions may be *common*, uncommon, *life-threatening*, or COMMON AND LIFE-THREATENING.

highly susceptible organisms. Disrupts protein synthesis in susceptible bacteria.

| Route | Onset | Peak | Duration |
|---|---|---|---|
| Topical | Unknown | Unknown | Unknown |

## INDICATIONS & DOSAGE
*Inflammatory acne vulgaris—*
**Adults and children:** apply to affected areas b.i.d.

## ADVERSE REACTIONS
**Skin:** sensitivity reactions, erythema, *burning, dryness, pruritus,* irritation, peeling, oily skin.

## INTERACTIONS
**Drug-drug.** *Clindamycin:* may antagonize clindamycin's effect. Separate administration times.
*Isotretinoin:* may cause cumulative dryness, resulting in excessive skin irritation. Use cautiously.
**Drug-lifestyle.** *Abrasive or medicated soaps or cleansers, acne products or other preparations containing peeling drugs (benzoyl peroxide, resorcinol, salicylic acid, sulfur, tretinoin), alcohol-containing products (aftershave, cosmetics, perfumed toiletries, shaving creams or lotions), astringent soaps or cosmetics, medicated cosmetics or cover-ups:* may cause cumulative dryness, resulting in excessive skin irritation. Use cautiously.

## EFFECTS ON DIAGNOSTIC TESTS
Drug may interfere with fluorometric determinations of urinary catecholamines.

## CONTRAINDICATIONS
Contraindicated in patients with hypersensitivity to drug or its components.

## NURSING CONSIDERATIONS
• Obtain cultures before beginning therapy.
• Before reconstitution, store drug at room temperature. After reconstitution, refrigerate drug; don't freeze. Expiration date is 2 to 4 months from date of reconstitution.
• Wash, rinse, and dry affected areas before application.
• Prolonged use may be needed when treating acne vulgaris, and may result in overgrowth of nonsusceptible organisms.

☑ **Patient teaching**
• Advise patient to avoid use near eyes, nose, mouth, or other areas bearing mucous membranes and to wash hands after applying.
• Tell patient to stop using drug and notify doctor if no improvement occurs or if condition worsens.
• Advise patient not to share towels or washcloths.
• Instruct patient to use each pledget once, then discard.
• Inform patient to keep drug away from heat and open flame.

## gentamicin sulfate
Garamycin, G-Myticin

*Pregnancy Risk Category C*

## HOW SUPPLIED
*Cream:* 0.1%
*Ointment:* 0.1%

## ACTION
Exact mechanism unknown. A bactericidal drug that disrupts bacterial protein synthesis by binding to ribosomes.

| Route | Onset | Peak | Duration |
|---|---|---|---|
| Topical | Unknown | Unknown | Unknown |

## INDICATIONS & DOSAGE
*Treatment and prophylaxis of superficial infections and superficial burns of the skin due to susceptible bacteria—*
**Adults and children over age 1:** rub in small amount gently t.i.d. or q.i.d., with or without gauze dressing.

## ADVERSE REACTIONS
**Skin:** minor skin irritation, possible photosensitivity, allergic contact dermatitis.

## INTERACTIONS
None significant.

## EFFECTS ON DIAGNOSTIC TESTS
None reported.

## CONTRAINDICATIONS
Contraindicated in patients with hypersensitivity to drug and its components and

in those who may exhibit cross-sensitivity with other aminoglycosides such as neomycin.

## NURSING CONSIDERATIONS
• **Alert:** Avoid use on large skin lesions or over a wide area because of possible systemic toxic effects.
• Restrict use of drug to selected patients; widespread use may lead to resistant organisms.
• Prolonged use may result in overgrowth of nonsusceptible organisms.

☑ **Patient teaching**
• Tell patient to clean affected area before applying drug and, to enhance absorption, have him remove crusts for impetigo before applying drug.
• Instruct patient to store drug in cool place.
• Tell patient to stop drug and notify doctor immediately if no improvement occurs or if condition worsens.

---

## ketoconazole
Nizoral

*Pregnancy Risk Category C*

### HOW SUPPLIED
*Cream:* 2%
*Shampoo:* 2%

### ACTION
Unknown. An imidazole that probably inhibits yeast growth by altering the permeability of the cell membrane.

| Route | Onset | Peak | Duration |
|-------|-------|------|----------|
| Topical | Unknown | Unknown | Unknown |

### INDICATIONS & DOSAGE
*Tinea corporis, tinea cruris, tinea pedis, tinea versicolor due to susceptible organisms; seborrheic dermatitis; cutaneous candidiasis—*
**Adults:** cover affected and immediate surrounding area once daily for at least 2 weeks; for seborrheic dermatitis, apply b.i.d. for 4 weeks. Patients with tinea pedis need 6 weeks of treatment. When using shampoo, wet hair, lather, and massage for 1 minute. Rinse and repeat, but leave drug on scalp for 3 minutes before rinsing. Shampoo twice weekly for 4 weeks, with at least 3 days between shampoos and then intermittently, p.r.n., to maintain control.

### ADVERSE REACTIONS
**Hepatic:** transient elevations in AST, ALT, and alkaline phosphatase levels.
**Metabolic:** transient alterations in serum cholesterol and triglyceride levels.
**Skin:** severe irritation, pruritus, stinging with cream use; increase in normal hair loss, irritation, abnormal hair texture, scalp pustules, pruritus, oiliness or dryness of hair and scalp with shampoo use.

### INTERACTIONS
**Drug-drug.** *Topical corticosteroids:* may cause increased absorption of corticosteroid. Avoid concomitant use.

### EFFECTS ON DIAGNOSTIC TESTS
None reported.

### CONTRAINDICATIONS
Contraindicated in patients with hypersensitivity to drug or its components.

### NURSING CONSIDERATIONS
• Use cautiously in breast-feeding women.
• Most patients show improvement soon after treatment begins.
• Treatment of tinea corporis or tinea cruris should continue for at least 2 weeks to reduce possibility of recurrence.
• **Alert:** Product contains sodium sulfite anhydrous, which may cause severe or life-threatening allergic reactions, including anaphylaxis, in asthmatic patients.

☑ **Patient teaching**
• Tell patient to stop drug and notify doctor if hypersensitivity reaction occurs.
• Advise patient to check with doctor if condition worsens; drug may have to be discontinued and diagnosis reevaluated.
• Warn patient that shampoo applied to permanent-waved hair removes curl.
• Warn patient to avoid contact of drug with eyes.

---

• Tell patient not to store drug above room temperature (77° F [25° C]); protect from light.

---

## mafenide acetate
Sulfamylon

*Pregnancy Risk Category C*

### HOW SUPPLIED
*Cream:* 8.5%

### ACTION
Unknown, although is known to interfere with bacterial cellular metabolism.

| Route | Onset | Peak | Duration |
|-------|-------|------|----------|
| Topical | Unknown | Unknown | Unknown |

### INDICATIONS & DOSAGE
*Adjunctive treatment of second- and third-degree burns to prevent infection due to susceptible organisms (especially* Pseudomonas aeruginosa)—
**Adults and children:** apply ¹⁄₁₆-inch thickness of cream daily or b.i.d. to clean debrided wounds. Reapply, p.r.n., to keep burned area covered.

### ADVERSE REACTIONS
**Hematologic:** eosinophilia, *bone marrow depression.*
**Metabolic:** *metabolic acidosis.*
**Respiratory:** *tachypnea.*
**Skin:** pain, *burning sensation,* rash, pruritus, swelling, urticaria, blisters, erythema.
**Other:** facial edema, *DIC.*

### INTERACTIONS
None significant.

### EFFECTS ON DIAGNOSTIC TESTS
None reported.

### CONTRAINDICATIONS
Contraindicated in patients with hypersensitivity to drug. Cross-sensitivity to other sulfonamides is unknown.

### NURSING CONSIDERATIONS
• Use cautiously in patients with acute renal failure or asthma.

• Clean area before applying drug; bathe patient daily, if possible.
• Use sterile gloves and instruments when applying cream to minimize risk of further wound contamination.
• Keep burn areas medicated at all times.
• Only a thin layer of dressing should be used, if indicated.
• *Alert:* Closely monitor acid-base balance, especially in patients with pulmonary and renal dysfunction. If acidosis occurs, discontinue drug for 24 to 48 hours and notify doctor.
• It's sometimes difficult to distinguish between adverse reactions and effects of severe burn.

### ☑ Patient teaching
• Explain purpose of drug and importance of keeping burned areas covered with drug at all times. Tell patient to alert nurse if drug rubs off in visible areas.
• Tell patient to report adverse reactions, especially pain or burning when drug is applied; these symptoms may indicate allergy. Instruct patient to notify doctor if pain is severe or prolonged; treatment may need to be temporarily stopped.
• Tell patient not to expose drug to excessive heat (above 104° F [40° C]).

---

## metronidazole (topical)
Metro-Cream, MetroGel, MetroGel-Vaginal

*Pregnancy Risk Category B*

### HOW SUPPLIED
*Topical cream:* 0.75%
*Topical gel:* 0.75%, 1%
*Vaginal gel:* 0.75%

### ACTION
Unknown. May cause bactericidal effect by interacting with bacterial DNA. It's active against many anaerobic gram-negative bacilli, anaerobic gram-positive cocci, *Gardnerella vaginalis,* and *Campylobacter fetus.*

| Route | Onset | Peak | Duration |
|-------|-------|------|----------|
| Topical | Unknown | Unknown | Unknown |
| Intravaginal | Unknown | 6-12 hr | Unknown |

---

## INDICATIONS & DOSAGE

*Inflammatory papules and pustules of acne rosacea—*
**Adults:** apply thin film to affected area b.i.d., morning and evening. Frequency and duration of therapy adjusted after response is seen.
*Bacterial vaginosis—*
**Adults:** 1 applicator intravaginally once daily or b.i.d. for 5 days. For once-daily dosing, administer h.s.

## ADVERSE REACTIONS

*Topical gel or cream:*
**EENT:** lacrimation, if applied around eyes.
**Skin:** rash, *transient redness, dryness, mild burning, stinging.*
*Vaginal form:*
**CNS:** dizziness, light-headedness, headache.
**GI:** cramps, pain, nausea, diarrhea, constipation, metallic or bad taste in mouth, decreased appetite.
**GU:** *cervicitis, vaginitis.*
**Hematologic:** increased or decreased WBC.
**Skin:** rash, *transient redness, dryness, mild burning, stinging.*
**Other:** overgrowth of nonsusceptible organisms.

## INTERACTIONS

**Drug-drug.** *Disulfiram:* disulfiram reaction may occur. Avoid concomitant use and wait 2 weeks following discontinuation of disulfiram before initiating metronidazole vaginal therapy.
*Oral anticoagulants:* may potentiate anticoagulant effect. Monitor patient for potential adverse reactions.
**Drug-lifestyle.** *Alcohol use:* disulfiram-like reaction may occur. Avoid concomitant use.

## EFFECTS ON DIAGNOSTIC TESTS
None reported.

## CONTRAINDICATIONS
Contraindicated in patients with hypersensitivity to drug or its ingredients, such as parabens, and other nitroimidazole derivatives.

## NURSING CONSIDERATIONS

• Use cautiously in patients with history or evidence of blood dyscrasia and in those with severe hepatic disease.
• Use vaginal gel cautiously in patients with history of CNS diseases. Seizures and peripheral neuropathy are associated with oral form.
• Topical therapy hasn't been linked to adverse effects observed with parenteral or oral therapy; however, some drug may be absorbed after topical use.
• Don't use vaginal gel in patients who have taken disulfiram within past 2 weeks.
• Oral form has been associated with psychotic reaction.

### ☑ Patient teaching
• Instruct patient to avoid use of topical gel around eyes.
• Advise patient to clean area thoroughly before use, and to wait 15 to 20 minutes after cleaning skin before applying drug to minimize risk of local irritation. Cosmetics may be used after applying drug.
• If local reactions occur, advise patient to apply drug less frequently or discontinue its use and contact doctor.
• Advise patient to avoid sexual intercourse while using vaginal preparation.
• Caution patient not to drink alcohol while being treated with vaginal preparation.

---

## miconazole nitrate
Daktarin§, Gyno-Daktarin§, Micatin◇, Monistat-Derm, Monistat 3, Monistat 7◇

*Pregnancy Risk Category B (vaginal); C (topical)*

## HOW SUPPLIED
*Cream:* 2%◇
*Powder:* 2%◇
*Spray:* 2%◇
*Vaginal cream:* 2%◇
*Vaginal suppositories:* 100 mg◇, 200 mg

---

## ACTION
A fungicidal imidazole that disrupts fungal cell membrane permeability.

| Route | Onset | Peak | Duration |
|-------|-------|------|----------|
| Topical, intravaginal | Unknown | Unknown | Unknown |

## INDICATIONS & DOSAGE
*Tinea corporis, tinea cruris, tinea pedis; cutaneous candidiasis; common dermatophyte infections—*
**Adults and children over age 1:** apply sparingly b.i.d. for 2 to 4 weeks. Powder or spray can be used liberally over affected area.
*Tinea versicolor—*
**Adults and children over age 1:** apply sparingly once daily for 2 weeks.
*Vulvovaginal candidiasis—*
**Adults:** 1 applicator or 100 mg suppository (Monistat 7) intravaginally h.s. for 7 days; course repeated, if needed. Or, 200 mg suppository (Monistat 3) intravaginally h.s. for 3 days.

## ADVERSE REACTIONS
**CNS:** headache.
**GU:** pelvic cramps; vulvovaginal burning, pruritus and irritation with vaginal cream.
**Hematologic:** transient decrease in hematocrit, increase or decrease in platelet count, RBC aggregation.
**Metabolic:** hyponatremia; hyperlipidemia; hypertriglyceridemia; abnormalities in lipoprotein and immunoelectrophoretic patterns due to polyoxyl 35 castor oil vehicle.
**Skin:** irritation, burning, maceration, allergic contact dermatitis.

## INTERACTIONS
None significant.

## EFFECTS ON DIAGNOSTIC TESTS
None reported.

## CONTRAINDICATIONS
Contraindicated in patients with hypersensitivity to drug or its components.

## NURSING CONSIDERATIONS
• Concurrent use (within 72 hours) of intravaginal forms and certain latex products, such as condoms or vaginal contraceptive diaphragms, isn't recommended because of possible interaction.
• Don't use occlusive dressings.

☑ **Patient teaching**
• Advise patient that drug is for perineal or intravaginal use only and to keep drug out of eyes.
• Caution patient that frequent or persistent yeast infections may be a symptom of a more serious medical problem such as AIDS.
• Tell patient to cautiously insert intravaginal form high into the vagina with applicator provided.
• Tell patient that drug may stain clothing.
• Warn patient to discontinue drug if sensitivity or chemical irritation occurs.
• Tell patient to use drug for full treatment period prescribed and to notify doctor if symptoms persist or worsen at end of therapy.
• Advise patient to avoid tampons and sexual intercourse during vaginal treatment.
• Instruct patient to apply sparingly in skin-fold areas and rub in well to prevent maceration.
• Tell patient to store vaginal product between 59° and 86° F (15° and 30° C).

---

## mupirocin
Bactroban, Bactroban Cream, Bactroban Nasal

*Pregnancy Risk Category B*

## HOW SUPPLIED
*Topical ointment:* 2%
*Topical cream:* 2%
*Intranasal ointment:* 2%

## ACTION
Unknown. Thought to inhibit bacterial protein and RNA synthesis.

| Route | Onset | Peak | Duration |
|-------|-------|------|----------|
| Topical, intranasal | Unknown | Unknown | Unknown |

## INDICATIONS & DOSAGE
*Impetigo—*
**Adults and children:** apply to affected areas t.i.d. for 1 to 2 weeks. Reevaluate patient in 3 to 5 days; may cover affected area with dressing.
*Secondarily infected traumatic skin lesions due to* Staphylococcus aureus *and* Streptococcus pyogenes—
**Adults and children:** apply thin film t.i.d. for 10 days; may cover with gauze dressing, if needed. Reevaluate patient if clinical improvement doesn't occur in 3 to 5 days.
*Eradication of nasal colonization with methicillin-resistant* S. aureus *in adult patients and health care workers—*
**Adults and children ages 12 and older:** divide ointment in single-use tube between nostrils (½ tube per nostril) b.i.d. for 5 days. After application, close nostrils by pressing together and releasing sides of nose repeatedly for 1 minute to spread ointment throughout nares.

## ADVERSE REACTIONS
**CNS:** headache.
**EENT:** rhinitis, pharyngitis, taste perversion, burning or stinging with intranasal use.
**Respiratory:** upper respiratory tract congestion, cough with intranasal use.
**Skin:** burning, pruritus, stinging, rash, pain, erythema with topical use.

## INTERACTIONS
None significant.

## EFFECTS ON DIAGNOSTIC TESTS
None reported.

## CONTRAINDICATIONS
Contraindicated in patients with hypersensitivity to drug or its components.

## NURSING CONSIDERATIONS
• Use cautiously in patients with burns or impaired renal function because serious renal toxicity may occur.
• Drug isn't for ophthalmic or internal use.
• Prolonged use may cause overgrowth of nonsusceptible bacteria and fungi.

• Local reactions appear to be caused by polyethylene glycol vehicle.
• *Alert:* Don't confuse Bactroban with bacitracin.

☑ **Patient teaching**
• Tell patient to notify doctor immediately if no improvement occurs in 3 to 5 days or if condition worsens.
• Tell patient not to use other nasal products with mupirocin.
• Warn patient about local adverse reactions associated with drug use.
• Caution patient not to use cosmetics or other skin products on treated area.

---

# naftifine hydrochloride
Naftin

*Pregnancy Risk Category B*

## HOW SUPPLIED
*Cream:* 1%
*Gel:* 1%

## ACTION
Unknown. A broad-spectrum fungicidal thought to inhibit sterol biosynthesis in susceptible fungi by blocking the enzyme squalene 2,3 epoxidase.

| Route | Onset | Peak | Duration |
|---|---|---|---|
| Topical | Unknown | Unknown | Unknown |

## INDICATIONS & DOSAGE
*Tinea corporis, tinea cruris, tinea pedis—*
**Adults:** apply cream to affected area once daily; or apply gel b.i.d. in morning and evening.

## ADVERSE REACTIONS
**Skin:** *burning, stinging,* dryness, pruritus, local irritation, erythema, rash.

## INTERACTIONS
None significant.

## EFFECTS ON DIAGNOSTIC TESTS
None reported.

## CONTRAINDICATIONS
Contraindicated in patients with hypersensitivity to drug or its components.

---

Reactions may be *common*, uncommon, *life-threatening*, or COMMON AND LIFE-THREATENING.

**NURSING CONSIDERATIONS**
• Therapy should be reevaluated if no improvement occurs after 4 weeks.
• Keep cream away from mucous membranes. Drug isn't for ophthalmic use.

☑ **Patient teaching**
• Tell patient not to use occlusive dressings unless directed otherwise by doctor.
• Instruct patient to wash hands after application.
• Instruct patient to discontinue therapy and notify doctor if irritation or sensitivity develops.

---

## neomycin sulfate
Myciguent ◊

*Pregnancy Risk Category C*

**HOW SUPPLIED**
*Cream:* 0.5% ◊
*Ointment:* 0.5% ◊

**ACTION**
Unknown. Thought to disrupt bacterial protein synthesis by binding to bacterial ribosomes.

| Route | Onset | Peak | Duration |
|-------|-------|------|----------|
| Topical | Unknown | Unknown | Unknown |

**INDICATIONS & DOSAGE**
*Prevention or treatment of superficial bacterial infections—*
**Adults and children:** rub fingertip-size dose into affected area once daily to t.i.d.

**ADVERSE REACTIONS**
**CNS:** *neuromuscular blockade.*
**EENT:** *ototoxicity.*
**GU:** *nephrotoxicity.*
**Skin:** *rash, contact dermatitis,* urticaria.

**INTERACTIONS**
None significant.

**EFFECTS ON DIAGNOSTIC TESTS**
None reported.

**CONTRAINDICATIONS**
Contraindicated in patients with hypersensitivity to drug or its components.

**NURSING CONSIDERATIONS**
• Don't use more than once daily on burns covering more than 20% of body surface.
• Prolonged use may result in overgrowth of nonsusceptible organisms.
• In products containing corticosteroids, use of occlusive dressings increases corticosteroid absorption and likelihood of systemic effects.
• Enhanced systemic absorption occurs on denuded or abraded areas.
• Watch for signs of hypersensitivity and contact dermatitis.
• *Alert:* Watch for signs of ototoxicity with prolonged or extended use.

☑ **Patient teaching**
• Tell patient to discontinue drug and notify doctor if no improvement occurs or if condition worsens.
• Tell patient to report adverse reactions, especially systemic reactions.
• Instruct patient not to use drug for more than 1 week, unless otherwise directed.

---

## nitrofurazone
Furacin

*Pregnancy Risk Category C*

**HOW SUPPLIED**
*Cream:* 0.2%
*Ointment:* 0.2% (soluble dressing)
*Topical solution:* 0.2%

**ACTION**
Unknown. A broad-spectrum antibiotic that probably inhibits bacterial enzymes involved in carbohydrate metabolism.

| Route | Onset | Peak | Duration |
|-------|-------|------|----------|
| Topical | Unknown | Unknown | Unknown |

**INDICATIONS & DOSAGE**
*Adjunctive treatment of second- and third-degree burns (especially when resistance to other antibiotics and sulfonamides occurs), prevention of skin allograft rejection—*
**Adults and children:** apply directly to lesion daily or q few days, depending on severity of burn. Drug may also be applied to dressings used to cover affected area.

---

**ADVERSE REACTIONS**
**Skin:** erythema, pruritus, burning, local edema, allergic contact dermatitis.

**INTERACTIONS**
None significant.

**EFFECTS ON DIAGNOSTIC TESTS**
None reported.

**CONTRAINDICATIONS**
Contraindicated in patients with hypersensitivity to drug.

**NURSING CONSIDERATIONS**
• Use cautiously in patients with known or suspected renal impairment. Monitor serum creatinine levels regularly, as ordered.
• Flushing dressing with sterile normal saline solution facilitates removal.
• Clean wound, as indicated by doctor, before reapplying dressings.
• Use sterile application technique to prevent further wound contamination.
• When using wet dressing, protect skin around wound with zinc oxide ointment.
• Dressings impregnated with drug shouldn't be stored for more than 24 hours.
• Drug may discolor in light but still retains its potency.
• Discard cloudy solutions if warming to 131° to 140° F (55° to 60° C) doesn't restore clarity.
• Store solution in tight, light-resistant container (brown bottle). Avoid exposure to direct light, prolonged heat, and alkaline materials.

☑ **Patient teaching**
• Tell patient to report irritation, sensitization, or infection.
• Explain all procedures to patient.
• Tell patient to notify doctor if condition worsens.

---

**nystatin**
Mycostatin, Nadostine†, Nilstat, Nystaform§, Nystan§

*Pregnancy Risk Category NR*

**HOW SUPPLIED**
*Cream:* 100,000 U/g

*Lozenges:* 200,000 U
*Ointment:* 100,000 U/g
*Oral suspension:* 100,000 U/ml
*Powder:* 100,000 U/g
*Vaginal tablets:* 100,000 U

**ACTION**
Disrupts integrity of fungal cell wall, promoting osmotic instability.

| Route | Onset | Peak | Duration |
|-------|-------|------|----------|
| P.O., topical, intravaginal | Unknown | Unknown | Unknown |

**INDICATIONS & DOSAGE**
*Cutaneous and mucocutaneous infections due to* Candida albicans—
**Adults and children:** apply to affected area up to several times daily until healing is complete. Apply cream: b.i.d. or as indicated; powder: b.i.d. or t.i.d.; lozenges: 1 or 2 four to five times daily until 48 hours after oral symptoms subside, but not more than 14 days; suspension: 4 to 6 ml q.i.d. (one-half of dose in each side of mouth); retain dose as long as possible before swallowing.
*Vulvovaginal candidiasis—*
**Adults:** 1 vaginal tablet daily for 14 days.

**ADVERSE REACTIONS**
**GI:** vomiting, with vaginal tablet.
**Skin:** occasional contact dermatitis from preservatives in some forms.

**INTERACTIONS**
None significant.

**EFFECTS ON DIAGNOSTIC TESTS**
None reported.

**CONTRAINDICATIONS**
Contraindicated in patients with hypersensitivity to drug or its components.

**NURSING CONSIDERATIONS**
• Don't use occlusive dressings.
• Preparation doesn't stain skin or mucous membranes.
• Cream is recommended for intertriginous areas; powder, for moist areas; ointment, for dry areas.

---

• Immunosuppressed patients may tolerate vaginal tablets orally for longer mucous membrane drug exposure.
• *Alert:* Don't confuse nystatin with Nilstat or Nitrostat.

☑ **Patient teaching**
• Show woman how to administer vaginal tablets and tell her to continue using vaginal tablets during menstrual period.
• Tell patient to insert drug high in vagina (except during pregnancy) and to refrain from sexual intercourse during vaginal treatment.
• Instruct patient to refrigerate tablets.
• Tell patient to use drug for full prescribed period even if condition improves and to continue drug at least 2 days after symptoms subside (for oral therapy). Immunosuppressed patients may use drug on long-term basis.
• Warn patient to avoid drug contact with eyes.
• Instruct patient not to use occlusive dressings with skin application.
• Tell patient to dissolve oral lozenges slowly in mouth.
• Demonstrate and stress importance of proper oral hygiene, especially for denture wearers.

---

### silver sulfadiazine
Flamazine†, Flint SSD, Silvadene, SSD AF, Thermazene

*Pregnancy Risk Category B*

**HOW SUPPLIED**
*Cream:* 1%

**ACTION**
A broad-spectrum sulfonamide that acts on cell membrane and cell wall; it's bactericidal for many gram-positive and gram-negative organisms.

| Route | Onset | Peak | Duration |
|---|---|---|---|
| Topical | Unknown | Unknown | Unknown |

**INDICATIONS & DOSAGE**
*Prevention and treatment of wound infection in second- and third-degree burns—*
**Adults:** apply ¹⁄₁₆-inch thickness to clean debrided wound daily or b.i.d.

**ADVERSE REACTIONS**
**Hematologic:** *leukopenia.*
**Metabolic:** altered serum osmolarity.
**Skin:** pain, burning, rash, pruritus, skin necrosis, erythema multiforme, skin discoloration.

**INTERACTIONS**
**Drug-drug.** *Topical proteolytic enzymes:* inactivation of enzymes. Don't use together.
**Drug-lifestyle.** *Sun exposure:* photosensitivity reactions may occur. Take precautions.

**EFFECTS ON DIAGNOSTIC TESTS**
None reported.

**CONTRAINDICATIONS**
Contraindicated in patients with hypersensitivity to drug and in those with G6PD deficiency. Also contraindicated in pregnant women at or near term and in premature or full-term neonates during first 2 months of life. Drug may increase possibility of kernicterus.

**NURSING CONSIDERATIONS**
• *Alert:* Use with caution in patients with hypersensitivity to sulfonamides.
• Use sterile application technique to prevent wound contamination.
• Use drug only on affected areas. Keep these areas medicated at all times.
• Bathe patient daily, if possible.
• Inspect patient's skin daily, and note any changes. Notify doctor if burning or excessive pain develops.
• Monitor serum sulfadiazine levels and renal function, as ordered, and check urine for sulfa crystals in patients with extensive burns.
• Tell doctor if hepatic or renal dysfunction occurs; drug may need to be stopped.
• Discard darkened cream, which indicates that drug is ineffective.

---

☑ **Patient teaching**
● Instruct patient to promptly report adverse reactions, especially burning or excessive pain with application.
● Inform patient of need for frequent blood and urine tests to watch for adverse effects.
● Tell patient that he may develop photosensitivity.
● Tell patient to continue treatment until satisfactory healing occurs or until site is ready for grafting.

## terbinafine hydrochloride
Lamisil

*Pregnancy Risk Category B*

### HOW SUPPLIED
*Cream:* 1%

### ACTION
A fungicidal that selectively inhibits an early step in synthesis of sterols used by fungi for cell-wall synthesis.

| Route | Onset | Peak | Duration |
|-------|-------|------|----------|
| Topical | Unknown | Unknown | Unknown |

### INDICATIONS & DOSAGE
*Interdigital tinea corporis, tinea cruris, tinea pedis; plantar tinea pedis—*
**Adults and children ages 12 and older:** cover affected area and immediate surrounding area b.i.d. for at least 1 week; use for 2 weeks for plantar tinea pedis.

### ADVERSE REACTIONS
**Skin:** irritation, burning, pruritus, dryness.

### INTERACTIONS
None significant.

### EFFECTS ON DIAGNOSTIC TESTS
None reported.

### CONTRAINDICATIONS
Contraindicated in patients with hypersensitivity to drug or its components.

### NURSING CONSIDERATIONS
● Observe patients for 2 to 6 weeks after therapy is complete to determine whether treatment was successful; review diagnosis if condition persists.
● Therapy shouldn't exceed 4 weeks.
● Drug isn't intended for oral, ophthalmic, or vaginal use.
● Drug isn't for use in breast-feeding women.
● *Alert:* Don't confuse terbinafine with terfenadine or terbutaline.

☑ **Patient teaching**
● Teach patient proper use of drug. Tell him to use only as directed for full recommended course, even if symptoms disappear, and not to apply near eyes, mouth, or mucous membranes or to use occlusive dressings unless so directed.
● Tell patient to discontinue drug and contact doctor if irritation or sensitivity develops.
● Tell patient to store drug between 41° and 86° F (5° and 30° C).

## terconazole
Terazol 3, Terazol 7

*Pregnancy Risk Category C*

### HOW SUPPLIED
*Vaginal cream:* 0.4%, 0.8%
*Vaginal suppositories:* 80 mg

### ACTION
Unknown. May increase fungal cell membrane permeability (*Candida* species only).

| Route | Onset | Peak | Duration |
|-------|-------|------|----------|
| Intravaginal | Unknown | Unknown | Unknown |

### INDICATIONS & DOSAGE
*Vulvovaginal candidiasis—*
**Adults:** 1 applicator of cream or 1 suppository inserted into vagina h.s.; 0.4% cream used for 7 consecutive days; 0.8% cream or 80-mg suppository for 3 consecutive days. Course repeated, if needed, after reconfirmation by smear or culture.

**ADVERSE REACTIONS**
**CNS:** *headache.*
**GI:** abdominal pain.
**GU:** dysmenorrhea, pain of female genitalia, vulvovaginal burning.
**Skin:** irritation, *pruritus,* photosensitivity.
**Other:** fever, chills, body aches.

**INTERACTIONS**
None significant.

**EFFECTS ON DIAGNOSTIC TESTS**
None reported.

**CONTRAINDICATIONS**
Contraindicated in patients with sensitivity to drug or its inactive ingredients.

**NURSING CONSIDERATIONS**
• Therapeutic effect of drug is unaffected by menstruation or oral contraceptive use.
• *Alert:* Don't confuse terconazole with tioconazole.

☑ **Patient teaching**
• Advise patient to continue treatment during menstrual period. However, tell her not to use tampons.
• Instruct patient to insert drug high in vagina (except during pregnancy).
• Tell patient to use for full treatment period prescribed. Explain how to prevent reinfection.
• Instruct patient to notify doctor and discontinue drug if fever, chills, other flulike symptoms, or sensitivity develops.
• Caution patient to refrain from sexual intercourse during treatment.
• Tell patient that drug base may react with latex, causing decreased effectiveness of condoms and diaphragms (for up to 72 hours after treatment is completed).
• Instruct patient to store drug at room temperature.

---

**tetracycline hydrochloride**
Achromycin, Topicycline

*Pregnancy Risk Category B*

**HOW SUPPLIED**
*Ointment:* 3%
*Topical solution:* 2.2 mg/ml

**ACTION**
Unknown. A broad-spectrum antibiotic that probably disrupts bacterial protein synthesis; usually bacteriostatic.

| Route | Onset | Peak | Duration |
|-------|-------|------|----------|
| Topical | Unknown | Unknown | Unknown |

**INDICATIONS & DOSAGE**
*Acne vulgaris—*
**Adults and children over age 11:** rub solution into affected areas b.i.d. until skin is thoroughly covered.
*Prevention or treatment of superficial skin infections due to susceptible bacteria—*
**Adults:** apply to affected area b.i.d. in morning and evening, or t.i.d.

**ADVERSE REACTIONS**
**Skin:** temporary stinging or burning on application; slight yellowing of treated skin, especially in patients with light complexions; severe dermatitis.

**INTERACTIONS**
**Drug-drug.** *Isotretinoin:* may cause cumulative dryness, resulting in excessive skin irritation. Use cautiously.
**Drug-lifestyle.** *Abrasive or medicated soaps or cleansers; acne products or other preparations containing peeling drugs (benzoyl peroxide, resorcinol, salicylic acid, sulfur, tretinoin); alcohol-containing products (aftershave, cosmetics, perfumed toiletries, shaving creams or lotions); astringent soaps or cosmetics; medicated cosmetics or cover-ups:* may cause cumulative dryness, resulting in excessive skin irritation. Use cautiously.
*Sun exposure:* photosensitivity reactions may occur. Take precautions.

**EFFECTS ON DIAGNOSTIC TESTS**
None reported.

**CONTRAINDICATIONS**
Contraindicated in patients with hypersensitivity to drug or its components.

**NURSING CONSIDERATIONS**
• Use cautiously in patients with hepatic or renal impairment and in breast-feeding women.

---

*Liquid contains alcohol.    **May contain tartrazine.    †Canada    ‡Australia    §U.K.    ◊ OTC

• **Alert:** Don't use in patients with sodium bisulfite sensitivity. Product may contain sulfites that can cause severe or life-threatening allergic reactions, including anaphylaxis and asthmatic episodes, in susceptible patients.
• Prolonged use may result in overgrowth of nonsusceptible organisms.
• Store drug at room temperature, away from excessive heat.
• Don't use ointment to treat acne vulgaris.

### ☑ Patient teaching
• Tell patient to wash area before applying.
• Explain that floating plug in bottle of Topicycline—an inert and harmless result of proper reconstitution of the preparation—shouldn't be removed.
• Teach patient how to increase or decrease applicator pressure against skin to control flow rate of solution.
• Instruct patient to apply generous amount of drug, avoiding eyes, nose, and mouth.
• Inform patient that drug application may cause stinging.
• Tell patient that she may continue normal use of cosmetics.
• Caution patient not to share drug with family members.
• Advise patient to use or discard drug within 2 months.
• Tell patient to discontinue drug and notify doctor if no improvement occurs or if condition worsens.
• Warn patient that yellowing of skin may occur; may be removed by washing.
• Warn patient that drug may stain clothing.
• Tell patient to avoid exposure to sunlight.

## tioconazole
Vagistat-1

*Pregnancy Risk Category C*

### HOW SUPPLIED
*Vaginal ointment:* 6.5%

### ACTION
A fungicidal imidazole that alters cell-wall permeability.

| Route | Onset | Peak | Duration |
|-------|-------|------|----------|
| Intravaginal | Unknown | Unknown | Unknown |

### INDICATIONS & DOSAGE
*Vulvovaginal candidiasis—*
**Adults:** 1 applicator (about 4.6 g) intravaginally h.s. one time only.

### ADVERSE REACTIONS
**GU:** *burning,* discharge, vaginal pain, genital pruritus, dysuria, dyspareunia, vulvar edema, irritation.

### INTERACTIONS
None significant.

### EFFECTS ON DIAGNOSTIC TESTS
None reported.

### CONTRAINDICATIONS
Contraindicated in patients with hypersensitivity to drug or other imidazole antifungal drugs (ketoconazole, miconazole).

### NURSING CONSIDERATIONS
• Not for use as self-medication in pregnant women or in patients with diabetes mellitus, HIV infection, or AIDS. Use only under direction of health care provider.
• It isn't known if drug appears in breast milk; women should temporarily stop breast-feeding while taking drug.
• Notify doctor if patient reports irritation or sensitivity.
• Drug shouldn't be used if patient has abdominal pain, high fever, odorous discharge, vomiting, or diarrhea unless directed by doctor.
• **Alert:** Don't confuse tioconazole with terconazole.

### ☑ Patient teaching
• Review proper use of drug with patient. Written instructions for patient are available with product. Tell patient to insert drug high into vagina (except during pregnancy).
• To avoid contamination of ointment, tell patient to open applicator just before use.

Reactions may be *common*, uncommon, *life-threatening*, or COMMON AND LIFE-THREATENING.

• Tell patient to use sanitary napkins, instead of tampons, to avoid staining clothing.
• Advise patient to avoid sexual intercourse on night after insertion.
• Tell patient that drug may be used during her menstrual period.
• Tell patient that drug base may react with latex, causing decreased effectiveness of condoms and diaphragms (for up to 72 hours after treatment is completed).
• Advise patient to see doctor before self-medicating if symptoms return within 2 months.

---

## tolnaftate

Absorbine Footcare, Aftate for Athlete's Foot◊, Aftate for Jock Itch◊, Athlete's Foot Powder◊, Dr. Scholl's Athlete's Foot◊, Genaspor◊, NP-27◊, Pitrex, Quinsana Plus, Tinactin◊, Ting◊, Zeasorb-AF◊

*Pregnancy Risk Category C*

### HOW SUPPLIED
*Aerosol liquid:* 1% (36% alcohol)◊
*Aerosol powder:* 1% (14% alcohol)◊
*Cream:* 1%◊
*Gel:* 1%◊
*Powder:* 1%◊
*Pump spray liquid:* 1% (36% alcohol)◊
*Topical solution:* 1%◊

### ACTION
Unknown, although has been shown to distort the hyphae and stunt mycelial growth in susceptible fungi.

| Route | Onset | Peak | Duration |
|---|---|---|---|
| Topical | Unknown | Unknown | Unknown |

### INDICATIONS & DOSAGE
*Superficial fungal infections of the skin; infections due to common pathogenic fungi; tinea pedis, tinea cruris, tinea corporis, tinea versicolor—*
**Adults and children:** apply ¼-inch to ½-inch (6-mm to 1.3-cm) ribbon of cream or 2 to 3 drops of solution to cover area; same amount of cream or solution to cover toes and interdigital webs of one foot;

or gel, powder, or spray to cover affected area. Apply drug and massage gently into skin b.i.d. for 2 to 6 weeks.

### ADVERSE REACTIONS
**Skin:** possible irritation.

### INTERACTIONS
None significant.

### EFFECTS ON DIAGNOSTIC TESTS
None reported.

### CONTRAINDICATIONS
Contraindicated in patients with hypersensitivity to drug or its components.

### NURSING CONSIDERATIONS
• Drug isn't used to treat fungal infections of hair or nails; tolnaftate is ineffective against these fungi.
• Drug is odorless and greaseless; it won't stain or discolor skin, hair, nails, or clothing.
• Powder or aerosol may be used inside socks and shoes of persons susceptible to tinea infections.
• Ointments, creams, and liquid are primarily used for treatment; powder and aerosol are adjuncts unless infection is very mild.
• *Alert:* Don't confuse tolnaftate with Tornalate.

### ✅ Patient teaching
• Teach patient to clean area and dry thoroughly before applying drug.
• Tell patient to use drug for full treatment period prescribed, even if condition has improved. Treatment should continue for at least 2 weeks after symptoms have resolved.
• Advise patient to use only small quantity of cream or lotion; treated area shouldn't be wet with solution.
• Tell patient to call doctor if no improvement occurs after 10 days.
• Tell patient to discontinue drug and notify doctor if condition worsens.
• Advise patient to wear shoes and cotton socks that fit well, and to change footwear daily.
• Tell patient to keep drug away from eyes.

---

*\*Liquid contains alcohol.    \*\*May contain tartrazine.    †Canada    ‡Australia    §U.K.    ◊OTC*

**crotamiton**
**lindane**
**permethrin**
**pyrethrins**

**COMBINATION PRODUCTS**
None.

---

### crotamiton
Eurax

*Pregnancy Risk Category C*

**HOW SUPPLIED**
*Cream:* 10%
*Lotion:* 10%

**ACTION**
Unknown.

| Route | Onset | Peak | Duration |
|-------|-------|------|----------|
| Topical | Unknown | Unknown | Unknown |

**INDICATIONS & DOSAGE**
*Parasitic infestation (scabies)—*
**Adults:** scrub entire body with soap and water. Remove scales or crusts. Then apply thin layer of cream over entire body, from chin down (with special attention to skin folds, creases, interdigital spaces, and genital area). Apply second coat in 24 hours. Wait additional 48 hours; then wash off. Treatment is repeated in 7 to 10 days if mites reappear or new lesions develop.
*Itching—*
**Adults:** apply locally, massaging gently into affected area until completely absorbed; repeat, p.r.n.

**ADVERSE REACTIONS**
**Skin:** *irritation,* allergic skin sensitivity.

**INTERACTIONS**
None significant.

**EFFECTS ON DIAGNOSTIC TESTS**
None reported.

**CONTRAINDICATIONS**
Contraindicated in patients with hypersensitivity to drug or its components and in those whose skin is raw or inflamed.

**NURSING CONSIDERATIONS**
• Estimate amount of cream needed per application; most patients tend to overuse scabicides. For most adults, a single tube of cream provides an amount sufficient for two applications.
• Don't apply drug to acutely inflamed or raw, weeping areas.
• Apply topical corticosteroids, as prescribed, if dermatitis develops from scratching.
• Make sure hospitalized patients are placed in isolation, with special linen-handling precautions, until treatment is completed.
• Monthly maintenance treatments may be needed in long-term care facilities, where infestation is a problem.
• *Alert:* Don't confuse Eurax with Serax or Urex.

☑ **Patient teaching**
• Teach patient or family member how to apply drug. Tell patient not to apply to face, eyes, mucous membranes, or urethral meatus. If accidental contact with eyes occurs, tell patient to flush with water and notify doctor.
• Tell patient to discontinue drug, wash it off skin, and notify doctor immediately if skin irritation or hypersensitivity develops.
• Instruct patient to change all clothing and bed linens and launder them in hot cycle of washing machine or dry clean after drug is washed off body.
• Instruct patient to reapply drug if it's washed off during treatment time.
• Tell patient to warn other family members and sexual contacts about infestation. Sexual contacts should be treated simultaneously.
• Reassure patient that, although itching may continue for several weeks, it will

---

Reactions may be *common,* uncommon, *life-threatening*, or COMMON AND LIFE-THREATENING.

stop; continued itching doesn't indicate that therapy is ineffective.

---

## lindane
GBH†, G-well, Kwell, Kwellada†, Scabene

*Pregnancy Risk Category B*

### HOW SUPPLIED
*Lotion:* 1%
*Shampoo:* 1%

### ACTION
Unclear. Appears to inhibit neuronal membrane function in arthropods, causing neuronal hyperactivity, seizures, and death after penetrating the parasite's exoskeleton.

| Route | Onset | Peak | Duration |
|-------|-------|------|----------|
| Topical | 190 min | Unknown | Unknown |

### INDICATIONS & DOSAGE
*Parasitic infestation (scabies, pediculosis)—*
**Adults and children:** Centers for Disease Control and Prevention recommends avoiding bathing before application on skin. If patient does bathe, let skin dry and cool thoroughly before using. For scabies, apply thin layer of cream or lotion over entire skin surface (with special attention to skin folds, creases, interdigital spaces, and genital area) and rub in thoroughly; for pediculosis, apply thin layer of cream or lotion to hairy areas. After 8 to 12 hours, wash off drug. Repeat process in 1 week if mites appear or new lesions develop.

Apply shampoo undiluted to dry hair and work into lather for 4 to 5 minutes; small amounts of water may enhance formation of lather. Apply 30 ml of shampoo for short hair, 45 ml for medium-length hair, or 60 ml for long hair. Rinse thoroughly and rub dry with towel. Comb with a fine-tooth comb.
**Elderly:** may need to reduce dosage because of increased skin absorption.

### ADVERSE REACTIONS
**CNS:** *dizziness, seizures.*

**Skin:** *irritation.*

### INTERACTIONS
**Drug-lifestyle.** *Oils:* may increase absorption of drug; if oil-based hair products are used, hair must be washed and dried before using lindane.

### EFFECTS ON DIAGNOSTIC TESTS
None reported.

### CONTRAINDICATIONS
Contraindicated in patients with hypersensitivity to drug or its components, in those with seizure disorders, and when skin is inflamed. Lotion form is contraindicated in premature neonates.

### NURSING CONSIDERATIONS
• Use cautiously in infants, young children, and elderly patients; all are at greater risk for CNS toxicity.
• Apply topical corticosteroids or administer oral antihistamines, as prescribed, for pruritus.
• Make sure that hospitalized patients are placed in isolation, with special linen-handling precautions, until treatment is completed.
• Modest amounts (6% to 13%) are absorbed through intact skin. Absorption is increased if applied to face, scalp, axillae, neck, scrotum, or irritated or broken skin.
• Avoid contact of drug with eyes.

☑ **Patient teaching**
• Teach patient or family member how to administer drug. Apply thin layer to cover body only once: 1 oz is used for children under age 6 and 1 to 2 oz for older children and adults. Drug shouldn't be left on for more than 12 hours and should be removed thoroughly by washing.
• Inform patient that drug can be poisonous when misused. Warn patient not to apply to open areas, acutely inflamed skin, or to face, eyes, mucous membranes, or urethral meatus. If accidental contact with eyes occurs, advise patient to flush with water and notify doctor.
• Tell patient to avoid inhaling vapors.
• Advise patient to wear gloves if applying to another person.

---

• Tell patient to wash drug off skin and to notify doctor immediately if skin irritation or hypersensitivity develops.
• Discourage repeated use, which can lead to skin irritation, systemic toxicity, or seizures. Advise patient to repeat use only if live lice or nits are found after 1 week.
• Warn patient not to use other creams or oils during treatment because of potential for enhanced absorption.
• Instruct patient to change all clothing and bed linens and launder them in hot water or dry clean after drug is washed off body.
• After application for lice infestation, tell patient to use fine-tooth comb or tweezers to remove nits from hairy areas.
• Advise patient to use lindane shampoo to clean combs or brushes and to wash them thoroughly afterward. Warn patient not to use lindane in such a way routinely.
• Warn patient that itching may continue for several weeks after effective treatment, especially in scabies.
• Instruct patient to reapply drug if it's washed off during treatment time.
• Tell patient to warn other family members and sexual contacts about infestation. Sexual contacts should be treated simultaneously.

---

## permethrin
### Elimite, Lyclear§, Nix

*Pregnancy Risk Category B*

### HOW SUPPLIED
*Topical liquid (cream rinse):* 1%
*Cream:* 5%

### ACTION
Acts on parasites' nerve cells to disrupt the sodium channel current, causing paralysis of parasites.

| Route | Onset | Peak | Duration |
|-------|-------|------|----------|
| Topical | 10-15 min | Unknown | 10 days |

### INDICATIONS & DOSAGE
*Infestation with* Pediculus humanus capitis *(head lice) and its nits*—
**Adults and children ages 2 and older:** use after hair has been washed with shampoo, rinsed with water, and towel-dried. Apply 25 to 50 ml of liquid to saturate the hair and scalp. Allow drug to remain on hair for 10 minutes before rinsing off with water.
*Treatment of* Sarcoptes scabiei—
**Adults and children ages 2 months and older:** thoroughly massage into the skin from the head to the soles. Infants should be treated on the hairline, neck, scalp, temple, and forehead. Cream should be removed after 8 to 14 hours by washing.

### ADVERSE REACTIONS
**Skin:** pruritus, *burning, stinging,* edema, tingling, numbness or scalp discomfort, mild erythema, scalp rash.

### INTERACTIONS
None significant.

### EFFECTS ON DIAGNOSTIC TESTS
None reported.

### CONTRAINDICATIONS
Contraindicated in patients with hypersensitivity to pyrethrins, chrysanthemums, or components of drug.

### NURSING CONSIDERATIONS
• A single treatment is usually needed. Combing of nits isn't needed for effectiveness, but drug package supplies a fine-tooth comb for cosmetic use, as desired.
• Retreat for lice, as prescribed, if lice are observed 7 days after initial application.

### ☑ Patient teaching
• Explain that treatment may temporarily worsen symptoms of head lice infestation, such as pruritus, erythema, and edema.
• Tell patient that headgear, comb and brush, scarves, coats, and bed linens should be disinfected by machine washing with hot water and machine drying for at least 20 minutes, using hot cycle. Nonwashable items should be sealed in plastic bag for 2 weeks, or sprayed with product designed to eliminate lice and their nits.
• Warn patient not to use drug on eyelashes or eyebrows.
• Tell patient to warn other family members and sexual contacts about infestation.

---

Reactions may be *common,* uncommon, *life-threatening,* or COMMON AND LIFE-THREATENING.

Sexual contacts should be treated simultaneously.

---

## pyrethrins
A-200, Barc◇, Blue, End Lice, Pronto, Pyrinyl◇, R & C, RID◇, Tisit◇, Triple X◇

*Pregnancy Risk Category C*

---

### HOW SUPPLIED
*Shampoo:* pyrethrins 0.2% and piperonyl butoxide 2%; pyrethrins 0.3% and piperonyl butoxide 3%; pyrethrins 0.33% and piperonyl butoxide 4%
*Topical gel:* pyrethrins 0.3% and piperonyl butoxide 3%
*Topical solution:* pyrethrins 0.18% and piperonyl butoxide 2%; pyrethrins 0.2%, piperonyl butoxide 2%, and deodorized kerosene 0.8%; pyrethrins 0.3% and piperonyl butoxide 3%; pyrethrins 0.3% and piperonyl butoxide 2%

### ACTION
Acts as contact poison that disrupts parasites' nervous system, causing paralysis and death of parasites.

| Route | Onset | Peak | Duration |
|---|---|---|---|
| Topical | Unknown | Unknown | Unknown |

### INDICATIONS & DOSAGE
*Infestations of head, body, and pubic (crab) lice and their eggs—*
**Adults and children:** apply to hair, scalp, or other infested areas until entirely wet. Allow to remain for 10 minutes but no longer. Wash thoroughly with warm water and soap or shampoo. Remove dead lice and eggs with fine-tooth comb. Treatment repeated, if needed, in 7 to 10 days to kill newly hatched lice; not to exceed two applications within 24 hours.

### ADVERSE REACTIONS
**Skin:** *irritation with repeated use.*

### INTERACTIONS
None significant.

### EFFECTS ON DIAGNOSTIC TESTS
None reported.

### CONTRAINDICATIONS
Contraindicated in patients with hypersensitivity to drug, ragweed, or chrysanthemums.

### NURSING CONSIDERATIONS
• Use cautiously in infants and small children.
• Apply topical corticosteroids or oral antihistamines, as prescribed, if dermatitis develops from scratching.
• Discard container by wrapping in several layers of newspaper.
• Inspect all family members daily for at least 2 weeks for infestation.
• Drug isn't effective against scabies.

### ✅ Patient teaching
• Instruct patient not to apply to open areas, acutely inflamed skin, eyebrows or eyelashes, or face, eyes, mucous membranes, or urethral meatus. If accidental contact with eyes occurs, advise patient to flush with water and notify doctor.
• Tell patient to discontinue drug, wash it off skin, and notify doctor immediately if skin irritation develops. All preparations contain petroleum distillates.
• Instruct patient to change and sterilize all clothing and bed linens after drug is washed off body. Washable items should be disinfected by machine washing in hot water and drying on hot cycle for at least 20 minutes. Other items can be dry cleaned and sealed in plastic bags for 2 weeks, or treated with products made for this purpose.
• Teach patient to remove dead parasites with a fine-tooth comb.
• Urge patient to warn other family members and sexual contacts about infestation. Sexual contacts should be treated simultaneously.

---

**betamethasone dipropionate**
**betamethasone valerate**
**clobetasol propionate**
**desonide**
**desoximetasone**
**dexamethasone**
**dexamethasone sodium phosphate**
**diflorasone diacetate**
**fluocinolone acetonide**
**fluocinonide**
**flurandrenolide**
**fluticasone propionate**
**halcinonide**
**hydrocortisone**
**hydrocortisone acetate**
**hydrocortisone butyrate**
**hydrocortisone valerate**
**mometasone furoate**
**triamcinolone acetonide**

### COMBINATION PRODUCTS
Corticosteroids for topical use are commonly combined with antibiotics and antifungals. (See Chapter 87, LOCAL ANTI-INFECTIVES.)

---

**betamethasone dipropionate**
Alphatrex, Diprolene,
Diprolene AF, Diprosone,
Maxivate

**betamethasone valerate**
Betacap§, Betatrex, Beta-Val,
Betnovate†‡, Luxiq, Valisone

*Pregnancy Risk Category C*

### HOW SUPPLIED
**betamethasone dipropionate**
*Aerosol:* 0.1%
*Cream:* 0.05%
*Gel:* 0.05%
*Lotion:* 0.05%
*Ointment:* 0.05%
**betamethasone valerate**
*Cream:* 0.01%, 0.1%
*Foam:* 0.12%

*Lotion:* 0.1%
*Ointment:* 0.1%

### ACTION
Unclear. Diffuses across cell membranes to form complexes with specific cytoplasmic receptors. Exhibits anti-inflammatory, antipruritic, vasoconstrictive, and antiproliferative activity. Considered a group III (medium-potency) drug according to vasoconstrictive properties.

| Route | Onset | Peak | Duration |
|-------|-------|------|----------|
| Topical | Unknown | Unknown | Unknown |

### INDICATIONS & DOSAGE
*Inflammation and pruritus associated with corticosteroid-responsive dermatoses—*
**Adults and children over age 12:** clean area; apply cream, ointment, lotion, aerosol spray, or gel sparingly. Dipropionate products are given once or twice daily; valerate products are given once daily to q.i.d. Maximum dose for Diprolene cream is 45 g/week and 50 ml/week for Diprolene lotion.
✳ *NEW INDICATION: Relief from inflammatory and pruritic manifestations of corticosteroid-responsive dermatoses of scalp (valerate only)—*
**Adults:** gently massage small amounts of foam into affected scalp areas b.i.d., in morning and evening, until control is achieved. If no improvement is seen within 2 weeks, reassess diagnosis.

### ADVERSE REACTIONS
**GU:** glycosuria with dipropionate.
**Metabolic:** hyperglycemia.
**Skin:** burning, pruritus, irritation, dryness, erythema, folliculitis, striae, acneiform eruptions, perioral dermatitis, hypopigmentation, hypertrichosis, allergic contact dermatitis; secondary infection, maceration, atrophy, miliaria with occlusive dressings.
**Other:** *hypothalamic-pituitary-adrenal axis suppression,* Cushing's syndrome.

---

Reactions may be *common*, uncommon, *life-threatening*, or COMMON AND LIFE-THREATENING.

**INTERACTIONS**
None significant.

**EFFECTS ON DIAGNOSTIC TESTS**
None reported.

**CONTRAINDICATIONS**
Contraindicated in patients with hypersensitivity to corticosteroids.

**NURSING CONSIDERATIONS**
• Gently wash skin before applying. To prevent skin damage, rub in gently, leaving a thin coat. When treating hairy sites, part hair and apply directly to lesions.
• Avoid applying near eyes or mucous membranes or in ear canal, groin area, or axillae.
• Don't dispense foam directly into warm hands because foam will begin to melt upon contact.
• Because of alcohol content of vehicle, gel products may cause mild, transient stinging, especially when used on or near excoriated skin.
• For patients with eczematous dermatitis whose skin may be irritated by adhesive material, hold dressing in place with gauze, elastic bandages, stockings, or stockinette.
• *Alert:* Don't use occlusive dressings.
• If antifungals or antibiotics are used concomitantly without prompt improvement, stop corticosteroid until infection is controlled, as ordered.
• Systemic absorption is likely with use of prolonged or extensive body surface treatment. Watch for symptoms.
• Avoid using plastic pants or tight-fitting diapers on treated areas in young children. Children may absorb larger amounts of drug and be more prone to systemic toxicity.
• Continue drug for a few days after lesions clear.
• *Alert:* Diprolene and Diprolene AF may not be substituted generically because other products have different potencies.

☑ **Patient teaching**
• Teach patient how to apply drug.
• Emphasize that drug is for external use only.

• Tell patient to stop drug and report signs of systemic absorption, skin irritation or ulceration, hypersensitivity, or infection.
• Instruct patient not to use occlusive dressings.
• Discuss personal hygiene measures to reduce chance of infection.

---

**clobetasol propionate**
Dermovate†, Temovate

*Pregnancy Risk Category C*

---

**HOW SUPPLIED**
*Cream:* 0.05%
*Gel:* 0.05%
*Solution:* 0.05%
*Ointment:* 0.05%

**ACTION**
Unclear. Diffuses across cell membranes to form complexes with specific cytoplasmic receptors. Exhibits anti-inflammatory, antipruritic, vasoconstrictive, and antiproliferative activity. Considered a group I (very high-potency) drug according to vasoconstrictive properties.

| Route | Onset | Peak | Duration |
|-------|-------|------|----------|
| Topical | Unknown | Unknown | Unknown |

**INDICATIONS & DOSAGE**
*Inflammation and pruritus associated with corticosteroid-responsive dermatoses—*
**Adults and children ages 12 and older:** apply thin layer to affected skin areas b.i.d., morning and evening, for maximum of 14 days. Total dose shouldn't exceed 50 g weekly.

**ADVERSE REACTIONS**
**GU:** glycosuria.
**Metabolic:** hyperglycemia.
**Skin:** burning, pruritus, irritation, dryness, erythema, folliculitis, perioral dermatitis, allergic contact dermatitis, hypopigmentation, hypertrichosis, acneiform eruptions.
**Other:** *hypothalamic-pituitary-adrenal (HPA) axis suppression,* Cushing's syndrome.

**INTERACTIONS**
None significant.

**EFFECTS ON DIAGNOSTIC TESTS**
None reported.

**CONTRAINDICATIONS**
Contraindicated in patients with hypersensitivity to corticosteroids and in those with primary scalp infections.

**NURSING CONSIDERATIONS**
• Gently wash skin before applying. To prevent skin damage, rub medication in gently and completely. When treating hairy sites, part hair and apply directly to lesions.
• Avoid applying near eyes or mucous membranes or in ear canal.
• *Alert:* Don't use occlusive dressings or bandage. Don't cover or wrap treated areas unless directed by doctor.
• If antifungals or antibiotics are used concomitantly and there isn't prompt improvement, stop corticosteroid until infection is controlled, as ordered.
• Discontinue drug and notify doctor if skin infection, striae, or atrophy occurs.
• HPA axis suppression occurs at doses as low as 2 g per day.

☑ **Patient teaching**
• Teach patient how to apply drug and to avoid contact with eyes.
• Tell patient to stop drug and report signs of systemic absorption, skin irritation or ulceration, hypersensitivity, or infection.
• Warn patient to use drug for no more than 14 consecutive days.

---

**desonide**
DesOwen, Tridesilon

*Pregnancy Risk Category C*

**HOW SUPPLIED**
*Cream:* 0.05%
*Ointment:* 0.05%
*Lotion:* 0.05%

**ACTION**
Unclear. Diffuses across cell membranes to form complexes with specific cytoplasmic receptors. Exhibits anti-inflammatory, antipruritic, vasoconstrictive, and antiproliferative activity. Considered a group IV (low-potency) drug according to vasoconstrictive properties.

| Route | Onset | Peak | Duration |
|-------|-------|------|----------|
| Topical | Unknown | Unknown | Unknown |

**INDICATIONS & DOSAGE**
*Inflammation and pruritus associated with corticosteroid-responsive dermatoses—*
**Adults:** clean area; apply sparingly b.i.d. to q.i.d.

**ADVERSE REACTIONS**
**GU:** glycosuria.
**Metabolic:** hyperglycemia.
**Skin:** burning, pruritus, irritation, dryness, erythema, folliculitis, perioral dermatitis, allergic contact dermatitis, hypertrichosis, hypopigmentation, acneiform eruptions; *maceration of skin, secondary infection, atrophy, striae, miliaria with occlusive dressings.*
**Other:** *hypothalamic-pituitary-adrenal axis suppression,* Cushing's syndrome.

**INTERACTIONS**
None significant.

**EFFECTS ON DIAGNOSTIC TESTS**
None reported.

**CONTRAINDICATIONS**
Contraindicated in patients with hypersensitivity to drug.

**NURSING CONSIDERATIONS**
• Gently wash skin before applying. Rub in gently, leaving a thin coat. When treating hairy sites, part hair and apply directly to lesions.
• Avoid applying near eyes or mucous membranes, or in ear canal.
• For patients with eczematous dermatitis whose skin may be irritated by adhesive material, hold dressing in place with gauze, stockings, or stockinette.
• Change dressing, as ordered. Stop drug and notify doctor if skin infection, striae, or atrophy occurs.
• If occlusive dressing has been applied and a fever develops, notify doctor and remove dressing.

---

• If antifungals or antibiotics are used concomitantly, stop corticosteroid until infection is controlled, as ordered.

• Systemic absorption is likely with use of occlusive dressings, prolonged treatment, or extensive body surface treatment. Watch for symptoms.

• Avoid using plastic pants or tight-fitting diapers on treated areas in young children. Children may absorb larger amounts of drug and be more prone to systemic toxicity.

• Continue treatment for a few days after lesions clear, as ordered.

☑ **Patient teaching**

• Teach patient how to apply drug.

• If an occlusive dressing is ordered, advise patient to leave dressing in place for no more than 12 hours each day, or as ordered, and not to use occlusive dressings on infected or exudative lesions.

• Tell patient to stop drug and report signs of systemic absorption, skin irritation or ulceration, hypersensitivity, or infection.

---

**desoximetasone**
Topicort

*Pregnancy Risk Category C*

**HOW SUPPLIED**
*Cream:* 0.05%, 0.25%
*Gel:* 0.05%
*Ointment:* 0.25%

**ACTION**
Unclear. Diffuses across cell membranes to form complexes with specific cytoplasmic receptors. Exhibits anti-inflammatory, antipruritic, vasoconstrictive, and antiproliferative activity. Considered a group III (medium-potency) drug according to vasoconstrictive properties.

| Route | Onset | Peak | Duration |
|-------|-------|------|----------|
| Topical | Unknown | Unknown | Unknown |

**INDICATIONS & DOSAGE**
*Inflammation associated with corticosteroid-responsive dermatoses—*
**Adults and children:** clean area; apply sparingly b.i.d.

**ADVERSE REACTIONS**
**GU:** glycosuria.
**Metabolic:** hyperglycemia.
**Skin:** burning, pruritus, irritation, dryness, erythema, folliculitis, hypertrichosis, acneiform eruptions, perioral dermatitis, hypopigmentation, allergic contact dermatitis; *maceration, secondary infection, atrophy, striae, miliaria with occlusive dressings.*
**Other:** *hypothalamic-pituitary-adrenal axis suppression,* Cushing's syndrome.

**INTERACTIONS**
None significant.

**EFFECTS ON DIAGNOSTIC TESTS**
None reported.

**CONTRAINDICATIONS**
Contraindicated in patients with hypersensitivity to drug or its components.

**NURSING CONSIDERATIONS**
• Gently wash skin before applying. To prevent skin damage, rub in gently, leaving thin coat. When treating hairy sites, part hair and apply directly to lesions.

• Avoid applying near eyes or mucous membranes, or in ear canal.

• For patients with eczematous dermatitis whose skin may be irritated by adhesive material, hold dressing in place with gauze, elastic bandages, stockings, or stockinette.

• Change dressing, as ordered. Stop drug and notify doctor if skin infection, striae, or atrophy occurs.

• If fever develops and occlusive dressing is in place, notify doctor and remove occlusive dressing.

• If antifungals or antibiotics are used concomitantly, stop corticosteroid until infection is controlled, as ordered.

• Systemic absorption is likely with use of occlusive dressings, prolonged treatment, or extensive body surface treatment. Watch for symptoms.

• Avoid using plastic pants or tight-fitting diapers on treated areas in young children. Children may absorb larger amounts of drug and be more prone to systemic toxicity.

---

• Continue drug for a few days after lesions clear, as ordered.

• Gel contains alcohol and may cause burning or irritation in open lesions.

• *Alert:* Don't confuse desoximetasone with dexamethasone.

### ☑ Patient teaching

• Teach patient how to apply drug.

• If an occlusive dressing is ordered, advise patient to leave dressing in place for no more than 12 hours each day and not to use occlusive dressings on infected or exudative lesions.

• Tell patient to stop drug and report signs of systemic absorption, skin irritation or ulceration, hypersensitivity, or infection.

---

### dexamethasone
Aeroseb-Dex

### dexamethasone sodium phosphate
Decadron Phosphate

*Pregnancy Risk Category C*

### HOW SUPPLIED
**dexamethasone**
*Aerosol:* 0.01%, 0.04%
**dexamethasone sodium phosphate**
*Cream:* 0.1%

### ACTION
Unclear. Diffuses across cell membranes to form complexes with specific cytoplasmic receptors. Exhibits anti-inflammatory, antipruritic, vasoconstrictive, and antiproliferative activity. Considered a group IV (low-potency) drug according to vasoconstrictive properties.

| Route | Onset | Peak | Duration |
|-------|-------|------|----------|
| Topical | Unknown | Unknown | Unknown |

### INDICATIONS & DOSAGE
*Inflammation associated with corticosteroid-responsive dermatoses—*
**Adults and children:** clean area; apply cream or aerosol sparingly t.i.d. or q.i.d.

For aerosol use on scalp, shake can well but gently, and apply to dry scalp after shampooing. Hold can upright or inverted and 6 inches away from area. Spray while moving container to all affected areas, which should take about 2 seconds. Don't massage drug into scalp or spray forehead or near eyes. When result is obtained, reduce dose gradually; then discontinue.

### ADVERSE REACTIONS
**GU:** glycosuria.
**Metabolic:** hyperglycemia.
**Skin:** burning, pruritus, irritation, dryness, erythema, folliculitis, hypertrichosis, acneiform eruptions, perioral dermatitis, hypopigmentation, allergic contact dermatitis; *maceration, secondary infection, atrophy, striae, miliaria with occlusive dressings.*
**Other:** *hypothalamic-pituitary-adrenal axis suppression,* Cushing's syndrome; altered growth and development in children.

### INTERACTIONS
None significant.

### EFFECTS ON DIAGNOSTIC TESTS
None reported.

### CONTRAINDICATIONS
Contraindicated in patients with hypersensitivity to drug or its components.

### NURSING CONSIDERATIONS
• Gently wash skin before applying. To prevent skin damage, rub cream in gently, leaving a thin coat. When treating hairy sites, part hair and apply directly to lesions.

• Avoid applying near eyes or mucous membranes or in ear canal, groin, or axillae.

• For patients with eczematous dermatitis whose skin may be irritated by adhesive material, hold dressing in place with gauze, stockings, or stockinette.

• Change dressing, as ordered. Stop drug and tell doctor if skin infection, striae, or atrophy occurs.

• If an occlusive dressing has been applied and a fever develops, notify doctor and remove dressing.

• When using aerosol around face, cover patient's eyes and warn against inhalation

---

of spray. Aerosol preparation contains alcohol and may produce irritation or burning in open lesions. To avoid freezing tissues, don't spray longer than 1 to 2 seconds or closer than 6 inches (15 cm).
• If antifungals or antibiotics are used concomitantly, stop corticosteroid until infection is controlled, as ordered.
• Systemic absorption is likely with use of occlusive dressings, prolonged treatment, or extensive body surface treatment. Watch for symptoms.
• Avoid using plastic pants or tight-fitting diapers on treated areas in young children. Children may absorb larger amounts of drug and be more prone to systemic toxicity.
• Continue treatment for a few days after lesions clear, as ordered.
• *Alert:* Don't confuse dexamethasone with desoximetasone.

☑ **Patient teaching**
• Teach patient and family how to apply drug.
• If an occlusive dressing is ordered, advise patient to leave in place for no longer than 12 hours each day and not to use occlusive dressings on infected or exudative lesions.
• Tell patient to stop drug and report signs of systemic absorption, skin irritation or ulceration, hypersensitivity, or infection.
• Tell patient to avoid scratching.

---

## diflorasone diacetate
Florone, Florone E, Maxiflor, Psorcon

*Pregnancy Risk Category C*

### HOW SUPPLIED
*Cream:* 0.05%
*Ointment:* 0.05%

### ACTION
Unclear. Diffuses across cell membranes to form complexes with specific cytoplasmic receptors. Exhibits anti-inflammatory, antipruritic, vasoconstrictive, and antiproliferative activity. Considered a group I or

II (very high- or high-potency) drug according to vasoconstrictive properties—

| Route | Onset | Peak | Duration |
|-------|-------|------|----------|
| Topical | Unknown | Unknown | Unknown |

### INDICATIONS & DOSAGE
*Inflammation and pruritus associated with corticosteroid-responsive dermatoses—*
**Adults and children:** clean area; apply sparingly in thin film. Apply cream b.i.d. to q.i.d. and emollient cream and ointment once daily to t.i.d. In children, use lowest dosage that promotes healing.

### ADVERSE REACTIONS
**CV:** hypertension.
**GU:** glycosuria.
**Metabolic:** hyperglycemia.
**Musculoskeletal:** osteoporosis.
**Skin:** burning, pruritus, irritation, dryness, erythema, folliculitis, perioral dermatitis, hypertrichosis, hypopigmentation, acneiform eruptions; *maceration, secondary infection, atrophy, striae, miliaria with occlusive dressings.*
**Other:** *hypothalamic-pituitary-adrenal axis suppression,* Cushing's syndrome.

### INTERACTIONS
None significant.

### EFFECTS ON DIAGNOSTIC TESTS
None reported.

### CONTRAINDICATIONS
Contraindicated in patients with hypersensitivity to drug or its components.

### NURSING CONSIDERATIONS
• Before applying, gently wash skin. To prevent skin damage, rub in gently, leaving a thin coat. When treating hairy sites, part hair and apply directly to lesions. Wear gloves to apply drug.
• Avoid applying near eyes, mucous membranes, or rectum or in ear canal, groin, or axillae.
• For patients with eczematous dermatitis whose skin may be irritated by adhesive material, hold dressing in place with gauze, elastic bandages, stockings, or stockinette.

---

• Change dressing, as ordered. Stop drug and notify doctor if skin infection, striae, or atrophy occurs.
• If occlusive dressing has been applied and a fever develops, notify doctor and remove dressing.
• If antifungals or antibiotics are used concomitantly, stop corticosteroid until infection is controlled, as ordered.
• Systemic absorption is likely with use of occlusive dressings, prolonged treatment, or extensive body surface treatment. Watch for symptoms.
• Avoid using plastic pants or tight-fitting diapers on treated areas in young children. Children may absorb larger amounts of drug and be more prone to systemic toxicity.

☑ **Patient teaching**
• Teach patient how to apply drug.
• Tell patient to wash hands after drug application.
• If an occlusive dressing is ordered, advise patient to leave it in place for no more than 12 hours each day and not to use occlusive dressings on infected or exudative lesions.
• Tell patient to stop drug and report signs of systemic absorption, skin irritation or ulceration, hypersensitivity, or infection.

---

## fluocinolone acetonide
Derma-Smoothe/FS, Fluonid, Flurosyn, FS Shampoo, Metosyn§, Synalar, Synemol

*Pregnancy Risk Category C*

### HOW SUPPLIED
*Cream:* 0.01%, 0.025%, 0.2%
*Oil:* 0.01%
*Ointment:* 0.025%
*Shampoo:* 0.01%
*Topical solution:* 0.01%

### ACTION
Unclear. Diffuses across cell membranes to form complexes with specific cytoplasmic receptors. Exhibits anti-inflammatory, antipruritic, vasoconstrictive, and antiproliferative activity. Considered a group III

(medium-potency) drug according to vasoconstrictive properties.

| Route | Onset | Peak | Duration |
|---|---|---|---|
| Topical | Unknown | Unknown | Unknown |

### INDICATIONS & DOSAGE
*Inflammation associated with corticosteroid-responsive dermatoses—*
**Adults and children:** clean area; apply cream, ointment, or topical solution sparingly b.i.d. to q.i.d.

### ADVERSE REACTIONS
**GU:** glycosuria.
**Metabolic:** hyperglycemia.
**Skin:** burning, pruritus, irritation, dryness, erythema, folliculitis, hypertrichosis, hypopigmentation, acneiform eruptions, perioral dermatitis, allergic contact dermatitis; *maceration, secondary infection, atrophy, striae, miliaria with occlusive dressings.*
**Other:** *hypothalamic-pituitary-adrenal axis suppression,* Cushing's syndrome.

### INTERACTIONS
None significant.

### EFFECTS ON DIAGNOSTIC TESTS
None reported.

### CONTRAINDICATIONS
Contraindicated in patients with hypersensitivity to drug or its components.

### NURSING CONSIDERATIONS
• Gently wash skin before applying. To prevent skin damage, rub in gently, leaving a thin coat. When treating hairy sites, part hair and apply directly to lesions.
• Avoid application near eyes or mucous membranes, in axillae, groin, rectal area, or ear canal if ear drum is perforated.
• For patients with eczematous dermatitis whose skin may be irritated by adhesive material, hold dressing in place with gauze, elastic bandages, stockings, or stockinette.
• Change dressing, as ordered. Stop drug and notify doctor if skin infection, striae, or atrophy occurs.
• If an occlusive dressing has been applied and a fever develops, notify doctor and remove dressing.

---

Reactions may be *common*, uncommon, ***life-threatening***, or COMMON AND LIFE-THREATENING.

• If antifungals or antibiotics are used concomitantly, stop corticosteroid until infection is controlled, as ordered.
• Systemic absorption is likely with use of occlusive dressings, prolonged treatment, or extensive body surface treatment. Watch for symptoms.
• Avoid using plastic pants or tight-fitting diapers on treated areas in young children. Children may absorb larger amounts of drug and be more prone to systemic toxicity.
• Fluonid solution on dry lesions may increase dryness, scaling, or pruritus; on denuded or fissured areas, it may produce burning or stinging. If these signs and symptoms persist and dermatitis hasn't improved, discontinue solution and notify doctor.
• *Alert:* Don't confuse fluocinolone with fluocinonide.

✓ **Patient teaching**
• Teach patient or family how to apply drug using gloves or sterile applicator.
• If an occlusive dressing is ordered, advise patient to leave in place for no more than 12 hours each day and not to use occlusive dressings on infected or exudative lesions.
• Tell patient to stop drug and report signs of systemic absorption, skin irritation or ulceration, hypersensitivity, or infection.

---

**fluocinonide**
Lidex, Lidex-E

*Pregnancy Risk Category C*

## HOW SUPPLIED
*Cream:* 0.05%
*Gel:* 0.05%
*Ointment:* 0.05%
*Topical solution:* 0.05%

## ACTION
Unclear. Diffuses across cell membranes to form complexes with specific cytoplasmic receptors. Exhibits anti-inflammatory, antipruritic, vasoconstrictive, and antiproliferative activity. Considered a group II

(high-potency) drug according to vasoconstrictive properties.

| Route | Onset | Peak | Duration |
|-------|---------|---------|----------|
| Topical | Unknown | Unknown | Unknown |

## INDICATIONS & DOSAGE
*Inflammation associated with corticosteroid-responsive dermatoses*—
**Adults and children:** clean area; apply cream, gel, ointment, or topical solution sparingly b.i.d. or q.i.d. In children, use lowest dosage that promotes healing.

## ADVERSE REACTIONS
**GU:** glycosuria.
**Metabolic:** hyperglycemia.
**Skin:** burning, pruritus, irritation, dryness, erythema, folliculitis, hypertrichosis, hypopigmentation, acneiform eruptions, perioral dermatitis, allergic contact dermatitis; *maceration, secondary infection, atrophy, striae, miliaria with occlusive dressings.*
**Other:** *hypothalamic-pituitary-adrenal axis suppression,* Cushing's syndrome.

## INTERACTIONS
None significant.

## EFFECTS ON DIAGNOSTIC TESTS
None reported.

## CONTRAINDICATIONS
Contraindicated in patients with hypersensitivity to drug or its components.

## NURSING CONSIDERATIONS
• Gently wash skin before applying. To prevent skin damage, rub in gently, leaving a thin coat. When treating hairy sites, part hair and apply directly to lesion.
• Avoid applying near eyes or mucous membranes, or in ear canal.
• For patients with eczematous dermatitis whose skin may be irritated by adhesive material, hold dressing in place with gauze, elastic bandages, stockings, or stockinette.
• Change dressing, as ordered. Stop drug and notify doctor if skin infection, striae, or atrophy occurs.

---

- If an occlusive dressing has been applied and a fever develops, notify doctor and remove dressing.
- If antifungals or antibiotics are used concomitantly, stop drug until infection is controlled, as ordered.
- Systemic absorption is likely with use of occlusive dressings, prolonged treatment, or extensive body surface treatment. Watch for symptoms.
- Avoid using plastic pants or tight-fitting diapers on treated areas in young children. Children may absorb larger amounts of drug and be more prone to systemic toxicity.
- Continue treatment for a few days after lesions clear, as ordered.
- *Alert:* Don't confuse fluocinolone with fluocinonide.

☑ **Patient teaching**
- Teach patient and family how to apply drug using gloves, sterile applicator, or careful hand washing.
- If an occlusive dressing is ordered, advise patient to leave in place no more than 12 hours each day and not to use occlusive dressings on infected or exudative lesions.
- Tell patient to stop drug and report signs of systemic absorption, skin irritation or ulceration, hypersensitivity, or infection.

## flurandrenolide
Cordran, Cordran SP, Drenison Tape†

*Pregnancy Risk Category C*

### HOW SUPPLIED
*Cream:* 0.025%, 0.05%
*Lotion:* 0.05%
*Ointment:* 0.025%, 0.05%
*Tape:* 4 mcg/cm²

### ACTION
Unclear. Diffuses across cell membranes to form complexes with specific cytoplasmic receptors. Exhibits anti-inflammatory, antipruritic, vasoconstrictive, and antiproliferative activity. Considered a group III

(medium-potency) drug according to vasoconstrictive properties.

| Route | Onset | Peak | Duration |
|-------|-------|------|----------|
| Topical | Unknown | Unknown | Unknown |

### INDICATIONS & DOSAGE
*Inflammation and pruritus associated with corticosteroid-responsive dermatoses*—
**Adults and children:** clean area; apply cream, lotion, or ointment sparingly b.i.d. or t.i.d.

Apply Cordran tape q 12 to 24 hours. Before applying tape, clean skin carefully, removing scales, crust, and dried exudate. Let skin dry for 1 hour before applying new tape. Shave or clip hair to allow good contact with skin and comfortable removal. If tape ends loosen prematurely, trim off and replace with fresh tape.

### ADVERSE REACTIONS
**GU:** glycosuria.
**Metabolic:** hyperglycemia.
**Skin:** burning, pruritus, irritation, dryness, erythema, folliculitis, hypertrichosis, hypopigmentation, acneiform eruptions, allergic contact dermatitis; *maceration, secondary infection, atrophy, striae, miliaria with occlusive dressings;* purpura, stripping of epidermis, furunculosis with tape.
**Other:** *hypothalamic-pituitary-adrenal axis suppression,* Cushing's syndrome.

### INTERACTIONS
None significant.

### EFFECTS ON DIAGNOSTIC TESTS
None reported.

### CONTRAINDICATIONS
Contraindicated in patients with hypersensitivity to drug or its components.

### NURSING CONSIDERATIONS
- Gently wash skin before applying. To prevent skin damage, rub in gently, leaving a thin coat. When treating hairy sites, part hair and apply directly to lesions.
- Avoid applying near eyes or mucous membranes, or in ear canal.
- *Alert:* Don't use tape for exudative lesions or lesions in intertriginous areas.

• Don't tear Cordran tape; cut it with scissors. Make sure skin is dry for 1 hour before applying tape.

• Replace tape q 12 hours or, if well tolerated and adherence is satisfactory, q 24 hours.

• For patients with eczematous dermatitis whose skin may be irritated by adhesive material, hold dressing in place with gauze, elastic bandages, stockings, or stockinette.

• Stop drug and tell doctor if skin infection, striae, or atrophy occurs.

• Notify doctor and remove occlusive dressing if fever develops.

• If antifungals or antibiotics are used concomitantly, stop drug until infection is controlled, as ordered.

• Systemic absorption is likely with use of occlusive dressings, prolonged treatment, or extensive body surface treatment. Watch for symptoms.

• Avoid using plastic pants or tight-fitting diapers on treated areas in young children. Children may absorb larger amounts of drug and be more prone to systemic toxicity.

• Continue treatment for a few days after lesions clear, as ordered.

☑ **Patient teaching**
• Teach patient or family how to apply drug.

• If an occlusive dressing is ordered, advise patient to leave in place for no more than 12 hours each day and not to use occlusive dressings on infected or exudative lesions.

• Tell patient to stop drug and report signs of systemic absorption, skin irritation or ulceration, hypersensitivity, or infection.

---

## fluticasone propionate
Cutivate

*Pregnancy Risk Category C*

**HOW SUPPLIED**
*Cream:* 0.05%
*Ointment:* 0.005%

**ACTION**
Exact mechanism unknown. Exhibits anti-inflammatory, antipruritic, and vaso-constrictive activity; considered a medium-potency drug.

| Route | Onset | Peak | Duration |
|-------|-------|------|----------|
| Topical | Rapid | Unknown | 10 hr |

**INDICATIONS & DOSAGE**
*Inflammatory and pruritic manifestations associated with corticosteroid-responsive dermatoses—*
**Adults:** apply sparingly to affected area b.i.d.; rub in gently and completely.
✻ *NEW INDICATION: Relief of inflammatory and pruritic manifestations of atopic dermatitis—*
**Children ages 3 months and older:** apply thin film (0.05%) to affected areas once daily or b.i.d. Rub in gently. Don't use for more than 4 weeks.
✻ *NEW INDICATION: Relief of inflammatory and pruritic manifestations of other corticosteroid-responsive dermatoses—*
**Children ages 3 months and older:** apply a thin film (0.05%) to affected areas b.i.d. Rub in gently. Don't use for more than 4 weeks.

**ADVERSE REACTIONS**
**CNS:** light-headedness.
**GU:** glycosuria.
**Metabolic:** hyperglycemia.
**Skin:** hives, burning, hypertrichosis, pruritus, irritation, erythema.
**Other:** *hypothalamic-pituitary-adrenal axis suppression,* Cushing's syndrome.

**INTERACTIONS**
None significant.

**EFFECTS ON DIAGNOSTIC TESTS**
None reported.

**CONTRAINDICATIONS**
Contraindicated in patients with hypersensitivity to drug or its components and in those with viral, fungal, herpetic, or tubercular skin lesions.

**NURSING CONSIDERATIONS**
• Don't mix drug with other bases or vehicles; this may affect potency.

---

*Liquid contains alcohol.   **May contain tartrazine.   †Canada   ‡Australia   §U.K.   ◇OTC

• If adverse reactions occur, doctor may order less potent drug.
• Discontinue drug, as ordered, if local irritation or systemic infection, absorption, or hypersensitivity occurs.
• Absorption of corticosteroid is enhanced when drug is applied to inflamed or damaged skin, eyelids, or scrotal area; lowest when applied to intact normal skin, palms of hands, or soles of feet.
• Don't use drug with an occlusive dressing or in diaper area.

☑ **Patient teaching**
• Teach patient or family member how to apply drug using gloves, sterile applicator, or careful hand washing.
• Tell patient to avoid prolonged use and contact with eyes. Warn him not to apply on face, in skin creases, or around eyes, genitals, axillae, or rectum.
• Instruct patient to notify doctor if condition persists or worsens or if burning or irritation develops.

---

## halcinonide
Halciderm Topical§, Halog, Halog-E

*Pregnancy Risk Category C*

### HOW SUPPLIED
*Cream:* 0.025%, 0.1%
*Ointment:* 0.1%
*Topical solution:* 0.1%

### ACTION
Unclear. Diffuses across cell membranes to form complexes with cytoplasmic receptors. Exhibits anti-inflammatory, antipruritic, vasoconstrictive, antiproliferative activity. Considered a group II (high-potency) drug according to vasoconstrictive properties.

| Route | Onset | Peak | Duration |
|-------|-------|------|----------|
| Topical | Unknown | Unknown | Unknown |

### INDICATIONS & DOSAGE
*Inflammation associated with corticosteroid-responsive dermatoses—*
**Adults and children:** clean area; apply cream, ointment, or topical solution sparingly b.i.d. or t.i.d. Rub cream in gently.

### ADVERSE REACTIONS
**GU:** glycosuria.
**Metabolic:** hyperglycemia.
**Skin:** burning, pruritus, irritation, dryness, erythema, folliculitis, hypertrichosis, hypopigmentation, acneiform eruptions, allergic contact dermatitis; *maceration, secondary infection, atrophy, striae, miliaria with occlusive dressings.*
**Other:** *hypothalamic-pituitary-adrenal axis suppression,* Cushing's syndrome.

### INTERACTIONS
None significant.

### EFFECTS ON DIAGNOSTIC TESTS
None reported.

### CONTRAINDICATIONS
Contraindicated in patients with hypersensitivity to drug or its components.

### NURSING CONSIDERATIONS
• Gently wash skin before applying. To prevent skin damage, rub in gently, leaving a thin coat. When treating hairy sites, part hair and apply directly to lesions.
• Avoid applying near eyes or mucous membranes or in ear canal, axillae, groin, or rectal area.
• Gently rub small amount of cream into lesion until it disappears. Reapply, leaving a thin coating on lesion, and cover with occlusive dressing, if ordered. Don't leave dressing in place for more than 12 hours each day.
• Don't use occlusive dressings on infected or exudative lesions.
• For patients with eczematous dermatitis whose skin may be irritated by adhesive material, hold dressing in place with gauze, stockings, or stockinette.
• Change dressing, as ordered. Stop drug and tell doctor if skin infection, striae, or atrophy occurs.
• Good results have been obtained by applying occlusive dressings in the evening and removing them in the morning, providing 12-hour occlusion. Then reapply drug; don't apply occlusive dressings during the day.
• If an occlusive dressing has been applied and a fever develops, notify doctor and remove dressing.

---

Reactions may be *common,* uncommon, *life-threatening*, or COMMON AND LIFE-THREATENING.

• If antifungals or antibiotics are used concomitantly, stop corticosteroid until infection is controlled, as ordered.

• Systemic absorption is especially likely with use of occlusive dressings, prolonged treatment, or extensive body surface treatment. Watch for symptoms.

• Avoid using plastic pants or tight-fitting diapers on treated areas in young children. Children may absorb larger amounts of drug and be more prone to systemic toxicity.

• Continue treatment for a few days after lesions clear, as ordered.

✅ **Patient teaching**

• Teach patient how to apply drug.

• If an occlusive dressing is ordered, advise patient to leave in place for no more than 12 hours each day and not to use occlusive dressings on infected or exudative lesions.

• Tell patient to stop drug and report signs of systemic absorption, skin irritation or ulceration, hypersensitivity, or infection.

## hydrocortisone

Acticort 100, Aeroseb-HC, Ala-Cort, Ala-Scalp, Anusol-HC, Bactine Hydrocortisone◊, Carmol-HC, Cetacort, Cort-Dome, Cortef◊, Cortenema, Cortizone-5◊, Cortril, Delacort, Dermacort◊, Dermolate Anti-Itch◊, Dermtex HC, Efcortelan§, Hi-Cor 2.5, Hycort, Hydrocortisyl§, Hydro-Tex, Hytone, LactiCare-HC, Nutracort, Orabase HCA, Penecort, Procort◊, Proctocort, Scalpicin◊, Squibb-HC‡, Synacort, Tegrin-HC◊, Texacort, T/Scalp, Unicort

## hydrocortisone acetate

Anu-Med HC, CaldeCORT Anti-Itch, CortaGel Extra Strength, Cortaid◊, Cortamed†, Cortef, Corticaine, Corticreme†, Cortifoam, Dermacort, Dermol HC, Epifoam, Gynecort, Hemril-HC Uniserts, Lanacort, ProctoCream-HC, Proctofoam-HC

## hydrocortisone butyrate
Locoid

## hydrocortisone valerate
Westcort

*Pregnancy Risk Category C*

## HOW SUPPLIED
**hydrocortisone**
*Cream:* 0.5%◊, 1%◊, 2.5%
*Enema:* 100 mg/60 ml
*Gel:* 1%
*Lotion:* 0.5%◊, 1%, 2%, 2.5%
*Ointment:* 0.5%◊, 1%◊, 2.5%
*Pledgets:* 0.5%
*Rectal cream:* 1%◊
*Rectal ointment:* 1%
*Stick roll-on:* 1%
*Topical solution:* 0.5%, 1%, 2.5%
**hydrocortisone acetate**
*Aerosol:* 1%
*Cream:* 0.5%◊, 1%
*Lotion:* 0.5%◊
*Ointment:* 0.5%◊, 1%
*Paste:* 0.5%
*Solution:* 1%
*Suppositories:* 25 mg, 30 mg
*Rectal foam:* 90 mg per application
**hydrocortisone butyrate**
*Cream:* 0.1%
*Ointment:* 0.1%
*Solution:* 0.1%
**hydrocortisone valerate**
*Cream:* 0.2%
*Ointment:* 0.2%

## ACTION
Unknown. Diffuses across cell membranes to form complexes with specific cytoplasmic receptors. Exhibits anti-inflammatory, antipruritic, vasoconstric-tive, and antiproliferative activity.

| Route | Onset | Peak | Duration |
|-------|-------|------|----------|
| Topical, P.R. | Unknown | Unknown | Unknown |

## INDICATIONS & DOSAGE
*Inflammation and pruritus associated with corticosteroid-responsive dermatoses, adjunctive topical management of seborrheic dermatitis of scalp—*
**Adults and children:** clean area; apply cream, gel, lotion, ointment, or topical so-

lution sparingly daily to q.i.d. Spray aerosol onto affected area daily to q.i.d. until acute phase is controlled; then reduce dosage to one to three times weekly, p.r.n. Children should receive lowest dose that provides positive results.

*Inflammation associated with proctitis—*
**Adults:** 1 applicator of rectal foam P.R. daily or b.i.d. for 2 to 3 weeks; then every other day, p.r.n. Enema is given once nightly for 21 days or until patient improves; may be used for 2 to 3 months if used every other night. Suppositories are inserted b.i.d. for 2 weeks.

## ADVERSE REACTIONS
*Topical use:*
**GU:** glycosuria.
**Metabolic:** hyperglycemia.
**Skin:** burning, pruritus, irritation, dryness, erythema, folliculitis, hypertrichosis, hypopigmentation, acneiform eruptions, allergic contact dermatitis; *maceration, secondary infection, atrophy, striae, miliaria with occlusive dressings.*
**Other:** *hypothalamic-pituitary-adrenal axis suppression,* Cushing's syndrome.
*Rectal use:*
**CNS:** *seizures, increased intracranial pressure,* vertigo, headache.
**CV:** hypertension.
**EENT:** cataracts, glaucoma.
**GI:** peptic ulcer, *pancreatitis,* abdominal distention.
**GU:** menstrual irregularities.
**Metabolic:** fluid or electrolyte disturbances (sodium and fluid retention, potassium loss, hypokalemic alkalosis, negative nitrogen balance due to catabolism of protein), menstrual irregularities, decreased carbohydrate tolerance.
**Musculoskeletal:** muscle weakness, osteoporosis, necrosis and fractures in bone.
**Skin:** impaired wound healing, fragile skin, petechiae, erythema, sweating.

## INTERACTIONS
None significant.

## EFFECTS ON DIAGNOSTIC TESTS
Drug may suppress skin reaction testing.

## CONTRAINDICATIONS
Contraindicated in patients with hypersensitivity to drug or its components.

## NURSING CONSIDERATIONS
● Gently wash skin before applying. To prevent skin damage, rub in gently, leaving a thin coat. When treating hairy sites, part hair and apply directly to lesions.
● Avoid applying near eyes or mucous membranes or in ear canal; may be safely used on face, groin, and armpits and under breasts.
● If an occlusive dressing is applied and a fever develops, notify doctor and remove dressing.
● Change dressing, as ordered. Stop drug and tell doctor if skin infection, striae, or atrophy occurs.
● When using aerosol near the face, cover patient's eyes and warn against inhalation of spray. Aerosol contains alcohol and may produce irritation or burning in open lesions. Don't spray longer than 3 seconds or closer than 6 inches (15 cm) to avoid freezing tissues. If spray is applied to dry scalp after shampooing, drug need not be massaged into scalp.
● If antifungals or antibiotics are used concomitantly, stop corticosteroid drug until infection is controlled, as ordered.
● Systemic absorption is likely with use of occlusive dressings, prolonged treatment, or extensive body surface treatment. Watch for symptoms.
● Avoid using plastic pants or tight-fitting diapers on treated areas in young children. Children may absorb larger amounts of drug and be more prone to systemic toxicity.
● Continue treatment for a few days after lesions clear, as ordered.
● *Alert:* Don't confuse hydrocortisone with hydroxychloroquine.

### ☑ Patient teaching
● Teach patient or family member how to apply drug.
● If an occlusive dressing is ordered, advise patient to leave in place for no more than 12 hours each day and not to use occlusive dressings on infected or exudative lesions.

---

Reactions may be *common*, uncommon, *life-threatening*, or COMMON AND LIFE-THREATENING.

• Tell patient to stop drug and report signs of systemic absorption, skin irritation or ulceration, hypersensitivity, or infection, or if there is no improvement.
• For enema administration, tell patient to lie on left side and retain fluid for 1 hour.
• Instruct patient to insert suppositories blunt end first after removing foil wrapper.
• For perianal application, instruct patient to place small amount of drug on a tissue and gently rub in.
• Tell patient to disassemble applicators or aerosol cap and clean with warm water after each use.

## mometasone furoate
Elocon

*Pregnancy Risk Category C*

### HOW SUPPLIED
*Cream:* 0.1%
*Ointment:* 0.1%
*Lotion:* 0.1%

### ACTION
Unclear. Diffuses across cell membranes to form complexes with specific cytoplasmic receptors. Exhibits anti-inflammatory, antipruritic, vasoconstrictive, and antiproliferative activity. Considered a group III (medium-potency) drug according to vasoconstrictive properties.

| Route | Onset | Peak | Duration |
|-------|-------|------|----------|
| Topical | Unknown | Unknown | Unknown |

### INDICATIONS & DOSAGE
*Inflammation and pruritus associated with corticosteroid-responsive dermatoses—*
**Adults:** apply to affected areas once daily.
**Children ages 2 and older:** apply to affected areas once daily for no more than 3 weeks.

### ADVERSE REACTIONS
**GU:** glycosuria.
**Metabolic:** hyperglycemia.
**Skin:** burning, erythema, pruritus, atrophy, irritation, acneiform eruptions, hypopigmentation, allergic contact dermatitis.
**Other:** *hypothalamic-pituitary-adrenal axis suppression,* Cushing's syndrome.

### INTERACTIONS
None significant.

### EFFECTS ON DIAGNOSTIC TESTS
None reported.

### CONTRAINDICATIONS
Contraindicated in patients with hypersensitivity to drug, its components, or other corticosteroids.

### NURSING CONSIDERATIONS
• Use cautiously in children ages 2 and older.
• Gently wash skin before applying. To prevent skin damage, rub in gently, leaving a thin coat. When treating hairy sites, part hair and apply directly to lesions.
• Don't apply near eyes or mucous membranes or in ear canal, axillae, groin, or rectal area.
• *Alert:* Don't use occlusive dressings.
• Systemic absorption is likely with use of occlusive dressings, prolonged treatment, or extensive body surface treatment. Watch for symptoms.
• If antimicrobials are used concomitantly, stop corticosteroid drug until infection is controlled, as ordered.
• Avoid using plastic pants or tight-fitting diapers on treated areas in young children; they may absorb larger amounts of drug and be more prone to systemic toxicity. Don't use cream or ointment on diaper area.

☑ **Patient teaching**
• Teach patient or family member how to apply drug.
• Tell patient to stop drug and report signs of systemic absorption, skin irritation or ulceration, hypersensitivity, or infection, or if there is no improvement in 2 weeks.

## triamcinolone acetonide
Adcortyl§, Aristocort, Delta-Tritex, Flutex, Kenalog, Kenalone‡, Triacet, Triderm

*Pregnancy Risk Category C*

### HOW SUPPLIED
*Aerosol:* 0.2 mg/2-second spray

*Cream:* 0.02%‡, 0.025%, 0.1%, 0.5%
*Lotion:* 0.025%, 0.1%
*Ointment:* 0.02%‡, 0.025%, 0.1%, 0.5%
*Paste:* 0.1%
*Solution:* 0.1%

## ACTION
Unclear. Diffuses across cell membranes to form complexes with specific cytoplasmic receptors. Exhibits anti-inflammatory, antipruritic, vasoconstrictive, and antiproliferative activity. Considered a group III (medium-potency) drug according to vasoconstrictive properties.

| Route | Onset | Peak | Duration |
|-------|-------|------|----------|
| Topical | Several hr | Unknown | ≥ 1 wk |

## INDICATIONS & DOSAGE
*Inflammation and pruritus associated with corticosteroid-responsive dermatoses—*
**Adults and children:** clean area; apply aerosol, cream, lotion, or ointment sparingly b.i.d. to q.i.d. Rub in lightly.
*Inflammation associated with oral lesions—*
**Adults and children:** apply paste h.s. and, if needed, b.i.d. or t.i.d., preferably after meals. Apply small amount without rubbing and press to lesion in mouth until thin film develops.

## ADVERSE REACTIONS
**CV:** syncope.
**GU:** glycosuria.
**Metabolic:** hyperglycemia.
**Skin:** burning, pruritus, irritation, dryness, erythema, folliculitis, hypertrichosis, hypopigmentation, acneiform eruptions, perioral dermatitis, allergic contact dermatitis; *maceration, secondary infection, atrophy, striae, miliaria with occlusive dressings.*
**Other:** *hypothalamic-pituitary-adrenal axis suppression,* Cushing's syndrome.

## INTERACTIONS
None significant.

## EFFECTS ON DIAGNOSTIC TESTS
None reported.

## CONTRAINDICATIONS
Contraindicated in patients with hypersensitivity to drug or its components.

## NURSING CONSIDERATIONS
● Gently wash skin before applying. To avoid skin damage, rub in gently, leaving a thin coat. When treating hairy sites, part hair and apply directly to lesions.
● Don't apply near eyes or in ear canal.
● Change dressing, as ordered. Stop drug and tell doctor if skin infection, striae, or atrophy occurs.
● When using aerosol near the face, cover patient's eyes and warn against inhalation of spray. Aerosol contains alcohol and may produce irritation or burning in open lesions. Don't spray longer than 3 seconds or closer than 6 inches (15 cm) to avoid freezing tissues.
● If antifungals or antibiotics are used concomitantly, stop corticosteroid until infection is controlled, as ordered.
● Systemic absorption is likely with the use of occlusive dressings, prolonged treatment, or extensive body surface treatment. Watch for symptoms.
● Avoid using plastic pants or tight-fitting diapers on treated areas in young children. Children may absorb larger amounts of drug and be more prone to systemic toxicity.
● *Alert:* Don't confuse triamcinolone with Triaminicin or Triaminicol.

☑ **Patient teaching**
● Teach patient or family member how to apply drug.
● If an occlusive dressing is ordered, advise patient to leave in place for no more than 12 hours each day and not to use occlusive dressings on infected or exudative lesions.
● Tell patient to stop drug and report signs of systemic absorption, skin irritation or ulceration, hypersensitivity, or infection, or if there is no improvement.

---

Reactions may be *common*, uncommon, *life-threatening*, or COMMON AND LIFE-THREATENING.

**vitamin A**
*vitamin B complex*
  cyanocobalamin
  folic acid
  hydroxocobalamin
  leucovorin calcium
  niacin
  niacinamide
  pyridoxine hydrochloride
  riboflavin
  thiamine hydrochloride
**vitamin C**
*vitamin D*
  cholecalciferol
  ergocalciferol
*vitamin D analogue*
  doxercalciferol
  paricalcitol
**vitamin E**
*vitamin K analogue*
  phytonadione
**sodium fluoride**
**sodium fluoride, topical**
*trace elements*
  chromium
  copper
  iodine
  manganese
  selenium
  zinc

## VITAMIN COMBINATION PRODUCTS
B complex vitamins ◇
B complex vitamins with iron ◇
B complex with vitamin C ◇
B vitamin combinations ◇
Calcium and vitamin products ◇
Fluoride with vitamins ◇
Geriatric supplements with multivitamins and minerals ◇
Miscellaneous vitamins and minerals ◇
Multivitamins ◇
Multivitamins and minerals with hormones ◇
Multivitamins with $B_{12}$ ◇
Vitamin A and D combinations ◇

## TRACE ELEMENT COMBINATION PRODUCTS
MULTIPLE TRACE ELEMENT PEDIATRIC: zinc sulfate 0.5 mg, copper sulfate 0.1 mg, manganese sulfate 0.03 mg, and chromium chloride 1 mcg per ml.
MULTIPLE TRACE ELEMENT NEONATAL: zinc sulfate 1.5 mg, copper sulfate 0.1 mg, manganese sulfate 0.025 mg, chromium chloride 0.85 mcg.
MULTIPLE TRACE ELEMENT WITH SELENI-UM: zinc sulfate 1 mg, copper sulfate 0.4 mg, manganese sulfate 0.1 mg, chromium chloride 4 mcg, and selenious acid 20 mcg.
NEOTRACE-4: zinc sulfate 1.5 mg, copper sulfate 0.1 mg, manganese sulfate 0.025 mg, and chromium chloride 0.85 mcg per ml.
PEDTRACE-4: zinc sulfate 0.5 mg, copper sulfate 0.1 mg, manganese sulfate 0.025 mg, and chromium chloride 0.85 mcg per ml.
PTE-4: zinc sulfate 1 mg, copper sulfate 0.1 mg, manganese sulfate 0.025 mg, and chromium chloride 1 mcg per ml.
PTE-5: zinc sulfate 1 mg, copper sulfate 0.1 mg, manganese sulfate 0.025 mg, chromium chloride 1 mcg, and selenium (as selenious acid) 15 mcg per ml.
TRACE METALS ADDITIVE: zinc chloride 0.8 mg, copper chloride 0.2 mg, manganese chloride 0.16 mg, and chromium chloride 2 mcg per ml.

---

## vitamin A (retinol)
Aquasol A, Del-Vi-A

*Pregnancy Risk Category C*

### HOW SUPPLIED
*Tablets:* 5,000 IU ◇, 10,000 IU
*Capsules:* 10,000 IU ◇, 25,000 IU, 50,000 IU
*Drops:* 30 ml with dropper (5,000 IU/ 0.1 ml, 50,000 IU/1 ml)
*Injection:* 2-ml vials (50,000 IU/ml with 0.5% chlorobutanol, polysorbate 80, buty-

lated hydroxyanisole, and butylated hydroxytoluene)

## ACTION
A coenzyme that stimulates retinal function, bone growth, reproduction, and integrity of epithelial and mucosal tissues.

| Route | Onset | Peak | Duration |
|-------|-------|------|----------|
| P.O. | Unknown | 3-5 hr | Unknown |
| I.M. | Unknown | Unknown | Unknown |

## INDICATIONS & DOSAGE
*Note:* RDAs have been converted to REs. One RE has the activity of 1 mcg *all-trans* retinol, 6 mcg beta carotene.
**Neonates and infants up to age 1:**
375 mcg RE or 1,250 IU.
**Children ages 1 to 3:** 400 mcg RE or 1,330 IU.
**Children ages 4 to 6:** 500 mcg RE or 1,665 IU.
**Children ages 7 to 10:** 700 mcg RE or 2,330 IU.
**Men over age 11:** 1,000 mcg RE or 3,330 IU.
**Women over age 11:** 800 mcg RE or 2,665 IU.
**Pregnant women:** 800 mcg RE or 2,665 IU.
**Breast-feeding women (first 6 months):** 1,300 mcg RE or 4,330 IU.
**Breast-feeding women (second 6 months):** 1,200 mcg RE or 4,000 IU.
*Severe vitamin A deficiency—*
**Adults and children over age 8:**
100,000 IU I.M. or 100,000 to 500,000 IU P.O. for 3 days; then 50,000 IU I.M. or P.O. for 2 weeks, followed by 10,000 to 20,000 IU P.O. for 2 months. Follow with adequate dietary nutrition and RE vitamin A supplements.
**Children ages 1 to 8:** 17,500 to 35,000 IU I.M. daily for 10 days.
**Infants under age 1:** 7,500 to 15,000 IU I.M. daily for 10 days.
*Maintenance dose to prevent recurrence of vitamin A deficiency—*
**Children ages 1 to 8:** 5,000 to 10,000 IU P.O. daily for 2 months; then adequate dietary nutrition and RE vitamin A supplements.

## ADVERSE REACTIONS
Adverse reactions usually occur only with toxicity.
**CNS:** irritability, headache, ***increased intracranial pressure,*** fatigue, lethargy, malaise.
**EENT:** papilledema, exophthalmos.
**GI:** anorexia, epigastric pain, vomiting, polydipsia.
**GU:** hypomenorrhea, polyuria.
**Hepatic:** jaundice, hepatomegaly, ***cirrhosis,*** elevated liver enzyme levels.
**Metabolic:** slow growth, decalcification, hypercalcemia, periostitis, premature closure of epiphyses, migratory arthralgia, cortical thickening over the radius and tibia.
**Skin:** alopecia; dry, cracked, scaly skin; pruritus; lip fissures; erythema; inflamed tongue, lips, and gums; massive desquamation; increased pigmentation; night sweats.
**Other:** splenomegaly, ***anaphylactic shock.***

## INTERACTIONS
**Drug-drug.** *Cholestyramine resin, mineral oil:* reduced GI absorption of fat-soluble vitamins. Avoid concomitant use.
*Isotretinoin, multivitamins containing vitamin A:* increased risk of toxicity. Avoid concomitant use.
*Neomycin (oral):* decreased vitamin A absorption. Avoid concomitant use.
*Oral contraceptives:* may increase plasma vitamin A levels. Monitor closely.
*Warfarin:* increased risk of bleeding. Monitor PT and INR closely.

## EFFECTS ON DIAGNOSTIC TESTS
Vitamin A therapy may falsely increase serum cholesterol levels by interfering with the Zlatkis-Zak reaction. It also has been reported to falsely elevate bilirubin determinations with Ehrlich's reagent.

## CONTRAINDICATIONS
Contraindicated orally in patients with malabsorption syndrome; if malabsorption is due to inadequate bile secretion, oral route may be used with concurrent administration of bile salts (dehydrocholic acid). Also contraindicated in patients with hypersensitivity to any ingredient in product and in those with hypervitaminosis A. I.V.

---

route contraindicated except for special water-miscible forms intended for infusion with large parenteral volumes. I.V. push of vitamin A of any type is also contraindicated (anaphylaxis or anaphylactoid reactions and death have resulted).

## NURSING CONSIDERATIONS
• *Alert:* Give parenteral form by I.M. route or continuous I.V. infusion (that is, in total parenteral nutrition infusion). Never give as I.V. bolus.
• Use cautiously in pregnant patients, avoiding doses exceeding RE.
• Assess patient's vitamin A intake from all sources.
• Liquid products are available for NG route. Preparation may be mixed with cereal or fruit juice.
• Vitamin may be administered I.M. for malabsorption syndrome or when oral administration isn't feasible.
• Adequate vitamin A absorption needs suitable dietary protein, fat, vitamin E, and zinc intake and bile secretion; give supplemental salts, as ordered. Zinc supplements may be needed in patients receiving long-term total parenteral nutrition.
• Watch for adverse reactions if dosage is high.
• Acute toxicity has resulted from single doses of 25,000 IU/kg of body weight; 350,000 IU in infants and over 2 million IU in adults have also proved acutely toxic. Doses that don't exceed RE are usually nontoxic.
• Chronic toxicity in infants (ages 3 to 6 months) has resulted from doses of 18,500 IU daily for 1 to 3 months. In adults, chronic toxicity has resulted from doses of 50,000 IU daily for over 18 months, 500,000 IU daily for 2 months, and 1 million IU daily for 3 days.
• Watch for skin disorders; high dosages may induce chronic toxicity.

☑ **Patient teaching**
• Tell patient not to take megadoses of vitamins without specific indications to avoid toxicity.
• Stress that prescribed vitamins shouldn't be shared with others.
• Instruct patient to protect drug from light.

• Teach patient about good food sources of vitamin A, such as green and yellow vegetables, cantaloupe, and liver (note that liver is also high in saturated fat).
• Advise patient that liquid product can be mixed with food, if desired.
• Tell patient to notify doctor of signs of overdose (nausea, vomiting, anorexia, malaise, dry and cracking skin and lips, irritability, hair loss, headache, visual disturbances, vertigo, bulging fontanelles in infants).

---

# cyanocobalamin (vitamin B$_{12}$)
Crystamine, Crysti-12, Cyanocobalamin, Cyanoject, Cyomin, Rubesol-1000, Rubramin PC

# hydroxocobalamin (vitamin B$_{12}$)
Hydrobexan, Hydro-Cobex, Hydro-Crysti 12, LA-12

*Pregnancy Risk Category C (if doses exceed RDA)*

---

## HOW SUPPLIED
**cyanocobalamin**
*Tablets:* 25 mcg ◊, 50 mcg ◊, 100 mcg ◊, 250 mcg ◊, 500 mcg ◊, 1,000 mcg ◊
*Injection:* 1,000 mcg/ml
**hydroxocobalamin**
*Injection:* 100 mcg, 1,000 mcg/ml

## ACTION
A coenzyme that stimulates metabolic function and is needed for cell replication, hematopoiesis, and nucleoprotein and myelin synthesis.

| Route | Onset | Peak | Duration |
|-------|-------|------|----------|
| P.O. | Unknown | 8-12 hr | Unknown |
| I.M., S.C. | Unknown | 1 hr | Unknown |

## INDICATIONS & DOSAGE
*RDA for cyanocobalamin—*
**Neonates and infants up to age 6 months:** 0.3 mcg.
**Infants ages 6 months to 1 year:** 0.5 mcg.
**Children ages 1 to 3:** 0.7 mcg.

---

**Children ages 4 to 6:** 1 mcg.
**Children ages 7 to 10:** 1.4 mcg.
**Adults and children ages 11 and older:** 2 mcg.
**Pregnant women:** 2.2 mcg.
**Breast-feeding women:** 2.6 mcg.
*Vitamin B$_{12}$ deficiency due to inadequate diet, subtotal gastrectomy, or other conditions, disorder, or disease except malabsorption related to pernicious anemia or other GI disease—*
**Adults:** 30 mcg hydroxocobalamin I.M. daily for 5 to 10 days, depending on severity of deficiency. Maintenance dose is 100 to 200 mcg I.M. once monthly. For subsequent prophylaxis, advise adequate nutrition and daily RDA vitamin B$_{12}$ supplements.
**Children:** 1 to 5 mg hydroxocobalamin given over 2 or more weeks in doses of 100 mcg I.M., depending on severity of deficiency. Maintenance dose is 30 to 50 mcg/month I.M. For subsequent prophylaxis, advise adequate nutrition and daily RDA vitamin B$_{12}$ supplements.
*Pernicious anemia or vitamin B$_{12}$ malabsorption—*
**Adults:** initially, 100 mcg cyanocobalamin I.M. or S.C. daily for 6 to 7 days; then 100 mcg I.M. or S.C. monthly.
**Children:** 30 to 50 mcg I.M. or S.C. daily over 2 or more weeks; then 100 mcg I.M. or S.C. monthly for life.
*Methylmalonicaciduria—*
**Neonates:** 1,000 mcg cyanocobalamin I.M. daily.
*Schilling test flushing dose—*
**Adults and children:** 1,000 mcg hydroxocobalamin I.M. as single dose.

## ADVERSE REACTIONS
**CV:** peripheral vascular thrombosis, pulmonary edema, *heart failure.*
**GI:** transient diarrhea.
**Skin:** itching, transitory exanthema, urticaria.
**Other:** *anaphylaxis, anaphylactoid reactions with parenteral administration;* pain, burning at S.C. or I.M. injection sites.

## INTERACTIONS
**Drug-drug.** *Aminoglycosides, anticonvulsants, colchicine, extended-release potassium products, aminosalicylic acid and*
*salts:* malabsorption of vitamin B$_{12}$. Don't use concomitantly.
**Drug-lifestyle.** *Alcohol use:* malabsorption of vitamin B$_{12}$. Don't use concomitantly.

## EFFECTS ON DIAGNOSTIC TESTS
Vitamin B$_{12}$ may cause false-positive results for intrinsic factor antibodies, which are present in the blood of half of all patients with pernicious anemia. Methotrexate, pyrimethamine, and most anti-infectives invalidate diagnostic blood assays for vitamin B$_{12}$.

## CONTRAINDICATIONS
Contraindicated in patients with hypersensitivity to vitamin B$_{12}$ or cobalt and in those with early Leber's disease.

## NURSING CONSIDERATIONS
• Use cautiously in anemic patients with coexisting cardiac, pulmonary, or hypertensive disease and in patients with severe vitamin B$_{12}$–dependent deficiencies.
• Use cautiously in premature infants; product may contain benzyl alcohol, which may cause "gasping syndrome."
• Determine reticulocyte count, hematocrit, vitamin B$_{12}$, iron, and folate levels before beginning therapy, as ordered.
• *Alert:* Avoid I.V. administration because of more rapid systemic elimination with resulting decreased utilization.
• Don't mix parenteral preparations in same syringe with other drugs.
• Drug is physically incompatible with dextrose solutions, alkaline or strongly acidic solutions, oxidizing or reducing agents, heavy metals, chlorpromazine, phytonadione, prochlorperazine, and other drugs.
• Hydroxocobalamin is approved for I.M. or deep S.C. use only. Its only advantage over cyanocobalamin is its longer duration.
• Don't give large oral doses of B$_{12}$ routinely; drug is lost through excretion.
• Closely monitor serum potassium levels for first 48 hours. Give potassium supplement, if ordered.
• Infection, tumors, or renal, hepatic, and other debilitating diseases may reduce therapeutic response.

---

Reactions may be *common,* uncommon, *life-threatening,* or COMMON AND LIFE-THREATENING.

• Deficiencies are more common in patients who are strict vegetarians and in their breast-fed infants.
• Vitamin $B_{12}$ deficiency may suppress symptoms of polycythemia vera.
• Protect vitamin $B_{12}$ from light. Don't refrigerate or freeze.

### ☑ Patient teaching
• Stress need for patient with pernicious anemia to return for monthly injections. Although total body stores may last 3 to 6 years, anemia will recur if not treated monthly.
• Stress importance of follow-up visits and laboratory studies.
• Teach patient healthy dietary habits.

---

## folic acid (vitamin $B_9$)
Folvite, Novo-Folacid†

*Pregnancy Risk Category A*

### HOW SUPPLIED
*Tablets:* 0.4 mg, 0.8 mg, 1 mg
*Injection:* 10-ml vials (5 mg/ml with 1.5% benzyl alcohol, 5 mg/ml with 1.5% benzyl alcohol and 0.2% EDTA)

### ACTION
Stimulates normal erythropoiesis and nucleoprotein synthesis.

| Route | Onset | Peak | Duration |
|---|---|---|---|
| P.O., I.M., S.C. | Unknown | 30-60 min | Unknown |

### INDICATIONS & DOSAGE
*RDA—*
**Neonates and infants up to age 6 months:** 25 mcg.
**Infants ages 6 months to 1 year:** 35 mcg.
**Children ages 1 to 3:** 50 mcg.
**Children ages 4 to 6:** 75 mcg.
**Children ages 7 to 10:** 100 mcg.
**Children ages 11 to 14:** 150 mcg.
**Men ages 15 and older:** 200 mcg.
**Women ages 15 and older:** 180 mcg.
**Pregnant women:** 800 mcg.
**Breast-feeding women:** 800 mcg.
*Megaloblastic or macrocytic anemia secondary to folic acid or other nutritional deficiency, hepatic disease, alcoholism, intestinal obstruction, excessive hemolysis—*
**Adults and children over age 4:** 0.4 to 1 mg P.O., S.C., or I.M. daily. After anemia secondary to folic acid deficiency is corrected, proper diet and RDA supplements are needed to prevent recurrence.
**Children under age 4:** up to 0.3 mg P.O., S.C., or I.M. daily.
**Pregnant and breast-feeding women:** 0.8 mg P.O., S.C., or I.M. daily.
*Prevention of megaloblastic anemia during pregnancy to prevent fetal damage—*
**Adults:** up to 1 mg P.O., S.C., or I.M. daily throughout pregnancy.
*Nutritional supplement—*
**Adults:** 0.1 mg P.O., S.C., or I.M. daily.
**Children:** 0.05 mg P.O. daily.
*Test for folic acid deficiency in patients with megaloblastic anemia without masking pernicious anemia—*
**Adults and children:** 0.1 to 0.2 mg P.O. or I.M. for 10 days while maintaining a diet low in folate and vitamin $B_{12}$.
*Tropical sprue—*
**Adults:** 3 to 15 mg P.O. daily.

### ADVERSE REACTIONS
**CNS:** altered sleep pattern, general malaise, difficulty concentrating, confusion, impaired judgment, irritability, overactivity.
**GI:** anorexia, nausea, flatulence, bitter taste.
**Respiratory:** *bronchospasm.*
**Skin:** allergic reactions including rash, pruritus, and erythema.

### INTERACTIONS
**Drug-drug.** *Aminosalicylic acid, chloramphenicol, methotrexate, oral contraceptives, sulfasalazine, trimethoprim:* antagonism of folic acid. Watch for decreased folic acid effect. Use together cautiously. *Phenytoin:* increased anticonvulsant metabolism causing decreased blood levels of the anticonvulsant. Monitor closely.

### EFFECTS ON DIAGNOSTIC TESTS
Drug alters serum and RBC folate levels; falsely low serum and RBC folate levels may occur with *Lactobacillus casei* assay in patients receiving anti-infectives such

as tetracycline that suppress growth of this organism.

### CONTRAINDICATIONS

Contraindicated in patients with undiagnosed anemia (it may mask pernicious anemia) and in those with $B_{12}$ deficiency.

### NURSING CONSIDERATIONS

• The U.S. Public Health Service recommends use of folic acid during pregnancy to decrease neural tube defects.
• Don't mix with other drugs in same syringe for I.M. injections.
• Patients with small-bowel resections and intestinal malabsorption may need parenteral administration.
• Protect drug from light and heat; store at room temperature.
• *Alert:* Don't confuse folic acid with folinic acid.

### ☑ Patient teaching

• Teach patient about proper nutrition to prevent recurrence of anemia.
• Stress importance of follow-up visits and laboratory studies.
• Teach patient about foods that contain folic acid: liver, oranges, whole wheat, broccoli, brussels sprouts.

---

## leucovorin calcium (citrovorum factor, folinic acid)
Wellcovorin

*Pregnancy Risk Category C*

### HOW SUPPLIED

*Tablets:* 5 mg, 10 mg, 15 mg, 25 mg
*Injection:* 1-ml ampule (3 mg/ml with 0.9% benzyl alcohol)
*Powder for injection:* 50-mg vial, 100-mg vial, 350-mg vial

### ACTION

A reduced form of folic acid that is readily converted to other folic acid derivatives.

| Route | Onset | Peak | Duration |
|-------|-------|------|----------|
| P.O. | 20-30 min | 2-3 hr | 3-6 hr |
| I.V. | 5 min | 10 min | 3-6 hr |
| I.M. | 10-20 min | < 1 hr | 3-6 hr |

### INDICATIONS & DOSAGE

*Overdose of folic acid antagonist (methotrexate or trimethoprim)—*
**Adults and children:** P.O., I.M., or I.V. dose equivalent to weight of antagonist given.
*Leucovorin rescue after high methotrexate dose in treatment of malignant disease—*
**Adults and children:** 10 mg/m² P.O., I.M., or I.V. q 6 hours until methotrexate levels fall below $5 \times 10^{-8}$ M.
*Megaloblastic anemia due to congenital enzyme deficiency—*
**Adults and children:** 3 to 6 mg I.M.; then 1 mg P.O. or I.M. daily for life.
*Folate-deficient megaloblastic anemia—*
**Adults and children:** up to 1 mg leucovorin I.M daily. Duration of treatment depends on hematologic response.
*Prevention of hematologic toxicity due to pyrimethamine or trimethoprim therapy—*
**Adults and children:** 400 mcg to 5 mg I.M. with each dose of folic acid antagonist.
*Hematologic toxicity due to pyrimethamine or trimethoprim therapy—*
**Adults and children:** 5 to 15 mg I.M. daily.
*Palliative treatment of advanced colorectal cancer—*
**Adults:** 20 mg/m² I.V.; then fluorouracil 425 mg/m² I.V. or 200 mg/m² I.V. (over 3 minutes or longer) followed by fluorouracil 370 mg/m² daily for 5 consecutive days. Repeated at 4-week intervals for two additional courses; then at intervals of 4 to 5 weeks, if tolerated.

### ADVERSE REACTIONS

**Skin:** urticaria.
**Other:** *hypersensitivity reactions, anaphylactoid reactions.*

### INTERACTIONS

**Drug-drug.** *Anticonvulsants:* may decrease effectiveness of these drugs. Monitor patient.
*Fluorouracil:* may enhance fluorouracil toxicity. Fluorouracil dose may need to be reduced.
*Methotrexate:* high doses of leucovorin may decrease efficacy of intrathecal methotrexate. Monitor effects.

---

Reactions may be *common*, uncommon, *life-threatening*, or COMMON AND LIFE-THREATENING.

## EFFECTS ON DIAGNOSTIC TESTS
Drug may mask diagnosis of pernicious anemia.

## CONTRAINDICATIONS
Contraindicated in patients with pernicious anemia and other megaloblastic anemias secondary to lack of vitamin $B_{12}$.

## NURSING CONSIDERATIONS
- I.V. route is preferred in patients with GI toxicity when doses exceed 25 mg.
- Follow leucovorin rescue schedule and protocol closely.
- Don't administer leucovorin with systemic methotrexate.
- Protect from light and heat; maintain protection and immediately administer reconstituted parenteral drug.
- *Alert:* Don't confuse leucovorin (folinic acid) with folic acid.

## ◗ I.V. administration
- When using powder for injection, reconstitute 50-mg vial with 5 ml, 100-mg vial with 10 ml, or 350-mg vial with 17 ml of sterile or bacteriostatic water for injection. When doses exceed 10 mg/m², don't use diluents containing benzyl alcohol.
- *Alert:* Don't exceed 160 mg/minute when giving by direct injection.

## ☑ Patient teaching
- Explain need for drug to patient and family, and answer any questions or concerns.
- Tell patient to report symptoms of hypersensitivity promptly.

---

## niacin (nicotinic acid, vitamin $B_3$)
Nia-Bid◇, Niacor◇, Niaspan, Nico-400, Nicobid◇, Nicolar**, Nicotinex, Slo-Niacin◇

## niacinamide (nicotinamide)◇

*Pregnancy Risk Category C*

## HOW SUPPLIED
**niacin**
*Tablets:* 25 mg◇, 50 mg◇, 100 mg◇, 250 mg◇, 500 mg

*Tablets (timed-release):* 250 mg◇, 375 mg◇, 500 mg◇, 750 mg◇, 1,000 mg◇
*Capsules (timed-release):* 125 mg◇, 250 mg◇, 300 mg◇, 400 mg◇, 500 mg
*Elixir:* 50 mg/5 ml◇
*Injection:* 100 mg/ml in 30-ml vials
**niacinamide**
*Tablets:* 50 mg◇, 100 mg◇, 125 mg◇, 250 mg◇, 500 mg◇

## ACTION
Stimulate lipid metabolism, tissue respiration, and glycogenolysis; niacin decreases synthesis of low-density lipoproteins and inhibits lipolysis in adipose tissue.

| Route | Onset | Peak | Duration |
|---|---|---|---|
| P.O. | Unknown | 45 min | Unknown |
| I.V., I.M., S.C. | Unknown | Unknown | Unknown |

## INDICATIONS & DOSAGE
*RDA—*
**Neonates and infants up to age 6 months:** 5 mg.
**Infants ages 6 months to 1 year:** 6 mg.
**Children ages 1 to 3:** 9 mg.
**Children ages 4 to 6:** 12 mg.
**Children ages 7 to 10:** 13 mg.
**Boys ages 11 to 14:** 17 mg.
**Boys ages 15 to 18:** 20 mg.
**Men ages 19 to 50:** 19 mg.
**Men ages 51 and older:** 15 mg.
**Women ages 11 to 50:** 15 mg.
**Women ages 51 and older:** 13 mg.
**Pregnant women:** 17 mg.
**Breast-feeding women:** 20 mg.
*Pellagra—*
**Adults:** 300 to 500 mg P.O., S.C., I.M., or I.V. daily in divided doses, depending on severity of deficiency.
**Children:** up to 300 mg P.O. or 100 mg I.V. daily, depending on severity of niacin deficiency.
*Hartnup disease—*
**Adults:** 50 to 200 mg P.O. daily.
*Niacin deficiency—*
**Adults:** up to 100 mg P.O. daily.

---

*Hyperlipidemias, especially with hyper-cholesterolemia—*
**Adults:** 1 to 2 g P.O. t.i.d. with or after meals, increased at intervals to 6 g daily.

### ADVERSE REACTIONS
**CV:** *excessive peripheral vasodilation, especially niacin;* hypotension, atrial fibrillation, ***arrhythmias, flushing.***
**EENT:** toxic amblyopia.
**GI:** *nausea, vomiting, diarrhea,* possible activation of peptic ulceration, epigastric or substernal pain.
**Hepatic:** elevated liver enzyme levels, ***hepatic dysfunction.***
**Metabolic:** hyperglycemia, hyperuricemia.
**Skin:** pruritus, dryness, tingling.

### INTERACTIONS
**Drug-drug.** *Antihypertensives (ganglionic or sympathetic blockers):* potential additive vasodilating effect, causing orthostatic hypotension. Use together cautiously and warn patient about orthostatic hypotension.
*Lovastatin (statin class):* may lead to rhabdomyolysis. Avoid concurrent use.
*Sulfinpyrazone:* uricosuric effects may be decreased by niacin. Avoid concurrent use.

### EFFECTS ON DIAGNOSTIC TESTS
Drug alters fluorometric test results for urine catecholamines and results for urine glucose tests that use cupric sulfate (Benedict's reagent).

### CONTRAINDICATIONS
Contraindicated in patients with hypersensitivity to drug and in those with hepatic dysfunction, active peptic ulcers, severe hypotension, or arterial hemorrhage.

### NURSING CONSIDERATIONS
• After symptoms of niacin deficiency subside, advise adequate nutrition and RDA supplements to prevent recurrence.
• Use cautiously in patients with gallbladder disease, diabetes mellitus, or unstable angina and in patients with history of liver disease, peptic ulcer, allergy, gout, or large alcohol intake.
• Most reactions are dose-dependent.

• Drug may cause dose-related rise in glucose intolerance; blood glucose level should be monitored carefully in diabetic patients.
• Give niacin with meals to minimize adverse GI effects.
• Administer aspirin (325 mg P.O. 30 minutes before niacin dose), as ordered, to possibly reduce flushing response to niacin.
• Timed-release niacin or niacinamide may prevent excessive flushing that occurs with large doses. However, timed-release niacin is linked to hepatic dysfunction, even at very low doses.
• Monitor hepatic function and blood glucose level early in therapy, as ordered.

### 🔋 I.V. administration
• Give slow I.V. (no faster than 2 mg/minute). Explain harmlessness of flushing syndrome.

### ☑ Patient teaching
• Stress that niacin is a potent drug, not just a vitamin, and may cause serious adverse effects. Explain importance of adhering to therapy.
• Tell patient flushing and warmth may subside with continued use and that concurrent use of alcohol may increase flushing.
• Tell patient to take with food to minimize stomach upset.
• Advise patient against self-medicating for hyperlipidemia.

---

## pyridoxine hydrochloride (vitamin B$_6$)
Nestrex ◇, Orovite
Complement B$_6$§ , Rodex

*Pregnancy Risk Category A*

### HOW SUPPLIED
*Tablets:* 10 mg ◇, 25 mg ◇, 50 mg ◇, 100 mg ◇, 200 mg ◇, 250 mg ◇, 500 mg ◇
*Capsules (timed-release):* 100 mg
*Capsules:* 500 mg
*Tablets (timed-release):* 100 mg
*Injection:* 100 mg/ml

---

Reactions may be *common*, uncommon, ***life-threatening***, or **COMMON AND LIFE-THREATENING**.

## ACTION
Acts as a coenzyme that stimulates various metabolic functions, including amino acid metabolism.

| Route | Onset | Peak | Duration |
|-------|-------|------|----------|
| P.O., I.V., I.M. | Unknown | Unknown | Unknown |

## INDICATIONS & DOSAGE
*RDA—*
**Neonates and infants up to age 6 months:** 0.3 mg.
**Infants ages 6 months to 1 year:** 0.6 mg.
**Children ages 1 to 3:** 1 mg.
**Children ages 4 to 6:** 1.1 mg.
**Children ages 7 to 10:** 1.4 mg.
**Boys ages 11 to 14:** 1.7 mg.
**Men ages 15 and older:** 2 mg.
**Girls ages 11 to 14:** 1.4 mg.
**Girls ages 15 to 18:** 1.5 mg.
**Women ages 19 and older:** 1.6 mg.
**Pregnant women:** 2.2 mg.
**Breast-feeding women:** 2.1 mg.
*Dietary vitamin $B_6$ deficiency—*
**Adults:** 10 to 20 mg P.O., I.M., or I.V. daily for 3 weeks; then 2 to 5 mg daily as supplement to proper diet.
*Seizures related to vitamin $B_6$ deficiency or dependency—*
**Adults and children:** 100 mg I.M. or I.V. in single dose.
*Vitamin $B_6$–responsive anemias or dependency syndrome (inborn errors of metabolism)—*
**Adults:** up to 600 mg P.O., I.M., or I.V. daily until symptoms subside, then 30 mg daily for life.
*Prevention of vitamin $B_6$ deficiency during drug therapy—*
**Adults:** 10 to 50 mg P.O. daily.
*Antidote for isoniazid poisoning—*
**Adults:** 4 g I.V.; then 1 g I.M. q 30 minutes until amount of pyridoxine administered equals amount of isoniazid ingested.

## ADVERSE REACTIONS
**CNS:** paresthesia, unsteady gait, numbness, somnolence, *seizures,* headache.

## INTERACTIONS
**Drug-drug.** *Levodopa:* decreased levodopa effect. Avoid concomitant use.

*Phenobarbital, phenytoin:* decreased anticonvulsant serum levels, increasing risk of seizures. Avoid concomitant use.
**Drug-lifestyle.** *Alcohol use:* no conclusive evidence, but delirium and lactic acidosis were reported after drinking alcohol. Avoid concomitant use.

## EFFECTS ON DIAGNOSTIC TESTS
Drug alters determinations of urobilinogen in spot test using Ehrlich's reagent, resulting in false-positive reaction.

## CONTRAINDICATIONS
Contraindicated in patients with hypersensitivity to drug.

## NURSING CONSIDERATIONS
• Drug isn't for I.V. use in patients with heart disease.
• *Alert:*Seizures have occurred after I.V. administration of large doses.
• Protect from light. Don't use solution if it contains a precipitate, although slight darkening is acceptable.
• When used to treat isoniazid toxicity, expect to also give anticonvulsants.
• If sodium bicarbonate is needed to control acidosis in isoniazid toxicity, don't mix in same syringe with pyridoxine.
• Patients taking high doses (2 to 6 g/day) may experience difficulty walking because of diminished proprioceptive and sensory function.
• Carefully monitor patient's diet. Excessive protein intake increases daily pyridoxine requirements.
• *Alert:*Don't confuse pyridoxine with pralidoxime or pyridium.

## I.V. administration
• Inject undiluted drug into I.V. line of free-flowing compatible solution. Or, infuse diluted drug over prescribed duration for intermittent infusion. Don't use for continuous infusion.

## Patient teaching
• Stress importance of compliance and of good nutrition if drug is prescribed for maintenance therapy to prevent recurrence of deficiency. Explain that pyridoxine, with isoniazid, has a specific therapeutic purpose and isn't just a vitamin.

---

• Advise patient taking levodopa alone to avoid multivitamins containing pyridoxine because of decreased levodopa effect.
• Warn patient that there may be burning at the injection site.

---

# riboflavin (vitamin B₂) ◇

*Pregnancy Risk Category A*

## HOW SUPPLIED
*Tablets:* 25 mg ◇, 50 mg ◇, 100 mg ◇
*Tablets (sugar-free):* 50 mg ◇, 100 mg ◇

## ACTION
Converts to two other coenzymes needed for normal tissue respiration. Drug is necessary for activation of pyridoxine.

| Route | Onset | Peak | Duration |
|-------|-------|------|----------|
| P.O. | Unknown | Unknown | Unknown |

## INDICATIONS & DOSAGE
*RDA—*
**Neonates and infants up to age 6 months:** 0.4 mg.
**Infants ages 6 months to 1 year:** 0.5 mg.
**Children ages 1 to 3:** 0.8 mg.
**Children ages 4 to 6:** 1.1 mg.
**Children ages 7 to 10:** 1.2 mg.
**Boys ages 11 to 14:** 1.5 mg.
**Boys ages 15 to 18:** 1.8 mg.
**Men ages 19 to 50:** 1.7 mg.
**Men ages 51 and older:** 1.4 mg.
**Women ages 11 to 50:** 1.3 mg.
**Women ages 51 and older:** 1.2 mg.
**Pregnant women:** 1.6 mg.
**Breast-feeding women (first 6 months):** 1.8 mg.
**Breast-feeding women (second 6 months):** 1.7 mg.
*Riboflavin deficiency or adjunct to thiamine treatment for polyneuritis or cheilosis secondary to pellagra—*
**Adults and children over age 12:** 5 to 25 mg P.O. daily, depending on severity.
**Children under age 12:** 3 to 10 mg P.O. daily, depending on severity.
  For maintenance, increase nutritional intake and supplement with vitamin B complex.

## ADVERSE REACTIONS
**GU:** bright yellow urine.

## INTERACTIONS
**Drug-drug.** *Probenecid:* reduced urinary excretion of riboflavin. Avoid concomitant use.
*Propantheline, other anticholinergics:* decreased rate and extent of absorption. Avoid concomitant use.

## EFFECTS ON DIAGNOSTIC TESTS
Drug alters urinalysis based on spectrophotometry or color reactions. Large doses of drug result in bright yellow urine. Riboflavin produces fluorescent substances in urine and plasma, which can falsely elevate fluorometric determinations of catecholamines and urobilinogen.

## CONTRAINDICATIONS
No known contraindications.

## NURSING CONSIDERATIONS
• Drug may be given I.M. or I.V. as a component of multiple vitamins.
• Riboflavin deficiency usually accompanies other vitamin B complex deficiencies and may require multivitamin therapy.
• Protect drug from air and light.
• *Alert:* Don't confuse riboflavin with ribavirin.

### ☑ Patient teaching
• Tell patient to take drug with meals; food increases its absorption.
• Stress proper nutritional habits to prevent recurrence of deficiency.
• Inform patient that riboflavin usually causes bright yellow or orange discoloration of urine.

---

# thiamine hydrochloride (vitamin B₁)
Betamin‡, Beta-Sol‡

*Pregnancy Risk Category A*

## HOW SUPPLIED
*Tablets:* 25 mg ◇, 50 mg ◇, 100 mg ◇, 250 mg ◇, 500 mg
*Tablet (enteric-coated):* 20 mg

---

*Elixir†:* 250 mcg/5 ml
*Injection:* 100 mg/ml

## ACTION
Combines with adenosine triphosphate to form a coenzyme needed for carbohydrate metabolism.

| Route | Onset | Peak | Duration |
|-------|-------|------|----------|
| P.O., I.V., I.M. | Unknown | Unknown | Unknown |

## INDICATIONS & DOSAGE
*RDA—*
**Neonates and infants up to age 6 months:** 0.3 mg.
**Infants ages 6 months to 1 year:** 0.4 mg.
**Children ages 1 to 3:** 0.7 mg.
**Children ages 4 to 6:** 0.9 mg.
**Children ages 7 to 10:** 1 mg.
**Boys ages 11 to 14:** 1.3 mg.
**Men ages 15 to 50:** 1.5 mg.
**Men ages 51 and older:** 1.2 mg.
**Women ages 11 to 50:** 1.1 mg.
**Women ages 51 and older:** 1 mg.
**Pregnant women:** 1.5 mg.
**Breast-feeding women:** 1.6 mg.
*Beriberi—*
**Adults:** depending on severity, 10 to 20 mg I.M. t.i.d. for 2 weeks; then dietary correction and multivitamin supplement containing 5 to 10 mg thiamine daily for 1 month.
**Children:** depending on severity, 10 to 50 mg I.M. daily for several weeks with adequate diet.
*Wet beriberi with myocardial failure—*
**Adults and children:** 10 to 30 mg I.V. t.i.d.
*Wernicke's encephalopathy—*
**Adults:** initially, 100 mg I.V.; then 50 to 100 mg I.V. or I.M. daily until patient is consuming a regular balanced diet.

## ADVERSE REACTIONS
**CNS:** restlessness, weakness.
**CV:** cyanosis, *CV collapse.*
**EENT:** tightness of throat.
**GI:** nausea, *hemorrhage.*
**Respiratory:** pulmonary edema.
**Skin:** feeling of warmth, pruritus, urticaria, diaphoresis.
**Other:** *angioedema,* tenderness, induration after I.M. administration.

## INTERACTIONS
None significant.

## EFFECTS ON DIAGNOSTIC TESTS
Drug may produce false-positive results in phosphotungstate method for determination of uric acid and in urine spot tests with Ehrlich's reagent for urobilinogen. Large doses of drug interfere with Schack and Waxler spectrophotometric determination of serum theophylline levels.

## CONTRAINDICATIONS
Contraindicated in patients with hypersensitivity to thiamine products.

## NURSING CONSIDERATIONS
• Use parenteral route only when P.O. route isn't feasible.
• Thiamine malabsorption is most likely in alcoholism, cirrhosis, or GI disease.
• Clinically significant deficiency can occur in about 3 weeks of totally thiamine-free diet.
• Thiamine deficiency usually requires concurrent treatment for multiple deficiencies.
• Dosages over 30 mg t.i.d. may not be fully utilized. After tissue saturation with thiamine, drug is excreted in urine as pyrimidine.
• In Wernicke's encephalopathy, administer thiamine before dextrose because dextrose increases thiamine requirement.
• *Alert:* Don't confuse thiamine with Thorazine.

### I.V. administration
• Dilute drug before use.
• *Alert:* Administer large I.V. doses cautiously; give patient a skin test before therapy if he has history of hypersensitivity reactions. Have epinephrine available to treat anaphylaxis.
• Don't use drug with materials that yield alkaline solutions. Thiamine is unstable in alkaline solutions.

### Patient teaching
• Inform breast-feeding woman that, if beriberi occurs in infant, both she and her child should be treated with thiamine.
• Stress proper nutritional habits to prevent recurrence of deficiency.

---

*Liquid contains alcohol.     **May contain tartrazine.     †Canada     ‡Australia     §U.K.     ◇ OTC

• Instruct patient to protect oral doses from light.

---

## vitamin C (ascorbic acid)
Ascorbicap ◇, Cebid Timecelles ◇, Cecon ◇, Cenolate ◇, Cevalin ◇, Cevi-Bid, Ce-Vi-Sol*, C-Span ◇, Dull-C ◇, Flavorcee ◇, N'ice w/Vitamin C Drops ◇, Redoxon†, Vita-C ◇

*Pregnancy Risk Category C*

### HOW SUPPLIED
*Tablets:* 25 mg ◇, 50 mg ◇, 100 mg ◇, 250 mg ◇, 500 mg ◇, 1,000 mg ◇
*Tablets (chewable):* 100 mg ◇, 250 mg ◇, 500 mg ◇, 1,000 mg ◇
*Tablets (timed-release):* 500 mg ◇, 1,000 mg ◇, 1,500 mg
*Capsules (timed-release):* 500 mg ◇
*Crystals:* 100 g (4 g/tsp) ◇, 500 g (4 g/tsp) ◇
*Lozenges:* 60 mg ◇
*Oral liquid:* 50 ml (35 mg/0.6 ml)* ◇
*Oral solution:* 100 mg/ml ◇
*Powder:* 100 g (4 g/tsp) ◇, 500 g (4 g/tsp) ◇
*Syrup:* 500 mg/5 ml ◇
*Injection:* 100 mg/ml, 250 mg/ml, 500 mg/ml

### ACTION
Stimulates collagen formation and tissue repair; involved in oxidation-reduction reactions.

| Route | Onset | Peak | Duration |
|---|---|---|---|
| P.O., I.V., I.M., S.C. | Unknown | Unknown | Unknown |

### INDICATIONS & DOSAGE
*RDA—*
**Neonates and infants up to age 6 months:** 30 mg.
**Infants ages 6 months to 1 year:** 35 mg.
**Children ages 1 to 3:** 40 mg.
**Children ages 4 to 10:** 45 mg.
**Children ages 11 to 14:** 50 mg.
**Adults and children ages 15 and older:** 60 mg.
**Pregnant women:** 70 mg.

**Breast-feeding women (first 6 months):** 95 mg.
**Breast-feeding women (second 6 months):** 90 mg.
*Frank and subclinical scurvy—*
**Adults:** depending on severity, 300 mg to 1 g P.O., S.C., I.M., or I.V. daily; then 70 to 150 mg daily for maintenance.
**Children:** depending on severity, 100 to 300 mg P.O., S.C., I.M., or I.V. daily; then at least 30 mg daily for maintenance.
**Premature infants:** 75 to 100 mg P.O., I.M., I.V., or S.C. daily.
*Extensive burns, delayed fracture or wound healing, postoperative wound healing, severe febrile or chronic disease states—*
**Adults:** 300 to 500 mg S.C., I.M., or I.V. daily for 7 to 10 days. 1 to 2 g daily for extensive burns.
**Children:** 100 to 200 mg P.O., S.C., I.M., or I.V. daily.
*Prevention of vitamin C deficiency in patients with poor nutritional habits or increased requirements—*
**Adults:** 70 to 150 mg P.O., S.C., I.M., or I.V. daily.
**Pregnant and breast-feeding women:** at least 70 to 150 mg P.O., S.C., I.M., or I.V. daily.
**Children:** at least 40 mg P.O., S.C., I.M., or I.V. daily.
**Infants:** at least 35 mg P.O., S.C., I.M., or I.V. daily.
*Potentiation of methenamine in urine acidification—*
**Adults:** 4 to 12 g P.O. daily in divided doses.

### ADVERSE REACTIONS
**CNS:** faintness, dizziness.
**GI:** diarrhea, heartburn, nausea, vomiting.
**GU:** acid urine, oxaluria, renal calculi.
**Other:** discomfort at injection site.

### INTERACTIONS
**Drug-drug.** *Aspirin (high doses):* increased risk of salicylate toxicity. Monitor patient closely.
*Contraceptives, estrogen:* increased serum levels of estrogen. Watch for adverse reactions.
*Oral iron supplements:* increased iron absorption. Give together.

---

Reactions may be *common,* uncommon, *life-threatening,* or COMMON AND LIFE-THREATENING.

*Warfarin:* decreased anticoagulant effect. Monitor closely.
**Drug-herb.** *Bearberry:* inactivation of bearberry in urine. Watch for effect.

**EFFECTS ON DIAGNOSTIC TESTS**
Ascorbic acid is a strong reducing agent; it alters results of tests that are based on oxidation-reduction reactions. Large doses (over 500 mg) may cause false-negative glucose determinations using glucose oxidase method or false-positive results using copper reduction method or Benedict's reagent.

Ascorbic acid shouldn't be used for 48 to 72 hours before an amine-dependent test for occult blood in the stool is conducted; a false-negative test may occur. Depending on reagents used, it may also interact with other diagnostic tests.

**CONTRAINDICATIONS**
Contraindicated in patients with an allergy to tartrazine or sulfites. Large doses are contraindicated during pregnancy.

**NURSING CONSIDERATIONS**
• When giving for urine acidification, check urine pH to ensure efficacy.
• Protect solution from light, and refrigerate ampules.

**⚠I.V. administration**
• Infuse cautiously in patients with renal insufficiency.
• *Alert:* Rapid infusion may cause faintness or dizziness.

**☑Patient teaching**
• For patient receiving vitamin C I.M., explain that I.M. route may promote better utilization.
• Stress proper nutritional habits to prevent recurrence of deficiency.
• Inform patient that vitamin C is readily absorbed from citrus fruits, tomatoes, potatoes, and leafy vegetables.

# vitamin D

## cholecalciferol (vitamin D₃)
Delta-D ◇, Vitamin D₃ ◇

## ergocalciferol (vitamin D₂)
Calciferol, Drisdol, Radiostol†, Vitamin D

*Pregnancy Risk Category C*

**HOW SUPPLIED**
*Tablets:* 1.25 mg (50,000 IU)
*Capsules:* 1.25 mg (50,000 IU)
*Oral liquid:* 8,000 IU/ml in 60-ml dropper bottle ◇
*Injection:* 12.5 mg (500,000 IU)/ml

**ACTION**
Promotes absorption and utilization of calcium and phosphate, helping to regulate calcium homeostasis.

| Route | Onset | Peak | Duration |
|---|---|---|---|
| P.O., I.M. | 2-14 hr | 4-12 hr | 2 days-6 mo |

**INDICATIONS & DOSAGE**
*RDA for cholecalciferol—*
**Neonates and infants up to age 6 months:** 300 IU.
**Infants ages 6 months to adults age 24:** 400 IU.
**Adults ages 25 and older:** 200 IU.
**Pregnant or breast-feeding women:** 400 IU.
*Rickets and other vitamin D deficiency diseases, renal osteodystrophy—*
**Adults:** initially, 12,000 IU P.O. or I.M. daily; usually increased, based on response, to maximum of 500,000 IU daily.
**Children:** 1,500 to 5,000 IU P.O. or I.M. daily for 2 to 4 weeks; repeated after 2 weeks, if needed. Or, give single dose of 600,000 IU.

After correction of deficiency, maintenance includes adequate diet and RDA supplements.
*Hypoparathyroidism—*
**Adults and children:** 50,000 to 200,000 IU P.O. or I.M. daily, with calcium supplement.

*Familial hypophosphatemia—*
**Adults:** 1 to 2 mg P.O. daily with phosphorus supplement, increased in 250- to 500-mcg increments at 3- to 4-month intervals.

## ADVERSE REACTIONS
Adverse reactions usually occur only in vitamin D toxicity.
**CNS:** headache, weakness, somnolence, decreased libido, overt psychosis, irritability.
**CV:** *calcification of soft tissues, including the heart;* hypertension; ***arrhythmias.***
**EENT:** rhinorrhea, conjunctivitis (calcific), photophobia.
**GI:** anorexia, nausea, vomiting, constipation, dry mouth, metallic taste, polydipsia.
**GU:** polyuria, albuminuria, hypercalciuria, nocturia, ***impaired renal function,*** reversible azotemia.
**Hepatic:** elevated AST and ALT levels.
**Metabolic:** *hypercalcemia,* hyperthermia, falsely increased serum cholesterol levels.
**Musculoskeletal:** bone and muscle pain, bone demineralization, weight loss.
**Skin:** pruritus.

## INTERACTIONS
**Drug-drug.** *Cardiac glycosides:* increased risk of arrhythmias. Monitor serum calcium levels.
*Cholestyramine, colestipol, mineral oil:* inhibited GI absorption of oral vitamin D. Space doses. Use together cautiously.
*Corticosteroids:* antagonized effect of vitamin D. Monitor vitamin D levels closely.
*Magnesium-containing antacids:* possible hypermagnesemia, especially in patients with chronic renal failure. Monitor serum magnesium levels.
*Phenobarbital, phenytoin:* increased vitamin D metabolism and decreased effectiveness. Monitor closely.
*Thiazide diuretics:* may cause hypercalcemia in patients with hypoparathyroidism. Monitor closely.
*Verapamil:* atrial fibrillation has occurred as a result of increased calcium. Monitor closely.

## EFFECTS ON DIAGNOSTIC TESTS
None reported.

## CONTRAINDICATIONS
Contraindicated in patients with hypercalcemia, hypervitaminosis D, malabsorption syndrome, decreased renal function, or renal osteodystrophy with hyperphosphatemia.

## NURSING CONSIDERATIONS
• Use ergocalciferol with extreme caution, if at all, in patients with heart disease, renal stones, or arteriosclerosis.
• Use cautiously in cardiac patients, especially those taking cardiac glycosides, and in patients with increased sensitivity to these drugs.
• Use I.M. injection of vitamin D dispersed in oil for patients unable to absorb oral form, as ordered.
• *Alert:* Monitor patient's eating and bowel habits; dry mouth, nausea, vomiting, metallic taste, and constipation may be early signs of toxicity.
• Monitor serum and urine calcium, phosphorus, potassium, and urea levels when high therapeutic dosages are used.
• Doses of 60,000 IU/day can cause hypercalcemia. Hypercalcemia may require I.V. hydration and aggressive diuresis.
• Malabsorption from inadequate bile or hepatic dysfunction may require addition of exogenous bile salts to oral form.
• Patients with hyperphosphatemia need dietary phosphate restrictions and binding drugs to avoid metastatic calcifications and renal calculi.
• Mineral oil interferes with absorption of fat-soluble vitamins.

☑ **Patient teaching**
• Teach patient that vitamin D is needed to absorb calcium. Instruct patient to read labels for vitamin D content.
• Advise that vitamin D is fat soluble and that mineral oil will interfere with absorption.
• Instruct patient to take only as directed and stress the dangers of excessive doses of fat-soluble vitamins.
• Instruct patient taking vitamin D to restrict intake of magnesium-containing antacids.
• Instruct patient to notify doctor if signs of toxicity occur, such as weakness, lethargy, headache, anorexia, weight loss, nau-

sea, vomiting, abdominal cramps, diarrhea, constipation, vertigo, polydipsia, polyuria, dry mouth, or muscle or bone pain.

**✱ NEW DRUG**

## doxercalciferol
Hectorol

*Pregnancy Risk Category B*

### HOW SUPPLIED
*Capsules:* 2.5 mcg

### ACTION
A vitamin D analogue that acts directly on the parathyroid glands to suppress parathyroid hormone (PTH) synthesis and secretion.

| Route | Onset | Peak | Duration |
|-------|-------|------|----------|
| P.O. | Unknown | 11-12 hr | Unknown |

### INDICATION & DOSAGE
*Reduction of elevated intact PTH levels in management of secondary hyperparathyroidism in patients undergoing long-term renal dialysis—*
**Adults:** initially, 10 mcg P.O. three times weekly at dialysis. Dosage adjusted as needed to lower intact PTH levels to 150 to 300 pg/ml. Dosage may be increased by 2.5 mcg at 8-week intervals if intact PTH level isn't decreased by 50% and fails to reach target range. Maximum dose is 20 mcg P.O. three times weekly. If intact PTH levels fall below 100 pg/ml, drug should be suspended for 1 week, then resumed at dose that is at least 2.5 mcg lower than last administered dose.

### ADVERSE REACTIONS
**CNS:** *dizziness, headache, malaise,* sleep disorder.
**CV:** *bradycardia, edema.*
**GI:** anorexia, dyspepsia, *nausea, vomiting,* constipation.
**Metabolic:** weight gain.
**Musculoskeletal:** arthralgia.
**Respiratory:** *dyspnea.*
**Skin:** pruritus.
**Other:** abscess.

### INTERACTIONS
**Drug-drug.** *Calcium-containing or non-aluminum-containing phosphate binders:* may cause hypercalcemia or hyperphosphatemia and decrease effectiveness of doxercalciferol. Use cautiously together and adjust dosage of phosphate binders, as appropriate.
*Cholestyramine, mineral oil:* reduced intestinal absorption of doxercalciferol. Avoid concomitant use.
*Glutethimide, phenobarbital, other enzyme inducers; phenytoin and other enzyme inhibitors:* may affect metabolism of doxercalciferol. Adjust dosage, as appropriate.
*Magnesium-containing antacids:* may cause hypermagnesemia. Avoid concomitant use.
*Vitamin D supplements:* may cause additive effects and hypercalcemia. Avoid concomitant use.

### EFFECTS ON DIAGNOSTIC TESTS
None reported.

### CONTRAINDICATIONS
Contraindicated in patients with recent history of hypercalcemia, hyperphosphatemia, or vitamin D toxicity.

### NURSING CONSIDERATIONS
• Use cautiously in patients with hepatic insufficiency.
• Monitor calcium, phosphorus, and intact PTH levels, as ordered.
• Doxercalciferol is administered with dialysis (about every other day). Dosing must be individualized and based on intact PTH levels, with monitoring of serum calcium and phosphorus levels before doxercalciferol therapy and weekly thereafter in the early phase of treatment.
• Management of secondary hyperparathyroidism may prevent bone disease in patients with renal failure.
• Calcium-based or non-aluminum-containing phosphate binders and a low-phosphate diet are used to control serum phosphorus levels in patients undergoing dialysis. Expect adjustments in dosages of doxercalciferol and concurrent therapies such as dietary phosphate binders in order to sustain PTH suppression and maintain

serum calcium and phosphorus levels within acceptable ranges.

• Progressive hypercalcemia secondary to vitamin D overdose may require emergency attention. Acute hypercalcemia may exacerbate arrhythmias and seizures, and affects action of digoxin. Chronic hypercalcemia can lead to vascular and soft-tissue calcification.

• If hypercalcemia, hyperphosphatemia, or a product of serum calcium × serum phosphorus (Ca × P) is greater than 70, immediately suspend administration of doxercalciferol, as ordered, until these parameters are lowered.

☑ **Patient teaching**
• Inform patient that dose must be adjusted over several months to achieve satisfactory PTH suppression.
• Tell patient to follow instructions regarding calcium supplementation and to adhere to a low-phosphorus diet.
• Tell patient to obtain doctor's approval before using OTC drugs, including antacids and vitamin products containing calcium or vitamin D.
• Inform patient that early signs and symptoms of hypercalcemia include weakness, headache, somnolence, nausea, vomiting, dry mouth, constipation, muscle pain, bone pain, and metallic taste. Late signs and symptoms include polyuria, polydipsia, anorexia, weight loss, nocturia, conjunctivitis, pancreatitis, photophobia, rhinorrhea, pruritus, hyperthermia, decreased libido, hypertension, and arrhythmias.

---

## paricalcitol
Zemplar

*Pregnancy Risk Category C*

### HOW SUPPLIED
*Injection:* 5 mcg/ml

### ACTION
A synthetic vitamin D analogue that reduces parathyroid hormone (PTH) levels.

| Route | Onset | Peak | Duration |
|-------|-------|------|----------|
| I.V. | Immediate | Unknown | 15 hr |

### INDICATIONS & DOSAGE
*Prevention and treatment of secondary hyperparathyroidism associated with chronic renal failure—*
**Adults:** 0.04 to 0.1 mcg/kg (2.8 to 7 mcg) I.V. no more frequently than every other day during dialysis. Doses as high as 0.24 mcg/kg (16.8 mcg) have been safely administered. If satisfactory response isn't observed, dosage may be increased by 2 to 4 mcg at 2- to 4-week intervals.

### ADVERSE REACTIONS
**CNS:** light-headedness, malaise.
**CV:** palpitation.
**GI:** dry mouth, GI bleeding, *nausea*, vomiting.
**Hepatic:** reduced serum total alkaline phosphatase level.
**Respiratory:** pneumonia.
**Other:** chills, edema, fever, flulike syndrome, *sepsis.*

### INTERACTIONS
None significant.

### EFFECTS ON DIAGNOSTIC TESTS
None reported.

### CONTRAINDICATIONS
Contraindicated in patients with hypersensitivity to drug or its ingredients and in those with evidence of vitamin D toxicity or hypercalcemia.

### NURSING CONSIDERATIONS
• Use cautiously in patients taking digitalis compounds. Patients taking digoxin are at greater risk for digitalis toxicity during drug therapy secondary to potential for hypercalcemia.
• Watch for ECG abnormalities.
• Monitor patient for symptoms of hypercalcemia, such as fatigue, muscle weakness, anorexia, depression, nausea, and constipation. Immediately notify doctor if hypercalcemia is suspected.
• Monitor serum calcium and phosphorus levels twice weekly when dosage is being adjusted, and then monitor monthly. PTH level should be measured every 3 months during therapy.
• As PTH level decreases, paricalcitol dose may need to be decreased. Acute overdose

---

Reactions may be *common*, uncommon, *life-threatening*, or COMMON AND LIFE-THREATENING.

of paricalcitol may cause hypercalcemia, which may require emergency attention.
• In patients with chronic renal failure, appropriate types of phosphate-binding compounds may be needed to control serum phosphorus levels, but excessive use of aluminum-containing compounds should be avoided.
• Store drug at room temperature (59° to 86° F [15° to 30° C]).

**I.V. administration**
• Drug is only administered as an I.V. bolus. Discard unused portion.
• Inspect drug for particulates and discoloration before use.

**Patient teaching**
• Stress importance of adhering to a dietary regimen of calcium supplementation and phosphorus restriction during drug therapy.
• Caution against use of phosphate or vitamin D–related compounds during drug therapy.
• Explain need for frequent laboratory tests.
• Instruct patient with chronic renal failure to take phosphate-binding compounds as prescribed but to avoid excessive use of aluminum-containing compounds. Alert patient to early symptoms of hypercalcemia and vitamin D intoxication, such as weakness, headache, somnolence, nausea, vomiting, dry mouth, constipation, muscle pain, bone pain, and metallic taste.
• Instruct patient to promptly report adverse reactions.
• Remind patient taking digoxin to watch for signs and symptoms of digitalis toxicity.

---

**vitamin E (tocopherols)**
Amino-Opti-E ◇, Aquasol E ◇, E-Complex-600 ◇, E-200 I.U. Softgels ◇, E-400 I.U. in a Water Soluble Base ◇, E-1000 I.U. Softgels, E-Vitamin Succinate ◇, Vita Plus E ◇

*Pregnancy Risk Category A*

**HOW SUPPLIED**
*Tablets (chewable):* 200 IU ◇, 400 IU ◇

*Capsules:* 100 IU ◇, 200 IU ◇, 400 IU ◇, 500 IU ◇, 600 IU ◇, 1,000 IU ◇, 73.5 mg, 147 mg, 165 mg, 330 mg
*Oral solution:* 50 mg/ml ◇

**ACTION**
Unknown. Thought to act as an antioxidant and protect RBC membranes against hemolysis.

| Route | Onset | Peak | Duration |
|-------|-------|------|----------|
| P.O. | Unknown | Unknown | Unknown |

**INDICATIONS & DOSAGE**
*Note:* RDAs for vitamin E have been converted to α-tocopherol equivalents (α-TE). One α-TE equals 1 mg of D-α tocopherol or 1.49 IU.
**Neonates and infants up to age 6 months:** 3 α-TE or 4 IU.
**Infants ages 6 months to 1 year:** 4 α-TE or 6 IU.
**Children ages 1 to 3:** 6 α-TE or 9 IU.
**Children ages 4 to 10:** 7 α-TE or 10 IU.
**Men ages 11 and older:** 10 α-TE or 15 IU.
**Women ages 11 and older:** 8 α-TE or 12 IU.
**Pregnant women:** 10 α-TE or 15 IU.
**Breast-feeding women (first 6 months):** 12 α-TE or 18 IU.
**Breast-feeding women (second 6 months):** 11 α-TE or 16 IU.
*Vitamin E deficiency in premature neonates and in patients with impaired fat absorption—*
**Adults:** depending on severity, 60 to 75 IU P.O. daily.
**Children:** 1 IU/kg daily.

**ADVERSE REACTIONS**
None reported with recommended dosages.

**INTERACTIONS**
**Drug-drug.** *Anticoagulants (oral):* hypoprothrombinemic effects may be increased, possibly causing bleeding. Monitor closely.
*Cholestyramine, colestipol, mineral oil:* inhibited GI absorption of oral vitamin E. Space doses. Use together cautiously.
*Iron:* may catalyze oxidation and increase daily requirements. Avoid concurrent use.

---

*Vitamin K:* antagonized effects of vitamin K possible with large doses of vitamin E. Avoid concurrent use.

## EFFECTS ON DIAGNOSTIC TESTS
None reported.

## CONTRAINDICATIONS
No known contraindications.

## NURSING CONSIDERATIONS
• Monitor patient with liver or gallbladder disease for response to therapy. Adequate bile is essential for vitamin E absorption.
• Water-miscible forms are more completely absorbed in GI tract.
• Requirements increase with rise in dietary polyunsaturated acids.
• Don't administer drug I.V.
• Hypervitaminosis E symptoms include fatigue, weakness, nausea, headache, blurred vision, flatulence, diarrhea.

☑ **Patient teaching**
• Tell patient not to crush tablets or open capsules. An oral solution and chewable tablets are commercially available.
• Warn patient against self-medicating with megadoses, which can cause thrombophlebitis. Vitamin is fat soluble and may accumulate.

---

## phytonadione (vitamin K₁)
AquaMEPHYTON, Konakion, Mephyton

*Pregnancy Risk Category A*

## HOW SUPPLIED
*Tablets:* 5 mg
*Injection (aqueous colloidal solution):* 2 mg/ml, 10 mg/ml
*Injection (aqueous dispersion):* 2 mg/ml, 10 mg/ml

## ACTION
An antihemorrhagic factor that promotes hepatic formation of active prothrombin.

| Route | Onset | Peak | Duration |
|---|---|---|---|
| P.O. | 6-12 hr | Unknown | Unknown |
| I.V., I.M., S.C. | 1-2 hr | Unknown | Unknown |

## INDICATIONS & DOSAGE
*RDA—*
**Neonates and infants up to age 6 months:** 5 mcg.
**Infants ages 6 months to 1 year:** 10 mcg.
**Children ages 1 to 3:** 15 mcg.
**Children ages 4 to 6:** 20 mcg.
**Children ages 7 to 10:** 30 mcg.
**Children ages 11 to 14:** 45 mcg.
**Boys ages 15 to 18:** 65 mcg.
**Men ages 19 to 24:** 70 mcg.
**Men ages 25 and older:** 80 mcg.
**Girls ages 15 to 18:** 55 mcg.
**Women ages 19 to 24:** 60 mcg.
**Women ages 25 and older:** 65 mcg.
**Pregnant and breast-feeding women:** 65 mcg.
*Hypoprothrombinemia secondary to vitamin K malabsorption, drug therapy, or excessive vitamin A dosage—*
**Adults:** depending on severity, 2.5 to 10 mg P.O., S.C., or I.M., repeated and increased up to 50 mg, if needed.
**Infants:** 2 mg P.O. or parenterally.
**Children:** 5 to 10 mg P.O. or parenterally.
*Hypoprothrombinemia secondary to effect of oral anticoagulants—*
**Adults:** 2.5 to 10 mg P.O., S.C., or I.M. based on PT, repeated if needed within 12 to 48 hours after oral dose or within 6 to 8 hours after parenteral dose. In emergency, 10 to 50 mg slow I.V., rate not to exceed 1 mg/minute, repeated q 4 hours, p.r.n.
*Prevention of hemorrhagic disease of newborn—*
**Neonates:** 0.5 to 1 mg I.M. within 1 hour after birth.
*Hemorrhagic disease of newborn—*
**Neonates:** 1 mg S.C. or I.M. Higher doses may be needed if mother has been receiving oral anticoagulants.
*Prevention of hypoprothrombinemia related to vitamin K deficiency in long-term parenteral nutrition—*
**Adults:** 5 to 10 mg I.M. weekly.
**Children:** 2 to 5 mg I.M. weekly.
*Prevention of hypoprothrombinemia in infants receiving less than 0.1 mg/L vitamin K in breast milk or milk substitutes—*
**Infants:** 1 mg I.M. monthly.

## ADVERSE REACTIONS
**CNS:** dizziness.

---

**CV:** transient hypotension after I.V. administration, rapid and weak pulse.
**Skin:** diaphoresis, flushing, erythema.
**Other:** *anaphylaxis, anaphylactoid reactions, usually after too-rapid I.V. administration;* pain, swelling, hematoma at injection site.

### INTERACTIONS
**Drug-drug.** *Anticoagulants:* temporary resistance to prothrombin-depressing anticoagulants may result, especially when larger doses of phytonadione are used. Monitor closely.
*Cholestyramine, mineral oil:* inhibited GI absorption of oral vitamin K. Space doses. Use together cautiously.

### EFFECTS ON DIAGNOSTIC TESTS
Drug may falsely elevate urine corticosteroid levels.

### CONTRAINDICATIONS
Contraindicated in patients with hypersensitivity to drug.

### NURSING CONSIDERATIONS
• Check brand name labels for administration route restrictions.
• Effects of I.V. injection are more rapid but shorter-lived than S.C. or I.M. injections.
• *Alert:* I.V. use has resulted in fatalities; use only when other routes of administration aren't feasible.
• For I.M. administration in adults and older children, administer in upper outer quadrant of buttocks; for infants, administer in anterolateral aspect of thigh or deltoid region.
• Anticipate order of weekly addition of 5 to 10 mg of phytonadione to total parenteral nutrition solutions.
• Monitor PT or INR to determine dosage effectiveness, as ordered.
• If severe bleeding occurs, don't delay other measures, such as fresh frozen plasma or whole blood.
• *Alert:* Watch for flushing, weakness, tachycardia, and hypotension; condition may progress to shock.
• Phytonadione therapy for hemorrhagic disease in infants causes fewer adverse reactions than other vitamin K analogues.

### ■I.V. administration
• Dilute with normal saline for injection, $D_5W$, or $D_5W$ in normal saline for injection. Give I.V. by slow infusion over 2 to 3 hours. Don't exceed rate of 1 mg/minute.
• Protect parenteral products from light. Wrap infusion container with aluminum foil.

### ☑Patient teaching
• Explain purpose of drug.
• Tell patient to avoid hazardous activities if dizziness occurs.
• Inform patient that drug is fat soluble; it should be taken only as prescribed.
• Teach patient that foods that provide vitamin K include cabbage, cauliflower, kale, spinach, fish, liver, eggs, meats, and dairy products.

## sodium fluoride
Fluor-A-Day†, Fluoritab, Fluorodex, Fluotic†, Flura, Flura-Drops, Flura-Loz, Karidium, Luride, Luride Lozi-Tabs, Luride-SF Lozi-Tabs, Pediaflor, Pedi-Dent†, Pharmaflur, Pharmaflur df, Pharmaflur 1.1, Phos-Flur

## sodium fluoride, topical
ACT◇, Fluorigard◇, Fluorinse, Gel-Kam, Gel-Tin◇, Karigel, Karigel-N, Minute-Gel, Point-Two, Prevident, Stop Gel◇, Thera-Flur, Thera-Flur-N

*Pregnancy Risk Category NR*

### HOW SUPPLIED
**sodium fluoride**
*Tablets:* 1 mg
*Tablets (chewable):* 0.25 mg, 0.5 mg, 1 mg
*Drops:* 0.125 mg/drop, 0.25 mg/drop, 0.2 mg/ml, 0.5 mg/ml
*Lozenges:* 1 mg
**sodium fluoride, topical**
*Gel:* 0.1%, 0.5%, 1.23%
*Gel drops:* 0.5%
*Rinse:* 0.01%◇, 0.02%◇, 0.09%

## ACTION
Stabilizes the apatite crystal of bone and teeth. Increases tooth resistance to acid breakdown.

| Route | Onset | Peak | Duration |
|-------|-------|------|----------|
| P.O. | Unknown | 30-60 min | Unknown |

## INDICATIONS & DOSAGE
*Prevention of dental caries—*
**Adults and children over age 6:** 5 to 10 ml of rinse or thin ribbon of gel applied to teeth with toothbrush or mouth trays for at least 1 minute h.s.
*If fluoride ion level in drinking water is below 0.3 ppm (parts per million):*
**Infants and children ages 6 months to 3 years:** 0.25 mg P.O. daily.
**Children ages 3 to 6:** 0.5 mg P.O. daily.
**Children ages 6 to 16:** 1 mg P.O. daily.
*If fluoride ion level in drinking water is 0.3 to 0.6 ppm:*
**Children ages 3 to 6:** 0.25 mg P.O. daily.
**Children ages 6 to 16:** 0.5 mg P.O. daily.

## ADVERSE REACTIONS
**CNS:** headache, weakness.
**GI:** gastric distress.
**Other:** staining of teeth, *hypersensitivity reactions.*

## INTERACTIONS
**Drug-drug.** *Aluminum hydroxide, calcium, iron, magnesium:* may decrease absorption. Separate administration times.
**Drug-food.** *Dairy products:* incompatibility may occur as a result of formation of calcium fluoride, which is poorly absorbed. Avoid concomitant use.

## EFFECTS ON DIAGNOSTIC TESTS
None reported.

## CONTRAINDICATIONS
Contraindicated in patients with hypersensitivity to fluoride or when intake from drinking water exceeds 0.6 ppm.

## NURSING CONSIDERATIONS
• Administer oral drops undiluted or mixed with fluids or food. Avoid simultaneous ingestion of dairy products.

• **Alert:** Chronic toxicity (fluorosis) may result from prolonged use of higher-than-recommended doses.

☑ **Patient teaching**
• Tell patient that tablets may be dissolved in mouth, chewed, or swallowed whole.
• Advise patient that topical rinses and gels shouldn't be swallowed by children under age 3 or used if water supply is fluorinated. Drug is most effective when used right after brushing teeth. Tell patient to rinse around and between teeth for 1 minute; then spit out.
• Tell patient not to eat, drink, or rinse mouth for 30 minutes after application.
• Tell patient to dilute drops or rinses in plastic, not glass, containers.
• Advise patient to notify dentist if tooth mottling occurs.
• Instruct patient not to exceed recommended dosage.

---

## trace elements

### chromium (chromic chloride)
Chroma-Pak, Chromic Chloride

### copper (cupric sulfate)
Cupric Sulfate

### iodine (sodium iodide)
Iodopen

### manganese (manganese chloride, manganese sulfate)

### selenium (selenious acid)
Sele-Pak, Selepen

### zinc (zinc sulfate)
Zinca-Pak

*Pregnancy Risk Category C*

## HOW SUPPLIED
**chromium**
*Injection:* 4 mcg/ml, 20 mcg/ml
**copper**
*Injection:* 0.4 mg/ml, 2 mg/ml
**iodine**
*Injection:* 100 mcg/ml
**manganese**
*Injection:* 0.1 mg/ml

---

**selenium**
*Injection:* 40 mcg/ml
**zinc**
*Injection:* 1 mg/ml, 5 mg/ml

## ACTION
Participates in synthesis and stabilization of proteins and nucleic acids in subcellular and membrane transport systems.

| Route | Onset | Peak | Duration |
|-------|-------|------|----------|
| I.V. | Immediate | Immediate | Unknown |

## INDICATIONS & DOSAGE
*Prevention of individual trace element deficiencies in patients receiving long-term total parenteral nutrition (TPN)—*
*Chromium—*
**Adults:** 10 to 15 mcg I.V. daily.
**Children:** 0.14 to 0.20 mcg/kg I.V. daily.
*Copper—*
**Adults:** 0.5 to 1.5 mg I.V. daily.
**Children:** 20 mcg/kg I.V. daily.
*Iodine—*
**Adults:** 1 to 2 mcg/kg I.V. daily.
**Children:** 2 to 3 mcg/kg I.V. daily.
*Manganese—*
**Adults:** 0.15 to 0.8 mg I.V. daily.
**Children:** 2 to 10 mcg/kg I.V. daily.
*Selenium—*
**Adults:** 20 to 40 mcg I.V. daily.
**Children:** 3 mcg/kg I.V. daily.
*Zinc—*
**Adults:** 2.5 to 4 mg I.V. daily.
**Full-term infants and children up to age 5:** 100 mcg/kg/day.
**Premature infants under 1,500 g to 3 kg (3.3 to 7 lb):** 300 mcg/kg/day.

## ADVERSE REACTIONS
None reported when used at recommended dosages except for hypersensitivity reactions to iodides.

## INTERACTIONS
None significant.

## EFFECTS ON DIAGNOSTIC TESTS
None reported.

## CONTRAINDICATIONS
Contraindicated in patients with hypersensitivity to iodine.

## NURSING CONSIDERATIONS
• Check serum levels of trace elements in patients who have received TPN for 2 months or longer, as ordered. Give supplement, if ordered. Report low serum levels of these elements.
• Normal serum levels are 1 to 5 mcg/L chromium; 80 to 163 mcg/dl copper; 6 to 12 mcg/dl manganese; 0.1 to 0.19 mcg/ml selenium; and 88 to 112 mcg/dl zinc.
• Solutions of trace elements are compounded by pharmacist for addition to TPN solutions according to various formulas.

### I.V. administration
• Cautiously infuse diluted solution through patent I.V. line over ordered duration.
• Don't administer undiluted because of potential for phlebitis.

### Patient teaching
• Explain need for zinc administration to patient and family.
• Tell patient to report signs of hypersensitivity promptly.
• Inform patient and family that trace elements are normally received from dietary intake and that, when patient begins eating well, supplements won't be needed.

amino acid infusions, crystalline
amino acid infusions in dextrose
amino acid infusions with
   electrolytes
amino acid infusions with
   electrolytes in dextrose
amino acid infusions for hepatic
   failure
amino acid infusions for high
   metabolic stress
amino acid infusions for renal
   failure
dextrose
fat emulsions
medium-chain triglycerides

### COMBINATION PRODUCTS
Various products contain dextrose or invert sugar in combination with electrolytes.

---

### amino acid infusions, crystalline
Aminosyn, Aminosyn II,
Aminosyn-PF, FreAmine III,
Novamine, Travasol, TrophAmine

### amino acid infusions in dextrose
Aminosyn II with Dextrose

### amino acid infusions with electrolytes
Aminosyn with Electrolytes,
Aminosyn II with Electrolytes,
FreAmine III with Electrolytes,
ProcalAmine with Electrolytes,
Travasol with Electrolytes

### amino acid infusions with electrolytes in dextrose
Aminosyn II with Electrolytes in
Dextrose

### amino acid infusions for hepatic failure
HepatAmine

### amino acid infusions for high metabolic stress
Aminosyn-HBC, BranchAmin,
FreAmine HBC

### amino acid infusions for renal failure
Aminess, Aminosyn-RF,
NephrAmine, RenAmin

*Pregnancy Risk Category C*

### HOW SUPPLIED
*Injection:* 250 ml, 500 ml, 1,000 ml,
2,000 ml containing amino acids in various concentrations
**amino acid infusions, crystalline**
Aminosyn: 3.5%, 5%, 7%, 8.5%, 10%
Aminosyn II: 3.5%, 5%, 7%, 8.5%, 10%,
15%
Aminosyn-PF: 7%, 10%
FreAmine III: 8.5%, 10%
Novamine: 11.4%, 15%
Travasol: 5.5%, 8.5%, 10%
TrophAmine: 6%, 10%
**amino acid infusions in dextrose**
Aminosyn II: 3.5% in 5% dextrose, 3.5%
in 25% dextrose, 4.25% in 10% dextrose,
4.25% in 20% dextrose, 4.25% in 25%
dextrose, 5% in 25% dextrose
Travasol: 2.75% in 5% dextrose, 2.75% in
10% dextrose, 2.75% in 25% dextrose
Travasol: 4.25% in 5% dextrose, 4.25% in
10% dextrose, 4.25% in 25% dextrose
**amino acid infusions with electrolytes**
Aminosyn: 3.5%, 7%, 8.5%
Aminosyn II: 3.5%, 7%, 8.5%, 10%
FreAmine III: 3%, 8.5%
ProcalAmine: 3%
Travasol: 3.5%, 5.5%, 8.5%
**amino acid infusions with electrolytes in dextrose**
Aminosyn II: 3.5% with electrolytes in
5% dextrose, 3.5% with electrolytes in
25% dextrose, 4.25% with electrolytes in
10% dextrose, 4.25% with electrolytes in
20% dextrose, 4.25% with electrolytes in
25% dextrose

---

Reactions may be *common*, uncommon, *life-threatening*, or COMMON AND LIFE-THREATENING.

Travasol: 2.75% with electrolytes in 5% dextrose, 2.75% with electrolytes in dextrose, 4.25% with electrolytes in 5% dextrose, 4.25% with electrolytes in 10% dextrose, 4.25% with electrolytes in 25% dextrose

**amino acid infusions for hepatic failure**
HepatAmine: 8%

**amino acid infusions for high metabolic stress**
Aminosyn-HBC: 7%
BranchAmin: 4%
FreAmine HBC: 6.9%

**amino acid infusions for renal failure**
Aminess: 5.2%
Aminosyn-RF: 5.2%
NephrAmine: 5.4%
RenAmin: 6.5%

## ACTION
Provides a substrate for protein synthesis or enhances conservation of existing body protein.

| Route | Onset | Peak | Duration |
|-------|-------|------|----------|
| I.V. | Immediate | Immediate | Unknown |

## INDICATIONS & DOSAGE
*Total parenteral nutrition (TPN) in patients who can't or won't eat—*
**Adults:** 1 to 1.5 g/kg I.V. daily.
**Children under 10 kg (22 lb):** 2 to 4 g/kg I.V. daily.
**Children over 10 kg:** 20 to 25 g I.V. daily for first 10 kg; then 1 to 1.25 g/kg I.V. daily for each kg over 10 kg.
*Nutritional support in patients with cirrhosis, hepatitis, and hepatic encephalopathy—*
**Adults:** 80 to 120 g of amino acids (12 to 18 g of nitrogen) I.V. daily of formulation for hepatic failure.
*Nutritional support in patients with high metabolic stress—*
**Adults:** 1.5 g/kg I.V. daily of formulation for high metabolic stress.
*Nutritional support in patients with renal failure—*
**Adults:** 0.3 to 0.5 g/kg I.V. daily (to total of 26 g daily). Patients on dialysis may need 1 to 1.2 g/kg daily.

## ADVERSE REACTIONS
**CV:** thrombophlebitis, edema, thrombosis, flushing.
**GI:** nausea.
**GU:** glycosuria, osmotic diuresis.
**Hepatic:** elevated liver enzyme levels.
**Metabolic:** *rebound hypoglycemia when long-term infusions are abruptly stopped,* hyperglycemia, metabolic acidosis, alkalosis, hypophosphatemia, *hyperosmolar hyperglycemic nonketotic syndrome,* hyperammonemia, electrolyte imbalances, fever, weight gain.
**Musculoskeletal:** osteoporosis.
**Other:** *hypersensitivity reactions,* tissue sloughing at infusion site due to extravasation, *catheter sepsis.*

## INTERACTIONS
**Drug-drug.** *Tetracycline:* may reduce protein-sparing effects of infused amino acids because of its antianabolic activity. Monitor patient.

## EFFECTS ON DIAGNOSTIC TESTS
None reported.

## CONTRAINDICATIONS
Contraindicated in patients with anuria and in those with inborn errors of amino acid metabolism, such as maple syrup urine disease and isovaleric acidemia.

## NURSING CONSIDERATIONS
• Use with extreme caution in children and neonates, especially those with low birth weight.
• Use cautiously in patients with renal insufficiency or failure, cardiac disease, or hepatic impairment.
• Administer cautiously to diabetic patients; insulin may be needed to prevent hyperglycemia. Also administer cautiously to patients with cardiac insufficiency; may cause circulatory overload. Patients with fluid restriction may tolerate only 1 to 2 L.
• Obtain baseline serum electrolyte, glucose, BUN, calcium, and phosphorus levels before therapy, as ordered; monitor these levels periodically throughout therapy.
• *Alert:*Infuse amino acids only in I.V. fluids or TPN solution.

• Safe and effective use of parenteral nutrition requires knowledge of nutrition as well as clinical expertise in recognizing and treating complications. Frequent evaluations of patient and laboratory studies are needed.

• Limit peripheral infusions to 2.5% amino acids and dextrose 10%. Check infusion site frequently for erythema, inflammation, irritation, tissue sloughing, necrosis, and phlebitis. Change peripheral I.V. sites routinely to prevent irritation and infection. If subclavian catheter is used, administer solution into midsuperior vena cava.

• Add vitamins, electrolytes, and trace elements, as ordered.

• Check fractional urine every 6 hours for glycosuria initially, then every 12 to 24 hours in stable patients. Abrupt onset of glycosuria may be an early sign of impending sepsis.

• Assess body temperature every 4 hours; elevation may indicate sepsis or infection.

• Watch for extraordinary electrolyte losses that may occur during NG suction, vomiting, diarrhea, or drainage from GI fistula.

• Be prepared to individualize dosage to metabolic and clinical response as determined by nitrogen balance and body weight corrected for fluid balance.

• If patient has chills, fever, or other signs of sepsis, replace I.V. tubing and bottle and send them to the laboratory to be cultured.

### I.V. administration
• Control infusion rate carefully with infusion pump. If infusion rate falls behind, notify doctor; don't increase rate to catch up.

### Patient teaching
• Explain need for use to patient and family, and answer any questions.
• Tell patient to report adverse reactions promptly.

## dextrose (d-glucose)

*Pregnancy Risk Category C*

### HOW SUPPLIED
*Injection:* 3-ml ampule (10%); 10 ml (25%); 25 ml (5%); 50 ml (5% and 50% available in vial, ampule, and Bristoject); 70-ml pin-top vial (70% for additive use only); 100 ml (5%); 150 ml (5%); 250 ml (5%, 10%); 500 ml (5%, 10%, 20%, 30%, 40%, 50%, 60%, 70%); 650 ml (38.5%); 1,000 ml (2.5%, 5%, 10%, 20%, 30%, 40%, 50%, 60%, 70%); 2,000 ml (50%, 70%)

### ACTION
A simple water-soluble sugar that minimizes glyconeogenesis and promotes anabolism in patients whose oral caloric intake is limited.

| Route | Onset | Peak | Duration |
|-------|-------|------|----------|
| I.V. | Immediate | Immediate | Unknown |

### INDICATIONS & DOSAGE
*Fluid replacement and caloric supplementation in patients who can't maintain adequate oral intake or who are restricted from doing so—*
**Adults and children:** dosage depends on fluid and caloric requirements. Peripheral I.V. infusion of 2.5%, 5%, or 10% solution or central I.V. infusion of 20% solution is used for minimal fluid needs. A 10% to 25% solution is used to treat acute hypoglycemia in neonate or older infant (2 ml/kg). A 50% solution is used to treat insulin-induced hypoglycemia (20 to 50 ml). Solutions of 10%, 20%, 30%, 40%, 50%, 60%, and 70% are diluted in admixtures, usually amino acid solutions, for total parenteral nutrition (TPN) given through a central vein.

### ADVERSE REACTIONS
**CNS:** confusion, *unconsciousness in hyperosmolar hyperglycemic nonketotic syndrome.*
**CV:** *pulmonary edema, exacerbated hypertension, heart failure with fluid overload in susceptible patients; phlebitis, venous sclerosis,* tissue necrosis with pro-

---

Reactions may be *common,* uncommon, *life-threatening,* or COMMON AND LIFE-THREATENING.

longed or concentrated infusions, especially when administered peripherally.

**GU:** glycosuria, osmotic diuresis.

**Metabolic:** hyperglycemia, dehydration, fever, hyperosmolarity with rapid infusion of concentrated solution or prolonged infusion, hypoglycemia from rebound hyperinsulinemia with rapid termination of long-term infusions, hypervolemia, hypovolemia.

**Skin:** sloughing, tissue necrosis if extravasation occurs with concentrated solutions.

### INTERACTIONS

**Drug-drug.** *Corticosteroids:* may cause salt and water retention and increased potassium excretion. Monitor glucose, sodium, and potassium levels.

### EFFECTS ON DIAGNOSTIC TESTS
None reported.

### CONTRAINDICATIONS
Contraindicated in patients in diabetic coma while blood glucose level remains excessively high. Use of concentrated solutions contraindicated in patients with intracranial or intraspinal hemorrhage, in dehydrated patients with delirium tremens, and in patients with severe dehydration, anuria, hepatic coma, or glucose-galactose malabsorption syndrome.

### NURSING CONSIDERATIONS
• Use cautiously in patients with cardiac or pulmonary disease, hypertension, renal insufficiency, urinary obstruction, or hypovolemia.

• Monitor serum glucose levels carefully. Prolonged therapy with $D_5W$ can cause depletion of pancreatic insulin production and secretion.

• *Alert:* Never stop hypertonic solutions abruptly. If needed, have $D_{10}W$ available to treat hypoglycemia if rebound hyperinsulinemia occurs.

• *Alert:* Use central veins to infuse dextrose solutions with concentrations above 10%.

• Take care to prevent extravasation. Check injection site frequently to prevent irritation, tissue sloughing, necrosis, and phlebitis.

• Check vital signs frequently. Report adverse reactions promptly.

• Monitor fluid intake and output and weight carefully, especially in patients with renal function impairment.

• Watch closely for signs and symptoms of fluid overload, especially if fluid intake is restricted.

### I.V. administration
• Control infusion rate carefully; maximum rate is 0.5 g/kg/hour. Use infusion pump when administering with amino acids for TPN.

• *Alert:* Never infuse concentrated solutions rapidly. Rapid infusion may cause hyperglycemia and fluid shift.

### Patient teaching
• Explain need for drug to patient and family, and answer any questions.

• Tell patient to report adverse reactions promptly.

---

### fat emulsions
Intralipid 10%, Intralipid 20%, Liposyn II 10%, Liposyn II 20%, Liposyn III 10%, Liposyn III 20%

*Pregnancy Risk Category C*

### HOW SUPPLIED
*Injection:* 50 ml (10%, 20%), 100 ml (10%, 20%), 200 ml (10%, 20%), 250 ml (10%, 20%), 500 ml (10%, 20%)

### ACTION
Provides neutral triglycerides, predominantly unsaturated fatty acids; acts as a source of calories and prevents fatty acid deficiency. When substituted for dextrose as a source of calories, fat emulsions decrease carbon dioxide production.

| Route | Onset | Peak | Duration |
|-------|-------|------|----------|
| I.V. | Immediate | Immediate | Unknown |

### INDICATIONS & DOSAGE
Intralipid:
*Source of calories as adjunct to total parenteral nutrition (TPN)—*
**Adults:** 1 ml/minute I.V. for 15 to 30 minutes (10% emulsion); 0.5 ml/minute

I.V. for 15 to 30 minutes (20% emulsion).
If no adverse reactions occur, rate increased to deliver 500 ml over 4 to 8 hours; total daily dose shouldn't exceed 3 g/kg.
**Children:** 0.1 ml/minute for 10 to 15 minutes (10% emulsion), 0.05 ml/minute I.V. for 10 to 15 minutes (20% emulsion). If no adverse reactions occur, rate increased to deliver 1 g/kg over 4 hours; daily dose shouldn't exceed 3 g/kg. Equals 40% of daily caloric intake; protein-carbohydrate TPN should supply remaining 60%.
*Fatty acid deficiency—*
**Adults and children:** 8% to 10% of total caloric intake I.V.
Liposyn:
*Prevention of fatty acid deficiency—*
**Adults:** 500 ml (10% emulsion) I.V. twice weekly. Infused initially at rate of 1 ml/minute for 30 minutes. Rate may be increased to, but shouldn't exceed, 500 ml over 4 to 6 hours.
**Children:** 5 to 10 ml/kg (10% emulsion) I.V. daily. Initially infused at rate of 0.1 ml/minute for 30 minutes. Rate may be increased to, but shouldn't exceed, 100 ml/hour.

## ADVERSE REACTIONS
*Early reactions:*
**CNS:** headache, sleepiness, dizziness.
**CV:** chest and back pains, flushing.
**EENT:** pressure over eyes.
**GI:** nausea, vomiting.
**Hematologic:** hypercoagulability.
**Metabolic:** hyperlipidemia, fever.
**Respiratory:** dyspnea, cyanosis.
**Skin:** diaphoresis.
**Other:** *hypersensitivity reactions;* irritation at infusion site.
*Delayed reactions:*
**CNS:** *focal seizures.*
**Hematologic:** *thrombocytopenia, leukopenia,* leukocytosis.
**Hepatic:** transient increases in liver function test results; altered results of serum bilirubin tests; hepatomegaly.
**Other:** fever, splenomegaly.

## INTERACTIONS
None significant.

## EFFECTS ON DIAGNOSTIC TESTS
Abnormally high mean corpuscular hemoglobin and mean corpuscular hemoglobin levels may be found in blood samples drawn during or shortly after fat emulsion infusion.

## CONTRAINDICATIONS
Contraindicated in patients with severe egg allergies, hyperlipidemia, lipid nephrosis, or acute pancreatitis accompanied by hyperlipidemia.

## NURSING CONSIDERATIONS
● Use cautiously in patients with severe hepatic disease, pulmonary disease, anemia, or blood coagulation disorders including thrombocytopenia, and in patients at risk for fat embolism.
● Use cautiously in jaundiced or premature infants.
● Drug may be mixed with amino acid solution, dextrose, electrolytes, and vitamins in same I.V. container. Check with pharmacist for acceptable proportions and compatibility information.
● Don't use fat emulsion if it separates or becomes oily.
● Because lipids support bacterial growth, change all I.V. tubing before each infusion. Check injection site daily. Report signs and symptoms of inflammation or infection promptly.
● Watch for adverse reactions, especially during first half of infusion.
● Monitor serum lipid levels closely when patient is receiving fat emulsion therapy. Lipemia must clear between doses.
● Monitor hepatic function carefully in long-term therapy.
● Check platelet count frequently in neonates receiving fat emulsions I.V.
● Carefully monitor serum triglyceride levels and free fatty acids in infants.
● Refrigeration of fat emulsions isn't needed.
● Intralipid and Liposyn differ mainly by their fatty acid components.

## ⚑I.V. administration
● *Alert:* Avoid rapid infusion, and use an infusion pump to regulate rate. Rapid infusion may cause fluid or fat overloading.

---

• An in-line filter with pores of 1.2 microns or larger is sometimes used to remove particulates.

### ☑ Patient teaching
• Explain need for fat emulsion therapy, and answer any questions.
• Tell patient to report adverse reactions promptly.

---

**medium-chain triglycerides**
MCT ◊

*Pregnancy Risk Category NR*

### HOW SUPPLIED
*Oil:* 960 ml (115 calories/15 ml) ◊

### ACTION
A source of rapidly hydrolyzable lipid.

| Route | Onset | Peak | Duration |
|-------|-------|------|----------|
| P.O. | Unknown | Unknown | Unknown |

### INDICATIONS & DOSAGE
*Inadequate digestion or absorption of food fats—*
**Adults:** 15 ml P.O. t.i.d. or q.i.d.

### ADVERSE REACTIONS
**CNS:** *reversible coma in susceptible patients.*
**GI:** *nausea, vomiting, diarrhea, abdominal distention, cramps.*

### INTERACTIONS
None significant.

### EFFECTS ON DIAGNOSTIC TESTS
None reported.

### CONTRAINDICATIONS
No known contraindications.

### NURSING CONSIDERATIONS
• Use cautiously in patients with hepatic cirrhosis and such complications as portacaval shunts or tendency to encephalopathy.
• To minimize GI adverse reactions, give smaller, more frequent doses with meals (mixed with salad dressing, in chilled fruit juice, or incorporated into sauces or when baking).
• Drug is more easily absorbed than long-chain fats; not dependent on bile salts for emulsification.
• Drug's rapid metabolism provides quick energy.
• Drug provides 7.7 calories/ml and no essential fatty acids.

### ☑ Patient teaching
• Instruct patient when and how to take drug to minimize GI adverse reactions.
• Tell patient to report persistent or severe adverse reactions promptly.
• Caution patient not to use plastic containers or utensils to give drug.

---

**allopurinol**
**colchicine**
**probenecid**
**sulfinpyrazone**

## COMBINATION PRODUCTS

COLBENEMID, PROBEN-C, PROBENECID WITH COLCHICINE: probenecid 500 mg and colchicine 0.5 mg.

### allopurinol

Apo-Allopurinol†, Capurate‡, Lopurin, Purinol†, Zyloprim, Zyloric§

*Pregnancy Risk Category C*

## HOW SUPPLIED

*Tablets (scored):* 100 mg, 200 mg†, 300 mg
*Capsules:* 100 mg‡, 300 mg‡
*Injection:* 500 mg/30 ml vial

## ACTION

Reduces uric acid production by inhibiting biochemical reactions preceding its formation.

| Route | Onset | Peak | Duration |
|-------|-------|------|----------|
| P.O. | Unknown | 0.5-2 hr | 1-2 wk |
| I.V. | Unknown | 0.5 hr | Unknown |

## INDICATIONS & DOSAGE

*Gout, primary or secondary to hyperuricemia; secondary to diseases such as acute or chronic leukemia, polycythemia vera, multiple myeloma, psoriasis—*
Dosage varies with severity of disease; can be given as single dose or divided, but doses above 300 mg should be divided.
**Adults:** mild gout, 200 to 300 mg P.O. daily; severe gout with large tophi, 400 to 600 mg P.O. daily. Same dosage for maintenance in secondary hyperuricemia. Maximum dose is 800 mg/day. Or, give 200 to 400 mg/m$^2$/day I.V. as a single infusion or equally divided dose q 6, 8, or 12 hours.

**Children:** initially 200 mg/m$^2$/day I.V. as single infusion or equally divided dose q 6, 8, or 12 hours.
*Hyperuricemia secondary to malignancies—*
**Children under age 6:** 50 mg P.O. t.i.d.
**Children ages 6 to 10:** 300 mg P.O. daily or divided t.i.d.
*Prevention of acute gouty attacks—*
**Adults:** 100 mg P.O. daily; increase at weekly intervals by 100 mg without exceeding maximum dose (800 mg), until serum uric acid falls to 6 mg/dl or less.
*Prevention of uric acid nephropathy during cancer chemotherapy—*
**Adults:** 600 to 800 mg P.O. daily for 2 to 3 days, with high fluid intake.
*Recurrent calcium oxalate calculi—*
**Adults:** 200 to 300 mg P.O. daily in single or divided doses.
*Adjust-a-dose:*For renally impaired patients, 200 mg P.O. or I.V. daily if creatinine clearance is 10 to 20 ml/minute; 100 mg P.O. or I.V. daily if below 10 ml/minute; and 100 mg P.O. or I.V. q 48 hours if below 3 ml/minute.

## ADVERSE REACTIONS

**CNS:** drowsiness, headache, paresthesia, peripheral neuropathy, neuritis.
**CV:** hypersensitivity vasculitis, necrotizing angiitis.
**EENT:** epistaxis.
**GI:** nausea, vomiting, diarrhea, abdominal pain, gastritis, taste loss or perversion, dyspepsia.
**GU:** *renal failure,* uremia.
**Hematologic:** *agranulocytosis,* anemia, *aplastic anemia, thrombocytopenia, leukopenia,* leukocytosis, eosinophilia.
**Hepatic:** *hepatitis, hepatic necrosis,* hepatomegaly, cholestatic jaundice, increased alkaline phosphatase, AST, and ALT levels.
**Musculoskeletal:** arthralgia, myopathy.
**Skin:** *rash*; exfoliative, urticarial, and purpuric lesions; *erythema multiforme;* severe furunculosis of nose; ichthyosis; alopecia; *toxic epidermal necrolysis.*
**Other:** ecchymoses, fever, chills.

Reactions may be *common*, uncommon, *life-threatening*, or COMMON AND LIFE-THREATENING.

## INTERACTIONS

**Drug-drug.** *Amoxicillin, ampicillin, bacampicillin:* increased possibility of rash. Avoid concomitant use.

*Anticoagulants except warfarin:* potentiation of anticoagulant effect. Dosage adjustments may be needed.

*Antineoplastics:* increased potential for bone marrow suppression. Monitor patient carefully.

*Chlorpropamide:* possible increased hypoglycemic effect. Avoid concomitant use.

*Diazoxide, diuretics, mecamylamine, pyrazinamide:* increased serum uric acid level. Adjust dosage of allopurinol.

*Ethacrynic acid, thiazide diuretics:* increased risk of allopurinol toxicity. Reduce dosage of allopurinol, and closely monitor renal function.

*Uricosurics:* additive effect. May enhance therapy.

*Urine-acidifying drugs (ammonium chloride, ascorbic acid, potassium or sodium phosphate):* may increase possibility of kidney stone formation. Monitor patient carefully.

*Xanthines:* increased serum theophylline levels. Adjust dosage of theophylline, as needed.

**Drug-lifestyle.** *Alcohol use:* increased serum uric acid levels. Avoid alcohol use.

## EFFECTS ON DIAGNOSTIC TESTS
None reported.

## CONTRAINDICATIONS
Contraindicated in patients with hypersensitivity to drug and in those with idiopathic hemochromatosis.

## NURSING CONSIDERATIONS
• Monitor serum uric acid levels to evaluate drug's effectiveness.
• Monitor fluid intake and output; daily urine output of at least 2 L and maintenance of neutral or slightly alkaline urine are desirable.
• Periodically monitor CBC and hepatic and renal function, especially at start of therapy, as ordered.
• Optimal benefits may need 2 to 6 weeks of therapy. Because acute gouty attacks may occur during this time, concurrent use of colchicine may be prescribed prophylactically.
• Don't restart drug in patients who experience a severe reaction.
• *Alert:* Don't confuse Zyloprim with ZORprin.

## I.V. administration
• Preparation of allopurinol includes reconstitution and dilution. Dissolve contents of each 30-ml vial with 25 ml of sterile water for injection. Solution should be diluted to desired concentration (no greater than 6 mg/ml) with normal saline injection or 5% dextrose for injection. Don't use sodium bicarbonate–containing solutions. Store solution at 68° to 77° F (20° to 25° C) and use within 10 hours. Don't use if particulates or discoloration is present. Refer to package insert for full list of drugs that are incompatible with allopurinol in solution.

## Patient teaching
• To minimize GI adverse reactions, tell patient to take drug with, or immediately after, meals.
• Encourage patient to drink plenty of fluids while taking drug unless otherwise contraindicated.
• Drug may cause drowsiness; tell patient not to drive or perform hazardous tasks requiring mental alertness until CNS effects of drug are known.
• If patient is taking allopurinol for treatment of recurrent calcium oxalate stones, advise him also to reduce his dietary intake of animal protein, sodium, refined sugars, oxalate-rich foods, and calcium.
• Tell patient to stop drug at first sign of rash, which may precede severe hypersensitivity or other adverse reactions. Rash is more common in patients taking diuretics and in those with renal disorders. Tell patient to report all adverse reactions.
• Advise patient to avoid alcohol during therapy.
• Teach patient importance of continuing drug even if asymptomatic.

## colchicine
Colgout‡

*Pregnancy Risk Category C (P.O.), D (I.V.)*

### HOW SUPPLIED
*Tablets:* 0.5 mg (1/120 grain), 0.6 mg (1/100 grain) as sugar-coated granules
*Injection:* 1 mg (1/60 grain)/2 ml

### ACTION
Unknown. As an antigout drug, apparently decreases WBC motility, phagocytosis, and lactic acid production, decreasing urate crystal deposits and reducing inflammation. As antiosteolytic drug, apparently inhibits mitosis of osteoprogenitor cells and decreases osteoclast activity.

| Route | Onset | Peak | Duration |
|-------|-------|------|----------|
| P.O. | ≤ 12 hr | 0.5-2 hr | Unknown |
| I.V. | 6-12 hr | Unknown | Unknown |

### INDICATIONS & DOSAGE
*Prevention of acute gout attacks as prophylactic or maintenance therapy—*
**Adults:** 0.5 or 0.6 mg P.O. daily. Patients who normally have one attack per year or less should receive drug only 1 to 4 days weekly; patients who have more than one attack per year should receive drug daily. In severe cases, 1.5 to 1.95 mg P.O. daily.
*Prevention of gout attacks in patients undergoing surgery—*
**Adults:** 0.5 to 0.6 mg P.O. t.i.d. 3 days before and 3 days after surgery.
*Acute gout, acute gouty arthritis—*
**Adults:** initially, 0.5 to 1.3 mg P.O.; then 0.5 or 0.6 mg q 1 to 2 hours until pain is relieved; nausea, vomiting, or diarrhea ensues; or maximum dose of 8 mg is reached. Or, 2 mg I.V.; then 0.5 mg I.V. q 6 hours if needed. (Note that some doctors prefer to give a single I.V. injection of 3 mg.) Total I.V. dose over 24 hours (one course of treatment) shouldn't exceed 4 mg.

### ADVERSE REACTIONS
**CNS:** peripheral neuritis.
**GI:** *nausea, vomiting, abdominal pain, diarrhea.*
**GU:** reversible azoospermia.
**Hematologic:** *aplastic anemia, thrombocytopenia, agranulocytosis with long-term use;* nonthrombocytopenic purpura.
**Hepatic:** increased alkaline phosphatase, AST, and ALT levels.
**Metabolic:** decreased serum carotene and cholesterol levels.
**Musculoskeletal:** myopathy.
**Skin:** alopecia, urticaria, dermatitis.
**Other:** severe local irritation if extravasation occurs, *hypersensitivity reactions.*

### INTERACTIONS
**Drug-drug.** *Vitamin B₁₂:* impaired absorption of oral vitamin $B_{12}$. Avoid concomitant use.
**Drug-lifestyle.** *Alcohol use:* may impair efficacy of colchicine prophylaxis. Don't use together.

### EFFECTS ON DIAGNOSTIC TESTS
Drug therapy may cause false-positive results of urine tests for RBCs or hemoglobin.

### CONTRAINDICATIONS
Contraindicated in patients with hypersensitivity to drug and in those with blood dyscrasias or serious CV disease, renal disease, or GI disorders.

### NURSING CONSIDERATIONS
• Use cautiously in elderly or debilitated patients and in those with early signs of CV, renal, or GI disease.
• Obtain baseline laboratory test results, including CBC, before therapy, as ordered; then periodically throughout therapy.
• *Alert:*Don't administer I.M. or S.C.; severe local irritation occurs.
• As maintenance therapy, give drug with meals to reduce GI effects. Drug may be used with uricosurics, as ordered.
• Monitor fluid intake and output; and keep output at 2 L daily.
• *Alert:*After full course of I.V. colchicine (4 mg), don't give colchicine by any route for at least 7 days. Colchicine is a toxic drug and death has resulted from overdose.
• First sign of acute overdose may be GI symptoms, followed by vascular damage, muscle weakness, and ascending paraly-

---

Reactions may be *common,* uncommon, *life-threatening,* or COMMON AND LIFE-THREATENING.

sis. Delirium and seizures may occur without patient losing consciousness.
• Discontinue drug as soon as gout pain is relieved or at first sign of GI symptoms, as ordered.

### I.V. administration
• Give by slow I.V. push over 2 to 5 minutes. Avoid extravasation because colchicine irritates tissues. Don't dilute colchicine injection with $D_5W$ injection or other fluids that might change pH of colchicine solution. If lower concentration of colchicine injection is needed, dilute with normal saline solution or sterile water for injection and give over 2 to 5 minutes by direct injection. Preferably, inject into the tubing of a free-flowing I.V. solution. Don't inject if diluted solution becomes turbid.

### Patient teaching
• Teach patient how to take drug and tell him to drink extra fluids.
• Tell patient to report adverse reactions, especially signs of acute overdose (nausea, vomiting, abdominal pain, diarrhea, unusual bleeding, bruising, tiredness, weakness, numbness, or tingling).
• Advise patient to avoid alcohol while taking drug.
• Tell patient with gout to limit intake of foods high in purine, such as anchovies, liver, sardines, kidneys, sweetbreads, peas, and lentils.

---

## probenecid
Benemid, Benuryl†, Probalan

*Pregnancy Risk Category B*

### HOW SUPPLIED
*Tablets:* 500 mg

### ACTION
Blocks renal tubular reabsorption of uric acid, increasing excretion, and inhibits active renal tubular secretion of many weak organic acids, such as penicillins and cephalosporins.

| Route | Onset | Peak | Duration |
|-------|-------|------|----------|
| P.O. | Unknown | 2-4 hr | Unknown |

### INDICATIONS & DOSAGE
*Adjunct to penicillin therapy—*
**Adults and children over 50 kg (110 lb):** 500 mg P.O. q.i.d.
**Children ages 2 to 14 or weighing 50 kg or less:** initially, 25 mg/kg P.O.; then 40 mg/kg/day in divided doses q.i.d.
*Gonorrhea—*
**Adults:** 3.5 g ampicillin P.O. with 1 g probenecid P.O. given together; or 1 g probenecid P.O. 30 minutes before dose of 4.8 million U of aqueous penicillin G procaine I.M., injected at two different sites.
*Hyperuricemia of gout, gouty arthritis—*
**Adults:** 250 mg P.O. b.i.d. for first week; then 500 mg b.i.d., to maximum of 2 g daily. Maintenance dose should be reviewed q 6 months and reduced by increments of 500 mg, if indicated.

### ADVERSE REACTIONS
**CNS:** *headache,* dizziness.
**CV:** flushing.
**GI:** anorexia, nausea, vomiting, sore gums.
**GU:** urinary frequency, renal colic, nephrotic syndrome.
**Hematologic:** *hemolytic anemia,* anemia, *aplastic anemia.*
**Hepatic:** *hepatic necrosis.*
**Skin:** dermatitis, pruritus.
**Other:** fever, exacerbation of gout, *hypersensitivity reactions including anaphylaxis,* fever.

### INTERACTIONS
**Drug-drug.** *Acyclovir, cephalosporins, ketamine, lorazepam, penicillin, thiopental:* may increase levels of these drugs. Use cautiously.
*Methotrexate:* decreased methotrexate excretion. Lower methotrexate dosage may be needed. Serum levels should be determined.
*Nitrofurantoin:* increased toxicity and reduced effectiveness. Reduce probenecid dose.
*NSAIDs:* may enhance toxicity. Avoid concomitant use.
*Sulfonylureas:* enhanced hypoglycemic effect. Monitor blood glucose levels closely. Dosage adjustment may be needed.
*Salicylates:* inhibited uricosuric effect of probenecid, causing urate retention. Don't use together.

---

*Liquid contains alcohol.     **May contain tartrazine.     †Canada     ‡Australia     §U.K.     ◇OTC

*Zidovudine:* may increase zidovudine levels and toxicity symptoms. Monitor patient.
**Drug-lifestyle.** *Alcohol use:* increased urate levels. Avoid use.

## EFFECTS ON DIAGNOSTIC TESTS
Drug causes false-positive test results for urinary glucose with tests using cupric sulfate reagent (Benedict's reagent, Clinitest, and Fehling's test); use glucose oxidase reagent (Diastix or Chemstrip uG) instead. Drug also decreases urinary excretion of 17-ketosteroids, sulfobromosulphthalein, aminohippuric acid, and iodine-related organic acids, interfering with laboratory procedures.

## CONTRAINDICATIONS
Contraindicated in patients with hypersensitivity to drug and in those with uric acid kidney stones or blood dyscrasias; also contraindicated in an acute gout attack and in children under age 2.

## NURSING CONSIDERATIONS
• Use cautiously in patients with peptic ulcer or renal impairment.
• Use cautiously in patients with sulfa allergy because probenecid is a sulfonamide derivative.
• To minimize GI distress, give drug with milk, food, or antacids. Continued disturbances might indicate need to lower dosage.
• Monitor BUN level and renal function tests periodically in long-term therapy.
• Force fluids to maintain minimum daily output of 2 to 3 L. Alkalinize urine with sodium bicarbonate or potassium citrate, as ordered. These measures will prevent hematuria, renal colic, urate stone development, and costovertebral pain.
• Therapy for treatment of gout isn't initiated until acute attack subsides. Drug doesn't contain an analgesic or anti-inflammatory, and it's of no value during acute gout attacks.
• Drug is suitable for long-term use; no cumulative effects or tolerance reported.
• Drug is ineffective in patients with chronic renal insufficiency (glomerular filtration rate below 30 ml/minute).

• Drug may increase frequency, severity, and length of acute gout attacks during first 6 to 12 months of therapy. Prophylactic colchicine or another anti-inflammatory is given during first 3 to 6 months.
• *Alert:* Don't confuse probenecid with Procanbid or Benemid with Beminal.

### ☑Patient teaching
• Instruct patient and family that, when prescribed as treatment for gout, drug must be taken regularly, as ordered, or gout attacks might occur.
• Tell patient to visit doctor regularly so that uric acid can be monitored and dosage adjusted, if needed. Lifelong therapy may be needed in patients with hyperuricemia.
• Advise patient with gout to avoid all drugs that contain aspirin, which may precipitate gout. Acetaminophen may be used for pain.
• Instruct patient to drink at least 6 to 8 glasses of water per day.
• Urge patient with gout to avoid alcohol; it increases urate level.
• Tell patient with gout to limit intake of foods high in purine, such as anchovies, liver, sardines, kidneys, sweetbreads, peas, and lentils. Also tell him to identify and avoid other foods that may trigger gout attacks.
• Instruct patient to take all medicine as prescribed when given with penicillin.

---

## sulfinpyrazone
Anturan†, Anturane

*Pregnancy Risk Category C*

## HOW SUPPLIED
*Tablets:* 100 mg
*Capsules:* 200 mg

## ACTION
Blocks renal tubular reabsorption of uric acid, increasing excretion, and inhibits platelet aggregation.

| Route | Onset | Peak | Duration |
|-------|-------|------|----------|
| P.O. | Unknown | 1-2 hr | 4-6 hr |

---

Reactions may be *common,* uncommon, *__life-threatening__,* or COMMON AND LIFE-THREATENING.

## INDICATIONS & DOSAGE
*Intermittent or chronic gouty arthritis—*
**Adults:** 200 to 400 mg P.O. b.i.d. first week; then 400 mg P.O. b.i.d. Maximum dose is 800 mg daily.

## ADVERSE REACTIONS
**GI:** *nausea, dyspepsia,* epigastric pain, reactivation of peptic ulcerations.
**GU:** altered renal function test results.
**Hematologic:** anemia, *leukopenia, agranulocytosis, thrombocytopenia, aplastic anemia.*
**Respiratory:** *bronchoconstriction in patients with aspirin-induced asthma.*
**Skin:** rash.

## INTERACTIONS
**Drug-drug.** *Aspirin, salicylates:* inhibited uricosuric effect of sulfinpyrazone. Don't use together.
*Oral anticoagulants:* increased anticoagulant effect and risk of bleeding. Use together cautiously.
*Oral antidiabetics:* increased effects. Monitor blood glucose.
*Probenecid:* inhibited renal excretion of sulfinpyrazone. Use together cautiously.
*Theophylline, verapamil:* increased clearance. Use cautiously.
**Drug-lifestyle.** *Alcohol use:* decreased effectiveness. Avoid concomitant use.

## EFFECTS ON DIAGNOSTIC TESTS
Drug decreases urinary excretion of aminohippuric acid and phenolsulfonphthalein.

## CONTRAINDICATIONS
Contraindicated in patients with hypersensitivity to pyrazole derivatives (including oxyphenbutazone and phenylbutazone) and in those with blood dyscrasias, active peptic ulcer, or symptoms of GI inflammation or ulceration.

## NURSING CONSIDERATIONS
• Use cautiously in patients with healed peptic ulcer and in pregnant women.
• Monitor BUN level, CBC, and renal function studies periodically during long-term use, as ordered.
• Monitor fluid intake and output closely. Therapy, especially at start, may lead to renal colic and formation of uric acid stones until acid levels are normal (about 6 mg/dl).
• Force fluids to maintain minimum daily output of 2 to 3 L. Alkalinize urine with sodium bicarbonate or other drug, as ordered.
• Drug doesn't contain an analgesic or anti-inflammatory, and is of no value during acute gout attacks.
• Drug may increase frequency, severity, and length of acute gout attacks during first 6 to 12 months of therapy. Prophylactic colchicine or another anti-inflammatory is given during first 3 to 6 months.
• Lifelong therapy may be needed in patients with hyperuricemia.
• *Alert:* Don't confuse Anturane with Artane or Antabuse.

### ☑ Patient teaching
• Instruct patient and family that drug must be taken regularly, as ordered, even during acute exacerbations.
• Tell patient to visit doctor regularly so blood levels can be monitored and dosage adjusted, if needed.
• Warn patient with gout not to take aspirin-containing drugs because these may precipitate gout. Acetaminophen may be used for pain.
• Tell patient with gout to avoid foods high in purine, such as anchovies, liver, sardines, kidneys, sweetbreads, peas, and lentils, and to identify and avoid any other foods that may trigger gout attacks.
• Instruct patient to drink at least 10 to 12 glasses of fluid daily.
• Advise patient to avoid alcohol during therapy.
• Instruct patient to report unusual bleeding or bruising or flulike symptoms.

**chymopapain**
**fibrinolysin and**
**desoxyribonuclease**
**hyaluronidase**

**COMBINATION PRODUCTS**
None.

---

### chymopapain
Chymodiactin

*Pregnancy Risk Category C*

**HOW SUPPLIED**
*Powder for injection:* 4,000 U/vial; each unit of chymopapain is also known as 1 picoKatal (pKat)

**ACTION**
Hydrolyzes noncollagenous proteins in the chondromucoprotein of the nucleus pulposus, lowering pressure within the disk.

| Route | Onset | Peak | Duration |
|-------|-------|------|----------|
| Intradisk | Unknown | Unknown | 1 wk |

**INDICATIONS & DOSAGE**
*Herniated lumbar disk—*
**Adults:** 2,000 to 4,000 U (pKat)/disk injected intradiskally. Maximum dose for multiple disk herniation is 8,000 U.

**ADVERSE REACTIONS**
**CNS:** *subarachnoid and intracerebral hemorrhage, seizures,* headache, paresthesia, dizziness.
**EENT:** conjunctivitis, vasomotor rhinitis.
**GI:** nausea.
**Musculoskeletal:** leg weakness, numbness of legs and toes, *back pain, stiffness, back spasm, soreness,* paraplegia, acute transverse myelitis.
**Skin:** erythema, rash, pruritic urticaria.
**Other:** *anaphylaxis, anaphylactoid reaction, angioedema.*

**INTERACTIONS**
**Drug-drug.** *Radiographic contrast media:* potential adverse reactions (increased risk of neurotoxicity) when injected with chymopapain. Avoid concurrent use.

**EFFECTS ON DIAGNOSTIC TESTS**
None reported.

**CONTRAINDICATIONS**
Contraindicated in patients with history of allergy to drug, papaya, or papaya derivatives such as meat tenderizers; in those who have previously received an injection of chymopapain; and in those with severe spondylolisthesis in addition to spinal stenosis, severe progressing paralysis, or evidence of spinal cord tumor or cauda equina lesion.

**NURSING CONSIDERATIONS**
• A ChymoFAST test can detect hypersensitivity to drug. Giving histamine-receptor antagonists before drug may lessen severity of anaphylactoid reactions (e.g., cimetidine 300 mg P.O. q 6 hours and diphenhydramine 50 mg P.O. q 6 hours for 24 hours before chymopapain administration).
• *Alert:*Drug should be used only by doctors qualified and experienced to perform laminectomy, diskectomy, or other spinal procedures, and who have received specialized training in chemonucleolysis. It shouldn't be injected in regions other than the lumbar spine; extremely toxic if injected into subarachnoid space.
• Use sterile water, not bacteriostatic water for injection, to reconstitute drug. Use within 1 hour after reconstitution. Discard unused drug.
• After wiping stopper with alcohol, allow to dry before drawing up drug because alcohol inactivates the enzyme.
• Watch very closely for anaphylactoid reaction (0.5% of patients). Reaction may be immediate or delayed up to 1 hour after injection and may last for minutes to several hours. Watch for hypotension and bronchospasm, possibly leading to laryn-

---

Reactions may be *common*, uncommon, *life-threatening*, or COMMON AND LIFE-THREATENING.

geal edema, arrhythmias, cardiac arrest, coma, and death. Other signs of allergic response include erythema, pilomotor erection, rash, pruritic urticaria, conjunctivitis, vasomotor rhinitis, angioedema, and various GI disturbances.

• Keep an I.V. line open to manage anaphylaxis quickly, if needed. Keep epinephrine and corticosteroids available.

☑ **Patient teaching**
• Instruct patient to anticipate delayed allergic reactions, such as rash, urticaria, or pruritus, which may occur up to 15 days after injection. Tell him to report these at once.
• Warn patient that he may experience back pain or involuntary muscle spasm in the lower back for several days after injection. Reassure him that this is common and isn't chronic.

## fibrinolysin and desoxyribonuclease
Elase, Elase-Chloromycetin

*Pregnancy Risk Category C*

### HOW SUPPLIED
*Powder for solution:* 25 U fibrinolysin and 15,000 U desoxyribonuclease in 30-ml vial
*Ointment:* 1 U fibrinolysin and 666.6 U desoxyribonuclease per gram in 10-g or 30-g tube (with applicator); or 1 U fibrinolysin, 666.6 U desoxyribonuclease, chloramphenicol 1% per gram

### ACTION
Attacks fibrin of blood clots and fibrinous exudates; desoxyribonuclease attacks DNA. Combined enzymatic action débrides wound surfaces and promotes healing.

| Route | Onset | Peak | Duration |
|-------|-------|------|----------|
| Intravaginal, transdermal | Unknown | Unknown | Unknown |

### INDICATIONS & DOSAGE
*Débridement of inflamed and infected lesions—*
**Adults and children:** ointment applied to lesions daily to t.i.d. for as long as en-

zyme action is desired. Or, solution prepared from powder applied topically as a liquid, spray, or wet dressing.

For wet-to-dry dressing, mix 1 vial of Elase powder with 10 to 50 ml of normal saline solution; saturate strips of fine gauze with solution. Pack ulcerated area with Elase gauze. Let gauze dry in contact with ulcerated lesion for 6 to 8 hours. Remove dried gauze and repeat t.i.d. or q.i.d.
*Mild to moderate cervicitis or vaginitis—*
**Adults:** 5 ml of ointment inserted intravaginally using applicator once daily h.s. for 5 days or until tube is empty. In more severe cases, instill 10 ml of solution intravaginally; wait 1 to 2 minutes for enzyme to disperse, then insert tampon and leave in overnight. Remove tampon next day. Continue therapy with ointment.
*Irrigation of infected wounds, empyema cavities, abscesses, otorhinolaryngologic wounds, subcutaneous hematomas—*
**Adults and children:** dilute prepared solution and irrigate wound, p.r.n., depending on extent and severity.

For solution as irrigating drug, drain cavity and replace Elase q 6 to 10 hours to reduce amount of by-product accumulation and to minimize loss of enzyme activity.

### ADVERSE REACTIONS
**CV:** hyperemia.
**Other:** *hypersensitivity reactions.*

### INTERACTIONS
None significant.

### EFFECTS ON DIAGNOSTIC TESTS
None reported.

### CONTRAINDICATIONS
Contraindicated in patients with hypersensitivity to drug or bovine products; it isn't for parenteral use.

### NURSING CONSIDERATIONS
• Dense, dry eschar is surgically removed before enzymatic débridement. Enzyme must be in constant contact with substrate. Necrotic debris is removed periodically; the enzyme is replenished at least once daily.

---

*Liquid contains alcohol.    **May contain tartrazine.    †Canada    ‡Australia    §U.K.    ◊OTC

• Prepare solution just before use and discard after 24 hours. Refrigerate unused portion.
• Clean and dry wound; cover with thin layer of Elase and nonadherent dressing.
• Ensure that aseptic wound-dressing techniques are used and that antibiotic therapy is instituted, as ordered.
• Change patient's dressing up to t.i.d. Flush away necrotic debris; then reapply ointment. Frequency of application may be more important than amount of drug used.

### ✔Patient teaching
• Explain drug use and administration to patient and family.
• Tell patient to report hypersensitivity reactions promptly.

---

## hyaluronidase
Hyalase§, Wydase

*Pregnancy Risk Category C*

### HOW SUPPLIED
*Injection:* 150 U/ml in 1-ml, 10-ml vials

### ACTION
Hydrolyzes hyaluronic acid, promoting diffusion of fluids in tissues.

| Route | Onset | Peak | Duration |
|-------|-------|------|----------|
| S.C. | Immediate | Unknown | 1-2 days |

### INDICATIONS & DOSAGE
*Adjunct to increase absorption and dispersion of other injected drugs—*
**Adults and children:** 150 USP U added to solution containing other drug.
*Hypodermoclysis—*
**Adults and children over age 3:**
150 USP U injected S.C. before clysis or injected into clysis tubing near needle for each 1,000-ml clysis solution.
*Excretory urography when contrast medium is given S.C.—*
**Adults and children:** with patient in a prone position, 75 USP U S.C. over each scapula; then injection of contrast medium at same sites.

### ADVERSE REACTIONS
None significant.

### INTERACTIONS
**Drug-drug.** *Local anesthetics:* increased potential for toxic local reaction. Use together cautiously.

### EFFECTS ON DIAGNOSTIC TESTS
None reported.

### CONTRAINDICATIONS
Contraindicated in patients with hypersensitivity to drug.

### NURSING CONSIDERATIONS
• Perform a skin test (0.02 ml of solution) for sensitivity. Don't inject into diseased areas. Watch for local reactions (wheal and pseudopods within 5 minutes and persisting, with itching, for 20 to 30 minutes). Erythema alone isn't considered a positive reaction.
• Don't inject into acutely inflamed or cancerous areas.
• *Alert:*Drug isn't recommended for I.V. use.
• For children, add 15 U to each 100 ml of solution. Drip rate shouldn't exceed 2 ml/minute.
• Don't add to solutions containing epinephrine and heparin.
• For hypodermoclysis, adjust dosage, rate of injection, and type of solution per patient's response, as ordered.
• If solution gets in eyes, flush with water.
• Protect from heat. Don't use cloudy or discolored solution. Store reconstituted solution below 86° F (30° C), and use within 14 days.

### ✔Patient teaching
• Explain need for drug to patient and family and describe how drug is given.
• Inform patient about possible adverse skin reactions.

---

**carboprost tromethamine**
**dinoprostone**
**methylergonovine maleate**
**oxytocin, synthetic injection**

**COMBINATION PRODUCTS**
None.

---

## carboprost tromethamine
Hemabate

*Pregnancy Risk Category C*

**HOW SUPPLIED**
*Injection:* 250 mcg/ml

**ACTION**
A prostaglandin that produces strong, prompt contractions of uterine smooth muscle, possibly mediated by calcium and cAMP.

| Route | Onset | Peak | Duration |
|-------|-------|------|----------|
| I.M. | Unknown | 15-60 min | 24 hr |

**INDICATIONS & DOSAGE**
*To abort pregnancy between weeks 13 and 20 of gestation—*
**Adults:** initially, 250 mcg deep I.M. Subsequent doses of 250 mcg administered at intervals of 1½ to 3½ hours, depending on uterine response. Dosage may be increased in increments to 500 mcg if contractility is inadequate after several 250-mcg doses. Total dose shouldn't exceed 12 mg.
*Postpartum hemorrhage due to uterine atony not managed by conventional methods—*
**Adults:** 250 mcg by deep I.M. injection. Repeat doses administered at 15- to 90-minute intervals, as needed. Maximum total dose is 2 mg.

**ADVERSE REACTIONS**
**CNS:** headache, anxiety, paresthesia, syncope, weakness.
**CV:** chest pain, *arrhythmias,* flushing.
**EENT:** blurred vision, eye pain.
**GI:** *vomiting, diarrhea, nausea.*
**GU:** endometritis, *uterine rupture,* uterine or vaginal pain, breast tenderness.
**Musculoskeletal:** backache, leg cramps.
**Respiratory:** coughing, wheezing.
**Skin:** rash, diaphoresis.
**Other:** *fever,* chills, hot flashes.

**INTERACTIONS**
**Drug-drug.** *Other oxytocics:* may potentiate action. Avoid concomitant use.

**EFFECTS ON DIAGNOSTIC TESTS**
None reported.

**CONTRAINDICATIONS**
Contraindicated in patients with hypersensitivity to drug and in those with acute pelvic inflammatory disease or active cardiac, pulmonary, renal, or hepatic disease.

**NURSING CONSIDERATIONS**
• Use cautiously in patients with history of asthma; hypotension; hypertension; CV, adrenal, renal, or hepatic disease; anemia; jaundice; diabetes; seizure disorders; or previous uterine surgery.
• Unlike other prostaglandin abortifacients, drug is administered by I.M. injection. Injectable form avoids risk of expelling vaginal suppositories that may occur in presence of profuse vaginal bleeding.
• Drug should be used only by trained personnel in a hospital setting.

☑ **Patient teaching**
• Explain use and administration of drug to patient and family.
• Instruct patient to report adverse reactions promptly.

## dinoprostone
Cervidil, Prepidil, Prostin E2

*Pregnancy Risk Category C*

### HOW SUPPLIED
*Vaginal suppositories:* 20 mg
*Endocervical gel:* 0.5 mg per application (2.5-ml syringe)
*Vaginal insert:* 10 mg

### ACTION
A prostaglandin that produces strong, prompt contractions of uterine smooth muscle, possibly mediated by calcium and cAMP.

| Route | Onset | Peak | Duration |
|---|---|---|---|
| Intravaginal (suppository) | 10 min | Unknown | 2-6 hr |
| Intravaginal (gel) | 15-30 min | Unknown | Unknown |
| Intravaginal (insert) | Unknown | Unknown | Unknown |

### INDICATIONS & DOSAGE
*To abort second-trimester pregnancy; to evacuate uterus in missed abortion, intrauterine fetal deaths up to 28 weeks' gestation, or benign hydatidiform mole (suppository only)—*
**Adults:** 20-mg suppository inserted high into posterior vaginal fornix; repeated q 3 to 5 hours until abortion is complete.
*Ripening of an unfavorable cervix in pregnant patients at or near term (gel or vaginal insert)—*
**Adults:** contents of one syringe administered intravaginally; if cervix remains unfavorable after 6 hours, dosage repeated. No more than 1.5 mg (three applications) should be given within 24-hour period.
*Vaginal insert—*
**Adults:** 10-mg vaginal insert placed transversely in posterior fornix of vagina immediately after removal from foil.

### ADVERSE REACTIONS
**CNS:** *headache, dizziness,* anxiety, paresthesia, weakness, syncope.
**CV:** chest pain, *arrhythmias.*
**EENT:** blurred vision, eye pain.
**GI:** *nausea, vomiting, diarrhea.*

**GU:** vaginal pain, vaginitis, endometritis, breast tenderness.
**Musculoskeletal:** *nocturnal leg cramps,* backache, muscle cramps.
**Respiratory:** coughing, dyspnea.
**Skin:** rash, diaphoresis.
**Other:** *fever, shivering, chills,* hot flashes.

### INTERACTIONS
**Drug-drug.** *Other oxytocics:* may potentiate action. Avoid concomitant use.
**Drug-lifestyle.** *Alcohol use:* inhibited effectiveness of dinoprostone with high doses. Avoid concomitant use.

### EFFECTS ON DIAGNOSTIC TESTS
None reported.

### CONTRAINDICATIONS
Gel form is contraindicated in patients with hypersensitivity to prostaglandins or constituents of gel and when prolonged contractions of the uterus are considered inappropriate. Also contraindicated in patients with placenta previa or unexplained vaginal bleeding during pregnancy and in whom vaginal delivery isn't indicated (because of vasa previa or active herpes genitalia).

Suppository form is contraindicated in patients with hypersensitivity to drug, acute pelvic inflammatory disease, and active cardiac, pulmonary, renal, or hepatic disease.

Insert form is contraindicated in patients with known hypersensitivity to drug. Also contraindicated when there is clinical suspicion or evidence of fetal distress where delivery isn't imminent; with unexplained vaginal bleeding during pregnancy or evidence or strong suspicion of marked cephalopelvic disproportion; when oxytocic drugs are contraindicated or when prolonged contraction of the uterus may be detrimental to fetal safety or uterine integrity; in patients already receiving oxytocic drugs; and in multipara with 6 or more previous term pregnancies.

### NURSING CONSIDERATIONS
• Use suppository form cautiously in patients with asthma, seizure disorders, anemia, diabetes, hypertension or hypoten-

---

*Reactions may be* common, *uncommon,* **life-threatening**, *or* COMMON AND LIFE-THREATENING.

sion, jaundice, scarred uterus, cervicitis, acute vaginitis, or CV, renal, or hepatic disease.

• Use gel form and insert forms cautiously in patients with asthma or in those with a history of asthma, glaucoma, or intraocular pressure; renal or hepatic dysfunction; or ruptured membranes.

• Administer only when critical care facilities are available.

• When using gel, warm to room temperature. After administration, patient should remain supine for 10 minutes.

• When using drug as an abortifacient, be prepared to pretreat patient with an antiemetic and antidiarrheal.

• For cervical ripening, have patient lie on her back; the cervix is examined using a speculum. Assist with insertion of gel, using aseptic technique: A catheter provided with drug is used to administer gel into cervical canal just below level of the internal os.

• When gel form is used, contents of syringe are used for one patient only. Discard syringe, catheter, and unused drug after administration; don't attempt to administer small amount of drug remaining in catheter.

• It isn't necessary to warm vaginal insert before administering. A minimal amount of water-soluble jelly may be used to aid insertion.

• Have patient remain supine for 2 hours following insertion of vaginal insert; thereafter, she may be ambulatory. Remove insert on onset of active labor or 12 hours after insertion.

• Treat dinoprostone-induced fever (self-limiting and transient and occurs in about 50% of patients) with water sponging and increased fluid intake, not with aspirin.

• Check vaginal discharge regularly.

• Abortion should be complete within 30 hours when suppository form is used.

• Freeze suppositories and inserts at –4° F (–20° C). Store gel in refrigerator at 36° to 46° F (2° to 8° C).

✓ **Patient teaching**
• Explain use and administration of drug to patient and family.
• Instruct patient to report adverse reactions promptly.

**methylergonovine maleate**
Methergine

*Pregnancy Risk Category C*

**HOW SUPPLIED**
*Tablets:* 0.2 mg
*Injection:* 0.2 mg/ml

**ACTION**
Increases motor activity of the uterus by direct stimulation of the smooth muscle.

| Route | Onset | Peak | Duration |
|---|---|---|---|
| P.O. | 5-10 min | 30 min | 3 hr |
| I.V. | Immediate | Unknown | 45 min |
| I.M. | 2-5 min | Unknown | 3 hr |

**INDICATIONS & DOSAGE**
*Prevention and treatment of postpartum hemorrhage due to uterine atony or subinvolution—*
**Adults:** 0.2 mg I.M. q 2 to 4 hours; for excessive uterine bleeding or other emergencies, 0.2 mg I.V. over 1 minute while blood pressure and uterine contractions are monitored. After initial I.M. or I.V. dose, 0.2 mg P.O. q 6 to 8 hours for 2 to 7 days. Dosage decreased if severe cramping occurs.

**ADVERSE REACTIONS**
**CNS:** dizziness, headache, *seizures,* hallucinations.
**CV:** hypertension, transient chest pain, palpitations, hypotension, thrombophlebitis, *CVA with I.V. use.*
**EENT:** tinnitus, nasal congestion.
**GI:** *nausea, vomiting,* diarrhea, foul taste.
**GU:** hematuria.
**Metabolic:** decreased serum prolactin levels.
**Musculoskeletal:** leg cramps.
**Respiratory:** dyspnea.
**Skin:** diaphoresis.

**INTERACTIONS**
**Drug-drug.** *Dopamine, I.V. oxytocin, regional anesthetics, vasoconstrictors*: excessive vasoconstriction. Use together cautiously.

## EFFECTS ON DIAGNOSTIC TESTS
None reported.

## CONTRAINDICATIONS
Contraindicated in patients with sensitivity to ergot preparations, in those with hypertension or toxemia, and during pregnancy.

## NURSING CONSIDERATIONS
• Use cautiously in patients with sepsis, obliterative vascular disease, or hepatic or renal disease, and during last stage of labor.
• Monitor and record blood pressure, pulse rate, and uterine response; report sudden change in vital signs, frequent periods of uterine relaxation, and character and amount of vaginal bleeding.
• Monitor contractions, which may continue 3 hours or more after P.O. or I.M. administration.
• Store tablets in tightly closed, light-resistant container. Discard if discolored.

### I.V. administration
• *Alert:* Drug shouldn't be routinely administered I.V. because of risk of severe hypertension and CVA. If it must be given I.V., administer slowly over 1 minute with careful blood pressure monitoring. I.V. dose may be diluted to 5 ml with normal saline solution before use. Contractions begin immediately after I.V. use and continue for up to 45 minutes.
• Store I.V. solution below 46° F (8° C). Daily stock may be kept at room temperature for 60 to 90 days.

### Patient teaching
• Explain use and administration of drug to patient and family.
• Instruct patient to report adverse reactions promptly.

---

## oxytocin, synthetic injection
Oxytocin, Pitocin

*Pregnancy Risk Category C*

## HOW SUPPLIED
*Injection:* 10 U/ml ampule, vial, or tubex

## ACTION
Causes potent and selective stimulation of uterine and mammary gland smooth muscle.

| Route | Onset | Peak | Duration |
|-------|-------|------|----------|
| I.V. | Immediate | Unknown | 1 hr |
| I.M. | 3-5 min | Unknown | 2-3 hr |

## INDICATIONS & DOSAGE
*Induction or stimulation of labor—*
**Adults:** initially, 1-ml (10 U) ampule in 1,000 ml of $D_5W$ injection or normal saline solution I.V. infused at 1 to 2 milliunits/minute. Rate increased in increments not exceeding 1 to 2 milliunits/minute at 15- to 30-minute intervals until normal contraction pattern is established. Rate decreased when labor is firmly established.
*Reduction of postpartum bleeding after expulsion of placenta—*
**Adults:** 10 to 40 U added to 1,000 ml of $D_5W$ or normal saline solution infused at rate needed to control bleeding, usually 20 to 40 milliunits/minute. Also, 1 ml (10 U) can be given I.M. after delivery of placenta.
*Incomplete or inevitable abortion—*
**Adults:** 10 U oxytocin I.V. in 500 ml of normal saline solution or dextrose 5% in normal saline solution. Infuse at rate of 10 to 20 milliunits (20 to 40 drops)/minute.

## ADVERSE REACTIONS
*Maternal:*
**CNS:** *subarachnoid hemorrhage, seizures, coma.*
**CV:** hypertension; increased heart rate, systemic venous return, and cardiac output; *arrhythmias.*
**GI:** nausea, vomiting.
**GU:** tetanic uterine contractions, *abruptio placentae,* impaired uterine blood flow, pelvic hematoma, increased uterine motility, *uterine rupture, postpartum hemorrhage.*
**Hematologic:** *afibrinogenemia possibly related to postpartum bleeding.*
**Other:** *hypersensitivity reactions, anaphylaxis.*
*Fetal:*
**CNS:** *infant brain damage.*

---

Reactions may be *common*, uncommon, *life-threatening*, or COMMON AND LIFE-THREATENING.

**CV:** *bradycardia,* PVCs, *arrhythmias.*
**EENT:** neonatal retinal hemorrhage.
**Hepatic:** neonatal jaundice.
**Respiratory:** *anoxia, asphyxia.*
**Other:** *low Apgar scores at 5 minutes.*

## INTERACTIONS
**Drug-drug.** *Cyclopropane anesthetics:*
less pronounced bradycardia and hypotension. Use together cautiously.
*Thiopental anesthetics:* possible delayed induction. Use together cautiously.
*Vasoconstrictors:* severe hypertension if oxytocin is given within 3 to 4 hours of vasoconstrictor in patients receiving caudal block anesthetic. Avoid concomitant use.

## EFFECTS ON DIAGNOSTIC TESTS
None reported.

## CONTRAINDICATIONS
Contraindicated in patients with hypersensitivity to drug and when vaginal delivery isn't advised (placenta previa or vasa previa), cephalopelvic disproportion is present, or delivery requires conversion, as in transverse lie. Also contraindicated in fetal distress when delivery isn't imminent, prematurity, or other obstetric emergencies and in patients with severe toxemia or hypertonic uterine patterns.

## NURSING CONSIDERATIONS
• Use with extreme caution during first and second stages of labor because cervical laceration, uterine rupture, and maternal and fetal death have been reported.
• Use with extreme caution, if at all, in patients with history of cervical or uterine surgery (including cesarean section), grand multiparity, uterine sepsis, traumatic delivery, or overdistended uterus and in invasive cervical cancer.
• Drug isn't recommended for routine I.M. use. However, 10 U may be given I.M. after delivery of placenta to control postpartum uterine bleeding.
• Never give oxytocin simultaneously by more than one route.
• Drug is used to induce or reinforce labor only when pelvis is known to be adequate, when vaginal delivery is indicated, when fetal maturity is assured, and when

fetal position is favorable. It should be used only in hospital where critical care facilities and doctor are immediately available.
• Monitor fluid intake and output. Antidiuretic effect may lead to fluid overload, seizures, and coma.
• Monitor and record uterine contractions, heart rate, blood pressure, intrauterine pressure, fetal heart rate, and character of blood loss every 15 minutes.
• Have magnesium sulfate (20% solution) available for relaxation of the myometrium.
• If contractions occur less than 2 minutes apart and if contractions over 50 mm Hg are recorded, or if contractions last 90 seconds or longer, stop infusion, turn patient on her side, and notify doctor.
• Drug isn't known to cause fetal abnormalities when used as indicated.
• *Alert:* Don't confuse Pitocin with Pitressin.

### I.V. administration
• Dilute drug by adding 10 U to 1 L of normal saline, lactated Ringer's, or $D_5W$ solution for induction or stimulation of labor, or by adding 10 U to 500 ml of normal saline, lactated Ringer's, or $D_5W$ solution to produce intense uterine contractions and reduce postpartum bleeding.
• Don't give drug by I.V. bolus injection. Administer by infusion only; give by piggyback infusion so drug may be discontinued without interrupting I.V. line. Use an infusion pump.

### Patient teaching
• Explain use and administration of drug to patient and family.
• Instruct patient to report adverse reactions promptly.

---

\*Liquid contains alcohol.   \*\*May contain tartrazine.   †Canada   ‡Australia   §U.K.   ◇OTC

**flavoxate hydrochloride**
**oxybutynin chloride**
**phenazopyridine hydrochloride**

**COMBINATION PRODUCTS**
None.

---

## flavoxate hydrochloride
Urispas

*Pregnancy Risk Category NR*

### HOW SUPPLIED
*Tablets:* 100 mg

### ACTION
Produces direct spasmolytic effect on smooth muscles of the urinary tract and provides some local anesthesia and analgesia.

| Route | Onset | Peak | Duration |
|-------|-------|------|----------|
| P.O. | Unknown | 2 hr | Unknown |

### INDICATIONS & DOSAGE
*Symptomatic relief of dysuria, urinary frequency and urgency, nocturia, incontinence, and suprapubic pain associated with urologic disorders—*
**Adults and children over age 12:** 100 to 200 mg P.O. t.i.d. to q.i.d. Dosage may be reduced with improvement of symptoms.

### ADVERSE REACTIONS
**CNS:** *confusion,* nervousness, dizziness, headache, drowsiness.
**CV:** tachycardia, palpitations.
**EENT:** *blurred vision,* disturbed eye accommodation, increased ocular tension.
**GI:** dry mouth, nausea, vomiting.
**GU:** dysuria.
**Hematologic:** eosinophilia, *leukopenia.*
**Skin:** urticaria, dermatoses.
**Other:** fever.

### INTERACTIONS
**Drug-lifestyle.** *Exercise, hot weather:* may precipitate heat stroke. Use cautiously.

### EFFECTS ON DIAGNOSTIC TESTS
None reported.

### CONTRAINDICATIONS
Contraindicated in patients with pyloric or duodenal obstruction, obstructive intestinal lesions or ileus, achalasia, GI hemorrhage, or obstructive uropathies of lower urinary tract.

### NURSING CONSIDERATIONS
• Use cautiously in patients suspected of having glaucoma and in pregnant or breast-feeding women.
• Safety and effectiveness of drug in children ages 12 and under are unknown.
• Check patient history for other drug use before giving drugs with anticholinergic adverse reactions. Such reactions may be intensified by flavoxate.
• *Alert:* Don't confuse Urispas with Urised.

☑ **Patient teaching**
• Warn patient to avoid hazardous activities, such as operating machinery or driving, until CNS effects of drug are known.
• Tell patient to contact doctor if adverse reactions occur or if symptoms aren't diminished.
• Caution patient that using drug during very hot weather may precipitate fever or heatstroke because it suppresses diaphoresis.

---

## oxybutynin chloride
Cystrin§, Ditropan, Ditropan XL

*Pregnancy Risk Category B*

### HOW SUPPLIED
*Tablets:* 5 mg
*Tablets (extended-release):* 5 mg, 10 mg
*Syrup:* 5 g/5 ml

### ACTION
Produces a direct spasmolytic effect and an antimuscarinic (atropine-like) effect on

urinary tract smooth muscles, increasing urinary bladder capacity and providing some local anesthesia and mild analgesia.

| Route | Onset | Peak | Duration |
|-------|-------|------|----------|
| P.O. | 30-60 min | 3-4 hr | 6-10 hr |
| P.O. (extended) | Unknown | 4-6 hr | 24 hr |

## INDICATIONS & DOSAGE
*Antispasmodic for uninhibited or reflex neurogenic bladder—*
**Adults:** 5 mg P.O. b.i.d. to t.i.d., to maximum of 5 mg q.i.d.
**Children over age 5:** 5 mg P.O. b.i.d., to maximum of 5 mg t.i.d.
✳ *NEW INDICATION: Overactive bladder—*
**Adults:** initially, 5 mg P.O. (Ditropan XL) once daily. Dosage adjustments may be made weekly in 5-mg increments, p.r.n., to maximum dose of 30 mg P.O. daily.

## ADVERSE REACTIONS
**CNS:** dizziness, insomnia, restlessness, hallucinations, asthenia.
**CV:** *palpitations, tachycardia,* vasodilation.
**EENT:** mydriasis, cycloplegia, decreased lacrimation, amblyopia.
**GI:** nausea, vomiting, *dry mouth, constipation,* decreased GI motility.
**GU:** impotence, *urinary hesitancy, urine retention,* suppression of lactation.
**Skin:** rash, decreased diaphoresis.
**Other:** fever.

## INTERACTIONS
**Drug-drug.** *Anticholinergics:* increased anticholinergic effects. Use cautiously.
*Atenolol, digoxin:* increased levels of these drugs. Monitor closely.
*CNS depressants:* increased CNS effects. Use cautiously.
*Haloperidol, levodopa:* decreased levels of these drugs. Monitor closely.
**Drug-lifestyle.** *Alcohol use:* increased CNS effects. Avoid concomitant use.
*Exercise, hot weather:* may precipitate heat stroke. Use cautiously.

## EFFECTS ON DIAGNOSTIC TESTS
None reported.

## CONTRAINDICATIONS
Contraindicated in patients with hypersensitivity to drug and in those with myasthenia gravis, GI obstruction, untreated narrow-angle glaucoma, adynamic ileus, megacolon, severe colitis, ulcerative colitis when megacolon is present, or obstructive uropathy. Also contraindicated in elderly or debilitated patients with intestinal atony and in hemorrhaging patients with unstable CV status.

## NURSING CONSIDERATIONS
• Use cautiously in elderly patients and in patients with autonomic neuropathy, reflux esophagitis, or hepatic or renal disease.
• Before giving drug, anticipate confirmation of neurogenic bladder by cystometry and rule out partial intestinal obstruction in patients with diarrhea, especially those with colostomy or ileostomy.
• If urinary tract infection exists, administer antibiotics, as ordered.
• Drug may aggravate symptoms of hyperthyroidism, coronary artery disease, heart failure, arrhythmias, tachycardia, hypertension, or prostatic hyperplasia.
• Periodically prepare patient for cystometry to evaluate response to therapy.
• *Alert:* Don't confuse Ditropan with Diazepam or Dithranol.

☑ **Patient teaching**
• Warn patient to avoid hazardous activities, such as operating machinery or driving, until CNS effects of drug are known.
• Caution patient that using drug during very hot weather may precipitate fever or heatstroke because it suppresses diaphoresis.
• Tell patient that Ditropan XL should be swallowed whole; don't chew or crush.
• Advise patient to store drug in tightly closed container at 59° to 86° F (15° to 30° C).
• Advise patient to avoid alcohol while taking drug.

---

# phenazopyridine hydrochloride (phenylazo diamino pyridine hydrochloride)

AZO-Standard◇, Baridium◇, Eridium◇, Geridium◇, Phenazo†, Phenazodine◇, Prodium◇, Pyridiate◇, Pyridium, Urodine◇, Urogesic◇, Viridium◇

*Pregnancy Risk Category B*

## HOW SUPPLIED
*Tablets:* 100 mg◇, 200 mg

## ACTION
Exerts local anesthetic action on urinary mucosa through unknown mechanism.

| Route | Onset | Peak | Duration |
|-------|-------|------|----------|
| P.O. | Unknown | Unknown | Unknown |

## INDICATIONS & DOSAGE
*Pain with urinary tract irritation or infection—*
**Adults:** 200 mg P.O. t.i.d. after meals for 2 days.
**Children:** 12 mg/kg P.O. daily in three equally divided doses after meals for 2 days.

## ADVERSE REACTIONS
**CNS:** headache.
**EENT:** staining of contact lenses.
**GI:** nausea, GI disturbances.
**Hematologic:** hemolytic anemia, methemoglobinemia.
**Skin:** rash, pruritus.
**Other:** *anaphylactoid reactions.*

## INTERACTIONS
None significant.

## EFFECTS ON DIAGNOSTIC TESTS
Drug may alter results of Diastix or Chemstrip uG, Acetest, and Ketostix. Clinitest should be used to obtain accurate urine glucose test results. Drug may also interfere with Ehrlich's test for urine urobilinogen, phenolsulfonphthalein excretion tests of kidney function, sulfobromophthalein excretion tests of liver function, and urine tests for protein, corticosteroids, or bilirubin.

## CONTRAINDICATIONS
Contraindicated in patients with hypersensitivity to drug and in those with glomerulonephritis, severe hepatitis, uremia, renal insufficiency, or pyelonephritis during pregnancy.

## NURSING CONSIDERATIONS
• When drug is used with an antibacterial, therapy shouldn't extend beyond 2 days.
• *Alert:* Don't confuse Pyridium with pyridoxine.

☑ **Patient teaching**
• Advise patient that taking drug with meals may minimize GI distress.
• Caution patient to stop drug and notify doctor immediately if skin or sclera becomes yellow-tinged, which may indicate drug accumulation due to impaired renal excretion.
• Inform patient that drug colors urine red or orange; it may stain fabrics or contact lenses.
• Tell diabetic patient that drug may alter Diastix or Chemstrip uG results. He should use Clinitest for accurate urine glucose test results. Also tell patient that drug may interfere with urinary ketone tests (Acetest or Ketostix).
• Advise patient to notify doctor if urinary tract pain persists. Tell him that drug shouldn't be used for long-term treatment.

---

Reactions may be *common,* uncommon, *life-threatening,* or COMMON AND LIFE-THREATENING.

**auranofin**
**aurothioglucose**
**gold sodium thiomalate**

**COMBINATION PRODUCTS**
None.

---

**auranofin**
Ridaura

*Pregnancy Risk Category C*

**HOW SUPPLIED**
*Capsules:* 3 mg

**ACTION**
Unknown. Anti-inflammatory effects are probably due to inhibition of sulfhydryl systems, which alters cellular metabolism. May also alter enzyme function and immune response and suppress phagocytic activity.

| Route | Onset | Peak | Duration |
|-------|-------|------|----------|
| P.O. | Unknown | 2 hr | Unknown |

**INDICATIONS & DOSAGE**
*Rheumatoid arthritis—*
**Adults:** 6 mg P.O. daily, either as 3 mg b.i.d. or 6 mg once daily. After 6 months, may be increased to 9 mg daily.
**Children:** initially, 0.1 mg/kg/day. Maintenance dose is 0.15 mg/kg/day; maximum dose is 0.2 mg/kg/day.

**ADVERSE REACTIONS**
**CNS:** confusion, hallucinations, *seizures.*
**EENT:** conjunctivitis.
**GI:** *diarrhea, abdominal pain, nausea, stomatitis,* glossitis, anorexia, metallic taste, dyspepsia, flatulence, constipation, dysgeusia, ulcerative colitis.
**GU:** proteinuria, hematuria, nephrotic syndrome, glomerulonephritis, *acute renal failure.*
**Hematologic:** *thrombocytopenia, aplastic anemia, agranulocytosis, leukopenia,* eosinophilia, anemia.

**Hepatic:** jaundice, elevated liver enzyme levels.
**Respiratory:** interstitial pneumonitis.
**Skin:** *rash, pruritus, dermatitis,* exfoliative dermatitis, urticaria, erythema, alopecia.

**INTERACTIONS**
**Drug-drug.** *Phenytoin:* may increase phenytoin blood levels. Watch for toxicity.

**EFFECTS ON DIAGNOSTIC TESTS**
Serum protein-bound iodine test, especially when done by the chloric acid digestion method, gives false readings during and for several weeks after gold therapy. May enhance tuberculin skin test.

**CONTRAINDICATIONS**
Contraindicated in patients with history of severe gold toxicity or toxicity due to previous exposure to other heavy metals and in those with necrotizing enterocolitis, pulmonary fibrosis, exfoliative dermatitis, bone marrow aplasia, or severe hematologic disorders. Also contraindicated in patients with urticaria, eczema, colitis, severe debilitation, hemorrhagic conditions, or systemic lupus erythematosus, and in patients who have recently received radiation therapy.

**NURSING CONSIDERATIONS**
• Use cautiously with other drugs that cause blood dyscrasias. Also use cautiously in patients with rash, history of bone marrow depression, or preexisting renal, hepatic, or inflammatory bowel disease.
• Monitor patient's platelet count monthly. Drug should be stopped if platelet count falls below 100,000/mm³, if hemoglobin drops suddenly, if granulocytes are below 1,500/mm³, or if leukopenia (WBC count below 4,000/mm³) or eosinophilia (eosinophils over 75%) exists.
• *Alert:* Monitor patient's urinalysis results monthly. If proteinuria or hematuria is detected, stop drug because it can cause

---

nephrotic syndrome or glomerulonephritis, and notify doctor.
• Monitor liver function tests.
• Warn women of childbearing potential of risks of drug therapy during pregnancy.

### ✓ Patient teaching
• Encourage patient to take drug as prescribed.
• Tell patient to continue concomitant drug therapy if prescribed.
• Remind patient to see doctor for monthly platelet counts.
• Suggest that patient has regular urinalysis.
• Tell patient to keep taking drug if mild diarrhea occurs but to immediately report blood in stool. Diarrhea is most common adverse reaction.
• Advise patient to report rash or other skin problems and to stop drug until reaction subsides. Pruritus may precede dermatitis; pruritic skin eruptions during drug therapy should be considered a reaction until proven otherwise.
• Inform patient that stomatitis may be preceded by a metallic taste; tell him to notify doctor if this occurs. Promote careful oral hygiene during therapy.
• Advise patient to report unusual bleeding or bruising.
• Inform patient that beneficial effect may be delayed as long as 3 months. If response is inadequate and maximum dose has been reached, expect doctor to discontinue drug.
• Warn patient not to give drug to others. Auranofin should be prescribed only for selected patients with rheumatoid arthritis.

---

## aurothioglucose
Gold-50‡, Solganal

## gold sodium thiomalate
Aurolate

*Pregnancy Risk Category C*

### HOW SUPPLIED
**aurothioglucose**
*Injection (suspension):* 50 mg/ml in sesame oil in 10-ml vial

**gold sodium thiomalate**
*Injection:* 50 mg/ml with benzyl alcohol

### ACTION
Unknown. Anti-inflammatory effects are probably due to inhibition of sulfhydryl systems, which alters cellular metabolism. May also alter enzyme function and immune response and suppress phagocytic activity.

| Route | Onset | Peak | Duration |
|-------|-------|------|----------|
| I.M. | Unknown | 3-6 hr | Unknown |

### INDICATIONS & DOSAGE
*Rheumatoid arthritis—*
**aurothioglucose**
**Adults:** initially, 10 mg I.M., followed by 25 mg for second and third doses at weekly intervals. Then, 50 mg weekly until 800 mg to 1 g has been given. If improvement occurs without toxicity, 25 to 50 mg is continued at 3- to 4-week intervals indefinitely.
**Children ages 6 to 12:** one-quarter usual adult dose. Don't exceed 25 mg per dose.
**gold sodium thiomalate**
**Adults:** initially, 10 mg I.M., followed by 25 mg in 1 week. Then, 25 to 50 mg weekly to total dose of 1 g. If improvement occurs without toxicity, 25 to 50 mg q 2 weeks for 2 to 20 weeks; then, 25 to 50 mg q 3 to 4 weeks as maintenance therapy. If relapse occurs, injections resumed at weekly intervals.
**Children:** initially, 10 mg I.M.; then, 1 mg/kg I.M. weekly, not to exceed 50 mg for a single injection. Follow adult spacing of doses.

### ADVERSE REACTIONS
**CNS:** confusion, hallucinations, *seizures.*
**CV:** *bradycardia*, hypotension.
**EENT:** corneal gold deposition, corneal ulcers.
**GI:** *diarrhea*, anorexia, abdominal cramps, nausea, vomiting, ulcerative enterocolitis, *metallic taste, stomatitis*.
**GU:** albuminuria, proteinuria, nephrotic syndrome, nephritis, acute tubular necrosis, hematuria, *acute renal failure.*
**Hematologic:** *thrombocytopenia, aplastic anemia, agranulocytosis, leukopenia*, eosinophilia, anemia.

---

Reactions may be *common*, uncommon, *life-threatening*, or COMMON AND LIFE-THREATENING.

**Hepatic:** *hepatitis,* jaundice, elevated liver function test results.
**Skin:** photosensitivity, *rash, dermatitis,* erythema, exfoliative dermatitis, diaphoresis.
**Other:** *anaphylaxis, angioedema.*

## INTERACTIONS
**Drug-lifestyle.** *Sun or ultraviolet light exposure:* photosensitivity reactions may occur. Take precautions.

## EFFECTS ON DIAGNOSTIC TESTS
Serum protein-bound iodine test, especially when done by chloric acid digestion method, gives false readings during and for several weeks after therapy.

## CONTRAINDICATIONS
Contraindicated in patients with hypersensitivity to drug and in those with history of severe toxicity from previous exposure to gold or other heavy metals. Also contraindicated in those with hepatitis, exfoliative dermatitis, severe uncontrollable diabetes, renal disease, hepatic dysfunction, uncontrolled heart failure, systemic lupus erythematosus, colitis, Sjögren's syndrome, urticaria, eczema, hemorrhagic conditions, or severe hematologic disorders and in those who have recently received radiation therapy.

## NURSING CONSIDERATIONS
• Use with extreme caution, if at all, in patients with rash, marked hypertension, compromised cerebral or CV circulation, or history of renal or hepatic disease, drug allergies, or blood dyscrasias.
• Warn women of childbearing potential about risks of gold therapy during pregnancy.
• *Alert:* Administer drug I.M. only.
• Give drug only under constant supervision of doctor thoroughly familiar with drug's toxicities and benefits.
• Give I.M., as ordered, preferably intragluteally. Drug is pale yellow; don't use if it darkens.
• Immerse aurothioglucose vial in warm water; shake vigorously before injecting.
• When injecting gold sodium thiomalate, have patient lie down for 10 to 20 minutes to minimize hypotension.

• Watch for anaphylactoid reaction for 30 minutes after administration.
• *Alert:* Keep dimercaprol available to treat acute toxicity.
• Analyze urine for protein and sediment changes before each injection.
• Monitor CBC, including platelet count, before every second injection.
• Monitor platelet counts if patient develops purpura or ecchymoses.
• Gold therapy may alter liver function studies.
• If adverse reactions are mild, some rheumatologists resume gold therapy after 2 to 3 weeks' rest.

### ☑ Patient teaching
• Inform patient that increased joint pain may occur for 1 to 2 days after injection but usually subsides.
• Advise patient to report rash or skin problems immediately and to stop drug until reaction subsides. Pruritus may precede dermatitis; pruritic skin eruptions during gold therapy should be considered a reaction until proven otherwise.
• Advise patient to report unusual bleeding or bruising.
• Instruct patient to report a metallic taste. Promote careful oral hygiene.
• Urge patient to avoid sunlight and artificial ultraviolet light.
• Tell patient that benefits may not appear for 3 to 4 months.
• Stress need for medical follow-up.

**activated charcoal**
**aminocaproic acid**
**ammonia spirit, aromatic**
**deferoxamine mesylate**
**digoxin immune Fab**
**dimercaprol**
**disulfiram**
**d-penicillamine**
**edetate calcium disodium**
**edetate disodium**
**flumazenil**
**ipecac syrup**
**naloxone hydrochloride**
**naltrexone hydrochloride**
**pralidoxime chloride**
**protamine sulfate**
**sodium polystyrene sulfonate**
**succimer**
(See also Chapter 38, ANTICHOLINERGICS.)
(See also Chapter 40, ADRENERGIC BLOCK-ERS [SYMPATHOLYTICS].)

**COMBINATION PRODUCTS**
None.

---

**activated charcoal**
Actidose◇, Actidose-Aqua◇,
CharcoAid◇, CharcoCaps◇,
Liqui-Char◇

*Pregnancy Risk Category C*

**HOW SUPPLIED**
*Tablets:* 250 mg◇
*Capsules:* 260 mg◇
*Powder:* 15 g◇, 30 g◇, 40 g◇, 50 g◇, 120 g◇, 240 g◇
*Oral suspension:* 15 g◇, 25 g◇, 30 g◇, 50 g◇

**ACTION**
An adsorbent that adheres to many drugs and chemicals, inhibiting their absorption from the GI tract.

| Route | Onset | Peak | Duration |
|-------|-------|------|----------|
| P.O. | Immediate | Unknown | Unknown |

**INDICATIONS & DOSAGE**
*Flatulence, dyspepsia—*
**Adults:** 600 mg to 5 g P.O. as single dose or 0.975 to 3.9 g P.O. t.i.d. after meals.
*Poisoning—*
**Adults and children:** initially, 1 to 2 g/kg (30 to 100 g) P.O. or 10 times the amount of poison ingested as a suspension in 120 to 240 ml (4 to 8 oz) of water.

Drug is commonly used for treating poisoning or overdose with acetaminophen, aspirin, atropine, barbiturates, dextropropoxyphene, digoxin, poisonous mushrooms, oxalic acid, parathion, phenol, phenylpropanolamine, phenytoin, propantheline, propoxyphene, strychnine, or tricyclic antidepressants.

Check with poison control center for use in other types of poisonings or overdoses.

**ADVERSE REACTIONS**
**GI:** *black stools,* nausea, constipation, intestinal obstruction.

**INTERACTIONS**
**Drug-drug.** *Acetylcysteine, ipecac:* drugs are inactivated by charcoal. Administer charcoal after vomiting has been induced by ipecac; remove charcoal by NG tube before giving acetylcysteine.
*Acetaminophen, barbiturates, carbamazepine, digitoxin, digoxin, furosemide, glutethimide, hydantoins, methotrexate, nizatidine, phenothiazines, phenylbutazones, propoxyphene, salicylates, sulfonamides, sulfonylureas, tetracyclines, theophyllines, tricyclic antidepressants, valproic acid:* charcoal may reduce absorption of these drugs. Administer charcoal at least 2 hours before or 1 hour after other drugs.

**EFFECTS ON DIAGNOSTIC TESTS**
None reported.

**CONTRAINDICATIONS**
No known contraindications.

---

## NURSING CONSIDERATIONS
• Although there are no known contra-indications, drug isn't effective in the treatment of all acute poisonings.
• Give after emesis is complete because activated charcoal absorbs and inactivates ipecac syrup.
• Mix powder (most effective form) with tap water to consistency of thick syrup. Adding a small amount of fruit juice or flavoring will make mix more palatable. Don't mix with ice cream, milk, or sherbet because these will decrease absorptive capacity of activated charcoal.
• Give by large bore NG tube after lavage, if needed.
• If patient vomits shortly after adminis-tration, be prepared to repeat dose.
• Space doses at least 1 hour apart from other drugs if treatment is for indications other than poisoning.
• Follow treatment with stool softener or laxative, as ordered, to prevent constipa-tion unless sorbitol is part of product in-gredients.
• Preparations made with sorbitol have a laxative effect that lessens risk of severe constipation or fecal impaction.
• Don't use charcoal with sorbitol in fruc-tose-intolerant patients or in children un-der age 1.
• *Alert:* Drug is ineffective for poisoning or overdose of cyanide, mineral acids, caustic alkalis, and organic solvents; not very effective with ethanol, lithium, methanol, and iron salts.

☑ **Patient teaching**
• Explain use and administration of drug to patient (if awake) and family.
• Warn patient that stools will be black.

---

## aminocaproic acid
Amicar

*Pregnancy Risk Category C*

## HOW SUPPLIED
*Tablets:* 500 mg
*Syrup:* 250 mg/ml
*Injection:* 250 mg/ml

## ACTION
Inhibits plasminogen activator substances and, to a lesser degree, blocks antiplasmin activity by inhibiting fibrinolysis.

| Route | Onset | Peak | Duration |
|-------|-------|------|----------|
| P.O. | 1 hr | 2 hr | Unknown |
| I.V. | 1 hr | Unknown | 3 hr |

## INDICATIONS & DOSAGE
*Excessive bleeding resulting from hyper-fibrinolysis—*
**Adults:** initially, 5 g P.O. or slow I.V. in-fusion; then 1 to 1.25 g hourly until bleed-ing is controlled. Maximum dose is 30 g daily.

## ADVERSE REACTIONS
**CNS:** dizziness, malaise, headache, delir-ium, *seizures,* hallucinations, weakness.
**CV:** hypotension, *bradycardia, arrhyth-mias.*
**EENT:** tinnitus, nasal congestion, con-junctival suffusion.
**GI:** nausea, cramps, diarrhea.
**GU:** *acute renal failure.*
**Hematologic:** generalized thrombosis.
**Hepatic:** increased CK, AST, and ALT levels.
**Musculoskeletal:** myopathy.
**Skin:** rash.

## INTERACTIONS
**Drug-drug.** *Estrogens, oral contracep-tives:* increased probability of hypercoag-ulability. Use together cautiously.

## EFFECTS ON DIAGNOSTIC TESTS
None reported.

## CONTRAINDICATIONS
Contraindicated in patients with hema-turia, active intravascular clotting, or pres-ence of DIC, unless heparin is used con-comitantly. Injectable form is contraindi-cated in newborns.

## NURSING CONSIDERATIONS
• Use cautiously in patients with cardiac, hepatic, or renal disease.
• *Alert:* Don't administer by bolus injec-tion because of risk of hypotension, bradycardia, and arrhythmias.

---

• *Alert:* Monitor coagulation studies, as ordered, and heart rhythm and blood pressure. Notify doctor of changes immediately.
• *Alert:* Don't confuse Amicar with Amikin.

### ⚡ I.V. administration
• Dilute solution with sterile water for injection, normal saline for injection, $D_5W$, or Ringer's injection. Infuse slowly. Arrhythmias may be precipitated by too rapid infusion. Don't give by direct or intermittent injection.

### ✅ Patient teaching
• Explain use and administration of drug to patient and family.
• Instruct patient to report adverse reactions promptly.

---

## ammonia spirit, aromatic ◊

*Pregnancy Risk Category NR*

### HOW SUPPLIED
*Solution:* 30 ml ◊, 60 ml ◊, 120 ml ◊; pints ◊; gallons ◊
*Inhalant:* 0.33 ml ◊, 0.4 ml ◊

### ACTION
Irritates the sensory receptors in the nasal membranes, producing reflex stimulation of the respiratory centers.

| Route | Onset | Peak | Duration |
|-------|-------|------|----------|
| P.O., inhalation | Immediate | Unknown | Unknown |

### INDICATIONS & DOSAGE
*Treatment or prevention of fainting—*
**Adults and children:** 1 broken capsule inhaled until awake or no longer faint; or 2 to 4 ml P.O. diluted in at least 30 ml of water.

### ADVERSE REACTIONS
**EENT:** irritation.

### INTERACTIONS
None significant.

### EFFECTS ON DIAGNOSTIC TESTS
None reported.

### CONTRAINDICATIONS
No known contraindications.

### NURSING CONSIDERATIONS
• Avoid inhaling vapors when administering drug.
• Monitor patient closely for response.

### ✅ Patient teaching
• Instruct patient how to use drug.
• Tell patient to store drug in refrigerator.

---

## deferoxamine mesylate
Desferal

*Pregnancy Risk Category C*

### HOW SUPPLIED
*Powder for injection:* 500 mg

### ACTION
Chelates iron by binding ferric ions.

| Route | Onset | Peak | Duration |
|-------|-------|------|----------|
| I.V., I.M., S.C. | Unknown | Unknown | Unknown |

### INDICATIONS & DOSAGE
*Adjunctive treatment of acute iron intoxication—*
**Adults and children:** 1 g I.M., followed by 500 mg I.M. for two doses q 4 hours; then 500 mg I.M. q 4 to 12 hours. Maximum dose is 6 g in 24 hours. Give I.V. by slow infusion (15 mg/kg/hour or less) only in CV collapse.
*Chronic iron overload from multiple transfusions—*
**Adults and children:** 500 mg to 1 g I.M. daily and 2 g by slow I.V. infusion in separate solution with each unit of blood transfused. Maximum dose is 6 g daily. Or, 20 to 40 mg/kg via S.C. infusion pump daily.

### ADVERSE REACTIONS
**CV:** tachycardia, *hypotension,* **severe hypotension.**
**EENT:** blurred vision, cataracts, hearing loss.

---

Reactions may be *common,* uncommon, *life-threatening,* or COMMON AND LIFE-THREATENING.

**GI:** diarrhea, abdominal discomfort with long-term use.
**GU:** dysuria with long-term use.
**Musculoskeletal:** leg cramps.
**Skin:** *erythema, urticaria,* cutaneous wheal formation, pruritus, rash, pain, induration at injection site; fever.
**Other:** *anaphylaxis.*

### INTERACTIONS
**Drug-drug.** *Ascorbic acid:* may enhance effects of deferoxamine and increase tissue toxicity of iron. Use together with extreme caution and close monitoring.

### EFFECTS ON DIAGNOSTIC TESTS
None reported.

### CONTRAINDICATIONS
Contraindicated in patients with severe renal disease, anuria, or primary hemochromatosis.

### NURSING CONSIDERATIONS
• Use cautiously in patients with impaired renal function.
• After reconstitution, administer I.M. or add to normal saline solution, $D_5W$, or lactated Ringer's solution and infuse at a rate not exceeding 15 mg/kg hour.
• *Alert:* Have epinephrine 1:1,000 available to treat hypersensitivity reaction.
• Monitor fluid intake and output carefully.
• *Alert:* Severe hypotension may result if drug is given by rapid bolus injection.

### ◻ I.V. administration
• To reconstitute, add 2 ml of sterile water for injection to each ampule. Make sure drug is completely dissolved. Reconstituted solution is good for 1 week at room temperature. Protect from light.

### ☑ Patient teaching
• Warn patient that urine may be red. Tell him to report persistent or serious adverse reactions promptly.
• Advise patient to have regular eye examinations during long-term therapy because cataract formation has been reported.

---

# digoxin immune Fab (ovine)
Digibind

*Pregnancy Risk Category C*

### HOW SUPPLIED
*Injection:* 38-mg vial

### ACTION
Binds molecules of unbound digoxin and digitoxin, making them unavailable for binding at site of action on cells.

| Route | Onset | Peak | Duration |
|-------|-------|------|----------|
| I.V. | 30 min | End of infusion | 15-20 hr |

### INDICATIONS & DOSAGE
*Potentially life-threatening digoxin or digitoxin intoxication—*
**Adults and children:** I.V. dosage varies according to amount of digoxin or digitoxin to be neutralized. Each vial binds about 0.5 mg of digoxin or digitoxin. Average adult dosage is 6 vials (228 mg). However, if toxicity resulted from acute digoxin ingestion and neither a serum digoxin level nor an estimated ingestion amount is known, 20 vials (760 mg) may be needed. For children under 20 kg (44 lb), a single vial is usually sufficient. See package insert for complete, specific dosage instructions.

### ADVERSE REACTIONS
**CV:** *heart failure,* rapid ventricular rate.
**Metabolic:** hypokalemia.
**Other:** *hypersensitivity reactions, anaphylaxis.*

### INTERACTIONS
None significant.

### EFFECTS ON DIAGNOSTIC TESTS
Drug alters standard cardiac glycoside determinations by radioimmunoassay procedures. Results may be falsely increased or decreased, depending on separation method used.

### CONTRAINDICATIONS
No known contraindications.

---

## NURSING CONSIDERATIONS

• Use cautiously in patients known to be allergic to ovine proteins and in those who have previously received antibodies. In these high-risk patients, skin testing is recommended because drug is derived from digoxin-specific antibody fragments obtained from immunized sheep.

• Drug is used only for life-threatening overdose in patients with anaphylaxis, severe hypotension, or cardiac arrest and in those with ventricular arrhythmias (such as ventricular tachycardia or fibrillation), progressive bradycardia (such as severe sinus bradycardia) or second- or third-degree AV block not responsive to atropine.

• Heart failure and rapid ventricular rate may result by reversal of cardiac glycoside's therapeutic effects.

• Monitor potassium level closely, as ordered.

• In most patients, signs of digitalis toxicity disappear within a few hours.

• Because drug interferes with digitalis immunoassay measurements, standard serum digoxin levels are misleading until drug is cleared from body (about 2 days).

**I.V. administration**

• Reconstitute drug in 38-mg vial with 4 ml of sterile water for injection. Gently roll vial to dissolve powder. Reconstituted solution contains 9.5 mg/ml. Drug may be given by direct injection if cardiac arrest seems imminent. Or, dilute with normal saline for injection to an appropriate volume and give by intermittent infusion over 30 minutes.

• Infuse drug through a 0.22-micron membrane filter.

• Refrigerate powder for injection. Reconstitute drug immediately before use. Reconstituted solutions may be refrigerated for 4 hours.

**✓ Patient teaching**

• Explain use and administration of drug to patient and family.

• Instruct patient to report adverse reactions promptly.

---

# dimercaprol
BAL in Oil

*Pregnancy Risk Category C*

## HOW SUPPLIED
*Injection:* 100 mg/ml

## ACTION
Forms complexes with heavy metals to create chelates that are renally excreted.

| Route | Onset | Peak | Duration |
|-------|-------|------|----------|
| I.M. | Unknown | 30-60 min | 4 hr |

## INDICATIONS & DOSAGE
*Severe arsenic or gold poisoning—*
**Adults and children:** 3 mg/kg deep I.M. q 4 hours for 2 days; then q.i.d. on third day; then b.i.d. for 10 days.
*Mild arsenic or gold poisoning—*
**Adults and children:** 2.5 mg/kg deep I.M. q.i.d. for 2 days; then b.i.d. on third day; then once daily for 10 days.
*Mercury poisoning—*
**Adults and children:** initially, 5 mg/kg deep I.M.; then 2.5 mg/kg daily or b.i.d. for 10 days.
*Acute lead encephalopathy or lead level over 100 mcg/ml—*
**Adults and children:** 4 mg/kg deep I.M.; then q 4 hours with edetate calcium disodium for 2 to 7 days. Use separate sites.

## ADVERSE REACTIONS
**CNS:** headache, paresthesia, muscle pain or weakness, anxiety.
**CV:** *transient increase in blood pressure, tachycardia.*
**EENT:** blepharospasm, conjunctivitis, lacrimation, rhinorrhea.
**GI:** *nausea; vomiting; burning sensation in lips, mouth, and throat;* excessive salivation; *abdominal pain.*
**Other:** *fever;* pain or tightness in throat, chest, or hands.

## INTERACTIONS
**Drug-drug.** *Iron:* toxic metal complex formed; concurrent therapy contraindicated. Wait 24 hours after last dimercaprol dose.

---

Reactions may be *common*, uncommon, *life-threatening*, or COMMON AND LIFE-THREATENING.

## EFFECTS ON DIAGNOSTIC TESTS
Drug therapy blocks thyroid uptake of $^{131}$I, causing decreased values.

## CONTRAINDICATIONS
Contraindicated in patients with hepatic dysfunction (except postarsenical jaundice) or iron, cadmium, or selenium poisoning; also contraindicated in those allergic to peanuts.

## NURSING CONSIDERATIONS
• Use cautiously in patients with hypertension, G6PD deficiency, or oliguria.
• Safe use in pregnancy hasn't been established; drug shouldn't be used unless judged by doctor to be needed to treat life-threatening acute poisoning.
• *Alert:* Don't give drug I.V.; give by deep I.M. route only.
• Don't let drug come in contact with skin because it may cause a skin reaction.
• Drug has an unpleasant, garliclike odor.
• Solution with slight sediment is usable.
• Use antihistamine, as ordered, to prevent or relieve mild adverse reactions.
• Keep urine alkaline to prevent renal damage.

☑ **Patient teaching**
• Explain use and administration of drug to patient and family.
• Instruct patient to report adverse reactions promptly.

---

## disulfiram
Antabuse

*Pregnancy Risk Category C*

---

## HOW SUPPLIED
*Tablets:* 250 mg, 500 mg

## ACTION
Blocks oxidation of ethanol at the acetaldehyde stage. Excess acetaldehyde produces a highly unpleasant reaction in the presence of even small amounts of ethanol.

| Route | Onset | Peak | Duration |
|---|---|---|---|
| P.O. | 1-2 hr | Unknown | 14 days |

## INDICATIONS & DOSAGE
*Adjunct in management of chronic alcoholism—*
**Adults:** 250 to 500 mg P.O. as single dose in morning for 1 to 2 weeks or in evening if drowsiness occurs. Maintenance dose is 125 to 500 mg P.O. daily (average dosage 250 mg) until permanent self-control is established. Treatment may continue for months or years.

## ADVERSE REACTIONS
**CNS:** drowsiness, headache, fatigue, delirium, depression, neuritis, peripheral neuritis, polyneuritis, restlessness, psychotic reactions.
**EENT:** optic neuritis.
**GI:** metallic or garlic aftertaste.
**GU:** impotence.
**Metabolic:** elevated serum cholesterol levels.
**Skin:** acneiform or allergic dermatitis, occasional eruptions.
**Other:** disulfiram reaction, precipitated by ethanol use, with possible flushing, throbbing headache, dyspnea, nausea, copious vomiting, diaphoresis, thirst, chest pain, palpitations, hyperventilation, hypotension, syncope, anxiety, weakness, blurred vision, confusion, arthropathy. *Severe disulfiram reaction: respiratory depression, CV collapse, arrhythmias, MI, acute heart failure, seizures, unconsciousness, death.*

## INTERACTIONS
**Drug-drug.** *Barbiturates:* prolonged duration of effect. Closely monitor patient.
*CNS depressants:* increased CNS depression. Use together cautiously.
*Coumarin anticoagulants:* increased anticoagulant effect. Adjust dosage of anticoagulant.
*Isoniazid:* ataxia or marked change in behavior. Don't use concomitantly.
*Metronidazole:* psychotic reaction. Don't use concomitantly.
*Midazolam:* increased plasma levels of midazolam. Use together cautiously.
*Paraldehyde:* toxic levels of acetaldehyde. Don't use concomitantly.
*Phenytoin:* increased blood levels of phenytoin. Monitor phenytoin blood lev-

---

els, and expect doctor to adjust phenytoin dosages.
*Tricyclic antidepressants, especially amitriptyline:* transient delirium. Closely monitor patient.
**Drug-herb.** *Herbal preparations containing alcohol:* may precipitate disulfiram reaction. Don't use concomitantly. Alcohol reaction may occur as long as 2 weeks after single disulfiram dose.
**Drug-food.** *Caffeine:* increased elimination half-life of caffeine. Watch for effects.
**Drug-lifestyle.** *Alcohol use (all sources, including back-rub preparations, cough syrups, liniments, shaving lotion):* may precipitate disulfiram reaction. Don't use concomitantly. Alcohol reaction may occur as long as 2 weeks after single disulfiram dose.

## EFFECTS ON DIAGNOSTIC TESTS
Drug may decrease urinary vanillylmandelic acid excretion and increase urinary levels of homovanillic acid. Decrease of radioactive iodine ($^{131}$I) uptake or protein-bound iodine levels may occur rarely.

## CONTRAINDICATIONS
Contraindicated in patients with hypersensitivity to disulfiram or other thiram derivatives used in pesticides and rubber vulcanization; in those with psychoses, myocardial disease, or coronary occlusion; in patients receiving metronidazole, paraldehyde, alcohol, or alcohol-containing products; and during alcohol intoxication or within 12 hours of alcohol ingestion.

## NURSING CONSIDERATIONS
● Don't give drug during pregnancy.
● Use with extreme caution in patients with diabetes mellitus, hypothyroidism, seizure disorder, cerebral damage, nephritis, or hepatic cirrhosis or insufficiency, and in those receiving concurrent phenytoin therapy.
● Never administer until patient has abstained from alcohol for at least 12 hours. He should clearly understand consequences of disulfiram therapy and give permission for its use. Use drug only in patients who are cooperative, well motivated, and receiving supportive psychiatric therapy.
● Complete physical examination and laboratory studies, including CBC, SMA-12, and transaminase level, should precede therapy and be repeated regularly, as ordered.
● The longer patient remains on drug, the more sensitive he becomes to alcohol.
● *Alert:* Don't confuse Antabuse with Anturane.

### ☑ Patient teaching
● *Alert:* Caution patient's family that disulfiram should never be given to patient without his knowledge; severe reaction or death could result if patient ingests alcohol.
● Tell patient to wear a medical identification bracelet or carry a card supplied by drug manufacturer identifying him as a disulfiram user.
● Mild reactions may occur in sensitive patient with blood alcohol levels of 5 to 10 mg/100 ml; symptoms are fully developed at 50 mg/100 ml; unconsciousness typically occurs at 125 to 150 mg/100 ml level. Reaction may last from 30 minutes to several hours or as long as alcohol remains in blood.
● Reassure patient that disulfiram-induced adverse reactions (unrelated to concomitant alcohol use), such as drowsiness, fatigue, impotence, headache, peripheral neuritis, and metallic or garlic taste, subside after about 2 weeks of therapy.
● Advise patient not to drink alcoholic beverages or use products containing alcohol, including topical preparations and mouthwash. Have patient verify content of OTC products with pharmacist before use.

---

## d-penicillamine
Cuprimine, Depen, D-Penamine‡

*Pregnancy Risk Category D*

---

**HOW SUPPLIED**
*Tablets:* 125 mg‡, 250 mg
*Capsules:* 125 mg, 250 mg

---

*Reactions may be* common, *uncommon,* ***life-threatening,*** or **COMMON AND LIFE-THREATENING.**

## ACTION
Chelates heavy metals and may inhibit collagen formation. Mechanism unknown for rheumatoid arthritis.

| Route | Onset | Peak | Duration |
|-------|-------|------|----------|
| P.O. | Unknown | 1 hr | Unknown |

## INDICATIONS & DOSAGE
*Wilson's disease—*
**Adults and children:** 250 mg P.O. q.i.d. 30 to 60 minutes before meals. Dosage adjusted to achieve urinary copper excretion of 0.5 to 1 mg daily.
*Cystinuria—*
**Adults:** 250 mg to 1 g P.O. q.i.d. before meals. Dosage adjusted to achieve urinary cystine excretion of less than 100 mg daily when renal calculi exist, or 100 to 200 mg daily when calculi don't exist. Maximum dose is 4 g daily.
**Children:** 30 mg/kg P.O. daily, divided q.i.d. before meals. Dosage adjusted to achieve urinary cystine excretion of less than 100 mg daily when renal calculi exist, or 100 to 200 mg daily when calculi don't exist.
*Rheumatoid arthritis—*
**Adults:** initially, 125 to 250 mg P.O. daily, with increases of 125 to 250 mg q 1 to 3 months, if needed. Maximum dose is 1.5 g daily.

## ADVERSE REACTIONS
**EENT:** tinnitus, *optic neuritis.*
**GI:** *anorexia, epigastric pain, nausea, vomiting, diarrhea, loss of or altered taste perception, stomatitis.*
**GU:** nephrotic syndrome, glomerulonephritis, proteinuria, hematuria.
**Hematologic:** *leukopenia,* eosinophilia, **thrombocytopenia,** monocytosis, **agranulocytosis, aplastic anemia,** lupus-like syndrome.
**Hepatic:** *hepatotoxicity.*
**Metabolic:** hypoglycemia.
**Musculoskeletal:** *arthralgia.*
**Respiratory:** *pneumonitis.*
**Skin:** alopecia, friability, especially at pressure spots; wrinkling, erythema, urticaria.
**Other:** myasthenia gravis syndrome with long-term use, *allergic reactions, lymphadenopathy,* ecchymoses.

## INTERACTIONS
**Drug-drug.** *Antacids, oral iron:* decreased effectiveness of d-penicillamine. Give at least 2 hours apart.
*Gold therapy, antimalarials, cytotoxic drugs, oxyphenbutazone, phenylbutazone:* associated with serious hematologic and renal reactions. Avoid concomitant use.
**Drug-food.** *Any food:* delayed and decreased absorption of drug. Administer drug 1 hour before or 3 hours after meals.

## EFFECTS ON DIAGNOSTIC TESTS
Drug may cause positive test results for antinuclear antibody with or without clinical systemic lupus-like syndrome.

## CONTRAINDICATIONS
Contraindicated in breast-feeding women, during pregnancy with cystinuria present, in patients with penicillamine-related aplastic anemia or granulocytosis, and in those with rheumatoid arthritis and renal insufficiency.

## NURSING CONSIDERATIONS
• Use with extreme caution, if at all, in patients with hypersensitivity to penicillin.
• Patients who have had a major toxic reaction to gold salt therapy may be at greater risk for serious adverse reactions.
• Patients should receive supplemental pyridoxine daily.
• If patients have a skin reaction, give antihistamines, as ordered. Handle patients carefully to avoid skin damage.
• Monitor CBC and renal and hepatic function every 2 weeks for first 6 months; then monthly, as ordered.
• Monitor urinalysis regularly for protein loss.
• *Alert:* Report rash and fever (important signs of toxicity) to doctor immediately.
• Withhold drug and notify doctor if WBC count falls below 3,500/mm³ or platelet count falls below 100,000/mm³. A progressive decline in platelet or WBC count in three successive blood tests may necessitate temporary cessation of therapy, even if such counts are within normal limits.
• *Alert:* Don't confuse d-penicillamine with penicillin, or Depen with Endep.

---

✅**Patient teaching**
- Tell patient that therapeutic effect may be delayed up to 3 months in treatment of rheumatoid arthritis.
- Tell patient to take drug on an empty stomach, at least 1 hour before or 3 hours after meals, and to maintain adequate fluid intake, especially at night.
- Advise patient to report early signs of granulocytopenia: fever, sore throat, chills, bruising, and prolonged bleeding time.
- Reassure patient that taste impairment usually resolves in 6 weeks without changes in dosage.

---

## edetate calcium disodium
Calcium Disodium Versenate,
Calcium EDTA

*Pregnancy Risk Category B*

### HOW SUPPLIED
*Injection:* 200 mg/ml

### ACTION
Forms stable, soluble complexes with metals, particularly lead.

| Route | Onset | Peak | Duration |
|---|---|---|---|
| I.V., I.M. | 1 hr | 24-48 hr | Unknown |

### INDICATIONS & DOSAGE
*Acute lead encephalopathy or blood lead levels above 70 mcg/dl—*
**Adults and children:** 1 to 1.5 g/m$^2$ I.V. or I.M. daily in two divided doses at 12-hour intervals for 3 to 5 days, usually with dimercaprol. A second course may be administered after at least 2-day drug-free interval.
*Lead poisoning without encephalopathy or asymptomatic with blood levels below 70 mcg/dl—*
**Children:** 1 g/m$^2$ I.V. or I.M. daily in divided doses for 5 days.

### ADVERSE REACTIONS
**CNS:** tremors, headache, numbness, tingling, malaise, fatigue.
**CV:** hypotension, rhythm irregularities.
**EENT:** histamine-like reactions including sneezing, congestion, and lacrimation.

**GI:** cheilosis, nausea, vomiting, anorexia, excessive thirst.
**GU:** proteinuria, hematuria; *nephrotoxicity with renal tubular necrosis leading to fatal nephrosis.*
**Hematologic:** *transient bone marrow suppression,* anemia.
**Hepatic:** increased AST and ALT levels.
**Metabolic:** zinc deficiency, hypercalcemia.
**Musculoskeletal:** myalgia, arthralgia.
**Skin:** rash.
**Other:** pain at I.M. injection site, fever, chills.

### INTERACTIONS
**Drug-drug.** *Zinc insulin:* interferes with action of insulin by binding with zinc. Monitor closely.

### EFFECTS ON DIAGNOSTIC TESTS
None reported.

### CONTRAINDICATIONS
Contraindicated in patients with anuria, hepatitis, or acute renal disease.

### NURSING CONSIDERATIONS
- Use with extreme caution in patients with mild renal disease. Expect dosages to be reduced.
- Add procaine hydrochloride, as ordered, to I.M. solution to minimize pain. Watch for local reactions.
- *Alert:* Because rapid I.V. use may increase intracranial pressure, I.M. route may be preferred for treating lead encephalopathy.
- Although I.M. route may be preferred for children and patients with lead encephalopathy, most experts recommend I.V. infusion whenever possible.
- Monitor fluid intake and output, urinalysis, BUN level, and ECG daily, as ordered.
- To avoid toxicity, use with dimercaprol, as ordered.
- *Alert:* Don't confuse edetate calcium disodium with edetate disodium.

### 💧I.V. administration
- Dilute drug with D$_5$W or normal saline for injection to concentration of 2 to 4 mg/ml. Infuse one-half of daily dose

---

over 1 hour in asymptomatic patients or 2 hours in symptomatic patients. Give rest of infusion at least 12 hours later. Or, give by slow infusion over at least 6 hours.

### ☑ Patient teaching
• Explain use and administration of drug to patient and family.
• Tell patients with lead encephalopathy to avoid excess fluids.

---

## edetate disodium
Disodium EDTA, Disotate, Endrate

*Pregnancy Risk Category C*

### HOW SUPPLIED
*Injection:* 150 mg/ml

### ACTION
Chelates with metals such as calcium to form a stable, soluble complex.

| Route | Onset | Peak | Duration |
|-------|-------|------|----------|
| I.V. | Unknown | Unknown | Unknown |

### INDICATIONS & DOSAGE
*Hypercalcemic crisis—*
**Adults:** 50 mg/kg/day by slow I.V. infusion over at least 3 hours. Maximum dose is 3 g/day.

### ADVERSE REACTIONS
**CNS:** circumoral paresthesia, numbness, headache.
**CV:** hypotension, thrombophlebitis.
**EENT:** erythema.
**GI:** nausea, vomiting, diarrhea.
**GU:** *nephrotoxicity with urinary urgency,* nocturia, dysuria, polyuria, proteinuria, renal insufficiency, *renal failure, tubular necrosis.*
**Metabolic:** severe hypocalcemia, decreased magnesium.
**Skin:** exfoliative dermatitis.
**Other:** pain at infusion site.

### INTERACTIONS
None significant.

### EFFECTS ON DIAGNOSTIC TESTS
Drug lowers serum calcium levels (when measured by oxalate or other precipitation methods and by colorimetry) and blood glucose levels in diabetic patients.

### CONTRAINDICATIONS
Contraindicated in patients with hypersensitivity to drug and in those with anuria, known or suspected hypocalcemia, significant renal disease, active or healed tubercular lesions, or history of seizures or intracranial lesions.

### NURSING CONSIDERATIONS
• Use cautiously in patients with limited cardiac reserve, heart failure, or hypokalemia.
• Keep I.V. calcium available to treat hypocalcemia.
• Keep patients in bed for 15 minutes after infusion to avoid orthostatic hypotension. Monitor blood pressure closely.
• Monitor ECG and renal function tests frequently, as ordered.
• Obtain serum calcium level after each dose, as ordered.
• Don't use to treat lead toxicity; edetate calcium disodium should be used instead.
• *Alert:* Don't confuse edetate disodium with edetate calcium disodium.

### ◨ I.V. administration
• Dilute drug in 500 ml of $D_5W$ or normal saline solution and infuse over 3 or more hours.
• *Alert:* Avoid rapid I.V. infusion; profound hypocalcemia may occur, leading to tetany, seizures, arrhythmias, and respiratory arrest. Drug isn't recommended for direct or intermittent injection. Avoid extravasation.
• Record I.V. site used, and avoid repeated use of same site, which increases likelihood of thrombophlebitis.

### ☑ Patient teaching
• Explain use and administration of drug to patient and family.
• Instruct patient to report adverse reactions promptly.

---

# flumazenil
Anexate§, Romazicon

*Pregnancy Risk Category C*

## HOW SUPPLIED
*Injection:* 0.1 mg/ml in 5- and 10-ml multiple-dose vials

## ACTION
A benzodiazepine antagonist that competitively inhibits the actions of benzodiazepines on the gamma-aminobutyric acid–benzodiazepine receptor complex.

| Route | Onset | Peak | Duration |
|-------|-------|------|----------|
| I.V. | 1-2 min | 6-10 min | Variable |

## INDICATIONS & DOSAGE
*Complete or partial reversal of sedative effects of benzodiazepines after anesthesia or short diagnostic procedures (conscious sedation)—*
**Adults:** initially, 0.2 mg I.V. over 15 seconds. If patient doesn't reach desired level of consciousness after 45 seconds, dose is repeated. Repeated at 1-minute intervals until cumulative dose of 1 mg has been given (initial dose plus four additional doses), if needed. Most patients respond after 0.6 to 1 mg of drug. For resedation, dosage may be repeated after 20 minutes; however, no more than 1 mg should be given at any one time and no more than 3 mg/hour.
*Suspected benzodiazepine overdose—*
**Adults:** initially, 0.2 mg I.V. over 30 seconds. If patient doesn't reach desired level of consciousness after 30 seconds, 0.3 mg is given over 30 seconds. If patient still doesn't respond adequately, 0.5 mg is given over 30 seconds; 0.5-mg doses are repeated, p.r.n., at 1-minute intervals until cumulative dose of 3 mg has been given. Most patients suffering from benzodiazepine overdose respond to cumulative doses between 1 and 3 mg; rarely, patients who respond partially after 3 mg may need additional doses, up to 5 mg total. If patient doesn't respond in 5 minutes after receiving 5 mg, sedation is unlikely to be caused by benzodiazepines. In case of resedation, dosage may be repeated after 20 minutes; however, no more than 1 mg should be given at any one time and no more than 3 mg/hour.

## ADVERSE REACTIONS
**CNS:** *dizziness, abnormal or blurred vision, headache,* **seizures,** *agitation, emotional lability, tremor, insomnia.*
**CV:** *arrhythmias,* cutaneous vasodilation, palpitations.
**GI:** *nausea, vomiting.*
**Respiratory:** dyspnea, hyperventilation.
**Skin:** *diaphoresis.*
**Other:** *pain at injection site.*

## INTERACTIONS
**Drug-drug.** *Antidepressants, drugs that can cause seizures or arrhythmias:* seizures or arrhythmias can develop after effect of benzodiazepine overdose is removed. Flumazenil shouldn't be used in mixed overdose, especially in cases in which seizures (from any cause) are likely to occur.

## EFFECTS ON DIAGNOSTIC TESTS
None reported.

## CONTRAINDICATIONS
Contraindicated in patients who are hypersensitive to flumazenil or benzodiazepines; those who show evidence of serious tricyclic antidepressant overdose; and those who have received benzodiazepines to treat a potentially life-threatening condition such as status epilepticus.

## NURSING CONSIDERATIONS
• Use cautiously in patients with head injury, psychiatric disorders, or alcohol dependency. Also use cautiously in patients at high risk for developing seizures; those who have recently received multiple doses of a parenteral benzodiazepine; those who display signs of seizure activity; and in those who may be at risk for unrecognized benzodiazepine dependence, such as intensive care unit patients.
• Safety and efficacy of drug in children haven't been established.
• Monitor patients closely for resedation that may occur after reversal of benzodiazepine effects because flumazenil's duration of action is shorter than that of all benzodiazepines. Duration of monitoring

period depends on specific drug being reversed. Monitor closely after long-acting benzodiazepines, such as diazepam, or after high doses of short-acting benzodiazepines, such as 10 mg of midazolam. In most cases, severe resedation is unlikely in patients who fail to show signs of resedation 2 hours after a 1-mg dose of flumazenil.

### I.V. administration
• Be sure airway is secure and patent.
• Administer drug into I.V. line in large vein with free-flowing I.V. solution over 15 to 30 seconds to minimize pain at injection site. Compatible solutions include $D_5W$, lactated Ringer's injection, and normal saline.
• Avoid extravasation into perivascular tissues.

### Patient teaching
• Warn patient not to perform hazardous activities within 24 hours of procedure because of resedation risk.
• Tell patient to avoid alcohol, CNS depressants, and OTC drugs for 24 hours.
• Give family necessary instructions or provide patient with written instructions. Patient won't recall information given in postprocedure period; drug doesn't reverse amnesic effects of benzodiazepines.

## ipecac syrup

*Pregnancy Risk Category C*

### HOW SUPPLIED
*Syrup\**: 70 mg powdered ipecac/ml (contains glycerin 10% and alcohol 1% to 2.5%) ◊

### ACTION
Induces vomiting by acting locally on the gastric mucosa and centrally on the chemoreceptor trigger zone.

| Route | Onset | Peak | Duration |
|-------|-------|------|----------|
| P.O. | 20-30 min | Unknown | 20-25 min |

### INDICATIONS & DOSAGE
*To induce vomiting in poisoning—*
**Adults and children over age 12:** 15 to 30 ml P.O.; then 3 to 4 glasses of water.

**Children ages 1 to 12:** 15 ml P.O.; then 240 to 480 ml (8 to 16 oz) of water. Dose may be repeated in patients over age 1 if vomiting doesn't occur within 20 minutes. If no vomiting occurs within 30 to 35 minutes after second dose, gastric lavage should be performed.
**Infants and children ages 6 months to 1 year:** 5 to 10 ml P.O.; then 120 to 240 ml (4 to 8 oz) of water.

### ADVERSE REACTIONS
**CNS:** depression, *drowsiness.*
**CV:** *arrhythmias, bradycardia,* hypotension; atrial fibrillation, *fatal myocarditis.*
**GI:** *diarrhea.*

### INTERACTIONS
**Drug-drug.** *Activated charcoal:* neutralized emetic effect. Don't give together; may give activated charcoal after vomiting.

### EFFECTS ON DIAGNOSTIC TESTS
None reported.

### CONTRAINDICATIONS
Contraindicated in semicomatose or unconscious patients and in those with severe inebriation, seizures, anaphylaxis, severe hypotension, or loss of gag reflex.

### NURSING CONSIDERATIONS
• *Alert:* Don't administer after ingestion of petroleum products or volatile oils because of potential for dangerous or lethal aspiration. Don't administer after ingestion of caustic substances such as lye because of potential for additional injury to the esophagus and mediastinum.
• Stomach is usually emptied completely; vomitus also may contain some intestinal material.
• If two doses don't induce vomiting, be prepared for gastric lavage.
• Ipecac syrup usually induces vomiting within 20 to 30 minutes.
• In antiemetic toxicity, ipecac syrup is usually effective if less than 1 hour has elapsed since ingestion of antiemetic.
• No systemic toxicity occurs with doses of 1 oz (30 ml) or less.
• Ipecac syrup is commonly abused by bulimics who binge, then purge.

## ✓ Patient teaching
• Advise patient or parent to consult doctor or poison control center in case of accidental ingestion.
• Recommend to parents that 1 oz (30 ml) of syrup be available in the home after child's first birthday for immediate use in case of emergency.
• Show parents how to administer drug and tell them what to do in case of accidental poisoning.
• Warn parents not to let child sleep on his back after taking drug. Use a pillow to prop child on his side.

---

**naloxone hydrochloride**
Narcan

*Pregnancy Risk Category B*

## HOW SUPPLIED
*Injection:* 0.02 mg/ml, 0.4 mg/ml, 1 mg/ml

## ACTION
Unknown. Thought to displace previously administered narcotic analgesics from their receptors (competitive antagonism); it has no pharmacologic activity of its own.

| Route | Onset | Peak | Duration |
|-------|-------|------|----------|
| I.V. | 1-2 min | 5-15 min | Variable |
| I.M., S.C. | 2-5 min | 5-15 min | Variable |

## INDICATIONS & DOSAGE
*Known or suspected narcotic-induced respiratory depression, including that caused by pentazocine and propoxyphene—*
**Adults:** 0.4 to 2 mg I.V., S.C., or I.M. repeated q 2 to 3 minutes, p.r.n. If no response is observed after 10 mg has been administered, diagnosis of narcotic-induced toxicity should be questioned.
**Children:** 0.01 mg/kg I.V.; then second dose of 0.1 mg/kg I.V., if needed. If I.V. route isn't available, drug may be administered I.M. or S.C. in divided doses.
**Neonates:** 0.01 mg/kg I.V., I.M., or S.C. Dose may be repeated q 2 to 3 minutes, p.r.n.
*Postoperative narcotic depression—*
**Adults:** 0.1 to 0.2 mg I.V. q 2 to 3 minutes, p.r.n. Dose may be repeated within 1 to 2 hours, if needed.

**Children:** 0.005 to 0.01 mg I.V. repeated q 2 to 3 minutes, p.r.n.
**Neonates (asphyxia neonatorum):**
0.01 mg/kg I.V. into umbilical vein. May be repeated q 2 to 3 minutes.

## ADVERSE REACTIONS
**CNS:** tremors, *seizures.*
**CV:** tachycardia, hypertension with higher-than-recommended doses; hypotension, *ventricular fibrillation.*
**GI:** nausea, vomiting.
**Respiratory:** *pulmonary edema.*
**Other:** withdrawal symptoms in narcotic-dependent patients with higher-than-recommended doses, diaphoresis.

## INTERACTIONS
None significant.

## EFFECTS ON DIAGNOSTIC TESTS
None reported.

## CONTRAINDICATIONS
Contraindicated in patients with hypersensitivity to drug.

## NURSING CONSIDERATIONS
• Use cautiously in patients with cardiac irritability and opiate addiction. Abrupt reversal of opiate-induced CNS depression may result in nausea, vomiting, diaphoresis, tachycardia, CNS excitement, and increased blood pressure.
• Duration of action of the narcotic may exceed that of naloxone, and patients may relapse into respiratory depression.
• Respiratory rate increases within 1 to 2 minutes.
• *Alert:* Drug is effective only in reversing respiratory depression caused by opiates, not against other drug-induced respiratory depression, including that caused by benzodiazepines.
• Patients who receive naloxone to reverse opioid-induced respiratory depression may exhibit tachypnea.
• Monitor respiratory depth and rate. Be prepared to provide oxygen, ventilation, and other resuscitation measures.
• *Alert:* Don't confuse naloxone with naltrexone.

---

Reactions may be *common*, uncommon, *life-threatening*, or COMMON AND LIFE-THREATENING.

## I.V. administration
• Be prepared to administer continuous I.V. infusion (needed in many instances to control adverse effects of epidurally administered morphine). If 0.02 mg/ml isn't available, adult concentration (0.4 mg) may be diluted by mixing 0.5 ml with 9.5 ml of sterile water for injection to make neonatal concentration (0.02 mg/ml).

## Patient teaching
• Inform family of use and administration of drug.
• Reassure family that patient will be monitored closely until effects of narcotic are alleviated.

---

## naltrexone hydrochloride
Nalorex§, ReVia, Trexan

*Pregnancy Risk Category C*

### HOW SUPPLIED
*Tablets:* 50 mg

### ACTION
Unknown. Probably reversibly blocks the subjective effects of opioids administered I.V. by competitively occupying opiate receptors in the brain.

| Route | Onset | Peak | Duration |
|-------|-------|------|----------|
| P.O. | 15-30 min | 12 hr | 24 hr |

### INDICATIONS & DOSAGE
*Adjunct for maintenance of opioid-free state in detoxified individuals—*
**Adults:** initially, 25 mg P.O. If no withdrawal signs occur within 1 hour, an additional 25 mg is given. Once patient has been started on 50 mg q 24 hours, flexible maintenance schedule may be used. From 50 to 150 mg may be given daily, depending on schedule prescribed.
*Alcohol dependence—*
**Adults:** 50 mg P.O. once daily.

### ADVERSE REACTIONS
**CNS:** *insomnia, anxiety, nervousness, headache,* depression, dizziness, fatigue, somnolence, *suicidal ideation.*
**GI:** *nausea, vomiting,* anorexia, *abdominal pain,* constipation, increased thirst.
**GU:** delayed ejaculation, decreased potency.
**Hematologic:** lymphocytosis.
**Hepatic:** altered liver function test results, *hepatotoxicity.*
**Musculoskeletal:** *muscle and joint pain.*
**Skin:** rash.
**Other:** chills.

### INTERACTIONS
**Drug-drug.** *Thioridazine:* increased somnolence and lethargy. Monitor closely.

### EFFECTS ON DIAGNOSTIC TESTS
None reported.

### CONTRAINDICATIONS
Contraindicated in patients with hypersensitivity to drug, in those receiving opioid analgesics, in opioid-dependent patients, in patients in acute opioid withdrawal, and in those with positive urine screen for opioids or acute hepatitis or liver failure.

### NURSING CONSIDERATIONS
• Use cautiously in patients with mild hepatic disease or history of recent hepatic disease.
• Treatment for opioid dependency shouldn't begin until patients receive naloxone challenge, a provocative test of opioid dependency. If signs and symptoms of opioid withdrawal persist after naloxone challenge, don't administer drug.
• Patient must be completely free from opioids before taking drug, or severe withdrawal symptoms may occur. Patients who have been addicted to short-acting opioids, such as heroin and meperidine, must wait at least 7 days after last opioid dose before starting drug. Patients who have been addicted to longer-acting opioids such as methadone should wait at least 10 days.
• In an emergency, anticipate that patients receiving naltrexone may be given an opioid analgesic, but dose must be higher than usual to surmount naltrexone's effect. Watch for respiratory depression from the opioid; it may be longer and deeper.
• For patients being treated because of history of opioid dependency and who are expected to be noncompliant, be prepared

to try a flexible maintenance dose regimen of 100 mg on Monday and Wednesday and 150 mg on Friday, as ordered.
• Drug should be used only as part of a comprehensive rehabilitation program.
• *Alert:* Don't confuse naltrexone with naloxone.

☑ **Patient teaching**
• Advise patient to carry a medical identification card and to tell medical personnel that he takes naltrexone.
• Give patient names of nonopioid drugs that he can continue to take for pain, diarrhea, or cough.

---

**pralidoxime chloride (2-PAM chloride; 2-pyridine-aldoxime methochloride)**
Protopam Chloride

*Pregnancy Risk Category C*

**HOW SUPPLIED**
*Injection:* 1 g/20 ml in 20-ml vial without diluent or syringe; 1 g/20 ml in 20-ml vial with diluent, syringe, needle, and alcohol swab (emergency kit); 600 mg/2 ml auto-injector, parenteral

**ACTION**
Reactivates cholinesterase inactivated by organophosphorus pesticides and related compounds, permitting degradation of accumulated acetylcholine and facilitating normal functioning of neuromuscular junctions.

| Route | Onset | Peak | Duration |
|-------|-------|------|----------|
| I.V. | Unknown | 5-15 min | Unknown |
| I.M. | Unknown | 10-20 min | Unknown |
| S.C. | Unknown | Unknown | Unknown |

**INDICATIONS & DOSAGE**
*Antidote for organophosphate poisoning—*
**Adults:** 1 to 2 g in 100 ml of normal saline solution by I.V. infusion over 15 to 30 minutes. Repeated in 1 hour if muscle weakness persists. Additional doses may be given cautiously. I.M. or S.C. injection may be used if I.V. isn't feasible.
**Children:** 20 to 40 mg/kg I.V., administered as for adults.

*Cholinergic crisis in myasthenia gravis—*
**Adults:** 1 to 2 g I.V.; then 250 mg I.V. q 5 minutes, p.r.n.

**ADVERSE REACTIONS**
**CNS:** dizziness, headache, drowsiness.
**CV:** tachycardia.
**EENT:** blurred vision, diplopia, impaired accommodation.
**GI:** nausea.
**Hepatic:** transient elevation of liver enzyme levels.
**Musculoskeletal:** muscular weakness.
**Respiratory:** hyperventilation.
**Other:** mild to moderate pain at injection site.

**INTERACTIONS**
*Barbiturates:* potentiated by anticholinesterases. Use cautiously in treatment of seizures.

**EFFECTS ON DIAGNOSTIC TESTS**
None reported.

**CONTRAINDICATIONS**
Contraindicated in patients with hypersensitivity to drug.

**NURSING CONSIDERATIONS**
• Use with extreme caution in patients with myasthenia gravis (overdose may trigger myasthenic crisis).
• Initially, remove secretions, maintain patent airway, and institute mechanical ventilation, if needed. After dermal exposure to organophosphate, remove patient's clothing and wash his skin and hair with sodium bicarbonate, soap, water, and alcohol as soon as possible. A second washing may be needed. When washing patient, wear protective gloves and clothes to avoid exposure.
• Draw blood for cholinesterase levels before giving drug.
• Drug should be used in hospitalized patients only; have respiratory and other supportive measures available. If possible, obtain accurate medical history and chronology of poisoning. Drug should be given as soon as possible after poisoning; treatment is most effective if initiated within 24 hours after exposure.

---

Reactions may be *common*, uncommon, *life-threatening*, or COMMON AND LIFE-THREATENING.

• To ameliorate muscarinic effects and block accumulation of acetylcholine associated with organophosphate poisoning, give atropine 2 to 4 mg I.V. with pralidoxine if cyanosis isn't present, as ordered. (If cyanosis is present, give atropine I.M.) Give atropine every 5 to 6 minutes, as ordered, until signs of atropine toxicity (flushing, tachycardia, dry mouth, blurred vision, excitement, delirium, and hallucinations) appear; atropinization should be maintained for at least 48 hours.

• Observe patient for 48 to 72 hours if poison was ingested. Delayed absorption may occur from lower bowel. It's difficult to distinguish between toxic effects produced by atropine or organophosphate compounds and those resulting from pralidoxime.

• Watch patient with myasthenia gravis who is being treated for overdose of cholinergic drugs for signs of rapid weakening. He can pass quickly from cholinergic crisis to myasthenic crisis and needs more cholinergic drugs to treat myasthenia. Keep edrophonium available for establishing differential diagnosis.

• Avoid use of aminophylline, morphine, phenothiazine-like tranquilizers, reserpine, succinylcholine, theophylline in patients with organophosphate poisoning.

• Drug isn't effective against poisoning due to phosphorus, inorganic phosphates, or organophosphates with no anticholinesterase activity.

• *Alert:* Don't confuse pralidoxime with pramoxine or pyridoxine.

🖐 **I.V. administration**
• Reconstitute by adding 20 ml of sterile water for injection to vial containing 1 g of drug. Further dilute by adding 100 ml of normal saline solution. Infuse over 15 to 30 minutes.

• If patient has pulmonary edema, give drug by slow I.V. push over 5 minutes. Don't exceed 200 mg/minute.

• *Alert:* If drug is infused too rapidly, tachycardia, laryngospasm, and muscle rigidity may result.

✅ **Patient teaching**
• Explain use and administration of drug to patient and family.

• Tell patient to report adverse effects.
• Caution patient treated for organophosphate poisoning to avoid contact with insecticides for several weeks.

## protamine sulfate
Prosulf§

*Pregnancy Risk Category C*

### HOW SUPPLIED
*Injection:* 10 mg/ml

### ACTION
A heparin antagonist that forms a physiologically inert complex with heparin sodium.

| Route | Onset | Peak | Duration |
|-------|-------|------|----------|
| I.V. | 30-60 sec | Unknown | 2 hr |

### INDICATIONS & DOSAGE
*Heparin overdose—*
**Adults:** dosage based on venous blood coagulation studies, usually 1 mg for each 90 to 115 U of heparin. Give by slow I.V. injection over 10 minutes in doses not to exceed 50 mg.

### ADVERSE REACTIONS
**CNS:** lassitude.
**CV:** fall in blood pressure, *bradycardia, circulatory collapse,* transitory flushing.
**GI:** nausea, vomiting.
**Respiratory:** dyspnea, *pulmonary edema, acute pulmonary hypertension.*
**Other:** feeling of warmth, *anaphylaxis, anaphylactoid reactions.*

### INTERACTIONS
None significant.

### EFFECTS ON DIAGNOSTIC TESTS
None reported.

### CONTRAINDICATIONS
Contraindicated in patients with hypersensitivity to drug.

### NURSING CONSIDERATIONS
• Postoperative dose is based on coagulation studies and a repeat PT 15 minutes after administration is advised.

---

• Calculate dosage carefully. One mg of protamine neutralizes 90 to 115 U of heparin depending on salt (heparin calcium or heparin sodium) and source of heparin (beef or pork).
• Risk of hypersensitivity reaction increases in patients with known hypersensitivity to fish; in vasectomized or infertile men; and in patients taking protamine-insulin products.
• Monitor patient continually.
• Watch for spontaneous bleeding (heparin rebound), especially in dialysis patients and in those who have undergone cardiac surgery.
• Protamine may act as an anticoagulant in very high doses.
• I.V. route may cause flushing.
• *Alert:* Don't confuse protamine with Protopam or Protropin.

**◖ I.V. administration**
• Administer slowly by direct I.V. injection. Have emergency equipment available to treat anaphylaxis or severe hypotension.
• *Alert:* Excessively rapid I.V. administration may cause acute hypotension, bradycardia, pulmonary hypertension, dyspnea, transient flushing, and feeling of warmth.

**☑ Patient teaching**
• Explain use and administration of drug to patient and family.
• Tell patient to report adverse effects.

---

**sodium polystyrene sulfonate**
Kayexalate, SPS

*Pregnancy Risk Category C*

**HOW SUPPLIED**
*Powder:* 1-lb jar (3.5 g/tsp)
*Suspension:* 15 g/60 ml*

**ACTION**
A potassium-removing resin that exchanges sodium ions for potassium ions in the intestine: 1 g of sodium polystyrene sulfonate is exchanged for 0.5 to 1 mEq of potassium. The resin is then eliminated. Much of the exchange capacity is used for cations other than potassium

(calcium and magnesium) and possibly for fats and proteins.

| Route | Onset | Peak | Duration |
|-------|-------|------|----------|
| P.O., P.R. | Unknown | Unknown | Unknown |

**INDICATIONS & DOSAGE**
*Hyperkalemia—*
**Adults:** 15 g P.O. daily to q.i.d. in water or sorbitol (3 to 4 ml/g of resin). Or, mix powder with appropriate medium—aqueous suspension or diet appropriate for renal failure—and instill through an NG tube.
Or, 30 to 50 g/100 ml of sorbitol q 6 hours as warm emulsion deep into sigmoid colon (20 cm).
**Children:** 1 g/kg of body weight/dose P.O. or P.R., p.r.n., to correct hyperkalemia.
Oral administration preferred because drug should remain in intestine for at least 30 minutes.

**ADVERSE REACTIONS**
**GI:** *constipation,* fecal impaction, anorexia, gastric irritation, nausea, vomiting, *diarrhea with sorbitol emulsions.*
**Metabolic:** hypokalemia, hypocalcemia, hypomagnesemia, sodium retention.

**INTERACTIONS**
**Drug-drug.** *Antacids and laxatives (nonabsorbable cation-donating types, including magnesium hydroxide):* systemic alkalosis and reduced potassium exchange capability. Don't use together.

**EFFECTS ON DIAGNOSTIC TESTS**
None reported.

**CONTRAINDICATIONS**
Contraindicated in patients with hypersensitivity to drug and in those with hypokalemia.

**NURSING CONSIDERATIONS**
• Use cautiously in patients with severe heart failure, severe hypertension, or marked edema.
• Don't heat resin; this impairs drug's effect. Mix resin only with water or sorbitol for P.O. administration. Never mix with orange juice (high potassium content) to disguise taste.

---

Reactions may be *common,* uncommon, *life-threatening,* or COMMON AND LIFE-THREATENING.

• Chill oral suspension for greater palatability.
• If sorbitol is given, mix with resin suspension.
• Consider solid form. Resin cookie and candy recipes are available; ask pharmacist or dietitian to supply.
• Premixed forms are available (SPS and others). If preparing manually, mix polystyrene resin only with water and sorbitol for rectal use. Don't use mineral oil for P.R. administration to prevent impaction; ion exchange needs aqueous medium. Sorbitol content prevents impaction.
• Prepare P.R. dose at room temperature. Stir emulsion gently during administration.
• Use #28 French rubber tube for rectal dose; insert 20 cm into sigmoid colon. Tape tube in place. Or, consider an indwelling urinary catheter with a 30-ml balloon inflated distal to anal sphincter to aid in retention. This is especially helpful for patients with poor sphincter control. Use gravity flow. Drain returns constantly through Y-tube connection. Place patient in knee-chest position or with hips on pillow for a while if back-leakage occurs.
• After P.R. administration, flush tubing with 50 to 100 ml of nonsodium fluid to ensure delivery of all drug. Flush rectum to remove resin.
• Prevent fecal impaction in elderly patients by administering resin P.R., as ordered. Give cleansing enema before P.R. administration. Have patient retain enema for 6 to 10 hours if possible, but 30 to 60 minutes is acceptable.
• Watch for constipation in oral or NG administration. Use sorbitol (10 to 20 ml of 70% syrup every 2 hours, as needed) to produce one or two watery stools daily.
• Monitor serum potassium levels at least once daily. Treatment may result in potassium deficiency and is usually stopped when potassium is reduced to 4 or 5 mEq/L.
• Watch for signs of hypokalemia: irritability, confusion, arrhythmias, ECG changes, severe muscle weakness, and sometimes paralysis, and digitalis toxicity in digitalized patients.
• When hyperkalemia is severe, polystyrene resin alone isn't adequate for lowering serum potassium. Dextrose 50% with regular insulin I.V. push may also be given.
• Watch for symptoms of other electrolyte deficiencies (magnesium, calcium) because drug is nonselective. Monitor serum calcium in patients receiving sodium polystyrene therapy for more than 3 days. Supplementary calcium may be needed.
• Watch for sodium overload. Drug contains about 100 mg sodium/g. About one-third of resin's sodium is retained.

☑ **Patient teaching**
• Explain use and administration of drug to patient.
• Advise patient to report adverse reactions promptly.
• Teach patient about low-potassium diet.

---

## succimer
Chemet

*Pregnancy Risk Category C*

### HOW SUPPLIED
*Capsules:* 100 mg

### ACTION
A chelating drug that forms water-soluble complexes with lead and increases its excretion in urine.

| Route | Onset | Peak | Duration |
|-------|-------|------|----------|
| P.O. | Unknown | 1-2 hr | Unknown |

### INDICATIONS & DOSAGE
*Lead poisoning in children with blood lead levels above 45 mcg/dl—*
**Children:** initially, 10 mg/kg or 350 mg/m² q 8 hours for 5 days. Dosage rounded as appropriate to nearest 100 mg (see chart). Then, frequency of administration decreased to q 12 hours for an additional 2 weeks.

| Weight in kg (lb) | Dose (mg) |
|-------------------|-----------|
| 8-15 (17-34) | 100 |
| 16-23 (35-51) | 200 |
| 24-34 (52-75) | 300 |
| 35-44 (76-98) | 400 |
| > 45 (> 99) | 500 |

---

*Liquid contains alcohol.  **May contain tartrazine.  †Canada  ‡Australia  §U.K.  ◇OTC

## ADVERSE REACTIONS

**CNS:** *drowsiness, dizziness, sensory motor neuropathy, sleepiness, paresthesia, headache.*
**CV:** *arrhythmias.*
**EENT:** plugged ears, cloudy film in eyes, otitis media, watery eyes, sore throat, rhinorrhea, nasal congestion.
**GI:** *nausea, vomiting, diarrhea, loss of appetite, abdominal cramps, hemorrhoidal symptoms, metallic taste in mouth, loose stools.*
**GU:** decreased urination, difficult urination, proteinuria.
**Hematologic:** increased platelet count, intermittent eosinophilia.
**Hepatic:** *elevated serum AST, ALT, alkaline phosphatase levels.*
**Metabolic:** *elevated cholesterol levels.*
**Musculoskeletal:** *leg, kneecap, back, stomach, rib, or flank pain.*
**Respiratory:** cough, head cold.
**Skin:** papular rash, herpetic rash, mucocutaneous eruptions, pruritus.
**Other:** *flulike syndrome,* candidiasis.

## INTERACTIONS

*Other chelation therapy (such as CaNa$_2$EDTA):* Unknown adverse effects. Separate administration by 4 weeks.

## EFFECTS ON DIAGNOSTIC TESTS

Drug may cause false-positive results for urinary ketones in tests using nitroprusside reagents (Ketostix). Falsely decreased levels of serum uric acid and CK have also been reported.

## CONTRAINDICATIONS

Contraindicated in patients with hypersensitivity to drug.

## NURSING CONSIDERATIONS

● Use cautiously in patients with compromised renal function.
● Measure severity of poisoning by initial blood lead level and by rate and degree of rebound of blood lead level. Severity should be used as a guide for more frequent blood lead monitoring.
● Monitor serum transaminase level before and at least weekly during therapy. Transient mild elevations of serum transaminase levels have been observed.

Monitor patients with history of hepatic disease.
● Monitor patients at least once weekly for rebound blood lead levels. Elevated levels and associated symptoms may return rapidly after drug is stopped because of redistribution of lead from bone to soft tissues and blood.
● Course of treatment lasts 19 days. Repeated courses may be needed if indicated by weekly monitoring of blood lead levels.
● Minimum of 2 weeks between courses is recommended unless high blood lead levels indicate need for immediate therapy.
● Concurrent administration with other chelating drugs isn't recommended. Patients who have received edetate calcium disodium with or without dimercaprol may use succimer as subsequent therapy after a 4-week interval.

### ✅ Patient teaching

● Explain use and administration of drug to parents and child. Stress importance of complying with frequently ordered blood tests.
● Tell parents of young child who can't swallow capsules that capsule can be opened and its contents sprinkled on a small amount of soft food. Or, beads from capsule may be poured on a spoon; follow with flavored beverage.
● Tell patient to maintain adequate fluid intake.
● Assist parents with identifying and removing sources of lead in child's environment. Chelation therapy isn't a substitute for preventing further exposure and shouldn't be used to permit continued exposure.
● Tell patient to notify doctor if rash occurs. Consider possibility of allergic or other mucocutaneous reactions each time drug is used.

---

alendronate sodium
alitretinoin
alprostadil
amifostine
aminoglutethimide
anagrelide hydrochloride
aprotinin
becaplermin
calcipotriene
capsaicin
cisapride
clomiphene citrate
etanercept
finasteride
imiglucerase
imiquimod
infliximab
isotretinoin
leflunomide
levocarnitine
mesalamine
mesna
minoxidil (topical)
nimodipine
olsalazine sodium
orlistat
pamidronate disodium
pilocarpine hydrochloride
raloxifene hydrochloride
riluzole
ritodrine hydrochloride
sevelamer hydrochloride
sildenafil citrate
sulfasalazine
tamsulosin hydrochloride
thalidomide
tiludronate disodium
tolterodine tartrate
tretinoin

**COMBINATION PRODUCTS**
None.

## alendronate sodium
Fosamax

*Pregnancy Risk Category C*

**HOW SUPPLIED**
*Tablets:* 5 mg, 10 mg, 40 mg

**ACTION**
Suppresses osteoclast activity on newly formed resorption surfaces, which reduces bone turnover. Bone formation exceeds resorption at remodeling sites, leading to progressive gains in bone mass.

| Route | Onset | Peak | Duration |
|-------|-------|------|----------|
| P.O. | Unknown | Unknown | Unknown |

**INDICATIONS & DOSAGE**
*Osteoporosis in postmenopausal women, prevention of fractures—*
**Adults:** 10 mg P.O. daily, taken with water only, at least 30 minutes before first food, beverage, or medication of day.
*Paget's disease of bone—*
**Adults:** 40 mg P.O. daily for 6 months, taken with water only, at least 30 minutes before first food, beverage, or medication of day.
*Prevention of osteoporosis in post-menopausal women—*
**Adults:** 5 mg P.O. daily, taken with water only, at least 30 minutes before first food, beverage, or medication of day.
✱ *NEW INDICATION: Glucocorticoid-induced osteoporosis in men and women receiving glucocorticoids in a daily dose equivalent to 7.5 mg or more of prednisone and who have low bone mineral density—*
**Adults:** 5 mg P.O. daily, taken with water only, at least 30 minutes before first food, beverage, or medication of day. For postmenopausal women not receiving estrogen, recommended dose is 10 mg P.O. daily taken with water only, at least 30 minutes before first food, beverage, or medication of day.

## ADVERSE REACTIONS
**CNS:** headache.
**GI:** abdominal pain, nausea, dyspepsia, constipation, diarrhea, flatulence, acid regurgitation, esophageal ulcer, vomiting, dysphagia, abdominal distention, gastritis, taste perversion.
**Musculoskeletal:** musculoskeletal pain.

## INTERACTIONS
**Drug-drug.** *Antacids, calcium supplements:* may interfere with drug absorption. Tell patient to wait at least 30 minutes after taking alendronate before taking other drugs.
*Aspirin, NSAIDs:* increased risk of upper GI adverse reactions with drug doses above 10 mg/day. Monitor patient closely.
*Hormone replacement therapy:* not recommended for use with alendronate in treating osteoporosis; evidence of effectiveness is lacking. Avoid concurrent use.
*Ranitidine:* increased availability of alendronate. Reduce dosage, as needed.
**Drug-food.** *Any food:* decreased absorption of drug. Administer with full glass of water at least 30 minutes before eating, drinking, or ingesting other drugs.

## EFFECTS ON DIAGNOSTIC TESTS
None reported.

## CONTRAINDICATIONS
Contraindicated in patients with hypersensitivity to drug and in those with hypocalcemia, severe renal insufficiency, or abnormalities of the esophagus that delay esophageal emptying.

## NURSING CONSIDERATIONS
• Use cautiously in patients with active upper GI problems (dysphagia, symptomatic esophageal diseases, gastritis, duodenitis, ulcers) or mild to moderate renal insufficiency.
• Hypocalcemia and other disturbances of mineral metabolism (such as vitamin D deficiency) should be corrected before therapy begins.
• When used to treat osteoporosis in postmenopausal women, disease may be confirmed by findings of low bone mass on diagnostic studies or by history of osteoporotic fracture.

• When used to treat Paget's disease, drug is indicated for patients with alkaline phosphatase level at least two times upper limit of normal, for those who are symptomatic, and for those at risk for future complications from the disease.
• **Alert:** Make sure patient doesn't lie down for at least 30 minutes after taking drug to facilitate delivery to stomach and to reduce potential for esophageal irritation.
• Monitor patient's serum calcium and phosphate levels throughout therapy, as ordered.
• **Alert:** Don't confuse Fosamax with Flomax.

☑ **Patient teaching**
• Stress importance of taking tablet only with a glass (6 to 8 ounces) of plain water at least 30 minutes before ingesting anything else, including food, beverages, and other drugs. Tell patient that waiting longer than 30 minutes will improve absorption.
• Warn patient not to lie down for at least 30 minutes after taking drug to facilitate delivery to stomach and to reduce potential for esophageal irritation.
• Advise patient to report adverse effects immediately, especially chest pain or difficulty swallowing.
• Advise patient to take supplemental calcium and vitamin D if dietary intake is inadequate.
• Tell patient about benefits of weight-bearing exercises in increasing bone mass. If applicable, explain importance of reducing or eliminating cigarette smoking and alcohol use.

✴ *NEW DRUG*

# alitretinoin
Panretin

*Pregnancy Risk Category D*

## HOW SUPPLIED
*Gel:* 0.1%

## ACTION
A retinoid that binds to and activates all intracellular retinoid receptors to control

cellular differentiation and proliferation; inhibits growth of Kaposi's sarcoma cells.

| Route | Onset | Peak | Duration |
|-------|-------|------|----------|
| Topical | Unknown | Unknown | Unknown |

## INDICATIONS & DOSAGE
*Topical treatment of cutaneous lesions in patients with Kaposi's sarcoma related to AIDS—*
**Adults:** initially, apply generous coating of gel b.i.d. to lesions only. Frequency may be increased to t.i.d. or q.i.d. based on patient tolerance.

## ADVERSE REACTIONS
**CNS:** *paresthesia.*
**Skin:** *burning pain at application site, rash, pruritus,* exfoliative dermatitis, excoriation, drainage, fissures, cracking, scabbing, crusting, oozing, edema.

## INTERACTIONS
**Drug-lifestyle.** *Exposure to DEET (N,N-diethyl-m-toluamide), a common component of insect repellent products:* increased DEET toxicity. Don't use insect repellents containing DEET during drug therapy.
*Sun exposure:* possible photosensitizing effect. Minimize exposure of treated areas to sunlight and sunlamps.

## EFFECTS ON DIAGNOSTIC TESTS
None reported.

## CONTRAINDICATIONS
Contraindicated in patients with known hypersensitivity to retinoids, drug, or its components; also contraindicated in pregnant women.

Don't use gel on patients requiring systemic anti–Kaposi's sarcoma therapy, such as those with more than 10 new Kaposi's sarcoma lesions in previous month, symptomatic lymphedema, symptomatic pulmonary Kaposi's sarcoma, or symptomatic visceral involvement.

## NURSING CONSIDERATIONS
• Use cautiously in women of childbearing age.
• Cover lesions with a generous coating of gel. Don't apply drug to normal skin

around lesions because it may irritate the skin, or to or near mucosal surfaces.
• Allow gel to dry for 3 to 5 minutes before covering with clothing.
• Don't use occlusive dressings with drug.
• If patient experiences a toxic reaction (intense erythema, edema, vesiculation) at application site, frequency of application may need to be reduced. If severe irritation occurs, drug may be discontinued for few days until symptoms subside.

### ✅ Patient teaching
• Tell woman of childbearing age to avoid getting pregnant during therapy.
• Inform patient that, although he may respond to drug within 2 weeks of starting treatment, most patients need a longer response time.
• Caution patient to minimize exposure of treated areas to sunlight and sunlamps.
• Instruct patient to cover lesions with generous coating of gel, but not to apply it to normal skin around lesions because it may irritate the skin, or to or near mucosal surfaces.
• Tell patient to allow gel to dry for 3 to 5 minutes before covering with clothing.
• Tell patient that drug has no systemic effect on internal Kaposi's sarcoma nor does it prevent new Kaposi's sarcoma lesions in areas where it hasn't been applied.

# alprostadil
Caverject, Muse, Viridal§

*Pregnancy Risk Category X*

## HOW SUPPLIED
*Injection:* 5 mcg/ml, 10 mcg/ml, and 20 mcg/ml after reconstitution
*Urogenital suppository:* 125 mcg, 250 mcg, 500 mcg, 1,000 mcg

## ACTION
A prostaglandin derivative that induces erection by relaxing trabecular smooth muscle and dilating cavernosal arteries. This leads to expansion of lacunar spaces and entrapment of blood by compressing venules against the tunica albuginea, a

---

process referred to as the corporal veno-occlusive mechanism.

| Route | Onset | Peak | Duration |
|-------|-------|------|----------|
| Intra-cavernous | 5-20 min | 5-20 min | 1-6 hr |
| Urogenital | 10 min | 16 min | 1 hr |

## INDICATIONS & DOSAGE

*Erectile dysfunction due to vasculogenic, psychogenic, or mixed etiology—*
**Adults:** dosages are highly individualized, with initial dose of 2.5 mcg intracavernously. If partial response occurs, second dose of 2.5 mcg is given; then increased further in increments of 5 to 10 mcg until patient achieves erection (one suitable for intercourse and not exceeding 1 hour's duration). If no response occurs to initial dose, second dose may be increased to 7.5 mcg within 1 hour; then increased further in increments of 5 to 10 mcg until patient achieves suitable erection. Patient must remain in doctor's office until complete detumescence occurs. Procedure shouldn't be repeated for at least 24 hours.
*For urogenital suppository:*
**Adults:** initial dose (125 to 250 mcg) given under supervision of doctor. Adjust dosage as needed until response is sufficient for sexual intercourse. Maximum of two administrations in 24 hours; maximum dose is 1,000 mcg.
*Erectile dysfunction of neurogenic etiology (spinal cord injury)—*
**Adults:** dosages are highly individualized, with initial dose of 1.25 mcg intracavernously. If partial response occurs, second dose of 1.25 mcg is given, followed by an increment of 2.5 mcg, to dose of 5 mcg; then in increments of 5 mcg until patient achieves erection (one suitable for intercourse and not exceeding 1 hour's duration). If no response occurs to initial dose, next higher dose may be given within 1 hour. Patient must remain in doctor's office until complete detumescence occurs. If there is a response, procedure shouldn't be repeated for at least 24 hours.
*For urogenital suppository:*
**Adults:** initial dose (125 to 250 mcg) given under supervision of doctor. Adjust dosage as needed until response is suffi-cient for sexual intercourse. Maximum of two administrations in 24 hours; maximum dose is 1,000 mcg.

## ADVERSE REACTIONS

**CNS:** headache, dizziness.
**CV:** hypertension.
**EENT:** sinusitis, nasal congestion.
**GU:** *penile pain;* prolonged erection; penile fibrosis, rash, or edema; penis disorder; prostatic disorder.
**Musculoskeletal:** back pain.
**Respiratory:** upper respiratory tract infection, flulike syndrome, cough.
**Other:** injection site hematoma or ecchymosis, localized trauma or pain.

## INTERACTIONS

**Drug-drug.** *Anticoagulants:* increased risk of bleeding from intracavernosal injection site. Monitor patient closely.
*Cyclosporine:* decreased cyclosporine levels. Monitor closely.
*Vasoactive drugs:* safety and efficacy of concomitant use haven't been studied. Avoid concomitant use.

## EFFECTS ON DIAGNOSTIC TESTS
None reported.

## CONTRAINDICATIONS
Contraindicated in patients with hypersensitivity to drug and in those with conditions associated with predisposition to priapism (sickle cell anemia or trait, multiple myeloma, leukemia) or penile deformation (angulation, cavernosal fibrosis, Peyronie's disease). Don't use drug in men with penile implants or for whom sexual activity is inadvisable or contraindicated. Also, drug shouldn't be used by sexual partners of pregnant women unless condoms are used. Drug isn't given to women or children.

## NURSING CONSIDERATIONS
• Regular follow-up care, with thorough examination of the penis, is strongly recommended to detect signs of penile fibrosis. Drug should be discontinued in patients who develop penile angulation, cavernosal fibrosis, or Peyronie's disease.

---

## ☑ Patient teaching
• Teach patient how to prepare and administer drug before he begins treatment at home. Stress importance of reading and following patient instructions in each package insert. Tell him to store unopened suppositories in refrigerator (36° to 46° F [2° to 8° C]) and store injection at room temperature (59° to 86° F [15° to 30° C]).
• Tell patient not to shake contents of reconstituted vial, and remind him that vial is designed for single use only. Tell him to discard vial if solution is discolored or contains precipitate.
• Review administration and aseptic technique.
• Inform patient that he can expect an erection 5 to 20 minutes after administration, with a preferable duration of no more than 1 hour. If his erection lasts more than 6 hours, tell him to seek medical attention immediately.
• Remind patient to take drug as instructed (generally, no more than three times weekly, with at least 24 hours between each use). Warn him not to change dosage without consulting doctor.
• Caution patient to use a condom if there is a chance his sexual partner is pregnant.
• Review possible adverse reactions. Tell patient to inspect his penis daily and to report redness, swelling, tenderness, curvature, priapism, unusual pain, nodules, or hard tissue.
• Urge patient not to reuse or share needles, syringes, or drug.
• Warn patient that drug doesn't protect against sexually transmitted diseases. Also, caution him that bleeding at injection site can increase risk of transmitting blood-borne diseases to his partner.
• Remind patient to keep regular follow-up appointments so doctor can evaluate drug effectiveness and safety.

---

## amifostine
Ethyol

*Pregnancy Risk Category C*

### HOW SUPPLIED
*Injection:* 500 mg anhydrous base and 500 mg mannitol in 10-ml vial

## ACTION
Dephosphorylated by alkaline phosphatase in tissue to a pharmacologically active free thiol metabolite. Free thiol in normal tissues binds and detoxifies reactive metabolites of cisplatin, reducing the toxic effects of cisplatin on renal tissue. Free thiol can also act as a scavenger of free radicals that may be generated in tissues exposed to cisplatin.

| Route | Onset | Peak | Duration |
|-------|-------|------|----------|
| I.V. | 5-8 min | Unknown | Unknown |

## INDICATIONS & DOSAGE
*Reduction of cumulative renal toxicity associated with repeated administration of cisplatin in patients with advanced ovarian cancer or non-small-cell lung cancer—*
**Adults:** 910 mg/m² daily as a 15-minute I.V. infusion, starting 30 minutes before chemotherapy. If hypotension occurs and blood pressure doesn't return to normal within 5 minutes after stopping treatment, subsequent cycles should use dose of 740 mg/m².
✷ *NEW INDICATION: Reduction of moderate to severe xerostomia in patients undergoing postoperative radiation treatment for head and neck cancer—*
**Adults:** 200 mg/m² daily as 3-minute I.V. infusion, starting 15 to 30 minutes before standard fraction radiation therapy.

## ADVERSE REACTIONS
**CNS:** dizziness, somnolence.
**CV:** *hypotension.*
**GI:** *nausea, vomiting.*
**Metabolic:** hypocalcemia.
**Other:** flushing or feeling of warmth, chills or feeling of coldness, hiccups, sneezing, ***allergic reactions ranging from rash to rigors.***

## INTERACTIONS
**Drug-drug.** *Antihypertensives, other drugs that could potentiate hypotension:* may cause profound hypotension. Monitor closely.

## EFFECTS ON DIAGNOSTIC TESTS
None reported.

---

## CONTRAINDICATIONS

Contraindicated in patients with hypersensitivity to aminothiol compounds or mannitol. Drug shouldn't be used in patients receiving chemotherapy for potentially curable malignancies (including certain malignancies of germ-cell origin), except for patients involved in clinical studies. Also contraindicated in hypotensive or dehydrated patients and in those receiving antihypertensives that can't be stopped during 24 hours preceding amifostine administration.

## NURSING CONSIDERATIONS

• Use cautiously in elderly patients and in patients with ischemic heart disease, arrhythmias, heart failure, or history of stroke or transient ischemic attacks.
• Use cautiously in patients for whom common adverse effects of nausea, vomiting, and hypotension are likely to have serious consequences.
• If possible and if ordered, stop antihypertensive therapy 24 hours preceding amifostine administration.
• Patients receiving drug should be adequately hydrated before administration. Monitor patient's blood pressure before and immediately after infusion, and periodically thereafter as clinically indicated.
• Antiemetics, including dexamethasone 20 mg I.V. and a serotonin 5HT$_3$-receptor antagonist, should be given before, and with, amifostine administration. Additional antiemetics may be needed, based on chemotherapeutic drugs given.
• Monitor patient's fluid balance if drug is used with highly emetogenic chemotherapy.
• Monitor serum calcium level in patients at risk for hypocalcemia, such as those with nephrotic syndrome. If needed, administer calcium supplements, as ordered.
• Safety and effectiveness of drug in children haven't been established.

## ⬛I.V. administration

• Reconstitute each single-dose vial with 9.5 ml of sterile normal saline injection. Using other solutions to reconstitute drug isn't recommended. Reconstituted solution (500 mg amifostine/10 ml) is chemically stable for 5 hours at room temperature (about 77° F [25° C]) or 24 hours if refrigerated (35° to 46° F [2° to 8° C]).
• Drug can be prepared in polyvinyl chloride bags in concentrations of 5 to 40 mg/ml and has same stability as when drug is reconstituted in single-use vial.
• Inspect vial for particulates and discoloration before use; discard drug if cloudiness or precipitation exists.
• Keep patient supine during infusion. Monitor blood pressure every 5 minutes. If hypotension occurs and requires interrupting therapy, notify doctor and keep patient supine with legs elevated. Then give infusion of normal saline solution, as ordered, using a separate I.V. line. If blood pressure returns to normal within 5 minutes and patient is asymptomatic, infusion may be restarted so full dose of drug can be given. If full dose can't be given, limit subsequent doses to 740 mg/m$^2$.
• Don't infuse for over 15 minutes; longer infusion has been associated with higher risk of adverse reactions.

### ☑ Patient teaching

• Instruct patient to remain in a supine position throughout infusion.
• Advise patient not to breast-feed; it's unknown if drug or its metabolites appear in breast milk.

---

## aminoglutethimide
Cytadren, Orimeten§

*Pregnancy Risk Category D*

## HOW SUPPLIED

*Tablets:* 250 mg

## ACTION

Blocks conversion of cholesterol to delta-5-pregnenolone in the adrenal cortex, inhibiting synthesis of adrenal corticosteroids.

| Route | Onset | Peak | Duration |
|-------|-------|------|----------|
| P.O. | Unknown | 1.5 hr | 1.5-3 days |

---

## INDICATIONS & DOSAGE
*Suppression of adrenal function in Cushing's syndrome and adrenal cancer—*
**Adults:** 250 mg q.i.d. at 6-hour intervals. Dosage may be increased in increments of 250 mg daily q 1 to 2 weeks to maximum daily dose of 2 g.

## ADVERSE REACTIONS
**CNS:** *drowsiness,* headache, dizziness.
**CV:** hypotension, tachycardia.
**GI:** *nausea, anorexia,* vomiting.
**GU:** decreased urinary aldosterone levels.
**Hematologic:** transient *leukopenia, agranulocytosis, thrombocytopenia.*
**Hepatic:** increased serum alkaline phosphatase and AST levels.
**Metabolic:** adrenal insufficiency, masculinization, hypothyroidism, decreased plasma cortisol and serum thyroxine levels, increased thyroid-stimulating hormone levels.
**Musculoskeletal:** myalgia.
**Skin:** *morbilliform rash,* hirsutism, pruritus, urticaria.
**Other:** fever.

## INTERACTIONS
**Drug-drug.** *Dexamethasone, medroxyprogesterone:* increased hepatic metabolism of these drugs. Monitor patient closely.
*Oral anticoagulants:* decreased anticoagulant effect. Monitor PT and INR.
*Theophylline:* reduced action of theophylline. Monitor patient closely.
**Drug-lifestyle.** *Alcohol use:* may potentiate effects of aminoglutethimide. Avoid concomitant use.

## EFFECTS ON DIAGNOSTIC TESTS
None reported.

## CONTRAINDICATIONS
Contraindicated in patients with hypersensitivity to drug or to glutethimide.

## NURSING CONSIDERATIONS
• Perform baseline hematologic studies, as ordered.
• Monitor blood pressure frequently.
• Monitor CBC periodically.
• Drug may cause adrenal hypofunction, especially under stressful conditions, such

as surgery, trauma, or acute illness. Patients may need mineralocorticoid supplements to treat hyponatremia and orthostatic hypotension. Glucocorticoid replacement may also be needed, especially in patients with breast cancer. Monitor such patients carefully.
• Drug may cause decreased thyroid hormone production. Monitor thyroid function studies.
• *Alert:* Don't confuse Cytadren with cytarabine.

### ☑ Patient teaching
• Warn patient to watch for signs of infection (fever, sore throat, fatigue) and bleeding (easy bruising, nosebleeds, bleeding gums, melena). Patient should take his temperature daily.
• Warn patient to avoid activities that require alertness and good motor coordination until CNS effects of drug are known.
• Advise patient to stand up slowly to minimize orthostatic hypotension.
• Tell patient to report rash that persists for more than 8 days. Reassure patient that drowsiness, nausea, and loss of appetite usually diminish within 2 weeks after start of therapy, but advise him to notify doctor if these symptoms persist.
• Inform patient that masculinizing effects are reversible.

---

## anagrelide hydrochloride
Agrylin

*Pregnancy Risk Category C*

## HOW SUPPLIED
*Capsules:* 0.5 mg, 1 mg

## ACTION
Reduces platelet production, possibly by decreasing megakaryocyte hypermaturation.

| Route | Onset | Peak | Duration |
|-------|-------|------|----------|
| P.O. | Immediate | 1 hr | 48 hr |

## INDICATIONS & DOSAGE
*Essential thrombocythemia to reduce the elevated platelet count and risk of throm-*

*bosis and to ameliorate associated symptoms—*
**Adults:** 0.5 mg P.O. q.i.d. or 1 mg P.O. b.i.d. for at least 1 week; then adjust dosage to lowest effective dose needed to maintain platelet count below 600,000/mm$^3$, and ideally to normal range. Don't increase dose by more than 0.5 mg/day in any 1 week; don't exceed 10 mg/day or 2.5 mg in single dose.

## ADVERSE REACTIONS
**CNS:** amnesia, *asthenia,* confusion, depression, *dizziness, headache,* syncope, insomnia, migraine, nervousness, pain, paresthesia, malaise, somnolence.
**CV:** *arrhythmias,* angina, *CVA,* chest pain, CV disease, *heart failure, hemorrhage,* hypertension, *palpitations,* orthostatic hypotension, vasodilatation, tachycardia, *edema.*
**EENT:** abnormal vision, amblyopia, diplopia, epistaxis, rhinitis, sinusitis, tinnitus, visual field abnormality.
**GI:** *abdominal pain,* aphthous stomatitis, constipation, *diarrhea,* dyspepsia, anorexia, eructation, *flatulence,* GI distress, *GI hemorrhage,* gastritis, melena, *nausea,* vomiting.
**GU:** dysuria, hematuria.
**Hematologic:** anemia, ecchymosis, lymphadenoma, *thrombocytopenia.*
**Metabolic:** dehydration.
**Musculoskeletal:** arthralgia, back pain, leg cramps, myalgia, neck pain.
**Respiratory:** asthma, bronchitis, *dyspnea,* pneumonia, respiratory disease.
**Skin:** alopecia, photosensitivity, pruritus, rash, skin disease, urticaria.
**Other:** chills, fever, flulike symptoms.

## INTERACTIONS
**Drug-drug.** *Sucralfate:* may interfere with anagrelide absorption. Monitor closely.
**Drug-food.** *Any food:* may decrease bioavailability. Give drug 1 hour before or 2 hours after meals.

## EFFECTS ON DIAGNOSTIC TESTS
None reported.

## CONTRAINDICATIONS
No known contraindications.

## NURSING CONSIDERATIONS
• Use with caution in patients with CV disease because drug may cause vasodilation, tachycardia, palpitations, and heart failure.
• Use with caution in patients with serum creatinine level over 2 mg/dl and in those with liver function tests exceeding 1.5 times upper limit of normal.
• During first 2 weeks of treatment, monitor blood counts and liver and renal function test results.
• Because it isn't known if drug appears in breast milk, use caution when administering drug to breast-feeding women.

### ✅ Patient teaching
• Instruct patient to report increased bleeding, bruising, or cardiac symptoms.
• Instruct woman of childbearing age to use contraception during therapy.

---

## aprotinin
Trasylol

*Pregnancy Risk Category B*

## HOW SUPPLIED
*Injection:* 10,000 KIU (kallikrein inactivator units)/ml (1.4 mg/ml) in 100-ml and 200-ml vials

## ACTION
A naturally occurring protease inhibitor that acts as a systemic hemostatic, decreasing bleeding and turnover of coagulation factors. Inhibits fibrinolysis by affecting kallikrein and plasmin, prevents triggering of the contact phase of the coagulation pathway, and increases the resistance of platelets to damage from mechanical injury and high plasmin levels that occur during cardiopulmonary bypass.

| Route | Onset | Peak | Duration |
|-------|-------|------|----------|
| I.V. | Unknown | Unknown | Unknown |

## INDICATIONS & DOSAGE
*To reduce blood loss or the need for transfusion in patients undergoing coronary artery bypass grafts—*
**Adults:** initially 10,000 U (1 ml) I.V. test dose at least 10 minutes before loading dose. If no allergic reaction is evident,

---

anesthesia may be induced while loading dose of 2 million U is given I.V. slowly over 20 to 30 minutes. When loading dose is complete, sternotomy may be performed. Before bypass is initiated, cardiopulmonary bypass circuit is primed with 2 million U of drug by replacing an aliquot of priming fluid with drug. A continuous infusion at rate of 500,000 U/hour is then given I.V. until patient leaves operating room. This is known as regimen A. Or second regimen, known as regimen B, may be given, which is half the dosage of regimen A (except for test dose).

## ADVERSE REACTIONS
**CV:** *cardiac arrest, heart failure, ventricular tachycardia, MI, heart block, atrial fibrillation, atrial flutter,* hypotension, supraventricular tachycardia.
**GU:** elevated serum creatinine levels, *nephrotoxicity, renal failure.*
**Hepatic:** altered liver function test results.
**Respiratory:** pneumonia, respiratory disorder, apnea, asthma, dyspnea.
**Other:** *hypersensitivity reactions, anaphylaxis,* fever, *shock, sepsis.*

## INTERACTIONS
**Drug-drug.** *Captopril:* decreased hypotensive effects. Monitor patient closely.
*Fibrinolytic drugs:* inhibits effects of fibrinolytics. Avoid concomitant use.
*Heparin:* prolonged activated clotting time. Monitor clotting time and PTT.

## EFFECTS ON DIAGNOSTIC TESTS
Because aprotinin inhibits contact activation of the intrinsic clotting system, drug therapy prolongs results of coagulation assays that depend on contact activation, including PTT and celite activation clotting time assays. It may increase CK and transaminase levels and may falsely prolong whole blood clotting times when determined by surface activation methods such as the Hemochron method.

## CONTRAINDICATIONS
Contraindicated in patients with hypersensitivity to beef because drug is prepared from bovine lung.

## NURSING CONSIDERATIONS
• *Alert:* Use drug cautiously and monitor patients closely for hypersensitivity reaction. Patients may experience anaphylaxis after full therapeutic dose even if they remain asymptomatic after test dose. If symptoms of hypersensitivity occur (skin eruptions, itching, dyspnea, nausea, tachycardia), discontinue infusion immediately, notify doctor, and provide supportive treatment.
• Obtain history of possible allergies. Patients with history of allergies to drugs or other substances may be at higher risk for developing an allergic reaction to aprotinin.
• To avoid hypotension, make sure patient is supine when loading dose is given. Monitor blood pressure.
• Monitor laboratory studies, including liver function tests, as ordered.
• Monitor patient for increased serum creatinine levels and other signs of nephrotoxicity. If nephrotoxicity occurs, it's usually mild and reversible.
• Store drug between 36° and 77° F (2° and 25° C). Protect drug from freezing.

### I.V. administration
• Drug is incompatible with amino acids, corticosteroids, fat emulsions, heparin, and tetracyclines. Don't add other drugs to I.V. container and use separate I.V. line.
• Be prepared to administer test dose. Test dose is particularly important in patients who have previously received drug because they have a higher risk of anaphylaxis. In such patients, pretreat with an antihistamine, as ordered.
• Administer all doses through a central line.

### Patient teaching
• Explain use and administration of drug to patient and family.
• Reassure patient and family that he will be monitored continuously throughout drug administration for adverse reactions.

---

## becaplermin
Regranex Gel

*Pregnancy Risk Category C*

### HOW SUPPLIED
*Gel:* 100 mcg/g in tubes of 2 g, 7.5 g, 15 g

### ACTION
Thought to promote chemotactic recruitment and proliferation of cells involved in wound repair and formation of new granulation tissue.

| Route | Onset | Peak | Duration |
|---|---|---|---|
| Topical | Unknown | Unknown | Unknown |

### INDICATIONS & DOSAGE
*Lower extremity diabetic neuropathic ulcers that extend into the subcutaneous tissue or beyond and have adequate blood supply—*
**Adults:** apply daily in ⅟₁₆-inch even thickness to entire surface of wound. The following table shows the length of gel to apply in inches (or centimeters) based on tube size and wound size.

| Tube size | (inches) | (cm) |
|---|---|---|
| 2 g | Ulcer length × ulcer width × 1.3 | (Ulcer length × ulcer width) ÷ 2 |
| 7.5, 15 g | Ulcer length × ulcer width × 0.6 | (Ulcer length × ulcer width) ÷ 4 |

### ADVERSE REACTIONS
**Musculoskeletal:** osteomyelitis.
**Skin:** erythematous rash.
**Other:** cellulitis, infection.

### INTERACTIONS
None significant.

### EFFECTS ON DIAGNOSTIC TESTS
None reported.

### CONTRAINDICATIONS
Contraindicated in patients with hypersensitivity to drug or its components (such as parabens or m-cresol) and in those with known neoplasms at application site.

### NURSING CONSIDERATIONS
• Use cautiously in breast-feeding women.
• *Alert:* Don't use drug in wounds that close by primary intention.
• Drug facilitates complete healing of diabetic ulcers when used as an adjunct to good ulcer care practices, which include initial sharp débridement, infection control, and pressure relief.
• Treatment efficacy hasn't been evaluated for diabetic neuropathic ulcers that don't extend through the dermis into subcutaneous tissue or for ischemic diabetic ulcers.
• To apply drug, calculate length of gel by measuring ulcer's greatest length and width, and use dosage formula. Squeeze calculated length of gel to apply onto clean measuring surface such as waxed paper. Use cotton swab or other application aid to transfer and spread drug over entire ulcer area in a ⅟₁₆-inch thick continuous layer. Place a saline-moistened dressing over site and leave in place for about 12 hours. After 12 hours, remove dressing and rinse away residual gel with normal saline or water, and apply a fresh moist dressing, without becaplermin, for rest of day.
• Monitor wound size and healing; recalculate amount of drug to be applied at least once weekly. If ulcer doesn't decrease in size by about one-third after 10 weeks, or if complete healing hasn't occurred within 20 weeks, treatment should be reassessed.
• Watch for application site reactions. Sensitization, or irritation caused by parabens or m-cresol, should be considered.
• Drug is for external use only.
• Safety and effectiveness of drug in children under age 16 haven't been established.

### ✓ Patient teaching
• Instruct patient to wash hands thoroughly before applying gel.
• Advise patient not to touch tip of tube against ulcer or any other surfaces.
• Instruct patient on proper procedure for wound care, including applying gel and changing dressings.

---

Reactions may be *common*, uncommon, *life-threatening*, or COMMON AND LIFE-THREATENING.

• Stress need to keep area covered with a wet dressing at all times.
• Tell patient to store drug in refrigerator (36° to 46° F [2° to 8° C]).
• Instruct patient not to use drug after expiration date.

---

## calcipotriene
Dovonex

*Pregnancy Risk Category C*

---

### HOW SUPPLIED
*Ointment:* 0.005%
*Cream:* 0.005%
*Solution:* 0.005%

### ACTION
A synthetic vitamin $D_3$ analogue that regulates the development and production of skin cells.

| Route | Onset | Peak | Duration |
|-------|-------|------|----------|
| Topical | Unknown | Unknown | Unknown |

### INDICATIONS & DOSAGE
*Moderate plaque psoriasis—*
**Adults:** apply thin layer to affected area b.i.d. Rub in gently and completely.

### ADVERSE REACTIONS
**Metabolic:** hypercalcemia.
**Skin:** *burning, pruritus, irritation,* atrophy, dermatitis, dry skin, erythema, folliculitis, hyperpigmentation, peeling, rash, worsening of psoriasis.

### INTERACTIONS
None significant.

### EFFECTS ON DIAGNOSTIC TESTS
None reported.

### CONTRAINDICATIONS
Contraindicated in patients with hypersensitivity to drug or its components and in those with hypercalcemia or evidence of vitamin D toxicity. Also contraindicated for use on the face.

### NURSING CONSIDERATIONS
• Use cautiously in breast-feeding women.

• Use cautiously in elderly patients; they may experience more severe adverse skin reactions.

### ☑ Patient teaching
• Advise patient to apply only thin layer of ointment. Transient elevations of serum calcium level can occur, especially when applied excessively.
• Advise patient not to use drug on face, in eyes, orally, or vaginally. Tell him to wash his hands after applying ointment.
• Tell patient to discontinue drug and call doctor if drug irritates lesions or surrounding, uninvolved skin.

---

## capsaicin
Axsain ◇ , Capzacin-P, Dolorac ◇ , Zostrix ◇ , Zostrix-HP ◇

*Pregnancy Risk Category NR*

---

### HOW SUPPLIED
*Cream:* 0.025% (Zostrix), 0.075% (Axsain), 0.25% (Dolorac)

### ACTION
Unknown. May increase release of substance P, a principal neurotransmitter for pain, from peripheral type C sensory fibers to central neurons.

| Route | Onset | Peak | Duration |
|-------|-------|------|----------|
| Topical | Unknown | Unknown | Unknown |

### INDICATIONS & DOSAGE
*Temporary relief from pain after herpes zoster infections; neuralgias, such as postoperative pain and painful diabetic neuropathy; pain associated with osteoarthritis or rheumatoid arthritis—*
**Adults and children over age 2:** apply to affected areas not more than q.i.d.
*Temporary relief from arthritis pain (Dolorac)—*
**Adults and children ages 12 and older:** apply thin film to affected area b.i.d.

### ADVERSE REACTIONS
**Respiratory:** cough, irritation.
**Skin:** redness, *stinging or burning on application.*

---

**INTERACTIONS**
None significant.

**EFFECTS ON DIAGNOSTIC TESTS**
None reported.

**CONTRAINDICATIONS**
Contraindicated in patients with hypersensitivity to drug.

**NURSING CONSIDERATIONS**
• Drug is for external use only.

☑ **Patient teaching**
• Warn patient to avoid getting drug in eyes or on broken skin.
• Advise patient not to bandage area tightly after applying drug.
• Tell patient to wash hands after applying drug.
• Inform patient that transient burning or stinging is usually evident at initial therapy but decreases with cautious use. This effect persists in patients who use drug less often than t.i.d.
• Tell patient who is self-medicating with capsaicin to contact doctor if symptoms persist beyond 2 to 4 weeks or resolve and shortly reappear.

---

**cisapride**
Propulsid

*Pregnancy Risk Category C*

**HOW SUPPLIED**
*Tablets:* 10 mg, 20 mg
*Suspension:* 1 mg/ml

**ACTION**
Stimulates serotonin-4 (5-HT$_4$) receptors, enhancing release of acetylcholine at the myenteric plexus and increasing GI motility.

| Route | Onset | Peak | Duration |
|-------|-------|------|----------|
| P.O. | 30-60 min | 1-2 hr | Unknown |

**INDICATIONS & DOSAGE**
*Symptoms of nocturnal heartburn due to gastroesophageal reflux disease that doesn't respond adequately to lifestyle*
modifications, antacids, and gastric acid–reducing drugs—
**Adults:** initially, 10 mg P.O. q.i.d. 15 minutes before meals and h.s. If response is inadequate, increase to 20 mg q.i.d.

**ADVERSE REACTIONS**
**CNS:** *headache,* insomnia, anxiety, nervousness.
**CV:** QT-interval prolongation.
**EENT:** rhinitis, sinusitis, abnormal vision.
**GI:** *diarrhea, abdominal pain,* nausea, constipation, flatulence, dyspepsia.
**GU:** frequency, urinary tract infection, vaginitis.
**Musculoskeletal:** arthralgia.
**Respiratory:** cough, upper respiratory tract infections.
**Skin:** rash, pruritus.
**Other:** pain, fever, viral infections.

**INTERACTIONS**
**Drug-drug.** *Antiarrhythmics (classes IA and III), bepridil, phenothiazines, sertindole, sparfloxacin, terodiline, tetracyclic antidepressants, tricyclic antidepressants:* increased likelihood of QT interval prolongation. Avoid concomitant use.
*Anticholinergics:* decreased effectiveness of cisapride. Avoid concomitant use.
*Anticoagulants:* may increase clotting times. Monitor closely.
*Benzodiazepines:* enhanced sedation. Avoid concomitant use.
*Cimetidine:* increased absorption of these drugs; cimetidine increases cisapride levels. Use together cautiously.
*Clarithromycin, erythromycin, fluconazole, indinavir, itraconazole, ketoconazole, miconazole, nefazodone, ritonavir, troleandomycin:* increased cisapride levels, which may cause ventricular arrhythmias. Concomitant use is contraindicated.
**Drug-lifestyle.** *Alcohol use:* enhanced sedation. Avoid concomitant use.

**EFFECTS ON DIAGNOSTIC TESTS**
None reported.

**CONTRAINDICATIONS**
Contraindicated in patients with hypersensitivity to drug and in those with history of prolonged QT intervals, ventricular

---

arrhythmia, ischemic heart disease, heart failure, renal failure, respiratory failure, and uncorrected electrolyte disorders, such as hypokalemia or hypomagnesemia. Also contraindicated in patients for whom increased GI motility may be harmful, such as those with mechanical obstruction, hemorrhage, or perforation of GI tract. Administration with macrolides, antifungals, protease inhibitors, and nefazodone is contraindicated.

### NURSING CONSIDERATIONS
• *Alert:* Before use, confirm with patient, pharmacist, and doctor that patient isn't taking other drugs that may interfere with cisapride metabolism. Serious ventricular arrhythmias may result.
• Use cautiously in breast-feeding women because small amounts of drug appear in breast milk.
• Consider ECG before initiation of cisapride.
• Protect 20-mg tablets from light; protect all products from moisture. Store at room temperature.

### ☑ Patient teaching
• Remind patient to avoid alcohol and sedatives during therapy.
• Advise patient to immediately report adverse effects.
• Tell patient to consult doctor or pharmacist before taking OTC products.

---

## clomiphene citrate
Clomid, Milophene, Serophene

*Pregnancy Risk Category X*

### HOW SUPPLIED
*Tablets:* 50 mg

### ACTION
Unknown. Appears to stimulate release of follicle-stimulating hormone, luteinizing hormone, and pituitary gonadotropins, resulting in maturation of the ovarian follicle, ovulation, and development of the corpus luteum.

| Route | Onset | Peak | Duration |
|-------|-------|------|----------|
| P.O. | Unknown | Unknown | Unknown |

### INDICATIONS & DOSAGE
*To induce ovulation—*
**Adults:** 50 mg P.O. daily for 5 days starting on day 5 of menstrual cycle (first day of menstrual flow is day 1) if bleeding occurs, or at any time if patient hasn't had recent uterine bleeding. If ovulation doesn't occur, may increase dose to 100 mg P.O. daily for 5 days as soon as 30 days after previous course. Repeated until conception occurs or until three courses of therapy are completed.

### ADVERSE REACTIONS
**CNS:** headache, restlessness, insomnia, dizziness, light-headedness, depression, fatigue.
**EENT:** blurred vision, diplopia, scotoma, photophobia.
**GI:** nausea, vomiting, bloating, distention.
**GU:** urinary frequency and polyuria; abnormal uterine bleeding; *ovarian enlargement,* cyst formation that regresses spontaneously when drug is stopped; *breast discomfort.*
**Metabolic:** weight gain.
**Skin:** reversible alopecia, urticaria, rash, dermatitis.
**Other:** *hot flashes.*

### INTERACTIONS
None significant.

### EFFECTS ON DIAGNOSTIC TESTS
Drug therapy may increase levels of serum thyronine, thyroxine-binding globulin, and sex hormone-binding globulin. It may also increase sulfobromophthalein retention and follicle-stimulating hormone and luteinizing hormone secretion.

### CONTRAINDICATIONS
Contraindicated during pregnancy and in patients with undiagnosed abnormal genital bleeding, ovarian cyst not due to polycystic ovarian syndrome, hepatic disease or dysfunction, uncontrolled thyroid or adrenal dysfunction, or presence of organic intracranial lesion (such as a pituitary tumor). Also contraindicated in patients with liver disease.

---

*Liquid contains alcohol.   **May contain tartrazine.   †Canada   ‡Australia   §U.K.   ◇OTC

## NURSING CONSIDERATIONS
• Monitor patient closely because of potentially serious adverse reactions.
• *Alert:* Don't confuse clomiphene with clomipramine or clonidine.

### ✅ Patient teaching
• Tell patient that risk of multiple births exists, which increases with higher doses.
• Teach patient to take and chart basal body temperature to ascertain if ovulation has occurred.
• Reassure patient that ovulation generally occurs after first course of therapy. If pregnancy doesn't occur, therapy may be repeated twice.
• Advise patient to stop drug and contact doctor immediately if pregnancy is suspected because drug may have teratogenic effect.
• *Alert:* Advise patient to stop drug and contact doctor immediately if abdominal symptoms or pain occur; these symptoms may indicate ovarian enlargement or ovarian cyst. Also tell patient to immediately notify doctor if signs and symptoms of impending visual toxicity occur, such as blurred vision, diplopia, scotoma, or photophobia.
• Warn patient to avoid hazardous activities, such as driving or operating machinery, until CNS effects are known. Drug may cause dizziness or visual disturbances.

---

## etanercept
Enbrel

*Pregnancy Risk Category B*

---

## HOW SUPPLIED
*Injection:* 25-mg single-use vial

## ACTION
Binds specifically to tumor necrosis factor (TNF) and blocks its action with cell surface TNF receptors, reducing inflammatory and immune responses found in rheumatoid arthritis.

| Route | Onset | Peak | Duration |
|-------|-------|------|----------|
| S.C. | Unknown | 72 hr | Unknown |

## INDICATIONS & DOSAGE
*Reduction in signs and symptoms of moderately to severely active rheumatoid arthritis in patients who demonstrate inadequate response to one or more disease-modifying antirheumatic drugs with methotrexate and who don't respond adequately to methotrexate alone—*
**Adults:** 25 mg S.C. twice weekly, 72 to 96 hours apart.
✳ *NEW INDICATION: Reduction in signs and symptoms of moderately to severely active polyarticular-course juvenile rheumatoid arthritis in patients who have had an inadequate response to one or more disease-modifying antirheumatic drugs—*
**Children ages 4 to 17:** 0.4 mg/kg (up to maximum of 25 mg per dose) S.C. twice weekly, 72 to 96 hours apart.

## ADVERSE REACTIONS
**CNS:** asthenia, *headache,* dizziness.
**EENT:** *rhinitis,* pharyngitis, sinusitis.
**GI:** abdominal pain, dyspepsia.
**Respiratory:** *upper respiratory tract infections,* cough, respiratory disorder.
**Skin:** *injection site reaction,* rash.
**Other:** *infections,* malignancies.

## INTERACTIONS
None significant.

## EFFECTS ON DIAGNOSTIC TESTS
None reported.

## CONTRAINDICATIONS
Contraindicated in patients with hypersensitivity to drug or its components and in those with sepsis.

## NURSING CONSIDERATIONS
• *Alert:* Anti-TNF therapies, including etanercept, may affect defenses against infection. Notify doctor and discontinue therapy, as ordered, if serious infection occurs.
• *Alert:* Drug is for S.C. injection only.
• *Alert:* Don't give live vaccines concurrently during therapy.
• Patients with juvenile rheumatoid arthritis should, if possible, be brought up-to-date with all immunizations in compliance with current immunization guidelines before initiating treatment.

---

Reactions may be *common,* uncommon, ***life-threatening,*** or COMMON AND LIFE-THREATENING.

• Reconstitute aseptically with 1 ml of supplied sterile bacteriostatic water for injection, USP (0.9% benzyl alcohol). Don't filter reconstituted solution during preparation or administration. Inject diluent slowly into vial. Minimize foaming by gently swirling during dissolution rather than shaking. Dissolution takes less than 5 minutes.

• Visually inspect solution for particulates and discoloration before use. Reconstituted solution should be clear and colorless. Don't use solution if it's discolored, cloudy, or if particulates exist.

• Don't add other drugs or diluents to reconstituted solution.

• Use reconstituted solution as soon as possible; may be refrigerated in vial for up to 6 hours at 36° to 46° F (2° to 8° C).

• Injection sites should be at least 1 inch apart; areas where skin is tender, bruised, red, or hard should never be used. Recommended sites include the thigh, abdomen, and upper arm. Rotate sites regularly.

• Patient may develop positive antinuclear antibody or positive anti-double-stranded DNA antibodies measured by radioimmunoassay and *Crithidia luciDae* assay.

• Drug isn't recommended for use in children under age 4.

• Needle cover of diluent syringe contains dry natural rubber (latex) and shouldn't be handled by persons sensitive to latex.

### ☑Patient teaching

• If patient will be self-administering, advise him about mixing and injection techniques, including rotation of injection sites.

• Instruct patient to use puncture-resistant container for disposal of needles and syringes.

• Tell patient that injection site reactions generally occur within first month of therapy and decrease thereafter.

• Inform patient of importance of avoiding live vaccine administration during therapy. Stress importance of alerting doctor or other health care providers of etanercept use.

• Instruct patient to promptly report signs and symptoms of infection to doctor.

• Advise breast-feeding woman to discontinue breast-feeding during therapy.

## finasteride
Propecia, Proscar

*Pregnancy Risk Category X*

### HOW SUPPLIED
*Tablets:* 1 mg, 5 mg

### ACTION
Competitively inhibits corticosteroid 5 alpha-reductase, an enzyme responsible for formation of potent androgen 5 alpha-dihydrotestosterone (DHT) from testosterone. Because DHT influences development of the prostate gland, decreasing levels of this hormone in adult men should relieve the symptoms associated with BPH. In male pattern balding, the balding scalp contains miniaturized hair follicles and increased amounts of DHT. Finasteride decreases scalp and serum DHT levels in such cases.

| Route | Onset | Peak | Duration |
|-------|-------|------|----------|
| P.O. | Unknown | 1-2 hr | 24 hr |

### INDICATIONS & DOSAGE
**Propecia**
*Male pattern hair loss (androgenetic alopecia) in men only—*
**Adults:** 1 mg P.O. daily.
**Proscar**
*Symptomatic BPH to improve symptoms and reduce risk of acute urine retention and need for surgery, including transurethral resection of prostate and prostatectomy—*
**Adults:** 5 mg P.O. daily.

### ADVERSE REACTIONS
**GU:** decreased libido, impotence, decreased volume of ejaculate.

### INTERACTIONS
None significant.

### EFFECTS ON DIAGNOSTIC TESTS
None reported.

### CONTRAINDICATIONS
Contraindicated in patients with hypersensitivity to drug. Although drug isn't

---

*Liquid contains alcohol.   **May contain tartrazine.   †Canada   ‡Australia   §U.K.   ◇OTC

used in women or children, manufacturer indicates pregnancy as a contraindication.

## NURSING CONSIDERATIONS
• Before therapy, patient should be evaluated for conditions that mimic BPH, including hypotonic bladder; prostate cancer, infection, or stricture; or relevant neurologic conditions.
• Carefully monitor patients who have a large residual urine volume or severely diminished urine flow; these patients may not be candidates for drug therapy.
• Carefully evaluate sustained increases in serum prostate-specific antigen levels, which could indicate noncompliance with therapy.
• Although drug's elimination rate is decreased in elderly patients, dosage adjustments aren't needed.
• Because it's impossible to identify which patients will respond to finasteride, minimum of 6 months of therapy may be needed.
• Long-term effects on complications of BPH, including acute urinary obstruction and risk of surgery, are unknown.

✓ **Patient teaching**
• Warn woman who is or may become pregnant not to handle crushed tablets because of risk of adverse effects on male fetus.
• Inform patient that 3 months or more of daily use is generally needed to see benefits when drug is used to treat hair loss.
• Tell patient to anticipate baseline and periodic digital rectal examinations.
• Reassure patient that drug may decrease volume of ejaculate but doesn't appear to impair normal sexual function. Impotence and decreased libido have occurred in less than 4% of patients.

---

**imiglucerase**
Cerezyme

*Pregnancy Risk Category C*

## HOW SUPPLIED
*Injection:* 200 U/vial

## ACTION
Catalyzes the hydrolysis of glucocerebroside to glucose and ceramide (part of the normal degradation pathway for lipids) and thus prevents the sequelae of Gaucher's disease, which normally occur as a result of the accumulation of glucocerebroside.

| Route | Onset | Peak | Duration |
|-------|-------|------|----------|
| I.V. | Unknown | 1 hr | Unknown |

## INDICATIONS & DOSAGE
*Long-term endogenous enzyme (glucosylceramidase) replacement therapy in confirmed type I Gaucher's disease—*
**Adults and children:** dosage individualized; initially, 2.5 to 60 U/kg I.V. administered over 1 to 2 hours. Frequency of dosing typically is once q 2 weeks, but may range from three times weekly to once monthly, based on severity of disease. Dosage may be reduced for maintenance therapy, at intervals of 3 to 6 months, while response parameters are carefully monitored.

## ADVERSE REACTIONS
**CNS:** headache, dizziness.
**CV:** mild hypotension.
**GI:** nausea, abdominal discomfort.
**GU:** decreased urinary frequency.
**Skin:** pruritus, rash.
**Other:** *hypersensitivity reactions.*

## INTERACTIONS
None significant.

## EFFECTS ON DIAGNOSTIC TESTS
None reported.

## CONTRAINDICATIONS
Contraindicated in patients with hypersensitivity to drug.

## NURSING CONSIDERATIONS
• Use with caution in patients who have previously been treated with drug and who have developed antibody to drug or have exhibited symptoms of hypersensitivity to drug.
• Monitor response parameters so that doctor can determine lowest effective dosage.

---

Reactions may be *common,* uncommon, *life-threatening,* or COMMON AND LIFE-THREATENING.

### I.V. administration
• Reconstitute drug in each vial with 5.1 ml of sterile water for injection USP. Inspect solution for particulates and discoloration before use; if either is present, don't use. Withdraw 5 ml (amount in vial after reconstitution is 5.3 ml) of reconstituted solution and dilute solution further with normal saline solution to final volume of 100 to 200 ml. Because drug is preservative-free, use immediately. Administer by I.V. infusion over 1 to 2 hours.
• When diluted to 50 ml, drug has been shown to be stable for up to 24 hours when stored at 36° to 46° F (2° to 8° C).

### ✅ Patient teaching
• Explain use and administration of drug to patient and family. Stress importance of compliance with administration schedule.
• Tell patient to report persistent or severe adverse reactions promptly.

---

## imiquimod
Aldara

*Pregnancy Risk Category B*

### HOW SUPPLIED
*Cream:* 5% in single-use packets containing 250 mg

### ACTION
Exact mechanism unknown. An immune response modifier; has no direct antiviral activity.

| Route | Onset | Peak | Duration |
|-------|-------|------|----------|
| Topical | Unknown | Unknown | Unknown |

### INDICATIONS & DOSAGE
*External genital and perianal warts—*
**Adults:** apply thin layer to affected area three times weekly before normal sleeping hours. Continue treatment until there is total clearance of the genital or perianal warts or for maximum of 16 weeks.

### ADVERSE REACTIONS
**CNS:** headache.
**Musculoskeletal:** myalgia.

**Skin:** local itching, burning, pain, soreness, erythema, ulceration, edema, erosion, induration, flaking, excoriation.
**Other:** flulike symptoms.

### INTERACTIONS
None significant.

### EFFECTS ON DIAGNOSTIC TESTS
None reported.

### CONTRAINDICATIONS
No known contraindications.

### NURSING CONSIDERATIONS
• Safety of drug in breast-feeding women is unknown.
• Safety and efficacy of drug in patients under age 18 haven't been established.
• Drug isn't recommended for treatment of urethral, intravaginal, cervical, rectal, or intra-anal human papilloma viral disease.
• Don't use until genital or perianal tissue is healed from previous drug or surgical treatment.
• Patient usually experiences local skin reactions at site of application or surrounding areas. Use nonocclusive dressings, such as cotton gauze, or cotton undergarments in management of skin reactions. Patient's discomfort or severity of the local skin reaction may require a rest period of several days. Resume treatment once reaction subsides.
• Drug isn't a cure; new warts may develop during therapy.

### ✅ Patient teaching
• Advise patient that effect of cream on transmission of genital or perianal warts is unknown. New warts may develop during therapy; drug isn't a cure.
• Tell patient to use cream only as directed and to avoid contact with eyes.
• Tell patient to wash hands before and after applying cream.
• Advise patient to apply cream in thin layer over affected area and rub in until cream isn't visible. Advise patient to avoid excessive use of cream. Tell patient not to occlude area after applying cream and to wash with mild soap and water 6 to 10 hours following application of cream.

---

• Advise patient that mild local skin reactions, such as erythema, erosion, excoriation, flaking, and edema at site of application or surrounding areas, are common. Tell patient that most skin reactions are mild to moderate. Advise him to report severe skin reactions promptly.

• Instruct uncircumcised man being treated for warts under the foreskin to retract foreskin and clean area daily.

• Advise patient that drug can weaken condoms and vaginal diaphragms and that concomitant use isn't recommended.

• Advise patient to avoid sexual contact while cream is on the skin.

• Tell patient to store drug at temperatures below 86° F (30° C) and to avoid freezing.

---

## infliximab
### Remicade

*Pregnancy Risk Category C*

### HOW SUPPLIED
*Injection:* 100-mg vial

### ACTION
A monoclonal antibody that binds to human tumor necrosis factor (TNF)-alpha to neutralize its activity and inhibit its binding with receptors, thereby reducing the infiltration of inflammatory cells and TNF-alpha production in inflamed areas of the intestine.

| Route | Onset | Peak | Duration |
|-------|-------|------|----------|
| I.V. | Unknown | Unknown | Unknown |

### INDICATIONS & DOSAGE
*Reduction of signs and symptoms in patients with moderately to severely active Crohn's disease with inadequate response to conventional therapy—*
**Adults:** 5 mg/kg single I.V. infusion over not less than 2 hours.
*Reduction in number of draining enterocutaneous fistulas in patients with fistulizing Crohn's disease—*
**Adults:** 5 mg/kg I.V. infused over not less than 2 hours. Additional doses of 5 mg/kg should be given at 2 and 6 weeks after initial infusion.

### ADVERSE REACTIONS
**CNS:** *headache, fatigue,* dizziness, malaise, insomnia.
**CV:** hypertension, hypotension, tachycardia, chest pain, flushing.
**EENT:** pharyngitis, rhinitis, sinusitis, conjunctivitis, toothache.
**GI:** *nausea, abdominal pain,* vomiting, constipation, dyspepsia, flatulence, intestinal obstruction, oral pain, ulcerative stomatitis.
**GU:** dysuria, increased micturition frequency.
**Hematologic:** anemia, hematoma.
**Hepatic:** elevated liver enzyme levels.
**Musculoskeletal:** myalgia, arthralgia, arthritis, back pain.
**Respiratory:** *upper respiratory tract infections,* bronchitis, coughing, dyspnea, flu syndrome, respiratory tract allergic reaction.
**Skin:** rash, pruritus, candidiasis, acne, alopecia, eczema, erythema, erythematous rash, maculopapular rash, papular rash, dry skin, increased sweating, urticaria.
**Other:** ecchymosis, *fever,* chills, pain, peripheral edema, hot flashes, abscess.

### INTERACTIONS
None significant.

### EFFECTS ON DIAGNOSTIC TESTS
None reported.

### CONTRAINDICATIONS
Contraindicated in patients with hypersensitivity to murine proteins or other components of drug.

### NURSING CONSIDERATIONS
• Use cautiously in elderly patients.
• *Alert:* Watch for infusion-related reactions, including fever, chills, pruritus, urticaria, dyspnea, hypotension, hypertension, and chest pain, during administration and for 2 hours following completion. If an infusion-reaction occurs, discontinue drug, notify doctor, and be prepared to give acetaminophen, antihistamines, corticosteroids, and epinephrine, as ordered.
• Watch for development of lymphomas and infection. Patients with chronic

---

Reactions may be *common,* uncommon, ***life-threatening,*** or COMMON AND LIFE-THREATENING.

Crohn's disease and long-term exposure to immunosuppressants are more likely to develop lymphomas and infections.
• Drug may affect normal immune responses. Patient may develop autoimmune antibodies and lupus-like syndrome; drug should be discontinued. Symptoms can be expected to resolve.
• Some patients test positive for antinuclear antibodies. Some have developed a lupus-like syndrome that resolved after drug was discontinued.

**I.V. administration**
• Drug is incompatible with plasticized polyvinyl chloride equipment or devices; prepare only in glass infusion bottles or polypropylene or polyolefin infusion bags. Administer through polyethylene-lined administration sets with an in-line, sterile, nonpyrogenic, low-protein-binding filter (pore size of 1.2 mm or less).
• Vials don't contain antibacterial preservatives; use reconstituted drug immediately. Reconstitute with 10 ml sterile water for injection, using syringe with 21G or smaller needle. Don't shake; gently swirl to dissolve powder. Solution should be colorless to light yellow and opalescent, and may develop a few translucent particles. Don't use if other particles or discoloration exists.
• Dilute total volume of reconstituted drug to 250 ml with normal saline injection. Infusion concentration range is 0.4 to 4 mg/ml. Infusion should begin within 3 hours of preparation and must be administered over not less than 2 hours.
• Don't infuse drug in same I.V. line with other drugs.

**Patient teaching**
• Tell patient about infusion-reaction symptoms and instruct him to report them.
• Inform patient of postinfusion adverse effects and instruct him to report them promptly.
• Inform breast-feeding woman to stop breast-feeding if drug is to be administered.

# isotretinoin
Accutane, Roaccutane‡

*Pregnancy Risk Category X*

## HOW SUPPLIED
*Capsules:* 10 mg, 20 mg, 40 mg

## ACTION
Unknown. Thought to normalize keratinization, reversibly decrease size of sebaceous glands, and alter composition of sebum to a less viscous form that is less likely to cause follicular plugging.

| Route | Onset | Peak | Duration |
|-------|-------|------|----------|
| P.O. | Unknown | 3 hr | Unknown |

## INDICATIONS & DOSAGE
*Severe recalcitrant nodular acne unresponsive to conventional therapy—*
**Adults and adolescents:** 0.5 to 2 mg/kg P.O. daily in two divided doses for 15 to 20 weeks.

## ADVERSE REACTIONS
**CNS:** headache, fatigue, *pseudotumor cerebri.*
**EENT:** *conjunctivitis,* corneal deposits, dry eyes, visual disturbances, *epistaxis, dry nose.*
**GI:** nonspecific GI symptoms, *nausea, vomiting,* anorexia, *abdominal pain, dry mouth,* gum bleeding and inflammation.
**Hematologic:** anemia, elevated platelet count.
**Hepatic:** elevated AST, ALT, and alkaline phosphatase levels.
**Metabolic:** *hypertriglyceridemia,* hyperglycemia, altered uric acid levels.
**Musculoskeletal:** *musculoskeletal pain.*
**Skin:** *cheilosis, rash, dry skin, facial skin desquamation,* peeling of palms and toes, *petechiae, nail brittleness,* thinning of hair, skin infection, photosensitivity, *cheilitis, pruritus, fragility.*
**Other:** *drying of mucous membranes.*

## INTERACTIONS
**Drug-drug.** *Carbamazepine:* decreased carbamazepine levels. Monitor levels.
*Tetracyclines:* increased risk of pseudotumor cerebri. Avoid concomitant use.

---

*Liquid contains alcohol.    **May contain tartrazine.    †Canada    ‡Australia    §U.K.    ◇OTC

*Vitamin A, products containing vitamin A:* increased toxic effects of isotretinoin. Don't use together without doctor's permission.

**Drug-food.** *Any food:* enhanced absorption of drug. Administer drug with milk, a meal, or shortly after a meal.

**Drug-lifestyle.** *Alcohol use:* increased risk of hypertriglyceridemia. Avoid concomitant use.

*Sun exposure:* increased photosensitivity reactions. Avoid prolonged or unprotected exposure to sun.

**EFFECTS ON DIAGNOSTIC TESTS**
None reported.

**CONTRAINDICATIONS**
Contraindicated in patients with hypersensitivity to parabens, which are used as preservatives, vitamin A, or other retinoids. Also contraindicated in woman of childbearing age unless patient has had a negative serum pregnancy test within 2 weeks before beginning therapy, will begin drug therapy on second or third day of next menstrual period, and will comply with stringent contraceptive measures for 1 month before therapy, during therapy, and for at least 1 month after therapy.

**NURSING CONSIDERATIONS**
• Monitor baseline serum lipid studies and liver function tests before therapy and at regular intervals.
• Monitor blood glucose level regularly and CK levels in patients who participate in vigorous physical activity, as ordered.
• Most adverse reactions appear to be dose-related, occurring at doses exceeding 1 mg/kg daily. Reactions are generally reversible when therapy is discontinued or dosage is reduced.
• *Alert:* Patient who experiences headache, nausea and vomiting, or visual disturbances should be screened for papilledema. Signs and symptoms of pseudotumor cerebri require immediate discontinuation of drug and prompt neurologic intervention.
• *Alert:* Severe fetal abnormalities may occur if drug is used during pregnancy.
• Anticipate a second course of therapy, if needed, not to start for at least 8 weeks after completion of first course because improvement may continue after withdrawal of drug.

✅ **Patient teaching**
• Advise patient to take drug with or shortly after meals to facilitate absorption.
• Tell patient to immediately report visual disturbances and bone, muscle, or joint pain.
• Warn patient that contact lenses may feel uncomfortable during therapy.
• Warn patient against using abrasives, medicated soaps and cleansers, acne preparations containing peeling drugs, and topical alcohol products (including cosmetics, aftershave, cologne) because these products cause cumulative irritation or excessive drying of skin.
• Tell patient to avoid prolonged sun exposure and to use sunblock. Drug may have additive effect if used with other drugs that cause photosensitivity.
• Advise patient of childbearing age to use two reliable forms of contraception simultaneously, unless abstinence is chosen method of birth control, for 1 month before, during, and 1 month after treatment.
• Advise patient not to donate blood during or for 30 days after therapy; severe fetal abnormalities may occur if a pregnant woman receives blood containing isotretinoin.

---

# leflunomide
## Arava

*Pregnancy Risk Category X*

---

**HOW SUPPLIED**
*Tablets:* 10 mg, 20 mg, 100 mg

**ACTION**
An immunomodulatory drug that inhibits dihydroorotate dehydrogenase, an enzyme involved in pyrimidine synthesis, and has antiproliferative activity and anti-inflammatory effects.

| Route | Onset | Peak | Duration |
|-------|-------|------|----------|
| P.O. | Unknown | 6-12 hr | Unknown |

---

Reactions may be *common*, uncommon, ***life-threatening***, or **COMMON AND LIFE-THREATENING**.

## INDICATIONS & DOSAGE

*Active rheumatoid arthritis to reduce signs and symptoms and to retard structural damage as evidenced by X-ray erosions and joint space narrowing—*
**Adults:** 100 mg P.O. q 24 hours for 3 days; then 20 mg (maximum daily dose) P.O. q 24 hours. Dose may be decreased to 10 mg daily if higher dose isn't well-tolerated.

## ADVERSE REACTIONS

**CNS:** asthenia, dizziness, headache, paresthesia, malaise, migraine, sleep disorder, vertigo, neuritis, anxiety, depression, insomnia, neuralgia.
**CV:** angina pectoris, *hypertension,* chest pain, palpitation, tachycardia, vasculitis, vasodilation, varicose vein, peripheral edema.
**EENT:** pharyngitis, rhinitis, sinusitis, epistaxis, mouth ulcer, oral candidiasis, enlarged salivary glands, stomatitis, tooth disorder, dry mouth, blurred vision, cataracts, conjunctivitis, eye disorder, gingivitis, taste perversion.
**GI:** anorexia, *diarrhea,* dyspepsia, gastroenteritis, nausea, abdominal pain, vomiting, cholelithiasis, colitis, constipation, esophagitis, flatulence, gastritis, melena.
**GU:** urinary tract infection, albuminuria, cystitis, dysuria, hematuria, menstrual disorder, pelvic pain, vaginal candidiasis, prostate disorder, urinary frequency.
**Hematologic:** anemia.
**Hepatic:** elevated liver enzyme levels.
**Metabolic:** diabetes mellitus, fever, hyperglycemia, hyperthyroidism, hypokalemia, hyperlipidemia, increased CK levels, weight loss.
**Musculoskeletal:** arthrosis, back pain, bursitis, muscle cramps, myalgia, bone necrosis, bone pain, arthralgia, leg cramps, joint disorder, neck pain, synovitis, tendon rupture, tenosynovitis.
**Respiratory:** bronchitis, increased cough, pneumonia, *respiratory infection,* asthma, dyspnea, lung disorder.
**Skin:** *alopecia,* eczema, pruritus, *rash,* dry skin, acne, contact dermatitis, fungal dermatitis, hair discoloration, hematoma, herpes simplex, herpes zoster, nail disorder, skin nodule, subcutaneous nodule, maculopapular rash, skin disorder, skin discoloration, skin ulcer.

**Other:** *allergic reaction,* flulike syndrome, injury or accident, pain, abscess, cyst, hernia, increased sweating, ecchymoses.

## INTERACTIONS

**Drug-drug.** *Charcoal, cholestyramine:* decreased plasma levels of leflunomide. Sometimes used for this effect in overdose.
*Methotrexate, other hepatotoxic drugs:* increased risk of hepatotoxicity. Monitor liver enzymes, as ordered.
*NSAIDs (diclofenac, ibuprofen):* increased levels of NSAIDs. Clinical significance is unknown.
*Rifampin:* increased active leflunomide metabolite level. Use caution with concomitant use.
*Tolbutamide:* increased tolbutamide levels. Clinical significance is unknown.

## EFFECTS ON DIAGNOSTIC TESTS

None reported.

## CONTRAINDICATIONS

Contraindicated in patients with hypersensitivity to drug or its components and in women who are or may become pregnant or who are breast-feeding. Drug isn't recommended for patients with hepatic insufficiency, hepatitis B or C, severe immunodeficiency, bone marrow dysplasia, or severe uncontrolled infections. Drug isn't recommended for use in patients under age 18 and in men attempting to father a child.

## NURSING CONSIDERATIONS

• Use cautiously in patients with renal insufficiency.
• Vaccination with live vaccines isn't recommended. The long half-life of drug should be considered when contemplating administration of a live vaccine after stopping drug treatment.
• *Alert:* Drug can cause fetal harm when administered to pregnant women; women planning pregnancy should discontinue drug therapy and consult doctor. Men planning to father a child should discontinue drug therapy and follow recommended leflunomide removal protocol (cholestyramine 8 g, P.O. t.i.d. for 11 days).
• Risk of malignancy, particularly lymphoproliferative disorders, is increased

with use of some immunosuppressants, including leflunomide.
• Monitor liver enzymes (ALT and AST) before starting therapy and monthly thereafter until stable. Frequency can then be decreased based on clinical situation.

### ✅ Patient teaching

• Explain need and frequency of required blood tests and monitoring.
• Instruct patient to use birth control during course of treatment and until it has been determined that drug is no longer active.
• Warn patient to immediately notify doctor if signs or symptoms of pregnancy occur (such as late menses or breast tenderness).
• Advise breast-feeding woman to discontinue breast-feeding during therapy.
• Inform patient that aspirin, other NSAIDs, and low-dose corticosteroids may be continued during treatment. However, use of drug with antimalarials, intramuscular or oral gold, penicillamine, azathioprine, or methotrexate hasn't been adequately studied.

---

## levocarnitine (L-carnitine)
Carnitor, VitaCarn

*Pregnancy Risk Category B*

---

### HOW SUPPLIED

*Tablets:* 330 mg
*Capsules:* 250 mg ◇
*Oral liquid:* 100 mg/ml
*Injection:* 1 g/5 ml

### ACTION

Facilitates transport of long-chain fatty acids into cellular mitochondria. The fatty acids are then used to produce energy.

| Route | Onset | Peak | Duration |
|-------|-------|------|----------|
| P.O., I.V. | Unknown | Unknown | Unknown |

### INDICATIONS & DOSAGE

*Primary and secondary systemic carnitine deficiency—*
**Adults:** 990 mg P.O. b.i.d. or t.i.d. Or, 10 to 30 ml (1 to 3 g) of oral liquid daily.

**Children:** 50 to 100 mg/kg/day P.O. in divided doses.

All doses depend on clinical response. Higher doses may be given. However, for children, maximum dose is 3 g/day.
*Immediate and long-term treatment of secondary carnitine deficiency—*
**Adults:** 50 mg/kg I.V. slowly over 2 to 3 minutes q 3 to 4 hours.

### ADVERSE REACTIONS

**GI:** *nausea, vomiting, cramps, diarrhea.*
**Other:** *body odor.*

### INTERACTIONS

**Drug-drug.** *D,L-carnitine (sold as vitamin $B_T$):* inhibition of levocarnitine and possible deficiency. Avoid concomitant use.
*Valproic acid:* increased requirement for carnitine. Adjust dosage, as ordered.
**Drug-food.** *Any food:* decreased GI upset. Dissolve drug in drink or liquid food or take with meals.

### EFFECTS ON DIAGNOSTIC TESTS

None reported.

### CONTRAINDICATIONS

No known contraindications.

### NURSING CONSIDERATIONS

• Give enteral liquid alone or dissolved in drinks or liquid food.
• Use entire or partial contents of containers of liquid immediately after opening; discard any unused contents.
• Monitor patient's tolerance during first week of therapy and after increasing dosage, as ordered.
• Monitor blood chemistry results and plasma carnitine levels periodically, as ordered, as well as vital signs and patient's overall clinical condition.

### 🔷 I.V. administration

• A loading dose frequently is given to patients with severe metabolic crisis, followed by an equivalent dose over next 24 hours.
• Drug is compatible and stable when mixed in solutions of normal saline or lactated Ringer's in concentrations ranging from 250 mg/500 ml to 4,200 mg/500 ml.

---

Reactions may be *common*, uncommon, *life-threatening*, or COMMON AND LIFE-THREATENING.

• Store mixed infusions at room temperature (77° F [25° C]) for up to 24 hours in polyvinyl chloride plastic bags.
• Don't refrigerate solution.

### ☑ Patient teaching
• Tell patient to consume oral liquid slowly to minimize GI distress. If GI intolerance persists, dosage may have to be reduced.
• Warn patient to avoid vitamin $B_T$ because it will interact with drug and render it ineffective.
• Caution patient not to share drug with others. Some people have used it to improve athletic performance.
• Warn patient about possible body odor.
• Space doses evenly every 3 to 4 hours and give drug with or after meals, if possible.
• Tell patient to store drug at room temperature.

---

## mesalamine
Asacol, Mesasal, Pentasa, Rowasa, Salofalk

*Pregnancy Risk Category B*

### HOW SUPPLIED
*Tablets (delayed-release):* 400 mg
*Capsules (controlled-release):* 250 mg
*Rectal suspension:* 4 g/60 ml
*Suppositories:* 500 mg

### ACTION
Unknown. An active metabolite of sulfasalazine; probably acts topically by inhibiting prostaglandin production in the colon.

| Route | Onset | Peak | Duration |
|-------|-------|------|----------|
| P.O., P.R. | Unknown | 3-12 hr | Unknown |

### INDICATIONS & DOSAGE
*Active mild to moderate distal ulcerative colitis, proctitis, or proctosigmoiditis—*
**Adults:** 800 mg P.O. (tablets) t.i.d. for total dose of 2.4 g/day for 6 weeks; or 1 g P.O. (capsules) q.i.d. for total dose of 4 g up to 8 weeks; or 500 mg P.R. (suppository) b.i.d.; or 4 g as retention enema once daily (preferably h.s.). Rectal dosage form

should be retained overnight (for about 8 hours). Usual course of therapy for rectal form is 3 to 6 weeks.

### ADVERSE REACTIONS
**CNS:** headache, dizziness, fatigue, malaise, asthenia, chills.
**CV:** chest pain.
**GI:** abdominal pain, cramps, discomfort, flatulence, diarrhea, rectal pain, bloating, nausea, *pancolitis,* vomiting, constipation, eructation.
**Musculoskeletal:** arthralgia, myalgia, back pain, hypertonia.
**Respiratory:** wheezing.
**Skin:** itching, rash, urticaria, hair loss.
**Other:** fever.

### INTERACTIONS
**Drug-drug.** *Lactulose:* may impair release of delayed or extended-release products. Monitor closely.
*Omeprazole:* increased absorption of mesalamine. Monitor closely.

### EFFECTS ON DIAGNOSTIC TESTS
None reported.

### CONTRAINDICATIONS
Contraindicated in patients with hypersensitivity to drug, its components, or salicylates.

### NURSING CONSIDERATIONS
• Use cautiously in patients with renal impairment. Problems haven't been documented, but nephrotoxic potential from absorbed mesalamine exists.
• Monitor periodic renal function studies in patients on long-term therapy, as ordered.
• Because the mesalamine rectal suspension contains potassium metabisulfite, it may cause hypersensitivity reactions in patients sensitive to sulfites.
• *Alert:* Don't confuse Asacol with Os-Cal.

### ☑ Patient teaching
• Instruct patient to carefully follow instructions supplied with drug and to swallow tablets whole.
• Advise patient to discontinue drug if fever or rash occurs. Patient intolerant of

---

sulfasalazine may also be hypersensitive to mesalamine.
• Teach patient about proper use of retention enema.

---

# mesna
Mesnex, Uromitexan§

*Pregnancy Risk Category B*

## HOW SUPPLIED
*Injection:* 100 mg/ml

## ACTION
Prevents ifosfamide-induced hemorrhagic cystitis by reacting with urotoxic ifosfamide metabolites.

| Route | Onset | Peak | Duration |
|-------|-------|------|----------|
| I.V. | Unknown | Unknown | Unknown |

## INDICATIONS & DOSAGE
*Prophylaxis of hemorrhagic cystitis in patients receiving ifosfamide—*
**Adults:** dosage varies with amount of ifosfamide administered; calculated as 20% of ifosfamide dose at time of ifosfamide administration. Usual dose is 240 mg/m$^2$ as an I.V. bolus with administration of ifosfamide; repeated at 4 and 8 hours after administration of ifosfamide.

## ADVERSE REACTIONS
**CNS:** *headache, fatigue.*
**CV:** *hypotension.*
**GI:** *soft stools, nausea, vomiting, diarrhea, dysgeusia.*
**Musculoskeletal:** *limb pain.*
**Other:** *allergy.*
   *Note:* Because mesna is used with ifosfamide and other chemotherapeutic drugs, it's difficult to determine adverse reactions attributable solely to mesna.

## INTERACTIONS
None significant.

## EFFECTS ON DIAGNOSTIC TESTS
Mesna may produce a false-positive test for urinary ketones. A red-violet color will return to violet with the addition of acetic acid.

## CONTRAINDICATIONS
Contraindicated in patients with hypersensitivity to mesna or thiol-containing compounds.

## NURSING CONSIDERATIONS
• Monitor urine samples for hematuria daily. Monitor BUN and creatinine levels and intake and output.
• Mesna isn't effective in preventing hematuria from other causes (such as thrombocytopenia).
• Although formulated to prevent hemorrhagic cystitis from ifosfamide, drug won't protect against other toxicities associated with drug therapy.
• Drug contains benzyl alcohol, which has been associated with fatal gasping syndrome in premature infants.

### 🖐 I.V. administration
• Prepare I.V. solution by diluting commercially available ampules with D$_5$W solution, dextrose 5% and normal saline for injection, normal saline for injection, or lactated Ringer's solution to obtain final solution of 20 mg mesna/ml.
• Although diluted solutions are stable for 24 hours at room temperature, it's recommended that they be refrigerated and used within 6 hours. After opening ampule, discard any unused drug.
• Mesna and ifosfamide are compatible in same I.V. infusion.
• Mesna I.V. is incompatible with cisplatin; don't mix them.

### ✅ Patient teaching
• Explain to patient and family or other caregiver need for drug and how it's administered.
• Instruct patient to report persistent or severe adverse reactions.
• Advise patient to promptly report blood in urine.

---

# minoxidil (topical)
Rogaine

*Pregnancy Risk Category C*

## HOW SUPPLIED
*Topical solution:* 2%

---

## ACTION
Unknown. Stimulates hair growth, possibly by dilating arterial microcapillaries around hair follicles.

| Route | Onset | Peak | Duration |
|---|---|---|---|
| Topical | Unknown | Unknown | Unknown |

## INDICATIONS & DOSAGE
*Androgenetic alopecia*—
**Adults:** 1 ml of 2% solution applied to affected area b.i.d. Maximum daily dose is 2 ml.

## ADVERSE REACTIONS
**CNS:** headache, dizziness, faintness, light-headedness.
**CV:** edema, chest pain, hypertension, hypotension, palpitations, increased or decreased pulse rate.
**EENT:** sinusitis.
**GI:** diarrhea, nausea, vomiting.
**GU:** urinary tract infection, renal calculi, urethritis.
**Metabolic:** weight gain.
**Musculoskeletal:** back pain, tendinitis.
**Respiratory:** bronchitis, upper respiratory infection.
**Skin:** *irritant dermatitis,* allergic contact dermatitis, eczema, hypertrichosis, *local erythema, pruritus, dry skin or scalp, flaking,* alopecia, exacerbation of hair loss.

## INTERACTIONS
**Drug-drug.** *Petroleum jelly, topical corticosteroids, topical retinoids, other drugs that may enhance skin absorption:* increased risk of systemic effects of minoxidil. Don't apply minoxidil with other drugs.

## EFFECTS ON DIAGNOSTIC TESTS
None reported.

## CONTRAINDICATIONS
Contraindicated in patients with hypersensitivity to drug or components of solution.

## NURSING CONSIDERATIONS
• Use cautiously in patients over age 50 and in those with cardiac, renal, or hepatic disease.
• Patients need to have normal, healthy scalps before beginning therapy because absorption of drug through irritated skin may cause adverse systemic effects.
• Treatment is most likely to succeed in patients with balding area smaller than 4 inches (10 cm) that developed within past 10 years.

## ☑ Patient teaching
• Teach patient how to apply topical minoxidil. Hair and scalp should be thoroughly dry before application, and drug shouldn't be applied to other body areas. Tell patient not to use drug on irritated or sunburned scalp or with other drugs on scalp. Tell him to thoroughly wash hands after application.
• Warn patient to avoid inhaling any spray or mist from drug and to avoid spraying around eyes because solution contains alcohol and may be irritating.
• Inform patient that more frequent applications or using more than 2 ml/day won't increase hair growth, but instead may increase adverse reactions. Don't attempt to double doses for missed applications.
• Teach patient to monitor pulse rate and body weight.
• Advise patient of need for medical follow-ups 1 month after therapy starts and every 6 months thereafter.
• Advise patient that therapy will be prolonged and will continue for at least 4 months before clinical effects appear and that drug must be used daily for optimal results. About 40% of patients will see moderate to dense hair growth.
• Tell patient that discontinuing drug may result in loss of new hair growth. New hair growth is usually fine and may be colorless, but will resemble existing hair after continued treatment.

---

## nimodipine
Nimotop

*Pregnancy Risk Category C*

## HOW SUPPLIED
*Capsules:* 30 mg

## ACTION
Inhibits calcium ion influx across cardiac and smooth-muscle cells, decreasing my-

---

ocardial contractility and oxygen demand, and dilates coronary and cerebral arteries and arterioles.

| Route | Onset | Peak | Duration |
|-------|-------|------|----------|
| P.O. | Unknown | 1 hr | Unknown |

## INDICATIONS & DOSAGE
*Improvement of neurologic deficits after subarachnoid hemorrhage from ruptured congenital aneurysms—*
**Adults:** 60 mg P.O. q 4 hours for 21 days. Begin therapy within 96 hours after subarachnoid hemorrhage.
*Adjust-a-dose:* For patients with hepatic failure, 30 mg P.O. q 4 hours for 21 days.

## ADVERSE REACTIONS
**CNS:** headache, psychic disturbances.
**CV:** decreased blood pressure, flushing, edema, tachycardia.
**GI:** nausea, diarrhea, abdominal discomfort.
**Musculoskeletal:** muscle cramps.
**Respiratory:** dyspnea.
**Skin:** dermatitis, rash.

## INTERACTIONS
**Drug-drug.** *Antihypertensives:* possible enhanced hypotensive effect. Monitor patient closely.
*Calcium channel blockers:* possible enhanced CV effects. Monitor patient closely.
*Cimetidine:* increased nimodipine bioavailability. Monitor closely.

## EFFECTS ON DIAGNOSTIC TESTS
None reported.

## CONTRAINDICATIONS
No known contraindications.

## NURSING CONSIDERATIONS
• Use cautiously in patients with hepatic failure.
• Reserve drug for patients who are in good neurologic condition (for example, Hunt and Hess grades I to III).
• Monitor blood pressure and heart rate in all patients, especially at start of therapy.
• If capsule can't be swallowed, make a hole in each end of capsule with an 18G needle, and extract contents into syringe. Empty syringe into patient's NG tube.

Flush tube with 30 ml of normal saline solution.
• *Alert:* If using a needle to extract contents of capsule, make sure that drug isn't then given I.V. instead of P.O. Label the syringe, "for oral use only" before withdrawing the contents of the capsule.

☑ **Patient teaching**
• Explain use of drug, and review administration schedule with patient and family. Stress importance of compliance for maximum drug effectiveness.
• Instruct patient to report persistent or severe adverse reactions promptly.

---

**olsalazine sodium**
Dipentum

*Pregnancy Risk Category C*

## HOW SUPPLIED
*Capsules:* 250 mg

## ACTION
Unknown. After oral administration, converts to 5-aminosalicylic acid (5-ASA or mesalamine) in the colon, where it has local anti-inflammatory effect.

| Route | Onset | Peak | Duration |
|-------|-------|------|----------|
| P.O. | Unknown | 1 hr | Unknown |

## INDICATIONS & DOSAGE
*Maintenance of remission of ulcerative colitis in patients intolerant of sulfasalazine—*
**Adults:** 500 mg P.O. b.i.d. with meals.

## ADVERSE REACTIONS
**CNS:** headache, depression, vertigo, dizziness, fatigue.
**GI:** *diarrhea,* nausea, *abdominal pain,* dyspepsia, bloating, anorexia.
**Musculoskeletal:** arthralgia.
**Skin:** rash, itching.

## INTERACTIONS
**Drug-drug.** *Anticoagulants, coumarin derivatives:* prolonged PT or INR. Monitor bleeding studies.
**Drug-food.** *Any food:* decreased GI irritation. Administer drug with food.

---

Reactions may be *common,* uncommon, *life-threatening,* or COMMON AND LIFE-THREATENING.

**EFFECTS ON DIAGNOSTIC TESTS**
None reported.

**CONTRAINDICATIONS**
Contraindicated in patients with hypersensitivity to salicylates.

**NURSING CONSIDERATIONS**
• Use cautiously in patients with preexisting renal disease. Although problems haven't been reported, possibility of renal tubular damage from absorbed drug or its metabolites must be considered.
• Regularly monitor BUN and creatinine levels and urinalysis in patients with pre-existing renal disease, as ordered.
• Some patients have reported diarrhea during therapy. Although diarrhea appears to be dose-related, it's difficult to distinguish from worsening of disease symptoms. Exacerbation of disease has been noted with similar drugs.
• *Alert:* Don't confuse olsalazine with olanzapine.

☑ **Patient teaching**
• Teach patient to take drug in evenly divided doses and with food to minimize adverse GI reactions.
• Instruct patient to report persistent or severe adverse reactions promptly.

✳ *NEW DRUG*

──────────────

**orlistat**
Xenical

*Pregnancy Risk Category B*

──────────────

**HOW SUPPLIED**
*Capsules:* 120 mg

**ACTION**
A reversible inhibitor of lipases that forms bond with active site of gastric and pancreatic lipases, inactivating them. Thus, enzymes can't hydrolyze dietary fat, in the form of triglycerides, into absorbable free fatty acids and monoglycerides. The undigested triglycerides aren't absorbed, resulting in caloric deficit.

| Route | Onset | Peak | Duration |
|-------|-------|------|----------|
| P.O. | Unknown | Unknown | Unknown |

**INDICATIONS & DOSAGE**
*Management of obesity, including weight loss and weight maintenance with a reduced-calorie diet; reduction of risk of weight gain after previous weight loss—*
**Adults:** 120 mg P.O. t.i.d. with each main meal containing fat (during or up to 1 hour after meals).

**ADVERSE REACTIONS**
**CNS:** *headache,* dizziness, fatigue, sleep disorder, anxiety, depression.
**CV:** pedal edema.
**EENT:** otitis, tooth and gingival disorders.
**GI:** *oily spotting, flatus with discharge, fecal urgency, fatty or oily stool, oily evacuation, increased defecation, abdominal pain,* fecal incontinence, nausea, infectious diarrhea, rectal pain, vomiting.
**GU:** menstrual irregularity, vaginitis, urinary tract infection.
**Musculoskeletal:** *back pain, pain in lower extremities,* arthritis, myalgia, joint disorder, tendonitis.
**Respiratory:** *influenza, upper respiratory tract infection,* lower respiratory tract infection.
**Skin:** rash, dry skin.

**INTERACTIONS**
**Drug-drug.** *Fat-soluble vitamins (such as vitamins A and E and beta-carotene):* decreased absorption of vitamins. Separate administration times by 2 hours.
*Pravastatin:* slightly increased pravastatin levels and additive lipid-lowering effects of drug. Monitor patient.
*Warfarin:* possible change in coagulation parameters. Monitor INR.

**EFFECTS ON DIAGNOSTIC TESTS**
None reported.

**CONTRAINDICATIONS**
Contraindicated in patients with hypersensitivity to drug or its components and in those with chronic malabsorption syndrome or cholestasis. Exclude organic causes of obesity such as hypothyroidism before starting drug therapy.

**NURSING CONSIDERATIONS**
• Use cautiously in patients with history of hyperoxaluria or calcium oxalate

──────────────

nephrolithiasis or risk of anorexia nervosa or bulimia.
• Use cautiously in patients receiving cyclosporine therapy because of potential changes in cyclosporine absorption related to variations in dietary intake.
• Drug is recommended for use in patients with an initial body mass index (BMI) of 30 kg/m² or more, or 27 kg/m² or more and other risk factors (such as hypertension, diabetes, or dyslipidemia).
• Advise patient to adhere to dietary guidelines. GI effects may increase when patient takes drug with high-fat foods, specifically when over 30% of total daily calories come from fat.
• Drug reduces absorption of some fat-soluble vitamins and beta-carotene. To ensure adequate nutrition, advise patient to take daily multivitamin supplements that contain fat-soluble vitamins during therapy.
• In diabetic patients, because improved metabolic control may accompany weight loss, dosage of oral antidiabetic or insulin may need to be reduced.
• As with other weight-loss drugs, potential for misuse in certain patients exists (such as those with anorexia nervosa or bulimia.
• *Alert:* Don't confuse Xenical with Xeloda.

☑ **Patient teaching**
• Advise patient to follow a nutritionally balanced, reduced-calorie diet that derives only 30% of its calories from fat. Daily intake of fat, carbohydrate, and protein should be distributed over three main meals. If a meal is occasionally missed or contains no fat, tell patient that dose of drug can be omitted.
• To ensure adequate nutrition, advise patient to take daily multivitamin supplements that contain fat-soluble vitamins at least 2 hours before or after administration of drug, such as at bedtime.
• Tell patient with diabetes that weight loss may improve his glycemic control, so dosage of his oral antidiabetic (such as sulfonylureas or metformin) or insulin may need to be reduced during drug therapy.

• Tell woman of childbearing age to inform doctor if pregnancy or breast-feeding is planned during therapy.

---

# pamidronate disodium
Aredia

*Pregnancy Risk Category C*

## HOW SUPPLIED
*Injection:* 30-mg, 60-mg, 90-mg vials

## ACTION
An antihypercalcemic that inhibits resorption of bone. Adsorbs to hydroxyapatite crystals in bone and may directly block dissolution of calcium phosphate. Blocks mature osteoclast formation. Apparently doesn't inhibit bone formation or mineralization.

| Route | Onset | Peak | Duration |
|-------|-------|------|----------|
| I.V. | Unknown | Unknown | Unknown |

## INDICATIONS & DOSAGE
*Moderate to severe hypercalcemia associated with cancer (with or without bone metastases)—*
**Adults:** dosage depends on severity of hypercalcemia. Serum calcium levels should be corrected for serum albumin. Corrected serum calcium (CCa) is calculated using this formula:

$$CCa = \text{serum calcium} + 0.8 \,(4 - \text{serum albumin})$$
$$\text{(mg/dl)} \quad \text{(mg/dl)} \quad \text{(g/dl)}$$

Patients with moderate hypercalcemia (CCa levels of 12 to 13.5 mg/dl) may receive 60 to 90 mg by I.V. infusion over 4 hours for 60-mg dose and over 24 hours for 90-mg dose. Patients with severe hypercalcemia (CCa levels over 13.5 mg/dl) may receive 90 mg by I.V. infusion over 24 hours. A minimum of 7 days should elapse before retreatment to allow for full response to initial dose.
*Moderate to severe Paget's disease—*
**Adults:** 30 mg I.V. as a 4-hour infusion on 3 consecutive days for total dose of 90 mg. Cycle repeated, p.r.n.

*Osteolytic bone metastases of breast cancer with standard antineoplastic therapy—*
**Adults:** 90 mg I.V. infusion over 2 to 4 hours q 3 to 4 weeks.

## ADVERSE REACTIONS
**CNS:** *seizures, fatigue,* somnolence, syncope.
**CV:** *atrial fibrillation,* tachycardia, *hypertension.*
**GI:** *abdominal pain, anorexia, constipation, nausea, vomiting,* **GI hemorrhage.**
**Hematologic:** *leukopenia, thrombocytopenia,* anemia.
**Metabolic:** *hypophosphatemia, hypokalemia, hypomagnesemia, hypocalcemia, fever.*
**Other:** *infusion-site reaction.*

## INTERACTIONS
None significant.

## EFFECTS ON DIAGNOSTIC TESTS
None reported.

## CONTRAINDICATIONS
Contraindicated in patients with hypersensitivity to drug or other bisphosphonates such as etidronate.

## NURSING CONSIDERATIONS
• Use with extreme caution, and consider risks versus benefits, in patients with renal impairment.
• Assess hydration status before treatment. Use drug only after patient has been vigorously hydrated with normal saline solution. In patients with mild to moderate hypercalcemia, hydration alone may be sufficient.
• Because drug can cause electrolyte disturbances, carefully monitor serum electrolyte levels, especially calcium, phosphate, and magnesium, as ordered. Short-term administration of calcium may be needed in patients with severe hypocalcemia. Also monitor creatinine level, CBC and differential count, and hemoglobin levels and hematocrit, as ordered.
• Carefully monitor patients with preexisting anemia, leukopenia, or thrombocytopenia during first 2 weeks of therapy.

• Monitor patient's temperature. Some patients experience an elevation of 1.8° F (1° C) for 24 to 48 hours after therapy.
• Solution is stable for 24 hours at room temperature.

### ◖ I.V. administration
• Reconstitute drug with 10 ml of sterile water for injection. After drug is completely dissolved, add to 1,000 ml of half-normal or normal saline for injection or D₅W. Don't mix with infusion solutions that contain calcium, such as Ringer's injection or lactated Ringer's injection. Visually inspect for precipitate before use.
• *Alert:* Give drug only by I.V. infusion. Nephropathy is possible when drug is given as bolus.

### ✓ Patient teaching
• Explain use and administration of drug to patient and family.
• Instruct patient to report adverse reactions promptly.

---

## pilocarpine hydrochloride
Salagen

*Pregnancy Risk Category C*

## HOW SUPPLIED
*Tablets:* 5 mg

## ACTION
A cholinergic parasympathomimetic that increases secretion of salivary glands, eliminating dryness.

| Route | Onset | Peak | Duration |
|-------|-------|------|----------|
| P.O. | 20 min | 1 hr | 3-5 hr |

## INDICATIONS & DOSAGE
*Xerostomia from salivary gland hypofunction due to radiotherapy for cancer of head and neck—*
**Adults:** 5 mg P.O. t.i.d.; may be increased to 10 mg P.O. t.i.d., p.r.n.
*Symptoms of dry mouth in patients with Sjögren's syndrome—*
**Adults:** 5 mg P.O. q.i.d.

---

## ADVERSE REACTIONS
**CNS:** *dizziness, headache,* tremor, *asthenia.*
**CV:** hypertension, tachycardia.
**EENT:** *rhinitis,* lacrimation, amblyopia, pharyngitis, voice alteration, conjunctivitis, epistaxis, *sinusitis, abnormal vision.*
**GI:** *nausea,* dyspepsia, diarrhea, abdominal pain, vomiting, dysphagia, taste perversion.
**GU:** *urinary frequency.*
**Musculoskeletal:** myalgia.
**Skin:** rash, pruritus.
**Other:** *sweating, chills, flushing,* edema.

## INTERACTIONS
**Drug-drug.** *Beta-adrenergic antagonists:* may increase risk of conduction disturbances. Use together cautiously.
*Drugs with anticholinergic effects:* may antagonize anticholinergic effects. Use together cautiously.
*Drugs with parasympathomimetic effects:* may result in additive pharmacologic effects. Monitor patient closely.

## EFFECTS ON DIAGNOSTIC TESTS
None reported.

## CONTRAINDICATIONS
Contraindicated in patients with hypersensitivity to pilocarpine, in those with uncontrolled asthma, and when meiosis is undesirable, such as in acute iritis or narrow-angle glaucoma.

## NURSING CONSIDERATIONS
• Use cautiously in patients with CV disease, controlled asthma, chronic bronchitis, chronic obstructive pulmonary disease, cholelithiasis, biliary tract disease, nephrolithiasis, or cognitive or psychiatric disturbances.
• Don't use drug in breast-feeding women.
• Safety and efficacy of drug in children haven't been established.
• Examine patient's fundus carefully before beginning therapy because retinal detachment has been reported in patients with retinal disease.
• Monitor patient for signs and symptoms of toxicity: headache, visual disturbance, lacrimation, sweating, respiratory distress, GI spasm, nausea, vomiting, diarrhea, atrioventricular block, tachycardia, bradycardia, hypotension, hypertension, shock, mental confusion, arrhythmia, and tremors. Immediately notify doctor of suspected toxicity.

☑ **Patient teaching**
• Warn patient that driving ability may be impaired, especially at night, by drug-induced visual disturbances.
• Advise patient to drink plenty of fluids to prevent dehydration.
• Inform elderly patient with Sjögren's syndrome that he may be especially prone to urinary frequency, diarrhea, and dizziness.

---

## raloxifene hydrochloride
Evista

*Pregnancy Risk Category X*

## HOW SUPPLIED
*Tablets:* 60 mg

## ACTION
A selective estrogen receptor modulator that reduces resorption of bone and decreases overall bone turnover. These effects on bone are manifested as reductions in serum and urine levels of bone turnover markers and increases in bone mineral density.

| Route | Onset | Peak | Duration |
|-------|-------|------|----------|
| P.O. | Unknown | Unknown | 24 hr |

## INDICATIONS & DOSAGE
*Prevention of osteoporosis in postmenopausal women—*
**Adults:** 60 mg P.O. once daily.

## ADVERSE REACTIONS
**CNS:** depression, insomnia, migraine.
**CV:** chest pain.
**EENT:** *sinusitis,* pharyngitis, laryngitis.
**GI:** nausea, dyspepsia, vomiting, flatulence, GI disorder, gastroenteritis, abdominal pain.
**GU:** vaginitis, urinary tract infection, cystitis, leukorrhea, endometrial disorder, vaginal bleeding.

---

**Metabolic:** weight gain, fever.
**Musculoskeletal:** *arthralgia*, myalgia, arthritis, leg cramps, breast pain.
**Respiratory:** increased cough, pneumonia.
**Skin:** rash, sweating.
**Other:** *infection, flu syndrome, hot flashes,* peripheral edema.

**INTERACTIONS**
**Drug-drug.** *Cholestyramine:* causes significant reduction in absorption of raloxifene. Avoid concomitant use.
*Highly protein-bound drugs (such as clofibrate, diazepam, diazoxide, ibuprofen, indomethacin, naproxen):* may interfere with binding sites. Use with caution.
*Warfarin:* may cause a decrease in PT. Monitor PT and INR closely.

**EFFECTS ON DIAGNOSTIC TESTS**
None reported.

**CONTRAINDICATIONS**
Contraindicated in women with hypersensitivity to drug or its components; in those with past history or currently active venous thromboembolic events, including deep vein thrombosis, pulmonary embolism, and retinal vein thrombosis; in pregnant women or those planning pregnancy; in breast-feeding women; and in children.

**NURSING CONSIDERATIONS**
• Use cautiously in patients with severe hepatic impairment.
• Watch for signs of blood clots. Greatest risk of thromboembolic events occurs during first 4 months of treatment.
• Discontinue drug at least 72 hours before prolonged immobilization and resume only after patient is fully mobilized.
• Report unexplained uterine bleeding because endometrial proliferation hasn't been associated with drug use.
• Watch for breast abnormalities that occur during treatment. No association between breast enlargement, breast pain, or an increased risk of breast cancer has been shown.
• The following laboratory changes may occur: increased apolipoprotein A levels; reduced serum total cholesterol, low-density lipoprotein cholesterol, fibrino-

gen, apolipoprotein B, and lipoprotein (a) levels; modest increases in hormone-binding globulin levels; small decreases in serum total calcium, inorganic phosphate, total protein, and albumin levels, and platelet count.
• Safety and efficacy of drug haven't been evaluated in men.
• Effect on bone mineral density beyond 2 years of drug treatment isn't known.
• Use with hormone replacement therapy or systemic estrogen hasn't been evaluated and, therefore, isn't recommended.

✅ **Patient teaching**
• Advise patient to avoid long periods of restricted movement (such as during traveling) because of increased risk of venous thromboembolic events.
• Inform patient that hot flashes or flushing may occur and that drug doesn't aid in reducing them.
• Instruct patient to practice other bone loss prevention measures, including supplemental calcium and vitamin D if dietary intake is inadequate, weight-bearing exercises, and discontinuing alcohol consumption and smoking.
• Tell patient that drug may be taken without regard to food.
• Advise patient to report unexplained uterine bleeding or breast abnormalities during therapy.
• Explain adverse reactions and instruct patient to read patient package insert before starting therapy and to reread it each time prescription is renewed.

---

**riluzole**
Rilutek

*Pregnancy Risk Category C*

**HOW SUPPLIED**
*Tablets:* 50 mg

**ACTION**
May protect motor neurons from excitotoxic effects of glutamate by inhibiting glutamate release, inactivating some sodi-

---

um channels, and interfering with transmitter binding.

| Route | Onset | Peak | Duration |
|-------|-------|------|----------|
| P.O. | Unknown | Unknown | Unknown |

## INDICATIONS & DOSAGE
*Amyotrophic lateral sclerosis—*
**Adults:** 50 mg P.O. q 12 hours, taken on empty stomach.

## ADVERSE REACTIONS
**CNS:** headache, aggravation reaction, *asthenia,* hypertonia, depression, dizziness, insomnia, malaise, somnolence, vertigo, circumoral paresthesia.
**CV:** hypertension, tachycardia, palpitation, orthostatic hypotension.
**EENT:** rhinitis, sinusitis.
**GI:** abdominal pain, *nausea,* vomiting, dyspepsia, anorexia, diarrhea, flatulence, stomatitis, tooth disorder, dry mouth, oral candidiasis.
**GU:** urinary tract infection, dysuria.
**Musculoskeletal:** back pain, arthralgia.
**Respiratory:** *decreased lung function,* increased cough.
**Skin:** pruritus, eczema, alopecia, exfoliative dermatitis.
**Other:** phlebitis, weight loss, peripheral edema.

## INTERACTIONS
**Drug-drug.** *Allopurinol, methyldopa, sulfasalazine:* increased risk of hepatotoxicity. Monitor patient closely.
*Inducers of CYP 1A2 (omeprazole, rifampin):* may increase riluzole elimination. Monitor closely.
*Potential inhibitors of CYP 1A2 (amitriptyline, caffeine, phenacetin, quinolones, theophylline):* may decrease riluzole elimination. Monitor closely.
**Drug-food.** *Any food:* decreased bioavailability. Administer 1 hour before or 2 hours after meals.
*Charbroiled foods:* may increase elimination of drug. Avoid concomitant use.
**Drug-lifestyle.** *Alcohol use:* may increase risk of hepatotoxicity. Avoid excessive use.
*Smoking:* may increase riluzole elimination. Avoid contact.

## EFFECTS ON DIAGNOSTIC TESTS
None reported.

## CONTRAINDICATIONS
Contraindicated in patients with history of severe hypersensitivity to drug or its components.

## NURSING CONSIDERATIONS
• Use cautiously in patients with hepatic or renal dysfunction, in elderly patients, and in women and Japanese patients (who may have lower metabolic capacity to eliminate drug than men and Caucasian patients, respectively).
• Elevations in baseline liver function studies (especially bilirubin) preclude drug use. Perform liver function studies periodically during therapy, as ordered. In many patients, drug may increase serum aminotransferase level; if level exceeds five times upper limit of normal or if clinical jaundice develops, notify doctor.
• Give drug at least 1 hour before or 2 hours after meals to avoid decreased bioavailability.

☑ **Patient teaching**
• Tell patient to take drug at same time each day. If a dose is missed, tell him to take next tablet when planned.
• Instruct patient to take drug on an empty stomach to facilitate full dose absorption.
• Instruct patient to report fever to doctor, who may order a WBC count.
• Warn patient to avoid hazardous activities until CNS effects of drug are known and to limit alcohol use during therapy.
• Tell patient to store drug at room temperature, protect from bright light, and keep out of children's reach.

---

**ritodrine hydrochloride**
Yutopar, Yutopar S.R.†

*Pregnancy Risk Category B*

---

## HOW SUPPLIED
*Tablets†:* 10 mg
*Capsules (extended-release)†:* 40 mg
*Injection:* 10 mg/ml, 15 mg/ml
*Injection for I.V. infusion:* 0.3 mg/ml
(150 mg in 500 ml $D_5W$)

---

## ACTION

A beta agonist that stimulates the beta$_2$-adrenergic receptors in uterine smooth muscle, inhibiting contractility.

| Route | Onset | Peak | Duration |
|-------|-------|------|----------|
| P.O.  | 30-60 min | 30-60 min | Unknown |
| I.V.  | 5 min | 60 min | Unknown |

## INDICATIONS & DOSAGE

*Preterm labor—*
**Adults:** usual initial dose is 0.05 mg/minute I.V., gradually increased by 0.05 mg/minute q 10 minutes until desired result is obtained or until maternal heart rate reaches 130 beats/minute. Effective dosage ranges from 0.15 to 0.35 mg/minute.

## ADVERSE REACTIONS

**CNS:** nervousness, anxiety, *headaches, tremors,* emotional upset, malaise.
**CV:** changes in blood pressure, palpitations, *pulmonary edema, dose-related tachycardia.*
**GI:** *nausea, vomiting.*
**Hematologic:** *leukopenia, agranulocytosis.*
**Metabolic:** *hyperglycemia,* hypokalemia.
**Other:** *erythema, anaphylactic shock.*

## INTERACTIONS

**Drug-drug.** *Atropine:* may potentiate systemic hypertension. Monitor blood pressure.
*Beta blockers:* may inhibit ritodrine's action. Avoid concurrent use.
*Corticosteroids:* may produce pulmonary edema in mother. Monitor patient closely.
*Diazoxide, inhalation anesthetics, magnesium sulfate, meperidine:* potentiated adverse cardiac effects, arrhythmias, and hypotension. Monitor patient closely.
*Sympathomimetics:* additive sympathomimetic effects. Use together cautiously.

## EFFECTS ON DIAGNOSTIC TESTS

None reported.

## CONTRAINDICATIONS

Contraindicated in patients with hypersensitivity to drug and in those with antepartum hemorrhage, eclampsia and severe preeclampsia, intrauterine fetal death, chorioamnionitis, maternal cardiac disease, pulmonary hypertension, maternal hyperthyroidism, or uncontrolled maternal diabetes mellitus. Also contraindicated in pregnant women before 20th week of pregnancy and in those with pre-existing maternal medical conditions, such as hypovolemia, pheochromocytoma, and uncontrolled hypertension, that would seriously be affected by pharmacologic properties of drug.

## NURSING CONSIDERATIONS

• Use cautiously in patients with a sulfite sensitivity.
• *Alert:* Because CV responses are common and more pronounced during I.V. administration, closely monitor CV effects, including maternal pulse rate and blood pressure, and fetal heart rate. Maternal tachycardia of more than 140 beats/minute or persistent respiratory rate of more than 20 breaths/minute may be a sign of impending pulmonary edema. Discontinue drug and notify doctor if pulmonary edema develops.
• Monitor blood glucose level during infusion, especially in diabetic mother.
• Monitor amount of fluids administered I.V. to prevent circulatory overload.
• Keep patient in left lateral position to minimize risk of hypotension.
• *Alert:* Don't confuse ritodrine with ranitidine.

## I.V. administration

• Dilute 150 mg in 500 ml D$_5$W to yield a concentration of 0.3 mg/ml.
• In patients whose condition contraindicates dextrose, dilute drug in normal saline, Ringer's, or lactated Ringer's solution to avoid risk of pulmonary edema.
• Don't use ritodrine I.V. if solution is discolored or contains precipitates.
• Continue I.V. infusion for 12 hours after contractions have stopped. Recurrence of preterm labor may be treated with repeated infusion of ritodrine.

## Patient teaching

• Explain to patient use and administration of drug.
• Instruct patient to report adverse reactions promptly.

---

*Liquid contains alcohol.   **May contain tartrazine.   †Canada   ‡Australia   §U.K.   ◇OTC

## sevelamer hydrochloride
Renagel

*Pregnancy Risk Category C*

### HOW SUPPLIED
*Capsules:* 403 mg

### ACTION
A phosphate binder that inhibits intestinal phosphate absorption and decreases serum phosphorus levels.

| Route | Onset | Peak | Duration |
|-------|-------|------|----------|
| P.O. | Unknown | Unknown | Unknown |

### INDICATIONS & DOSAGE
*Reduction of serum phosphorus in patients with endstage renal disease—*
**Adults:** initially, 2 to 4 capsules P.O. t.i.d. with meals, depending on severity of hyperphosphatemia. Gradually adjust dosage based on serum phosphorus level with goal of lowering serum phosphorus to 6 mg/dl or less. If serum phosphorus level is 9 mg/dl or more, 4 capsules P.O. t.i.d. with meals; if serum phosphorus level is between 7.5 and 9 mg/dl, 3 capsules P.O. t.i.d. with meals; if serum phosphorus level is between 6 and 7.5 mg/dl, 2 capsules P.O. t.i.d. with meals.

### ADVERSE REACTIONS
**CNS:** *headache, pain.*
**CV:** hypertension, *hypotension, **thrombosis.***
**GI:** *vomiting,* nausea, constipation, *diarrhea,* flatulence, *dyspepsia.*
**Respiratory:** increased cough.
**Other:** *infection.*

### INTERACTIONS
None significant.

### EFFECTS ON DIAGNOSTIC TESTS
None reported.

### CONTRAINDICATIONS
Contraindicated in patients with hypersensitivity to drug or its components and in those with hypophosphatemia or bowel obstruction.

### NURSING CONSIDERATIONS
• Use cautiously in patients with dysphagia, swallowing disorders, severe GI motility disorders, or major GI tract surgery.
• Monitor serum calcium, bicarbonate, and chloride levels, as ordered.
• Watch for symptoms of thrombosis (numbness or tingling of extremities, chest pain, shortness of breath), and notify doctor if they occur.
• Although no known drug interactions have been studied, drug may bind to concomitantly administered drugs and decrease their bioavailability. Administer other drugs 1 hour before or 3 hours after sevelamer.
• Don't crush or break capsules, and administer only with meals.

### ☑ Patient teaching
• Instruct patient to take with meals and adhere to prescribed diet.
• Inform patient that capsules must be taken whole because contents expand in water; caution him not to open or chew capsules.
• Tell patient to take other drugs as directed, but they must be taken either 1 hour before or 3 hours after sevelamer.
• Inform patient about common adverse reactions and instruct him to report them immediately. Teach patient signs and symptoms of thrombosis (numbness, tingling extremities, chest pain, changes in level of consciousness).

## sildenafil citrate
Viagra

*Pregnancy Risk Category B*

### HOW SUPPLIED
*Tablets:* 25 mg, 50 mg, 100 mg

### ACTION
Has no direct relaxant effect on isolated human corpus cavernosum, but enhances effect of nitric oxide (NO) by inhibiting phosphodiesterase type 5 ($PDE_5$), which is responsible for degradation of cyclic guanosine monophosphate (cGMP) in the corpus cavernosum. When sexual stimulation causes local release of NO, inhibi-

tion of PDE$_5$ by sildenafil causes increased levels of cGMP in the corpus cavernosum, resulting in smooth-muscle relaxation and inflow of blood to the corpus cavernosum.

| Route | Onset | Peak | Duration |
|-------|-------|------|----------|
| P.O. | Unknown | 0.5-2 hr | 4 hr |

## INDICATIONS & DOSAGE
*Erectile dysfunction—*
**Adults under age 65:** 50 mg P.O., p.r.n., about 1 hour before sexual activity. Dosage range is 25 to 100 mg based on effectiveness and toleration. Maximum is one dose daily.
**Elderly (ages 65 and older):** 25 mg P.O., p.r.n., about 1 hour before sexual activity. Dosage may be adjusted based on patient response. Maximum is one dose daily.
*Adjust-a-dose:* For adults with hepatic or severe renal impairment: 25 mg P.O. about 1 hour before sexual activity. Dosage may be adjusted based on patient response. Maximum is one dose daily.

## ADVERSE REACTIONS
**CNS:** anxiety, *headache,* dizziness, *seizures,* somnolence, vertigo.
**CV:** *MI, sudden cardiac death, ventricular arrhythmias, cerebrovascular hemorrhage, transient ischemic attack,* hypertension, flushing.
**EENT:** diplopia, temporary vision loss, decreased vision, ocular redness or bloodshot appearance, increased intraocular pressure, retinal vascular disease, retinal bleeding, vitreous detachment or traction, paramacular edema, photophobia, color-tinged vision, blurred vision, ocular burning, swelling, pressure.
**GI:** *dyspepsia,* diarrhea.
**GU:** hematuria, prolonged erection, priapism, urinary tract infection.
**Musculoskeletal:** arthralgia, back pain.
**Respiratory:** respiratory tract infection.
**Skin:** rash.
**Other:** flulike syndrome.

## INTERACTIONS
**Drug-drug.** *Beta blockers, loop and potassium-sparing diuretics:* increased blood levels of major metabolite of sildenafil, N-desmethyl sildenafil. Clinical

significance of these interactions isn't known. Monitor patient.
*CYP3A4 inducers, rifampin:* reduced sildenafil plasma levels. Monitor effect.
*Hepatic isoenzyme inhibitors (such as cimetidine, erythromycin, itraconazole, ketoconazole):* may reduce clearance of sildenafil. Avoid concomitant use.
*Nitrates:* sildenafil enhances hypotensive effects. Don't use together.
**Drug-food.** *High-fat meal:* reduced rate of absorption and decreased peak serum levels. Separate administration time from meals.

## EFFECTS ON DIAGNOSTIC TESTS
None reported.

## CONTRAINDICATIONS
Contraindicated in patients with hypersensitivity to drug or its components and in those with underlying CV disease. Concomitant use of organic nitrates at any frequency and in any form is also contraindicated.

## NURSING CONSIDERATIONS
• Use cautiously in patients ages 65 and older; in patients with hepatic or severe renal impairment, retinitis pigmentosa, bleeding disorders, or active peptic ulcer disease; in those who have suffered an MI, stroke, or life-threatening arrhythmias within last 6 months; in those with history of cardiac failure, coronary artery disease, uncontrolled high or low blood pressure, or anatomic deformation of the penis (such as angulation, cavernosal fibrosis, or Peyronie's disease); and in those with conditions that may predispose them to priapism (such as sickle cell anemia, multiple myeloma, leukemia).
• *Alert:* Drug increases risk of cardiac events. Systemic vasodilatory properties of drug cause transient decreases in supine blood pressure and cardiac output (about 2 hours after ingestion). With the potential cardiac risk of sexual activity, drug increases risk for patients with underlying CV disease.
• *Alert:* Serious CV events, including MI, sudden cardiac death, ventricular arrhythmias, cerebrovascular hemorrhage, transient ischemic attack, and hypertension

have been reported in temporal association with drug use. Most, but not all, of these incidents involved preexisting CV risk factors. Many events occurred during or shortly after sexual activity; a few occurred shortly after drug use without sexual activity; and others occurred hours to days after drug use and sexual activity.
• There is no indication for use of drug in newborns, children, or women.

✓ **Patient teaching**
• Advise patient that drug shouldn't be regularly or intermittently used with nitrates.
• Advise patient of potential cardiac risk of sexual activity, especially in presence of preexisting CV risk factors. Instruct patient to notify doctor of such symptoms as angina pectoris, dizziness, or nausea on initiation of sexual activity and tell him to refrain from further activity.
• Warn patient that erections lasting more than 4 hours and priapism (painful erections lasting longer than 6 hours) can occur and should be reported immediately. Penile tissue damage and permanent loss of potency may result if priapism isn't treated immediately.
• Inform patient that drug doesn't offer protection against sexually transmitted diseases; protective measures such as condoms should be used.
• Instruct patient to take drug 30 minutes to 4 hours before sexual activity; maximum benefit can be expected less than 2 hours after ingestion.
• Advise patient that drug is most rapidly absorbed if taken on an empty stomach.
• Inform patient that impairment of color discrimination (blue, green) may occur and to avoid hazardous activities that rely on color discrimination.
• Instruct patient to notify doctor of visual changes.
• Advise patient that drug is effective only in presence of sexual stimulation.
• Caution patient to take drug only as prescribed.

# sulfasalazine (salazosulfapyridine, sulphasalazine)
Azulfidine, Azulfidine EN-Tabs, PMS-Sulfasalazine E.C.†, Salazopyrin††‡, Salazopyrin EN-Tabs††‡

*Pregnancy Risk Category B*

## HOW SUPPLIED
*Tablets:* 500 mg with or without enteric coating

## ACTION
Unknown.

| Route | Onset | Peak | Duration |
|-------|-------|------|----------|
| P.O. | Unknown | 3-12 hr | Unknown |

## INDICATIONS & DOSAGE
*Mild to moderate ulcerative colitis, adjunctive therapy in severe ulcerative colitis, Crohn's disease—*
**Adults:** initially, 3 to 4 g P.O. daily in evenly divided doses; usual maintenance dose is 2 g P.O. daily in divided doses q 6 hours. Dosage may be started with 1 to 2 g, with gradual increase in dosage to minimize adverse effects.
**Children over age 2:** initially, 40 to 60 mg/kg P.O. daily, divided into three to six doses; then 30 mg/kg daily in four doses. Dosage may be started at lower dose if GI intolerance occurs.
*Rheumatoid arthritis in patients who have responded inadequately to salicylates or NSAIDs—*
**Adults:** 2 g P.O. daily in evenly divided doses. Dosage may be started at 0.5 to 1 g daily to reduce possible GI intolerance.

## ADVERSE REACTIONS
**CNS:** headache, depression, *seizures,* hallucinations.
**GI:** *nausea, vomiting, diarrhea,* abdominal pain, anorexia, stomatitis.
**GU:** *toxic nephrosis with oliguria and anuria,* crystalluria, hematuria, oligospermia, infertility.
**Hematologic:** *agranulocytosis,* aplastic anemia, megaloblastic anemia, *thrombocytopenia, leukopenia,* hemolytic anemia.

---

Reactions may be *common,* uncommon, *life-threatening,* or COMMON AND LIFE-THREATENING.

**Hepatic:** elevated liver function test results, jaundice, *hepatotoxicity.*
**Skin:** *erythema multiforme, Stevens-Johnson syndrome, generalized skin eruption,* epidermal necrolysis, **exfoliative dermatitis,** photosensitivity, urticaria, pruritus.
**Other:** *hypersensitivity reactions, serum sickness, drug fever, anaphylaxis.*

## INTERACTIONS
**Drug-drug.** *Antibiotics:* may alter action of sulfasalazine by altering internal flora. Monitor closely.
*Digoxin:* may reduce absorption of digoxin. Monitor closely.
*Folic acid:* absorption may be decreased. No intervention needed.
*Iron:* lowered blood levels of sulfasalazine caused by iron chelation. Monitor closely.
*Oral anticoagulants:* increased anticoagulant effect. Watch for bleeding.
*Oral antidiabetics:* increased hypoglycemic effect. Monitor blood glucose levels.
*Oral contraceptives:* decreased contraceptive effectiveness and increased risk of breakthrough bleeding. Suggest nonhormonal form of contraception.

## EFFECTS ON DIAGNOSTIC TESTS
Drug alters results of urine glucose tests that use cupric sulfate (Benedict's reagent or Clinitest).

## CONTRAINDICATIONS
Contraindicated in patients with hypersensitivity to drug or its metabolites, in those with porphyria or intestinal and urinary obstruction, and in children under age 2.

## NURSING CONSIDERATIONS
• Use cautiously and in reduced doses in patients with impaired hepatic or renal function, severe allergy, bronchial asthma, or G6PD deficiency.
• Although therapeutic response in rheumatoid arthritis has been noted as soon as 4 weeks after starting therapy, it may take 12 weeks of therapy before some patients show benefit.
• Drug colors alkaline urine orange-yellow.

• Administer drug with food to decrease GI irritation.
• *Alert:* Discontinue drug immediately and notify doctor if patient shows signs and symptoms of hypersensitivity.
• *Alert:* Don't confuse sulfasalazine with sulfisoxazole, salsalate, or sulfadiazine.

## ☑ Patient teaching
• Instruct patient to take drug after food intake and to space doses evenly.
• Warn patient to avoid ultraviolet light.
• Advise patient that drug may produce an orange-yellow discoloration of skin and urine.
• Instruct patient to notify doctor immediately if discoloration of skin or urine occurs.
• Advise patient to make sure fluid intake is adequate and to swallow tablets intact.

## tamsulosin hydrochloride
Flomax

*Pregnancy Risk Category B*

## HOW SUPPLIED
*Capsules:* 0.4 mg

## ACTION
Selectively blocks alpha receptors in the prostate, leading to relaxation of smooth muscles in the bladder neck and prostate, improving urine flow and reduction in symptoms of BPH.

| Route | Onset | Peak | Duration |
|-------|-------|------|----------|
| P.O. | Unknown | 4-5 hr | 9-15 hr |

## INDICATIONS AND DOSAGE
*BPH—*
**Adults:** 0.4 mg P.O. once daily, administered 30 minutes after same meal each day. If no response after 2 to 4 weeks, dose may be increased to 0.8 mg P.O. once daily.

## ADVERSE REACTIONS
**CNS:** asthenia, *dizziness, headache,* insomnia, somnolence, syncope, vertigo.
**CV:** chest pain, orthostatic hypotension.
**EENT:** amblyopia, pharyngitis, *rhinitis,* sinusitis.
**GI:** diarrhea, nausea, tooth disorder.

**GU:** abnormal ejaculation, decreased libido.
**Musculoskeletal:** back pain.
**Respiratory:** increased cough.
**Other:** *infection.*

## INTERACTIONS
**Drug-drug.** *Alpha blockers:* may interact with tamsulosin. Avoid concomitant use.
*Cimetidine:* decreased clearance of tamsulosin. Use with caution.

## EFFECTS ON DIAGNOSTIC TESTS
None reported.

## CONTRAINDICATIONS
Contraindicated in patients with hypersensitivity to drug or its components.

## NURSING CONSIDERATIONS
• Monitor patient for decreases in blood pressure.
• Symptoms of BPH and carcinoma of the prostate are similar; rule out carcinoma before starting therapy.
• If treatment is interrupted for several days or more, restart therapy at 1 capsule daily.
• *Alert:* Don't confuse Flomax with Fosamax.

### ☑ Patient teaching
• Instruct patient not to crush, chew, or open capsules.
• Tell patient to rise slowly from chair or bed during initiation of therapy and to avoid situations in which injury could occur as a result of syncope. Advise him that drug may cause sudden drop in blood pressure, especially after first dose or when changing doses.
• Instruct patient not to drive or perform hazardous tasks for 12 hours following initial dose or changes in dose until response can be monitored.
• Tell patient to take drug about 30 minutes after same meal each day.

# thalidomide
Thalomid

*Pregnancy Risk Category X*

## HOW SUPPLIED
*Capsules:* 50 mg

## ACTION
Exact mechanism unknown. An immunomodulatory drug.

| Route | Onset | Peak | Duration |
|-------|-------|------|----------|
| P.O. | Unknown | 3-6 hr | Unknown |

## INDICATIONS & DOSAGE
*Immediate treatment of cutaneous manifestations of moderate to severe erythema nodosum leprosum (ENL)—*
**Adults:** 100 to 300 mg P.O. daily h.s.
*Note:* If patient weighs below 50 kg (110 lb), start dosing at lower end of range.
*Maintenance therapy for prevention and suppression of cutaneous manifestations of ENL recurrence—*
**Adults:** up to 400 mg P.O. daily h.s. or in divided doses.

## ADVERSE REACTIONS
**CNS:** *asthenia, drowsiness, somnolence, dizziness,* peripheral neuropathy, *headache,* agitation, insomnia, malaise, nervousness, *paresthesia,* tremor, vertigo.
**CV:** orthostatic hypotension, ***bradycardia,*** peripheral edema.
**EENT:** dry mouth, oral candidiasis, pharyngitis, sinusitis.
**GI:** abdominal pain, anorexia, constipation, *diarrhea,* flatulence, *nausea.*
**GU:** albuminuria, *hematuria,* impotence.
**Hematologic:** ***neutropenia, increased HIV viral load,*** anemia, *lymphadenopathy,* LEUKOPENIA.
**Hepatic:** abnormal liver function test results, increased AST levels.
**Musculoskeletal:** back pain, neck pain or rigidity.
**Metabolic:** hyperlipidemia.
**Skin:** acne, fungal dermatitis, nail disorder, pruritus, *rash,* ***maculopapular rash,*** *sweating.*

---

Reactions may be *common,* uncommon, *life-threatening,* or COMMON AND LIFE-THREATENING.

**Other:** *human teratogenicity, hypersensitivity reactions,* facial edema, fever, chills, accidental injury, infection, pain.

## INTERACTIONS
**Drug-drug.** *Barbiturates, chlorpromazine, reserpine:* enhanced sedative activity. Use cautiously together.
*Drugs associated with peripheral neuropathy:* increased risk of peripheral neuropathy. Use cautiously together.
**Drug-food.** *Any food:* decreased absorption of drug. Take 1 hour after meals.
**Drug-lifestyle.** *Alcohol use:* increased sedation. Avoid concomitant use.

## EFFECTS ON DIAGNOSTIC TESTS
None reported.

## CONTRAINDICATIONS
Contraindicated in patients with hypersensitivity to drug or its components; in pregnant women; and in those capable of becoming pregnant, except when alternative therapies are inappropriate and patient meets all conditions listed in the System for Thalidomide Education and Prescribing Safety (S.T.E.P.S.) program.

## NURSING CONSIDERATIONS
• *Alert:* Administer drug only in compliance with all terms outlined in the S.T.E.P.S. program; drug may be prescribed and dispensed only by doctors and pharmacists registered with the S.T.E.P.S. program.
• All sexually mature patients (men and women) capable of reproduction must meet rigid S.T.E.P.S. program requirements, including ability to understand and carry out instructions, ability and willingness to comply with mandatory contraceptive measures (use of at least two highly effective means of contraception), and written acknowledgment of understanding of all warnings concerning hazards of fetal exposure to drug and risk of contraception failure.
• Sexually mature women who haven't undergone a hysterectomy or who haven't been postmenopausal for at least 24 consecutive months (that is, who have had menses at some time in preceding 24 consecutive months) are considered to be women of childbearing potential even with history of infertility.
• Perform mandatory pregnancy test within 24 hours before starting drug therapy in women of childbearing potential, then weekly during first month of therapy, then monthly for women with regular menstrual cycles. If menstrual cycles are irregular, pregnancy testing continues every 2 weeks during therapy. Retesting is performed if menstrual changes occur, including missed menses.
• Immediately report suspected fetal exposure to FDA via MedWATCH, at 1-800-FDA-1088, and to manufacturer.
• Corticosteroids may be administered concomitantly in patients with moderate to severe neuritis associated with severe ENL reaction. Corticosteroids can be tapered and discontinued when neuritis improves.
• Patient with history of requiring prolonged treatment to prevent recurrence of cutaneous ENL or who experiences flare during tapering, should use minimum effective dose. Tapering should be attempted every 3 to 6 months at dose reduction rate of 50 mg every 2 to 4 weeks.
• Perform WBC and differential before initiating therapy and periodically thereafter, as ordered. Patients with an absolute neutrophil count falling below 750/mm$^3$ during treatment should be reevaluated.
• Monitor patient for signs and symptoms of neuropathy at least once monthly during first 3 months of therapy, then periodically. If such symptoms as numbness, tingling, or pain in hands or feet occur, immediately notify doctor.

☑ **Patient teaching**
• Warn patient of dangers of fetal exposure to any amount of thalidomide. Ascertain that patient understands and follows the S.T.E.P.S. program.
• Stress that blood and sperm donations are prohibited during therapy.
• Explain that at least two highly reliable means of contraception must be used simultaneously and continuously from at least 1 month before initiation to 1 month after completion of therapy.
• Instruct patient to report signs or symptoms of pregnancy immediately without regard to chances of pregnancy.

---

*Liquid contains alcohol.   **May contain tartrazine.   †Canada   ‡Australia   §U.K.   ◇OTC

• Inform woman of childbearing potential of mandatory pregnancy testing schedule.
• Inform patient that, if pregnancy occurs, drug must be discontinued immediately.
• Caution patient that it isn't known whether drug is present in ejaculate of men receiving thalidomide, and that men receiving drug must always use a latex condom when engaging in sexual activity with women of childbearing potential.
• Advise patient to read package insert carefully.
• Instruct woman taking drugs (such as HIV-protease inhibitors, griseofulvin, rifampin, rifabutin, phenytoin, carbamazepine) that reduce the effect of hormonal contraceptive drugs to use two other effective means of contraception.
• Tell breast-feeding woman to discontinue breast-feeding during therapy.
• Stress importance of storing drug at room temperature, protected from light, and out of reach of children or others who may mistakenly take drug.
• Instruct patient to take drug only as prescribed.
• Caution patient against sharing drug with others, including those who also have a thalidomide prescription.
• Warn patient of potential for dizziness and orthostatic hypotension; instruct him to change position slowly when rising.
• Inform patient that drug frequently causes drowsiness and somnolence. Advise patient to avoid hazardous activities and alcohol or other drugs that might cause drowsiness.
• Tell patient to take drug at bedtime with glass of water, at least 1 hour after the evening meal.
• Teach patient signs and symptoms of peripheral neuropathy and to report their occurrence immediately.
• Tell patient to notify doctor if hypersensitivity reactions, such as erythematous macular rash, fever, tachycardia, and hypotension, or other adverse reactions occur.

---

# tiludronate disodium
Skelid

*Pregnancy Risk Category C*

## HOW SUPPLIED
*Tablets:* 240 mg (equivalent of 200 mg of tiludronic acid)

## ACTION
A bisphosphonate analogue. Thought to suppress bone resorption by reducing osteoclastic activity.

| Route | Onset | Peak | Duration |
|-------|-------|------|----------|
| P.O. | Unknown | 2 hr | Unknown |

## INDICATIONS & DOSAGE
*Paget's disease of bone in patients who have serum alkaline phosphatase level at least twice the upper limit of normal, who are symptomatic, or who are at risk for future complications of their disease—*
**Adults:** 400 mg P.O. once daily for 3 months, taken with full glass of plain water (6 to 8 oz) 2 hours before or after meals.

## ADVERSE REACTIONS
**CNS:** anxiety, dizziness, headache, insomnia, involuntary muscle contractions, paresthesia, somnolence, vertigo.
**CV:** chest pain, hypertension.
**EENT:** cataracts, conjunctivitis, glaucoma, pharyngitis, rhinitis, sinusitis.
**GI:** anorexia, constipation, diarrhea, dyspepsia, flatulence, gastritis, nausea, vomiting, dry mouth, tooth disorder.
**Metabolic:** vitamin D deficiency.
**Musculoskeletal:** arthralgia, arthrosis, back pain, *whole body pain.*
**Respiratory:** bronchitis, coughing.
**Skin:** pruritus, rash.
**Other:** edema, sweating, infection, hyperparathyroidism.

## INTERACTIONS
**Drug-drug.** *Aluminum antacids, calcium supplements, magnesium antacids:* may dramatically reduce bioavailability of tiludronate. Don't administer within 1 hour of each other.

---

Reactions may be *common,* uncommon, *life-threatening,* or COMMON AND LIFE-THREATENING.

*Aspirin:* may decrease bioavailability of tiludronate. Don't administer within 2 hours of drug.

*Indomethacin:* may increase bioavailability of tiludronate. Use cautiously; drug shouldn't be taken within 2 hours of indomethacin.

**Drug-food.** *Any food:* delayed drug absorption. Don't give within 2 hours of meals.

*Beverages other than plain water:* may reduce drug absorption. Don't give with drug.

**EFFECTS ON DIAGNOSTIC TESTS**
None reported.

**CONTRAINDICATIONS**
Contraindicated in patients with hypersensitivity to drug or its components and in those with severe renal failure (creatinine clearance below 30 ml/minute).

**NURSING CONSIDERATIONS**
• Use cautiously in patients with upper GI disease, such as dysphagia, esophagitis, esophageal ulcer, or gastric ulcer.
• Correct hypocalcemia and other disturbances of mineral metabolism (such as vitamin D deficiency) before initiating therapy.
• Administer drug for 3 months to assess response.
• It isn't known if drug appears in breast milk. Use caution when administering drug to breast-feeding women.

☑ **Patient teaching**
• Tell patient to take drug with 6 to 8 oz (180 to 240 ml) of plain water.
• Instruct patient that drug shouldn't be taken within 2 hours of food.
• Advise patient to maintain adequate vitamin D and calcium intake.
• Advise patient not to take calcium supplements, aspirin, or indomethacin within 2 hours of taking drug.
• Tell patient that antacids containing aluminum or magnesium can be taken 2 hours after taking drug.

## tolterodine tartrate
Detrol

*Pregnancy Risk Category C*

**HOW SUPPLIED**
*Tablets:* 1 mg, 2 mg

**ACTION**
A competitive muscarinic receptor antagonist. Both urinary bladder contraction and salivation are mediated via cholinergic muscarinic receptors.

| Route | Onset | Peak | Duration |
|-------|-------|------|----------|
| P.O. | Unknown | 1-2 hr | Unknown |

**INDICATIONS & DOSAGE**
*Overactive bladder in patients with symptoms of urinary frequency, urgency, or urge incontinence—*
**Adults:** 2 mg P.O. b.i.d. Dose may be lowered to 1 mg P.O. b.i.d. based on patient response and tolerance.
*Adjust-a-dose:* For adults with significantly reduced hepatic function or in those who are currently taking drug that inhibits cytochrome P-450 3A4 isoenzyme system, 1 mg P.O. b.i.d.

**ADVERSE REACTIONS**
**CNS:** *dry mouth,* fatigue, paresthesia, vertigo, dizziness, *headache,* nervousness, somnolence.
**CV:** hypertension, chest pain.
**EENT:** abnormal vision, xerophthalmia, pharyngitis, rhinitis, sinusitis.
**GI:** abdominal pain, constipation, diarrhea, dyspepsia, flatulence, nausea, vomiting.
**GU:** dysuria, micturition frequency, urine retention, urinary tract infection.
**Metabolic:** weight gain.
**Musculoskeletal:** arthralgia, back pain.
**Respiratory:** bronchitis, coughing, upper respiratory tract infection.
**Skin:** pruritus, rash, erythema, dry skin.
**Other:** flulike syndrome, falls, fungal infection, infection.

**INTERACTIONS**
**Drug-drug.** *Antifungal drugs (itraconazole, ketoconazole, miconazole), cyto-*

---

*chrome P-450 3A4 inhibitors (such as macrolide antibiotics [clarithromycin, erythromycin]):* effects haven't been studied. However, tolterodine doses above 1 mg b.i.d. shouldn't be given concurrently. *Fluoxetine:* increased tolterodine levels. Avoid concomitant use.

### EFFECTS ON DIAGNOSTIC TESTS
None reported.

### CONTRAINDICATIONS
Contraindicated in patients with hypersensitivity to drug or its components and in those with uncontrolled narrow-angle glaucoma or urine or gastric retention.

### NURSING CONSIDERATIONS
• Use with caution in patients with significant bladder outflow obstruction, GI obstructive disorders (such as pyloric stenosis), controlled narrow-angle glaucoma, and hepatic or renal impairment.
• Assess baseline bladder function and monitor therapeutic effects.
• Safety and effectiveness of drug in children haven't been established.

### ☑Patient teaching
• Tell patient that sugarless gum, hard candy, or saliva substitute may help relieve dry mouth.
• Advise patient to avoid driving or other potentially hazardous activities until visual effects of drug are known.
• Advise breast-feeding woman to discontinue breast-feeding during therapy.
• Instruct patient to immediately report signs of infection, urine retention, or GI problems.

---

## tretinoin (retinoic acid, vitamin A acid)
Renova, Retin-A, Stieva-A†

*Pregnancy Risk Category C*

### HOW SUPPLIED
*Cream:* 0.025%, 0.05%, 0.1%
*Gel:* 0.01%, 0.025%
*Solution:* 0.05%

### ACTION
Inhibits comedones by increasing epidermal cell mitosis and turnover.

| Route | Onset | Peak | Duration |
|-------|-------|------|----------|
| Topical | Unknown | Unknown | Unknown |

### INDICATIONS & DOSAGE
*Acne vulgaris—*
**Adults and children:** clean affected area and lightly apply once daily h.s.
*Adjunct therapy to skin care and sun avoidance program—*
**Adults:** apply to affected area once daily h.s.

### ADVERSE REACTIONS
**Skin:** *feeling of warmth, slight stinging,* local erythema, peeling, chapping, swelling, blistering, crusting, temporary hyperpigmentation or hypopigmentation.

### INTERACTIONS
**Drug-drug.** *Topical drugs containing resorcinol, salicylic acid, or sulfur:* increased risk of skin irritation. Don't use together.
*Topical minoxidil or photosensitizing drugs:* increased risk of skin irritation. Don't use together.
**Drug-lifestyle.** *Abrasive cleansers, medicated cosmetics, skin preparations containing alcohol:* increased risk of skin irritation. Don't use together.
*Sun exposure:* increased photosensitivity reactions. Avoid prolonged or unprotected exposure to sun.

### EFFECTS ON DIAGNOSTIC TESTS
None reported.

### CONTRAINDICATIONS
Contraindicated in patients with hypersensitivity to drug or its components.

### NURSING CONSIDERATIONS
• Use cautiously in patients with eczema.
• Relapses generally occur within 3 to 6 weeks after therapy is stopped.
• *Alert:* Don't confuse tretinoin with trientine.

---

Reactions may be *common,* uncommon, *life-threatening,* or COMMON AND LIFE-THREATENING.

### ✅ Patient teaching

• Instruct patient to clean area thoroughly before application and to avoid getting drug in eyes, mouth, or mucous membranes.

• Tell patient to wash face with mild soap no more than b.i.d. or t.i.d. Warn patient against using strong or medicated cosmetics, soaps, or other skin cleansers. Also advise him to avoid topical products containing alcohol, astringents, spices, and lime because they may interfere with drug's actions.

• Tell patient that normal use of cosmetics is allowed.

• Advise patient not to discontinue drug if transient exacerbation of inflammatory lesions occurs. If severe local irritation develops, advise patient to discontinue drug temporarily and notify doctor. Dosage will be readjusted when application is resumed. Some redness and scaling are normal reactions.

• Warn patient that he may experience increased sensitivity to wind or cold temperatures.

• Instruct patient to minimize exposure to sunlight or ultraviolet rays during treatment. If he becomes sunburned, he should delay therapy until sunburn subsides. Tell patient who can't avoid exposure to sunlight to use SPF-15 sunblock and to wear protective clothing.

• Warn patient that he may have a temporary increase in lesions, which will improve in 2 to 3 weeks.

aloe
angelica
bilberry
capsicum
cat's-claw
chamomile
echinacea
eucalyptus
fennel
feverfew
flax
garlic
ginger
ginkgo
ginseng
goldenseal
grapeseed; pinebark
kava
milk thistle
nettle
passion flower
primrose, evening
saw palmetto
St. John's wort
valerian

---

### aloe
aloe vera, Barbados aloe, Cape aloe, Curacao aloe, lily of the desert

#### COMMON FORMS
Available in capsules or as cream, hair conditioner, gel, juice, liniment, lotion, ointment, shampoo, skin cream, soap, sunscreen, and in facial tissues. Also as an ingredient in Benzoin Compound Tincture.
*Capsules:* 75 mg, 100 mg, 200 mg aloe vera extract or aloe vera powder
*Gel:* 98%, 99.5%, 99.6% aloe vera gel
*Juice:* 99.6%, 99.7% aloe vera juice

#### ACTION
When taken internally, aloin produces a metabolite that irritates the large intestines and stimulates colonic activity. It also causes active secretion of fluids and electrolytes and inhibits reabsorption of fluids from the colon, resulting in a feeling of distention and increased peristalsis. The cathartic effect occurs 8 to 12 hours after ingestion.

When applied externally, besides acting as a moisturizer on burns and other wounds, aloe reduces inflammation. Antipruritic effect may result from blockage of the conversion of histidine to histamine. Wound healing may result from increased blood flow to the wound area.

#### USES
Used externally as a topical gel for minor burns, sunburn, cuts, frostbite, skin irritation, and other wounds and abrasions.

Used internally as a stimulant laxative. Also used to treat amenorrhea, asthma, colds, seizures, bleeding, and ulcers.

Aloe products also used to treat acne, AIDS, arthritis, asthma, blindness, bursitis, cancer, colitis, depression, diabetes, glaucoma, hemorrhoids, multiple sclerosis, peptic ulcers, and varicose veins.

#### DOSAGE
*Pruritus, skin irritation, burns, other wounds (external forms)—*
Applied liberally, p.r.n. Although internal use isn't recommended, some sources suggest 100 to 200 mg aloe or 50 to 100 mg aloe extract P.O., taken in the evening. Information about dosages for aloe juice is lacking.

#### ADVERSE REACTIONS
**GI:** painful intestinal spasms, damage to intestinal mucosa that may be irreversible, harmless brown discoloration of intestinal mucous membranes, severe hemorrhagic diarrhea.
**GU:** *kidney damage,* red discoloration of urine with frequent use; reflex stimulation of uterine musculature possibly causing spontaneous abortion or premature birth during late pregnancy.
**Metabolic:** fluid and electrolyte loss with frequent use, loss of potassium from in-

---

testine, leading to reduced serum potassium level.

**Skin:** contact dermatitis, delayed healing of deep wounds with topical use.

**Other:** accumulation of blood in the pelvic region, with large doses; *death from overdose.*

## INTERACTIONS

**Herb-drug.** *Antiarrhythmics, cardiac glycosides, corticosteroids, loop diuretics, thiazides, other potassium-wasting drugs:* increased effects when aloe used internally. Avoid internal use of aloe when taking these drugs.

## CONTRAINDICATIONS

External aloe products contraindicated in patients with hypersensitivity to aloe and in those with history of allergic reactions to plants in the Liliaceae family (such as garlic, onions, and tulips).

Internal use contraindicated in menstruating, pregnant, or breast-feeding women, in children, and in patients with cardiac or kidney disease.

## NURSING CONSIDERATIONS

• Oral use can cause severe abdominal discomfort and serious hypokalemia and electrolyte imbalance.

• Internal use can cause hypokalemia and disturbance of cardiac rhythm.

• Unapproved use of aloe vera injections for cancer has been associated with death.

• Injectable aloe vera products or chemical constituents of aloe vera aren't recommended.

☑ **Patient teaching**

• Caution patient against use of aloe vera gel or aloe vera juice for internal use.

---

### angelica

angelica root, angelique, dong quai, garden angelica, tang-kuei, wild angelica

## COMMON FORMS

Available as fluid extract, tincture, essential oil, or cut, dried, or powdered root.

## ACTION

Root extracts may have antitumor properties; may also have anti-inflammatory and analgesic actions.

Isolated substances extracted from the root inhibit platelet aggregation, exert antimicrobial action, and decrease myocardial injury and risk of PVCs and arrhythmias induced by myocardial reperfusion.

## USES

Used to treat gynecologic disorders, postmenopausal symptoms, menstrual discomfort, regulation of the menstrual cycle, and anemia. Also used to treat headaches and backaches, improve circulation in the extremities, and relieve osteoporosis, hay fever, asthma, and eczema.

## DOSAGE

No consensus exists.

## ADVERSE REACTIONS

**CV:** hypotension.
**Skin:** photodermatitis, phototoxicity.

## INTERACTIONS

**Herb-drug.** *Heparin:* increased risk of bleeding. Avoid concomitant use.
*Warfarin:* significantly prolonged PT when used with warfarin. Avoid concomitant use.

## CONTRAINDICATIONS

Contraindicated in pregnant or breast-feeding women because of potential stimulant effects on the uterus.

## NURSING CONSIDERATIONS

• Use cautiously in diabetic patients because various species of this plant contain polysaccharides that may disrupt blood glucose level control.

• Watch for signs of bleeding in patients taking angelica—especially those already receiving anticoagulants.

• Improved pulmonary function and decreased mean arterial pulmonary pressures occurred when angelica compounds were used with nifedipine in patients with COPD and pulmonary hypertension.

☑ **Patient teaching**

• Advise patient that use of herb poses a cancer risk.

• Warn patient to watch for signs of allergic reactions to herb and to report such reactions promptly to doctor.
• Advise patient to take precautions against direct sun exposure while taking angelica products.

## bilberry
bilberries, bog bilberries, European blueberries, huckleberries, whortleberries

### COMMON FORMS
*Capsules:* 60 mg, 80 mg, 120 mg, 450 mg. Also available in liquid, tincture, fluid extract, and dried root, leaves, and berries.

### ACTION
Herb may reduce vascular permeability and tissue edema. Also may aid blood flow. It exerts potent antioxidant effects and a protective effect on low-density lipoproteins.

Chemical components of bilberry may exert changes in the retina, allowing better adaptation to darkness and light, decrease excessive platelet aggregation, and exert preventative and curative antiulcer actions.

### USES
Used to treat visual and circulatory problems, glaucoma, cataracts, diabetic retinopathy, macular degeneration, varicose veins, and hemorrhoids. Also used to improve night vision.

### DOSAGE
Suggested doses vary considerably. Most herbalists recommend using standardized products consisting of 25% anthocyanoside content.
*To improve night vision—*
60 to 120 mg of bilberry extract P.O. daily.
*Visual and circulatory problems—*
240 to 480 mg P.O. daily in two or three divided doses.

### ADVERSE REACTIONS
**Other:** *toxic reactions.*

*Note:* Long-term consumption of large doses of bilberry leaves can be poisonous. Doses of 1.5 g/kg/day or more may be fatal.

### INTERACTIONS
**Herb-drug.** *Anticoagulants, other antiplatelet drugs:* inhibition of platelet aggregation, potentially enhancing risk of bleeding if used concurrently. Monitor patient. *Disulfiram:* disulfiram reaction if patient takes form containing alcohol. Avoid concurrent use.

### CONTRAINDICATIONS
Contraindicated in pregnant and breast-feeding women.

### NURSING CONSIDERATIONS
• Use cautiously in patients taking anticoagulants.
• Monitor for signs and symptoms of bleeding if patient is taking an anticoagulant.

### ☑Patient teaching
• Warn patient taking disulfiram not to take bilberry product containing alcohol.

## capsicum
bell pepper, capsaicin, cayenne pepper, chili pepper, hot pepper, paprika, red pepper, tabasco pepper

### COMMON FORMS
*Cream:* 0.025%, 0.075%, 0.25%
*Gel:* 0.025%
*Lotion:* 0.025%, 0.075%
*Roll-on:* 0.075%
*Self-defense spray:* 5%, 10%
Also available as the vegetable, pepper.

### ACTION
Topical capsicum produces an extremely intense irritation at the contact point. Initial dose causes profound pain; however, repeated applications cause desensitization, with anti-inflammatory and analgesic effects.

Juices from the fruits may have antibacterial properties in vitro.

### USES
Used to treat bowel disorders, chronic laryngitis, and peripheral vascular disease. Various preparations of capsicum are applied topically as counterirritants and ex-

---

Reactions may be *common*, uncommon, *life-threatening*, or COMMON AND LIFE-THREATENING.

ternal analgesics. Topical products also used to treat pain associated with postherpetic neuralgia, rheumatoid arthritis, osteoarthritis, diabetic neuropathy, postsurgical pain (including postmastectomy and postamputation pain), and other neuropathic pain and complex pain syndromes. Also used to treat refractory pruritus and pruritus associated with renal failure, and as a nonlethal self-defense spray.

## DOSAGE
Concentrations of topical products range from 0.025% to 0.25%. Preparations are most effective when applied t.i.d. or q.i.d. and have a duration of action of about 4 to 6 hours. Applications given less frequently typically result in incomplete analgesia.

## ADVERSE REACTIONS
**EENT:** blepharospasm, extreme burning pain, lacrimation, conjunctival edema, hyperemia, burning pain in nose, sneezing, serous discharge. (Ocular complications are rare and are usually due to eye rubbing.)
**GI:** discomfort that is minimized if seeds are removed before ingestion.
**Respiratory:** transient bronchoconstriction, cough, retrosternal discomfort.
**Skin:** transient skin irritation, itching, stinging, erythema without vesicular eruption that diminish with repeated use.

## INTERACTIONS
**Herb-drug.** *Centrally acting adrenergics:* may reduce effectiveness of antihypertensives, such as clonidine or methyldopa. Avoid concomitant use.
*MAO inhibitors:* may promote toxicity (hypertensive crisis) when used together. Avoid concomitant use.

## CONTRAINDICATIONS
Contraindicated in patients with hypersensitivity to capsicum or chili pepper products. Also contraindicated in pregnant women.

## NURSING CONSIDERATIONS
• Don't use herb in pregnant women because of possible uterine stimulant effects.
• Intensity of adverse reactions is dose-related and concentration-dependent.

• After topical application, relief occurs as early as 3 days, but may take as long as 14 to 28 days, depending on condition requiring analgesia.
• Evidence that topical application causes permanent neurologic injury is lacking.

### ☑ Patient teaching
• Tell patient to avoid contact with eyes, mucous membranes, and broken skin.
• If incidental contact occurs, inform patient to flush exposed area with cool running water for as long as necessary.
• Caution patient taking MAO inhibitors or centrally acting adrenergic against use of this herb.
• Advise a woman to avoid use of herb during pregnancy or when breast-feeding.

## cat's-claw
life-giving vine of Peru, samento, una de gato

## COMMON FORMS
Available in tablets and capsules; also as teas or tinctures and the cut, dried, or powdered bark, roots, and leaves.
*Tablets, capsules:* 25 mg, 150 mg, 175 mg, 300 mg, 350 mg (standard extract); 400 mg, 500 mg, 800 mg, 1 g, 5 g (raw herb)

## ACTION
Some chemical components stimulate immune system function and exert antitumor activity. Other components may inhibit platelet aggregation and the sympathetic nervous system, reduce the heart rate, decrease peripheral vascular resistance, and lower blood pressure. They also may exhibit antiviral activity and antioxidant properties in vitro. One component has weak diuretic properties.

## USES
Used to treat systemic inflammatory diseases, such as arthritis and rheumatism, and inflammatory GI disorders, such as diverticulitis, gastritis, Crohn's disease, dysentery, and ulcerations. Also used as a contraceptive.

## DOSAGE
No consensus exists. Herbalists recommend 500 to 1,000 mg P.O. t.i.d.

## ADVERSE REACTIONS
**CV:** potential hypotension.

## INTERACTIONS
**Herb-drug.** *Antihypertensives:* may potentiate effects. Avoid concomitant use.

## CONTRAINDICATIONS
Contraindicated in patients undergoing skin grafts and organ transplants and in those with coagulation disorders or receiving anticoagulants.

## NURSING CONSIDERATIONS
• Monitor patient for signs of bleeding, such as petechiae or epistaxis, unusual bruising, or bleeding gums.
• Avoid use of herb in pregnant or breast-feeding women; effects are unknown.

### ☑ Patient teaching
• Recommend another method of contraception if herb is being used for this purpose.
• Tell patient to rise slowly from a sitting or lying position to avoid dizziness from possible hypotension.
• Advise patient to watch for signs of bleeding, especially if anticoagulants are also being taken.
• Advise a woman to avoid use of herb during pregnancy or when breast-feeding.

---

## chamomile
common chamomile, English chamomile, German chamomile, Hungarian chamomile, sweet false chamomile

## COMMON FORMS
Available as capsules, liquid, tea, and in many cosmetic products.
*Capsules:* 354 mg, 360 mg

## ACTION
Herb exhibits anti-inflammatory, antiallergenic, antidiuretic, sedative, antibacterial, and antifungal properties. It may lower serum urea levels. Some compounds may stimulate liver regeneration following oral administration; others exhibit in vitro antitumor activity. One component may have antiulcer effects.

## USES
Used to treat stomach disorders, such as GI spasms and other GI inflammatory conditions, insomnia, menstrual disorders, migraine, epidermolysis bullosa, eczema, eye irritation, throat discomfort, and hemorrhoids. Also used as a topical bacteriostat, sleep inducer, and mouthwash.

## DOSAGE
Usually taken as a tea, prepared by adding 3 g (1 tablespoon) of the flower head to hot water and steeping for 10 to 15 minutes; it's then taken up to q.i.d.

## ADVERSE REACTIONS
**EENT:** allergic conjunctivitis.
**GI:** emesis.
**Skin:** contact dermatitis.
**Other:** *anaphylaxis.*

## INTERACTIONS
**Herb-drug.** *Anticoagulants:* may potentiate effects. Avoid concomitant use.
*Other drugs taken concurrently:* potential for decreased absorption of these drugs secondary to chamomile's antispasmodic activity in GI tract. Avoid concomitant use.

## CONTRAINDICATIONS
Avoid use in pregnant or breast-feeding women. Chamomile is believed to be an abortifacient, and some of its components have shown teratogenic effects.

## NURSING CONSIDERATIONS
• Monitor patient for allergic reactions.
• Use cautiously in patients with hypersensitivity to components of volatile oils and in those at risk for contact dermatitis.

### ☑ Patient teaching
• Caution patient with history of allergies against use of this herb.
• Advise a woman to avoid use of herb during pregnancy or when breast-feeding.

---

Reactions may be *common,* uncommon, *life-threatening,* or COMMON AND LIFE-THREATENING.

## echinacea
American cone flower, black sampson, black susans, coneflower, echinacea care liquid, Indian head

### COMMON FORMS
Available as capsules and tablets; also as hydroalcoholic extracts, fresh-pressed juice, glycerite, lozenges, and tinctures.
*Capsules:* 125 mg, 355 mg (85 mg herbal extract powder), 500 mg
*Tablets:* 335 mg

### ACTION
Herb extract stimulates the immune system and reduces growth of bacteria responsible for vaginal infections. Components may exert local anesthetic effects and anti-inflammatory activities. Essential oil components produce a tingling sensation on the tongue. Some compounds also exhibit direct antitumor activity and defense against infectious diseases. Conjugates in the plant activate adrenal cortex activity. The fresh-pressed juice of the aerial portion and the extract of the roots may inhibit influenza, herpes infections, and vesicular stomatitis virus.

### USES
Used as a wound-healing agent for abscesses, burns, eczema, varicose ulcers of the leg and other skin wounds, and as a nonspecific immunostimulant for the supportive treatment of upper respiratory and urinary tract infections.

### DOSAGE
*Expressed juice:* 6 to 9 ml P.O. daily. *Capsules containing powdered herb:* equivalent to 900 mg to 1 g P.O. t.i.d.; doses can vary. *Tincture:* 0.75 to 1.5 ml (15 to 30 gtt) P.O. two to five times daily. The tincture has been given as 60 gtt P.O. t.i.d. *Tea:* 4 g (2 teaspoons) of coarsely powdered herb simmered in 240 ml (1 cup) of boiling water for 10 minutes. Avoid this method of administration because some active compounds are water-insoluble.

### ADVERSE REACTIONS
Adverse effects are uncommon. Allergic reactions may occur in patients allergic to plants belonging to the daisy family.

### INTERACTIONS
None significant.

### CONTRAINDICATIONS
Contraindicated in patients with severe illness, such as HIV infection, collagen disease, leukosis, multiple sclerosis, and tuberculosis or other autoimmune diseases.

### NURSING CONSIDERATIONS
• Avoid use of herb in pregnant or breast-feeding women; effects are unknown.
• Many tinctures contain significant concentrations of alcohol (from 15% to 90%) and may not be suitable for children, alcoholic patients, those with liver disease, or those taking disulfiram or metronidazole.
• Watch for immune suppression in patients who have used herb excessively.

### ☑ Patient teaching
• Advise patient taking herb for prolonged time that overstimulation of immune system and possible immune system suppression may occur. Echinacea shouldn't be used for more than 8 weeks; therapy lasting 10 to 14 days is probably sufficient.
• Advise patient not to delay treatment for an illness that doesn't resolve after taking herb.
• Advise a woman to avoid use of herb during pregnancy or when breast-feeding.

## eucalyptus
fever tree, gum tree, Tasmanian blue gum

### COMMON FORMS
Available as an oil, lotion and a fluid extract.

### ACTION
Herb produces a stimulant effect on nasal cold receptors. Acts as a counterirritant and causes an increase in cutaneous blood flow. It also exhibits antimicrobial, antifungal, and anti-inflammatory effects.

## USES
Used to relieve nasal congestion.

## DOSAGE
*Various uses—*
Typical oral dosages include 0.05 to
0.2 ml (eucalyptol), 0.05 to 0.2 ml (eucalyptus oil), or 2 to 4 g (fluid extract).
*Topical use—*
30 ml oil mixed with 500 ml water.

## ADVERSE REACTIONS
**CNS:** delirium, dizziness, *seizures.*
**EENT:** miosis.
**GI:** epigastric burning, nausea, vomiting.
**Musculoskeletal:** muscular weakness.
**Respiratory:** cyanosis.

## INTERACTIONS
None significant.

## CONTRAINDICATIONS
Eucalyptus oil is contraindicated in patients receiving hypoglycemic therapy and
in pregnant or breast-feeding women.

## NURSING CONSIDERATIONS
• Watch for adverse reactions, and institute seizure precautions where appropriate.

☑ **Patient teaching**
• Instruct patient to dilute herb before internal or external use.
• Advise patient to keep herb away from
children and pets.
• Advise a woman to avoid use of herb
during pregnancy or when breast-feeding.

---

## fennel
bitter fennel, carosella, common
fennel, fenchel, fenouil, fenouille,
sweet fennel

## COMMON FORMS
*Volatile oil in water:* 2% (sweet fennel),
4% (bitter fennel)

## ACTION
Herb may exhibit stimulant and antiflatu-
lent properties. Fennel oil with methyl-
paraben inhibits the growth of *Salmonella*

*enteritidis* and, to a lesser extent, *Listeria monocytogenes.*

## USES
Used to increase milk secretion, promote
menses, facilitate birth, and increase libido.

## DOSAGE
*GI complaints—*
Herbalists recommend 0.1 to 0.6 ml P.O. of
the oil daily, or 5 to 7 g of the fruit daily.

## ADVERSE REACTIONS
**CNS:** *seizures.*
**GI:** nausea, vomiting.
**Skin:** contact dermatitis, photodermatitis.
**Other:** potential for tumors.

## INTERACTIONS
None significant.

## CONTRAINDICATIONS
Avoid use of herb in pregnant women.

## NURSING CONSIDERATIONS
• Use cautiously in patients allergic to
other members of the Umbelliferae family, such as celery, carrots, or mugwort.
• Monitor patient for allergic reactions.

☑ **Patient teaching**
• Inform patient that herb can't be recommended for any use because of insufficient evidence.
• Remind patient that risks of herb's long-
term use are unknown.
• Advise patient to avoid sun exposure if
photodermatitis occurs.
• Advise a woman to avoid use of herb
during pregnancy or when breast-feeding.

---

## feverfew
altamisa, bachelor's button,
chamomile grande, featherfew,
featherfoil, midsummer daisy

## COMMON FORMS
Available as capsules, liquid, and tablets.
The leaves are commonly used to make
infusions or teas.
*Capsules:* 250 mg (leaf extract), 380 mg
(pure leaf)

---

## ACTION

Herb's main active ingredients may inhibit serotonin release by human platelets. Extracts of feverfew contain chemicals that inhibit activation of leukocytes and the synthesis of leukotrienes and prostaglandins.

## USES

Used as an antipyretic and to treat psoriasis, toothache, insect bites, rheumatism, asthma, stomachache, menstrual problems, and threatened miscarriage. Also used for migraine prophylaxis.

## DOSAGE

*Treatment of migraine—*
Average dosage: 543 mcg P.O. parthenolide (a component of feverfew) daily.
*Migraine prophylaxis—*
25 mg of freeze-dried leaf extract P.O. daily, or 50 mg of leaf P.O. daily with food, or 50 to 200 mg of aerial parts of plant P.O. daily.

## ADVERSE REACTIONS

**GI:** mouth ulcerations commonly with crude herb.
**Other:** *hypersensitivity reactions,* post–feverfew syndrome (moderate to severe pain and joint and muscle stiffness).

## INTERACTIONS

None significant.

## CONTRAINDICATIONS

Contraindicated in pregnant or breast-feeding women.

## NURSING CONSIDERATIONS

• Monitor patient for allergic reaction.
• Monitor for mouth ulcerations. Encourage proper oral hygiene.
• Feverfew potency is frequently based on parthenolide content in product, which is variable.

### ☑ Patient teaching

• Instruct patient not to withdraw herb abruptly, but to taper its use gradually because of risk of post–feverfew syndrome.
• Assure patient that several other strategies for migraine treatment and prophylaxis exist and that these should be attempted before taking products with unknown benefits and risks.
• Remind patient to promptly report unusual signs and symptoms, such as mouth sores or skin ulcerations.

---

## flax
flaxseed, linseed, lint bells, linum

## COMMON FORMS

Available as a powder, capsules, softgel capsules, and an oil.
*Capsules (softgel):* 1,000 mg

## ACTION

Herb decreases total cholesterol and low-density lipoprotein levels. It may decrease thrombin-mediated platelet aggregation. Flax contains lignans, which may have weak estrogenic, antiestrogenic, and corticosteroid-like activity. Diets high in flax may lower risk of breast and other hormone-dependent cancers. Linolenic acid supplement, derived from flax, arginine, and yeast RNA, may improve weight gain in some patients with HIV.

## USES

Used to treat constipation, functional disorders of the colon resulting from laxative abuse, irritable bowel syndrome, and diverticulitis. Also used as a supplement to decrease risk of hypercholesterolemia and atherosclerosis. Flax has been made into a poultice and used to treat areas of local inflammation.

## DOSAGE

*All systemic uses—*
15 to 30 ml of oil or mature seeds daily in two or three divided doses. Average dose is 30 ml of oil or mature seeds daily.
*Topical use—*
30 to 50 g of flax meal applied as a hot, moist poultice or compress, p.r.n.

## ADVERSE REACTIONS

**GI:** diarrhea, flatulence, nausea.
**Other:** symptoms of overdose, such as shortness of breath, tachypnea, weakness, and unstable gait, progressing to paralysis and *seizures.*

## INTERACTIONS
**Herb-drug.** *Laxatives, stool softeners:* possible increase in laxative actions of flax. Avoid concurrent use.
*Oral drugs:* possible diminished absorption of oral drugs. Avoid taking flax and other drugs concurrently.

## CONTRAINDICATIONS
Contraindicated in pregnant and breast-feeding women. Avoid use in patients with suspected or actual ileus or prostate cancer.

## NURSING CONSIDERATIONS
• Don't use in pregnant or breast-feeding women because herb's hormonal effects may cause teratogenicity or spontaneous abortion.
• Monitor patient for potential toxicity related to oral ingestion of herb; cyanosis is a symptom of flax toxicity.
• Immature seedpods are especially poisonous.

### ☑ Patient teaching
• Encourage patient to drink plenty of fluids to minimize risk of flatulence.
• Instruct patient to refrigerate flaxseed oil to prevent breakdown of essential fatty acids.
• Remind patient that other cholesterol-lowering therapies exist that have been proven to improve survival and lower risk of cardiac disease; flax has no such clinical support.
• Instruct patient never to ingest immature seeds and to keep flax away from children and pets.
• Remind patient that risks of taking flax on long-term basis are unknown.
• Tell patient to report decreased effects of other drugs being taken.

---

## garlic
allium, camphor of the poor, da-suan, la-suan, nectar of the gods, poor man's treacle, stinking rose

## COMMON FORMS
Available as tablets, fresh bulb, antiseptic oil, fresh extract, powdered garlic, freeze-dried garlic powder, and garlic oil (essential oil).

*Tablets (garlic extract):* 100 mg, 320 mg, 400 mg, 600 mg
*Tablets (allicin total potential):* 2 to 5 mg
*Dried powder:* 400 to 1,200 mg
*Fresh bulb:* 2 to 5 g

## ACTION
Garlic may exhibit antithrombotic, lipid-lowering, cholesterol-lowering, antitumor, and antimicrobial effects. It may have hypoglycemic activity and hypotensive properties as well as antibacterial, antifungal, larvicidal, insecticidal, amebicidal, and antiviral activities. A component in garlic oil may inhibit adenosine diphosphate–induced platelet aggregation. It also may decrease a type of carcinogen and nitrite accumulation.

## USES
Used to treat asthma, diabetes, inflammation, heavy metal poisoning, constipation, and athlete's foot and to improve serum lipid profiles in some patients and reduce morbidity in patients with AIDS. Also used as an antimicrobial.

## DOSAGE
*Lipid-lowering action—*
600 to 900 mg daily, or average of 4 g (fresh garlic) or 8 mg (garlic oil) daily.

## ADVERSE REACTIONS
**CNS:** dizziness.
**GI:** nausea, vomiting, irritation of mouth, esophagus, and stomach.
**Hematologic:** decreased hemoglobin production and lysis of RBCs with chronic use or excessive doses.
**Respiratory:** asthma.
**Skin:** contact dermatitis, diaphoresis, hypothyroidism, rash.
**Other:** garlic odor.

## INTERACTIONS
**Herb-drug.** *Anticoagulants:* may increase risk of bleeding when used concomitantly. Monitor patient.
*Antiplatelets:* may enhance effects of antiplatelet therapy. Monitor patient.

## CONTRAINDICATIONS
Contraindicated in patients sensitive to garlic or other members of the Lilaceae

---

Reactions may be *common*, uncommon, *life-threatening*, or COMMON AND LIFE-THREATENING.

family and in those with GI disorders, such as peptic ulcer or reflux disease. Also contraindicated in pregnant women.

## NURSING CONSIDERATIONS
• Don't give to pregnant women because of herb's oxytocic effects.
• Perform periodic CBCs on patients taking garlic in high doses or using herb long-term.

### ✓ Patient teaching
• Advise patient that cholesterol-lowering drugs are commonly used for hypercholesterolemia because of their proven survival data and ability to lower cholesterol levels more effectively than garlic.
• Instruct patient to watch for signs of bleeding (bleeding gums, easy bruising, tarry stools, petechiae) if garlic supplements are taken with hemostatic drugs.
• Remind patient to report such symptoms as burning of the mouth or gums, recurring heartburn, chest pain, or stomach ulcer–like pain.
• Tell patient that, although rare, cases of anaphylaxis have been reported.

## ginger
zingiber

### COMMON FORMS
Available as root, extract, liquid, powder, capsules, tablets, and teas.
*Root:* 530 mg
*Extract:* 250 mg
*Liquid, powder, capsules:* 100 mg, 465 mg
*Tablets (chewable):* 67.5 mg

### ACTION
Ginger inhibits platelet aggregation induced by adenosine diphosphate and epinephrine. It may exhibit positive inotropic and anti-inflammatory effects. Specific components of ginger produce varying CV effects.

### USES
Used as an antiemetic, GI protectant, anti-inflammatory for arthritis treatment, CV stimulant, antitumor drug, and antioxidant, and for microbial and parasitic infestations. Also used to treat morning, motion, or sea sickness and postoperative nausea and vomiting, and to provide relief from pain and swelling due to rheumatoid arthritis, osteoarthritis, or muscular discomfort.

### DOSAGE
Dosage forms and strengths vary with each disease state.
*As an antiemetic—*
500 to 1,000 mg powdered ginger P.O., or 1,000 mg fresh ginger root P.O.

### ADVERSE REACTIONS
**CNS:** CNS depression with overdose.
**CV:** *arrhythmias* with overdose.

### INTERACTIONS
**Herb-drug.** *Anticoagulants:* may enhance risk of bleeding. Monitor patient.

### CONTRAINDICATIONS
Contraindicated in pregnant women; effects are unknown.

### NURSING CONSIDERATIONS
• Use only under medical supervision in patients receiving anticoagulants because ginger may affect bleeding time by inhibiting platelet function.
• Monitor patient for bleeding.

### ✓ Patient teaching
• Advise a woman to avoid use of ginger during pregnancy.
• Instruct patient to watch for signs and symptoms of bleeding when taking ginger.
• Explain that no consensus exists with respect to dosing and monitoring.

## ginkgo
EGB 761, GBE, GBE 24, GBX, ginkgo biloba, ginkogink, LI 1370, rokan, sophium, tanakan, tebonin

### COMMON FORMS
Available as ginkgo biloba extract in capsules, tablets, and sublingual sprays (standardized to contain 24% flavone glycosides and 6% terpenes) and as concentrated alcoholic extract of fresh leaf.

*Tablets, capsules:* 30 mg, 40 mg, 60 mg, 120 mg, 260 mg, 420 mg
*Capsules (ginkgo biloba extract [24% standardized extract] bound to phosphatidylcholine):* 80 mg
*Sublingual sprays:* 15 mg/spray, 40 mg/spray

## ACTION
Herb produces arterial vasodilation and arterial and venous vasoactive changes that increase tissue perfusion and cerebral blood flow. It inhibits arterial spasms, decreases capillary permeability and blood viscosity, and reduces capillary fragility and erythrocyte aggregation. Ginkgo biloba extract acts as an antioxidant, and ginkgolide B (a component of gingko) may be a potent inhibitor of platelet activating factor.

## USES
Used to treat cerebrovascular disease, peripheral vascular insufficiency, arrhythmias, asthma, impotence secondary to serotonin reuptake inhibitors, premenstrual syndrome, senile macular degeneration, hearing loss, and vestibular disorders. Also used to improve mental alertness and overall brain function.

## DOSAGE
*Dementia syndromes—*
120 to 240 mg P.O. daily in two or three divided doses.
*Peripheral arterial disease, vertigo, tinnitus—*
120 to 160 mg P.O. daily in two or three divided doses.

## ADVERSE REACTIONS
**CNS:** headache; *seizures in children following ingestion of more than 50 seeds.*
**GI:** diarrhea, flatulence, nausea, vomiting.
**Skin:** *contact hypersensitivity reactions;* dermatitis if contact with fruit occurs.

## INTERACTIONS
**Herb-drug.** *Anticoagulants, antiplatelets:* inhibits platelet activating factor. Use ginkgo biloba extract with careful monitoring in patients taking anticoagulants or antiplatelets.

## CONTRAINDICATIONS
Contraindicated in patients with history of allergy to ginkgo products. Also contraindicated in children and pregnant women.

## NURSING CONSIDERATIONS
● Use cautiously in patients taking anticoagulants.
● Monitor patient for bleeding or unusual bruising.
● Fruit pulp and seed coats contain ginkgolic acid and bilobin, which are structurally related to the urushiols found in poison ivy, mango fruit rind, and cashew nut shells.

### ☑ Patient teaching
● Advise patient to report unusual bleeding or bruising.
● Instruct patient to keep seeds out of reach of children because of potential risk of seizures with ingestion.
● Advise patient to avoid contact with the fruit pulp or seed coats because of the risk of contact dermatitis. More potent preparations may cause irritation or blistering of skin or mucous membranes if applied externally.

## ginseng
American ginseng, Asiatic ginseng, Chinese ginseng, G115, Japanese ginseng, jintsam, Korean ginseng

## COMMON FORMS
Available as capsules, teas, extract, root powder, whole root (by the pound), and oil.
*Capsules:* 100 mg, 250 mg, 500 mg
*Tea bags:* 1,500 mg ginseng root
*Extract:* 2-oz root extract (in alcohol base)
*Root powder:* 1 oz, 4 oz

## ACTION
Ginseng compounds may exert opposing effects. For example, one compound has CNS-depressant, anticonvulsant, analgesic, and antipsychotic effects and stress-ulcer preventing action. Another compound has CNS-stimulating, anti-

fatigue, hypertensive, and stress-ulcer aggravating effects. Some components enhance cardiac performance, whereas others depress cardiac function.

Oral ginseng may reduce cholesterol and triglyceride levels, decrease platelet adhesiveness, impair coagulation, and increase fibrinolysis. It may also reduce stress by acting on the adrenal gland.

Extracts of ginseng may exhibit antioxidant activity.

## USES

Used to minimize or reduce the activity of the thymus gland. Also used as a sedative, demulcent (soothes irritated or inflamed internal tissues or organs), aphrodisiac, antidepressant, sleep aid, and diuretic. May be used to improve stamina, concentration, healing, stress resistance, vigilance, and work efficiency and to improve well-being in elderly patients with debilitated or degenerative conditions.

Also used to decrease fasting blood glucose level and hemoglobin $A^{1c}$ in diabetic and nondiabetic patients and to treat hyperlipidemia, hepatic dysfunction, and impaired cognitive function.

## DOSAGE

Dosages vary with the disease state; usually, 0.5 to 2 g dry ginseng root daily or 200 to 600 mg ginseng extract daily, in one or two equal doses.
*Improved well-being in debilitated elderly patients—*
0.4 to 0.8 g root P.O. daily on a continual basis.

## ADVERSE REACTIONS

**CNS:** headache, insomnia, nervousness.
**CV:** chest pain, palpitations, hypertension.
**EENT:** epistaxis.
**GI:** diarrhea, nausea, vomiting.
**GU:** impotence, vaginal bleeding.
**Skin:** pruritus, skin eruptions (with ginseng abuse).
**Other:** breast pain.

Ginseng abuse syndrome occurs when large doses of the herb are taken with other psychomotor stimulants, such as tea and coffee; symptoms include diarrhea, hypertension, restlessness, insomnia, skin eruptions, depression, appetite suppression, euphoria, and edema.

## INTERACTIONS

**Herb-drug.** *Antidiabetics, insulin:* use cautiously because of ginseng's hypoglycemic effect.
*MAO inhibitors, such as hypericin, phenelzine, selegiline, tranylcypromine:* adverse reactions, including headache, tremors, mania. Avoid concomitant use.

## CONTRAINDICATIONS

Avoid use in pregnant or breast-feeding women; effects are unknown.

## NURSING CONSIDERATIONS

• Use cautiously in patients with CV disease, hypertension, hypotension, or diabetes, and in those also receiving corticosteroid therapy.
• Monitor patient for signs and symptoms of ginseng abuse syndrome.
• Monitor diabetic patient for signs and symptoms of hypoglycemia.

☑**Patient teaching**
• Advise patient not to take herb for a prolonged time.
• Tell patient with preexisting medical conditions to check with doctor before taking ginseng.
• Advise diabetic patient to check glucose levels closely until effects of herb are known.
• Instruct patient to watch for unusual symptoms (nervousness, insomnia, palpitations, diarrhea) because of risk of ginseng toxicity.
• Advise pregnant or breast-feeding woman to consult doctor before taking herb because safety hasn't been established.

## goldenseal

eye balm, eye root, goldsiegel, ground raspberry, Indian dye, Indian turmeric, jaundice root

## COMMON FORMS

Available as capsules and tablets and as ethanol and water extracts, dried ground root powder, tinctures, and teas.

*Capsules, tablets:* 250 mg, 350 mg, 400 mg, 404 mg, 470 mg, 500 mg, 535 mg, 540 mg

## ACTION
Herb may have anti-inflammatory, astringent, oxytocic, antihemorrhagic, and laxative properties and inhibits muscular contractions. It decreases anticoagulant effect of heparin and acts as a cardiac stimulant (at lower dosages), increases coronary perfusion, and inhibits cardiac activity (at higher dosages).

It may exhibit antipyretic activity (greater than aspirin) and antimuscarinic, antihistaminic, antitumor, antimicrobial, antiparasitic, and hypotensive effects. Herb also causes vasoconstriction and produces significant changes in blood pressure.

## USES
Used to treat GI disorders, gastritis, peptic ulceration, anorexia, postpartum hemorrhage, dysmenorrhea, eczema, pruritus, tuberculosis, cancer, mouth ulcerations, otorrhea, tinnitus, and conjunctivitis; also used as a wound antiseptic, diuretic, laxative, and anti-inflammatory.

Used to shorten duration of acute *Vibrio cholera* diarrhea and diarrhea due to some species of *Giardia, Salmonella, Shigella,* and some Enterobacteriaceae. May be used to improve biliary secretion and function in patients with hepatic cirrhosis.

## DOSAGE
*Ethanol and water extract:* 250 mg P.O. t.i.d. *Dried rhizome:* 0.5 to 1 g t.i.d.

## ADVERSE REACTIONS
**CNS:** CNS depression, paralysis with higher doses, paresthesia, *seizures.*
**CV:** *asystole, bradycardia, heart block.*
**GI:** diarrhea, GI cramping and pain, mouth ulceration, nausea, vomiting.
**Hematologic:** leukocytosis.
**Respiratory:** *respiratory depression with high doses.*
**Skin:** contact dermatitis.
**Other:** *death with large alkaloid doses;* symptoms of overdose, including GI upset, nervousness, depression, exaggerated reflexes, and *seizures that progress to respiratory paralysis and CV collapse.*

## INTERACTIONS
**Herb-drug.** *Anticoagulants:* may offset the beneficial effects of therapeutic anticoagulants. Avoid concomitant use.
*Antihypertensives:* may interfere or enhance hypotensive effects when taken with goldenseal or its extracts. Don't use together.
*Beta blockers, calcium channel blockers, digoxin:* may enhance or interfere with the cardiac effects of these drugs. Don't use together.
*Benzodiazepines, other CNS depressants:* may enhance sedative effects when taken with goldenseal. Avoid use with goldenseal.
**Herb-lifestyle.** *Alcohol use:* may enhance sedative effects when taken with goldenseal. Avoid use together.

## CONTRAINDICATIONS
Contraindicated in patients with CV disease, particularly hypertension, heart failure, or arrhythmia, and in pregnant women.

## NURSING CONSIDERATIONS
• Monitor cardiac rate and rhythm.
• Monitor patient for signs and symptoms of vitamin B deficiencies (megaloblastic anemia, peripheral neuropathy, seizures, cheilosis, glossitis, angular stomatitis, seborrheic dermatitis, and infertility).

### ☑ Patient teaching
• Tell patient to avoid hazardous activities until CNS effects of herb are known.
• Instruct patient to avoid consumption of herb because of risk of serious adverse reactions.

---

## grapeseed; pinebark
muskat, Pinus maritima, Pinus nigra, Vitis coignetiae, Vitis vinifera

## COMMON FORMS
*Tablets, capsules:* 25 mg to 300 mg

## ACTION
Herb demonstrates antilipoperoxidant activity and xanthine oxidase inhibition. It inhibits enzymes responsible for skin

---

Reactions may be *common,* uncommon, *life-threatening,* or COMMON AND LIFE-THREATENING.

turnover. Extract exhibits therapeutic effects in Ehrlich ascites carcinoma and inhibits growth of *Streptococcus mutans*.

## USES
Used as an antioxidant to treat circulatory disorders (hypoxia from atherosclerosis, inflammation, and cardiac or cerebral infarction). Also used to treat pain, limb heaviness, and swelling in patients with peripheral circulatory disorders and to treat inflammatory conditions, varicose veins, and cancer.

## DOSAGE
*Tablets, capsules:* 25 to 300 mg P.O. daily for up to 3 weeks; then a maintenance dose of 40 to 80 mg P.O. once daily.

## ADVERSE REACTIONS
None reported.

## INTERACTIONS
None significant.

## CONTRAINDICATIONS
No known contraindications.

## NURSING CONSIDERATIONS
• Evaluate underlying condition for which patient claims to be using herb.

## ☑ Patient teaching
• Instruct patient with a circulatory disorder not to delay seeking medical attention if signs and symptoms worsen (changes in sensation, color, or temperature of extremity).

## kava
ava, awa, kava-kava, kawa, kew, sakau, tonga, yagona

## COMMON FORMS
As a drink made from pulverized roots, tablets, capsules, or extract.

## ACTION
Components of root may cause local anesthetic activity that is similar to cocaine but lasts longer than benzocaine. Some components show fungistatic properties against several fungi.

Induces muscular relaxation and inhibits the limbic system, an effect associated with suppression of emotional excitability and mood enhancement. Produces mild euphoria with no effect on thoughts and memory during the intoxication. Other effects include analgesia, sedation, hyporeflexia, impaired gait, and pupil dilation.

## USES
Used in attenuating spinal seizures, as an antipsychotic, and for seizure control in epileptic patients. Also used to treat anxiety disorders, depression, insomnia, asthma, pain, rheumatism, venereal disease, and muscle spasms and to promote wound healing.

## DOSAGE
*Anxiety—*
90 to 110 mg dried kava extract t.i.d.
*Freshly prepared kava beverages:* 400 to 900 g weekly.

## ADVERSE REACTIONS
**CNS:** changes in motor reflexes and judgment.
**EENT:** visual disturbances.
*With chronic, heavy use:*
**EENT:** reddened eyes.
**Hematologic:** decreased platelet and lymphocyte count.
**Metabolic:** weight loss.
**Respiratory:** shortness of breath, pulmonary hypertension.
**Skin:** dry, flaking discolored skin.
**Other:** dopamine antagonism, increased patellar reflexes, reduced plasma protein, urea, and bilirubin levels.

## INTERACTIONS
**Herb-drug.** *Alprazolam:* may cause coma. Avoid concomitant use.
*Benzodiazepines, other CNS depressants:* additive sedative effects. Avoid concomitant use.
*Levodopa:* increased parkinsonian symptoms. Avoid concomitant use.
*Pentobarbital:* may cause additive effects. Avoid concomitant use.
**Herb-lifestyle.** *Alcohol use:* increased kava toxicity. Avoid concomitant use.

## CONTRAINDICATIONS

Avoid use in pregnant or breast-feeding women and in children under age 12; effects are unknown.

## NURSING CONSIDERATIONS

• Use cautiously in patients with renal disease, thrombocytopenia, or neutropenia.
• Avoid use with psychotropic drugs.
• Monitor patient for adverse effects with long-term use.

### ✓ Patient teaching

• Inform patient that significant adverse reactions may occur with long-term use.
• Tell patient to avoid alcohol and other CNS depressants while taking kava because they enhance herb's sedative and toxic effects.
• Inform patient that absorption of kava may be enhanced if taken with food.
• Advise a woman to avoid taking herb during pregnancy or when breast-feeding.

---

## milk thistle

Carduus marianus L., Cnicus marianus, holy thistle, Lady's thistle, Marian thistle, Mary thistle, St. Mary thistle

## COMMON FORMS

Available as capsules, tablets, and extract.
*Capsules:* 50 mg, 100 mg, 175 mg, 200 mg, 505 mg
*Tablets:* 85 mg (standardized to contain 80% silymarin with the flavonoid silibinin)

## ACTION

Herb exerts hepatoprotective and antihepatotoxic actions over liver toxins by altering the outer liver membrane cell structure so that toxins can't enter the cell. It also leads to activation of the regenerative capacity of the liver through cell development.

## USES

Used as a liver-cleansing agent. Extracts have been used as an antidote after ingestion of *Amanita phalloides* and other poisonous mushrooms and to treat acute and chronic liver disease and hepatitis C. Also used to improve liver function test results and blunt hepatotoxicity in patients with psychotic drug–induced hepatic damage.

## DOSAGE

420 to 800 mg P.O. daily as single dose or two or three divided doses; or 200 to 400 mg of silymarin component P.O. daily, calculated as the silibinin component.

## ADVERSE REACTIONS

**GI:** mild laxative effect with standardized extracts.
**GU:** uterine stimulant effect.

## INTERACTIONS

None significant.

## CONTRAINDICATIONS

Contraindicated in pregnant or breast-feeding women.

## NURSING CONSIDERATIONS

• Use cautiously in patients with hypersensitivity to plants belonging to the Asteraceae family.
• Monitor liver function test results during therapy.

### ✓ Patient teaching

• Advise patient to consult doctor specializing in liver disease before pursuing herbal therapy.
• Advise a woman to report planned or suspected pregnancy.
• Instruct patient to report unusual symptoms immediately.

---

## nettle

common nettle, greater nettle, stinging nettle

## COMMON FORMS

Available as capsules and dried leaf, root extract, or tincture.
*Capsules:* 150 mg, 300 mg

## ACTION

Herb acts primarily as a diuretic by increasing urine volume and decreasing systolic blood pressure. It may stimulate uterine contractions. Extract reduces urine flow, nocturia, and residual urine.

---

Reactions may be *common,* uncommon, *life-threatening*, or COMMON AND LIFE-THREATENING.

## USES
Used as an antispasmodic and expectorant and to treat rheumatism, asthma, cough, tuberculosis, hypertension, heart failure, and urinary, bladder, and kidney disorders. Also used to treat nosebleeds, uterine bleeding, diabetes, gout, cancer, and eczema, and for wound healing.

Used for bladder irrigation in treatment of prostatic adenoma and to reduce postoperative blood loss, bacteriuria, and inflammation. Used for early treatment of BPH and for treating allergic rhinitis. Juice may be applied to the scalp to stimulate hair growth.

## DOSAGE
*Allergic rhinitis—*
150 to 300 mg capsules P.O. *Tea:* mix 5 to 10 ml dried herb in 240 ml boiling water; take up to 480 ml daily. *Tincture:* 2.5 to 5 ml up to b.i.d.

## ADVERSE REACTIONS
**CV:** edema.
**Skin:** urticaria from contact with leaves.
*With internal use:*
**GI:** diarrhea, gastric irritation, stomach irritation.
**GU:** decreased urine volume, oliguria.

## INTERACTIONS
**Herb-drug.** *Diuretics:* may potentiate effects. Avoid concomitant use.

## CONTRAINDICATIONS
Contraindicated in pregnant and breast-feeding women because of its diuretic and uterine stimulation properties and in children under age 2.

## NURSING CONSIDERATIONS
• Use cautiously, and in reduced dosages, in older children and adults over age 65.
• Monitor patient's urine output.
• Monitor for adverse skin reactions if leaves contact skin.

☑ **Patient teaching**
• Advise patient to eat foods high in potassium, such as bananas and fresh vegetables, to replenish electrolytes lost through diuresis.

• Caution patient against self-medicating with nettle for BPH or to relieve fluid accumulation associated with heart failure without medical approval and supervision.
• Tell patient to wash thoroughly with soap and water, use antihistamines and corticosteroid creams, and to wear heavy gloves if plant is to be handled. If rubbed against skin, nettles can cause intense burning for 12 hours or more.

---

## passion flower
apricot vine, granadilla, Jamaican honeysuckle, maypop, passion fruit, water lemon

## COMMON FORMS
Available as liquid extract, crude extract, tincture, and dried herb, and in several homeopathic remedies.
*Liquid extract:* 1:1 in 25% alcohol
*Tincture:* 1:8 in 45% alcohol, or containing 0.7% flavonoids

## ACTION
Herb exerts both stimulatory and depressant CNS effects. It may have anticonvulsant effects and may reduce spontaneous motor activity.

## USES
Used as a sedative and to treat nervousness.

## DOSAGE
*Parkinson's disease—*
10 to 30 gtt P.O. (0.7% flavonoids) t.i.d.
*Dried herb:* 0.25 to 1 g P.O. t.i.d. *Liquid extract:* 0.5 to 1 ml P.O. t.i.d. *Tea:* 4 to 8 g daily in divided doses. *Tincture:* 0.5 to 2 ml P.O. t.i.d.

## ADVERSE REACTIONS
**CNS:** CNS depression with large doses.

## INTERACTIONS
**Herb-drug.** *MAO inhibitors:* may potentiate action. Monitor patient.
*Other CNS depressants:* possible additive effects. Use cautiously.

## CONTRAINDICATIONS
Contraindicated in pregnant and breast-feeding women; harman alkaloids may act as a uterine stimulant.

## NURSING CONSIDERATIONS
• Monitor patient for possible adverse CNS effects.

☑ **Patient teaching**
• Advise a woman to report planned or suspected pregnancy.
• Advise woman to avoid use of herb during pregnancy or when breast-feeding.
• Warn patient considering consumption of herb of its potential sedative effects.

---

## primrose, evening
king's-cure-all

## COMMON FORMS
*Capsules:* 50 mg, 500 mg, 1,300 mg
*Gelcaps:* 500 mg, 1,300 mg

## ACTION
Herb aids prostaglandin synthesis.

## USES
An infusion of the whole plant is used for sedative and astringent properties. Used to treat asthmatic coughs, GI disorders, whooping cough, psoriasis, multiple sclerosis, asthma, Raynaud's disease, and Sjögren's syndrome. Poultices made with evening primrose oil may be used to speed wound healing.

Herb used to treat pruritic symptoms of atopic dermatitis and eczema, breast pain and tenderness associated with premenstrual syndrome, benign breast disease, and diabetic neuropathy.

Also used in rheumatoid arthritis to improve symptoms and reduce need for pain medication; and to lower serum cholesterol, improve hypertension, and decrease platelet aggregation.

May be used to calm hyperactive children and to reduce mammary tumors from baseline size.

## DOSAGE
The following dosages are based on a standardized gamma linoleic acid content of 8%.
*Eczema—*
**Adults:** 320 mg to 8 g P.O. daily.
**Children ages 1 to 12:** 160 P.O. mg to 4 g P.O. daily; continue for 3 months.
*Breast pain—*
3 to 4 g P.O. daily.
No consensus exists for all other disorders.

## ADVERSE REACTIONS
**CV:** thrombosis.
**CNS:** headache, temporal lobe epilepsy (most common in schizophrenic patients or in those taking drugs such as phenothiazines).
**GI:** nausea.
**Skin:** rash.
**Other:** inflammation, possible immunosuppression after use for over 1 year.

## INTERACTIONS
**Herb-drug.** *Phenothiazines:* may increase risk of seizures. Avoid concomitant use.

## CONTRAINDICATIONS
Avoid use of herb in pregnant women; effects are unknown.

## NURSING CONSIDERATIONS
• Use cautiously, if at all, in schizophrenic patients and in those taking seizure drugs.
• Monitor patient for adverse effects, especially with long-term use.

☑ **Patient teaching**
• Instruct patient with seizure disorders to reconsider using herb.
• Caution parents to use herb for a hyperactive child only under medical supervision.

---

## saw palmetto
American dwarf palm tree, cabbage palm, IDS 89, LSESR, sabal

## COMMON FORMS
Available as tablets, capsules, teas, berries (fresh or dried), and liquid extract.

---

Reactions may be *common,* uncommon, *life-threatening,* or COMMON AND LIFE-THREATENING.

## ACTION
Herb has an anti-inflammatory effect and inhibits prolactin and growth factor-induced prostatic cell proliferation. May inhibit hormonally induced prostate enlargement.

## USES
Used as a mild diuretic; also used to treat GU problems such as BPH and to increase sperm production, breast size, and sexual vigor.

## DOSAGE
*BPH—*
320 mg P.O. daily in two divided doses for 3 months. Other recommendations include 1 to 2 g fresh saw palmetto berries or 0.5 to 1 g dried berry in decoction P.O. t.i.d.

## ADVERSE REACTIONS
**CNS:** headache.
**CV:** hypertension.
**GI:** abdominal pain, constipation, diarrhea, nausea.
**GU:** dysuria, impotence, urine retention.
**Musculoskeletal:** back pain.
**Other:** decreased libido.

## INTERACTIONS
None significant.

## CONTRAINDICATIONS
Contraindicated during pregnancy and in women of childbearing age because of herb's potential hormonal effects.

## NURSING CONSIDERATIONS
• Use cautiously in conditions other than BPH because of lack of data regarding herb's effects.
• Obtain baseline prostate-specific antigen (PSA) before starting treatment because of concern that herb causes a false-negative PSA result. However, saw palmetto probably doesn't alter size of prostate.
• Herb should be taken with the morning and evening meal to minimize GI effects.

☑ **Patient teaching**
• Inform patient wishing to use herb for BPH symptoms to do so only after a diagnosis has been made, and on doctor's advice.
• Advise a woman to avoid use of herb during pregnancy or when breast-feeding.
• Advise patient to take herb with meals to minimize GI upset.

# St. John's wort
amber, devil's scourge, goatweed, grace of God, Hypericum, klamath weed

## COMMON FORMS
Available as capsules, sublingual capsules, and liquid tinctures.
*Capsules:* 100 mg, 300 mg, 500 mg (standardized to 0.3% hypericin); 250 mg (standardized to 0.14% hypericin)

## ACTION
Herb inhibits stress-induced increase in corticotropin-releasing hormone, corticotropin, and cortisol. It also has antiviral activity, including action against retroviruses.

## USES
Used to treat depression, hypothyroidism, bronchial inflammation, insomnia, cancer, enuresis, burns, hemorrhoids, insect bites and stings, kidney disorders, gastritis, and scabies, and has been used as a wound-healing agent. Herb can be used to treat HIV infection and can be used topically for phototherapy of skin diseases, including psoriasis, cutaneous T-cell lymphoma, warts, and Kaposi's sarcoma.

## DOSAGE
*Depression—*
300 mg standardized extract preparations (standardized to 0.3% hypericin) P.O. t.i.d. for 4 to 6 weeks; or 2 to 4 g tea that has been steeped in 240 to 480 ml of water for about 10 minutes and taken P.O. daily for 4 to 6 weeks.
*Burns, skin lesions—*
Cream applied topically; strength isn't standardized.

## ADVERSE REACTIONS
Adverse effects are uncommon.

**CNS:** dizziness, restlessness, sleep disturbances.
**GI:** constipation, dry mouth, GI distress.
**Other:** allergic hypersensitivity; rarely, phototoxicity.

## INTERACTIONS
**Herb-drug.** *Indinavir:* significant decrease of indinavir plasma concentrations. Avoid concomitant use.
*MAO inhibitors, narcotics, OTC cold and flu products, sympathomimetics:* may enhance MAO inhibition activity. Avoid concurrent use.
*Paroxetine:* may result in sedative-hypnotic intoxication with ingestion of herb. Avoid concurrent use.
*Serotonergic drugs, such as amphetamines, serotonin reuptake inhibitors, trazodone, tricyclic antidepressants:* serotonin syndrome may occur when used with these drugs. Use cautiously together.
**Herb-food.** *Tyramine-containing foods:* may enhance MAO inhibition activity. Avoid concurrent use.
**Herb-lifestyle.** *Alcohol use:* may enhance MAO inhibition activity. Avoid concurrent use.

## CONTRAINDICATIONS
Contraindicated in patients with history of allergy to St. John's wort or its components. Avoid use in children and in pregnant or breast-feeding women; effects are unknown.

## NURSING CONSIDERATIONS
• Patient's depression should be medically evaluated. Conventional therapy may be prudent for a more moderate to severe disorder.

☑ **Patient teaching**
• Tell patient to purchase herbs only from a reputable source, and that products and their contents may vary among different manufacturers.
• Caution patient against using herb with alcohol and OTC cold and flu products.
• Advise patient to take precautions against sun exposure.

# valerian
all heal, amantilla, herba
benedicta, katzenwurzel, phu
germanicum, phu parvum

## COMMON FORMS
Available as standardized capsules, tablets, and tinctures; as tinctures and teas containing crude dried herb; and with other dietary supplements.
*Standardized capsules, tablets (0.8% valerenic acid):* 250 mg, 400 mg, 450 mg, 493 mg, 530 mg, 550 mg
*Standardized tinctures:* 2% essential oil

## ACTION
Herb may exhibit a sedative effect and weak anticonvulsant and antidepressant properties. It also has antispasmodic effects on GI smooth muscle, produces coronary dilation, and has antiarrhythmic activity.

## USES
Used as a sedative and antispasmodic and as a daytime sedative for restlessness and tension. Also used to treat restlessness and nervous disturbances of sleep.

## DOSAGE
Composition and purity of valerian preparations vary greatly.
*Sleep disorders—*
400 to 900 mg standardized valerian extract ½ to 1 hour before bedtime. *Tea:* 2 to 3 g of crude dried herb several times daily. *Tincture:* 3 to 5 ml several times daily.

## ADVERSE REACTIONS
*With acute overdose or chronic use:*
**CNS:** excitability, headache, insomnia.
**CV:** cardiac disturbance.
**EENT:** blurred vision.
**GI:** nausea.
**Hepatic:** *hepatotoxicity* from combination products containing valerian, and from overdose averaging 2.5 g.
**Other:** *hypersensitivity reactions.*

## INTERACTIONS
**Herb-drug.** *CNS depressants:* potential additive effects. Avoid concomitant use.

---

Reactions may be *common,* uncommon, *life-threatening*, or COMMON AND LIFE-THREATENING.

*Disulfiram:* disulfiram reaction may occur if herbal extract or tincture contains alcohol. Avoid concomitant use.

**Herb-lifestyle.** *Alcohol use:* potential additive effects. Avoid concomitant use.

## CONTRAINDICATIONS
Contraindicated in patients with history of allergy to valerian. Avoid use in patients with hepatic impairment because of risk of hepatotoxicity. Avoid use in pregnant or breast-feeding women; effects are unknown.

## NURSING CONSIDERATIONS
• Monitor periodic liver function tests in patients with preexisting hepatic disease and in those who have used herb on long-term basis.

☑ **Patient teaching**
• Inform patient that many extract products contain 40% to 60% alcohol and may not be appropriate for all patients.
• Warn patient taking disulfiram not to take herbal form containing alcohol.
• Counsel patient about herb's sedative effects and to avoid hazardous activities until CNS effects of herb are known.
• Advise a woman to avoid use of herb during pregnancy or when breast-feeding.
• Inform patient that safety and efficacy of herb in children haven't been established.

# Most common drug errors

Listed below are 25 of the most common drug errors and steps you can take to prevent them.

## Drug orders

Prescribing and filling drug orders must be done carefully to avoid potential problems.

### Pharmacy computer systems

*Error:* The Institute for Safe Medication Practices (ISMP) performed a field test on 307 pharmacy computer systems; only four detected all unsafe orders. Many didn't detect potentially lethal orders, including doses that exceeded safe limits, drug ingredient duplications, and orders to administer oral solutions I.V.

*Best practice or prevention:* Don't rely on the pharmacy computer system to detect all unsafe orders. Before administering a drug, understand the correct dosage, indications, and adverse effects; if necessary, refer to a current drug reference.

### Drug name confusion

*Error:* Health care professionals have been repeatedly warned about the potential for confusing amrinone (Inocor), an inotrope, with amiodarone (Cordarone), an antiarrhythmic that has negative chronotropic effects. However, patient injuries, including death, continue because of name confusion.

A doctor ordered amrinone for a woman with a history of MI and stroke who had severe hypotension from bradycardia. The nurse who phoned the order to the pharmacy couldn't pronounce the drug name. The pharmacist asked to speak with the doctor, who also had trouble pronouncing it. Finally, the pharmacist used a brand name to ask if the doctor was requesting Cordarone. The doctor said yes and ordered Cordarone. The patient received the drug and died.

*Best practice or prevention:* To prevent such a problem, confirm the patient's diagnosis before administering either drug.

### Abbreviations

*Error:* Abbreviating drug names is risky. A cancer patient with anemia may receive epoetin alfa, commonly abbreviated EPO, to stimulate RBC production. In one case, when a cancer patient was admitted to a hospital, the doctor wrote, "May take own supply of EPO." However, the patient wasn't anemic. Sensing that something was wrong, the pharmacist interviewed the patient, who confirmed that he was taking "EPO"—evening primrose oil—to lower his cholesterol level.

*Best practice or prevention:* Ask all prescribers to spell out drug names.

### Unclear orders

*Error:* A patient was supposed to receive one dose of the antineoplastic lomustine to treat brain cancer. (Lomustine is typically given as a single oral dose once every 6 weeks.) The doctor's order read "Administer h.s." Because this was misinterpreted to mean every night, the patient received nine daily doses, developed severe thrombocytopenia and leukopenia, and died.

*Best practice or prevention:* If you're unfamiliar with a drug, check a drug book before administering it. If a prescriber uses "h.s." but doesn't specify the frequency of administration, call him to clarify the order. When documenting orders, note "h.s. nightly" or "h.s. × one dose today."

### Misinterpretation of orders

*Error:* Several reports to the ISMP involved errors related to insulin orders. In one case, an order was written as "add 10U of regular insulin to each TPN bag," and the pharmacist preparing the solution misinterpreted the dose as 100 units. In another case, a pharmacy technician entering orders misinterpreted a sliding scale when the insulin order used "u" for units, an error that could have caused a 10-fold overdose if a nurse hadn't caught it. Yet another report involved a nurse who received a verbal order to resume an insulin drip but wrote "resume heparin drip." Fortunately, the pharmacist caught the error.

*Best practice or prevention:* Before administering drugs such as insulin or heparin, which are ordered in units, always check the prescriber's written order against the provided order. Never abbreviate "units." If you must accept a verbal order, have another nurse listen in; then transcribe that order directly onto an order form and repeat it to ensure that you've transcribed it correctly.

### Inadvertent overdose

*Error:* The inadvertent prescribing of harmful acetaminophen doses has become a disturbing trend. To relieve pain, prescribers may write orders for combined acetaminophen and opioid analgesic tablets (Lortab, Tylox, Darvocet-N) without realizing that the total acetaminophen dose could be toxic.

Consider this order: "Tylox, 1 to 2 tablets every 4 hours, as needed, for pain." By taking the higher dose, the patient would receive 1,000 mg of acetaminophen every 4 hours, exceeding the maximum recommended dose of 4 g/day.

*Best practice or prevention:* To prevent an acetaminophen overdose from combined analgesics, note the amount in each drug. Beware of substitutions by the pharmacy because the amount of acetaminophen may vary.

### Lipid-based drugs

*Error:* Serious drug errors, some fatal, have occurred because of confusion between certain lipid-based (liposomal) drugs and their conventional counterparts. The drugs involved include:
- lipid-based amphotericin B (Abelcet, Amphotec, AmBisome) and conventional amphotericin B for injection (available generically and as Fungizone)
- the pegylated liposomal form of doxorubicin (Doxil) and its conventional form, doxorubicin hydrochloride (Adriamycin, Rubex)
- a liposomal form of daunorubicin (DaunoXome, daunorubicin citrate liposomal) and conventional daunorubicin hydrochloride (Cerubidine).

*Best practice or prevention:* Lipid-based products have different dosages than their conventional counterparts. Check the original order and labels carefully to avoid mix-ups.

### Drug preparation

When preparing a drug for administration, be alert for potential problems.

### Syringe tip caps and children

*Error:* A syringe tip cap poses a potential choking hazard to a small child: If you forget to remove the cap from an oral syringe before administering a drug, the cap could blow off into the child's mouth when you press the plunger. If a cap from an oral or a hypodermic syringe gets lost in the linens, the child may find it later and swallow or aspirate it.

*Best practice or prevention:* Remove and discard the cap in a secured sharps container before administering the drug; don't place it in a trash can where the child may find it later.

Teach parents about the potential danger of syringe tip caps. Tell them to store a capped syringe where children can't reach it and to remove the cap before giving the drug.

### Inattentiveness

*Error:* When a hospital pharmacy received an order for Fludara (fludarabine), a pharmacy technician asked the pharmacist if Navelbine (vinorelbine) was the same as Fludara (both are antineoplastics). The preoccupied pharmacist said "yes." The technician prepared the Navelbine, but labeled it as Fludara. The pharmacist checked the preparation but didn't notice the error, and the patient received the wrong drug.

*Best practice or prevention:* To prevent errors of this type, the hospital posted tables of antineoplastics and their dosing guidelines in the pharmacy. As an added safeguard, the pharmacy now sends the empty drug vial or box top with the prepared solution for the nurse to double-check before infusing the drug.

### Injectable solution color changes

*Error:* In two cases, alert nurses noticed that antineoplastics prepared in the pharmacy didn't look the way they should.

The first error involved a 6-year-old child who was to receive 12 mg of methotrexate intrathecally. In the pharmacy, a 1-g vial was mistakenly selected instead of a 20-mg vial, and the drug was reconstituted with 10 ml of normal saline. The vial containing 100 mg/ml was incorrectly labeled as containing 2 mg/ml, and 6 ml of the solution was drawn into a syringe. Although the syringe label indicated 12 mg of drug, the syringe actually contained 600 mg of drug.

When the nurse received the syringe and noted that the drug's color didn't appear right, she returned it to the pharmacy for verification. The pharmacist retrieved the vial used to prepare the dose and drew the remaining solution into another syringe. The solutions in both syringes matched, and no one noticed the vial's 1-g label. The pharmacist concluded that a manufacturing change caused the color difference.

The child received the 600-mg dose and experienced seizures 45 minutes later. A pharmacist responding to the emergency detected the error. The child received an antidote and recovered.

A similar case involved a 20-year-old patient with leukemia who received mitomycin instead of mitoxantrone. The nurse had questioned the drug's unusual bluish tint, but the pharmacist assured her that the color difference was due to a change in manufacturer. Fortunately, the patient didn't suffer any harm.

*Best practice or prevention:* If a familiar drug seems to have an unfamiliar appearance, investigate the cause. If the pharmacist cites a manufacturing change, ask him to double-check whether he has received verification from the manufacturer. Document the appearance discrepancy, your actions, and the pharmacist's response in the patient record.

### Dropper confusion

*Error:* Ordering drugs such as liquid ferrous sulfate by the dropperful is a dangerous practice. One person might correctly consider the dropper full when the liquid meets the upper calibration mark; another might incorrectly fill the entire length of the dropper. Also, parents administering the drug at home may use a different dropper, which could significantly alter the dose given.

*Best practice or prevention:* Dosing directions for liquid drugs should always be expressed as weight per volume, such as 15 mg/0.6 ml. Verify the correct dose and teach parents to use only the dropper provided. Show them the mark on the dropper that indicates a full dose and ask them to demonstrate the proper technique.

### Incorrect allergy history

*Error:* After a patient was admitted to the hospital, a nurse faxed a list of the patient's allergies to the pharmacy. The pharmacist couldn't read it, so he accessed the files from the patient's previous admission. However, these records didn't reflect an allergy to the anti-infective cefazolin that the patient had recently developed.

A consulting doctor ordered cefazolin, and the pharmacy processed the order. The medication administration record (MAR) generated by the pharmacy's database didn't indicate the allergy, and the nurse didn't know about it either.

The patient received cefazolin and became hypotensive and unresponsive. The nurse immediately notified the doctor and administered the antihistamine diphenhydramine. The patient recovered and was discharged the next day.

*Best practice or prevention:* Perform a new allergy history with each admission. If the patient's history must be faxed, name the drugs, note how many are included, and follow the facility's faxing safeguards. If the pharmacy also adheres to strict guidelines, the computer-generated MAR should be accurate.

## Drug administration

When administering a drug, be careful to avoid the following problems.

### Patient misidentification

*Error:* Two common errors for nurses who are administering drugs are inadver-

tently failing to check the patient's identification and confusing patients with similar names. Using a tactic that helps prevent wrong-site surgery—involving the patient in the identification process—could also help prevent these drug errors.
*Best practice or prevention:* Urge the patient to clearly state his full name, even without being asked, at admission and before accepting drugs, procedures, or treatments. Teach him to offer his identification bracelet for inspection when anyone arrives with drugs and to insist on having it replaced if it's removed.

### Herbal medicines
*Error:* Surveys suggest that about one-third of Americans use herbal products as medicine. Some people take them with conventional drugs; others use them as replacements. Herbal products are available without a prescription. Because government quality assurance standards don't apply to herbal products' manufacturing and labeling, their ingredients may be misrepresented or contaminated.

Research on the effects of herbal products is limited. Because these products may contain a mixture of chemicals, their use carries risks.
*Best practice or prevention:* Ask the patient about his use of alternative therapies, including herbal products, and record your findings in his medical record. Monitor the patient carefully and report unusual events. Ask the patient to keep a diary of all therapies he uses and to take the diary for review each time he visits a health care professional.

### Calculation errors
*Error:* A physician assistant wrote the following order for a woman being admitted to the hospital for neck surgery: "methyl-prednisolone 10.6 g (30 mg/kg) over 1 hour IVPB before surgery" to minimize inflammation. The patient weighed 154 lb (70 kg), so the dose should have been 2.1 g, and not 10.6 g. However, neither the pharmacist nor the nurse independently checked the calculation, and the patient received an overdose. She developed significant hyperglycemia and hypokalemia but recovered without injury.

*Best practice or prevention:* Writing the mg/kg or mg/m$^2$ dose and the calculated dose provides a safeguard against calculation errors. Whenever a prescriber provides the calculation, double-check it and document that the dose was verified.

### Eyedrops for two or more
*Error:* Using one bottle of eyedrops to treat several patients may seem like a good way to prevent waste, control cost, and save time. Some facilities, for example, administer shared drugs to multiple patients undergoing outpatient cataract surgery. But this practice has risks.

Although eyedrops contain preservatives to prevent bacterial growth, contaminants may remain on the bottle top's inner surfaces or outer grooves. The dropper can also become contaminated if it accidentally touches an infected eye. (Cross-infections have been reported.)

Administering the wrong drug or wrong concentration is more likely because patient names don't appear on the containers. A patient may receive the wrong drops because the nurse can't check the bottle label against his patient identification.
*Best practice or prevention:* Just as sharing any drug is poor practice, eyedrops shouldn't be used for more than one patient. If unit doses aren't available for surgical patients, each patient should fill his prescriptions before admission and bring his drugs with him.

### Interactions with cisapride
*Error:* The pharmaceutical company has changed the labeling on cisapride (Propulsid), a drug used to treat nocturnal heartburn caused by gastroesophageal reflux disease. Among the changes, a warning states that serious cardiac arrhythmias may occur when patients taking Propulsid also take other drugs that may inhibit cisapride metabolism.

The warning was added because ventricular tachycardia, ventricular fibrillation, torsades de pointes, and prolongation of the QT interval have been reported in patients taking Propulsid with clarithromycin (Biaxin), erythromycin, fluconazole (Diflucan), indinavir (Crixivan), itraconazole (Sporanox), ketoconazole (Nizoral), nefazodone (Serzone), ritonavir (Norvir), or troleandomycin (Tao). Cardiac arrhythmias have also been reported in patients taking Propulsid without the contraindicated drugs.

*Best practice or prevention:* Before administering Propulsid, make sure the patient isn't taking any of the contraindicated drugs. If so, don't give Propulsid and immediately alert the doctor.

Because of inappropriate use of this drug in the United States, the FDA and the manufacturer of Propulsid have decided to limit its use. Anyone with questions can call (800)-JANSSEN.

### Celexa, Celebrex, and Cerebyx confusion

*Error:* An 80-year-old woman mistakenly received 20 mg of Celexa (citalopram), a selective serotonin reuptake inhibitor (SSRI), b.i.d. for 1 month for arthritis pain. She should have received 100 mg of Celebrex (celecoxib), an NSAID. A member of the pharmacy staff had confused the drug names when pulling the product from the shelf. Although the patient wasn't harmed, the potential for harm was great because she was already taking an SSRI.

*Best practice or prevention:* Help prevent errors related to Celebrex, Celexa, and the anticonvulsant Cerebyx (fosphenytoin) by asking prescribers to use the generic name and by confirming the drug's indication if the order doesn't clearly state it. For verbal orders, repeat the drug name and your understanding of its indication to the prescriber.

### Labels and toxicity

*Error:* A container of 5% acetic acid, used to clean tracheostomy tubing, was left near nebulization equipment in the room of a 10-month-old infant. A respiratory therapist mistook the liquid for normal saline solution and used it to dilute albuterol for the child's nebulizer treatment. During treatment, the child experienced bronchospasm, hypercapnic dyspnea, tachypnea, and tachycardia.

*Best practice or prevention:* Leaving potentially dangerous chemicals near patients is extremely risky, especially when the container labels don't indicate toxicity. To prevent such problems, read the label on every drug you prepare and never administer anything that isn't labeled.

### Dosage equations

*Error:* A 13-month study at Albany (N.Y.) Medical Center examined 200 prescribing errors arising from the use of dosage equations. Almost 70% involved pediatric patients, for whom dosage equations are commonly used. Mistakes in decimal point placement, mathematical calculation, or expression of the regimen accounted for over 50% of the errors. Examples include prescribing the entire day's drug as a single dose instead of at intervals or using an entire day's dose at each interval. Use of dosage equations invites drug errors.

*Best practice or prevention:* Alternatives to dosage equations include using preestablished ranges or tables, incorporating a calculator into a computer order entry system, and requiring both the calculated dose and dosage equation on orders to facilitate independent checks.

After calculating drug dosages, always have another nurse calculate them independently to double-check your results. If doubts or questions remain or if the calculations don't match, ask a pharmacist to calculate the dose before administering the drug.

### Misread orders

*Error:* Two reports concerned incorrect dosing of the tricyclic antidepressant nortriptyline (Pamelor, Aventyl, or, in Australia, Allegron) when ordered for neuropathic pain syndromes. The cases involved 10-mg and 20-mg orders that were misread as 100 mg and 200 mg, respectively. One patient receiving an incorrect dose required hospitalization; the other developed sedation and orthostatic hypotension after two doses, which led to recognition of the error.

*Best practice or prevention:* Nortriptyline and other tricyclic antidepressants aren't prescribed as frequently as they once were. To make sure you're familiar with recommended dosages, refer to a drug handbook and then ask a pharmacist, if necessary.

### Air bubbles in pump tubing

*Error:* After starting an I.V. drip to administer insulin, 2 U/hour, to a 9-year-old patient, a nurse noted air bubbles in the tubing and pump chamber. To remove them and promote proper flow, she disconnected the tubing and increased the pump rate to 200 ml/hour. When the bubbles were cleared, she reconnected the tubing and restarted the infusion without resetting the rate. The child received about 50 U of insulin before the error was detected. Fortunately, the child wasn't harmed.

*Best practice or prevention:* To clear bubbles from I.V. tubing, never increase the pump's flow rate to flush the line. Instead, remove the tubing from the pump, disconnect it from the patient, and use the flow-control clamp to establish gravity flow. When the bubbles have been removed, return the tubing to the pump, restart the infusion, and recheck the flow rate.

### Misplaced decimals

*Error:* A patient in the intensive care unit was to receive the opioid fentanyl, 12.5 to 25 mcg I.V. every 4 to 6 hours, as needed, for pain. Unit stock consisted of 5-ml ampules of fentanyl 0.05 mg/ml, so each ampule contained 0.25 mg (250 mcg). A nurse preparing a dose confused the volume needed when she converted from milligrams to micrograms and administered 5 ml thinking it contained 25 micrograms. The patient suffered respiratory arrest but was resuscitated.

*Best practice or prevention:* Numerous serious fentanyl errors have been reported, and a misplaced decimal point caused many of them. A safer alternative for intermittent dosing is I.V. morphine. Fentanyl doses are best prepared in the pharmacy rather than in the unit. If a fentanyl dose must be prepared, refer to dosing charts, follow the facility's protocols, and ask another nurse to check your calculations.

### Incorrect administration route

*Error:* A nurse was caring for a patient who had a jejunostomy tube for oral drugs and a central I.V. line for hyperalimentation and I.V. drugs. At the bedside was a stock bottle of digoxin elixir. After checking the concentration, the nurse used a syringe to withdraw 2.5 ml of elixir for a 0.125-mg dose. She then mistakenly administered the elixir through the central line rather than the jejunostomy tube.

Using an incorrect route put the patient at risk for overdose and secondary infection from unsterile I.V. administration. Fortunately, he was receiving antibiotics for a preexisting infection and suffered no adverse reactions.

*Best practice or prevention:* This case emphasizes the need to ensure that the right route is being used to administer any drug. When the patient has multiple lines, label the distal end of each line. Using a parenteral syringe to prepare oral liquid drugs increases the chance for error because the syringe tip fits easily into I.V. ports. To safely administer an oral drug through a feeding tube, use a dose prepared by the pharmacy and a syringe with the appropriate tip.

### Stress

*Error:* A nurse-anesthetist administered the sedative midazolam (Versed) to the wrong patient. When she discovered the error, she grabbed what she thought was a vial of the antidote flumazenil (Romazicon), withdrew 2.5 ml, and administered it. When the patient didn't respond, she realized she'd grabbed a vial of ondansetron (Zofran), an antiemetic, instead. Another practitioner assisted with proper I.V. administration of flumazenil, and the patient recovered without harm.

*Best practice or prevention:* Committing a serious error can cause enormous stress and cloud your judgment. If you're involved in a drug error, ask another professional to administer the antidote.

# Therapeutic drug monitoring guidelines

| DRUG | LABORATORY TEST MONITORED | THERAPEUTIC RANGES OF TEST |
|---|---|---|
| aminoglycoside antibiotics (amikacin, gentamicin, tobramycin) | Serum amikacin peak<br>  trough<br>Serum gentamicin/tobramycin<br>  peak<br>  trough<br>Serum creatinine | 20 to 25 mcg/ml<br>5 to 10 mcg/ml<br><br>4 to 8 mcg/ml<br>1 to 2 mcg/ml<br>0.6 to 1.3 mg/dl |
| amphotericin B | Serum creatinine<br>BUN<br>Serum electrolytes (especially potassium and magnesium)<br><br><br><br>Liver function tests<br>CBC with differential and platelets | 0.6 to 1.3 mg/dl<br>7 to 18 mg/dl<br>Potassium: 3.5 to 5 mEq/L<br>Magnesium: 1.7 to 2.1 mEq/L<br>Sodium: 135 to 145 mEq/L<br>Chloride: 98 to 106 mEq/L<br>*<br>***** |
| antibiotics | WBC with differential<br>Cultures and sensitivities | ***** |
| biguanides (metformin) | Serum creatinine<br>Fasting serum glucose<br>Glycosolated hemoglobin<br>CBC | 0.6 to 1.3 mg/dl<br>65 to 110 mg/dl<br>5.5% to 8.5% of total hemoglobin<br>***** |
| clozapine | WBC with differential | ***** |
| digoxin | Serum digoxin<br>Serum electrolytes (especially potassium, magnesium, and calcium)<br><br><br><br>Serum creatinine | 0.5 to 2 ng/ml<br>Potassium: 3.5 to 5 mEq/L<br>Magnesium: 1.7 to 2.1 mEq/L<br>Sodium: 135 to 145 mEq/L<br>Chloride: 98 to 106 mEq/L<br>Calcium: 8.6 to 10 mg/dl<br>0.6 to 1.3 mg/dl |
| diuretics | Serum electrolytes<br><br><br><br><br>Serum creatinine<br>BUN<br>Uric acid<br>Fasting serum glucose | Potassium: 3.5 to 5 mEq/L<br>Magnesium: 1.7 to 2.1 mEq/L<br>Sodium: 135 to 145 mEq/L<br>Chloride: 98 to 106 mEq/L<br>Calcium: 8.6 to 10 mg/dl<br>0.6 to 1.3 mg/dl<br>7 to 18 mg/dl<br>2 to 7 mg/dl<br>65 to 110 mg/dl |
| erythropoietin | Hematocrit | Female: 36% to 48%<br>Male: 42% to 52% |
| ethosuximide | Serum ethosuximide | 40 to 75 mcg/ml |

Note: ***** For those areas marked with asterisks, the following values can be used:

Hemoglobin: Female: 12 to 16 g/dl
  Male: 14 to 18 g/dl
Hematocrit: Female: 37% to 48%
  Male: 42% to 52%
RBCs: 4 to 5.5 x 10$^6$/mm$^3$
WBCs: 5 to 10 x 10$^3$/mm$^3$

Differential: Neutrophils: 45% to 74%
  Bands: 0% to 4%
  Lymphocytes: 16% to 45%
  Monocytes: 4% to 10%
  Eosinophils: 0% to 7%
  Basophils: 0% to 2%

## MONITORING GUIDELINES

Wait until the administration of the third dose to check drug levels. Obtain blood for peak level 30 minutes after I.V. infusion or 60 minutes after I.M. administration. For trough levels, draw blood just before next dose. Notify doctor of drug levels so that dosage may be adjusted accordingly. Recheck after three doses. Monitor serum creatinine and BUN levels and urine output for signs of decreasing renal function.

Monitor serum creatinine, BUN, and serum electrolyte levels at least weekly during therapy. Also, regularly monitor blood counts and liver function tests during therapy.

Specimen cultures and sensitivities will determine the cause of the infection and the best treatment. Monitor WBC with differential weekly during therapy.

Check renal function and hematologic parameters before initiating therapy and at least annually thereafter. If the patient has impaired renal function, don't use metformin because it may cause lactic acidosis. Monitor response to therapy by periodically evaluating fasting glucose and glycosolated hemoglobin levels. A patient's home monitoring of blood glucose levels helps monitor compliance and response.

Obtain WBC with differential before initiating therapy, weekly during therapy, and 4 weeks after discontinuing the drug.

Check serum digoxin levels at least 12 hours, but preferably 24 hours, after the last dose is administered. To monitor maintenance therapy, check drug levels at least 1 to 2 weeks after therapy is initiated or changed. Make any adjustments in therapy based on entire clinical picture, not solely on drug levels. Also, check electrolyte levels and renal function periodically during therapy.

To monitor fluid and electrolyte balance, perform baseline and periodic determinations of serum electrolyte, serum calcium, BUN, uric acid, and serum glucose levels.

After therapy is initiated or changed, monitor the hematocrit twice weekly for 2 to 6 weeks until stabilized in the target range and a maintenance dose determined. Monitor hematocrit regularly thereafter.

Check drug level 10 to 13 days after therapy is initiated or changed.

*(continued)*

* For those areas marked with one asterisk, the following values can be used:

ALT: 7 to 56 U/L
AST: 5 to 40 U/L
Alkaline phosphatase: 17 to 142 U/L
LD: 60 to 220 U/L
GGTP: < 40 U/L
Total bilirubin: 0.2 to 1 mg/dl

| DRUG | LABORATORY TEST MONITORED | THERAPEUTIC RANGES OF TEST |
|------|---------------------------|----------------------------|
| gemfibrozil | Serum lipids | Total cholesterol: < 200 mg/dl<br>LDL: < 130 mg/dl<br>HDL: Female: 40 to 85 mg/dl<br>　　　Male: 37 to 70 mg/dl<br>Triglycerides: 40 to 160 mg/dl |
| heparin | Activated partial thromboplastin time (APTT) | 1.5 to 2 times control |
| HMG-CoA reductase inhibitors (fluvastatin, lovastatin, pravastatin, simvastatin) | Serum lipids<br><br><br><br><br>Liver function tests | Total cholesterol: < 200 mg/dl<br>LDL: < 130 mg/dl<br>HDL: Female: 40 to 85 mg/dl<br>　　　Male: 37 to 70 mg/dl<br>Triglycerides: 40 to 160 mg/dl<br>* |
| insulin | Fasting serum glucose<br>Glycosylated hemoglobin | 65 to 110 mg/dl<br>5.5% to 8.5% of total hemoglobin |
| lithium | Serum lithium<br>Serum creatinine<br>CBC<br>Serum electrolytes (especially potassium and sodium)<br><br><br>Fasting serum glucose<br>Thyroid function tests | 0.8 to 1.2 mEq/L<br>0.6 to 1.3 mg/dl<br>*****<br>Potassium: 3.5 to 5 mEq/L<br>Magnesium: 1.7 to 2.1 mEq/L<br>Sodium: 135 to 145 mEq/L<br>Chloride: 98 to 106 mEq/L<br>65 to 110 mg/dl<br>TSH: 0.2 to 5.4 microU/ml<br>$T_3$: 80 to 200 ng/dl<br>$T_4$: 5.4 to 11.5 mcg/dl |
| methotrexate | Serum methotrexate<br><br><br>CBC with differential<br>Platelet count<br>Liver function tests<br>Serum creatinine | Normal elimination:<br>　< 10 micromol 24 hours postdose<br>　< 1 micromol 48 hours postdose<br>　< 0.2 micromol 72 hours postdose<br>*****<br>140 to 400 × $10^3$/mm³<br>*<br>0.6 to 1.3 mg/dl |
| phenytoin | Serum phenytoin<br>CBC | 10 to 20 mcg/ml<br>***** |
| potassium chloride | Serum potassium | 3.5 to 5 mEq/L |
| procainamide | Serum procainamide<br>Serum N-acetylprocainamide<br><br>CBC | 4 to 8 mcg/ml (procainamide)<br>5 to 30 mcg/ml (combined procainamide and NAPA)<br>***** |

Note: ***** For those areas marked with asterisks, the following values can be used:

| | |
|---|---|
| Hemoglobin: Female: 12 to 16 g/dl<br>　Male: 14 to 18 g/dl<br>Hematocrit: Female: 37% to 48%<br>　Male: 42% to 52%<br>RBCs: 4 to 5.5 x $10^6$/mm³<br>WBCs: 5 to 10 x $10^3$/mm³ | Differential: Neutrophils: 45% to 74%<br>　Bands: 0% to 4%<br>　Lymphocytes: 16% to 45%<br>　Monocytes: 4% to 10%<br>　Eosinophils: 0% to 7%<br>　Basophils: 0% to 2% |

## MONITORING GUIDELINES

Therapy is usually withdrawn after 3 months if response is inadequate. Patient must be fasting to measure triglyceride levels.

When drug is given by continuous I.V. infusion, check APTT every 4 hours in the early stages of therapy. When drug is given by deep S.C. injection, check APTT 4 to 6 hours after injection.

Perform liver function tests at baseline, 6 to 12 weeks after therapy is initiated or changed, and periodically thereafter. If adequate response isn't achieved within 6 weeks, consider changing the therapy.

Monitor response to therapy by evaluating serum glucose and glycosolated hemoglobin levels. Glycosolated hemoglobin level is a good measure of long-term control. A patient's home monitoring of blood glucose levels helps measure compliance and response.

Checking blood lithium levels is crucial to the safe use of the drug. Obtain serum lithium levels immediately before next dose. Monitor levels twice weekly until stable. Once at steady state, levels should be checked weekly; when the patient is on the appropriate maintenance dose, levels should be checked every 2 to 3 months. Monitor serum creatinine, serum electrolyte, and fasting serum glucose levels; CBC; and thyroid function tests, as ordered, before therapy is initiated and periodically during therapy.

Monitor methotrexate levels according to dosing protocol. Monitor CBC with differential, platelet count, and liver and renal function tests more frequently when therapy is initiated or changed and when methotrexate levels may be elevated, such as when the patient is dehydrated.

Monitor serum phenytoin levels immediately before next dose and 2 to 4 weeks after therapy is initiated or changed. Obtain a CBC at baseline and monthly early in therapy. Notify doctor if toxic effects appear at therapeutic levels. Adjust the measured level for hypoalbuminemia or renal impairment, which can increase free drug levels.

Check level weekly after oral replacement therapy is initiated until stable and every 3 to 6 months thereafter.

Measure procainamide levels 6 to 12 hours after a continuous infusion is started or immediately before the next oral dose. Combined (procainamide and NAPA) levels can be used as an index of toxicity when renal impairment exists. Obtain CBC periodically during longer-term therapy.

*(continued)*

* For those areas marked with one asterisk, the following values can be used:

ALT: 7 to 56 U/L
AST: 5 to 40 U/L
Alkaline phosphatase: 17 to 142 U/L
LD: 60 to 220 U/L
GGTP: < 40 U/L
Total bilirubin: 0.2 to 1 mg/dl

| DRUG | LABORATORY TEST MONITORED | THERAPEUTIC RANGES OF TEST |
|---|---|---|
| quinidine | Serum quinidine | 2 to 6 mcg/ml |
| | CBC | ***** |
| | Liver function tests | * |
| | Serum creatinine | 0.6 to 1.3 mg/dl |
| | Serum electrolytes (especially potassium) | Potassium: 3.5 to 5 mEq/L |
| | | Magnesium: 1.7 to 2.1 mEq/L |
| | | Sodium: 135 to 145 mEq/L |
| | | Chloride: 98 to 106 mEq/L |
| sulfonylureas | Fasting serum glucose | 65 to 110 mg/dl |
| | Glycosylated hemoglobin | 5.5% to 8.5% of total hemoglobin |
| theophylline | Serum theophylline | 10 to 20 mcg/ml |
| thyroid hormone | Thyroid function tests | TSH: 0.2 to 5.4 microU/ml |
| | | $T_3$: 80 to 200 ng/dl |
| | | $T_4$: 5.4 to 11.5 mcg/dl |
| vancomycin | Serum vancomycin | 20 to 40 mcg/ml (peak) |
| | | 5 to 10 mcg/ml (trough) |
| | Serum creatinine | 0.6 to 1.3 mg/dl |
| warfarin | INR | For an acute MI, atrial fibrillation, treatment of pulmonary embolism, prevention of systemic embolism, tissue heart valves, valvular heart disease, or prophylaxis or treatment of venous thrombosis: 2 to 3 |
| | | For mechanical prosthetic valves or recurrent systemic embolism: 3 to 4.5 |

Note: ***** For those areas marked with asterisks, the following values can be used:

Hemoglobin: Female: 12 to 16 g/dl
    Male: 14 to 18 g/dl
Hematocrit: Female: 37% to 48%
    Male: 42% to 52%
RBCs: 4 to 5.5 x $10^6$/mm$^3$
WBCs: 5 to 10 x $10^3$/mm$^3$

Differential: Neutrophils: 45% to 74%
    Bands: 0% to 4%
    Lymphocytes: 16% to 45%
    Monocytes: 4% to 10%
    Eosinophils: 0% to 7%
    Basophils: 0% to 2%

## MONITORING GUIDELINES

Obtain levels immediately before next oral dose and 30 to 35 hours after therapy is initiated or changed. Periodically obtain blood counts, liver and kidney function tests, and serum electrolyte levels.

Monitor response to therapy by periodically evaluating fasting glucose and glycosolated hemoglobin levels. A patient's home monitoring of blood glucose levels helps measure compliance and response.

Obtain serum quinidine levels immediately before next dose of sustained-release oral product and at least 2 days after therapy is initiated or changed.

Monitor thyroid function tests every 2 to 3 weeks until appropriate maintenance dose is determined.

Serum vancomycin levels may be checked with the third dose administered, at the earliest. Draw peak levels ½ hour after the I.V. infusion is completed. Draw trough levels immediately before the next dose is administered. Renal function can be used to adjust dosing and intervals.

Check INR daily, beginning 3 days after therapy is initiated. Continue checking it until therapeutic goal is achieved, and monitor it periodically thereafter. Also, check levels 7 days after any change in warfarin dose or concomitant, potentially interacting therapy.

* For those areas marked with one asterisk, the following values can be used:

ALT: 7 to 56 U/L
AST: 5 to 40 U/L
Alkaline phosphatase: 17 to 142 U/L
LD: 60 to 220 U/L
GGTP: < 40 U/L
Total bilirubin: 0.2 to 1 mg/dl

# Selected local and topical anesthetics

| DRUG, INDICATIONS, DOSAGE | ADVERSE REACTIONS |
|---|---|

## Local

**bupivacaine hydrochloride**
(Marcain‡, Marcaine, Sensorcaine)
Dosages given are for the drug without epinephrine and for adults.
Volume listed below refers to the total volume of anesthetic given,
sometimes in incremental doses of 2 to 6 ml.
*Epidural block—*
0.25% solution: 10 to 20 ml (25 to 50 mg)
0.5% solution: 10 to 20 ml (50 to 100 mg)
0.75% solution: 10 to 20 ml (75 to 150 mg), single-dose only
*Caudal block—*
0.25% solution: 15 to 30 ml (37.5 to 75 mg)
0.5% solution: 15 to 30 ml (75 to 150 mg)
*Spinal block—*
0.75% solution (in dextrose 8.25%): 1 to 1.6 ml (7.5 to 12 mg)
*Peripheral nerve block—*
0.25% solution: 5 ml (12.5 mg)
0.5% solution: 5 ml (25 mg)

**CV:** edema.
**Skin:** dermatologic reactions.
**Respiratory:** *status asthmaticus.*
**Other:** *anaphylactoid reactions,
anaphylaxis*
Systemic effects from high blood
levels of the drug—
**CNS:** anxiety, nervousness,
*seizures* followed by drowsiness.
**CV:** *arrhythmias, bradycardia,
cardiac arrest,* hypotension, my-
ocardial depression.
**EENT:** blurred vision, tinnitus.
**GI:** nausea, vomiting.
**Respiratory:** *respiratory arrest.*

---

**chloroprocaine hydrochloride**
(Nesacaine, Nesacaine-MPF)
Dosages given are for the drug without epinephrine and for adults.
Volume listed below refers to the total volume of anesthetic given,
sometimes in incremental doses of 2 to 6 ml.
*Infiltration and nerve block—*
1% solution: 3 to 20 ml (30 to 200 mg)
2% solution: 2 to 40 ml (40 to 800 mg)
*Caudal and epidural block—*
2% to 3% solution: 15 to 25 ml (300 to 750 mg)
   May be repeated with smaller doses q 40 to 50 minutes. Dose
and interval may be increased when given with epinephrine. Maximum adult dose is 800 mg; when given with epinephrine, maximum dose is 1 g.

**CV:** edema.
**Respiratory:** *status asthmaticus.*
**Skin:** dermatologic reactions.
**Other:** *anaphylactoid reactions,
anaphylaxis.*
Systemic effects from high blood
levels of the drug—
**CNS:** anxiety, nervousness,
*seizures* followed by drowsiness.
**CV:** *arrhythmias, bradycar-
dia, cardiac arrest,* hypotension,
myocardial depression.
**EENT:** blurred vision, tinnitus.
**GI:** nausea, vomiting.
**Respiratory:** *respiratory arrest.*

---

**etidocaine hydrochloride**
(Duranest, Duranest-MPF)
Dosages given are for the drug without epinephrine and for adults.
   Dose limit is 4 mg/kg or 300 mg per injection. When given with
epinephrine, dose limit is 5.5 mg/kg or 400 mg per injection. May
be repeated q 2 to 3 hours.
*Peripheral nerve block—*
1% solution: 5 to 40 ml (50 to 400 mg)
*Central neural block (lower limbs, cesarean section, lumbar,
epidural)—*
1% solution: 10 to 30 ml (100 to 300 mg)
*Transvaginal block—*
1% solution: 5 to 20 ml (50 to 200 mg)
*Caudal block—*
1% solution: 10 to 30 ml (100 to 300 mg)

**CV:** edema.
**Respiratory:** *status asthmaticus.*
**Skin:** dermatologic reactions.
**Other:** *anaphylactoid reactions,
anaphylaxis.*
Systemic effects from high blood
levels of the drug—
**CNS:** anxiety, apprehension, ner-
vousness, *seizures* followed by
drowsiness.
**CV:** *arrhythmias, bradycardia,
cardiac arrest,* hypotension, my-
ocardial depression.
**EENT:** blurred vision, tinnitus.
**GI:** nausea, vomiting.
**Respiratory:** *respiratory arrest.*

---

Reactions may be *common*, uncommon, *life-threatening*, or COMMON AND LIFE-THREATENING.

| INTERACTIONS | NURSING CONSIDERATIONS |
|---|---|
| *Beta blockers:* enhanced sympathomimetic effects when used with bupivacaine and epinephrine. Use with caution.<br>*Butyrophenones, phenothiazines:* may reduce or reverse pressor effect of epinephrine. Monitor patient.<br>*Chloroprocaine:* may lessen bupivacaine's action. Don't use together.<br>*CNS depressants:* may cause additive CNS effects. Reduce dosage of CNS depressants.<br>*Cyclic antidepressants, MAO inhibitors:* severe, sustained hypertension when used with bupivacaine and epinephrine. Use with extreme caution.<br>*Enflurane, halothane, isoflurane, related drugs:* arrhythmias when used with bupivacaine and epinephrine. Use with extreme caution. | • Contraindicated in patients with history of hypersensitivity reactions to local amide-type anesthetics and in children younger than age 12 for spinal or topical anesthesia or paracervical block.<br>• Some solutions contain sulfites and should be avoided in patients with sulfite hypersensitivity.<br>• Don't use for I.V. regional anesthesia (Bier block, Bier's local anesthesia).<br>• Don't use 0.75% solution for obstetric surgery; lower percentages are effective and less hazardous.<br>• Use cautiously in debilitated, elderly, or acutely ill patients and in patients with severe hepatic disease or drug allergies.<br>• Use solutions with epinephrine cautiously in patients with CV disorders and in body areas with limited blood supply (ears, nose, fingers, toes).<br>• Keep resuscitation equipment and drugs available.<br>• Don't use solution with preservatives for caudal or epidural block.<br>• Discard partially used vials without preservatives.<br>• Check solution for particles.<br>• Protect solutions containing epinephrine from light. |
| *Bupivacaine:* chloroprocaine may lessen bupivacaine's action. Monitor for effect.<br>*CNS depressants:* may cause additive CNS effects. Reduce dosage of CNS depressants.<br>*Sulfonamides:* chloroprocaine inhibits the action of sulfonamides. Don't use in conditions in which a sulfonamide drug is required. | • Contraindicated in patients with hypersensitivity to procaine, tetracaine, or other PABA derivatives and for spinal or topical anesthesia. Epidural and caudal blocks are contraindicated in patients with CNS disease.<br>• Use cautiously in debilitated, elderly, or acutely ill patients; in children; and in patients with drug allergies, paracervical block, or CV disease.<br>• Keep resuscitation equipment and drugs available.<br>• Don't use solution with preservatives for caudal or epidural block.<br>• Don't use discolored solution.<br>• Check solution for particles.<br>• Discard partially used vials without preservatives. |
| *Cyclic antidepressants, MAO inhibitors:* severe, sustained hypertension or hypotension with etidocaine and epinephrine. Use with extreme caution.<br>*Enflurane, halothane, isoflurane, related drugs:* arrhythmias when used with etidocaine and epinephrine. Use with extreme caution.<br>*CNS depressants:* may cause additive CNS effects. Reduce dosage of CNS depressants. | • Contraindicated in patients with inflammation or infection in puncture region, septicemia, severe hypertension, spinal deformities, or neurologic disorders; in children younger than age 14; and for spinal anesthesia.<br>• Contraindicated in patients with known history of hypersensitivity to local anesthetics of the amide type.<br>• Some solutions contain sulfites and should be avoided in patients with sulfite hypersensitivity.<br>• Use cautiously in debilitated, elderly, or acutely ill patients; in patients with severe shock, heart block, general drug allergies, or hepatic and renal disease; and as epidural block in pregnant women.<br>• Use solutions with epinephrine cautiously in patients with CV disease and in body areas with limited blood supply (ears, nose, fingers, toes).<br>• Don't use solution with preservatives for caudal or epidural block; check solution for particles.<br>• Keep resuscitation equipment and drugs available. |

*(continued)*

| DRUG, INDICATIONS, DOSAGE | ADVERSE REACTIONS |
|---|---|

**Local** (continued)

**lidocaine hydrochloride**
[lignocaine hydrochloride]
(Dilocaine, Lidoject-1, Lidoject-2, Nervocaine, Xylocaine)
Dosages given are for drug without epinephrine and for adults. Volume listed below refers to total volume of anesthetic given, sometimes in incremental doses of 2 to 6 ml.
*For anesthesia other than spinal—*
Maximum single dose is 4.5 mg/kg or 300 mg. With epinephrine, maximum dose is 7 mg/kg or 500 mg.
*Caudal (obstetric) or epidural (thoracic) block—*
1% solution: 20 to 30 ml (200 to 300 mg)
*Epidural (lumbar anesthesia) block—*
1% solution: 25 to 30 ml (250 to 300 mg)
1.5% solution: 15 to 20 ml (225 to 300 mg)
2% solution: 10 to 15 ml (200 to 300 mg)
*Spinal surgical anesthesia—*
5% (with 7.5% dextrose): 1.5 to 2 ml (75 to 100 mg)
*Caudal (surgery) block—*
1.5% solution: 15 to 20 ml (225 to 300 mg)

**CV:** edema.
**Respiratory:** *status asthmaticus.*
**Skin:** dermatologic reactions.
**Other:** *anaphylactoid reactions, anaphylaxis.*
Systemic effects from high blood levels of the drug—
**CNS:** anxiety, nervousness, *seizures* followed by drowsiness.
**CV:** *arrhythmias, bradycardia, cardiac arrest,* myocardial depression, hypotension.
**EENT:** blurred vision, tinnitus.
**GI:** nausea, vomiting.
**Respiratory:** *respiratory arrest.*

**procaine hydrochloride**
(Novocain)
*Spinal anesthesia—*
**Adults:** initial dose shouldn't exceed 1 g. Before using, dilute 10% solution with normal saline injection, sterile distilled water, or CSF. For hyperbaric technique, use dextrose solution.
*Perineum:* 0.5 ml of 10% solution (50 mg) and 0.5 ml diluent injected at the L4 interspace.
*Perineum and lower extremities:* 1 ml of 10% solution (100 mg) and 1 ml diluent injected at the L3 or L4 interspace.
*Up to costal margin:* 2 ml of 10% solution (200 mg) and 1 ml diluent injected at the L2, L3, or L4 interspace.
*Peripheral nerve block—*
1% solution: 50 ml (500 mg)
2% solution: 25 ml (500 mg)
*Infiltration—*
350 to 600 mg in 0.25% to 0.5% solution. Maximum initial dose is 1 g.

**CV:** edema.
**Respiratory:** *status asthmaticus.*
**Skin:** dermatologic reactions.
**Other:** *anaphylactoid reactions, anaphylaxis.*
Systemic effects from high blood levels of the drug—
**CNS:** anxiety, nervousness, *seizures* followed by drowsiness.
**CV:** *arrhythmias, bradycardia, cardiac arrest,* hypotension, myocardial depression.
**EENT:** blurred vision, tinnitus.
**GI:** nausea, vomiting.
**Respiratory:** *respiratory arrest.*

**ropivacaine hydrochloride**
(Naropin)
Dosages given are for adults. Avoid rapid injection of large volume of local anesthetic and use incremental doses. Use smallest dose and concentration required to produce desired result.
*Lumbar epidural block in surgery—*
0.5% solution: 15 to 30 ml (75 to 150 mg)
0.75% solution: 15 to 25 ml (119 to 188 mg)
1.0% solution: 15 to 20 ml (150 to 200 mg)
*Lumbar epidural block for cesarean section—*
0.5% solution: 20 to 30 ml (100 to 150 mg)
*Thoracic epidural administration to establish block for postoperative pain relief—*
0.5% solution: 5 to 15 ml (25 to 75 mg)
*Major nerve block (brachial plexus)—*
0.5 % solution: 35 to 50 ml (175 to 250 mg)
*Field block (minor nerve blocks and infiltration)—*
0.5% solution: 1 to 10 ml (5 to 200 mg)

**CNS:** anxiety, dizziness, headache, hypoesthesia, pain, paresthesia.
**CV:** *bradycardia,* chest pain, hypotension, hypertension, tachycardia.
**GI:** nausea, vomiting.
**GU:** oliguria, urine retention.
**Hematologic:** anemia.
**Musculoskeletal:** back pain.
**Skin:** pruritus.
**Other:** fever, chills, postoperative complications.
*Neonatal*—vomiting, jaundice, tachypnea, respiratory distress.
*Fetal*— *bradycardia,* fever, tachycardia, distress.

---

Reactions may be *common,* uncommon, *life-threatening,* or COMMON AND LIFE-THREATENING.

| INTERACTIONS | NURSING CONSIDERATIONS |
|---|---|

*Beta blockers:* enhanced sympathomimetic effects. Don't use with lidocaine and epinephrine.
*Butyrophenones, phenothiazines:* may reduce or reverse the pressor effect of epinephrine. Monitor patient.
*CNS depressants:* may cause additive CNS effects. Reduce dosage of CNS depressants.
*Cyclic antidepressants, MAO inhibitors:* severe, sustained hypertension when used with lidocaine and epinephrine. Use with extreme caution.
*Enflurane, halothane, isoflurane, related drugs:* arrhythmias when used with lidocaine and epinephrine. Use with extreme caution.

• Contraindicated in patients with inflammation or infection in puncture region, septicemia, severe hypertension, spinal deformities, and neurologic disorders.
• Also contraindicated in patients with known history of hypersensitivity to local anesthetics of the amide type.
• Use cautiously in debilitated, elderly, or acutely ill patients; in patients with severe shock, heart block, or general drug allergies; in obstetric patients; and for paracervical block.
• Dose and interval are increased with epinephrine.
• Use solutions with epinephrine cautiously in patients with CV disorders and in body areas with limited blood supply (ears, nose, fingers, toes).
• Don't use solution with preservatives for spinal, epidural, or caudal block.
• Keep resuscitation equipment and drugs available.
• Discard partially used vials without preservatives.
• Check solution for particles.

---

*CNS depressants:* may cause additive CNS effects. Reduce dosage of CNS depressants.
*Echothiophate iodide:* reduced hydrolysis of procaine. Use together cautiously.
*Succinylcholine:* prolonged neuromuscular blockade. Use cautiously together.
*Sulfonamides:* procaine inhibits the action of sulfonamides. Don't use when a sulfonamide is required.

• Contraindicated in patients with hypersensitivity to chloroprocaine, tetracaine, or other PABA derivatives and in those with traumatized urethras.
• Also contraindicated in pregnant women with cephalopelvic disproportion, placenta previa, abruptio placentae, floating fetal head, and intrauterine manipulation.
• Use cautiously in hyperexcitable patients; in those with CNS disease, infection at puncture site, shock, profound anemia, cachexia, sepsis, hypertension, hypotension, GI hemorrhage, bowel perforation or strangulation, peritonitis, cardiac decompensation, massive pleural effusion, or increased intra-abdominal pressure; and in pregnant women.
• Keep resuscitation equipment and drugs available.
• Use preservative-free solution for epidural block.
• Discard partially used vials without preservatives.

---

*Amide-type anesthetics:* additive effects if given with ropivacaine. Use with caution.
*CNS depressants:* may cause additive CNS effects. Reduce dosage of CNS depressants.
*Fluvoxamine, imipramine, theophylline, verapamil:* may interact with ropivacaine. Use with caution.

• Contraindicated in patients with known hypersensitivity to drug or local amide-type anesthetics.
• Use cautiously (especially when giving repeat doses) in debilitated, elderly, acutely ill, or breast-feeding patients and in patients with hypotension, hypovolemia, impaired CV function, heart block, or hepatic disease.
• Don't inject drug rapidly.
• Aspiration for blood should be done before all doses to avoid intravascular or subarachnoid injection.
• Drug should only be used by personnel familiar with use of drug. Have emergency equipment and personnel available.
• Don't use drug in emergency situations.
• Don't use drug for the production of obstetric paracervical block anesthesia, retrobulbar block, or spinal anesthesia (subarachnoid block).
• Don't use drug for I.V. regional anesthesia (Bier block).
*(continued)*

---

*Liquid contains alcohol.   **May contain tartrazine.   †Canada   ‡Australia   §U.K.   ◊OTC

| DRUG, INDICATIONS, DOSAGE | ADVERSE REACTIONS |
|---|---|

### Local (continued)

**ropivacaine hydrochloride** (continued)
*Lumbar epidural block in labor—*
Initially, 0.2% solution: 10 to 20 ml (20 to 40 mg); then 6 to 14 ml/hour (12 to 28 mg/hour) as continuous infusion or 10 to 15 ml/hour (20 to 30 mg/hour) as incremental "top-up" injections
*Lumbar epidural block in postoperative pain management—*
0.2% solution: 6 to 10 ml/hour (12 to 20 mg/hour) as continuous infusion
*Thoracic epidural block in postoperative pain management—*
0.2% solution: 4 to 8 ml/hour (8 to 16 mg/hour) as continuous infusion
*Infiltration (minor nerve block) in postoperative pain management—*
0.2% solution: 1 to 100 ml (2 to 200 mg)
0.5% solution: 1 to 40 ml (5 to 200 mg)

---

**tetracaine hydrochloride**
(Pontocaine)
Dosage for adults varies according to extent of block.
*Low spinal (saddle) block in vaginal delivery—*
2 to 5 mg as hyperbaric solution (in 10% dextrose)
*Perineum and lower extremities:* 5 to 10 mg
*Up to costal margin:* 15 to 20 mg

**CV:** edema.
**Respiratory:** *status asthmaticus.*
**Skin:** dermatologic reactions.
**Other:** *anaphylactoid reactions, anaphylaxis.*
Systemic effects from high blood levels of the drug—
**CNS:** anxiety, nervousness, *seizures* followed by drowsiness.
**CV:** *arrhythmias, bradycardia, cardiac arrest,* hypotension, myocardial depression.
**EENT:** blurred vision, tinnitus.
**GI:** nausea, vomiting.
**Respiratory:** *respiratory arrest.*

### Topical

**proparacaine hydrochloride**
(AK-Taine, Alcaine, Ophthetic)
*Anesthesia for tonometry, gonioscopy—*
**Adults and children:** 1 or 2 gtt of 0.5% solution instilled in eye just before procedure.
*Anesthesia for cataract extraction, glaucoma surgery—*
**Adults and children:** 1 or 2 gtt of 0.5% solution instilled in eye q 5 to 10 minutes for five to seven doses.
*Removal of foreign bodies or sutures—*
**Adults and children:** 1 or 2 gtt 2 to 3 minutes before procedure or q 5 to 10 minutes for one to three doses.

**EENT:** conjunctival redness, transient eye pain.
**Other:** *hypersensitivity reactions.*

---

**tetracaine**
(Pontocaine Solution)
**tetracaine hydrochloride**
(Pontocaine)
*Anesthesia for tonometry, gonioscopy; removal of corneal foreign bodies, suture removal from cornea; other diagnostic and minor surgical procedures—*
**Adults and children:** 1 to 2 gtt of 0.5% or 1%† in eye just before procedure.

**EENT:** transient stinging in eye 30 seconds after initial instillation, epithelial damage with excessive or long-term use.
**Other:** sensitization with repeated use (allergic skin rash, urticaria).

---

Reactions may be *common*, uncommon, *life-threatening*, or COMMON AND LIFE-THREATENING.

| INTERACTIONS | NURSING CONSIDERATIONS |
|---|---|

● Use an adequate test dose (3 to 5 ml of short-acting local anesthetic solution containing epinephrine) before induction of complete block.
● Restlessness, anxiety, incoherent speech, light-headedness, numbness and tingling of mouth and lips, metallic taste, tinnitus, dizziness, blurred vision, tremors, twitching, depression, or drowsiness may be early warning signs or symptoms of CNS toxicity.
● Don't use drug in ophthalmic surgery.

---

*CNS depressants:* may cause additive CNS effects. Reduce dosage of CNS depressants.
*Sulfonamides:* tetracaine inhibits the action of sulfonamides. Don't use in conditions in which a sulfonamide is required.

● Safety and efficacy in children haven't been established.
● Contraindicated in patients with hypersensitivity to procaine or related drugs and in those with infection at injection site or CNS disease.
● Saddle block is contraindicated in patients with cephalopelvic disproportion, placenta previa, abruptio placentae, intrauterine manipulation, and floating fetal head.
● Use cautiously in patients with shock, profound anemia, cachexia, hypertension, hypotension, peritonitis, cardiac decompensation, massive pleural effusion, increased intracranial pressure, and infection.
● Keep resuscitation equipment and drugs available.
● When CSF is added to powdered drug or drug solution during spinal anesthesia, solution may be cloudy. Don't use discolored or crystallized solutions.
● Protect drug from light; store in refrigerator.

---

None significant.

● Contraindicated in patients with hypersensitivity to ester-type local anesthetics, PABA or its derivatives, or to other ingredients in these preparations.
● Use cautiously in patients with cardiac disease and hyperthyroidism.
● Drug isn't for long-term use; it may delay wound healing.
● Warn patients not to rub or touch eye while cornea is anesthetized.
● Warn patients with corneal abrasion that pain is relieved only temporarily.
● Don't use discolored solution.
● Store drug in tightly closed container. Refrigerate opened containers.
● Check solution for particles.

---

*Anticholinesterases:* prolonged ocular anesthesia and increased risk of toxic reaction. Use with caution.
*Sulfonamides:* interference with sulfonamide antibacterial activity. Wait 30 minutes after anesthesia before instilling sulfonamide.

● Contraindicated in patients with hypersensitivity to drug or similar drugs (such as ester-type local anesthetics), PABA or its derivatives, or other ingredients in these preparations.
● Avoid long-term use.
● Drug doesn't dilate the pupil, paralyze accommodation, or increase intraocular pressure.
● Don't use discolored solution. Keep container tightly closed.
● Warn patient not to touch or rub eye while cornea is anesthetized.

---

*Liquid contains alcohol.    **May contain tartrazine.    †Canada    ‡Australia    §U.K.    ◇OTC

# Diagnostic skin tests

## DRUG, INDICATIONS, DOSAGE

**coccidioidin**
BioCox, Spherulin

*Suspected coccidioidomycosis—*
**Adults and children:** 0.1 ml of 1:100 dilution I.D. into flexor surface of forearm. In patients who don't react to this form, repeat test using 1:10 dilution. Use 1:1,000 or 1:10,000 dilution if erythema nodosum is evident.

**histoplasmin**
Histolyn-CYL, Histoplasmin Diluted

*To differentiate histoplasmosis from coccidioidomycosis, tuberculosis, sarcoidosis, and other mycotic or bacterial infections—*
**Adults and children:** 0.1 ml into flexor surface of forearm.

**mumps skin test antigen**
MSTA

*Detection of delayed hypersensitivity to mumps antigens and assessment of cell-mediated immunity—*
**Adults and children:** 0.1 ml I.D. into flexor surface of forearm.

**tuberculin purified protein derivative (Mantoux, PPD, TST)**
Aplisol, PPD-Stabilized Solution (Mantoux test), Selavo-PPD Solution, Tubersol

*Diagnosis of tuberculosis—*
**Adults and children:** initially, 1 tuberculin unit (TU; for patients suspected of being highly sensitized) or 5 TU (for patients not expected to be highly sensitized) I.D. into flexor surface of forearm. If patient has a negative reaction, retest him with 250 TU.

**tuberculosis multiple-puncture tests**
Aplitest (dried purified protein derivative [PPD]), Mono-Vacc Test (liquid Old Tuberculin [OT]), Tine Test (dried OT, dried PPD)

*Screening for tuberculosis—*
**Adults and children:** clean skin thoroughly with alcohol and allow to dry; make skin taut on flexor surface of forearm and press points firmly into selected site. Hold device at injection site for about 3 seconds to ensure depositing of dried tuberculin B in tissue lymph.

| ADVERSE REACTIONS | NURSING CONSIDERATIONS |
|---|---|
| **Other:** *hypersensitivity reactions* (vesiculation, ulceration, necrosis), *anaphylaxis,* Arthus reaction. | • Pregnancy Risk Category C.<br>• Contraindicated in patients with hypersensitivity to thimerosal or erythema nodosum.<br>• Read test at 24 and 48 hours. |
| **Skin:** urticaria, ulceration, vesiculation, or necrosis in highly sensitive patients.<br>**Other:** *angioedema, anaphylaxis.* | • Pregnancy Risk Category C.<br>• Contraindicated in patients with a history of positive reaction to this test.<br>• Read test within 48 to 72 hours.<br>• For cell-mediated immunity with other antigens, reaction should be examined in 24 to 48 hours. |
| **Other:** *hypersensitivity reactions* (vesiculation, ulceration), *anaphylaxis,* Arthus reaction. | • Pregnancy Risk Category C.<br>• Contraindicated in patients with hypersensitivity to eggs, egg products, or thimerosal.<br>• Read test at 48 and 72 hours. |
| **CNS:** pain.<br>**Skin:** pruritus, vesiculation.<br>**Other:** *hypersensitivity reactions, anaphylaxis,* Arthus reaction, ulceration, necrosis. | • Pregnancy Risk Category C.<br>• Contraindicated in patients with a history of positive reaction to tuberculin tests; severe reactions may occur.<br>• Read test within 48 to 72 hours. If repeat test using 250 TU shows no response, patient is nonreactive.<br>• A patient who doesn't show a positive reaction to 1 TU or 5 TU on the first test may be retested with 5 TU. If second test reaction is negative, patient may be tested with 250 TU. Perform any repeat testing on the other forearm. Don't use 250 TU for the initial injection. |
| **Other:** *hypersensitivity reactions* (vesiculation, ulceration, necrosis), *anaphylaxis*. | • Pregnancy Risk Category C.<br>• Contraindicated in patients with a history of positive reaction to tuberculin tests.<br>• Read test within 48 to 72 hours. Verify questionable or positive reactions with the Mantoux test. |

Reactions may be *common*, uncommon, *life-threatening*, or COMMON AND LIFE-THREATENING.

# Cancer chemotherapy: Acronyms and protocols

This chart lists commonly used chemotherapy acronyms and protocols, including standard dosages for specific cancers.

| ACRONYM & INDICATION | GENERIC DRUG NAME | TRADE DRUG NAME | DOSAGE |
|---|---|---|---|
| **ABVD** (Hodgkin's disease) | doxorubicin | Adriamycin | 25 mg/m$^2$ I.V., days 1 and 15 |
| | bleomycin | Blenoxane | 10 U/m$^2$ I.V., days 1 and 15 |
| | vinblastine | Velban | 6 mg/m$^2$ I.V., days 1 and 15 |
| | dacarbazine | DTIC-Dome | 350 to 375 mg/m$^2$ I.V., days 1 and 15 *Repeat cycle q 28 days.* |
| **AC** (Bony sarcoma) | doxorubicin | Adriamycin | 75 to 90 mg/m$^2$ (total dose) by 96-hour continuous I.V. infusion |
| | cisplatin | Platinol | 90 to 120 mg/m$^2$ intra-arterial or I.V., day 6 *Repeat cycle q 28 days.* |
| **AC** (Breast cancer) | doxorubicin | Adriamycin | 60 mg/m$^2$ I.V., day 1 |
| | cyclophosphamide | Cytoxan | 400 to 600 mg/m$^2$ I.V., day 1 *Repeat cycle q 21 days.* |
| **ACE (CAE)** (Small-cell lung cancer) | doxorubicin | Adriamycin | 45 mg/m$^2$ I.V., day 1 |
| | cyclophosphamide | Cytoxan | 1,000 mg/m$^2$ I.V., day 1 |
| | etoposide (VP-16) | VePesid | 50 mg/m$^2$ I.V., days 1 to 5 *Repeat cycle q 21 days.* |
| **AP** (Endometrial cancer) | doxorubicin | Adriamycin | 50 to 60 mg/m$^2$ I.V., day 1 |
| | cisplatin | Platinol | 50 to 60 mg/m$^2$ I.V., day 1 *Repeat cycle q 21 days.* |
| **BEP** (Testicular cancer) | bleomycin | Blenoxane | 30 U I.V., days 2, 9, and 16 |
| | etoposide (VP-16) | VePesid | 100 mg/m$^2$, days 1 to 5 |
| | cisplatin | Platinol | 20 mg/m$^2$ I.V., days 1 to 5 *Repeat cycle q 21 days.* |
| **CAF (FAC)** (Breast cancer) | cyclophosphamide | Cytoxan | 100 mg/m$^2$ P.O., days 1 to 14 |
| | doxorubicin | Adriamycin | 30 mg/m$^2$ I.V., days 1 and (optional) 8 |
| | fluorouracil (5-FU) | Adrucil | 400 to 500 mg/m$^2$ I.V., days 1 and 8 *Repeat cycle q 28 days.* |
| *or* | cyclophosphamide | Cytoxan | 500 mg/m$^2$ I.V., day 1 |
| | doxorubicin | Adriamycin | 50 mg/m$^2$ I.V., day 1 |
| | fluorouracil (5-FU) | Adrucil | 500 mg/m$^2$ I.V., day 1 *Repeat cycle q 21 days.* |
| **CAP** (Non-small-cell lung cancer) | cyclophosphamide | Cytoxan | 400 mg/m$^2$ I.V., day 1 |
| | doxorubicin | Adriamycin | 40 mg/m$^2$ I.V., day 1 |
| | cisplatin | Platinol | 60 mg/m$^2$ I.V., day 1 *Repeat cycle q 28 days.* |

| ACRONYM & INDICATION | GENERIC DRUG NAME | TRADE DRUG NAME | DOSAGE |
|---|---|---|---|
| **CAV (VAC)** (Small-cell lung cancer) | cyclophosphamide | Cytoxan | 750 to 1,000 mg/m$^2$ I.V., day 1 |
| | doxorubicin | Adriamycin | 40 to 50 mg/m$^2$ I.V., day 1 |
| | vincristine | Oncovin | 1.4 mg/m$^2$ (2 mg maximum) I.V., day 1 *Repeat cycle q 21 days.* |
| **CC** (Ovarian cancer, epithelial) | carboplatin | Paraplatin | 300 mg/m$^2$ I.V., day 1 |
| | cyclophosphamide | Cytoxan | 600 mg/m$^2$ I.V., day 1 *Repeat cycle q 28 days.* |
| **CF** (Head and neck cancer) | cisplatin | Platinol | 100 mg/m$^2$ I.V., day 1 |
| | fluorouracil (5-FU) | Adrucil | 1,000 mg/m$^2$ daily by continuous I.V. infusion, days 1 to 5 *Repeat cycle q 21 to 28 days.* |
| *or* | carboplatin | Paraplatin | 400 mg/m$^2$ I.V., day 1 |
| | fluorouracil (5-FU) | Adrucil | 1,000 mg/m$^2$ daily by continuous I.V. infusion, days 1 to 5 *Repeat cycle q 21 to 28 days.* |
| **CFM (CNF, FNC)** (Breast cancer) | cyclophosphamide | Cytoxan | 500 mg/m$^2$ I.V., day 1 |
| | fluorouracil (5-FU) | Adrucil | 500 mg/m$^2$ I.V., day 1 |
| | mitoxantrone | Novantrone | 10 mg/m$^2$ I.V., day 1 *Repeat cycle q 21 days.* |
| **CHOP** (Malignant lymphoma) | cyclophosphamide | Cytoxan | 750 mg/m$^2$ I.V., day 1 |
| | doxorubicin | Adriamycin | 50 mg/m$^2$ I.V., day 1 |
| | vincristine | Oncovin | 1.4 mg/m$^2$ (2 mg maximum) I.V., day 1 |
| | prednisone | Deltasone | 100 mg P.O., days 1 to 5 *Repeat cycle q 21 days.* |
| **CHOP-Bleo** (Malignant lymphoma) | cyclophosphamide | Cytoxan | 750 mg/m$^2$ I.V., day 1 |
| | doxorubicin | Adriamycin | 50 mg/m$^2$ I.V., day 1 |
| | vincristine | Oncovin | 2 mg I.V., days 1 and 5 |
| | prednisone | Deltasone | 100 mg P.O., days 1 to 5 |
| | bleomycin | Blenoxane | 15 U I.V., days 1 and 5 *Repeat cycle q 14 to 21 days.* |
| **CISCA** (Genitourinary cancer) | cisplatin | Platinol | 70 to 100 mg/m$^2$ I.V., day 2 |
| | cyclophosphamide | Cytoxan | 650 mg/m$^2$ I.V., day 1 |
| | doxorubicin | Adriamycin | 50 mg/m$^2$ I.V., day 1 *Repeat cycle q 21 to 28 days.* |
| **CMF** (Breast cancer) | cyclophosphamide | Cytoxan | 100 mg/m$^2$ P.O., days 1 to 14, or 400 to 600 mg/m$^2$ I.V., day 1 |
| | methotrexate | Folex | 40 mg/m$^2$ I.V., days 1 and 8 |
| | fluorouracil (5-FU) | Adrucil | 400 to 600 mg/m$^2$ I.V., days 1 and 8 *Repeat cycle q 28 days.* |
| **COP** (Malignant lymphoma) | cyclophosphamide | Cytoxan | 750 to 1,000 mg/m$^2$ I.V., day 1 |
| | vincristine | Oncovin | 1.4 mg/m$^2$ (2 mg maximum) I.V., day 1 |
| | prednisone | Deltasone | 60 mg/m2 P.O., days 1 to 5 Repeat cycle q 21 days. |

*(continued)*

| ACRONYM & INDICATION | GENERIC DRUG NAME | TRADE DRUG NAME | DOSAGE |
|---|---|---|---|
| **COPP** (Hodgkin's disease and malignant lymphoma) | cyclophosphamide | Cytoxan | 500 to 650 mg/m² I.V., days 1 and 8 |
| | vincristine | Oncovin | 1.4 mg/m² (2 mg maximum) I.V., days 1 and 8 |
| | procarbazine | Matulane | 100 mg/m² P.O., days 1 to 10 or 1 to 14 |
| | prednisone | Deltasone | 40 mg/m² P.O., days 1 to 14 *Repeat cycle q 28 days.* |
| **CP** (Ovarian cancer) | cyclophosphamide | Cytoxan | 600 to 1,000 mg/m² I.V., day 1 |
| | cisplatin | Platinol | 50 to 100 mg/m² I.V., day 1 *Repeat cycle q 21 days.* |
| **CVP** (Leukemia— CLL) | cyclophosphamide | Cytoxan | 400 mg/m² P.O., days 1 to 5 |
| | vincristine | Oncovin | 1.4 mg/m² (2 mg maximum) I.V., day 1 |
| | prednisone | Deltasone | 100 mg/m² P.O., days 1 to 5 *Repeat cycle q 21 days.* |
| **CVPP** (Hodgkin's disease) | lomustine (CCNU) | CeeNu | 75 mg/m² P.O., day 1 |
| | vinblastine | Velban | 4 mg/m² I.V., days 1 and 8 |
| | procarbazine | Matulane | 100 mg/m² P.O., days 1 to 14 |
| | prednisone | Deltasone | 30 mg/m² P.O., days 1 to 14 (cycles 1 and 4 only) *Repeat cycle q 28 days.* |
| **CYVADIC** (Soft-tissue sarcoma) | cyclophosphamide | Cytoxan | 500 to 600 mg/m² I.V., day 1 |
| | vincristine | Oncovin | 1.4 mg/m² (2 mg maximum) I.V., days 1 and 5 |
| | doxorubicin | Adriamycin | 50 mg/m² I.V., day 1 |
| | dacarbazine | DTIC-Dome | 250 mg/m² I.V., days 1 to 5 *Repeat cycle q 21 days.* |
| **DCBT** (Dartmouth regimen) (Melanoma) | dacarbazine | DTIC-Dome | 220 mg/m² I.V., days 1 to 3, days 22 to 24 |
| | cisplatin | Platinol | 25 mg/m² I.V., days 1 to 3, days 22 to 24 |
| | carmustine (BCNU) | BiCNU | 150 mg/m² I.V., day 1 |
| | tamoxifen | Nolvadex | 10 mg P.O. b.i.d., starting day 4 |
| **DVP** (Leukemia— ALL, adult induction) | daunorubicin | Cerubidine | 45 mg/m² I.V., days 1 to 3 and day 14 |
| | vincristine | Oncovin | 2 mg I.V., days 1, 8, 15, and 22 |
| | prednisone | Deltasone | 45 mg/m² P.O., for 28 to 35 days |
| **EP** (Small-cell or non-small-cell lung cancer) | cisplatin | Platinol | 75 to 100 mg/m² I.V., day 1 |
| | etoposide (VP-16) | VePesid | 75 to 100 mg/m² I.V., days 1 to 3 *Repeat cycle q 21 to 28 days.* |
| **FAC (CAF)** (Breast cancer) | fluorouracil (5-FU) | Adrucil | 500 mg/m² I.V., days 1 and 8 |
| | doxorubicin | Adriamycin | 50 mg/m² I.V., day 1 |
| | cyclophosphamide | Cytoxan | 500 mg/m² I.V., day 1 *Repeat cycle q 21 days.* |
| **FAM** (Adenocarcinoma, gastric cancer) | fluorouracil (5-FU) | Adrucil | 600 mg/m² I.V., days 1, 8, 29, and 36 |
| | doxorubicin | Adriamycin | 30 mg/m² I.V., days 1 and 29 |
| | mitomycin | Mutamycin | 10 mg/m² I.V., day 1 *Repeat cycle q 8 weeks.* |

| ACRONYM & INDICATION | GENERIC DRUG NAME | TRADE DRUG NAME | DOSAGE |
|---|---|---|---|
| **F-CL** (Colorectal cancer) | fluorouracil (5-FU) | Adrucil | 600 mg/m$^2$ I.V., 1 hour after initiating leucovorin infusion weekly for 6 weeks |
| | leucovorin calcium | Wellcovorin | 500 mg/m$^2$ over 2 hours weekly for 6 weeks *Repeat cycle after 2-week break.* |
| *or* | fluorouracil (5-FU) | Adrucil | 370 to 400 mg/m$^2$ I.V., days 1 to 5, following leucovorin |
| | leucovorin calcium | Wellcovorin | 200 mg/m$^2$ daily I.V., days 1 to 5 *Repeat cycle q 28 to 35 days.* |
| *or* | fluorouracil (5-FU) | Adrucil | 425 mg/m$^2$ I.V., days 1 to 5, following leucovorin |
| | leucovorin calcium | Wellcovorin | 20 mg/m$^2$ I.V., days 1 to 5 *Repeat q 28 to 35 days.* |
| **5 + 2** (Leukemia—AML, induction) | cytarabine (ara-C) | Cytosar-U | 100 to 200 mg/m$^2$ by continuous I.V. infusion, days 1 to 5 |
| | daunorubicin | Cerubidine | 45 mg/m$^2$ I.V., days 1 and 2 |
| **FL** (Prostate cancer) | flutamide | Eulexin | 250 mg P.O. t.i.d. |
| | leuprolide acetate | Lupron | 1 mg S.C. daily |
| *or* | flutamide | Eulexin | 250 mg P.O. t.i.d. |
| | leuprolide acetate | Lupron Depot | 7.5 mg I.M. q 28 days *Repeat cycle q 28 days.* |
| **FLe** (Colorectal cancer) | levamisole | Ergamisol | 50 mg P.O. q 8 hours for days 1 to 3, repeated q 2 weeks for 1 year |
| | fluorouracil (5-FU) | Adrucil | 450 mg/m$^2$ I.V. for days 1 to 5 and day 28; weekly thereafter for 48 weeks |
| **FZ** (Genitourinary, prostate cancer) | flutamide | Eulexin | 250 P.O. q 8 hours |
| | goserelin acetate | Zoladex | 3.6 mg implant S.C. q 28 days |
| **HDMTX** (high-dose methotrexate) (Bony sarcoma) | methotrexate | Folex | 8 to 12 g/m$^2$ I.V. weekly for 2 to 12 weeks |
| | leucovorin calcium | Wellcovorin | 15 to 25 mg/m$^2$ I.V. or P.O. q 6 hours for 10 doses, beginning 24 hours after methotrexate dose (serum methotrexate levels must be monitored) *Repeat cycle q 7 days for 2 to 4 weeks.* |
| **MACOP-B** (Malignant lymphoma) | methotrexate | Folex | 400 mg/m$^2$ I.V., weeks 2, 6, and 10 |
| | leucovorin calcium | Wellcovorin | 15 mg/m$^2$ P.O. q 6 hours for six doses, beginning 24 hours after methotrexate dose |
| | doxorubicin | Adriamycin | 50 mg/m$^2$ I.V., weeks 1, 3, 5, 7, 9, and 11 |
| | cyclophosphamide | Cytoxan | 350 mg/m$^2$ I.V., weeks 1, 3, 5, 7, 9, and 11 |
| | vincristine | Oncovin | 1.4 mg/m$^2$ (2 mg maximum) I.V., weeks 2, 4, 6, 8, 10, and 12 |
| | bleomycin | Blenoxane | 10 U/m$^2$ I.V., weeks 4, 8, and 12 |
| | prednisone | Deltasone | 75 mg P.O. daily for 12 weeks; taper dose over last 2 weeks Repeat cycle as indicated in protocol. |

*(continued)*

| ACRONYM & INDICATION | GENERIC DRUG NAME | TRADE DRUG NAME | DOSAGE |
|---|---|---|---|
| **MAID** (Soft-tissue sarcoma) | mesna | MESNEX | Uroprotection 1.5 to 2.5 g/m²/day by continuous I.V. infusion, days 1 to 3 |
| | doxorubicin | Adriamycin | 15 to 20 mg/m² by continuous I.V. infusion, days 1 to 3 |
| | ifosfamide | Ifex | 1.5 to 2.5 g/m² I.V., days 1 to 3 |
| | dacarbazine | DTIC-Dome | 250 to 300 mg/m² by continuous I.V. infusion days 1 to 3 *Repeat cycle q 28 days.* |
| **MBC** (Head and neck cancer) | methotrexate | Folex | 40 mg/m² I.V., days 1 and 15 |
| | bleomycin | Blenoxane | 10 U/m² I.M. or I.V., days 1, 8, and 15 |
| | cisplatin | Platinol | 50 mg/m² I.V., day 4 *Repeat cycle q 21 days.* |
| **MC** (Leukemia— AML, induction) | mitoxantrone | Novantrone | 12 mg/m² I.V. daily, days 1 to 3 |
| | cytarabine (ara-C) | Cytosar-U | 100 to 200 mg/m² daily by continuous I.V. infusion, days 1 to 7 *Repeat cycle q 28 days.* |
| **MICE (ICE)** (Non-small-cell lung cancer) | mesna | MESNEX | Dosage is 20% of ifosfamide dose given I.V. immediately before and at 4 and 8 hours after ifosfamide infusion |
| | ifosfamide | Ifex | 2,000 mg/m² I.V., days 1 to 3 |
| | carboplatin | Paraplatin | 300 to 350 mg/m² I.V., day 1 |
| | etoposide (VP-16) | VePesid | 60 to 100 mg/m² I.V., days 1 to 3 *Repeat cycle q 28 days.* |
| **MOPP** (Hodgkin's disease) | mechlorethamine (nitrogen mustard) | Mustargen | 6 mg/m² I.V., days 1 and 8 |
| | vincristine | Oncovin | 1.4 mg/m² (2 mg maximum) I.V., days 1 and 8 |
| | procarbazine | Matulane | 100 mg/m² P.O., days 1 to 14 |
| | prednisone | Deltasone | 40 mg/m² P.O., days 1 to 14 *Repeat cycle q 28 days.* |
| **MOPP** (ABV hybrid) (Hodgkin's disease) | mechlorethamine (nitrogen mustard) | Mustargen | 6 mg/m² I.V., day 1 |
| | vincristine | Oncovin | 1.4 mg/m² I.V., day 1 (2 mg maximum) |
| | procarbazine | Matulane | 100 mg/m² P.O., days 1 to 7 |
| | prednisone | Deltasone | 40 mg/m² P.O., days 1 to 14 |
| | doxorubicin | Adriamycin | 35 mg/m² I.V., day 8 |
| | bleomycin | Blenoxane | 10 U/m² I.V., day 8 |
| | vinblastine | Velban | 6 mg/m² I.V., day 8 *Repeat cycle q 28 days.* |
| **MP** (Multiple myeloma) | melphalan (L-phenylalanine mustard) | Alkeran | 8 to 10 mg/m² P.O., days 1 to 4 |
| | prednisone | Deltasone | 40 to 60 mg/m² P.O., days 1 to 7 *Repeat cycle q 28 to 42 days.* |

| ACRONYM & INDICATION | GENERIC DRUG NAME | TRADE DRUG NAME | DOSAGE |
|---|---|---|---|
| **MVAC** (Genitourinary cancer) | methotrexate | Folex | 30 mg/m$^2$ I.V., days 1, 15, and 22 |
| | vinblastine | Velban | 3 mg/m$^2$ I.V., days 2, 15, and 22 |
| | doxorubicin | Adriamycin | 30 mg/m$^2$ I.V., day 2 |
| | cisplatin | Platinol | 70 mg/m$^2$ I.V., day 2 *Repeat cycle q 28 days.* |
| **MVPP** (Hodgkin's disease) | mechlorethamine (nitrogen mustard) | Mustargen | 6 mg/m$^2$ I.V., days 1 and 8 |
| | vinblastine | Velban | 6 mg/m$^2$ I.V., days 1 and 8 |
| | procarbazine | Matulane | 100 mg/m$^2$ P.O., days 1 to 14 |
| | prednisone | Deltasone | 40 mg/m$^2$ P.O., days 1 to 14 *Repeat cycle q 4 to 6 weeks.* |
| **PCV** (Brain tumors) | procarbazine | Matulane | 60 mg/m$^2$ P.O., days 8 to 21 |
| | lomustine (CCNU) | CeeNu | 110 mg/m$^2$ P.O., day 1 |
| | vincristine | Oncovin | 1.4 mg/m$^2$ (2 mg maximum) I.V., days 8 and 29 *Repeat cycle q 6 to 8 weeks.* |
| **ProMACE** (Malignant lymphoma) | prednisone | Deltasone | 60 mg/m$^2$ P.O., days 1 to 14 |
| | methotrexate | Folex | 1.5 g/m$^2$ I.V., day 14 |
| | leucovorin calcium | Wellcovorin | 50 mg/m$^2$ I.V. q 6 hours for five to six doses, beginning 24 hours after methotrexate dose |
| | doxorubicin | Adriamycin | 25 mg/m$^2$ I.V., days 1 and 8 |
| | cyclophosphamide | Cytoxan | 650 mg/m$^2$ I.V., days 1 and 8 |
| | etoposide (VP-16) | VePesid | 120 mg/m$^2$ I.V., days 1 and 8 |
| **ProMACE/ cytaBOM** (Malignant lymphoma) | cyclophosphamide | Cytoxan | 650 mg/m$^2$ I.V., day 1 |
| | doxorubicin | Adriamycin | 25 mg/m$^2$ I.V., day 1 |
| | etoposide (VP-16) | VePesid | 120 mg/m$^2$ I.V., day 1 |
| | prednisone | Deltasone | 60 mg/m$^2$ P.O., days 1 to 14 |
| | cytarabine (ara-C) | Cytosar-U | 300 mg/m$^2$ I.V., day 8 |
| | bleomycin | Blenoxane | 5 U/m$^2$ I.V., day 8 |
| | vincristine | Oncovin | 1.4 mg/m$^2$ (2 mg maximum) I.V., day 8 |
| | methotrexate | Folex | 120 mg/m$^2$ I.V., day 8 |
| | leucovorin calcium | Wellcovorin | 25 mg/m$^2$ P.O. q 6 hours for six doses beginning 24 hours after methotrexate dose *Repeat cycle q 21 to 28 days.* |
| **7 + 3 (A + D)** (Leukemia— AML, induction) | cytarabine (ara-C) | Cytosar-U | 100 or 200 mg/m$^2$/day by continuous I.V. infusion, days 1 to 7 |
| | daunorubicin | Cerubidine | 45 mg/m$^2$ I.V., days 1 to 3 |

*(continued)*

| ACRONYM & INDICATION | GENERIC DRUG NAME | TRADE DRUG NAME | DOSAGE |
|---|---|---|---|
| **VAC Standard** (Soft-tissue sarcoma) | vincristine | Oncovin | 2 mg/m$^2$ (2 mg/week maximum) I.V. weekly for 12 weeks |
| | dactinomycin (actinomycin D) | Cosmegen | 0.015 mg/kg/day (0.5 mg/day maximum) continuous I.V. infusion, days 1 to 5 q 3 months |
| | cyclophosphamide | Cytoxan | 2.5 mg/kg daily P.O. for 2 years |
| **VAD** (Multiple myeloma) | vincristine | Oncovin | 0.4 mg by continuous I.V. infusion, days 1 to 4 |
| | doxorubicin | Adriamycin | 9 to 10 mg/m$^2$ by continuous I.V. infusion, days 1 to 4 |
| | dexamethasone | Decadron | 40 mg P.O. on days 1 to 4, 9 to 12, and 17 to 20 *Repeat cycle q 4 to 5 weeks.* |
| **VBP** (Genitourinary, testicular cancer) | vinblastine | Velban | 46 mg/m$^2$ I.V., days 1 and 2 |
| | bleomycin | Blenoxane | 30 U I.V., days 1, 8, 15, and (optional) 22 |
| | cisplatin | Platinol | 20 mg/m$^2$ I.V., days 1 to 5 *Repeat cycle q 21 to 28 days.* |
| **VC** (Non-small-cell lung cancer) | vinorelbine | Navelbine | 30 mg/m$^2$ I.V. weekly |
| | cisplatin | Platinol | 120 mg/m$^2$ I.V., days 1 and 29 *Repeat cycle q 6 weeks.* |
| **VDP** (Malignant melanoma) | vinblastine | Velban | 5 mg/m$^2$ I.V., days 1 and 2 |
| | dacarbazine | DTIC-Dome | 150 mg/m$^2$ I.V., days 1 to 5 |
| | cisplatin | Platinol | 75 mg/m$^2$ I.V., day 5 *Repeat cycle q 21 to 28 days.* |
| **VIP** (Genitourinary, testicular cancer) | vinblastine | Velban | 0.11 mg/kg I.V., days 1 and 2 |
| | ifosfamide | Ifex | 1.2 g/m$^2$/day continuous I.V. infusion, days 1 to 5 |
| | cisplatin | Platinol | 20 mg/m$^2$ I.V. over 1 hour, days 1 to 5 |
| | mesna | MESNEX | 400 mg I.V. 15 minutes before ifosfamide day 1; then 1.2 g daily by continuous I.V. infusion, days 1 to 5 *Repeat cycle q 21 days.* |
| *or* | etoposide (VP-16) | VePesid | 75 mg/m$^2$ I.V., days 1 to 5 |
| | ifosfamide | Ifex | 1.2 g/m$^2$/day continuous I.V. infusion, days 1 to 5 |
| | cisplatin | Platinol | 20 mg/m$^2$, days 1 to 5 |
| | mesna | MESNEX | 400 mg I.V. 15 minutes before ifosfamide day 1; then 1.2 g daily by continuous I.V. infusion, days 1 to 5 *Repeat cycle q 21 days.* |

# Selected drugs used for conscious sedation

Defined as the induction of a minimally depressed level of consciousness (LOC), conscious sedation is used during certain short medical procedures to relieve pain and anxiety, produce a hypnotic state, cause short-term amnesia, or achieve a combination of these effects. Over the last decade, conscious sedation has gained widespread popularity and is now performed in gastroenterology, radiology, pulmonology, and cardiac catheterization suites as well as in critical care settings.

## Required safeguards

Conscious sedation must occur in a controlled environment with emergency resuscitative equipment readily available. During the procedure, the patient must be able to maintain a patent airway independently and respond appropriately to physical or verbal commands. To avoid deep sedation and cardiopulmonary depression, the sedative dose is titrated to decrease the patient's LOC only to the point of slurred speech and nystagmus.

## Drug options

Drugs used for conscious sedation include analgesics, hypnotics, and amnestic drugs. Nurses who administer them must demonstrate an understanding of their pharmacology, familiarity with facility policy, and knowledge of and clinical competency in preprocedure patient assessment, procedural monitoring (including ECG, blood pressure, pulse oximetry, and LOC), airway management, postprocedure monitoring, and discharge criteria.

This table gives general dosing guidelines and key nursing considerations for the drugs most commonly used to produce conscious sedation in adults. Administered alone or in combination, these agents produce varying levels of sedation and commonly have potent synergistic effects.

| DRUG | DOSAGE | KEY CONSIDERATIONS |
|---|---|---|
| **fentanyl citrate (Sublimaze)** Drug is an opioid agonist that's 100 times more potent than morphine sulfate. Its analgesic activity of 100 mcg is equivalent to 10 mg morphine or 75 mg meperidine. | *Adults:* 0.5 to 1 mcg/kg I.V. titrated in 25-mcg increments over several minutes. *Elderly or debilitated patients with renal or hepatic disease:* individualize and reduce dosage. | • Watch for bradycardia, hypotension, apnea, respiratory depression, and chest wall rigidity. <br>• Drug may cause nausea and vomiting. <br>• Contraindicated in patients with elevated intracranial pressure or head trauma. <br>• If overdose occurs, maintain patent airway and provide respiratory and CV support. <br>• Use naloxone (Narcan), as ordered, to reverse respiratory and CV depressant effects. Low doses (1 to 4 mcg/kg) have been used to reverse respiratory depression associated with conscious sedation procedures. Patient may require additional doses (0.1 to 0.2 mg) based on total dosage and time elapsed since last narcotic dose. |
| **diazepam (Valium)** Drug is a benzodiazepine with anxiolytic, amnestic, | *Adults:* up to 10 mg I.V. given slowly immediately before the procedure is usually adequate. If | • Individualize doses and titrate to achieve desired effect. |

*(continued)*

| DRUG | DOSAGE | KEY CONSIDERATIONS |
|------|--------|--------------------|
| **diazepam (Valium)** *(continued)* anticonvulsant, skeletal muscle relaxant, and sedative-hypnotic properties. | opiates aren't given concomitantly, up to 20 mg I.V. may be required. Or, 5 to 10 mg I.M. given 30 minutes before the procedure. | • Drug is a potent respiratory depressant, particularly when given with opioids. <br> • Hypotension and bradycardia may occur in patients premedicated with a narcotic. <br> • For I.V. administration, give directly into a large vein at a rate not exceeding 5 mg/minute. <br> • For pharmacologic reversal of sedative effects, administer flumazenil (Romazicon). Individualize dosage; generally, 0.2 mg I.V. over 15 seconds. May repeat p.r.n. Don't exceed 3 mg in any 1-hour period. |
| **lorazepam (Ativan)** Drug is a benzodiazepine with sedative-hypnotic and anxiolytic properties. | *Adults:* 2 mg I.V. 15 to 20 minutes before the procedure. For greater amnestic effect, give up to 4 mg I.V. <br> *Elderly:* use reduced dosage and wait several minutes to evaluate pharmacologic effect before administering additional sedative doses. Don't exceed 2 mg I.V. total for patients over age 50. | • Individualize doses and titrate to achieve desired effect. <br> • Before I.V. administration, dilute drug with an equal volume of compatible solution and inject directly into the vein or into the tubing of an existing I.V. infusion at a rate not exceeding 2 mg/minute. <br> • Have emergency resuscitation equipment available when administrating drug I.V. <br> • For pharmacologic reversal of sedative effects, administer flumazenil (Romazicon). Individualize dosage; generally, 0.2 mg I.V. over 15 seconds. May repeat p.r.n. Don't exceed 3 mg in any 1-hour period. |
| **midazolam (Versed)** Drug is an ultrashort-acting, water-soluble benzodiazepine with amnestic, anxiolytic, sedative, muscle relaxant, and anticonvulsant properties. | *Healthy adults:* 0.5 mg I.V. over a 2-minute period. For the initial dose, don't exceed 2.5 mg. Some patients may respond to as little as 0.5 to 1 mg. <br> *Adults ages 60 and over or debilitated patients with decreased pulmonary reserve:* incremental 0.25- to 0.5-mg doses administered over a 2-minute period. Wait several minutes to evaluate pharmacologic effect before administering additional sedative doses. | • Individualize doses and titrate to achieve desired effect. <br> • Bolus administration isn't recommended for conscious sedation procedures. <br> • Drug is potent respiratory depressant, particularly when given with opioids. <br> • Hypotension and bradycardia may occur in patients premedicated with a narcotic. <br> • Excessive doses or development of hypoxia may lead to agitation, involuntary movement, hyperactivity, and combativeness. <br> • For pharmacologic reversal of sedative effects, administer flumazenil (Romazicon). Reversal dosage is individualized; generally, 0.2 mg is given I.V. over 15 seconds. May repeat dose to achieve desired effect; however, don't exceed 3 mg in any 1-hour period. |

| DRUG | DOSAGE | KEY CONSIDERATIONS |
|------|--------|--------------------|
| **meperidine (Demerol)** Drug is an opioid analgesic that's also used as an adjunct to anesthesia. | *Adults:* 50 to 100 mg I.M. or S.C. 30 to 90 minutes before anesthesia. | • Watch for bradycardia, hypotension, respiratory depression, and apnea.<br>• Drug may cause nausea and vomiting.<br>• If I.V. administration is necessary, decrease dosage and administer commercially available injections slowly, preferably as a diluted solution.<br>• Use naloxone (Narcan) to reverse respiratory and CV depressant effects. |
| **propofol (Diprivan)** Drug is a sedative-hypnotic. It produces rapid hypnosis through nonspecific cortical depression. It possesses intrinsic antiemetic properties and has no analgesic properties. | *Adults:* 10-mg incremental doses administered I.V. to augment effects of benzodiazepines and opioids.<br>*Elderly or debilitated patients:* reduce dosage. | • To avoid deep sedation or general anesthesia, use extreme caution when administering drug. Give incremental doses slowly over several minutes and allow adequate circulation time to assess full pharmacologic effect.<br>• Watch for dose-dependent respiratory depression, which may lead to apnea.<br>• Drug potentiates CNS and cardiopulmonary depressant effects of concomitantly administered narcotics and sedatives.<br>• If overdose occurs, maintain patent airway and provide respiratory and CV support. |

# Table of equivalents

## Metric system equivalents

**Metric weight**

| | | |
|---|---|---|
| 1 kilogram (kg or Kg) | = | 1,000 grams (g or gm) |
| 1 gram | = | 1,000 milligrams (mg) |
| 1 milligram | = | 1,000 micrograms (µg or mcg) |
| 0.6 g | = | 600 mg |
| 0.3 g | = | 300 mg |
| 0.1 g | = | 100 mg |
| 0.06 g | = | 60 mg |
| 0.03 g | = | 30 mg |
| 0.015 g | = | 15 mg |
| 0.001 g | = | 1 mg |

**Metric volume**

| | | |
|---|---|---|
| 1 liter (l or L) | = | 1,000 milliliters (ml)* |
| 1 milliliter | = | 1,000 microliters (µl) |

| Household | | Metric |
|---|---|---|
| 1 teaspoon (tsp) | = | 5 ml |
| 1 tablespoon (T or tbs) | = | 15 ml |
| 2 tablespoons | = | 30 ml |
| 8 ounces | = | 240 ml |
| 1 pint (pt) | = | 473 ml |
| 1 quart (qt) | = | 946 ml |
| 1 gallon (gal) | = | 3,785 ml |

## Temperature conversions

| FAHRENHEIT DEGREES | CENTIGRADE DEGREES | FAHRENHEIT DEGREES | CENTIGRADE DEGREES | FAHRENHEIT DEGREES | CENTIGRADE DEGREES |
|---|---|---|---|---|---|
| 106.0 | 41.1 | 100.6 | 38.1 | 95.2 | 35.1 |
| 105.8 | 41.0 | 100.4 | 38.0 | 95.0 | 35.0 |
| 105.6 | 40.9 | 100.2 | 37.9 | 94.8 | 34.9 |
| 105.4 | 40.8 | 100.0 | 37.8 | 94.6 | 34.8 |
| 105.2 | 40.7 | 99.8 | 37.7 | 94.4 | 34.7 |
| 105.0 | 40.6 | 99.6 | 37.6 | 94.2 | 34.6 |
| 104.8 | 40.4 | 99.4 | 37.4 | 94.0 | 34.4 |
| 104.6 | 40.3 | 99.2 | 37.3 | 93.8 | 34.3 |
| 104.4 | 40.2 | 99.0 | 37.2 | 93.6 | 34.2 |
| 104.2 | 40.1 | 98.8 | 37.1 | 93.4 | 34.1 |
| 104.0 | 40.0 | 98.6 | 37.0 | 93.2 | 34.0 |
| 103.8 | 39.9 | 98.4 | 36.9 | 93.0 | 33.9 |
| 103.6 | 39.8 | 98.2 | 36.8 | 92.8 | 33.8 |
| 103.4 | 39.7 | 98.0 | 36.7 | 92.6 | 33.7 |
| 103.2 | 39.6 | 97.8 | 36.5 | 92.4 | 33.6 |
| 103.0 | 39.4 | 97.6 | 36.4 | 92.2 | 33.4 |
| 102.8 | 39.3 | 97.4 | 36.3 | 92.0 | 33.3 |
| 102.6 | 39.2 | 97.2 | 36.2 | 91.8 | 33.2 |
| 102.4 | 39.1 | 97.0 | 36.1 | 91.6 | 33.1 |
| 102.2 | 39.0 | 96.8 | 36.0 | 91.4 | 33.0 |
| 102.0 | 38.9 | 96.6 | 35.9 | 91.2 | 32.9 |
| 101.8 | 38.8 | 96.4 | 35.8 | 91.0 | 32.8 |
| 101.6 | 38.7 | 96.2 | 35.7 | 90.8 | 32.7 |
| 101.4 | 38.6 | 96.0 | 35.6 | 90.6 | 32.6 |
| 101.2 | 38.4 | 95.8 | 35.4 | 90.4 | 32.4 |
| 101.0 | 38.3 | 95.6 | 35.3 | 90.2 | 32.3 |
| 100.8 | 38.2 | 95.4 | 35.2 | 90.0 | 32.2 |

## Weight conversions

| | | |
|---|---|---|
| 1 oz = 30 g | 1 lb = 453.6 g | 2.2 lb = 1 kg |

*1 ml = 1 cubic centimeter (cc); however, ml is the preferred measurement term today.

# Estimating surface area in children

Pediatric drug dosages should be calculated on the basis of body surface area or body weight. If your pediatric patient is average size, find his weight and corresponding surface area in the box. Otherwise, to use the nomogram, lay a straightedge on the correct height and weight points for your patient, and observe the point where it intersects on the surface area scale. *Note:* Don't use drug dosages based on body surface area in premature or full-term newborns. Instead, use body weight.

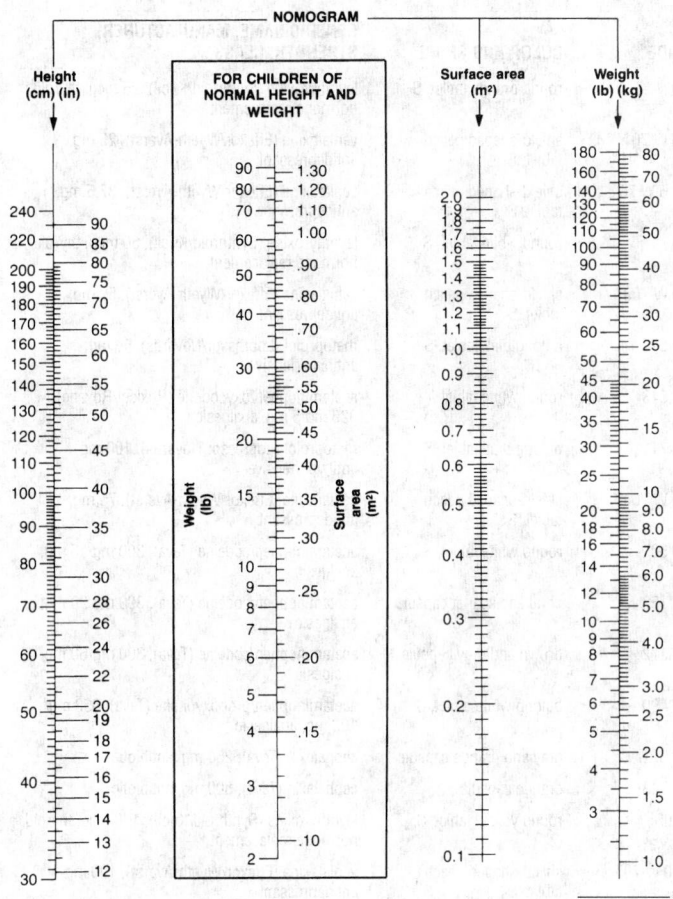

Behrman, R.E., et al. *Nelson Textbook of Pediatrics,* 16th edition. 1999. Courtesy W.B. Saunders Co., Philadelphia.

# Common drug imprint codes

When administering drugs, you may come across some tablets and capsules that you don't recognize. A reliable method for identifying them is to check the drug imprint code on the tablet or capsule.

Below are drug imprint codes and descriptions for some of the most commonly prescribed tablets and capsules. Column 1 lists the drug code in numeric and alphabetical order. Column 2 describes the pill's shape, color, type (tablet or capsule), and additional characteristics (C = coated; S = scored). Column 3 lists the generic drug name, trade name, manufacturer, strength, and class.

| CODE | COLOR AND SHAPE | GENERIC NAME, MANUFACTURER, STRENGTH, CLASS |
|------|-----------------|---------------------------------------------|
| 25 | round orange tablet, S | levothyroxine (Synthroid/Knoll), 25 mcg, thyroid hormone replacement |
| 25 W 701 | shield-shaped peach tablet, S | venlafaxine (Effexor/Wyeth-Ayerst), 25 mg, antidepressant |
| 37.5 W 781 | shield-shaped peach tablet, S | venlafaxine (Effexor/Wyeth-Ayerst), 37.5 mg, antidepressant |
| 50 | round white tablet, S | levothyroxine (Synthroid/Knoll), 50 mcg, thyroid hormone replacement |
| 50 W 703 | shield-shaped peach tablet, S | venlafaxine (Effexor/Wyeth-Ayerst), 50 mg, antidepressant |
| 51 51 | oblong pink tablet, S | metoprolol (Lopressor/Novartis), 50 mg, antihypertensive |
| 54 543 | round white tablet | acetaminophen/oxycodone (Roxicet/Roxane), 325 mg/5 mg, analgesic |
| 71 71 | oblong blue tablet, S | metoprolol (Lopressor/Novartis), 100 mg, antihypertensive |
| 75 W 704 | shield-shaped peach tablet, S | venlafaxine (Effexor/Wyeth-Ayerst), 75 mg, antidepressant |
| 93 50 | round white tablet, S | acetaminophen/codeine (Teva), 300 mg/15 mg, analgesic |
| 93 152 | coral and scarlet capsule | acetaminophen/codeine (Teva), 300 mg/30 mg, analgesic |
| 93 172 | brown and gray capsule | acetaminophen/codeine (Teva), 300 mg/60 mg, analgesic |
| 93 490 | oblong white tablet, C | acetaminophen/propoxyphene (Teva), 650 mg/100 mg, analgesic |
| 93 541 | gray and orange capsule | cephalexin (Teva), 250 mg, antibiotic |
| 93 543 | orange capsule | cephalexin (Teva), 500 mg, antibiotic |
| 100 | round yellow tablet, S | levothyroxine (Synthroid/Knoll), 100 mcg, thyroid hormone replacement |
| 100 W 705 | shield-shaped peach tablet, S | venlafaxine (Effexor/Wyeth-Ayerst), 100 mg, antidepressant |
| 150 | round blue tablet, S | levothyroxine (Synthroid/Knoll), 150 mcg, thyroid hormone replacement |
| 200 | round pink tablet, S | levothyroxine (Synthroid/Knoll), 200 mcg, thyroid hormone replacement |

S = scored        C = coated

| CODE | COLOR AND SHAPE | GENERIC NAME, MANUFACTURER, STRENGTH, CLASS |
|------|-----------------|---------------------------------------------|
| 884 MILES 30 | round pink tablet | nifedipine (Adalat CC/Bayer), 30 mg, antihypertensive |
| 885 MILES 60 | round salmon tablet | nifedipine (Adalat CC/Bayer), 60 mg, antihypertensive |
| 886 MILES 90 | round dark red tablet | nifedipine (Adalat CC/Bayer), 90 mg, antihypertensive |
| 3170 | blue and gray capsule | loracarbef (Lorabid/Lilly), 200 mg, antibiotic |
| 5513 | round white tablet | carisoprodol (Schein), 350 mg, muscle relaxant |
| A 49 | round white tablet, S | atenolol (Lederle), 50 mg, antihypertensive |
| A 71 | round white tablet | atenolol (Lederle), 100 mg, antihypertensive |
| A KT KT | oval yellow tablet, C | clarithromycin (Biaxin/Abbott), 250 mg, antibiotic |
| AMB 5 5401 | capsule-shaped pink tablet, C | zolpidem (Ambien/Searle), 5 mg, sedative |
| AMB 10 5421 | capsule-shaped white tablet, C | zolpidem (Ambien/Searle), 10 mg, sedative |
| A MO | round white tablet; C, S | metoprolol (Toprol-XL/Astra), 50 mg, antihypertensive |
| A MS | round white tablet; C, S | metoprolol (Toprol-XL/Astra), 100 mg, antihypertensive |
| A MY | oval white tablet; C, S | metoprolol (Toprol-XL/Astra), 200 mg, antihypertensive |
| B 11 | round light green tablet | ethinyl estradiol/levonorgestrel (Tri-Levlen/Berlex), placebo, oral contraceptive |
| B 95 | round brown tablet | ethinyl estradiol/levonorgestrel (Tri-Levlen/Berlex), 0.030 mg/0.05 mg, oral contraceptive |
| B 96 | round white tablet | ethinyl estradiol/levonorgestrel (Tri-Levlen/Berlex), 0.040 mg/0.075 mg, oral contraceptive |
| B 97 | round light yellow tablet | ethinyl estradiol/levonorgestrel (Tri-Levlen/Berlex), 0.030 mg/0.125 mg, oral contraceptive |
| BARR 514 | gray and orange capsule | cephalexin (Barr), 250 mg, antibiotic |
| BARR 515 | orange capsule | cephalexin (Barr), 500 mg, antibiotic |
| BARR 545 | capsule-shaped orange tablet | cephalexin (Barr), 250 mg, antibiotic |
| BARR 546 | capsule-shaped dark orange tablet | cephalexin (Barr), 500 mg, antibiotic |
| BIOCRAFT 01 | caramel and buff capsule | amoxicillin (Teva), 250 mg, antibiotic |
| BIOCRAFT 03 | buff capsule | amoxicillin (Teva), 500 mg, antibiotic |
| BIOCRAFT 33 | oval white tablet, S | sulfamethoxazole/trimethoprim (Teva), 800 mg/160 mg, antibiotic |
| BIOCRAFT 115 | gray and orange capsule | cephalexin (Teva), 250 mg, antibiotic |
| BIOCRAFT 117 | orange capsule | cephalexin (Teva), 500 mg, antibiotic |
| BL 32 | round white tablet, S | sulfamethoxazole/trimethoprim (Teva), 400 mg/80 mg, antibiotic |
| BMS 7720 250 | oval light orange tablet, C | cefprozil (Cefzil/Bristol-Myers Squibb), 250 mg, antibiotic |

*(continued)*

S = scored    C = coated

| CODE | COLOR AND SHAPE | GENERIC NAME, MANUFACTURER, STRENGTH, CLASS |
|------|-----------------|---------------------------------------------|
| BMS 7721 500 | oval white tablet, C | cefprozil (Cefzil/Bristol-Myers Squibb), 500 mg, antibiotic |
| BRISTOL 7278 | pink and maroon capsule | amoxicillin (Apothecon), 250 mg, antibiotic |
| BRISTOL 7279 | pink and maroon capsule | amoxicillin (Apothecon), 500 mg, antibiotic |
| C | oval white tablet, S | medroxyprogesterone (Cycrin/ESI Lederle), 2.5 mg, progestin |
| CARDURA | oval white tablet | doxazosin (Cardura/Pfizer), 1 mg, antihypertensive |
| CARDURA | oval yellow tablet | doxazosin (Cardura/Pfizer), 2 mg, antihypertensive |
| CARDURA | oval orange tablet | doxazosin (Cardura/Pfizer), 4 mg, antihypertensive |
| CARDURA | oval green tablet | doxazosin (Cardura/Pfizer), 8 mg, antihypertensive |
| CIBA 3 | round pale green tablet, S | methylphenidate (Ritalin/Novartis), 10 mg, psychotherapeutic drug |
| CIBA 7 | round yellow tablet | methylphenidate (Ritalin/Novartis), 5 mg, psychotherapeutic drug |
| CIBA 34 | round pale yellow tablet, S | methylphenidate (Ritalin/Novartis), 20 mg, psychotherapeutic drug |
| COTRIM 93 93 | round white tablet, S | trimethoprim/sulfamethoxazole (Cotrim/Teva), 80 mg/400 mg, antibiotic |
| COTRIM DS 93 | oval white tablet, S | trimethoprim/sulfamethoxazole (Cotrim DS/Teva), 93 160 mg/800 mg, antibiotic |
| CYCRIN | oval light purple tablet, S | medroxyprogesterone (Cycrin/ESI Lederle), 5 mg, progestin |
| CYCRIN | oval peach tablet, S | medroxyprogesterone (Cycrin/ESI Lederle), 10 mg, progestin |
| DAN 5442 DAN | round white tablet, S | prednisone (Geneva), 10 mg, anti-inflammatory |
| DAN 5443 DAN | round peach tablet, S | prednisone (Danbury), 20 mg, anti-inflammatory |
| DAN 5490 DAN | round white tablet, S | prednisone (Schein), 50 mg, anti-inflammatory |
| DAYPRO 1381 | capsule-shaped white tablet; C, S | oxaprozin (Daypro/Searle), 600 mg, anti-inflammatory |
| DP 301 | oval white tablet, S | methylprednisolone (Duramed), 4 mg, anti-inflammatory |
| DYAZIDE SB | red and white capsule | triamterene/hydrochlorothiazide (Dyazide/SK Beecham), 37.5 mg/25 mg, antihypertensive |
| E 647 | yellow capsule | phentermine (Eon Labs), 30 mg, anorexant |
| EC | rectangular pink tablet | erythromycin base (Ery-Tab/Abbott), 250 mg, antibiotic |
| ED | oval pink tablet | erythromycin base (Ery-Tab/Abbott), 500 mg, antibiotic |
| EH | rectangular white tablet | erythromycin base (Ery-Tab/Abbott), 333 mg, antibiotic |
| ES | round pink tablet, C | erythromycin stearate (Erythrocin/Abbott), 250 mg, antibiotic |
| ET | oval pink tablet, C | erythromycin stearate (Erythrocin/Abbott), 500 mg, antibiotic |
| FOSAMAX MRK 212 | triangular white tablet | alendronate (Fosamax/Merck), 40 mg, antiosteoporotic |

S = scored    C = coated

| CODE | COLOR AND SHAPE | GENERIC NAME, MANUFACTURER, STRENGTH, CLASS |
|---|---|---|
| FOSAMAX MRK 936 | oval white tablet | alendronate (Fosamax/Merck), 10 mg, antiosteoporotic |
| G 0556 | round peach tablet | hydrochlorothiazide (Zenith), 25 mg, antihypertensive |
| G 800 | capsule-shaped white tablet, C | ibuprofen (Greenstone), 800 mg, anti-inflammatory |
| G 3719 | oval white tablet, S | alprazolam (Greenstone), 0.25 mg, anxiolytic |
| G 3720 | oval peach tablet, S | alprazolam (Greenstone), 0.5 mg, anxiolytic |
| G 3721 | oval blue tablet, S | alprazolam (Greenstone), 1 mg, anxiolytic |
| G 3722 | oval white tablet, S | alprazolam (Greenstone), 2 mg, anxiolytic |
| G 3725 | round white tablet, S | glyburide (Greenstone), 1.25 mg, antidiabetic |
| G 3726 | round pink tablet, S | glyburide (Greenstone), 2.5 mg, antidiabetic |
| G 3727 | round blue tablet, S | glyburide (Greenstone), 5 mg, antidiabetic |
| G 3740 | round orange tablet, S | medroxyprogesterone (Greenstone), 2.5 mg, progestin |
| G 3741 | hexagonal white tablet, S | medroxyprogesterone (Greenstone), 5 mg, progestin |
| G 3742 | round white tablet, S | medroxyprogesterone (Greenstone), 10 mg, progestin |
| GG 172 | round yellow tablet, S | triamterene/hydrochlorothiazide (Geneva), 75 mg/50 mg, antihypertensive |
| GG 263 | round white tablet; C, S | atenolol (Geneva), 50 mg, antihypertensive |
| GG 264 | round white tablet, C | atenolol (Geneva), 100 mg, antihypertensive |
| GG 580 | red capsule | triamterene/hydrochlorothiazide (Geneva), 50 mg/25 mg, antihypertensive |
| GG 606 | white capsule | triamterene/hydrochlorothiazide (Geneva), 37.5 mg/25 mg, antihypertensive |
| GL 500 | cylindrical white tablet, C | metformin (Glucophage/Bristol-Myers Squibb), 500 mg, antidiabetic |
| GL 850 | cylindrical white tablet, C | metformin (Glucophage/Bristol-Myers Squibb), 850 mg, antidiabetic |
| GLAXO 387 | capsule-shaped light blue tablet, C | cefuroxime axetil (Ceftin/Glaxo Wellcome), 250 mg, antibiotic |
| GLAXO 394 | capsule-shaped dark blue tablet, C | cefuroxime axetil (Ceftin/Glaxo Wellcome), 500 mg, antibiotic |
| GLAXO 395 | capule-shaped white tablet, C | cefuroxime axetil (Ceftin/Glaxo Wellcome), 125 mg, antibiotic |
| GLYBUR 364 364 | round blue tablet | glyburide (Copley), 5 mg, antidiabetic |
| GLYBUR 433 433 | round pink tablet, S | glyburide (Copley), 2.5 mg, antidiabetic |
| GLYBUR 477 477 | round white tablet, S | glyburide (Copley), 1.25 mg, antidiabetic |
| HH | gray capsule | terazosin (Hytrin/Abbott), 1 mg, antihypertensive |
| HK | red capsule | terazosin (Hytrin/Abbott), 5 mg, antihypertensive |
| HN | blue capsule | terazosin (Hytrin/Abbott), 10 mg, antihypertensive |

*(continued)*

S = scored    C = coated

| CODE | COLOR AND SHAPE | GENERIC NAME, MANUFACTURER, STRENGTH, CLASS |
|------|-----------------|---------------------------------------------|
| HY | yellow capsule | terazosin (Hytrin/Abbott), 2 mg, antihypertensive |
| I25 | round white tablet, C | sumatriptan (Imitrex/Glaxo Wellcome), 25 mg, antimigraine drug |
| IBU 600 | oval white tablet, C | ibuprofen (Boots), 600 mg, anti-inflammatory |
| IBU 800 | oval white tablet, C | ibuprofen (Boots), 800 mg, anti-inflammatory |
| JANSSEN P 10 | round white tablet, S | cisapride (Propulsid/Janssen), 10 mg, GI stimulant |
| JANSSEN P 20 | oval blue tablet | cisapride (Propulsid/Janssen), 20 mg, GI stimulant |
| JANSSEN R 1 | oval white tablet, S | risperidone (Risperdal/Janssen), 1 mg, antipsychotic |
| JANSSEN R 2 | oval orange tablet | risperidone (Risperdal/Janssen), 2 mg, antipsychotic |
| JANSSEN R 3 | oval yellow tablet | risperidone (Risperdal/Janssen), 3 mg, antipsychotic |
| JANSSEN R 4 | oval green tablet | risperidone (Risperdal/Janssen), 4 mg, antipsychotic |
| KL | oval yellow tablet, C | clarithromycin (Biaxin/Abbott), 500 mg, antibiotic |
| LANOXIN T9A | round green tablet, S | digoxin (Lanoxin/Glaxo Wellcome), 0.5 mg, antiarrhythmic |
| LANOXIN X3A | round white tablet, S | digoxin (Lanoxin/Glaxo Wellcome), 0.25 mg, antiarrhythmic |
| LANOXIN Y3B | round yellow tablet, S | digoxin (Lanoxin/Glaxo Wellcome), 0.125 mg, antiarrhythmic |
| LASIX HOECHST | oval white tablet | furosemide (Lasix/Hoechst Marion Roussel), 20 mg, diuretic |
| LL HEART B12 | round yellow tablet | hydrochlorothiazide/bisoprolol (Ziac/Lederle), 6.25 mg/2.5 mg, antihypertensive |
| LL HEART B13 | round pink tablet | hydrochlorothiazide/bisoprolol (Ziac/Lederle), 6.25 mg/5 mg, antihypertensive |
| LL HEART B14 | round white tablet | hydrochlorothiazide/bisoprolol (Ziac/Lederle), 6.25 mg/10 mg, antihypertensive |
| M 32 | round pink tablet, S | metoprolol (Mylan), 50 mg, antihypertensive |
| M 37 | round purple tablet | amitriptyline (Mylan), 75 mg, antidepressant |
| M 47 | round blue tablet; C, S | metoprolol (Mylan), 100 mg, antihypertensive |
| M 53 | pentagonal green tablet, C | cimetidine (Mylan), 200 mg, antiulcerative |
| M 77 | round white tablet, C | amitriptyline (Mylan), 10 mg, antidepressant |
| M 241 | round white tablet, S | atenolol (Mylan), 50 mg, antihypertensive |
| M 321 | round white tablet | lorazepam (Mylan), 0.5 mg, anxiolytic |
| M 537 | round blue tablet, C | naproxen (Mylan), 275 mg, anti-inflammatory |
| M 751 | round orange tablet, C | cyclobenzaprine (Mylan), 10 mg, muscle relaxant |
| M 757 | round white tablet | atenolol (Mylan), 100 mg, antihypertensive |
| MACROBID | black and yellow capsule | nitrofurantoin (Macrobid/Procter & Gamble), 100 mg, antibiotic |
| MCNEIL 659 | capsule-shaped white tablet, C | tramadol (Ultram/Ortho-McNeil), 50 mg, analgesic |
| MD 530 | round green-blue tablet, S | methylphenidate (MD Pharm), 10 mg, psychotherapeutic |

S = scored    C = coated

| CODE | COLOR AND SHAPE | GENERIC NAME, MANUFACTURER, STRENGTH, CLASS |
|------|-----------------|---------------------------------------------|
| MD 531 | round yellow tablet | methylphenidate (MD Pharm), 5 mg, psychotherapeutic |
| MEVACOR 730 MSD | octagonal peach tablet | lovastatin (Mevacor/Merck), 10 mg, antihyperlipidemic |
| MEVACOR 731 MSD | octagonal blue tablet | lovastatin (Mevacor/Merck), 20 mg, antihyperlipidemic |
| MEVACOR 732 MSD | octagonal green tablet | lovastatin (Mevacor/Merck), 40 mg, antihyperlipidemic |
| MJ 021 | round white tablet | estradiol (Estrace/Bristol-Myers Squibb), 0.5 mg, estrogen replacement |
| MJ 755 | round lavender tablet | estradiol (Estrace/Bristol-Myers Squibb), 1 mg, estrogen replacement |
| MJ 756 | round turquoise tablet | estradiol (Estrace/Bristol-Meyers Squibb), 2 mg, estrogen replacement |
| MRK 951 | teardrop-shaped light green tablet | losartan (Cozaar/Merck), 25 mg, antihypertensive |
| MRK 952 | teardrop-shaped green tablet | losartan (Cozaar/Merck), 50 mg, antihypertensive |
| MSD 963 | U-shaped beige tablet, C | famotidine (Pepcid/Merck), 20 mg, antiulcerative |
| MSD 964 | U-shaped light brown tablet, C | famotidine (Pepcid/Merck), 40 mg, antiulcerative |
| MYLAN 130 | capsule-shaped reddish orange tablet, C | propoxyphene/acetaminophen (Mylan), 65 mg/650 mg, analgesic |
| MYLAN 152 | round white tablet, S | clonidine (Mylan), 0.1 mg, antihypertensive |
| MYLAN 185 | round white tablet, S | clonidine (Mylan), 0.2 mg, antihypertensive |
| MYLAN 199 | round white tablet, S | clonidine (Mylan), 0.3 mg, antihypertensive |
| MYLAN 216 40 | round white tablet, S | furosemide (Mylan), 40 mg, diuretic |
| MYLAN 232 80 | round white tablet, S | furosemide (Mylan), 80 mg, diuretic |
| MYLAN 271 | round white tablet, S | diazepam (Mylan), 2 mg, anxiolytic |
| MYLAN 345 | round orange tablet, S | diazepam (Mylan), 5 mg, anxiolytic |
| MYLAN 457 | round white tablet, S | lorazepam (Mylan), 1 mg, anxiolytic |
| MYLAN 477 | round green tablet, S | diazepam (Mylan), 10 mg, anxiolytic |
| MYLAN 521 | capsule-shaped white tablet | propoxyphene/acetaminophen (Mylan), 100 mg/650 mg, analgesic |
| MYLAN 733 | oval light blue tablet, C | naproxen (Mylan), 550 mg, anti-inflammatory |
| MYLAN 777 | round white tablet, S | lorazepam (Mylan), 2 mg, anxiolytic |
| MYLAN 4010 | peach capsule | temazepam (Mylan), 15 mg, sedative |
| MYLAN 5050 | yellow capsule | temazepam (Mylan), 30 mg, sedative |
| MYLAN 7250 | pink and white capsule | cefaclor (Mylan), 250 mg, antibiotic |
| MYLAN 7500 | pink and gray capsule | cefaclor (Mylan), 500 mg, antibiotic |
| MYLAN A | round white tablet, S | alprazolam (Mylan), 0.25 mg, anxiolytic |

*(continued)*

S = scored    C = coated

| CODE | COLOR AND SHAPE | GENERIC NAME, MANUFACTURER, STRENGTH, CLASS |
|------|-----------------|---------------------------------------------|
| MYLAN A1 | round blue tablet, S | alprazolam (Mylan), 1 mg, anxiolytic |
| MYLAN A3 | round peach tablet, S | alprazolam (Mylan), 0.5 mg, anxiolytic |
| MYLAN A4 | round white tablet, S | alprazolam (Mylan), 2 mg, anxiolytic |
| MYLAN G1 | round white tablet, S | glipizide (Mylan), 5 mg, antidiabetic |
| MYLAN G2 | round white tablet, S | glipizide (Mylan), 10 mg, antidiabetic |
| NR | oval peach tablet | divalproex (Depakote/Abbott), 250 mg, anticonvulsant |
| NS | oval lavender tablet | divalproex (Depakote/Abbott), 500 mg, anticonvulsant |
| NT | oval salmon tablet | divalproex (Depakote/Abbott), 125 mg, anticonvulsant |
| ORTHO 75 | round light peach tablet | ethinyl estradiol/norethindrone (Ortho-Novum 7/7/7/Ortho-McNeil), 35 mcg/0.75 mg, oral contraceptive |
| ORTHO 135 | round peach tablet | ethinyl estradiol/norethindrone (Ortho-Novum 7/7/7/Ortho-McNeil), 35 mcg/1 mg, oral contraceptive |
| ORTHO 180 | round white tablet | ethinyl estradiol/norgestimate (Ortho Tri-Cyclen/Ortho-McNeil), 35 mcg/0.18 mg, oral contraceptive |
| ORTHO 215 | round light blue tablet | ethinyl estradiol/norgestimate (Ortho Tri-Cyclen/Ortho-McNeil), 35 mcg/0.215 mg, oral contraceptive |
| ORTHO 250 | round blue tablet | ethinyl estradiol/norgestimate (Ortho Cyclen/Ortho-McNeil), 35 mcg/0.25 mg, oral contraceptive |
| ORTHO 535 | round white tablet | ethinyl estradiol/norethindrone (Ortho-Novum 7/7/7/Ortho-McNeil), 35 mcg/0.5 mg, oral contraceptive |
| ORTHO D 150 | round orange tablet | ethinyl estradiol/desogestrel (Ortho-Cept/Ortho-McNeil), 30 mcg/0.15mg, oral contraceptive |
| P 57 | round white tablet, S | lorazepam (Purpac), 0.5 mg, anxiolytic |
| P 59 | round white tablet, S | lorazepam (Purpac), 1 mg, anxiolytic |
| PAR 161 300 | round white tablet | ibuprofen (Par), 300 mg, anti-inflammatory |
| PAR 467 | capsule-shaped white tablet, C | ibuprofen (Par), 400 mg, anti-inflammatory |
| PAR 468 | capsule-shaped white tablet, C | ibuprofen (Par), 600 mg, anti-inflammatory |
| P-D 362 | orange-banded white capsule | phenytoin sodium (Dilantin Kapseals/Parke-Davis), 100 mg, anticonvulsant |
| P-D 365 | pink-banded white capsule | phenytoin sodium (Dilantin Kapseals/Parke-Davis), 30 mg, anticonvulsant |
| P-D 532 20 | round brown tablet, C | quinapril (Accupril/Parke-Davis), 20 mg, antihypertensive |
| P-D 535 40 | oval brown tablet, C | quinapril (Accupril/Parke-Davis), 40 mg, antihypertensive |
| P-D 916 | round green tablet | ethinyl estradiol/norethindrone (Loestrin [Fe]/Parke-Davis), 30 mcg/1.5 mg, oral contraceptive |

S = scored        C = coated

| CODE | COLOR AND SHAPE | GENERIC NAME, MANUFACTURER, STRENGTH, CLASS |
|------|----------------|---------------------------------------------|
| PFIZER 305 | red capsule | azithromycin (Zithromax/Pfizer), 250 mg, antibiotic |
| PFIZER 308 | oval white tablet | azithromycin (Zithromax/Pfizer), 600 mg, antibiotic |
| PFIZER 550 | round off-rectangular white tablet, C | cetirizine (Zyrtec/Pfizer), 5 mg, antihistamine |
| PFIZER 551 | round off-rectangular white tablet, C | cetirizine (Zyrtec/Pfizer), 10 mg, antihistamine |
| PPP 785 | oval white tablet, S | cefadroxil (Duricef/Bristol-Myers Squibb), 1,000 mg, antibiotic |
| PREMPRO | oval peach tablet, C | conjugated estrogens/medroxyprogesterone (Prempro/Wyeth-Ayerst), 0.625 mg/2.5 mg, estrogen replacement |
| PRINIVIL 207 MSD | shield-shaped peach tablet | lisinopril (Prinivil/Merck), 20 mg, antihypertensive |
| PRINIVIL 237 MSD | shield-shaped red tablet | lisinopril (Prinivil/Merck), 40 mg, antihypertensive |
| PROPACET | oblong white tablet, C | propoxyphene/acetaminophen (Propacet/Teva), 100 mg /650 mg, analgesic |
| R 001 3 | round white tablet, S | acetaminophen/codeine (Purepac), 300 mg/30 mg, analgesic |
| R 003 4 | round white tablet, S | acetaminophen/codeine (Purepac), 300 mg/60 mg, analgesic |
| R 027 | round white tablet, S | alprazolam (Purepac), 0.25 mg, anxiolytic |
| R 029 | round peach tablet, S | alprazolam (Purepac), 0.5 mg, anxiolytic |
| R 031 | round blue tablet, S | alprazolam (Purepac), 1.0 mg, anxiolytic |
| R 063 | round white tablet, S | lorazepam (Purepac), 2 mg, anxiolytic |
| RUGBY 3367 | blue capsule | dicyclomine (Rugby), 10 mg, antispasmodic |
| RUGBY 3377 | round blue tablet | dicyclomine (Rugby), 20 mg, antispasmodic |
| SEARLE 151 | round white tablet | ethinyl estradiol/ethynodiol diacetate (Demulen 1/35/Searle), 35 mcg/1 mg, oral contraceptive |
| SGP 1/35 | round pale blue tablet | ethinyl estradiol/norethindrone (Genora 1/35/Rugby), 35 mcg/1 mg, oral contraceptive |
| SQUIBB 181 | orange and gray capsule | cephalexin (Apothecon), 250 mg, antibiotic |
| SQUIBB 239 | orange capsule | cephalexin (Apothecon), 500 mg, antibiotic |
| SQUIBB 603 | oblong pink tablet, C | tetracycline (Sumycin/Apothecon), 500 mg, antibiotic |
| SQUIBB 648 | round white tablet, C | penicillin V potassium (Veetids 500/Apothecon), 500 mg, antibiotic |
| SQUIBB 663 | pink tablet, C | tetracycline (Sumycin/Apothecon), 250 mg, antibiotic |
| SQUIBB 684 | round peach tablet, C | penicillin V potassium (Veetids 250/Apothecon), 250 mg, antibiotic |
| SQUIBB 971 | red and gray capsule | ampicillin (Principen/Apothecon), 250 mg, antibiotic |
| SQUIBB 974 | red and gray capsule | ampicillin (Principen/Apothecon), 500 mg, antibiotic |
| TEGRETOL 27 | capsule-shaped pink tablet, S | carbamazepine (Tegretol/Novartis), 200 mg, anticonvulsant |

*(continued)*

S = scored     C = coated

| CODE | COLOR AND SHAPE | GENERIC NAME, MANUFACTURER, STRENGTH, CLASS |
|---|---|---|
| TEGRETOL 52 | round pink and red speckled tablet, S | carbamazepine (Tegretol/Novartis), 100 mg, anticonvulsant |
| TENORMIN 101 | round white tablet | atenolol (Tenormin/Zeneca), 100 mg, antihypertensive |
| TENORMIN 105 | round white tablet | atenolol (Tenormin/Zeneca), 50 mg, antihypertensive |
| TR 5/ORGANON | round white tablet | ethinyl estradiol/desogestrel (Desogen/Organon), 30 mcg/0.15 mg, oral contraceptive |
| VASOTEC 14 MSD | barrel-shaped yellow tablet, S | enalapril (Vasotec/Merck), 2.5 mg, antihypertensive |
| VASOTEC 712 MSD | barrel-shaped white tablet, S | enalapril (Vasotec/Merck), 5 mg, antihypertensive |
| VASOTEC 713 MSD | barrel-shaped salmon tablet | enalapril (Vasotec/Merck), 10 mg, antihypertensive |
| VASOTEC 714 MSD | barrel-shaped peach tablet | enalapril (Vasotec/Merck), 20 mg, antihypertensive |
| W 641 | round brown tablet | ethinyl estradiol/levonorgestrel (Triphasil/Wyeth-Ayerst), 30 mcg/0.05 mg, oral contraceptive |
| W 642 | round white tablet | ethinyl estradiol/levonorgestrel (Triphasil/Wyeth-Ayerst), 40 mcg/0.075 mg, oral contraceptive |
| W 643 | round light yellow tablet | ethinyl estradiol/levonorgestrel (Triphasil/Wyeth-Ayerst), 30 mcg/0.125 mg, oral contraceptive |
| W 650 | round light green tablet | ethinyl estradiol/levonorgestrel (Triphasil/Wyeth-Ayerst), placebo, oral contraceptive |
| WATSON 540 | oval blue tablet, S | hydrocodone/acetaminophen (Watson), 10 mg/500 mg, analgesic |
| WC 084 | oval white tablet, C | gemfibrozil (Warner Chilcott), 600 mg, antihyperlipidemic |
| WYETH 78 | round white tablet | ethinyl estradiol/norgestrel (Lo/Ovral/Wyeth-Ayerst), 30 mcg/0.3 mg, oral contraceptive |
| Z 2984 | light blue and white capsule | doxycycline (Zenith), 50 mg, antibiotic |
| Z 2985 | light blue capsule | doxycycline (Zenith), 100 mg, antibiotic |
| Z 4280 | capsule-shaped white tablet; C, S | verapamil (Verapamil SR/Zenith), 240 mg, antihypertensive |
| Z 4286 | oval white tablet; C, S | verapamil (Verapamil SR/Zenith), 180 mg, antihypertensive |
| ZOCOR 726 MSD | shield-shaped buff tablet | simvastatin (Zocor/Merck), 5 mg, antihyperlipidemic |
| ZOCOR 735 MSD | shield-shaped peach tablet | simvastatin (Zocor/Merck), 10 mg, antihyperlipidemic |
| ZOCOR 740 MSD | shield-shaped tan tablet | simvastatin (Zocor/Merck), 20 mg, antihyperlipidemic |
| ZOCOR 749 MSD | shield-shaped red tablet | simvastatin (Zocor/Merck), 40 mg, antihyperlipidemic |

S = scored        C = coated

# Dialyzable drugs

The amount of a drug removed by dialysis differs among patients and depends on several factors, including the patient's condition, drug's properties, length of dialysis and dialysate used, rate of blood flow or dwell time, and purpose of dialysis. This table indicates the effect of hemodialysis on selected drugs.

| DRUG | LEVEL REDUCED BY HEMODIALYSIS | DRUG | LEVEL REDUCED BY HEMODIALYSIS |
|------|-------------------------------|------|-------------------------------|
| acetaminophen | Yes (may not influence toxicity) | ceftizoxime | Yes |
| | | ceftriaxone | No |
| acyclovir | Yes | cefuroxime | Yes |
| allopurinol | Yes | cephalexin | Yes |
| alprazolam | No | cephalothin | Yes |
| amikacin | Yes | cephapirin | Yes |
| aminoglutethimide | Yes | cephradine | Yes |
| amiodarone | No | chloral hydrate | Yes |
| amitriptyline | No | chlorambucil | No |
| amoxicillin | Yes | chloramphenicol | Yes |
| amoxicillin/clavulanate potassium | Yes | chlordiazepoxide | No |
| amphotericin B | No | chloroquine | No |
| ampicillin | Yes | chlorpheniramine | No |
| ampicillin/clavulanate potassium | Yes | chlorpromazine | No |
| | | chlorthalidone | No |
| aspirin | Yes | cimetidine | Yes |
| atenolol | Yes | ciprofloxacin | Yes (only by 20%) |
| azathioprine | Yes | cisplatin | No |
| aztreonam | Yes | clindamycin | No |
| bretylium | Yes | clofibrate | No |
| captopril | Yes | clonazepam | No |
| carbamazepine | No | clonidine | No |
| carbenicillin | Yes | clorazepate | No |
| carmustine | No | cloxacillin | No |
| cefaclor | Yes | codeine | No |
| cefadroxil | Yes | colchicine | No |
| cefamandole | Yes | cortisone | No |
| cefazolin | Yes | co-trimoxazole | Yes |
| cefonicid | Yes (only by 20%) | cyclophosphamide | Yes |
| cefoperazone | Yes | diazepam | No |
| cefotaxime | Yes | diazoxide | No |
| cefotetan | Yes (only by 20%) | diclofenac | No |
| cefoxitin | Yes | dicloxacillin | No |
| ceftazidime | Yes | | |

*(continued)*

| DRUG | LEVEL REDUCED BY HEMODIALYSIS | DRUG | LEVEL REDUCED BY HEMODIALYSIS |
|---|---|---|---|
| digoxin | No | insulin | No |
| diltiazem | No | isoniazid | Yes |
| diphenhydramine | No | isosorbide | No |
| dipyridamole | No | isradipine | No |
| disopyramide | Yes | kanamycin | Yes |
| doxazosin | No | ketoconazole | No |
| doxepin | No | ketoprofen | Yes |
| doxorubicin | No | labetalol | No |
| doxycycline | No | lidocaine | No |
| enalapril | Yes | lithium | Yes |
| erythromycin | Yes (only by 20%) | lomustine | No |
| ethacrynic acid | No | lorazepam | No |
| ethambutol | Yes (only by 20%) | mechlorethamine | No |
| ethchlorvynol | Yes | mefenamic acid | No |
| ethosuximide | Yes | meperidine | No |
| famotidine | No | mercaptopurine | Yes |
| fenoprofen | No | methadone | No |
| flecainide | No | methicillin | No |
| fluconazole | Yes | methotrexate | Yes |
| flucytosine | Yes | methyldopa | Yes |
| fluorouracil | Yes | methylprednisolone | No |
| fluoxetine | No | metoclopramide | No |
| flurazepam | No | metolazone | No |
| fosinopril | No | metoprolol | No |
| furosemide | No | metronidazole | Yes |
| ganciclovir | Yes | mexiletine | Yes |
| gentamicin | Yes | mezlocillin | Yes |
| glipizide | No | miconazole | No |
| glutethimide | Yes | midazolam | No |
| glyburide | No | minocycline | No |
| guanfacine | No | minoxidil | Yes |
| haloperidol | No | misoprostol | No |
| heparin | No | morphine | No |
| hydralazine | No | nadolol | Yes |
| hydrochlorothiazide | No | nafcillin | No |
| hydroxyzine | No | naproxen | No |
| ibuprofen | No | netilmicin | Yes |
| imipenem/cilastatin | Yes | nifedipine | No |
| imipramine | No | nitroglycerin | No |
| indomethacin | No | nitroprusside | Yes |

| DRUG | LEVEL REDUCED BY HEMODIALYSIS | DRUG | LEVEL REDUCED BY HEMODIALYSIS |
|------|-------------------------------|------|-------------------------------|
| nizatidine | No | ranitidine | Yes |
| norfloxacin | No | rifampin | No |
| nortriptyline | No | streptomycin | Yes |
| omeprazole | No | sucralfate | No |
| oxacillin | No | sulbactam | Yes |
| oxazepam | No | sulfamethoxazole | Yes |
| penicillin G | Yes | sulindac | No |
| pentamidine | No | temazepam | No |
| pentazocine | Yes | theophylline | Yes |
| phenobarbital | Yes | ticarcillin | Yes |
| phenylbutazone | No | timolol | No |
| phenytoin | No | tobramycin | Yes |
| piperacillin | Yes | tocainide | Yes |
| piroxicam | No | tolbutamide | No |
| prazosin | No | trazodone | No |
| prednisone | No | triazolam | No |
| primidone | Yes | trimethoprim | Yes |
| procainamide | Yes | valproic acid | No |
| propoxyphene | No | vancomycin | No |
| propranolol | No | verapamil | No |
| protriptyline | No | warfarin | No |
| quinidine | Yes | | |

# English-Spanish drug phrase translator

## Medication history

**Do you take any medications?**
– Prescription?
– Over-the-counter?
– Other?

**¿Toma Ud. medicamentos?**
– ¿De receta?
– ¿Sin necesidad de receta?
– ¿Otro?

**Which prescription medications do you take routinely?**
– How often do you take them?
    Once daily?
    Twice daily?
    Three times daily?
    Four times daily?
    More often?

**¿Qué medicamentos de receta toma Ud. por rutina?**
– ¿Con qué frecuencia los toma?
    ¿Una vez al día?
    ¿Dos veces al día?
    ¿Tres veces al día?
    ¿Cuátro veces al día?
    ¿Con más frecuencia?

**Which over-the-counter medications do you take routinely?**
– How often do you take them?
– Once daily?
– Twice daily?
– Three times daily?
– Four times daily?
– More often?

**¿Qué medicamentos que no necesitan receta toma Ud. por rutina?**
– ¿Con que frecuencia los toma?
– ¿Una vez al día?
– ¿Dos veces al día?
– ¿Tres veces al día?
– ¿Cuatro veces al día?
– ¿Con más frecuencia?

**Which medications do you take periodically?**

**¿Qué medicamentos toma Ud. periódicamente?**

**Why do you take these medications?**

**¿Por qué toma Ud. estos medicamentos?**

**What is the dosage for each medication?**

**¿Cuál es la dosis para cada uno de los medicamentos?**

**How does each medication make you feel?**

**¿Cómo le hace sentirse cada medicamento?**

**Are you allergic to any medications?**

**¿Está Ud. alérgico(a) a algúnos medicamentos?**

– Which medications?
– What happens when you have an allergic reaction?

– ¿A qué medicamentos?
– ¿Qué pasa cuando Ud. tiene una reacción alérgica?

## Medication teaching

### PURPOSE OF THE MEDICATION
**This medication will:**
– elevate your blood pressure.
– improve circulation to your _____.

– lower your blood pressure.
– lower your blood sugar.

**Este medicamento hará que:**
– su presión sanguínea suba.
– la circulación por (la región del cuerpo) mejore.

– su presión sanguínea baje.
– el nivel de azucar en la sangre baje.

– make your heart rhythm more even.
– raise your blood sugar.
– reduce or prevent the formation of blood clots.
– remove fluid from your body.
– remove fluid from your feet, ankles, or legs.
– remove fluid from your lungs so that they work better.
– remove fluid from your pancreas so that it works better.

**This medication will help your body to:**

– kill the bacteria in your _____.

– slow down your heart rate.
– soften your bowel movements.
– speed up your heart rate.
– use insulin more efficiently.

**This medication will help you to:**

– breathe better.
– fight infections.
– relax.
– sleep.
– think more clearly.

**This medication will relieve or reduce:**

– the acid production in your stomach.
– anxiety.
– bladder spasms.
– burning in your stomach or chest.
– burning when you urinate.
– diarrhea.
– muscle cramps.
– nausea.
– pain in your _____.

**This medication will help your body to produce more or less:**
– antibodies.
– clotting factors.
– insulin.
– platelets.
– red blood cells.
– white blood cells.

**This medication or treatment will destroy:**
– antibodies.
– bacteria.
– cancer cells.
– clotting factors.
– platelets.

– el ritmo del corazón sea más uniforme.
– su nivel de azucar en la sangre suba.
– se reduzca o evite la formación de coágulos de sangre.
– se le quite fluido en el cuerpo.
– se le quite fluido de los pies, tobillos o piernas.
– se le quite fluido de los pulmones para que funcionen mejor.
– se le quite fluido de la páncreas para que funcione mejor.

**Este medicamento le ayudará a su cuerpo a:**
– destruir la bacteria de la (región infectada).
– reducir el latir del corazón.
– ablandar sus evacuaciones.
– acelerar el latir del corazón.
– usar la insulina más eficazmente.

**Este medicamento le ayudará a Ud. a:**
– respirar con mayor facilidad.
– luchar contra infecciones.
– relajarse.
– dormir.
– pensar con mayor claridad.

**Este medicamento le aliviará o disminuirá:**
– la producción de acido en el estómago.
– la angustia.
– espasmos en la vejiga.
– sensación ardiente en el estómago o tórax.
– sensación ardiente al orinar.
– diarrea.
– espasmos en los músculos.
– nausea.
– dolor en la (el) _____.

**Este medicamento le ayudará a su cuerpo a producir más o menos:**
– anticuerpos.
– factores o agentes coagulantes.
– insulina.
– plaquetas.
– células rojas de sangre.
– células blancas de sangre.

**Este medicamento o tratamiento destruirá:**
– anticuerpos.
– bacteria.
– células cancerosas.
– factores o agentes coagulantes.
– plaquetas.

– red blood cells.
– white blood cells.

– células rojas de sangre.
– células blancas de sangre.

## MEDICATION ADMINISTRATION

**I would like to give you:**
– an injection.
– an I.V. medication.
– a liquid medication.
– a medicated cream or powder.
– a medication through your epidural
  catheter.
– a medication through your rectum.
– a medication through your _____ tube.
– a medication under your tongue.
– some pill(s).
– a suppository.

**Quisiera darle a Ud. un(a):**
– inyección.
– medicamento por vía intravenosa.
– medicamento en forma líquida.
– medicamento en pomada o polvo.
– medicamento por el catéter epidural.

– medicamento por el recto.
– medicamento por su _____ tubo.
– medicamento debajo de la lengua.
– píldoras.
– supositorio.

**This is how you take this medication.**

**Así se toma este medicamento.**

**If you can't swallow this pill, I can crush
it and mix it in some food or liquid
such as:**
– applesauce.
– pudding.
– yogurt.

**Si Ud. no se puede tragar esta píldora,
puedo aplastarla y mezclarla en un ali-
mento/líquido, tal como:**
– puré de manzana.
– pudín.
– yogur.

**If you can't swallow this pill, I can get it
in another form.**

**Si Ud. no puede tragarse esta píldora,
puede obtenerla en otra forma.**

**If you can't swallow a pill, you can crush
it and mix it in soft food.**

**Si Ud. no se puede tragar la píldora, la
puede moler y mezclarla en un alimento
blando.**

**I need to mix this medication in juice or
water.**

**Tengo que mezclar este medicamento en
jugo (zumo) o agua.**

**I need to give you this injection in your:**
– abdomen.
– buttocks.
– hip.
– outer arm.
– thigh.

**Tengo que ponerle esta inyección:**
– en el abdomen.
– en las nalgas.
– en la cadera.
– en el brazo.
– en el muslo.

**I need to give you this medication I.V.**

**Tengo que darle este medicamento por
via intravenosa (I.V.).**

**Place it under your tongue.**

**Póngaselo debajo de la lengua.**

**You should feel some burning when it is
under your tongue.**

**Ud. debiera sentir un ardor cuando se lo
pone debajo de la lengua.**

**This indicates that it is working.**

**Esto indica que está tomando efecto.**

**Some medications are coated with a spe-
cial substance to protect your stomach
from getting upset.**

**Algunos medicamentos están cubiertos
con una sustancia especial para prote-
gerle contra un trastorno estomacal.**

**Do not chew:**
- enteric-coated pills.
- long-acting pills.
- capsules.
- sublingual medication.

**No masque Ud.:**
- píldoras con recubrimientoentérico.
- píldoras de efecto prolongado.
- cápsulas.
- medicamentos sublinguales.

**Ask your doctor or pharmacist whether you can:**
- mix your medication with food or fluids.
- take your medication with or without food.

**Pregúntele Ud. a su doctor o farmacéutico si debiera:**
- mezclar su medicamento con un alimento o con líquidos.
- tomar su medicamento con o sin alimento.

**You need to take your medication:**
- after meals.
- before meals.
- on an empty stomach.
- with meals or food.

**Ud. tiene que tomarse el medicamento:**
- después de las comidas.
- antes de las comidas.
- con el estómago vacío.
- con las comidas o con un alimento.

**SKIPPING DOSES**
**If you skip or miss a dose:**
- Take it as soon as you remember it.
- Wait until the next dose.
- Call the doctor if you are not sure.
- Do not take an extra dose.

**Si Ud. omite o se salta una dosis:**
- Tómesela encuanto se acuerde.
- Espérese hasta la siguiente dosis.
- Llame al doctor si Ud. no está seguro(a).
- No se tome una dosis extra.

**ADVERSE EFFECTS**
**Some common adverse effects of _____ are:**
- constipation
- diarrhea
- difficulty sleeping
- dry mouth
- fatigue
- headache
- itching
- light-headedness
- nausea
- poor appetite
- rash
- upset stomach
- weight loss or gain
- frequent urination.

**Unos efectos adversos comunes a _____ son:**
- estreñimiento
- diarrea
- dificultad en dormir
- boca seca
- fatiga
- dolor de cabeza
- comezón (picazón)
- mareo
- nausea
- poco apetito
- erupción
- trastorno estomacal
- perdida o aumento de peso
- orinar con frecuencia.

**These adverse effects:**
- will go away after your body gets used to the medication.
- may persist as long as you take the medication.

**Estos efectos adversos:**
- desaparecerán una vez que su cuerpo se acostumbre al medicamento.
- puede continuar mientras Ud. tome el medicamento.

**If they bother you, speak to your doctor about changing your medication.**

**Si le molestan a Ud., hable con su doctor acerca de que le cambie el medicamento.**

**If you have an adverse reaction to your medication, call your doctor right away.**

**Si Ud. tiene una reacción adversa a su medicamento, llame a su doctor inmediatamente.**

## OTHER CONCERNS

**Tell your doctor if you are pregnant or breast-feeding.**

**Dígale a su doctor si Ud. está ebarazada o si cría a los pechos.**

**While you are taking this medication, ask your doctor if:**
– you can safely take other over-the-counter medications.
– you can drink alcoholic beverages.
– your medications interact with each other.

**Mientras Ud. tome este medicamento, pregúntele a su doctor si:**
– puede tomar otros medicamentos que no necesitan receta.
– puede tomar bebidas alcohólicas.
– sus medicamentos interaccionan uno con el otro.

## STORING MEDICATION

**You should keep your medication:**
– in a cool, dry place.
– in the refrigerator.
– at room temperature.
– out of direct sunlight.
– away from heat.
– away from children.

**Ud. debiera guardar sus medicamentos:**
– en un lugar fresco, seco.
– en el refrigerador.
– al tiempo.
– fuera de la luz de sol.
– lejos de la calefacción.
– lejos del alcance de los niños.

**Do not keep your medication:**
– in a warm place or near heat.

– in the sun.
– in your pocket.
– in the bathroom medicine cabinet.

**No guarde Ud. su medicamento:**
– en un lugar caliente ni cerca de la calefacción.
– en el sol.
– en su bolsillo.
– en el botiquín del baño.

## TEACHING A PATIENT TO GIVE A SUBCUTANEOUS INJECTION

**To give yourself an injection, follow these steps:**
– Draw up the medication.
– Replace the cap carefully.
– Decide where you are going to give the injection.
– Clean the skin area with alcohol.
– Gently pinch up a little skin over the area.
– Using a dartlike motion, stab the needle into your skin.
– Gently pull back on the plunger to see if there is any blood in the syringe.
– Steadily push the medication into your skin.
– Pull the needle out.
– Apply gentle pressure with the alcohol wipe.
– Dispose of the needle in a proper receptacle.

**Así es como uno se pone una inyección a sí mismo(a):**
– Saque el medicamento.
– Coloque de nuevo la tapa con cuidado
– Decida Ud. donde va a ponerse la inyección.
– Limpie el área de la piel con alcohol.
– Suavemente pellizque un poco de piel sobre el área.
– Con un movimiento rápido, penetre la aguja en su piel.
– Con cuidado retire el émbolo para ver si hay sangre en la jeringa.
– Constantemente empuje el medicamento dentro de su piel.
– Saque la aguja.
– Ejerza presión suavemente con un limpión de alcohol.
– Deshagase de la aguja en un recipiente apropiado.

## INSULIN PREPARATION AND ADMINISTRATION
**The doctor has ordered insulin for you.** | **El doctor ha recetado insulina para Ud.**

**To draw up insulin, follow these steps:**

– Wipe the rubber top of the insulin bottle with alcohol.
– Remove the needle cap.
– Pull out the plunger until the end of the plunger in the barrel aligns with the number of units of insulin that you need.

– Push the needle through the rubber top of the insulin bottle.
– Inject the air into the bottle.
– Without removing the needle from the bottle, turn it upside down.
– Withdraw the plunger until the end of the plunger aligns with the number of units you need.
– Gently pull the needle out of the bottle.

**Para extraer la insulina siga las siguientes pasos:**

– Limpie la tapa de hule (goma) de la botella de la insulina con alcohol.
– Quítele el capuchón a la aguja.
– Saque el émbolo hasta el otro extremo del émbolo en la cuba esté al nivel de la dosis de insulina (número de unidades) que Ud. necesita.

– Empuje la aguja por la tapa de hule (goma) de la botella de insulina.
– Inyecte el aire dentro de la botella.
– Sin sacar la aguja de la botella, póngala al revés.
– Retire el émbolo hasta que llegue la insulina al número de unidades que Ud. necesita.
– Retire Ud. la aguja de la botella suavemente.

**To mix insulin, follow these steps:**

– Wipe the rubber tops of the insulin bottles with alcohol.
– Gently roll the cloudy insulin between your palms.
– Remove the needle cap.
– Pull out the plunger until the end of the plunger in the barrel aligns with the number of units of NPH or Lente insulin that you need.

– Push the needle through the rubber top of the cloudy insulin bottle.
– Inject the air into the bottle.
– Remove the needle.
– Pull out the plunger until the end of the plunger in the barrel aligns with the number of units of clear regular insulin that you need.

– Push the needle through the rubber top of the clear insulin bottle.
– Inject the air into the bottle.
– Without removing the needle, turn the bottle upside down.
– Withdraw the plunger until it aligns with the number of units of clear regular insulin that you need.
– Gently pull the needle out of the bottle.

**Para mezclar la insulina siga los siguientes pasos:**

– Limpie la tapa de hule (goma) de las botellas de insulina con alcohol.
– Suavemente mueva la insulina turbia entre las palmas de la mano.
– Retire el capuchón de la aguja.
– Saque el émbolo hasta que el otro extremo del émbolo en el barril esté al nivel con la dosis de insulina turbia (NPH o insulina Lente) (número de unidades) que Ud. necesita.

– Empuje la aguja por la tapa de goma (hule) de la botella de insulina turbia.
– Inyecte el aire dentro de la botella.
– Saque la aguja.
– Retire el émbolo hasta que el otro extremo del émbolo en el barril esté al nivel con la dosis de insulina clara (regular) (número de unidades) que Ud. necesita.

– Empuje Ud. la aguja por la tapa de goma de la botella de insulina clara.
– Inyecte el aire dentro de la botella.
– Sin sacar la aguja, vuelva la botella al revés.
– Retire el émbolo hasta que llegue a la dosis de insulina (regular) clara (número de unidades) que Ud. necesita.
– Suavemente saque Ud. la aguja de la botella.

– Push the needle into the cloudy (NPH or Lente) insulin without injecting it into the bottle.

– Empuje la aguja en la insulina turbia (NPH o insulina Lente) sin inyectarla dentro de la botella.

– Withdraw the plunger until you reach your total dosage of insulin in units (regular combined with NPH or Lente).

– Retire el émbolo hasta que llegue a su dosis total de insulina en unidades (regular y NPH/Lente conbinadas).

– We will practice again.

– Practicaremos juntos(as) otra vez.

## Home care phrases

Wash your hands before touching medications.

Lávese Ud. las manos antes de tocar los medicamentos.

Check the medication bottle for name, dose, and frequency (how often it's supposed to be taken).

En el envase del medicamento verifique Ud. el nombre, la dosis y la frecuencia (con que frequencia se debe tomar).

Check the expiration date on all medications.

Verifique Ud. la fecha en la que el medicamento expira.

Store medications according to pharmacy instructions.

Guarde Ud. los medicamentos según las instrucciones de la farmacia.

Under adequate lighting, read medication labels carefully before taking doses.

Bajo luz adecuada, lea Ud. la etiqueta del medicamento con mucho cuidado antes de tomar las dosis.

Don't crush medication without first asking the doctor or pharmacist.

No machaque Ud. el medicamento sin antes preguntárselo al doctor o al farmacéutico.

Contact your doctor if a new or unexpected symptom or another problem appears.

Póngase Ud. en contacto con su doctor si un síntoma nuevo o inesperado u otros problemas aparecen.

Do not stop taking medication unless instructed by your doctor.

No deje Ud. de tomar el medicamento sólo que se lo ordene su doctor.

Discard outdated medications.

Deshágase Ud. de medicamentos caducos.

Never take someone else's medications.

Nunca tome Ud. los medicamentos de otra persona.

Keep a record of your current medications.

Apunte Ud. (tome nota de) sus medicamentos actuales.

## General drug therapy phrases

**DRUG CLASSES**

| | |
|---|---|
| Analgesic | Analgésico |
| Anesthetic | Anestético |
| Antacid | Antiácido |
| Antianginal agent | Agente antianginal |
| Antianxiety agent | Agente ansiolítico |
| Antiarrhythmic agent | Agente antiarrítmico |
| Antibiotic | Antibiótico |
| Anticancer agent | Agente anticarcinógeno |

| | |
|---|---|
| Anticoagulant | Anticoagulante |
| Anticonvulsant | Anticonvulsivante |
| Antidepressant | Antidepresivo |
| Antidiarrheal | Antidiarreico |
| Antifungal agent | Agente antifúngico |
| Antigout agent | Agente antigota |
| Antihistamine | Antihistamínico |
| Antihyperlipemic agent | Agente hiperlipémico |
| Antihypertensive agent | Agente antihipertenso |
| Anti-inflammatory agent | Agente antiinflamatorio |
| Antimalarial agent | Agente antimalárico |
| Antiparkinsonian agent | Agente antiparkinsoniano |
| Antipsychotic agent | Agente antipsicótico |
| Antipyretic | Antipirético |
| Antiseptic | Antiséptico |
| Antispasmodic | Antiespasmódico |
| Antithyroid agent | Agente antitiroideo |
| Antituberculosis agent | Agente antituberculoso |
| Antitussive agent | Agente antitusígeno |
| Antiviral agent | Agente antiviral |
| Appetite stimulant | Estimulante para el apetito |
| Appetite suppressant | Supresor de apetito |
| Bronchodilator | Broncodilatador |
| Decongestant | Descongestivo |
| Digestant | Digestivo (agente que estimula la digestión) |
| Diuretic | Diurético |
| Emetic | Emético |
| Fertility agent | Agente para la fertilidad |
| Hypnotic | Hipnótico |
| Insulin | Insulina |
| Laxative | Laxante |
| Muscle relaxant | Relajante de músculos |
| Oral contraceptive | Anticonceptivo oral |
| Oral hypoglycemic agent | Agente hipoglucémico oral |
| Sedative | Sedante |
| Steroid | Esteroide |
| Thyroid hormone | Hormona de la glándula tiroides |
| Vaccine | Vacuna |
| Vasodilator | Vasodilatador |
| Vitamin | Vitamina |

## ROUTES

| Intradermal | Intradérmica |
|---|---|
| Intramuscular | Intramuscular |
| Intravenous | Intravenosa |
| Oral | Oral |
| Rectal | Rectal |
| Subcutaneous | Subcutánea |
| Topical | Tópica |
| Vaginal | Vaginal |

## PREPARATIONS

| Capsule | Cápsula |
|---|---|
| Cream | Pomada |
| Drops | Gotas |
| Elixir | Elixir |
| Injection | Inyección |
| Inhaler | Inhalador |
| Lotion | Loción |
| Lozenge | Pastilla |
| Powder | Polvo |
| Spray | Atomizador |
| Suppository | Supositorio |
| Suspension | Suspensión |
| Syrup | Jarabe |
| Tablet | Tableta |

## FREQUENCY

| Once daily | Una vez al día |
|---|---|
| Twice daily | Dos veces al día |
| Three times daily | Tres veces al día |
| Four times daily | Cuatro veces al día |
| In the morning | Por la mañana |
| With meals | Con las comidas |
| Before meals | Antes de las comidas |
| After meals | Después de las comidas |
| Before bedtime | Antes de acostarse |
| When you have_____ | Cuando Ud. tome_____ |
| Only when you need it | Sólo cuando lo necesite |
| Every four hours | Cada cuatro horas |
| Every six hours | Cada seis horas |
| Every eight hours | Cada ocho horas |

# Acknowledgments

*We would like to thank the following companies for granting us permission to include their drugs in the full-color photoguide.*

**Abbott Laboratories**
Biaxin®
Depakote®
Depakote® Sprinkle
E.E.S.®
Ery-Tab®
Erythrocin Stearate Filmtab®
Erythromycin Base Filmtab®
Hytrin®
PCE®

**AstraZeneca LP**
Nolvadex®
Prilosec®
Tenormin®
Toprol XL®
Zestril®

**Aventis**
Allegra®
Carafate®
Cardizem®
Cardizem® CD
DiaBeta®
Lasix®
Slo-bid™ Gyrocaps®
Trental®

**Bayer Corporation**
Adalat® CC
Cipro®

**Bristol-Myers Squibb Company**
BuSpar®
Capoten®
Cefzil®
Duricef®
Estrace®
Glucophage®
Monopril®
Pravachol®
Serzone®
Sumycin®
Trimox®
Veetids®

**DuPont Pharmaceuticals Company**
Coumadin®

**Endo Pharmaceuticals, Inc.**
Percocet®

**ESI Lederle Division of American Home Products Corporation**
atenolol

**Ethex Corporation**
potassium chloride

**Forest Pharmaceuticals, Inc.**
Lorcet® 10/650

**Glaxo Wellcome, Inc.**
Ceftin®
Lanoxin®
Zantac®
Zantac® EFFERdose®
Zovirax®

**Janssen Pharmaceutica, Inc.**
Propulsid®
Risperdal®

**Jones Pharma**
Levoxyl®

**King Pharmaceuticals, Inc.**
Altace®
Lorabid®

**KV Pharmaceutical Company**
Micro-K Extencaps®

**Eli Lilly and Company**
Axid®
Ceclor®
Darvocet-N® 100
Prozac®

**McNeil-PPC, Inc.**
Motrin®

**Medeva Pharmaceuticals**
methylphenidate hydrochloride

**Merck & Co., Inc.**
Cozaar®
Fosamax®
Mevacor®
Pepcid®
Prinivil®
Sinemet®
Sinemet® CR
Vasotec®
Vioxx®
Zocor®

**Mylan Pharmaceuticals, Inc.**
amitriptyline hydrochloride
cimetidine
cyclobenzaprine hydrochloride
doxepin hydrochloride
furosemide
glipizide
naproxen
propoxyphene napsylate with acetaminophen

**Novartis Pharmaceuticals Corporation**
Fiorinal® with Codeine
Lotensin®
Pamelor®

**Novopharm USA, Inc., Division of Novopharm Limited**
amoxicillin trihydrate

**Ortho-McNeil Pharmaceutical**
Floxin®
Levaquin®
Tylenol® with Codeine No. 3
Ultram®

**Pfizer, Inc.**
Cardura®
Diflucan®
Glucotrol®
Glucotrol XL®
Norvasc®
Procardia XL®
Viagra®
Zithromax®
Zoloft®
Zyrtec®

**Pharmacia & Upjohn**
Deltasone®
Glynase®
Micronase®
Provera®
Xanax®

**Proctor and Gamble Pharmaceuticals, Inc.**
Macrobid®

**Roche Laboratories, Inc.**
Bumex®
Klonopin®
Naprosyn®
Ticlid®
Toradol®
Valium®

**Roxane Laboratories, Inc.**
Roxicet™

**Schein Pharmaceutical, Inc.**
nortriptyline hydrochloride

**Schering Corporation and Key Pharmaceuticals, Inc.**
Claritin®
K-Dur®
Theo-Dur®

**Schwarz Pharma**
Verelan®

**G.D. Searle & Company**
Ambien®
Calan®
Celebrex®
Daypro®

**SmithKline Beecham Pharmaceuticals**
Amoxil®
Augmentin®
Compazine®
Coreg®
Dyazide®
Paxil®
Relafen®
Tagamet®

**Tap Pharmaceuticals, Inc.**
Prevacid®

**Teva Pharmaceuticals, USA**
cephalexin

**Warner-Lambert Company**
Accupril®
Dilantin® Infatabs®
Dilantin® Kapseals®
Lipitor®
Lopid®
Nitrostat®

**Watson Laboratories, Inc.**
hydrocodone bitartrate and acetaminophen

**Wyeth-Ayerst Laboratories**
Ativan®
Cordarone®
Effexor®
Inderal®
Lodine®
Oruvail®
Premarin®

**Zenith Goldline Pharmaceuticals**
verapamil hydrochloride

# Index

t refers to a table; **boldface** refers to full-color photographs

t refers to a table; **boldface** refers to full-color photographs

---

t refers to a table; **boldface** refers to full-color photographs

t refers to a table; **boldface** refers to full-color photographs

t refers to a table; **boldface** refers to full-color photographs

Lung cancer
  doxorubicin for, 907-908
  etoposide for, 939
  gemcitabine for, 941
  mechlorethamine for, 879
  porfimer for, 949
  topotecan for, 954-955
  vinorelbine for, 962
Lupron, 927
Lupron Depot, 927
Lupron Depot-Ped, 927
Lupron Depot-3 Month, 927
Lupron Depot-4 Month, 927
Lupron for Pediatric Use, 927
Lupus erythematosus, hydroxy-chloroquine for, 49
Luride, 1155
Luride Lozi-Tabs, 1155
Luride-SF Lozi-Tabs, 1155
Lustral, 442
Lutrepulse, 747
Luvox, 516
Luxiq, 1122
Lyclear, 1120
Lyme disease
  ceftriaxone for, 120
  cefuroxime for, 122
Lyme disease vaccine, 990-991
LYMErix, 990
lymphocyte immune globulin, 969-971
Lymphogranuloma venereum
  chloramphenicol for, 203
  sulfamethoxazole for, 140
  sulfisoxazole for, 141
Lymphoma
  doxorubicin for, 908
  rituximab for, 952
  thiotepa for, 885
Lymphosarcoma
  bleomycin for, 902
  chlorambucil for, 872
  mechlorethamine for, 879
  methotrexate for, 898
Lysodren, 943

**M**

Maalox Antacid Caplets, 645
Maalox Anti-Diarrheal Caplets, 655
Maalox Daily Fiber Therapy, 669
Maalox Extra Strength Tablets, 643
Maalox Plus, 643
Maalox Tablets, 643
Maalox Therapeutic Concentrate Suspension, 643
Macrobid, 201, 208, **C9**
Macrodantin, 208
Macrodex, 821
Macrolide anti-infectives, 194-200
Madopar, 498
Madopar HBS, 498
Madopar Q, 498
mafenide acetate, 1107

magaldrate, 646-647
Magan, 344
Magnaprin, 337
Magnaprin Arthritis Strength, 337
magnesium chloride, 823-824
magnesium citrate, 665-666
magnesium hydroxide, 665-666
magnesium oxide, 647-648
magnesium salicylate, 344-345
magnesium sulfate, 413-414, 665-666, 823-824
Magnesium supplementation, magnesium salts for, 823
Magnesium toxicity, calcium salts for, 818
Mag-Ox 400, 647
Malaria
  chloroquine for, 47
  doxycycline for, 130
  hydroxychloroquine for, 48-49
  mefloquine for, 50
  primaquine for, 51
  pyrimethamine for, 52
  pyrimethamine with sulfadox-ine for, 52
  quinidine for, 238
  sulfadiazine for, 138
  tetracycline for, 134
Male infertility, menotropins for, 750
Male pattern hair loss
  finasteride for, 1217
  minoxidil for, 1227
Malignant effusions
  bleomycin for, 902
  mechlorethamine for, 879
  thiotepa for, 885
Malignant hypertension, fenoldopam for, 278
Malignant hyperthermia crisis, dantrolene for, 563
Malignant lymphoma
  carmustine for, 870
  chlorambucil for, 872
  cyclophosphamide for, 875
  vinblastine for, 959
  vincristine for, 960
Malignant melanoma. *See also* Melanoma.
  dacarbazine for, 937
  interferon alfa-2b, recombi-nant, for, 1032
Mallamint, 817
Malogen, 721
manganese, 1156-1157
manganese chloride, 1156-1157
manganese sulfate, 1156-1157
Mania
  divalproex for, 422
  lithium for, 518
mannitol, 809-810
Mantoux test, 1284t
Maox, 647
Mapap, Children's, 338

Mapap Infant Drops, 338
Marax, 597
Marax-DF Syrup, 597
Marcain, 1278t
Marcaine, 1278t
Marinol, 675
Marnal, 337
Marvelon, 736
Mastocytosis
  cimetidine for, 684
  cromolyn for, 631
Matulane, 951
Mavik, 308
Maxair, 614
Maxair Autohaler, 614
Maxalt, 525
Maxalt-MLT, 525
Maxaquin, 148
Maxenal, 553
Maxeran, 678
Maxidex Ophthalmic, 1051
Maxidex Ophthalmic Suspen-sion, 1051
Maxiflor, 1127
Maximum Strength, 648
Maxipime, 102
Maxitrol Ointment/Ophthalmic Suspension, 1041
Maxivate, 1122
Maxolon, 678
Maxzide, 259, 797
Maxzide-25mg, 797
MCT, 1163
measles, mumps, and rubella virus vaccine, live, 991-992
Measles exposure, immune globulin for, 1015
Measles outbreak control, measles virus vaccine, live attenuated, for, 994
measles and rubella virus vac-cine, live attenuated, 993
measles virus vaccine, live at-tenuated, 993-995
mebendazole, 28
Mechanical ventilation, facilitat-ing
  atracurium for, 567
  cisatracurium for, 569
  mivacurium for, 572
  pancuronium for, 574
  rocuronium for, 578
  succinylcholine for, 580
  tubocurarine for, 581
  vecuronium for, 583
mechlorethamine hydrochloride, 879-881
meclizine hydrochloride, 677-678
meclozine hydrochloride, 677-678
Meda Cap, 338
Medigesic, 337
Medihaler Ergotamine, 556
Medihaler-Iso, 607

---

t refers to a table; **boldface** refers to full-color photographs

t refers to a table; **boldface** refers to full-color photographs

t refers to a table; **boldface** refers to full-color photographs

t refers to a table; **boldface** refers to full-color photographs

t refers to a table; **boldface** refers to full-color photographs

---

t refers to a table; **boldface** refers to full-color photographs

t refers to a table; **boldface** refers to full-color photographs

# About NDH2001*Plus!*

NDH2001*Plus!* mini-CD lets you:
- take 10 continuing education tests (and earn up to 35.5 contact hours)
- customize and print patient-teaching instructions for 200 of the most commonly prescribed drugs, in regular or large print
- use the drug imprint code translator to identify common drugs
- learn about potentially dangerous drug interactions
- link directly to **NDHnow.com** for drug updates and important drug news.

## Windows system requirements
- Windows 95 or higher
- Pentium 90 or higher
- 16 MB RAM
- 10 MB free hard-disk space
- 256 color-display adapter (16-bit color recommended)
- CD-ROM drive and mouse

## Macintosh system requirements
- Mac OS 8.0 or higher
- 32 MB RAM
- 10 MB free hard-disk space
- 256 color-display adapter (16-bit color recommended)
- CD-ROM drive and mouse

---

**CAUTION:** Do not attempt to use this mini-CD in a floppy disk drive, Zip drive, slot drive, or car stereo. Do not insert the mini-CD into a CD-ROM drive that requires the mini-CD to be in a vertical position. Placing the CD into such a drive may result in jamming.

Before installing this program, make sure your monitor is set up to display 256 colors or greater. If it isn't, consult your user's manual for instructions about changing the display settings.

---

## To install on Windows 95 or higher:
- Place the mini-CD on the inner ring of the CD-ROM drive tray. Close the tray.
- In a few moments, the CD should automatically start. Once it starts, click the "Install NDH2001*Plus!*" button to install on your computer.
- Click "Start" and select "Run" if the CD doesn't start automatically.
- Type **d:\setup** (where **d** is the letter of your CD-ROM drive), and click *OK*. Follow on-screen instructions for installing the CD.

## To install on Mac OS 8.0 or higher:
- Place the mini-CD on the inner ring of the CD-ROM drive tray. Close the tray.
- In a few moments, the CD icon should appear on your desktop. Double-click the CD icon.
- Double-click "Setup" to install on your computer.

**Special note:** Before using NDH2001*Plus!* read the file *Readme.txt* for important information about operating the program.

For technical support, call toll free 1-877-872-7748, Monday through Friday, 8 am to 5 pm Eastern Standard Time.

For information about obtaining a network license for NDH2001*Plus!*, call 1-800-346-7844 ext. 1500.

The clinical information and tools in NDH2001*Plus!* are based on research and consultation with nursing, medical, and legal authorities. To the best of our knowledge, this program reflects currently accepted practice; nevertheless, it can't be considered absolute and universal. For individual application, all recommendations must be considered in light of your institution's policies and procedures, the patient's clinical condition and, before administration of new or infrequently used drugs, in light of the latest package-insert information. The authors and publisher disclaim responsibility for adverse effects resulting directly or indirectly from the suggested procedures, from undetected errors, or from the reader's misunderstanding of the program.